Analyte	Conventional Units			SI Units		
	EXPECTED ADULT REFERENCE OR THERAPEUTIC RANGE					
Blood gases and	**Parameter**	**Arterial**	**Venous**	**Arterial**	**Venous**	
oxygen saturation	pH	7.35-7.45	7.33-7.43	7.35-7.45	7.33-7.43	
(B)	P_{CO_2}	35-45 mm Hg	38-50 mm Hg	263-338	285-	
	P_{O_2}	80-100 mm Hg	30-50 mm Hg	600-750	225-375 kPa	
	O_2 saturation	95%-100%	60%-80%			
C-reactive protein	<10 mg/L			<85 pmol/L		566
Caffeine (S, P)	8-20 µg/mL			40-100 µmol/L		1073
Calcium (S)	80-105 mg/L			2.0-2.6 mmol/L		507
(U)	<275 mg/24 hr males			<6.87 mmol/24 hr males		
	<250 mg/24 hr females			<6.25 mmol/24 hr females		
Carbohydrate screen (U)	Undetectable			—		907
Carbon dioxide total (S, P)	21-31 mmol/L			21-31 mmol/L		462
Carcinoembryonic	<2.5 ng/mL (method dependent)			—		960
antigen (S)						
	<5.0 ng/mL smokers			—		
Ceruloplasmin (S)	M 220-400 mg/L			1.3-2.5 µmol/L		907
	F 250-600 mg/L			1,5-3.6 µmol/L		
Chloride (S)	101-111 mEq/L			101-111 mmol/L		441
(U)	110-250 mEq/L (or 24 hr)			110-250 mmol/24 hr		
Cholesterol total						603
Desirable	<200 mg/dL			<5.1 mmol/L		
Borderline high	200-239 mg/dL			5.1-6.2 mmol/L		
High risk	≥240 mg/dL			>6.2 mmol/L		
High-density lipoprotein, HDL						
Low risk	<40 mg/dL			<1 mmol/L		
High risk	>60 mg/dL			>1.6 mmol/L		
Low-density lipoprotein, LDL	Optimal <100 mg/dL					603
	High risk >160 mg/dL					
Cholinesterase	Age, sex, and phenotype dependent					907
Chorionic gonadotropin, human (hCG)	<20 mIU/mL					753, 849
Creatine kinase total (S)	130-253 U/L (method dependent)			2.17×10^{-6} katal/L		566
Creatine kinase isoenzymes (S)	<10 µg/L for CK-MB			—		566, 1064
	<3% of total CK activity for CK-MB					
Creatinine (S)	6.4-10.4 mg/L male			57-92 µmol/L		477
	5.7-9.2 mg/L female			50-81 µmol/L		
(U)	1.0-2.0 g/day male			8.8-17.7 mmol/day		
	0.8-1.8g/day female			7.1-15.9 mmol/day		
Creatinine clearance	97-137 mL/min male					477
	88-128 mL/min female					
Cyclosporin A (B)	Dependent on organ and time after transplant					972, 1013
	250-375 ng/mL renal <6 mo			0.20-0.30 µmol/L		
	100-250 ng/mL renal >6 mo			0.08-0.20 µmol/L		
Digoxin (S, P)	0.9-2.0 ng/mL			1.1-2.4 nmol/L		566
Drug screen (U)	Not present					989
Estradiol						753, 849
	Women					
	Follicular	28-166 pg/mL		103-592 pmol/L		
	Pre-ovulatory peak	187-382 pg/mL		685-1404 pmol/L		
	Luteal phase	32-201 pg/mL		120-738 pmol/L		
	Postmenopausal	4.6-32 pg/mL		17-120 pmol/L		
	Men	5.4-17 pg/mL		20-65 pmol/L		

B, Whole blood; P, plasma; S, serum; U, urine.
*A more complete list and description of methods of analysis can be found in
Clinical chemistry: a managerial and scientific infobase, Cincinnati, 2003, Pesce-Kaplan Publishers, v 5.0.

Continued on back endpaper.

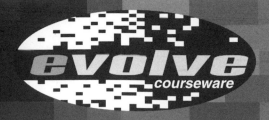

The Latest *Evolution* in Learning.

Congratulations!

You now have access to EVOLVE for *Clinical Chemistry: Theory, Analysis, Correlation, fourth edition* by Lawrence A. Kaplan, Amadeo J. Pesce, and Steven C. Kazmierczak!

Visit the Web address listed below to start your learning evolution today!

▶▶ LOGIN: *http://evolve.elsevier.com/Kaplan/chemistry*

A website just for you as you learn clinical chemistry with the new fourth edition of *Clinical Chemistry: Theory, Analysis, Correlation*

- **What you will receive:**

Whether you're a student, an instructor, or a practitioner, you'll find information just for you.

Things like:

- Content Updates

- Links to Related Products

- Author Information

- And More!

Think outside the book...*evolve.*

Clinical Chemistry

Theory, Analysis, Correlation

Clinical Chemistry

Theory, Analysis, Correlation

Lawrence A. Kaplan, PhD, DABCC, FACB
Clinical Professor Pathology
New York University
Director, Clinical Chemistry
Bellevue Hospital
New York, New York

Amadeo J. Pesce, PhD, DABCC, FACB
Professor, Department of Pathology and Laboratory Medicine
University of Cincinnati, College of Medicine
Cincinnati, Ohio
Laboratory Director
Adams County Hospital
West Union, Ohio
Laboratory Director
Drake Center
Cincinnati, Ohio

Steven C. Kazmierczak, PhD, DABCC, FACB
Department of Pathology
Oregon Health and Sciences University
Portland, Oregon

Fourth Edition

with 500 illustrations

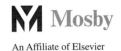

An Affiliate of Elsevier

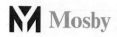

An Affiliate of Elsevier

11830 Westline Industrial Drive
St. Louis, Missouri 63146

CLINICAL CHEMISTRY: THEORY, ANALYSIS, CORRELATION   ISBN 0-323-01716-9

NOTICE

Pharmacology is an ever-changing field. Standard safety precautions must be followed, but as new research and clinical experience broaden our knowledge, changes in treatment and drug therapy may become necessary or appropriate. Readers are advised to check the most current product information provided by the manufacturer of each drug to be administered to verify the recommended dose, the method and duration of administration, and contraindications. It is the responsibility of the licensed prescriber, relying on experience and knowledge of the patient, to determine dosages and the best treatment for each individual patient. Neither the publisher nor the author assumes any liability for any injury and/or damage to persons or property arising from this publication.

Library of Congress Cataloging-in-Publication Data

Clinical chemistry: theory, analysis, correlation / [edited by] Lawrence A. Kaplan, Amadeo J. Pesce, Steven C. Kazmierczak. – 4th ed.
 p.; cm.
Includes bibliographical references and index.
ISBN 0-323-01716-9
1. Clinical chemistry. I. Kaplan, Lawrence A., 1944- II. Pesce, Amadeo J. III. Kazmierczak, Steven C.
[DNLM: 1. Chemistry, Clinical. QY 90 C6415 2003]
RB40 .C58 2003
616.07′56–dc21

                  2002028818

Publisher: Andrew Allen
Acquisitions Editor: Karen Fabiano
Developmental Editor: Ellen Wurm
Publishing Services Manager: Linda McKinley
Project Manager: Jennifer Furey
Designer: Julia Dummitt
Cover Designer: Sheilah Barrett

RT/MVY

Printed in the United States of America

Last digit is the print number: 9 8 7 6 5 4 3 2

Contributors

Nancy W. Alcock, PhD
Retired
(Contributor to a previous edition)

Rita R. Alloway, PharmD, BCPS
Research Professor
Director, Transplant Clinical Research
University of Cincinnati, College of Medicine
Division of Nephrology and Hypertension
Cincinnati, Ohio

Carmelita Alvares, MD
Assistant Professor
Department of Pathology and Laboratory Medicine
University of Cincinnati
Cincinnati, Ohio

David J. Anderson, PhD
Associate Professor
Director of Clinical Chemistry
Department of Chemistry
Cleveland State University
Cleveland, Ohio

Victor W. Armstrong, PhD
Department of Clinical Chemistry/Central Laboratory
Centre of Internal Medicine
George August University
Goettingen, Germany

Kenneth E. Blick, PhD, ABCC, FACB, ACS
Professor
Department of Pathology
University of Oklahoma Health Science Center and OU
    Medical Center
Oklahoma City, Oklahoma

John M. Brewer, PhD
Professor of Biochemistry
Department of Biochemistry and Molecular Biology
University of Georgia
Athens, Georgia

Elizabeth Ann Byrne, MS, CLS
Retired
(Contributor to a previous edition)

Cathy Cao, MD
University of Cincinnati Medical Center
Cincinnati, Ohio

R. Neill Carey, PhD
Clinical Chemist
Peninsula Regional Medical Center
Salisbury, Maryland

John F. Chapman, Jr., DrPH
Professor, Department of Pathology and Laboratory
    Medicine
University of North Carolina
Chapel Hill, North Carolina

I-Wen Chen, PhD
Retired
(Contributor to a previous edition)

David Chou, MD, MS
Department of Laboratory Medicine
University of Washington Academic Medical Centers
Seattle, Washington

Robert H. Christenson, PhD, DABCC, FACB
Professor of Pathology
Professor of Medical and Research Technology
University of Maryland School of Medicine
Director, Rapid Response, Clinical Chemistry and
    Toxicology
University of Maryland Medical Center
Baltimore, Maryland

Niel T. Constantine, PhD
Professor of Pathology
Director, Clinical Immunology
University of Maryland School of Medicine
Institute of Human Virology
Baltimore, Maryland

Lawrence J. Crolla, PhD
Consulting Clinical Chemist
Alexian Brothers Medical Center
Elk Grove Village, Illinois

Laurence M. Demers, PhD, DABCC, FACB
Distinguished Professor of Pathology and Medicine
Director, Clinical Chemistry, Automated Testing
    Laboratory, Specimen Processing and Core Endocrine
    Laboratory, University Hospital
Departments of Pathology and Medicine
The Pennsylvania State University College of Medicine
The M.S. Hershey Medical Center
Hershey, Pennsylvania

Richard F. Dods, PhD
Illinois Mathematics and Science Academy
Aurora, Illinois

James G. Donnelly, PhD, FACB, FCACB
Associate Professor of Clinical Pathology
New York University School of Medicine
New York, New York

D. Robert Dufour, MD
Professor of Pathology
The George Washington School of Medicine
Adjunct Professor of Pathology
Uniformed Services University of the Health Sciences
Chief, Pathology
Veterans Affairs Medical Center
Washington DC

Barry N. Elkins, PhD
Chief of Chemistry
Saint Vincent Catholic Medical Centers of New York
St. Vincent's Hospital Manhattan
New York, New York

Carolyn S. Feldkamp, PhD
Division Head, Clinical Chemistry Division
Department of Pathology
Henry Ford Hospital
Detroit, Michigan

Mariano Fernandez-Ulloa, MD
Professor of Clinical Radiology
University of Cincinnati, College of Medicine
Cincinnati, Ohio

Martin Roy First, MD
Professor of Medicine
Director, Section of Transplantation
University of Cincinnati Medical Center
Cincinnati, Ohio

Kenneth J. Friedman, PhD
Assistant Professor
Department of Pathology and Laboratory Medicine
University of North Carolina
Chapel Hill, North Carolina

Christopher S. Frings, PhD
President, Chris Frings and Associates
Clinical Professor
Departments of Pathology and Allied Health Sciences
University of Alabama
Birmingham, Alabama
(Contributor to a previous edition)

Carl C. Garber, PhD
Director, Technical Statistics Applications
Quest Diagnostics
Teterboro, New Jersey

Jack Gauldie, PhD
Associate Professor
Department of Pathology
McMaster University
Hamilton, Ontario, Canada
(Contributor to a previous edition)

Lewis Glasser, MD
Retired
(Contributor to a previous edition)

R. Jeffrey Goldsmith, PhD
Department of Psychiatry
University of Cincinnati Medical Center
Cincinnati, Ohio

Catherine A. Hammett-Stabler, PhD, DABCC, FACB
Department of Pathology and Laboratory Medicine
University of North Carolina
Chapel Hill, North Carolina

William R. Heineman, PhD
Distinguished Research Professor
Department of Chemistry
University of Cincinnati
Cincinnati, Ohio

W. Edward Highsmith, Jr., PhD
Associate Professor of Pathology
Director, Molecular Diagnostics Laboratory
University of Maryland
Baltimore, Maryland

David C. Hohnadel, PhD, FACB
Technical Director
ACM Medical Laboratories, Inc.
Park Ridge Hospital
Unity Health System
Rochester, New York

Oussama Itani, MD, FAAP
Assistant Professor of Pediatrics and Human Development
Michigan State University
Kalamazoo, Michigan

Ellis Jacobs, PhD
Director, Clinical Laboratory Evaluation Program
New York Department of Health
New York, New York

Mark A. Jandreski, PhD, DABCC, FACB
Manufacturing Development Manager, Nucleic Acid
    Diagnostics
Bayer Diagnostics
East Walpole, Massachusetts

Sarah H. Jenkins, PhD
Laboratory Director
The Children's Medical Center
Dayton, Ohio
(Contributor to a previous edition)

Stephen E. Kahn, PhD, DABCC, FACB
Professor, Pathology, Cell Biology, Neurobiology and
    Anatomy
Associate Director, Clinical Laboratories
Section Chief and Director, Chemistry, Toxicology and
    Near Patient Testing
Loyola University Medical Center
Maywood, Illinois

Marcia Kaplan, MD
Associate Professor of Psychiatry
University of Cincinnati Medical Center
Cincinnati, Ohio

Jon R. Kirchhoff, PhD
Associate Professor
Department of Chemistry
University of Toledo
Toledo, Ohio
(Contributor to a previous edition)

Leonard I. Kleinman, MD (in memorlam, 1998)
Professor and Director of Newborn Services
Department of Pediatrics
State University of New York at Stony Brook School of
    Medicine
Stony Brook, New York

Michael Lehrer, PhD
Associate Professor of Pathology
Albert Einstein College of Medicine
Bronx, New York
Senior Scientific Consultant
LabOne, Inc.
Lenexa, Kansas

Cheryl Lesar
Nurse Practitioner
Outpatient Substance Dependence Program
Opiate Substitution Program
Coordinator of Nicotine Dependent Services
Cincinnati VA Medical Center
Cincinnati, Ohio

John M. Lorenz, MD
Professor of Clinical Pediatrics
College of Physicians and Surgeons
Columbia University
New York, New York

Craig E. Lunte, PhD
Associate Professor
Department of Chemistry
University of Kansas
Lawrence, Kansas

Fermina M. Mazzella
Department of Pathology and Laboratory Medicine
Medical College of Georgia
Augusta, Georgia

Herbert K. Naito, PhD, MBA
Chief, Ancillary Testing and Satellite Facilities
Pathology and Laboratory Medicine Service
Lewis Stokes Cleveland Veterans Affairs Medical Center
Cleveland, Ohio

Elisabeth Nye, PhD, MBBS FRACP
Endocrinologist
Department of Chemical Pathology
Princess Alexandra Hospital
Wooloongabba, Australia

Michael Oellerich, MD, Hon MD
Professor, Department of Clinical Chemistry
George August University
Goettingen, Germany

Richard B. Passey, PhD
Professor of Pathology
Director, Clinical Chemistry Laboratory
University of Oklahoma
Director, Clinical Chemistry
University Hospital
Oklahoma City, Oklahoma
(Contributor to a previous edition)

Michael A. Pesce, PhD
Director of the Specialty Laboratory
Columbia-Presbyterian Medical Center
Associate Professor of Clinical Pathology
Columbia University
College of Physicians and Surgeons
New York, New York

Jane E. Phillips, PhD
Scientific Advisor
Department of Scientific Affairs and Business Development
Roche Diagnostics Corporation
Indianapolis, Indiana

Alphonse Poklis, PhD
Professor, Department of Pathology
Affiliate Professor, Department of Pharmacology &
    Toxicology
Medical College of Virginia Campus at Virginia
    Commonwealth University
Affiliate Professor, Chemistry & Forensic Science
Department of Chemistry
College of Humanities & Sciences
Virginia Commonwealth University
Richmond, Virginia

Michael D. Privitera, MD
Professor and Vice-Chair, Department of Neurology
Director, Comprehensive Epilepsy Treatment Program
Medical Director, UC Physicians
University of Cincinnati Medical Center
Cincinnati, Ohio

Morris R. Pudek, PhD, FCACB
Clinical Professor, Department of Pathology
University of British Columbia
Head, Division of Clinical Chemistry
Vancouver General Hospital
Vancouver, British Columbia, Canada

Lisa Reninger, MT, ASCP
Laboratory Administrative Director
Alexian Brothers Medical Center
Elk Grove Village, Illinois

Wolfgang A. Ritschel, MD, PhD
Professor of Pharmacokinetics and Biopharmaceutics
Head, Division of Pharmaceutics and Drug Delivery Systems
University of Cincinnati Medical Center
Cincinnati, Ohio
(Contributor to a previous edition)

Jeri D. Ropero-Miller, PhD, BA
Clinical Assistant Professor
Department of Pathology and Laboratory Medicine
University of North Carolina
Deputy Chief Toxicologist
North Carolina Office of the Chief Medical Examiner
Chapel Hill, North Carolina

Donald L. Rucknagel, PhD
Director, Sickle Center
Children's Hospital Medical Center
Cincinnati, Ohio

Wendy R. Sanhai, PhD
Technology Licensing Specialist/Patent Advisor
Office of Technology Transfer
National Institutes of Health
Bethesda, Maryland

Edward A. Sasse, PhD
Associate Professor, Department of Pathology
Medical College of Wisconsin
Chief, Chemistry Section
Pathology and Laboratory Medicine Service
Milwaukee Veterans Affairs Medical Center
Milwaukee, Wisconsin
(Contributor to a previous edition)

William E. Schreiber, MD
Professor, Department of Pathology and Laboratory
    Medicine
The University of British Columbia
Consultant Pathologist, Department of Pathology and
    Laboratory Medicine
Vancouver Hospital and Health Sciences Center
Vancouver, British Columbia, Canada

Harold R. Schumacher, MD
Director, Hematology Division
Department of Pathology and Laboratory Medicine
University of Cincinnati Medical Center
Cincinnati, Ohio

Bette Seamonds, PhD, DABCC
Clinical Chemist
Director of Point-of-Care Services
Mercy Health Laboratory
Darby, Pennsylvania

John E. Sherwin, PhD
Chief
Genetic Disease Laboratory
Department of Health Services
State of California
Berkeley, California

Paul W. Stiffler, PhD
Microbiology Consultant
LaGrange Memorial Hospital
LaGrange, Illinois
(Contributor to a previous edition)

M. Wilson Tabor, PhD
Associate Professor of Environmental Health
Director of Environmental Analytical Chemistry
Institute of Environmental Health
University of Cincinnati Medical Center
Cincinnati, Ohio
(Contributor to a previous edition)

Stephan G. Thompson, PhD
Senior Research Manager
ThauMDx LLC
Santa Barbara, California

Reginald C. Tsang, MD
Children's Hospital of Cincinnati
University of Cincinnati
Department of Pediatrics
Cincinnati, Ohio

Richard Wenstrup, MD
Associate Professor of Pediatrics
University of Cincinnati
Director, Molecular Genetics Laboratory
Cincinnati Children's Hospital Medical Center
Cincinnati, Ohio

John F. Wheeler, PhD
Assistant Professor
Department of Chemistry
Furman University
Greenville, South Carolina
(Contributor to a previous edition)

Ruth E. Winecker, PhD
Chief Toxicologist
North Carolina-Office of the Chief Medical Examiner
Clinical Assistant Professor
Pathology and Laboratory Medicine
University of North Carolina
Chapel Hill, North Carolina

Remarkably, nearly two decades have passed since we published the first edition of this textbook. Remarkable because we still enjoy the process of creation. Remarkable because we can still find stimulating colleagues willing to participate in this process with us, and remarkable because teachers and students still find our efforts worthwhile. And, more remarkable still, is the enduring patience of our wives. This edition is dedicated to all these remarkable people.

Lawrence A. Kaplan
New York City

Amadeo J. Pesce
Cincinnati

To my wife Diana, and children, Caitlin and Connor, for their patience, love, and support. Thanks to my mentors, John Lott and Fred Van Lente, for their guidance and encouragement when it was needed most. Finally, thanks to Drs. Kaplan and Pesce, two extraordinary individuals whose foresight, imagination, and inspiration have made the production of this textbook possible.

Steven C. Kazmierczak
Portland, Oregon

This is one of the first clinical chemistry textbooks to be published in the current millennium. The purpose of this textbook remains the same: we wish to educate students about the discipline of clinical chemistry and provide an extensive reference for clinical chemistry professionals. Much has changed in this field, as well as in the field of publishing. It is a challenge and a privilege to be asked to prepare another edition at the dawn of the new millennium. We are very pleased to have been able to work with the publishers to create a suitable textbook for students and professionals of this millennium.

This edition takes advantage of the remarkable changes in the science of clinical chemistry and the world around us. Some of the most significant changes to be found in this edition are listed below.

INTERNET

At the time of the third edition the Internet had yet to achieve the power that we see today. The wealth of information that is available on the Web is almost beyond belief. While we realize that most young students know more than the editors do about the Web, we have researched many Internet sites and have listed about 300 Web addresses that we believe are worth investigating as additional learning resources. They are listed after the references of most chapters and, in activated forms, in the CD-ROM (see below). While we recognize that the life span of many websites can be short and of variable content, we encourage students of this textbook to browse the Web for clinical chemistry sites, beginning with the sampling that we have provided for you. All of our sites were active in the autumn of 2002.

CD-ROM TECHNOLOGY

We are using the power of CD-ROM technology to greatly expand the amount and types of material that we can present to students. We have moved all the material on methodology from the textbook and placed it on the accompanying CD-ROM. In doing so we have increased the number of methods described to more than 115 and greatly expanded the content of each method. The methods are presented in the same format used in our previous text editions, with summary tables and complete descriptions of many techniques. However, the references are now inserted as popups.

We have added a full *Urinalysis manual*, complete with more than 60 colored photomicrographs of urine sediment and many summary charts.

We are connecting our text and CD-ROM to the Internet in several ways. First, we have assembled all the references in the textbook in an EndNote file format. This will allow readers to connect to the PubMed Internet site in order to obtain additional information on many of these references, as well as related articles. Please review the ReadMe file on the CD-ROM for instructions for using the EndNote files. Second, we have provided a compendium of active Internet sites to help students find additional learning resources. They are listed by chapter and by subject matter.

We have included a number of *algorithms* in Microsoft Excel format that can be used to make calculations such as converting from one unit to another and performing creatinine clearance calculations.

We have added an updated version of our very popular *Workbook and Study Guide*. This book contains 36 experiments. 52 case histories serve as excellent practical reviews of pathophysiology, biochemistry, and laboratory management. As a further aid to students, there are more than 700 questions to help prepare for examinations. Answers to both the case histories and the review questions are provided, along with page references to either the textbook or the CD-ROM. The Table of Contents for the CD-ROM may be found on p. xiv.

As a useful aid to both instructors and students, everything in the CD-ROM can be printed.

THE TEXTBOOK

Most of the chapters have been updated and expanded. Of course, the Urinalysis chapter (Chapter 57) can be found in a greatly expanded form on the CD-ROM. Many of the more important revisions to the textbook reflect new tests and a better understanding of old tests.

Chapter 17 contains much information about recent technology and regulations for point-of-care testing.

Chapter 18 includes information on HIPPA and recent concepts of LIS technology.

Chapter 28 deals extensively with recent findings related to bone disease and women's health.

Chapter 31 has an up-to-date description of the use of troponin to detect cardiac ischemia and new diagnostic testing for cardiac failure.

Chapter 33 has the latest NCEP guidelines for cholesterol screening and treatment.

Chapter 40 includes new discussions of fetal lung maturity testing and screening for gestational diabetes.

Chapter 47 discusses the Human Genome Project, which has greatly expanded our knowledge of genetic-based disease, while Chapter 48 provides a description of the techniques used to detect these diseases.

Chapter 51 has been greatly expanded and includes a new section on Bioterrorism.

We hope that our readers will enjoy this edition of our textbook.

The preparation of this work could not have been accomplished without the help of the following individuals: Fanta Davis and Stefanie Kaplan of New York City; Jennifer Webb, Gerrado Perrotta, and Michael Nolting of Cincinnati; and Becky Hawkins and Shawn Gill of Adams County, Ohio. We acknowledge Dr. Meyer Horowitz of Cincinnati who has always been kind enough to lend his expertise to our efforts. We thank Dr. Paul Horn for reviewing the chapter on reference intervals. We also acknowledge the passing of one of our most important contributors: a friend and colleague, Lennie Kleinman, in 1998.

We thank the Chairpersons of our University Departments for their support that allowed us to complete this work: Vittorio Devendi and Robert Boortstein, New York University, Bellevue Hospital; Cecilia Fenoglio-Preiser, University of Cincinnati; and Don Houghton and Jim MacLowry, Oregon Health and Sciences University, Portland, Oregon. We are very pleased to have the opportunity to have worked with a new set of very professional editors from Elsevier: Karen Fabiano, Ellen Wurm, and Jennifer Furey.

Lawrence A. Kaplan
Amadeo J. Pesce
Steven C. Kazmierczak

Table of Contents for Accompanying CD-ROM

Contents

PART I

Laboratory Techniques

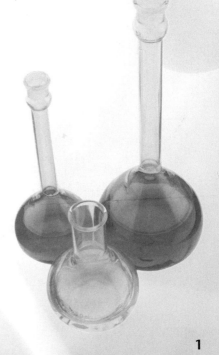

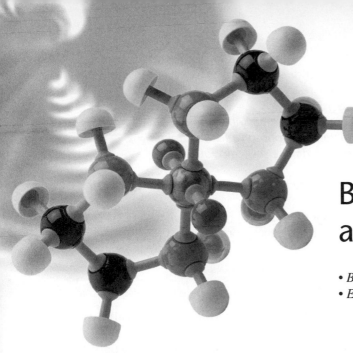

CHAPTER 1

Basic Laboratory Principles and Techniques

• *Bette Seamonds*
• *Elizabeth Ann Byrne*

Chapter Outline

Objectives

- Describe the methods used for water purification and the specifications, uses, and storage and handling procedures associated with the different grades of reagent water.
- Describe the quality control and impurity testing procedures used for different grades of reagent water.
- List commonly used laboratory supplies and describe their proper use, quality control, cleaning, and maintenance procedures.
- Compare and contrast the use and care of glass and plastic supplies.

- Describe the specifications associated with the quality of reagent chemicals and solvents.
- Know the proper procedures for using pipets.
- Describe the operation and maintenance of balances, centrifuges, water baths, and heating blocks in the clinical laboratory.
- Describe the use and calibration of thermometers.
- Know general laboratory safety regulations, the components of the OSHA-mandated Chemical Hygiene Plan, and the plan for protection against blood-borne pathogens.

Key Terms

balances   Mechanical or electronic instruments used to measure weight accurately.

beakers   Laboratory utensils used to contain liquids or solids.

blood-borne pathogens   Potentially infectious agents in blood and body fluids.

buret (burette)   Laboratory utensil used to deliver a wide range of volumes accurately.

centrifuge   Instrument used to separate materials from solution by application of increased gravitational force by rotating or spinning samples rapidly.

Chemical Hygiene Plan   A laboratory plan that follows OSHA-mandated regulations, to protect employees against chemical hazards.

chemical purity   Degree of purity or homogeneity as designated by various scientific agencies, such as the American Chemical Society and National Institute of Standards and Technology (NIST).

desiccant   Material used in a dessicator to absorb water from the air.

desiccator   Large container used to store material in a water-free environment.

dilution   Process of preparing less concentrated solutions from a solution of greater concentration.

Erlenmeyer flask   Laboratory utensil used to contain liquids.

funnel   Laboratory utensil used to transfer liquids or solids into a container; also used for extraction of liquids.

graduated cylinder   Laboratory utensil used to measure a volume of liquid.

heating block   A temperature-controlled device used to warm and maintain materials at a specified temperature.

metric system   A system of measurement of weights, distances, and volumes.

Occupational Safety and Health Administration (OSHA)   Government agency responsible for mandating regulations to ensure safety in the workplace.

pipet (pipette)   Laboratory utensil used to transfer a specific or varying volume of liquid.

sanitization   The process used to maintain cleanliness in a water-purification system.

syringe   A device used for drawing up a specified quantity of liquid and then dispensing it volumetrically.

Système International d'Unités (SI)   An internationally accepted system of measurements.

thermometer   A device, physical, electronic, or optical, that is used to measure temperature.

volumetric flask   Laboratory utensil used to contain a specific volume of liquid.

water bath   A temperature-controlled device filled with water, used to warm and maintain materials at a specified temperature.

water purification   A treatment process (distillation, deionization, reverse osmosis, ultraviolet irradiation, ultrafiltration, or ozonolysis) used to remove water contaminants.

water purity   Three levels of purity are defined, based on the amount of biological and dissolved organic and inorganic material present in the water.

Part 1: Basic Laboratory Principles and Techniques

BETTE SEAMONDS

To provide accurate and precise clinical data, the clinical chemistry laboratory must be concerned with the analytical components used to provide this information. Familiarity with the purity of chemicals, solvents, and reagent water is essential. In addition, selection and use of appropriate analytical equipment and safe work practices are essential.

WATER AS A REAGENT

Water is one of the most important and commonly used reagents in the clinical laboratory. Because of its importance as a laboratory reagent and because it is often "produced" within each laboratory, water is discussed more fully in the following section.

Reagent Grade Water

Organic and inorganic impurities in the reagent water can introduce significant error into an analysis. Some impurities are easy to detect, but others are far more difficult. The need for high-purity reagent water in the clinical laboratory cannot be overemphasized.

Water systems that are improperly designed or inadequately maintained may actually add contaminants not originally found in the source water (feedwater). Thus the quality of reagent water produced by different purification systems can differ greatly. In general, systems that continually recirculate the water provide protection against stagnation and consequently minimize bacterial growth. However, the system must be decontaminated at regular intervals. The material used for the construction of pipes is important; plastics such as polyvinyl chloride (PVC) are commonly used but are not necessarily the best choice. PVC, in particular, leaches organic impurities into the purified water. In addition, it has a porous surface that tends to harbor bacteria and other biological impurities. For more detailed information, the reader is referred to the guideline "Preparation and Testing of Reagent Water in the Clinical Laboratory" published by the National Committee for Clinical Laboratory Standards (NCCLS).[1]

Water quality is *not* defined solely by the purification process used. Different types of purification processes may be employed, and in many laboratories multiple processes are used. The quality of the feedwater is important, often dictating the purification processes to be used and ultimately the types of contaminants likely to remain. Many of the characteristics of feedwater are affected by geographical and seasonal variations. The seasonal variability depends on rainfall, ground drainage, sewage, and industrial waste, whereas geographic location determines the hardness (mineral content) of the feedwater. Table 1-1 summarizes the types of purification processes available and their relative effectiveness in removing contaminants from feedwater. The laboratory should work closely with a reputable manufacturer to design a water-purification system to meet its specific needs.

Purification Process

Distillation. Distillation of water in glass effectively removes bacteria, pyrogens, particulate matter, dissolved ionized solids, and to a lesser extent dissolved organic contaminants. It is not useful for elimination of dissolved ionized gases such as ammonia, carbon dioxide, and chlorine or low–boiling point organic compounds.

Deionization. In the deionization process, water is passed through a bed of mixed cation- and anion-exchange resins. Hydrogen and hydroxyl ions on the surface of the resins are displaced by cationic and anionic impurities. This process is excellent for removal of dissolved ionized gases and solids but is ineffective for all other contaminants. In addition, the resin must be frequently replaced or regenerated. Deionization is used in conjunction with *carbon adsorption,* which is very effective in removal of dissolved organic compounds. The characteristics of the carbon employed dictate the efficacy of removal of the different organic contaminants. Neither deionization nor carbon adsorption will remove particulate matter, bacteria, or pyrogens.

Reverse osmosis. In reverse osmosis, water is forced under pressure through a semipermeable membrane, leaving behind remnants of the dissolved organic, ionic, and suspended impurities, including microbial and viral contaminants. Reverse osmosis, however, does not remove dissolved gases effectively. This method is frequently used to pretreat water before purification by deionization.

Ultrafiltration. In ultrafiltration, water is passed through semipermeable membranes of pore size $\leq 0.2\ \mu m$, removing particulate matter, emulsified solids, most bacteria, and pyrogens. Increasingly, $0.1\ \mu m$ postmembrane filters are being used to achieve an improved bacteria-free and pyrogen-free product. Ultrafiltration does not effectively remove dissolved ionized solids, gases, and most organic contaminants.

Ultraviolet oxidation and sterilization. Ultraviolet (UV) oxidation and sterilization are used after other purifi-

TABLE 1-1 A COMPARISON OF WATER-PURIFICATION PROCESSES

| | MAJOR CLASSES OF CONTAMINANTS | | | | | |
Purification Process	Dissolved Ionized Solids	Dissolved Ionized Gases	Dissolved Organics*	Particulate Matter	Micro-organisms*	Pyrogens/Endotoxins
Distillation	E[†]	G/P	G	E	E	E
Deionization	E	E	P	P	P	P
Reverse osmosis	G[‡]	P	G	E	E	E
Carbon adsorption/absorption	P	P[§]	E/G[‖]	P	P	P
Filtration (0.22 μm)	P	P	P	E	E	P
Ultrafiltration	P	P	P	E	E	E
Nanofiltration	G/P	P	G[¶]	E	E	E
Chemical oxidation	P	P	P	P	E/G	E/G
Ultraviolet oxidation•	P	P	G[#]	P	G/P	P
Ultraviolet sterilization•	P	P	P	P	G[**]	P

Note: This chart is offered only as a general guideline. Because of the variability of performance within each process and feedwater supply, potential users are urged to contact a reputable manufacturer of pure water equipment for applications assistance before selecting a system for the laboratory.
E, Excellent (capable of complete or near-total removal); G, Good (capable of removing large percentages); P, Poor (little or no removal).
*Treatment with ozone, although currently not commonly used in clinical laboratory water purification systems, has been shown preliminarily to be very effective in oxidizing bacteria, viruses, and their organic metabolites.
†The resistivity of water purified by distillation is an order of magnitude less than that of water purified by deionization because of the presence of CO_2 and sometimes H_2S, NH_3, and other ionized gases in the feedwater.
‡The residual concentration of dissolved ionized solids depends partly on the original concentration in the feedwater.
§Activated carbon will remove chlorine by adsorption.
‖When used in combination with other purification processes, special grades of activated carbon and other synthetic adsorbents exhibit excellent capabilities for removing organic contaminants. Their use, however, is targeted toward specific compounds and applications; consult with the manufacturer before use.
¶Ultrafilters are useful for reducing specific feedwater organic contaminants based on the rated molecular weight cutoff of the membrane.
•Ultraviolet light kills microorganisms but does not remove them. Another process is required to remove them.
#185 nm UV oxidation (batch process systems) is effective in removing trace organic contaminants when used after treatment. Feedwater makeup plays a crucial role in the performance of these batch processors. They should not be confused with in-line UV sterlllizers, which use 254 nm UV radiation to inactivate bacteria.
**254 nm UV sterilizers, although not physically removing bacteria, may have bactericidal or bacteriostatic capabilities limited by intensity, contact, time, and flow rate.
Reproduced with permission from Preparation and testing of reagent water in the clinical laboratory, ed 3, Approved Guideline C3-A3, Wayne, PA, 1997, NCCLS.

cation processes to remove trace amounts of organic contaminants (oxidation) and bacteria (sterilization). Different wavelengths are used for these processes—185 nm for oxidation and 254 nm for sterilization. UV treatment is limited by intensity, contact time, and flow rate. Sterilization is the more commonly used procedure, but is frequently referred to as *UV oxidation.*

Ozone. Ozone treatment, used primarily in industrial settings, effectively removes organic contaminants. However, smaller, less expensive ozone generators are becoming available and will possibly begin finding their way into clinical laboratory settings. After it is introduced into the pretreated water, the ozone kills bacteria by rupturing the cell membrane almost instantaneously (~2 sec). Chlorine, on the other hand, simply diffuses into the cell and requires approximately half an hour to achieve its effect. The actual rate of lysis depends on the ozone level: higher ozone concentrations are used for highly contaminated systems, whereas lower concentrations are used for maintenance. After the microorganisms are lysed, the cytoplasmic constituents are oxidized by the ozone. The ozone is then removed by UV irradiation at 254 nm. Removal is crucial because ozone is incompatible with the deionization resins. Ozone treatment can be effectively used to combat microbial contamination in pipes and purified water.

Grades of Water Purity

Three levels of **water purity** (types I, II, and III) plus a special reagent water category have been defined by the NCCLS. The College of American Pathologists (CAP) has also defined three grades of reagent water, which are essentially equivalent to those of the NCCLS. Table 1-2 summarizes the NCCLS specifications for the three levels of water quality. Waters falling into the "Special" category may require additional treatment to meet more specific requirements and applications.

Water conforming to specifications published by other agencies such as the American Society for Testing and Materials (ASTM), the American Chemical Society (ACS), and the United States Pharmacopeia (USP) may or may not be equivalent to water conforming to NCCLS specifications. ASTM water most closely resembles NCCLS type II water, whereas USP specifications are designed to ensure safety for *in vivo* and *in vitro* applications. USP water must pass a series of designated tests, such as those that document the absence of pyrogens, rather than meet definitive contaminant concentrations.

Storage and Handling of Reagent Water

Type I water should be used immediately after it is produced. It cannot be stored because its resistivity will rapidly decrease

TABLE 1-2   REAGENT WATER SPECIFICATIONS

	Type I	Type II	Type III
Maximum **microbial** content, colony forming units per mL (CFU/mL)	10*	1000	NS
pH	NS	NS	5.0 to 8.0
Minimum **resistivity**, megohm • centimeter (mΩ • cm 25° C)	10 (inline)	1.0	0.1
Maximum **silicate** mg/L SiO_2	0.05	0.1	1.0
Particulate matter[†]	0.22-µm filter[†]	NS	NS
Organic contaminants[‡]	Activated[†] carbon or distillation or reverse osmosis	NS	NS

NS, *Not specified.*
Preferably, type I water should be bacteria free.
[†]*This specification is a process specification and is not measured by the end user.*
[‡]*At a minimum, some form of activated carbon should be included in a reagent water system as pretreatment to help remove organic contaminants found in raw water supplies. Furthermore, additional treatment with special grades of carbon may be indicated for applications requiring extremely low levels of organic contaminants. Because the performance of carbon used in pretreatment and posttreatment is site specific, consult with the manufacturer for recommended replacement intervals. (See also footnote ||, Table 1-1.)*
Reproduced with permission from Preparation and testing of reagent water in the clinical laboratory, *ed 3, Approved Guideline C3-A3, Wayne, PA, 1997, NCCLS.*

as carbon dioxide is absorbed. In addition, ionic and organic contaminants will be leached from the storage container, and microbial contamination will occur.[2] Type II water can be stored for short periods. The storage and distribution systems should be constructed of materials that minimize bacterial and chemical contamination. When water is removed from a storage tank into a secondary vessel for routine use, the secondary vessel and the water must be replaced at least daily. Water should not be stored in carboys for routine use because this leads to degradation of the water quality.[2]

Under some conditions, purchased stored water may be used. One example is water that is provided as a diluent by the manufacturer of a specific analytic system. In this case the water has been validated by the manufacturer for use as stated in the product insert. *Under no conditions can such a product be substituted for reagent water.* Similarly, sterile water is not equivalent to reagent-grade water and therefore is not an acceptable substitute. As already stated, USP water meets specifications for particular tests and not for specific contaminants. Other purchased products may include those for use in high-performance liquid chromatographic (HPLC) procedures in facilities where the quality of in-house reagent water is not satisfactory for that purpose.

If water must be purchased, several important issues should be considered. The purchased product should define silica content, bacterial contamination, and conductivity at the time of manufacture. The water should be purchased in quantities appropriate to usage. The packaged water should be protected from environmental contamination and from the leaching effects of the container. When the container is opened, the bacterial count and conductivity should be measured for assessment of quality degradation since manufacture. The limits of acceptability should be similar to those of type II water. When required analytically, the water should be poured into an appropriate secondary container from which it will be sampled. Care must be taken to avoid touching the inside lid

or dipping a pipet directly into the primary vessel. Unused portions of water must not be returned to the primary container. Water from the primary container should be discarded after a period of no more than 1 week.

Purchased water provides an ideal supply of feedwater for benchtop purification systems. Such systems, and even those capable of purifying tap water, are available and allow even the smallest laboratory to produce limited quantities of type I water.

Suggested Uses

The scientific literature contains little documentation of the analytical difficulties caused by poor quality water. However, many users of the NCCLS document on reagent water have reported specific instances of analytic problems attributed to water quality. These include difficulty with coagulation and hematologic analyses, interference with some immunoassay procedures, instrumentation problems (including background absorbance difficulties), leaching of contaminants from improperly regenerated deionization resins, and absorption of perfume into highly purified water causing difficulty with cell culture procedures. In addition, bacteria, silicate, and other ion contamination have been shown to interfere with enzyme and bilirubin analyses.[3] Undoubtedly as techniques become more sensitive, more definitive information may become available.

Type I water should be used in all quantitative and most qualitative laboratory procedures, for electrophoretic analyses, for toxicology screening procedures, and in the preparation of buffers, standards, and controls. Further treatment of type I water may be necessary for trace element and heavy metal analyses. Type II water is acceptable for use in reagents with preservatives or reagents that are sterilized, and in most stains. Type III water is acceptable for washing and preliminary rinsing of glassware. It may also serve as source water for further purification.

Special purpose reagent water may be necessary for specific procedures such as HPLC, chromosome analyses, human leukocyte antigen (HLA) testing, and *in vitro* fertilization (IVF) and gamete intrafallopian transfer (GIFT) procedures. Systems can be designed to produce water that meets specific requirements, or type I water can be purified further.

Quality Control and Impurity Testing

Water must be monitored at regular intervals to evaluate the performance of a water purification system. Because of the variety of contaminants found in water, no single test can measure water purity. The schedule for regular evaluations may vary with the season and with the contaminants found. In addition to ensuring that the purification system is functioning acceptably under routine conditions, monitoring ensures the purity of the water after a component or components of the system have been changed. At a minimum, frequent bacterial surveillance and resistivity determinations are necessary. The monitoring of other parameters such as pH, silicate content, pyrogens, organic contamination, and particulate matter depends on many factors. Each laboratory should determine frequency guidelines based on the history, system design, and use of its water purification system. In general, if the source water and the purification system produce a product that is consistently negative for a particular contaminant, the laboratory may test for that contaminant infrequently. Some of the tests must be performed by the laboratory, and other tests may be referred out.

Microbial monitoring. Bacteria can inactivate reagents by metabolizing certain components. In addition, they contribute to the total organic contamination and can alter optical properties of test solutions. Although microbial monitoring is retrospective, it provides the laboratory with useful information and may be helpful in detecting impending problems. *Weekly* testing should be performed. Several acceptable methods are available, although no single method can be assumed to quantitate all bacteria in a water sample. Therefore the number of viable bacteria may be higher than the number of colony-forming units determined in any given method. Several criteria may be applied to choosing a method, but regardless of the method selected, the first step in obtaining a reliable result is the collection of an appropriate sample.

Before collection, the spigot should be fully opened for at least 1 minute. This procedure flushes the system adequately, and should also be employed when drawing water to use in reagent preparation. One of the most common causes of rapid bacterial contamination in water is inadequate flushing. The volume of water collected for analysis varies with the procedure used. An amount from 1 mL (for bacteriologic samplers) to 100 mL (standard plate count or filtration methods) may be collected. After collection, the sample should be processed as soon as possible. The sample should not be stored more than 1 hour at room temperature or 6 hours in the refrigerator. For certain procedures the sample must be vortexed vigorously to ensure distribution of organisms within the sample. The most commonly found organisms are gram-negative rods.

Resistivity. Resistivity measurements are used to assess the ionic content of purified water. The higher the ion concentration, the lower the resistivity. Ion-exchange tanks should be equipped with an in-line "resistivity" light that is calibrated to go off when the resistivity falls below 2 mΩ•cm, at which point the capacity of the tanks is exhausted. Systems that supply type I water *must* have an in-line resistivity meter that is capable of reading to 18 mΩ•cm. The resistivity must be 10 mΩ•cm at a minimum (preferably 15 to 18 mΩ•cm) in order to meet type I specifications. Off-line measurements may be used for resistivity monitoring of type II and type III water; however, in-line measurements are easier and more accurate and are therefore recommended for systems producing type II water. Procedures for off-line measurements are available.[1] The frequency of monitoring is *daily*.

pH. Monitoring of the pH of purified (particularly type I) water is generally not necessary, but methods are available if a pH problem is suspected.[1] Anecdotal reports have suggested that in some facilities, source water pH problems have led to product water pH problems. Some systems now allow in-line pH measurements, but they are not yet used in clinical laboratories.

Pyrogens. Pyrogens are not monitored routinely in the clinical laboratory. However, anecdotal reports from manufacturers indicate that some immunoassay reagents are affected by interference from pyrogens. Therefore testing for this contaminant may become more important with time. Procedures for pyrogen testing are readily available.[4,5]

Silica. Silica in the water supply can be a major problem in some geographical areas. Silica can interfere with trace metal and electrolyte analyses, enzyme determinations, and some spectrophotometrical assays, and removal of this contaminant is essential. Colloidal silica is readily removed by distillation and certain reverse osmosis membranes. Soluble silica may be measured by spectrophotometrical analysis.[1] However, the procedure requires the use of a narrow-bandpass instrument, preferably capable of reading at ~800 nm. Frequently the reagent blanks generate absorbances higher than those of the water being tested. For this reason it may be preferable to refer samples for analysis by inductively coupled plasma (ICP) spectrometry.

Organic contaminants. Bacteria can multiply in the resin beds, significantly increasing the organic contamination of water. Methods for routinely assessing contamination, though plentiful, are either not sufficiently specific (permanganate) or impractical (e.g., requiring research grade spectrophotometers and HPLC). If the laboratory has access to HPLC, the measurement is easily accomplished.[6] The best approach to dealing with organic contamination is to design and maintain the system optimally. Semiannual **sanitization** (or more frequently if quality control data dictate) helps control bacteria levels. Use of carbon adsorption and UV treatment also help remove organic contaminants. Constant surveillance of the system ensures the production of reagent water of the desired quality.

System Documentation and Record Keeping

A procedure manual should be developed for the water-purification system that includes the following[1,7]:

1. A quality assurance plan defining responsibilities of personnel
2. Procedures for preventive maintenance
3. Quality control checklists
4. Worksheets for documenting daily, weekly, monthly, and other testing
5. Documentation of corrective action taken

CHEMICAL LABORATORY SUPPLIES
Chemicals

Chemicals are available in varying degrees of purity, and in many instances the types and concentrations of impurities are known. Less pure grades of chemicals include *chemically pure*, *practical grade*, *technical grade*, and *commercial grade*. Such chemicals are unsuitable for use in analytical work. Certain chemicals, especially pharmaceuticals, are produced to meet the specifications defined in *The United States Pharmacopoeia (USP)*, *The National Formulary*, and *The Food Chemical Index*. These specifications define impurity tolerances that are not injurious to health.

Most qualitative and quantitative analyses in the clinical laboratory require the use of chemicals that meet the specifications of the ACS; such chemicals are described as either *analytical grade* or *reagent grade*. ACS specifications establish the maximum quantities of impurities allowed in each chemical or provide impurity contents on a lot-to-lot basis. Some manufacturers sell certified or very pure materials when specifications have not been established by the ACS.

Additional standards of purity for certain chemicals have been specified by the International Union for Pure and Applied Chemistry (IUPAC). These include atomic weight standards (grade A); ultimate standards (grade B); primary standards (grade C), which are commercially available and have less than 0.002% impurities; working standards (grade D), which are commercially available and have less than 0.05% impurities; and secondary substances (grade E), which are defined or standardized by an acceptable reference method using a primary standard (grade C) as the reference material.

Primary Standards

Primary standards are supplied with certificates of analysis for each lot. These preparations must be stable, nonhygroscopic substances of definite composition that can be dried without changing composition.

Standard Reference Materials

Standard Reference Materials (SRMs) are available from the National Institute of Standards and Technology (NIST). Not all SRMs are as pure as primary standards; however, NIST defines their chemical and physical properties and provides a certificate documenting results of characterization. These standards may then be used to characterize other materials. SRMs are available in solid, liquid, or gaseous form. The solids may be crystalline, powder, or lyophilized products.

Organic Solvents

Classification of organic solvents follows the same guidelines as those used for other chemicals. Thus for many analyses, in particular those involving spectroscopy and chromatography, reagents of even higher purity than reagent grade are required. These solvents frequently are referred to as *spectrograde*, *nanograde*, or *HPLC grade*, and information about the presence of contaminants is supplied with the solvent. The purity ensures minimal spectral interference and minimal residual contamination after extraction and evaporation of the solvent in the analytic procedure. In general these solvents are more than 99% pure (as determined by gas chromatography) and no single impurity exceeds 0.2%.

Gases

Gases, particularly those used in gas chromatography and atomic absorption analyses, must be extremely pure. Helium purity must be 99.9999% for gas chromatographic procedures. As with other reagents, information regarding contaminants and their concentrations is of utmost importance. (See Appendix D for more specific information.)

Chemical Safety

Many chemicals and solvents are flammable, teratogenic, and carcinogenic. Therefore all chemicals should be handled with the utmost care, and inhalation of fumes or dust should be avoided. Similarly, the handling of gas cylinders requires adherence to specific regulations. The specifics of safe practices are discussed in the laboratory safety section.

Desiccants

A **desiccant** is a material used to absorb and remove water from the air or from another substance (Table 1-3). Some desiccants are deliquescent and therefore lose their efficiency after liquefaction occurs. Others produce dust and should therefore be avoided. The most commonly used desiccants are manufactured with a moisture-sensitive indicator salt, such as cobalt chloride, to indicate exhaustion. Silica gel and anhydrous calcium sulfate (Drierite) are examples. These agents can be regenerated by heat, making them cost efficient.

LABORATORY PLASTIC AND GLASSWARE COMPOSITION AND CLEANING

Laboratory supplies that are used for the preparation, measurement, and storage of fluids and other products of reactions include tubing, glassware, and plasticware. Glass must be used for procedures involving HPLC and gas-liquid chromatography (GLC) because solvents readily attack plastics. On the other hand, many solutions with a pH above 6.0 can attack glassware, and alkaline solutions should be stored in plastic.[8] Glass also tends to adsorb metal ions, possibly altering significantly the concentrations of standard solutions.

Tubing

Natural latex rubber tubing is durable and can be used for glass connections. It is, however, affected by contact with

TABLE 1-3   SOME COMMON DRYING AGENTS (DESICCANTS)

Desiccant	Properties	Uses
Anhydrous $CaCl_2$	High capacity, slow acting, works well below 30° C	Most conditions, very inexpensive
Anhydrous $MgSO_4$	Neutral, rapid action	Most conditions, inexpensive
Anhydrous Na_2SO_4	Neutral, high capacity, works only below 32° C, slow action	Can remove large volume of water
Anhydrous $CaSO_4$	Extremely rapid action, chemically inert, limited capacity to absorb water (6% to 10% of its weight in water)	More expensive than $MgSO_4$ and Na_2SO_4; sold commercially as Drierite; can be easily regenerated by heating at 230° to 240° C for 3 hours
Al_2O_3 (activated alumina)	Can absorb 15% to 20% of its weight in water	Can be repeatedly reactivated by heating at 175° C for 7 hours

oils, alkalis, corrosives, and hot water. Neoprene (synthetic) rubber tubing may be substituted for latex tubing in most situations. It should not be used with chlorinated or aromatic hydrocarbons.

More expensive than rubber tubing, synthetic plastic Tygon tubing is the most useful. Tygon is resistant to chemicals and inert to chemicals. It can be used in many applications such as peristaltic pumps; it can also be joined to other tubing using a heat welding process. Over time it tends to discolor and become slightly brittle. Polytetrafluoroethylene (Teflon) tubing is also available; it is more expensive than Tygon tubing but serves as a substitute in certain situations.

Types of Glass

Many types of glass are available. They differ in their tensile strength, resistivity to certain agents, and heat or light resistance. Most reusable glassware in the clinical laboratory is made from borosilicate glass, which is available under the brand names of Pyrex (Corning Glass Works, Corning, NY) and Kimax (Kimble Glass Company, Vineland, NJ). Borosilicate glass has a low alkaline earth content and is free of contaminants such as heavy metals. Therefore liquids can be heated in borosilicate glass with minimal contamination. This type of glass can be safely heated to approximately 600° C for short periods. Table 1-4 lists additional types of glass and their uses.

TABLE 1-4   TYPES OF COMMONLY USED GLASS AND THEIR PROPERTIES

Glass	Properties	Purpose
Kimax/Pyrex	Relatively inert borosilicate glass, high resistance to heat and cold shock	All purpose
Vycor	Good resistance to drastic conditions of heat, shock, chemical treatment, and high temperature; acid and alkali resistant	Ashing, ignition techniques
Corex	Aluminosilicate glass, about six-fold stronger than borosilicate glass; scratch resistant; resistant to alkaline etching	Used under conditions of stress
High silica	>96% silicate; comparable to fused quartz; heat, chemical, and electrical tolerance; excellent optical properties	For high-precision analytical work, optical reflectors, and mirrors
Boron-free	Alkali resistant; poor heat resistance; soft; <0.2% boron	Highly alkaline solutions
Low actinic	Amber or red color reduces light exposure of contents	For use with light-sensitive materials in range of 300 to 500 nm (e.g., bilirubin, vitamin A, carotene)
Flint	Soda-lime glass containing oxides of sodium, silicon, and calcium; poor resistance to high temperature or temperature changes, poor chemical resistance; may also leach organic contaminants	Used for disposable glassware items (e.g., pipets)
Coated	Thin, metallic oxide fire-bonded to glass surface	Conducts electricity, acts as electrostatic shield; protects against infrared
Optical	Made of soda lime, lead, and borosilicate	Prisms, lenses, and optical mirrors
Pyroceram	High thermal resistance, chemically stable, corrosion resistant	Hot plates, heat exchangers

Types of Plastic

Plastic laboratory utensils are made from polymerized organic monomers. The properties of the plastics depend on the nature of the monomer and the final polymer forms used to prepare the plastic materials. The most commonly used plastics include the polyolefins (i.e., polyethylene, polypropylene), polystyrene, polycarbonate, Teflon, and PVC.

Polyolefins, which are relatively chemically inert, are resistant to most acids, alkalis, and salt solutions. Organic acids and hydrocarbons cause swelling and penetration of the plastic. Concentrated sulfuric acid attacks polyethylene at room temperature. Polyethylene is used in most disposable plasticware and cannot be sterilized. Polypropylene may be sterilized.

Polycarbonate is stronger than polypropylene and has better temperature tolerances. Its chemical resistance is not as good as that of the polyolefins. Its primary characteristics are its clarity and resistance to shattering, making it the material of choice for items such as centrifuge tubes.

Teflon is an extremely inert plastic with excellent temperature tolerance ($-270°$ to $+255°$ C) and chemical resistivity. Because of its nonwettable surface and antiadhesive properties, it is an excellent material for stir bars, bottle-cap liners, stopcocks, and tubing. It is one of the most desirable materials for use in water distribution systems; however, it is considerably more costly than other plastics used for this purpose. Although it is easy to clean and dry, it scratches and warps readily.

PVC plastic is soft and flexible but porous. It is used frequently in the form of tubing, particularly in reagent water systems. Its drawbacks have been discussed in the section on reagent water.

Table 1-5 reviews the characteristics of some plastics commonly encountered in laboratory products.

In many instances, plastic utensils should be used instead of glass because plastic utensils do not release ions into solution and they are unbreakable. However, some plastics such as polyethylene are porous, and evaporation may be a problem. Therefore long-term storage in partially filled plastic containers is undesirable. In addition, polyethylene and other plastics can adsorb proteins and other compounds such as dyes, stains, and some salts, resulting in analytical problems. Nevertheless, plastic containers are preferable for use in trace-metal analyses. One can remove the small quantities of trace metals in the plastic by soaking the plastic in 1 M HCl and rinsing with water purified to eliminate trace metal contamination. Long-term soaking (>8 hr) in acid should be avoided because it makes the plastic brittle. Plastic can also be cleaned with alcohol, alkalis, or alcoholic alkalis to remove trace organic contaminants that contribute to trace metal adsorption.

Cleaning of Glass and Plastic Utensils

Glassware must be thoroughly clean before it is used in any analytical procedure. Unclean glassware results in chemical contamination. In addition, if glassware is not clean, the surface of the glass does not wet uniformly, and volume errors result, caused by incomplete drainage of dispensing devices or distortion of the meniscus.

Dirty utensils should be rinsed immediately after use and soaked in either a weak detergent solution or in a tenfold dilution of household bleach. Any vessels in which hazardous materials were contained should be handled separately to prevent unintentional exposure to the hazardous agent. Numerous effective cleaning agents are available for washing laboratory glassware and plasticware. Some items, such as pipets, require additional soaking before washing. In many institutions washing is done by an automatic glassware washer. The manufacturers of automatic washers usually recommend or require specific detergents. In general, metal-free, nonionic detergents that are not highly alkaline are used. The washer must be equipped with the appropriate purified water rinse cycles to prevent contamination. If utensils are washed manually, they must be thoroughly rinsed with tap water and then rinsed three to five times with purified, preferably type I, water. When glassware is clean, purified water drains as a continuous film, whereas unclean vessels will have small drops of water clinging to the surface. After drying, the appearance of spots indicates unclean glassware, possibly the result of inadequate rinsing. This procedure is not appropriate for nonwettable plastics. Incomplete detergent removal can be detected by rinsing a vessel with a dilute (20 mg/L) aqueous solution of sulfobromophthalein (Bromsulphalein) dye or some other acid-base indicator, or by measuring the pH of purified water added to the glassware.

As previously mentioned, acid washing may be necessary in some instances. Dilute HCl (1 M) or dilute HNO_3 (1 M) is preferred. Chromic acid is no longer used for this procedure because of residual contamination and the hazards of handling and preparing the solutions.

Ultrasonic cleaners may also be used to supplement the action of detergents. These may be particularly helpful in cleaning protein-coated utensils.

Both glassware and plasticware should be dried either at room temperature or at temperatures below $100°$ C. This prevents degradation of the plastic and changes in the volume designations of glassware. If solvents are used to assist in drying, they should be of high quality and water miscible. Any gases used should also be of high purity.

LABORATORY UTENSILS
Beakers

Beakers (Fig. 1-1, *4*) are wide-mouthed, straight-sided, cylindrical vessels available in both glass and plastic. Beaker volumes vary from 5 mL to several liters. They are used for general mixing and preparation of nonvolumetric liquid reagents.

Funnels

Funnels are most commonly used to transfer liquids or solids into containers. *Filtering funnels* (Fig. 1-1, *7*) are usually 58- or 60-degree angled funnels with either short or long, thin stems. They are used with filter paper to remove particles from solution. Many funnels have ridges to increase the surface area available for filtering. *Powder funnels* for use in transferring solids (Fig. 1-1, *8*) have wide-mouthed stems to

TABLE 1-5 SUMMARY OF THE CHEMICAL RESISTANCE (AT 20° C) AND PHYSICAL PROPERTIES OF VARIOUS PLASTICS

Classes of Substances				TYPES OF RESINS*						
	LDPE	HDPE	PP, PA	PET, PETC	PMP	FEP, TFE, ETFE	PC	PSF	PVC Bottles†	PS
Chemical Resistance										
Acids, dilute or weak	E	E	E	E	E	E	E	E	E	E
Acids‡ strong and concentrated	E	E	E	N	E	E	N	G	E	F
Alcohols, aliphatic	E	E	E	E	E	E	G	G	E	E
Aldehydes	G	G	G	N	G	E	F	F	N	N
Bases	E	E	E	N	E	E	N	E	E	E
Esters	G	G	G	N	G	E	N	N	N	N
Hydrocarbons, aliphatic	F	G	G	E	F	E	F	G	E	N
Hydrocarbons, aromatic	F	G	F	N	F	E	N	N	N	N
Hydrocarbons, halogenated	N	F	F	N	N	E	N	N	N	N
Ketones	G	G	G	N	F	E	N	N	N	N
Oxidizing agents, strong	F	F	F	N	F	E	N	G	G	N
Physical Properties				*PET* *PETC*						
Maximum-use temperature (° C)	80	120	135 (PP) 130 (PA)	150 70	175	205 (FEP) 150 (ETFE)	135	165	70¶	–
Brittleness temperature (° C)	–100	–100	0 (PP) –40 (PA)	–60 –40	20	–270 (FEP) –100 (ETFE)	–135	–100	–30	–
Sterilization§										
Autoclaving	No	No	Yes	No No	No	Yes	Yes‖	Yes	No¶	–
Gas	Yes	Yes	Yes	Yes Yes	Yes	Yes	Yes	Yes	Yes	–
Dry heat	No	No	No	No No	Yes‖	Yes	No	Yes	No	–
Chemical	Yes	Yes	Yes	Some Yes	Yes	Yes	Yes	Yes	Yes	–
Microwavability•	Yes	No	Yes	Yes Yes	Yes	Yes	No	Yes	Yes	No
Noncytotoxicity#	Yes	Yes	Yes	Yes Yes	Yes	Yes	Yes	Yes	Yes	Yes

*Resin codes: ETFE, *Tefzel ETFE (ethylene tetrafluoroethylene)*; FEP, *Teflon FEP (fluorinated ethylene propylene)*; HDPE, *high-density polyethylene*; LDPE, *low-density polyethylene*; PA, *polyallomer*; PC, *polycarbonate*; PMP, *polymethylpentene ("TPX")*; PP, *polypropylene*; PS, *polystyrene*; PSF, *polysulfone*; PVC, *polyvinyl chloride*; TFE, *Teflon TFE (tetrafluoroethylene)*; PET, *polyethylene terephthalate*; PETC, *polyethylene terephthalate copolyester*.

Chemical resistance classification: *E, 30 days of constant exposure cause no damage. Plastic may even tolerate it for years. G, Little or no damage after 30 days of constant exposure to the reagent. F, Some effect after 7 days of constant exposure to the reagent. Depending on the plastic, the effect may be crazing, cracking, loss of strength, or discoloration. Solvents may cause softening, swelling, and permeation losses with LDPE, HDPE, PP, PA, and PMP. The solvent effects on these five resins are normally reversible; the part will usually return to its normal condition after evaporation. N, Not recommended for continuous use. Immediate damage may occur. Depending on the plastic, the effect will be a more severe crazing, cracking, loss of strength, discoloration, deformation, dissolution, or permeation loss.*

† For polyvinyl chloride tubing, see the current Nalgene Labware Catalog.

‡ Except for oxidizing acids. For oxidizing acids, see "Oxidizing agents, strong."

§ Sterilization: Autoclaving: Clean and rinse item with distilled water-before autoclaving. Certain chemicals that have no appreciable effect on resin at room temperature may cause deterioration at autoclaving temperatures unless removed with distilled water beforehand. Gas: ethylene oxide. Dry heat: At 160° C. Chemical: Benzalkonium chloride, formalin, ethanol, and so on.

‖ Sterilization reduces mechanical strength. Do not use polycarbonate vessels for vacuum applications if they have been autoclaved.

¶ Except for the polyvinyl chloride in tubing, which will withstand temperatures to 121° C and can be autoclaved. Refer to "The Use and Care of Plastic Labware" in the current Nalgene Labware Catalog for detailed information on sterilization.

• Ratings based on 5-minute tests using 600 watts of power on exposed, empty labware. Labware should not be exposed to chemicals that attack or are absorbed by the plastic due to heating. Do not exceed maximum temperature.

#"Yes" indicates the resin has been determined to be noncytotoxic, based on USP and ASTM biocompatibility testing standards utilizing an MEM elution technique on a W138 human diploid long cell line.

Interpretation of chemical resistance: *This summary is a general guide only. Because so many factors can affect the chemical resistance of a given product, you should test under your own conditions. If any doubt exists about specific applications of Nalgene products, please contact Technical Service, Nalge Nunc International; 75 Panorama Creek Drive, Rochester, NY 14625-2385, or call (800) 625-4327, or e-mail nntech@nalgenunc.com, or visit the website at www.nalgenunc.com.*

Effects of chemicals on plastics: *Chemicals can affect the strength, flexibility, surface appearance, color, dimensions, or weight of plastics. The basic modes of interaction that cause these changes are (1) chemical attack on the polymer chain, resulting in reduction in physical properties, including oxidation; reaction of functional groups in or on the chain; and depolymerization; (2) physical change, including absorption of solvents, resulting in softening and swelling of the plastic; permeation of solvent through the plastic; dissolution in a solvent; and (3) stress cracking from the interaction of a "stress-cracking agent" with molded-in or external stresses. The reactive combination of compounds of two or more classes may cause a synergistic or undesirable chemical effect. Other factors affecting chemical resistance include temperature, pressure, and internal or external stresses (such as centrifugation), length of exposure, and concentration of the chemical. As temperature increases, resistance to attack decreases.*

CAUTION: *Do not store strong oxidizing agents in plastic labware except that made of Teflon FEP. Prolonged exposure causes embrittlement and failure. Although prolonged storage may not be intended at the time of filling, a forgotten container will fail in time and result in leakage of contents. Do not place plastic labware in a flame or on a hot plate.*

Modified from Nalgene labware catalog, *Rochester, NY, 2000, Nalge Nunc International; An apogent Company.*

allow easy passage of the solids. The inner surface of these funnels is smooth. Both filtering and powder funnels are available in plastic and glass. *Separatory funnels* (Fig. 1-1, *2*) are constructed with a ground-glass stoppered opening at one end and a stopcock opening at the other end. These devices are used for manual liquid-liquid extractions of relatively large volumes of samples. The lower phase is separated from the upper phase through the stopcock, allowing salvage of one or both phases.

Desiccators

Desiccators (Fig. 1-1, *10*) are used to dry, or keep dry, solid or liquid materials. The desiccant is usually placed in the bottom of the desiccator and a shelf placed above the desiccant. The material is then stored on top of the shelf. The top of the desiccator has a wide, flat, ground-glass lip that fits snugly against an opposing lip on the bottom part of the desiccator. Stopcock grease is usually placed on the surface of the lips to provide an airtight seal. Many desiccators also have a stopcock outlet on the upper portion to allow the desiccator to be evacuated. Laboratories often have several desiccators to allow for storage at different temperatures, including ambient, refrigerator, and freezer temperatures. The types of desiccants available are described in Table 1-3.

Graduated Cylinders

Graduated cylinders are narrow, straight-sided vessels that are used to measure specific volumes (Fig. 1-1, *5*). They are available in plastic and glass in sizes ranging from 5 mL to several liters. They may be calibrated *to deliver* (TD) or *to contain* (TC) the volume indicated at specific temperatures, and they are graduated into subdivisions of approximately 100 portions of the total volume of the cylinder. Sometimes they are equipped with stoppers and are used to prepare solutions requiring less accuracy than those prepared volumetrically.

Burets

Traditional **burets** are long, graduated glass tubes with a stopcock at one end (Fig. 1-1, *9*). These devices are used to deliver, accurately, known amounts of liquid into a container. By measurement from graduated line to graduated line, fractional volumes of less than 1 mL may be dispensed with a high degree of accuracy. Microprocessor-controlled automatic burets are now available with an accuracy as high as 0.1%. The dispensed volumes are monitored on a digital display capable of reading to 0.001 mL.

Flasks

Flasks of many types are used in the clinical laboratory; the most commonly used are the **volumetric** and **Erlenmeyer flasks** shown in Fig. 1-1, *1* and *6*. **Round-bottom** flasks are often used to evaporate a sample to dryness. The sizes of laboratory flasks vary from 1 mL to several liters.

Volumetric flasks. Volumetric flasks are essential for the accurate preparation of solutions of known concentration. Class A specifications for volumetric flasks are defined by the NIST and imprinted on the glass (Fig. 1-2). These specifi-

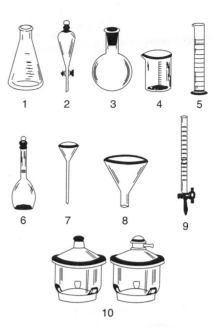

Fig. 1-1 Examples of commonly used laboratory utensils. *1*, Erlenmeyer flask. *2*, Separatory funnel. *3*, Round-bottom flask. *4*, Beaker. *5*, Graduated cylinder. *6*, Volumetric flask. *7*, Long-stem funnel (filtering). *8*, Powder funnel. *9*, Buret. *10*, Desiccators.

TABLE 1-6 ACCURACIES OF VOLUMETRIC FLASKS

Capacity (mL)	Limit of Error (mL)	Percent Error
25	0.03	0.1
50	0.05	0.1
100	0.08	0.08
250	0.11	0.04
500	0.15	0.03
1000	0.30	0.03

cations are accurate only at the temperature specified on the flask (Table 1-6). Volumetric flasks are used to contain (TC) an exact volume when the flask is appropriately filled to the indicator line. Such flasks therefore do not deliver an exact volume and cannot be used as transfer devices. The top of the volumetric flask is capped by a tight-fitting ground-glass or Teflon stopper. This allows the flask to be inverted without loss of liquid. Under no circumstances should a volumetric flask be heated because heating can distort the shape and volume of the flask. *Volumetric flasks should not be used for reagent storage.*

Syringes

Syringes may be used for accurate volumetric work such as the injection of small volumes of a sample, liquid or gas, for chromatographic analysis. Syringes are available in a range of sizes from 1 to 500 μL. They are constructed of glass and

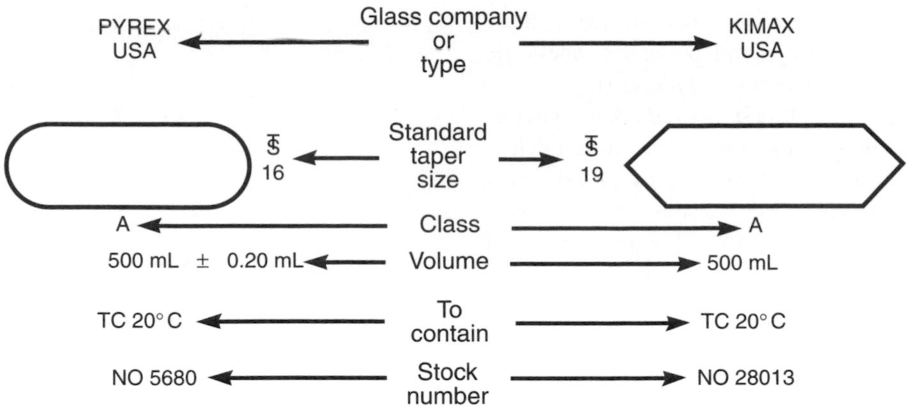

Fig. 1-2 Example of NIST specifications found imprinted on Class A volumetric flasks.

TABLE 1-7 ACCURACIES (IN mL) OF MANUAL PIPETS

Type of Pipet	1.0 mL	5.0 mL	10.0 mL	25.0 mL
NBS standard	—	0.01	0.02	0.025
Class A volumetric	0.006	0.01	0.02	0.03
Mohr	0.01	0.02	0.03	0.10
Mohr long tip	0.02	0.04	0.06	—
Serological	0.01	0.02	0.03	0.10
Serological large opening	0.05	0.10	0.10	0.20
Serological long tip	0.02	0.04	0.06	—

have a precision-bore hole into which a tight-fitting plunger is placed. The dispensing tip of the syringe is a very fine diameter metal needle that is able to pierce the septum of the injection port. For syringes of greater than $5\,\mu L$ volume, manufacturers claim that inaccuracy will not exceed 1% of the total syringe volume and repeated measurements will not differ by more than 1% of the dispensed volume. For devices of less than $5\,\mu L$ volume, 2% inaccuracy is the best that is achievable. In general, syringes are not calibrated because internal standards are employed in chromatographic procedures, allowing for correction of transfer errors. For gas chromatographic work with volatile samples, the syringes must be airtight.

Automatic syringes are also used to deliver reagents and samples in automated laboratory instruments (see p. 293, Chapter 16).

Pipets

Most pipets are made of glass, although plastic serological pipets are available. Two general categories of manual pipets are defined: transfer (volumetric) and measuring. Within these categories, three further subclassifications exist: to contain (TC), to deliver (TD), and to deliver/blow-out (TD/blow-out).

TC or *rinse-out* pipets must be refilled or rinsed with the appropriate solvent after the initial liquid has been drained from the pipet. These pipets contain or hold an exact amount of liquid that must be completely transferred for accurate measurement. Some examples of TC pipets are Sahli hemoglobin, transfer micro, and Lang-Levy pipets. None of these devices meets Class A specifications.

TD/blow-out pipets are filled and allowed to drain, after which the remaining fluid in the tip is blown out. These devices thus transfer or deliver an exact amount of liquid and are not rinsed out. Pipets belonging to this group include Ostwald-Folin and serological devices. They are easily identified by the two frosted bands near the mouthpiece of the pipet (Fig. 1-3). Serological pipets are long glass (or plastic) tubes of uniform diameter. They have volume graduations extending to the delivery tip of the pipet. Thus the last drop of liquid blown out is included in the delivery volume. These pipets come with long tapered tips and variable tip openings to allow for controlled delivery. Pipets with large-tipped openings are used for delivery of viscous fluids.

TD pipets are filled and allowed to drain by gravity. To ensure complete drainage, the flow rates are set to specifications defined by the NIST. The pipet must be held vertically and the tip placed against the side of the accepting vessel but not touching the liquid in it. Pipets classified in this group include volumetric transfer, Mohr, and serological pipets (see Figs. 1-3 and 1-4). TD pipets meet class A standards.

Volumetric (TD) pipets (see Fig. 1-4) have an open-ended bulb, which holds the bulk of the liquid; a long glass tube at one end with a line (mark) indicating the extent to which the pipet is to be filled; and a tapered delivery portion. After draining, these devices deliver the exact volume specified with a high degree of accuracy (Table 1-7). Ostwald-Folin (TD) pipets are similar in appearance to volumetric pipets but have their bulbs closer to the delivery tip. They are used for accurate measurement of viscous liquids such as blood or serum and require that the contents be blown out. Thus they have etched bands near the top. To ensure complete delivery of the viscous fluid, the liquid is blown out after the pipet is allowed to drain freely to the last drop.

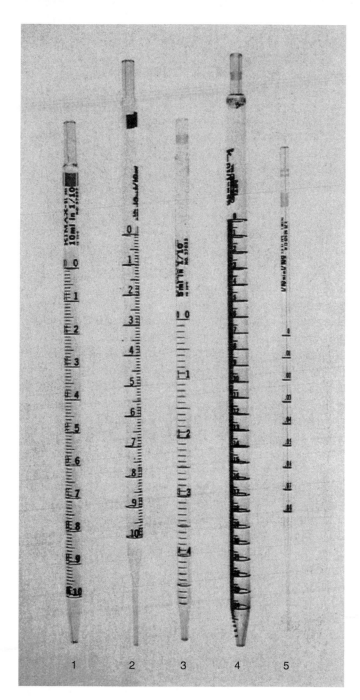

Fig. 1-3 Examples of transfer to deliver (TD) pipets. *1,* Mohr. *2,* Mohr long tip. *3,* Serological. *4,* Serological large opening. *5,* Serological long tip.

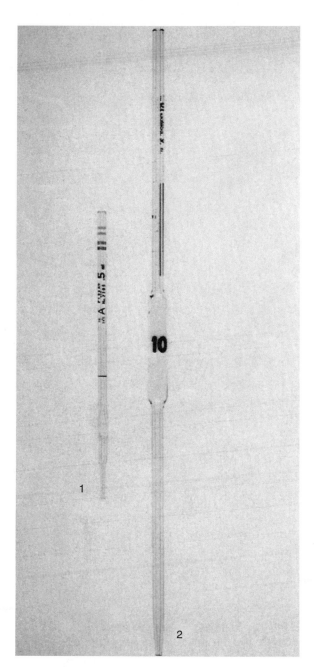

Fig. 1-4 Examples of to deliver (TD) pipets. *1,* Ostwald-Folin. *2,* Class A volumetric.

Micropipets

Micropipets contain or deliver small volumes of liquid ranging from 1 to 1000 µL. Reusable glass micropipets are no longer used in the clinical laboratory; however, their characteristics are described elsewhere.[9] Inexpensive disposable tubes with specific volume demarcations are available. They are filled by capillary action, and the liquid is blown out of the tube by a device that is similar to a medicine dropper.

The most common type of micropipet is a semiautomated device that uses either air displacement or positive displacement to dispense the contained liquid. Some models with a digital volume adjustment are also available. There are many brands of *air-displacement* pipets, but all are piston-operated

Mohr (TD) pipets are uniform in diameter with tapered delivery tips. Graduations are incised on the stem at uniform intervals so that the calibration occurs above but not on the tip. The accuracy listed for these pipets is valid only when the pipet is filled. If smaller volumes are dispensed, the accuracy decreases proportionally. Mohr pipets with long tips are used for dispensing liquids into small vials. They are less accurate than the standard tapered-tip variety. Mohr pipets are never used as blow-out devices. The accuracy of Mohr and other pipets is summarized in Table 1-7.

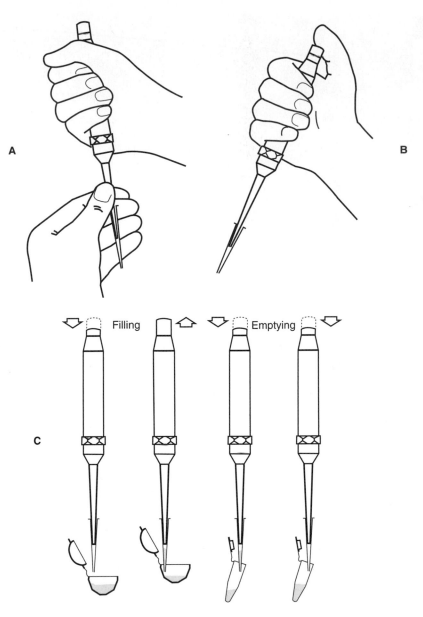

Fig. 1-5   Steps in using Eppendorf type of micropipet. **A,** Attaching proper tip size for range of pipet volume and twisting tip as it is pushed onto pipet to give an airtight, continuous seal. **B,** Holding pipet before use. **C,** Detailed instructions for filling and emptying pipet tip. Follow manufacturer's complete instructions for care and use of micropipets.

devices. A disposable and exchangeable polypropylene tip is attached to the pipet barrel, and liquid is drawn into and dispensed from this disposable tip (Fig. 1-5). Some instruments can automatically eject the used pipet tip and reload a new one, minimizing analytical contamination. Several brands of *positive-displacement* pipets are also available. The capillary tips, which may be made of siliconized glass, glass, or plastic, can be reused. These devices are particularly useful for handling reagents that react with plastics. Positive-displacement pipettors deliver liquid by means of a Teflon-tipped plunger that fits snugly inside the capillary. Carryover of liquid is negligible in properly maintained instruments. In some instances, a washing step is used between samples.

The precision and accuracy of these devices are excellent if they are properly maintained. Sample recovery is at least 99%, with reproducibility errors of 0.6% to 0.3% for volumes between 10 and 500 μL. For volumes less than 10 μL the errors are significantly larger. For this reason manual procedures involving small volumes should be avoided.

Dilutors and Dispensers

Manual dispensers and pipettors are frequently used in the laboratory to add repeatedly a specified volume of reagent or diluent to a solution (Fig. 1-6). Several types are commercially available, but all consist of a reagent bottle to which a plunger with a valve system is attached. The dispenser is fitted with a

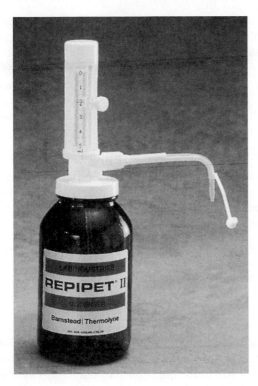

Fig. 1-6   Example of manual dispenser or repipettor. *(Courtesy Barnstead International, Dubuque, IA.)*

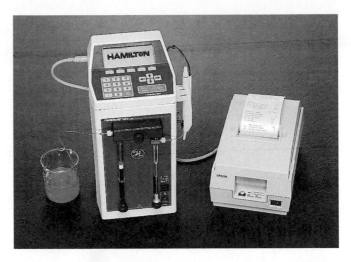

Fig. 1-7   Example of dual-syringe type of dilutor-dispenser. *(Courtesy Hamilton, Reno, NV.)*

tube or straw that reaches to the bottom of the bottle. The device must be primed with liquid to ensure removal of any air bubbles. Once primed, depression of the plunger delivers a selected amount of liquid. Return of the plunger to the original position refills the dispenser chamber. Manufacturers claim an error rate of 1% and a reproducibility rate of 0.1% for these devices at full deflection of the plunger. Manual dispensers require frequent cleaning to remove material that can hamper piston action.

Repetitive dispensing pipettors are useful for the serial dispensing of relatively small volumes of the same liquid. The volume dispensed is determined by the pipettor setting and by the size of the disposable syringe tip, which also acts as the liquid reservoir.

Automated diluter-dispensers are frequently used to prepare many samples for analysis. Such devices can be an integral part of an automated chemistry analyzer. The dispensers pipet a preset volume of sample and diluent into a receiving vessel or instrument. The frequently used dual-piston dispenser allows adjustment of both sample and diluent volumes (Fig. 1-7). One motor-driven syringe processes the sample, the other the diluent. The syringes are activated by a microprocessor, allowing each piston to fill the syringes simultaneously. A second signal repositions the valves to allow diluent to flow through the sample syringe. This displaces the sample, forcing it through the pipet tip and rinsing it in preparation for the next sample. Variable ratios of sample to diluent can be selected. However, a tenfold volume of diluent ensures adequate rinsing and negligible carryover.

The inaccuracy is considered to be less than 0.5% of dispensed volume, and reproducibility is on the order of 0.05% of full-syringe volume, or 0.1% when at least 10% of the syringe volume is dispensed.

VOLUMETRIC TECHNIQUES
Class A Pipets

Clinical chemistry analytical procedures require exact volumetric measurements and transfers to ensure accurate results, and Class A glassware is therefore required. In fact, the CAP specifies that volumetric pipets must be of certified accuracy (Class A) or the volumes of the devices must be verified (for example, by a gravimetric procedure). In addition, automatic pipets and diluting devices must be periodically checked for accuracy and precision. Therefore most laboratories routinely use Class A glassware. In addition, the glassware must be scrupulously clean; beads of liquid cling to the sides of dirty vessels and pipets and volume measurements are inaccurate. Borosilicate glass pipets must be inspected frequently. Pipets with broken tips or etched glass should be discarded.

Class A pipets are filled with the aid of a rubber bulb or similar device. *Under no circumstances is mouth pipetting permissible.* The bulb is used to fill the pipet above the calibration mark. The pipet is grasped by the thumb and middle finger, with the index finger placed over the upper opening, controlling the flow of liquid (Fig. 1-8). After the pipet is filled above the mark, the tip is wiped with a lint-free tissue to remove excess fluid. The liquid is then allowed to drain so that the lowest part of the meniscus, sighted at eye level, is lined up with the mark, after which the pipet is transferred to the receiving vessel. Next, the pipet is held in a vertical position with the tip against the side of the receiving vessel, and the liquid is drained as the index finger is removed from the pipet orifice. TD pipets must be held in position long enough (~2 sec) to permit delivery of the specified volume. With TC or blow-out pipets, the rubber bulb is used to blow out the last remaining solution after drainage is complete.

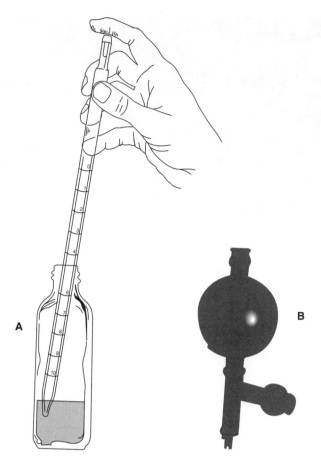

Fig. 1-8   **A**, Proper pipetting technique as described in text. **B**, Example of rubber pipetting bulb used to aspirate sample into pipet.

Micropipets

Air-displacement micropipets may be used in either of two modes, the *forward mode* or the *reverse mode.* The reverse mode is used with two-component stroke mechanism systems only. The precision of these devices in the forward mode depends on the precise draining caused by the air pressure, and they are relatively sensitive to the physical character-istics of the liquid being pipetted. Reverse-mode operation, on the other hand, is considerably less sensitive to the type of liquid being dispensed. In the forward mode the piston is depressed to the first stop position on a two-stroke device, the tip is placed in the liquid, and the piston is slowly allowed to rise back to the original position. This fills the tip with the designated volume of liquid. The pipet tip is then drawn up the sidewall of the vessel so that any adhering liquid is removed. If any extraneous droplets are visible, the tip is wiped carefully with a lint-free tissue, with care being taken not to "wick" out any sample from the pipet tip. The tip is then placed on the wall of the receiving vessel, and the piston is depressed smoothly to the first stop position on a two-stroke device, allowing the liquid to drain. After 1 second, the piston is depressed to the second stop, blowing out the remaining liquid. When the reverse mode is used, the liquid is aspirated after depressing to the second stop position. This overfills the

pipet with sample. To dispense the liquid, the piston is depressed to the first stop and, after 1 second, the pipet is removed.

Positive-displacement micropipets are used in the same manner as forward mode air-displacement devices. Again, careful wiping of the tip is crucial in order not to wick out a sample from the tip. The need for maintenance of the Teflon tip cannot be overemphasized. More detailed information on this technique is published elsewhere.[10]

General Procedures for Solution Preparation

Solution preparation requires accurate measurement of the solute and solvent. The degree of accuracy required dictates the specific glassware to be used. The following procedure may be used for solution preparation:

1. Measure the solute by weighing, pipetting, or dispensing from a graduated cylinder or pipettor (as examples).
2. Prepare volumetric solutions by quantitatively transferring the solute to the receiving flask. If the solute exists as a stock solution, a volumetric pipet is used for transfer.
3. Add sufficient solvent to dissolve the solute where necessary.
4. If the receiving flask is a volumetric flask, add the solids or liquids to the flask and then add diluent to approxi-mately two thirds the volume of the flask. Dissolution of the solid or liquid can be effected by swirling the liquid. After dissolution, continue adding diluent until the meniscus, sighted at eye level, reaches the line etched into the neck of the flask. Completely mix the solution by placing a cover on the opening of the flask, holding the neck of the flask in your hand and swirling the liquid while simul-taneously inverting the flask. Alternatively the dilution or dissolving of a solid in diluent can be achieved in an Erlenmeyer flask. The solution is then transferred to a volumetric flask, followed by several washes of the Erlenmeyer flask with diluent, transferring the liquid used for the washes to the volumetric flask.
5. Bring the solution to volume after the solute is completely dissolved.
6. If the use of a magnetic stir bar is necessary, remove the bar and rinse it with solvent before bringing the solution to volume.
7. Bring the solution to volume at room temperature *only.*
8. Mix the solution well to ensure homogeneity.
9. Transfer the solution to an appropriate reagent-storage container (amber/clear, plastic/glass).

Quality Control of Micropipets, Dispensers, and Dilutors

General. The accuracy and precision of each manual micropipet should be verified on acquisition and monitored during the course of the year. The frequency of verification depends on the amount of use. Heavily used devices may need monthly verification, whereas rarely used devices may need to be checked only once or twice per year unless more frequent validation is mandated by an inspection agency. Manufacturers of newer micropipets are claiming a 2-year calibration stability; however, more frequent calibrations may be required by inspection agencies.

Routine maintenance is crucial. Air-displacement pipets have a fixed stroke length that must be maintained. In addition, such pipets have seals to prevent air from leaking into the pipet when the piston is moved, and these must be greased to maintain proper operation. The manufacturer will provide guidelines for performing this maintenance. Any worn parts must be replaced and devices that do not meet specifications for precision or accuracy generally require servicing by the manufacturer.

Positive-displacement pipets, in general, require similar maintenance with regard to spring checks and replacement of Teflon tips. Many of these devices also are supplied with a slide wire that is used to quickly check the plunger setting. This device cannot be used in place of routine performance checks. Again, the manufacturer provides guidelines for performing routine maintenance.

Quality control validation. The primary method for validating performance of micropipets is a gravimetric technique.[10] A secondary method is a spectrophotometrical procedure with potassium dichromate. The latter method is unacceptable for volumes of less than 10 μL. The following protocol describes the gravimetric method of verification and is based on the procedure described in the NCCLS guideline, *Determining Performance of Volumetric Equipment:*[10]

1. Make sure all items used (water, weighing vials, and pipets) are at room temperature.
2. All measurements require the use of Type I water.
3. Measure and record the barometric pressure and the ambient temperature (*t*) of the water to 0.1° C.
4. To minimize evaporation errors, place a small amount of water in the weighing vessel (between 2 and 30 sample volumes, or a minimum of 0.5 mL). Cover with a square of Parafilm or a stopper. Ensure all manipulations are performed without direct handling of the vial.
5. Weigh the vial (water and cover) and record the weight to the nearest 0.1 mg (W_v), or preferably set to zero the weight of the vial, water, and cover.
6. Transfer the aliquot of water to be measured to the weighing vial using the pipet to be tested. Recover the vial.
7. Reweigh the vial to the nearest 0.1 mg and record the weight (W_t).
8. Repeat these measurements (W_v and W_t) to obtain 10 readings in order to evaluate both accuracy and precision. (A "quick check" method using four samplings allows rough assessment of precision.)
9. Calculate the mean weight ($\overline{W}_t$) as follows:

$$\overline{W} = \Sigma \frac{W_t}{n} - \Sigma \frac{W_v}{n}$$

where *n* is the number of repetitive weighings.
10. Refer to *The Handbook of Chemistry and Physics*[11] to obtain the correction factor for the water temperature. Assess the conversion factor z (μL/mg), incorporating the density of water at the test temperature and pressure.
11. Calculate the volume measured as follows:

Mean volume, $\overline{V}_t$ = Mean weight, $\overline{W}_t \cdot z$
where $\overline{W}_t$ is calculated from #9 above

12. The *accuracy* is then computed by evaluating the difference between the actual mean volume measured and the nominal volume as stated by the manufacturer, expressed as %:

$$\frac{\text{Mean volume}}{\text{Nominal volume}} \times 100\%$$

13. The *precision* is derived from the distribution of the individual weighings about their mean and expressed as percent coefficient of variation (%CV).

In general, an error of 0.1% or less in the accuracy may be ignored when using the pipet. Larger errors may have to be evaluated more critically and the pipet adjusted, if necessary, to achieve a more accurate volume. Manufacturers may use mercury in place of water to assess performance. This practice is not acceptable in a routine laboratory setting.

The practice of using radioisotopes and enzymes is unacceptable because of large inherent errors and poor standardization. Other methods such as acid-base titration and coulometry have been suggested, but adequate documentation is not available to validate these methods.

The accuracy of a dispenser can also be evaluated by a gravimetric procedure. The volume to be tested is set and the device is primed to ensure that no air bubbles are present. The water is then carefully dispensed into a preweighed test tube or other container and the resulting volume determined by the same equation used for pipet testing. A graduated cylinder can be used to make a rough assessment of the dispenser's performance. This procedure is helpful when making adjustments to the dispenser volume and provides a mechanism for daily verification. The gravimetric procedure should be performed at regular intervals (monthly, quarterly), depending on the use of the pipettor.

Automatic dilutors are best evaluated by use of a potassium dichromate spectrophotometrical method. A series of dilutions (*n* = 20) are prepared by the dilutor, measured spectrophotometrically, and then compared with a manual dilution made in the same volume ratios. The manual dilution must be prepared in volumetric flasks with sufficiently large volumes of sample (no less than 1 mL) to ensure accuracy. The absorbance of the sample prepared using the automatic dilutor is then compared with that of the sample diluted manually, and the accuracy of the automatic dilutor is computed as previously described. Agreement should be within 2%. Similarly, the precision is computed using the distribution of individual absorbances about the mean, expressed as %CV. The %CV should be no more than 1%. This procedure can be used to evaluate some dilutor systems incorporated into automated instruments. Again procedures involving the use of enzymes are unacceptable. The frequency of verification is determined by the amount of use. Monthly determinations are sufficient for most devices, including dilutors incorporated into automated equipment.

Pipets, dilutors, and dispensers must be reevaluated whenever the devices are serviced or repaired. All procedures must be documented and records maintained according to federal, state, and local inspection agency guidelines.

TABLE 1-8 BASIC QUANTITIES AND UNITS OF THE SYSTÈME INTERNATIONAL D'UNITÉS (SI)

Quantity	Basic Unit	Symbol
Length	Meter	m
Mass	Kilogram	kg
Time	Second	s
Electric current	Ampere	A
Temperature	Kelvin	K
Luminous intensity	Candela	cd
Amount of substance	Mole	mol

TABLE 1-9 SI-DERIVED UNITS USED IN MEDICINE

Derived Quantity	Derived Unit	Symbol
Area	Square meter	m^2
Volume	Cubic meter	m^3
Speed	Meter per second	m/s or $m \cdot s^{-1}$
Substance concentration	Mole per cubic meter	mol/m^3, or $mol \cdot m^{-3}$
Pressure	Pascal	Pa
Work energy or quantity of heat	Joule	J
Celsius temperature	Celsius degree	°C
Activity (radionuclide)	Becquerel	Bq
Power	Watt	W
Electric charge or quantity	Coulomb	C
Electric potential	Volt	V
Resistance		Ω
Conductance	Siemens	S

TABLE 1-10 SI PREFIXES

Prefix*	Factor	Symbol
atto	10^{-18}	a
femto	10^{-15}	f
pico	10^{-12}	p
nano	10^{-9}	n
micro	10^{-6}	μ
milli	10^{-3}	m
centi	10^{-2}	c
deci	10^{-1}	d
deka	10^{1}	da
hecto	10^{2}	h
kilo	10^{3}	k
mega	10^{6}	M
giga	10^{9}	G
tera	10^{12}	T
peta	10^{15}	P
exa	10^{18}	E

*It is recommended that only one prefix be used.

UNITS OF MEASUREMENT
SI Units

The **Système International d'Unités (SI)** system, which is based on the **metric system,** has seven basic units[12] (Table 1-8). Two or more basic units may be combined by multiplication or division to form SI-derived units (Table 1-9). Basic and derived units may be too large or too small for convenient use. Prefixes that form decimal multiples or submultiples of the units are permissible (Table 1-10). A few non-SI units have been retained because of difficulties encountered in converting them to SI units or because of their widespread use. Non-SI units relevant to clinical chemistry and their symbols are time, expressed in minutes (min), hours (h), or days (d); and volume, expressed as liters (L) or deciliters (dL). The General Conference of Weights and Measures (*Conférence Générale des Poids et Mésures,* CGPM) has approved l, *l,* or L as the volume designation; however, L is the official abbreviation accepted in the United States.

SI Units in the Clinical Laboratory[12-15]

The SI unit describes the concentration of body constituents in terms of the number of dissolved molecules, measured in moles (mol, μmol, and so on) rather than the amount of dissolved mass (mg, g, and so on).[12-15] A *mole* of a chemical contains the number of grams equivalent to its formula mass (see p. 35). The SI unit of enzyme activity is the *katal*, which is defined as the amount of enzyme that will catalyze the transformation of 1 mole of substrate per second in an assay system. This terminology has been approved by the Joint Commission on Biochemical Nomenclature of the International Union of Biochemistry (IUB) and the IUPAC but has not been approved by CGPM. Thus the use of International Units (IU or U) for describing enzyme activity will undoubtedly continue (see Chapter 54). There is a constant relationship between the katal and IU (1 katal = 16.67 IU) when measured under identical conditions of temperature, pH, substrate, and coenzyme concentration.

Often SI units are not used when the molecular weight of a protein is uncertain. However, even under these conditions it is possible to express substance concentration rather than mass concentration provided that the approximate molecular weight is included in the documentation. Such an approach also applies to hormones. IU are used to express enzyme activity, whereas SI units are used for reporting osmolality. The SI unit for reporting pressure is the *pascal.* However, the numerical values expressed in pascals for blood pressure and blood gas partial pressures are too large, and therefore the kilopascal is the preferred unit. For further information regarding the SI system, the reader should refer to the NIST publication *Guide for the Use of the International System of Units.*[13]

MEASUREMENT OF MASS

Mass may be defined as the quantity of matter. Weight is a function of mass under the influence of gravity as expressed by the equation:

Weight = Mass × Gravity

Thus two objects of equal mass that are subject to the same gravitational force have equal weights. The gram (g) is a unit of mass. Measurement of mass or weight is achieved through use of a balance. The type of balance selected depends on the function being performed. Different balances are required for measuring kilogram (kg) weights (for example, for fecal fat analysis) and microgram weights (for example, for preparation of drug standards for toxicology analyses). Laboratories are equipped with different balances so that all necessary weight measurements can be performed.

Types of Balances

Most laboratories today have replaced mechanical balances with electronic ones. These are either top loading or analytical in design. The electronic balance is a single pan balance that uses an electromagnetic force instead of weights to counterbalance the load placed on the pan (Fig. 1-9). The pan is attached directly to a coil suspended in the field of a permanent magnet. A current is passed through the coil, producing an electromagnetic force that keeps the pan in a constant position. When a load is placed on the pan, a photoelectric-cell scanning device attached to the lever arm changes position and transmits a current to an amplifier that increases the current flow through the coil and restores the pan to its original position. This current is proportional to the weight of the load on the pan and produces a measurable voltage that is converted by a microprocessor to a numeric display or data output that gives the mass of the load. The accuracy of an electronic balance depends on the linearity of both the torque motor and the digital voltmeter. Some electronic balances have a built-in electronic vibration damper. Excessive vibration can be detected when variation of the pointer or oscillation of numbers in the last decimal place of the digital display is observed. Most electronic balances have built-in taring ability allowing the weight of the weighing vessel to be "zeroed." This is a great convenience when performing multiple weighings, such as for pipet calibrations. In addition, electronic balances can be interfaced with data-processing equipment, thus providing calculations such as weight averaging and statistical analysis of multiple weighings. Electronic balances allow weighings to be completed in 5 seconds or less. Table 1-11 summarizes the performance characteristics of balances.

Requirements for Operation

All balances should be located away from direct sunlight and drafts that can interfere with the weighing process. Analytical balances should be placed in a vibration-free location, preferably on an isolated heavy (such as marble) table. The more sensitive the balance, the more crucial these requirements are. Before a balance is used, it should be leveled by adjusting the foot screws and centering the bubble in the spirit level. The optical zero should also be verified. All weighings must be performed using weighing paper, plastic boats, beakers, or some other container. Under no conditions should chemicals be placed directly on the pan. After completion of the weighing process, all loose chemical crystals must be removed from the balance area. Similarly, any liquid spills, particularly of corrosive chemicals, must be cleaned

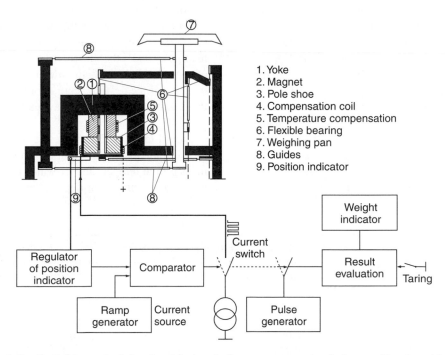

1. Yoke
2. Magnet
3. Pole shoe
4. Compensation coil
5. Temperature compensation
6. Flexible bearing
7. Weighing pan
8. Guides
9. Position indicator

Fig. 1-9 Switching principle of an electronic force compensator balance. *(Courtesy Mettler Toledo, Inc., Columbus, OH.)*

TABLE 1-11 CHARACTERIZATION OF TYPES OF BALANCES IN RELATIONSHIP TO THEIR OPERATING RANGES

Type of Balance	Weighing Capacity (g)	Readability	Reproducibility
Precision balances	32,000	0.1 g	±0.1 g
	16,000	0.1 g	±0.05 g
	6000	0.01 g	±0.01 g
	2000	0.01 g	±0.005 g
	1200	0.001 g	±0.001 g
	110	0.001 g	±0.0005 g
Analytical balances	210	0.1 mg	±0.1 mg
	205	0.01 mg	±0.03 mg
	50	0.1 mg	±0.1 mg
	20	2 µg	±3 µg
Microbalances	5.1	1 µg	±0.9 µg
	2.1	0.1 µg	±0.25 µg

up immediately to prevent permanent damage to the pans. Weights should be handled using forceps, never bare hands. Direct contact with skin deposits oils, salts, and moisture on the weights. The smaller the weight, the more significant the effect.

Maintenance Procedures

In addition to the requirements already described, balances should be serviced at least annually, more frequently if they are heavily used. Service must be performed by the manufacturer or its representative. Periodic checks to verify weight accuracy are also required, and records must be kept documenting quality control and maintenance procedures. Verification procedures should be performed at least monthly and before any crucial analytical procedure. Verification of performance requires the use of NIST Class S weights. The CAP also requires that approved laboratories validate balance performance using Class S weights.[16] A 100-g weight should weigh 100 g ±0.5 mg. Class S weights should be checked to verify that their apparent weights are within NIST specifications (Table 1-12). Unacceptable performance indicates the need for service. Some newer analytical balances have a single built-in weight for performing this function. Such balances still require verification of the entire measuring range.

THERMOMETRY
Types of Thermometers

Water baths and heating blocks must be maintained at constant temperature when temperature-sensitive assays are performed. Refrigerators and freezers must be maintained at constant temperature when used to store temperature-sensitive materials. Liquid-in-glass thermometers, thermistors, and electronic digital thermometers are used to monitor the temperature of these devices.

The temperature of every temperature-controlled device must be checked and recorded,* along with any corrective action, every day as part of the quality control procedures performed in the laboratory. The accuracy of the thermometers used to monitor the heating baths should be verified regularly, usually every 6 to 12 months. It has been recommended[17] that the thermometer have an accuracy range of one half that of the desired temperature range. For instance, if the desired accuracy for a heating bath is ±0.1° C, the thermometer should have a maximum uncertainty of ±0.05° C.

Liquid-in-glass thermometers are available for partial or total immersion. Partial immersion thermometers are used to measure the temperature of water baths, heating blocks, and ovens. The immersion depth is engraved on the stem and is

TABLE 1-12 INDIVIDUAL NIST TOLERANCES FOR CLASS S WEIGHTS

Nominal Mass	Individual Tolerance (mg)	Maintenance Tolerance (mg)
1, 2, 3, 4, 10, 20, 30, 50 mg	±0.014	±0.014
100, 200, 300, 500 mg	±0.025	±0.05
1, 2, 3, 5 g	±0.054	±0.11
10, 20, 30 g	±0.074	±0.148
50 g	±0.12	±0.22
100 g	±0.25	±0.5

usually located about 76 mm from the bulb. Total immersion thermometers are generally used to check refrigerator and freezer temperatures but can be substituted for partial immersion thermometers if they are verified at the same immersion depth that they will be used in the laboratory. Mercury-containing thermometers are now being replaced with other liquid-in-glass thermometers for general laboratory use.

Calibration of Liquid-in-Glass Thermometers

Calibration of thermometers requires the use of an NIST-certified or NIST-traceable thermometer. As part of the NIST SRM program, certified thermometers are available that can be used to calibrate thermometers at 0° C and in the range of 24° to 38° C. The NIST-traceable thermometers have wider operating ranges. The following procedure outlines the necessary steps to validate noncertified thermometers; it is based on the NCCLS standard *Temperature Calibration of Water Baths, Instruments, and Temperature Sensors*[17]:

1. Check the liquid column for separation or gas bubbles. (If any are present, refer to the NCCLS standard for procedures to correct the problem.)
2. Perform an ice-point determination.[17] This will check for changes in bulb volume. After completion, set the thermometer aside for a few days to ensure recovery of the bulb.
3. Adjust the heating bath to the temperature required for analysis. It is important that the volume of the bath be at least 100 times greater than the volume of the fluid in which the thermometer being calibrated is placed. This ensures maintenance of a uniform temperature throughout the bath.
4. Place the reference and noncertified thermometers in test tubes filled with water to the appropriate depth. The thermometers should be placed close to one another but with sufficient space between to ensure adequate circulation in the bath.
5. If a total-immersion thermometer is being calibrated for use as a partial-immersion device, it must be immersed in the heating bath to the same depth used for test applications. Proper immersion of the thermometer is essential.
6. After thermal equilibrium is reached (this will require several minutes for liquid-in-glass thermometers), determine the temperature reading for both thermometers.
7. Electronic thermometers that use thermistor probes may be calibrated similarly. Thermal equilibrium of these devices occurs in a few milliseconds.

Thermometers differing from the reference thermometer by more than 1° C should be discarded or returned to the supplier. Agreement within 0.1° C is required for critical laboratory purposes such as enzyme analyses. If discrepancies are between 0.2° and 1° C, the thermometer can be used for less critical functions such as monitoring ovens, refrigerators, and freezers. Each thermometer should be assigned a log number and the results of the calibration documented in a thermometer log book; this is useful for inspection purposes.

Also available from NIST is a gallium melting point cell, which can be used to calibrate electronic thermistor probes to a temperature of 29.772° C. These probes can then be used to verify the accuracy of liquid-in-glass thermometers in the 20° to 40° C range.[17]

WATER BATHS, HEATING BLOCKS, AND OVENS

Water baths may be either circulating or noncirculating in design. For clinical chemistry applications, noncirculating baths are, in general, unacceptable because temperature control is inadequate (±1° C). Circulating water baths, which have a tighter temperature control, are necessary. Such baths are equipped with an external or internal circulating pump that maintains adequate thermal equilibrium. In some instances the pump may be coupled to a refrigeration unit to provide temperature control below room temperature. The bath liquid should be type II (or type I) reagent water to which is added a bactericidal agent such as thimerosal (Merthiolate) at a dilution of 1:1000. The bactericidal agent controls bacterial growth, reducing the frequency with which the bath water must be changed. The use of high-quality water is necessary to control salt deposits on the heat exchangers; such deposits interfere with maintenance of adequate temperature control.

Metal heating blocks are somewhat less efficient in maintaining a constant temperature and usually operate within ±0.5° C. Blocks that are incorporated into the cuvette compartment of a spectrophotometer operate with greater accuracy, usually ±0.2° C or better.

The temperature of water baths and heating blocks should be measured daily with a thermometer calibrated against an NIST thermometer or NIST-certified thermometer. All measurements must be recorded and any corrective action documented.

Laboratory ovens may be used to dry chemicals, extracts, electrophoretic support media, thin-layer chromatography plates, and glassware. For most purposes a temperature control of ±1° C is adequate. Thermometers used to monitor oven temperature should be checked for accuracy at least annually. The temperature of the oven should be measured daily to check for malfunction of the heating elements or thermistor controls. All gaskets should also be checked to verify integrity. Worn gaskets require replacement to ensure adequate temperature control. All measurements must be recorded and any corrective action documented.

CENTRIFUGES
Types

Three general types of centrifuge are available: *swinging-bucket,* or *horizontal-head, centrifuges; fixed-angle,* or *angle-head, centrifuges;* and *ultracentrifuges.* These are available as floor or table models, allowing the laboratory to purchase the instrument that best suits its needs.

Centrifuges are used in the clinical laboratory to separate substances of significantly different masses or densities. The two substances to be separated can be a solid (particles) and a liquid or two liquids of different densities. Centrifuges are used in the chemistry laboratory primarily to separate clotted blood or cells from serum or plasma and body fluids. Although the choice of a specific relative centrifugal force (RCF) to carry out these separations is not crucial, a force of 1000 to

$1200 \times g$ for 10 ± 5 min is recommended.[18] In some instances, more time may be necessary (see Chapter 3).

Swinging bucket, or horizontal-head, rotors hold the tubes in a vertical position when the centrifuge is at rest; the tubes move to and remain in a horizontal position when the rotor is in motion. During centrifugation, particles constantly move along the tube while it is in the horizontal position, distributing the sediment uniformly against the bottom of the tube. After centrifugation is complete and the rotor has ceased turning, the surface of the sediment is flat with a column of liquid above it.

Fixed-angle rotors keep the tubes at a specified angle, 25 to 52 degrees to the vertical axis of rotation. During centrifugation, particles move along the side of the tube to form a sediment that packs against the side and bottom of the tube. The surface of the sediment in this case is parallel to the shaft of the centrifuge. As the rotor slows and then stops, gravity may cause the sediment to slide down the tube, forming a poorly packed pellet. Fixed-angle rotors are used when rapid sedimentation of small particles is required. The design of these rotors is more aerodynamic, allowing operation at speeds higher than those achievable with a swinging-bucket rotor. This capability allows microhematocrit centrifuges to operate at 11,000 to 15,000 revolutions per minute (rpm), with an RCF as high as $14,000 \times g$.

Ultracentrifuges are high-speed centrifuges that use fixed-angle or swinging-bucket rotors. They are often refrigerated to counter the heat generated as a result of friction. A small air-driven ultracentrifuge, the Airfuge (Beckman Coulter Inc., Spinco Division, Palo Alto, CA) is a miniature air turbine with a small rotor operating at 90,000 to 100,000 rpm, generating a maximum RCF of $178,000 \times g$. This type of centrifuge has been used to separate chylomicrons from serum, allowing accurate analyses to be performed on the clear infranatant. It has also been used to fractionate lipoproteins, perform drug-binding assays, and prepare tissue for hormone-receptor assays. Analytical ultracentrifuges are used to determine sedimentation coefficients of proteins, allowing assessment of molecular weights.

Centrifuge Components

All centrifuges have a motor, drive shaft, and head or rotor, which may be in the form of a chamber with a cover. A power switch, timer, speed control, tachometer, and brake are the components that control the centrifuge. When necessary, refrigeration units are included. Some centrifuges are equipped with an alarm that sounds when a malfunction such as a tube imbalance occurs. Some centrifuges automatically shut down under these conditions, preventing tube breakage and the potential for exposure to biohazardous agents. All modern centrifuges have a required safety latch that prevents the operator from opening the instrument before the rotor has stopped.

Swinging-bucket rotors use pairs of buckets or carriers that swing freely. The carriers are designed to accept a variety of cushioned inserts, allowing centrifugation of small tubes or large bottles. Different fixed-angle rotors are required for different-sized containers.

The motor in a large centrifuge is usually a direct-current, heavy-duty, high-torque, electric motor. In smaller centrifuges the current is usually alternating. Power is transmitted to the rotor by the commutator and brushes. The rotor shaft is usually driven by a gyro system, and the bearings are usually sealed, minimizing vibration and the need for lubrication. Centrifuge speed is controlled by a potentiometer that modulates the voltage supplied to the motor. Speed is also determined by the mass of the load in the rotor. The tachometer measures rotor speed in rpm. The brake decelerates the rotor by reversing the polarity of the current to the motor. The timer permits the rotor to reach a preprogrammed speed; the rotor then decelerates without braking after a set time has elapsed.

Refrigerated centrifuges are used when the heat generated during centrifugation could cause evaporation or denaturation of protein or leakage of cellular components in the sample. The temperature can be controlled between $-15°$ and $25°$ C, allowing centrifugation at higher speeds and for prolonged periods.

The selection of centrifuge tubes and bottles is of importance. Plastic tubes (polystyrene, polypropylene) have a higher speed tolerance and can withstand RCFs as high as $5000 \times g$. Tubes with tapered bottoms, which form more compact pellets, may be required under certain conditions such as preparing urine sediment for microscopic analysis and some radioimmunoassay procedures. The tubes must fit snugly in the carriers; small tubes in too large a carrier result in improperly packed pellets. The top of the tube must not protrude so far above the carrier that the rotor is impeded. Balancing of tubes within the carriers is crucial. Newer centrifuges automatically decelerate and shut down when carriers are improperly balanced. Fig. 1-10 demonstrates appropriate balancing. Improper balancing can cause the centrifuge to vibrate, disrupting the formed pellet. Whenever possible, tubes containing biohazardous materials should be centrifuged with the caps or stoppers in place to minimize aerosols.

Maintenance and Quality Assurance

Daily cleaning of the inside surfaces of the centrifuge with a tenfold dilution of household bleach or an equivalent disinfectant is crucial. When tube breakage occurs, the portions of the centrifuge in contact with the blood or other potentially infectious agent must be immediately decontaminated. The centrifuge bowl should be cleaned with a germicidal disinfectant, and the rotor heads and buckets should be autoclaved. All broken glass or plastic must be carefully removed and disposed of appropriately.

Centrifuge speeds that are routinely used should be checked periodically using a reliable photoelectric or strobe tachometer in accordance with CAP inspection guidelines.[19] The measured and rated speeds should not differ by more than 5% under specified conditions. The accuracy of the centrifuge timer should also be checked and verified according to CAP inspection guidelines.[19] The temperature of refrigerated centrifuges should be checked at least monthly (daily is preferred) under standardized conditions. The agreement between the

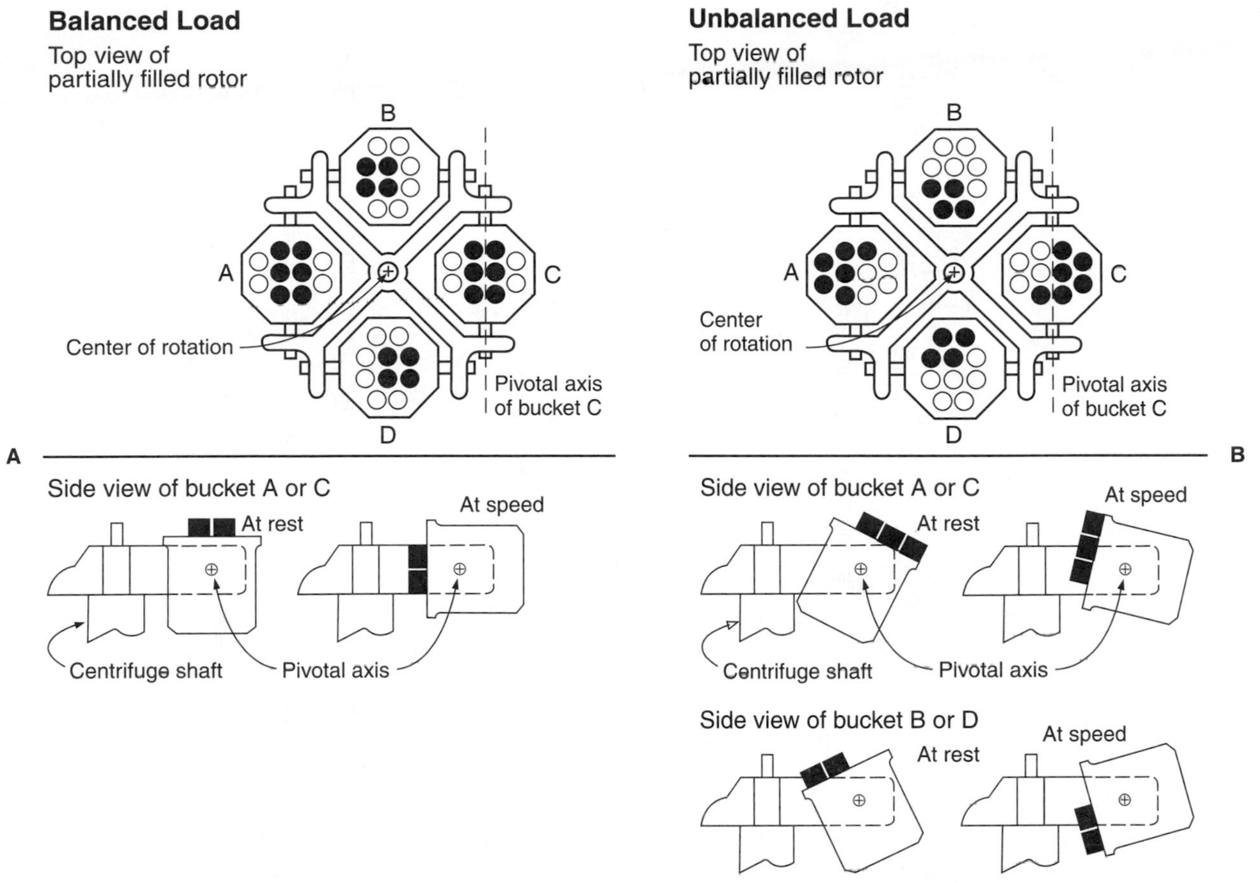

Balanced Load

Top view of
partially filled rotor

Unbalanced Load

Top view of
partially filled rotor

Fig. 1-10 Examples of balanced and unbalanced loads. **A,** Assuming all tubes have been filled with an equal amount of liquid, this rotor load is balanced. The opposing bucket sets *A-C* and *B-D* are loaded with an equal number of tubes and are balanced across the center of rotation. Each bucket is also balanced with respect to its pivotal axis. **B,** Even if all the tubes are filled equally, this rotor is improperly loaded. None of the bucket loads are balanced with respect to their pivotal axes. At operating speed, buckets *A* and *C* will not reach the horizontal position. Buckets *B* and *D* will pivot past the horizontal. Also note that the tube arrangement in the opposing buckets *B* and *D* is not symmetrical across the center of rotation. *(From A centrifuge primer, Palo Alto, CA, 1980, Spinco Div. Beckman Instruments, Inc. [out of print].)*

measured and expected (or programmed) temperature should be within 2° C.

Manufacturer's instructions for lubrication, maintenance, and replacement of brushes should be followed. (Centrifuges of recent manufacture do not have brushes.) Failure to replace worn brushes may cause the motor to fail and require replacement. All maintenance function checks must be recorded, and all corrective actions documented.

Principles of Centrifugation

The speed of a centrifuge is expressed in rpm, whereas the RCF generated is expressed as a number times the gravitational force, *g*. The relationship between rpm and RCF is expressed by the equation

$$RCF = 1.12 \times 10^{-5} \times r \times (rpm)^2$$

where *r* is the radius of the centrifuge expressed in centimeters and is equal to the horizontal distance from the center of the centrifuge bucket to the rotor shaft, and 1.12×10^{-5} is

an empirical factor. Fig. 1-11 shows a nomogram for determination of the RCF when the radius and rpm are known. The RCF applied to a tube in a swinging-bucket rotor may be considerably greater than that applied to the same tube in a fixed-angle rotor because the tube never reaches a horizontal position under the latter condition. For this reason, it is preferable to process serum separator tubes with swinging-bucket horizontal rotors, which operate at higher RCFs.

At times it may be necessary to duplicate centrifugation conditions in two different instruments. This may be achieved by applying the following equations.

Calculation of adjusted speed[20]:

$$\text{rpm (new rotor)} = 1000 \times \frac{\text{RCF (original rotor)}}{1.12 \times r \text{ (cm, original rotor)}}$$

Calculation of adjusted time[20]:

$$\text{Time (new rotor)} = \frac{\text{Time (old rotor)} \times \text{RCF (original rotor)}}{\text{RCF (new rotor)}}$$

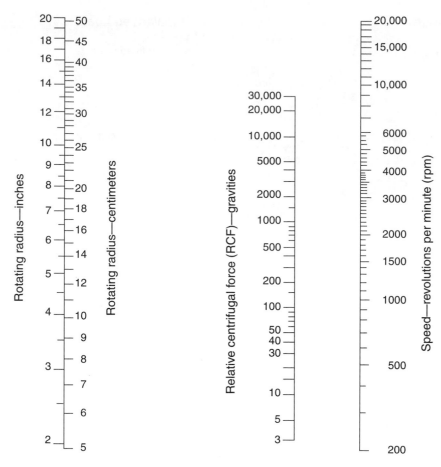

Fig. 1-11 Nomogram for relating relative centrifugal force (RCF) to revolutions per minute (rpm).

These calculations do not take into account the differences between the instruments in the time necessary to reach full speed or to decelerate. Therefore some additional adjustments are necessary.

LABORATORY SAFETY

The Occupational Safety and Health Administration (OSHA) has mandated three programs to ensure the safety of laboratory and other healthcare personnel. The first deals with occupational exposure to chemical hazards[21] and became law in January 1991. The second deals with occupational exposure to blood-borne pathogens[22] and became law in March 1992. The third, which became law in April 2001, concerns the use of safer needle devices and is a revision of the earlier blood-borne pathogen standard.[23] In addition to these mandated programs, the laboratory is responsible for the practice of general safety procedures.

Each clinical laboratory is responsible for designating a safety officer. This individual may also function as the chemical hygiene officer and program coordinator for the blood-borne pathogen program. The responsibilities of this employee include the preparation and updating of manuals that address safety policies and procedures, maintenance of records of training and continuing education, and maintenance of records of exposure to hazardous materials. The safety officer may also be responsible for ensuring that protective devices are available and are being properly and consistently used and that the laboratory is functioning as a safe working environment. In a large facility these functions are shared by several employees; however, the safety officer still plays a key role in ensuring that all regulations are followed.

General Safety Practices

Fire safety is of utmost importance in the clinical laboratory. All equipment used for fire protection should meet the standards set by the National Fire Protection Association (NFPA). The equipment, which should be accessible to laboratory workers, may include fire extinguishers, fire blankets, cabinets for storage of flammable solvents and chemicals, fire alarms, smoke detectors, and sprinkler systems. The selection of the appropriate type of extinguisher is important, as is frequent inspection to ensure that it is in good working order. Tables 1-13 and 1-14 classify types of fires and compare types of fire extinguishers. Halotron extinguishers are generally used for areas in which computers are housed. Warning signs must be posted in these areas, and self-contained breathing equipment must be provided. Several extinguishers are necessary in a larger laboratory, and different types may be appropriate. All employees must be familiar with their use, and annual retraining is mandatory.

Electrical safety is also crucial because the potential for both electrical shock and fire exists. All equipment must be Underwriters Laboratories (UL) approved. This also includes extension cords, which should be used as temporary solutions only. All electrical outlets and equipment must be grounded, and wires should be checked for fraying or wear. Regular inspection decreases the likelihood of electrical accidents. Laboratory workers should document these inspections.

Any equipment used in an area where organic solvents are present must be equipped with explosion-free fittings such as plugs and outlets.

General safety equipment includes safety showers and eyewashes in each large work area. The safety program must also include measures for routinely verifying that this equipment is operational, and maintenance records must be kept. Asbestos (heat-resistant) gloves are required for handling hot equipment, hot glassware, and dry ice. Other personal protective equipment is discussed in the sections involving chemical and biological hazards.

The Chemical Hygiene Plan

OSHA has mandated that as of January 31, 1991, laboratories must develop a Chemical Hygiene Plan for the protection and education of employees.[21] This plan should contain the elements indicated in the box.

Standard Operating Procedures

Standard operating procedures include protocols for handling accidents and chemical spills. In general, if chemicals have come into contact with eyes or skin, the contact areas require

TABLE 1-13	CLASSES OR TYPES OF FIRES
Class	**Hazard**
A	Cloth, wood, paper, ordinary combustibles
B	Flammable liquids (greases, solvents), flammable gases (natural or manufactured)
C	Operating electrical equipment (if electricity is turned off, fire is reclassified as A or B)

ELEMENTS OF A CHEMICAL HYGIENE PLAN

1. A description of standard operating procedure
2. Material Safety Data Sheets (MSDSs)
3. A list of chemicals in inventory
4. Information on appropriate chemical storage
5. Labeling requirements
6. A description of required engineering controls
7. A list of required personal protective equipment
8. Information on waste removal and disposal
9. Information on mandated environmental monitoring where appropriate
10. Housekeeping requirements
11. Requirements for employee physicals and medical consultations
12. Training requirements
13. Record-keeping requirements
14. Designation of a chemical hygiene officer and committee
15. Other information deemed necessary for safety assurance

TABLE 1-14 COMPARISON OF FIRE EXTINGUISHER TYPES

Type	Advantages	Disadvantages	Notes
Halotron (class A, B, C, or B, C)	• Quick fire knockdown • Will reach hidden fires • No damage to equipment • Good discharge range • Heat absorber • Rechargeable	• Requires rapid discharge • More expensive • Not for deep-seated fires	• Most common system for electrical/electronics • Maximum effectiveness requires rapid detection
Triclass dry chemical (class A, B, C)	• Good on oil/grease • Good knockdown • Low cost • Rechargeable	• Limited personnel hazard • Equipment damage likely • Clean-up required • Not suitable for hidden fires	• Compatible with other agents • Subject to equipment interference
Carbon dioxide (class B, C)	• Good fire suppression and cooling capability • Will reach hidden fires • No equipment damage • No messy clean-up/odor • Rechargeable	• May be toxic to personnel • May cause thermal/static (shock) damage • Heavy vapor settles out limiting total discharge range	• Secondary choice to Halotron when fighting class B and C fire
Dry chemical regular (class B, C)	• Won't bake on • Easy clean-up • Good knockdown • No odor • Nonconductive • Rechargeable	• Not suitable for hidden fires • Slight respiratory hazard	• Secondary choice to Halotron when fighting class B and C fires

flushing with copious amounts of water followed by medical attention when necessary. The eye-washing procedure requires 15 minutes of washing; portable eyewash stations are therefore unacceptable. Clean-up procedures should be individually defined for specific chemicals when necessary and should specifically designate the protective clothing to be used during the clean-up procedure.

Rules for avoiding unnecessary chemical exposure must also be defined. Smoking, eating, drinking, and applying cosmetics must be prohibited in all work areas. Long hair and loose clothing should be secured; sandals and canvas shoes should be prohibited. Contact lenses should not be worn in the laboratory because they prevent proper washing of the eyes in the event of a splash. In addition, plastic lenses may be damaged by organic vapors, leading to chronic eye infections. Hand-washing after handling chemicals and before leaving the laboratory for the purposes of eating or drinking should be emphasized.

Cracked or chipped glassware should be immediately discarded because it can break during use. All glassware that has been in contact with a toxic or corrosive substance should be rinsed well with water or alcohol (depending on the solubility) before being placed with other soiled glassware.

The laboratory is required to maintain an alphabetized, up-to-date file of MSDSs to comply with local, state, and federal Right-to-Know laws. MSDSs are required for all chemicals, reagents, and kits used by the laboratory but not for any pharmaceutical agents such as aspirin.[24] The MSDS contains information about the physical and health hazards of each product. The file must be accessible to all employees and outside contractors working in the laboratory.

Inventory

A *chemical inventory* is performed annually, listing all hazardous agents used or stored in the laboratory. A substance can be classified as hazardous by the Department of Transportation (DOT), the Environmental Protection Agency (EPA), or by the NFPA diamond (see the following section on labeling). The inventory should be arranged alphabetically and should include the manufacturer and manufacturing address, physical state, quantity stored, Chemical Abstract Service (CAS) number if known, location of storage, and any hazard classification for health risks, fire, reactivity, or corrosivity. A separate list must be maintained for carcinogens or suspected carcinogens.

Storage of Chemicals

The quantities of chemicals stored in the laboratory should be as small as practical. All refrigerators used for chemical storage must be clearly marked. Under no conditions may food or drink be stored, even temporarily, in a refrigerator used for chemical storage. Explosion-proof refrigerators, clearly labeled, are necessary for storage of solvents with a low flash point.

Toxic chemicals, including carcinogens, must be stored in unbreakable, chemically resistant secondary containers in well-ventilated areas. The containers must be labeled to indicate that the compound is a CANCER SUSPECT AGENT or has HIGH CHRONIC TOXICITY.

Large amounts of volatile solvents must be stored in special safety cabinets approved by the NFPA. Where possible, these cabinets should be vented to the outside. Bench storage of volatile solvents is limited based on the OSHA classification of the solvent. The classification is determined by flash point and boiling point, with Class IA and IB solvents being the most combustible. Bench storage of such solvents may be limited to as little as 1 pint; however, some local fire departments may require compliance with more stringent regulations. Larger quantities must be transferred to safety cans with spring-loaded spouts. All cabinets where in-use solvents are kept should be appropriately labeled.

Large cylinders of *compressed gas* may be used in the laboratory. The most commonly used gases are oxygen, hydrogen, nitrogen, helium, carbon dioxide, and, to a lesser extent, acetylene and propane. Usually the tanks are color-coded and the contents labeled by the NFPA diamond label system. OSHA regulations governing gas cylinders are based on publications of the Compressed Gas Association, Inc.[25] Cylinders should be stored away from the laboratory in a secure, upright position, preferably in a locked, ventilated, fire-resistant space with the empty cylinders well separated from the full ones. The cylinder must always be secured on a dolly or hand truck during transport. The protective cap must be left in place until the cylinder is connected. Gas cylinders (even when empty) must be securely fastened to a wall or bench or placed in a floor retainer because a fall can rupture the outlet valve, allowing the cylinder to be propelled like a torpedo. The laboratory worker should mark each cylinder with a tag that lists the date it was put into use. An exhausted cylinder should be replaced before it is completely empty to avoid contamination with foreign materials; it should be labeled with an EMPTY sign. In general, empty cylinders are recycled by suppliers. Small cylinders containing propane, however, are not. These should be disposed of according to local fire codes.

Reduction valves for different types of gases are not interchangeable. Never substitute one regulator, with or without an adaptor, for another. Laboratory personnel should never attempt to force or free stuck or frozen regulator valves. All connections should be tested for leaks with soapy water. Very small leaks of oxygen or nitrogen are of little consequence, but leaks of hydrogen, acetylene, and other flammable gases are unacceptable. When a cylinder of flammable gas is shut down, it should be turned off at the main intake valve and the gas allowed to burn out. The reduction valves are then closed. A cylinder valve is not turned on unless the reduction valve is off. It is important to remember that propane is heavier than air, and therefore a small quantity of leaking gas can flow along the top of the bench and be ignited by a flame elsewhere. For this reason, small, single-use cylinders of propane are more convenient and safer to use.

Labeling and Handling Requirements

OSHA regulation 29 CFR 1910.1450[21] defines specific labeling requirements. The labels of chemicals in the original containers must not be removed or defaced. For chemicals not in the original container, the labeling information must include the following:

1. Identity of the hazardous chemical
2. Route of body entry (eyes, nose, mouth, skin)
3. Health hazard
4. Physical hazard
5. Target organ affected

Labeling requirements apply to all substances with a rating of 2 or greater according to the Hazards Identification System developed by the NFPA. This system consists of four small, diamond-shaped symbols grouped into a larger diamond shape (Fig. 1-12). The left diamond is *blue* and indicates a *health hazard*, the top is *red* and identifies a *flammability hazard*, the right diamond is *yellow* and indicates a *reactivity-stability hazard* (used for substances that are capable of explosion or violent chemical change), and the bottom *white* diamond is used for provision of *special hazard information* such as water reactivity. The degree of the hazard is rated using a scale of 0 to 4, with 4 indicating the most severe risk.

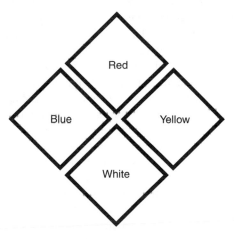

Fig. 1-12 Identification system of the National Fire Protection Association. *(From Bauer JD:* Clinical laboratory methods, *ed 9, St Louis, 1982, Mosby.)*

Such common items as isopropanol (isopropyl alcohol) or diluted bleach in squirt bottles therefore require regulatory labels. In addition, it may be desirable to use additional warning labels such as those used by the DOT, shown in Fig. 1-13. Labels must also indicate any available antidote or treatment modes.

The handling of hazardous chemicals requires great care. A discussion of the handling and disposal of radioactive chemicals is presented in Chapter 9. All flammable and toxic liquids must be used in an area with good ventilation, preferably in a fume hood. A properly operating fume hood should have a minimum air flow of 150 linear ft^3/min. Corrosive solutions such as acids, alkalis, and mercury salts should also be used in a fume hood. Stock bottles of concentrated acids should be transported in acid carriers to prevent and contain breakage. The use of personal protective equipment must be enforced. When reagents are prepared with concentrated acid, the acid must be *slowly* added to the water. Precautions for the handling of powdered carcinogens include the use of disposable equipment and a respirator, in addition to all other standard safety measures. After the compound is handled, the area should be carefully cleaned and the glassware rinsed with strong acid or an organic solvent before regular washing.

Engineering controls are an important part of the daily operation of the laboratory. In addition to the provision, inspection, and documentation of functionality of fire extinguishers, eyewashes, and safety showers, other aspects of the laboratory environment must be monitored and validated. The quality and quantity of ventilation (4 to 12 air changes per hour) must be documented on a quarterly basis; airflow through the laboratory must also be monitored. All areas where hazardous substances are handled or stored such as storerooms, glove boxes, and cold rooms must have adequate ventilation and exhaust ducting. All fume hoods must be inspected after installation, and then annually by a reputable company. The inspection should include an evaluation of flow patterns and a flow-velocity profile. Any hood that fails inspection must be taken out of service immediately. A weekly safety checklist should be maintained that includes the following items: adequate air flow, no unnecessary items in the

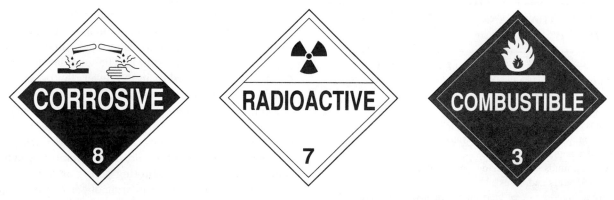

Fig. 1-13 Department of Transportation (DOT) labels. *(Courtesy Lab Safety Supply, Inc., Janesville, WI.)*

hood, baffle settings correct, and guard window documented. Before a hood is used, acceptable hood performance should be confirmed by the technologist. This can be accomplished by using a permanent flowmeter or observing the disappearance of smoke or fumes produced after carefully bringing together two applicator sticks whose cotton tips have been dipped in strong ammonia and hydrochloric acid respectively. (The tips are drenched with running water before disposal.) Alternatively, a paper wipe such as Kimwipe (Kimberly-Clark, Roswell, Georgia) may be held firmly under a baffle in the down position and the force of the exhaust evaluated. *Care must be taken not to release the tissue into the exhaust system.*

OSHA has defined the *personal protective equipment* required for laboratory operations involving chemical hazards. (Much of this equipment is identical to that required for protection against blood-borne pathogens, as will be described on p. 31 in the following section.) Handling of hazardous chemicals requires the use of gloves (the type to be used depends on the type of chemical hazard). Laboratory coats protect clothing; if chemical splashes are probable, an impervious full-body apron offers additional protection. Masks, safety glasses with side shields, or full-face shields are necessary if a potential for eye, nose, or mouth contamination exists. Respirators must be provided and used according to the requirements listed in 29 CFR 1910.134. All personal protective equipment should be removed before a laboratory worker leaves a work area.

Waste and Chemical Control

Chemical waste and hazardous chemical disposal procedures must comply with all local and state regulations. Most laboratories are considered small-quantity generators by the EPA and are required to secure a generation number from the regional EPA office. Certain chemicals can be disposed of in the sanitary sewer system. Specific information must be obtained from local sources, but only those chemicals that are reasonably soluble (at least 3%) in water can be poured down the drain, and these must be flushed with at least 100 volumes of excess water. Compounds that should never be poured down a drain are listed in the box.

COMPOUNDS THAT CANNOT BE DISPOSED OF IN A DRAIN

Organic solvents with a boiling point of less than 50° C
Hydrocarbons
Halogenated hydrocarbons
Nitro compounds
Mercaptans
Most oxygenated compounds that contain more than five
   carbon atoms (such as Freon)
Organic compounds such as azides and peroxides
Concentrated acids and bases
Highly toxic, malodorus, or lacrimatory (tear-producing)
   compounds

The laboratory is responsible for determining the disposition of chemical waste that is removed from the premises. The MSDS sheets and other sources may provide useful information for disposal of specific chemicals.[24,26] Incineration in an environmentally acceptable manner is common for combustible liquids. *Placing volatile chemicals in a hood for the purpose of evaporation is unacceptable.* The laboratory staff must familiarize itself with the rules and regulations governing storage and disposition of toxic chemicals such as solvents and formaldehyde. Records of disposal must be maintained.

Sodium azide, another troublesome chemical, is still used as a bacteriostatic agent. Azides form explosive salts with many metals, including copper and iron. These salts are readily detonated by mechanical shock. Although the amount of sodium azide used as a preservative is relatively small, continued use can result in a buildup of the metallic salts in sewer pipes. These salts are extremely explosive; even the use of a wrench on such a drain line can result in a violent explosion. The removal of azides from pipes is difficult. One method involves closing the lower end of a section of pipe and allowing a 10% solution of sodium hydroxide to remain in contact with the pipe for at least 16 hours. The pipe is then rinsed with copious amounts of water for at least 15 minutes. The use of azides should be avoided or minimized because in addition to their explosive potential they are carcinogenic.

Mercury, a neurotoxin (see p. 718, Chapter 38) and common environmental pollutant, is increasingly seen as a pollution problem in hospitals. An agreement between the EPA and the American Hospital Association in 1998 requires hospitals to minimize the production of mercury-containing pollutants and reduce the amount of products that contain mercury. This includes replacing mercury-containing thermometers. Some colorimetric methods that use mercury salts in the reagent may still be in use, although mercury-free procedures have mostly replaced them. However, many common laboratory reagents, supplies, and even medicinals still use mercury-containing preservatives (such as thimerosal). The disposal of large amounts of spent reagent produced by automated analyzers that use those methods may be a problem; the solution should not be disposed of in the sewer system. The waste material should be collected in large plastic containers and made slightly acidic with acetic acid. If necessary, thioacetamide (about 10 g/L) is added. The solution is then stored in a well-ventilated area (small amounts of hydrogen sulfide may be liberated), and over time the mercury precipitates as mercuric sulfide. The supernatant may then be decanted and disposed of in the sewer; the mercuric sulfide should be disposed of by burial.

Environmental monitoring may be necessary if the laboratory uses any chemical defined in the OSHA publication 29 CFR 1910 Subpart Z three or more times per week. Included in this list is formaldehyde. Monitoring consists of semiannual room air monitoring during an 8-hour period as well as individual badge monitoring of one or more employees exposed to the chemical. In the event that permissible exposure limits are exceeded, monitoring is required more frequently (quarterly) until acceptable exposure levels are achieved. Although xylene is not officially included on the list, a similar procedure should be followed for this chemical. Glutaraldehyde is also a potent sensory irritant that has the ability to precipitate proteins; excessive exposure may cause necrotic or inflammatory lesions of the upper respiratory tract.

Housekeeping such as floor cleaning and general laboratory cleaning should be done regularly according to a defined schedule; housekeeping personnel must be informed of the risks associated with working in the laboratory. The laboratory should be maintained as a clutter-free environment. Hallways and stairwells should be free from obstruction, waste must be handled appropriately, laboratory supplies should be stored appropriately, and all spills should be cleaned appropriately. *Spill clean-up kits* must be readily available for use. Multipurpose products such as sand and soda ash are useful, as are commercial products such as those marketed by chemical companies and safety product suppliers. The laboratory can assemble a kit containing equivalent supplies (rubber gloves, towels, scoop, and various chemicals for neutralizing and absorbing organic solvents and corrosive chemicals). Kits must be labeled and highly accessible. Spills should be cleaned up immediately by laboratory workers using appropriate personal protective equipment. Special clean-up kits are available for handling formaldehyde and mercury spills. The formaldehyde kits neutralize the spill and allow the contents to be disposed of in the regular trash under most conditions. Spilled mercury tends to break up into very small droplets, which are difficult to pick up. Even after collection, disposal tends to be a problem because metallic mercury must not be incinerated or burned. Many mercury kits are available that contain a material that absorbs mercury droplets, producing a less toxic substance, which may be disposed of by burial. Some kits may also include waste disposal through the kit manufacturer. The benches and floors in older laboratories may contain fine cracks in which mercury droplets can lodge. These droplets are difficult to remove, but the cracks should be cleaned, if possible, because mercury is somewhat volatile at room temperature. Rubbing powdered sulfur or sodium polysulfide into the cracks may help to change the mercury into the less volatile sulfide salt.

OSHA regulations mandate that personnel exposed to hazardous chemicals be provided with *medical consultations* and *examinations* on a regular basis (such as annually). The extent of the physical examination is determined by the amount and type of exposure. In addition to regular examinations, personnel should be medically evaluated whenever a major spill occurs, when environmental monitoring indicates exposure above action levels, or when signs and symptoms of toxicity develop. Employees should then be continuously monitored and counseled until a medical clearance is given. *Medical records must be maintained for 30 years after the employee leaves the workplace.*

Training is a necessary and important part of the Chemical Hygiene Plan. Refresher training sessions or competency examinations must be given at least annually and attendance records documented. Training should ensure that the employee knows the extent of chemical exposure, understands the labeling system, knows the meaning of and location of the laboratory's MSDS book, is familiar with the required personal protective equipment, and knows how to react to and handle spills. Many training methods may be used such as videotapes, handouts, and demonstrations.

Record keeping is a crucial component of the laboratory safety program. The laboratory must maintain records of (1) accident and incident reports, (2) inventory and usage records for high-risk substances, (3) environmental monitoring where appropriate, (4) medical consultations, (5) training attendance records, (6) housekeeping procedures, and (7) safety inspections.

Protection against Biohazards and Medical Wastes

Universal precautions. OSHA promulgated a final rule on December 6, 1991, that dealt with occupational exposure to blood and other potentially infectious materials. The program for protection against biohazards was to be fully instituted by July 6, 1992.[22] Many of the requirements of the program are similar to those contained in the Chemical Hygiene Plan, including development of a document describing the following:

1. The extent of exposure for all employees
2. Engineering and work practice controls
3. Personal protective equipment
4. Task assessment
5. Housekeeping procedures
6. Spill cleanup procedures
7. Laundry requirements
8. Labeling requirements
9. Waste disposal
10. Provision of vaccinations
11. Medical consultations
12. Training
13. Record keeping

Some *occupational exposure* to blood-borne pathogens is probably inherent in every task in the chemistry laboratory. Therefore all personnel are at risk. Even though this is the case, it is necessary to define the extent of exposure.

Universal precautions, as defined by the Centers for Disease Control and Prevention (CDC) and adopted by OSHA, are observed to prevent contact with blood and other potentially infectious materials.[27] The general recommendations include the following:

1. All personnel must routinely use barrier precautions to prevent skin and mucous membrane exposure when contact with blood or body fluids from any patient is expected. Gloves must be worn during the performance of venipuncture and when handling blood, body fluids, or items soiled with blood or fluids. Protective eyewear or face shields must be worn during procedures that are likely to cause splashing, to prevent exposure of the mucous membranes of the mouth, nose, and eyes to droplets of blood or body fluids. Gowns and aprons must be worn during procedures that are likely to generate splashing.

2. If the hands or skin become contaminated with blood or other body fluids, they should be washed immediately and thoroughly. Hands should be washed immediately after gloves are removed.

3. Healthcare workers must avoid injuries from needles, scalpels, and other sharp devices. Needles must *not* be recapped, bent, broken, or removed from disposable syringes. After use, disposable syringes, needles, scalpel blades, and other sharp items must be placed in puncture-resistant containers.

4. Healthcare workers who have exudative skin lesions or weeping dermatitis must avoid direct patient care and contact with blood and other potentially infectious materials until the condition is resolved.

5. Pregnant women are particularly cautioned to follow these rules.

Other work practice controls include the following:

1. Specimens of blood and other potentially infectious materials must be transported in leakproof containers. The laboratory worker should take care to avoid contaminating the outside of the container and any accompanying laboratory requisition.

2. Biological safety cabinets should be used for procedures such as blending, sonicating, and vigorous mixing, which can generate droplets.

3. Mouth pipetting is prohibited. Mechanical devices are used to pipet *all* liquids.

4. Eating, drinking, smoking, applying cosmetics or lip balm, and handling contact lenses are prohibited in biohazardous work areas, just as they are prohibited in areas where chemicals are used.

5. Only authorized personnel are permitted in the laboratory. Casual visitors are discouraged. Any visitor to the work area, including instrument service personnel, should be provided with personal protective equipment to the extent necessary.

6. Instruments requiring service should be decontaminated before repair.

7. Chemistry analyzers that generate fine sprays of sample from the sample probe should be equipped with shields, if possible.

8. All employees must wash their hands and remove laboratory coats and other personal protective equipment before leaving the work area.

A revision of the Bloodborne Pathogen Standard 29 CFR 1910.1030 went into effect in April 2001. This revision includes the Needlestick Safety and Prevention Act,[23] which requires that needles used for withdrawing blood must have a "built-in safety feature or mechanism that effectively reduces the risk of an exposure incident." The standard requires that the laboratory must not only provide the devices, but also must monitor the use of the devices as part of a quality improvement program. The Bloodborne Pathogen Manual must reflect these changes in technology; in addition, input should be documented from non-managerial employees, such as

physicians and technologists, responsible for direct patient care. Such individuals are at high risk for injuries from contaminated sharps.

Personal protective equipment. Safety equipment must be provided in the appropriate size by the employer at no cost to the employee. Laboratory coats must be impervious to fluids, offering optimal protection against biohazardous agents. Aprons may be used to provide additional protection. Safety glasses, masks, or full-face shields are used to protect the eyes, mouth, and nose.

Task assessment. Safety policies should be established for each task performed by the laboratory. These policies should include engineering and work practice controls and requirements for personal protective equipment. For much of the work performed in the chemistry laboratory, coats, glasses, and gloves are necessary. For some tasks, additional protection is required.

Housekeeping procedures. Following a written schedule, laboratory workers must decontaminate all equipment and work surfaces with a chemical germicide such as a 1:10 dilution of household bleach (1) after completing specified procedures, (2) when surfaces are overtly contaminated, (3) immediately after any spill of a potentially infectious material, and (4) at the end of the work shift.

Routine cleaning procedures should be instituted for items such as waste cans and other receptacles. Broken glassware that may be contaminated is handled using mechanical means and disposed of appropriately.

Spills of biological material are decontaminated as soon as possible by absorbing the spilled fluid with disposable absorbent material such as paper towels or gauze, flooding the contaminated area with bleach or wiping it with bleach-soaked towels, and then wiping the area with clean, dry towels or gauze. All contaminated items are placed in a biohazard bag and disposed of according to laboratory policy. Spill clean-up requires the use of personal protective equipment.

Contaminated laundry must be packed in red bags at the location where it is used or labeled with a biohazard sign if placed in another type of bag. All laundering and repair of laboratory coats are provided by the employer. *Under no conditions may employees launder their own laboratory coats.* When handling soiled laundry, personnel must wear gloves. Storage of clean and dirty coats must be well separated.

Warning labels (Fig. 1-14) must be used to identify (1) the entrance to work areas; (2) refrigerators and freezers that contain blood and other potentially infectious agents; (3) all containers used to store, transport, or ship potentially infectious materials; and (4) containers of regulated waste (other than red bags). Areas where food is stored should be labeled as nonbiohazard (clean) areas.

Disposal. Regulated medical waste (infectious waste) must be disposed of in accordance with local and state regulations.[28] Contaminated materials should be segregated at the point of use into categories such as needles or sharps and other infectious waste. Containers must be leakproof and should be disposed of when three-fourths full. Any biohazardous waste

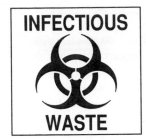 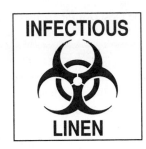

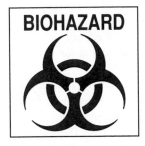

Fig. 1-14   Biohazard labels. *(Courtesy Lab Safety Supply, Inc., Janesville, WI.)*

that is decontaminated by a procedure such as autoclaving is exempt from these regulations and may be disposed of by standard processes. Several types of systems are now available for waste treatment that render the treated product unrecognizable; these include pulverizing or high heat processes. The legality of these devices is determined on a state-by-state basis.

Vaccination. Vaccinations against hepatitis B virus (HBV) must be offered to all employees without cost. Any employee who declines the vaccination must sign a form indicating that the continued risk of exposure to blood-borne pathogens is understood. These employees are at liberty to change their minds at any time. The vaccine is administered in a series of three doses over 6 months. Protective levels of antibodies are induced in 90% to 99% of adults; however, follow-up studies 3 to 5 years after vaccination have shown that in many individuals, titers are no longer measurable. These individuals should receive a single booster vaccination. No time frame for further follow up has been suggested.

Medical consultations and evaluations must be provided if an employee is exposed to a biohazardous agent through a needlestick, a cut, a mucous membrane exposure (eyes, nose, or mouth), or an exposure involving skin contact with large amounts of blood. The source patient is requested to consent to testing for both HBV and human immunodeficiency virus (HIV), if necessary by law. If consent is not required, testing is performed and the employee is informed of the results. The employee's blood is collected and tested as soon as possible. If the employee does not consent to HIV testing, the sample must be preserved for at least 90 days to allow for a change of mind.

High-risk exposures from patients known to be HIV positive or patients at risk of being HIV positive are handled as emergencies. Medication such as azidothymidine (AZT)

must be administered, preferably within 4 hours of the exposure.

Follow-up study of the exposed employee, including antibody or antigen testing, counseling, and postexposure prophylaxis, is conducted. The employee is retested at 6, 12, and 26 weeks after exposure if the patient is HIV positive or is a high-risk subject.

Training. All new employees require specific training sessions to ensure that they understand the epidemiology of blood-borne diseases and the modes of transmission. Explanation of the types and appropriate use of personal protective equipment is essential, as is explanation of emergency procedures to be followed in the event of exposure. All employees must be familiar with the laboratory's policies for protection against transmission of blood-borne pathogens. Adherence to all policies must be monitored regularly; counseling or retraining should be provided when failures are evident.

Records of the employee's HBV vaccination status are mandatory. In addition, results of physical examinations and consultations must be maintained. *All such records must be maintained for the duration of employment plus 30 years.*

Documentation of all training sessions is kept for 3 years and includes dates of all programs, a summary of each program's content, names and qualifications of all instructors, and an attendance list, including names and job titles.

Quality control of all safety procedures as defined by OSHA is a major issue in today's laboratory. All necessary records covering chemical hygiene and biohazard protection should be readily available and carefully maintained to meet current government regulations.

Latex allergy. Since 1991, when OSHA required employers to provide gloves and other protective measures for their employees,[22] laboratory workers have shown a marked increase in the development of latex allergy. The allergy may be in response to either proteins from the rubber tree itself or to the chemicals used in the production of latex. Latex products can produce three types of responses:

1. Irritant contact dermatitis, which is the most common reaction but not a true allergy
2. Allergic contact dermatitis (delayed hypersensitivity with a rash usually appearing 24 to 48 hours after contact), which results from the chemicals added to latex during harvesting, processing, and manufacturing
3. Latex allergy, which is more serious and can cause severe reactions such as respiratory symptoms (see Chapter 25)

The amount of latex exposure required to produce sensitization or an allergic response is unknown. However, the proteins responsible for latex allergies can be adsorbed onto the powder used on many latex gloves, resulting in increased skin exposure. In addition, the removal of powdered gloves can produce an aerosol of latex-contaminated powder, which can increase the risk for respiratory symptoms. Therefore, powder-free gloves should be used whenever possible to minimize the amounts of allergy-causing proteins.[29] Moreover, wearing latex gloves during episodes of dermatitis of the hands may increase skin exposure and the risk of developing latex allergy. The risk of progression from rash to a more serious reaction is unknown, but a rash could be the first sign of allergy.[30]

Recommendations from the National Institute of Occupational Safety and Health (NIOSH) include the provision that reduced protein, powder-free gloves should be available to every employee. Employees should also be provided with continuing education programs and training materials about latex allergy, and high-risk workers should be periodically screened for allergy symptoms. Some hospitals have adopted a program to screen newly hired employees for a latex allergy or sensitization. Employees should be aware that "hypoallergenic" gloves do not decrease the risk of latex allergy. They may, however, reduce the reactions to the chemical additives used in the production of latex (allergic contact dermatitis). Appropriate work practices also include the following:

- Do not use oil-based hand creams or lotions (they cause deterioration of the gloves) unless they have been shown to reduce latex-associated problems and maintain barrier protection.
- Wash hands with mild soap after glove removal and dry thoroughly.
- Keep work area clean to minimize latex dust.
- Be aware of procedures for preventing latex allergy.
- Learn to recognize the symptoms of latex allergy, including rashes, hives, flushing, itching, nasal and eye symptoms, asthma, and shock.
- Report these symptoms to your employee health service.
- Avoid direct contact with latex gloves and other latex-containing products until seen by a physician; if a latex allergy is demonstrated, use a medical alert bracelet.

Part 2: Calculations in Clinical Chemistry[31]
ELIZABETH ANN BYRNE

DILUTION

In several areas of the medical laboratory, an employee must dilute blood or body fluids to prepare a measurable concentration. Accurate preparation of these dilutions is mandatory for reporting the actual concentrations of body-fluid constituents. Diagnosis, prognosis, and therapy depend on these test results.

Dilution can be defined as expressions of concentrations. Dilutions express the amount, either volume or weight, of a substance in a specified total final volume. A 1:5 dilution contains 1 volume (weight) in a *total* of 5 volumes (weights)—that is, 1 volume and 4 volumes.

Expression of a 1:5 dilution can be stated as the common fraction $\frac{1}{5}$. This fraction enables a technician to calculate the actual concentration of a diluted solution.

Example. A 100 mg/mL nitrogen standard is diluted 1:10. The concentration of the resulting solution is $100 \times \frac{1}{10} = 10$ mg/mL.

The most commonly used equation for preparing dilutions is:

$$V_1 \times C_1 = V_2 \times C_2 \qquad \textit{Eq. 1–1}$$

where V_1 is the volume, C_1 is the concentration of solution 1, and V_2 and C_2 are the volume and concentration of the diluted solution. These may be expressed as % (weight/volume, w/v), molarity, or normality concentration. V_2 and C_2 are similarly related. This basic equation can be expressed as:

$$\frac{V_1}{V_2} = \frac{C_1}{C_2} \qquad \textit{Eq. 1–2}$$

The most common error in setting up any equation of this type is *not placing* the related volumes or concentrations in the proper place and having the units cancel out, leaving the final, uncanceled units.

One helpful practice for successfully solving laboratory calculations is to label all numbers in any equation with their respective units of measurement. This may take an extra minute but will save many minutes of reviewing calculations when the final result appears illogical or incorrect. A problem that does *not* properly cancel out units cannot be successfully solved. A second helpful practice is to reduce fractions to their least common denominators before calculating the results.

Example. Prepare 500 mL of 0.5 M NaCl (molecular weight of NaCl = 58.5 g/mol):

$$500 \text{ mL} \times \frac{\text{Liter}}{1000 \text{ mL}} \times \frac{0.5 \text{ mol}}{\text{Liter}} \times \frac{58.5 \text{ g}}{\text{mol}} = \frac{0.5 \times 58.5 \text{ g}}{2}$$

$$= \frac{29.25 \text{ g}}{2} = 14.6 \text{ g}$$

14.6 g of NaCl dissolved in 500 mL = 0.5 M NaCl

Example. Preparation of 250 mL of 0.1 M HCl from stock 1 M HCl:

$$\text{Using } C_1 \times V_1 = C_2 \times V_2$$

Where V_1 is the unknown $V_2 = 250$ mL
$C_1 = 1.0$ mol/L $C_2 = 0.1$ mol/L
1.0 mol/L $\times V_1 = 250$ mL $\times 0.1$ mol/L
$V_1 = 25$ mL

Measure 25 mL of 1 M HCl; dilute to 250 mL with distilled water. This diluted solution has a 0.1 M HCl concentration. (Mathematical reasoning indicates that a 1:10 dilution of stock 1 M HCl results in a 0.1 M concentration, and 25 mL diluted to 250 mL equals a 1:10 dilution.)

Another Application of Dilutions

So that a 24-hour urine creatinine concentration could be assayed, the specimen had to be diluted 1:5 before measurement. Calculate the 24-hour excretion if the 24-hour urine volume is 1800 mL and the measured creatinine concentration is 260 mg/L:

$$\text{Total excretion} = 1800 \frac{\text{mL}}{24 \text{ hr}} \times 260 \frac{\text{mg}}{\text{L}} \times 5 \times \frac{1 \text{ L}}{1000 \text{ mL}}$$

Total excretion = Total urine volume × Concentration × Dilution
Total excretion = 2340 mg/24 hr or 2.34 g/24 hr

Exercises

Calculate the concentrations (answers are at the end of this chapter).

1. 10 M NaOH, which is diluted 1:20 = _____ M?
2. 2 M HCl, which is diluted 1:5 = _____ M?
3. 1000 mg/L glucose, diluted 1:10 and then 1:2 = _____ mg/L?

Serial dilutions are those in which all the dilutions after the first one are the same. Exceptions to this general description of preparation of serial dilutions are included with certain techniques in serology, such as the antistreptolysin titer.

Serial dilution example. To determine the anti-Rh_0 (D) titer, serum is diluted 1:5 by addition of 0.2 mL of serum to 0.8 mL of saline solution, in tube 1. Tubes 2 through 8 contain 0.5 mL of saline as diluent. Dilution is performed by transferring 0.5 mL of tube 1 to tube 2, mixing, and then transferring 0.5 mL of tube 2 to tube 3, continuing through the tubes to tube 8, mixing after each transfer. The concentration of serum in the tubes decreases by a factor of 2 with each dilution: 1:5, 1:10, 1:20, 1:40, 1:80, 1:160, 1:320, and 1:640.

4. For an ABO titer, tube 1 contains 0.9 mL of diluent, tubes 2 to 8 contain 0.5 mL of diluent, 0.1 mL of serum is added to tube 1, and serial dilutions using 0.5 mL are carried out in the remaining tubes. If the last tube showing agglutination with A cells is tube 6, what is the anti-A titer of the serum? (This is equal to the dilution in tube 6 = 1:?)

5. All tubes for a serial dilution contain 0.5 mL of saline solution, 0.5 mL of serum is added to tube 1, and 0.5 mL is transferred through the row of tubes. Sheep cells are added to the tubes, and agglutination is demonstrated through tube 7. What is the titer of sheep cell agglutinations?

WEIGHTS AND CONCENTRATIONS
Definitions and Examples

Percent concentrations. Percent concentrations are generally expressed as parts of solute per 100 parts of total solution; hence the expression *percent*, or *per one hundred*. The use of percent concentration is derived historically from the early pharmaceutical chemists. Although these terms are still commonly used in the United States, major organizations (American Association for Clinical Chemistry [AACC], CAP) are attempting to use unified SI units. Concentrations in SI units are described in moles per liter when the molecular weight of the substance is known. If the molecular weight is unknown, weight (mass) per milliliter or weight per liter is used. Throughout the text, SI units are used where possible.

The three basic forms of concentration are as follows:

Weight per unit weight (w/w). Both solute and solvent are weighed, the total equaling 100 g.

Example. 5% w/w of NaCl contains 50 g of NaCl + 950 g of diluent.

Volume per unit volume (v/v). The volume of liquid solute per total volume of solute and solvent is expressed.

Example. 1% of HCl (v/v) contains 1 mL of HCl per 100 mL (or 1 dL) of solution.

Weight per unit volume (w/v). The most frequently used expression, concentrations of w/v are reported as grams percent (g%) or g/dL, as well as mg/dL and µg/dL. When percent concentration is expressed without a specified form, it is assumed to be weight per unit volume. The use of weight percent to describe concentration is being discouraged by professional organizations and, with few exceptions, is not used in this book. SI units express w/v in terms of weight per microliters (µL), milliliters (mL), or liters (L).

Example. To prepare 100 mL of 100 g/L of NaCl, weigh 10 g of NaCl and dilute to volume in a 100 mL volumetric flask.

Molarity. Molarity expresses concentration as the number of moles per liter of solution. One mole is the molecular weight of the substance in grams. A millimole is 1/1000 of a mole. A molar solution contains 1 gram–molecular weight of a substance per liter.

$$1 \text{ mol} = 1000 \text{ mmol}$$
$$1 \text{ mmol} = 1000 \text{ µmol}$$
$$1 \text{ µmol} = 1000 \text{ nmol}$$

Examples. 1 M NaOH (molecular weight, or MW = 40.0 g/mol) contains 1 gram–equivalent molecular weight per liter, or 40 g diluted to 1000 mL with distilled water. A millimolar (1 mM) solution, or 0.001 molar (0.001 M), contains 1 mmol/L. 1 mM of NaOH is 1/1000 of 40 g, that is, 0.040 g (or 40 mg). When diluted to 1000 mL, the concentration of the solution is 0.001 M.

Normality. Normality expresses concentration in terms of equivalent weights of substances. Equivalent weights are determined by the valence, which reflects the number of combining or replaceable units. A 1 normal (1 N) solution contains 1 equivalent weight per liter. The equivalent weight of an element or compound is equal to the molecular weight divided by the valence.

Normality and *molarity* relationships can be readily calculated if their definitions are understood.

Examples

1 M HCl = 1 N HCl, since 1 mole of H^+ or Cl^- reacts for every mole of HCl.

1 M H_2SO_4 = 2 N H_2SO_4, since 2 moles of H^+ (that is, equivalents) react for every mole of H_2SO_4.

1 M H_3PO_4 = 3 N H_3PO_4, since 3 moles of H^+ react for every mole of H_3PO_4.

1 M $CaCl_2$ = 2 N $CaCl_2$, since 2 Cl$^-$ can react for every mole of $CaCl_2$.

1 M $CaSO_4$ = 2 N $CaSO_4$, since 2 mole volume electrons are available for reaction with either Ca^{++} or $SO_4^=$.

Equivalent weights are known as the number of grams of an element (or compound) that will react with another element (or compound). This so-called law of combining weights is operable for all chemical compounds.

To simplify chemistry procedures and reports, factors can be used to express a quantity of one compound as an equivalent quantity of another compound. This process can be termed *equivalency.*

Example. Calculate the amount of urea if a patient's urea nitrogen level is 800 mg/L. The formula for urea is NH_2—CO—NH_2, and its molecular weight is 60 g/mol. The molecular equivalent weight for nitrogen in the mole is 14 g/mol $\times$ 2 molecules = 28. *The urea/nitrogen factor* is determined by the following equation:

$$\frac{MW\ of\ urea\ (60)}{2 \times MW\ of\ nitrogen\ (28)} = \frac{x\ g\ of\ urea}{1\ g\ of\ urea\ nitrogen}$$

$28x = 60$
$x = 2.14$ (factor)

This factor states that 2.14 g of urea equivalently represents 1 g of urea nitrogen, so 800 mg/L urea nitrogen $\times$ 2.14 equals 1712 mg/L of urea. Laboratory results today are reported as urea nitrogen because historical methods for this particular test are based on measurement of the urea nitrogen.

Competent laboratory personnel should be able to convert mg/dL to mEq/L. Electrolyte equivalents can be calculated from the equation:

$$mg/dL \times 10 = 10\ mg/L$$

because mg/mEq weight is the millimolar weight in milligrams divided by the valence

$$\frac{mg/L}{mg/mEq} = mEq/L$$

or

$$\frac{mg/dL}{mg/mEq} \times 10\ \frac{dL}{L} = mEq/L$$

Example. What is the mEq/L concentration of serum chloride reported as 250 mg/dL? Since the millimolecular weight of chloride is 35.5 (that is, 1 mmol = 35.5 mg), the milliequivalent weight of chloride is

$$\frac{MW}{Valence} = \frac{35.5\ g/mol}{1}$$

$$\frac{250\ mg/dL}{35.5\ mg/mEq} \times 10\ \frac{dL}{L} = 70\ mEq/L$$

Specific gravity. Specific gravity can be used to determine the mass (weight) of solutions. It relates the weight of 1 mL of the solution and the weight of an equal volume of pure water at 4° C (1 g). One particular use of specific gravity is in preparation of dilutions from concentrated commercial acids, the equation being:

Specific gravity $\times$ Percent assay = Grams of compound per milliliter

Example. Concentrated HCl has a specific gravity of 1.25 g/mL and is assayed as being 38% HCl. What is the amount of HCl per milliliter?

$$1.25\ g/mL \times 0.38 = 0.475\ g\ of\ HCl\ per\ mL$$

One common error is neglecting to change the percent assay to its proper decimal; in the previous example, 38% = 0.38!

Exercise

6. How many milliliters of concentrated HCl are needed to prepare 1 L of a 0.1 N HCl solution if the molecular weight of HCl = 36.5?

Water of hydration. Some salts are available in forms both anhydrous (no water) and hydrated (with water molecules). The form of the available salt, including the water of hydration, is listed on the manufacturer's label. To prepare accurate weight concentrations of these salts, calculations must include the molecules of water present in the compound. This is most easily done by calculating the percentage of the compound that is in the anhydrous form. With this percentage, the weight of the hydrated form can be corrected to that of the anhydrous form.

The advantage of using molar concentrations is that the water of hydration does *not* have to be accounted for in the calculations. For example, 1 mol of $CuSO_4$ = 160 g, and 1 mol of $CuSO_4 \cdot 5H_2O$ = 250 g. One gram–equivalent molecular weight of each compound contains 1 mol of $CuSO_4$—that is:

250 g $CuSO_4 \cdot 5H_2O$ = 1 mol of $CuSO_4$ = 160 g of $CuSO_4$

Example. How many grams of $MgCl_2$ are there in 1 g of $MgCl_2 \cdot 3H_2O$?

Mg	24		Mg	24
Cl$_2$	71		Cl$_2$	71
	95 MW		3 H$_2$O	54
				149 MW

$$\frac{95}{149} = \frac{x}{1}$$

$149\ x = 95$
$x = 63.8\%$

One gram of $MgCl_2 \cdot 3H_2O$ contains 0.638 g of $MgCl_2$.

Mole fraction. Mole fraction refers to the ratio of the amount of a component to the total mixture of components. Mole fraction is a derived unit that is expressed as either a percent or a decimal.

Example. What percent Mg is contained in $MgCl_2 \cdot 3H_2O$?

Mg = 24
Cl = 35.5 $\frac{24}{149} = 16.1\%$
$MgCl_2 \cdot 3H_2O$ = 149

Mg is 16.1% of the molecule $MgCl_2 \cdot 3H_2O$.

Example. To determine mole percent calcium in calcium carbonate (MW = 100), 1 mol of $CaCO_3$ contains 100 g, comprising 40 (Ca) + 12 (C) + 48 (3 $\times$ O), of which 40 is calcium. The mole fraction of calcium in 1 L of 1 mol of calcium carbonate equals 40%.

Example. How much $CuSO_4 \cdot 5H_2O$ must be weighed to prepare 1 L of a solution containing 80 mg of $CuSO_4$?

Total MW of $CuSO_4 \cdot 5H_2O$ = 250
MW of $CuSO_4$ = 160

The proportion of $CuSO_4 \cdot 5H_2O$ that is $CuSO_4$ is 160/250 = 0.64. Therefore, 1 g of $CuSO_4 \cdot 5H_2O$ contains 1 g $\times$ 0.64 = 0.64 g of $CuSO_4$. The rest, 0.36 g, is water. Thus:

$$\frac{80}{0.64} = 125 \text{ mg of CuSO}_4 \cdot 5\text{H}_2\text{O}$$

Examples of Calculations

a. What is the normality of concentrated HCl that has a specific gravity of 1.19 g/mL and a 38% assay?

Specific gravity × Percent = Grams/milliliter
1.19 × 0.38 = 0.452 g/ml = 452 g/L
1 equivalent weight of HCl = 36.5 g

$$\frac{452 \text{ g/L}}{36.5 \text{ g/Eq}} = 12.4 \text{ N}$$

b. If 24.5 g of H_2SO_4 (MW = 98 g/mol) are dissolved in a 1 L solution
1. What is its molarity?
2. What is its normality?
(Answer 1) 1 mol of H_2SO_4 = 98 g; therefore 24.5 g equals

$$\frac{1 \text{ mol}}{98 \text{ g}} = \frac{x}{24.5}$$

$$x = 0.25 \text{ mol}$$
$$0.25 \text{ mol in 1 L} = 0.25 \text{ mol/L} = 0.25 \text{ M}$$

(Answer 2) The valence of H_2SO_4 equals 2; therefore the equivalent weight of H_2SO_4 is expressed as follows:

$$\text{Equivalent weight} = \frac{\text{Molecular weight}}{\text{Valence}} = \frac{98 \text{ g}}{2}$$

Equivalent weight = 49 g
To solve for number of equivalents in 24.5 g

$$\frac{1 \text{ equivalent}}{49 \text{ g}} = \frac{x}{24.5 \text{ g}}$$

$$x = 0.5 \text{ equivalent}$$
$$0.5 \text{ equivalent in 1 L} = 0.5 \text{ Eq/L} = 0.5 \text{ N}$$

c. The molecular weight of $CaCO_3$ is 100 g/mol, and the atomic weight of calcium is 40 g/mol; how many grams or milligrams of $CaCO_3$ are needed to prepare:
1. 1 L of 0.1 M $CaCO_3$?
2. 10 mL of 100 mg/dL of Ca^{++} using $CaCO_3$?
3. 50 mg/L of $CaCO_3$?
4. 0.2 mEq/L of Ca^{++} using $CaCO_3$?
(Answer 1) 10 grams; 1 mol of $CaCO_3$ = 100 g; therefore 0.1 mol = 10 g, since 0.1 molar = 0.1 mol/L = 10 g/L
(Answer 2) The percentage weight Ca^{++} in $CaCO_3$ is

$$\frac{\text{Atomic weight Ca}^{++}}{\text{Molecular weight CaCO}_3} = \frac{40}{100} = 40\%$$

In 10 mL, 10 mg of Ca^{++} is needed or

$$\frac{10 \text{ mg}}{\% \text{ Ca in CaCO}_3} = \frac{10 \text{ mg}}{40\%} = \frac{10 \text{ mg}}{0.4} = 25 \text{ mg of CaCO}_3$$

Therefore 25 mg of $CaCO_3$ = 10 mg Ca^{++}
(Answer 3) For 1 L, 50 mg of $CaCO_3$ is needed.
(Answer 4) 1 equivalent weight of $CaCO_3$ equals

$$\frac{\text{Molecular weight of CaCO}_3}{\text{Valence}} = \frac{100 \text{ g/mol}}{2 \text{ Eq/mol}} = 50 \text{ g/Eq}$$

To convert to milliequivalents

$$1 \text{ mEq} = \frac{1 \text{ Eq}}{1000}$$

$$\therefore \frac{50 \text{ g}}{1 \text{ Eq}} \times \frac{1 \text{ Eq}}{1000 \text{ mEq}} = 50 \text{ mg/mEq}$$

To calculate amount to prepare 1 L of 0.2 mEq

$$\frac{1 \text{ mEq wt}}{50 \text{ mg}} = \frac{0.2 \text{ mEq wt}}{x}$$

$$x = 10 \text{ mg of CaCO}_3$$

Exercises

7. 3 M $CaCl_2$ (MW 111.1) = _____ N $CaCl_2$
8. 2 N H_3PO_4 (MW 98) = _____ M H_3PO_4
9. 2 M H_2SO_4 (MW 98) = _____ N H_2SO_4
10. 250 mL of 5% NaCl contains _____ g of NaCl
11. How much $CuSO_4 \cdot 5H_2O$ must be weighed to prepare 100 mL of 5% $CuSO_4$? (MW $CuSO_4$ = 159.61; MW H_2O = 18)
12. What percent of $CuSO_4 \cdot 5H_2O$ is water? _____ %

CALCULATIONS BASED ON PHOTOMETRIC MEASUREMENTS (BEER'S LAW)

Refer to Chapter 4 for a description of the relationship between percent transmittance, absorbance, and concentration.

Colorimetry

Colorimetry is the measurement of the kind and amount of light absorbed or transmitted by a solution. These measurements of absorbance or transmittance are logarithmically related. Beer's law reflects the relationships between the absorbance and concentration of a known standard solution with that of solutions with unknown concentrations, the patients' samples. Beer's law states that the absorbance of a solution is directly related to its concentration. If Beer's law is true, then:

$$C_u = \frac{A_u}{A_s} \times C_s \qquad \textit{Eq. 1-3}$$

C_u and A_u represent concentration and absorbance of the unknown samples, whereas C_s and A_s reflect that of the standard solution. When preparing a colorimetric method for clinical chemistry analysis, the technician must be sure that Beer's law is followed or this formula cannot be used. In other words, this formula can only be used if the absorbance and concentration are directly related—that is, if the absorbance doubles with a doubling of concentration. A *standard curve* can be used to determine concentration values graphically. Standard-curve preparations are described on p. 40.

Absorbance and Transmittance

Absorbance measures the amount of light that is blocked or absorbed by a solution. Absorbance is also termed *optical density* (OD), a term found in the older literature and not in common use today.

Transmittance measures the amount of light that passes through a solution. The transmittance is usually expressed as a percentage, or *%T*. The %T scale is linear, as noted on a colorimeter readout scale.

As discussed in Chapter 4, the absorbance and percent transmittance are logarithmically related because absorbance is a logarithmic function. Interconversion of the absorbance and percent transmittance is commonly expressed by the following formula:

$$A = -\log \frac{\%T}{100} \qquad \textit{Eq. 1-4}$$

This equation can be algebraically converted to the following form:

$$A = -(\log \%T - \log 100)$$
$$A = -(\log \%T - 2)$$
$$A = -\log \%T + 2$$
$$A = 2 - \log \%T \qquad \textit{Eq. 1-5}$$

A laboratory worker can obtain absorbance from a hand calculator using this formula by punching in the numbers for %T, converting to the log form, placing a minus sign, and adding 2.

Examples. Determining concentrations using absorbance (A, or OD) readings.

a. If absorbance of an unknown is 0.25 and the concentration of a standard is 4 mg/L with an absorbance of 0.40, the concentration of the unknown can be calculated using:

$$C_u = \frac{A_u}{A_s} \times C_s$$

$$C_u = \frac{0.25}{0.40} \times 4 \text{ mg/L}$$

$$C_u = 2.5 \text{ mg/L}$$

b. To calculate the concentration of glucose if the following information is known:

$$C_s = 2000 \text{ mg/L, } A_s = 0.40, A_u = 0.25$$

Using the same formula above

$$C_u = \frac{0.25}{0.40} \times 2000 \text{ mg/L}$$

$$C_u = 1250 \text{ mg/L}$$

c. To calculate glucose concentration of unknown (C_u) if the %T is given. If the 1000 mg/L glucose standard (C_s) reads 49% T, and the unknown reads 55% T, the %T must be converted to absorbance because only absorbance is linearly proportional to concentration:

$$A_s = 2 - \log \%T \qquad A_u = 2 - \log \%T$$
$$A_s = 2 - 1.690 \qquad A_u = 2 - 1.740$$
$$A_s = 0.31 \qquad\qquad A_u = 0.26$$
$$49\% \text{ T} = 0.31 \ A = A_s$$
$$55\% \text{ T} = 0.26 \ A = A_u$$
$$C_s = 1000 \text{ mg/L, } A_u = 0.26, A_s = 0.31$$

Using the formula as in (a) and (b) previously:

$$C_u = \frac{0.26}{0.31} \times 1000 \text{ mg/L} = 839 \text{ mg/L}$$

Molar Extinction Coefficient

Molar extinction coefficients are used in the clinical laboratory to calculate concentrations and activities of enzymes in IU

and to determine the purity of dissolved substances. Specific applications include checking standard solutions such as hemoglobin or bilirubin. The molar extinction coefficient, or molar absorbance coefficient, or $\in$, is defined as the absorbance at a given wavelength of a 1 M solution of the substance in a 1 cm cuvette at 25° C. It is related to absorbance by the formula

$$A = \in cl \qquad \textit{Eq. 1-6}$$

where A = absorbance at a specified wavelength, c = concentration of the substance being measured in moles/L, and l = the path length in cm.

A suitable bilirubin standard, as a 1 M solution in chloroform, would have a theoretical absorbance of 60,700 (mean) ± 800 at 453 nm, when measured in a 1 cm cuvette at 25° C. Logical reasoning suggests that if this standard were diluted to 1:60,700 the absorbance would read 1.

Example. 1 M bilirubin standard is diluted to 1:60,700 and then 1:2, with the final dilution being 1:121,400. The absorbance of this dilution reads 0.495 in a 1 cm cuvette. What is the extinction coefficient of this bilirubin standard?

$$\in = \frac{0.495 \ (121,400)}{1 \text{ mol/L (1 cm)}}$$

$$\in = 60,093 \text{ liters} \cdot \text{mol}^{-1} \cdot \text{cm}^{-1}$$

A major application of $\in$ is the measurement of concentrations of substances. If the $\in$ of a substance is known and a 1 cm cuvette is used, Beer's law is simplified to the following:

$$c = \frac{A}{\in}$$

Example. The $\in$ of NADH at 340 nm is 6.22×10^3 $L \cdot \text{mol}^{-1} \cdot \text{cm}^{-1}$. If the absorbance of NADH at 340 nm reads 0.350, what is the concentration?

$$c = \frac{0.350}{622 \times 10^3 \text{ L} \cdot \text{mol}^{-1}}$$

$$c = 5.6 \times 10^{-5} \text{ mol/L}$$

Exercises

13. NADH has a molar absorptivity of 3.3×10^3 at a wavelength of 366 nm. Calculate the concentration of a solution that has an A (absorbance) of 0.175 at 366 nm.

14. A chemistry technologist is checking a bilirubin standard. What is the molar absorptivity of a 1 M solution diluted to 1:60,700 and reading 0.70 in a 7 mm cuvette?

15. The chemistry technologist has a solution of NADH with a concentration of 0.05×10^{-3} mol/L. Calculate the molar absorptivity if it measures 0.300 at 334 nm.

BUFFERS

Buffers resist changes in acidity by forming a weakly ionized acid or base with the added H^+ or OH^- ions. For example, when HCl is added to a solution of Na^+Ac^- (sodium acetate) plus H^+Ac^- (acetic acid), the H^+ of HCl will react with the Ac^- forming more HAc, which is only slightly ionized. The acetate–acetic acid effectively buffers by removing H^+ from the solution.

The Henderson-Hasselbalch equation is used to express acid-base relationships. Several forms of this equation can be used. They will not be delineated at this time but can be used for calculating acid-base problems. The simplest equation is:

$$pH = pK + \log \frac{\text{Concentration of conjugate base}}{\text{Concentration of weak acid}} \qquad \textit{Eq. 1-7}$$

The pK value depends on a specific set of conditions, including degree of dissociation, temperature, and pH. The pK for the bicarbonate buffer system in serum or plasma is 6.10 at 37° C. Chemical reference books such as the *Handbook of Chemistry and Physics* contain pK values. Capable medical technologists should grasp the basic calculations of the Henderson-Hasselbalch equations even though laboratory instruments provide direct "read-out" values on patients' acid-base tests.

Examples

a. Calculate the pH of an acetate buffer composed of 0.20 M sodium acetate and 0.05 M acetic acid. (The pK for acetic acid is 4.76.)

$$\begin{aligned} pH &= pK + \log \frac{[\text{Salt}]}{[\text{Acid}]} \\ &= 4.76 + \log \frac{0.20}{0.05} \\ &= 4.76 + \log 4 \\ &= 5.3621 \\ pH &= 5.36 \end{aligned}$$

b. Now for a complicated example. Prepare 1 L of an acetate buffer whose acetate concentration is 0.2 M and has a pH of 5.0. (The pK of acetic acid is 4.76; the molecular weight of acetic acid is 60; the molecular weight of sodium acetate is 82.)

$$\begin{aligned} pH &= 4.76 + \log \frac{[\text{Salt}]}{[\text{Acid}]} \\ \log \frac{[\text{Salt}]}{[\text{Acid}]} &= 5.0 - 4.76 \\ [\text{Salt}]/[\text{Acid}] &= \text{antilog } 0.24 \\ [\text{Salt}]/[\text{Acid}] &= 1.7 \end{aligned}$$

The number 1.7 is the ratio of the moles per liter of salt to the moles per liter of acid. Any molar concentrations of salt to acid yielding a ratio of 1.7 will result in a 5.0 pH acetate buffer. *Note:* The problem specifies a concentration of 0.2 M solution, or $HAc + Ac^- = 0.2$ M.

If

$$Ac^-/HAc = 1.7$$

then

$$Ac^- = 1.7 \; HAc$$

or

$$HAc + 1.7 \; HAc = 0.2 \text{ M}$$

and

$$\begin{aligned} 2.7 \; HAc &= 0.2 \\ HAc &= 0.074 \text{ mol/L of acid} \\ MW \times M &= g/L \\ 60 \times 0.074 &= 4.44 \text{ g/L of acid needed} \end{aligned}$$

To calculate the weight of salt needed for 1 L use:

$$\begin{aligned} \text{Moles of salt} &= \text{Total moles} - \text{Moles of acid} \\ &= 0.2 - 0.074 \\ &= 0.126 \text{ moles of salt} \end{aligned}$$

As done for the acid:

$$\begin{aligned} MW \text{ of salt} \times M &= \text{Grams of salt/liter} \\ 82 \text{ g/mol} \times 0.126 \text{ mol/L} &= 10.33 \text{ g of salt/L} \end{aligned}$$

When 4.44 g of acid and 10.33 of salt are dissolved in a total volume of 1 L, the resulting buffer concentration is 0.2 M at a pH of 5.0.

ENZYME CALCULATIONS

Expressing enzyme activity in U has been generally accepted since its recommendation by the IUB in the early 1960s. One U of an enzyme is defined as the amount that will catalyze the transformation of 1 mmole of the substrate per minute under standard conditions. Activity is expressed in terms of enzyme units per liter of serum, or milliunits per milliliter, in the following relationship:

$$1 \text{ U/L} = \mu\text{mole/minute/liter of serum}$$

Explanation of the basic equation for the conversion of absorbance data to U is not provided in this portion of laboratory calculation. Suffice it to state that any change in factors such as temperature or volume must be accounted for in the following basic equation (see Chapter 54):

$$U/L = \frac{\Delta A/\text{min} \times V_t \times 10^6 \; (\mu\text{mol/mol})}{\in \times V_s \times l} \qquad \textit{Eq. 1-8}$$

$\Delta A/\text{min}$ = Absorbance change per minute
 V_t = Total reaction volume, including sample, reagent, and diluent
 V_s = Serum volume
 l = Cuvette path length
 $\in$ = Extinction coefficient

The factor of 10^6 µmol/mol is added to convert the answer to µmol/min/L (U/L).

Example. What is the lactate dehydrogenase (LD) activity of 0.1 ml of serum + 3 mL of substrate if the NADH being formed showed a 0.002 ΔA/min at 340 nm? $\in$ for NADH = $6.22 \times 10^3 \cdot L \cdot mol^{-1} \cdot cm^{-1}$. Using the previously provided formula:

$$U/L = \frac{0.002 \; (10^6 \; \mu\text{mol/mol}) \; (3.1 \text{ mL})}{1 \text{ min} \left(6.22 \times 10^3 \; \dfrac{L}{mol \cdot cm} \right) (0.1 \text{ mL}) (1 \text{ cm})}$$

$$U/L = 9.9$$

Example. Calculation of U units per liter of alkaline phosphatase activity using *p*-nitrophenol standard requires attention to all factors of the formula:

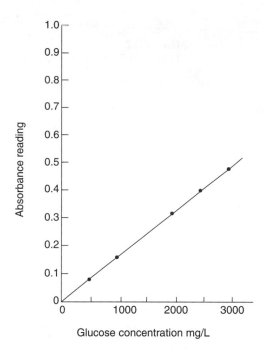

Fig. 1-15 Standard curve for glucose analysis: absorbance versus concentration on linear-linear graph paper.

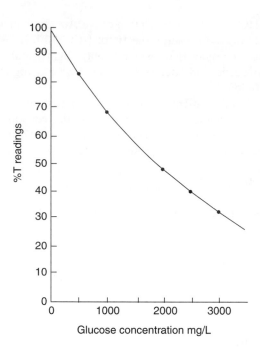

Fig. 1-16 Standard curve for glucose analysis: percent transmittance (%T) versus concentration on linear-linear graph paper.

$$U/L = \frac{\Delta A/min \times V_t \times 10^6 \, (\mu mol/mol)}{\in \times V_s \times l}$$

If ΔA of sample = 0.070, the $\in$ for *p*-nitrophenol is 50,000 L/mol · cm; timing = 15 min; V_t = 5.5 mL; V_s = 0.005 mL.

$$U/L = \frac{0.070 \left(10^6 \, \frac{\mu mol}{mol}\right)(5.5 \, mL)}{15 \, min \left(50,000 \, \frac{L}{mol \cdot cm}\right)(0.005 \, mL)(1 \, cm)}$$

$$U/L = \frac{0.070 \times 5.5 \times 1000}{50 \times 0.075}$$

103 U/L = Alkaline phosphatase activity

STANDARD CURVES

Preparing standard curves on graph paper is an essential way of examining data for validity. Often calculations or computers do not reveal abnormalities of the system, but calculate averages of results. Therefore graphing of data is an important way to validate assays.

Previously in this chapter, Beer's law was defined as the direct relationship of the absorbance and concentration of a solution. This means that if a 2% solution reads 0.1 *A*, then a 4% concentration will read 0.2 *A*, and an 8% solution will read 0.4 *A*. Most solutions obey Beer's law; that is, concentration and absorbance are directly proportional only over specified ranges of concentrations.

Graphs

Fig. 1-15 indicates that absorbances of glucose standard concentrations plotted on linear paper result in a straight line,

confirming that Beer's law is followed for the concentrations up to 3000 mg/L. The Fig. 1-16 graph, which plots the %T values of the same glucose concentrations used in Fig. 1-15 on linear paper, features a semicurved line; %T values are not linear versus concentrations. (Recall the logarithmic relationship of absorbance and %T.) Plotting %T values on semilog paper results in a straight line, which can be used to interpolate the concentrations of glucose from %T values (Fig. 1-17).

Exercises

Find glucose concentrations for the following readings using Figs. 1-15 and 1-17.

16. 0.3 *A* = _____ mg/L
17. 0.39 *A* = _____ mg/L
18. 49% *T* = _____ mg/L
19. 52% *T* = _____ mg/L

Exercises Using One Known Standard Value to Determine Concentrations of Unknowns

What are the glucose concentrations of the following patients' samples if the 2000 mg/L standard reads 0.32 *A*?

We can employ either:

$$C_u = \frac{A_u}{A_s} \times C_s$$

or

$$\frac{C_u}{C_s} = \frac{A_u}{A_s}$$

20. 0.22 *A* = _____ mg/L
21. 0.14 *A* = _____ mg/L
22. 0.46 *A* = _____ mg/L

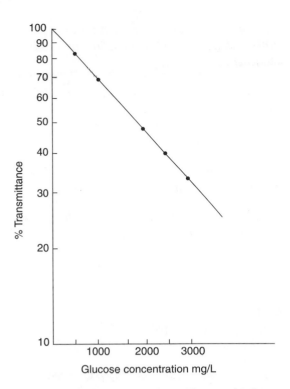

Fig. 1-17 Standard curve for glucose analysis: percent transmittance (%T) versus concentration on log-linear graph paper.

Renal Clearance Test Calculations

Renal clearance tests are used to assess kidney function. Renal clearance is a rate measurement that expresses the volume of blood cleared of the substance being studied (typically creatinine or urea) per unit of time. Therefore the unit for the clearance test is milliliters per minute.

To calculate creatinine clearance, the following information is required:

Serum concentration (S)

Urine concentration (U) (*Caution:* the serum and urine concentrations must be in the same units, e.g., mg/L or mg/dL)

Volume of urine excreted per minute (V) (volume of urine collected divided by time period in minutes)

$$\text{Clearance (uncorrected)} = \frac{U \times V}{S}$$

This calculation does not account for the patient's body surface area. If the physician requests a corrected value, the equation must be multiplied by 1.73/A, where 1.73 equals the average body surface area in square meters and A equals the patient's body surface area:

$$\text{Clearance (corrected)} = \frac{U \times V}{S} \times \frac{1.73}{A}$$

The patient's body surface area is computed from a nomogram, using the patient's height and weight or calculated using the following formula:

$$\log A = (0.425 \times \log W) + (0.725 \times \log H) - 2144$$

where A is the body surface area in square meters, W is the patient's weight in kilograms, and H is the patient's height in centimeters.

Examples

a. Determine the uncorrected creatinine clearance for a patient with a serum creatinine of 25 mg/L. The urine creatinine was 500 mg/L and the urine volume was 312 mL/4 hr.

$$312 \text{ mL}/240 \text{ min} = 1.3 \text{ mL/min}$$

$$C = \frac{U}{S} \times V = \frac{500}{25} \times 1.3 = 26 \text{ mL/min}$$

b. Calculate the corrected creatinine clearance for a child who weighed 22.7 kg, was 95 cm long, and passed 500 mL of urine during a 24-hour period. Serum and urine creatinine values were 0.14 mmol/L and 4.75 mmol/L, respectively.

$$\begin{aligned}
\log A &= (0.425 \times \log 22.7) \\
&\quad + (0.725 \times \log 95) \\
&\quad - 2144 \\
\log A &= 0.576 + 1434 - 2144 = 0.134 \\
A &= 0.734 \\
500 \text{ ml}/1440 &\text{ min} = 0.35 \text{ mL/min}
\end{aligned}$$

$$C = \frac{U}{X} \times V \times \frac{1.73}{A}$$

$$= \frac{4.75}{0.14} \times 0.35 \times \frac{1.73}{0.734}$$

$$= 28.0 \text{ mL/min}$$

Timed Urine Tests

Results of urine tests may be reported in several ways. Values can be reported as concentration units, quantity per total volume, and quantity per unit of time. The clinical usefulness of urine tests is increased when quantitative results are expressed as amount per total volume or amount excreted in a given period. Good laboratory practice dictates that the urine total volume and the beginning and end time period of collection be recorded.

When urine test results are reported as quantity per total volume, the concentration is measured and the results are corrected as follows:

$$\frac{\text{Amount}}{\text{Total volume}} = \text{Measured concentration} \times \text{Total volume}$$

This calculation requires that both the urine and the instrument concentration be reported using the same volume units.

Examples

a. Calculate the amount of protein in 2400 mL of urine having a concentration of 30 mg/dL.

$$\frac{\text{Amount}}{\text{Total volume}} = \frac{30 \text{ mg}}{100 \text{ mL}} \times 2400 \text{ mL} = 720 \text{ mg}$$

b. Determine the amount of sodium in 1800 mL of urine with a sodium concentration of 35 mEq/L.

$$\frac{\text{Amount}}{\text{Total volume}} = \frac{35 \text{ mEq}}{1000 \text{ mL}} \times 1800 \text{ mL} = 63 \text{ mEq}$$

When results are reported as quantity per time period of collection, the calculation of amount of substance per total volume must be performed first and the result reported for the length of time instead of for total volume.

ADDITIONAL EXERCISES

23. The hemoglobin standard solution contains 200 g/L. What amounts would be used to prepare 6 mL of the following concentrations?
200 g/L?
150 g/L?
100 g/L?
50 g/L?

24. a. What fraction of urea is nitrogen? Urea is $CO(NH_2)_2$.
Atomic weights:
C = 12
O = 16
N = 14
H = 1
b. What percent of urea is nitrogen?

25. There is available concentrated HCl having a 38% assay and a specific gravity of 1.170.
a. What is the weight of HCl present in 1 mL?

_____

b. For the preparation of 100 mL of 10% wt/vol HCl, _____ mL of HCl would be diluted to a total volume of _____ mL.

26. Normal saline solution is 0.85% concentration. What is its molarity? (NaCl molecular weight is 58.5.)

27. If a protein standard reads 0.48 A, and a patient's sample reads 0.36 A, what is the patient's protein concentration? Select one of the following answers:
a. Twice the standard concentration
b. Equal to the standard concentration
c. Three fourths of the standard concentration
d. Not enough data for calculation

28. A patient in a diabetic coma has high blood glucose levels; serum from this patient is diluted 1:2 and again 1:2 before it is readable from the glucose chart as 1900 mg/L. What is the actual concentration in (a) mg/L, (b) mg/dL and (c) g/L?

29. How many mEq/L are there in a solution containing 27.7 mg/dL of potassium? (Atomic weight of K = 39.)

30. How many milliliters of 0.4 N NaOH can be made from 20 mL of 2 N solution?

31. What is the normality of a solution containing 40 mEq of NaOH per 50 mL?

32. What is the dilution of serum in a tube containing 200 µL of serum, 500 µL of saline, and 300 µL of reagent?

33. Calculate the alkaline phosphatase activity in U/L for the following:
$\in$ of standard (p-nitrophenol) = 5×10^4 L·mol^{-1}·cm^{-1}
ΔA_{sample} = 0.150
V_{sample} = 0.2 mL
V_{total} = 2.2 mL
Timing = 15 minutes

34. What is the extinction coefficient for the following:
Solution concentration = 1.2 molar
Dilution of solution = 1/121,400
Reading in a 1 cm cuvette = 0.6

35. A 0.01 M Na_2HPO_4 solution needs to be prepared (MW of Na_2HPO_4 = 141.98). Only the hydrated salt, $Na_2HPO_4 7H_2O$ (MW = 267.98) is available. How many grams are needed to prepare 250 mL?

36. If a 50 mg/mL solution of Na_2HPO_4 needs to be prepared, how many grams of the hydrated salt described in question 35 need to be weighed to make a 1 L solution?

37. A medical technologist desires to prepare 50 mL of a 10 mg/mL solution of NADH (MW = 663.44). To do this accurately, the technologist first prepares a stock solution containing approximately 50 mg/mL. The absorbance of a 1:1000 dilution of the stock solution is measured at 340 nm and from the known molar absorbance of NADH at this wavelength (6.22×10^3), the actual concentration is calculated. A suitable dilution is then made to prepare the 50 mL of the desired 10 mg/mL solution. Presume that the technologist, following these directions, has prepared a dilution of the stock solution with an absorbance of 0.562. Calculate the concentration of NADH in this stock solution as mmol/L and mg/L. What dilution should be made to prepare the 10 mg/mL of NADH solution?

38. A patient's serum calcium level is 3.5 mEq/L. The expected normal range is 90 to 110 mg/L. Is the patient's calcium level lower than, within, or higher than the expected normal range?

39. A sodium concentration is reported as 3500 mg/L. What is the concentration in mEq/L? (Atomic weight of sodium = equivalent weight = 23 g/mol or 23 mg/mmol.)

40. If the cyanmethemoglobin standard, with a concentration of 200 g/L, reads 0.426 A, and a patient's blood sample reads 0.297 A, what is the concentration of hemoglobin in the sample?

41. A 200 mg/L urea nitrogen standard reads 0.30 A and a patient's sample reads 0.40 A. The concentration of the standard compared with the patient's level is
    a. Higher
    b. Twice as much
    c. 3/4 as much
    d. 4/3 as much

42. A glucose standard of 2000 mg/L reads 0.4 A and a patient's sample reads 1.0 A. The technologist should:
    a. Report the result as 500 mg/dL
    b. Repeat test before reporting
    c. Repeat test on diluted sample
    d. Prepare fresh glucose standard

APPENDIX: ANSWERS TO PROBLEMS

1. 0.5 M
2. 0.4 M
3. 50 mg/L
4. 1:320
5. 1:128
6. 8.55 mL
7. 6
8. 0.667
9. 4
10. 12.5
11. 7.82
12. 36.05
13. $c = 53 \times 10^{-6}$ mol/L
14. $\epsilon = 60,700$ L·mol^{-1}·cm^{-1}
15. 6.0×10^3 L·mol^{-1}·cm^{-1}
16. 1900 mg/L
17. 2400 mg/L
18. 1920 mg/L
19. 1740 mg/L
20. 1375 mg/L
21. 875 mg/L
22. 2875 mg/L
23. 200 g/L = 6 mL + 0 mL of diluent
    150 g/L = 4.5 mL + 1.5 mL of diluent
    100 g/L = 3.0 mL + 3 mL of diluent
    50 g/L = 1.5 mL + 4.5 mL of diluent
24. a. 28/60 = 7/15
    b. 46.6%
25. a. 0.445 g
    b. 22.5 mL will be diluted to 100 mL
26. 0.145 mol/L
27. c
28. a. 7600 mg/L
    b. 760 mg/dL
    c. 7.6 g/L
29. 7.1 mEq/L
30. 100 mL
31. 0.8 N
32. 1:5
33. 2.2 U/L
34. 6.07×10^4
35. 0.67 g
36. 94.4 g
37. Concentration of NADH in stock solution is 90.4 mmol/L, or 60 mg/mL. Take 8.3 mL of the stock and dilute to 50 mL to prepare the 10 mg/ML of solution.
38. 70 mg/L; lower than the expected range
39. 152 mEq/L
40. 139 g/L
41. c. 3/4 as much
42. c

References

1. *Preparation and testing of reagent water in the clinical laboratory,* ed 3, NCCLS Approved Guideline C3-A3, Villanova, PA, 1997, NCCLS.
2. Gabler R, Hegde R, Hughes D: Degradation of high purity water on storage, *J Liquid Chromatog* 6:2565, 1983.
3. Winstead M: *Reagent grade water: how, when and why?,* Austin, TX, 1967, American Society of Medical Technologists.
4. Jorgenson JH, Smith RF: Rapid detection of contaminated intravenous fluids using the Limulus in vitro endotoxin assay, *Appl Microbiol* 26:521, 1973.
5. Sullivan JD, Jr, Valoes FW, Watson SW: Endotoxins: the Limulus amebocyte lysate system. In Bernheimer AW, editor: *Mechanisms in bacterial toxicology,* New York, 1976, John Wiley and Sons.
6. Bristol DW: Detection of trace organic impurities in binary solvent systems. A solvent purity test, *J Chromatog* 188:193, 1980.
7. *Clinical laboratory technical procedure manuals,* ed 3, NCCLS Approved Standard GP2-A3, Villanova, PA, 1996, NCCLS.
8. Statement from the Quadrennial Symposium on Measurable Properties (Quantities) and Units in Clinical Chemistry, Gaithersburg, MD, August 5 and 6, 1976, *Am J Clin Pathol* 71:465, 1979.
9. Kaplan LA, Pesce AJ, editors: *Clinical chemistry: theory, analysis, correlation,* ed 2, St Louis, 1989, Mosby.
10. *Determining performance of volumetric equipment,* NCCLS Proposed Standard I8-P, Villanova, PA, 1984, NCCLS.
11. Lide DR, editor: *Handbook of chemistry and physics,* ed 81, Boca Raton, FL, 2001, CRC Press.
12. Lashor TW, Macurdy LB: *Precision laboratory standards of mass and laboratory weights,* National Bureau of Standards Circular 547, Washington, DC, 1954, United States Department of Commerce.
13. McCoubrey AO: *Guide for the use of the International System of Units. The modernized metric system,* National Institute of Standards and Technology Special Publication 811, Washington, DC, 1991, United States Department of Commerce.
14. The National Committee for Clinical Laboratory Standards Position Paper (PPC-11): Quantities and Units (SI), *Clin Chem* 25:657, 1979.
15. Committee on Hospital Care, American Academy of Pediatrics: Metrication and SI units, *Pediatrics* 65:659, 1980.
16. *Laboratory instrument maintenance manual,* Skokie, IL, 1989, College of American Pathologists.
17. *Temperature calibration of water baths, instruments, and temperature sensors,* ed 2, NCCLS Approved Standard I2-A2, Villanova, PA, 1990, NCCLS.
18. *Procedures for the handling and processing of blood specimens,* ed 2, NCCLS Approved Guideline H18-A2, Villanova, PA, 1999, NCCLS.
19. *Laboratory instrument evaluation and verification manual,* Skokie, IL, 1989, College of American Pathologists.

20. *A centrifuge primer,* Palo Alto, CA, 1980, Spinco Div. Beckman Instruments, Inc. (out of print).
21. *Occupational exposures to hazardous chemicals in laboratories,* final rule, Federal Register, 29 CFR Part 1910.1450, Washington, DC, 1990, Department of Labor, Occupational Safety and Health Administration.
22. *Occupational exposure to bloodborne pathogens,* final rule, Federal Register, 29 CFR Part 1910.1030, Washington, DC, 1991 Department of Labor, Occupational Safety and Health Administration.
23. *Needlestick and other sharps injuries,* final rule, Federal Register, 29 CFR Part 1910, Washington, DC, 2001, Department of Labor, Occupational Safety and Health Administration.
24. *Sigma-Aldrich library of chemical safety data,* St Louis, Sigma Chemical Co. (available in printed or CD-ROM format).
25. Compressed Gas Association, Inc.: *Handbook of compressed gases,* ed 2, New York, 1981, Reinhold Publishing.
26. Lan G, Sansone EB: *Destruction of hazardous chemicals in the laboratory,* New York, 1990, John Wiley & Sons.
27. United States Department of Health and Human Services: Recommendations for prevention of HIV transmission in health care setting, *MMWR* 56(25):1, 1987.
28. Rutale WA, Weber DJ: Infectious waste – mismatch between science and policy: soundboard, *N Eng J Med* 325:578, 1991.
29. Tarlo SM et al: Control of airborne latex by use of powder-free latex gloves, *J Allergy Clin Immunol* 93:985, 1994.
30. Kelly KJ, Sussman G, Fink JN: Stop the sensitization, *J Allergy Clin Immunol* 98:857, 1996.
31. Campbell JM, Campbell JB: *Laboratory mathematics: medical and biological applications,* ed 5, St Louis, 1997, Mosby.

Internet Sites

www.physchem.ox.ac.uk/MSDS—Oxford University safety

www.admiralmetals.com/metric_conv.htm—See also the calculation algorithm on CD

www.mhhe.com/biosci/genbio/dolphin5e/labprep.mhtml—A number of sections on practical lab technique, including calculations

www.practicingsafescience.org—Online safety course

www.pp.okstate.edu/ehs/HAZMAT/labman.htm—Oklahoma State University laboratory safety manual

http://www.osha-slc.gov/OshStd_data/1910_1450.html—Occupational Safety and Health Administration (OSHA) Regulations (Standards – 29 CFR): Occupational exposure to hazardous chemicals in laboratories—1910.1450

www.nccls.org/—National Committee for Clinical Laboratory Standards

http://www.epa.gov/—Environmental Protection Agency

http://www.epa.state.oh.us/opp/hospital.html—Mercury pollution

www.medal.org—The Medical Algorithms Project; has a calculations program

http://www.phys.ksu.edu/area/jrm/safety/msds.html—Link for MSDS

http://omni.ac.uk/browse/mesh/detail/C0600201L086383.html—BIOME, Greenfield Medical Library, Queens Medical Centre, Nottingham; target audience is the UK learning, teaching, and research community

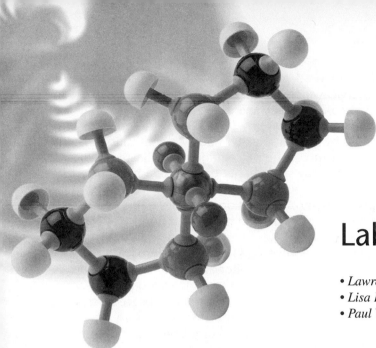

CHAPTER 2

Laboratory Management

• *Lawrence J. Crolla*
• *Lisa Reninger*
• *Paul W. Stiffler*

Chapter Outline

Regulations
CLIA '88
  OSHA
  Laboratory compliance
Hospital management structure
  Organization of a hospital
  Organization of a clinical chemistry laboratory
Good management skills and personal characteristics
Communication management
  Communication within the total organization
  Communication within the laboratory
Personnel management
  Staff
  Job or position description
  Work scheduling
  Continuing education and employee competency

  Alternative positions
Resource management
Financial management
  Budgeting
  Capital justification
  Purchasing
  Cost accounting
  Overview of reimbursement issues
Information management
  Financial performance
  Productivity
  Test utilization
  Turnaround time
Performance improvement
  Quality assurance monitors

Objectives

• Discuss the basic organizational structure of hospitals and clinical laboratories.
• Describe the core regulations governing clinical laboratories and how laboratories can comply with these regulations.
• Discuss how to apply managerial tools to the

operation of the laboratory.
• Discuss how to manage technical and financial resources.
• Outline quality monitors that can be used for laboratory improvement.

Key Terms

CAP College of American Pathologists.
CLIA '88 Clinical Laboratory Improvement Amendments of 1988.
complexity model The seven criteria used for categorizing test systems, assays, and examinations

based on assigning scores of 1, 2, or 3 within each category.
deemed status Equivalency between accreditation/state requirements and CLIA standards.

demographics   Personal data about a specific population.

empowerment   When managers create a nurturing environment in which their staff can learn, grow, improve, and function effectively.

Federal Register   Provides a uniform system for making regulations and legal notices issued by federal agencies available to the public.

full-time equivalent (FTE)   Full-time employee scheduled to work 8 hours per work day for 260 days; or 10 hours per work day for 208 days; or 2080 hours per year.

HCFA   Health Care Financing Administration.

HHS   Department of Health and Human Services.

high-complexity test   One that scores 13 or higher by the complexity model categorization system described in CLIA '88.

HIPPA   Health Insurance Portability & Accountability Act of 1996. Major aspects of this federal law are standardization of electronic patient health transactions, providing for unique health identifiers for employers, health plans, and health care providers; and establishing security and privacy standards (www.hep-c-alert.org/links/hippa.html).

hospital information system   Also known as miniframe or mainframe computers.

JCAHO   Joint Commission on Accreditation of Healthcare Organizations.

laboratory information system (LIS)   Miniframe or mainframe computers.

Medicaid   A program sponsored by federal, state, and local governments providing medical benefits to the medically indigent regardless of age.

Medicare   A program of medical care and hospital services sponsored by the federal government for persons 65 years and older.

moderate-complexity test   Test with a score of 12 or less by the complexity model categorization system.

patient mix   The percentage of Medicare, Medicaid, private pay, and charity patients in a hospital's patient population.

productivity   Production efficiency expressed as units of work divided by defined hours or defined positions.

quality assurance (QA) program   Program designed to (1) monitor and evaluate the ongoing and overall quality of the total testing process and the effectiveness of its policies and procedures; (2) identify and correct problems and ensure the accurate, reliable, and prompt reporting of test results; and (3) ensure the adequacy and competency of the staff.

quality control (QC)   Procedures for monitoring and evaluating the quality of the analytical testing process of each method to ensure the accuracy and reliability of patient test results and reports.

service level demands   Specimen collection and test turnaround time requirements for the laboratory.

waived test   Test systems or simple laboratory examinations and procedures that are cleared by the Food and Drug Administration (FDA) for home use; they employ methodologies that are so simple and accurate as to render the likelihood of erroneous results negligible and pose no reasonable risk of harm to the patient if the test is performed incorrectly. See also Chapter 17.

By performing analyses on various human specimens, the personnel of a clinical chemistry laboratory provide information to physicians that they can use to diagnose and treat human diseases. The laboratory must not only comply with legal operating regulations, but also perform tests in a cost-effective manner. Balancing these requirements is the responsibility of the laboratory management staff. The production of patient results requires a complex infrastructure comprised of testing systems (e.g., analyzers, reagents, test procedures), staff to perform the analyses, administrative staff, and systems for the integration of laboratory results with a hospital or other information system.

Much of the way a laboratory must operate is delineated in great detail by federal regulations. One of the most important of these is the Clinical Laboratory Improvement Amendments of 1988 (**CLIA '88**). The goal of these regulations is to ensure the quality of laboratory test results regardless of where the tests are performed. In addition, laboratory management must keep abreast of other federal and state regulations, including guidelines on compliance and appropriate billing, blood-borne pathogen exposure, and chemical exposure and waste disposal, as well as a growing number of employee safety regulations (see Chapter 1) and the **Health Insurance Portability & Accountability Act of 1996 (HIPPA)** (see Chapter 18). Therefore, this chapter begins by reviewing the regulatory concerns of laboratories.

REGULATIONS

A large part of managing a laboratory today involves ensuring that the laboratory is in compliance with all of the federal, state, and city regulations that now abound. A hospital laboratory must be certified by the Health Care Financing Administration (**HCFA**), by a private certifying agency, or by a state regulatory agency that has received **"deemed status."** These certifying agencies inspect laboratories to determine whether they are in compliance with federal regulations, including CLIA '88. The College of American Pathologists (**CAP**) and the Joint Commission on

Accreditation of Healthcare Organizations (**JCAHO**) are two of the private certifying agencies that have received deemed status to act on behalf of the federal government. Blood banks require inspections by different certifying agencies.

CLIA '88

The CLIA '88 regulations apply to almost every laboratory in the United States performing laboratory testing for assessment of the health of human beings. The regulations are broken into various subparts, the most important of which include the following:

Subpart H—*Participation in Proficiency Testing* is required for laboratories performing tests of moderate complexity (including the subcategory), high complexity, or any combination of these tests.

Subpart I—*Proficiency Testing Programs* provide unknown samples for tests of moderate complexity (including the subcategory), high complexity, or any combination of these tests to laboratories performing these tests on human specimens.

WHAT EVERY PROCEDURE MANUAL MUST INCLUDE

The procedure manual must include the following, when applicable to the test procedure:

1. Requirements for specimen collection and processing and criteria for specimen rejection
2. Procedures for microscopic examinations, including the detection of inadequately prepared slides
3. Step-by-step performance of the procedure, including test calculations and interpretation of results
4. Preparation of slides, solutions calibrators, controls, reagents, stains, and other materials used in testing
5. Calibration and calibration-verification procedures
6. The reportable range for patient test results as established or verified in CLIA '88 Section 493.1213
7. Control procedures
8. Remedial action to be taken when calibration or control results fail to meet the laboratory's criteria for acceptability
9. Limitations in methodologies, including interfering substances
10. Reference range (normal values)
11. Imminent life-threatening laboratory results or "panic" (critical) values
12. Pertinent literature references
13. Appropriate criteria for specimen storage and preservation to ensure specimen integrity until testing is completed
14. The laboratory's system for reporting patient results, including (when appropriate) the protocol for reporting critical values
15. Description of the course of action to be taken in the event that a test system becomes inoperable
16. Criteria for the referral of specimens, including procedures for specimen submission and handling as described in CLIA '88 Section 493.1103

Subpart J—*Patient Test Management* deals with test requisition; patient preparation; collection, identification, transportation, and processing of samples; and reporting test results. This subpart also specifies how long records must be kept and outlines the documentation necessary for any problems that may have occurred in the reporting process.

Subpart K—*Quality Control (QC)* specifies how QC is to be done and how often. It also covers procedure manuals (see box) and the documentation required to bring a new test into the laboratory.

Subpart M—*Personnel* defines the responsibilities, education, training, and experience required for each of the personnel positions at a testing site where **moderate-complexity testing** or **high-complexity testing** is performed.

Subpart P—*Quality Assurance (QA) Programs* deal with the various *monitors* that should be evaluated to ensure that the laboratory is producing quality work. If all monitors are evaluated in a consistent program, according to the guidelines presented in this section, laboratories will be in compliance with most regulations and should not have to fear unannounced inspections.

Subpart Q—*Inspection* describes requirements applicable to all CLIA '88–certified and CLIA '88–exempt laboratories. Failing an inspection or failing to permit an inspection has severe consequences.

Subpart R—*Enforcement Procedures* provide for intermediate sanctions that may be imposed on laboratories performing clinical diagnostic tests on human specimens when those laboratories are found to be noncompliant with one or more of the conditions for Medicare coverage of their services.

Subpart T—*Consultations* will be available from the federal Clinical Laboratory Advisory Committee. This committee advises and makes recommendations on technical and scientific aspects of the provisions of CLIA '88.

OSHA (see pp. 27-34, Chapter 1)

Another federal regulation that is very important to laboratories is the Occupational and Safety Health Act of 1970. This act authorizes the Occupational Safety and Health Administration (OSHA) to implement regulations that ensure the operation of a safe laboratory. OSHA covers all forms of safety, from the physical environment to working with chemicals and blood-borne pathogens. OSHA mandates that laboratories have documented plans for occupational exposure to hazardous chemicals (Chemical Hygiene Plan), blood-borne pathogens (Exposure Control Plan), and prevention of needle stick and other "sharps" injuries. In addition, the Department of Health and Human Services (**HHS**), Centers for Disease Control and Prevention (CDC) requires laboratories to have documented Tuberculosis Control Plans. Chapter 1 discusses many aspects of OSHA regulations and additional information on these regulations can be found on the OSHA web site at www.osha.gov.

Laboratory Compliance

In the August 24, 1998, *Federal Register* 63 FR 45076, the HHS Office of Inspector General (OIG) released Compliance Guidelines for Clinical Laboratories. These guidelines provide a framework for hospital laboratories to develop *compliance programs* to help ensure acceptable ethical and legal conduct by their employees and prevent fraud, abuse, and waste. Each laboratory should develop compliance programs that are applicable to its particular configuration, taking into consideration the scope of services and available resources. The OIG guidelines highlight seven program elements that laboratories should adopt to be in compliance:

1. Written standards of conduct for employees, including policies and procedures
2. Designation of a compliance officer
3. Compliance training programs for all employees
4. Maintenance of a process such as a hotline to receive complaints while protecting the anonymity of the complainant
5. System to respond to allegations of misconduct and enforce disciplinary action against violators
6. Use of audits to monitor compliance
7. Investigation and remediation of identified problems and policies regarding non-employment of sanctioned individuals

More information on laboratory compliance can be obtained by reviewing the *Federal Register*.

Several organizations have issued guidelines regarding the length of time that laboratory records must be retained (Table 2-1). Because the agencies that issue these guidelines also

TABLE 2-1   LABORATORY RECORDS RETENTION SCHEDULE

Type of Records	Length of Record Retention (Years)	Sources and Notes
General		
Test requisitions	2 years	1, 2, 3
Test printout/works sheets	2 years	1, 2
Patient laboratory results and sendouts	2 years	1, 3 From date of report
Pathology test reports	20 years	1 From date of report
Accession logs	2 years	1
Bone marrow reports	20 years	1
Controlled substances	3 years	DEA
Radioactive materials	3 years	NRC
Quality control	2 years	1, 2, 3
Test procedure	2 years	1, 2, 3 After discharge and date of initial use
Proficiency tests	2 years	1, 2 From date of performance
Proficiency test failure—corrective action	2 years	1
Instrument maintenance	Life of instrument	
Environmental exposure measurement	30 years	5 Post-employment
Training records	3 years	5
Specimens		
Blood/body fluid smears	7 days	1
Bone marrow smears	20 years	2
Microbiology—stained smears	7 days	1
Blood Bank		
Autologous donor records	10 years	4
Unit disposition records/logbooks	10 years	4
Records of employee signatures	10 years	4
Test records	5 years	1, 2
Test reports	5 years	1, 2
Quality control/maintenance	5 years	1, 2
Permanently deferred donors	Indefinitely	4
Patient transfusion record	10 years	4
HCV/HIV lookback records	10 years	4
Therapeutic phlebotomy records	10 years	4
Investigation of transfusion transmitted disease reports	10 years	4

(1) *College of American Pathologists (CAP)*
(2) *Clinical Laboratory Improvement Amendments of 1988 (CLIA '88)*
(3) *American Hospital Association (AHA)*
(4) *American Association of Blood Banks (AABB)*
(5) *Occupational Safety and Health Administration (OSHA)*
DEA, *Drug Enforcement Agency*; NRC, *Nuclear Regulatory Commission.*

accredit hospitals and laboratories, these guidelines have the force of law.

Laboratories should devote time to these compliance issues. Severe fines can be levied for violation of any of the federal CLIA '88 or OSHA regulations, as well as for any identified fraudulent billing practices. CLIA '88 certification is also required for Medicare reimbursement, providing strong motivation for compliance.

One of the most important actions the laboratory can take to ensure compliance with regulations is to obtain copies of the regulations and make them available to laboratory personnel. Forming a regulatory committee made up of representatives from each laboratory section also helps to ensure that a laboratory is in compliance with all regulations. The committee can help formulate needed policies and procedures for compliance issues and conduct in-service education and inspections to keep the laboratory aware of its responsibilities. Managers can achieve compliance with regulations only by having everyone involved.

HOSPITAL MANAGEMENT STRUCTURE
Organization of a Hospital

The size, **patient mix,** market, and affiliations of a hospital affect its organizational structure. Fig. 2-1 illustrates a common organizational structure for many hospitals. Hospital vice presidents each have several departments reporting to them. Because they cannot be experts in all areas, they must work closely with the managers of each reporting department. Each department has its own internal structure, depending on its specific functions. In general, the flow of responsibility is from least senior managers to more senior managers and then to the department head. The importance of fiscal concerns is so great that most departments have a real or assumed line of responsibility to the finance department to manage billings, research funds, and purchasing.

A discrete computer section is usually located within both the hospital and the laboratory. The hospital information system consists of miniframe or mainframe computers. The hospital computer section processes patient demographic and billing information, whereas the laboratory computer processes laboratory data. Ideally, these systems are interfaced for maximum efficiency and billing accuracy (see Chapter 18).

Organization of a Clinical Chemistry Laboratory

Pathology departments should have a generalized organizational chart that shows the reporting relationship between staff member positions in each laboratory or section. This helps everyone involved to understand the chain of command (authority). This organizational chart should show the lines of "courtesy" reporting as well as direct reporting; it should also show any outside factors that strongly affect the organizational reporting structure. A typical schema of a department of pathology is illustrated in Fig. 2-2.

Each clinical laboratory should also have a detailed organizational chart depicting the way each laboratory section is structured. A schema of a "typical" chemistry laboratory is shown in Fig. 2-3. Subdividing a clinical laboratory into departments, sections or units, and then into shifts should be done in a manner that enables the individual laboratory to use space, equipment, reagents, and personnel efficiently and flexibly to meet its expected service demands. Therefore, the laboratory is not likely to be made up of departments corresponding to the specialties and subspecialties described in the final regulations for CLIA '88 published in the *Federal Register*. All laboratory testing must be performed and supervised by qualified and properly trained employees (see the Personnel Management section on p. 53).

CLIA '88 explicitly delineates the education, certification, and experience requirements for the *laboratory director* of a laboratory performing moderately and highly complex testing (sections 493.1405, 493.1406, and 493.1443). These requirements are summarized in Figs. 2-4 and 2-5. A state-licensed MD, DO, DPM, or a board-certified PhD may also serve as the laboratory's clinical consultant, who can interpret both moderate- and high-complexity testing laboratory data for the clinical staff. If the laboratory performs only moderate-complexity testing, it must have a staff technical consultant and testing personnel. If high-complexity testing is performed,

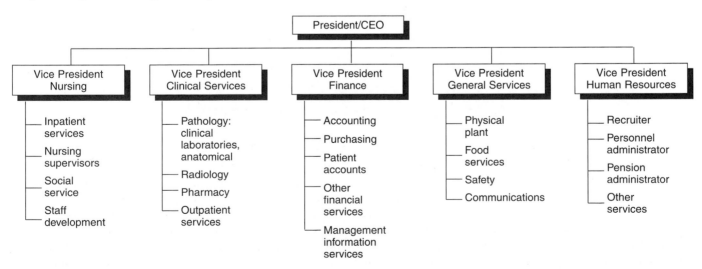

Fig. 2-1   Chart of a hospital organizational structure.

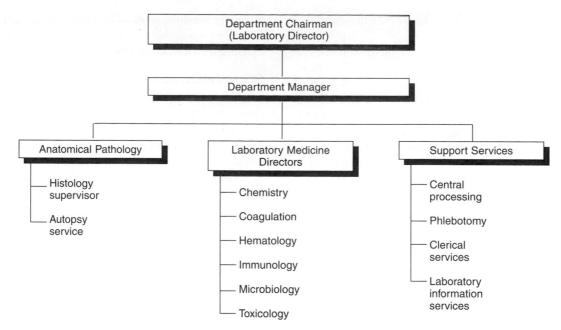

Fig. 2-2 Organizational chart for a department of pathology.

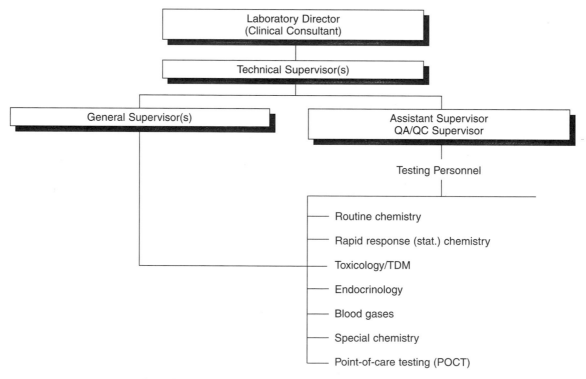

Fig. 2-3 Organizational chart for a chemistry laboratory.

GOOD MANAGEMENT SKILLS AND PERSONAL CHARACTERISTICS

the laboratory must also have a designated technical supervisor and a general supervisor. CLIA '88 defines a technical supervisor as one who acts as the principal laboratory supervisor, whereas a general supervisor acts as the immediate bench supervisor, reviewing daily work and QC. Personnel requirements under CLIA '88 are constantly being modified. The reader should consult the most current regulation for personnel requirements before making any personnel decisions.

The management skills and personal characteristics of the laboratory manager determine the day-to-day work environment of the clinical laboratory. A motivated professional team not only is able to provide the level of service expected by the medical staff, hospitalized patients, and patients from outpatient and outreach services, but also is able to establish and accomplish its strategic goals.

Personnel Qualifications
Laboratory Director
Moderate Complexity Testing
42 CFR 493.1405

A qualified laboratory director must meet the requirements stated in one of the boxes below.

MD or DO and certified by ABP or AOBP or MD or DO or DPM and one of the following: • 1 year directing or supervising nonwaived lab testing • As of 1/19/93, 20 CMEU in lab practice • Lab training in Medical Residency equivalent to 20 CMEU	PhD in chemical, physical, biological, or clinical lab sciences and one of the following: • Certified by ABMM, ABCC, ABB, or the ABMLI • 1 year directing or supervising nonwaived lab testing	Master's degree in chemical, physical, biological, or clinical lab sciences or medical technology and 1 year of lab training or experience or both and 1 year supervisory lab experience

This chart is a paraphrased and abridged version of the Code of Federal Regulations, Chapter 42, Section 493. Please consult the Code of Federal Regulations for exact wording. See *Federal Register* for job responsibilities and more detailed information.	Bachelor's degree in chemical, physical, or biological science or medical technology and 2 years of lab training or experience or both and 2 years of supervisory lab experience or be serving as a laboratory director and meet qualifications on or before 2/28/92 as laboratory director under CFR 493.1406 or be qualified on or before 2/28/92 under state law to direct a lab in state in which lab is located

MD or DO or DPM always needs to be licensed in the state in which the lab is located.

State may require other degrees and experience to be licensed.

All degrees must be from an accredited institution.

Fig. 2-4 Summary chart of CLIA '88 personnel qualifications for a laboratory director for moderate-complexity testing.

Many positive management skills and personal characteristics are listed in Box 2-1. Laboratory managers should concentrate on those skills and characteristics that fit their own personalities and the personalities of their employees.

In addition to working with their strengths, good laboratory managers must identify their weaknesses so that these, in turn, can be strengthened by formal education and training or by finding the resources (plans and people) to balance these weaknesses. Although the technical staff of laboratories receives training for the specific tasks they perform, laboratory managers rarely receive management training in advance. They should be provided with both formal and on-the-job training. The laboratory manager's personal style, which is the result of the integration of management skills and personal characteristics, strongly determine how easily and how well the laboratory achieves its goals.

The mix of management skills and personal characteristics differs for each successful laboratory manager for three basic reasons. The first is that each hospital's administration management team and laboratory staff have unique personalities. The second is that each hospital has a different strategic plan with specific goals for the laboratory to achieve in addition to maintaining its established service level. The third reason is that the amount and type of resources allocated to the laboratory for maintaining its day-to-day operations varies from institution to institution.

COMMUNICATION MANAGEMENT
Communication within the Total Organization

The laboratory manager must communicate effectively and frequently with appropriate departmental and hospital administrators, hospital departments, hospital committees, and medical staff to keep them informed of the laboratory's role in achieving the hospital's goals. This is also a good way for the laboratory manager to keep informed of any changes in the strategic plan or goals or in the priority of the goals. All interdepartmental communications should be formally documented. When a problem exists, the laboratory manager should gather the facts and assess the relative effect of the problem on patients and service level. Then the manager weighs possible solutions and develops a plan of corrective action. The problem, action plan, and outcome must be docu-

Personnel Qualifications
Laboratory Director
High Complexity Testing
CFR 493.1443

A qualified laboratory director must meet the requirements stated in one of the boxes below.

| MD or DO and certified by ABP or AOBP or MD or DO or DPM and one of the following: • 2 years directing or supervising high-complexity testing • 1 year of lab training during medical residency | PhD in chemical, physical, biological, or clinical lab sciences and one of the following: • Certified by ABMM, ABCC, ABB, or the ABMLI • 1 year directing or supervising nonwaived lab testing | Be serving as a lab director and must have previously qualified or been eligible to qualify under 42CFR 493.1415 (published 3/14/90 at 55 FR 9538) on or before 2/28/92 or On or before 2/28/92 be qualified under state law to direct a lab in this state in which the lab is located |

This chart is a paraphrased and abridged version of the Code of Federal Regulations, Chapter 42, Section 493. Please consult the Code of Federal Regulations for exact wording. See *Federal Register* for job responsibilities and more detailed information.

MD or DO or DPM always needs to be licensed in the state in which the lab is located.

State may require other degrees and experience to be licensed.

All degrees must be from an accredited institution.

Fig. 2-5 Summary chart of CLIA '88 personnel qualifications for a laboratory director for high-complexity testing.

mented. After an appropriate time, everyone involved must review and reevaluate the original problem and solution.

In addition to solving problems as they arise, the lab manager should use frequent, formal communication modes to maintain a professional, cooperative relationship with the medical staff. Modes of communication can include participation in daily medical rounds, participation in departmental and hospital grand rounds, and publication of newsletters. These devices allow the laboratory to keep the medical staff apprised of changes in the field of laboratory science and in the laboratory itself (such as new methods, new tests, or test availability) and, ideally, allow the medical staff to have input into prospective changes. When change in laboratory policy is made without appropriate medical staff review and input, that change is at risk for failure.

The laboratory manager must also be adept at using political skills to represent the interests and concerns of the laboratory staff to the entire hospital, especially when resources are limited and additional supplies, space, and staff are needed. Political skill is also required to negotiate agreements and promote understanding and cooperation in the total organization. The laboratory manager, while being an advocate for the laboratory, is above all a loyal member of the administrative staff.

Communication within the Laboratory

Today's successful laboratory manager fosters a staff of "knowledge workers," that is, empowered staff members who participate in management decisions. This manager combines **empowerment** and participative management with the added value that comes from experience and judgment gained as information is gathered and distributed. When staff combines experience and judgment with information, information becomes knowledge. Therefore, to develop and maintain empowered knowledge workers, the laboratory manager provides accurate and timely information to staff so they can use this information to participate in planning and implementation (participative management). This process is especially helpful in setting and implementing the short-term and long-term goals of the strategic plan. In addition, the staff must be valued for their experience and judgment, which is based, in part, on their performance and **productivity**, competency, entrepreneurial skills, risk taking, and creativity.

For the laboratory staff to be empowered, they must have a clear understanding of the human and financial resources necessary to meet service level expectations (based on the work load, test mix, and turnaround time goals) and customer service expectations (based on the need to satisfy both the

DESIRABLE MANAGEMENT SKILLS AND PERSONAL CHARACTERISTICS FOR LABORATORY MANAGERS

Analytical	Compassionate
Communicative	Giving feedback
Fair	Considerate
Understanding	Listening
Objective	Responsible
Accurate	Rational
Visionary	Credible
Competent	Trustworthy
Articulate	Financially astute
Informed	LIS literate
Political	Organized
Punctual	Respectful
Providing leadership	Able to delegate
Resourceful	Goal setting

LIS, *Laboratory information system.*

customer and the patient). With this information, the empowered laboratory staff can participate in helping the laboratory manager set the objectives and plan the implementation process needed to reach the short-term and long-term goals of the strategic plan as well as solve daily problems. Because the perspective of the technical staff, supervisors, and nontechnical staff is clearly different from that of a laboratory manager, each can contribute uniquely to the overall planning process. Their input also helps ensure that the process of planning the objectives and the process to reach laboratory goals is reasonable and effective. To prevent overwhelming the staff when implementing plans to achieve higher levels of technical and customer service, the manager should prioritize goals and select one goal at a time as the focus. By empowering the laboratory staff and having them participate in the management of the laboratory, the laboratory manager establishes visibility, accessibility, and credibility. The staff gains trust and respect for its manager. Also, when the manager gives and receives feedback, both positive and negative, this helps focus the laboratory staff to stay on-target to achieve goals.

The laboratory manager should not assume that the laboratory staff has unlimited capacity and no burnout threshold. With the use of positive feedback on a regular basis, dedicated staff members can occasionally achieve Herculean goals under unusual circumstances. However, a good manager recognizes that operating a laboratory this way routinely does not work. The good manager knows that a laboratory operating with the appropriate number of knowledge workers plus the necessary reagents and equipment to process the routine workload is more likely to achieve the technical and customer service goals of the laboratory's strategic plan.

The manager needs to stay in constant touch with the staff, either directly or through the supervisory staff, to monitor the progression of assigned tasks. This may take the form of informal meetings in the laboratory or formal meetings with one or more staff members. Formal meetings should always have an agenda. The laboratory manager can also communicate with the staff by memorandum, bulletin board postings, computer mailboxes, e-mail, telephone, or facsimile transmission. Minutes should always be taken when meeting with personnel, either individually or in groups. The minutes should clearly state the purpose and the outcome of the meeting, including goals that have been set and/or actions that need to be taken. Meeting minutes should be distributed to everyone who attended or usually attends a meeting. Frequent communication shortens the period of time the staff or manager is "off target" for achieving the goals and allows for a constant reassessment of the suitability and effectiveness of the plan of action.

PERSONNEL MANAGEMENT
Staff

CLIA '88 has created job categories for all clinical laboratory technical and testing positions. It has also established uniform requirements that include the minimum education and experience a person must have to direct, consult, supervise, or perform each specific test on human specimens. Under CLIA '88 the education and experience requirements for each job category depend on the complexity rating of the tests being performed in the laboratory. The test **complexity model** assigns all tests to one of four categories: waived, physician-performed microscopy, moderately complex, or highly complex. The HCFA classifies each test by method, instrument, reagent, and complexity. These test classifications change and are published periodically in the *Federal Register*. Laboratory managers must keep abreast of the changes in test complexities in order to assign staff appropriately. Until a test is classified, it is considered highly complex. No education or experience requirements are needed for personnel who perform and report the results of **waived tests.**

If the tests performed by the laboratory are classified as moderately complex (with no highly complex tests being performed), the laboratory must have a laboratory director, technical consultant, clinical consultant, and testing personnel. The requirements for education, experience, and training for each of these positions are less stringent than those for the positions required when highly complex tests are performed.

If highly complex testing is performed (regardless of whether moderately complex tests are performed too), the laboratory must have a laboratory director, technical supervisor, clinical consultant, general supervisor, and testing personnel. Laboratory managers must review additions, changes, and deletions to the personnel qualifications for each of these positions as HCFA makes them.

The laboratory manager must identify each test performed in the laboratory as waived, moderately complex, or highly complex, so that adequately trained and supervised personnel can perform the tests. The test mix, test volume, and service level, including test frequency and turnaround time, then determine the actual number and types of supervisory and testing personnel positions needed to be in compliance with CLIA '88 and to provide adequate service.

Job or Position Description

Every technical and testing staff position should have a clearly written job or position description. The job description should state, at a minimum, the education and experience or training required by CLIA '88 for the position along with any additional requirements formulated by the laboratory. It should also indicate the specific job functions the laboratory worker is expected to perform. CLIA '88 requires that technical and testing personnel be evaluated against the requirements for moderate- or high-complexity testing and found to meet the qualifications of those duties. CLIA '88 and other accrediting bodies also mandate that specific information be maintained in an employee's personnel file. Box 2-2 lists the information that should be kept in each analyst's personnel file.

Work Scheduling

The actual staff schedule for a particular laboratory may not conform to the standard three 8-hour shifts per day, with staff members working five 8-hour days per week. Alternative scheduling formats include the use of 10-hour shifts, flex time, and staggered shifts. Many laboratories use a combination of all these formats to achieve complete coverage. This provides overlap between shifts and enhances intershift communication and continuity of workflow.

Laboratory managers must take into account the strengths and weaknesses of individual technologists when planning a work schedule, including the balance of weaker and stronger technologists in each shift. By carefully reviewing workload statistics, the laboratory manager can determine whether the workload is distributed equitably (within a shift as well as between shifts) and schedule staff accordingly. Some work areas such as an intensive care laboratory, are "fixed" positions; that is, they do not depend on productivity or volume and must always be staffed.

Laboratory staffing must take into account the number of days off allowed for sick leave, personal leave, holiday leave, and vacation leave. Therefore for one "fixed" position, between 1.5 and 2.0 individuals must be hired for each shift to provide coverage 7 days a week.

Because the largest single cost for a laboratory is labor, most laboratories attempt to increase productivity (billable tests/**full-time equivalents [FTE]**) by automation or by combining work stations to increase efficiency (see Chapter 16). Further discussion of productivity is found on p. 55 (resource management).

Continuing Education and Employee Competency

Continuing education. The final regulations of CLIA '88 state that the laboratory director or technical consultant in a moderately complex testing laboratory and the laboratory director or technical supervisor in a highly complex testing laboratory must identify needs for remedial training or continuing education to improve skills. Managers must also identify the training needs for each workstation and ensure that each individual performing tests receives regular in-service training and education appropriate for the type and complexity of the laboratory services performed. Therefore the laboratory should maintain and post a current list of the continuing education programs available both in house and through professional organizations that meet these needs for laboratory personnel.

The laboratory can offer programs on general topics such as laboratory management, laboratory information systems, government regulations for laboratories, OSHA, safety, technology of the future, as well as on specific technical topics such as pathophysiology, current in-house testing, and instrumentation. Attendance at state, regional, and national meetings should be encouraged when topic and exhibits are pertinent. Attendance at all continuing education programs must be documented and a record of attendance maintained in the employee's personnel file.

Employee competency. The laboratory director has the ultimate responsibility for ensuring the competency and continuing education of all testing personnel under the final regulations of CLIA '88. The Feb. 28, 1992, *Federal Register* states that the director (493.1407 and 493.1445), technical consultant (493.1413), technical supervisor (493.1451), or general supervisor (493.1463) are

Responsible for: (8) evaluating the competency of all testing personnel and assuring that the staff maintain their competency to perform and report test results promptly, accurately, and proficiently. The procedures for evaluation of the competency of the staff must include, but are not limited to (i) Direct observations of routine patient test performance, including patient preparations, if applicable; specimen handling, processing and testing; (ii) Monitoring the recording and reporting of test results; (iii) Review

---

BOX 2-2

USEFUL INFORMATION TO KEEP IN EACH EMPLOYEE'S PERSONNEL FILE

- Performance standards
- Employee application, including working experience
- Relevant education and certification
- Level of CLIA '88 test complexity employee can perform
- Whether employee requires direct supervision
- Areas of the laboratory employee is competent to staff
- Periodic evaluations for competency
- In-service education record
- Record of training in health and safety measures
- Training courses attended
- Record of vaccinations, such as for hepatitis B, or a signed statement declining the vaccination

of intermediate test results or worksheets, quality control records, proficiency testing results, and preventive maintenance records; (iv) Direct observation of performance of instrument maintenance and function checks; (v) Assessment of test performance through testing previously analyzed specimens, internal blind testing samples or external proficiency testing samples; and (vi) Assessment of problem solving skills; and (9) Evaluating and documenting the performance of individuals responsible for moderate-complexity testing (technical consultant) and high-complexity testing (technical supervisor) at least semiannually during the first year the individual tests patient specimens. Thereafter, evaluation must be performed at least annually unless test methodology or instrumentation changes, in which case, prior to reporting patient test results, the individual's performance must be reevaluated to include the use of the new test methodology or instrumentation.

The frequency of reviews may be greater, according to local regulations. Besides evaluating employee competency under CLIA '88, the manager needs to discuss routine assessments for productivity, professionalism, and general goal achievement with each individual employee. Personnel should know why they have performed less well than, as well as, or better than expected, and each should be given positive ways to achieve better performance. The employee must be given an opportunity to comment on the review. The entire assessment process must be documented, with copies sent to the employee and the employee's file. Documentation of fair and frequent assessments is important for the development of the employee (see discussion later in this chapter), as well as to provide a framework for necessary disciplinary actions.

Alternative Positions

The process of continuously training and motivating the laboratory staff is a significant part of the manager's job. Routine technical work coupled with limited opportunity for advancement can lead to high staff turnover. The use of a system of alternative positions can help overcome these obstacles to staff retention. In this system, the credentials and experience required to advance to another position are clearly delineated.

New positions with responsibilities that are intermediate between those of a technologist and those of a supervisor may need to be created. In addition, whenever possible the laboratory manager should promote from within. This type of practice tends to produce dedicated and loyal employees who can move both horizontally and vertically within the organization.

The final regulations of CLIA '88 state that anyone with at least a high school diploma or equivalent can be trained to perform moderately complex tests (493.1423). Appropriate training and proficiency must be documented before the staff member is permitted to analyze patient specimens. This allows certain non-testing personnel such as phlebotomists and aides to be trained to function as testers. Criteria should be established for the promotion of testing personnel to supervisory positions within the laboratory. Similarly, management positions or ancillary positions such as laboratory information systems coordinator, phlebotomy trainer, outreach programs coordinator, and off-site or off-shift supervisor should be identified. The education and training requirements and job responsibilities for all positions must be recorded in writing. The benefits of promotion to the employees are greater job satisfaction, additional education, recognition for achievement by feedback, a basis for a more objective performance appraisal, and monetary compensation.

Cross-training, which allows staff members to be rotated into several departments, is another option for alternative positions. Cross-training helps relieve the monotony of specialization, where an analyst performs the same job function day after day. Cross-training can broaden and sharpen a worker's skills, allowing that staff member to work with more people and develop a better understanding of the entire laboratory operation. In some laboratories, cross-training may be a necessity, providing increased staffing flexibility so that the laboratory can meet service demands. A specialist in an area can promote continuity and competently train new staff members. However, specialization can cause staffing problems by decreasing laboratory flexibility.

RESOURCE MANAGEMENT

The laboratory manager is responsible for managing laboratory resources, which include laboratory staff, reagents, supplies, and capital equipment. All these are crucial for providing various laboratory services for patients, as defined in the strategic plan. The laboratory's service level expectations should be developed during discussions with the hospital or system's management and laboratory users, based on available laboratory resources.

The laboratory manager must accept the hospital or system's strategic plan on behalf of the laboratory and must use all laboratory resources to fulfill the laboratory's goals within the plan. The laboratory manager must be able to look at the hospital or system's strategic plan as a whole and understand how the laboratory is interconnected to the other departments/services and the effect each component has on the whole. Competent managers motivate and empower the laboratory staff to plan and implement the tasks necessary to achieve the laboratory's goals within the strategic plan. Therefore the manager must promote an atmosphere of freedom and creativity that values employee involvement. In addition to introducing new diagnostic tests to maintain service levels at the highest possible standards, the laboratory manager, when appropriate, seeks new business for the laboratory. If successful, the manager must motivate the laboratory staff to realize that these opportunities are in their best professional interest.

Practically speaking, resource management is used to carry out the day-to-day laboratory operation. To manage these responsibilities successfully, the laboratory manager must prepare one set of agenda for the short term (day-to-day) operation plan and a second set of agenda for the long-term (strategic) plan, which sets goals for the next 5 years. These plans should be updated yearly.

Resources need to be allocated based on current data, historical data, and predictions regarding the effect of current trends on the laboratory's operation. In the short term, sudden increases in the workload can be accommodated if the laboratory has equipment with the capacity to handle higher volumes or backup equipment and cross-trained staff. Use of overtime, reassigning work to another workstation, or sending low-volume testing to a reference laboratory may also help. Moving work to another shift that has the capacity to absorb the extra work is another option. If the trend is sustained and permanent increases are seen in the routine workload, appropriate measures must be taken to obtain additional staff, reagents and supplies, and equipment if necessary. If the workload suddenly decreases, workstations can be shut down or consolidated with other workstations that have the capacity to handle additional work. Laboratory staff members also can be encouraged to use earned vacation time, take personal time off, or cut back on hours.

Long-term planning is concerned with the laboratory's operation a year or more into the future. The laboratory manager must review the short-term plans and closely follow the current day-to-day operation of the laboratory, predicting the effects of current trends on laboratory operations in the future. Specifically, the effect of projected changes in test volume and test mix on staffing, reagents, supplies, and equipment must be evaluated so that future **service level demands** can be adequately met. When planning for the future, the manager should consider the following significant factors:

- The possibility of new government regulations
- The opportunity for reimbursement
- The need for cost control
- Cost accounting
- The existence of markets for laboratory services
- Customer satisfaction
- Employee satisfaction
- Existing competition

In addition, the laboratory manager must be aware of technological advances that have the potential to increase the laboratory's productivity while reducing costs and improving test result turnaround times.

The laboratory manager must communicate regularly with the laboratory staff about changes that strongly influence the day-to-day operation of the laboratory, as well as changes that may influence the laboratory in the future. All staff members should participate in the process of making provisional or final plans to accommodate these changes.

FINANCIAL MANAGEMENT
Budgeting

The laboratory manager is responsible for preparing the laboratory's operating budget and ensuring that the laboratory operates within that budget. Supervisors and section heads should participate in preparing the budget by taking responsibility for the budgets of their respective sections.

The budget is prepared by using actual figures from the laboratory's current operating expenses, revenues, utilization data, and patient **demographics**. Any factors that may have a material effect on the financial operation of the laboratory during the current and next budget years must be taken into account during budget preparation. The greater the service level demands, the greater the basic operating expenses because more personnel, reagents, and equipment are needed. Increases in basic expenses must be considered during analysis of the profitability of increasing testing volume. After the budget has been approved by the administration, the laboratory manager must verify that all provisions are accurate. The actual verification of the budget should be done by those in the laboratory most familiar with each component of the operation. The supporting detailed documents used to prepare the budget are also used for this process.

The budget should be easy to read and understand so that it can be regularly monitored and variations beyond established limits can be readily identified and investigated. The expense, revenue, and utilization line items for each laboratory unit should be individually defined so they can be closely monitored to ensure the budget is being followed. The line items for each financial and operational laboratory unit may include labor and benefits, testing supplies, non-testing supplies, reagents, equipment rental and lease contracts, service contracts, repairs and maintenance, payment for tests sent to reference laboratories, individual test utilization, inpatient/outpatient/other charges and revenue (billed and collected), and bad debt.

The records used to prepare the current budget should be retained so that variations within each line item can be readily investigated. Monthly reports should compare each unit's actual performance to that predicted in the budget. The laboratory should establish criteria for investigating variances from the budget. Explanations for each unacceptable line item variance should describe the variance as a trend, a random fluctuation, or an actual change caused by periodic ordering or payment patterns, changes in workload, personnel-related matters, or operational changes. The explanation should include any corrective actions to be taken. Notes kept during the corrective action investigation help in preparation of the next budget.

Comparisons of year-to-date actual performance with both the budget predictions and the previous year's actual figures show trends in specific line items. Sometimes these trends are only in the budget of a particular item and not in the budget of the entire laboratory. Monthly and year-to-date comparison studies allow the laboratory manager to review each unit's specific variances and take corrective action to adjust the budget for the individual unit or total laboratory. An understanding of the reasons for the variances from budget enables the laboratory manager to prepare future budgets that reflect revenue and expense items more accurately.

Two types of budget analysis can be done—static and flexible. A comparison of the current month's actual dollars spent versus the budgeted dollars is a static one. This comparison excludes variances attributable to increases or decreases in test volumes. A comparison of the current month's actual dollars spent per test with the budgeted

STATIC VERSUS FLEXIBLE BUDGET ANALYSIS			
	Actual	*Budget*	*Variance*
Test supply costs	$960	$1000	($40)
Billable tests	90	100	(10)
Supply cost/test	$10.60	$10.00	$.60

dollars per test is a flexible reporting system. This comparison allows for budget variances related to volume changes. See the example in the table above.

At first glance, the manager would see the static negative variance of $40 and might be tempted to justify it by noting the number of billable tests. However, looking at the supply cost per test would show that further investigation is required because the supply cost per test is $.60 per test unit over budget.

Capital Justification

Most laboratories require capital justification for one-time purchases costing more than a designated amount. The amount can be as low as $500 or as high as $100,000. The level of detail required to justify a purchase may vary with the cost of the purchase. If equipment is purchased for laboratory testing, the justification must clearly detail the costs of the item, installation, supplies, reagents, controls, standards, and a service contract. The laboratory manager should calculate the cost per reportable result, taking into account the frequency and size of runs, frequency of calibrations, whether the equipment will be used for urgent or routine testing (or both), whether single or duplicate samples will be tested, and the number of repeat, control, and standard samples analyzed per run. The labor cost per test must also be accurately calculated. An operational and financial comparison of the proposed method with the existing method should underscore and substantiate the capital justification. The formal financial justification is called a *proforma*. A proforma is financial analysis of a future

condition. The proforma is made up from the elements listed in Box 2-3.

The proforma uses the concept of discounted cash flow, a system that evaluates a purchase by considering the future value of money. The yearly return on investment is the value obtained by subtracting expenses from revenues. Essentially, if positive discounted cash flow remains after expenses, the investment is positive. The proforma calculation employs data on the cost of capital, which can be obtained from the institution's finance department. Please see Table 2-2 for an example of the proforma calculation using ProformIT software (World-Wide Healthcare Consulting, Ltd., Highland Park, Illinois).

When acquiring a piece of capital equipment, the laboratory manager may wish to maximize flexibility for obtaining "state of the art" technology by minimizing the time that the laboratory is obligated to use a specific instrument. Therefore the laboratory manager must carefully evaluate the costs of purchasing, leasing, renting, or reagent renting an instrument. When an instrument is acquired through a reagent rental plan, the laboratory is billed for the reagents only (the vendor includes the equipment price in the reagent pricing) at an agreed price. The laboratory contracts to purchase a minimum amount of testing materials, based on current and future needs. Table 2-3 compares reagent rental costs with outright purchase. The type of buying decisions described in Table 2-3 are based on cash flow. If lump sum capital dollars are not available, reagent rental can be used to acquire a piece of equipment. However, buying capital equipment using reagent rental programs may cost the hospital more real dollars than a lump sum purchase. The reason is that the hospital normally gets some reimbursement from Medicare and other payers for capital expenditure. If reagent rental is used, no capital reimbursement is allowed. If cash flow is an issue, a true lease can be used. In this vehicle a monthly capital cost is billed along with the reagent cost. This capital cost can usually be submitted for reimbursement.

Manufacturers sometimes offer additional incentives when more than one unit is to be obtained. As stated previously, the manager must perform a cost analysis for each test being considered and prepare a proforma financial statement for the equipment being acquired. Managers also need to take into account the cost of evaluating and setting up the method chosen. In all cases the test cost analysis and proforma financial statement must be clearly written and carefully documented with supporting data attached to the written report. A copy of the manufacturer's contract should also be included.

Purchasing

Supplies, reagents, and equipment are purchased with funds allocated in the department budget. To stay within this budget, the laboratory manager, staff, and purchasing department must work as a team, securing the lowest prices available from vendors, national contracts, and various buying groups. Price, location of distribution centers, availability of items, and a vendor's customer service should be evaluated

BOX 2-3

ELEMENTS OF A PROFORMA

- Expenses
  Capital
  Indirect
  Direct
- Other costs (to be included with expenses)
- Revenues
  Existing
  Future
- Savings

TABLE 2-2   EXAMPLE OF A FINANCIAL PROFORMA CALCULATION

5 YEARS CASH FLOW ANALYSIS
FOR CAPITAL BUDGETING

Project: Proform IT™ Se v 1.3

Project Name	Initial Capital Investment	Year 1	Year 2	Year 3	Year 4	Year 5 (a)	Total Years 1 to 5 (a)
Income Statement							
Test Revenues:							
Inpatient test revenue		$ 9,500,000	$ 9,785,000	$ 10,078,550	$ 10,380,907	$ 10,692,334	$ 50,436,790
Outpatient test revenue		$ 2,350,000	$ 2,420,500	$ 2,493,115	$ 2,567,908	$ 2,644,946	$ 12,476,469
Gross patient test revenue		$ 11,850,000	$ 12,205,500	$ 12,571,665	$ 12,948,815	$ 13,337,279	$ 62,913,259
Contractual allowances for tests		$ 5,925,000	$ 6,102,750	$ 6,285,833	$ 6,474,407	$ 6,668,640	$ 31,456,630
Net patient test revenue		$ 5,925,000	$ 6,102,750	$ 6,285,833	$ 6,474,407	$ 6,668,640	$ 31,456,630
Other test related revenue	$ –	$ –	$ –	$ –	$ –	$ –	$ –
Revenue from sale of existing equipment	$ –						$ –
Residual value of capital investment						$ –	$ –
Net revenue		$ 5,925,000	$ 6,102,750	$ 6,285,833	$ 6,474,407	$ 6,668,640	$ 31,456,630
Operating Expenses to Perform Tests:							
Wages and salaries		$ 740,000	$ 769,600	$ 800,384	$ 832,399	$ 865,695	$ 4,008,079
Employee benefits		$ 148,000	$ 153,920	$ 160,077	$ 166,480	$ 173,139	$ 801,616
Supplies, consum., reagents, expend.		$ 3,115,000	$ 3,208,450	$ 3,304,704	$ 3,403,845	$ 3,505,960	$ 16,537,958
Equipment service contract		$ –	$ –	$ –	$ –	$ –	$ –
Equipment depreciation		$ 200,000	$ 200,000	$ 200,000	$ 200,000	$ 200,000	$ 1,000,000
Construction depreciation		$ 1,600	$ 1,600	$ 1,600	$ 1,600	$ 1,600	$ 8,000
Software/Interface depreciation		$ 1,200	$ 1,200	$ 1,200	$ 1,200	$ 1,200	$ 6,000
Other test related expenses		$ 10,000	$ 10,000	$ 10,000	$ 10,000	$ 10,000	$ 50,000
Indirect expenses		$ 1,303,500	$ 1,342,605	$ 1,382,883	$ 1,424,370	$ 1,467,101	$ 6,920,459
Total operating expenses for tests		$ 5,519,300	$ 5,687,375	$ 5,860,847	$ 6,039,893	$ 6,224,695	$ 29,332,111
Net Operating Cash Flow		$ 405,700	$ 415,375	$ 424,985	$ 434,514	$ 443,945	$ 2,124,519
Depreciation Add Back		$ 202,800	$ 202,800	$ 202,800	$ 202,800	$ 202,800	$ 1,014,000
Net Cash Flow	$ (1,014,000)	$ 608,500	$ 618,175	$ 627,785	$ 637,314	$ 646,745	$ 3,138,519
Cumulative Cash Flow		$ 608,500	$ 1,226,675	$ 1,854,460	$ 2,491,774	$ 3,138,519	
Discounted Cash Flow		*$ 563,426*	*$ 529,985*	*$ 498,356*	*$ 468,445*	*$ 440,164*	*$ 2,500,376*

Financial Analysis:

Total Capital Investment	$ (1,014,000)	Discounted Payback Period 1.9 Years
		versus
Total Discounted Cash Flow	2,500,376	Depreciated Life of Equipment 5.0 Years
Net Present Value @ 8.00%	$ 1,486,376 Acceptable	
Internal Rate of Return	54% Acceptable	
Hurdle Rate	11%	
Return on Investment	68%	

before the placement of a specific or standing order. The laboratory may need to purchase a more expensive reagent or supply instead of a lower-price generic item to be certain that test results are accurate and test systems function properly. The purchasing department should aid in negotiating volume discounts and in obtaining the same lot numbers over time for longer consistency of results.

One of the biggest problems most hospitals face is cash flow—that is, collecting sufficient funds in time to pay expenses. For this reason, alternative purchasing options have become common in the laboratory setting. However, when making these transactions, management and the purchasing department must always consider the cost of borrowing money.

TABLE 2-3 COMPARISON OF OUTRIGHT PURCHASE* VERSUS REAGENT RENTAL	
Outright Purchase	*Reagent Rental*
Instrument price	Reagent cost/test[†,‡] × Test volume/year × 5 years
Loss interest on money for 5 years	Total cost for 5 years
Service contract for 4 years	
Instrument cost for 5 years	
Instrument cost for 5 years	
Reagent cost†/test × Test volume/year × 5 years	
Total cost for 5 years	

*Add individual lines to sum up costs.
†Includes volume of calibrators and controls.
‡Assumes service is included for 5 years.

Cost Accounting

Cost accounting is a method by which all costs associated with the production or acquisition of a particular item are identified. In the clinical laboratory, this is primarily applied to calculation of the cost per billable test result. The more detailed and complete the analysis, the more accurate and useful the cost determination. Box 2-4 supplies a list of costs to be included in the analysis. An example of the calculation of the direct costs for a test can be found on p. 409, Chapter 22. A complete analysis may highlight overlooked cost factors that significantly influence the true cost per reportable result. A significant advantage lies in understanding which factors have the greatest effect on test costs and which factors are affected by equipment or methodologies within the manager's laboratory. This type of analysis is also advantageous when comparing a new test method or procedure with an existing one to calculate more accurately the true cost per reportable test result. The ultimate goal of cost accounting is the determination of the actual cost for a billable test. This allows the laboratory manager to set the price of tests aggressively in a competitive marketplace. The simplest way to perform cost accounting is to use software, such as SumNet (World-Wide Healthcare Consulting, Ltd., Highland Park, Illinois), which is specifically designed for laboratory cost accounting. SumNet is available as a web application at www.CLMA.org.

Overview of Reimbursement Issues

Reimbursement in a hospital setting refers to the process by which payments are received from payers such as **Medicare** and **Medicaid**, private insurance companies, health maintenance organizations, and patients. Private patient billing is the smallest billing component in most institutions and the only ones that pays the full amount of the hospital bill. Most other payers negotiate a discount rate with the hospital or laboratory. Medicare pays a flat rate per diagnosis. This flat rate is based on a 1983 system called the Diagnosis Related Group (DRG). The flat payment is fixed for each diagnosed disease and covers all inpatient services, including laboratory tests performed during a patient's hospital stay.

BOX 2-4

DIRECT VERSUS INDIRECT COSTS

Direct Costs
Reagents
Labor
Equipment costs
Service costs
Collection supplies
Testing supplies
Quality control material
Depreciation

Indirect Costs
Building depreciation
Hospital overhead
Laboratory overhead
Accounting expenses
Regulatory expenses
Management labor
LIS expenses

LIS, *Laboratory information system.*

Medicare reimbursement is broken into two categories: Part A and Part B. Most simply stated, Part A billings provide payment for inpatient hospital services, whereas Part B billings pay for physician services and outpatient laboratory tests. If outpatient laboratory tests are performed within 72 hours of admission, hospitals are required to include them for coverage under the DRG payment rather than bill for them separately. All outpatient tests are reimbursed according to a code number. These numbers, called Common Procedure Terminology (CPT) codes, are constantly updated and modified. The laboratory must always have a current copy of CPT codes for billing.

Medicare's reimbursement plan has the effect of forcing a laboratory to operate more like a business. Reimbursements are based on a capital payment of approximately $400 per

TABLE 2-4	EXAMPLES OF LABORATORY MANAGEMENT REPORTS PROVIDED BY AN LIS	
Type of Report	*Function*	*Frequency*
Total workload	Monitors adequacy of the total number of personnel in the laboratory Monitors workload trends	Quarterly
Shift workload	Monitors adequacy of the number of staff in each shift	Quarterly
Employee workload	Monitors the workload of one analyst; compares productivity with others in shift and between shifts	Quarterly
Routine quality control	Monitors short-term accuracy and precision	Bimonthly
Turnaround time	Monitors the adequacy of service	Monthly

discharge. Fewer patients means less money available for capital expenditures. Also, if a hospital does not make a capital purchase, it still receives the same amount of money.

INFORMATION MANAGEMENT

Chapter 18, Laboratory Information Systems, reviews the use of a **laboratory information system (LIS)** to manage information and increase a laboratory's productivity. Financial and utilization reports generated by the LIS are some of the tools used to manage information. Table 2-4 lists many of the utilization reports that a laboratory manager should routinely review. A list of work production reports can be found on p. 323 in Chapter 18.

When setting up a management system to evaluate laboratory performance, the manager should ensure that the system, at a minimum, gathers data that can be used to monitor the laboratory's financial performance, productivity, utilization, and test result turnaround time.

The following section briefly summarizes several key indicators for each of the monitors. The management system should be able to evaluate these monitors for each section (such as chemistry, hematology, and microbiology) and for the laboratory as a whole.

Financial Performance

Financial reports by the LIS should provide accurate, up-to-date, detailed information about the way actual laboratory expenses compare with those in the budget. However, these financial reports do not inform the laboratory manager about how well the laboratory is performing compared with laboratories of similar size, patient acuity (a measurement that indicates how sick the patient is), location, and service level. Subscribing to a commercially available database system such as Labtrends (Health Care Development Services, Northbrook, Illinois) or LMIP (College of American Pathologists, Northfield, Illinois) allows such comparisons to be made. Specific laboratory areas can be compared and significant differences evaluated so that corrective action can be taken to improve productivity, expenses, and revenue. The average cost per performed test is an exceptionally important measure of operational performance. Because labor and supplies usually constitute about 70% to 75% of most laboratories' budgets (including employee benefits, depreciation expense, and pathologist compensation), these elements must be closely monitored. Repair, preventative mainte-

---

FINANCIAL PERFORMANCE MONITORS

Cost/on-site performed test
Compensation and benefit expense/performed test
Compensation and benefit expense/hour
Supply expense/performed test
Cost/referred test
Repair and preventive maintenance expense/performed test
Pathologist compensation as a percentage of total laboratory expense

---

nance, and referred testing usually represent 3% to 10% of most hospital laboratory budgets. Monitors for these costs are shown in the box.

Productivity

Measuring the overall productivity of the laboratory and of each laboratory section should be part of any operational performance system developed. The following indicators should be included in the review of productivity:

> Number of performed tests/testing FTE (including supervisor time) assigned to an individual work station
> Number of performed tests/total FTE
> Number of performed tests/worked hour
> Worked hours as a percentage of paid hours

Using these parameters and comparing the laboratory with a database such as Labtrends or LMIP, the laboratory manager can see how efficient the laboratory is compared with similar laboratories. This comparison can then be used to help justify additional personnel if the laboratory is operating with insufficient staff (higher than average productivity) compared with the mean of the comparative database.

Test Utilization

A medical staff's use of laboratory tests varies greatly from hospital to hospital and is not driven exclusively by patient acuity or programmatic demands. Laboratory test use at hospitals with similar inpatient acuity and programs (such as organ transplant or acquired immunodeficiency syndrome [AIDS]) has substantially different rates. Systems used to monitor operational performance should include the following key utilization indicators:

- Number of inpatient performed tests/patient day
- Number of inpatient performed tests/patient discharge

Some hospitals may perform test utilization reviews for individual areas or for individual physicians in an attempt to control overuse of laboratory resources.

Turnaround Time

Test result turnaround time (TAT) statistics can help laboratory managers better understand and evaluate operational performance. Because service demands can greatly affect staffing patterns, instrumentation choice, and labor costs, managers should measure actual TATs to determine whether the TAT expectations of the hospital's medical staff are met. The TAT monitoring system should include the 20 to 30 tests most commonly performed in the laboratory, as well as those requiring an especially short TAT (such as urgent [stat.] tests and pregnancy tests).

Several approaches are available for monitoring TAT by test name. A common methodology identifies and tracks the distribution of TATs based on the length of time elapsed from the time the test was ordered until the result was available. Evaluation of TAT should take into account its three time components: the pre-analytic, analytic, and post-analytic phases. To monitor TAT in this manner, LIS software needs to identify specimen collection time, specimen accession time (or time that the specimen is received in the laboratory), and the time the result was available to a physician.

PERFORMANCE IMPROVEMENT

Performance improvement is a method of measuring and improving a laboratory's total effectiveness and contribution to the organization. Although performance improvement can be approached in many ways, the following core elements are always present:

- Planning
- Process design
- Performance measurement
- Performance assessment
- Performance improvement

The laboratory should evaluate its core processes and develop performance measures that support the strategic plan or mission of the hospital. Performance measures may also be chosen as a result of an identified problem (risk management activities) or as a result of customer (physician) feedback. Measures may include but are not limited to QA or operational excellence monitors, customer service goals (e.g., TAT), financial performance goals (such as cost per procedure), human resource goals (retention or decreased turnover rates of workers), and compliance monitors (billing accuracy).

After choosing the measures, the manager must next decide how often to examine them. Some (such as TAT) might be evaluated monthly until the target time is repeatedly met.

The next step is to establish target goals for the measures through a system of internal or external benchmarking. With these benchmarks the laboratory can begin not only

to measure but also to assess the process in a routine, continuous manner. If the results of the monitor are stable but do not meet the target goal, the manager can put a plan of action into place to correct the deficiency.

Measurement of the monitor again determines whether the process has been improved. If not, a new plan and audit are put in place until the performance of the indicator is satisfactory.

In addition to performance improvement monitors, CLIA '88 demands that, at a minimum, the monitors listed in its Quality Assurance Monitors be evaluated. An example of a form for performance monitoring is found in Fig. 2-6. The reader can obtain copies of the *Federal Register* for a complete description of the QA process under CLIA '88.

Quality Assurance Monitors

QA is a process the laboratory uses to ensure the correct result for the right patient at the right time. The following monitors should be included in a QA program.

Patient test management. Based on the results of its evaluations, the laboratory must monitor, evaluate, and revise (if necessary) the following elements:

1. The criteria established for patient preparation and for specimen collection, labeling, preservation, and transportation
2. The information solicited and obtained on the laboratory's test requisition for its completeness, relevance, and necessity for testing patient specimens
3. The use and appropriateness of the criteria established for specimen rejection
4. The completeness, usefulness, and accuracy of the test report information necessary for the interpretation or use of test results
5. The timely reporting of test results based on testing priorities (e.g., stat., routine), as well as the accuracy and reliability of test reporting systems, appropriate storage of records, and retrieval of test results

Quality control assessment. The laboratory must have an ongoing QC mechanism to evaluate the corrective actions taken under the Remedial Actions section of CLIA '88 (493.1219). The outcome of the evaluation determines what ineffective policies and procedures must be revised. The mechanism must reevaluate and review the effectiveness of corrective actions taken for the following:

1. Problems identified during the evaluation of calibration and control data for each test method
2. Problems identified during the evaluation of patient test values for the purpose of verifying the reference range of a test method
3. Errors detected in reported results

Proficiency testing assessment. Under Subpart H of the Proficiency Testing part of CLIA '88, the corrective actions taken for any unacceptable, unsatisfactory, or unsuccessful proficiency testing result(s) must be evaluated for effectiveness.

Comparison of test results. If a laboratory performs the same test using different methodologies or instruments,

```
Name of Institution: Sunland Hospital
Name of Laboratory or Section: Chemistry


Quality Assurance Monitor Report

Test Name: Stat. pregnancy test, serum
Monitor: Turnaround time
Evaluation criteria and/or threshold:
     95% of stat. serum pregnancy tests are completed within:
     (a)   30 minutes within receipt in the laboratory.
     (b)   90 minutes from the time of collection.

Time period of monitor:    Month, Year:   July, 1995 OR
                           Quarter:    1st  2nd  3rd  4th

Status of monitor:         MET    NOT MET     (underline)

Data for monitor:
     (a)   96.3% of all requests completed within 30 minutes of receipt in laboratory.
     (b)   95.9% of all requests completed within 90 minutes of collection.




Review of action:  There was 1 outlier that was completed 2 hours after collection. Sample lost
in accessioning area, clerk was advised.


Further action or comments: Three samples outside laboratory turnaround times. Samples
entered laboratory during lunch periods. Will speak with supervisor about maintaining coverage
during this time.


Comparison with previous monitors:  Give % within limits

Previous:                              Two previous:
Date:_____ %:_____         Date:_____%:_____


Laboratory Director:    _____
Technical Supervisor: _____
```

Fig. 2-6   Forms for quality assurance monitoring.

or performs the same test at multiple testing sites, it must have a system in place to evaluate and define the relationship between test results using different methodologies, instruments, or testing sites; this evaluation should be performed twice a year. If a laboratory performs tests that are not included under Subpart I of the Proficiency Testing part of CLIA '88, the laboratory must have a system for verifying the accuracy of its test results at least twice a year.

Relationship of patient information to patient test results. For internal QA, the laboratory must have a mechanism to identify and evaluate patient test results that appear inconsistent with clinically relevant criteria. These include patient age; gender; diagnosis or pertinent clinical data, when provided; distribution of patient test results when available; and relationship with other test parameters, when available within the laboratory.

Personnel assessment. The laboratory must have an ongoing mechanism to evaluate the effectiveness of its policies and procedures for ensuring employee competence and, if applicable, consultant competence.

Communications. The laboratory must have a system in place to document problems that occur as a result of breakdowns in communication between the laboratory and the individual authorized to order or receive the results of test procedures or examinations. Corrective actions must be taken to resolve the problems and minimize communication breakdowns.

Complaint investigation. The laboratory must have a system for documenting all complaints and problems reported to the laboratory. Investigations of complaints must be made and corrective actions instituted as necessary and appropriate.

QA review with staff. The laboratory must have a mechanism for documenting and assessing problems identified during QA reviews and discussing them with the staff. The laboratory must take any corrective actions necessary to prevent recurrences.

QA records. The laboratory must maintain documentation of all QA activities, including problems identified and corrective actions taken. All QA records must be available to the HHS and maintained for 2 years.

Bibliography

General

Davidson JP: Are you entrepreneurial material? *Clin Lab Manage Rev* 4(3):192, 1990.

Fritz R: I'm your new boss . . . why are you laughing? *Clin Lab Manage Rev* 6(2):162, 1992.

Harty-Golder B: Lab portion of OSHA exposure control plan for bloodborne pathogens, *MLO* 10, June 2001.

Holland C, Lien J: Systems thinking: managing the pieces as part of the whole, *Clin Leadersh Manag Rev* 15(3):157, 2001.

Leebov W: How to help your staff strengthen customer service: a do-able approach, *Clin Leadersh Manag Rev* 15(3):192, 2001.

Snyder JR: Managing knowledge workers in clinical systems, *Clin Leadersh Manag Rev* 15(2):120, 2001.

Regulations

Federal Register 56(235): 64175-64182, Dec 6, 1991.

Federal Register 57(40): 7001-7186, Feb 28, 1992.

Federal Register 58(11): 5211-5237, Jan 19, 1993.

Federal Register 58(139): 39154-39156, July 22, 1993.

Federal Register 60(78): 20035, Apr 24, 1995.

Federal Register 60: 25944-25976, May 15, 1995.

Hospital Management Structure
Communication management

Baytos LM: Launching successful diversity initiatives, *HR Magazine* 37(3):91, 1992.

Haynes ME: How to conduct quality meetings, *Clin Lab Manage Rev* 4(1):29, 1990.

Hunt LB: Here's how you can harness the positive energy of conflict, *Clin Lab Manage Rev* 6(5):456, 1992.

Ketchum SM: Overcoming the four toughest management challenges, *Clin Lab Manage Rev* 5(4):246, 1991.

Lussier RN: Assigning tasks effectively using a model, *Clin Lab Manage Rev* 6(2):150, 1992.

Miner FC: If two heads are better than one, why do I have bruises on my forehead? *Clin Lab Manage Rev* 5(5):386, 1991.

Pfeiffer IL, Dunlap JB: Empowered employees—a good personnel investment, *Clin Lab Manage Rev* 6(2):154, 1992.

Rinke WJ: Establishing a shared vision in your organization, *Clin Lab Manage Rev* 3(2):95, 1989.

Veninga RL: Crisis management: strategies for building morale in uncertain times, *Clin Lab Manage Rev* 6(5):449, 1992.

Young S: Developing your political skills, *Clin Lab Manage Rev* 3(2):100, 1989.

Personnel management

Comer DR: Improving group productivity by reducing individual loafing, *Clin Lab Manage Rev* 6(3):232, 1992.

Dawson KM, Dawson SN: The cure for employee malaise—motivation, *Clin Lab Manage Rev* 5(4):296, 1991.

Fritz R: How to keep your best people for the '90s, *Clin Lab Manage Rev* 4(4):306, 1990.

Petrick JA, Manning GE: Work morale and assessment and development for the clinical laboratory manager, *Clin Lab Manage Rev* 6(2):141, 1992.

Surber JA, Wallhermfechtel M: A comprehensive career ladder for the clinical laboratory, *Clin Lab Manage Rev* 4(6):441, 1991.

Resource management

Hinterhuber HH, Popp W: Are you a strategist or just a manager? *Harvard Bus Rev* 70(1):105, 1992.

Reeves PN: Strategic planning for every manager, *Clin Lab Manage Rev* 4(4):272, 1990.

Financial management

Brase SJ, Matysik MK: Laboratory manager's financial handbook, *Clin Lab Manage Rev* 6(2):164, 1992.

Carpenter RB: Laboratory cost analysis: a practical approach, *Clin Lab Manage Rev* 4(3):168, 1990.

Getzen TE: Laboratory manager's financial handbook: what is value? *Clin Lab Manage Rev* 6(3):237, 1992.

Kisner HJ: Laboratory manager's financial handbook: expense management—supplies, *Clin Lab Manage Rev* 6(4):341, 1992.

Melbin JE: One for all, *MT Today*, p 8, Dec 7, 1992.

Patterson PP: Cost accounting in hospitals and clinical laboratories: part II, *Clin Lab Manage Rev* 3(1):26, 1989.

Portugal B: Factors influencing relative financial performance of hospital laboratories, *Clin Lab Manage Rev* 3(2):81, 1989.

Continuous quality improvement

Bull G, Maffetone MA, Miller SK: As we see it: implementing TQM, *Clin Lab Manage Rev* 6(3):256, 1992.

Clark GB: Quality assurance, an administrative means to a managerial end, *Clin Lab Manage Rev* 6(5): Part I, 4(1):7, 1990; Part II, 4(4):224, 1991; Part III, 5(6):463, 1991; Part IV, 6(5):426, 1992.

Westgard JO, Barry PL, Tomar RH: Implementing total quality management (TQM) in health-care laboratories, *Clin Lab Manage Rev* 5(5):353, 1991.

General Resources

Lifshitz MS, De Cresce RP: *Understanding, selecting, and acquiring clinical laboratory analyzers,* New York, 1986, Alan R. Liss.

Martin BG, editor: *The CLMA guide to managing a clinical laboratory,* Malvern, Pennsylvania, 1991, Clinical Laboratory Management Association.

Rubenstein NM: *Handbook of clinical laboratory management,* Rockville, MD, 1986, Aspen Publishers.

Sattler J, Smith A: *A practical guide to financial management of the clinical laboratory,* ed 2, Oradell, NJ, 1986, Medical Economics Books.

Snyder JR, Senhauser DA, editors: *Administration and supervision in laboratory medicine,* Philadelphia, 1989, JB Lippincott.

Internet Sites

http://www.ascp.org—ASCP

http://www.asmusa.org—ASM

http://www.cap.org—CAP

http://www.cdc.gov—CDC

http://www.hcfa.gov/medicaid/clia/cliahome.htm—CLIA '88

http://www.clma.org—CLMA

http://www.fda.gov—FDA

http://www.access.gpo.gov/nara/cfr/index.html—*Federal Register*

http://www.hcfa.gov—HCFA

http://www.jcaho.org—JCAHO

http://www.nccls.org—NCCLS

http://www.nist.gov—NIST

http://oig.hhs.gov—OIG

http://www.osha.gov—OSHA

http://www.itaa.org/isec/ehealth/hippa.htm—HIPPA

http://www.cap.org/html/lip/lmip.html—College of American Pathologists Laboratory Improvement Program; Laboratory Management Index Program (LMIP)

http://www.ascld-lab.org/aslab015.html—American Society of Crime Laboratory Directors (ASCLD), a nonprofit professional society devoted to the improvement of crime laboratory operations through sound management practices

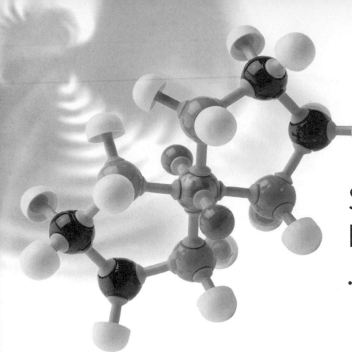

CHAPTER 3

Sources and Control of Preanalytical Variation

• *D. Robert Dufour*

Objectives

- Describe the three major categories of preanalytical variation; for each category, outline the steps that can be taken by laboratories to minimize variation.
- Outline the differences among arterial, capillary, and venous blood and the common laboratory tests that are significantly affected by these differences.
- Discuss the appropriate uses of anticoagulants and preservatives and their effects on common laboratory tests. Recognize the causes and pattern of EDTA contamination.

- Categorize the types of tests affected by hemoconcentration, the causes of hemoconcentration, and the control techniques to limit its occurrence.
- Discuss the sequence of changes occurring in specimens after specimen collection and the control techniques to limit the resulting alterations in analyte concentration.
- Define delta checks and summarize their utility in detection of preanalytical errors.

Key Terms

additive   A chemical added to a specimen that changes one or more of its physical or chemical properties.

adsorb   Attachment of a chemical substance to a solid surface.

aerosol   A fine mist produced by atomization of a liquid.

analyte   A substance that can be measured by an analytical technique.

anastomotic   Connecting two blood vessels.

anticoagulant   A substance that can suppress, delay, or prevent coagulation of blood by preventing formation of fibrin.

antiseptic   A chemical that reduces the number of bacteria.

arterial   Related to or derived from arteries, the vessels delivering blood from the heart to the tissues of the body.

artifactual   Changed state of a material resulting from artificial, rather than natural, processes or conditions.

bar code   A system of using varying-width bars as a way to provide identification information.

capillary   Related to tiny blood vessels in tissues, through which nutrients are delivered and waste products are removed by the blood.

catheter   A hollow plastic or rubber tube that connects a body cavity with the surface of the body.

chelation   The process of an organic molecule binding multiple metal ions.

chronobiology   The science of study of cyclic variation in living organisms.

circadian (pronounced ser-ca-dé-un)   Changes in concentration of analytes that occur over the course of a single day.

clot   An aggregation of blood cells held together by fibrin, a polymerized protein.

cyclic variation   Changes in concentration of analytes that occur repetitively in a predictable fashion over a given period of time.

delta check   Comparison of analyte concentration in one specimen from a person with that in the previous specimen from the same person.

EDTA   Ethylenediaminetetraacetic acid, a commonly used chemical that chelates calcium. It acts as an anticoagulant and preservative by binding calcium and other cations, thus inactivating several enzymes needed for clot formation and for breaking down protein and lipid analytes in blood.

evaporation   Transformation of water to vapor.

extracellular   Outside of cells.

glycolytic   Relating to the process of metabolism of glucose.

hemoconcentration   The process of increasing concentration of cells, proteins, and occasionally other analytes in blood through loss of water, either in vitro or in vivo.

hemolysis   Rupture of red blood cells, releasing analytes found in cells into the serum or plasma.

heparin   An anticoagulant that directly inhibits formation of fibrin.

infradian (pronounced infra-dé-un)   Changes in concentration of analytes that occur less frequently than once a day.

intraindividual   Within a single person.

intravenous   Within a vein; usually refers to intravenous fluid in which water containing medications, glucose, or electrolytes is given to a patient through a catheter inserted into a vein.

in vitro   Literally, "in glass"; occurring in an artificial situation, as in a test tube.

in vivo   Occurring in a living organism.

nonlaminar   Not in an orderly, layered fashion with smooth gradations from one layer to another. With liquids, nonlaminar flow produces shearing forces where different layers or laminae come into contact.

phlebotomy   Puncturing a vein with a needle for the purpose of obtaining a sample of blood.

plasma   The liquid part of blood in the bloodstream; obtained as a specimen by collecting blood with an anticoagulant and centrifuging the specimen.

postprandial   After a meal, also *postcibal*.

preanalytical variation   Factors that alter results of a laboratory test and that occur before the process of performing that test.

preservatives   Chemicals that prevent a change in the concentration of analytes in a sample of blood, urine, or other body fluid.

proteolysis   The process of degradation of proteins, which may occur by chemical reactions or enzymatic processes.

serum   The liquid part of blood remaining after a clot has formed.

serum separator   A mechanical device that physically separates serum from cells (plasma separators separate plasma from cells), preventing changes in concentration of serum analytes as the result of cell metabolism.

stasis   A decrease in flow of blood to or from a part of the body.

TBEP   Tris(2-butoxyethyl) phosphate, a chemical found in some types of rubber, which may leak from stoppers and bind to proteins, displacing chemicals and altering their serum (or plasma) concentrations.

tourniquet   A mechanical device (such as a wide rubber band) used on the surface of an extremity to compress veins, enlarging them by preventing the return of blood to the heart and lungs.

ultradian (pronounced ultra-dé-un)   Changes in concentration of analytes that occur over a period of time much less than 1 day.

venous   Related to veins, the vessels returning blood from tissues to the heart and lungs.

Laboratory tests, which measure an **analyte** in a specimen of blood or other body fluid, are ordered by physicians to evaluate the status of a patient. The concentration of many analytes in the blood is a good reflection of the physiological state of the patient, as discussed in later chapters. It is assumed that the analytical results obtained are representative of the actual analyte concentration in the patient and, thus, of his or her physiological state. Unfortunately, several factors may invalidate this assumption. Errors may occur because of analytical bias; traditional quality control is aimed at minimizing measurement errors. However, many nonanalytical factors can actually change the concentration of one or more analytes in a specimen so that results do not reflect the patient's physiological condition. These are collectively termed *preanalytical* sources of error. Just as control of temperature, wavelength, and time of incubation will limit analytical error, preanalytical error can also be controlled. The purpose of this chapter is to detail the common sources of preanalytical error and the methods that can be used to control them.

Laboratories are responsible for taking steps to minimize sources of error by developing standard procedures that govern patient preparation, sample collection, methods of sample transport, and preservation of samples. Agencies that accredit laboratories, including the College of American Pathologists (CAP) and the Joint Commission on Accreditation of Healthcare Organizations (JCAHO), require each laboratory to provide a detailed manual that documents the proper method for specimen collection. Ideally, such a document should include the procedures used to minimize errors at each of the points where variation may develop.

A number of guides to good laboratory practice are available to help determine and control sources of preanalytical error. Many of these can be obtained from the National Committee for Clinical Laboratory Standards (NCCLS); see box for a partial listing.

PRECOLLECTION CAUSES OF VARIATION
Cyclic Biological Variables

Cyclic variation refers to changes in concentration of analytes that occur in a predictable fashion at certain times of the day, week, or month. The study of such cyclic changes is termed **chronobiology**.[1] Rhythmic variation is typical of many biological functions; diurnal variation in drug metabolism and incidence of myocardial infarction are but two examples of the importance of this field.[2] The most reproducible cyclic variation is **circadian**, which occurs during the course of a single day. Melatonin, a peptide produced by the pineal gland in response to darkness, is known to influence the function of many parts of the hypothalamic-pituitary axis.[3] As a result, the concentration of most pituitary hormones increases at night and falls during the day. Those hormones whose concentrations are affected by pituitary stimulation show a similar diurnal variation. Diurnal changes seem to be influenced by sleeping and waking, rather than simply by the time on the clock. People who work irregular shifts or who have recently arrived in a

---

> ## STANDARDS FROM THE NATIONAL COMMITTEE FOR CLINICAL LABORATORY STANDARDS (NCCLS, WWW.NCCLS.ORG/CLINCHEM.HTM)
>
> H1-A4, Evacuated Tubes and Additives for Blood Specimen Collection
>
> H3-A4, Procedures for the Collection of Diagnostic Blood Specimens by Venipuncture
>
> H4-A4, Procedures for the Collection of Diagnostic Blood Specimens by Skin Puncture
>
> H18-A2, Procedures for the Handling and Processing of Blood Specimens
>
> H21-A3, Collection, Transport, and Processing of Blood Specimens for Coagulation Testing and General Performance of Coagulation Assays
>
> C38-A, Control of Preanalytical Variation in Trace Element Determinations
>
> H11-A3, Procedures for the Collection of Arterial Blood Specimens
>
> GP16-A2, Urinalysis and Collection, Transportation, and Preservation of Urine Specimens

---

new time zone typically have some delay in adjusting their diurnal cycle; however, eventually the concentration of pituitary hormones will be highest during sleep, gradually falling after awakening.[4] When one is interpreting hormonal tests, therefore, it is necessary to consider the time of waking of the patient for sample collection. Several other commonly measured substances, such as iron[5] and acid phosphatase,[6] also show a prominent circadian variation. Urinary excretion of most electrolytes, such as sodium, potassium, and phosphate, shows considerable circadian variation.[7] The excretion rates of these analytes determined in specimens obtained at different times of the day may differ by as much as 50%. Both serum and urine levels of bone turnover markers such as osteocalcin and collagen telopeptides show values that differ by 50% to 100% between highest and lowest values.[8-10] For such tests, it is advisable to recommend to physicians that tests be collected only at certain times of the day, and reference limits should be based on those collection times.

Most pituitary hormones are not released into the circulation in a constant fashion but are secreted in episodic bursts. This **ultradian** variation is typical of most pituitary hormones, as shown in Fig. 3-1. The concentration during such a burst of secretion may be several times the basal level. A single specimen, therefore, is unlikely to be representative of total hormone production. For such tests, it may be necessary to collect multiple specimens and either analyze them separately to determine an integrated secretory rate or pool multiple specimens and analyze the pool.

Cyclic variation over a period greater than 1 day (**infradian**) may also affect laboratory test results. In women, the menstrual cycle is associated with significant changes in the concentrations of ovarian hormones. Related to this are monthly fluctuations in the concentrations of

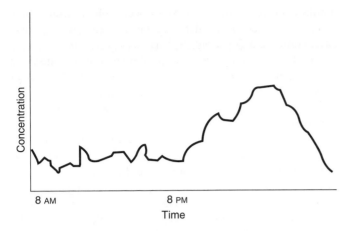

Fig. 3-1 Diurnal and ultradian pattern of hormone release. Most pituitary hormones show pronounced diurnal variation, with levels generally higher during sleep than during the day. Some, such as growth hormone (illustrated here), are released in episodic bursts during the day. A randomly obtained result is difficult to interpret because it may represent a peak, a trough, or some point between.

TABLE 3-1 INTRAINDIVIDUAL VARIATION FOR COMMON LABORATORY TESTS

Test Serum	Average (%)	Range (%)
Alanine aminotransferase	20	5 to 30
Albumin	2.5	1.5 to 4
Alkaline phosphatase	7	5 to 10
Amylase	9	5 to 12
Aspartate aminotransferase	8	5 to 12
Bilirubin, total	19	13 to 30
Calcium, total	2	1 to 3
Chloride	1.2	1.1 to 1.3
Cholesterol, total	6	5 to 9
Cholesterol, HDL	6	3 to 9
Creatinine	5	3 to 8
Ferritin	10	5 to 18
Glucose, fasting	10	5 to 13
Iron	15	10 to 25
Lactate dehydrogenase	10	8 to 13
Magnesium	4	3 to 5
Osmolality	1	1 to 2
Phosphate	8	5 to 10
Potassium	3	1 to 5
Protein, total	2	2 to 3.5
Sodium	0.6	0.5 to 1
Thyrotropin (TSH)	18	15 to 20
Thyroxine	5	4 to 7
Triglycerides	20	15 to 30
Urea (BUN)	10	5 to 17
Uric acid	7	5 to 10

From Rosen JF, Chesney RW: Circulating calcitriol concentrations in health and disease, J Pediatr *103:1, 1983; Fraser CG: Biological variation in clinical chemistry—an update: collated data, 1988,* Arch Pathol Lab Med *116:916, 1992; Fraser CG:* Arch Pathol Lab Med *112:404, 1988; Dufour DR: Reference values in endocrinology. In Becker KL, editor: Principles and practice of endocrinology, ed 3, Philadelphia, 2001, Raven-Lippincott.*

other analytes such as calcium, magnesium, cholesterol, parathyroid hormone, renin, aldosterone, and antidiuretic hormone.[11] *Circannual* variation, which has been reported for some substances, is related to seasonal changes in the diet or climatic variation. For example, serum 1,25-dihydroxy-vitamin D concentration is higher in the summer than in the winter,[12] and urinary oxalate is higher in the summer than in other seasons (oxalate is present in high concentrations in strawberries).[13] Bone alkaline phosphatase also shows significant annual variation.[14] For other analytes, such as the higher thyroid-stimulating hormone (TSH) response to thyroid-releasing hormone in summer,[15] the cause of variation is not clear.

In addition to such predictable variability, random fluctuations can cause pronounced changes in concentration from one day to the next. Although many analytes such as electrolytes, proteins, and alkaline phosphatase show less than 5% **intraindividual** variation, day-to-day variation may be over 20% for substances such as bilirubin, creatine kinase, triglycerides, and most steroid hormones. Urinary excretion of creatinine varies by approximately 10% in a given individual, but most other substances excreted in the urine show fluctuations of 25% to 50% over relatively short periods of time.[16] Table 3-1 lists the long-term biological variability for many common analytes.

Patient-Related Physical Variables

Exercise is a common, controllable cause for variation in laboratory test results. Among routine chemistry tests, potassium, phosphate, creatinine, and serum proteins are significantly altered by a brief period of exercise.[17] Chronic aerobic exercise at a fairly constant level is associated with lower plasma activities of muscle enzymes (such as CK, AST, ALT, and LDH) than is seen in sedentary individuals.[18]

Strenuous exercise, such as strength training, is associated with increases in muscle enzymes, uric acid, and bilirubin (Fig. 3-2). Short-term intensive exercise, such as marathon running, produces rapid increases in potassium, uric acid, bilirubin, and muscle enzymes, whereas glucose and phosphate concentrations fall significantly.[19] In persons training for distance events, serum gonadotropin and sex steroid concentrations are greatly decreased, whereas prolactin concentration is increased.[20]

Diet-related changes in laboratory tests are pronounced for many analytes; most are transient and easily controlled. After food ingestion, there is an increase in concentration of substances absorbed from food, such as glucose and triglycerides. The increase in glucose is not marked in normal individuals, since glucose is released slowly from starches present in food. In addition, sodium, uric acid, iron, and lactate dehydrogenase concentrations are significantly altered after a meal,[17] showing a **postprandial** rise. Hormones that are secreted in response to eating, such as gastrin and insulin, will also show a postprandial rise. The plasma concentration of substances, such as potassium and phosphate,

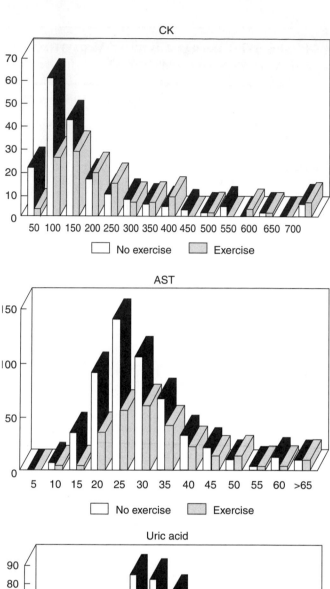

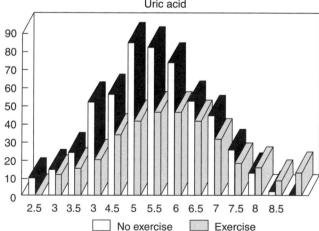

Fig. 3-2   Effect of exercise on laboratory test results. Data from 750 medical students show that exercise is associated with shifting of the distribution of results to higher values (displayed on *x axis*; *y axis* represents number of students).

which shift into cells under the influence of insulin, will fall after meals. Substances present in food may interfere chemically with test results. For example, vanillin interferes in chemical assays for vanillylmandelic acid, and dietary serotonin can increase urine concentration of 5-hydroxy-

indoleacetic acid (5-HIAA). Stool occult blood tests, which detect heme, are affected by intake of meat and, in some cases, iron and horseradish.[21] Dietary variation can also induce longer-lasting changes in laboratory tests; alteration in dietary protein intake is associated with reversible changes in urine creatinine excretion and in creatinine clearance.[22]

Stress, whether mental or physical, can reversibly alter results of many laboratory tests. It is well known that stress induces production of ACTH, cortisol, and catecholamines. Even mild stress, which can result from a needle stick, preparing for an examination (even a driver's license exam), or an elective hospital admission, may be enough to cause changes.[23,24] Although total cholesterol may increase with mild stress,[25] high-density-lipoprotein cholesterol falls by about 15%.[26] Preparation of the antecubital fossa for venipuncture will result in a pronounced increase in plasma catecholamines. More severe stress causes more profound changes. After acute myocardial infarction, cholesterol begins to fall by 24 hours and may reach a nadir of 60% of baseline value, returning to typical values for the patient after about 3 months.[27] Patients in intensive care units have suppression of production of many pituitary hormones[28,29] and aldosterone.[30] Because of these changes, unless no acceptable alternative exists, elective evaluation of endocrine function and lipid status should not be performed during a hospital admission for some other cause.

Posture is a readily controllable cause of **preanalytical variation**. In the upright position, increased hydrostatic pressure causes leakage of water and electrolytes from the intravascular fluid compartment, resulting in an increase in concentration of proteins. If **phlebotomy** is performed before a patient is seated for at least 15 minutes after a period of standing, **hemoconcentration** as great as 5% to 8% occurs.[31] This increase can produce clinically important differences in concentrations of calcium, cholesterol, and lipoproteins. In the supine position, water and electrolytes return to the vascular space, resulting in a fall in protein concentrations of a similar magnitude. The difference in the measured hemoglobin concentration between the time of admission to a hospital (when the patient may have had phlebotomy performed after a period of standing) and the next morning (when blood may have been drawn while the patient was lying in bed) could lead the physician to suspect that the patient had developed internal hemorrhage or **hemolysis**.

Procedures to Minimize Patient Variables

Important ways to control patient variables include asking the health care provider to take a complete patient history, providing the phlebotomist or patient with clear instructions, and taking steps to determine that all protocols have been followed.

Biological cyclic variables. The laboratory should determine which of the tests performed have significant cyclic or food-related changes in concentration; the two boxes on p. 69 list the most important tests affected in this manner. Optimally, the specimens for these tests should be collected shortly after the patient awakens, with the patient still in the fasting state. If there is an ultradian pattern of variation, as there is for most pituitary hormones, several specimens should be collected at intervals extending over the usual cycle to provide an accurate picture of hormone production.[32] For example, for gonadotropins, it is advisable to collect three or four specimens, waiting at least a half hour between specimen collections, and to pool the serum before analysis. A more sophisticated method is to place an indwelling **catheter** in the patient and obtain specimens hourly over a day. Each specimen is analyzed separately, and the concentration is plotted against the time of day the specimen was obtained. The area under the curve is reported as an integrated measure of hormone production.

Physical variables. If samples are being collected for analytes that will be affected by exercise, it is prudent to inquire whether the patient has engaged in strenuous exercise in the past 24 to 48 hours. Any history of strenuous exercise should be noted on the requisition form and included in the final report. Alternatively, the patient may be asked to return at a later time for specimen collection. Stress before collection is difficult to control; physicians should, however,

be apprised of those tests that are thus affected and of the magnitude of change induced by physical and mental stress. It may be advisable for the laboratory to require special consultation before the collection of samples for tests that are severely affected by patient stress, such as adrenal or pituitary function tests, catecholamine metabolites, lipid analysis, and glucose tolerance tests. The effects of posture can be minimized if one requires ambulatory patients to be seated for at least 15 minutes before blood is drawn. For assays that are subject to pronounced dietary effects, including measurements of glucose tolerance, urine hydroxyproline, 5-HIAA, and catecholamine metabolites, it is advisable to provide the patient with specific guidelines before the day scheduled for sample collection. If a test requires special patient preparation, such as measurement of renin and aldosterone, glucose tolerance tests, 24-hour urine analysis, or 72-hour fecal fat, it is good practice to schedule the test in advance and to give the patient a printed instruction sheet at that time.

BLOOD COLLECTION CAUSES OF VARIATION
Blood Collection Technique

The use of improper procedures for obtaining specimens can introduce significant error in the final results of laboratory tests; in the author's laboratory, collection-related errors are the most common cause of erroneous results. Several publications[33-35] detail appropriate procedures for performing phlebotomy to obtain blood specimens, and certification programs in phlebotomy have established standards for the training and education of phlebotomists. In teaching hospitals, phlebotomy is often performed by a variety of individuals (such as nurses, physicians' assistants, and students) who have limited or no formal training in phlebotomy techniques. Patient care assistants, who perform multiple patient care functions (including phlebotomy), are being used increasingly to reduce the need for dedicated phlebotomists. Hospitals that give this responsibility to such individuals have often noted an increased frequency of mislabeled, improperly collected, or contaminated specimens.[36-38] Continuing education by laboratory personnel, feedback on causes of rejected specimens, and oversight by the laboratory of phlebotomy performance has been shown to reduce the frequency of errors.

In most laboratories, specimens are collected using evacuated tubes and specially designed needles that allow simultaneous puncture of the vein and the tube's stopper. Collection tubes are typically made of glass, though plastic tubes are being used more frequently to reduce the risk of blood-borne pathogen exposure by laboratory and housekeeping staff. Specimens collected in plastic and glass tubes are equally suitable for most assays.[39] Many tubes are coated with silicone, which reduces adhesion of **clot**, allowing better separation of serum and cells. Stoppers are typically made of rubber. In older formulations, tris(2-butoxyethyl) phosphate (**TBEP**) was used as a plasticizer; this compound is capable of displacing many drugs from their transport proteins. The drugs then diffuse into red cells, lowering the serum

---

TESTS SUBJECT TO DIURNAL VARIATION

Acid phosphatase*
ACTH
Catecholamines
Cortisol (and other adrenal steroids)
Gastrin*
Growth hormone*
Glucose tolerance
Iron
Osteocalcin*
Parathyroid hormone*
Prolactin*
Renin/aldosterone
TSH*

Higher in the afternoon and evening; all others higher in the morning.

TESTS AFFECTED BY MEALS

Chloride*
Gastrin
Glucagon
Glucose
Growth hormone
Insulin
Ionized calcium
Phosphate*
Potassium*
Triglycerides
Urine pH

Lower after meals; all others higher.

concentration of the drug. TBEP has been removed from most currently used stoppers. Some tubes have special protective caps over the stoppers that are not in direct contact with the blood, lowering the risk of transmission of infectious agents.

In some cases, blood is drawn into a syringe and then transferred to tubes for transport to the laboratory. If this procedure is used, there is a risk of infection for the phlebotomist during the specimen transfer. Injection of blood into evacuated tubes also increases the risk of skin puncture by the needle and the risk of producing a hemolyzed specimen (p. 73); therefore this technique is *not* recommended.

In infants and in adults with poor venous access, skin puncture may be used to obtain specimens. Special microtubes that contain **anticoagulants** are filled by **capillary** action. If capillary tubes are to be transported to the laboratory, they should contain a small piece of metal, which can be moved through the specimen by means of a magnet to mix the blood immediately after collection and before centrifugation or analysis (Fig. 3-3). If testing is to be done immediately near the site of collection, as is typical for many point-of-care testing instruments, mixing devices are usually not needed. Contamination of the sample with fluid from tissue is a potential cause of concern in all capillary blood collection procedures. Tissue fluid contains virtually no protein and therefore no protein-bound analytes; contamination decreases the concentration of such analytes in the specimen. One may minimize tissue fluid contamination by using only freely flowing blood from puncture sites. It is therefore unacceptable to "milk" blood by applying pressure to the tissue near the puncture site.

Types of Blood Samples

Differences between arterial, capillary, and venous blood are an occasional cause for misleading test results. *Arterial blood* is the source of nutrients for all body tissues and is the best sample to use for evaluation of adequate delivery of necessary substances such as oxygen to the body tissues. *Venous blood* differs from arterial blood in that it has lower concentrations of substances used in metabolism, such as oxygen and glucose, and higher concentrations of waste products, such as organic acids, ammonia, and carbon dioxide. The extent of the difference in analyte concentration

between arterial and venous blood is dependent on tissue perfusion; with poor perfusion, the difference increases. Some have suggested measuring the difference in blood-gases between arterial and central venous blood as a measure of generalized tissue perfusion for monitoring patients in shock.[40] *Capillary blood* is, in general, closer in composition to arterial than to venous blood. Specimens of capillary blood that closely resemble arterial blood are obtained by warming specific sites, such as the earlobe or the foot. In states of poor tissue perfusion and in neonates, however, there is a significant difference in the Po_2 of capillary and arterial blood. Fingerstick glucose may be as much as 50% lower than venous plasma glucose in patients in shock[41]; at least some of the difference is caused by the lower Po_2 in capillary blood in shock cases, which affects whole blood glucose oxidase methods. For some substances, the difference between venous and capillary blood concentrations depends on hormonal factors that affect tissue extraction. For example, in the fasting state, capillary blood glucose concentration is similar to that of venous blood. In postprandial specimens, when insulin concentration is increased, the difference between capillary and venous blood glucose concentrations may be as high as 15%.[42]

Errors Related to Preservatives and Anticoagulants

Preservatives and anticoagulants are widely used for collecting specimens of blood, urine, and other body fluids. When blood is removed from the body and allowed to clot, it separates into a solid clot containing blood cells and fibrin and a liquid phase termed *serum*. If an anticoagulant such as **heparin** is added, the liquid phase is termed *plasma*. Serum and heparinized plasma are similar in most respects; however serum differs from plasma in that it lacks fibrinogen, lowering total protein by an average of 3 g/L. Platelets release potassium into serum during clot formation; plasma potassium is typically about 0.2 to 0.3 mmol/L lower than that of serum potassium. For unknown reasons, phosphate concentration is lower in plasma by an average of 2 mg/L.[43] In patients with some hematological disorders and increased numbers of white blood cells or platelets, these differences are exaggerated. With these few exceptions, serum and heparinized plasma are routinely used interchangeably for laboratory tests. The choice of specimen type is dependent on instrumentation, assay methods, and need for rapid results.

Heparinized plasma can be separated from cells immediately after collection, and thus plasma specimens are suitable for rapid analysis in emergency situations. Although heparin is an effective anticoagulant, in some serum specimens from patients receiving heparin, fibrin formation continues after separation, which may cause coating and plugging of sampling probes and tubing. In patients admitted for unstable angina, heparin-related fibrin formation in serum may trap the indicator antibody, causing falsely elevated CK-MB and troponin. This has led the National Academy for Clinical Biochemistry to recommend in its guidelines that heparinized plasma, rather than serum, be used for cardiac marker measurement.[44] Heparin also

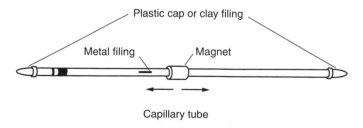

Plastic cap or clay filing

Metal filing   Magnet

Capillary tube

Fig. 3-3 Schematic of heparinized capillary tubes. Magnet is used to move metal filing back and forth through the sealed tube to mix the blood sample with heparin and, later, to remix the sample before analysis.

displaces thyroxine from its binding proteins, causing falsely elevated free thyroxine results.[45] The cation used in heparin salts (such as lithium or ammonium) will cause contamination of specimens used for these analytes. For these reasons, some laboratories prefer not to use heparinized blood.

In addition to heparin, other anticoagulants and preservatives are often used for various specimens. Table 3-2 lists some of the most commonly used substances and some typical indications for the use of these **additives**. Although these compounds are essential for certain tests, they may be totally inappropriate for other tests. **EDTA**, which is used for hematology specimens, is also used for some chemistry assays because **chelation** of divalent cations inactivates several enzymes that lead to **in vitro** changes in lipids, nucleic acids, and peptide hormones. Chelation of cations such as iron, magnesium, and calcium, however, falsely lowers results in most colorimetric assays for these analytes and reduces the activity of enzymes that require cation activators (including alkaline phosphatase and creatine kinase). Coagulation specimens contaminated with EDTA may have falsely prolonged clotting times as a result of calcium chelation. Contamination of specimens with anticoagulants, especially EDTA, is a common problem in many laboratories. In the author's laboratory, approximately two or three EDTA-contaminated specimens are received each month. The pattern of abnormalities seen with EDTA contamination is shown in the following box.

To avoid contamination, tubes without anticoagulants or preservatives should be filled first, followed by tubes containing preservatives and anticoagulants. Because of the potential for EDTA interference in many assays, tubes containing EDTA should be drawn last. If liquid anticoagulants are used, it is important to ensure that the proportion of blood and anticoagulant used is constant. In specimens with

---

EFFECTS OF EDTA CONTAMINATION

Increased potassium
Reduced calcium, magnesium (colorimetric assays)
Reduced alkaline phosphatase, creatine kinase

---

inadequate blood volume ("short draw"), there may be significant dilution of blood by the anticoagulant solution. Since most anticoagulants do not enter into cells, alterations in hematocrit will affect the ratio of anticoagulant to plasma. For example, patients with a high hematocrit will have a relative excess of the anticoagulant and a resulting dilution of the plasma, whereas in anemic individuals there may be insufficient anticoagulant.

Errors Related to Serum Separator Tubes

Serum and plasma separator tubes are used by many laboratories to simplify the process of separating serum (or plasma) from cellular elements. If separation does not occur, metabolism continues in the cellular phase, producing a variety of changes that are discussed later in this chapter. Serum and plasma separator tubes contain a relatively inert, impenetrable gel that has a density intermediate between cellular elements and normal plasma or serum. During centrifugation, the gel rises from the bottom of the tube and forms a mechanical barrier that prevents metabolic changes from affecting plasma concentrations (Fig. 3-4). It is critical that centrifugation of tubes containing gels be performed using "swinging bucket" rotors (see p. 24). Use of fixed-angle centrifuge rotors often leads to incomplete separation of red cells from serum or plasma and allows metabolic changes to affect the sample. Tubes containing such gels can

---

TABLE 3-2   COMMONLY USED ANTICOAGULANTS AND PRESERVATIVES AND INDICATIONS FOR THEIR USE

Samples	Type of Anticoagulant or Additive	Chemical Basis of Anticoagulant or Additive	Application
Whole blood	EDTA*	Binds calcium	Hematology
	Na heparin	Lead-free	Lead
Plasma	Na citrate	Binds calcium	Coagulation
	Heparin ± separator gel[†]	Inhibits thrombin	Chemistry
	Oxalates	Binds calcium	Coagulation
Serum	None	None	Chemistry
	None	Contaminant-free	Trace elements
	Serum separator	Gel barrier	Chemistry
	Thrombin	Increased rate of clotting	Stat. chemistries
Antiglycolytic agents			
Serum	Iodoacetate	Inhibits glyceraldehyde-3-phosphate dehydrogenase	Glucose, lactic acid
Partial plasma	Fluoride/oxalate	Inhibits enolase	Glucose

Comes as Na^+ or K^+ salt forms.
[†]*Comes as Na^+, Li^+, or NH^{4+} salt forms.*

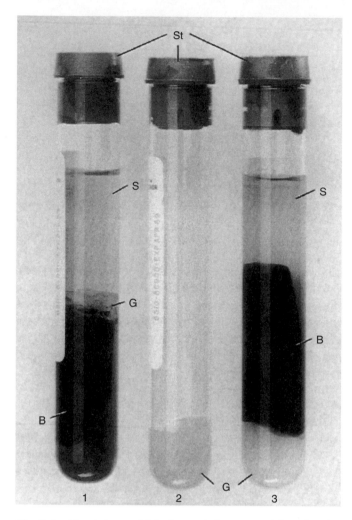

Fig. 3-4 Vacutainer phlebotomy tubes containing barrier gel (red/gray tops). *1*, Tube filled with blood and centrifuged; *2*, unfilled tube; *3*, tube filled with blood and not centrifuged. Notice positions of gel before (*3*) and after (*1*) centrifugation. *B*, Clotted blood; *St*, red/gray stoppers; *G*, barrier gel; *S*, serum.

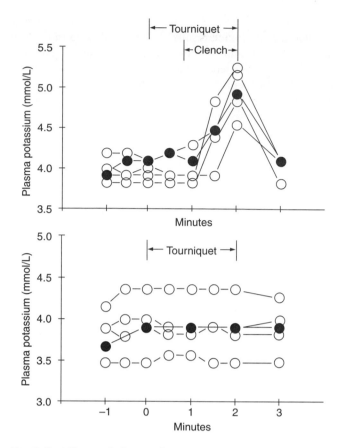

Fig. 3-5 Effects of the application of a tourniquet plus fist clenching (*upper panel*) and tourniquet alone (*lower panel*) on plasma potassium concentrations. *Solid circles* represent the patient, and *open circles* denote the control subjects. The application of a tourniquet alone had no effect on plasma potassium levels, whereas clenching the fist as well resulted in a strong increase in these levels in both the patient and the control subjects. (*From Don BR et al: Pseudohyperkalemia caused by fist clenching during phlebotomy,* N Engl J Med *322:1291, 1990. Copyright 1990 Massachusetts Medical Society. All rights reserved.*)

be centrifuged and stored without removal of the stopper, reducing the risk of producing infectious **aerosols** and preventing evaporation. Some therapeutic agents **adsorb** onto the gel, falsely lowering the concentrations of phenytoin, tricyclic antidepressants and certain antiarrhythmic drugs, such as flecainide. With these exceptions, most substances in plasma are unaffected by the use of separator gels.

Errors Related to Faulty Collection Techniques

Tourniquets. **Tourniquet** use is an important, controllable cause of variation in laboratory test results. Tourniquets are widely used in phlebotomy to block venous return, causing dilatation of the veins and making identification of an appropriate site for venipuncture easier. Tourniquets are often left on during the process of venipuncture, under the assumption that continued venous dilation will allow faster specimen collection and prevent "collapse" of the vein. Although tourniquets do make the process of phlebotomy easier, the **stasis** they induce causes predictable changes

in laboratory test results. Within 1 minute after applying a tourniquet, the increased pressure causes loss of water and electrolytes from plasma to the **extracellular** fluid space, producing a rise in the concentration of proteins, cells, and substances bound to cells and proteins. After 3 minutes, there is generally a 5% to 8% increase in concentration of proteins. If a tourniquet is left on for 15 minutes, the increase in concentration may reach 15%. The magnitude of this effect may differ from the first tube to the last tube drawn, with later specimens showing greater hemoconcentration. An additional concern with tourniquet use is relative stasis of blood flow. Concentrations of metabolic byproducts such as lactate and hydrogen ion increase in tissue, and restoration of blood flow after removal of a tourniquet causes a rise in the venous lactate concentration. When blood is collected during use of a tourniquet, the patient is often advised to alternately clench and relax the fist to increase the speed of collection. Not only is there little evidence of the efficacy of this procedure, but it may also be the cause of **artifactual** hyperkalemia[46] (Fig. 3-5).

Hemolysis. Hemolysis occurs whenever there is trauma to the relatively fragile red blood cells, either during collection or, less commonly, after phlebotomy is completed. Failure to allow drying of skin disinfectants, such as alcohol, before phlebotomy, is an uncommon cause of hemolysis. More frequently, hemolysis is caused by turbulent, **non-laminar** flow during the process of collection. Within the range of calibers commonly used, hemolysis is not caused by using a needle that is too small or too large. Nonlaminar flow is a common occurrence when blood moves too slowly or too rapidly through a needle. If blood is drawn with a syringe, drawing the plunger back forcefully or injecting blood into evacuated tubes by using pressure on the plunger frequently produces hemolysis. Similarly, a slow flow rate into an evacuated tube from a collapsed vein often produces a hemolyzed specimen. Turbulence in a tube containing blood can also cause hemolysis after collection is completed; faulty mechanical transporters and centrifuges are rare causes of hemolysis, as discussed later in the chapter.

Hemolysis alters laboratory test results in two ways. Most important, the contents of the red blood cells are released, increasing the concentration of intracellular substances such as lactate dehydrogenase (LD), potassium, and magnesium while lowering the concentration of extracellular solutes such as sodium. Since the activity of LD is approximately 150 times higher and potassium concentration is 30 times higher within red blood cells, hemolysis falsely elevates the serum or plasma levels of these analytes. Because hemoglobin absorbs light over much of the visible and near-ultraviolet spectrum, hemolysis can interfere with results of many spectrophotometric assays. The box below gives the tests most commonly affected by hemolysis and the nature of the interference in each assay.

Intravenous fluid contamination. Intravenous fluid contamination can be an important cause of variation in test results. Many inpatients are given intravenous fluids, which typically have higher concentrations of glucose, drugs, and some electrolytes than those found in blood. Intravenous fluid contamination occurs when blood is drawn from a vein that is connected to the vein containing the catheter. Although it may appear that a vein in the forearm is sufficiently distant from the catheter, there are extensive **anastomotic** connections. Any blood drawn from a vein on the same side of a tourniquet as a catheter runs the risk of fluid contamination. In many cases, blood is drawn through a connector or port in a catheter. It has been shown that, for most analytes, removing and discarding a volume of blood equal to the volume of the catheter is adequate for preventing contamination. In the case of drugs administered through a catheter (including heparin and potassium), it may take a volume of more than five times that of the catheter to prevent incorrect results. In patients receiving intravenous fluids on a long-term basis, a multilumen catheter is commonly used to provide a port for collection of blood. Even if blood is drawn through this separate port, contamination can still occur if intravenous fluid is being administered simultaneously through a different lumen.

The most common pattern of intravenous fluid interference is a sharp increase in the blood concentration of the substances contained in the fluid. Potassium concentration of intravenous fluid can be as much as 10-fold higher than that of blood, and the glucose concentration of intravenous fluid is 50,000 mg/L. Drug concentrations are typically over 100-fold higher than those of blood when fluid is administered as a slow infusion. Less frequently, there may be enough fluid present to actually dilute the concentration of normal blood constituents, including solutes such as urea and creatinine; in most cases of fluid contamination, these are only minimally altered.

Errors Related to Patient and Sample Identification

Because there is no way to prove that an unlabeled specimen came from a given patient, proper specimen identification is essential. Although labeling may seem the simplest part of specimen collection, in most laboratories it is the single most common cause of erroneous laboratory results. In our hospital, approximately 1% of the specimens that are not drawn by the laboratory are received with inadequate identification. Approximately 0.05% are received with incorrect patient identification. Although errors can be made when one is labeling the specimens from patients with similar names, the most common cause of inaccurate specimen identification is the phlebotomist's failure to label the specimen before leaving the patient's bedside. In our laboratory, over 99% of mislabeled specimens occur in this setting.

Chain of Custody

In certain situations, as in forensic testing, positive specimen identification is required at every step in the process of collection, transport, and analysis. For such specimens, an appropriate chain-of-custody form (Fig. 3-6) should be used. According to guidelines published by the National Institute of Drug Abuse,[47] positive identification begins with placing a tamperproof seal on the specimen container before it leaves the donor's sight; the label is typically initialed by the donor and sometimes by the witness. After the donor certifies on the chain-of-custody form that the specimen was obtained from him or her, each person who takes possession of the specimen signs the form and notes the date and time the

---

EFFECTS OF HEMOLYSIS ON CHEMISTRY TESTS

Increase caused by release from red blood cells
    Potassium, magnesium, lactate dehydrogenase, aspartate
      aminotransferase, total protein, iron, phosphate,
      ammonium
Increase caused by interference in assay
    Cholesterol, triglycerides, creatine kinase, CK-MB
      (immunoinhibition)
Decrease caused by interference in assay
    Bilirubin (direct spectrophotometry), carotene, insulin,
      albumin

TOXICOLOGY LABORATORY

Chain of Evidence Form

SUBJECT NAME _____   SUBJECT SOCIAL SEC. # _____

DATE/TIME OF COLLECTION _____   COLLECTED BY _____

NUMBER OF SPECIMENS _____   TYPE OF SPECIMEN: _____ BLOOD _____ SERUM _____ URINE

WITNESS _____

Sent by Name/Date/Time	Received by Name/Date/Time	Condition of Seals
1.		
2.		
3.		
4.		
5.		

Specimen Opened for Testing Name/Date/Time	Witnessed by Name/Date/Time	Condition of Seals
A. Outside Package 6.		
B. Specimen 7.		

LABORATORY ACCESSION NUMBER:

This form must remain with the specimen until line #7 is completed. At that time the form should be turned over to the laboratory supervisor or the designate for filling.

Fig. 3-6   Example of a chain-of-custody form. *(From Pesce AJ, Kaplan LA:* Methods in clinical chemistry, *St Louis, 1987, Mosby.)*

specimen was transferred to the next person in the testing process. Commonly, each person certifies that the specimen was kept in a secure condition during the time it was in that person's custody. This ensures that the result will be legally admissible in court, since it can be traced directly to the person from whom it was obtained.

Procedures to Minimize Phlebotomy-Related Variation

Generally, procedures to minimize collection-related variation are directly under the control of the laboratory. Therefore the laboratory should work closely with the phlebotomy team, nursing administration, and physicians to produce clear written guidelines to help minimize all errors. Phlebotomy guidelines for *each* test that the laboratory performs should be included in the laboratory manual. Guidelines should specify the type of specimen to collect, the volume of specimen needed, and for blood, whether arterial, capillary,

or venous blood is required. The frequency of phlebotomy errors should be monitored, as suggested by CLIA '88 regulations (see Chapter 2).

Patient identification. The initial step in preventing collection errors is the accurate identification of the patient before specimen collection. When working with an outpatient, ask for a name, including correct spelling of the last name, and any identification number needed (such as patient registration or insurance number). A hospital inpatient should be asked for a name, and identification should be confirmed by comparison with that written on the hospital wrist band. The patient's hospital identification number should be checked against the number on the request slip to ensure that both are the same. If the patient has more than one identification band, all bands should be checked to ensure that they contain the same information; there is a relatively high frequency of errors in patients with more than one band.

With children, or adults with neurological or mental illnesses, a more positive form of identification, such as a hospital card or picture identification, may be necessary. Handwritten specimen labels should be clearly and legibly written before the phlebotomist leaves the patient's bedside; the label should include the name and identification number of the patient and the date and time of collection.

To assist in making proper identification, laboratory computer systems usually provide preprinted labels along with collection lists (see Chapter 18). Many hospitals use a **bar code** system on these labels to increase the accuracy of positive patient identification.[48] The complexity of bar-coded labels varies. Some simply have the patient's name and hospital number, whereas others contain a list of all tests to be performed on the specimen, the time the specimen was obtained, and the name of the person performing the phlebotomy. Portable bar code readers may be taken to the patient's bedside to compare the specimen label bar code with the patient's wrist band bar code to verify specimen identification. Bar codes also reduce clerical error, identifying samples to be introduced onto instruments for analysis. They can also be used to automate test requests on random-access instruments; in addition, bar codes facilitate sampling from the collection tube on many currently used instruments, further reducing the likelihood of specimen identification errors (see Chapter 18). In one study using bar codes, not a single specimen identification error occurred in the analysis of over 300,000 specimens. Because of the many types of bar codes available, laboratories should carefully review manufacturer's specifications before starting to use a bar code label system. Chapters 16 and 18 discuss the use of bar codes in greater detail.

Preservatives and anticoagulants. Any anticoagulants or preservatives that are needed should be specified, and allowable alternatives should also be itemized. Since many laboratories prefer to use plasma or serum from separator tubes for the majority of chemistry analyses, those tests for which these *cannot* be used should be clearly listed; a short list is provided in the box. Use of a specific order of specimen collection will prevent specimen contamination; tubes without anticoagulants or additives are always collected first, followed in order by tubes with separator gels, heparin tubes, other anticoagulants, and finally EDTA.

Sample collection. Guidelines for phlebotomy procedures on patients with indwelling catheters should be included in the phlebotomy manual. If the patient has an intravenous line, blood should not be drawn from the same side of a tourniquet as the intravenous line and preferably not from the same arm. Instructions on the amount of blood to be withdrawn before sampling from an intravenous or intra-arterial line must be provided. Since removal of a volume of blood equal to the volume of the catheter is adequate for most analytes, the volume of the most commonly used catheters should be provided in the manual. Those tests that are more severely affected by fluid contamination, such as therapeutic drugs, should carry the caution *not* to draw specimens through an indwelling catheter.

TESTS FOR WHICH SEPARATOR GELS ARE INAPPROPRIATE

Analyte adsorbs to gel
  Flecainide, tricyclic antidepressants, haloperidol
Whole blood needed
  Red blood cell enzymes, hemoglobin A_{1c}, lead, cyclosporin A
Possible contaminants in gel
  Trace metals
Preservatives needed
  Most peptide hormones, renin, catecholamines

Although many veins can be used for venipuncture, the antecubital fossa in the arm is the most widely used site. Because tourniquets are used in most instances of venipuncture, specific instructions on appropriate tourniquet use are needed. The phlebotomist can identify the phlebotomy site and clean the skin before applying the tourniquet; alternatively, the tourniquet should be released after a suitable vein is identified. The tourniquet should be kept on for as short a period as possible, preferably less than 1 minute, before phlebotomy is actually performed. Any **antiseptic** used should be allowed to dry before specimen collection to minimize the likelihood of hemolysis. Specimens should be collected only if blood is free-flowing; otherwise, venous blood samples may hemolyze, and capillary blood specimens will be diluted with tissue fluid. Because chemistry tests are usually most affected by hemoconcentration, the specimens for these tests should be the first drawn. The patient should *not* be advised to clench and loosen his or her fist during collection, since this action will stimulate the release of muscle metabolites into the vein.

POSTCOLLECTION CAUSES OF VARIATION

Postcollection causes of variation are more easily controlled by the laboratory than phlebotomy-related variations, since it is possible to develop criteria for acceptable conditions for storage and handling of specimens after collection, at a time when the specimens are usually in the laboratory's possession. Among the specimen-handling variables that may affect test results are transportation, separation of serum from cellular elements, and storage conditions.

Sample Transportation

Errors related to sample transportation. Specimens are usually transported manually by phlebotomists or couriers. A reasonable delay in transportation is usually well tolerated for most analytes, since metabolic changes occur relatively slowly at room temperature. In general, delays of up to an hour will not change the concentration of most analytes. Glucose, often considered one of the more labile substances in blood, falls by approximately 2% to 3% per hour at normal room temperature in tubes without **glycolytic** inhibitors, such as fluoride.[49] An arterial blood-gas sample is probably the specimen most subject to handling error. Table 3-3 lists the common causes of changes in arterial blood-gas

TABLE 3-3	EFFECT OF SPECIMEN-HANDLING VARIABLES ON BLOOD GAS MEASUREMENTS		
Factor Not Controlled	**pH**	**PO₂**	**PCO₂**
Not submersing specimen in ice slurry	Decrease up to 0.01 in 10 minutes	Decrease up to 5% in 10 minutes	Minimal change
Air bubbles not removed	Increased if sample agitated	Increase slightly, decrease in patients with high initial PO_2	Decrease
Excess liquid heparin added	Decrease with some forms; usually no effect	Increase slightly, decrease in patients with high initial PO_2	Decrease

results and the direction and relative magnitude of the changes induced. Products of metabolism (such as lactate, ammonia, and hydrogen ion) accumulate in the sample after collection unless enzymatic reactions are slowed. Other metabolic processes, such as **proteolysis**, also occur at room temperature. Peptides, which are susceptible to degradation by plasma proteases, will generally decrease in concentration; however renin precursor (prorenin) will be converted to enzymatically active renin if plasma is allowed to cool slowly.[50]

Procedures to minimize sample-transportation errors

SAMPLE PRESERVATION DURING TRANSPORTATION. To minimize postcollection variation, specimens should be delivered and stored promptly after collection. Analytes that are subject to in vitro change in concentration at room temperature should be promptly transported to the laboratory in an ice slurry. Handling instructions should be clear; in many cases, specimens are improperly placed on top of ice, or they are transported protruding from a container of ice or immersed in ice without water. Since a solid conducts heat less rapidly than a liquid, specimens handled in this way will not cool as rapidly and may show artifactual changes. Although cooling samples during transport minimizes many artifactual changes in analyte concentration, cooling increases the release of potassium from cells.

For a substance whose concentration changes with in vitro metabolism, a specific time of delay that can be tolerated should be specified. The two most common techniques for preventing metabolism of glucose are the use of glycolytic inhibitors, such as fluoride and iodoacetate, and chilling specimens in ice water. If plain or **serum separator** tubes are used, at least a half hour should pass before centrifugation to allow clot formation to become complete. Tubes with clot accelerators or anticoagulants can be centrifuged immediately. After centrifugation, specimen collection tubes without barrier gels should have the plasma or serum separated from the cells as quickly as possible to prevent artifacts.

USE OF MECHANICAL TRANSPORTERS. Transportation of specimens to the laboratory often significantly delays processing. A CAP Q-Probe on emergency department laboratory tests showed that specimen transport by couriers adds a median of 60% to 100% to the total turnaround time for stat specimens.[51] Mechanical transport systems, typically using pneumatic tubes, are used by some laboratories to expedite specimen delivery. Carefully designed systems can greatly reduce the time needed for specimens to reach the laboratory. In contrast to the average delay of approximately 30 minutes for manual transport, the average delay with pneumatic tube systems in one hospital system was 2 minutes. Thus pneumatic tube systems have the potential to reduce the need for satellite laboratories and near-patient testing devices. However, the pneumatic tube system may produce trauma to the red blood cells. The risk of hemolysis is increased by use of specimen tubes that are less than fully filled, sudden deceleration, and sharp turns in the tube system. Lack of adequate packing can increase the number of tubes that are broken during transit. Pneumatic tube systems should be periodically monitored to ensure that tube velocity does not increase beyond acceptable limits. Monitoring of the prevalence of hemolyzed samples can be used for this purpose.

TRANSPORTATION TO REMOTE SITES. When specimens are transported to remote testing sites, such as reference laboratories, changes can occur in the concentration of many substances. In general, unless the assay specifically calls for whole blood testing, it is best to separate plasma or serum physically from cells before preparing specimens for shipping. Serum or plasma separator tubes can also be used for this purpose; the collection site performs centrifugation, then sends the tube to the laboratory. When separator gels are used, the collection site must use centrifuges that have swinging buckets to avoid the problem of incomplete separation by the gel. To avoid breakage during transit, it is preferable to use tightly capped plastic tubes. Precautions must be taken to prevent the thawing of frozen specimens. Although most referral laboratories suggest the use of insulated containers packed with dry ice, overnight delivery services have become reliable enough that most specimens can be adequately preserved by the use of reusable "ice packs." Specimens must be packaged securely to prevent leakage and labeled as potentially infectious.

Sample Processing

Errors arising from incorrect sample processing. Centrifugation is the method commonly used for the initial separation of serum and cells. The principles of centrifugation are covered in Chapter 1. In general, centrifugation of samples for 5 to 10 minutes at 1000 to 2000 G is adequate for complete separation of serum and red blood cells, including specimens containing serum or plasma separator gels. Serum specimens should not be centrifuged until clot formation is completed (at least 20 to 30 minutes after the specimen is collected). When separator gels are used, centrifuges with horizontal rotors produce better separation, as discussed earlier. In our laboratory, we store samples with separator gels up to 72 hours with no significant changes in the concentrations of most analytes as long as there were no visible points of contact between the serum and cells.

Caution should be taken to ensure that clotting has, in fact, been completed because there can be physiological reasons for extended clotting times. For example, specimens from patients undergoing dialysis or patients in cardiac care units may continue to clot for hours after collection because of heparin received by the patient. In such cases, recentrifugation, serum filters, and wooden sticks can be used to remove additional fibrin. With tubes that do not contain separator gels, an additional step is necessary to complete the separation. Before centrifugation, substances such as glass beads, plugs, or other mechanical devices may be added to tubes to perform the same function as the gel. After centrifugation, hollow cylinders containing filters or one-way valves at one end can be inserted into the collection tube to provide a physical barrier, and pipets can be used to remove the serum manually. The serum yield when these alternative separation methods are used is often less than that achieved with gels. The use of such alternative procedures instead of serum separator gels increases the risk of spillage and concomitant infection and thus often increases laboratory costs.

As discussed previously, serum must be separated from cells because hematological cells will continue to perform their metabolic functions and alter specimen composition. Although this occurs most rapidly and most dramatically for blood-gas measurements, more subtle changes occur with delayed separation of other specimens. At room temperature, glycolysis continues slowly, with glucose falling by an average of 3% per hour. After approximately 24 hours, the lack of glucose causes leakage of potassium and smaller proteins, such as enzymes, from the cells; and breakdown of organic phosphate compounds causes a rise in inorganic phosphate. After several days, visible hemolysis becomes apparent. If specimens are refrigerated without separation, glycolysis is inhibited, but leakage of potassium and enzymes occurs.

In persons with high white blood cell or platelet counts, dramatic changes can occur in vitro following phlebotomy. Platelets release potassium from their cytoplasm during clot formation; this causes potassium concentration to be higher in serum than in plasma. Although normal individuals have a difference of 0.2 to 0.3 mmol/L between serum and plasma potassium, this difference increases by an average of 0.15 mmol/L for each increment in the platelet count of 100,000/mm^3.[52] Because white blood cells are more active metabolically than are red blood cells, changes resulting from delayed separation are exaggerated in patients with leukemia. Glucose concentration may fall and potassium concentration may begin to rise in as little as 30 minutes,[53] and pH may decrease by as much as 0.6 in 10 minutes if the specimen is not rapidly chilled in an ice slurry. In patients with lymphocytic leukemia, heparin appears to induce

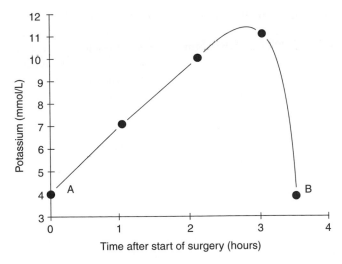

Fig. 3-7 Effect of heparin on potassium in lymphocytic leukemia. The graph represents serum potassium concentration obtained during surgery to remove the spleen in a patient with chronic lymphocytic leukemia and a white blood count of about 350,000/mm^3. Point *A* represents preoperative serum potassium. The next three points represent specimens obtained through an arterial catheter containing heparin at 1, 2, and 3.25 hours into the surgery. Point *B* represents serum potassium obtained from the arm opposite the arterial catheter 15 minutes after the previous specimen with serum potassium of 11.2 mmol/L.

degeneration of lymphocytes in vitro, leading to rapid rises in plasma (but not serum) potassium concentration[54] as shown in Fig. 3-7.

Procedure to minimize sample-processing errors. The most effective way to minimize sample-processing errors is to centrifuge samples requiring separation as soon as possible. If plain tubes are used, centrifugation should not be performed until at least a half hour after blood collection to allow complete clot formation. Tubes with clot accelerators or anticoagulants can be separated immediately. After centrifugation, in specimens without gels, plasma or serum should be separated from the cells as quickly as possible to prevent changes to the sample.

Sample storage

Errors arising from improper sample storage. Once serum or plasma has been separated from cells, most substances show little change in concentration over a 2- or 3-day period when kept at 4° C. For labile analytes, including enzymes such as creatine kinase and lactate dehydrogenase, most polypeptide hormones, and some other substances, the specimen must be frozen to prevent storage-related changes. Analytes that may be intrinsically stable on storage may change in the presence of other compounds. For example, triglyceride concentration falls in serum obtained from patients taking heparin, apparently because of the activation of lipoprotein lipase.[55] Aminoglycoside antibiotics, such as tobramycin and gentamicin, are stable when stored at refrigerator temperatures unless the serum also contains certain synthetic penicillins, most notably piperacillin; aminoglycoside concentrations can fall to less than 50% of baseline value at 72 hours when both drugs are present.[56]

Evaporation can increase sample concentration. When a sample is uncovered, the rate of evaporation is affected by temperature, humidity, air movement, and the surface area of the sample.[57] If humidity is low, a situation often found in air-conditioned laboratories, there is a direct linear relationship between temperature and rate of evaporation; however at high humidities, temperature changes have a minimal effect on evaporation rate. One of the most important factors affecting evaporation is the rate of air movement over the surface of a liquid. For any given rate of air flow, increasing the height of the column of air over the specimen or decreasing the area of opening in the specimen container will decrease the rate of evaporation by decreasing air movement over the specimen. Small, fully filled sample cups may show as much as 50% loss of water in a few hours. As with any other form of hemoconcentration, this will lead to an increase in concentration of proteins and protein-bound substances; however evaporation also increases the concentration of other solutes.

Procedures to minimize storage errors. Storage errors can be prevented by the proper selection of time, temperature, and storage conditions. Most analytes are stable when stored at refrigerator temperatures for up to 72 hours. If an analyte is not stable, specimens should be frozen until analysis. Most specimens can be stored at −70° C without affecting analyte concentrations, even when frozen for many years.[58] Alkaline phosphatase activity will increase with freezing, apparently as a result of the destruction of an inhibitor. At standard freezer temperatures of −10° to −20° C, most substances will be stable for shorter periods. Care must be taken to prevent repeated thawing and refreezing of specimens; this is especially problematic with newer frost-free freezers, which periodically increase freezer temperature to allow the melting of frost. Analytes that are susceptible to repeated freeze/thaw cycles, such as complement, should be stored in other types of freezers. Frozen samples should be allowed to thaw slowly at room temperature or in a 37° C water bath and should then be mixed thoroughly before analysis.

To prevent specimen evaporation, specimens should be covered while stored and kept, if at all possible, away from areas of rapid air flow. Whenever possible, containers with a small surface area and a large column of air over the specimen should be used to minimize evaporation. The identification of each sample should be confirmed at each step of the operation to minimize the likelihood of specimen confusion. Direct sampling from the collection tube is the best way to minimize such errors, especially if bar-coded labels and bar code readers are available.

OTHER PREANALYTICAL COLLECTION CONCERNS
Urine Collection: Sources of Variation

Biological variables. Preanalytical variation in urine is somewhat difficult to control. Although changes in serum concentration are primarily related to degree of hemoconcentration, urine variation can be caused by several factors. The most important variable in determining urine concentration of a substance is the relative amount of water excreted. The body is capable of greatly altering urine concentration to meet the need for water excretion or water conservation. Since most of the solute in urine is composed of waste products such as urea and creatinine, urine osmolality is a measure of relative water excretion. Normal individuals may have urine osmolality as low as 75 mOsm/kg and as high as 1200 mOsm/kg; the relative concentration of other solutes may thus vary over a 15-fold range in concentration. As mentioned earlier in the discussion of random variation, intraindividual variation in urinary concentration is, on the average, several times higher than intraindividual variation for the same analytes in serum.[11] Controlling the hydration status of the patient during the urine collection process can minimize this source of variability.

Other causes of preanalytic variation also affect urine measurements. *Diurnal variation* independent of relative concentration is observed for many urine substances, notably protein, sodium, potassium, phosphate, and hormones. Part of the diurnal variation in protein excretion is posture-related since the relative concentration of protein compared to creatinine increases in the upright position.[59] *Stress* increases protein excretion; both exercise and fever have been shown to cause transient increase in urinary protein.[60] *Dietary changes* in intake of a substance will often alter urinary excretion. Hydroxyproline, a component of collagen, is often used to measure bone turnover; gelatin, a component of many processed foods, contains collagen and can be a major source of urinary hydroxyproline excretion.[61] Creatine supplements, increasingly used by body-builders, also increase urine creatinine excretion.[62] Creatinine excretion is often used to evaluate the adequacy of collection of a timed urine. However short-term fluctuation in dietary protein intake alters the excretion of creatinine in the urine.[22]

Time of collection. Variation in urine measurements can be the result of improperly collected 24-hour urine specimens. Such specimens are among the most difficult to collect properly. As mentioned above, urine creatinine is often used as a measure of the completeness of urine collection, and specimens with too much or too little creatinine are considered to indicate an improperly timed collection. Because excretion of creatinine is relatively reproducible in a given individual on a stable diet (average day-to-day variation of 10% with little diurnal variation), the ratio of the concentration of the substance of interest to that of creatinine has also been advocated as a means to provide an accurate estimate of total urinary excretion.[63,64] This is especially important for pediatric specimens because it is often difficult to get children to cooperate with timed urine collections.

Sample stability. Many compounds stable in serum are unstable in urine. Both bacterial contamination and low pH can produce in vitro changes in the concentration of many analytes. Collection of urine into containers with various preservatives, acids, or bases is commonly needed to prevent such variation; a more complete discussion of urine preservatives is given in Chapter 57 and in the CD-ROM. In general, stable substances such as electrolytes, protein, and creatinine can be measured in urine samples without the use of preservatives. Addition of concentrated acids or bases does not usually affect electrolyte or creatinine measurements; however, a specimen containing an appropriate preservative for the measurement of one analyte may be unsuitable for use in the measurement of a different substance. Storage of urine specimens during collection may also alter analyte concentration. For example, porphyrins are unstable when exposed to light, whereas calcium may precipitate at low temperatures. Most formed elements in urine, such as cells and casts, are unstable when stored. Refrigeration is often used to prevent bacterial growth in urine specimens. Refrigeration, however, promotes the formation of crystals that would not have been found at body temperature and lowers the concentrations of those substances that have precipitated.

Preanalytical variation in other body fluids. Preanalytical variation in other body fluids has not been extensively studied. Many factors that affect other samples, such as hemoconcentration, tourniquet use, and stress, do not affect the composition of cerebrospinal, pleural, peritoneal, and synovial fluids. A delay in transport of specimens to the laboratory usually causes little change in normal fluid composition, since these specimens are virtually cell-free. If measurements of unstable analytes such as lactate, glucose, or pH are requested, specimens should be transported to the laboratory in an ice slurry to prevent artifactual change in concentration. For fluids other than cerebrospinal fluid, use of an anticoagulant is advisable to prevent the formation of fibrin clots, which can falsely lower cell counts.

Specimen Collection from Infants

Capillary sampling. Venipuncture in infants and small children is usually not an acceptable method for obtaining blood, both because of the difficulty in finding a vein and the importance of preserving available veins for use in administration of intravenous fluid. Capillary blood is the specimen usually available for testing in these children. In neonates, the outer aspects of the sole of the foot are the preferred sites for skin puncture, whereas earlobes or fingers are acceptable in older infants and small children. The skin surface is often warmed to produce "arterialized" capillary blood; as mentioned earlier, however, agreement with arterial blood-gases is poor in neonates, particularly in premature infants. It is essential to allow any topical antiseptics to dry before skin puncture, since the collected blood will freely mix with any remaining liquid on the surface. Contamination with antiseptics can falsely dilute specimens and may cause hemolysis. It may be helpful to apply mild pressure after the skin is punctured, but squeezing or "milking" the puncture site will contaminate the sample with tissue fluid.

Because of the small volume of sample obtained and, in neonates, the high hematocrit, relatively little serum or plasma is available for testing. Special capillary tubes containing appropriate anticoagulants or preservatives are available to facilitate collection of required specimens (see p. 70). Use of pediatric serum separator tubes or heparinized plasma will result in a greater amount of sample for the same amount of blood obtained. However the small sample size often results in a relatively large surface area, making evaporation an even more important consideration. Control of factors causing evaporation is especially important for pediatric specimens. Hemoconcentration, posture, and diet-related changes are relatively less important for neonates than with older children or adults. The extent of cyclic variations in infants and children is largely unknown.

Blood collection for metabolic diseases. When infants are screened for inborn metabolic errors, specimens are often collected on filter paper and transported to a specialized laboratory as dried blood spots. There is little information on specific preanalytic factors related to dried blood spots; however some factors do affect the results of such tests.[65] Because such specimens are collected as capillary blood, care must be taken to avoid contamination with antiseptics, which may interfere in the assays. The paper must be fully saturated in the area of collection to provide an adequate amount of sample. For many metabolic errors, screening must not be done until at least 24 hours after the infant has begun feeding, since the metabolic product that accumulates is derived from ingested food. Obtaining specimens before this time can produce false-negative results. For tests that require measurement of enzyme activity, care must be taken to prevent exposure of the specimens to excess heat during the shipping process; if specimens are mailed, temperatures in outdoor mail boxes can be high enough to produce falsely low results. All the general precautions discussed previously, such as prevention of evaporation and mislabeling, must be carefully followed.

Computer-Based Aids for Error Detection

Computer-based systems that aid in error detection can reduce the number of erroneous results that are reported.[66] In many laboratory and hospital computer systems, it is possible to compare the results from the current specimen with those from previous samples on the same patient (see Chapter 18). Such result comparisons are termed **delta checks.**[67] A delta check can test for results that vary by a set amount or set percentage; on some systems, it is possible to use one type of check for values at a certain level and another for higher or lower concentrations. Tests that are particularly appropriate for monitoring with delta checks are those that normally change little from one day to the next. Some of these are listed in Table 3-4. Measuring the rate of analyte change may also add to the sensitivity of error detection.[68] Delta checks should not be used for substances that are subject to pronounced intraindividual variation (see Table 3-4). A list of delta check values used in the author's laboratory is given in Table 3-5. Although fluctuations in one test result may be seen in as many as 1% of all specimens, multiple test results that fail delta checks are usually the result of either a significant change in the patient's condition or a nonrepresentative specimen. Selection of tests that

TABLE 3-4 DELTA CHECKS FOR ANALYSIS

Appropriate	Inappropriate
Electrolytes: Na, K, Cl	Glucose
Total protein	Phosphate
Albumin	Lactate dehydrogenase
Urea	Creatine kinase
Creatinine	Aspartate aminotransferase
Alkaline phosphatase	Alanine aminotransferase
Hemoglobin and hematocrit; mean cell volume and red blood cell distribution width index	

TABLE 3-5 DELTA CHECK VALUES

Test	Delta Check Value
Albumin	10 g/L
Anion gap	10 mmol/L
Calcium	10 mg/L
Chloride	5 mmol/L
Cholesterol	± 30%
CO_2 content	5 mmol/L
Creatinine	± 50%
Direct bilirubin	± 50%
Glucose (fasting only)	± 30%
Magnesium	0.25 mmol/L
Mean corpuscular volume	4 μm^3
Mean platelet volume	1.5 μm^3
Osmolality	15 mOsm/kg
Potassium	1 mmol/L
Red blood cell distribution width	2% (absolute change)
Sodium	5 mmol/L
Total bilirubin	± 50%
Total protein	10 g/L
Urea nitrogen	± 50%
Uric acid	15 mg/L

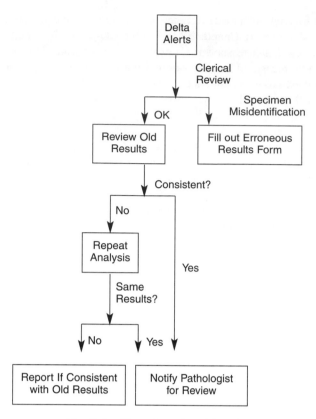

Fig. 3-8 Flow chart for delta alerts.

typically change in parallel, such as AST and ALT or urea and creatinine, may improve delta check utility (see Table 3-4).[69] Common causes of failed delta checks include specimens drawn above intravenous lines, contaminated specimens, and misidentified specimens. Review of such results before release can lead to a significant reduction in the reporting of erroneous results. A method that can be used for the evaluation of specimens failing delta checks is outlined in Fig. 3-8. The laboratory information system can automatically perform the delta check review, also allowing so-called autoverification of results (see Chapter 18).

Criteria for Rejection of Specimens

To prevent the reporting of misleading results, each laboratory must establish criteria for specimen rejection. A specimen must be rejected when the results obtained by analysis of that specimen will not be representative of the patient's condition. The most common cause for specimen rejection is inadequate identification. Specimens *must* have the patient's name and identification number on both the sample and the accompanying request slip. Specimens that are not drawn by laboratory personnel should be checked carefully before they are accepted by the laboratory. For specimens requiring special handling, improper collection and transportation are the most common causes for rejection. In most laboratories that process blood-gas specimens, an average of 5% of the specimens have not been collected correctly and must be rejected.[70] Specimens are often collected in the incorrect tube for the assay requested. Each laboratory must have a list of acceptable alternative specimens for each test; for example, a laboratory manual may suggest collection of serum for a particular test, but heparinized plasma is an acceptable alternative. If the specimen contains another anticoagulant or preservative, it should be rejected (though it may be used for other analyses). For tubes containing preservatives or anticoagulants, there must be a proper ratio of specimen to preservative. This is most critical with liquid solutions of preservatives but may also occur with powdered anticoagulants. Tubes that do not have the appropriate ratio should not be accepted for analysis. For tests that require special patient preparation, the absence of such preparation should cause rejection. If a test is affected by hemolysis, hemolyzed specimens should be rejected. If a test result is affected by lipemia (and the specimen cannot be cleared by ultracentrifugation before analysis), test results should not be reported. Finally, any specimens with results that fail delta checks or results that are considered unlikely to be valid (e.g., potassium over 10 mmol/L, calcium less than 40 mg/L, and so on) should be reported to the laboratory

director for review before the results are reported. Although many physicians complain when the laboratory does not report results for tests ordered, if there is any question about the validity of a result, it should not be reported. Erroneous results can lead to inappropriate treatment of the patient.

References

1. Arendt J, Minors DS, Waterhouse JM, editors: *Biological rhythms in clinical practice*, Boston, 1989, Wright.
2. Liskowsky DR: Biological rhythms and shift work, *JAMA* 268:3047, 1992.
3. Utiger RD: Melatonin: the hormone of darkness, *N Engl J Med* 327:1377, 1992.
4. Fevre-Montage M et al: Effects of "jet lag" on hormonal patterns. II. Adaptation of melatonin circadian periodicity, *J Clin Endocrinol Metab* 52:642, 1978.
5. Tietz NW: *Clinical guide to laboratory tests*, ed 3, Philadelphia, 1995, Saunders.
6. Benvenuti M et al: Circadian rhythm in prostatic acid phosphatase (PAP): a potential tumor marker rhythm in prostatic cancer (PCa), *Chronobiologia* 10:383, 1983.
7. Kemp GJ, Blumsohn A, Morris BW: Circadian changes in plasma phosphate concentration, urinary phosphate excretion, and cellular phosphate shifts, *Clin Chem* 38:400, 1992.
8. Aoshima H et al: Circadian variation of urinary type I collagen crosslinked C-telopeptide and free and peptide-bound forms of pyridinium crosslinks, *Bone* 22:73, 1998.
9. Gertz BJ et al: Application of a new serum assay for type I collagen cross-linked N-telopeptides: assessment of diurnal changes in bone turnover with and without alendronate treatment, *Calcif Tissue Int* 63:102, 1998.
10. Panteghini M, Pagani F: Biological variation in bone-derived biochemical markers in serum, *Scand J Clin Lab Invest* 55:609, 1995.
11. Dufour DR: Reference values in endocrinology. In Becker KL, editor: *Principles and practice of endocrinology*, ed 3, Philadelphia, 2001, Raven-Lippincott.
12. Rosen JF, Chesney RW: Circulating calcitriol concentrations in health and disease, *J Pediatr* 103:1, 1983.
13. Elomaa I et al: Seasonal variation of urinary calcium and oxalate excretion, serum $25(OH)D_3$, and albumin level in relation to renal stone formation, *Scand J Urol Nephrol* 16:155, 1982.
14. Douglas AS et al: Seasonal differences in biochemical parameters of bone remodeling, *J Clin Pathol* 49:284, 1996.
15. Harrup JS, Ashwell K, Hopton MR: Circannual and within-individual variation of thyroid function tests in normal subjects, *Ann Clin Biochem* 22 (4):371, 1985.
16. Fraser CG: Biological variation in clinical chemistry—an update: collated data, 1988, *Arch Pathol Lab Med* 116:916, 1992.
17. Statland BE, Winkel P, Bokelund H: Factors contributing to intra-individual variation of serum constituents: 2. Effects of exercise and diet on variation of serum constituents in healthy subjects, *Clin Chem* 19:1380, 1973.
18. Robinson D, Whitehead TP: Effect of body mass and other factors on serum liver enzyme levels in men attending for well population screening, *Ann Clin Biochem* 26:393, 1989.
19. Stansbie D, Bedley JP: Biochemical consequences of exercise, *JIFCC* 3:87, 1991.
20. Ronkainen H: Depressed follicle-stimulating hormone, luteinizing hormone, and prolactin responses to luteinizing hormone-releasing hormone, thyrotropin-releasing hormone, and metoclopramide test in endurance runners in the hard training season, *Fertil Steril* 44:755, 1985.
21. Ahlquist DA et al: HemoQuant, a new quantitative assay for fecal hemoglobin: comparison with hemoccult, *Ann Intern Med* 101:297, 1984.
22. Perrone RD, Madias NE, Levey AS: Serum creatinine as an index of renal function: new insights into old concepts, *Clin Chem* 38:1933, 1992.
23. Dugue B et al: The driving license examination as a stress model: effects on blood picture, serum cortisol and the production of interleukins in man, *Life Sci* 69:1641, 2001.
24. Armario A et al: Acute stress markers in humans: response of plasma glucose, cortisol and prolactin to two examinations differing in the anxiety they provoke, *Psychoneuroendocrinology* 21:17, 1996.
25. Muldoon MF et al: Acute cholesterol responses to mental stress and change in posture, *Arch Intern Med* 152:775, 1992.
26. Genest JJ et al: Effect of elective hospitalization on plasma lipoprotein cholesterol and apolipoproteins AI, B, and LP(a), *Am J Cardiol* 65:677, 1990.
27. Gore JM et al: Validity of serum total cholesterol level obtained within 24 hours of acute myocardial infarction, *Am J Cardiol* 54:722, 1984.
28. Gebhart SP et al: Reversible impairment of gonadotropin secretion in critical illness: observations in postmenopausal women, *Arch Intern Med* 149:1637, 1989.
29. Kaptein EM et al: Thyroxine metabolism in the low thyroxine state of critical nonthyroidal illnesses, *J Clin Endocrinol Metab* 53:764, 1981.
30. Davenport MW, Zipser RD: Association of hypotension with hyperreninemic hypoaldosteronism in the critically ill patient, *Arch Intern Med* 143:735, 1983.
31. Statland BE, Bokelund H, Winkel P: Factors contributing to intra-individual variation of serum constituents: 4. Effects of posture and tourniquet application on variation of serum constituents in healthy subjects, *Clin Chem* 20:1513, 1974.
32. Van Cauter E: Endocrine rhythms. In Becker KL, editor: *Principles and practice of endocrinology*, ed 3, Philadelphia, 2001, Lippincott-Williams and Wilkins.
33. National Committee for Clinical Laboratory Standards: *Approved Standard Procedures for the Collection of Diagnostic Blood Specimens by Skin Puncture*, Villanova, PA, 1982, NCCLS.
34. College of American Pathologists: *So you're going to collect a blood specimen*, ed 5, Danville, IL, 1992, Interstate Printers.
35. Pendergraph GA: *Handbook of phlebotomy*, ed 2, Philadelphia, 1988, Lea & Febiger.
36. Jones BA, Meier F, Howanitz PJ: Complete blood count acceptability: a College of American Pathologists Q-Probes study of 703 laboratories, *Arch Pathol Lab Med* 119:203, 1995.
37. Schiffman RB et al: Blood culture contamination: a College of American Pathologists Q-Probes study involving 640 institutions and 497,134 specimens from adult patients, *Arch Pathol Lab Med* 122:216, 1998.
38. Jones BA, Calam RR, Howanitz PJ: Chemistry specimen acceptability: a College of American Pathologists Q-Probes study of 453 laboratories, *Arch Pathol Lab Med* 121:19, 1997.
39. Hill BM et al: Comparison of plastic vs. glass evacuated serum-separator (SST) blood-drawing tubes for common clinical chemistry determinations, *Clin Chem* 38:1474, 1992.
40. Adrogue HJ et al: Assessing acid-base status in circulatory failure: differences between arterial and central venous blood, *N Engl J Med* 320:1312, 1989.
41. Atkin S et al: Fingerstick glucose determination in shock, *Ann Intern Med* 114:1020, 1991.
42. Irjala K et al: Interpretation of oral glucose tolerance test: capillary-venous difference in blood glucose and the effect of analytical method, *Scand J Clin Lab Invest* 46:307, 1986.
43. Doumas BT et al: Differences between values for plasma and serum in tests performed in the Ektachem 700 XR analyzer, and evaluation of "plasma separator tubes (PST)," *Clin Chem* 35:151, 1989.
44. Wu AH et al: National Academy of Clinical Biochemistry Standards of Laboratory Practice: recommendations for the use of cardiac markers in coronary artery disease, *Clin Chem* 45:1104, 1999.
45. Midgley JE: Direct and indirect free thyroxine assay methods: theory and practice, *Clin Chem* 47:1353, 2001.
46. Don BR et al: Pseudohyperkalemia caused by fist clenching during phlebotomy, *N Engl J Med* 322:1290, 1990.

47. National Institute on Drug Abuse: *Urinalysis Collection Handbook for Federal Drug Testing Programs*, Washington, DC, 1988, US Department of Health and Human Services.
48. Weilert M, Tilzer LL: Putting bar codes to work for improved patient care, *Clin Lab Med* 11:227, 1991.
49. Sazama K, Robertson EA, Chesler RA: Is routine antiglycolysis required for routine glucose analysis? *Clin Chem* 25:1086, 1979.
50. Sealey JE: Plasma renin activity and plasma prorenin assays, *Clin Chem* 37:1811, 1991.
51. Howanitz PJ et al: Emergency department stat test turnaround times: a College of American Pathologists' Q-Probes study for potassium and hemoglobin, *Arch Pathol Lab Med* 116:122, 1992.
52. Graber M et al: Thrombocytosis elevates serum potassium, *Am J Kidney Dis* 12:116, 1988.
53. Ringelhann B, Laszlo E, Vajda L: Pseudohyperkalaemia in acute myeloid leukemia, *Lancet* 1:928, 1974.
54. Dufour DR, Mesonero C, Miller K: Artifactual hyperkalemia induced by heparin in patients with extreme leukocytosis, *Clin Chem* 33:914, 1987.
55. Hortin G et al: Decreased stability of triglycerides and increased free glycerol in serum from heparin-treated patients, *Clin Chem* 34:1847, 1988.
56. Pickering LK, Rutherford I: Effect of concentration and time upon inactivation of tobramycin, gentamicin, netilmicin, and amikacin by azlocillin, carbenicillin, mecillinam, mezlocillin and pi-peracillin, *J Pharmacol Exp Ther* 217:345, 1981.
57. Burtis CA: The effects of temperature and evaporation on analytical error in the clinical laboratory, *Clin Lab Annu* 1:1, 1982.
58. DiMagno EP et al: Effect of long-term freezer storage, thawing, and re-freezing on selected constituents of serum, *Mayo Clin Proc* 64:1226, 1989.
59. Howey JEA, Browning MCK, Fraser CG: Selecting the optimum specimen for assessing slight albuminuria, and a strategy for clinical investigation: novel uses of data on biological variation, *Clin Chem* 33:2034, 1987.
60. Clerico A et al: Exercise-induced proteinuria in well-trained athletes, *Clin Chem* 36:562, 1990.
61. Yoneyama K et al: The day to day variations of urinary hydroxyproline and creatinine excretions, and dietary protein intake, *Nippon Eiseigaku Zasshi* 39:587, 1984.
62. Ropero-Miller JD et al: Effect of oral creatine supplementation on random urine creatinine, pH, and specific gravity measurements, *Clin Chem* 46:296, 2000.
63. Ginsberg JM et al: Use of single voided urine samples to estimate quantitative proteinuria, *N Engl J Med* 309:1543, 1983.
64. Huikeshoven FJM, Zuiderhoudt FMJ: Hypocalciuria in hypertensive disorder in pregnancy and how to measure it, *Eur J Obstet Gynecol Reprod Biol* 36:81, 1990.
65. Buist NRM: Laboratory aspects of newborn screening for metabolic disorders, *Lab Med* 19:145, 1988.
66. Ladenson JH: Patients as their own controls: use of the computer to identify "laboratory error," *Clin Chem* 21:1648, 1975.
67. Sher PP: An evaluation of the detection capacity of a computer-assisted real-time delta check system, *Clin Chem* 25:870, 1979.
68. Lacher DA, Connelly DP: Rate and delta checks compared for selected chemistry tests, *Clin Chem* 34:1966, 1988.
69. Lacher DA: Relationship between delta checks for selected chemistry tests, *Clin Chem* 36:2134, 1990.
70. Shapiro BA et al: *Clinical application of blood gases*, ed 4, St Louis, 1989, Mosby.

Internet Sites

www.upstate.edu/phlebotomy/—State University of New York-Upstate: a comprehensive overview of blood drawing

http://www.srbr.org/—The Society for Research on Biological Rhythms

www.nccls.org/—NCCLS Approved Guideline: contains guidelines for patient preparation, specimen collection

http://www.westgard.com/qcapp18.htm—Six Sigma: Test Interpretation Guidelines as Tolerance Limits, by Dr. James O. Westgard

http://www.acclc.es/invitroveritas/vol2/art20.html—Associació Catalana de Ciènces del Laboratori Clínic (ACCLC)

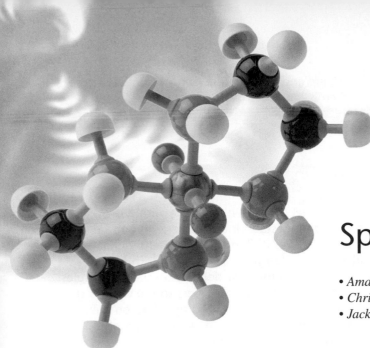

CHAPTER 4

Spectral Techniques

- *Amadeo J. Pesce*
- *Christopher S. Frings*
- *Jack Gauldie*

Chapter Outline

Objectives

- Describe the relationships among wavelength, frequency, energy, and color of the ultraviolet and visible spectra.
- Describe the relationship between percent transmittance (%T) and absorbance (A) and how this relationship affects the color of a solution.
- Describe the Beer-Lambert law and its limitations.
- Illustrate the construction and operation of photometric monochromators and detectors and explain the advantages or disadvantages associated with the use of each in spectral instruments. Further

describe the principles of spectral isolation and band pass.
- Draw a block diagram of the essential components of the atomic absorption spectrophotometer and the fluorometer and state the principle of the operation of each, highlighting similarities and differences. Explain the interferences associated with each.
- Describe how the instrumentation and basic principles of photometry are modified with the applications of turbidimetry, nephelometry, or

- fluorometry and identify any unique interferences or sources of error associated with each.
- Describe one of the chemical reactions that result in chemiluminescence.

- Compare and contrast the principles of absorption and emission spectroscopy.

Key Terms

absorbance   Defined as 2 - log %T, it is directly proportional to concentration of absorbing species if Beer's law is followed.

absorption spectrum   The range of electromagnetic energy that is used for spectroanalysis, including both visible light and ultraviolet radiation; also graph of spectrum for a specific compound.

absorptivity   Absorbance divided by the product of the concentration of a substance and the sample path length.

angle of detection   The angle at which scattered light is measured in nephelometry.

atomic absorption spectrophotometry   A quantitative spectroscopic measurement in which the emitted light from a source composed of one element is absorbed by the same element in a vapor phase. The amount of light absorbed is directly related to the concentration of the element in a sample.

band pass   The range of wavelengths that reaches the exit slit of a monochromator; usually referred to as the range of wavelengths transmitted at a point equal to half the peak intensity transmitted.

Beer-Lambert law (most commonly referred to as **Beer's law**)   The concentration of a substance is directly proportional to the amount of radiant energy absorbed.

bioluminescence   An enzyme-catalyzed reaction that uses complex organic molecules and adenosine triphosphate (ATP) to yield light.

blank   A solution consisting of all the components including solvents and solutes except the compound to be measured. This solution is used to set I_o, the original light intensity.

chemiluminescence   A chemical reaction usually involving oxidation in which one of the products is light.

cuvette   The receptacle in a photometer in which the sample is placed.

diode array   A two-dimensional matrix of light-sensitive semiconductors, the response of which allows recording of a complete absorption spectrum in milliseconds.

electrochemiluminescence   A chemical reaction in which an electrochemically activated molecule oxidizes a second molecule, which emits light.

electronic transition   The change in the orbital position of an electron of an atom or molecule. In the case of the absorption of a photon of light, the electron usually goes from the ground or the lowest energy level to some higher one with a consequent higher energy state (increased energy) of the molecule. Basis of fluorescence phenomena.

emission wavelength   The wavelength of light (λ_{em}) that is used to monitor decay of excited molecules into fluorescence; usually refers to the wavelength of output photons measured by a fluorometer.

excitation wavelength   The wavelength of radiant energy (λ_{ex}) that is absorbed by a molecule and causes it to be raised to a higher energy state; usually refers to the wavelength of incident energy of a fluorometer.

filter   An optical device (usually glass) that allows only a portion of **polychromatic**, incident light to pass through. The amount of transmitted light is related to the band pass of the filter.

flameless atomic absorption   An atomic absorption technique in which the element is converted to a vapor phase without the use of a flame.

fluorescence   The light emitted by an atom or molecule after absorption of a photon. This light is at longer wavelengths (less energy) than the absorbed light and is usually emitted in less than 10^{-8} sec. However, some compounds emit the photon at a slower rate.

grating   An optical device consisting of a reflecting, ruled surface that disperses polychromatic light into a uniform, continuous spectrum. Dispersion of light is attributable to interference phenomena at the ruled surface.

hollow-cathode lamp   A lamp consisting of a metal cathode and an inert gas. When an electric current is passed through the cathode, the metal is sputtered free and, after colliding with the gas in the lamp, emits a line spectrum of specific wavelengths related to the metal of the cathode.

infrared radiation   The region of the electro-magnetic spectrum extending from about 780 to 300,000 nm.

internal standard   An element or compound added in a known amount to yield a signal against which an instrument or an analyte to be measured can be calibrated.

light scattering   The interaction of light with particles that cause the light to be bent away from its original path (cause of turbidity).

line spectrum   Discontinuous emission spectrum of elements in which the emitted light bands cover a very narrow (0.1 nm) range of wavelengths.

luminescence   Light emitted at low temperatures, often as the result of a chemical reaction (*chemiluminescence*).

molar absorptivity ($\in$)   The absorbance of light, at a specific wavelength, divided by the product of concentration in moles per liter and the sample path length in centimeters. Molar absorptivity is expressed as L/mol·cm.

monochromatic   Light of one color (wavelength). In practice this refers to radiant energy composed of a very narrow range of wavelengths.

monochromator   Device used to isolate a certain wavelength or range of wavelengths. Usually refers to prisms or grating.

nephelometry   A technique that measures the amount of light scattered by particles suspended in a solution.

phosphorescence   Similar to fluorescence, the light emitted by an atom or molecule after absorption of a photon. The light is usually emitted at a time greater than 10^{-3} sec after absorption of the photon.

photodetector   A device that responds to light (photons) usually in a manner proportional to the number of photons striking its light-sensitive surface. Commonly a current that is proportional to the incident light intensity is generated.

photometer   An instrument that measures light intensity; composed of a source of radiant energy, filter for wavelength selection, cuvette holder, detector, and a readout device.

photon   A particle consisting of a discrete packet of radiant energy.

polarized fluorescence   The orientation of the emitted fluorescent light, which can be calculated from the polarization formula.

polychromatic   Light of many colors (wavelengths), usually referring to white light, or that encompassing a defined portion of the spectrum.

Rayleigh scatter   The reflection of light at different angles by particles suspended in a solution. This scattering occurs when the wavelength of incident light is greater than the size of the particles.

reflectance spectrophotometry   A quantitative spectrophotometric technique in which the light reflected from the surface of a colorimetric reaction is used to measure the amount of the reaction product.

refraction   A process by which the path of incident light is bent after the light passes obliquely from one medium to another of different density.

refractive index   The ratio of the speed of light in two different media; usually the reference medium is air.

refractometer   An instrument for measuring the refractive index (refractivity) of various substances, especially of solutions.

spectrophotometer   An instrument that measures light intensity. It is composed of a source of radiant energy, entrance slit, monochromator, exit slit, cuvette holder, detector, and readout device. Measurements in these instruments can be made over a continuous range of available spectrum.

stray light   Radiant energy reaching the detector and consisting of wavelengths other than those defined by the filter or monochromator.

time-delayed fluorescence   A technique in which the fluorescence of slowly emitting compounds such as metal chelates is measured. Usually the time between 400 and 1000 msec is monitored.

ultraviolet radiation   The region of the electromagnetic spectrum from about 180 to 390 nm.

visible light   The radiant energy in the electromagnetic spectrum visible to the human eye (approximately 390 to 780 nm).

wavelength   The linear distance traversed by one complete wave cycle of electromagnetic energy.

LIGHT AND MATTER[1-3]
Properties of Light and Radiant Energy

Electromagnetic radiant energy is a form of energy that can be described in terms of its wavelike properties. Electromagnetic waves travel at high velocities and do not require the existence of a supporting medium for propagation.

The **wavelength,** λ, of a beam of electromagnetic radiant energy is the linear distance traversed by one complete wave cycle and is usually given in nanometers (nm, 10^{-9} m). The frequency, ν, is the number of cycles occurring per second and is obtained by the relationship

$$\nu = \frac{c}{\lambda}$$

The velocity, c, varies with the medium through which the radiant energy is passing ($c = 3 \times 10^{10}$ cm/sec when measured in a vacuum).

Radiant energy can be shown to behave as if it were composed of discrete packets of energy called **photons**. The energy of a photon is variable and depends on the frequency or wavelength of the radiant energy. The relationship between the energy, E, of a photon and frequency is given by the formula

$$E = h\nu$$

in which h is Planck's constant and has a numerical value of 6.62×10^{-27} erg·sec. The equivalent expression involving wavelength is

TABLE 4-1 ELECTROMAGNETIC SPECTRUM

	Gamma Rays	X-Rays	Ultraviolet (UV)	Visible	Infrared (IR)	Microwaves
Wavelength (nm)*	0.1	1	180	390	780	400×10^3

This is the wavelength interval at which the lowest type of respective radiant energy occurs.

TABLE 4-2 COLORS AND COMPLEMENTARY COLORS OF VISIBLE SPECTRUM

Wavelength* (nm)	Color Absorbed†	Complementary or Solution Color Transmitted
350 to 430	violet	yellow
430 to 475	blue	orange
475 to 495	blue-green	red-orange
495 to 505	blue-green	orange-red
505 to 555	green	red
555 to 575	yellow-green	violet-red
575 to 600	yellow	violet
600 to 650	orange	blue
670 to 700	red	green

From Brown TL, Lemay HE: Chemistry: the central science, *Englewood Cliffs, 1977, Prentice-Hall.*
**Because of the subjective nature of color, the wavelength ranges are only approximations.*
†If a solution absorbs light of the color listed in the second column, the observed color of the solution, that is, the transmitted complementary light, is given in the third column.

$$E = \frac{hc}{\lambda}$$

This equation shows that shorter wavelengths have a higher energy than longer wavelengths have.

The electromagnetic spectrum covers a very large range of wavelengths, as shown in Table 4-1. The areas of the electromagnetic spectrum that are commonly used in the clinical laboratory are the **ultraviolet** (UV) **radiation** and **visible light** regions. The visible region is generally specified as the region between 390 and 780 nm, whereas the UV spectrum usually referred to in the clinical chemistry laboratory falls between 180 and 390 nm. Sunlight or light emitted from a tungsten filament is a mixture of radiant energy of different wavelengths that the eye recognizes as "white." The breakdown of the visible region into color absorbed and color reflected is shown in Table 4-2. If a solution absorbs radiant energy (light) between 400 and 480 nm (blue), it will *transmit* all other colors and appear yellow to the eye. Therefore yellow is the complementary color of blue. If white light is focused on a solution that absorbs energy between 505 and 555 nm (green), the transmitted light and thus the solution will appear red. If a red light is focused on a red solution, red light will be transmitted because this solution cannot absorb red light. On the other hand, if green light is focused on the red solution,

no light is transmitted, because the solution absorbs all light but red. The human eye responds to radiant energy between 390 and 780 nm, but laboratory instrumentation permits measurements at both shorter wavelengths, such as UV, and longer wavelengths, such as **infrared** (IR), of the spectrum.

Interactions of Light with Matter

Absorption process. When an atom, ion, or molecule absorbs a photon, the added energy results in an alteration of state, and the species is said to be excited. Excitation may involve any of the following processes:

1. Transition of an electron to a higher energy level
2. A change in the mode of vibration of the molecule's covalent bonds
3. Alteration of its mode of rotation about the covalent bonds

Each of these transitions requires a definite quantity of energy, a specific **excitation wavelength;** the probability of occurrence for a particular transition is greatest when the photon absorbed supplies this exact quantity of energy.

The energy requirements for these transitions vary widely. Usually elevation of electrons to higher energy levels requires greater energy absorption than is needed to cause vibrational changes. Rotational alterations usually have the lowest energy requirements. Therefore absorption of energy in the microwave and far-infrared regions results in shifts in the rotational energy levels, because the energy of the radiant energy is insufficient to cause other types of transitions. Changes in vibrational levels are caused by absorption in the near-infrared and visible regions. Promotion of an electron to a higher energy level occurs after energy absorption in the visible, ultraviolet, and x-ray regions of the spectrum. The energy content of the electrons of covalent bonds varies with the nature of the bonds. The energy of a photon of light needed to excite an electron therefore varies with the bond, and each type of bond has its own characteristic pattern of optimum wavelengths of light that can be absorbed by that bond. Table 4-3 gives the electronic absorption bands for many organic groups.[4]

The absorption pattern of a complex organic molecule containing tens of thousands of bonds must therefore describe the cumulative sum of the absorption of *all* the individual covalent bonds.

The absorption of radiant energy by a solution can be described by means of a plot of the **absorbance** as a function of wavelength. This graph is called an **absorption spectrum** (Fig. 4-1). The absorption spectrum reflects the sum of the energy transitions characteristic for a molecule at each

TABLE 4-3	ELECTRON ABSORPTION BANDS FOR REPRESENTATIVE CHROMOPHORES						
Chromophore	*System*	λ_{max}	$\in_{max}$	λ_{max}	$\in_{max}$	λ_{max}	$\in_{max}$
Ether	—O—	185	1000				
Thioether	—S—	194	4600	215	1600		
Amine	—NH$_2$	195	2800				
Thiol	—SH	195	1400				
Disulfide	—S—S—	194	5500	255	400		
Sulfone	—SO$_2$—	180	–				
Ethylene	—C=C—	190	8000				
Ketone	>C=O	195	1000	270 to 285	18 to 30		
Ester	—COOR	205	50				
Aldehyde	—CHO	210	strong	280 to 300	11 to 18		
Carboxyl	—COOH	200 to 210	50 to 70				
Nitro	—NO$_2$	210	strong				
Azo	—N=N—	285 to 400	3 to 25				
Nitrate	—ONO$_2$	270 (shoulder)	12				
	—(C=C)$_2$— (acyclic)	210 to 230	21,000				
	—(C=C)$_3$—	260	35,000				
	—(C=C)$_5$—	330	118,000				
	C=C—C≡C	219	6500				
Benzene		184	46,700	202	6900	255	170
Anthracene		252	199,000	375	7900		
Quinoline		227	37,000	270	3600	314	2750
Isoquinoline		218	80,000	266	4000	317	3500

From Willard HH, Merritt LL, Dean JA: Instrumental methods of analysis, ed 4, Princeton, NJ, 1965, Van Nostrand.

wavelength of light. Absorption spectra are often helpful for qualitative identification purposes. This is particularly true for low-energy absorptions such as those found in the IR region. Irrespective of the amount of energy absorbed, an excited species tends to return spontaneously to its unexcited, or ground, state; in the process it releases energy as kinetic (movement), vibrational, or light (see the later discussion of **fluorescence**) energy.

Emission process. Some elements and compounds can be excited in such a fashion that when the electrons return from the excited state to the ground state, the energy is dissipated as radiant energy. The radiant energy may consist of one or more than one energy level and therefore may consist of different **emission wavelengths.** This principle is used in flame photometry and fluorometric methods and is further discussed with these topics.

ABSORPTION SPECTROSCOPY[4-11]
Radiant-Energy Absorption

Consider a beam of radiant energy with an original intensity, I_0, impinging on and passing through a square cell (whose sides are perpendicular to the beam) containing a solution of a compound that absorbs radiant energy of a certain wavelength (Fig. 4-2). The intensity of the transmitted radiant energy, I_s, will be less than I_0. Some of the incident radiant energy may be reflected by the surface of the cell or

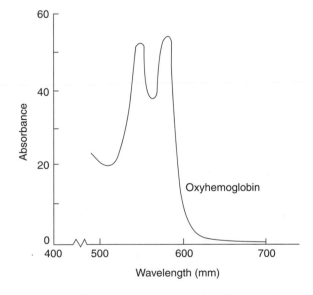

Fig. 4-1 Absorption spectrum of oxyhemoglobin.

absorbed by the cell wall or the solvent. Therefore these factors must be eliminated if *only* the absorption of the compound of interest is to be considered. This is done by use of a **blank** or reference solution containing everything but the compound to be measured. The amount of light passing through the blank solution is set as the new I_0 (relative to

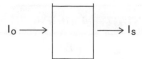

Fig. 4-2 Transmittance of radiant energy through a cuvette. I_0 is the incident radiation; I_s is the transmitted radiation.

the reference cell and solution). The transmittance for the compound in solution is defined as the proportion of the incident light that is transmitted:

$$\text{Transmittance} = T = I_s / I_0$$

Usually this ratio is described as a percentage:

$$\text{Percentage} = \%\text{T} = I_s / I_0 \times 100\%$$

The concept of transmittance is important because only transmitted light can be measured.

As the concentration of the compound in solution increases, more light is absorbed by the solution and less light is transmitted. Percent T varies inversely and logarithmically with concentration. However, it is more convenient to use absorbance, *A,* which is directly proportional to concentration. Therefore

$$A = -\log I_s / I_0 = -\log T = \log \frac{1}{T}$$

To convert *T* to %T, the denominator and numerator are multiplied by 100%:

$$A = \log \frac{1}{T} \times \frac{100\%}{100\%} = \log \frac{100\%}{\%T}$$

This can be rearranged to

$$A = \log 100\% - \log \%T$$

or

$$A = 2 - \log \%T$$

It is important to remember that absorbance is not a directly measurable quantity but can be obtained only by mathematical calculation from transmittance data.

The relationship between absorbance and %T is shown in Fig. 4-3, in which the linear %T scale runs from 0 to 100%, whereas the logarithmic absorbance scale runs from infinity to 0.

Beer-Lambert Law

The **Beer-Lambert law** (most commonly referred to simply as **Beer's law**) states that the concentration of a substance is directly proportional to the amount of radiant energy absorbed or inversely proportional to the logarithm of the transmitted radiant energy. If the concentration of a solution is constant and the path length through the solution that the

light must traverse is doubled, the effect on the absorbance is the same as doubling the concentration, because twice as many absorbing molecules are now present in the radiant-energy path. Thus the absorbance is also directly proportional to the path length of the radiant energy through the cell.

Beer's law states the mathematical relationship that connects absorbance of radiant energy, concentration of a solution, and path length:

$$A = abc$$

A is absorbance; *a,* **absorptivity**; *b,* light path of the solution in centimeters; and *c,* concentration of the substance of interest.

This equation forms the basis of quantitative analysis by absorption photometry or absorption spectroscopy. Absorbance values have no units. The absorptivity is a proportionality constant related to the chemical nature of the solute and has units that are reciprocal of those for *b* and *c.*

When *c* is expressed in moles per liter and *b* is expressed in centimeters, the symbol $\in$, called the **molar absorptivity**, is used in place of *a* and is a constant for a given compound at a given wavelength under specified conditions of solvent, pH, temperature, and so on. It has units of L/mol·cm. A compound with a higher molar absorptivity has a higher absorbance for the same molar concentration than a compound with a lower molar absorptivity. Therefore, when selecting a chromogen for spectrophotometric methods, the chromogen with a higher molar absorptivity should be used, to impart a greater sensitivity to the measurement.

Once a chromogen is proved to follow Beer's law at a specific wavelength (that is, a linear plot of *A* versus *c* with a zero intercept; Fig. 4-4, *A*), the concentration of an unknown solution can be determined by measurement of its absorbance and interpolation of its concentration from the graph of the standards. In contrast, when %T is plotted versus concentration (on linear graph paper), a curvilinear relationship is obtained (Fig. 4-4, *B*). Because of the linear relationship between absorbance and concentration, it is possible to relate unknown concentrations to a single standard by a simple proportional equation. Therefore

$$\frac{A_s}{A_u} = \frac{C_s}{C_u}$$

and

$$C_u = \frac{A_u}{A_s} \times C_s$$

in which C_u and C_s are the concentration of the unknown and standard, respectively, and A_u and A_s are the absorbance of the unknown and standard.

These equations are valid *only* if the chromogen obeys Beer's law and both standard and unknown are measured

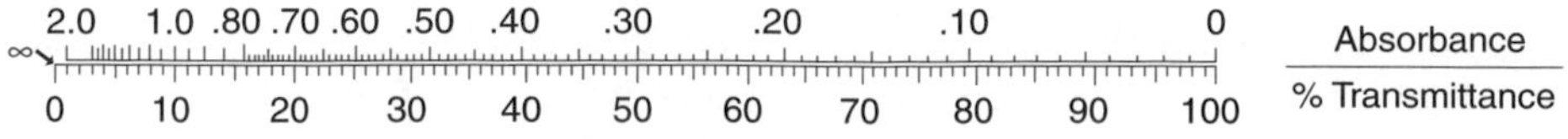

Fig. 4-3 Scale showing relationship between absorbance and percent transmittance.

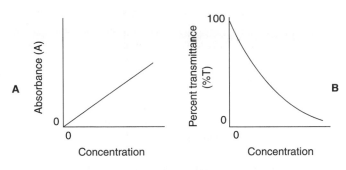

Fig. 4-4 Relationships of absorbance (**A**) and percent transmittance (**B**) to concentration.

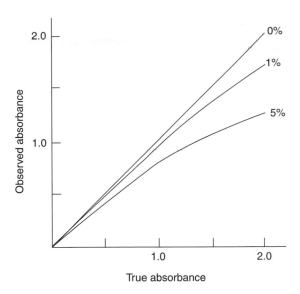

Fig. 4-5 Effect of stray radiation on true absorbance. *(From Frings CS, Broussard LA: Calibration and monitoring of spectrometers and spectrophotometers,* Clin Chem *25:1013, 1979.)*

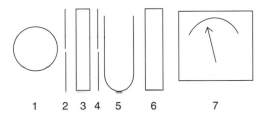

Fig. 4-6 Components of a spectrophotometer. *1,* Source of radiant energy; *2,* entrance slit; *3,* wavelength selector; *4,* exit slit; *5,* cuvette and cuvette holder; *6,* detector; *7,* readout device.

in the same cell. The concentration range over which a chromogen obeys Beer's law must be determined for each set of analytical conditions.

Beer's law is an ideal mathematical relationship that contains several limitations. Deviations from Beer's law, that is, variations from the linearity of the absorbance versus concentration curve (Fig. 4-5), occur when (1) very elevated concentrations are measured, (2) incident radiant energy is not monochromatic, (3) the solvent absorption is significant compared with the solute absorbance, (4) radiant energy is transmitted by other mechanisms (stray light), and (5) the sides of the cell are not parallel. If two or more chemical species are absorbing the wavelength of incident radiant energy, each with a different absorptivity, Beer's law will not be followed. If the absorbance of a fluorescent solution is being measured, Beer's law may not be followed.

Stray radiation (**stray light**) is radiant energy that reaches the detector at wavelengths other than those indicated by the **monochromator** setting. All radiant energy that reaches the detector, with or without having passed through the sample, will be recorded. Fig. 4-5 shows the effects of stray light on Beer's law. As the amount of stray light increases (or monochromicity decreases), deviation from Beer's law also increases (that is, linearity decreases).

Instrumentation

Single-beam spectrophotometer. The major components of a single-beam spectrophotometer are shown in Fig. 4-6. The apparatus needed can be divided into seven basic components: (1) a stable source of radiant energy; (2) an entrance slit to focus the light; (3) a wavelength selector; (4) an exit slit to focus the light; (5) a device to hold the transparent container (**cuvette**), which contains the solution to be measured; (6) a radiant-energy detector; and (7) a device to read out the electrical signal generated by the detector. If a **filter** is used as the wavelength selector, **monochromatic** light at only discrete wavelengths is available, and the instrument is called a **photometer**. If a monochromator is used (that is, a prism or grating, see later discussion) as the wavelength selector, the instrument can provide monochromatic light over a continuous range of wavelengths and is called a *spectrometer* or *spectrophotometer.* Spectrophotometers can be double-beam instruments with two

cuvette holders, one for the sample and the other for the blank, or reference sample. Advantages of the double-beam instrument include the capability of making simultaneous corrections for changes in light intensity, grating efficiency, slit-width variation, and so on. It is particularly useful for obtaining spectral curves.

Sources of radiant energy. A tungsten-filament lamp is useful as the source of a continuous spectrum of radiant energy from 360 to 950 nm (Fig. 4-7). Tungsten iodide lamps are often used as sources of visible and near-UV radiant energy. The tungsten halide filaments are longer lasting, produce more light at shorter wavelengths, and emit a higher intensity radiant energy than tungsten filaments do.

Hydrogen and deuterium discharge lamps emit a continuous spectrum and are used for the UV region of the spectrum (220 to 360 nm) (Fig. 4-8). The deuterium lamp has more intensity than the hydrogen lamp does. Mercury-vapor lamps emit a discontinuous or line spectrum (313, 365, 405, 436, and 546 nm) (see Fig. 4-8). This is useful for wavelength-calibration purposes but is not used in many spectrophotometers. The mercury lamp is used in photometers or

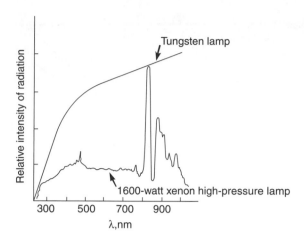

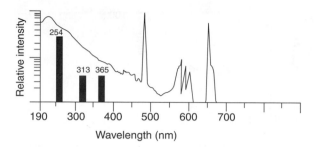

Fig. 4-8   Intensity of radiant energy versus wavelength for a mercury lamp *(solid bars)* and a deuterium lamp *(continuous line)*. For illustrative purposes, the intensity of the mercury emission lines has been reduced several hundredfold, and only those lines (wavelengths are *numbers above bars*) in the ultraviolet region of the spectra have been depicted.

Fig. 4-7   Intensity of radiant energy versus wavelength for a tungsten filament and a 1600-watt xenon light source. Tungsten lamp intensity has been magnified approximately a hundredfold to place it on the same scale as the xenon lamp. *(Modified from Brewer JM et al, editors:* Experimental techniques in biochemistry, *Englewood Cliffs, NJ, 1974, Prentice-Hall.)*

spectrophotometers employed for high-performance liquid chromatography (HPLC). Recently, light-emitting diodes have been employed as light sources.

It is important to understand that the amount of light emitted from a light source is not constant over a continuous range of wavelengths. Thus a typical lamp has a complex transmittance spectrum with maxima and minima (see Figs. 4-7 and 4-8). Lamps of different types and even from different manufacturers can vary. Therefore care must be taken in choosing a lamp for a particular analysis, because the amount of light emitted at the desired wavelength may be too little or too much. For example, hydrogen or deuterium lamps, used for UV analysis, have a maximum output of UV radiation in the 250 to 300 nm range. The output of radiant energy at longer wavelengths (greater than 340 nm) is considerably less and can be too weak for many analyses.

Wavelength selectors. Isolation of the required wavelength or range of wavelengths can be accomplished by use of a filter or monochromator. Filters are the simplest devices, consisting of only a material that selectively transmits the desired wavelengths and absorbs all other wavelengths. In a monochromator, a **grating** or *prism* disperses radiant energy from the source lamp into a spectrum from which the desired wavelength is isolated by mechanical slits.

Filters. There are two types of filters: (1) those with selective transmission characteristics, including glass and Wratten filters, and (2) those based on the principle of interference (interference filters). The Wratten filter consists of colored gelatin between clear glass plates; glass filters are composed of one or more layers of colored glass. Both types of filters transmit more radiant energy in some parts of the spectrum than in others.

Interference filters work on a different principle. The principle is the same as that underlying the play of colors from a soap film, namely, interference. When radiant energy

strikes the thin film, some is reflected from the front surface, but some of the radiant energy that penetrates the film is reflected by the surface on the other side. The latter rays of radiant energy have now traveled farther than the first by a distance two times the film thickness. If the two reflected rays are in phase, their resultant intensity is doubled, whereas, if they are out of phase, they destroy each other. Therefore, when white light strikes the film, some reflected wavelengths will be augmented and some destroyed, resulting in colors.

Monochromators. Monochromators can give a much narrower range of wavelengths than filters can and are easily adjustable over a wide spectral range. The dispersing element may be a prism or a grating.

Dispersion by a prism is nonlinear, becoming less linear at longer wavelengths (over 550 nm). Therefore, to certify wavelength calibration three different wavelengths must be checked. Prisms give only one order of emerging spectrum and thus provide higher optical efficiency, because the entire incident energy is distributed over the single emerging spectrum.

A grating consists of a large number of parallel, equally spaced lines ruled on a surface. Dispersion by a grating is linear; therefore only two different wavelengths must be checked to certify the wavelength accuracy.

Band pass. Except for laser optical devices, the light obtained by a wavelength selector is not truly monochromatic (that is, of a single wavelength) but consists of a range of wavelengths. The degree of monochromicity is defined by the following terms. **Band pass** is that range of wavelengths that passes through the exit slit of the wavelength-selecting device. The *nominal wavelength* of this light beam is the wavelength at which the peak intensity of light occurs. For a wavelength selector such as a filter or a monochromator whose entrance and exit slits are of equal width, the nominal wavelength is the middle wavelength of the emerging spectrum.

The range of wavelengths obtained by a filter producing a symmetrical spectrum is usually noted by its *half-band width* (or *half-band pass*). This describes the wavelengths obtained

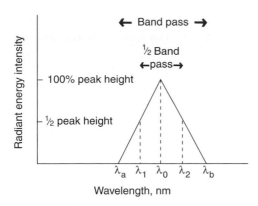

Fig. 4-9 Idealized distribution of radiant energy emerging from exit slit of wavelength selector. For a filter or a monochromator with entrance and exit slits of equal width, a symmetrical distribution of transmitted energy occurs, as shown.

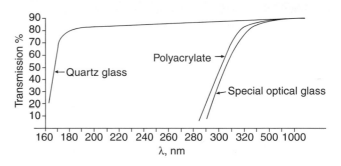

Fig. 4-10 Transmission characteristics of several types of optical materials used for cuvettes. *(From Keller H: Optical methods of measurement. In Richterich R, Colombo JP, editors: Clinical chemistry, New York, 1981, Wiley & Sons.)*

between the two sides of the transmittance spectrum at a transmittance equal to one half the peak transmittance (Fig. 4-9). For monochromators, the degree of monochromicity is described by the *nominal band width,* which corresponds to those wavelengths that are centered about the peak wavelengths and transmit 75% of the total radiant energy present in the emerging beam of light. For monochromators with variable exit slits, the band pass will also vary.

Slits. There are two types of slits present in monochromators. The first, at the entrance, focuses the light on the grating or prism where it can be dispersed with a minimum of stray light. The second slit, at the exit, determines the band width of light that will be selected from the dispersed spectrum. By increasing the width of the exit slit, the band width of the emerging light is broadened, with a resultant increase in energy intensity but a decrease in spectral purity. In diffraction-grating monochromators, the exit slit may be of fixed width, resulting in a constant band pass. In contrast, prism monochromators have variable exit slits. The purpose of both slits in filter photometers is to make the light parallel and reduce stray radiation.

Cuvettes. The receptacle in which a sample is placed for spectrophotometric or photometric measurement is called a *cuvette,* or *cell.* Glass cuvettes are satisfactory for use in the range of 320 to 950 nm. For measurement below 320 nm it is necessary to use quartz (silica) cells. Such cells can be used at higher wavelengths also. Fig. 4-10 shows the transmission pattern of several types of cuvettes. Cuvettes with a square cross section and with a circular cross section (i.e., test tubes) are available. Greater accuracy is achieved by square cuvettes with parallel sides made of *optical glass.* Although cuvettes usually have internal dimensions (that is, path lengths) of 1 cm, cuvettes with other dimensions are available.

Detectors

Barrier layer (photovoltaic) cells. Barrier layer cells are detectors consisting of a plate of copper or iron on which a semiconducting layer of cuprous oxide or selenium is placed.

This layer is covered by a light-transmitting layer of metal that serves as a collector electrode. As illumination passes through the electrode to the semiconducting layer, an electron flow is induced in the semiconducting layer, and this flow can be sensed by an ammeter. These detectors are rugged, relatively inexpensive, and sensitive from the UV region up to about 1000 nm. No external power is required, and the photocurrent produced is directly proportional to the radiant-energy intensity.

Barrier layer cells exhibit the fatigue effect, which means that on illumination, the current rises above the apparent equilibrium value and then gradually decreases.

Photomultiplier tubes. A photomultiplier tube is an electron tube that is capable of significantly amplifying a current. The cathode is made of a light-sensitive metal that can absorb radiant energy and emit electrons in proportion to the radiant energy that strikes the surface of the light-sensitive metal. These surfaces vary in their response to light of different energies (wavelengths) and so also in the sensitivity of the photomultiplier tube (Fig. 4-11). The electrons produced by the first stage go to a secondary surface, where each electron produces between four and six additional electrons. Each of the electrons from the second stage goes on to another stage, again producing four to six electrons. As many as 15 stages (or dynodes) are present in today's photomultiplier tubes (Fig. 4-12). Photomultiplier tubes have rapid response times, do not show as much fatigue as other detectors, and are very sensitive.

Photodiodes. Photodiodes are semiconductors that change their charged voltage (usually 5 V) upon being struck by light. The change is converted to current and is measured. A **diode array** is a two-dimensional matrix composed of hundreds of thin semiconductors spaced very closely together. Light from the instrument is dispersed by either a grating or prism onto the photodiode array. Each position or diode on the array is calibrated to correspond to a specific wavelength. Each diode is scanned, and the resultant electronic change is calculated to be proportional to absorption. The entire spectrum is essentially recorded within milliseconds.

Instrument Performance

The sensitivity of response of a spectrophotometer is a combination of lamp output, efficiency of the filter or monochromator in the transmission of light, and response of the photomultiplier. Because these factors are all functions of

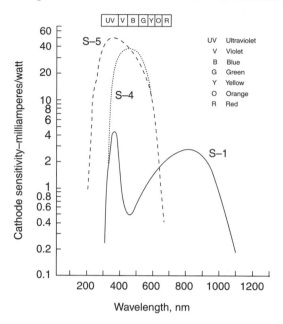

Fig. 4-11 Response of cathodes of several photomultiplier tubes to energy of different wavelengths. Sensitivity is expressed as milliamperes of current generated per watt of incident radiation.

wavelength, it is clear that the instrument must be reset when wavelength is changed. This resetting most often takes the form of adjustment of the blank solution to read 100% T (zero absorbance) by changing the photomultiplier gain.

A series of recommendations on instrument specifications that covers many aspects of instrumentation used for photometric analysis has been proposed.[12] These specifications are listed in Table 4-4.

Selection of Optimum Conditions and Limitations

When establishing a new spectrophotometric procedure, it is important to record the absorption spectrum of the material that is being measured. This absorption spectrum should be recorded in relation to either water or a reagent blank, depending on the actual method of analysis chosen. Examples of such spectra are presented throughout the sections of this text. This spectrum will help to determine the best wavelength for the spectrophotometric analysis. The optimum wavelength for a specific analysis depends on several factors, including the absorption maxima of the chromogen, the slope of the absorption peak, and the absorption spectra of possible interfering chromogens.

An example of an absorption spectrum is shown in Fig. 4-13. According to Beer's law, the higher the molar absorptivity, the greater the absorption at a given concentration and wavelength and the higher the sensitivity of the analysis. In this spectrum there are three peaks of absorption (highest absorption coefficient): λ_1, λ_2, and λ_3 nm. The

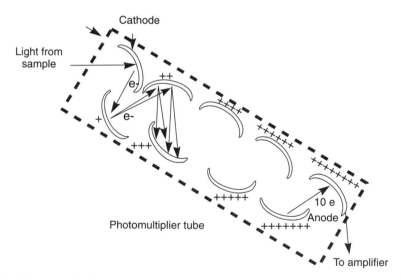

Fig. 4-12 Schema of photomultiplier tube. Each dynode (electrode used to generate secondary emissions of electrons) is represented by a *crescent*. Light impinges on each cathode and frees an electron. Electron is drawn toward first dynode (stage) by applied voltage. Secondary electrons are released and pass on to successive dynodes, which are at increasingly higher voltages, as depicted by the + symbols. Increasing numbers of secondary electrons are generated at each stage. In this diagram a tenfold amplification of the initial signal is produced at the anode. A photomultiplier tube may increase the signal several thousandfold. *(From Simonson MG: The application of a photon-counting fluorometer for the immunofluorescent measurement of therapeutic drugs. In Kaplan LA, Pesce AJ, editors: Nonisotopic alternatives to radioimmunoassay, New York, 1981, Marcel Dekker. Reprinted from Ref. [02], p 103, by courtesy of Marcel Dekker, Inc.)*

absorptivity at λ_2 is too low, and the use of λ_2 can be ruled out immediately.

If an absorption peak is narrow, as it is for λ_1, any small error in the setting of the spectrophotometer at this wavelength results in a large change in absorbance. With spectrophotometers using manually set wavelengths, this can cause large run-to-run imprecision and analytical error. A filter photometer requires a high-quality, accurate filter to ensure accuracy when monitoring at a narrow absorption peak.

These problems can be avoided by use of a wider absorption peak (λ_3). With this absorption peak, small changes in wavelength adjustment result in only small changes in absorptivity, and precision and accuracy will be high.

The sensitivity of many methods may be improved by use of absorption bands at shorter wavelengths (such as UV), because very often these are more intense. However, often there is additional nonspecific absorption from buffers or other chemical moieties in the solution at shorter wavelengths. Therefore appropriate blanks must be used to obtain accurate measurements. In some techniques the analyte is purified before analysis, and detection at short wavelengths (UV) is feasible and provides optimum sensitivity.

Knowledge of the wavelengths at which the commonly interfering chromogens absorb light also helps determine the wavelength of choice. A general rule for selecting the optimum wavelength at which to monitor a spectrophotometric reaction includes three criteria: (1) Choose an absorption peak with the greatest possible molar absorptivity. (2) Choose a relatively broad peak. (3) Choose a peak that is as far as possible from the absorption peaks of commonly interfering chromogens.

Quality Control Checks of Spectrophotometers[13]

Several quality control checks should be performed to certify that spectrophotometers are functioning within specifications. These checks are wavelength accuracy, linearity of detector response, stray radiation (stray light), and photometric accuracy. Details of the spectrophotometer performance checks can be found in references 5 and 13.

Wavelength accuracy. If the wavelength calibration of an instrument changes, the measured absorbance will change. The magnitude of the absorbance error attributable to inaccurate wavelength calibration depends on the relative location of the point on the absorption spectrum of the chromophore to be measured. That is, the absorbance error relative to the wavelength error is greater when the absorbance measurement is on the slope of the absorbance band than when the absorbance measurement is on or near the peak of the absorbance band. Maintenance of wavelength calibration is especially important for analyses such as spectrophotometric enzyme assays.

The most accurate method of checking the wavelength accuracy involves the replacement of the source lamp with a radiant energy source that has strong emission lines at well-defined wavelengths. Useful radiant energy sources are (1) the mercury vapor lamp, which has strong emission lines at 313, 365, 405, 436, and 546 nm, and (2) the deuterium or

---

TABLE 4-4   GUIDELINES FOR PHOTOMETRIC ENZYME INSTRUMENTS

Parameter	Error or Range (95% Confidence, ±2 SD)
Carry-over	
Sample to sample	<0.3%
Temperature accuracy	±0.1° C
Equilibration time	20 sec
Sample handling	
Accuracy	1%
Precision	0.5%
Size	50 μL or less
Reagent handling	
Mixing time	≤10 sec
Photometric performance (at a rate of 0.1 A/min)	
Initial absorbance 0 to 1 A	<3%
Initial absorbance 1 to 2 A	<5%
Wavelength accuracy	±2 nm
Band width	<8 nm
Wavelength range	Variable
Absorbance range	0 to 2 A
Linearity	<2%
Cell path/placement	<0.6%
Absorbance drift (10 to 60 min)	<2%
Absorbance accuracy	<2%
Absorbance reproducibility	
Low 0 to 1 A	±2%
High 1 to 2 A	±4%

From Instrumentation Guidelines Study Group, Subcommittee on Enzymes: Clin Chem 23:2160, 1977.

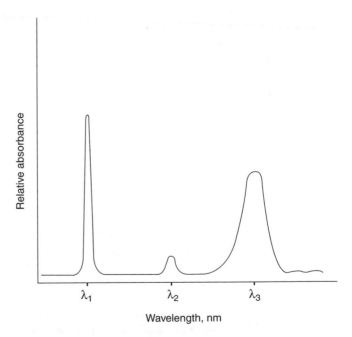

Fig. 4-13 Schema of idealized absorption spectrum. λ_1, λ_2, and λ_3 represent the absorption bands of a chromophore.

hydrogen lamp, which has useful emission lines at 486 and 656 nm (see Fig. 4-8). Spectrophotometers equipped with a hydrogen or deuterium radiant-energy lamp have built-in sources for checking wavelength accuracy.

A second method for checking wavelength calibration involves the use of rare-earth glass filters such as holmium oxide and didymium. Holmium oxide has strong absorption lines at approximately 241, 279, 287, 333, 361, 418, 453, 536, and 636 nm. Didymium has much broader absorption bands at approximately 573, 586, 685, 741, and 803 nm. Because of the possibility of filter deterioration, this wavelength accuracy should be periodically checked.

A third method for checking wavelength calibration involves the use of solutions. A solution of a stable chromogen can be used as a secondary wavelength calibration standard to determine whether the wavelength accuracy of an instrument has changed after the wavelength accuracy has been certified by a primary wavelength calibration standard such as a mercury or deuterium lamp. Disadvantages of using chemical solutions for wavelength calibration are that the absorption peaks are generally broad and spectral shifts may result from contamination, aging, or preparation errors.

Irrespective of the method, calibration at two wavelengths is necessary for grating instruments, and calibration at three wavelengths is necessary for prism instruments.

Linearity of detector response. A properly functioning spectrophotometer must exhibit a linear relationship between the radiant energy absorbed and the instrument readout. Instrument linearity is a prerequisite for spectrophotometric accuracy and analytical accuracy. Solid glass filters may be used to check instrument linearity. The most common method for certifying linearity of detector response is through the use of solutions of varying concentrations of a compound known to follow Beer's law. Some compounds used for this purpose are oxyhemoglobin at 415 nm, *p*-nitrophenol at 405 nm, cobalt ammonium sulfate at 512 nm, copper sulfate at 650 nm, and green food coloring at 257, 410, and 630 nm.

The absorbances of solutions containing increasing concentrations of one such compound are plotted against the known concentration. A nonlinear plot of absorbance versus concentration indicates either an error in dilution or an instrument problem. Besides a faulty detector, stray radiation or too wide a slit may cause a nonlinear response.

Stray radiation. An increase in stray radiation is often observed at the extreme ends of the spectral range, where detector response or source energy is at its lowest. Stray radiation usually causes a negative deviation from Beer's law. Methods used to detect stray radiation employ filters or solutions that are highly transmitting over a portion of the spectrum but are essentially opaque below an abrupt "cutoff" wavelength. Several solutions have been used to check for stray radiation, including Li_2CO_3 below 250 nm, NaBr (0.1 mol/L) below 240 nm, and acetone below 320 nm. The exact wavelength at which the cutoff occurs is a function of concentration, cell path length, and temperature; thus the wavelengths reported may vary somewhat. Many filters can

detect stray radiation. If solutions or filters that transmit no radiant energy at the measurement wavelength are used, the measured transmittance is the amount of stray radiation present. Multiplication of this transmittance by 100 gives the percentage of stray radiation. An instrument malfunction is indicated whenever the amount of stray radiation exceeds 1%.

Action taken to eliminate stray radiation includes changing the light source, verifying wavelength calibration, sealing light leaks, realigning instrument components, and cleaning optical surfaces.

Photometric accuracy. When performing analyses that do not use chemical standards, absorbance accuracy is essential. An absorbance standard should have a constant, stable absorbance at a suitable wavelength that is insensitive to the spectral band width of the instrument and to variations in the configuration of the light beam. Such standards should be easy to use and readily available. The National Institute of Standards and Technology (NIST) has a set of three neutral-density glass filters (SBM 930) that have known absorbances at four wavelengths for each filter. These filters are not completely stable and must be recalibrated by the NIST periodically.

Potassium dichromate solution, cobalt ammonium sulfate solution, and potassium nitrate solution have been used as standards for checking photometric accuracy. Standard solutions are subject to absorbance changes with time, temperature, and pH, which make them unsuitable as long-term calibration standards for photometric accuracy.

Reflectance Spectrophotometry

In **reflectance spectrophotometry**, a beam of light is directed at a flat surface and the reflected light is quantified. The light reflected from the surface is focused onto a photomultiplier tube. The instrumentation can be similar to that of a single-beam filter spectrophotometer (Fig. 4-14). A lamp generates light that passes through a filter and a series of slits and is focused on the test surface. Some of the light incident to a test sample is absorbed by the chromophores on the surface, and the remainder is reflected. (This is analogous to light passing through a solution, for in this case also, some light is absorbed and the remainder passes through.) The reflected light is then passed through a series of slits and lenses and on to a **photodetector**. The signal is then converted to an appropriate readout. The term *reflection density* is used to describe the absorption of light by chromophores at the surface. Reflection density is related to the intensity of light reflected by the sample.[14] The reflection density, D_R, of the test sample is related to the ratio of the light reflected by the standard reflector (usually a barium sulfate–coated surface), R_0, to the light reflected by the test sample, R_{test}, as described by the equation

$$D_R = \log (R_0/R_{test})$$

This is analogous to the equation that relates %T (and thus absorbance) to incidental transmitted light (see equation, p. 88). In general, the optical properties of different surfaces vary considerably. The optical properties of test paper or

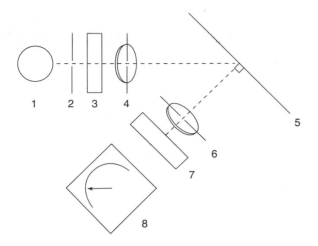

Fig. 4-14 Diagram of reflectance spectrophotometer. *1,* Light source; *2,* slit; *3,* filter or wavelength selector; *4,* collimating lens or slit; *5,* test surface; *6,* collimating lens or slit; *7,* detector; *8,* readout device.

plastic strips differ from those of dry film. Therefore, to calibrate an instrument for the measurement of reflection density, a standard with the specific surface employed by the test system must be used. The D_R value in the equation on p. 94 may be corrected for stray reflectance. A black standard with the same surface characteristics as the test sample can be used to give a value for maximum absorbance. Any reflection read by the instrument under these conditions is stray reflection. This value can be subtracted from the test value to correct for this variable. The use of reflectance allows quantitative measurement of reactions on surfaces such as a dipstick or dry film.

Disadvantages of the procedure include the problem of standardization. The amount of light reflected and subsequently measured is instrument dependent. The angle at which the reflection is measured, the surface area monitored, and so on are variables. In addition, test-surface variations (caused during the manufacturing or handling process) can alter surface reflectance properties.

Recording or Spectral Spectrophotometry

The recording of entire absorption spectra is used either for the identification of compounds or to convert the spectra mathematically to their first or second derivative. Recording of spectra can be done by spectrophotometers of the type described earlier or by diode-array detection systems, in which there is a spatial relationship between the spectral lines spread by a prism or grating and the diode light detector. First- and second-derivative spectroscopy is the mathematical conversion of the absorption curve into the derivative function. These derivatives are used to eliminate interference to the observed absorption spectral lines and permit more accurate analyses.

Multiwavelength Spectrophotometry[15]

The previous examples have described simple cases of light measurement assuming that the color or fluorescence of the analyte of interest was predominant at the chosen

wavelength. Commonly there is a spectral background in test solutions. One way to correct for this background is to subtract it out by measuring light at a second wavelength somewhat removed and at a longer wavelength from the first peak measurement. The difference between the two is considered to be the true absorption value. This is termed a bichromic measurement. Measurement at more than one wavelength is used to quantify several components that have spectral overlap. For this purpose the extinction coefficient of each component at each measured wavelength must be known. In the case of blood hemoglobin, not all of the analyte is in one form, and the spectra of these forms (reduced hemoglobin, oxyhemoglobin, carboxyhemoglobin, methemoglobin, and sulfhemoglobin) overlap each other. The predominant forms of hemoglobin can be quantified taking measurements at a series of wavelengths. Because the extinction coefficients of each form of hemoglobin are well established at each of these wavelengths, a matrix equation can be set up so that the measurements at six wavelengths (535, 560, 577, 622, 636, and 670 nm) can be used to calculate each component. This principle is used in most cooximeters.

Similar multiple wavelength measurements can be used for examination of fluorescence emission spectra to differentiate multiple fluorescent labels from each other.

ATOMIC ABSORPTION[16,17]

Atomic absorption (AA) **spectrophotometry** is used in the clinical laboratory for determining calcium, magnesium, lithium, lead, copper, zinc, and other metals.

Principle

Vaporized atoms in the ground state absorb light at very narrowly defined wavelengths. These absorption bands are on the order of 0.001 to 0.01 nm in width, and thus the entire absorption spectrum of atoms is called a **line spectrum**. If these atoms in the vapor state are excited, they can return to the ground state by emitting light of the same discrete wavelengths as the line spectrum. In AA spectrophotometry the ionic form of the element is not excited in the flame but is dissociated from its chemical bonds and, by attracting free electrons produced by the combustion process, is placed in the atomic ground state. In this form it is capable of absorbing light at the specific wavelengths of its line spectrum.

In AA a beam of radiant energy containing the line spectrum of the element to be measured is passed through a flame containing the vaporized metal to be determined. The source emitting such radiant energy is called a **hollow-cathode lamp**. The wavelength of the absorbed radiant energy is the same as would be emitted if the element were excited. With the aid of a monochromator, the attenuation of one of the wavelengths of the incident light is measured. This attenuation is caused by the photons interacting with ground-state atoms in the flame. Beer's law is valid for relating the concentration of atoms in the flame and transmission or absorption of light. Only a small percentage of atoms in the flame are excited, and most atoms are in a form capable of absorbing radiant energy emitted by the hollow-cathode lamp.

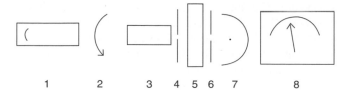

Fig. 4-15 Essential components of atomic absorption spectrophotometer. *1,* Hollow-cathode lamp; *2,* chopper; *3,* flame and burner assembly; *4,* entrance slit; *5,* wavelength selector; *6,* exit slit; *7,* detector; *8,* readout device.

Instrumentation

Fig. 4-15 shows the major components of an AA spectrophotometer.

Hollow-cathode lamp. The hollow-cathode lamp is the most practical means of generating a line spectrum of the required spectral purity. The lamps have a hollow or cuplike cathode that is lined with the pure metal of the element to be determined or with an appropriate alloy. A separate lamp is used for each element, except for a few instances in which the cathode can be constructed in such a manner that a single lamp serves for two or three elements (such as calcium and magnesium). The lamp is filled with an inert monatomic gas, usually argon or neon, at low pressure. The inert gas selected for the lamp can vary with the analyte to be measured. For example, lead and iron can be better analyzed with neon-filled lamps, whereas lithium analysis is better performed with argon-filled lamps. For other measured elements, the choice of inert gas is not critical. Quartz or a special glass that allows transmission of the proper wavelength is used as the window. A current is supplied to the cathode, and metal atoms are continually released (sputtered) from the inner surface of the cathode, filling the lamp with an atomic vapor. Atoms in this vapor undergo electronic excitation by collisions with the inert gas, and the resulting excited atoms emit their characteristic radiant energy when returning to the ground-state electron level. This results in a beam of radiant energy with the correct wavelength for absorption by ground-state atoms in the flame.

Burner. In AA spectrophotometry, the sample solution must be converted into the vapor phase. One technique converts the sample into a fine spray or aerosol while it is being introduced into the flame. This process is called *nebulization.* The nebulizer is usually considered part of the burner. Within the flame, solvent evaporates from the aerosol, leaving microscopic particles that disintegrate under the influence of heat to yield atoms. This phenomenon is termed *atomization.* Acetylene is the commonly used fuel in the burner. Temperatures of 2300° C are usually achieved in flame AA.

Two kinds of burners have been used in most clinical applications. One is the total-consumption burner, within which the gases and the sample mix within the flame. The flame in this type of burner can be made hot enough to cause molecular dissociations, which may be desirable for some chemical systems. The second type of burner is the premix burner (laminar-flow burner), in which larger droplets from the atomization go to waste and not into the flame. The path length through the premix burner is longer than that of the total-consumption burner, which provides greater sensitivity. The flame temperature is not as hot as that of the total-consumption burner.

Flameless AA. The purpose of the flame is to convert the sample into an atomic vapor. Other atomization processes can replace the flame. One process applicable to mercury analysis uses chemical reactions to convert mercury into an atomic vapor. The sample is decomposed by digestion with acids, then a reducing agent is added to convert mercury to the elemental state, and finally a stream of gas is bubbled through the apparatus, pushing mercury vapor into a sealed cell with quartz windows in the path of the optical beam. Absorbance measurements are made at 253.7 nm.

In a more frequently employed atomization technique, the sample is dried on a carbon support platform or tube. The sample is vaporized in an inert atmosphere when an electric current is passed through the support to create instantaneously a temperature sufficiently elevated to vaporize the analyte. These atomizers occupy the space normally occupied by the flame in flame AA instruments. The temperatures achieved by **flameless atomic absorption** (up to 2700° C) are necessary to vaporize heavier metals. Flameless AA instruments have a greater sensitivity than flame AA instruments.

Monochromator and detector. Monochromators (grating or prisms) and photomultiplier tubes can isolate a pure radiant-energy signal and measure the intensity of that signal. Extraneous radiant energy, both from other wavelengths of the line spectrum and from light generated by the flame, is kept from reaching the photomultiplier tube by the monochromator. The photomultiplier tube converts the radiant energy that was *not* absorbed in the flame into a signal and amplifies this signal to drive a recorder or meter.

Sources of Error

Chemical, ionization, matrix, and burner interferences can occur in AA measurements. Additional factors that may cause variable behavior from sample to sample or between unknowns and standards include temperature, solvent composition, salt content, viscosity, and surface tension.

Chemical interference. With some elements the presence of certain anions in the sample results in the formation of compounds that are not completely dissociated in the flame. The result is a decrease in the number of ground-state atoms present in the flame. The most common example of chemical interference in atomic absorbance is the formation of a tight complex of calcium with anions, especially phosphate ions. The effect of tightly complexing anions can be minimized or eliminated when lanthanum is added to the sample to displace calcium from the complex. Lanthanum forms a more stable complex with phosphate than calcium does.

In flameless AA, chemical interference may arise from compounds that vaporize with the element to be measured. The addition of "matrix modifiers" to the sample permits the vaporization of the element to occur at higher temperatures, allowing interfering compounds to be burned off at lower temperatures.

Ionization interference. When atoms in the flame become ionized (A^+) instead of remaining in the ground state (A^0), they will not absorb the incident light. This is termed *ionization interference,* and this effect results in an apparent decrease in analyte concentration. Ionization interference can be corrected by adding an excess of a substance that is more easily ionized, thus providing free electrons. The excess free electrons thus shift the reaction:

$$A^+ + e^- \rightarrow A^0$$

to the formation of ground-state atoms. Ionization interference is minimized by operation of the flame at the lower temperatures of acetylene-air combustion.

Matrix interference. Differences in the matrix between the sample and the standard can result in errors. Protein is sometimes included in the standards when the serum dilution factor is small. The matrix effects are minimized as compositional differences between the standard and the sample become negligible. Calcium standards must contain physiological concentrations of sodium, because sodium causes a negative interference.

The "standard-addition" technique has been employed to minimize matrix differences in the measurement of aluminum and other elements by flameless AA. In this technique, multiple levels of standard are added to diluted samples, and all are measured by flameless AA. The negative intercept of the regression line of signal versus amount of aluminum added is equal to the amount of aluminum in the sample.

Burner problems. The most critical component in the flame AA spectrophotometer is the flame and its associated nebulizer. A steady flame is essential, and controlled gas flows are required for both oxidant and fuel. A clean burner head is essential for precise and accurate analysis. Similarly, in flameless AA, the carbon platform must be changed after some number of firings to give reproducible results.

Emission interference. Many analyte atoms introduced into the flame become excited and emit a photon to return to the ground state. The light emitted is, of course, at the same wavelengths as the incident light being measured. The emitted light enhances the signal being received by the photodetector. The increased signal is translated as a decreased absorption and therefore a falsely lower concentration of analyte. This interference can be eliminated by use of a *chopper* (see Fig. 4-15) to create a pulsed beam of incident light from the hollow-cathode lamp. The light caused by emission interference, however, is a constantly produced beam. This steady emission can be electronically differentiated from the pulsed beam of transmitted light and thus eliminated as a source of interference.

FLAME PHOTOMETRY[18,19]

Flame photometry was widely used in the clinical laboratory to determine sodium, potassium, and lithium concentrations in biological fluids. This technique is now rarely used.

Principle

Atoms of some metals, when given sufficient heat energy as supplied by a hot flame, become excited and reemit this energy at wavelengths characteristic for the element as described previously. The reactions undergone by ions in the flame are as follows:

$$A^+ + e^- \rightarrow A^0$$
$$A^0 + \text{Heat} \rightarrow A^*$$
$$A^* \rightarrow A^0 + h\nu$$

A^* represents the excited atom in the flame, A^0 an atom with ground-state electron energy, and $h\nu$ a photon. Alkali metals are relatively easy to excite in a flame. Lithium produces a red emission; sodium, a yellow emission; and potassium, a red-violet color in a flame. These colors are characteristic of the metal atoms that are present as cations in solution.

The intensity of the characteristic wavelength of radiant energy produced by the atoms in the flame is directly proportional to the number of atoms excited in the flame, which is directly proportional to the concentration of the substance of interest in the sample. The actual number of atoms present in the excited state is a small fraction of the total number of atoms present in the flame. For reproducible quantitation, an internal standard such as cesium is used. A review of the technique of flame photometry can be found in reference 19.

FLUOROMETRY[20-22]
Principle

Fluorescence may be considered one of the results of the interaction of light with matter. When light impinges on matter, it can simply pass through, as in a transparent solution, it can be scattered by the interaction, or it can be absorbed. When light is transmitted, there is no loss of energy. When light is scattered, there is no change of energy; the light is the same wavelength before and after it interacts with matter. But when light is absorbed, the light energy is converted into any one of a number of forms, including radiationless **electronic transitions** (converting the energy into heat) and others, such as fluorescence and **phosphorescence**, in which photons are emitted (Fig. 4-16). Absorption of the light can be used, of course, to determine the concentration of compounds as is done in absorption spectroscopy. If the absorbed light is reemitted, the emitted photons can be used to quantitate the amount of the light-emitting compound (fluor). Quantitation is also possible with use of scattered light, because the amount of scattered light is related to the number and size of particles in solution. Methods that use light scattering are termed **nephelometry** and *turbidity* (see p. 101).

Fluorescent light is the result of the absorbance of a photon of radiant energy by a molecule. Once the molecule absorbs a photon, the molecule has an increased energy level, and because the molecular energy is greater than that of its environment, it seeks to eject the excess energy. When the

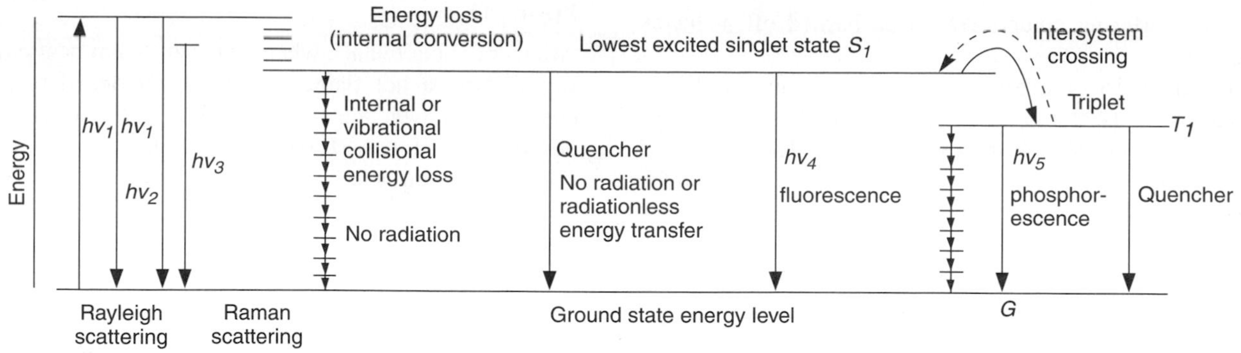

Fig. 4-16 on the top of the page shows an energy level schema with the following labels:

Energy loss (internal conversion) — Lowest excited singlet state S_1 — Intersystem crossing — Triplet — T_1 — hv_1 hv_1 — hv_2 — hv_3 — Internal or vibrational collisional energy loss — No radiation — Quencher No radiation or radiationless energy transfer — hv_4 fluorescence — hv_5 phosphorescence — Quencher — Energy — Rayleigh scattering — Raman scattering — Ground state energy level — G

Fig. 4-16 Schema showing conversion of light energy into different forms of molecular and radiant energy. *(From Pesce AJ et al, editors:* Fluorescence spectroscopy, *New York, 1971, Marcel Dekker. Reprinted from Ref. [02], p 108, by courtesy of Marcel Dekker, Inc.)*

energy is lost as an ejected photon, the result is fluorescence or phosphorescence emission.

For fluorescence to occur, there must be a high probability that the energy of the excited state can be converted to the ground state by the ejection of a photon. Not all compounds fluoresce; indeed, only a very few fluoresce. In those that do fluoresce, not every single photon absorbed is converted to fluorescent light. Some excited compounds lose energy by radiationless transitions, that is, by transfer of the energy to the solvent. For the same amount of light absorbed, molecules with higher fluorescence efficiency have brighter or more intense fluorescence. In solutions, when a molecule returns to the ground state by emitting a photon, there is less energy in the emitted photon than was present in the one initially absorbed. In other words, the emitted fluorescent light is at a longer wavelength than the exciting or absorbed radiation (Fig. 4-17).

Instrumentation

The basic components of a fluorometer are similar to those of an absorption spectrophotometer. The major difference is the introduction of a set of filters or a monochromator before

and after the cell to isolate the emitted light. A diagram of a fluorometer is presented in Fig. 4-18.

The principal components are the excitation light, filters or monochromators to separate the exciting light from the emitted light, and a sensitive detector. Most often, the measurement of fluorescent light is made at an angle of 90 degrees to the exciting light. This is done to maximize the sensitivity of the instrument by minimizing the amount of excitation light that can reach the photodetector. The detector is a photomultiplier or similar device that can quantitate the very small fluorescent light signal and thus achieve the desired level of sensitivity. Because the spectrum of absorption and emission varies from one compound to another, the instrument must be optimized for every analyte measured. This is done by adjusting the exciting wavelength to achieve the maximum absorption of photons, which usually means setting the instrument to the absorption maximum of the compound. By the same token, the wavelength of maximum emission of the fluorescent photons must also be ascertained, and this is the wavelength at which the fluorescence signal is most often recorded.

Limitations

The fluorescence signal of a compound is affected by many variables, including (1) solvent, (2) pH, (3) temperature, (4) absorbance of the solution, and (5) presence of interfering or specifically quenching compounds. Standardization is not usually done by an absolute procedure as in absorption spectroscopy because the fluorescence varies depending on (1) the intensity of the incident light on the sample, (2) the amount of light intercepted by the detector as controlled by the slits, (3) the band width of light analyzed, and (4) the efficiency of the detector. The quantum yield or efficiency of light emission of a photon is constant if solvent, pH, temperature, and so on are kept constant, but in general the instrument will not be constant on a daily basis. Therefore relative fluorescence yield is used for most measurements. For a reagent blank in a fluorometric assay, only the zero, or null, fluorescence can be set. There is no equivalent to the 100% scale of transmission. Therefore the electronic signal

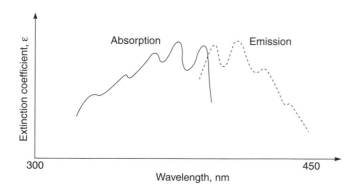

Fig. 4-17 Absorption (excitation) and emission (fluorescence) spectra of a fluorescent compound. *(From Pesce AJ et al, editors:* Fluorescence spectroscopy, *New York, 1971, Marcel Dekker. Reprinted from Ref. [02], p 108, by courtesy of Michael Dekker, Inc.)*

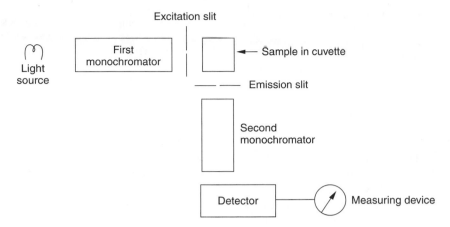

Fig. 4-18 Essential components of a fluorometer. *(From Brewer JM et al, editors: Experimental techniques in biochemistry, Englewood Cliffs, NJ, 1974, Prentice-Hall.)*

varies from instrument to instrument for the same concentration of analyte.

To enable a series of fluorescent standards to form a curve that is linear with concentration, the absorbance of the solutions should not exceed 0.1. Above this absorbance, all portions of the solution are not uniformly illuminated; that is, the initially illuminated layer of the solution absorbs more light than the final layer, and thus the initial layer fluoresces more than the final layer. In dilute solutions, such as those with absorbance of less than 0.1, this does not occur. However, certain assays employ the inverse quantitative relationship between fluorescence intensity and the amount of light absorbed by a solution whose absorbance is greater than 0.1. Such assays are termed *fluorescence attenuation assays*. In these systems a constant amount of fluorescent dye is placed in each test and control solution. In the test solution, the analyte causes a reaction in which a light-absorbing compound is produced. The greater the amount of colored reaction product formed by the analyte, the smaller the amount of light absorbed by the fluorescent dye. Thus the decrease in light passing through the solution results in a proportionate decrease in fluorescence intensity that can be related to the concentration of the analyte.

Time-Delayed Fluorescence[23]

One approach that can be used to improve the sensitivity of fluorescence techniques is the use of **time-delayed** or *time-resolved* **fluorescence**. The fluorescence emission time of most fluorescent molecules, such as fluorescein, is in the range of nanoseconds (nsec); that is, the fluorescence signal decays within 100 nsec. Some compounds such as the metal chelate diketone-europium have very long fluorescence lifetimes, 10 to 1000 microseconds (μsec). By measuring the fluorescence after 400 μsec, over a period of an additional 400 μsec, the fluorescence intensity of these compounds can be obtained without interference from light scattering or from any other molecules that may fluoresce. Aside from increasing the specificity of analysis, this technique provides greatly increased sensitivity.

Specialized instruments that use this technique illuminate the sample for a time, stop the illumination, and measure the emitted fluorescence over a specified time from 400 to 800 μsec after the illumination (Fig. 4-19). A limitation of this technique is the requirement for separation steps because the chelates cannot be measured directly in body fluids (see Chapter 13 for more details).

Chemiluminescence[23-25]

A **chemiluminescence** reaction is any chemical reaction in which one of the products of the reaction is light. The enzyme peroxidase can react with molecules such as luminol (5-amino-2,3-dihydro-1,4-phthalazinedione) to yield light as part of the reaction product. The luminol reaction results in photon emission in the range of 400 to 450 nm. The low photon yield of this reaction has limited its sensitivity and its application. However, by adding enhancer molecules (luciferin, 6-hydroxybenzothiazole) the reaction can be followed for many minutes (30 or more) with a several thousand–fold increase in photon output. The products of

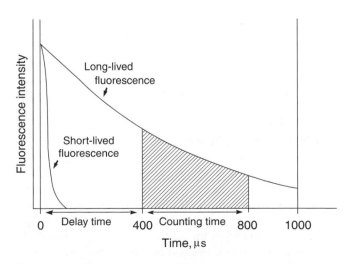

Fig. 4-19 Schema showing difference between short- and long-lived fluorescence.

these reactions are not known. A partial reaction may be written as follows:

$$2\ H_2O_2 + \text{Luminol and enhancer} \xrightarrow{\text{Peroxidase}} 2\ H_2O + h\nu + \text{Oxidized luminol}$$

The peroxidase is often part of an enzyme-labeled immunoassay system in which peroxidase is the label. The reaction can be measured by very sensitive photomultiplier tubes. The advantage of this technique is that it can be very sensitive. One molecule of peroxidase can turn over several million molecules of substrate per minute. Thus detection can be more sensitive than that achievable with radio-isotopes. A disadvantage of the system is that the reaction is performed in a heterogeneous system in which the peroxidase is attached to a solid phase. The H_2O_2 and luminol must be in a system free from common biological matrices, such as serum, and therefore a separation step is necessary.

Other dye systems resulting in quantitative chemilumines-cent reactions use the aromatic acridinium esters and the dioxetanes. The acridinium esters are most often oxidized by hydrogen peroxide to yield light, whereas the dioxetanes are made into stable phosphate ester derivatives that, when hydrolyzed, become spontaneously degraded, yielding light as one of the products.

Bioluminescence, the naturally occurring chemilumines-cence phenomenon, has been extensively studied, and the reaction involving the molecule luciferin, adenosine tri-phosphate (ATP), and luciferase in the presence of oxygen is the best understood.

$$\text{Luciferin} + \text{ATP} + O_2 \xrightarrow{\text{Luciferase}} \text{Oxyluciferin} + \text{Light}$$

The reaction is quantitative because one photon of light is released for every ATP consumed. The sensitivity of the reaction is limited only by the photodetector's ability to count photons.

Electrochemiluminescence[26]

The electrochemiluminescence process is based on the for-mation of an excited-state chemical intermediate that returns to the ground state by emitting a photon. This technique of excitation is different from those in which an excited state is achieved by absorption of a photon. In this case the excited state is reached by a chemical reaction. One commercially successful system is based on the chemiluminescent properties of ruthenium complexes when they encounter free radicals. In this system a ruthenium(II)-tris(bipyridyl) [$Ru(bpy)_3^{2+}$] complex is oxidized from the 2^+ state to a 3^+ state by interaction with the cathode. This 3^+ complex reacts with a free radical, reducing the complex to a highly excited 2^+ state. The excited complex then emits a photon to return to the ground state. The complex may be recycled to undergo these same reactions. It is this reaction with the free radical that powers the excited state. The free radicals in the Igen system are generated by the reaction of tripropylamine (TPA) with the anode, which yields a positively charged TPA free radical. This species gives up a hydrogen ion to form the TPA free radical. This free radical reacts with the 3^+ complex.

$$\text{Ru (complex)}^{2+} \xrightarrow{\text{electrode}} e^- + \text{Ru (complex)}^{3+}$$

$$\text{TPA} \xrightarrow{\text{electrode}} e^- + \text{TPA}^{\bullet+} \rightarrow \text{TPA}^\bullet + H^+$$

$$\text{Ru (complex)}^{3+} + \text{TPA}^{\bullet+}\ e^- \rightarrow \text{TPA degradation products} + \text{excited Ru (complex)}^{2+}$$

$$\text{excited Ru (complex)}^{2+} \rightarrow \text{Ru (complex)}^{2+} + h\nu \text{ (light at 620 nm)}$$

The light from the excited Ru (complex)$^{2+}$ is released over about 0.6 seconds. Therefore this is a luminescent process. The ruthenium complex can be attached to proteins, nucleic acids, and ligands. These labeled molecules are used in a variety of immunoassay formats.

Fluorescence Polarization[21,27,28]

Light is considered to be composed of an electronic vector and a magnetic vector. If the light is polarized, all the electronic vectors have the same orientation.

When light is absorbed by a fluorescent molecule, it excites the chromophore that has specific orientations, result-ing in the transition of an electron to a higher energy level. The excited molecule emits light as the electron (fluorescent oscillator) returns to a lower energy level. Fluorescence polarization measurements require a dye with an electronic orientation such that the emitted light retains the initial orientation of the incident beam. An example of such a molecule is fluorescein. If polarized light is used to excite fluorescein molecules, the reemitted fluorescent light can also be polarized. However, molecules in solution rotate, and so this orientation and the fluorescence polarization can be lost. In fluorescence polarization, the dye must be selected so that its molecular rotation is so great between the times of light absorption and emission that the molecule becomes randomly oriented during this time and the fluorescence is minimally polarized. The quantity that is measured is the intensity of the oriented light or the difference between the oriented and nonoriented light.

To measure polarized light, several options are available. One approach is to excite the test solution with light polarized in one dimension and to record the amount of the emitted fluorescence. The polarizer is placed immediately after the first monochromator as shown in the diagram of a fluorometer given in Fig. 4-18. The solution is then excited by light that is polarized at 90 degrees to the light used in the first excitation, and the emitted fluorescence is recorded. Polarization (*P*) can be determined from the following equation:

$$P = \frac{I_{vv} - I_{hv}}{I_{vv} + I_{hv}}$$

in which I_{vv} equals the signal recorded when the vertically polarized light is used to excite the sample, and I_{hv} is the response when the horizontally polarized light is used to excite the sample. Emitted light is measured from the vertical polarizer at a 90-degree orientation from the incident light by use of a second polarizer that is placed before the second monochromator.

Numerous processes affect the final polarization. For many fluorescent dyes, including the most popular one, fluorescein, orientation of light is retained if the molecule is held rigid. When the molecule randomly rotates by the process of brownian motion, polarization is lost. The ability of a molecule in solution to rotate partially depends on the viscosity of the solution and on the molecular volume of the molecule. When the viscosity of the solution or the molecular volume increases, the fluorescent molecules rotate slower and the polarization increases. In the case of the fluorescence polarization immunoassay, when the drug-fluorescein derivative is bound by antibody, the molecular volume increases. Therefore the **polarized fluorescence** increases. When the derivative is unbound, the molecular volume is low and the fluorescence polarization is low (see Chapter 13).

Fluorescence polarization measurements can be made very accurately, and they are less affected by variations in fluorescence intensity than standard fluorescence measurements are (see previous equation). Thus precision on the order of 1% or greater of measurement is readily achieved, which translates into more precise assay measurements. Another advantage of fluorescence polarization is that the technique can be used as a homogeneous assay. Disadvantages include the fact that the technique is limited to assays that can use fluorescent dyes, the instrumentation required for performing fluorescence polarization measurement is often very specialized and may measure only fluorescence intensity or polarization, and the system is less flexible than absorption spectroscopy. In addition, when performing fluorescence polarization measurements, it is crucial to control temperature and viscosity.

NEPHELOMETRY AND TURBIDIMETRY[29-31]
Principle

Interaction of light with particles. To understand the principle of nephelometric or turbidimetric assays, we must first examine the concept of light scattering. When a collimated (that is, parallel, nondivergent) beam of light strikes a particle in suspension, some light is reflected, some is scattered, some is absorbed, and some is transmitted. Nephelometry is the measurement of the light scattered by a particulate solution. Turbidity measures **light scattering** as a decrease in the light transmitted through the solution.

In considering nephelometry, the question of how light is scattered by a *homogeneous* particle suspension must be examined. Three types of scatter can occur. If the wavelength, λ, of light is much larger than the size of the particle ($d < 0.1\ \lambda$), the light is symmetrically scattered around the particle, with a minimum in the intensity of the scatter occurring at 90 degrees to the incident beam, as described by Rayleigh (Fig. 4-20, *A*).

If the wavelength of the incident light is much smaller than the size of the particle ($d > 10\lambda$), most of the light appears to be scattered forward because of destructive out-of-phase backscatter, as described by the Mie theory (Fig. 4-20, *B*).

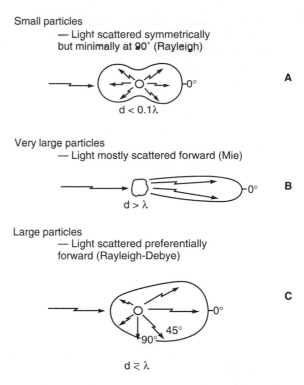

Fig. 4-20 Effect of particle size on scattering of incident light in a homogeneous solution. *(From Gauldie J: Principles and clinical applications of nephelometry. In Kaplan LA, Pesce AJ, editors:* Nonisotopic alternatives to radioimmunoassay, *New York, 1981, Marcel Dekker. Reprinted from Ref. [02], p 109, by courtesy of Marcel Dekker, Inc.)*

If, however, the wavelength of light is approximately equal to the size of the particles, more light appears scattered in a forward direction than in a backward direction (Fig. 4-20, *C*), as described by Rayleigh-Debye scatter.[27]

One of the most common uses of light-scattering analyses is the measurement of antigen-antibody reactions. Because most antigen-antibody complex systems are heterogeneous with particle diameters of 250 to 1500 nm and the wavelengths used in most light-scattering analyzers are 320 to 650 nm, the scatter seen is essentially Rayleigh-Debye, with the blank scatter being primarily described by **Rayleigh scatter**. Thus the ability to detect light scatter in a forward direction ($\theta = 15$ to 90 degrees) leads to greater sensitivity for nephelometric determinations. Such is the case in the newer rate and laser nephelometers.

Detection of scattered light

Turbidimetry. Turbidimetry measures the reduction in the light transmission caused by particle formation, and it quantifies the residual light transmitted (Fig. 4-21). The instrumentation required for turbidimetric measurements ranges from a simple manual spectrophotometer available in most laboratories to a sophisticated discrete analyzer. Because this technique measures a decrease in a large signal of transmitted light, the photometric accuracy and sensitivity of the instrument primarily limit the sensitivity of turbidimetry. Instruments used for turbidimetry can be used for many other assays, such as enzyme assays and those assays based on color development.

Nephelometry. Nephelometry, on the other hand, detects a portion of the light that is scattered at a variety of angles (Fig. 4-22). The sensitivity of this method primarily depends on the absence of blank or background scatter, because the instruments are detecting a small increment of signal at a scatter angle, θ, on a supposedly black, or null, background. Ideally, no light is detected in the absence of a scattering species, and so subsequent scatter in samples is measured against this black background. The signal is magnified by

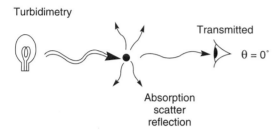

Fig. 4-21 Schema of turbidity measurement. θ, Angle of detection. *(From Gauldie J: Principles and clinical applications of nephelometry. In Kaplan LA, Pesce AJ, editors: Nonisotopic alternatives to radioimmunoassay, New York, 1981, Marcel Dekker. Reprinted from Ref. [02], p 109, by courtesy of Marcel Dekker, Inc.)*

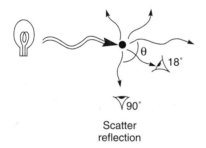

Fig. 4-22 Schema of nephelometric measurements. θ, Angle of detection. *(From Gauldie J: Principles and clinical applications of nephelometry. In Kaplan LA, Pesce AJ, editors: Nonisotopic alternatives to radioimmunoassay, New York, 1981, Marcel Dekker. Reprinted from Ref. [02], p 109, by courtesy of Marcel Dekker, Inc.)*

the use of a photomultiplier, and so the detection range is increased. However, such measurements require the committed use of a nephelometer, which has limited use in other assays.

Instrumentation

Schematic layout of instruments. A schematic layout of the basic components of a nephelometer is shown in Fig. 4-23. Typical systems consist of a light source, a collimating system, a wavelength selector such as a filter (the last two items are unnecessary with laser light sources), a sample cuvette, a stray light trap, and a photodetector.

Light source. Fluoronephelometers use a medium-pressure mercury-arc lamp as a light source, which serves both for nephelometry and fluorometry. The relatively high-intensity light and short-wavelength emission bands make this a good source. Other light sources range from simple low-voltage tungsten-filament lamps and light-emitting diodes to sophisticated low-power lasers. Lasers produce stable, highly collimated, and intense beams of light (typically 1 milliradian divergence) that require no additional optical collimators as other light sources do. In optical systems using laser light, it is easier to reduce stray light, which contributes to background scatter, and to mask the transmitted beam, thus allowing measurement of forward scatter. The increase in light intensity achievable with lasers also results in an improvement of signal-to-noise ratio, but this is limited somewhat by detector saturation. Disadvantages of laser sources include cost, safety problems, and the restricted availability of limited fixed wavelengths. Because particle size may continually change during the course of reaction analysis, as during immune precipitate formation, light scatter at a single wavelength may change while the average light scatter over many wavelengths remains relatively constant. The Beckman Array employs a broad-band filter for selection of a wavelength region from a normal tungsten lamp source to overcome this problem, which is obviously more acute in rate methods when the size of the particle is changing most rapidly.

In all cases, the photodetector system must be matched to the wavelength or wavelengths of the scattered light, which, for nephelometry and turbidimetry, corresponds to the incident light wavelength or wavelengths.

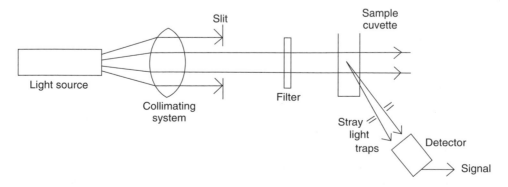

Fig. 4-23 Schema of basic components of a nephelometer.

Angle of detection.[32] Because particles the size of antigen-antibody complexes appear to scatter light more in the forward direction, there is an increased signal-to-noise ratio as the detector is placed nearer the transmitted path (0 degrees).

The blank signal, described best by Rayleigh scatter (see Fig. 4-20, *A*), is not so affected by an altered **angle of detection.** Thus, although most early nephelometers detected light scattered at 90 degrees for reasons of manufacturing ease, which limited low-angle measurement capability, the detection of forward light scatter should provide theoretically greater sensitivity. The newer instruments tend to operate with lower detection angles, optimized in many cases to give the highest signal-to-noise ratio for the particular instrument's optics. Obviously, detection at 0 degrees is not possible because of the high intensity of the transmitted beam, but some laser-equipped fast analyzers using a mask to block the transmitted beam are able to operate at very low angles. Instruments employing low-angle detectors tend to have greater sensitivity than the 90-degree type of instruments.

Limitations: Turbidimetry Versus Nephelometry

Although the principle of nephelometry—detection of a small signal (amplifiable) on a black background—should lend this method high sensitivity, the sophistication and specifications of the instruments available do not achieve this promise. Turbidimetry—detection of a small decrease in a large signal—should be limited in sensitivity; however, current instruments have excellent discrimination and can quantify small changes in signal, thereby allowing turbidimetric measurements to achieve high sensitivity.

Turbidimetry and nephelometry have similarities to absorption spectrophotometry, and many sources of interference and errors are common to all these systems. Many techniques, discussed in Chapter 23, that can be used to minimize absorption interferences are also applicable to turbidimetry and nephelometry. Nevertheless, sample turbidity can be an interference for both techniques. Because of the uniqueness of nephelometric measurements, especially in the case of antibody-antigen reactions, some specific applications are discussed in this chapter.

Endogenous color and choice of wavelength. Basic light-scattering theory predicts that the intensity of scattered light increases as shorter wavelengths of incident light are used. Most immunological assay reactions employ serum protein reactions requiring the choice of a wavelength at which neither the proteins nor the colored serum components absorb appreciably. Because proteins absorb strongly at wavelengths shorter than 300 nm and serum has an absorption peak at 400 to 425 nm because of porphyrins, instruments tend to operate in the 320 to 380 or 500 to 650 nm ranges. Reduction of the protein concentration by dilution decreases background absorption. Most immunochemical reactions measured by nephelometry use high-affinity antibodies that allow for large dilutions of protein and consequent improvement of sensitivity.

Comparison of sensitivity. Sensitivity in nephelometers is largely controlled by the amount of background scatter from sample and reagents. Because background scatter can be high relative to specific scatter, instruments do not reach their full potential of sensitivity. This limitation, coupled with the higher wavelengths generated in laser instruments, accounts for the fact that laser instruments show no great increase in sensitivity over conventional nephelometers.

Sensitivity in turbidimetric measurements depends on the ability of the detector to resolve small changes in light intensity. Using low wavelengths and high-quality spectrophotometers with their high-precision detection systems, sensitivity in turbidimetry is usually adequate for many measurements and in many cases compares well to nephelometry. Theoretically, with additional refinements nephelometry ultimately should provide higher sensitivity than turbidimetry does.

End-point versus kinetic analysis. Examination of light scattered as a function of time, after there is mixture of an antibody and antigen, shows that after an initial delay there is an almost linear increase in scatter followed by a slower attainment of plateau scatter. The secondary reaction occurs much more slowly than the first because larger particles form and begin to flocculate, and they distort the scatter intensity seen at forward angles. Both turbidity and nephelometry measurements behave in this manner.

There are two basic ways of measuring light scatter caused by this reaction, end-point analysis and rate analysis. End-point analysis requires blank (reagent) determinations and a reasonable amount of elapsed time before final measurement. Fig. 4-24 shows the forward scatter developed at 70 degrees of a rate nephelometric analyzer.[31] Comparing the two graphs, the differences between an end-point analysis (blank value versus reading at $t = x$) and a rate or kinetic analysis (increase in scattered intensity over a set time interval) can be seen. The kinetic approach, which electronically subtracts any blank signal, does not require a separate reagent blank to be run. Both kinetic and end-point analysis can be applied equally to turbidimetry and nephelometry.

REFRACTIVITY
Principle

When a beam of light impinges on a boundary surface, it can be reflected, absorbed, or, if the material is transparent, pass into the boundary and emerge on the other side. When light passes from one medium into another, the path of the light beam changes direction at the boundary surface if its speed in the second medium is different from that in the first (Fig. 4-25). This bending of light is called **refraction.**[33]

Because the degree of refraction of a light beam depends on the difference in the speed of light between two different media, the *ratio* of the two speeds has been expressed as the *index of refraction*, or **refractive index**. The relative ability of a substance to bend light is called *refractivity.* The expression of a refractive index, *n,* is always relative to air with the convention that *n* of air = 1. The measurement of the

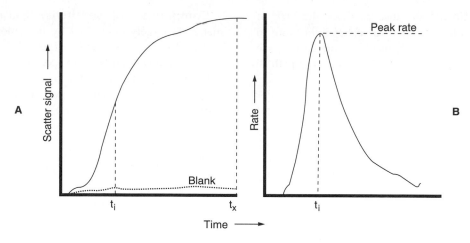

Fig. 4-24 Kinetic analysis of light scattering. **A,** Intensity of scattered light signal versus time. **B,** Rate of change of scattered light signal versus time.

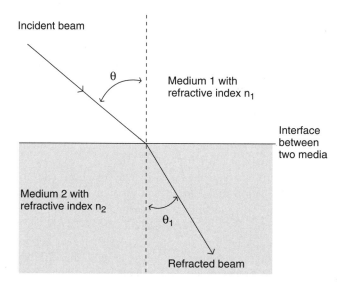

Fig. 4-25 Schema illustrating bending of light when it passes from a medium of one density into a medium of a different density, with an angle of deflection, θ_1.

refractive index is the measurement of angles, because the light is bent at an angle proportional to the relationship of n in the medium through which the light is passing:

$$\frac{n}{n_1} = \frac{\sin \theta}{\sin \theta_1}$$

The refractivity of a liquid depends on (1) the wavelength of the incident light, (2) the temperature, (3) the nature of the liquid, and (4) the total mass of solid dissolved in the liquid. If the first three factors are held constant, the refractive index of a solution is a direct measure of the total mass of dissolved solids.

Applications

Refractometry has been applied to the measurement of total serum protein concentration.[34] The assumption of this analysis is that the serum matrix (that is, the concentration of

electrolytes and small organic molecules) remains essentially the same from patient to patient. Because the mass of protein is normally so much greater than the mass of other serum constituents, small variations of these other substances have no significant effect on the refractive index of serum. **Refractometers** are calibrated against "normal" serum, and total protein concentrations are read directly from a scale.

Refractometry is also used to estimate the specific gravity of urine samples. The refractive index is linearly related to the total mass of dissolved solids and thus to specific gravity. This remains valid over most of the range normally encountered for urine (that is, up to 1.035 g/mL).

Interference

When the concentration of small molecular weight compounds or particulate matter greatly increases, positive interference results. This interference occurs in the presence of

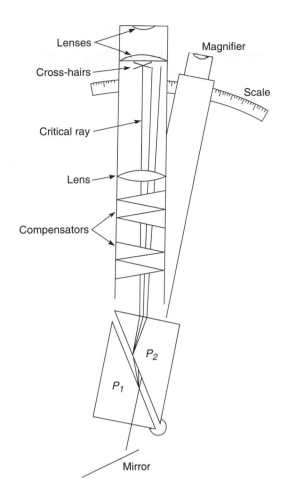

Lenses

Magnifier

Cross-hairs

Scale

Critical ray

Lens

Compensators

P_2

P_1

Mirror

Fig. 4-26 Schema of an Abbé refractometer. *(From Shugar GJ, Shugar RA, Bauman L: Chemical technicians' ready reference book, New York, 1973, McGraw-Hill. Reproduced by permission of the McGraw-Hill Companies.)*

hyperglycemia, hyperbilirubinemia, azotemia (increased serum urea), lyophilized samples, and hyperlipidemia. Hemolysis also results in false-positive values for total serum protein.

Instrumentation

Most clinical refractometers are based on the Abbé refractometer (Fig. 4-26), marketed by American Optical Corporation. This refractometer consists of two prisms and a series of lenses. Light passes through the first prism where the light beam is dispersed. The dispersed light passes into and through the thin layer of the liquid sample where it is refracted. The light beam passes through a second prism where the light is again dispersed and on leaving is again refracted. The boundary at the edge of the refracted light beam is aligned perpendicularly to the scale on which serum protein concentrations or specific gravity can be read. The scale for reading serum protein (g/dL or g/L) is established by calibration of the instrument against a "normal" serum solution. This type of refractometer is extraordinarily simple, having no moving or electrical parts. Thus it is easily reproducible, measuring protein with a precision of ±1% and an accuracy of ±1 g/L. The sample size is on the order of 50 μL.

More complex refractometers are used to monitor column effluents for high-performance liquid chromatography analysis (see Chapter 6).

References

1. Richards WG, Scott RR: *Structure and spectra of molecules,* New York, 1985, Wiley & Sons.
2. Clayton RK: *Light and living matter: the physical part,* New York, 1970, McGraw-Hill.
3. Jaffe HH, Orchin M: *Theory and applications of ultraviolet spectroscopy,* New York, 1966, Wiley & Sons.
4. Willard HH, Merritt LL, Dean JA: *Instrumental methods of analysis,* ed 4, Princeton, NJ, 1965, Van Nostrand.
5. Frings CS, Broussard LA: Calibration and monitoring of spectrometers and spectrophotometers, *Clin Chem* 25:1013, 1979.
6. Brewer JM, Pesce AJ, Ashworth RB, editors: *Experimental techniques in biochemistry,* Englewood Cliffs, NJ, 1974, Prentice-Hall.

7. Keller H: Optical methods of measurement. In Richterich R, Colombo JP, editors: *Clinical chemistry,* New York, 1981, Wiley & Sons.

8. Ward KM, Harris E: Spectrophotometry. In Ward KM, Lehmann CA, Leiken AM, editors: *Clinical laboratory instrumentation and automation: principles, application, and selection,* Philadelphia, 1994, WB Saunders.

9. Narayanan S: *Principles and applications of laboratory instrumentation,* Chicago, 1989, ASCP Press.

10. Khazanie P: Spectrophotometry. In Anderson SC, Cockagne S, editors: *Clinical chemistry: concepts and applications,* Philadelphia, 1993, WB Saunders.

11. *Federal Register* 57(4):7164-7165, 1992.

12. Instrumentation Guidelines Study Group, Subcommittee on Enzymes: Guidelines for photometric instruments for measuring enzyme reaction rates, *Clin Chem* 23:2160, 1977.

13. Alexander LR, Barnhart ER: *Photometric quality assurance instrument check procedures,* Atlanta, 1980, U.S. Department of Health and Human Services, Centers for Disease Control, Bureau of Laboratories.

14. Curme HG et al: Multilayer film elements for clinical analysis: general concepts, *Clin Chem* 24:1335, 1978.

15. Zijlstr WG, Buursma A, Zwart A: Performance of an automated six-wavelength photometer (Radiometer OSM3) for routine measurement of hemoglobin derivatives, *Clin Chem* 34:149, 1988.

16. Rubeska I: *Atomic absorption spectroscopy,* Cleveland, 1969, Chemical Rubber Co. Press.

17. Robinson JW: *Atomic absorption spectroscopy,* ed 2, New York, 1973, Marcel Dekker.

18. Winefordner JD, editor: *Spectrochemical methods of analysis,* New York, 1977, Wiley & Sons, Wiley Interscience.

19. Dvorak J, Rubeska I, Rezak Z: *Flame photometry: laboratory practice,* Cleveland, 1971, Chemical Rubber Co. Press.

20. Simonson MG: The application of a photon-counting fluorometer for the immunofluorescent measurement of therapeutic drugs. In Kaplan LA, Pesce AJ, editors: *Nonisotopic alternatives to radioimmunoassay,* New York, 1981, Marcel Dekker.

21. Pesce AJ, Rosen CG, Pasby TL, editors: *Fluorescence spectroscopy,* New York, 1971, Marcel Dekker.

22. Wehry FL, editor: *Modern fluorescence spectroscopy,* New York, 1976, Plenum Press.

23. Hemmilä I: Fluoroimmunoassays and immunofluorometric assays, *Clin Chem* 31:359, 1985.

24. *Enhanced luminescence: a practical immunoassay system,* Medicine Publishing Foundation Symposium Series 18, Oxford, UK, 1986, Medicine Publishing Foundation.

25. Scholmerich J et al, editors: *Bioluminescence and chemiluminescence: new perspectives,* New York, 1987, Wiley & Sons.

26. Blackburn GF et al: Electrochemiluminescence detection for development of immunoassays and DNA probe assays for clinical diagnostics, *Clin Chem* 37:1534, 1991.

27. Spencer RD: Fluorescence polarization. In Kaplan LA, Pesce AJ, editors: *Nonisotopic alternatives to radioimmunoassay,* New York, 1981, Marcel Dekker.

28. Jolly MD et al: Fluorescence polarization immunoassay. I. Monitoring aminoglycoside antibiotics in serum and plasma, *Clin Chem* 27:1190, 1981.

29. Ritchie RF, editor: *Automated immunoanalysis,* parts 1 and 2, New York, 1978, Marcel Dekker.

30. Deverill I, Reeves WG: Light scattering and absorption developments in immunology, *J Immunol Methods* 38:191, 1980.

31. Gauldie J: Principles and clinical applications of nephelometry. In Kaplan LA, Pesce AJ, editors: *Nonisotopic alternatives to radio-immunoassay,* New York, 1981, Marcel Dekker.

32. Kusnetz J, Mansberg HP: Nephelometry. In Ritchie RF: *Automated immunoanalysis,* part 1, New York, 1978, Marcel Dekker.

33. Glover FA, Gaulden JDS: Relationship between refractive index and concentration of solutions, *Nature* 200:1165, 1963.

34. Rubini MD, Wolf AV: Refractometric determination of total solids and water of serum and urine, *J Biol Chem* 225:868, 1957.

Bibliography

Skoog DA, Holler JF, Nieman TA: *Principles of instrumental analysis,* 1998, Brooks/Cole.

Internet Sites

http://depts.washington.edu/spectral

http://www.nist.gov/srd/analy.htm—National Institute of Standards and Technology (NIST)

http://www.aist.go.jp/RIODB/SDBS/menu-e.html—SDBS Integrated Spectral Data Base System for Organic Compounds; National Institute of Advanced Industrial Science and Technology, Tsukuba, Ibaraki, Japan

http://www.bertholf.net/rlb/Lectures/Lectures/Review%20of%20Analytical%20Methods%20I.pps—PowerPoint lecture by Robert L. Bertholf PhD, Associate Professor of Pathology, Chief of Clinical Chemistry and Toxicology

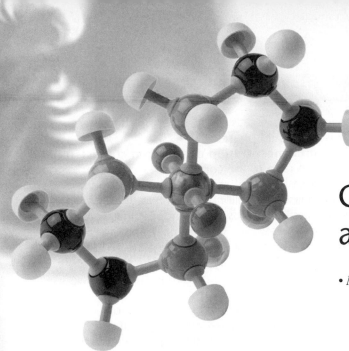

CHAPTER 5

Chromatography: Theory and Practice

• *M. Wilson Tabor*

Chapter Outline

Branches of chromatography
General principles
Resolution
  Theoretical plates
  Retention
  Selectivity
  Improving peak resolution
Polarity
  Solvent polarity and solvent strength
  Stationary-phase polarity and selectivity
Mechanisms of chromatography
  Adsorption

Partition
Ion exchange
Gel-permeation (molecular or size exclusion)
  chromatography
Sample preparation for chromatography
  Nature of problem
  Mechanical methods for initial isolation of analyte
  Chromatographic methods for initial isolation of analyte
  Extraction methods for analyte isolation
  Processing of sample extracts

Objectives

- State the general principles of chromatography and describe their application to the divisions and subdivisions of chromatography, supporting each description with an illustration of mechanism.
- State the effect of each of the following chromatographic parameters on the resolution of a chromatographic separation:
  1. Height equivalent to a theoretical plate
  2. Retention time
  3. Mobile phase polarity
  4. R_f
- Describe the separation processes involved with the following types of chromatography and list

the class of molecules that can be separated by each type:
  1. Adsorption
  2. Partition
  3. Ion exchange
  4. Gel permeation
- Describe four physicochemical forces that are central to polarity and explain how polarity affects the chromatographic behavior of compounds in normal-phase and reversed-phase chromatography.
- List three basic techniques for sample preparation for chromatography and provide the basis of purification for each technique.

Key Terms

adsorption   Process whereby one substance adheres to another because of attractive forces between surface atoms of the two substances. (See Fig. 5-13.)

analyte   The substance or component in a sample that is being measured.

band   A chromatographic zone; that is, a region where the separated substance is concentrated.

capacity factor   The ratio of the elution volume of a substance to the void volume in the column. (See Equation 5-6 and Fig. 5-9, *A*.) Also called *retention factor* (*k*).

chromatogram   A series of separated bands or zones detected either visually, as in some paper chromatographic or thin-layer chromatographic separations, or indirectly by a detection system. In the latter case, the detection system usually outputs an electrical signal, which is graphically plotted through time, to display the series of separated bands or zones.

chromatography   A method of analysis in which the flow of a mobile phase (gas or liquid) containing the sample promotes the separation of sample components, which are differentially distributed between this phase and a stationary phase. The stationary phase may be a solid or a liquid coated or bonded onto a solid.

dipole   The attractive force of compounds with centers of both positive and negative charges that are the result of an unequal sharing of bonding electrons between two elements of the compound with large differences in electronegativity. (See Fig. 5-11, *B*.)

dispersive force   The attractive force, sometimes termed *van der Waals forces,* of compounds that results from the induction of a temporary dipole within an individual compound. (See Fig. 5-11, *A*.)

efficiency   A measure of chromatographic performance usually related to the sharpness of the peaks in the chromatogram and quantitated by the number, *N*, of theoretical plates of a column. (See Equation 5-3, Figs. 5-6 and 5-7, and Table 5-1.)

electrostatic interaction   The attractive force between compounds with formal positive or negative charges. (See Fig. 5-11, *D*.)

eluotropic series   Series of solvents or solvent mixtures arranged in the order of their ability to elute a solute from an adsorbent.

elution   Removal of a solute from a stationary phase by passage of a suitable mobile phase.

elution volume (V_e)   The volume of mobile phase required to elute a solute from a chromatographic column. (See Equation 5-6 and Fig. 5-9, *A*.)

emulsion   For a liquid-liquid extraction, a mixture formed when one of the immiscible liquid phases becomes dispersed as fine droplets in the other immiscible liquid phase.

equilibrium concentration distribution coefficient (K_D)   The ratio of the concentration of a sample component in one phase to its concentration in a second phase at equilibrium. The two phases may be two immiscible liquids or the mobile phase and the stationary phase. (See Equation 5-1 and Fig. 5-3.)

height equivalent to a theoretical plate (HETP)   The number obtained by dividing the column length by the theoretical plate number. (See Equation 5-4 and Fig. 5-7.)

hydrogen bonding   The attractive force of compounds formed when a hydrogen atom covalently linked to an electronegative element, like oxygen, nitrogen, or sulfur, has a large degree of positive character relative to the electronegative atom, thereby causing the compound to possess a large dipole. (See Fig. 5-11, *C*.)

partition   Process by which a solute is distributed between two immiscible phases. (See Fig. 5-15.)

peak   A band or zone in a chromatogram showing a maximum of concentration between two minima.

pK_a   The pK of an acid is the pH at which it is half-dissociated.

polarity (*P'*)   The attractive forces encompassing the total interaction of solvent molecules with sample molecules and of solvent or sample molecules with the stationary phase.

R_f   A ratio used in paper chromatography and thin-layer chromatography that is the distance from the origin to the center of the separated zone divided by the distance from the origin to the solvent front. (See Equation 5-9.)

resolution (*R* or *R_s*)   The degree of separation between two components by chromatography. (See Equations 5-2, 5-8, and 5-10 and Fig. 5-5.)

retention time (t_R)   The time that has elapsed from the injection of the sample into the chromatographic system to the recording of the peak maximum of the component in the chromatogram. (See Fig. 5-7.)

selectivity (*α*)   The ratios of the capacity factors for two substances measured under identical chromatographic conditions; sometimes termed *separation factor* or *chromatographic selectivity*. (See Equation 5-7 and Fig. 5-9, *B*.)

theoretical plate number (*N*)   A number defining the efficiency of the chromatographic column. (See Equation 5-3 and Fig. 5-7.)

void volume (V_0)   The interstitial volume of the chromatographic column, that is, the volume of mobile phase imbided in the pores and around the stationary phase in a column. (See Equation 5-8 and Fig. 5-9, *A*.)

The need for fast, reproducible, and accurate analyses for many classes of analytes present in small amounts is being met today in the clinical laboratory largely as a result of the developments in chromatography during the past two decades.

Chromatography is a collective term referring to a group of separation processes whereby a mixture of solutes, dissolved in a common solvent, are separated from one another by a differential distribution of the solutes between two phases. One phase, the solvent, is mobile and carries the mixture of solutes through the other phase, the fixed or stationary phase. Chromatographic methods encompass a great number of variations in technique in which the mobile phase ranges from liquids to gases and the stationary phase ranges from sheets of cellulose paper to capillary glass tubes as fine as a human hair that are internally coated with a covalently bonded complex or complex organic polymers. A cursory examination of the scientific literature shows that both the numbers of chromatographic methods published and their applications have been growing exponentially.[1-4]

Modern chromatography began in 1906, when Michael S. Tswett detailed his separation of chlorophylls using a column of calcium carbonate (chalk)[5] and introduced a system of nomenclature that is now universally applied to chromatography ('color writing,' from the Greek words *khrōma, khrōmatos,*, meaning 'color,' and *graphē,* meaning 'drawing, writing'). This is but the first of the many published accounts of the colorful history of chromatography.[6]

BRANCHES OF CHROMATOGRAPHY

Chromatographic methods are generally classified according to the physical state of the solute carrier phase, that is, the mobile phase. These branches are represented in Figs. 5-1 and 5-2 as solution and gas chromatography, referring to the respective liquid and gaseous states of the mobile phase. In Fig. 5-1 these branches are further classified according to how the stationary-phase matrix is contained for a particular chromatographic method. For example, solution chromatography is divided into flat and column methods, depending on whether the stationary phase is a thin layer mechanically

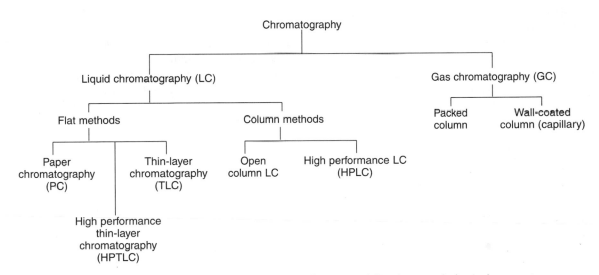

Fig. 5-1   Branches of chromatography according to mobile phase and physical apparatus.

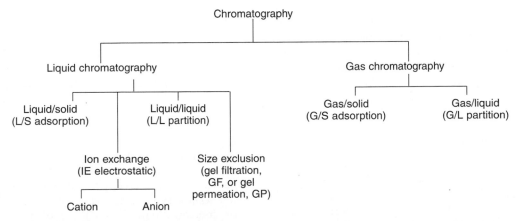

Fig. 5-2   Branches of chromatography according to mechanism of separation on stationary phase.

supported on a sheet or is packed into a column. The flat method of support may involve use of a sheet of paper, such as cellulose, or a thin layer on a mechanical backing, such as glass or plastic.

Column methods are classically referred to as *liquid chromatography.* Furthermore, *column methods* is a term generally used to subdivide solution chromatography wherein the stationary phase is packed into a glass or metal tube. However, it is noted that gas chromatography is strictly a column method because a column must be used for containment of the stationary phase (see Chapter 7).

The main divisions of chromatography, based on mobile phase, may also be subdivided according to the mechanism of solute interaction with the stationary phase (see Fig. 5-2). Two mechanisms, **adsorption** and **partition**, are the most commonly encountered for both solution and gas mobile-phase separations. Adsorption chromatography (liquid-solid [L/S] or gas-solid [G/S]) is a process whereby solutes of a sample are separated by their differences in *attraction* to the stationary versus the mobile phase. Partition chromatography (liquid-liquid [L/L] or gas-liquid [G/L]) is a process whereby the solutes of a sample are separated by differences in their *distribution* between two liquid phases (L/L) or between a gas and a liquid phase (G/L). In both cases of partition chromatography, the stationary phase is liquid, and the mobile phase is a liquid or a gas.

Other mechanistic divisions of solution chromatography are ion exchange and gel permeation. Ion-exchange chromatography (IE) uses an insoluble matrix containing covalently linked ionic groups for the stationary phase, which can reversibly exchange either cations or anions with the mobile phase. Gel-filtration (GF) chromatography refers to a stationary phase of a solvent-swollen hydrophilic gel in the form of porous beads that is used with an aqueous-solvent mobile phase. Gel-permeation (GP) chromatography refers to a stationary phase of solvent-swollen hydrophobic gel in the form of porous beads that is used with an organic-solvent mobile phase. Both GF and GP chromatography are sometimes referred to as *molecular exclusion* (or *inclusion*) *chromatography* (see p. 123).

The boundaries between these mechanistically different types of chromatography are not finite, since for some chromatographic separations more than one mechanism may be operating. For example, in GF chromatography adsorptive interactions between the solute molecules and the stationary phase are common, in addition to the prevailing size-exclusion mechanism. More discussion of these mechanisms is presented after a brief discussion of chromatographic theory and principles.

GENERAL PRINCIPLES

The theoretical basis of chromatography is well developed, with both solution and gas-phase methods sharing the same foundation.[7] Only a few general concepts of this theory are discussed in this section. For more extensive discussions and additional reference leads, refer to representative reviews and books[8-14] and the *Analytical Chemistry*

compendium reviews[1-5,15] on specialized chromatographic techniques.

The separation of a mixture containing two or more components is an operation with the goal of producing fractions, with each fraction having an increased concentration of one component relative to the other components contained in the original mixture. The physicochemical basis of chromatographic separation techniques is principally distribution equilibrium.[12] Distribution equilibrium refers to the differences in solubility and adsorption of a component in two immiscible phases.

Separation equilibrium can be visualized as the distribution of a solute, S, between two immiscible phases, upper phase (u) and lower phase (l), at constant temperature and pressure. The ratio of the solute concentrations in the two phases determines the separation, which can be defined by an **equilibrium concentration distribution coefficient (K_D)** for the molar concentration, C_u and C_l, of solute in the upper and lower phases respectively:

$$K_D = \frac{C_u}{C_l} \qquad \textit{Eq. 5-1}$$

Molar concentration is defined in the classical sense as the number of moles of solute per unit volume of solvent. The distribution coefficient is sometimes referred to as a *partition ratio*. In practical terms, a K_D of 1.0 means that 50% of the solute is distributed in the upper phase and 50% is distributed in the lower phase (Fig. 5-3, *A*). Likewise, a K_D of 9.0 means

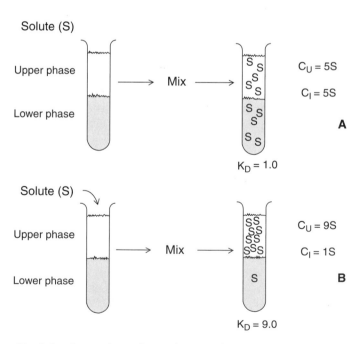

Fig. 5-3 Separation of a solute, S, by partition into two different solvent systems. In the first system, **A**, solute has a distribution coefficient, K_D, of 1.0, indicating an equal partitioning between upper and lower phases after mixing. In the second system, **B**, solute has a K_D of 9.0, indicating a partitioning of nine parts of the solute in the upper phase and one part of the solute in the lower phase after mixing. C_u, Upper-phase concentration; C_l, lower-phase concentration.

that 90% of the solute is distributed in the upper phase and 10% is in the lower phase (Fig. 5-3, *B*).

For a more generalized application of distribution coefficients to chromatography, let $C_l = C_m$, where C_m refers to the amount of the solute distributed into a unit amount of mobile phase, and let $C_u = C_s$, where C_s refers to the amount of the solute distributed into a unit amount of stationary phase. In this more generalized case, the distribution equilibriums for a solute being separated in a given chromatographic system at constant temperature (that is, *isothermal*) can be graphically illustrated by a plot of solute concentration in the mobile phase, C_m, versus the concentration in the stationary phase, C_s. This is called an *adsorption-distribution isotherm plot* (Fig. 5-4, *A*). The slope of the isotherm is equal to the distribution equilibrium coefficient, K_D.

The resulting shape of a distribution isotherm plot (see Fig. 5-4, *A*) depends on several factors. Since solute move-

ment between the mobile phase and the stationary phase is a thermodynamic equilibrium process, the distribution equilibrium coefficient, K_D, is both temperature- and pressure-dependent. However, the earlier assumption that temperature and pressure are not contributing factors in the situation under discussion is usually made for most routine chromatographic procedures. This assumption and the overall thermodynamic basis of solute-solvent interaction theory[11,13] hold true only for dilute solutions of the solute in the mobile phase. This type of situation exists in conventional gas chromatography and high-performance liquid chromatography (HPLC). For these separations, the distribution isotherms approach linearity (see Fig. 5-4, *A*), and the solute-concentration profiles resemble a discrete circular spot (Fig. 5-4, *B*) or a symmetric bell-shaped (that is, *gaussian*) **elution** peak (Fig. 5-4, *C1*). However, it must be noted that one cannot predict the behavior of any given sample in any given chromatographic system.

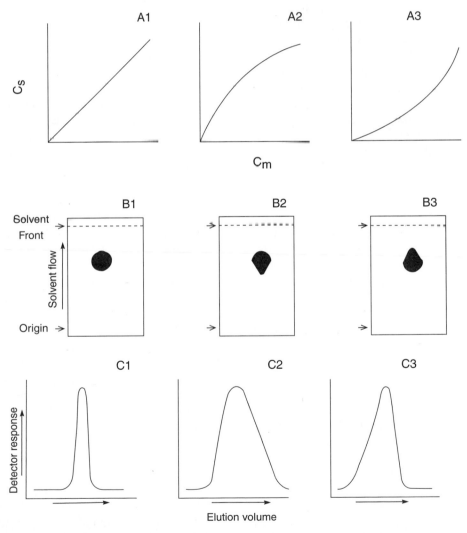

Fig. 5-4 Relationship between equilibrium distribution isotherm (*A1 to A3*) and solute shape, position, and elution profile in a PC/TLC chromatogram (*B1 to B3*) or a GC/HPLC chromatogram (*C1 to C3*). C_s, Concentration of solute in stationary phase; C_m, concentration of solute in mobile phase.

Linearity of distribution isotherms, as in Fig. 5-4, *A1,* is the exception rather than the norm. In most cases, convex or concave distribution isotherms are observed for solute-stationary phase interactions (Fig. 5-4, *A2* and *A3,* respectively). Several factors influence the degree to which nonlinearity is observed. At higher concentrations of solute in the mobile phase, nonlinearity results, since the thermodynamic basis of solute-solvent interactions holds only for dilute solutions. Another factor is the complexity of the sample, that is, the presence of multiple solutes. Interaction of these components with each other will cause a deviation from linearity.

If dilute solutions are used or there are no solute-solute interactions, a Langmuir, or convex, isotherm (Fig. 5-4, *A2*) may be observed. This isotherm shows that the limited number of adsorptive sites on the stationary phase become occupied by solute with increasing solute concentration, thereby losing their capacity to adsorb in proportion to the overall increase in solute concentration. Therefore the resulting solute-elution profile (Fig. 5-4, *B2* and *C2*) is characterized by a sharp front or leading edge, which indicates a high-solute concentration. The rear boundary of the solute-elution pattern decreases asymmetrically from the peak.

When the solute is poorly adsorbed to the stationary phase, preferring the mobile phase, the anti-Langmuir, or concave, isotherm (Fig. 5-4, *A3*) is observed. In this situation, the resulting solute-elution profile (Fig. 5-4, *B3* and *C3*) is characterized by sloping (i.e., low-solute concentration) front boundaries and sharp (i.e., high-solute concentration) rear boundaries. Also, the **elution volume** for the solute is a function of sample size.

RESOLUTION

The ultimate goal of any given chromatographic technique is to separate the components of a given sample within a reasonable time. The purpose of such a separation is to detect or quantitate a particular component or group of components of interest in pure form. The ability to resolve the components from one another and the degree to which this **resolution** is accomplished are measures of the adequacy of the chromatographic separation. The question of what is adequate resolution for a given sample has been detailed by Snyder.[16] One can answer this question by defining the objectives of the chromatographic separation. Generally, objectives for the analyst in a chemical laboratory depend on the following questions: (1) Is a particular substance present in a sample; that is, should a qualitative analysis be followed? (2) How much of a particular substance is present in a sample; that is, should a quantitative analysis be followed?[17] In the following discussion of the theory of resolution, the principal emphasis (and corresponding illustrations) will be on column techniques, gas or liquid, rather than on flat methods.

Note that, by convention, the concentrations of solutes separated in a chromatographic system are plotted out versus time, units of elution volume, or distance. The **bands** or zones of analytes separated are usually referred to as a **peak**.

An actual chromatographic separation of a three-component mixture by high-performance liquid chromatography is shown in Fig. 5-5, indicating important parameters for assessment of resolution, *R*. The quantity *R* for any two components is defined as the distance, *d*, between the peak centers of two peaks divided by the average base width, *W*, of the peaks:

$$R = \frac{d_2 - d_1}{\frac{1}{2}(W_1 + W_2)} \qquad \text{Eq. 5-2}$$

For this calculation, both the distance, *d*, and the peak width, *W*, are measured in the same units. This method of calculating resolution is based on the assumption that the distribution isotherms for the components being separated approach linearity (see Fig. 5-4, *A*) under specified conditions. The set of specified conditions are mobile phase, stationary phase, and solute-concentration range.

A resolution value of 1.25 or greater is required for good quantitative or qualitative chromatographic analyses. If the resolution is 0.4 or less, the peak shape does not clearly show the presence of two or more components. The actual value of the resolution depends on two factors: width of the peak and the distance between the peak maxima for column separations or diameter of the circular spots and the distance between these spots for flat-method separations.

These determinant factors of resolution also are indicative of the **efficiency** of the chromatographic process. Efficiency is decreased by the broadening of a solute band as it migrates through the stationary phase. If broadening occurs to any significant extent during the chromatographic process, the resulting peaks will be wide or the resulting spots will be diffuse. The separation of components is then poor, and the sensitivity with which they can be detected is reduced. An example of high- versus low-efficiency separation is illustrated in Fig. 5-6 for both column and flat-method separations.

Solute-band broadening occurs during the actual chromatographic process and may be described as follows for a column separation. The sample, in a small volume of solvent, is introduced into the mobile phase at a point near the inlet end of the column. Once entering the column, the sample begins to disperse by thermal diffusion processes, which continue as it passes through the column. The longer the time a solute band spends in a column (i.e., the longer the **retention time**), the greater the opportunity for thermal diffusion and the greater the band dispersion. The result is broader but gaussian (symmetrical, as in Fig. 5-4, *C1*) elution peaks for the more retained solutes. This process is similar in flat methods of chromatography, resulting in larger diameter but symmetrical spots, as in Fig. 5-4, *B1*, for the more retained solutes. Several additional factors contribute to solute-band broadening.[18,19] These include nonuniform regions of the stationary phase, nonuniform particle-size distribution, and nonuniform column packing, which may result in nonuniform passage of solute molecules. In the latter case, some molecules spend more time in the separa-

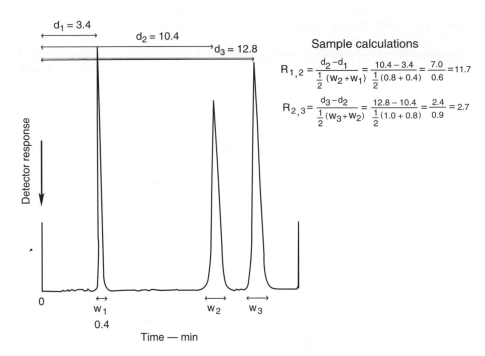

Sample calculations

$$R_{1,2} = \frac{d_2 - d_1}{\frac{1}{2}(w_2 + w_1)} = \frac{10.4 - 3.4}{\frac{1}{2}(0.8 + 0.4)} = \frac{7.0}{0.6} = 11.7$$

$$R_{2,3} = \frac{d_3 - d_2}{\frac{1}{2}(w_3 + w_2)} = \frac{12.8 - 10.4}{\frac{1}{2}(1.0 + 0.8)} = \frac{2.4}{0.9} = 2.7$$

Fig. 5-5   Calculation of resolution of sample components actually separated by HPLC. The distances d_1 to d_3 are the actual amounts of time from injection ($\downarrow$) to apex of eluting peak for each component, *1* to *3*, respectively. Peak widths w_1 to w_3 are measured by triangulation at base of each peak for components *1* to *3*, respectively. Both d and w must be measured the same way from the time of injection, that is, in units of time (minutes or seconds), length (inches or centimeters), or elution volume (milliliters). Resolution, *R*, is unitless.

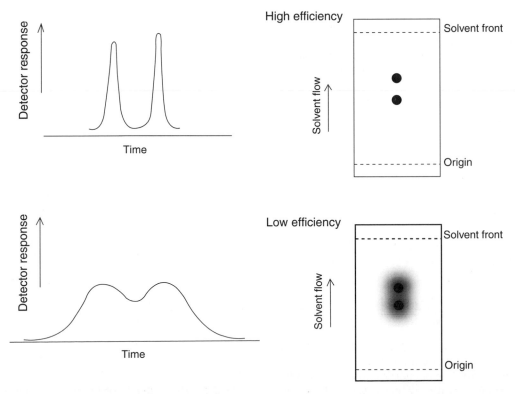

Fig. 5-6   Model chromatograms exemplifying high-efficiency separations and low-efficiency separations.

tion system than others do; that is, they have a longer path. These processes result in broader, nongaussian dispersion of solute bands, such as asymmetrical eluting peaks or trailing spots, as in Fig. 5-4, *C2* and *B2* respectively.

Therefore one way to maximize column efficiency (i.e., decrease the extent of band broadening) is to use a well-packed chromatography column containing a stationary-phase packing that is not only small but also uniform in size distribution of particles. Columns meeting these criteria are readily obtainable today from numerous commercial sources.

Theoretical Plates

One can obtain a numerical assessment of column efficiency by calculating the number of theoretical plates for a given column. A theoretical plate is a microscopic segment of a column where a perfect equilibrium is assumed to exist between the solute in the mobile and stationary phases. Theoretically, it is the smallest unit of separation in a column. The theory originated with Martin and Synge[20] in their mathematical treatment of the chromatographic process. The **theoretical plate number (N)** can be calculated for a column directly from a **chromatogram** (Fig. 5-7) by the following:

$$N = 16\left(\frac{t_R}{W}\right)^2 \qquad \textit{Eq. 5-3}$$

In this expression, W is the base width of the chromatographic peak, and t_R is the retention time of the solute, that is, the time from introduction of the sample onto the column to the apex of the eluting solute peak. Both t_R and W must be measured in the same units, such as time or distance. (Note that N is dimensionless.) A larger number of theoretical plates indicates relatively narrow peaks, that is, an efficient column and better resolution.

Related to the number of theoretical plates is the column **height equivalent to a theoretical plate (HETP)**, which can be calculated by the following:

$$HETP = \frac{L}{N} \qquad \textit{Eq. 5-4}$$

In this equation, L equals the column length, usually in millimeters. Maximum column efficiency is obtained when HETP is as small as possible.

In addition to the factors affecting column efficiency, N is affected by the flow rate of the mobile phase. The mobile-phase linear velocity, μ, can be calculated by

$$\mu = \frac{L}{t_o} \qquad \textit{Eq. 5-5}$$

In this equation, L is column length, and t_o is the time it takes a discrete portion of the solvent to flow through the column. A plot of HETP versus μ shows the experimental relationship of these two variables in gas chromatography (GC) (Fig. 5-8, *A*) and in liquid chromatography (LC) (Fig. 5-8, *B*). At the minimum HETP, the optimum flow velocity, μ_{opt}, is obtained. For gas chromatography (see Fig. 5-8, *A*) this plot is the well-known van Deemter plot.[21]

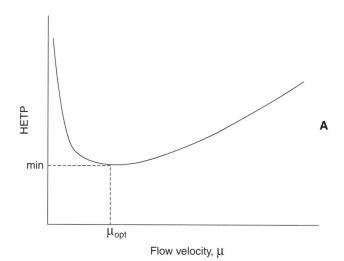

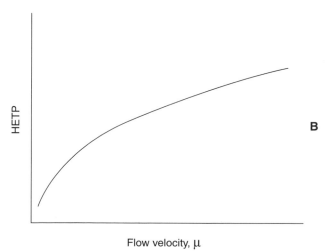

Fig. 5-8 Dependence of theoretical plate height, HETP, on mobile-phase velocity, μ, in gas chromatography, **A**, and in liquid chromatography, **B**.

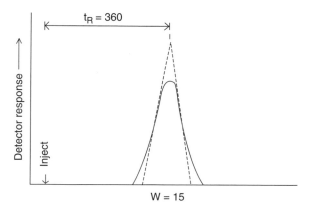

Fig. 5-7 Calculation of number of theoretical plates, *N*, from an HPLC or gas chromatogram. Elution or retention time, t_R, is measured from time of injection to apex of eluting peak for component. Peak width, *W*, is measured at the base of the peak by triangulation, as shown. Both t_R and *W* are measured in the same units.

At high mobile-phase velocities, HETP varies linearly with μ for gas chromatography (see Fig. 5-8, *A*), but in liquid chromatography (see Fig. 5-8, *B*) a minimum in HETP is seldom observed, and the HETP tends to level off at high values for μ. In practice, GC mobile-phase velocities are usually between one and two orders of magnitude greater than those of LC. For LC, lower velocities and column efficiencies are necessary because of the active role the mobile phase plays in the chromatographic separation process. Therefore, to improve separation efficiency in LC, use smaller stationary-phase particles, usually one-tenth to one-hundredth the size of those used in GC.

Retention

Resolution depends on factors in addition to theoretical plates. One of these is the ratio of the volumes of mobile and stationary phases in the column, that is, the **capacity factor**, *k* (which used to be designated *k'*), which can be calculated from the chromatogram (Fig. 5-9, *A*) by the equation:

$$k = \frac{V_e - V_0}{V_0} = \frac{t_R - t_0}{t_0} \qquad \text{Eq. 5-6}$$

The volumes in this equation are the **void volume**, V_0, of the column, that is, the volume of the mobile phase in the column, and the elution volume, V_e, of a solute retained by the stationary phase and undergoing chromatography. The HPLC chromatogram for Fig. 5-9, *A*, was obtained by injection of a sample containing two solutes undergoing chromatography, the first of which was not retained by the stationary phase and the second of which was retained. The volumes, V_0 and V_e, were then measured from the injection point to the apex of the peak of each component. As indicated previously, the capacity factor can be calculated also by the measurement of the times, t_0 and t_R, from sample injection to the apex of the peak of the component not retained and of the peak of the component retained, respectively.

Small values of *k* indicate that the sample components are little retained by the stationary phase and elute close to the unretained peak. Large values of *k* indicate that the sample components are well retained by the stationary phase and that long analysis times are required. For this latter situation, one must remember that solute-band broadening increases with residence time on the column because of an increased diffusion of the solute. Therefore the resulting peaks on elution will be wide and diffuse, decreasing sensitivity and making detection difficult.

The *k* value for a particular solute is constant for any given chromatography system at constant mobile-phase compositions and stationary-phase size and composition. Within these limits, the capacity factor varies neither with flow rate of the mobile phase nor with column dimensions, that is, length and diameter.

Selectivity

Another parameter on which resolution depends is the **selectivity** factor, α (alpha), a term that describes the ability of a chromatographic system to separate two solutes. The selectivity factor is the ratio of the capacity factors for two solutes:

$$\alpha = \frac{k_2}{k_1} \qquad \text{Eq. 5-7}$$

The capacity factors for two solutes are determined as shown in Fig. 5-9, *B*, from which the resultant selectivity of the system can be calculated. The selectivity of any given column for the sample is a function of the process of solute exchange between the mobile phase and the stationary phase.[11] Therefore, to affect selectivity, one can change the chemical composition of either the mobile phase or the stationary phase to increase the preference of the solute for one phase or the other. In LC, changes either in the stationary or in the mobile phases are usually made to improve selectivity. However, in GC, changes in stationary-phase chemistry are used for selectivity improvement.

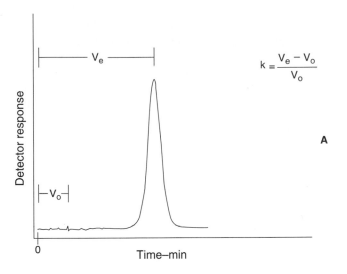

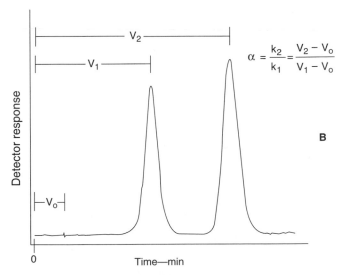

Fig. 5-9 **A,** Calculation of capacity factor, *k*, from an HPLC chromatogram. Sample was retained by stationary phase and underwent chromatography. **B,** Calculation of selectivity factor, α, from HPLC chromatogram. Solutes *A* and *B* were retained by stationary phase and underwent a chromatographic separation as indicated.

Improving Peak Resolution

General peak resolution. With the definition of the factors affecting resolution established, a more fundamental equation can now be written:

$$R = \left(\frac{N^{0.5}}{4}\right)\left(\frac{\alpha - 1}{\alpha}\right)\left(\frac{k_2}{1 + k_1}\right) \qquad \textit{Eq. 5-8}$$

Therefore the resolution of any two solutes in a given chromatographic system is a function of three factors: (1) theoretical plate number N, a column-efficiency factor; (2) a selectivity factor, α; and (3) a capacity factor, k.

A similar relationship can be derived for flat methods of chromatography.[11] However, a major difference exists between flat and column methods of chromatography. In a column method of chromatography, the solutes in a given sample pass completely through the bed of the stationary phase. But in a flat method of chromatography, the separation process is stopped when the mobile phase has reached the end of the bed of the stationary phase, thereby resulting in the solute bands having migrated through only a portion of the bed (Fig. 5-10). For this type of separation, solute retention is measured in terms of the $\boldsymbol{R_f}$ value, which is the distance, d_2, migrated by the solute divided by the distance, d_1, migrated by the mobile phase, or solvent front. This relationship can be expressed as

$$R_f = \frac{d_2}{d_1} \qquad \textit{Eq. 5-9}$$

In consideration of this major feature of flat methods of chromatography, the resolution equation for the separation of two solutes becomes as follows:

$$R = \left(\frac{N^{0.5}}{4}\right)\left(\frac{\alpha - 1}{\alpha}\right)\left(\frac{k_2}{(1 + k_2)^{2/3}}\right) \qquad \textit{Eq. 5-10}$$

The terms of this equation are as previously defined. The question of the practical significance of the resolution equations can now be addressed. Specifically, how do these equations relate resolution to the actual experimental condi-tions of the chromatographic separation and the physical design of a particular chromatographic device? The three fundamental parameters, N, α, and k, of resolution can be adjusted more or less independently of one another.

Variation of *N* to optimize resolution. The dynamics or rates of the various physical processes that occur during the separation determine N. Experimentally one can change N by adjusting or varying a variety of parameters or conditions. Remember that a doubling of the value for N will increase the resolution by a factor of 1.4. (Notice that in the resolution equation R is proportional to the square root of N.) Experimental parameters that can be changed to optimize N are summarized in Table 5-1.

Variation of capacity factor *k* to optimize resolution. Temperature is one parameter that is varied to effect a change in the capacity factor. Since the solute-stationary phase interactions are temperature-dependent, a change in this parameter will affect solute retention. This is especially important in GC, but it is also important, though to a much lesser extent, for other chromatographic techniques.

A second way to vary the capacity factor is by effecting changes in the strength of the stationary phase. For partition chromatography, increasing the percentage of liquid-phase coating on the matrix support will effect an increase in k. Most GLC analyses are done on columns containing 2% to 10% ratios of liquid-phase coating to stationary-phase matrix support.[22,23] Since retention time is proportional to the amount of liquid phase present, lower percentage ratios mean shorter analysis times. However, higher percentages of stationary phase for partition chromatography mean higher resolution. Therefore the final selection of the percentage of stationary phase must be a compromise between analysis time and resolution.

Additionally, one can vary the capacity factor, k, to improve resolution by changing the solvent strength of the mobile phase, but this is applicable only to LC methods (see

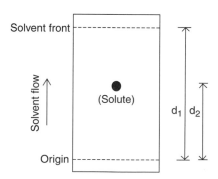

Fig. 5-10 Calculation of R_f (solvent-front ratio) value for a sample component from a paper or thin-layer chromatogram. The distance d_1 from origin to solvent front and distance d_2 from origin to center of spot of separated component are measured, as shown, in terms of same units; that is, length (centimeters or millimeters). Resulting R_f value, d_2 divided by d_1, is unitless.

TABLE 5-1   EXPERIMENTAL PARAMETERS AFFECTING *N*

Parameters	Direction of Change Necessary To Increase N
Mobile-phase flow rate	Decrease
Column length	Increase
Average particle size of stationary phase	Decrease
Particle-size distribution	Decrease
Volume of sample introduced	Decrease
Viscosity of sample introduced	Increase
Viscosity of mobile phase	Increase
Temperature (as it controls mobile-phase viscosity)	Decrease
Extracolumnar effects (i.e., dead volumes, excessive connective tubing)	Decrease

p. 119). In GC the mobile phase is an inert gas such as helium or nitrogen, but in LC the mobile phase is an active component of the chromatographic procedure, ranging from very nonpolar, such as hexane, to polar, such as water, in solvent strength.

For the adsorption and partition modes of LC (see Fig. 5-2), the chromatographic process involves a continual distribution of the solute molecules between the mobile and the stationary phases. Any shift in the equilibrium concentration distribution coefficient (K_D) affects the capacity factor; that is, the elution volume per time of a particular solute in the given sample. One way to shift this coefficient is to increase or decrease the **polarity** of the mobile phase relative to the stationary phase. Numerous examples of mobile-phase alterations could be given. This is a powerful technique for varying the k of solutes being separated (see pp. 139-141, Chapter 6).

Variation of selectivity to optimize resolution. After optimization of the k values, the selectivity, or separation factor, α, can then be adjusted to maximize the resolution. In general, the separation factor is varied by changes in the chemistries of the mobile phase, the stationary phase, or the sample. These changes may be accomplished as follows.

Derivatization. The chemical form of the sample can be altered in a variety of ways to affect selectivity. The most common method is derivatization. Knapp[24] has summarized an extensive variety of derivatization reactions for samples to be separated by GC. Derivatization is not only used in GC to improve sample volatility or solute detection limits, but is also used to improve selectivity.[25] In LC, derivatization techniques are generally used to improve detection,[19,21,26] with the most extensive collection of methods presented in a book by Frei and Lawrence.[27]

Alterations in mobile-phase chemistry. Another method for improving the separation factor in LC is altering the mobile-phase chemistry.[28] Solvent polarity changes can be used to improve the capacity factor, k. For improving the separation factor, solvents of similar polarity (strength) but different chemical natures are interchanged without affecting the overall polarity of the mobile phase, resulting in changes in the solvent selectivity. For example, the resolution of an HPLC separation initially developed with a mobile phase of methylene chloride to hexane, 50/50 by volume, could be improved by substitution of tetrahydrofuran for methylene chloride without changing the solvent strength.[13,29,30] The reason for improvement in resolution would be that tetrahydrofuran has a quite different selectivity toward certain classes of compounds, such as lipids, than methylene chloride does. In this case, with substitution of an ether for an organic halide, the functional groups of the mobile phase have been altered. Changing solvent functionality without changing solvent strength is a powerful technique for improving selectivity and thereby resolution in LC. Depending on the sample and chromatographic and detector requirements, the choice of solvent or solvents that can be used to effect changes in selectivity is extensive, as detailed by Snyder[31] in his compendium of properties of 911 solvents. A further discussion of the properties of solvents is presented in a later section.

Alterations in stationary-phase chemistry. As adjustments in the functionality of the mobile phase are used to improve the separation factor in LC, similar changes in the functionality of the stationary phase are commonly used to improve the separation factor in GC. For example, many polyester stationary phases, such as ethylene glycol succinate, can be replaced by the cyanopropyl silicone stationary phases, such as Silar 10C, allowing for a change in functionality with little or no change in polarity. For relatively nonpolar stationary phases, the hydrocarbon phases, such as Apiezon N, can be readily replaced by the alkyl silicone phases, such as OV-1, for a functionality change. These changes in stationary phase afford an improvement in selectivity, thereby leading to an optimization in resolution. Details concerning the initial choice of phase are discussed in the following sections.

POLARITY

In previous sections, the importance of solvent strength and stationary-phase strength was discussed in relationship to the effect on resolution. Both factors affect chromatographic resolution by altering the capacity factor and the separation factor as described earlier in Equations 5-6 and 5-7. These parameters are linked by the *principle of polarity*.

The role of polarity is central to the interaction of molecules in the liquid or gaseous state, and polarity is a major determinant property in the overall chromatographic process. The concept of polarity can be interpreted several ways[19,29,30] but generally is considered to encompass the total interaction of solvent molecules with sample molecules and of solvent or sample molecules with the stationary phase. The physicochemical basis for polarity is the interaction of attractive forces that exist between molecules. These four attractive forces are more specifically referred to as *dispersive*, *dipolar*, *hydrogen-bonding*, and *dielectric interactions*. As illustrated in Fig. 5-11 and discussed below, all four of these interactions involve the attraction of induced, partial, or formal positive and negative charges.

Dispersion interactions of molecules, sometimes termed *van der Waals forces*, refer to the induced attraction between two molecules. This temporary separation of opposite charges (**dipole**) in one molecule induces the polarization of electrons in an adjacent molecule, thereby causing the two molecules to be attracted to each other by **electrostatic interactions** (Fig. 5-11, *A*). The formation of temporary dipoles in molecules is the physical basis for existence in the liquid state of many compounds composed of elements with small differences in electronegativity, for example, the elements carbon and hydrogen. Generally, dispersive interactions are an important determinant in polarity only when other forces are lacking or when some elemental constituents of molecules are electron-rich species (such as halogens in halohydrocarbons).

Some molecules possess permanent rather than temporary dipoles (Fig. 5-11, *B*). These compounds have centers of positive and negative charge that are the result of an unequal sharing of bonding electrons between two elements with

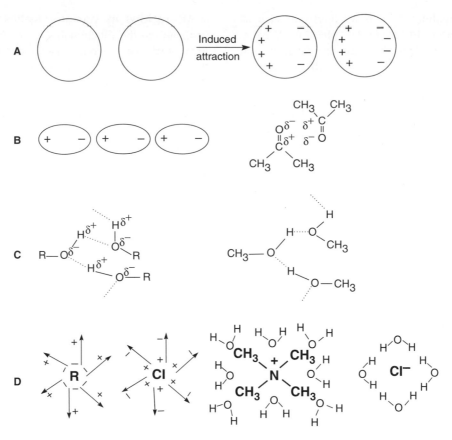

Fig. 5-11 Physicochemical interactions between molecules that constitute concept of polarity. **A,** Dispersive or van der Waals interactions. **B,** Dipole interactions. **C,** Hydrogen bonding. **D,** Electrostatic interactions.

large differences in electronegativity within the same molecule. This overall molecular dipole is enhanced by the presence of elemental nonbonding electron pairs within a compound. These are outer shell electrons within an element that are spin paired. Elements such as oxygen, sulfur, halogens, and nitrogen possess nonbonding electrons when covalently linked to other atoms in compounds. The resulting permanent dipole is directional, with one end of the molecule being partially positive and the other being partially negative.

One special category of dipolar molecules is composed of those with hydrogen covalently linked to an electronegative element such as oxygen, nitrogen, or sulfur. In these molecules the hydrogen has a large degree of positive character relative to the electronegative atom to which it is bonded. Because of the small size of the hydrogen atom compared with other atoms, this positive end of the dipole can approach close to the negative end of a neighboring dipole. The force of attraction between the two is quite large, about 10 times that of normal dipolar interactions. This special case of dipole-dipole interactions is termed **hydrogen bonding** and is one of the most important types of weak attractive forces. This bonding is illustrated in Fig. 5-11, *C,* for the alcohol methanol.

The fourth type of attractive force is the electrostatic or dielectric interaction. In this case, the solute molecule of

the stationary phase is a charged ionic species having either a formal positive or a formal negative charge. A small counterion, such as H^+ or Cl^-, is present but is generally separated from the charged solute or stationary phase because of solvation by the mobile phase (Fig. 5-11, *D*). These ionic species increase the dipolar character of the solvent by an enhancement of polarization. Dielectric interactions are quite strong and favor the dissolution of ionic or ionizable sample molecules in strongly dipolar solvents such as water or methanol.

The polarity of a solute molecule is the result of the four attractive forces described above. The polarity of a molecule will affect its interactions with the mobile and stationary phases. The more polar molecules have this property primarily because of strong dipoles, an ionic character, an ability to form strong hydrogen bonds, or a combination of the three forces. The less polar (nonpolar) molecules have dispersive forces as a primary basis of interaction with a very weak ability to interact through dipolar, hydrogen bonding, or dielectric forces. The practical aspects of these interactive forces and the degree of polarity or nonpolarity form the basis for the mechanisms of chromatography. The role of polarity in these mechanisms is discussed below for each of the three chromatographic constituents—the solute, the solvent or mobile phase, and the stationary phase.

Solvent Polarity and Solvent Strength

Solvent strength in liquid chromatography is a measure of the ability of the mobile phase to compete with the solute molecules for active sites (i.e., interaction or attraction sites) on the stationary phase. When the stationary phase is silica gel, the active sites are the highly polar hydroxyl groups (Si—OH). Therefore, in this case, solvent strength increases with solvent or mobile-phase polarity. However, when the stationary phase is nonpolar, such as a polydivinylbenzene (such as XAD-2), the solvent strength decreases with increases in solvent or mobile-phase polarity. The strength of a solvent is directly related to its polarity.

Solvent polarity has been described and quantitated in various ways.[29-35] The four most common solvent polarity-classification schemes are (1) the Hildebrand solubility parameter, which is based on thermodynamic properties of the compound in question[34]; (2) the Rohrschneider polarity scale of P' values, which is based on the measurement of solvent properties through the use of model solutes[31]; (3) the **eluotropic series**, which ranks solvents in order of their eluting power for removing solutes from a polar stationary phase, such as alumina[36]; and (4) the solvent selectivity grouping of Snyder and Karger, which is a blend of the three previous approaches and incorporates specific solubility parameters for dispersion, dipole, and hydrogen-bonding interactions. A listing of the solvent selectivity groups is given in Table 5-2 along with representative classes of compounds and specific examples for each group.

Solvents within any one group exhibit the same types of attractive forces. For example, the compounds of group 1 (I) are all strong hydrogen-bonding acceptors and weak hydrogen-bonding donors and have intermediate dipole moments. The solvents in group 5 (V) are compounds whose dipole interactions predominate over any hydrogen-bonding interactions. However, the solvents in group 0 are compounds in which only dispersion interactions (i.e., temporary dipoles) are the predominant force. These solvents do not have permanent dipoles, nor do they interact through hydrogen bonding.

The overall degree of the interactive forces of the solvent is quantitated in the polarity index, P'.[29,30] A list of solvents commonly used in chromatography is presented in Table 5-3 with values for their polarity indices and their solvent selectivity group classifications. It is noted that solvents within any one group may vary widely in their overall degree of polarity. For example, the solvents listed for group 6 (VIA) vary more than three polarity units. In group 2 (II), the polarity index varies more than two units. Even though these variations are relatively large, one must remember that solvents within the same group exhibit the same kinds of chemical interactions.

This information can be used as a basis for solvent selections and can be used to vary the mobile-phase selectivity, α, to improve resolution. The first important step in solvent selection is to maximize solute solubility in a given solvent. For a solvent to be an effective mobile phase in chromatography, it should dissolve the sample over the range of expected solute concentrations.

The most significant factor affecting solute solubility is solvent polarity. One can vary liquid mobile-phase polarity systematically over a wide range of P' values by using a combination of two solvents, since solvent polarities are additive according to:

$$P' \text{ (of combined solvents A + B)} = \phi_A P'_A + \phi_B P'_B \quad \textbf{\textit{Eq. 5-11}}$$

In this expression, ϕ_A and ϕ_B are the volume fractions of solvents A and B, which have solvent polarities of P'_A and P'_B, respectively. The two solvents should differ in P' values so that maximization of sample solubility can be achieved. It is important that the two solvents are miscible in all proportions. Usually a solvent that is too weak (A) to dissolve the sample is mixed with a solvent that is too strong (B). The two solvents are now chosen from the solvent groups (see Table 5-3) according to the compatibility of interactive forces with sample solutes and stationary-phase chemical functionalities. For example, to calculate P' for solvent mixtures of isooctane (solvent A) and chloroform (solvent B), their individual polarity values are obtained from Table 5-3. Any mixtures of these two solvents would range in polarity from -0.4 to 4.3, that is, weakest (100% isooctane) to strongest (100% chloroform). A 50%:50% mixture of these two solvents would have a P' of $(0.5 \times -0.4) + (0.5 \times 4.3)$, or 1.95. Also, for each 10% change in solvent composition, the polarity of the mixture would change by 0.47 unit:

$$0.1(P'_B - P'_A) = 0.1(4.3 - [-0.4]) = 0.47$$

Once a suitable solvent mixture has been found to dissolve the sample, it is then applied to a chromatographic system such as a silica HPLC column. As previously discussed, the retention index k for the solutes in the sample is maximized to a value between 2 and 8. This is accomplished by adjustment of the solvent polarity by small changes in the relative proportions of the two solvents.

TABLE 5-2 SOLVENT CLASSIFICATION BY SELECTIVITY GROUPS

Solvent Group	Representative Classes or Examples of Compounds
0	*n*-Alkanes, cyclohexane, saturated fluorochlorohydrocarbons
1 (I)	Aliphatic ethers, trialkylamines
2 (II)	Aliphatic alcohols
3 (III)	Pyridine derivatives, tetrahydrofuran, amides
4 (IV)	Glycols, benzyl alcohol, acetic acid
5 (V)	Methylene chloride, ethylene chloride, bis(2-ethoxyethyl) ether
6 (VIA)	Aliphatic ketones and esters, nitriles, dioxane, sulfoxides
7 (VIB)	Nitrocompounds, phenyl alkyl ethers, aromatic hydrocarbons, carbon tetrachloride
8 (VII)	Halobenzenes, diphenyl ether
9 (VIII)	Fluoroalkanols, chloroform, water

TABLE 5-3 REPRESENTATIVE SOLVENT POLARITY INDICES

Solvent	Polarity Index	Solvent Group
Isooctane	-0.4	0
Hexane	0.0	0
Carbon tetrachloride	1.7	7
Dibutyl ether	1.7	1
Triethylamine	1.8	1
Toluene	2.3	7
Chlorobenzene	2.7	8
Diphenyl ether	2.8	8
Diethyl ether	2.9	1
Benzene	3.0	7
Ethyl bromide	3.1	6
Methylene chloride	3.4	5
1,2-Dichloroethane	3.7	5
Bis(2-ethoxyethyl) ether	3.9	5
n-Propanol	4.1	2
Tetrahydrofuran	4.2	3
Chloroform	4.3	9
Ethyl acetate	4.3	6
Isopropanol	4.3	2
2-Butanone	4.5	6
Dioxane	4.8	6
Ethanol	5.2	2
Nitroethane	5.3	7
Pyridine	5.3	3
Acetone	5.4	6
Benzyl alcohol	5.5	4
Methoxyethanol	5.7	4
Acetic acid	6.2	4
Acetonitrile	6.2	6
Dimethylformamide	6.4	3
Dimethyl sulfoxide	6.5	6
Methanol	6.6	2
Nitromethane	6.8	7
Water	9.0	9

TABLE 5-4 PREFERRED STATIONARY PHASES

Phase Type	Examples
Dimethylsilicone	OV-1, OV-101, SE-30, SP-2100
50% phenylmethylsilicone	OV-17, SP-2750
Trifluoropropylmethylsilicone	OV-210, SP-2401
Polyethylene glycol	Carbowaxes
Diethylene glycol succinate	DEGS, EGSS-X, EGA
3-Cyanopropylsilicone	Silar 10C, SP-2340, Apolar 10C

From Hawkes S et al: J Chromatogr Sci 13:115, 1975.

volved in the chromatographic separation process. The latter is discussed in the following sections on the role of stationary-phase polarity and the mechanisms of chromatography.

Stationary-Phase Polarity and Selectivity

The stationary phase is the fundamental component of the chromatographic separation (Table 5-4). The role of the stationary phase depends on its selectivity, which, in turn, is determined by the polarity of the phase. The forces constituting stationary-phase polarity are the same interactions responsible for mobile-phase (solvent) polarity: dispersion, dipole, hydrogen bonding, and dielectric.

The relative strength of polarity of stationary phases is more difficult to ascertain than the relative strength of polarity of liquid mobile phases, as previously described. Most attention has been directed to the stationary phases used in GC, wherein the two major variables determining the separation are the stationary phase itself and the temperature of the column. In this mode of chromatography, studies of the affinity of solute molecules of varying polarities have led to a classification system for stationary phase according to polarity. Details on the Rohrschneider[37] and McReynolds[38] classifications can be found in Chapter 7.

MECHANISMS OF CHROMATOGRAPHY

The mechanisms by which a chromatographic method can separate sample components are generally based on polar interactions and physical interactions (interactions resulting from the size and shape of the solute molecules). The latter interaction is principally the mechanism for gel-permeation chromatography, though molecular size plays a minor role in other modes of chromatography. The other broad mechanistic classes of chromatography are adsorption, partition, and ion exchange. Each is briefly discussed in the following sections.

Adsorption

The interactions of solute or mobile-phase molecules at the surface of a solid particle form the basis of the adsorption mechanism. There are fundamentally two types of adsorbents, nonpolar and polar. The latter category includes those that

Resolution is then maximized for the solute separation by adjustments in chromatographic selectivity, α. This is done by exchanging one of the mobile-phase solvents with a solvent in another solvent selectivity group (see Table 5-2) but with the *same polarity* of the overall mixture being kept. For example, chloroform, $P' = 4.3$, could be exchanged with isopropanol, $P' = 4.3$, in the previously described isooctane-chloroform mixture. The net effect of this exchange would be to go from a solvent that is a strong hydrogen-bonding donor, chloroform, to a solvent that is both a strong hydrogen-bonding donor and hydrogen-bonding acceptor. Other examples of such changes were given earlier in the discussion on selectivity. Further discussions of solvent selection and optimization are given by Snyder and associates.[19,30]

In principle, this approach is a general guide to solvent choice both for dissolving the sample and for optimizing a mobile phase in LC (HPLC, thin-layer chromatography, and so on). It does, however, require knowledge of the forces in-

TABLE 5-5 SELECTED GROUPS OF SOLUTES IN ORDER OF INCREASED RETENTION IN NORMAL-PHASE AND REVERSED-PHASE CHROMATOGRAPHY		
Reversed Phase	**Solute Type**	**Normal Phase**
Most retained	Fluorocarbons	Least retained
	Saturated hydrocarbons	
	Unsaturated hydrocarbons	
↓	Halides and esters	↓
	Aldehydes and ketones	
	Alcohol and thiols	
Least retained	Acids and bases	Most retained

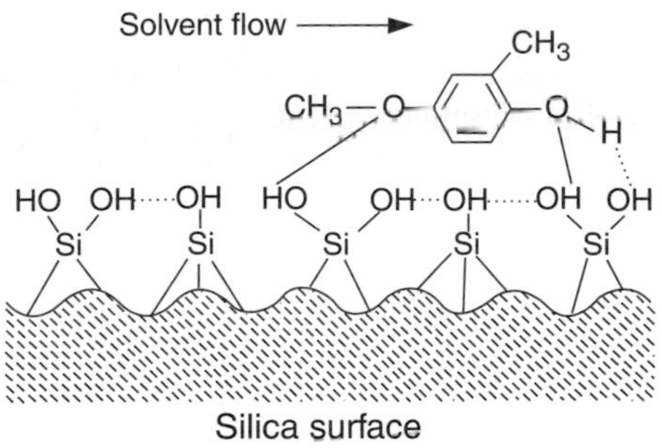

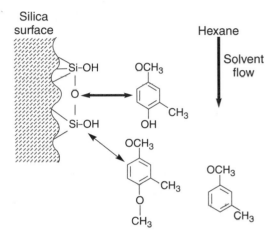

Fig. 5-12 Mechanism of separation of a metabolite of methylanisole by silica gel chromatography. Hydrogen bonds, ·····; covalent bonds, ——.

are acidic (i.e., having electron-accepting surfaces) and those that are basic (i.e., having electron-donating surfaces).

The nonpolar adsorbents have limited application in gas-solid chromatography (GSC)[22] (see Chapter 7). The mechanism for adsorption of the solute to nonpolar stationary phases is principally by dispersive interactions. Retention is determined by the adsorption energy and the surface volume of the stationary phase. A decrease in temperature or an increase in pressure increases adsorption. The converse is also true; that is, an increase in desorption can be accomplished by an increase in temperature or a decrease in pressure.

Polar adsorbents are the most widely used stationary phases in liquid-solid chromatography (LSC), with applications in both flat and column methods. Limited applications are found in GSC. The most common stationary phases are silica and alumina for LSC and silica or porous glass and aluminosilicates (zeolites or molecular sieves) for GSC. This latter group also has application in LC for gel-permeation chromatography, in which the separation is principally through the mechanism of molecular exclusion. This is discussed later in the section on the mechanism of gel permeation.

The principal polar adsorbents used in LC are silica and alumina, accounting for more than 95% of the applications in HPLC[19] and thin-layer chromatography (TLC).[14,39,40] Both hydrogen bonding and dipole interactions between the solute and the surface hydroxyl (silica and acid-washed alumina) or the oxygen anionic (base-washed alumina) groups of the stationary phases constitute the mechanisms of separation by this method (Fig. 5-12). The number and topographic arrangement of these groups, along with the total surface area, determine the activity and strength of the adsorption. Retention of solutes on these phases increases with increasing polarity of the compound class (Table 5-5). Retention of a solute molecule requires displacement of adsorbed solvent molecules (Fig. 5-13). Adjustments in solvent polarity, as previously described, ultimately determine the strength of adsorption of the solute to the stationary phase and the retention characteristics of the system.

Fig. 5-13 Mechanism of adsorption chromatography by separation of 3-methylanisole and two of its biochemical metabolites. The most polar sample components, such as 3-methyl-4-hydroxyanisole, are retained the most by polar silica gel stationary phase (*heavy arrow*). Sample components of intermediate polarity, such as 2,5-dimethoxytoluene, are retained to a much lesser degree (*light arrow*), whereas relatively nonpolar components, such as 3-methylanisole, are not retained and prefer the nonpolar mobile phase, hexane.

Adsorption chromatography offers many advantages for use in LC separations. First, an extensive literature is available to the investigator for the separation of many types and classes of compounds by TLC. These methods are readily transferable to adsorption HPLC. Second, the flexibility, speed, and low cost of TLC allow its use in experimental development, particularly for selection of mobile phases. Once the optimum separation has been achieved, the transfer of the method to HPLC is straightforward. Third, TLC has a great value for use in the preliminary investigation of samples of unknown constituents, particularly when one considers the advantages noted above. Finally, adsorption chromatography, particularly with silica gel, has been widely used for the separation of drugs in both the HPLC and TLC modes.

Partition

Partition chromatography is based on the separation of solutes by use of differences in their distribution between two immiscible phases. In liquid-liquid chromatography (LLC), the phase support is usually coated with a polar substance (normal phase), with separations accomplished by use of an immiscible mobile phase. A normal-phase partition system would consist of silica coated with a monolayer of water or some other polar liquid and a relatively nonpolar solvent system. Separations in this system are based on solute polarity, with the least polar compounds eluting first and the most polar substances retained the longest (Fig. 5-14). A

similar separation system operates in paper chromatography, in which the cellulose is coated with an aqueous monolayer, and immiscible solvents are used as the mobile phase.

In 1969, Halasz and Sebestian[41] introduced a variation in the stationary phase for LLC, in which the silica support was chemically modified to produce a monolayer of a nonpolar organic substituent. These chemically bonded stationary-phase supports are available with a variety of functional groups. The most commonly used bonded phases are hydrocarbon phases such as octadecyl or octyl groups bonded to silica (Fig. 5-15). The organic nature of the bonded phases imparts a nonpolar character to the stationary phase. There-

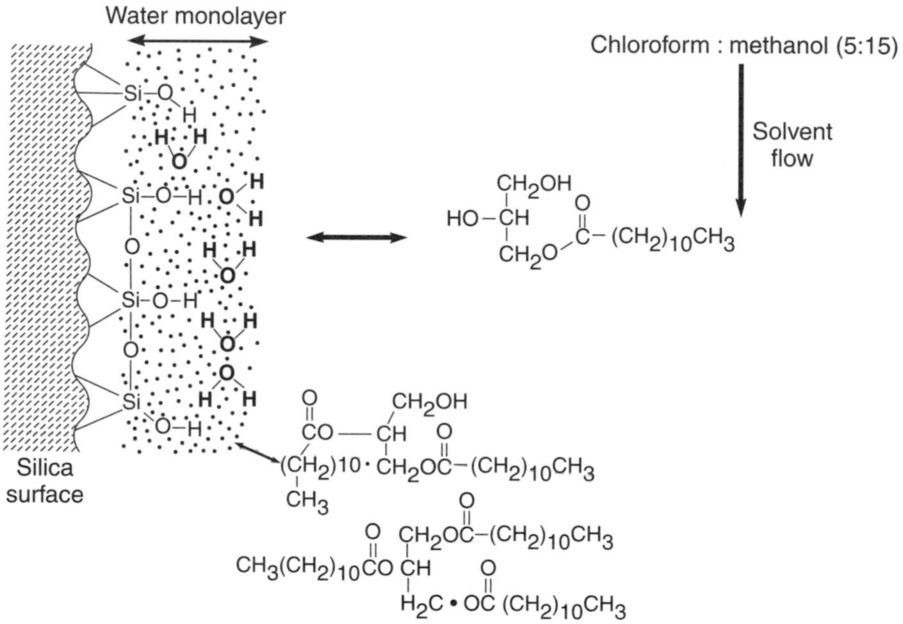

Fig. 5-14 Mechanism of liquid/liquid chromatography as exemplified by the separation of the monoglycerides, diglycerides, and triglycerides of lauric acid. Silica gel stationary phase has a monolayer of water strongly held by hydrogen bonding. Solute molecules are partitioned between the liquid mobile phase (chloroform:methanol) and liquid stationary phase, or water monolayer. The most polar sample components, the monoglycerides, are retained most by the polar stationary phase (*heavy arrow*). Sample components of intermediate polarity, such as the diglycerides, are retained to a much lesser degree (*light arrow*), whereas relatively nonpolar components, such as the triglycerides, are not retained and prefer the relatively nonpolar stationary phase.

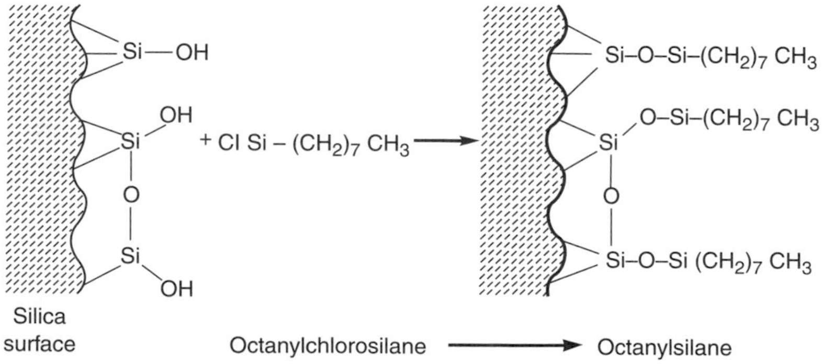

Fig. 5-15 Chemical preparation of bonded, stationary phase (reversed phase). Organochlorosilane reacts with nucleophilic hydroxyl (OH) groups of silica gel, forming siloxane covalent bond (Si—O—Si).

fore the mobile phases commonly used are highly polar, such as water, methanol, or acetonitrile (see Table 5-3). Solutes are separated by their relatively nonpolar character (i.e., the most polar eluting first), whereas the nonpolar solutes are retained longer. From this type of separation characteristic, the use of bonded phases in LLC is termed *reversed-phase chromatography.* A further discussion and examples of normal-phase and reversed-phase LC are given in Chapter 6.

Another example of chromatography in which a partition mechanism operates is gas-liquid chromatography (GLC). The forces of interaction between solute molecules and the liquid-coated stationary phase are as previously discussed for LLC. However, for GC, the mobile phase serves as an inert carrier for the sample constituents, whereas in LLC the mobile phase is an active, interacting component in the partition mechanism.

Ion Exchange

Ion-exchange chromatography uses stationary phases that possess formal positive or negative charges. The most common retention mechanism is the exchange of sample ions, A, and mobile-phase ions, B, with the charged groups, R, of the stationary phase:

$$A^- + R^+ B^- \rightarrow B^- + R^+ A^- \quad \textit{Anion exchange} \qquad \textit{Eq. 5-12, A}$$

$$A^+ + B^+ R^- \rightarrow B^+ + A^+ R^- \quad \textit{Cation exchange} \qquad \textit{Eq. 5-12, B}$$

In the first case, anion exchange is occurring, whereas cation exchange is shown for the second; sample ions compete with mobile-phase ions for ionic sites on the stationary phase. The sample ions that interact weakly with the stationary phase will be retained least, whereas those that interact strongly will be retained the most and will be eluted later. The principal force of these interactions is electrostatic, or the attraction of opposite charges.

To effect a separation of sample constituents, the extent of ionization of sample molecules is controlled by variations in pH of the mobile phase. Since the solutes are predominantly weak acids, HA, or weak bases, B, a change in pH will shift the following ionization equilibriums either to the right or to the left:

$$\textbf{pH}\!\downarrow \qquad \textbf{pH}\!\uparrow$$

$$HA \rightleftharpoons H^+ + A^- \qquad \textit{Eq. 5-13, A}$$

$$BH^+ \rightleftharpoons H^+ + B \qquad \textit{Eq. 5-13, B}$$

An increase in ionization leads to an increased retention of the sample. Factors other than pH controlling solute retention in ion-exchange chromatography are (1) charge strength of the solute ion, (2) ionic strength of the mobile phase, and (3) charge strength of the counterion on the stationary phase. One can decrease the retardation of solutes by increasing the ionic strength of the mobile phase and decreasing the strength of the counterion, such as use of Na^+ instead of H^+ for cation-exchange phases, or by adjusting the pH of the mobile phase in a manner to decrease dissociation of either the solute, the counterion on the packing, or both.

Gel-Permeation (Molecular or Size Exclusion) Chromatography[42]

In contrast to the previous mechanisms and modes of chromatography, gel-permeation chromatography (GPC) separation is strictly based on molecular size. The stationary phase for GPC contains pores of a particular average size, and if the sample molecules are too large to enter the pores, they are not retained (excluded) by the stationary phase and are eluted from the column first. Small sample molecules permeate deeply into the pores and are retained the longest. They ultimately diffuse from the pores and are swept away by the flow of the mobile phase. Intermediate-sized sample molecules enter the pores to some extent but are not retained as easily as the small sample molecules because they do not penetrate as deeply into the pores. They are eluted from the column in volumes between those needed to elute the largest solute (small V_e) and smallest solutes (large V_e). This mechanism is illustrated in Fig. 5-16.

The major advantage of this mode of chromatography is that the LC method can be used to separate virtually any sample, as long as it is soluble in a mobile phase. Additionally, it is applicable to soluble species with an average molecular weight of 50 to more than 10 million. Since molecular size is the property of interest, representative calibration curves should be obtained by use of calibration standards of known molecular weight. Likewise, stationary phase choice is based on the expected molecular-weight range of the solute molecules in the sample and compatibility with the mobile phase. A mobile phase for GPC should be chosen first on the basis of sample solubility, and then a

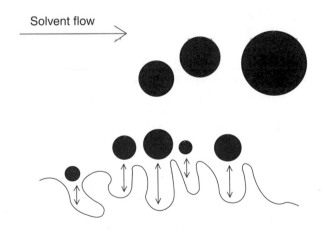

Solvent flow

Surface of stationary phase

Fig. 5-16 Mechanism of size-exclusion chromatography. Stationary phase, in form of porous beads, contains pores of varying diameter. Mobile phase outside and inside pores is the same, except the liquid inside is immobilized. When a sample containing solutes varying from small to large molecules elutes through column, small molecules penetrate all pores and are retained, thus being eluted later than large molecules, which move only in mobile phase. Molecules of intermediate size penetrate only some pores, thereby being retained to a lesser degree than small molecules.

compatible stationary phase is selected. Most stationary phases are compatible with aqueous or proton-donating (such as methanol) solvents. However, there are available stationary phases that are compatible only with organic solvents. Lists of the available phases for GPC are tabulated in the manufacturers' literature, in reviews,[43] and in books.

SAMPLE PREPARATION FOR CHROMATOGRAPHY
Nature of Problem

Few chromatographic analyses are conducted on the sample as submitted to the clinical laboratory. For any given sample, the goal of the chromatographic analysis is either a qualitative or a quantitative determination of its components. To achieve this objective, one should separate the components of interest as discrete zones with the same peak or spot distributions and k or R_f values as the standards under identical chromatographic conditions. However, the complexity of a biological sample matrix usually renders the chromatographic separation ineffectual by: (1) interaction of sample impurities with the stationary phase, causing a reduction in the resolving power of the system; (2) saturation of most chromatographic detector systems, tending to raise the noise level and thereby decreasing sensitivity; (3) interaction of the component of interest with other matrix components, leading to irreproducibility of the separation from sample to sample; and (4) poorly resolved components that interfere with the analysis. To minimize these sample effects in the chromatographic separation, a strategy for separation of the analyte from interfering components (*sample cleanup*) is required.

Any separation method employed in the laboratory must meet the criteria of yield, separation, capacity, and cost-effectiveness. The advantages of having high yield in any sample manipulation step are obvious, but if recovery is quantitative with little purification, the method is unsatisfactory. The corollary is also true: if the separation from impurities is excellent, but there is a low yield, the method is of little value. Many separation methods are readily applied on a large scale, where large amounts of sample are available, but others are applicable only to small-scale separations. The criterion of cost-effectiveness, which includes time, equipment, reagents, and labor, may render a separation method impracticable.

The strategy of sample preparation for chromatographic analysis should include consideration of whether the objective of the analysis is to qualitatively detect or to quantitate the substance under investigation.[44]

Mechanical Methods for Initial Isolation of Analyte

The type of sample matrix received by the analyst in a clinical chemistry laboratory varies from a simple homogeneous-appearing liquid such as perspiration to a complex heterogeneous solid such as feces. However, the most commonly received sample matrices are urine and blood (or plasma). The initial step in analyte preparation for chromatography will vary according to matrix.

Solid samples, such as tissues or feces, are first disrupted or treated for preparation of a homogeneous solution or suspension from which the analyte can be isolated. Homogenization of tissues in a blender such as a Polytron (Brinkmann Instruments, Inc., Westbury, NY) with an appropriate solvent may solubilize the desired analyte. The use of a Potter-Elvehjem tissue grinder is also effective. Tissue can also be extracted in a mortar with a pestle and a small amount of solvent. In addition to these grinding or shearing techniques, solid samples can be disrupted by sonication in solvent or hydrolyzed by acid, base, or enzymes. A procedure for preparing homogeneous powders of feces for subsequent extraction has been developed for the investigation of drug metabolism. It involves grinding the sample with a stainless steel ball mill in the presence of anhydrous sodium sulfate.[45]

Liquid samples may also require an initial treatment for removal of analytes sequestered by matrix components. Mild base hydrolysis has been used to release sequestered polychlorinated biphenyls from blood lipid components.[46] Whole blood can be diluted with sterile water to disrupt blood cells osmotically before analyte isolation. Another initial treatment applied to blood or urine samples is to remove proteins and other macromolecules through precipitation. Two of the more commonly used protein-precipitating agents are trichloroacetic acid and barium sulfate.

In other mechanical methods of matrix disruption, such as homogenization in a solvent or buffer, centrifugation is commonly employed to remove cell debris, particulate matter, or other large contaminants. An alternative method for the removal of insolubles is filtration, either through an inert material, such as glass wool, or through a nitrocellulose or nylon membrane.

Chromatographic Methods for Initial Isolation of Analyte

A common method for the initial isolation of components of interest from aqueous solutions, such as urine or blood, is the use of XAD-2 resin chromatography.[47] This stationary phase of polydivinylbenzene has a large surface area and is of a nonionic character, making it capable of adsorbing many classes of organic compounds from aqueous solution, principally by dispersive and dipole interactions. The adsorbed organics are eluted from the XAD-2 by organic solvents such as methanol, acetone, diethyl ether, hexane, methylene chloride, or combinations of these solvents.[48] The XAD-2 method has been applied most often to urine- or blood-screening methods for drugs of abuse and their metabolites, but it can also be applied to isolate trace amounts of many types of compounds.

Another very common chromatographic technique for initial analyte isolation is the use of small columns of silica or of octadecylsilyl-bonded phase.[49,50] The analytes from a relatively large volume of samples are adsorbed from aqueous solution by forces similar to those operating in the XAD-2 procedure. Desorption is accomplished when a small volume of an appropriate solvent is passed through the silica or reversed-phase cartridge; the sample may then be processed for any mode of chromatography. Many additional resins, of the type just described, are currently available for the isolation of compounds of interest to the clinical chemist.[51]

Other types of chromatographic methods have been used in the preparation of samples for analysis. Ion-exchange chromatography has been widely used to isolate charged analytes. Anion exchange, first suggested by Horning and Horning,[52] has been widely used for the isolation of acidic constituents from biological fluids. Although DEAE-Sephadex is the most widely used ion-exchange stationary phase for sample cleanup, other anion exchangers, such as AGIX and Dowex 3, have been used.

Extraction Methods for Analyte Isolation

Liquid-liquid and liquid-solid partition methods have been widely used for both primary and secondary extraction steps in a wide variety of clinical chemistry analyses before the chromatographic quantitation step. The reasons for the use of extraction procedures are numerous, including the isolation of the analyte from large quantities of contaminating materials and its concentration into a small volume of solvent, making detection easier. Liquid-liquid extraction procedures are easily accomplished, usually permitting the workup of multiple samples simultaneously.

The success of an extraction step depends on knowledge of the polarity of the analyte. This information is used to select an extracting solvent that will effectively remove the analyte from the sample. A general rule of solvent selection is that compounds tend to favor solvents having the same polarity interaction forces. It is critical that the chosen solvent be immiscible with the sample matrix.

Other points must be considered in solvent selection. The solvent must be chemically compatible with the analyte; that is, no chemical reaction should be possible between the two. The solvent must be compatible with all subsequent operations after the extraction. For example, a solvent with a high boiling point would be difficult to remove, and so the analyte solution would be difficult to concentrate by evaporation. The solvent should not introduce any contaminants that would make the analysis difficult. Many laboratory supply companies offer common solvents of high-purity grades, such as: (1) *HPLC-grade solvents*, which are compatible with most detector systems and do not contain particulate matter that would foul the HPLC equipment; (2) *pesticide-grade solvents,* which are compatible with electron-capture GC detectors because they do not introduce any contaminating substances; and (3) *lipograde-grade solvents,* which do not contain any greases or other substances that would interfere with the analysis of lipids. These are but a few of the types of quality solvents available. If the solvent is not available in the required purity, a purification of the solvent must be done before use in any sample cleanup procedure. Most commonly, a distillation of the solvent will suffice, but sometimes more extensive purification measures are required. Methods of more rigorous purification procedures for most solvents are described in Weissberger's text.[53] Even with the use of the highest quality solvents commercially available or prior purification of solvents, impurities may still be a problem. The most common contaminant is plasticizers, usually coming from cap liners and other plastic materials.[54] These contaminants, various alkyl phthalates, can interfere with some analyses, particularly when electron-capture gas chromatography is used. Foil-lined screw caps of extraction tubes or sample vials have been shown to be the source of contaminants that interfered with GC.[55] These contamination problems can be eliminated by using screw-cap liners made of Teflon.

Once a decision on the solvents for extraction has been made, the actual operations in extraction must be considered. In general, a repeated series of extractions with smaller volumes of solvent will be more efficient than a single extraction with a large volume. For solid samples, the solvent may be introduced during the mechanical disruption step as previously mentioned. The cycle of grinding, sonication, and so on is repeated several times with several volumes of solvent. However, doing so sometimes does not effectively extract the desired analyte. In this case, the pulverized solid sample may have to be extracted with a Soxhlet extractor or a continuous infusion extractor. Both of these methods are more efficient than manual operations for extracting substances from a solid matrix. However, the requirements for these methods include a reasonably volatile extracting solvent and stability of the analyte at the boiling point of the solvent.

To extract an analyte with ionizable groups, it is best to first solubilize the solid sample in an aqueous solution. The pH of the sample solution is then adjusted below the **pK$_a$** of acidic components or above the pK$_a$ of basic components with the addition of acid or base, respectively, to convert the analyte, 95% or greater, into its extractable (nonionized) form. A nomogram relating pK$_a$ values of acids to percent ionization at various pH values has been published by Hopgood.[56] If the pK$_a$ of the analyte is not known, a lowering of the pH of the aqueous solution to a pH of 2.0 by the addition of acid is usually sufficient to permit the extraction of most acidic analytes. Likewise, raising the pH to 12 is usually sufficient to permit the extraction of most basic analytes of unknown pK$_a$.

For liquid-liquid extraction, an increase in the ionic strength of the aqueous layer will enhance the ease of extraction of the analyte, causing it to favor the extracting solvent. An ionic neutral salt, such as sodium chloride or potassium bromide, is commonly used for this purpose.

One of the problems frequently encountered in liquid-liquid extractions is the formation of **emulsions**, that is, one of the immiscible phases becomes dispersed as fine droplets in the other. To avoid emulsion formation, several precautions can be taken during the actual extraction process: (1) If the two liquid layers have a large contact surface, avoid vigorous mixing of the phases. The use of gentle agitation will accomplish the extraction. (2) Filter all finely divided particulate matter before extraction. (3) Use solvent pairs with large differences in density.

If an emulsion does form, there are several steps that will possibly break it. First, try to get the dispersed droplets to achieve coalescence by mechanically disrupting their surfaces. Stirring with a glass rod or filtration through a loose bed of glass wool will sometimes break the emulsion. Second, if the densities of the two solvents are sufficiently different, centrifugation will sometimes effect separation. Third, cooling or freezing the mixture sometimes causes a coalescence of droplets. Fourth, an increase in ionic strength, by the addition of salt or a small amount of an alcohol, such as ethanol or 2-ethyl-1-hexanol, may cause a decrease in the forces stabilizing the emulsion. Fifth, a change in the ratio of the two solvents by addition of more extraction solvent or a partial evaporation of solvent may break the emulsion. Finally, filtration through phase-separation filter paper will break many emulsions commonly encountered.

In most cases, one of these procedures will be successful in breaking the emulsion. For examples of the use of solvent extraction techniques, see the procedures for the analysis of drugs on the CD-ROM.

Processing of Sample Extracts

Many analyte extracts are too dilute for direct chromatographic analysis or for derivatization reactions before chromatography and are usually concentrated by evaporation of the extracting solvent.

Any solvent-evaporation procedure must be conducted with care to avoid loss of the analyte. Such a loss of analyte can occur if traces of water are present in the extract. These can be removed by use of an anhydrous salt, such as sodium carbonate or sodium sulfate. Alternative desiccating salts, such as calcium oxide or magnesium sulfate, can also be used. Other purposes for drying an extract may be to subsequently conduct a derivatization procedure, such as acetylation or silylization, or to prevent interference with the chromatography step.

During concentration of an extract, take care to avoid losses of the analyte. The analyte may be lost by irreversibly binding to the walls of the concentration vessel during concentration. This can be avoided by prior silylization of the glassware. Some substances are sufficiently volatile to form azeotrope mixtures with the solvent and be lost during evaporation. To avoid this, many gentle concentration methods or apparatuses are available. MicroSynder or Kurderna-Danish concentrators evaporate solvent under mild conditions. If the analyte is heat- or oxygen-sensitive, evaporation of the solvent under a stream of purified inert gas, such as nitrogen or argon, can be employed. In this case, warm the vessel to a range of 35° to 50° C to expedite the evaporation process. The use of a rotary evaporator under reduced pressure is also a gentle method for solvent evaporation. A comparison of solvent reduction methods has been made by Constable et al,[57] wherein recoveries of analytes varied from 41% to 140%, depending on the method employed. These results emphasize the importance of method validation and the key role that quality assurance samples, such as samples spiked with analyte, play in the use of a specific approach to cleanup.

Another method for concentrating the analyte is the back-extraction of the compound of interest from the solvent. For example, Kossa and associates[58] have published a variety of methods whereby the analyte, in the original extracting solvent, is back-extracted into a small volume of analyte-derivatizing solvent before gas chromatography. Methods of this type expedite the analysis, since solvent-evaporation steps are not required. Other examples of analyte cleanup procedures for preparing samples for chromatography are detailed in the review by Ko and Petzold[59] and Sunshine.[60] Additional examples are given in Chapters 6 and 7 on HPLC and GC and for individual analytes on the CD-ROM.

References

1. Anderson DJ et al: Clinical chemistry, *Anal Chem* 63:165R, 1991.
2. Eiceman GA, Clement RE, Hill HH, Jr: Gas chromatography, *Anal Chem* 64:170R, 1992.
3. Dorsey JG et al: Liquid chromatography: theory and methodology, *Anal Chem* 64:353R, 1992.
4. Sherma J: Planar chromatography, *Anal Chem* 64:134R, 1992.
5. Tswett MS: Chromatographic absorption analysis: selected works. In Berezken VG, compiler; Masson MR, translation editor: *Ellis Horwood Series in Analytical Chemistry*, New York, 1990, E. Horwood Publishing.
6. Heftman E: History of chromatography. In Heftman E, editor: *Chromatography: fundamentals and applications of chromatography and related differential migration methods*, ed 5, Journal of Chromatography Library, vol 51Aa, New York, 1992, Elsevier Science Publishers.
7. Strain HH, Svec WA: Differential methods of analysis. In Heftman E, editor: *Chromatography: a laboratory handbook of chromatography methods*, ed 3, New York, 1975, Van Nostrand Reinhold Co.
8. Kalasz H, Ettre LS: *Chromatography: the state of the art*, Wellingborough, UK, 1984, Collets.
9. Ettre LS: The development of chromatography, *Anal Chem* 43:20A, 1971.
10. Laitinen HA, Ewing GW, editors: *A history of analytical chemistry*, Washington, DC, 1977, Analytical Chemistry Division of American Chemical Society.
11. Giddings JC: Reduced plate height equation: a common link between chromatographic methods, *J Chromatogr* 13:301, 1964.
12. Schoenmakers OJ: *Optimization of chromatographic selectivity: a guide to method development*, New York, 1986, Elsevier.
13. Wong HY: *Therapeutic drug monitoring and toxicology*, Chromatographic Science Series, vol 32, New York, 1985, Marcel Dekker.
14. Snyder LR, Glajch JL, Kirkland JJ: *Practical HPLC method development*, New York, 1988, Wiley & Sons.
15. Sherma J, Fried B, editors: *Thin layer chromatography*, Chromatographic Science Series, vol 55, New York, 1990, Marcel Dekker.
16. Snyder LR: A rapid approach to selecting the best experimental conditions for high speed liquid column chromatography. 1. Estimating initial sample resolution and the final resolution required by a given problem, *J Chromatogr Sci* 10:200, 1972.
17. Katz E: *Quantitative analysis using chromatographic techniques*, New York, 1987, Wiley & Sons.
18. Giddings JC: Non-equilibrium and diffusion: a common basis for theories of chromatography, *J Chromatogr* 2:44, 1959.
19. Snyder LR, Kirkland JJ: *Introduction of modern liquid chromatography*, ed 2, New York, 1979, Wiley & Sons.
20. Martin AJP, Synge RLM: A new form of chromatogram employing two liquid phases. I. A theory of chromatography. II. Application to the micro-determinations of the higher monoaminoacids in proteins, *Biochem J* 35:1358, 1941.

21. Van Deemter JJ, Zuiderweg FJ, Klinkenberg A: Longitudinal diffusion and resistance to mass transfer as causes of nonideality in chromatography, *Chem Engl Sci* 5:271, 1956.

22. Grob RL: *Modern practice of gas chromatography,* ed 2, New York, 1985, Wiley & Sons.

23. Rotzsche H: *Stationary phases in gas chromatography,* Journal of Chromatography Library, vol 48, New York, 1991, Elsevier Science Publishers.

24. Knapp DR: *Handbook of analytical derivatization reactions,* New York, 1979, Wiley & Sons.

25. McMahon DH: Methods development guidelines for chemical derivatization in gas chromatography, *J Chromatogr Sci* 23:426, 1985.

26. Lawrence JF: Advantages and limitations of chemical derivatization for trace analysis by liquid chromatography, *J Chromatogr Sci* 23:484, 1985.

27. Lingeman H, Underberg WJM, editors: *Detection-oriented derivatization techniques in liquid chromatography,* Chromatographic Science Series, vol 48, New York, 1990, Marcel Dekker.

28. West SD: The prediction of reversed-phase HPLC retention indices and resolution as a function of solvent strength and selectivity, *J Chromatogr Sci* 25:122, 1987.

29. Keller RA, Snyder LR: Relation between the solubility parameter and the liquid-solid solvent strength parameter, *J Chromatogr Sci* 9:345, 1971.

30. Karger BL, Snyder LR, Eon C: An expanded solubility parameter treatment for classification and use of chromatographic solvents and absorbents: parameters for dispersion, dipole, and hydrogen bonding interactions, *J Chromatogr* 125:71, 1976.

31. Snyder LR: Solvent selection for separation processes. In Perry ES, Weissberger A, editors: *Techniques of chemistry: separation and purification,* ed 3, vol 12, New York, 1978, Wiley & Sons.

32. Glajch JL et al: Optimization of solvent strength and selectivity for reverse-phase liquid chromatography using an interactive mixture-design statistical technique, *J Chromatogr* 199:57, 1980.

33. Snyder LR: Classification of the solvent properties of common liquids, *J Chromatogr* 92:223, 1974.

34. Hildebrand JH, Scott RI: *The solubility of non-electrolytes,* ed 3, New York, 1964, Dover Publications; and Hildebrand JH, Scott RI: *Regular solutions,* Englewood Cliffs, NJ, 1962, Prentice-Hall.

35. Snyder LR: Solvent selection for separation processes. In Perry ES, Weissberger A, editors: *Techniques of chemistry: separation and purification,* ed 3, vol 12, New York, 1978, Wiley & Sons.

36. Trappe W: Die Trennung von biologischen Fettstoffen aus ihren natürlichen Gemischen durch Anwendung von Adsorptionssäulen. 1. Mitteilung: Die eluotrope Reihe der Lösungsmittel, *Biochem Z* 305:150, 1940.

37. Rohrschneider L: Eine Methode zur Charakterisierung von gaschromatographischen Trennflüssigkeiten, *J Chromatogr* 22:6, 1966.

38. McReynolds WO: Characterization of some liquid phases, *J Chromatogr Sci* 8:685, 1970.

39. Zlatkin A, Kaiser RE: *HPTLC: high performance thin-layer chromatography,* Journal of Chromatography Library Series 9, New York, 1977, Elsevier Scientific Publishing.

40. Touchstone JC: *Practice of thin layer chromatography,* ed 3, New York, 1992, Wiley & Sons.

41. Halasz I, Sebastian I: New stationary phase for chromatography, *Angew Chem, Int Ed* 8:453, 1969.

42. Anderson DMW: Gel permeation chromatography. In Simpson CF, editor: *Practical high performance liquid chromatography,* Philadelphia, 1978, Heyden & Sons.

43. Hunt BJ, Holding SR, editors: *Size exclusion chromatography,* New York, 1989, Chapman & Hall.

44. Tabor MW: Chemical analysis for assessment and evaluation of environmental pollutants: fact or artifact, *Environ Sci Res* 38:205, 1990.

45. Smith CC, Khalil A, Tabor MW: Fractionation of urinary and fecal metabolites of the antimalarial drug WR-158,122 following oral doses in rats and rhesus monkey, *Toxicologist* 3:52, 1983.

46. Que Hee SS et al: Screening method for Aroclor 1254 in whole blood, *Anal Chem* 55:157, 1983.

47. Stolman A, Pranitis PA: XAD-2 resin drug extraction methods for biological samples, *Clin Toxicol* 10:49, 1977.

48. Weissman N et al: Screening method for detection of drugs of abuse in human urine, *Clin Chem* 17:875, 1971.

49. Shackleton CHL, Whitney JD: Use of Sep-Pak cartridges for urinary steroid extraction: evaluation of the method for use prior to gas chromatographic analysis, *Clin Chim Acta* 107:231, 1980.

50. Heikkinen R, Fotsis T, Adlercreutz H: Reversed-phase C18 cartridge for extraction of estrogens from urine and plasma, *Clin Chem* 27:1186, 1981.

51. Tabor MW, Loper JC: Analytical isolation, separation and identification of mutagens from nonvolatile organics of drinking water, *Int J Environ Anal Chem* 19:281, 1985.

52. Horning EC, Horning MG: Metabolic profiles: gas-phase methods for analysis of metabolites, *Clin Chem* 17:802, 1971.

53. Riddick JA, Bunger WB: Organic solvents. In Weissberger A, editor: *Techniques of chemistry,* vol 2, ed 3, New York, 1978, Wiley & Sons.

54. DeZeeuw RA, Jonkman JHG, van Mansvelt FJW: Plasticizers as contaminants in high purity solvents: a potential source of interference in biological analysis, *Anal Biochem* 67:339, 1975.

55. Denney DW, Karsek FW: Detection and identification of contaminants from foil-lined screw-cap sample vials, *J Chromatogr* 151:75, 1978.

56. Hopgood MF: Nomogram for calculating percentage ionization of acids and bases, *J Chromatogr* 47:45, 1970.

57. Constable DJC, Smith SR, Tanaka J: Comparison of solvent reduction methods for concentration of polycyclic aromatic hydrocarbon solutions, *Environ Sci Technol* 18:975, 1984.

58. Kossa WC et al: Pyrolytic methylation/gas chromatography: a short review, *J Chromatogr Sci* 17:177, 1979.

59. Kö H, Petzold EN: Isolation of samples prior to chromatography. In Tsuji K, Morozowich W, editors: *GLC and HPLC determination of therapeutic agents,* part 1, New York, 1978, Marcel Dekker.

60. Sunshine I: *Manual of analytical toxicology,* Boca Raton, Fla, 1971, CRC Press.

Bibliography

Books

American Society of Testing Materials: *ASTM standards on chromatography,* ed 2, ASTM Subcommittee E19.07 on Compilation of Chromatographic Methods, Philadelphia, 1989, ASTM.

Cazes J: *Encyclopedia of chromatography* (Den New Dekker Encyclopedias), New York, 2001, Marcel Dekker.

Fried B, Sherma J: *Practical thin-layer chromatography: a multidisciplinary approach,* New York, 1996, CRC Press.

Fritz JS, Gjerdec DT: *Ion chromatography,* ed 3, New York, 2000, John Wiley & Sons.

Grob RL: *Modern practice of gas chromatography,* ed 3, New York, 1995, Wiley & Sons.

Heftman E: *Chromatography: fundamentals and applications of chromatography and related differential migration methods,* ed 5, Journal of Chromatography Library, vol 51 A and B, New York, 1992, Elsevier Science Publishers.

Hermanson GT, Mallia AK, Smith PK: *Immobilized affinity ligand techniques,* New York, 1997, Academic Press

McNair HM, Miller JM: *Basic gas chromatography* (techniques in analytical chemistry), New York, 1991, John Wiley & Sons.

Papadoyannis IN: *HPLC in clinical chemistry,* Chromatographic Science Series, vol 54, New York, 1990, Marcel Dekker.

Sherma J, Fried B, editors: *Thin layer chromatography,* Chromatographic Science Series, vol 55, New York, 1990, Marcel Dekker.

Snyder LR, Glajch JL, Kirkland JJ: *Practical HPLC method development,* New York, 1988, Wiley & Sons.

Snyder LR, Kirkland J, Glajch J: *Practical HPLC method,* New York, 2002, John Wiley & Sons.

Weston A, Brown PR: *HPLC and CE: principles and practice,* New York, 1997, Academic Press.

Comprehensive Abstracts, Journals, and Series in Chromatography

Advances in Chromatography, New York, Marcel Dekker, Inc.

Analytical Abstracts, London, Royal Society of Chemistry.

Chemical Abstracts, Columbus, Ohio, American Chemical Society.

Chromatographia, New York, Pergamon Press.

Chromatographic Reviews, Amsterdam, Elsevier Scientific Publishing Co.

Chromatographic Science Series, New York, Marcel Dekker, Inc.

Chromatography Symposium Series, New York, Elsevier Scientific Publishing Co.

Gas and Liquid Chromatography Abstracts, Barking, Essex, Applied Science Publishers.

Gas Chromatography Abstracts, London, Butterworth & Co.

Journal of Chromatography, New York, Elsevier Scientific Publishing Co.

Journal of Chromatography Library, New York, Elsevier Scientific Publishing Co.

Journal of Chromatographic Science, Niles, Ill, Preston Publications.

Journal of High Resolution Chromatography and Chromatography Communications, Heidelberg, NY, Muthing Press.

Journal of Liquid Chromatography, New York, Marcel Dekker, Inc.

Progress in Thin-Layer Chromatography and Related Methods, Ann Arbor, Mich, Lewis Publishers.

Internet Sites

http://www.home4u.de/niven/rn_know1.htm—Niven's chromatographic terms

http://ull.chemistry.uakron.edu/chemsep/chrom_theory/—University of Akron web site

http://www.fda.gov/cder/guidance/cmc3.pdf—Center for Drug Evaluation and Research (need Adobe Acrobat)

http://www.dq.fct.unl.pt/QOF/hplcts.html—Troubleshooting guide

http://www.chromatography.co.uk/TECHNIQS/Default.htm—Troubleshooting guide

http://www.accessexcellence.org/TSN/SS/chromatography_background.html

http://www.netaccess.on/ca/~dbc/cic_hamilton/chrom.html—Chromatography resources

http://www.metabase.net/docs/unibe/01164.html—Spanish language site

www.icfes.gov.co/revistas/recolqui/972601/972601~7.htm—Colombian government web site

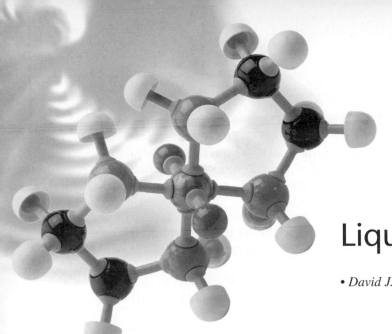

CHAPTER 6

Liquid Chromatography*

• *David J. Anderson*

Chapter Outline

Resolution, efficiency, and speed of analysis
  Resolution
  Chromatographic efficiency
  Speed of analysis
Quantitation
  Approaches
  Standardization
General elution problem
Selection of a chromatographic mode
  Size-exclusion chromatography
  Ion-exchange chromatography
  Adsorption chromatography
  Partition and bonded-phase chromatography
  Reversed-phase chromatography
  Ion-pair chromatography

  Affinity chromatography
  Chromatography of enantiomers
Different types of HPLC packing materials
  *Different supports addressing problems of silica
    supports*
  Restricted access media
  Pore size considerations
  High-speed analysis
Instrumentation
  Solvent-delivery systems
  Sample-introduction systems
  Columns and connectors
  Detection systems
Applications

Objectives

- Describe the advantage of using peak height or peak area to quantitate an analyte using liquid chromatography.
- Define external standardization, internal standardization, and standard addition; explain how unknown concentrations are determined with each standardization process; state the requirements for internal standard selection and use.
- Discuss the various liquid chromatographic modes used to separate molecules and discuss the factors to consider in choosing the appropriate mode.
- Describe the different types of packing material that

are commercially available, detailing the advantages and disadvantages of each.
- Diagram the basic column liquid chromatographic system; list four basic components of a high-performance liquid chromatography (HPLC) separation system and state the purpose of each.
- List four types of detector systems used in HPLC and, for each, describe the principle of operation, its practical use, and the advantages or disadvantages associated with its use.
- Summarize the applications of HPLC in the analysis of clinically relevant compounds.

---

*With acknowledgment of the previous contributor, Larry D. Bowers.

Key Terms

bonded phase　A chromatographic packing material in which the stationary phase is covalently bound to the surface of the support.

efficiency　Characteristic of a column or packing material that describes the extent of broadening of the chromatographic peak. Higher efficiencies lead to narrower chromatographic peaks.

effluent　Mobile phase that has left the column.

eluant　Mobile phase.

eluate　A compound or mixture that has been separated in the column and left it.

gradient elution　An elution system in which the solvent composition is varied during the run.

H　Height equivalent to one theoretical plate (HETP).

isocratic elution　Elution with a solvent mixture of constant composition.

L　Length of the chromatographic column, usually in millimeters.

mobile phase　The mixture of solvents that is percolated through the column.

μ　Solvent velocity in the column ($\mu = L/t_0$).

N　Number of theoretical separating plates in a chromatographic column.

normal phase　A chromatographic mode in which the mobile phase is less polar than the stationary phase.

packing material　Term referring to the material that is placed ("packed") into the chromatographic column, consisting of both the stationary phase and the support.

permeability　A measure of the ease with which the mobile phase can be forced through the column.

R_s　Resolution; the degree of separation between two **eluates**.

reversed phase　Chromatographic mode in which the mobile phase is more polar than the stationary phase.

stationary phase　The portion of the separation system that is immobilized in the column.

support　The particles on which the stationary phase is held.

t_R　Retention time; the time required to elute a compound from a chromatographic column.

V_0　Volume of solvent required to elute an unretained compound; also called *void volume*.

V_R　Retention volume; the volume of the mobile phase required to elute a compound from a chromatographic column at t_R.

A glossary of 500 terms, abbreviations, and equation variables for liquid chromatography/separation techniques has been published[1] (also available at www.chromatographyonline.com).

Liquid chromatography is a form of separation science in which a liquid mobile phase is percolated through a column or thin layer of particles. Fig. 6-1 shows a schematic diagram of a column chromatograph used in liquid chromatography. The liquid **mobile phase** is taken from the reservoir and moved through the column, usually by a pump. A method of introducing the sample into the chromatographic system is also required. The most important constituent of a chromatographic instrument is the column. The column is filled with **packing material**, which consists of small particles **(support)** on which specific sites or a layer of solvent (both referred to as **stationary phase**) is held. The differential equilibration of the analytes between the mobile and the stationary phases results in their separation. All chromatographic modes (see Chapter 5) can be used in liquid chromatography. Finally, the column **effluent** can either be collected for further analysis or analyzed with an on-line detector, such as a photometer. Aliquots of the liquid phase can be collected if subsequent analysis is desired. The recording of any parameter that allows the analyte or analytes to be monitored as a function of elution volume or time is called a *chromatogram.*

Liquid chromatography is well suited for use in the clinical laboratory. Because the retention of a compound is determined by equilibria, the position of the peak in the chromatogram (i.e., the retention volume) can be helpful in analytical identification. If a substance coelutes with a known compound, it may be the same material; an identical retention, however, does not *prove* identity. In addition, measurement of the height or area of the peak can provide quantitative information. Because the components of a mixture are separated, quantitation of several compounds in a single analysis is possible. Such quantitation is useful in the measurement of drugs or intermediates in a metabolic pathway (such as porphyrins). Another advantage of liquid chromatography is that the relatively polar compounds present in body fluids readily dissolve in commonly used mobile-phase solvents. This is in contrast to gas chromatography, which requires volatile analytes. Proteins and peptides are readily separated by liquid chromatography.

Despite the fact that liquid chromatography was discovered before gas chromatography, it was used in only a very small number of analytical applications in the clinical laboratory. Classical liquid chromatography typically required hours or days to complete a separation, whereas gas chromatography required only minutes. With the development of small (10 μm) totally porous particles in the early 1970s, liquid chromatography was able to achieve speed and resolution comparable to packed-column gas chromatography (GC). The introduction of covalently bonded stationary phases resulted in the further popularization of HPLC. Develop-

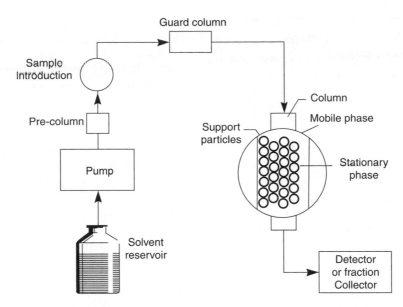

Fig. 6-1 Schematic diagram of a column liquid chromatographic system. *(From Bowers LD, Carr PW: Quantitative aspects of HPLC workshop, Minneapolis, 1983.)*

ments such as microprocessor automation have made both analytical and preparative chromatography easier to perform and more appealing. At present, HPLC is recognized as a true complement to GC in chromatographic analysis.

Good up-to-date books on HPLC at the beginning[2] and more advanced[3] levels have been published. A comprehensive 7000 page encyclopedia on the theory, techniques, and applications of separation techniques has also been published.[4] The internet serves as a major resource for up-to-date information, and some examples are provided after the references at the end of this chapter.

RESOLUTION, EFFICIENCY, AND SPEED OF ANALYSIS

The object of any chromatographic technique is to separate, or resolve, the species of interest from other compounds of interest or from interferences in the sample matrix. Analysts must also be concerned about the speed of the analytical scheme, including any sample preparation steps, the separation itself, and the calculation and reporting of results. Not surprisingly, speed of analysis and resolving power are related. The evolution of HPLC was based on an understanding and optimization of the factors that affect resolution.

Resolution

The relative separation of two chromatographic peaks is measured by a parameter known as *resolution*, or, R_s. A further definition of R_s and an example of the calculation of R_s can be found on p. 112 of Chapter 5. It is dependent on the positions of the centers of the peaks that correspond to each compound and on the width of the peak between the points at which it is indistinguishable from the background signal. If the peak tracing reaches the background level before rising for the second peak, baseline resolution has been achieved. If the first peak shown in the bottom panel of Fig. 6-2 were

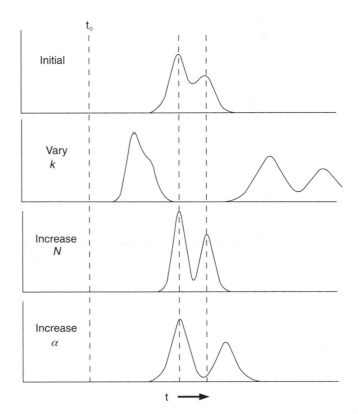

Fig. 6-2 Effect of varying k, N, and α on a resolution. t, Time. *(From Snyder LK, Kirkland JJ: Introduction to modern liquid chromatography, ed 2, New York, 1979, Wiley & Sons. This material is used by permission of John Wiley & Sons, Inc.)*

collected up to the minimum in the valley between the two peaks, the compound in that peak would be 100% free of the compound making up the second peak. When the baseline resolution is not achieved (Fig. 6-2, top), some of the compound present in the second peak is collected along with the

TABLE **6-1** EFFECT OF RESOLUTION ON VARIOUS PEAK PARAMETERS*

Resolution	Purity[†]	% Error in Area[‡]	% Error in Peak Height[‡]
0.6	90	>-25	~15
0.8	95	-10	1
1.0	98	-3	<1
1.25	99.5	<-1	0
1.5	100	0	0

*Assuming a peak-height ratio of 1:1 for the two components.
[†]Purity of major peak, assuming collection is stopped at the lowest point of the valley between the peaks.
[‡]Error for the smaller peak.

compound in the first peak. Table 6-1 shows the relative impurity in the first peak for various resolution values when both peaks are the same size. Snyder and Kirkland have covered this topic more completely.[5] Resolution of peaks also affects quantitation, as discussed later.

Because resolution depends on peak widths, resolution must be controlled by the factors that govern the peak width, namely, **efficiency** (N, number of theoretical plates) and relative peak retention. Peak retention is determined by the retention factor (k) and selectivity (α) as discussed in Chapter 5. Equation 6-1 gives an expression for calculating resolution from these factors.

$$R_s = \left(\frac{\sqrt{N}}{4}\right)\left(\frac{\alpha - 1}{\alpha}\right)\left(\frac{k}{1 + k}\right) \qquad \textit{Eq. 6-1}$$

The effect of changes in each of these parameters on resolution is illustrated in Fig. 6-2.

Chromatographic Efficiency

Chromatographic efficiency (p. 112 of Chapter 5) is a characteristic of a column or packing material describing the extent of broadening of the chromatographic peak. Higher efficiencies lead to narrower peaks, increased resolution, and increased sensitivity. The efficiency of a column can be estimated quantitatively from the van Deemter equation:

$$H = A + B / \mu + C\mu \qquad \textit{Eq. 6-2}$$

in which H is the height of the theoretical plate, μ is the mobile phase velocity, and A, B, and C are constants, the values of which depend on fundamental parameters of the chromatographic system as given below:

$$A = 2\lambda d_p \qquad \textit{Eq. 6-3}$$

$$B = 2\lambda D_m \qquad \textit{Eq. 6-4}$$

$$C = \frac{(1 + 6k + 11k^2)d_p^2}{24(1 + k)^2 D_m} + \frac{8kd_f^2}{\pi^2(1 + k)^2 D_s} \qquad \textit{Eq. 6-5}$$

in which d_p is the particle diameter of the packing material, d_f is the thickness of the stationary- phase layer, D_m and D_s are diffusion coefficients of the analyte in the mobile and stationary phase respectively, k is the retention factor, and

λ and γ are correction factors taking into account column packing nonhomogeneity. Each term in equation 6-2 is descriptive of different processes in liquid chromatography that lead to band spreading, with the A, B, and C terms giving the contributions of the multipath effect (eddy diffusion), longitudinal diffusion, and mass transfer (both in the mobile and stationary phases), respectively. Other expressions quantitating efficiency have been suggested; however, the van Deemter equation appears to be the most appropriate to use.[6] Several books giving more details on theoretical aspects of efficiency as they apply to chromatography have been published.[6-8]

The important conclusions to be drawn from equations 6-2 to 6-5 are that efficiency increases (H decreases) with: (1) decreased particle diameter of the packing material, (2) decreased flow velocity of the mobile phase, and (3) increased diffusion coefficient of the analyte. It should be noted that the role of longitudinal diffusion (B term in equation 6-2) is significant only at low flow velocities, lower than the flow velocities commonly used in HPLC. The major design feature employed for increasing efficiency of HPLC systems has been the use of small-diameter packing materials. HPLC techniques typically use packing materials having diameters of 10, 5, and 3 µm. Packing materials of particle diameter less than 3 µm are not normally used because of the high pressure that would be generated with the pumping of mobile phase through the column. Also evident from equations 6-2 to 6-5 is the effect of the analyte's diffusion coefficient on efficiency. As seen from equation 6-5, macromolecules, which have smaller diffusion coefficients, give broader peaks than smaller molecules, which have larger diffusion coefficients. In general, modern HPLC columns have about 50,000/m theoretical plates for smaller molecules.

For the practicing chromatographer, four final points about efficiency are worthy of mention. First, a new column should always be tested upon receipt to be sure that reasonable efficiency is obtained with that column. An initial efficiency value also serves as a benchmark for measuring the decline in column performance as it is used. Second, the column should be tested under the manufacturer's flow and mobile-phase conditions. The buyer should be aware that a column tested at 0.1 mL/min to obtain a high number of theoretical plates may not be the best column to use at more practical flow rates. Third, N is in reality a measure of system efficiency. Thus a poorly designed detector can make the best column look bad. To achieve the high efficiencies reported by some column manufacturers, the entire system must be optimized. Finally, remember that to enhance resolution twofold, N must be increased fourfold. Thus adjustment of N is normally used to fine-tune a relatively good separation.

The retention of a compound on a column is often described by using its *retention factor, k* (see p. 115 of Chapter 5). The retention factor k is a normalizing factor that allows retention on different-sized columns, or columns operated at different flow rates, to be compared because the k, by definition, is related to the equilibrium of the analyte between the mobile and stationary phases. In terms of resolution, k values over 5 do not increase resolution much and can, in fact, slow analysis and deteriorate the limit of detection. In liquid chromatography, k is adjusted primarily by changes in mobile-phase composition, though it is also inversely related to the temperature.

The difference in retention of two compounds as measured by the ratio of their retention factors is called the *separation factor*, or α (see p. 115 of Chapter 5), which is a measure of selectivity. Note that if α is large there is a large difference in the retention volumes of the two compounds, and the separation can be performed with few plates and little column retention. Selectivity is frequently adjusted by changes in mobile-phase composition. One of the major advantages of liquid chromatography is the wide range of selectivity achievable by varying the composition of the mobile phase. For example, an ion-exchange separation depends on the number of charges on the analytes. We can change the selectivity by varying the mobile-phase pH, ionic strength, or salt composition (NaCl versus LiCl). Selection of a mobile-phase system requires an understanding of the separation mechanisms and a great deal of experience. A change in the stationary phase can also be used to adjust selectivity because the equilibrium achieved between the stationary phase and the mobile phase is the basis of any chromatographic separation. If the retention of the analytes is adequate ($1.5 \leq k \geq 6$), the resolution can be improved most readily by changing the selectivity.

Speed of Analysis

So far, we have discussed retention only in terms of mobile-phase volume, V_R, because (1) the volume of mobile phase used is a direct reflection of cost and (2) changes in the flow rate do not affect the V_R. In contrast, the retention time, t_R, is a function of flow rate and retention volume, that is:

$$t_R = \frac{V_R}{F} \qquad \textit{Eq. 6-6}$$

in which F is the flow rate in milliliters per minute. For example, if the diameter of the column were doubled, its volume and thus the retention volume would increase by a factor of 4. Then t_R could be kept constant by increasing the flow rate by a factor of 4, but solvent consumption would increase accordingly.

The optimization of analysis speed depends on several factors. The most important relationships in achieving a rapid separation are given in the box. Guichon has discussed these factors in great detail.[9] The minimum time possible for a separation is the product of the time required for an analyte to pass one plate and the number of plates required for adequate resolution. The smaller the height of a theoretical plate, H, the faster the separation. Retention time is also increased by the need for more resolution; by small separation factors, α; and by large retention factors, k. Again, to obtain the fastest separations, a mobile phase must be selected to maximize α at relatively small values of k. Under optimal conditions for a separation requiring 3000 plates, an

---

PRACTICAL CONSIDERATIONS IN SPEED OF ANALYSIS

$$t_R = N \cdot \frac{H}{\mu} \cdot (1 + k)$$

$$L = NH$$

$$\Delta P = NH\mu \cdot \frac{\eta}{K_0}$$

μ, Solvent velocity in the column ($= L/t_0$); η, solvent viscosity; K_0, column **permeability**. (See reference 9 for more detail.) ΔP, Column back-pressure.

---

analysis time of 100 sec is feasible with HPLC. One of the problems in translating theory to practice in the clinical laboratory is that the analyte may have to be separated from an unknown metabolite or interferent, and hence α is not known during the development of the separation. In this case, a slower separation time is acceptable, and the selectivity of the detector must be relied upon to indicate a potential problem.

QUANTITATION
Approaches

Quantitation in liquid chromatography is achieved when either the peak height or the peak area is related to the concentration of analyte in the sample. The chromatographic trace is a recording of the concentration of the analyte or analytes as sensed by the detector. At the peak height maximum

$$C_{\max} = \frac{C_S V_S}{V_R} \sqrt{\frac{N}{2\pi}} \qquad \textit{Eq. 6-7}$$

C_S and V_S are the concentration and volume of sample injected, respectively, V_R is the retention volume, and N is the number of theoretical plates. The greater the peak height for any given concentration, the more sensitive is the method. Thus minimizing the retention volume and maximizing the number of theoretical plates results in the most sensitive assay. The factors that decrease the retention volume are a small column void volume (V_o) and a small retention factor. Low flow rates and small support-particle diameters lead to large plate counts. Also note that, unlike the sensitivity of gas chromatography, liquid chromatographic sensitivity is improved by injection of larger sample volumes. The peak height can be related to the concentration in the sample by a sensitivity factor, S. The sensitivity factor changes if the retention volume changes, making day-to-day operation without standardization difficult but not impossible.

Example. If identical samples were injected onto a 4.6 mm internal diameter (ID) and a 2.1 mm ID column, what would be the relative size of the peaks if all else were unchanged?

$$C_{\max} = \frac{1}{V_R}[C_S V_S \sqrt{\frac{N}{2\pi}}] = \frac{1}{\Phi \pi r^2 L}[\overline{C}] \qquad \textit{Eq. 6-8}$$

in which Φ is the void fraction, r is the radius, and L is the length (15 cm) of the column; C is the mass injected into the column. If Φ and L are the same for the two columns, then:

$$\frac{C_{max}\,(2.1)}{C_{max}\,(4.6)} = \frac{(2.3)^2}{(1.05)^2} = 4.8 \qquad \textit{Eq. 6-9}$$

Therefore the peak from the 2.1 mm column would be almost five times as large. This sensitivity advantage is causing increased interest in microbore and capillary columns. Another advantage of using columns with smaller diameters is a decrease in the amount of mobile phase used, thus decreasing cost, minimizing negative environmental impact, and increasing compatibility with on-line mass spectrometry detection by minimizing solvent introduced into the mass spectrometer.

The second approach to quantitation of an analyte is measurement of the peak area. Most liquid chromatography detectors are concentration dependent; that is, they measure a concentration in the flow cell. (This is in contrast to most GC detectors, which are mass-flow dependent.) The peak area obtained from a concentration-dependent detector is inversely proportional to flow rate. Therefore significant variation in peak area can occur if the flow rate changes during a chromatographic run. In addition, less resolution is required for an equal degree of accuracy when peak heights rather than peak areas are used because the overlap of peaks, even with a resolution of 1.0, affects peak area but does not affect the peak maximum.[5] A rough rule of thumb is: use peak *height* when there are interfering peaks or when maximum accuracy is required, but use peak area when precision is the main requirement. For peaks barely above the baseline noise, peak heights should always be used.

Standardization

Standardization in liquid chromatography (LC) can be accomplished in any of three ways: external standardization, internal standardization, or standard addition. For external standardization, a calibration curve is constructed from the peak height (or peak area) values obtained with known concentrations of analyte and a constant injection volume. The slope of the curve is the sensitivity factor, *S,* in peak-height units per concentration unit (such as mm/mM). The concentration of the unknown is then simply its peak height divided by the sensitivity factor. Notice that, if the calibration curve is linear, the sensitivity factor can be obtained from a single standard. It would be important in this case to check several control specimens to verify the validity of the sensitivity factor. The principal sources of error in external calibration are variable losses in the preparative steps before LC analysis and sample-injection variability. It is thus important to treat the standards and samples in the same way. It should be possible to achieve 1% precision with external calibration, but up to 5% is commonly observed.

Internal standardization uses a compound that is usually structurally similar to the analyte to correct for losses during sample preparation and injection imprecision. The same amount of internal standard is added to each sample and

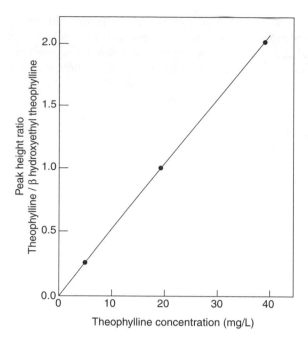

Fig. 6-3 Calibration curve for theophylline using internal standard technique.

standard before sample pretreatment and chromatography. The calibration curve is then constructed from the ratio of the peak heights (or areas) of the standard and the internal standard at various standard concentrations (Fig. 6-3). Again, unknown concentrations can be measured by using the sensitivity factor or interpolating the value from the calibration curve. It is hoped that any losses or variations that occur will affect the analyte and internal standard equivalently. In practice, this is difficult to achieve. An internal standard can be used not only to improve accuracy and precision but also as a quality control check because its peak height should be the same in all chromatograms. Several requirements must be met in the selection of an internal standard. These are summarized in the box below. In some cases internal standards do not improve precision and accuracy and may reduce precision because of the imprecision involved in measuring two peaks.

REQUIREMENTS FOR INTERNAL STANDARD (IS) SELECTION AND USE

1. The internal standard must be completely resolved from all peaks in the sample.
2. It must be eluted near the analyte, with $k \pm 30\%$ being preferable.
3. It must behave similarly to the analyte in pretreatment if losses are to be corrected. This may require more than one internal standard.
4. It must have a peak height or area approximately equal to a standard in the concentration range desired.
5. It must not normally be present in the sample.
6. It should be commercially available in pure form.
7. It should be added as a liquid.

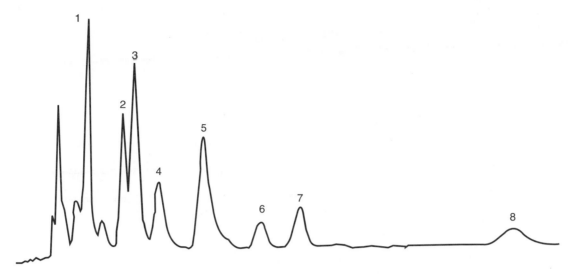

Fig. 6-4 Separation of common human bile acid conjugates by reversed-phase HPLC. Peaks correspond to taurocholate, *1*; taurochenodeoxycholate, *2*; taurodeoxycholate, *3*; taurolithocholate, *4*; glycocholate, *5*; glycochenodeoxycholate, *6*; glycodeoxycholate, *7*; and glycolithocholate, *8*. *(From Roberts G, Bowers LD, unpublished data.)*

The final calibration method, standard addition, requires two analyses to be performed on each sample and thus is not as popular as the other methods. After a sample is analyzed once, a known amount of the compound of interest is added in a very small amount of liquid so that little dilution occurs, and the sample is reanalyzed. To correct for extraction variability, the addition should be made to the biological fluid and the entire analytical scheme repeated. Quantitative data can be obtained from the ratio of the peak height (or area) before and after addition of the standard. Addition of the standard can also help to verify the identity of the peak because the standard must coelute for the unknown to be the same compound. The converse is not true, however, because more than one compound may elute at the same retention volume.

GENERAL ELUTION PROBLEM

The chromatographer is sometimes required to separate compounds that, though structurally related, behave quite differently in the separation system. In Fig. 6-4, a separation of bile acid conjugates demonstrates the problem. When the mobile-phase composition is adjusted to achieve resolution of peaks 2 and 3, peak 8 is retained for over 30 min. Because there are no other peaks near peak 8, the excessive baseline value present between peaks 7 and 8 is a waste of valuable analysis time. Use of a mobile phase with a constant composition is referred to as **isocratic elution**. The alternative to this is to change the mobile-phase composition during the chromatographic run. This can be done as a single change from one mobile phase to another (step gradient) or as a continuous change in any of a variety of shapes (such as linear, segmented linear, or exponential gradient). A complete treatment of **gradient elution** can be found in references 10 to 12. In brief, the peak retention volume,

width, and resolution are determined primarily by the rate of solvent-composition change. Thus many of the concepts discussed earlier are not valid in gradient elution. Any quantitative analyses developed using gradient elution should be carefully documented. In HPLC, the ability to vary mobile-phase composition can be purchased as a part of the solvent-delivery system. It generally increases the cost of the system significantly.

A disadvantage of gradient elution is that the column requires equilibration with the original mobile-phase conditions before the next run. This can take considerable time, particularly with **reversed-phase** analyses. Thus isocratic techniques are predominantly used in the clinical laboratory.

SELECTION OF A CHROMATOGRAPHIC MODE

In Chapter 5 the various mechanisms of chromatography were discussed, including ion exchange, size exclusion (gel permeation or steric exclusion), adsorption, and partition (reversed and **normal phase**). As mentioned previously, all these modes are available in liquid chromatography. The selection of the "best" mode is a problem of significant magnitude for the chromatographer. The choice is made based on an understanding of the mechanism of each mode and its strengths and weaknesses, and frequently it is accomplished by experience. Fig. 6-5 illustrates one method of selecting a chromatographic mode using mechanistic considerations. In addition to these modes, more specialized techniques have been employed, including affinity chromatography and chromatographic techniques for the determination of enantiomers.

Size-Exclusion Chromatography

One of the chromatographer's first considerations is the size of the molecules to be separated. If the molecules are

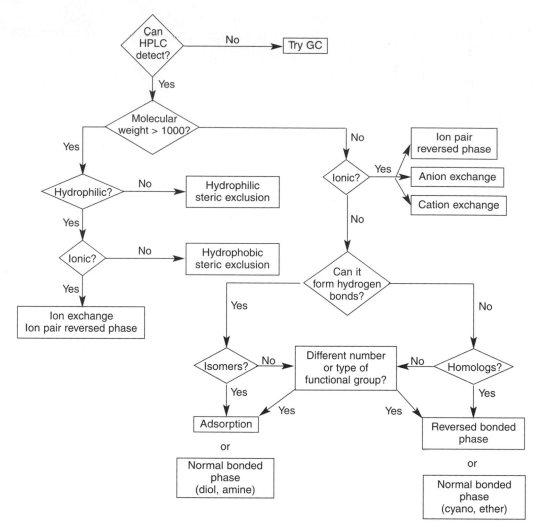

Fig. 6-5 Selection guide for chromatographic modes. *(From Bowers LD, Carr PW:* Quantitative aspects of HPLC workshop, *Minneapolis, 1983.)*

relatively large (>100,000 daltons [D]), *size* (or *steric*) exclusion (SEC) is a logical first choice (see Chapter 5). If, on the other hand, the molecular weights are less than 1000 D, size exclusion is probably not the mode of choice.

Ion-Exchange Chromatography

Another key factor that affects the choice of a separation mode is if the analyte is an ion or if an ionizable group is present on the molecule. Ion exchange is a logical choice for molecules that can be charged, regardless of molecular size. Ion exchange is based on the interaction of analyte charges with an oppositely charged group bound to the chromatographic support. Retention can be varied by varying pH or ionic strength. The greater the number of charges on the analyte, the greater is the retention. Increasing ionic strength, and with it the number of charged groups (such as Na^+) competing with the analyte for the exchange sites on the support, reduces retention. *Ion-pair* chromatography, which uses reversed-phase packing materials, can also be used to separate ionic compounds (see p. 140). An updated review

of biological compounds determined by ion-exchange chromatography has been published.[13]

Adsorption Chromatography

If the molecule has a molecular weight less than 1000 and is not ionizable, another characteristic of the compound must be used to achieve the separation. One such characteristic is the ability of the compound to form hydrogen bonds. Adsorption chromatography is based on the interaction of the analyte with a three-dimensional binding site on the support matrix, which may involve hydrogen bonding. Thus the structure and polarity of the solute are important in determining retention. For example, it is relatively easy to separate *p*-dinitrobenzene from *o*-dinitrobenzene using adsorption chromatography because of the structural differences between the two compounds. On the other hand, separating caproic acid (with six carbon atoms) from caprylic acid (with eight carbon atoms) is very difficult because the parts of the molecules that interact with the stationary phase are identical.

In adsorption chromatography, compounds are eluted from the column because of competition between the analyte and the solvent for the binding site. A solvent that elutes compounds more rapidly and therefore competes better for the chromatographic sites is called a *strong solvent*. Water is a strong solvent for silica adsorbents because it interacts strongly with the silanol (SiOH) groups responsible for the adsorption mechanism. A solvent that does not compete well for sites is called a *weak solvent*. Hexane is a weak solvent for silica adsorbents. Solvent strength can be adjusted by using mixtures of solvents. Snyder[14] has developed a scale of solvent strength called the *eluotropic series* and has extended the solvent strength theory to binary and ternary[15] mixtures. Interestingly, solvent mixtures of the same strength can show differences in selectivity because Snyder's theory considers only the adsorption process, whereas in reality the solute can also interact with the solvent.

One final consideration in adsorption chromatography is the control of the "activity" of the adsorbent. Silica contains several types of silanol groups, which interact differently with various types of compounds. A small amount of water, methanol, acetonitrile, isopropanol, or other strong solvent is used to block the strongest sites and give a more reproducible adsorption surface. This problem has caused some chromatographers to avoid adsorption systems, probably unnecessarily. A separation that involves nonpolar to intermediate-polarity compounds that can form hydrogen bonds or that have isomeric components will probably be easily achieved with adsorption chromatography.

Partition and Bonded-Phase Chromatography

The interactions between solute and stationary phase in partition chromatography are not nearly so well defined as those for adsorption systems. Any chemical forces that exist between molecules can be used in partition-based separations, including hydrogen bonding, van der Waals forces, ion-ion interactions, and so on (see Chapter 5). The basis of partition systems is the distribution of a solute between two liquid solvent layers, one stationary and the other mobile. It is essentially analogous to thousands of liquid extractions taking place in a column. In classical partition chromatography, a polar liquid, such as β, β'-oxydipropionitrile (β, β'-ODPN), was coated onto the support particles, and an immiscible solvent such as hexane was used as the mobile phase. Because solvent-solute interactions involve the entire molecule, a typical partition system as given here would separate a homologous series (C6, C7, and C8 carboxylic acids) and some positional isomers. A partition system with a polar stationary phase and a nonpolar mobile phase is called *normal phase* because it was the first type of system developed. Later, a system with a nonpolar stationary phase, such as squalane, and a polar mobile phase, such as a water-acetonitrile mixture, was developed and called *reversed phase*. Both types of liquid-liquid partition chromatography had many problems related to the finite solubility of all solvents in each other. For example, the β, β'-ODPN would slowly dissolve in the hexane and slowly change the amount of stationary phase, which in turn would change the retention volumes of the analytes. The temperature had to be very closely controlled, and gradient elution was impossible with partition chromatography. These problems made partition chromatography difficult to use in the clinical laboratory.

All of this changed with the development of chemically bonded stationary phases. These materials are prepared by covalent bonding of an organic moiety onto the surface of the support particle, usually silica. The organic groups include nonpolar functions, such as octadecylsilane (ODS, or C18) or octylsilane (C8), and polar groups, such as cyanopropyl (CN), aminopropyl (NH_2), or glycidoxypropyl (diol) silanes. The advantages of **bonded phases** are that: (1) polar and ionic compounds are readily separated, (2) the stationary phase does not strip off, (3) a gradient elution can be used, and (4) the columns are easy to use and take care of. The main disadvantage of bonded phases is that at pH values below 2 the bonded group is cleaved from the support and at pH values above 8 the silica support particles dissolve, although packing materials with supports other than silica have been developed that can be used up to pH 12 to 14 (see later discussion). Because most separations for clinical laboratory applications can be performed within this workable pH window, bonded phases are very popular. The following section has been included to discuss the variety of separations feasible with reversed-phase systems.

Reversed-Phase Chromatography[16]

The discussion is expanded here for the reversed-phase chromatographic technique because of its popularity in use. In a survey of HPLC users, approximately 50% of the HPLC separations were performed on reversed-phase columns.[17] The most popular reversed-phase packing material is the ODS, or C18 packing material. The mobile phase in reversed phase is most commonly water containing an organic modifier such as methanol, acetonitrile, or tetrahydrofuran. In general, retention of an analyte on the reversed-phase column depends on the relative amounts of polar and nonpolar character of the analyte, as shown in Fig. 6-6 for the amino acid tyrosine. Retention on the reversed-phase packing material is favored by increased nonpolar content of the analyte, whereas residence in the mobile phase leading to early elution from the column is favored by an increased content of polar functionalities present on the analyte. The organic modifier component of the mobile phase competes with the stationary phase for the nonpolar part of the analyte molecule, and thus retention is decreased with an increased organic modifier in the mobile phase.

The simplified description of retention mechanism given is important to a basic understanding of reversed-phase mechanism. However, there are complex intricacies to retention mechanism as presented elsewhere.[18, 19] Although a partition mechanism is proposed by some (in which solute is fully encompassed by the stationary phase), an adsorption mechanism (in which the solute is retained on the stationary phase through surface contact only), or a combination of both, has also been proposed.

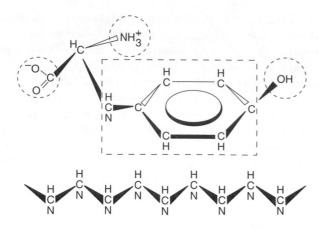

Fig. 6-6 Retention in reversed-phase chromatography is the result of the interaction of the nonpolar portion of the compound such as tyrosine *(enclosed in box)* with the non-polar stationary phase. Hydrophilic groups *(circled)* tend to decrease retention.

Stationary-phase considerations. As noted earlier, the separation obtained for any group of analytes is a function of both the stationary phase and the mobile phase. The analyst has the ability to vary mobile-phase conditions but is dependent on manufacturers for the stationary phase, particularly for bonded-phase packings. If chromatography is to be reproducible, the behavior of the stationary phase toward nonpolar, polar, and ionic compounds must be the same from column to column and from lot to lot. In addition, the durability of columns is important because of their expense. Significant improvements in these features have occurred in recent years, but there are some limitations in producing a column with absolutely reproducible reversed-phase column packings.

The preparation of an octadecylsilane (ODS, C18) stationary phase is usually accomplished when the silanol (SiOH) groups on the silica gel are reacted with an ODS such as octadecyldimethylchlorosilane. The resulting surface contains octadecyl groups bound to the surface by siloxone (Si-O-Si) bonds as shown in Fig. 6-7. Most manufacturers of columns use silanes with only one chloride group, and the resulting stationary phase is called *monomeric*. Because of the stereochemistry of the silica gel surface, only about one third of the silanol groups can react with the ODS groups. The remaining silanol groups are polar and can interact with polar analytes, changing the selectivity of the stationary phase. Trimethylchlorosilane can react with about an additional 20% of the surface silanol groups with a resultant increase in the nonpolar character of the support (see Fig. 6-7). This process is called *end capping* and is used in many commercially available packing materials. As might be expected, differences in the surface morphology of the silica gel, reaction conditions in the ODS-bonding step, and the presence or absence of end capping make columns purchased from different manufacturers perform differently. In fact, variations from lot to lot of packing material may be quite noticeable in the separations obtained for certain analyses. Thus it is not surprising that in adapting a method to a laboratory significant changes in the mobile phase may be required if a C18 column from a manufacturer other than that named in the original report is used. Choice of a reversed-phase column still requires trial and error. For the novice, use of the brand of column reported in a publication is probably warranted to obtain acceptable chromatograms in a reasonable amount of time. The situation with respect to columns is improving as a better understanding of the silica backbone is achieved. A report has been prepared that compares 60 commonly used C18 phases from different manufacturers according to specifications, hydrophobicity, polarity, column efficiency, chromatography of basic compounds, and residual silanol activity[20].

The most utilized reversed-phase functionalities are C18 and C8 (straight chain hydrocarbons of 18 and 8 carbons, respectively). Functionalities from C1 to C30 are available. Other functionalities that have recently been developed include C30 phases, fluorinated alkyl phases, amide-alkyl phases, and polar embedded phases. C30 phases have unique selectivity for certain isomers, carotenoids, chlorophyll, and flavonoids, and have among the highest hydrophobic content of any reversed-phase ligand. Fluorinated alkyl phases have unique selectivity for halogenated organics, compounds with a carbonyl functionality, and hydrophobic compounds such as fat-soluble vitamins and phospholipids. This type of reversed-phase packing material is more hydrophilic than the usual reversed-phase packing material of similar chain length. Polar embedded phases consist of alkyl-bonded

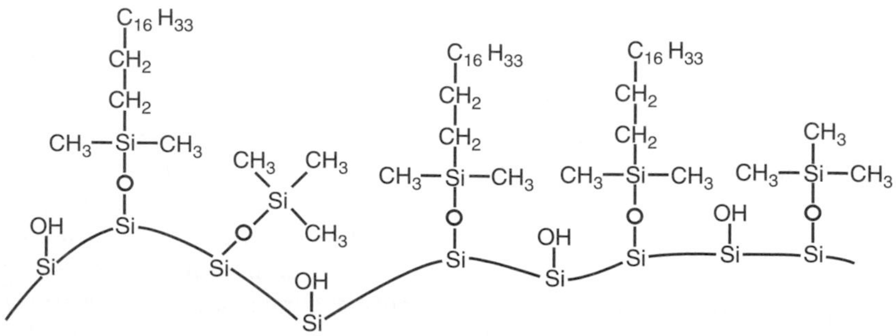

Fig. 6-7 Schematic diagram of a silica-based octadecyl reversed-phase support that has been end capped. Notice presence of residual silanol groups on surface.

phases (usually C18, C8) and either contain a polar functionality within the alkyl chain or use a hydrophilic endcapping reagent; they display stable retention in highly aqueous mobile phases that have little or no organic modifier present, and are useful for basic compounds.

Mobile-phase considerations. The real power in liquid chromatography arises from the fact that changes in mobile-phase composition can have major effects on selectivity and thus on resolution. In reversed-phase systems, two types of changes can be made: (1) changing the type of organic solvent used and (2) additions to the mobile phase that affect its pH, ionic strength, or complexing ability. It has been recognized for some time that the type of organic solvent used has an effect on retention and selectivity. In some cases, a change from methanol to acetonitrile actually alters the elution order of the compounds. Unfortunately at this time the use of solvents to vary selectivity is largely empirical, and the exact role of each solvent in a separation is poorly defined. However, the relative strength of solvents is well defined with solvent strength, and therefore the ability to elute solutes, increasing in the following order: methanol < DMSO < ethanol ≤ acetonitrile < tetrahydrofuran < dioxane < isopropanol. As a rule, when adjusting the retention of a solute, a 10% increase in the fraction of organic solvent (such as methanol or acetonitrile) in water causes a twofold or threefold decrease in the k value.

Ion suppression. Mobile-phase modifications that change retention by introducing a second chemical equilibrium process in the mobile phase have been used since the inception of reversed-phase chromatography.[21] The first approach was control of pH to effect retention. If, for example, ascorbic acid was to be separated by HPLC, there would be a strong influence of pH on retention. At pH values above the pK_a of ascorbic acid, the acid would be deprotonated and charged and therefore would not partition itself strongly into the nonpolar stationary phase. Retention would be relatively low. On the other hand, at pH values below the pK_a, the acid would be protonated and uncharged and so would be much more strongly retained. In the area about one pH unit on either side of the pK_a, the retention changes rapidly as a function of pH, as shown in Fig. 6-8. The use of pH control to increase retention for acids has been termed *ion suppression.* It is a very useful method of adjusting retention behavior. Buffers are normally used to control the pH. It is important to remember that an acid-base pair is a good buffer only within one pH unit of the pK_a. Table 6-2 lists some useful buffers for reversed-phase HPLC.

Chromatography of basic compounds on conventional reversed-phase packing material. Basic compounds can be chromatographed on conventional reversed-phase packing materials by making modifications in the mobile phase. The biggest difficulty in chromatographing basic compounds on silica reversed-phase packing materials is the presence of silanol groups on the silica surface. As mentioned previously, approximately 50% of the silanol groups remain on the silica support after synthesis of the reversed-phase packing material. A small percentage of these

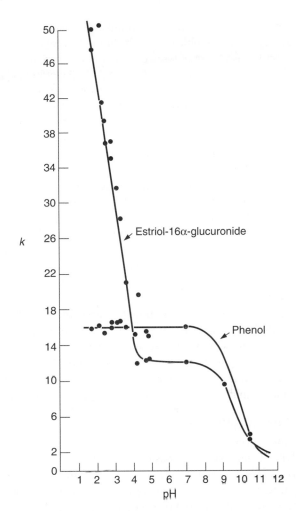

Fig. 6-8 Change in k as a function of pH for estriol-16α-glucuronide and phenol. Decrease in k at pH 2 is attributable to ionization of glucuronic acid; decrease at pH 10 is attributable to ionization of phenolic group, *(From Oliphant C, Bowers LD, unpublished data.)*

TABLE 6-2 USEFUL BUFFERS FOR REVERSED-PHASE HPLC

Buffer Pair	pK_a
Phosphoric acid/dihydrogen phosphate	2.12
Chloracetic acid/chloracetate	2.87
Succinic acid/monohydrogen succinate	4.23
Acetic acid/acetate	4.77
Piperazine phosphate	5.33
Monohydrogen succinate/succinate	5.65
Tetramethylethylenediamine phosphate	6.13
Dihydrogen phosphate/monohydrogen phosphate	7.20
Tris(hydroxymethyl)aminomethane	8.19

remaining silanol groups are strongly reactive, leading to adverse chromatographic effects, including severe tailing and irreversible adsorption of basic compounds and variable retention for different reversed-phase columns. At the mobile phase pH values normally used in reversed-phase analysis (neutral pH) a basic analyte is positively charged. The highly reactive silanol groups on the silica surface, which are acidic and thus negatively charged, interact with the positively charged basic compound through an ion-exchange mechanism. Addition of amine modifiers (such as triethylamine) to the mobile phase prevents adverse chromatographic effects of silanol on basic analytes through a mechanism by which the positively charged amine modifier binds to the silanol ion-exchange sites on the reversed-phase packing material, thus blocking the silanol sites from interaction with the basic analyte. Low pH and high ionic-strength mobile phases, which drive the equilibrium of the silanol groups to the protonated or counterion-associated form (which does not interact with positively charged basic compounds), are additional strategies used in conventional reversed-phase chromatography of basic compounds. In addition to the silanol ion-exchange mechanism mentioned above, silanol hydrogen bonding and metal impurities present within the silica have been implicated in the adverse chromatography effects seen for silica supports.

Ion-Pair Chromatography[16]

The most popular method for chromatographing ionizable analytes (such as weak bases or weak acids) and ionic analytes on a reversed-phase column is by ion-pair chromatography. Ion-pair chromatography has advantages over ion-suppression and ion-exchange chromatography. Use of ion suppression employing silica-based, reversed-phase packing material is limited by the range of pH stability of the silica support (which is stable from pH 2 to 8). Thus the requirement of a low-pH mobile phase for the ion-suppression chromatography of weak acids limits the column lifetime, whereas ion suppression of weak bases is not possible on silica-based, reversed-phase materials, because the pH requirement is too high. The advantage of ion-pair chromatography over ion-exchange chromatography is that it can separate both ionic and nonionic compounds simultaneously.

In ion-pair chromatography, a hydrophobic ionic species *(counterion)* that has the opposite charge to the analyte is added to the mobile phase, which is pumped through a reversed-phase column. The complex of the counterion and ionic analyte is called an *ion pair.* Several retention mechanisms have been proposed for ion-pair chromatography with the exact mechanism still a matter of debate. Retention is most commonly explained by one of two basic models. One model depicts the role of the counterion as a neutralizing agent, combining with the analyte ion in the mobile phase to form a neutral species that is retained on the reversed-phase column. The other model depicts the role of the counterion in terms of a modifier of the stationary phase, with the adsorption of the counterion on the reversed-phase packing material, changing the packing material into an ion exchanger that retains the ionic analyte.

Optimization of the separation in ion-pair chromatography is achieved through the manipulation of several mobile-phase variables, including type and concentration of ion-pair reagent, pH, type and concentration of organic modifier, ionic strength, and temperature.

The most common types of ion-pairing reagents used are alkyl (or aryl) sulfonates (RSO_3^-), alkyl sulfates ($ROSO_3^-$), and perchlorate (ClO_4^-), which are anionic counterions used for the chromatography of cationic species, and quaternary amines (NR_4^+), which are cationic counterions for the chromatography of anionic species. As would be expected, retention of analyte (which binds to the counterion) is increased with increased alkyl chain length of the ion-pairing reagent. Retention is also increased with increased concentration of ion-pair reagent. These two effects are shown in Fig. 6-9, in which the retention of epinephrine is shown to increase when: (1) the chain length is increased from butyl sulfonate to decyl sulfonate and (2) when the concentration of any ion-pairing reagent is increased (up to a point at which there is limited solubility of the ion-pairing reagent or there is a saturation effect, in which the concentration of the ion-pairing agent adsorbed onto the reversed-phase packing material is limited). It should be noted that analytes that do not bind to the counterion have decreased retention with increased concentration of the ion-pairing reagent (neutral species show a slight decrease in retention, whereas ionic analytes having the same charge as the counterion show a pronounced decrease in retention).

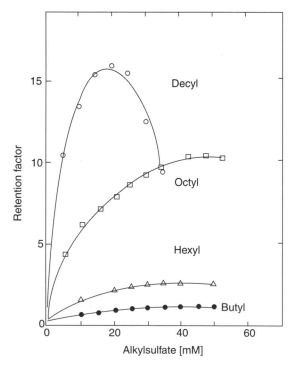

Fig. 6-9   Variation of retention factor, *k*, of epinephrine as a function of ion-pairing reagent concentration for several *n*-alkylsulfonates. *(From Horvath C et al: Enhancement of retention by ion-pair formation in liquid chromatography with nonpolar stationary phases,* Anal Chem *49:2295, 1977.)*

Adjustment of pH is also critical to ion-pair chromatography. Mobile-phase pH affects retention by controlling the charge state of analytes and counterions that are weak acids or weak bases. In general, retention is greatest at pH values at which the counterion and analyte are fully charged, which occurs at intermediate pH values. For example, for chromatography of a weak acid compound using a weak base counterion (or vice versa, a weak base analyte and a weak acid counterion), the pH must be between the pK_a of the acid and the base, such that both are charged. For analytes that have different pK values, the separation of analytes can be affected by adjusting the pH.

Retention can also be adjusted through manipulation of organic modifier (such as acetonitrile) concentration, ionic strength, and temperature. A decreased retention is seen for increased organic modifier content, which is attributable to the decreased strength of adsorption of the ion-pair reagent to the reversed-phase column. Increased ionic strength decreases retention because of reduced formation of ion pairs between the analyte and counterion as the result of competitive binding of the salt component to the counterion or analyte ion, or to both. The effect of temperature on retention is not predictable, being dependent on the particular ion pair.

Selection of the type of reversed-phase column to use is not a critical factor affecting selectivity of separation in ion-pair chromatography. The chain length and carbon content of the packing material are important to the determination of the concentration of the ion-pair reagent and organic modifier required for reasonable retention times. However, there is little to be gained in terms of optimization of separation by changing types of reversed-phase columns. C18 columns are most often employed in ion-pair chromatography.

Affinity Chromatography[22,23]

Affinity chromatography is a powerful tool in the analysis of biochemicals. In affinity chromatography the principle of specifically interacting biochemical pairs is employed. Examples of biochemical pairs used in affinity chromatography are given in Table 6-3. In affinity chromatography one of the components of the pair (termed the *affinity ligand*) is immobilized onto a support and packed into a column, making it a very specific chromatographic technique for the complementary component of the pair.

There are three stages to the affinity chromatographic separation process. The first stage is the injection of the sample into the aqueous *application buffer* (usually pH 7) pumped through the column, with all species passing through the column nonretained, except for the complementary analyte, which is retained by the column. After all the nonretained components pass through the column, the second stage of the chromatographic process is initiated and the mobile phase is switched to an aqueous *elution buffer,* which causes disruption of the binding forces between the analyte and affinity ligand, leading to elution of the analyte from the column. There are two categories of elution buffers, biospecific and general. Biospecific elution buffers contain a species that specifically interacts with the affinity ligand or analyte to affect elution. Biospecific elution thus adds a second step of specificity to the chromatographic process because there is specificity not only in retention, but also in elution of the analyte. Examples of biospecific elution include addition of sugars to the mobile phase in affinity chromatography by using lectin supports, and enzyme inhibitors to the mobile phase in the affinity chromatography of enzymes. General elution buffers affect elution by nonspecific means, through disruption of the electrostatic, hydrogen bonds, van der Waals, and hydrophobic forces. Strategies for general elution include changing mobile-phase pH or ionic strength, adding organic modifiers to the mobile phase, or using denaturing conditions in the mobile phase (5 to 8 M urea or 6 M guanidine). The disadvantage of general elution schemes is that species that nonspecifically adsorb to the support may elute with the analyte. The third stage of the affinity chromatographic process is reequilibration of the column with application buffer before injection of the next sample.

Traditionally affinity chromatography has been relegated to purification roles, because only large–particle diameter polysaccharide-based hydrophilic supports were available in the past (hydrophilic supports are required in affinity

---

TABLE 6-3   BIOCHEMICAL PAIRS USED IN AFFINITY CHROMATOGRAPHY

Affinity Ligand	Complementary Component
Inhibitors, cofactors, substrate analogs	Enzymes
Immunoglobulins	Antigens, haptens
Receptors	Hormones
Nucleic acid components	Complementary nucleic acid components, polynucleotide-binding proteins
Lectins	Carbohydrates, glycoproteins
m-Aminophenylboronic acid	*cis*-diol–containing compounds (carbohydrates, nucleic acid components, catecholamines, glycoproteins)
Protein A, protein G	Immunoglobulin G
Heparin	Coagulation proteins
Dye molecules	Various proteins and enzymes
Metal chelators	Proteins, peptides, nucleic acid components

chromatography to minimize nonspecific adsorption or denaturation of biomacromolecules). These low-performance supports have low efficiency and do not have the mechanical strength to withstand the high pressures that are generated from the high flow rates used in HPLC. The broad peaks and long analysis times precluded conventional affinity chromatography from being used as an analytical tool. This changed with the development of high-performance silica supports in which the surface was modified by the covalent attachment of a hydrophilic layer. In addition, hydrophilic high-performance polymeric supports have been developed. *High-performance affinity chromatography (HPAC)* is done by incorporation into normal HPLC setup columns containing high-performance packing material with covalently attached affinity ligands. A review covering the determination of various clinically relevant analytes by HPAC has been published[24].

Affinity chromatography using *m*-aminophenylboronic acid columns is commonly employed in the clinical laboratory in the determination of glycated hemoglobins, which are used in the assessment of treatment of diabetics. The affinity ligand *m*-aminophenylboronic acid is a general ligand that binds compounds that contain a *cis*-diol functional group, which is present in compounds such as catechols, carbohydrates, and the carbohydrate portion of many glycoproteins. In the determination of glycated hemoglobins, hemolysate of red blood cells is injected onto an *m*-aminophenylboronic acid column, which retains the glycated hemoglobin, allowing the nonglycated hemoglobins to pass through the column. Changing the mobile phase to one containing the sugar alcohol sorbitol and monitoring the eluant at 415 nm elutes the glycated hemoglobin.

Affinity chromatography has limitless flexibility through the use of antibodies as affinity ligands, a subclassification of affinity chromatography referred to as *immunoaffinity chromatography.*

Chromatography of Enantiomers[25-27]

Separation of enantiomers (chiral compounds) has its greatest application in the determination of pharmaceuticals, because approximately 50% of the most frequently used drugs exist as enantiomer pairs. A compound that has one chiral center (which is most commonly a carbon atom that has four different groups bonded) exists in two isomeric forms differing from one another in the spatial arrangement of the atoms around the chiral center. Each of the enantiomer pairs has identical physical properties (making separation difficult) but differs in reactivities toward chiral reagents and in their reactivity in biological systems. The activity, metabolism, and sometimes the toxicity of a drug depend on the enantiomeric form, and thus the separation of drug enantiomers is critical in pharmaceutical analysis. HPLC is the method of choice for the determination of enantiomers.

There are three general ways of determining enantiomers by HPLC: chromatography on conventional columns after derivatization with a chiral reagent, chromatography on conventional columns using mobile phases containing chiral complexing reagents, and chromatography on columns containing a *chiral stationary phase.*

Derivatization of the enantiomer analyte with a chiral reagent leads to the formation of a diastereomer. One diastereomer isomer is formed when a particular enantiomer reacts with the derivatizing agent, whereas a different diastereomer isomer is formed when the other enantiomer reacts. Diastereomer isomers have different physical properties, which facilitate their separation on conventional HPLC columns. In a similar manner, the presence of chiral reagents in the mobile phase leads to the formation of a different diastereomer isomer complex for each component of a particular enantiomer pair. Conventional HPLC columns can readily separate these diastereomer isomer complexes.

Specialized packing material containing a chiral compound as a stationary phase separates enantiomers as a result of differential spatial interaction of each enantiomer with the chiral support. Determination of enantiomers using chiral stationary-phase columns is advantageous compared to the derivatization or mobile-phase complexation methods because these previously described methods require reagents that have a high degree of optical purity. Chiral stationary phases include both biological and synthetic stationary phases. Biological stationary phases include the covalent attachment to support of the following: (1) derivatized biological polymers such as polysaccharides, proteins, and peptides; (2) modified small biological molecules, such as amino acids and alkaloids, and (3) macrocyclic antibiotics. In addition there are native biological-like polymer supports such as cellulose triacetate and cellulose tribenzoate. Synthetic stationary phases include brush-type (Pirkle) phases, poly(meth)acrylates, polysiloxanes and polysiloxane copolymers, and imprinted polymers. In addition, chiral ligand exchange is used, which consists of a ligand with a bound transition metal immobilized onto a support. There are many different types of chiral stationary phases that are commercially available, the suitability of which for a particular enantiomer separation must largely be determined empirically. Thus there is not one universal chiral stationary phase applicable to all enantiomer separations; the choice of column is dependent on the enantiomer compound determined. A database of chiral separations is found at www.chirbase.u-3mrs.fr/chirbase/.

DIFFERENT TYPES OF HPLC PACKING MATERIALS

A useful reference has been published giving information on HPLC packing materials,[28] with updated information summarized in another reference.[29] A database giving characteristics of approximately 90,000 columns, involving 3600 trade names from over 100 suppliers is given at www.sciquest.com. Tables 6-4 to 6-6 contain a summary of general information and list the types of packing material commercially available for the different HPLC modes. Advances in packing materials have been along three lines: (1) development of packing materials that are designed to alleviate the problems of silica supports; (2) development of packing materials, known as restricted access media, that allow direct chromatography of serum (or plasma); and (3) development of higher efficiency supports for macromolecules. In Table 6-6, adsorption and polar-bonded packing materials are grouped together under normal-phase chromatography, which is consistent with a classification made by others, because both are polar packing materials.

Different Supports Addressing Problems of Silica Supports

Problems associated with the use of silica supports include a limited pH range (2< pH <8), poor performance in the reversed-phase chromatography of basic compounds, and problems with reproducibility. An ideal support material would have the high performance and pressure capabilities of silica supports but would be able to withstand a larger pH range, be inert, and have reproducible retention characteristics. Supports that are better than silica supports in some aspects but inferior to silica in other aspects have been developed.[30] These are described next.

High-performance polymeric supports.[31,32] Significant advances have been made in the last several years in upgrading polymeric supports from a low-performance status (low-pressure operation; low-efficiency packing materials; purification uses) to a high-performance status (high-pressure operation; high-efficiency packing materials; analytical and purification uses). Polymeric supports can be classified as

---

TABLE 6-4   REVERSED-PHASE HPLC: GENERAL INFORMATION AND PACKING MATERIALS

Mode	Reversed Phase
General Information	
Compounds determined	Low-and medium-polarity compounds
Comments	Most widely used chromatographic mode in clinical analysis
	Mobile-phase ion suppression or ion pairing is required for ionic or ionizable compounds
Commercially Available Packing Materials	
Bonded phase	n-Octadecyl (C18), n-octyl (C8) (Most widely used reversed-phase functionalities)
	n-Butyl (C4) (Preferred functionality for protein separations; however, less stable in acidic mobile phases [such as TFA] than C8, C18)
	Phenyl (Preferred functionality for compounds containing an aromatic group or groups)
	Cyano [-$(CH_2)_3CN$] (Used for retention of more polar compounds)
	C30 (See text)
	Fluorinated alkyl (See text)
	Polar embedded (See text)
	Others: Mixed phases such as C18/phenyl, amide/alkyl, and C18/ion-exchange functionalities
	Other chain lengths (C1-C30)
	(These functional groups can be attached to the following supports: silica, polybutadiene modified/PM/ alumina, PS-DVB, PVA, PM, hybrid organic-inorganic, octadecylphenyl modified carbon-coated zirconia)
Polymer covered	Silica modified with alkyl polysiloxanes, multifunctional alkyl silanes, alkyl PVA
	Alumina modified with polybutadiene (with or without attached alkyl groups)
	Polystyrene-coated zirconia or titanium dioxide
	Polybutadiene-coated or carbon-coated zirconia
Base support (native)	PS-DVB
	PAM
	Porous graphite
	Poly (divinylbenzene-methacrylate)
High speed	
Nonporous	PS-DVB (native), PM and silica (reversed-phase functionalities)
Perfusion	PS-DVB (native) (Applied Biosystems)
Monolithic	Silica (C18 functionality) (Merck Eurolab, Kyoto Jushi-Seiko)
Poroshell	Silica (solid core with porous outer shell, C18 functionality) (Agilent Technologies)
Styros	PS-DVB (native) (OraChrom)
Restricted access media	Internal surface reversed phase (ISRP) (Regis Technologies)
	(Glycine-L-phenylalanine-L-phenylalanine [GFF] on silica)
	Semipermeable surface (SPS) (Regis Technologies)
	(C8, C18, cyano and phenyl within polyoxyethylene bonded to silica)
	Shielded hydrophobic phase (SHP) (Supelco) (phenyl groups embedded in a hydrophilic network of poly[ethylene]oxide bonded to silica)
	Mixed functionalities
	• Capcell Pak MF (Phenomenex) (C1/C8/phenyl on polymer-coated silica)
	• Diol-C8 silica (Merck KGaA)

PS-DVB, *Poly(styrene-divinylbenzene)*; PAM, *poly(alkylmethacrylate)*; PM, *polymethacrylate*; PVA, *poly(vinyl alcohol)*; TFA, *trifluoroacetic acid.*

TABLE 6-5 ION-EXCHANGE HPLC: GENERAL INFORMATION AND PACKING MATERIALS

| Mode | ION EXCHANGE* | |
	Anion	Cation
General Information		
Compounds determined	Negatively charged compounds, acidic compounds, protein with pI <8	Positively charged compounds, basic compounds, proteins with pI >6
Comments	The charge of the stationary phase will vary with mobile phase pH (near pK_a of support functionality) for weak ion exchangers but not for strong ion exchangers	
Commercially Available Packing Material		
Bonded phase	*Weak*	*Weak*
	Primary, secondary, tertiary amines ($-NH_2$, $-NHR$, $-NR_2$)	Carboxylic acid [$-COO^-$] (Weak acid functionalities with pK_a = 4–6; most utilized is carboxymethyl (CM) [CH_2-COO^-])
	(Weak base functionalities with pK_a = 5–9; most utilized is DEAE [$O-CH_2-CH_2-N-(C_2H_5)_2$])	
	Strong	*Strong*
	Quaternary amine [$-NR_3^+$] (Strong base functionality with pK_a >13)	Sulfonic acid [$-SO_3^-$] (Strong acid functionalities with pK_a <1)
	(Note that various functional groups given above can be attached to silica, PS-DVB, PM, PVA, porous graphite)	*Intermediate*
		Sulfoalkyl [$-(CH_2)_n-SO_3^-$] (Most utilized is SE and SP [pK_a for SP = 2.3])
		(Note that functional groups given above can be attached to silica, PS-DVB, and PM)
Polymer covered	*Weak*	*Weak*
	Polyethyleneimine (PEI)-coated supports (silica, PS-DVB, and zirconia)	Latex with carboxylic acid functionally coated onto poly(ethylvinyl-divinylbenzene) or PS-DVB supports
		Polybutadiene-maleic acid copolymer on silica
	Strong	*Strong*
	Latex with quaternary amine functionality coated onto poly(ethylvinyl-divinylbenzene) or PS-DVB supports	Polymer-coated silica with sufonic acid functionality
	Quaternized PEI on zirconia	
Base support (native)	None	None
High speed		
Nonporous	PM (PEI, DEAE, and NR_3^+ functionalities)	PM (carboxyl and SP functionalities)
	Poly (dimethylaminopropylmethacrylamide) (dimethylaminopropyl functionality)	Silica (various functionalities)
	Silica (various functionalities)	
Perfusion	PS-DVB with polyethyleneimine (weak), quaternized polyethyleneimine (strong) (Applied Biosystems)	PS-DVB with polyhydroxylated polymer [CM (weak) and SE and SP (strong) functionalies] (Applied Biosystems)
Monolithic	Polymer [such as polyglycidylmethacrylate-co-ethyleneglycoldimethacrylate (BIA Separations)] (DEAE, ethylenediamine, quaternary amine functionalities) (BIA Separations, Bio Rad)	Polymer [such as polyglycidylmethacrylate-co-ethyleneglycoldimethacrylate (BIA Separations)] (sulfonyl and CM functionalities) (BIA Separations, Bio Rad)
Styros	PS-DVB (quaternary aminomethyl, polyamine, DEAE functionalities) (OraChrom)	PS-DVB (SP and SE functionalities) (OraChrom)
Others		Phosphonic acid and phosphonic acid derivative of EDTA adsorbed to zirconia

PS-DVB, *Poly(styrene-divinylbenzene)*; PM, *polymethacrylate*; PVA, *poly(vinyl alcohol)*; PEI, *polyethyleneimine*; DEAE, *diethylaminoethyl*; SE, *sulfoethyl*; SP, *sulfopropyl*.
*Mixed anion-cation packing exchange materials also exist, such as sulfonyl-quaternary amine on ethylvinylbenzene cross-linked with DVB.

either hydrophobic or hydrophilic. Poly(styrene-divinyl-benzene) (PS-DVB) was the first polymeric HPLC support developed and is the predominant hydrophobic polymeric support used. Poly(alkyl methacrylate) (PAM) is another hydrophobic support, as is polymethacrylate (PM), which includes poly(hydroxylalkyl methacrylate or acrylate). The major hydrophilic polymeric supports that are commercially available are poly(vinyl alcohol) (PVA) and cross-linked agarose. The uses of these supports are given in Tables 6-4 to 6-6. Ligands are covalently attached to these supports to

TABLE 6-6 NORMAL-PHASE AND SIZE-EXCLUSION HPLC: GENERAL INFORMATION AND PACKING MATERIALS

Mode	Normal Phase	Size Exclusion
General Information		
Compounds determined	Hydrophilic compounds (such as saccharides; complements reversed phase, which does not retain hydrophilic compounds) Isomers (such as steroids) Class separation	Compounds >1000 daltons
Comments	Low-performance normal-phase cleanup of sample is often done before HPLC or immunoassay procedure Bonded normal phases compared to native silica and alumina: • Sharper peaks, no tailing • Less strength of retention • Faster mobile-phase equilibration, making gradient chromatography possible	Hydrophilic SEC (all packing materials listed below except PS-DVB) is used in clinical analysis
Commercially Available Packing Material		
Bonded phase	Diol [$-(CH_2)_3OCH_2CH(OH)CH_2(OH)$] Cyano [$-(CH_2)_3CN$] (also referred to as nitrile) Amino [$-(CH_2)_nNH_2$] (where n = 3 or 5) Fluorinated aromatic Dinitro-aromatic Polarity: amino > cyano > diol Almost all bonded phase supports are silica based, with a few exceptions such as aminopropyl on PS-DVB	Diol on silica [$-(CH_2)_3OCH_2CH(OH)CH_2(OH)$]
Polymer covered	Polyamine on PVA	Polyether and PVA on silica
Base support (native)	Silica Alumina Porous graphite Zirconia Titania (mixed adsorption/ion exchange properties)	PM, PVA, cross-linked agarose, PS-DVB
Monolithic	Silica (Kyoto Jushi-Seiko)	

PS-DVB, Poly(styrene-divinylbenzene); PM, polymethacrylate; PVA, poly(vinyl alcohol); SEC, size exclusion.

produce reversed-phase, ion-exchange, and normal-phase packing materials. No modification of the polymer support is required for size-exclusion chromatography. It should be noted that PS-DVB reversed-phase packing materials are most often used without modification of the surface. These native PS-DVB packing materials, however, have selectivities different from those of conventional alkyl-bonded reversed-phase packing materials. PS-DVB supports require hydrophilic surface modification to be utilized in modes other than reversed-phase.

Polymeric supports have two advantages over silica supports. The first is the extended pH range of polymeric supports. All polymeric supports listed in the preceding paragraph have a pH range of at least 2 to 12 (up to 14). This allows reversed-phase determination of a basic compound without the necessity of adding ion-pairing reagents. High-pH mobile phases can be used with polymeric supports, allowing basic compounds to be chromatographed as neutral species and thus retained on the reversed-phase column.

The second advantage of polymeric supports is that they do not have reactive functional groups such as silanols on the surface and thus do not show adverse peak tailing and recovery effects when basic analytes are chromatographed.

The major disadvantage of polymeric supports is that they are less efficient than silica supports. PS-DVB supports also require at least 10% to 20% organic content in the mobile phase to prevent shrinkage of the support material. In comparison, the hydrophilic polymeric supports are less susceptible to shrinkage and swelling effects when the concentration of the organic modifier is changed, and these supports are thus compatible with completely aqueous mobile phases. A disadvantage of the hydrophilic polymeric supports is that they are subject to pressure limitations, which can preclude their use at very high flow rates. Upper pressure limits are 4500 to 6000 psi for PS-DVB supports, 2000 to 2900 psi for PM and PVA supports, and 200 to 400 psi for the cross-linked agarose supports (compared to a pressure rating of greater than 6000 psi for most silica packing materials). For

PM and PVA supports, flow rates up to 1.5 to 2.0 mL/min can be employed (15 cm × 4.6 mm column). Cross-linked agarose gels have more severe flow rate restrictions.

Polymeric packing materials have yet to be extensively characterized with respect to reproducibility.

Other high-performance packing materials. There have been other packing materials developed, in addition to polymeric packing materials, that address the problems associated with silica supports. Deactivated reversed-phase silica packing materials have been developed by various manufacturers and do not require the presence of amine modifiers in the mobile phase so that chromatography of basic compounds can be performed. These packing materials employ high-purity silica with low trace metal content. One or more of the following strategies may be used to further deactivate the silica: excessive end capping, attaching a dense surface coverage of alkyl ligand, covering the silica surface with a polymer layer, employing proprietary treatments to modify the reactivity and distribution of the silanols on the surface, attaching novel ligands, and electrostatically shielding the silica surface. As with conventional silica packing materials these packing materials are limited to a mobile-phase pH range of 2 to 8, though some manufacturers claim an increase in upper pH limit to pH 10 for some polymer-covered silica supports.

A hybrid organic-inorganic reversed-phase packing material is available from Waters.[33] The base support is formed by polymerizing two organosilanes, one that forms the silica portion and the other that forms the methylsiloxane portion of the support. This hybrid character is distributed throughout the interior and exterior of the matrix. Reversed-phase functionalities are then covalently attached to form the bonded phases. These supports have advantages of increased pH stability to as high as pH 11.5, decreased silanol concentration for less peak tailing of basic compounds, and a longer lifetime at elevated temperatures. Another type of reversed-phase silica that has high stability in alkaline pH is available from Agilent Technologies (Zorbax Extend-C18). This packing material employs a bidentate C18-bonded phase that protects the silica surface from degradation at high pH.

Other packing materials are also commercially available. Alumina-based reversed-phase packing materials have an operating pH range of 2 to 13. Recently, zirconia supports (ZirChrom Separations) have been introduced that combine the advantages of high efficiency and rigidity of silica (3 μm zirconia supports give plate counts of over 100,000/m) and a pH range stability for reversed-phase packing materials of 1 to 14. Zirconia-based packing materials include reversed-phase, ion-exchange, and normal phase.

Porous graphite[34] is a material that has reversed-phase retention characteristics, with the additional characteristics of being able to separate geometric isomers and retain hydrophilic compounds, an increased pH range (1 to 14), and better performance with basic solutes. Porous graphite is considerably more hydrophobic than conventional reversed-phase silica, requiring a higher concentration of organic modifier in the mobile phase.

Restricted Access Media[35]

It is normally necessary to remove proteins from plasma and serum samples before reversed-phase and normal-phase chromatography because the organic composition of the mobile phases used in these modes causes the denaturation and precipitation of proteins, which adsorb onto the packing material, leading to pressure buildup, decreased column efficiency, and decreased column capacity. Packing materials known as *restricted access media* allow direct injection of serum or plasma samples onto the column without any sample pretreatment. The different types of restricted-access media that are commercially available are listed in Table 6-4. These packing materials consist of the stationary phase of a reversed-phase functionality on silica covered by a hydrophilic barrier, (or in the case of mixed-phase packing materials a stationary phase consisting of weak hydrophobic [or hydrophilic] groups alongside C8 or C18 reversed-phase functionalities). The hydrophilic barrier allows the passage of small molecules into the interior stationary phase while sterically preventing larger molecules, such as proteins, from interacting with the stationary phase. Because restricted access techniques require no sample preparation, they are simpler and faster than conventional HPLC. Disadvantages include poorer detection limits (μg/mL) and an inherent difficulty in determining compounds that are tightly bound to proteins or other macromolecules.

Pore Size Considerations

Conventionally, macromolecules are chromatographed on supports that have pores large enough for the macromolecule to enter them (pore diameters ranging from 30 to 400 nm), and smaller molecules are chromatographed on supports with smaller pore sizes (diameters of 5 to 15 nm). When HPLC analysis is performed on macromolecules, peaks that are broader than those seen with HPLC analysis of smaller molecules are obtained. This decrease in efficiency is seen because macromolecules, which have smaller diffusion coefficients, move more slowly into and out of the pores of the packing material. This phenomenon leads to decreased sensitivity, decreased resolution, and increased analysis time. Alternatively, macromolecules can be chromatographed on packing materials that minimize pore diffusional effects, such as *nonporous*, *perfusion*, or *monolithic packing materials*, as described later.

High-Speed Analysis

Short columns design is one strategy to speeding up chromatographic analysis. Columns ≤ 5 cm have been used to decrease analysis time. Packing materials of decreased size (≤ 3 μm diameter) must be used for these short columns to achieve the same resolution as columns of conventional length. However, a further gain in time saving by increasing the flow rate cannot be realized with porous packing materials because of increased band spreading resulting from the long distances that the molecules have to diffuse in the pores. In addition, there is increased pressure in columns packed with smaller packing material (pressure increases by an exponential factor of a decrease in particle diameter). Columns packed with small-diameter packing material have reduced column life because of the high pressures generated and problems with plugging. Thus use of short columns packed with porous small-diameter packing materials has its limitations

Nonporous packing materials are one solution addressing the detrimental effects of pores at increased flow rates. Narrow peaks can be achieved at high flow rates with these packing materials because there are no pores present. The disadvantages of these packing materials are diminished capacity (1% to 10% of that of conventional supports) and high back pressures (resulting from the small particle diameter [1 to 3 µm] of the supports). The reason for the diminished capacity of a nonporous packing material is the decreased surface area of the support, because most of the surface area in a chromatographic support is in the pores. High pressures are generated on these columns because of the small-diameter packing materials, thus limiting the upper flow rates that can be used, which puts an upper limit to the speed of analysis that can be achieved. However, reductions in separation times by a factor of five to ten are realized with nonporous compared to porous packing materials. Example separations include the following: all 20 PTH derivatives of amino acids in 7 min,[36] seven proteins in 7 sec,[37] and 40 tryptic digest peptide components in 2 to 3 min.[37] Nonporous packing materials that are commercially available are polymeric and silica supports with reversed-phase, ion-exchange, and affinity functionalities.

Perfusion packing materials[38] (from PerSeptive Biosystems), which have a greater loading capacity than that of the nonporous packing materials, consist of a PS-DVB core, a hydrophilic cross-linked copolymer layer bonded to the PS-DVB support, and the stationary phase. The support contains two types of pores, suprapores measuring 600 to 800 nm in diameter, and a family of smaller pores measuring 50 to 150 nm in diameter. Analyte transport in these pores occurs through convection in the suprapores (i.e., the pores are large enough that the mobile phase actually flows through these pores) and by diffusion in the smaller pores. The higher capacity of the perfusion packing materials (in comparison to that of the nonporous packing materials) results from the increased surface area created by the 50 to 150 nm pores, the pores in which retention of the analyte occurs. The high efficiencies for these supports in the chromatography of macromolecules can be explained by the fact that the 50 to 150 nm pores generally measure 1 µm or less in length, limiting the space that the analyte has to diffuse in the pores. Perfusion packing materials for reversed-phase, ion-exchange, normal-phase, and affinity chromatography have been developed.

Monolithic packing materials are like perfusion packing materials having macropores and smaller pores. The difference is that the monolithic supports are a continuous interconnected bed, not discrete particles. The continuous matrix consists of a base material of either silica or a polymer with attached functional groups forming the stationary phase.

The macropores (1 to 2 µm in silica monoliths) form channels through the bed that give the packing material a greater degree of porosity than conventional packing materials (80% compared to 65%). Silica monoliths have efficiencies equivalent to 5 µm silica packing materials. The combination of increased porosity (30% to 40% lower pressure drops compared to 5 µm silica packing material) and decreased flow rate–dependent diffusional band-broadening allows for high flow rates and thus increased speed of analysis. Reversed-phase, ion-exchange, normal-phase, and affinity monoliths are currently available.

INSTRUMENTATION

As mentioned previously, modern HPLC requires relatively sophisticated instrumentation to achieve difficult separations in less than 10 min. There are four basic components in the separation system itself: (1) a solvent-delivery system to provide the driving force for the mobile phase, (2) a sample introduction system, (3) the column, and (4) the detector (Fig. 6-1). In addition, a recorder or integrator, often used with computer data acquisition, is used to display or calculate the results. Books detailing proper operation, maintenance, and troubleshooting for all the components of an HPLC system have been published.[39,40]

Solvent-Delivery Systems

The most common delivery system is based on the reciprocating piston pump. Other types, including pneumatic amplification and diaphragm pumps, are mainly of historical interest. In the first pumps used in HPLC, solvent delivery occurred during less than half the cycle time. This meant that flow through the column was erratic. The stoppage of flow and the compression of the solvent that occurred when the pump head refilled also resulted in a signal at the detector, which limited the detection of analyte. In the jargon of chromatography, the stoppage is known as a "pulse." Pump pulsations are a source of detector noise.

The central mechanics of a reciprocating pump is a piston moving back and forth in a cylinder chamber. When the piston is moving forward, solvent is delivered, with the flow rate determined by the frequency of the piston cycle. When the piston is moving backward, solvent is drawn into the cylinder chamber from the solvent reservoir (refill phase). There is also a third phase of the pumping cycle: compression of the liquid during the initial forward movement of the piston. This compression phase does not deliver fluid. Most present-day HPLC pumps have two design characteristics to minimize pulsations. One is a dual-piston reciprocating design (two pistons in two cylinder chambers out-of-phase with one another [i.e., one piston is refilling while the other is delivering solvent]). The other is microprocessor control of the delivery, refill, and compression phase times to minimize pulsations and compensate for the compression of mobile-phase solvent. The microprocessor speeds up the backward piston movement during the refill phase, to minimize the time of pulsation. It also adjusts for the compressibility of the liquid by slightly increasing the frequency of pump cycle by an amount appropriate for a particular solvent and uses compensation circuits to minimize detector noise. Some HPLC pumps also employ pulse dampeners to further minimize pulses.

It must be emphasized, however, that although pulses can be minimized in a reciprocating piston pump, they can never be eliminated. Syringe pumps (Eldex, Isco) are the only HPLC pumps that produce pulse-free mobile phase delivery, important for detectors sensitive to pulsations, such as electrochemical, conductivity, and refractive index detectors. Syringe pumps operate by a large piston pushing liquid (after solvent compression) contained in a large cylinder chamber (100 to 1000 mL). There are no refill strokes during the chromatography (only as needed between sets of chromatographic runs). Syringe HPLC pumps are the best pumps for producing low flow rates (down to 10 nL/min), useful for capillary HPLC. Most good reciprocating pumps are rated down to 1 to10 µL/min; however, a recent advance has pushed the lower limit to 100 nL/min (Micro-Tech Scientific). The main disadvantage of syringe pumps is their high cost.

Gradient elution can be attained when the solvents are mixed after they pass through the HPLC pumps. The gradient can be produced by a continual adjustment of the flow rate of the multiple HPLC pumps, each pumping one solvent while keeping the total flow rate constant, to adjust the composition of the mobile phase (called *high-pressure mixing*). Alternatively, the solvents are mixed before they enter a single HPLC pump, with the gradient produced by a continual adjustment of the times that a proportioning valve allows a particular solvent to be pumped by the HPLC pump from one of several solvent reservoirs (called *low-pressure mixing*). High-pressure mixing gradient systems are considered the best with respect to performance. Low-pressure mixing gradient systems are disadvantageous because of the high dead volume before the column; this is especially disadvantageous for microbore and capillary HPLC techniques because it leads to long delay times for the gradient to reach the column. In addition, low-pressure mixing has a greater susceptibility to outgassing of dissolved gases, which can occur with the mixing of different solvents (not thoroughly degassed) at low pressures before the column. The disadvantage of high-pressure mixing gradient systems is the increased cost associated with the multiple HPLC pumps and controller instrumentation.

Sample-Introduction Systems

The most widely used method of introducing a sample into the chromatographic system is the fixed-loop injection valve. A sample aliquot is loaded into an external loop of stainless steel tubing. The valve is then rotated so that the sample loop is flushed onto the column by the mobile phase from the pump. Returning the valve to the original position allows loading of the next sample. Fixed-loop valves can be used in two ways: partial-fill method and full-loop method. In the latter the entire loop (such as 20 µL) is filled with sample and injected. It is the most precise method. It should be recognized, however, that accurate results require flushing of

the loop with 5 to 10 loop volumes before loading. In the partial-fill mode, the sample loop is not filled with sample. In this case, the loading syringe determines the precision of the injection volume.

In addition to the manual valve injector described above, many automatic sampling devices are also available. These autosamplers allow unattended operation of the HPLC system, making 24 hr/day use possible. They are usually quite reliable and precise because of mechanical advances and computerization. The devices may cost $5,000 to $10,000 but play an important role in busy laboratories.

Columns and Connectors

The column is of course the most important part of the separation system. The packing material for columns has been discussed at length. The usual HPLC column has an inside or internal diameter of 4.1 or 4.6 mm and a length of 100 to 250 mm. Column-end fittings are required at both ends to connect the column to the other system components and to hold the packing material inside. The frits used should have pores less than one fourth the average diameter of the packing material. In addition to the analytical (or preparative) column, which actually performs the separation, two types of protector columns might be used. A *guard column* (Fig. 6-1) is located between the injector and the analytical column and is 1/15 to 1/25 the volume of the latter. It is packed with a material similar to that of the analytical column. Its function is to collect any particulate matter or any strongly retained components of the sample and therefore to protect the expensive analytical column. A *precolumn* is positioned between the pump and the injection valve for HPLC techniques employing silica-based packing materials. It is always packed with silica, the purpose of which is to saturate the mobile phase with silicate and thus prevent dissolution of the packing material in the analytical column. This has reportedly allowed operation of silica columns at pH values of 10, far beyond the normal pH for dissolution of silica.

The analytical column has been described previously. The high efficiencies obtained with current HPLC columns result from the use of small (3, 5, or 10 µm), totally porous particles. To obtain efficient columns and reasonable operating pressures, the range between the largest and smallest particle must be as small as possible. Although irregularly shaped packing materials were produced in the past, almost all present HPLC packing materials are spherical.

Capillary (0.1 to 0.5 mm), microbore (1 mm ID) and smallbore (2 mm ID) columns are used because of the increase in sensitivity (as described previously) and because of the conservation of mobile phase in comparison to conventional HPLC columns, which is advantageous for cost, environmental, and detector compatibility reasons. Concerning detector compatibility, capillary/microbore columns are required for mass spectrometric detection. The reason is that mass spectrometers require the removal of as much mobile phase as possible, mandating the use of capillary/microbore columns, which introduce smaller amounts of mobile phase into the detector than conventional HPLC designs.

In addition to the columns, the connections made between system components are critical because the fittings should introduce as little peak spreading as possible. They should be of the zero dead volume or at least low dead volume type. An excellent article on the intricacies of HPLC plumbing is available.[41]

Detection Systems

The final component in the chromatographic system is responsible for detecting the compounds as they elute from the column. Ideally a detector would respond to any compound, would detect picograms or less of the analytes, would be immune to any solvent-related phenomena, and would respond linearly to a wide range of concentrations. Unfortunately, liquid chromatography does not have such a detector. Three types of HPLC detectors routinely used in the clinical laboratory are absorbance, fluorescence, and electrochemical detectors. Mass spectrometric detection is important in clinical research. The selection of the appropriate detector depends on the required selectivity and sensitivity. Several books giving a detailed description of various HPLC detection methods have been published.[42-44] Derivatization methods, though not covered in the following discussion, are an important means of enhancing sensitivity or specificity of detection in HPLC analysis.[45,46]

Absorbance detection. The most frequently used HPLC detection mode is absorbance spectrophotometry. The advantage of absorbance detectors over fluorescence or electrochemical detectors is that they can be used to detect a greater variety of compounds. However, absorbance detectors have poorer detection limit capabilities by a factor of 1000 compared with fluorescence and electrochemical detectors. The detection limit for absorbance detectors is approximately 5×10^{-10} g/mL. Wavelengths longer than 200 nm are required for absorbance detectors because mobile-phase solvents absorb appreciably at the low-ultraviolet wavelength region of the spectrum (<200 nm). In general, the number of compounds that can be detected increases as wavelength

decreases. However, at shorter wavelengths there is also increased detection of interfering compounds and an increase in baseline shifts when gradient chromatography is used. It is thus desirable to use the longest wavelength at which a compound absorbs to increase the specificity of the technique.

There are three types of absorbance detectors that are used: fixed-wavelength, variable-wavelength, and multiple-wavelength absorbance detectors. These detectors, as described in the next paragraphs, differ in the number of wavelengths available for monitoring and whether multiple wavelengths can be monitored simultaneously.

Fixed-wavelength detectors. This detector is popular because of its low cost. Fixed-wavelength detectors are limited in the choice of wavelengths that can be used. The choice is determined by the specific light source that is used. Each kind of arc lamp emits specific spectral lines. The wavelengths of various lamps are given in Table 6-7. The low-pressure mercury vapor lamp is the most widely used lamp, with the 254 nm wavelength used most often. The cadmium and zinc lamps are used for shorter ultraviolet (UV) wavelengths. Phosphor-coated mercury lamps produce different wavelengths, increasing the number of wavelengths available for use.

Variable-wavelength detectors. These detectors are advantageous because a continuous-spectrum light source and a monochromator are used to allow unlimited choice of visible and UV wavelengths. However, these detectors are more complex and expensive than the fixed-wavelength detectors. Deuterium and tungsten lamps are used to provide UV and visible wavelengths, respectively. Some detectors use a deuterium source for both the UV and the visible region; however, these detectors have decreased precision in the visible range in comparison with detectors with a tungsten light source.

Multiple-wavelength detectors. These detectors are variable-wavelength detectors that have the capability of monitoring multiple wavelengths simultaneously. This class of detectors includes detectors that differ greatly in complexity and sophistication; from those detectors that have dual-channel capability, in which two wavelengths can be monitored simultaneously, to those detectors that can record an entire spectrum in fractions of a second. All multiple-wavelength detectors (dual channel, spectrum recording) are advantageous for several reasons. One reason is the optimization of analyte detection, because the detector allows the monitoring of each analyte at the particular wavelength at which there is a maximum analyte/interferent response ratio. Another reason is that the multiple-wavelength detector can be used for verification of peak purity.

The principal HPLC detector used for continual recording of the spectra of the effluent is the photodiode array (PDA) detector. A book on the use of PDA in HPLC analysis has been published.[47] PDA detectors employ a reverse-optics scheme (i.e., the diffraction grating is placed after the sample cell instead of before it) in which the entire spectrum of light (usually from a deuterium lamp) is directed through the

---

TABLE 6-7   WAVELENGTHS EMITTED BY ARC SOURCES USED IN FIXED-WAVELENGTH DETECTORS

Source	Mercury	Phosphor Mercury	Cadmium	Zinc
Emission lines (nm)	254	280	229	214
	313	300	326	308
	365	320		
	405	340		
	436	470		
	546	510		
	578	610		
		660		

From Yeung ES, editor: Detectors for liquid chromatography, *New York, 1986, Wiley & Sons.*

flow cell to a diffraction grating, which disperses the light into component wavelengths. The dispersed wavelengths are directed to an array consisting of 32 to 512 diodes (higher-resolution PDAs have the larger number of diodes). When light strikes a diode, it produces a current proportional to the intensity of the light. Because the light hitting the array is spatially dispersed according to wavelength, each diode has a particular range of wavelengths that is striking it, and thus the detector records the entire spectrum simultaneously. The fastest PDAs can record a spectrum every 10 msec (specifications for one representative company are a spectrum acquisition rate of 12.5 msec for a wavelength range of 190 to 600 nm, with a 4 nm band width, and a noise level during the scan of less than $\pm 2.5 \times 10^{-5}$ absorbance unit, or AU [at 254 nm]).

Fluorescence detection. The technique of fluorescence is based on the ability of a molecule to emit light after it has been excited by light radiation. For a description of fluorescence spectroscopy, refer to Chapter 4. The main differences in fluorometer performance between manufacturers arise from differences in the lamp intensity and the detection efficiency. Commercially available instruments use emission from either deuterium or xenon arc lamps for exciting light. Because the fluorescent intensity is directly proportional to the excitation light intensity, there has been a great deal of interest recently in laser sources. Fluorescence is a highly sensitive detection method for those compounds that fluoresce, but because many molecules do not fluoresce, numerous methods for derivatizing compounds have been developed. Epinephrine and other amine compounds can react with dimethylaminonaphthalenesulfonyl (dansyl) chloride or *o*-phthalaldehyde to produce highly fluorescent compounds.

Electrochemical detection.[48] For a select group of compounds electrochemical detection is the method of choice because of its superior detection limit capability (femtomole to picomole). The types of compounds that can be determined by liquid chromatography–electrochemical detection (LCEC detection) are compounds that undergo reversible electron transfer reactions. Characteristics of a small oxidation (or reduction) potential and fast kinetics are most desirable for sensitive and selective detection. The classes of organic compounds that have these characteristics are phenols (such as hydroquinones, catechols, and catecholamines), aromatic amines, thiols, nitro compounds, and quinones. Compounds such as aldehydes and ketones require too high a reduction potential, whereas alkyl amines and carboxylic acid functionalities require too high an oxidation potential for direct determination by LCEC detection. Highly conjugated compounds such as α,β-unsaturated ketones and imines may be determined by LCEC detection; however, UV detection techniques are better. The most common LCEC analyses done in the clinical laboratory, in which LCEC detection has a decided advantage because of its superior detection limit capabilities, are the determination of catecholamines, catecholamine metabolites, serotonin, and 5-hydroxyindoleacetic acid.

Amperometric and coulometric detection. In general, electrochemical detection of an analyte occurs through an electron transfer between the electrode surface and the analyte molecule, with subsequent measurement of the current. The oxidizing strength of the electrode surface (increasingly positive potential for stronger oxidizing capability), or reducing strength of the electrode surface (increasingly negative potential for stronger reducing capability), is determined by the potential applied. The potential thus establishes the selectivity of the detector. Operation at lower oxidative potentials (or less negative reductive potentials) provides greater selectivity. The name of this detection technique is *controlled potential amperometry.* In this technique, the detector cells consist of three electrodes: a working electrode (at which the redox reaction occurs), a reference electrode, and an auxiliary electrode (see p. 282, Chapter 15). The potential is applied between the reference and working electrodes, and the current is passed between the auxiliary (or counter) and working electrodes.

Detectors are classified as either *amperometric*, in which 1% to 10% of the analyte reacts at the electrode, or *coulometric,* in which 100% of the analyte reacts. Increasing the electrode surface area or slowing the flow rates to increase the percentage of electroconversion does not increase detection limits because there is a concomitant increase in background electrolysis and hence noise. Thus coulometric detectors have no detection limit advantage over amperometric detectors. Factors such as variations in temperature, flow rate, and mobile-phase impurities, which are important contributors to noise, need to be controlled to achieve the lowest detection limits. For this reason gradients are not usually employed in LCEC detection. Three amperometric detector designs are used, which are diagrammed in Fig. 6-10: thin layer, wall jet, and tubular. The most common amperometric electrode is the thin-layer electrode, in which column effluent passes through a very small volume flat channel (<1 μL) in which the working electrode is contained on one side of the channel and the reference and auxiliary electrodes are contained on the other side. The coulometric detector consists of porous material through which the mobile phase passes, providing the large surface area required for complete electroconversion of the analyte species. It should also be noted that a conductive mobile phase is required for electro-

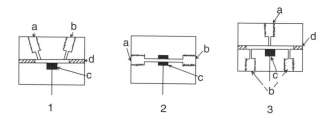

Fig. 6-10 Schematic diagram of thin layer or channel *(1),* tubular *(2),* and wall-jet *(3)* electrochemical flow cell designs. *(Reprinted with permission from Weber SG: Eng Chem Prod Res Develop 20:593, 1981. Copyright 1981, American Chemical Society.)*

chemical detection, with a concentration of electrolyte or buffer of 0.01 to 0.1 M normally employed.

The best choice of material for the active surface of the electrode depends on the compound to be measured and the conditions of analysis. The glassy carbon electrode is the most widely used material because of its wide potential range (+1.2 to -0.8 V versus Ag/AgCl), its mechanical stability with high flow rates, and its chemical stability with non-aqueous solvents. For substances requiring high reduction potentials, a mercury film on gold is used (+0.2 to -1.2 V versus Ag/AgCl). Mercury electrodes are used in the determination of thiols, because the association of thiol to mercury lowers the oxidation potential of complexed mercury to +0.1 V.

For cathodic reactions, several problems associated with oxygen reduction restrict the limit of detection to the nanogram range. To make the reductive mode more sensitive, all oxygen needs to be removed from the mobile phase.

***Pulsed amperometric detection (PAD).*[49]** A significant development in electrochemical detectors that allowed sensitive detection of carbohydrates occurred in the early 1980s. Before this, derivatization of carbohydrates with fluo-rophoric or chromophoric reagents was needed for sensitive detection. Carbohydrate detection was accomplished by use of electrodes consisting of noble metals such as platinum or gold, which catalyze oxidation reactions of carbohydrate compounds, reactions that do not occur at reasonable potentials when other materials are used for the electrode. Electrodes made with noble metals, however, present unique problems that result from the formation of metal oxides at positive potentials and the irreversible absorption of compounds onto the surface. These problems were solved by the development of a triple-pulse waveform scheme. *Pulsed amperometric detection* (PAD) refers to the electrochemical detection technique that uses this triple-pulse waveform on platinum or gold electrodes. In this technique, a cycle of three potentials is applied over a 600 to 1000 msec period. These potentials, which are needed for the analytical process, are: (1) a reducing potential, at which metal oxides on the electrode's surface are reduced and at which adsorption of the analyte occurs; (2) an oxidizing potential, at which the analyte is measured (the current resulting from the oxidation of hydrogen atoms that were removed catalytically by the metal surface); and (3) a yet higher oxidizing potential, at

TABLE 6-8 CLINICALLY RELEVANT COMPOUNDS DETERMINED BY HPLC

	COMPOUND	
Class	*Subclass*	*Most Prevalent HPLC Mode or Modes Used*
Amino acids		Reversed phase, ion exchange
Anions	Oxalate, citrate, sulfate, phosphate, iodide, bromide, chloride, thiocyanate, nitrate, nitrite	Ion exchange
Bile acids		Reversed phase
Bilirubins		Reversed phase
Bioamines	Catecholamines and catecholamine metabolites	Reversed phase, ion pair
	Serotonin and serotonin metabolites	Reversed phase, ion pair
Carbohydrates	Monosaccharides and oligosaccharides	Reversed phase, ion exchange, ion-moderated partition, normal phase
Drug and drug metabolites		Reversed phase
Fatty acids and organic acids	Fatty acids	Reversed phase
	Organic acids	Ion exchange, ion-moderated partition, reversed phase
Hemoglobins		
	Glycated hemoglobins	Ion exchange, affinity
	Hemoglobin variants	Ion exchange
Isomers, positional		Normal phase
Lipoproteins		Size exclusion
Nucleic acid compounds		
	Nucleic acid bases, nucleosides, nucleotides	Reversed phase, ion pair
	Oligonucleotides	Reversed phase, ion exchange
	DNA restriction fragments	Reversed phase, ion exchange
Phospholipids		Normal phase
Porphyrins		Reversed phase
Prostaglandins		Reversed phase
Steroids		Reversed phase
Vitamins	Biotins, folates, nicotinamides, pantothenic acids, retinoids (vitamin A), riboflavins, thiamines, tocopherols (vitamin E), vitamin B_6, vitamin B_{12}, vitamin C, vitamin D, vitamin K	Reversed phase

which desorption of molecules previously adsorbed to the electrode surface occurs. Besides carbohydrates, alcohols and amino acids have been determined by this technique.

Conductivity detection. Like the LCEC techniques described previously, measurement of conductivity is also considered to be an electrochemical detection method. The HPLC determination of inorganic anions uses anion-exchange chromatography with conductivity detection. Conductivity is a measure of conductance when a constant alternating potential is applied at a platinum electrode surface. The amount of current generated increases with increased solution conductance. Current in these electrodes is temperature dependent, and thus temperature must be strictly controlled.

Mass spectrometric detection.[50] Mass spectrometry (MS) has become a premier detection technique in HPLC because of its combined sensitivity/detection limit (down to femtomole amounts) and specificity (molecular mass determination) capabilities. The advent of two ionization technologies, electrospray ionization (ESI) (also called *ionspray*) and atmospheric pressure chemical ionization (APCI), has revolutionized MS capabilities in bioanalysis by allowing the determination of ionic, polar, and nonvolatile compounds. This has paved the way for the direct interfacing of MS to HPLC. ESI is used for the ionization of highly polar/ionic compounds, whereas APCI is used for the ionization of compounds having comparatively lower polarity, although there is an overlap in compounds that can be determined by both ionization techniques. HPLC effluent (or a split portion of the effluent) from microbore/capillary columns can be directly fed into ESI and APCI ionization sources of a variety of mass analyzers, including quadrupole, quadrupole-quadrupole, time-of-flight, quadrupole-time-of-flight, ion trap, and Fourier transform ion cyclotron resonance. Important applications of the HPLC-MS techniques in clinical analysis include determination of inborn errors of metabolism, drug analysis, and proteomics. See Chapter 8 for a more detailed discussion of MS.

APPLICATIONS

Several books on HPLC of clinical and biochemical analytes have been published.[51-61] Table 6-8 contains a comprehensive list of the classes of clinically relevant compounds in which HPLC plays a significant role in analysis. The HPLC modes given in Table 6-8 for each compound class are the modes most prevalently used (as determined by a survey of recent literature). A database of thousands of chromatograms organized by compound, detector type, and column is available at www.sciquest.com.

References

1. Majors RE, Carr PW: Glossary of liquid-phase separation terms, *LCGC* 19:124, 2001.
2. Meyer VR: *Practical high-performance liquid chromatography*, ed 3, New York, 1998, Wiley & Sons.
3. Katz E et al, editors: *Handbook of HPLC*, New York, 1998, Marcel Dekker.
4. Wilson ID, editor: *Encyclopedia of separation science*, San Diego, 2000, Academic Press.
5. Snyder LR, Kirkland JJ: *Introduction to modern liquid chromatography*, ed 2, New York, 1979, Wiley & Sons.
6. Scott RPW: *Liquid chromatography column theory*, New York, 1992, Wiley & Sons.
7. Karger BL, Snyder LR, Horvath C: *An introduction to separation science*, New York, 1973, Wiley & Sons.
8. Giddings JC: *Dynamics of chromatography*, New York, 1965, Marcel Dekker.
9. Guichon GG: Optimization in liquid chromatography. In Horvath C, editor: *High performance liquid chromatography: advances and perspectives*, vol 2, New York, 1980, Academic Press.
10. Ghrist BFD, Cooperman BS, Snyder LR: Design of optimized high-performance liquid chromatographic gradients for the separation of either small or large molecules. I. Minimizing errors in computer simulations, *J Chromatogr* 459:1, 1988.
11. Ghrist BFD, Snyder LR: Design of optimized high-performance liquid chromatographic gradients for the separation of either small or large molecules. II. Background and theory, *J Chromatogr* 459:25, 1988.
12. Ghrist BFD, Snyder LR: Design of optimized high-performance liquid chromatographic gradients for the separation of either small or large molecules. III. An overall strategy and its application to several examples, *J Chromatogr* 459:43, 1988.
13. Swadesh JK, editor: *HPLC practical and industrial applications*, ed 2, Boca Raton, FL, 2001, CRC Press.
14. Snyder LR: *Principles of adsorption chromatography*, New York, 1963, Marcel Dekker.
15. Snyder LR, Glajch JL, Kirkland JJ: Theoretical basis for a systematic optimization of mobile phase selectivity in liquid-solid chromatography, *J Chromatogr* 218:299, 1981.
16. Szepesi G: *How to use reverse-phase HPLC*, New York, 1992, VCH.
17. Majors RE: Trends in HPLC column usage, *LCGC* 9:686, 1991.
18. Dorsey JG, Dill KA: The molecular mechanism of retention in reversed-phase liquid chromatography, *Chem Rev* 89:331, 1989.
19. Forgács E, Cserháti T: *Molecular basis of chromatographic separation*, Boca Raton, FL, 1997, CRC Press, pp 132-181.
20. *Comparison guide to C18 reversed phase HPLC columns*, MAC-MOD Analytical, Chadds Ford, PA (www.mac-mod.com).
21. Karger BL, LePage JN, Tanaka N: Secondary chemical equilibria in high-performance liquid chromatography. In Horvath C, editor: *High performance liquid chromatography: advances and perspectives*, vol 1, New York, 1980, Academic Press.
22. Turkova J: *Bioaffinity chromatography*, ed 2, Amsterdam, 1993, Elsevier.
23. Scouten WH: *Affinity chromatography: bioselective adsorption on inert matrices*, St Louis, 1992, Sigma-Aldrich.
24. Hage DS: Affinity chromatography: a review of clinical applications, *Clin Chem* 45:593, 1999.
25. Special review edition devoted to enantiomer separation: *J Chromatogr A* 906:1, 2001.
26. Allenmark S: *Chromatographic enantioseparation: methods and applications*, ed 2, New York, 1991, Ellis Horwood.
27. Krstulovic AM: *Chiral separations by HPLC*, New York, 1989, Ellis Horwood.
28. Unger KK, editor: *Packings and stationary phases in chromatographic analysis*, New York, 1990, Marcel Dekker.
29. Majors RE: Advances in the design of HPLC packings, *LCGC* 18:586, 2000.
30. Anderson DJ: High-performance liquid chromatography (advances in packing materials), *Anal Chem* 67:475R, 1995.
31. Mikes O, Coupek J: Organic supports. In Gooding KM, Regnier FE, editors: *HPLC of biological macromolecules*, New York, 1990, Marcel Dekker, pp 25-46.
32. Tanaka N, Araki M: Polymer-based packing materials for reversed-phase chromatography, *Adv Chromatogr* 30:81, 1989.
33. Cheng Y-F et al: Hybrid organic-inorganic particle technology: breaking through traditional barriers of HPLC separations, *LCGC* 18:1162, 2000.
34. Ross P: The role of porous graphitic carbon in HPLC, *LCGC* 18:14, 2000.

35. Anderson DJ: High-performance liquid chromatography (direct injection techniques), *Anal Chem* 65:434R, 1993.

36. Boros B, Kovacs K, Ohmacht R: Fast separation of amino acid phenylthiohydantoin derivatives by HPLC on a non-porous stationary phase, *Chromatographia* 51(suppl):S202, 2000.

37. Issaeva T, Kourganov A, Unger K: Super-high-speed liquid chromatography of proteins and peptides on non-porous Micra NPS-RP packings, *J Chromatogr A* 846:13, 1999.

38. Afeyan NB, Fulton SP, Regnier FE: Perfusion chromatography packing materials, *J Chromatogr* 544:267, 1991.

39. Dolan JW, Snyder LR: *Troubleshooting LC systems: a comprehensive approach to troubleshooting LC equipment and separations*, Clifton, NJ, 1989, Humana Press.

40. Sadek PC: *Troubleshooting HPLC systems*, New York, 2000, Wiley & Sons.

41. Dolan J, Upchurch P: *Interchangeability of HPLC fittings*, Oak Harbor, WA, 1983, Upchurch Scientific; also *LC* 2:20, 1984, and 3:92, 1985.

42. Parriott D, editor: *A practical guide to HPLC detection*, San Diego, 1993, Academic Press.

43. Yeung ES, editor: *Detectors for liquid chromatography*, New York, 1986, Wiley & Sons.

44. Scott RPW: *Chromatographic detectors; design, function, and operation*, New York, 1996, Marcel Dekker.

45. Lingeman H, Underberg WJM, editors: *Detection-oriented derivatization techniques in liquid chromatography*, New York, 1990, Marcel Dekker.

46. Lunn G, Hellwig LC: *Handbook of derivatization reactions for HPLC*, New York, 1998, Wiley & Sons.

47. Huber L, George SA, editors: *Diode array detection in HPLC*, New York, 1993, Marcel Dekker.

48. Anderson DJ: High-performance liquid chromatography, *Anal Chem* 63:213R, 1991.

49. Johnson DC, LaCourse WR: Liquid chromatography with pulsed electrochemical detection at gold and platinum electrodes, *Anal Chem* 62:589A, 1990.

50. Tomer KB: Separations combined with mass spectrometry, *Chem Rev* 101:297, 2001.

51. Heftmann E, editor: *Chromatography: fundamentals and applications of chromatography and related differential migration methods*, part B: *Applications*, ed 5, Amsterdam, 1992, Elsevier.

52. Hanai T, editor: *Liquid chromatography in biomedical analysis*, Amsterdam, 1991, Elsevier.

53. Papadoyannis IN: *HPLC in clinical chemistry*, New York, 1990, Marcel Dekker.

54. Hearn MTW, editor: *HPLC of proteins, peptides and polynucleotides, contemporary topics and applications*, New York, 1991, VCH.

55. Gooding KM, Regnier FE, editors: *HPLC of biological macromolecules*, New York, 1990, Marcel Dekker.

56. Fallon A, Booth RFG, Bell LD, editors: *Applications of HPLC in biochemistry*, Amsterdam, 1987, Elsevier.

57. Lim CK, editor: *HPLC of small molecules*, Oxford, UK, 1986, IRL Press (Oxford University Press).

58. Henschen A et al, editors: *High performance liquid chromatography in biochemistry*, Weinheim, Federal Republic of Germany, 1985, VCH.

59. Katz ED, editor: *High performance liquid chromatography: principles and methods in biotechnology*, New York, 1996, Wiley & Sons.

60. Lunn G, Schmuff N: *HPLC methods for pharmaceutical analysis*, New York, 1997, Wiley & Sons.

61. De Leenheer AP, Lambert WE, Van Bocxlaer JF, editors: *Modern chromatographic analysis of vitamins*, ed 3, New York, 2000, Marcel Dekker.

Internet Sites

www.chromatographyonline.com
http://www.chirbase.u-3mrs.fr/chirbase/
www.sciquest.com
htp://hplc.chem.shu.edu—Seton Hall University Online Textbook
http://hplc.chem.shu.edu/NEW/HPLC_Book/—Chemiluminescent reactions HPLC

http://www.ntri.tamuk.edu/hplc/hplc.html—Introduction to HPLC
http://www.home4u.de/niven/rn_hplc.htm—Niven's chromatographic terms
http://biobenchelper.hypermart.net/tech/hplc.htm
http://www.fda.gov/cder/guidance/cmc3.pdf—Center for Drug Evaluation and Research (Requires Adobe Acrobat)

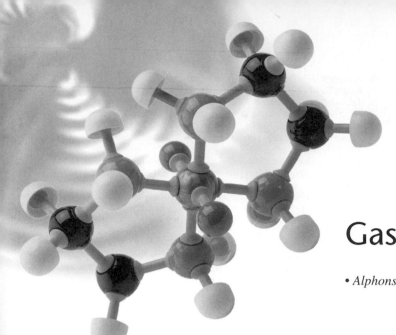

CHAPTER 7

Gas Chromatography

• *Alphonse Poklis*

Objectives

• Diagram the basic components of a gas
chromatographic system, describe the function of
each component, and outline the mechanisms of
gas-liquid and gas-solid chromatography.
• Explain the significance of temperature dependence
in gas chromatography and tell why temperature is
the most important single parameter.
• Name four common carrier gases and state the

function of a carrier gas, summarizing the criteria
for selection of an appropriate carrier gas for
chromatographic separation.
• Define derivatization and state why the process is
used in gas chromatography.
• Describe the operation of the six types of detectors
that may be used in gas chromatography.

Key Terms

active sites   Places, usually on the stationary phase,
   that reversibly bind the compound to be separated.
capillary column   An open tubular column with an
   inside diameter of 0.20 to 0.35 mm.
chemical ionization   The component molecule to
   be analyzed is mixed with an ionized gas, such as

methane or isobutane. A positive charge is
transferred to the molecule, the $M + 1$ charged
molecule and its fragments are separated by the
mass spectrometer, and their size and relative
abundance are measured. (*M* is "mass.")
corrected retention time   The amount of time a

compound is retained on a column minus the gas-holdup time.

derivative   A molecule chemically altered from the original one. Usually in gas chromatography, it refers to chemical groups added to increase the volatility of the initial compound.

diffusivity   The ability of molecules to diffuse or spread because of the thermal energy inherent in the molecule.

effective plate (number of effective plates)   The number of partitions that are practically available on a column.

electron-capture detector   A device that releases beta particles into the carrier-gas stream, producing low-energy electrons, which are captured by eluted compounds and change in current measured. This type of detector is very sensitive and specific for compounds with chemical groups of high electronegativity, such as halogens.

electron impact   Fragmentation of molecules into specific charged fragments by collision with high-energy electrons.

flame ionization detector   A device in which eluted components are mixed with hydrogen and burned in the air to produce a flame, which ionizes these components. A pair of electrodes measures the number of ions.

flow regulator   A system of valves that is set to yield a desired gas pressure and thus control the rate of gas movement (flow) through a gas chromatographic system.

Fourier-transform infrared spectrometer   A device that may be considered as a gas chromatographic detector. The infrared spectral lines of compounds are obtained as the compounds elute from the chromatograph.

gas chromatography   A physical technique that separates components based on their distribution between a gas and a stationary phase.

gas-holdup time   The amount of time it takes for the carrier gas to move from the injection port to the detector, analogous to the void volume of liquid chromatography.

gas-liquid chromatography   A separation technique in which the stationary phase is a liquid.

gas-solid chromatography   A separation technique in which the stationary phase is a solid.

injection port   A device usually having a septum and a heating block to volatilize the compounds to be separated. This is placed before the column.

Kovats index   This index relates the logarithm of the retention time of a compound, regardless of its chemical nature, to those of the *n*-paraffins.

liquid phase   The nonvolatile fluid that coats the immobile support medium. These fluids have the property of acting as solvents for the compounds to be separated.

mass fragment   A degraded portion of a molecule containing one or more charges.

mass spectrometer   A device that may be considered a gas chromatographic detector. Compounds are fragmented into specific groups of charged molecules, which are separated into their mass and charge components, and their relative abundance is measured.

mass transfer   The movement of mass from one phase to another.

McReynolds constant   A constant describing a system that classifies the stationary phase in terms of its ability to separate various compounds.

negative chemical ionizations   Similar to chemical ionization except that the gas is oxygen or hydrogen, which produces primarily negative ions of the form $M - 1$. (M is "mass.")

nitrogen-phosphorus detector   A device similar to a flame ionization detector but into which alkaline metals are introduced. When nitrogen- or phosphorus-containing compounds are burned, the rate of release of alkaline metal vapor and thus of current flow is increased.

nonpolar   Usually applied to molecules that have a hydrophobic affinity, that is, those that are "water hating." Nonpolar substances tend to dissolve in nonpolar solvents.

nonvolatile liquid   A fluid that does not vaporize or have a form that is readily gaseous in nature.

open tubular column   A gas chromatographic column in which the stationary phase coats the inside walls of the column.

overloading   When too much of a compound is presented for adsorption by the stationary phase, nonequilibrium between the two phases occurs.

packed column   A gas chromatographic column in which the stationary-phase support consists of particulate material filling the column.

phase ratio   The ratio of mobile-phase (gas) volume to stationary-phase (column) volume. Usually indicated by the term "β."

plate   A chromatographic term that refers to a single partitioning unit of the chromatographic system.

polar   Usually applied to molecules that have a hydrophilic affinity, that is, those that are "water loving." Polar substances tend to dissolve in polar solvents.

relative retention time   The ratio of the corrected retention time of the reference compound to that of the sample compound.

retention index   A system relating the retention time to a standard.

Rohrschneider constant   Similar to the McReynolds constant.

selected-ion chromatogram   A technique in which only mass fragments of a preselected size are recorded and quantified by the mass spectrometer.

separator A device that removes large portions of the carrier gas and concentrates the solutes before entrance to the mass spectrometer.

septum A device that separates the chromatographic column from the laboratory environment. Usually it is a small disk of silicone rubber through which the solution to be separated is injected into the column.

silanization The chemical process of converting the SiOH moiety of a stationary phase to the ester form.

sorbent A material that has the property of interacting with the compound of interest, usually to make it bind.

thermal compartment The temperature-regulated oven in which the chromatographic column is placed.

thermal-conductivity detector A device that measures the difference between the heat conductivities of the carrier gas and that of the sample-gas effluents. A sample carried in gas increases the heat conductivity.

van Deemter equation Relates the HETP (height equivalent to the theoretical plate) to the linear velocity of the carrier gas.

wide-bore column An open tubular column with an inside diameter of 0.50 to 0.75 mm.

Chromatography is a physical technique that separates two or more compounds based on their distribution between two phases, a stationary and a mobile one. Review Chapter 5 for a description of the basic theory and practice of chromatographic separations. The stationary phase may be a liquid or a solid, and in **gas chromatography** (GC) the mobile phase is a gas that percolates over the stationary phase. When separation of sample components is accomplished by use of a mobile-gas phase and a stationary phase consisting of a thin layer of **nonvolatile liquid** held on a solid support, the technique is called **gas-liquid chromatography** (GLC). **Gas-solid chromatography** (GSC) employs a solid **sorbent** as the stationary phase. Both GLC and GSC may be further differentiated based on the stationary-phase support. When the **liquid phase** in GLC is coated over the surface of small particles, or the solid sorbent in GSC consists of small particles, the column acts as a container for the stationary phase. This technique is known as *packed-column GC*. When liquid-phase GLC or the solid sorbent coats the inner wall of the column, the column itself acts as a support for the stationary phase. This technique is known as *open-tubular GC*, or *capillary GC*. Regardless of the type of mobile or stationary phase, separation is achieved by the difference in partitioning of the various molecules of the sample between the two phases.

Gas chromatographic separation is illustrated by the following example: A sample containing the components to be separated is injected into a heated block in which they are immediately vaporized and swept by a stream of carrier gas through a column of stationary phase. The components are adsorbed onto the stationary phase at the head of the column and then are gradually desorbed by fresh carrier gas. The partitioning between the two phases occurs repeatedly as carrier gas sweeps the components toward the column outlet.

As the components are eluted, they enter a detector, where their presence is converted to an electric signal, which is then measured, usually by a strip chart recorder that produces a series of peaks charted versus time (Fig. 7-1). The appearance time, height, width, and area of these chromatogram peaks may be measured to yield valuable qualitative and quantitative data.

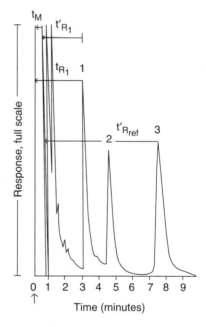

Fig. 7-1 Example of gas chromatogram showing detector response versus time. *Vertical arrow* (time = 0) indicates time of injection, and initial peak is "dead time," t_M. t_R designates uncorrected retention time, whereas t'_R is corrected retention time. $t'_{R_{ref}}$ is corrected retention time for internal standard or reference compound. Relative retention time for peak 1: $r = t'_{R_1}/t'_{R_{ref}}$. *(Reprinted from Mackell MA, Poklis A: Determination of pentazocine and tripelennamine in blood of T's and Blues addicts by gas-liquid chromatography with a nitrogen detector,* J Chromatogr *235(2):445, 1982.)*

MOLECULES THAT CAN BE SEPARATED BY GAS CHROMATOGRAPHY

Theoretically, any compound that can be vaporized or converted to a volatile **derivative** may be analyzed by gas chromatography. Compounds as small as carbon monoxide and methane and as large as 800 daltons have been successfully analyzed. Compounds larger than 800 daltons lack sufficient volatility. Generally, a compound must be stable as a vapor to produce a single identifiable chromatographic peak. Unstable compounds may be converted to stable, volatile derivatives. However, if a compound degrades to known products or a consistent number of products, the resultant pattern of multiple compounds may be used as a means of tentative identification.

Inorganic compounds, or the inorganic salts of organic acids and bases, lack sufficient volatility for gas chromatographic analysis. Thus the technique is generally applied to analysis of organic molecules in their neutral nonionic forms. Before chromatographic analysis, compounds are generally isolated and concentrated by means of solvent extraction and evaporation to dryness. The residues containing the analytes are dissolved in small amounts of volatile organic solvents. The solvent-analyte solution is then chromatographed. The analyte vapor should not interact with the solvent. The solvent should have greater volatility and much less affinity for the stationary phase than the analyte compounds do, thereby eluting far ahead of the analyte and not interfering with the chromatogram.

THEORY OF GAS CHROMATOGRAPHIC SEPARATION

The following is a brief discussion of the basic chromatographic theory as it applies to gas-liquid chromatography. See Chapter 5 for a review of general chromatography theory. For a more complete treatment of the many complex variables that influence gas chromatographic separations, consult Willett[1] and Grob.[2]

Partition Coefficient (K_D)

The general concepts of sample *partitioning* and the *partition coefficient (K_D)* have been described in Chapter 5 (see equation 5-1 and pp. 110 and 122). Similarly, definitions of *retention* and *retention time* and *capacity factor* (or capacity rates) have been described in Chapter 5 on p. 115 and Fig. 7-1. These basic concepts apply to both liquid chromatography (LC) (Chapter 6) and GC. The transit time required for the carrier gas to move from the point of injection to the end of the column is called the **gas-holdup time**, or *dead time*, t_M (see Fig. 7-1). It arises from the internal volumes of the injector, column, and detector and is equivalent to the void volume in high performance liquid chromatography (HPLC). A compound that does not partition into the stationary phase ($K_D = 0$) will be eluted from the column at t_M.

Because the "dead time" is a characteristic of both the particular gas chromatograph used for analysis (injector and detector volumes) and the column volume, it is the same for all sample components and is of no significance in identification. The difference between the uncorrected retention time and the dead time is called the **corrected retention time**, t'_R

$$t'_R = t_R - t_M \qquad \text{Eq. 7-1}$$

Partitioning in GC Systems

The K_D, or corrected time, t'_R, of a solute in a specific system must be determined experimentally; it cannot be predicted easily. Both the partition coefficient and retention time of a solute are directly related and depend on the affinity of solute for the stationary phase. The old rule "like dissolves like" offers a simple guide to solute affinity. **Polar** solutes will have greater partition coefficients, K_D, hence longer retention times on hydrophilic (polar) phases than hydrophobic (**nonpolar**) stationary phases. Likewise, hydrophobic solutes exhibit greater K_D's and longer retention times on the nonpolar rather than the polar stationary phase. If both a hydrophobic and a polar solute are chromatographed together on a polar stationary phase, the hydrophobic solute will have less affinity for the phase than the polar solute ($K_{D \text{ hydrophobic}} < K_{D \text{ polar}}$) and will be eluted before the polar solute ($t'_{R \text{ hydrophobic}} < t'_{R \text{ polar}}$).

The K_D of a solute is expressed as a concentration (amount/volume) ratio and therefore may be written as

$$K_D = [W_S / V_S] / [W_M / V_M] = \frac{V_M}{V_S} \cdot \frac{W_S}{W_M}$$

W_S = Weight of the sample in the stationary phase
W_M = Weight of the sample in the mobile phase
V_S = Volume of the stationary phase
V_M = Volume of the mobile phase

The ratio of the mobile-phase (gas) and stationary-phase (column) volumes (V_M/V_S) is called the **phase ratio** (β). The ratio of sample weights (W_S/W_M) in each phase is equal to the capacity ratio, k. Therefore, the partition coefficient can be expressed as

$$K_D = \beta k$$

The phase ratio and capacity ratio are characteristics for a particular column. However, their product, K_D, is independent of the particular column. Therefore, the higher the phase ratio (and smaller the volume of stationary phase), the smaller is the capacity ratio (less time for elution, t_R). In general, the smaller the capacity ratio (shorter t_R), the more difficult it is to achieve a particular separation. The amount of solute analyzed on a column without **overloading** is dependent on the amount of stationary phase that influences β. The greater the amount of stationary phase, the smaller the β and the larger the k (greater t_R).

Temperature Dependence

Temperature is the most important single parameter in a gas chromatograph separation. This is attributable to the great dependence of the partition coefficient, K_D, on temperature. The inverse relationship between K_D and temperature is given by the equation

$$\log K_D = \frac{\Delta H}{2.3R \cdot T_c} + \text{Constant} \qquad \text{Eq. 7-2}$$

ΔH is the partial molar heat of solution of the solute in the liquid state, R is the gas constant, and T_c is the column temperature.

This equation demonstrates that, in a given system, the higher the column temperature, the lower is the K_D, which means a lower capacity ratio, k (shorter retention time). Therefore, the retention times of solute molecules may be

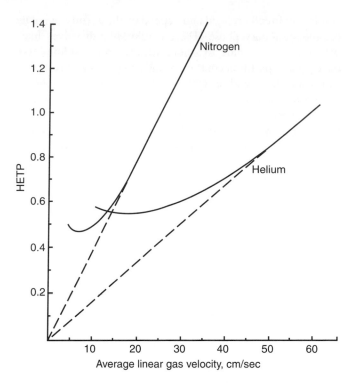

Fig. 7-2 Relationship between height equivalent to a theoretical plate (HETP) and average linear gas velocity for two different carrier gases: nitrogen and helium. *(From Ettre LS: Practical gas chromatography, Norwalk, CT, 1973, Perkin-Elmer Corp.)*

readily altered when one changes the column temperatures. Roughly, a 30° C decrease in column temperature will approximately double the retention time. Conversely, a 30° C increase in column temperature will approximately halve the retention time. The influence of temperature on separation is discussed later.

Column Performance

The ability of a column to produce optimum separations is measured by two quantities: *efficiency*, which is the ability to produce narrow peaks, and *resolution*, which is the ability to separate two adjacent peaks.

The general concepts of *resolution, theoretical plates*, and *height equivalent to a theoretical plate* (HETP), all used to describe the efficiency of a column, have been defined in Chapter 5 (pp. 114 to 115). HETP (or *H*) uses the uncorrected retention time, t_R. If the corrected retention time, t'_R, is employed instead, the expression *height equivalent to an effective plate*, or HEEP (*h*), is used. The term *HETP* defines not only the efficiency of the column, but also the overall efficiency of the system because of the gas-holdup times of the injector, column, and detector. Because the gas-holdup time varies in different instruments, the column efficiency is best expressed by the **number of effective plates** (HEEP, or *h*).

The relationship of the HETP to the linear gas velocity, μ, is complex. The factors affecting gas flow are expressed by the **van Deemter equation**:

TABLE 7-1	DIFFERENCES BETWEEN PACKED AND CAPILLARY COLUMNS	
Parameter	**Packed**	**Capillary**
Length, meters	1.5 to 6.0	5 to 100
Inner diameter, millimeters	2 to 4	0.2 to 0.7
Specific permeability, (10^{-7}) cm^2	1 to 10	10 to 1000
Flow, mL/min	10 to 60	0.5 to 15.0
Pressure drop, psi	10 to 40	3 to 40
Total effective plates (2 meters, 50 meters)	5000	150,000
Effective plates per meter	2500 (ID 2 mm)	3000 (ID 0.25)
Capacity	10 μg/peak	<50 ng/peak
Liquid film thickness, μm	1 to 10	0.05 to 0.5

$$HETP = A + B/\mu + C\mu$$

In **packed column** GC, *A* is the eddy diffusion term, which relates the effect of support-particle diameter and the column-packing procedure to the distance that a streamline of carrier gas persists before its velocity is drastically changed by the support. *B* is the longitudinal gas diffusion term, which relates peak broadening to the effect of diffusion in the flowing gas along the direction of flow. *C* is the resistance-to-mass transfer term, which relates the diffusion processes in the gas and liquid phases. The relationship of the HETP to linear velocity, when graphed, corresponds to a hyperbola (Fig. 7-2). If the slope of the rising part of the curve is extended down, it intercepts the *y*-axis, yielding the value of the *A* term (the contribution of the obtrusion of the gas flow to the HETP). In **open tubular columns** where the gas path is not inhibited, the *A*-term intercept is zero and the van Deemter equation is reduced to

$$HETP = B/\mu + C\mu$$

Thus open tubular columns have much lower HETPs and much greater efficiency than packed columns[3] (Table 7-1). Eventually the van Deemter curve reaches a minimum, which is the optimum velocity (μ_{opt}) yielding the smallest HETP. For open tubular columns the minimum HETP is determined solely by flow rate and the resistance to **mass transfer**, C_μ. The descending part of the curve (from μ_{opt} to the *y*-axis) represents the longitudinal diffusion term *B*. Because there are no support or sorbent particles hindering diffusion along the column in open tubular columns, the carrier-gas velocity must be much greater than that in packed columns (see Table 7-1). Thus the van Deemter plot is greatly shifted to the right (increased μ_{opt}) for open tubular columns.

The optimum velocity is ideal for only one compound; however, similar compounds have closely related optimum velocities, and a single flow rate is suitable for their separation. At higher flow rates, the gas sweeps the diffusing molecules from the liquid before all have emerged, thus broadening the peak.

TABLE 7-2 COMMON CARRIER GASES			
Gas	Molecular Weight	Density (g/L)	Impurities (ppm)
Argon	39.944	1.784	
Helium	4.007	0.177	Hydrocarbons (1 to 100)
Hydrogen	2.018	0.089	
Nitrogen	28.014	1.251	Oxygen (20)

MOBILE-PHASE CONSIDERATIONS

The most commonly used carrier gases are presented in Table 7-2. The carrier gas must be inert so as not to react with the sample components. Large quantities of relatively pure gas must be commercially available because appreciable amounts of carrier gas are used for analysis. Common impurities in carrier gases are moisture, oxygen, and hydrocarbons. Each of these contaminants may adversely affect various detectors, producing unstable recorder baseline or extraneous peaks. In certain situations, carrier-gas impurities may interact with sample components and prevent their analysis. For example, prepurified-grade nitrogen contains up to 20 ppm of oxygen. If high column temperatures are necessary to separate compounds that are readily oxidized, the oxygen impurity in nitrogen carrier gas may degrade the compounds on the column and prevent their detection or may produce multiple extraneous peaks of the degradation products. In such a situation, helium, which contains less oxygen contamination, should replace nitrogen as the carrier gas.

The choice of carrier gas does influence column performance (efficiency and resolution) and time required for analysis (retention time). As presented by the van Deemter equation, the height equivalent to a theoretical plate (HETP) is related to the linear gas velocity (μ) of the carrier gas. This interaction is highly complex, but the following brief discussion presents the basic effects of carrier gas upon separation.

In a flowing system (column) where the gas is compressible, the density, pressure, and velocity of the gas are different at each point in the column. The carrier gas is compressible, and the value of the carrier-gas velocity must be corrected to average conditions. The average linear gas velocity (μ) is determined by two factors: (1) the time necessary for an unretained solute to pass through the column (dead time, t_M) (p. 157) and (2) the length of the column, L. These factors determine μ by the following equation:

$$\mu = L/t_M \qquad \qquad \textit{Eq. 7-3}$$

In a given column, the optimum linear gas velocity (μ_{opt}) is proportional to the **diffusivity** of the vapors of the substances being chromatographed. However, the kinetic theory of gases states that the diffusivity in gas is inversely proportional to the square root of the molecular weight or density of the gas (see Table 7-2). Thus the μ_{opt} will be lower for high-density gases (low solute diffusivity), such as nitrogen and argon, and higher for low-density gases (high solute diffusivity), such as helium and hydrogen. Therefore in the same column different values of μ_{opt} will be obtained for different gases. Fig. 7-2 shows the relationship between the μ of two different carrier gases and the resultant HETP. Nitrogen has a minimum HETP of 0.465 at a μ_{opt} of 7 cm/sec, whereas helium has a minimum HETP of 0.55 at a μ_{opt} of 17.5 cm/sec. This demonstrates that in the same length of column, a high-density gas (nitrogen or argon) will produce better efficiency (more theoretical plates per unit length, lower HETP) than a low-density gas (helium or hydrogen). For a given system, the maximum resolution will be obtained at minimum h, which is determined at the μ_{opt} of the carrier gas. Also, for a given length of column, better resolution will be obtained by the carrier gas producing the lowest h value.

For a low-density gas, the diffusivity of the solute and the μ_{opt} in a given column are greater than those of a high-density gas. Therefore, shorter retention times (smaller t_R) are obtained with helium or hydrogen than with nitrogen or argon.

STATIONARY-PHASE CONSIDERATIONS
Gas-Solid Stationary Phases

In gas-solid chromatography the column is packed or the inner wall is coated with an adsorptive solid material on which the sample components are partitioned by adsorption on the surface of the solid. This material should possess a large surface area per unit volume to ensure rapid equilibrium between the stationary and gas phases. It should possess uniform particle size and pore structure and be strong enough to resist breakdown during handling and column packing. Theoretically, the smaller the particle size of support, the greater the efficiency of the column. However, the smaller the particles, the greater the resistance to flow and the greater the necessary carrier-gas pressure.

The most common chromatographic solids for adsorption phases are made from diatomaceous earth (kieselguhr). The processed white kieselguhr is sold under many trade names: Chromosorb W, Celite, Gas Chrom, and Anakron. The diatomite may also be crushed, blended, pressed into brick, and processed so that mineral impurities form oxides and silicates, which give the material a pink color. It is marketed as crushed firebrick, or Chromosorb P. This material has greater density and is less fragile than the white material. The pore size of the pink material is only 2 mm compared with 9 mm for the white; therefore, greater efficiency is obtained with the pink material.

Each support possesses individual properties that may enhance or hinder its use for a particular application. The white material is slightly alkaline and will interact with acidic compounds. Its surface, however, is nonadsorptive, a property that favors its application for analysis of polar compounds. The pink material adsorbs polar compounds; thus it is best suited for the separation of nonpolar molecules like hydrocarbons.

Another type of solid stationary phase consists of porous polymer beads, which allow the analyte molecules to go into partition directly from the gas phase into the amorphous polymer. Porapak, a polymer of ethylvinylbenzene cross-linked with vinylbenzene, is the most popular polymer phase. The material may be modified by copolymerization with various polar monomers to produce beads of varying polarity. Porapak columns are thermally stable up to 250° C. At temperatures above 250° C the column material will be degraded and eluted, a phenomenon called *column bleed*. These degradation products can be observed by the detector. Water and highly polar molecules are rapidly eluted from the polymer. Porapak is especially useful for baseline separation of aqueous samples containing low–molecular-weight alcohols, esters, halogens, hydrocarbons, ketones, and mercaptans (Table 7-3).

Gas-Liquid-Solid Supports for GLC

The stationary phase in gas-liquid chromatography is a thin film of liquid held on an inert support. In capillary chromatography, the liquid is coated on the walls of the tubing. In packed columns, the liquid is held in a thin-layer film across the surface of an inert support (Fig. 7-3). Many materials that act as stationary phases for GSC are also supports for the liquid phase in GLC. Both the pink and white solid phases described earlier are popular liquid supports. Although the support should be inert and should not influence separation, both pink and white materials have **active sites** because of metallic impurities and silanol (-SiOH) and siloxane (SiOSi-) groups, which form hydrogen bonds with polar compounds. This interaction gives rise to distorted (asymmetrical) peaks in the resultant GLC chromatogram. These active sites may be removed by acid washing of the mineral impurities from the support and by conversion of the silanol groups to silyl esters (**silanization**) of dimethyldichlorosilane or hexa-methyldisilazone. Silanization reduces surface activity but also reduces the surface area of the support so that no more than 10% (v/w) of the liquid stationary phase to total column weight may be applied. In certain instances, special additives are mixed with the liquid phase to block the active sites of untreated support material. Two such examples are the incorporation of stearic acid in silicone oil used in separation of fatty acids and the addition of potassium hydroxide to polar liquid phases used to separate amines.

In open tubular chromatography, the liquid is coated on the walls of the tubing. The cohesive forces of most liquid phases are greater than the adhesive or wetting forces between

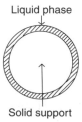

Liquid phase

Solid support

Fig. 7-3 Schema of solid support particle for gas chromatography with liquid stationary-phase coating.

the liquid and the glass surface of the column. Therefore, to create a uniform thin film the column is treated to produce an adhesive surface.[4] Several techniques are used: deposition of fumed silica, a microlayer of fine particles of salts such as barium carbonate or sodium chloride, quartz powder, or etching the glass with dry acid gas. These treatments increase the "roughness" of the surface, allowing the liquid to fill the holes and crevices and spread across the surface of the column. The character of the column surface may also be altered by treatment with wetting agents, such as Carbowax 20M, which are strongly attached to absorptive sites and deactivate the surface. After treatment, residual Carbowax 20M is washed from the column, and the liquid phase of choice is applied to the surface. Informative data describing preparation, applications, and limitations of support materials are readily available from commercial manufacturers and suppliers.

Liquid Phases

The universal popularity of GLC as a separation method is attributable to the large variety of liquid phases with differing solution properties and therefore different affinities for various classes of analytes. The range of liquids used as stationary phases is limited only by their volatility, thermal stability, and ability to wet the support. No single stationary phase will achieve all desired separations. Commercial suppliers typically offer 100 to 200 liquid phases; however, many of these phases are duplicates sold under various trade names or are so similar in character as to have little difference in their separation abilities. In fact, few laboratories require the use of more than a half dozen different liquid phases. Successful separation of 80% of a wide range of organic compounds may be achieved using only four to seven phases: OV-101, OV-17, Carbowax 20M, OV-225, DEGS, OV-275, and OV-210.[5,6] Examples of liquid phases, characteristics, and applications are presented in Table 7-3.

Liquid phases may be generally classified into five categories: (1) Nonpolar phases, which are hydrocarbon liquids such as squalane, silicone greases, Apiezon L, and silicone gum rubber. Generally, compounds are eluted from these phases in order of increasing boiling point. (2) Intermediate polarity phases that include polar or polarizable groups attached to a long nonpolar skeleton, such as esters of high molecular weight or alcohols such as diisodecyl-phthalate. Both polar and nonpolar compounds are separated by these phases, with the more polar ones eluted first. (3) Polar phases, which contain a high concentration of polar groups, such as carbowaxes. These phases differentiate between polar and nonpolar compounds by interacting strongly only with polar compounds, separating these from the earlier eluting, less polar compounds. (4) Hydrogen-bonding phases, which contain many hydrogen atoms readily available for hydrogen bonding, such as glycol phases. Polar compounds have greater affinity for the stationary phase and are eluted more slowly. (5) Special-purpose phases that can be prepared to use a specific chemical interaction between the sample and the stationary phase. An example of a special-

TABLE 7-3   Examples of Commonly Used Stationary Phases and Their Applications

Stationary Phase	Structures	Activity	Temperature (°C Min/Max)	Application	Specific Compounds
Silicone OV-1 (100% methyl)	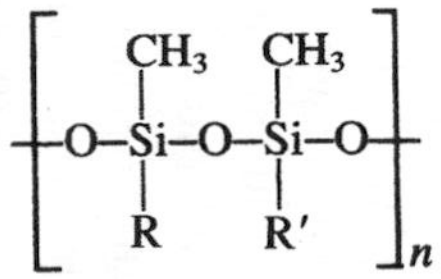 Silicone backbone: $-O-Si(CH_3)-O-Si(CH_3)(R)(R')-$ repeating unit n	Nonpolar	100/350	Bacteria, drugs	Fatty acid methyl esters, benzodiazepines
Silicone OV-17 (50% phenyl)	R and R′ = CH$_3$ in above structure; R and R′ = Phenyl in above structure	Intermediate polarity	20/350	Drugs, steroids	Tricyclic antidepressants, barbiturates, cholesterol
Silicone OV-210 (50%, 3,3,3-trifluoropropyl)	R and R′ = $-CH_2-CH_2-CF_3$ in above structure	Polar	20/300	Drugs, pesticides	Basic drugs, lindane, aldrin, DDT
Silicone OV-225 (25% cyanopropyl, 25% phenyl)	R = Phenyl, R′ = $-CH_2-CH_2-CH_2-CN$ in above structure	Polar	20/275	Steroids	TMS derivatives of 17-ketosteroids
10% Apiezon L 2% KOH	Undefined mixture of high-boiling hydrocarbons	Nonpolar	50/225 50/240	Amines Volatile fatty acids	Amphetamine Acetic through caproic acids
NPGS (neopentyl glycol succinate)	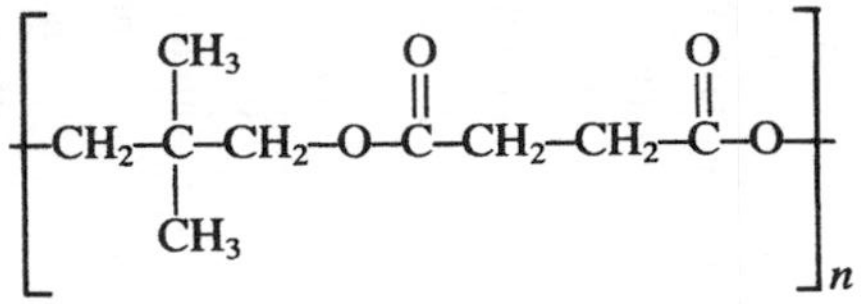 $-CH_2-C(CH_3)_2-CH_2-O-C(=O)-CH_2-CH_2-C(=O)-O-$ repeating unit n				
Carbopack B/5%	$(CH_2-CH_2-O)_n$	Polar		Alcohols, aldehydes, ketones	Methanol, ethanol, acetaldehyde acetone
DEGS (diethylene glycol succinate)	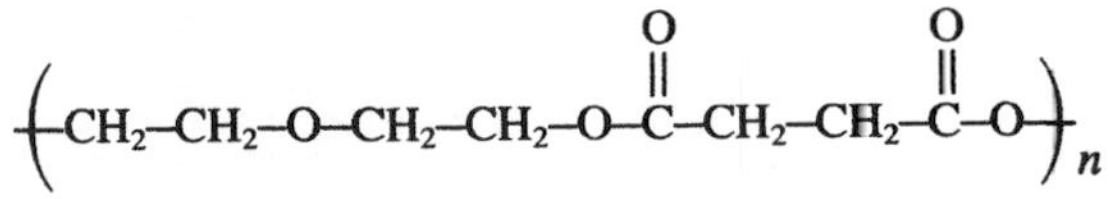 $(CH_2-CH_2-O-CH_2-CH_2-O-C(=O)-CH_2-CH_2-C-O)_n$	Polar	20/200	Bacteria	Fatty acid methyl esters
EGA (ethylene glycol adipate)	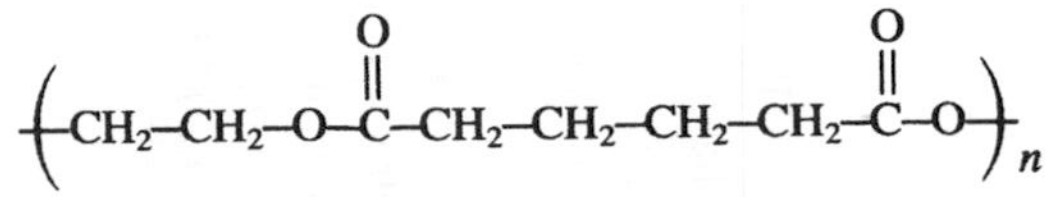 $(CH_2-CH_2-O-C(=O)-CH_2-CH_2-CH_2-CH_2-C-O)_n$		100/210	Amino acids	NBTFA derivatives of amino acids
Chromosorb 102 (styrene divinyl benzene polymer)	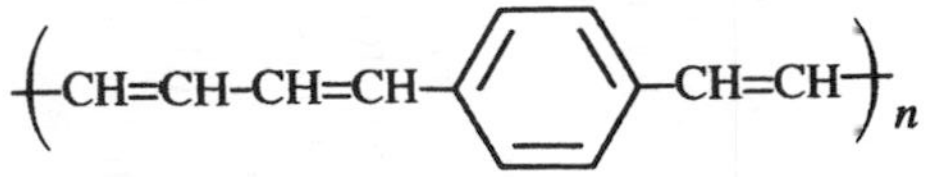 $(CH=CH-C_6H_4-CH=CH)_n$		<250° C	Alcohol, aldehydes	Methanol, ethanol, acetaldehyde
Porapak Q (ethylvinyl benzene + divinyl benzene polymer mixture)	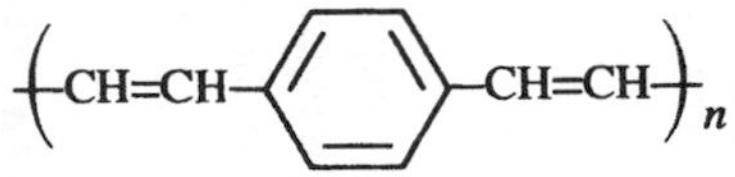 $(CH=CH-C_6H_4-CH=CH)_n$		<250° C	Low molecular weight	Chlorinated hydrocarbons

NBTFA, *Nitroblue tetrazolium fatty acid.*

purpose phase is silver nitrate dissolved in glycol to enhance separation of unsaturated hydrocarbons by charge-transfer interactions.

Each liquid phase has a specific temperature range for efficient use (see Table 7-3). The maximum temperature at which a phase may be used is determined by its volatility. Beyond this temperature the phase is lost because of decomposition or volatilization and is carried into the detector producing extensive background noise (column bleed). A column may be heated above the maximum temperature for brief periods of time as in temperature programming, but the maximum temperature must never be exceeded for isothermal (constant-temperature) analysis. Below the minimum temperature the increased viscosity or solidification of the liquid does not allow reproducible analysis.

The amount of stationary phase in the column is expressed in percentage by weight of the liquid phase on the support. In general, packed columns contain 3% to 10% liquid phase. Deviations from these values may occur in specific applications: very low liquid loads for high–molecular-weight compounds and high loads for small, highly volatile compounds such as hydrocarbons containing one to four carbon atoms. The amount of stationary phase directly affects the sample capacity and efficiency of the column. The greater the amount of liquid phase, the larger the amount of sample that may be chromatographed.

The manufacturers of open tubular columns often use trade names for the liquid phases presented in Table 7-3. However, the name usually retains a numerical designation so that the chromatographer can recognize the composition of the liquid phase as given in the table. For example, a **capillary column** of HP-1 or DB-1 is a 100% dimethyl polysiloxane (simethicone) comparable to OV-1 (see Table 7-3) produced by Hewlett-Packard and J&W Scientific, respectively.

Open tubular columns contain small amounts of stationary phase that significantly reduce the capacity of the column. Capillary columns with inside diameters (ID) of 0.2 mm have capacities of less than 100 ng of sample component. The sample capacity is increased by increasing the column ID. For example, columns with 0.32 mm will accept up to 500 ng of sample component, and columns with 0.53 mm up to 2000 ng of sample component. Columns with IDs of 0.75 mm approach the capacity of packed columns (15,000 ng). Such columns with increased IDs (0.50 to 0.75 mm) are referred to as "wide-bore" columns.

DERIVATIZATION

Often it is desirable to modify a molecule chemically to form a new product with properties that are preferable to those of its precursors. For example, you may need to derivatize a compound to make it volatile and stable as a gas and thus analyzable by GC. Derivatives are also prepared to achieve increased sensitivity, selectivity, or specificity for a given separation. Derivatives may be eluted from the column sooner, have less tailing, produce sharper peaks, provide stability to thermally labile compounds, and increase resolution. Derivatization involves a chemical reaction between some functional group on the sample molecule (usually a polar group, which reduces volatility or interacts with the stationary phase to increase retention time) and a smaller molecule (derivatizing agent), which forms a new product of increased volatility with a smaller partition coefficient (K_D). The derivatization may be carried out before sample injection or may occur in the **injection port** of the chromatograph ("on column" or "flash derivatization"). A few derivatization techniques are briefly presented, but for a more complete discussion consult the literature.[7,8]

A popular GC derivatization technique is the replacement of an active hydrogen by a trimethylsilyl (TMS) group. The resultant *silyl* derivatives are usually less polar and more volatile and display greater thermal stability than their parent compounds. Silylizing reagents react vigorously with water or alcohol-containing solvents; therefore, the conversion reactions are carried out in anhydrous solvents such as acetonitrile or tetrahydrofuran. TMS reagents are flammable, and some are highly corrosive. They should be handled with care.

$$\underset{\textbf{Alcohol}}{\text{ROH}} \quad + \quad \underset{\textbf{Trimethylchlorosilane}}{(CH_3)_3SiCl} \rightarrow ROSi(CH_3)_3 \quad + \quad HCl$$

Esterification is often used for GC analysis of compounds containing a carboxylic acid group. Methyl esters possess the greatest volatility and hence are most popular. Alkylation reactions with quaternary alkylammonium hydroxides or dimethylformamide-dialkyl acetals have become popular as "flash-derivatizing" reagents. Fig. 7-4 presents the derivatization reaction of tetramethylammonium hydroxide and barbiturate drugs. To increase sensitivity, use derivatizing reagents that produce halogen- or nitrogen-containing compounds with **electron-capture detectors**.

SELECTION OF A SEPARATION SYSTEM
Choosing the Mobile Phase

The mobile phase or carrier gas has one major function in gas chromatography: to carry the vaporized sample through the column and into the detector. As previously described, selection of the proper carrier gas depends on three considerations: (1) the operating principles of the detector through which the gas will be continuously flowing, (2) the presence of impurities in the carrier gas, and (3) the desired speed of analysis and performance of the column. Compounds that are negligibly partitioned into a stationary phase cannot be separated from each other. Similarly, compounds with too great an affinity for the stationary phase will have unacceptably long retention times or may be irreversibly retarded.

Stationary-Phase Selection

Liquid phases with the same physical properties as the sample will retain the sample and generally effect a separation. However, this general rule does not aid in determining which specific stationary phase is potentially the best for a particular separation. Several approaches to the choice of liquid-phase selection for a desired separation are briefly presented.

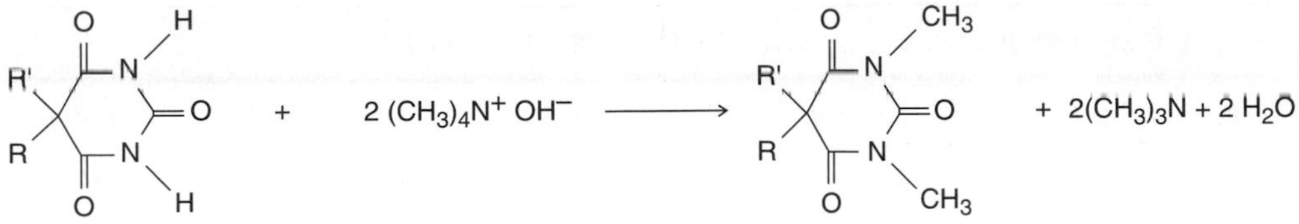

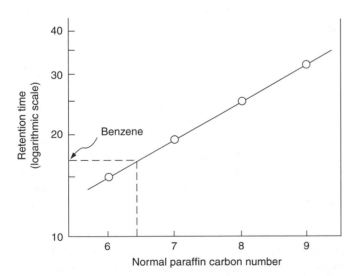

Fig. 7-4   Tetramethyl derivatization of barbiturate drugs.

Many sources of irreproducibility can affect GC analysis. These include variations in assay conditions and variations in stationary-phase packaging (lot to lot, company to company, and so on). **Relative retention times** are converted to indices or constants to ensure reproducible identification of peaks of interest regardless of exact assay conditions. These values can then be used to compare data between analyses, within a laboratory, or between laboratories.

Kovats index. If the components of the sample are known, the most likely stationary phase that will effect a separation may be selected by use of the Kovats **retention index**.[9,10] Retention indices relate the retention time of a compound, regardless of its chemical nature, to those of the *n*-paraffins (straight-chain hydrocarbons) eluted directly before and after it. Chromatographing the *n*-paraffins on a given column under set conditions yields a nearly linear relationship between the log of their retention time, t_R, and the number of carbon atoms in each paraffin, as shown in Fig. 7-5.

Each *n*-paraffin is given a retention index, *I*, that equals 100 times the number of carbon atoms. The retention index of all other compounds is calculated from the following relationship:

$$I = 100z + 100[(\log t_{R_x} - \log t_{R_z})/(\log t_{R_{(z+1)}} - \log t_{R_z})] \quad \textit{Eq. 7-4}$$

z equals the number of carbon atoms in the unknown compound; t_{R_x} is the retention time of the unknown substance *x*; t_{R_z} is the retention time of the *n*-paraffin eluted immediately before *x*; and $t_{R_{(z+1)}}$ is the retention time of the *n*-paraffin eluted immediately after *x*. For example, assume that the data presented in Table 7-4 and graphically represented in Fig. 7-5 were obtained by chromatography from a series of *n*-paraffins and benzene on a given liquid phase. The retention index, *I*, benzene (*z* = 6) on that liquid phase is calculated to be 650.

$$I = 100(6) + 100(0.052 / 0.104) = 600 + 50 = 650$$

The calculated *I* applies only to the particular stationary phase and temperature conditions. However, the effects of flow rate of the mobile phase and the percent loading (quantity of liquid phase) will change the retention time proportionally for all *n*-paraffins, and thus the calculated *I* values are unchanged. Extensive lists of retention indices of numerous compounds on liquid phases are available in the *ASTM Gas Chromatography Data Compilation Catalog AMD 25A*[11] and in a supplement catalog *AMD 25A S-1.*[12] If several compounds of a different chemical nature are to be separated simultaneously, the compounds of interest are located in the table and their respective *I* values for various stationary phases noted. A difference of at least 30 *I* units between the compounds indicates that a particular phase will efficiently separate them. The *I* values are based on peak apex only and give no indication of peak width. Therefore *I* values do not indicate the resolution of the compounds. However, since the retention times increase with the retention index, *I*, the retention indices indicate the order in which compounds will be eluted from the column. A clinical application of *I* values has been the qualitative identification of drugs on standard liquid phases under both isothermal and temperature-programmed conditions.[13] Retention index databases for packed columns may be used for preliminary identification of peaks eluting from open tubular columns.[14]

Rohrschneider and McReynolds constants. **Rohrschneider** and **McReynolds constants** are related systems that classify stationary phases in terms of their separating power.[15,16] The *I* values of a set of reference compounds of varying polarity are determined on the liquid phase being tested and compared against the *I* values for

Fig. 7-5   Linear relationship between log of retention time and number of carbon atoms in a series of paraffin hydrocarbons. *(From Rowland FW: The practice of gas chromatography, Palo Alto, CA, 1974, Hewlett-Packard Co.)*

TABLE 7-4   DATA USED FOR CALCULATION OF RETENTION INDEX

Compound	Carbon Atoms	Symbol	t_R (min)	log t_R (min)	Retention Index (I)
Hexane	6	z	14.96	1.175	600 (by definition)
Benzene	6	x	16.86	1.227	650 (by experiment)
Heptane	7	z + 1	19.01	1.279	700 (by definition)
Octane	8		24.15		800 (by definition)
Nonane	9		30.76		900 (by definition)

TABLE 7-5   REFERENCE COMPOUNDS USED TO DETERMINE MCREYNOLDS CONSTANTS

Reference Compound	Abbreviation	I*	Organic Compound Expected To Display Similar Behavior on Liquid Phase
Benzene	x′	650	Aromatics, olefins
Butanol	y′	590	Alcohols, phenols, weak acids
2-Pentanone	z′	627	Aldehydes, esters, ketones
Nitropropane	u′	652	Nitrogenous and nitrile compounds
Pyridine	s′	699	Nitrogenous aromatic heterocyclics, bases

Absolute value of retention indices observed on squalene.

TABLE 7-6   MCREYNOLDS CONSTANT OF VARIOUS LIQUID PHASES

Liquid Phase	McREYNOLDS CONSTANT				
	x′	y′	z′	u′	s′
1. DEGS	**496**	746	**590**	837	835
2. Carbowax 20M	**322**	536	**368**	572	510
3. Emulphor ON-870	202	395	251	395	344
4. Triton X-100	203	399	268	402	362
5. XE-60	204	381	340	493	367

x′, Benzene; y′, butanol; z′, 2-pentanone; u′, nitropropane; s′, pyridine.
Numbers in **boldfaced** type are McReynolds constants that are much higher for DEGS than for Carbowax 20M.

the same compounds obtained on a reference liquid phase. Squalene, a nonpolar liquid, is used as the reference phase. The constants are then calculated as indicated in the following equations:

$$\text{Rohrschneider constant } (x) = 1/100\ (I_{testphase} - I_{squalene}) \qquad Eq.\ 7\text{-}5$$

$$\text{McReynolds constant } (x') = I_{testphase} - I_{squalene} \qquad Eq.\ 7\text{-}6$$

Table 7-5 presents data related to five reference compounds used to determine the McReynolds constants. Both Rohrschneider and McReynolds constants may be used for two purposes: to select a liquid phase for a particular application and to classify liquid phases as to how similar or different they are in the ability to perform chromatographic separations.[17] An example of the use of McReynolds

constants for selection of a liquid phase for a given application would be the separation of saturated and unsaturated fatty acid methyl esters. If you have available liquid phases 1 (DEGS) and 2 (Carbowax 20M), presented in Table 7-6, you can choose the best phase for the separation by examining their McReynolds constants. For the ability to separate saturated and unsaturated fatty acid esters, consider the constants x′ (olefinic compounds, unsaturated esters) and z′ (esters) (see Table 7-6). The McReynolds constants for x′ and z′ (in bold face in Table 7-6) are much higher for DEGS than for Carbowax 20M; therefore DEGS is better suited for the separation of the fatty acid esters.

The characterization of liquid phases as to their ability to perform separations by use of McReynolds constants is demonstrated by examination of phases 3 (Emulphor ON-870), 4 (Triton X-100), and 5 (XE-60) in Table 7-6. All liquid phases are commercially available, and you can determine differences or similarities in separating power as illustrated in Table 7-6. Liquid phases 3 and 4 are almost identical in their ability to separate the reference compounds. Therefore, if used as a liquid phase, they would yield very similar chromatograms. Liquid phase 5 is similar to phases 3 and 4 for constants x′ and y′. Therefore separation of compounds characterized by these constants (see Table 7-6) on phase 5 (XE-60) would be essentially the same on phases 3 (Emulphor EN-870) and 4 (Triton X-100). The constants z′ and u′ are higher for phase 5, and the separation of the compounds listed in Table 7-6 for these constants would be better on XE-60 than on the other two phases. However, although keto compounds (constant z′) are better separated on phase 5, the separation of alcohols (constant y′) would be practically

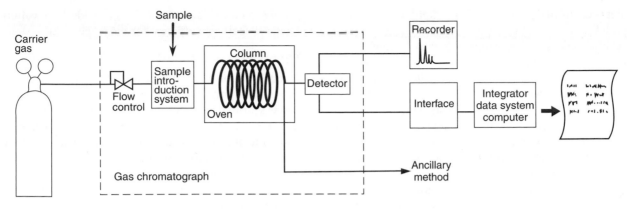

Fig. 7-6 Basic components of a gas chromatographic system. *(From Ettre LS:* Practical gas chromatography, *Norwalk, CT, 1973, Perkin-Elmer Corp.)*

identical on phases 3, 4, and 5. When using packed columns, differences in McReynolds constants of 20 or less are insignificant. Differences of 100 McReynolds units indicate significantly better separating ability of one phase compared with the other.

COMPONENTS OF GAS CHROMATOGRAPH

Basically, a gas chromatograph consists of six components (Fig. 7-6): (1) a pressurized carrier gas with ancillary pressure and **flow regulators**, (2) a sample-injection port, (3) a column, (4) a detector, (5) an electrometer and signal recorder, and (6) thermostated compartments encasing the column, detector, and injection port.

Carrier Gas

The efficiency of a gas chromatograph depends on a constant flow of carrier gas. The carrier gas from a pressurized tank flows through a toggle valve, a flowmeter (range 1 to 1000 L/min), metal restrictors, and a pressure gauge (1 to 4 atmospheres). The flow is adjusted by a needle valve mounted at the base of the flowmeter. The gas moves more slowly at the head of the column than at the outlet because of a pressure drop in the column. Thus the flow rates are measured as the gas leaves the column. This is done with a soap-film flowmeter. A simple sidearm buret with a rubber bulb filled with soap solution is connected to the detector outlet. One determines the flow rate by noting the time required for a film (bubble) to pass between two calibrated volume marks on the buret.

Carrier gas should be inert, dry, and pure. The most common carrier gases are inert, but they may contain contaminants that affect column performance and the response of ionization detectors. Hydrocarbon gases and water are removed from the carrier gas by a molecular sieve trap between the gas cylinder and the chromatograph.

Sample-Injection Port

Most GC analyses are performed on nonaqueous, liquid samples that are injected by a glass microsyringe. A needle is inserted through a **septum** into a heated block, where the sample is vaporized and swept by carrier gas into the column. The pressure inside the injection port is usually well above atmospheric pressure, and the stream of carrier gas sweeps away the sample and aids in vaporization. Thus a sample may be vaporized at temperatures below its atmospheric boiling point. However, the injection port temperature is usually set at 25° to 50° C higher than the boiling point of the highest boiling components in the sample. This ensures that immediate vaporization will occur and that the components will not be diluted by carrier gas and will enter the head of the column as a single band. The time required for vaporization is dependent on the amount and volatility of the sample. Dilute samples vaporize faster than concentrated samples. High-boiling or temperature-sensitive compounds may be diluted with volatile solvents, which lower injection temperatures significantly.

Because heated metal may catalyze the degradation of many biological compounds, many injection ports are equipped with a glass liner or a glass column that extends through the injectors flush to the septum. The latter approach is called *on-column injection*. For maximum efficiency it is imperative that the sample be the smallest possible volume (0.5 to 10 μL) consistent with detector sensitivity and be injected as a single, uniform band ("slug injection"). Insertion, injection, and withdrawal of the needle should be performed quickly and smoothly. Gaseous samples are injected by a gas-tight syringe or a calibrated bypass loop. The loop consists of a glass system of three stopcocks, between two of which a standard volume of gas is trapped and introduced into the carrier gas stream when the stopcocks are switched.

Because of the low capacity of capillary columns, injection of undiluted samples will often overload the column. This problem is avoided with capillary systems by splitting the carrier gas flow after vaporization. In the split-injection technique after vaporization of the sample, the carrier gas flow is divided into two parts with a variable ratio of flows. The smaller part of the gas/sample mixture enters the column while the larger flow bypasses the column inlet and leaves the system. The ratio of flow to the column and the outlet is controlled by a needle valve. Splitting ratios may be adjusted over a wide range (1:5 to 1:250).

A septum separates the chromatographic column from the laboratory environment. Septums are small disks of silicone rubber, and numerous types are available, depending on analytic requirements. Silicone rubber septums may absorb certain types of samples. Special septums (such as Teflon R coated) will alleviate this problem. Low–molecular-weight solvents used in the manufacture of septums may be released as the injection port is heated. This "bleed" of solvent may produce unwarranted peaks (ghost peaks) in chromatograms, and it increases the background level of the detector. Low-bleed septums from which the solvents have been extracted are available. Repeated injections through the septum will gradually destroy its mechanical strength, causing leakage. As a result, the retention time and sensitivity decrease as the carrier gas and part of the sample are released back through the septum into the atmosphere. This problem is easily avoided by regular insertion of new septums.

Various specialized injection systems are commercially available. If you are performing large numbers of similar analyses, consider using automatic sampling units.

Column Tubing

The column tubing is a container for the stationary phase (packing material) and directs the carrier gas flow. It should be inert and should not affect the separation by reaction with the stationary phase or the sample. Depending on the gas chromatograph used, the columns may be shaped as a U-tube or coiled in an open spiral or flat pancake shape.

Stainless steel and copper columns are often used for analyses requiring temperatures greater than 250° C. However, for the analysis of drugs, steroids, or other biological compounds, metal columns may absorb these analytes or catalyze their degradation; thus glass is the tubing of choice for the majority of clinical analyses. One disadvantage of glass, though, is its fragility and inflexibility. If the columns are not properly handled, they are easily broken during transport or installation. Nickel has been recommended as a substitute for glass. Nickel tubing has been effectively used in the analysis of specific drugs, pesticides, and cholesterol, which previously required glass tubing.[18] However, the application of nickel tubing to the broad range of biological compounds has not yet been established. Until such time, glass tubing remains the best choice for primary support when performing a clinical analysis.

The inside diameters of columns vary from capillary (0.2 mm) to packed columns of 4 mm. Packed columns of 4 mm ID contain four times the stationary phase as 2 mm ID columns of the same length and therefore possess a greater sample capacity. However, the same separation will require higher temperatures and a longer analysis time on the wider column. In addition, columns should be only as long as necessary to effect the desired separation. A short column provides a short analysis time, low temperatures, long column life, and less background in the detector. Packed

columns of 0.7 to 2 m (2 to 6 feet) or **wide-bore columns** of 15 m (45 feet) are sufficient for most chemical separations.

Thermal Compartment

Precise control of column temperature is imperative in gas chromatography. The column oven is controlled by a system that is sensitive to changes of 0.01 Celsius degree and maintains the column temperature to ± 0.1 Celsius degree of the desired temperature. The column oven, injection block, and detectors should have separate heaters and controls. Analysis may be performed at a constant oven temperature (isothermal), or the temperature may be varied during the analysis (temperature programming). The temperature change during analysis can be programmed to vary with time according to predetermined, reproducible patterns, giving linear, convex, or concave curves when column temperature is plotted against time (Fig. 7-7). Temperature programming is often used in separating a complex mixture, the components of which have widely varying affinity for the stationary phase. Initially the column temperature is set low to permit separation and elution of the compounds with little affinity for the stationary phase. The temperature is then raised to elute compounds of higher stationary-phase affinity. Many chromatographs are equipped with specialized oven controls that uniformly raise the column temperature after each sample injection.

Detectors

As the carrier gas exits from the column, a detector senses the separated components of the sample and provides a corresponding electrical signal. Any physical device that accomplishes this may be used as a detector; however, only a

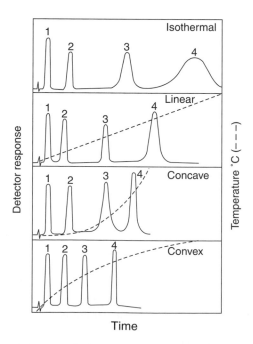

Fig. 7-7 Schema of theoretical separation of four compounds showing varying elution patterns with different temperature programming.

TABLE 7-7 DETECTORS AND APPROPRIATE GASES

Detector	Carrier Gas	Detector Gas
Thermal conductivity (TCD)	Helium, hydrogen	
Flame ionization (FID)	Helium, nitrogen	Air and hydrogen
Nitrogen-phosphorus (NPD)	Helium, nitrogen	Air and hydrogen
		Air and 8% hydrogen in helium
Electron capture	Nitrogen	5% methane in argon
	5% methane in argon	

few are commonly used. For proper operation or optimum response, each type of detector requires a specific carrier gas (Table 7-7). The most widely used detectors are discussed in the following section.[19,20]

Thermal-conductivity detector. A **thermal-conductivity detector** (TCD) measures the difference in ability to conduct heat (thermal conductivity) between pure carrier gas and the carrier with sample mixture. A sample carried in the gas increases the thermal conductivity. Usually four heat-sensing elements, thermistors or wires, are mounted in a brass or stainless steel heat sink and connected to form the arms of a Wheatstone bridge (Fig. 7-8). An electric current is passed through the wires. Two filaments in opposite arms of the bridge are cooled by carrier gas (reference), and the other two by the column effluent (sample). The heat lost over both sets of wires is balanced by adjusting the flow rate of the pure carrier gas. Emerging components from the column increase the rate of cooling of the sample wires because of the increased thermal conductivity of the gas mixture. This changes the electrical resistance of the sample wire pattern, causing the Wheatstone bridge to be out of balance. This imbalance causes a response on the recorder. Important variables in TCD response are carrier gas, flow rate, filament current, and detector temperature. TCDs lack selectivity because any compound cooling the wire will cause a response. Also they are not as sensitive as other detectors, with minimum detection ranging from 0.1 to 0.5 mg of analyte per microliter.

Flame-ionization detector (FID). In a **flame-ionization detector**, eluted components in the carrier gas are mixed with hydrogen and burned in air to produce a very hot flame to ionize organic compounds. A pair of electrodes, charged by a polarizing voltage, collects the ions and generates a current proportional to the number of ions collected. The resultant current is amplified by an electrometer, producing a response on the recorder. The response of an FID is directly proportional to the number of carbons in a molecule bound to hydrogen or other carbon atoms. It is insensitive to water, carbon monoxide, carbon dioxide, and most inorganic compounds. The FID is the most popular detector for the determination of organic compounds. Sensitivity depends on chemical structure; therefore, the detector response must be determined for each compound analyzed. At optimal conditions the minimal detectable quantity of organic compound is 1 ng. A cross section of an FID is shown in Fig. 7-9.

Nitrogen-phosphorus detector (NPD). A **nitrogen-phosphorus detector** is similar to an FID except that ions of an alkali metal (rubidium) are introduced into the hydrogen flame. When a compound containing nitrogen or phosphorus is burned in the flame, the rate of release of alkali metal vapor is increased. The alkali metal vapor readily ionizes in the flame and increases the current flow, which results in enhanced sensitivity for nitrogen and phosphorus. The optimum response is greatly dependent on the flow of

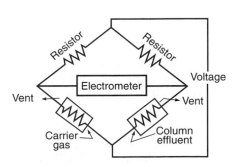

Fig. 7-8 Schema of thermal-conductivity detector. *(From Werner M, Mohrbacher RJ, Riendeau CJ: In Baer DM, Dito WR, editors:* Interpretation of therapeutic drug levels, *Chicago, 1981, American Society of Clinical Pathologists.)*

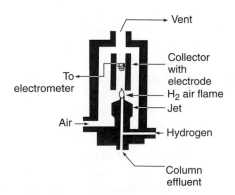

Fig. 7-9 Schema of flame-ionization detector. *(From Werner M, Mohrbacher RJ, Riendeau CJ: In Baer DM, Dito WR, editors:* Interpretation of therapeutic drug levels, *Chicago, 1981, American Society of Clinical Pathologists.)*

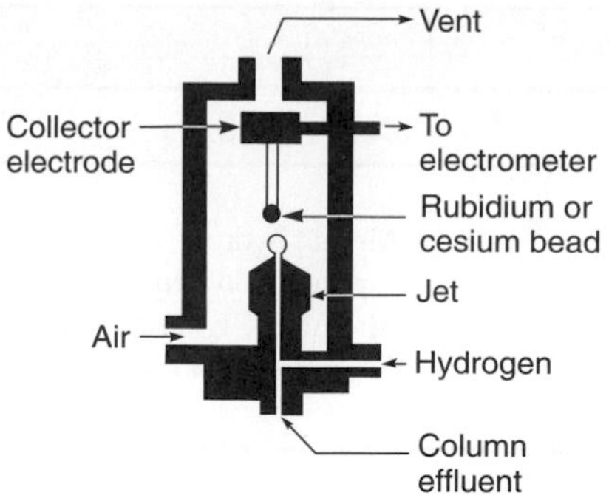

Fig. 7-10 Schema of alkali metal flame detector. *(From Werner M, Mohrbacher RJ, Riendeau CJ: In Baer DM, Dito WR, editors:* Interpretation of therapeutic drug levels, *Chicago, 1981, American Society of Clinical Pathologists.)*

hydrogen. The selective interaction of alkali metal ions with these compounds is complex and poorly understood. However, the sensitivity to organonitrogen compounds and lack of response to other organics make the NPD highly advantageous for the analysis of biological samples. At optimum conditions, the minimum detectable quantity of nitrogenous organic compounds is less than 1 ng. A cross section of an NPD is presented in Fig. 7-10.

Electron-capture detector. In an **electron-capture detector** (ECD), a radioactive isotope releases beta particles that collide with the carrier gas molecules, producing many low-energy electrons. The electrons are collected on electrodes and produce a small, measurable, *standing current.* As sample components that contain chemical groups with high electron affinity (electrophilic species), particularly halogen atoms, are eluted from the column, they capture the low-energy electrons generated by the isotope to form negatively charged ions. The detector measures the loss of cell current because of the recombination of the electrons. Three techniques are used for the collection of the electrons: (1) direct current (DC), (2) pulsed method, and (3) linear method. In the DC method, a constant voltage is applied to the cell electrodes, and the electrons are collected continuously to produce a steady current. The sensitivity of the method is less than that of other ECD methods because both negative ions and free electrons are collected by the electrodes. The reduction in current is smaller than it would be if only free electrons were collected. In the pulsed method, a voltage is applied in continuous pulses of short duration; therefore the heavy negative ions do not have time to respond, and only free electrons are captured. Between pulses, the electron concentration in the detector builds up to levels exceeding those of the DC method. Thus the pulse method has greater sensitivity. The DC and pulsed methods inherently produce a nonlinear response over a wide range of sample concentrations. Such a response is attributable to the finite amount of beta radiation emitted by the detector source per unit time. Because a decrease in current is measured, once a concentration of eluting solute captures a majority of the available low-energy electrons, only small changes in current (detector

response) will be observed with increasing concentrations of solute. The linear range is usually 400 to 500 times the detection limit of a solute for a tritium source and 100 times for a nickel-63 source. However, the linearized method uses electronic modifications that operate the detector in a pulsed mode such that constant cell current is produced. The linear range is thus expanded to ranges of 10,000:1 for a nickel-63 source. The sources of beta particles in an ECD are usually tritium or nickel-63. The ECD is the most sensitive detector available, since as little as 1 picogram of halogen-containing compound may be measured. Laboratories using electron-capture detectors must be licensed by the Nuclear Regulatory Commission and are subject to all regulations concerning employee safety and possible environmental contamination set forth by the commission.

Mass spectrometer as a detector. The **mass spectrometer** (MS) is a specialized chromatographic detector that provides extremely sensitive detection (picogram quantities) and specific analyte identification. GC and MS are presented in Chapter 8.

Fourier-transform infrared spectrometer (FTIR). The **Fourier-transform infrared spectrometer (FTIR)** obtains the infrared spectra of a compound as it elutes from the GC column. The report format of FTIR detectors is similar to that of MS detectors (Chapter 8). A GC/FTIR produces chromatograms measured at specific IR bands similar to SIM mode GC/MS, or records the entire IR spectrum of the compound just as an MS records the mass spectrum of a compound. Recent developments in narrow-range IR photon detectors and photo sample cells now give GC/FTIR sensitivity and specificity that rivals that of GC/MS.[21] There are two types of interface for the GC to the FTIR detector: "vapor phase" and "cryogenic deposition." In vapor phase, a heated fused-silica line directs the GC effluent through a long narrow IR gas cell known as a "lightpipe." An IR beam transmits through the lightpipe, which is sealed at each end with IR-transparent windows. In cryogenic deposition, the column effluent is directed into a vacuum chamber (10^{-5} torr) that ends with a fused-silica restrictor positioned above a ZnSe IR-transparent plate. The effluent is deposited on the **plate**, which is held at liquid nitrogen temperatures. The plate with the frozen eluent is continuously exposed to the IR beam.

Both methods continuously collect the IR spectra of the eluted compounds. The detector does not destroy the compound, and the effluent for the FTIR may be directed into another detector system such as an MS(GC/FTIR/MS). GC/FTIR/MS is an extremely powerful identification technique. At present GC/FTIR is not routinely applied in the clinical chemistry laboratory; however, it is gaining popularity in forensic toxicology laboratories.[22]

Readout. Strip-chart recorders are the most common readout devices in gas chromatography. Recorder sensitivity is usually 1 to 10 mV, with a full-scale response of 1 second or less. Quantitative determinations of separate compounds are performed in two ways: peak-height or peak-area measurements. Both the peak height and peak area of the detector response to the effluent sample are proportional to its concentration. Peak-height measurements are useful in repetitive analyses that are performed by the same operator in a fixed system, that require extensive calibration, or that only partially resolve compounds, making peak-area determinations difficult. In general, peak-area measurements are more precise. Peak area can be determined by manual or automated methods. Electronic integration of the peak area produces both the most precise and the most accurate measurements. Today, detectors may be connected to micro-processor units or to a computerized data system that automatically records the response, identifies the sample components, integrates the signals, performs calculations, stores all data, and prints out the analytical results in final form.

GC APPLICATIONS IN CLINICAL CHEMISTRY

GC is an extremely versatile and powerful analytical methodology. Numerous sample components may be simultaneously separated, identified, and quantitated. By choosing the appropriate stationary phase, one can analyze any mixture of compounds that may be vaporized or converted to volatile derivatives. Selectivity and high sensitivity may be added by varying detectors. Yet, despite these advantages, application of GC in most clinical chemistry laboratories is limited to a few special areas of testing: therapeutic drug monitoring (TDM), toxicology, and testing for inborn errors of metabolism. Even in these areas, GC is applied to specific tests in only a relatively few laboratories because of the specialized training required for maintenance. GC is used to perform TDM analysis of psychoactive drugs, particularly those having active metabolites, which must be measured with the parent drug.

The determination of drugs or toxicants offers the widest potential arena for clinical laboratory use of GC because it provides a rapid, simple, reliable method for the simultaneous determination of volatile poisons such as methanol, ethanol, isopropanol, acetone, and acetaldehyde. GC coupled

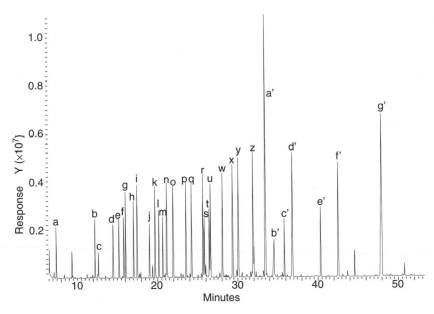

Fig. 7-11 Capillary GLC separation of metabolic organic acids and strong organic acid drugs as trimethylsilyl derivatives. *Gas chromatograph conditions:* Hewlett-Packard 6890, injection port splitless HP 5973A Mass Selective Detector (ms), HP ChemStation software. Initial temperature, 40° C; initial time, 4 minutes; ramp rate, 4° C/minute; final temperature, 280° C; final time, 0 minutes; injection port temperature, 170° C; transfer temperature, 170° C; equilibration time, 0.10 minute; run time, 54 minutes. *Column conditions:* Carrier gas, helium (99.95%); head pressure, 4.70 psi; column flow, 1 to 1.5 minutes; total flow, 20 mL/min; split ratio, 25:1. *Analytical column:* 12 m × 0.2 mm × 0.33 m HP-1 capillary (cross-linked methylsilicon). *Guard column:* 5 m column with connection injector liner: 4 mm splitless packed with glass wool. *a,* Isovaleric-TMS-1; *b,* lactic-TMS-2; *c,* glycolic-TMS-2; *d,* oxalic-TMS-2; *e,* valproic acid; *f,* 3-hydroxybutyric-TMS-2; *g,* 2-hydroxyisovaleric-TMS-2; *h,* malonic-TMS-2; *i,* methylmalonic-TMS-2; *j,* ethosuximide; *k,* ethylmalonic-MS-2; *l,* maleic-TMS-2; *m,* succinic-TMS-2; *n,* methylsuccinic; *o,* fumaric-TMS-2; *p,* L-glyceric-TMS-3; *q,* glutaric-TMS-2; *r,* 3-methylglutaric-TMS-2; *s,* mandelic-TMS-2; *t,* 3-hydroxy-3-methyl-glutaric-TMS-3; *u,* salicylic acid-TMS; *w,* 2-hydroxyphenylactic-TMS-2; *x,* 1,7-hepanedioc-TMS-2 (pimelic); *y,* 4-hydroxyphenlacetic-TMS-2; *z,* octanedioc-TMS-2 (suberic)/phenylpruvic-TMS-2; *a',* ortic-TMS-3; *b',* hippuric-TMS-1; *c',* citric-TMS-4; *d',* decanedioc-TMS-2 (sebacic); *e',* hexadeconoic-TMS-1 (palmitic); *f',* heptadecanoic-TMS-1; *g',* N-tetracan (C24).

with mass spectrometry is required when performing urine testing for drugs of abuse that are regulated by government agencies such as the Department of Defense, the Department of Transportation, and the Nuclear Regulatory Agency. Laboratories performing such testing must be certified by the Department of Health and Human Services. Up to now about 80 laboratories, some associated with clinical laboratories, are so accredited.

GC is applied in highly specialized procedures of clinical chemistry, such as the testing for inborn errors of meta-bolism. As a result of inherited defects in metabolism, unusual or inappropriate amounts of organic acids and other byproducts of metabolism accumulate in serum and are excreted in urine. The determination of organic acids and their concentrations in urine or serum is a valuable tool for these rare defects (Fig. 7-11).[23] Aciduria profiles are easily obtained with GC/FID, whereas serum profiles require more specific and sensitive GC/MS methods. At present, such testing is performed only in commercial reference laboratories or university medical centers.

References

1. Willett J, Kealey D: *Gas chromatography*, New York, 1987, John Wiley & Sons.
2. Grob RL: *Modern practice of gas chromatography*, ed 2, New York, 1985, Wiley & Sons.
3. Freeman RR: *High resolution gas chromatography*, ed 2, Palo Alto, CA, 1981, Hewlett-Packard Co.
4. Schomburg F: *Gas chromatography, a practical course*, Weinheim, Germany, 1990, VCH Publishers.
5. Delley R, Friedrich K: System CG72 von bevorzugten Trennflüssigkeiten für die Gas-chromatographie, *Chromatographia* 10:593, 1971.
6. Hawkes S et al: Preferred stationary liquids for gas chromatography, *J Chromatogr Sci* 13:115, 1975.
7. Siggia S: *Instrumental methods of organic functional group analysis*, New York, 1972, Wiley & Sons.
8. Ahuja S: Derivatization in gas chromatography, *J Pharm Sci* 65:163, 1976.
9. Kovats E: The Kovats' retention index system, *Anal Chem* 36:31A, 1964.
10. Lorenz LJ, Roger LB: Specification of gas chromatographic behavior using Kovats' indices and Rohrschneider constants, *Anal Chem* 43:1593, 1971.
11. American Society for Testing and Materials: *Gas chromatographic data compilation catalog AMD 25A*, Philadelphia, 1967, ASTM.
12. American Society for Testing and Materials: *Gas chromatographic data compilation catalog (suppl 25A S-1)*, Philadelphia, 1971, ASTM.
13. Perrigo BJ, Peel HW: The use of retention indices and temperature-programmed gas chromatography in analytical toxicology, *J Chromatogr Sci* 19:219, 1981.
14. Japp M, Gill R, Osselton MD: Comparison of drug retention indices determined on packed, wide bore capillary and narrow bore capillary columns, *J Forensic Sci* 32:1574, 1987.
15. Supina WR, Rose LP: The use of Rohrschneider constants for classification of GLC columns, *J Chromatogr Sci* 8:217, 1970.
16. McReynolds WO: Characterization of some liquid phases, *J Chromatogr Sci* 8:685, 1970.
17. Ettre LS: *Basic relationships of gas chromatography*, ed 2, Norwalk, CT, 1979, Perkin-Elmer Corp.
18. Fenimore DC et al: Nickel gas chromatographic columns: an alternative to glass for biological samples, *J Chromatogr* 140:9, 1977.
19. David DJ: *Gas chromatographic detectors*, New York, 1974, Wiley & Sons.
20. Sevcik J: *Detectors in gas chromatography*, New York, 1975, Elsevier/North-Holland.
21. Bourne S et al: Performance characteristics of a real-time direct deposition gas chromatography/Fourier transform infrared spectrometry system, *Anal Chem* 62:2448, 1990.
22. Kalasinsky KS, Levine B, Smith ML: Feasibility of using GC/FTIR for drug analysis in the forensic toxicology laboratory, *J Anal Toxicol* 16:332, 1991.
23. Forman DT: Role of the laboratory in diagnosis of organic acidurias, *Ann Clin Lab Sci* 21:85, 1991.

Bibliography

Jennings W, Mittlefehldt E, Stremple P, editors: *Analytical gas chromatography*, San Diego, 1997, Academic Press.
McNair HM, Miller JM: *Basic gas chromatography*, New York, 1997, John Wiley & Sons.

Miller JM: *Chromatography: concepts and contrasts*, New York, 1988, John Wiley & Sons.

Internet Sites

http://www.shu.ac.uk/schools/sci/chem/tutorials/chrom/gaschrm.htm—Gas chromatography tutorial
http://gc.discussing.info/alphabetical_index.html#K—Alphabetical index of over 500 key words
http://ull.chemistry.uakron.edu/chemsep/gc/—University of Akron tutorial
http://www.anc.univie.ac.at/scripts/gc2.pdf—University of Vienna tutorial

www.nysaes.cornell.edu/flavornet/instructions.html
http://gc.discussing.info/gs/b_theory/qualitative_analysis.html
http://cvadana.50megs.com/phytonet3.html
http://www.chem.vt.edu/chem-ed/sep/gc/gc.html—The Chemistry Hyper-media Project at Virginia Tech
http://hendrix.pharm.uky.edu/che626/GC/GC.htm

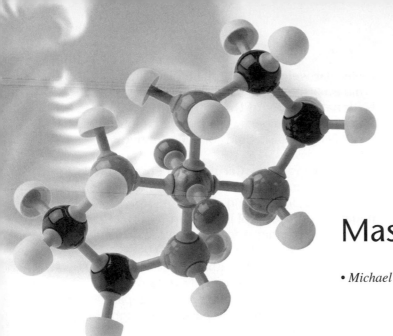

CHAPTER 8

Mass Spectrometry

• *Michael Lehrer*

Chapter Outline

Basic principles
Mass spectrometer
  Ion source
  Mass filter
  Detectors
  Computers
Creation of ion fragments
  Electron ionization (EI)
  Chemical ionization (CI)
Mass fragmentation
Comparison of electron ionization and chemical
  ionization
Use of the mass spectrometer

  Full-scan analysis
  Selected ion monitoring
  Quantitation
Separation techniques
  Gas chromatography/mass spectrometry
  Liquid chromatography/mass spectrometry
  Solids probe
Other mass spectrometers
  Ion trap detectors (ITD)
  Time-of-flight (TOF) MS
  Tandem mass spectrometry (MS/MS)
Forensic drug testing

Objectives

• Define the concepts of mass, charge, and mass
  fragmentation of molecules.
• Describe the basic components of a mass
  spectrometer.
• State how an ion source and mass filter are used to
  separate ions.

• Describe the key elements of a mass-fragmentation
  pattern.
• State the principles of how the mass-fragmentation
  pattern is used to identify molecules.
• Describe applications of mass spectrometry.

Key Terms

accelerating voltage A voltage potential in the ion
source that helps propel charged ion fragments
toward the detector.
atmospheric pressure ionization (API) Ionization
technique to allow large molecules and other
nonvolatile compounds to be analyzed by mass
spectrometry.

base peak The most intense peak in the mass spectrum.
chemical ionization (CI) Low-energy ionization
technique based on charge-transfer collision with an
inert reagent gas.
collision-induced dissociation (CID) The process in
which ions break apart as a result of collisions with
other molecules.

daughter ions The ionic output of the second mass spectroscopy (MS) analyzer of an MS/MS system.

electron ionization (EI) High-energy electron bombardment transforming molecules into fragment ions.

fingerprint The unique fragmentation patterns of organic compounds.

fragmentation pattern A display of the intensity of ion fragments formed versus mass-to-charge ratio.

full scan A mass spectrometric scanning sequence in which all ions in the entire mass range of interest are detected.

GC/MS Gas chromatograph interfaced with a mass spectrometer.

ionization potential The amount of energy required to displace an electron from the outer shell of a compound.

ionization source Area within the mass spectrometer where molecules are ionized by an electron beam.

ion-molecule reaction The product of a collision between an ion fragment and an intact molecule within the ion source.

IonSpray A variation of thermospray technique used to introduce liquid chromatograph eluent into the ion source of the mass spectrometer at ambient temperature.

ion trap detector (ITD) Mass spectrometer that operates on the principle of ion accumulation over time.

isotope dilution Quantitation of chemicals different only in their isotope composition.

LC/MS Liquid chromatograph (LC) interfaced with a mass spectrometer (MS).

magnetic sector Mass spectrometer that separates ion fragments based on their passage through a magnetic field.

mass filter The electronic or magnetic device that separates ions based on their mass-to-charge ratio.

mass fragmentation The breakdown of a large unstable molecular ion, usually in a defined pattern unique to the test molecule.

mass spectrometer A device to separate ions based on their mass-to-charge ratio.

mass spectrum The output of a mass spectrometer displaying mass-to-charge (m/z) ratios versus intensity of the ion fragment.

mass-to-charge (m/z) A ratio of the mass of a given ion fragment divided by its ionic charge.

molecular ion (M^+) The initial ion fragment corresponding to the molecular weight of the compound.

molecular weight The total molecular mass of a molecule.

National Institute of Drug Abuse (NIDA) A governmental agency charged with regulating and certifying forensic drugs of abuse testing laboratories.

National Laboratory Certification Program (NLCP) The governmental certification program for forensic workplace drug testing.

negative-ion chemical ionization (NICI) Chemical ionization technique focusing on the generation of negatively charged ions.

parent ion The ionic output of the first mass spectrometer analyzer of an MS/MS system.

quadrupole Mass spectrometer that separates ion fragments based on their passage through an electronic field.

quasimolecular ion The ion fragment often formed by transfer of a proton in chemical ionization corresponding to the molecular weight plus one.

reagent gas A gas, such as methane or isobutane, used to produce chemical ionization in the ion source.

selected ion monitoring (SIM) Selective scanning of a few preselected ion fragments by the detector.

selected ion profile Selective scanning and area integration in the SIM mode of a significant ion fragment.

soft ionization A low-energy ionization technique such as chemical ionization.

solids probe A probe used to introduce crystalline material directly into the mass spectrometer.

Substance Abuse and Mental Health Services Administration (SAMHSA) The agency within the Department of Health and Human Services (DHHS) that regulates NLCP laboratories.

tandem mass spectrometry (MS/MS) The coupling of two or more mass analyzers.

thermospray A technique used to introduce liquid chromatography eluent into the ion source of the mass spectrometer.

time-of-flight (TOF) mass spectrometer A spectrometer that separates ion fragments based on their transit time through a given path.

total ion current (TIC) Chromatographic integration and display of ion currents in GC/MS applications.

triple-stage quadrupole (TSQ) Instrumental configuration of a quadrupole MS/MS system.

unimolecular decomposition The high energy disintegration of an ion into smaller ion fragments.

BASIC PRINCIPLES

Mass spectrometry uses the creation and analysis of ions to analyze a wide variety of molecules. **Mass spectrometers** are devices that operate on the principle that charged particles moving through a magnetic or an electric field can be separated from other charged particles according to their **mass-to-charge (m/z)** ratios. Because molecules do not have a net charge, mass spectrometers induce them by an ionization process. Charged molecules are not stable and can break down into fragments and lose their charge by interacting with other molecules or surfaces. Implicit in the use of a mass spectrometer is the assumption that the ionized (including fragmented) products are formed in a reproducible manner if the ionization, separation, and detection systems are kept constant.

Each of the resulting ions has a specific molecular mass and charge, which the mass spectrometer separates and detects. Because the mass of each ion is discrete to greater than a thousandth of an atomic weight unit, the resulting separation of the ion masses is displayed as spectral lines of intensity versus the mass-to-charge ratio. The intensity of each ion is in proportion to the number of that ion reaching the detector.

Most ions have a single unit charge; consequently it is common practice to describe ions in terms of "mass" alone. However, doubly charged ions can occur and such ion fragments have a mass value that is one half of their true mass spectrometric value. The m/z value for each ion is plotted on the x-axis, and the ion's intensity is plotted on the y-axis to yield a line graph output (Fig. 8-1). The most intense ion in the spectrum is termed the **base peak** and is arbitrarily assigned an abundance value of 100%. The intensity of other peaks is then normalized to the base peak intensity. The record of all ions formed and the relative abundance of each constitute the **mass spectrum** of that compound. This unique

fragmentation pattern of the molecule is reproducible, and sample identification can be achieved when an unknown compound's ion values and intensities are compared against reference spectra. A match constitutes the chemical identification of the unknown compound.

MASS SPECTROMETER

All mass spectrometers include a system to create and maintain a vacuum; a device to introduce the samples (such as gas-liquid chromatography (GLC), liquid chromatography (LC), and solids probe); an **ionization source**, which serves to ionize the sample; a **mass filter** or analyzer where charged particles are separated according to their m/z ratios; and ion collection, amplification, and detection devices (Fig. 8-2). Contemporary mass spectrometers also incorporate computer systems for control of the instrument and for the acquisition, display, manipulation, and interpretation of data.

Ion Source

The ion source is maintained in a high-vacuum environment to enhance collision efficiency and ion formation. High-efficiency vacuum pumps maintain the ionization source pressure in the 10^{-5} to 10^{-7} torr range, which not only minimizes **ion-molecule reactions** (which complicate the analysis), but also optimizes the detection, resolution, and transmission of the ions generated.

Ions are generated in the ion chamber or ion source of the mass spectrometer (Fig. 8-3). The source may be viewed as a small closed box containing several pinhole orifices that serve as inlets and outlets. Variable positive and negative electronic potentials are induced on specific metallic surfaces. An electron beam is directed into the source. Compounds undergoing analysis enter the ion source and are bombarded by the ionization beam operating at 70 eV (by convention). Some of the compounds are converted into positive and

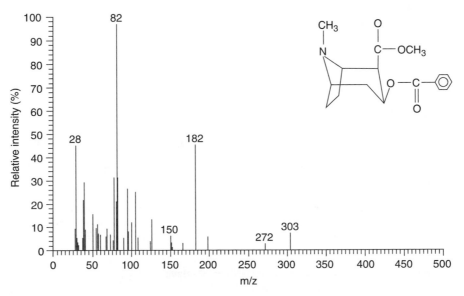

Fig. 8-1 Electron-impact mass spectrum of cocaine. *(From Saferstein R:* Forensic science handbook, *Englewood Cliffs, NJ, 1982, Prentice Hall.)*

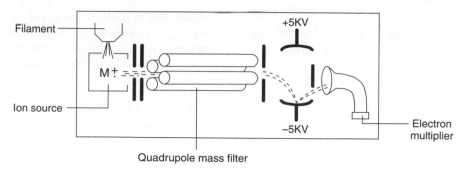

Fig. 8-2 A quadrupole mass spectrometer.

negative ions, and these ions are either attracted or repelled by the electronic potentials; that is, opposite charges attract, like charges repel. Electronic voltage programming optimizes the preservation of ions of a given polarity (either positive or negative ions). For example, the negative potential maintains the positive ions in motion within the volume defined by the source. If an ion comes into physical contact with the metallic surface, it is instantly grounded and eliminated. By manipulating the magnitude and polarity of the electronic potentials, the ions within the source can be stored, accelerated, and directed in space to the outlets that lead to the mass filter.

Mass Filter

Electronic separation. The mass filter separates the ions of interest according to their m/z ratios and allows these ions ultimately to reach the detector. Separation of the ions by the mass filter can occur electronically as is the case in a **quadrupole** mass spectrometer. A quadrupole filter consists

of a quadrant of four parallel hyperbolic or circular rods that provide a specific radio frequency field (Fig. 8-4). Opposite rods are electrically connected. The applied voltage consists of a constant direct current component U and a radio frequency component V_0 (cos wt); $w = 2\pi f$, in which f is the radio frequency, and t, the time during which the cycles are applied.[1] The potential difference between the two sets of rods is thus $U \pm V_0$ cos wt. This creates a unique oscillating field where a positive ion injected into the quadrupole region will oscillate between the adjacent electrodes of opposite polarity. At specified radio frequency, ions of a given mass undergo stable oscillation between the electrodes. Ions of lower or higher mass undergo oscillation of increasing amplitude until they are grounded on the quadrupole electrodes. Within the quadrupole field, no force is exerted in the longitudinal direction, and so an ion with stable oscillation continues at its original velocity down the flight path to the detector. With 5 to 30 V of ion acceleration potential, the ions undergo a sufficient number of oscilla-

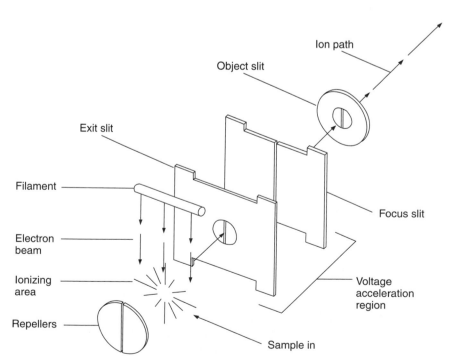

Fig. 8-3 Schema of an ion source. *(From Saferstein R: Forensic science handbook, Englewood Cliffs, NJ, 1982, Prentice Hall.)*

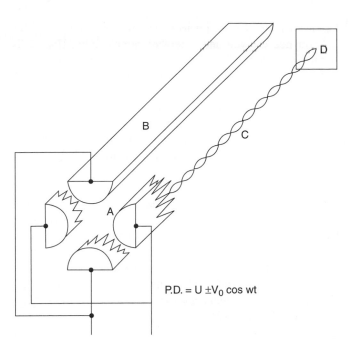

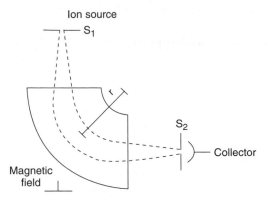

Fig. 8-5 Schema of 90-degree magnetic sector showing direction focusing of divergent ion beam. *(From McFadden WH: Techniques of combined gas chromatography/mass spectrometry, New York, 1973, Wiley & Sons. This material is used by permission of John Wiley & Sons, Inc.)*

Fig. 8-4 Schema of quadrupole mass filter. *A,* Ion injection; *B,* quadrupole rods; *C,* oscillating ion beams; *D,* collector. *(From McFadden WH: Techniques of combined gas chromatography/mass spectrometry, New York, 1973, Wiley & Sons. This material is used by permission of John Wiley & Sons, Inc.)*

tions during the flight period to provide reasonable mass separation.

Magnetic separation. Alternatively the mass filter can separate the ions magnetically, as is the case in **magnetic sector** mass spectrometers. Ions formed in the source are accelerated toward a homogeneous magnetic field (Fig. 8-5). For ions with an electronic charge, *z*, and mass, *m*, the kinetic energy will be related to the **accelerating voltage**, *V*, by the equation

$$V_z = \frac{1}{2} mv^2$$

in which *v* is the ion velocity. As the ions enter the magnetic field, *H*, they experience a force orthogonal to the field, which results in a curvature of the ion path. This accelerating force, *Hev*, is balanced by the centripetal force, so that

$$Hev = mv^2/r$$

in which *r* is the radius of the curvature. Elimination of the velocity term gives the equation

$$m/z = H^2r^2/2V$$

Thus, at a fixed radius, *r*, and for a singly charged ion, the mass focused at S_2 and collected by the detector is proportional to the square of the magnetic field and inversely proportional to the accelerating voltage. By varying either of these two parameters, ions of different mass-to-charge ratio can be deflected to the detector, and in this fashion the mass spectrum is scanned.[1]

For most applications it is preferable to vary the magnetic field and maintain constant accelerating voltage. When the

voltage is varied over a course of a mass scan (with constant magnetic field), the efficiency of transmitting ions of low mass is much greater than that for ions of high mass. This mass discrimination is attributable to the fact that an ion of mass 400 will have one tenth the accelerating voltage of an ion of mass 40. Because the higher mass region is the more important part of the spectrum, voltage scanning is used only for special cases in which magnetic scanning is impractical.

Magnetic sector mass spectrometry. Magnetic sector instruments offer high resolution and consequently are more complex and expensive than either quadrupole or ion trap systems. Resolution requirement is an important consideration in choosing among systems. Resolution is defined by the following equation:

$$\text{Resolution} = M/\Delta M$$

M is the mass of the ion, and Δ*M* is the difference in mass between *M* and its adjacent ion. High-resolution systems have a resolution of 10,000 or greater. Such systems can separate an ion of mass 200.00 from an ion of mass 200.02. Systems with resolution of less than 1000 are considered low-resolution systems. An instrument with a resolution of 800 will separate an ion of mass 800 from 801. Most clinical, environmental, and forensic applications can readily be achieved with the less-expensive lower-resolution instruments.

Detectors

Almost all mass spectrometers detect ions by using electron multipliers. The impacting ion signal is amplified in the same manner as that described by Fig. 4-12 on p. 92.

Computers

Modern mass spectrometers use computer interfaces and data-handling capacity to operate, record, and analyze the data generated by the mass spectrometer.

CREATION OF ION FRAGMENTS
Electron Ionization (EI)

Electron ionization (EI, electronic impact) is the most widely used method of ionization. For ionization to occur, the bombarding electrons must possess sufficient energy to displace an electron from the molecule's outer electron shell during the initial collision. The **ionization potential** of a molecule is the amount of energy required to displace that outer shell electron; most organic compounds have ionization potentials in the 7 to 13 eV range. Thus the energy of the incoming ionization beam must exceed the ionization potential of the molecule being analyzed to displace the molecule's valence electron successfully. Mass spectrometers are generally standardized on an ionization beam at 70 eV. At that setting, the electron beam always has sufficient energy to ionize incoming sample molecules efficiently. Additionally, bombardment at 70 eV results in collisions that impart excess energy to the ions generated, which enhances their decomposition to secondary fragments resulting in more structural information.

As gaseous sample molecules enter the ion source (Fig. 8-3), the electron beam originating from a heated rhenium or tungsten filament bombards them. A small positive potential on the repeller plate focuses and repels the positive ions generated through the exit slit toward the mass analyzer. A much higher voltage potential is placed on one or more of the plates and is used to accelerate the velocity of the ions as they leave the exit slit. A focus slit is used to direct the ion's trajectory toward the mass analyzer. Negative ions are also formed in the source. Such ions can be analyzed by reversing the voltage potentials of the repeller and accelerating plates.

Compounds that can readily accommodate an extra electron such as halogen-containing drugs (or drugs derivatized with halogen-containing derivatives), polycyclic aromatics, and substituted phenols can generate significant negative ions, which allow sensitive detection by negative ion mass spectrometry. However, the resulting negative ion mass spectrum has fewer ion fragments, and they are usually at relatively low masses; consequently negative-ion EI provides less structural information than its positive-ion counterpart, and as a result most applications center on positive-ion mass spectrometry.

Chemical Ionization (CI)

Chemical ionization (CI) is another ionization technique that has found great utility because it imparts the ability to exercise control over the site and degree of ion fragmentation. CI relies on an indirect approach to achieve sample molecule ion formation. A **reagent gas** is introduced into the source before the sample molecules enter. The 70 eV ionization beam ionizes the reagent gas to generate reagent gas ions. When sample molecules enter the source, they collide with reagent gas ions, resulting in a charge transfer from the reagent gas ion to the sample molecule. This "gentle" ionization process results in ionized sample molecules that are relatively stable and hence long lived. The versatility of

CI stems from the ability to select different reagent gases to influence the site and extent of sample ionization. This flexibility allows for the exercise of control over the complexity of the resulting spectrum and hence the degree of structural information derived. Methane, isobutane, water, and ammonia are some of the more commonly encountered CI reagent gases; fragments generated can differ depending on both the reagent gas used and on the chemical characteristics of the compound being analyzed. Choice of a particular reagent gas influences the ionization process. Several different mechanisms for charge transfer, such as proton transfer, charge exchange, or negative ionization, can occur. Proton transfer reactions and, to a lesser extent, negative ionization have received the most attention and widespread application.

Methane reagent gas exemplifies the proton transfer process. High-energy electron bombardment generates an abundance of CH_4^+ and CH_3^+ ions (Eq. 8-1), which quickly react with excess methane gas to form stable CH_5^+ and $C_2H_5^+$ ions[2] (Eqs. 8-2 and 8-3).

$$2CH_4 + 2e^- \rightarrow CH_4^+ + CH_3^+ + H\bullet + 4e^- \qquad \textit{Eq. 8-1}$$
$$CH_4^+ + CH_4 \rightarrow CH_5^+ + CH_3\bullet \qquad \textit{Eq. 8-2}$$
$$CH_3^+ + CH_4 \rightarrow C_2H_5^+ + H_2 \qquad \textit{Eq. 8-3}$$

CH_5^+ and $C_2H_5^+$ are relatively stable adducts and constitute nearly 90% of the total methane ionization by the time the sample molecules enter the source. They react as Brönsted acids with most incoming sample molecules (M), protonating them to yield the **quasimolecular ion** (MH)$^+$ corresponding to their molecular weight plus one (Eqs. 8-4 and 8-5).

$$M + CH_5^+ \rightarrow MH^+ + CH_4 \qquad \textit{Eq. 8-4}$$
$$M + C_2H_5^+ \rightarrow MH^+ + C_2H_4 \qquad \textit{Eq. 8-5}$$

In a similar fashion, isobutane reagent gas yields a predominant number of *tert*-butyl reagent gas ions that protonate the sample molecules as follows:

$$M + C_4H_9^+ \rightarrow MH^+ + C_4H_8 \qquad \textit{Eq. 8-6}$$

CI is considered a **soft ionization** technique because of its low-energy transfer ionization process when compared to EI. Consequently the quasimolecular ion produced is relatively stable and long lived when compared to the molecular ion produced in EI spectra. Because of this stability, the quasimolecular ion does not undergo as extensive fragmentation into secondary ion fragments as the molecular ion does in EI spectra. However, CI ionization does involve some energy transfer, because proton transfer reaction between the reagent gas ions and the sample molecule is an exothermic energy-producing process. The amount of energy transferred to the newly formed MH$^+$ ion is proportional to the exothermic reaction and determines the stability and hence survival of MH$^+$ in the source. The higher the exothermicity of the reaction the more likely is MH$^+$ to decompose.

MASS FRAGMENTATION

During the collision, energy is transferred from the ionization beam to the sample molecule. This resulting

$$M + e^- \longrightarrow M^+ + 2e^-$$
$$M^+ \longrightarrow F_1 + F_2 + F_3^+ \dots$$

Fig. 8-6 Electron ionization. *F*, Fragment; *M*, molecule; *M*⁺, molecular ion.

moiety can dissipate some of its excess energy by freeing its outer shell electron to give rise to a positively charged **molecular ion (M⁺)** corresponding to the **molecular weight** of the compound (Fig. 8-6). The molecular weight is one of the more important pieces of information obtained from a mass spectrum. The peak intensity of this molecular ion is directly proportional to the life span of the ion. A stable molecular ion lasts longer and hence generates an intense peak, whereas a short-lived ion generates a small peak. Most molecular ions are short lived because of their high energy level. Often they are so unstable and short-lived that they don't exist long enough to be detected. In such cases the mass spectrum does not exhibit the molecular ion at all. In general, ions that can easily dissipate their excess energy internally, such as extensively conjugated fragments, are more stable and hence longer lived.

EI ionization can be accomplished only when sample molecules exist in a gaseous state. Several suitable means for vaporizing and delivering the gaseous molecules into the ion source are available, as discussed later in this chapter.

In general, molecular ions are highly energized and thus inherently unstable. They dissipate their excess energy by breaking internal bonds and undergoing **unimolecular decompositions** that result in secondary ion fragments (F⁺). Simultaneously, secondary fragments are also formed by means of ion-molecule and ion-ion collisions that are occurring randomly in the ion source. Secondary fragments have lower masses; such fragments continue the process of dissipating their energy by further decomposition and by random collisions with other molecules and ions. The resulting effect is the formation of a large number of fragment ions with m/z values ranging from the molecular weight of the compound at the high end of the spectrum down to the lowest m/z values scanned. These fragments are detected and plotted according to their m/z ratios versus intensity to generate the mass spectrum of the compound. Fragmentation patterns provide a wealth of structural information about the molecule of interest. They provide the **"fingerprint"** specificity to enable mass spectrometrists to make compound identification certain.

When conducting molecular structure elucidation of an unknown that cannot be identified by a spectral library match, the mass spectrum displaying the fragmentation patterns needs to be examined, because it can yield extensive structural information. The initial focus centers on identifying the molecular ion that arises by the loss of the first electron and corresponds to the molecular weight of the compound of interest. Knowledge of the compound's molecular weight is extremely helpful in identifying the unknown. Subsequent fragmentation attributable to unimolecular decomposition and ion-molecule reactions yields other characteristic fragments that can help identify the chemical moieties present in the compound. In general, the higher m/z ion fragments are more helpful in compound identification than the lower ones. The reason is that higher m/z fragments represent the fragmentation of the molecule of interest at the earlier stages of its breakdown in the ion source. Consequently these fragments are closer to the molecule's original structure and are thus more "unique" than the lower m/z fragments. The lower m/z fragments are smaller parts of the molecule, and, although they can provide structural information, this information is less specific information. Unfortunately the most abundant ions in the EI mass spectra generally occur at low mass and may not necessarily be unique to the compound of interest. Low m/z ion data are still useful, provided that the compound being analyzed is pure. With either **GC/MS** or **LC/MS** this requires good chromatographic separation and the avoidance of coeluting interfering components.

Fig. 8-7 shows the postulated EI fragmentation decomposition of cocaine.[3] The molecular ion is m/z 303, and, although weak, it is readily seen in the mass spectrum (see Fig. 8-1). The charge of the molecular ion is localized on the nitrogen atom and to a lesser extent on the two carbonyl oxygen atoms. Decomposition of the molecular ion occurs by several different pathways. Breakup of the molecular ion's six-membered ring with the loss of benzoic acid generates a relatively stable carbonium ion at m/z 182, which is seen as an intense fragment. The loss of the methoxyl moiety from the molecular ion generates the smaller fragment at m/z 272, and the aromatic carbonyl fragment at m/z 105 is also formed by cleavage from the molecular ion. The base peak is m/z 82 and represents the formation of a substituted pyrrole ring, which is very stable because of its highly resonant ring structure.

Certain elements that are often present in a wide variety of molecules, including drugs and their metabolites, have unique mass spectrometric behavior that imparts additional information. Nitrogen, for example, is the only commonly encountered element that has an even atomic mass and an odd valence. Thus, if the molecular ion has an even mass, it can be deduced that the compound of interest has either no nitrogen atom or an even number of nitrogen atoms. Additional structural information can be obtained from the mass spectrum when the compound of interest contains two or more abundant natural isotopes. Ion fragments containing halogen atoms have characteristic isotope clusters arising from the two different isotopes present. For example, chlorine's natural isotopes are chlorine-35 and chlorine-37 with a relative abundance of 75.8% and 24.2%, respectively. Consequently, any fragments containing chlorine atoms always generate a characteristic pattern consisting of a doublet peak two atomic mass units (AMU) apart with a 3:1 ratio. Chlorine, bromine, and to a smaller degree silicon and sulfur are the only elements with sufficiently abundant natural isotopes to generate useful information with low-resolution mass spectrometers. Another useful fact to remember is that carbon-13 to carbon-12 abundance is approximately 1.1%. Increasing the number of carbon atoms

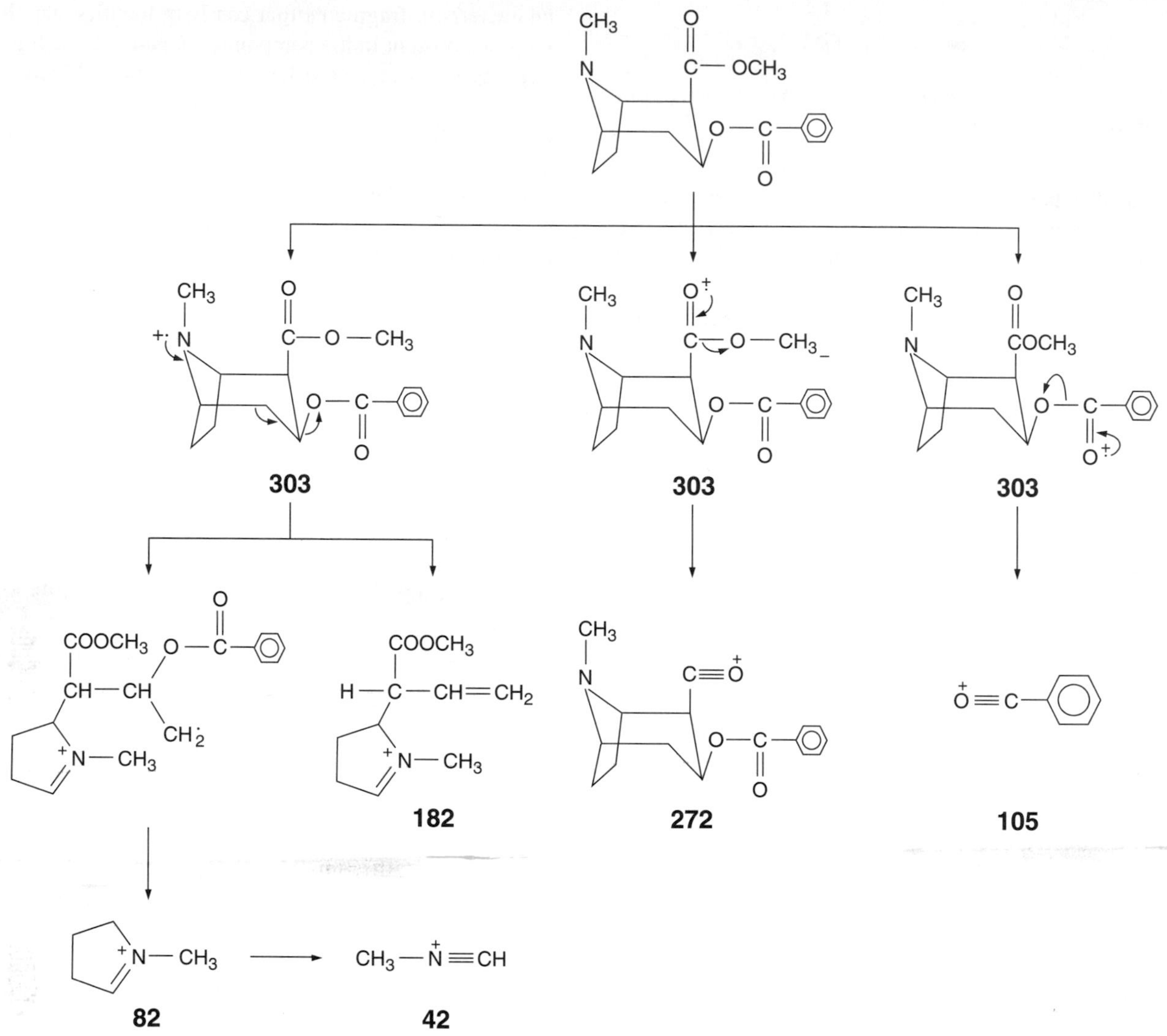

Fig. 8-7 Fragmentation pattern of cocaine.

in an ion increases the probability that one of these atoms will be a ^{13}C isotope. The (M + 1)$^+$/M$^+$ ratio for a 10-carbon ion will thus exhibit 10 times the probability for ^{13}C, or $10 \times 1.1\% = 11\%$. Although an approximation, this provides a means of determining the number of carbon atoms, which is paramount in interpreting the spectral lines of unknown organic compounds. To obtain more precise elemental composition, a high-resolution mass spectrometer is necessary.

Basic molecular structure and side chains of organic compounds can often be correlated to specific ion fragments in the mass spectrum. Metabolites frequently have similar structures and the same side chains as the parent compounds. Consequently, their mass spectra often contain similar or identical fragment ions. Chemically changing parent compounds either by metabolism or derivatization leads to anticipated fragment ions in the spectrum, making identification simpler. Such empirical observations are useful in the identification process. This pattern recognition is especially helpful in the identification of drug metabolites and

known poisons. There are numerous molecular decomposition patterns of various chemical moieties that have been systematically applied to interpreting fragmentation patterns. A discussion of such interpretations is beyond the scope of this chapter; publications on this subject are available.[4-6]

A major advantage of CI spectra is their relative simplicity compared to the corresponding EI spectra. A comparison of CI isobutane spectrum of cocaine (Fig. 8-8) to that obtained by EI (see Fig. 8-1) demonstrates this. Compared with the complex EI fragmentation patterns the CI mass spectrum is simpler and contains only a few ions. The isobutane CI spectrum of cocaine is dominated by the quasimolecular ion that readily reveals the sample's molecular weight. As was discussed earlier, the molecular weight is one of the most important pieces of information that may be obtained from the mass spectrum. Hence, CI is useful in obtaining molecular weight information that may not be always readily available by EI techniques. Other major CI fragmentations arise from the loss of protonated acid-labile groups from the quasi-

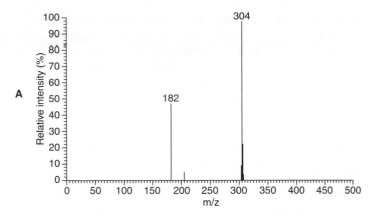

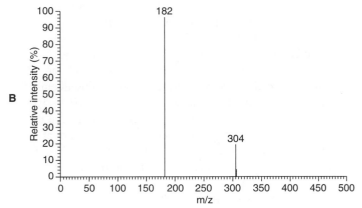

Fig. 8-8   **A,** Isobutane chemical ionization spectrum of cocaine. **B,** Methane chemical ionization spectrum of cocaine.

molecular ion. For example, benzoate esters (such as cocaine) may show the loss of benzoic acid, acetate esters the loss of acetic acid, and aliphatic alcohols the loss of water.

COMPARISON OF ELECTRON IONIZATION AND CHEMICAL IONIZATION

Sensitivity is another important factor that is affected by the ionization process. Typically, CI sensitivity can exceed that of EI by several orders of magnitude. This is attributable to CI's ability to concentrate total ion current into a small number of ions (because of the minimal fragmentation). Compare the cocaine CI fragmentation pattern with that obtained by EI. The CI spectrum (see Fig. 8-8) demonstrates that m/z 304 and 182 account for almost all the CI fragments generated. This is in stark contrast to the EI fragmentation (see Fig. 8-1) in which m/z 182 and 303 constitute only a small portion of the total number of fragments generated. As can be readily seen, the prominent CI ions typically have a higher response per unit weight of sample and hence greater sensitivity (compared to abundant EI ions). Additionally, such CI ions tend to have higher m/z values and hence are more unusual than the abundant EI ions, which tend to have a low m/z value. Notice that in the case of cocaine the base peak in EI is at a low mass (m/z 82), whereas it is at higher masses with CI (m/z 182 with methane CI and m/z 304 with isobutane CI). This example also serves to demonstrate that the selection of CI reagent gas has a pronounced influence on

the extent of fragmentation and the ultimate sensitivity of the analysis. Compounds that have different molecular weights generally give CI spectra with minimal overlap, enabling accurate identification of targeted compounds even when gas-liquid chromatography (GLC) fails to separate components of interest adequately.[7]

Chemical ionization data can supply significant mass spectral information that can be used by itself, or to supplement EI data. CI techniques should be viewed as complimentary to EI, because they help minimize EI specificity gaps that may be encountered. Because of these EI complimentary characteristics, it has been recommended that the International Olympics Committee (IOC) require chemical ionization analysis for every positive sample.[8] Instrumental advances during the past few years have made CI practical and easy to use. Incorporation of CI analyses in drugs of abuse testing laboratories can also be cost effective, because it can speed analytical analysis time by rapidly providing greater certainty of identification.

Negative ions produced under CI conditions are far more useful than under EI; significant **negative-ion chemical ionization (NICI)** applications exist. Whereas negative ions in EI tend to have low mass fragments that impart little structural information, negative ions in CI tend to have more useful high-mass fragments. Information from NICI can also serve to complement information gained from positive-ion mass spectra generated under CI and EI conditions. The formation of negative sample ions under CI conditions occurs through three primary pathways: electron capture, proton abstraction, and association. Of the three primary pathways, the electron capture (EC) process offers the most feasible approach for examining drugs and clinical samples. The EC ionization process takes place when the sample molecule captures a thermal or low-energy electron in the reagent gas plasma. For this to be the dominant process the reagent gas must be one that generates low-energy electrons upon electron bombardment. Additionally, the gas itself must not form negative ions capable of reacting with the sample molecule. Methane fulfills these criteria. Upon ionization, methane forms CH_4^+ and CH_3^+ (see Eq. 8-1) and low-energy electrons. The capture of these electrons by sample molecules and the subsequent decomposition of the resultant negative ions produce the NICI fragmentation pattern. An intense $(M - 1)^-$ ion fragment is often generated. Very high sensitivity is characteristic of NICI. In many cases, the intensity of the base negative CI ion is 30 to 100 times greater than the base positive CI ion.[2] This can effectively extend routine detection levels to the femtogram level.

USE OF THE MASS SPECTROMETER
Full-Scan Analysis

Full-scan mass spectrometric analysis in the EI mode is probably the best mass spectrometric technique for the unequivocal identification of a drug or its metabolite or metabolites. In the full-scan mode, the entire mass range of interest is repeatedly scanned. Scanning is programmed to start at the high m/z range and end at the low m/z value at the range of interest. In each scan every ion fragment generated is monitored and displayed. The scan rate must be slow enough so that the detector can register a given fragment but fast enough so that multiple scans can occur during a given analysis. Multiple scans are necessary for the resulting ion statistics to be meaningful. The resulting mass spectrum, consisting of all ion fragments generated, offers a very high degree of specificity. In combination with mass spectrometry's high sensitivity, this full-scan "fingerprint" is extremely effective in providing positive identification of organic compounds such as drugs and their metabolites.[9] Modern systems often rely on computer matching programs to identify unknown compounds. This is done by comparison of the acquired mass spectrum with an existing stored reference spectrum. A variety of different commercially available libraries exist. There are also many different library search algorithms to compare the unknown spectrum to existing stored reference spectra. Ten peak search, probability-based matching, forward or reverse search, purity search, and fit and reverse fit search algorithms are commonly used. Although a detailed description of the search algorithms and libraries is beyond the scope of this chapter, reference 10 offers a good discussion of the topic.

Full-scan techniques are more demanding in terms of sample cleanliness. Interfering or coeluting compounds must be avoided. The presence of interfering compounds generates extraneous ions and complicates the resulting spectra. This can make identification difficult or even impossible. Consequently most samples are purified before analysis. Samples are purified by recrystallizing solids, performing organic cleanup extraction of samples using biological fluids or particulate matter (such as organics in soil), and chromatographic separation by GC or LC before mass spectrometric analysis.

A total ion current (TIC) chromatogram is commonly generated when chromatographic separation is used. The total ion current is integrated, and the resulting chromatographic output resembles the appearance of a conventional GLC chromatogram. The full-scan mass spectrum is typically generated at the top of the chromatographic peak to maximize sensitivity. However, multiple mass spectral lines can be generated from any part of the peak, which is helpful in assessing the purity and chromatographic resolution. Coeluting components can be easily detected even in situations in which TIC peak shape is fully symmetrical. Although full-scan analysis offers the highest specificity, its sensitivity is limited. Scanning each fragment in the spectrum means that the detector spends significant time in regions where fragments give low-intensity adducts. Consequently the same characteristics that make full-scan techniques highly specific are also responsible for limiting its sensitivity. Aspects greatly influencing sensitivity are discussed in greater detail later in this chapter.

Selected Ion Monitoring

Greater EI sensitivity can be obtained when the mass spectrometer is operated in the **selected ion monitoring (SIM)** mode, in which it monitors ion currents at only a few preselected intense masses characteristic of the compound of interest. Use of few ion fragments for compound identification is less specific than use of a full scan, because all other ion fragments are discarded. This technique is frequently used for target compound identification applications such as forensic or clinical drugs of abuse analyses and is known by several names (such as SIM, selected, selective, or simultaneous ion monitoring; MID, multiple ion detection; and SMS, selective mass storage). Historically, the use of SIM techniques arose from sensitivity limitations of full-scan techniques in magnetic sector and quadrupole systems. In the full-scan mode, mass spectrometers do not always have sufficient sensitivity to detect low drug levels in complex matrices such as biological fluids. By focusing on just a few preselected intense ion fragments, sensitivity can be enhanced because the detector can spend all its time on those few ions rather than dividing its time on the several hundred ions scanned in the typical full-scan mode. Consequently, SIM techniques tend to enhance sensitivity by 10 to 100 times. This enhanced sensitivity, however, is obtained at the expense of decreased specificity, because the vast amount of data from the mass spectrum is lost and unavailable. In summary, SIM affords higher sensitivity but provides a less specific identification.

Most SIM applications use only a few ions (generally three intense ions) from the mass spectrum to identify the drug. For example, SIM analysis of cocaine can use ion fragments m/z 303, 182, and 82 (see Fig. 8-1). Selection of these three ions is preferred because of their relatively high intensity or uniqueness. The molecular ion at m/z 303 has a high m/z value and is considered unique, which helps increase the analytical specificity. The pyrrole ring with m/z 82 is a likely choice because of its high intensity (base peak). Although its relatively low m/z value makes it less specific, its intensity helps the SIM analysis achieve sensitivity at lower levels. It should be stressed that in SIM mode all other ion fragments in the spectrum are lost, reducing the overall specificity of analysis. Consequently, other compounds may interfere if they generate ions with the same m/z value.

Often, SIM methods attempt to minimize specificity shortcomings by comparing to each other the relative ion intensities of major ions being monitored. This practice has been widely used in drugs of abuse testing and requires that the ratios of the ion intensities in the unknown match, within ±20%, the corresponding ratios in an extracted standard. One limitation of this approach is that ion intensities and therefore ratios can vary depending on the amount of drug or metabolite present in the ion source. Consequently the ion ratios of an unknown sample may not be consistent with those of the extracted standard, especially when the drug or metabolite concentrations are either much higher or lower than those in the standard.[11]

Although identification in SIM techniques is less specific than in full-scan mode, it is adequate for many applications. However, care must be used because it is possible to incorrectly identify compounds when conditions are not optimized. For example, some drugs of abuse testing laboratories analyze amphetamine by means of GC/MS using m/z 44 as a quantification ion and m/z 58 as a qualifying ion following a protocol published by Hewlett-Packard.[12] One problem with this method is the choice of ions. These ions have low m/z values and are subject to potential interference from a variety of other compounds and background ion currents that may be present in the sample. For example, in addition to amphetamine, many other sympathomimetic amine compounds exhibit a large peak at m/z 58, and carbon dioxide (a common background component) exhibits a peak at m/z 44. Consequently, significant problems can arise because commonly encountered legal drugs (such as ephedrine, phentermine, phenylpropanolamine, and other common over-the-counter [OTC] medications) have the same ion fragments as those selected to characterize illicit amphetamine. Such legal medications and OTC compounds are generally coextracted in the sample-preparation step and their chromatographic retention times can be close to those of the illicit drugs.

Under suboptimal conditions, SIM methods such as the described amphetamine procedure can essentially amount to identification based on incremental differences in chromatographic retention times. Because chromatographic retention times often shift, the possibility of a false-positive or a false-negative result exists. The probability of inaccurate drug confirmations may be further increased in laboratories where GC/MS operators, who sometimes have little knowledge of the principles of mass spectrometry, may be swamped under excessive workloads with demanding turnaround times. Some **National Institute of Drug Abuse (NIDA)**-certified forensic drugs of abuse testing laboratories have lost their testing accreditation because of false-positive amphetamine or methamphetamine results generated by such SIM analyses. In conclusion, it can be surmised that SIM techniques have specificity pitfalls and that these hold the potential for serious errors for the unsuspecting. Employing MS techniques offering greater specificity, such as full-scan EI or CI, or both, can help minimize analytical and interpretational errors. It is also possible to increase both mass spectral sensitivity and specificity by noninstrumental techniques. However, such a discussion is beyond the scope of this chapter, and this discussion primarily focuses on the instrumental MS means for enhancing sensitivity and specificity.

Quantitation

SIM techniques are well suited for quantitative analysis because several different ion fragments can be monitored simultaneously. This mass spectral output is frequently referred to as a **selected ion profile**, or a *selected ion chromatogram.* In MS, quantitative accuracy is best achieved by incorporating an internal standard, which is added at the beginning of the analytical process. The addition of a known quantity of internal standard compensates for material lost at any stage of the analysis including the extraction, derivatization, and analytical steps. Consequently, the internal standards selected should chemically resemble the compounds of

interest as closely as possible so that their physical and chemical behavior matches those of the unknown. For this reason, deuterated compounds are widely used as internal standards. The technique of quantitation using chemicals different only in their isotope composition is termed **isotope dilution.** In the case of drug analysis a deuterated internal standard is used that is identical to the drug being assayed except that one or more hydrogen atoms have been substituted by deuterium atoms. The number and position of the deuterated atoms are chosen by ease of synthesis and position in the fragmenting ion pattern. This results in an internal standard that has very close characteristics in terms of polarity, extraction partition coefficient, derivatization, and chromatography compared to the drug itself. In fact, the internal standard will have a chromatographic retention time that is almost identical to that of the drug itself because of its structural similarity (Fig. 8-9). In conventional GLC, a deuterated internal standard cannot be used because it must be chromatographically resolved from the compound of interest. In MS, this is not a problem because the atomic mass of a deuterium atom is 1 AMU greater than hydrogen. The deuterated internal standard has a different molecular weight and hence is differentiated from the drug by the difference in masses rather than by chromatographic retention time. Its fragmentation pattern will mimic that of the drug, but the fragments containing deuterium atoms will have a correspondingly higher m/z value.

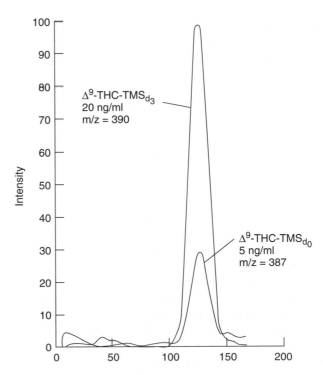

Fig. 8-9 Selected ion monitoring plot for quantitation of Δ^9-tetrahydrocannabinol in plasma. Undeuterated (d_0) and deuterated (d_3) drugs were monitored. *(From Saferstein R: Forensic science handbook, Englewood Cliffs, NJ, 1982, Prentice Hall.)*

The mass spectral SIM output displays only the ions exhibiting the m/z fragments being monitored. SIM quantitation simultaneously monitors the ion fragments of the compound and that of the internal standard. Fig. 8-9 shows selected ion profiles for two isotopes of silylated D^9-tetrahydrocannabinol analyzed by GC/MS. The internal standard contains the deuterated isotope (d_3), which is monitored at m/z 390. The ion profile of the compound of interest is the unlabeled analog, which is monitored at m/z 387. Chromatographic retention times of the two isotopes are essentially the same, and their detection is accomplished by taking advantage of the difference in the molecular weights of the ion fragments. A quantitative value is obtained when the peak area or intensity of the compound of interest is compared to that of the internal standard. This ratio is then used to generate a quantitative value from a previously established calibration curve.

SEPARATION TECHNIQUES

The mass spectrometer ionizes and separates all compounds entering the ion source. If there is more than one compound present, this results in a **mass fragmentation** pattern composed of all the components. For this reason, the clearest fragment patterns are those in which only one compound is analyzed at one time. Thus the mass spectrometer is usually coupled to a separation procedure such as gas or liquid chromatography.

Gas Chromatography/Mass Spectrometry

GLC is one of the most versatile instrumental techniques for performing separation of complex mixtures because of its sensitivity, speed of analysis, and versatility. Capillary columns enable chromatographers to devise separation procedures for virtually every compound of interest in clinical chemistry. The combination of GLC separation versatility coupled with specificity and sensitivity of MS makes GC/MS one of the most powerful techniques available for the identification of organic compounds. The same methods as described in Chapter 7 are used to prepare compounds for analysis by GC/MS.

The main technical issue in coupling these techniques arose from the incompatibility of pressure requirements. GLC requires a carrier gas flow at approximately atmospheric pressure to move the sample through the column. Mass spectrometers, on the other hand, require high vacuum (10^{-5} to 10^{-7} torr) to operate effectively. Molecular jet separators combined with differential vacuum pumps have been used to evacuate the carrier gas selectively just before the GLC effluent entry into the ion source of the mass spectrometer.[1] The more recent advent of capillary columns simplified the interface requirements because capillary columns function effectively at much lower carrier gas flow rates, which are within the pumping capacity of the mass spectrometer. Consequently, capillary column effluents can flow directly into the ion source.

Two different mass spectrometer data outputs are commonly obtained in GC/MS. The first, the TIC chromatogram, represents the integration of total ion current versus time of elution from the GLC column. That is, all the ions detected are summed together, and the total current is recorded. Its pattern resembles a conventional GLC chromatogram of detector response versus time. The full-scan mass spectrum is the second output. This analysis resolves the detected ions of the TIC into their mass fragment pattern. Mass spectral lines generated at different parts of the TIC peak can readily reveal whether the peak is pure or whether it contains multiple components. Additionally, the mass spectrum of a shoulder or minor peak can often reveal the identity of the component generating that ion current. The mass spectrum generated can either be a full scan or an SIM. In either case, sensitivity is maximized when the mass spectrum is generated at the apex of the TIC peak. TIC can also be monitored exclusively in the SIM mode, which generates a selective ion chromatogram. This is a common practice in target compound identification applications. The output is then composed of only the ions with the m/z value being monitored. SIM quantitations rely on this technique by simultaneously monitoring the ion fragments of the compound of interest and that of the internal standard.

Liquid Chromatography/Mass Spectrometry

Another potentially useful combination is high-performance liquid chromatography (HPLC) and MS. LC/MS is quickly becoming the preferred tool of liquid chromatographers. It is a powerful analytical technique that combines the resolving power of LC with the detection specificity of MS. LC/MS is suitable for the analysis of large, polar, ionic, thermally unstable, and nonvolatile compounds. It eliminates the need for time-consuming chemical modifications often required for gas chromatographic separation.

The barriers to interfacing LC are even greater than in the case of GC because the mobile phase used to propel the components through the HPLC column is less volatile and hence more difficult for selective removal (before mass spectrometric analysis) than the gaseous mobile phase used in GLC. Furthermore, LC is often used to separate components that are either not particularly volatile or are thermally labile. This further compounds the incompatibility because samples must first be volatilized into the gaseous state before they can be analyzed by MS. The difficulty of converting relatively nonvolatile molecules solvated in a liquid into the gaseous form without inducing excessive decomposition has always been the basis for the incompatibility; it is the reason why the evolution of LC/MS has been slower than GC/MS.

Thermospray is one approach to LC analysis, and this process creates charged droplets. The tip of the capillary tube from which the HPLC eluate emerges is heated by application of a high voltage. By optimizing the temperature, small droplets can be made to be ejected (spray) from the end of the tube into the ion source.

Thermospray relies on an "ion-evaporation" process in which ions are emitted from a liquid into the gas phase.[13] In theory, a charged droplet contains the solvent plus positive and negative ions, with ions of one polarity being dominant.

The difference is the net charge; it has been postulated that the excess charge resides at the surface of the droplet. As the solvent evaporates, the electric field at the surface of the droplet increases because of the decreasing radius. If the droplet evaporates far enough, a critical field is reached at which ions from the surface are emitted. Fig. 8-10 illustrates the ion-evaporation process. **IonSpray**[14] (also known as electrospray) is a related technique suited to the introduction of thermally labile compounds into the mass spectrometer. It differs from thermospray in that it does not use heat to produce the spray, and it can readily occur at atmospheric pressure. Thermospray is generally operated in high vacuum, though it can be used at pressures up to atmospheric. Elevated temperatures are required for thermospray. IonSpray allows the introduction of complex and polar compounds into the mass spectrometer. It also generates a quasimolecular ion and is especially suitable for polar and thermally labile compounds. In addition to HPLC, IonSpray can be interfaced with other separation techniques such as capillary zone electrophoresis to allow the analysis of complex biological samples.[15]

Atmospheric pressure ionization (API)-electrospray **(ES)** is useful for analyzing samples that have multiple charges, such as proteins, peptides, and oligonucleotides, as well as analyzing samples that are singly charged. It can be used to measure the molecular weights of most polymers, peptides, proteins, and oligonucleotides up to 150,000 D quickly and with high mass accuracy. In biopharmaceutical applications, chemists use API-ES to speed protein characterization, to accurately identify and characterize posttranslational modifications to proteins, and to quickly confirm the molecular weight of synthetic peptides. The ability to analyze these biological compounds by LC/MS and LC/MS/MS techniques is playing a key role in the field of genomics and in the rapid advance of innovations in proteomic technology.[16,17] Computerized MS using LC separation and flexible ionization techniques is the primary tool in the rapid progress of gene sequencing.[18,19]

Solids Probe

Direct MS using solids probe sample introduction has been used by toxicologists for many years to rapidly identify targeted compounds.[20,21] This technique is advantageous for compounds of low volatility, which can be introduced directly into the ion source. Another advantage of solids probe MS is that it eliminates the chromatographic separation step allowing for very rapid analysis. MS analysis probing solids has been used extensively both in the EI and CI modes with pure compounds. For biological specimens CI is especially practical, because compound identification can be done based on molecular weight.

OTHER MASS SPECTROMETERS
Ion Trap Detector (ITD)

Mass spectrometers based on **ion trap detector** technology are different in design from other MS systems. All current commercial instruments are relatively inexpensive bench top systems. Ion trap mass spectrometers combine the functions of an ion source and a mass analyzer. This is done in a simple three-electrode assembly consisting of a ring electrode and two end caps (Fig. 8-11). This simplicity is in sharp contrast to the complex mechanical assemblies commonly found in quadrupole and magnetic sector mass spectrometers. Electrons from a heated filament are pulsed by a gate electrode into the central cavity where they ionize the sample molecules, resulting in conventional EI fragmentation patterns characteristic of the compound. The unique feature of ion trap mass spectrometers is that they "trap" and "store" the ions generated over time within the ion source cavity. This is done by application of a radio frequency voltage to the central ring electrode, which causes ions of interest to be trapped and accumulated over time in the ion source. The trapped ions are then mass-selectively ejected from the cavity according to their m/z ratio onto the electron multiplier where they are detected. The effective trapping and accumulation of ions results in concentrating the ions of interest; consequently very high sensitivities are obtained with ITD. The ion trap's superior sensitivity allows the user to obtain full-scan mass spectra with limits of detection comparable to SIM analyses in conventional quadrupole detectors.

Time-of-Flight (TOF) MS

The **time-of-flight (TOF) mass spectrometer** is based on the requirement that ions generated in the source must travel

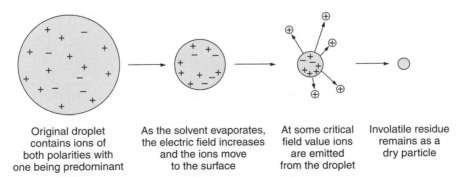

| Original droplet contains ions of both polarities with one being predominant | As the solvent evaporates, the electric field increases and the ions move to the surface | At some critical field value ions are emitted from the droplet | Involatile residue remains as a dry particle |

Fig. 8-10 Diagram of ion evaporation process. *(From* The API book, *Eden Prairie, MN, 1992, Perkin-Elmer Sciex.)*

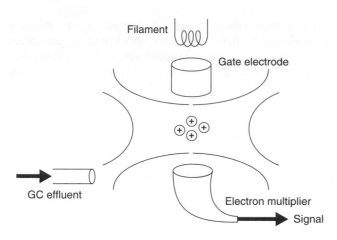

Fig. 8-11   The ion trap mass spectrometer.

a fixed distance to reach the detector. The accelerating voltage propels the ions into a "drift tube" that is typically 1 m long. The velocity of ions is proportional to their mass. Consequently different mass ions travel at different speeds and reach the detector at different times. The m/z value of any given ion can be determined mathematically when an accurate measurement is made of the time that the ion takes to traverse the distance and reach the detector. Currently this type of mass spectrometer is used in research for the analysis of complex biopolymers at the picomole level. This type of instrument using laser desorption ionization is suited for the measurement of high-mass molecules and can determine the molecular weights of peptides, intact proteins, and glycoproteins 300,000 D in size. TOF systems play a significant role in advancing the science of gene sequencing.

Tandem Mass Spectrometry (MS/MS)

In general, improving selectivity and detection limits of instrumental techniques can be achieved by extensive sample pretreatment (extraction, derivatization, chromatographic separation, and so on) before mass spectrometry. An alternative approach to improve detection limits and enhance selectivity is the coupling of two or more analytical techniques in tandem.[22] GC/MS, GC/MS/IR, MS/MS, and GC/MS/MS are examples (as compared to MS alone).

The acceptance of applications of **tandem mass spectrometry (MS/MS)** is attributable to the technique's ability to provide (1) increased speed of analysis; (2) decreased cost per sample; (3) improved limits of detection in complex mixtures; and (4) rapid, sensitive, and selective analysis of complex mixtures rapidly, often with minimal or no sample cleanup.[23-25] Solids probe MS/MS can be performed on drugs that are difficult to chromatograph and hence cannot be run on conventional GC/MS. In tandem MS/MS a mixture is introduced into the ion source of the first MS where ionization of the mixture produces ions characteristic of the individual drug components, termed **parent ions.** A characteristic parent ion of the targeted drug of interest is then selected and identified. This "separates" the analyte of interest from the other mixture components and can be thought of as analogous to the chromatographic separation step of GC/MS. The targeted parent ion is then subjected to second MS analysis where it is further fragmented into secondary ion fragments termed **daughter ions.** This step is analogous to the fragmentation that occurs during the ionization step in GC/MS. Mass analysis of the daughter ions by the second mass analyzer provides a unique and highly specific identification of the targeted parent ion.

Fig. 8-12 demonstrates the schema of a tandem mass spectrometer. It consists of two mass analyzers connected sequentially. A collision chamber for fragmentation of selected ions is situated between the two mass analyzers. Although different types of mass spectrometers can be combined, the triple-stage quadruple configuration is one of the more popular. Many applications use CI techniques for the initial ionization to generate an intense quasimolecular ion fragment. The ion selected should be as specific and as intense as possible. This ion is then subjected to collisions with inert gas in the collision chamber. The second mass analyzer then separates the resulting daughter ions. Daughter ions' spectral lines resemble conventional EI spectral lines and are used for the actual compound identification. MS/MS effectively generates highly characteristic fragmentation of a specific ion.

In summary, the first MS analysis is used to achieve separation of mixture into components, a process performed by the GC in conventional GC/MS. With MS/MS, however, this separation process is instantaneous, whereas with GC/MS it can take 5 to 15 minutes. This time advantage is the feature that gives MS/MS the potential for very rapid analysis. Whereas the throughput of samples in conventional GC/MS may typically be 4 to 6 samples per hour, in MS/MS it can be 60 samples per hour. Additional time efficiency is

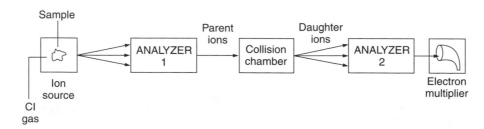

Fig. 8-12   Schema of a tandem mass spectrometer (MS/MS). *CI,* Chemical ionization. *(From Yinon Y: Forensic mass spectrometry, Boca Raton, FL, 1987, CRC Press.)*

gained, because sample extraction and derivatization can be drastically minimized and in some cases totally avoided.

FORENSIC DRUG TESTING (see Chapter 51)

In 1987, the Department of Health and Human Services (DHHS) charged the NIDA to develop and implement a laboratory accreditation program for laboratories testing government workers for drugs of abuse. The need for regulation arose from the fact that different laboratories were using different testing methodologies and different performance standards to designate a result as positive for drugs of abuse. The quality and reliability of results varied greatly. The regulations[26] were issued in 1988 and covered all aspects of the drugs of abuse testing. These included personnel requirements, security of facilities, chain-of-custody (COC), specimen handling, record keeping, confidentiality of results, proficiency testing, quality control (QC), independent inspection of facilities, and analytical testing requirements. The NIDA project, later called the Substance Abuse and Mental Health Services Administration (SAMHSA) program, has successfully implemented a rigorous accreditation program propagating these standards. Certified laboratories that fail to meet the standards have been decertified from the program. As of early 2002, 61 laboratories were certified by SAMHSA's National Laboratory Certification Program (NLCP). The goal of the program is to ensure that labs do not generate false-positive results and that the results generated can stand up to legal challenges. Consequently, the term *forensic* drugs-of-abuse testing is used. The NIDA analytical protocols for the detection of drugs of abuse in urine are based upon the use of two independent analytical techniques as follows:

1. A sensitive initial screening procedure to identify negative specimens and to select presumptive positive specimens for further testing. Screening had to be done using an FDA-registered immunoassay technique.
2. A highly specific confirmatory technique that is at least as sensitive as the initial screen for confirmation of presumptive positive results. The confirmation method was limited to GC/MS.

Both screening and confirmation steps are incorporated into a forensic urine drug detection program in which the consequences of such an analysis will be the basis of actions taken against the individual who supplied the sample.[27] Because of the potential negative effect on the individual, only rigorous and conclusive procedures are used. GC/MS is generally accepted as a rigorous confirmation technique, because it provides the best level of confidence in the result. A survey of experts, industrial arbitrators, and forensic toxicologists on the legal defensibility of laboratory analyses concluded that "most forensic experts believe that GC/MS is the gold standard and experts who must defend analytical data are of the opinion . . . that GC/MS confirmation is held to be the most defensible confirmation procedure by a considerable margin."[28] Other forensic drug workplace testing programs have also been instituted by some states such as Florida and New York. The College of American Pathologists (CAP) together with the American Association of Clinical Chemists have also implemented a voluntary forensic urine drug testing accrediting program. Analytically, all follow the SAMHSA model requiring GC/MS confirmation of an initial positive immunoassay screen.

It is worthwhile to remember that GC/MS is a technique combining GLC separation with mass spectrometric detection. This means that good GC/MS results are highly dependent on good chromatographic separations. Although it may seem self-evident, many users encounter GC/MS problems that could be readily avoided by optimizing chromatographic parameters. In fact, most GC/MS problems in the clinical and forensic toxicology laboratory are probably chromatographic. Thus it is important to consider chromatographic, as well as urine sample cleanup and derivatization issues, in any discussion of the application of GC/MS to drug testing in biological fluids. For several of the SAMHSA regulated drugs, derivatization is necessary to increase the compound's volatility and optimize the chromatographic process. Reactive groups such as hydroxyl, carboxylic acids, and amine moieties are converted to less-reactive functional groups by means of derivatization. This enhances their volatility and minimizes their chromatographic reactivity, resulting in better chromatographic performance and more rapid separation. Derivatization also increases the molecular weight of the compounds and hence increases specificity by generating more desirable higher m/z ion fragments. Several good in-depth discussions of derivatization techniques and related issues are readily available.[11,29-31] Deuterated internal standards should be used and should be added to the biological samples being assayed before the extraction process.

Two widespread misconceptions about mass spectrometry are (1) that GC/MS is a specific "method" and (2) that GC/MS is 100% accurate. GC/MS is in fact an instrumental analytical technique with many variations and a diverse variety of instrumental configurational possibilities. There are countless methods based on GC/MS techniques, each with its own set of advantages and disadvantages. Some GC/MS methods may be appropriate for a given analyte, whereas others may not be. Although forensic testing laboratories are required to use GC/MS, they have great flexibility and freedom in selecting instrumentation, mode of operation, and the actual analytical methodologies. When a correct method is performed correctly, it will result in the positive identification of a drug or metabolite. The result will be legally defensible if appropriate QC is part of the laboratory's analysis. The QC program should include the analysis of threshold-cutoff standards, drug-free samples, blind controls, and known controls containing drugs below and above the threshold value with each batch of samples. In addition, forensic requirements call for strict COC and laboratory security. Such requirements are part of the forensic package and are necessary because of the implications of laboratory results for job applicants, employees, and companies and because of the potential legal challenges of the laboratory's results. When all these aspects of testing are incorporated, the lab results are legally defensible.

References

1. McFadden WH: *Techniques of combined gas chromatography/mass spectrometry*, New York, 1973, Wiley & Sons.
2. Saferstein R: *Forensic science handbook*, Englewood Cliffs, NJ, 1982, Prentice-Hall.
3. Jindal SP, Vestergaard P: Quantitation of cocaine and its principal metabolite, benzoylecgonine, by GLC/mass spectrometry using stable isotope labeled analogues as internal standards, *J Pharm Sci* 67:811, 1978.
4. McLafferty FW: *Interpretation of mass spectra*, ed 3, Mill Valley, CA, 1980, University Science Book.
5. Silverstein RM, Bassler CG: *Spectrometrical identification of organic compounds*, New York, 1967, Wiley & Sons.
6. Budzikiewicz H, Djerassi C, Williams DH: *Mass spectrometry of organic compounds*, San Francisco, 1967, Holden-Day.
7. Lehrer M: Application of gas chromatography/mass spectrometry instrument techniques to forensic urine drug testing, *Clin Lab Med* 10:271, 1990.
8. deJong EG, Maes RA, van Rossum JM: *Why do doping control labs need MS/MS?* Presented at the International Symposium on Applied Mass Spectrometry in the Health Sciences, Barcelona, Sept 28, 1987.
9. Deutsch DG: *Analytical aspects of drug testing, chemical analysis series*, New York, 1989, Wiley & Sons.
10. Pfleger K, Maurer H, Weber A: *Mass spectral and GC data of drugs, poisons, and their metabolites*, New York, 1985, VCH.
11. Peat MA: Analytical and technical aspects of testing for drug abuse: confirmatory procedures, *Clin Chem* 34(3):471, 1988.
12. Hewlett-Packard technical application: *GC/MS confirmation of amphetamines*, publication #23-5954-8146, Waltham, MA, 1987, Hewlett-Packard.
13. Iribane JV, Thomson BA: On the evaporation of small ions from charged droplets, *J Chem Physiol* 64:2287, 1976.
14. Bruins AP, Covey TR, Henion JD: IonSpray interface for combined liquid chromatography/atmospheric pressure ionization mass spectrometry, *Anal Chem* 59:2642, 1987.
15. *The API book*, Eden Prairie, MN, 1992, Perkin-Elmer Sciex.
16. Andregg RJ: Comprehensive on-line LC/LC/MS of proteins, *Anal Chem* 69(8):1518, 1997.
17. Premstaller A et al: High performance liquid chromatography-electrospray ionization mass spectrometry using monolithic capillary columns for proteomic studies, *Anal Chem* 73(11):2390, 2001.
18. Chong BE et al: Differential screening and mass mapping of proteins from premalignant and cancer cell lines using nonporous reversed-phase HPLC coupled with mass spectrometric analysis, *Anal Chem* 73(6):1219, 2001.
19. Udiavar S et al: The use of multidimensional liquid-phase separations and mass spectrometry for the detailed characterization of posttranslational modifications in glycoproteins, *Anal Chem* 70(17):3572, 1998.
20. Lehrer M, Karmen A: Chemical ionization mass spectrometry for rapid assay of drugs in serum, *J Chromatogr* 126:615, 1976.
21. Saferstein R: Drug detection in urine by chemical ionization mass spectrometry, *J Forensic Sci* 23:29, 1978.
22. Yost RA, Johnson JV: Tandem mass spectrometry for trace analysis, *Anal Chem* 57(7):758A, 1985.
23. Glish GL, Shaddock VM, Harmon K: Rapid analysis of complex mixtures by mass spectrometry, *Anal Chem* 52:165, 1980.
24. Lee MS, Yost RA: Rapid identification of drug metabolites with tandem mass spectrometry, *Biomed Environ Mass Spectrometry* 15:193, 1988.
25. Weiss MD: Chemistry is winning the war against crime, *Industrial Chemist* 15:28-34, 1988.
26. Federal Register: *Mandatory guidelines for federal workplace drug testing: final guidelines*, April 11, 1988.
27. Lehrer M: Drug screening in the workplace, *Clin Lab Med* 7(2):389, 1987.
28. Hoyt DW et al: Drug testing in the workplace—are methods legally defensible? *JAMA* 258(4):504, 1987.
29. Blau K, King GS, editors: *Handbook of derivatives for chromatography*, Philadelphia, 1978, Heyden & Sons.
30. Foltz RL, Fentiman AF, Foltz RB: *GC/MS assays for abused drugs in body fluids*, National Institute of Drug Abuse monograph no 32, DHHS publ no (ADM) 80-1014, Washington, DC, 1980.
31. Hawks RL, Chiang CN: *Urine testing for drugs of abuse*, National Institute of Drug Abuse monogr no 73, DHHS publ no (ADM) 87-1481, Washington, DC, 1987.

Bibliography

Barker J: *Mass spectrometry (analytical chemistry by open learning series)*, London, 1999, Wiley & Sons.
Kinter M, Sherman NE: *Protein sequencing and identification using tandem mass spectrometry*, New York, 2000, Wiley-Interscience.
Watson JT: *Introduction to mass spectrometry*, ed 3, New York, 1997, Lippincott Williams & Wilkins.

Internet Sites

http://www.organicworldwide.net/mass.html
www.spectroscopynow.com/Spy/basehtml/SpyH/1,2466,4-4-770-0-770-directories—0,00.html
http://www.ionsource.com/links/ms_links.htm
www.asms.org/—American Society for Mass Spectrometry
http://ms.mc.vanderbilt.edu/tutorials/ms/ms.htm—Tutorial written by Vanderbilt University Mass Spectroscopy Research Center
http://www3.interscience.wiley.com/cgi-bin/itoc?ID=6043—Journal for Mass Spectrometry by Wiley Interscience

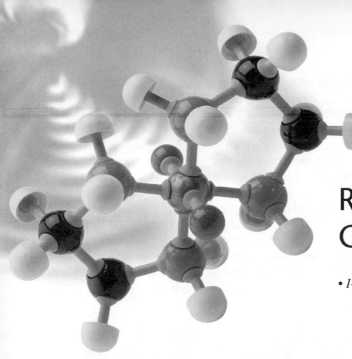

CHAPTER 9

Radioisotopes in Clinical Chemistry

• *I-Wen Chen*

Chapter Outline

Basic structure of an atom
  Fundamental particles of an atom
  Atomic structure nomenclature
Principles of radiation and radioactivity
  Nuclear radiation
  Radiation energy
  Rate of radioactive decay
  Properties of radiation and interaction with matter

Measurement of nuclear radiation
  Gas-filled detectors
  Scintillation detectors
Radiation health safety
  Monitoring
  Contamination control
  Waste disposal

Objectives

• Describe the basic structure of the atom. Explain the significance of the atomic number and atomic mass number as they relate to the existence of isotopes.
• Describe the modes of radioactive decay associated with tritium, carbon-14, and iodine-125 and name the particles emitted.
• Define and explain the importance of decay constants, decay factors, half-life, and specific activity.

• Summarize the operation of scintillation detectors. Diagram and explain the use of the crystal and liquid scintillation counters and describe the operation of each component. Define quenching and outline correction methods.
• Describe the use of isotopes in the clinical laboratories and list radiation safety considerations for monitoring personnel and work areas, contamination control, and waste disposal.

Key Terms

anticoincident circuit   A circuit used in the pulse-height analyzer of a radioactive-particle counter for setting window width (see **window**). It transmits a pulse arriving at its input from the lower discriminator only if there is no pulse arriving from the upper discriminator at the same time (see **discriminator**).

becquerel (Bq)   Système International d'Unités (SI) unit of radioactivity corresponding to a decay rate of $1/sec$ ($1\ Bq = 1\ sec^{-1} = 2.7 \times 10^{-11}\ Ci$) (see **curie**).

chemiluminescence   Production of light photons by an interaction of the sample material with the solute or solubilizer added to the scintillation solution in liquid scintillation counting.

coincidence resolving time   A time interval within which the output pulses from each photomultiplier tube of a liquid scintillation counter have to arrive at the coincident circuit to be counted.

coincident circuit   A circuit used in a liquid scintillation counter to eliminate the electronic noise. It determines whether a pulse from one photomultiplier tube is accompanied by a corresponding pulse from the other within the allowed time interval (see **coincidence resolving time**).

curie (Ci)   Unit of radioactivity. One curie is defined as an activity of a sample decaying at a rate of 3.7×10^{10} disintegrations per second (dps).

decay constant   A constant unique to each radioactive nuclide (see **nuclide**) representing the proportion of the atoms in a sample of that radionuclide undergoing decay in unit time.

decay factor   The fraction of radionuclides remaining after a time, t.

discriminator   Device used in the pulse-height analyzer of a radioactive-particle counter for setting upper (upper-level discriminator) and lower (lower-level discriminator) voltage limits for counting.

electron capture   One mode of radioactive decay in which the neutron-poor nuclides decay by capturing electrons from orbits closest to the nucleus to transform a proton to a neutron. The orbital vacancy created by the electron capture is filled by the electron from a higher orbit, resulting in emission of characteristic x rays.

electron volt (eV)   Basic unit of energy commonly used in radiation, defined as the amount of energy acquired by an electron when it is accelerated through an electrical potential of 1 volt.

half-life ($t_{1/2}$)   Time required for a given number of radionuclides in the sample to decrease to one half their original value.

isobar   Nuclides (see **nuclide***)* with the same atomic mass number but different atomic number.

isotope   Nuclides (see **nuclide**) with the same atomic number but different atomic mass number.

isotopic abundance   Amounts of isotopes present for a given element.

nucleon   A collective term for protons and neutrons in the nucleus.

nuclide   A nucleus with a particular atomic number and atomic mass number.

radiation absorbed dose (rad)   A measure of local energy deposition per unit mass of material irradiated. One rad is equal to 100 ergs of absorbed energy per gram of absorber. (No plural form.)

roentgen equivalent, man (rem)   That dose of any ionizing radiation causing the same amount of biological injury to human tissue as 1 rad of x, gamma, or beta radiation. In the case of x, gamma, or beta radiation, rem is equal to the absorbed dose in rad; in the case of alpha radiation; however, the dose in rem equals the dose in rad multiplied by 20, because only 0.05 rad of alpha radiation is needed to produce the same biological effect as 1 rad of x, gamma, or beta radiation. (No plural form.)

roentgen (R)   A unit of x rays or gamma rays representing the quantity of ionization produced by photon radiation in a given sample of air. One roentgen equals that quantity of photon radiation capable of producing one electrostatic unit of ions of either sign in 0.001293 g of air.

specific activity   Activity of the radionuclide per unit mass of the radioactive sample, expressed as curies (Ci) per µg, µCi per µmole, and so on.

specific ionization   Number of ion pairs produced per unit path length of ionizing radiation.

summation circuit   A circuit used in a liquid scintillation counter to sum all coincident pulses to improve counting efficiency for low-energy beta-particle emitters.

transmutation   A radioactive decay process that results in a change in nuclear constitution, such as electron capture decay (see **electron capture**).

wavelength shifter   The secondary scintillator added to scintillation liquid for shifting the wavelength of light emitted by the primary scintillator for more efficient detection by the photocathodes of photomultiplier tubes in liquid scintillation counting.

window   The voltage limit set by the upper-level and lower-level discriminators (see **discriminator**) of the pulse-height analyzer of a radioactive-particle counter for differential counting.

The use of **isotopes**, both stable and radioactive, has provided a great body of information in the medical sciences, much of which could not have been obtained in any other way. The usefulness of isotopes depends on the fact that isotopes of an element have identical chemical properties but different isotopic properties, such as radioactivity and increased mass, and on the fact that the isotopic properties and chemical properties of an element are independent of one another. Therefore, substitution of an atom in the molecule of a substance by other isotopes will not chemically alter that substance, and the isotopic properties of the isotopes incorporated into that substance will remain unchanged. The isotopic properties will make that substance more easily identifiable. For example, thyroxine is a thyroid hormone containing four atoms of iodine. One or all of these iodine atoms may be replaced by radioactive iodine without appreciable alteration of its chemical properties, and the radioiodine atoms incorporated into the thyroxine molecules will maintain their characteristic radioactivity. The radioiodine-labeled thyroxine molecules can be identified and quantified easily by virtue of their radioactivity. Radioiodine-labeled thyroxines are used in various thyroid-function tests.

The application of radioisotopically labeled compounds in clinical chemistry has greatly expanded since the advent of radioimmunoassays, in which the quantity of antigen bound to antibody is determined by measurement of radioactivity (see Chapters 12 and 13). The use of radioisotopes in clinical laboratories, however, has been decreasing in recent years because of the emergence of automated nonisotopic immunoassay technology, and radioimmunoassays will have more limited roles in the field of immunoassays for routine disease diagnosis. In this chapter, some basic principles involved in the measurement of isotopes are discussed.

BASIC STRUCTURE OF AN ATOM
Fundamental Particles of an Atom

An atom is the smallest unit of matter that still exhibits the chemical properties of an element. The primary building blocks of atoms, the electron, the proton, and the neutron, are termed *elementary particles.* According to the planetary model of the atom developed by Rutherford in 1911, the atom consists of a central, small, positively charged body (the nucleus, composed of protons and neutrons) around which the negatively charged electrons move in defined orbits. Although the Rutherford model is oversimplified, it can be used to explain many atomic phenomena satisfactorily. The planetary model of an atom of carbon is illustrated in Fig. 9-1.

The nucleus of carbon contains six protons and six neutrons. Since complete atoms are electrically neutral, six orbiting electrons are present in the carbon atom to match the six protons in the nucleus. They move around the nucleus in a series of orbits or shells, at varying distances from the nucleus, much as the planets of the solar system travel in different orbits at varying distances from the sun. The orbits, or shells, are called *K, L, M,* and so on, starting from the inner one. Only two electrons can be accommodated in the K shell; the L shell of the carbon atom contains the remaining

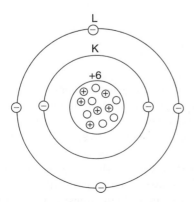

Fig. 9-1 Planetary model of carbon atom.

four. See the Periodic Table of Elements on the end sheets of this book, as well as Internet sites such as http://www.webelements.com/webelements/elements/text/periodic-table/radio.html, for additional information on the atomic structure of the elements.

The physical and chemical differences between the atoms of different elements depend on the number of protons and neutrons contained in an atomic nucleus, which determines both the mass and charge of the nucleus, and the number and arrangements of the electrons, which determine the chemical properties of elements.

Atomic Structure Nomenclature

Several important terms are helpful in understanding atomic structure:

nucleon   A collective term for protons and neutrons in the nucleus.

atomic number (Z)   The number of protons in the nucleus.

atomic mass number (A)   The total number of nucleons in the nucleus.

neutron number (N)   The number of neutrons in the nucleus.

nuclide   A nucleus with particular Z and A numbers.

element (E)   A nucleus with a given Z number.

isotope   Nuclides with the same Z but different A numbers (various nuclear species of the same element).

isobar   Nuclides with the same A but different Z numbers (different elements with the same atomic mass).

The atomic mass number is represented as a left superscript and the atomic number as a left subscript to the chemical symbol. Thus an element, *E,* is written as $^A_Z E$. The most abundant, naturally occurring, stable isotope of carbon has six protons and six neutrons in the nucleus. The atomic number, *Z,* is therefore 6; the atomic mass number, *A,* is 12 ($A = Z + N$); and the whole atom may be written as $^{12}_6 C$. The other naturally occurring but less abundant isotope of carbon is $^{13}_6 C$, which contains seven neutrons in the nucleus. $^{12}_6 C$ and $^{13}_6 C$ are both stable isotopes of carbon, and neither is radioactive. The best-known radioactive isotope of carbon is $^{14}_6 C$, which contains six protons and eight neutrons. Examples of other groups of isotopes of elements commonly used in clinical chemistry are $^1_1 H$, $^2_1 H$, and $^3_1 H$ and $^{125}_{53} I$, $^{127}_{53} I$, and $^{131}_{53} I$. $^1_1 H$ is the most abundant naturally occurring isotope of hydrogen and has one proton but no neutron in the nucleus. $^2_1 H$ is a stable isotope of hydrogen and is known as *deuterium* because its nucleus contains two nuclear particles, one proton and one neutron. $^3_1 H$, called *tritium,* is a radioactive isotope of hydrogen, the nucleus of which is formed by a combination of a proton and two neutrons. All isotopes of hydrogen have a single circling electron and therefore have identical chemical properties; however, their physical properties are different. For example, they have different boiling and freezing points. The tritium nucleus is unstable and will undergo radioactive transitions to become a different and stable nucleus—the nucleus of helium. The naturally occurring stable isotope of iodine is $^{127}_{53}$I. The other two isotopes of iodine mentioned here are radioactive isotopes with different numbers of neutrons in their nucleus, as indicated by their atomic mass numbers. In many cases the atomic number subscript is redundant because the atomic number and the chemical symbol both identify the chemical species. Therefore, except in some equations describing nuclear reactions, the subscript is normally omitted (such as ^{14}C, ^{3}H, and ^{125}I).

PRINCIPLES OF RADIATION AND RADIOACTIVITY
Nuclear Radiation

The release of energy or matter during the transformation of an unstable atom to a more stable atom is termed *nuclear radiation.* The numbers and arrangement of protons and neutrons in the nucleus of an atom determine whether the nucleus is stable or unstable.

Nuclear stability. There are favored neutron-to-proton ratios among stable **nuclides**. The ratio is equal to or close to unity for the light nuclides. When the atomic mass number exceeds 40, no stable nuclides exist with equal numbers of neutrons and protons because, as the number of protons increases, the repulsive coulombic forces between the protons increase at a greater rate than the attractive nuclear force does. Therefore, the addition of extra neutrons is necessary to increase the average distance between protons in the nucleus to reduce the coulombic force. For heavy nuclei the neutron-to-proton ratio is 1.5 or greater. For example, the heaviest stable isotope of lead, ^{208}Pb, has a neutron-to-proton ratio of 1.53.

Fig. 9-2 illustrates the relationship between the neutron and proton numbers of the stable nuclides. An imaginary line, called the *line of stability,* represented by a dashed line in the graph, can be obtained from the neutron-proton plot; the stable nuclides are clustered around this line. Nuclides

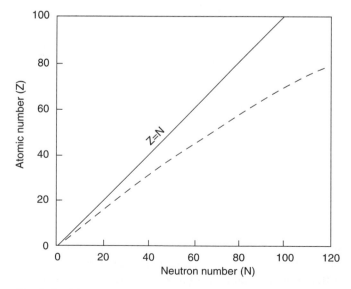

Fig. 9-2 Neutron-proton ratios for stable isotopes (*dashed line*).

deficient in protons lie below the line of stability and are unstable. Nuclides deficient in neutrons lie above the line and are also unstable. The graph also illustrates the fact that, as nuclides become heavier, more neutrons are required to maintain stability.

In addition to the favored neutron-to-proton ratio, the stable nuclides tend to favor even numbers. For example, 168 out of approximately 280 known stable nuclides have even numbers of both protons and neutrons, reflecting the tendency of nuclides to achieve stable arrangements by pairing up **nucleons** in the nucleus.

Modes of radioactive decay. Unstable nuclides are generally transformed into stable nuclides by one of the radioactive-decay processes described in the following text.

Decay by alpha-particle emission. An alpha (α) particle consists of two neutrons and two protons and is essentially a helium nucleus. Heavy nuclides that must lose mass to achieve nuclear stability frequently decay by alpha-particle emission because this is an effective way to reduce the mass number. The emission of one alpha particle removes two neutrons and two protons from the nucleus, resulting in the reduction of an atomic number by 2 and a mass number by 4. Very heavy radioactive nuclides that decay with alpha-particle emission are of little interest in clinical chemistry. An example of alpha-particle decay is as follows:

$$^{226}_{88}\text{Ra} \rightarrow {}^{222}_{86}\text{Rn} + {}^4_2\text{He (alpha particle)}$$

Decay by beta-particle emission. Beta (β) particles are either negatively charged electrons (negatrons, β^-) or positively charged electrons (positrons, β^+). Proton-deficient nuclides lying below the line of stability, shown in Fig. 9-2, usually decay by negatron emission, because this mode of decay transforms a neutron into a proton, moving the nucleus closer to the line of stability. Neutron-deficient nuclides lying above the line of stability usually decay by positron emission, since this mode transforms a proton into a neutron.

In beta-particle decay processes the mass number does not change because the total number of nucleons in the nucleus remains the same. Such decay processes are known as **isobaric** transitions. However, the atomic number increases by 1 in the negatron emission and decreases by 1 in the positron emission, resulting in a **transmutation** of elements (conversion of one element to another). Examples of decay by beta emission are as follows:

$$^{11}_6\text{C} \rightarrow {}^{11}_5\text{B} + \beta^+ + \nu \text{ (positron emission)}$$

$$^3_1\text{H} \rightarrow {}^3_2\text{He} + \beta^- + \nu \text{ (negatron emission)}$$

The neutrino *(ν)* is a particle with no mass or electrical charge and virtually does not interact with matter. The only practical consequence of its emission from the nucleus is that it carries away some energy released in the decay process.

Decay by electron capture. In addition to the decay by positron emission, the neutron-deficient nuclides may decay by **electron capture** to transform a proton to a neutron. Thus the electron capture is sometimes called *inverse negatron decay.* It is also an isobaric transition leading to a transmutation of elements. In the electron-capture process the electron is captured from orbits closest to the nucleus, that is, the K and L shells (K and L capture; see Fig. 9-1). The orbital vacancy created by the electron capture is quickly filled by the electron from a higher orbit, resulting in emission of a characteristic x ray.

The daughter nucleus formed by this mode of decay is frequently in an excited or metastable state and may further undergo decay by gamma (γ)-ray emission, as described in the following paragraph.

Decay by gamma-ray emission. In some cases the isobaric transitions previously mentioned (negatron emission, positron emission, electron capture) result in a daughter nucleus in an excited or metastable state, which means that it possesses excess energy above its minimum possible ground-state energy. Such an excited or metastable nuclide decays promptly to a more stable nuclear arrangement by emitting gamma rays, electromagnetic radiation of very short wavelength:

$$^{125}_{53}I \xrightarrow[\text{capture}]{\text{Electron}} {}^{125}_{52}Te^* \rightarrow {}^{125}_{52}Te + \gamma$$

*The nuclide is in an excited or metastable state.

Notice that gamma emission is not accompanied by any change in mass number, proton number, or neutron number. This is called an *isomeric transition*.

Radiation Energy

In any of the radioactive decay processes mentioned previously, a fixed amount of energy is released with each disintegration. Most or all of the released energy will appear as the kinetic energy of the emitted particles or photons. The basic unit of energy commonly used in radiation is the **electron volt (eV)**. One electron volt is defined as the amount of energy acquired by an electron when it is accelerated through an electrical potential of 1 V. Basic multiples are the kiloelectron volt (keV; 1 keV = 1000 eV) and the megaelectron volt (MeV; 1 MeV = 1000 keV= 1,000,000 eV). In general, the energy of beta particles emitted from radionuclides in clinical use ranges from 18 keV to 3.6 MeV, and that of gamma rays ranges from 27 keV to 2.8 MeV.

Rate of Radioactive Decay

Decay constant, decay factor, and half-life. Radioactive decay is a spontaneous process; that is, it is not possible to predict when a given radioactive atom will decay, and the probability of decay in a large number of atoms can be given only on a statistical basis. For a sample containing N radioactive nuclei, the number of nuclei decaying at any given moment (dN/dt) can be given by the following:

$$dN/dt = -\lambda N \qquad \textit{Eq. 9-1}$$

In this equation, λ is the **decay constant** of the radioactive nuclide, and the minus sign indicates that the number of radioactive nuclides is decreasing with time. Each radionuclide has a characteristic decay constant that represents the proportion of the atoms in a sample of that radionuclide undergoing decay per unit time. The decay constant, λ, is

measured in units of (time)$^{-1}$. Therefore, the equivalence $\lambda = 0.05$ sec^{-1} means that, on the average, 5% of the radionuclides are disintegrating per second. On integration of this equation, we obtain

$$N = N_o e^{-\lambda t} \qquad \textit{Eq. 9-2}$$

where N_0 is the number of radionuclides present at time $t = 0$, and e is the base of the natural logarithm. Therefore, the number of radionuclides remaining after a time, $t(N)$, is equal to the number of radionuclides at a time, $t = 0$ (N_0), multiplied by the factor ($e^{-\lambda t}$). This factor is the fraction of radionuclides remaining after a time, t, and is termed the **decay factor**. The decay factor, $e^{-\lambda t}$, is an exponential function of time, t; that is, a constant fraction of the number of radionuclides present in the sample disappears during a given time interval. A given time interval is customarily expressed as the time required for a given number of radionuclides in the sample to decrease to one half its original value. This time interval is termed the **half-life ($t_{1/2}$)**. The half-life of a radionuclide is related to its decay constant as follows:

$$t_{1/2} = 0.693/\lambda \qquad \textit{Eq. 9-3}$$

Units of radioactivity. The average rate of decay of a sample (see Eq. 9-2), that is, the average number of nuclides disintegrating per second (dps) or per minute (dpm), is the activity of the sample and is used to determine the amount of radioactivity present in the sample.

Radioactivity is measured in **curie (Ci)** units. One curie is defined as the activity of a sample decaying at a rate of 3.7×10^{10} dps (2.22×10^{12} dpm), which is very close to the activity of 1 g of ^{226}Ra (3.656×10^{10} dps/g). In fact, the curie was originally defined as the activity of 1 g of ^{226}Ra. The basic multiples of the curie are as follows:

1 Ci = 10^3 millicurie (mCi) = 10^6 microcurie (μCi) = 10^9 nanocurie (nCi) = 10^{12} picocurie (pCi)

In clinical chemistry the amounts of radioactivity used are usually in the range of nanocuries to microcuries; occasionally, picocurie quantities are measured. The use of Système International d'Unités (SI) units in radioactivity measurements has been introduced. The basic unit of this system is the **becquerel (Bq)**, in which 1 Bq = 1 dps. Thus

1 μCi = 3.7×10^4 Bq

This system has not gained widespread acceptance in the United States. In Eq. 9-2, N_0 and N are the numbers of radionuclides present at times 0 and t, respectively. These quantities are extremely difficult to measure. However, the effects of the nuclear disintegrations can be measured more easily with use of one of the radioactive detectors described on pp. 195 to 197. In this way the total number of disintegrations per second occurring within the radioactive sample, or the radioactivity, at any given time can be estimated. Since the radioactivity, A, is proportional to the number of atoms, N, Eq. 9-2 can be written as

$$A = A_o e^{-\lambda t} \qquad \textit{Eq. 9-4}$$

TABLE 9-1	Decay Factors for ^{125}I			
	DAYS			
Days	*0*	*4*	*8*	*12*	*16*
0	—	0.955	0.912	0.871	0.831
20	0.794	0.758	0.724	0.691	0.660
40	0.630	0.602	0.574	0.548	0.524
60	0.500	0.477	0.456	0.435	0.416

Therefore, the decay constant, the decay factor, and the half-life are also applicable to activity versus time.

Decay factors of commonly used radionuclides can be obtained from decay-factor tables, which are available from most radiopharmaceutical companies and instrument manufacturers. An example of such a table for ^{125}I is Table 9-1. The decay factor can be used to calculate the amount of radioactivity remaining after a certain time. For example, the decay factor for ^{125}I 28 days after the manufacturer's calibration date is 0.724 according to Table 9-1. This number, multiplied by the initial amount of radioactivity, gives the level of radioactivity left at 28 days.

It is often necessary to know the **specific activity** of a radioactive sample. This is the activity of the radionuclide per unit mass of the radioactive sample and thus is measured in microcuries per microgram, microcuries per micromole, and so on or submultiples thereof. The specific activity of the nuclide is inversely proportional to the half-life of the radionuclide and is an important factor in determining the sensitivity of radioimmunoassay. A list of nuclides commonly used in clinical chemistry and some of their radiation characteristics are presented in Table 9-2. The low decay rates of ^{3}H and ^{14}C with long half-lives give them low specific activity and make them less suitable for radio-

immunoassay work. The specific activities of nuclides listed in Table 9-2 are calculated under the assumption that all nuclides present are radioactive (carrier-free). This assumption does not always hold true. For example, the **isotopic abundance** of available ^{131}I preparations seldom exceeds 20%; that is, only about 20% of iodine atoms present in the ^{131}I preparation are ^{131}I—the rest are ^{127}I (stable iodine). Therefore, the actual specific activity of ^{131}I preparations is only about one fourth of the theoretical specific activity shown in Table 9-2. Similarly, the specific activity of molecules depends on the isotopic abundance of the radionuclides present in the molecules. A thyroxine molecule contains four iodine atoms, and thus the specific radioactivity of radioiodine-labeled thyroxine preparations depends not only on the kind of radioactive iodine used for labeling but also on how many of the stable iodines are replaced by the radioactive iodine.

Properties of Radiation and Interaction with Matter

An understanding of the properties of radiation and the mechanism of the energy loss of radiation as it passes through matter is important, because the operation of every detecting device for any type of radiation depends on one or more of the particular properties of the radiation that is being measured and the interactions of radiation with matter. Further, the safe manipulation of radioactive substances requires a knowledge of the nature of radiation and its ability to penetrate matter. The harmful effects of radiation on tissues are highly dependent on the ability of the radiation to ionize matter and on the energy of the incident radiation.

The interactions of radiation with matter result in the transfer of energy from a radioactive nucleus to the surrounding material. This transfer is accomplished through processes of excitation and ionization; therefore, radiation emitted from radionuclides is frequently termed *ionizing radiation.*

TABLE 9-2	Radiation Characteristics of Radionuclides Commonly Used in Clinical Chemistry				
		MAIN RADIATION		**SPECIFIC ACTIVITY***	
Nuclide	*Half-Life*	*Type*	*Energy (keV)*	*mCi/µg*	*mCi/µmole*
^{3}H	12.3 years	β–	18	9.7	29
^{14}C	5760 years	β–	158	0.0044	0.062
^{32}P	14.3 days	β–	1700	285	9120
^{35}S	87.1 days	β–	167	42.8	1500
^{51}Cr	27.8 days	EC†	γ320	92	4690
^{59}Fe	45 days	β–/γ	460/1099	49.1	2900
^{57}Co	270 days	EC†	γ122	8.5	480
^{125}I	60 days	EC†	γ35	17.3	2200
^{131}I	8.1 days	β–/γ	807/364	123	16,100

*Carrier free.
†Electron capture.

TABLE 9-3 BASIC PROPERTIES OF RADIATION

Radiation	Charge	Energy Range	APPROXIMATE RANGE OF TRAVEL IN		Relative Specific Ionization*
			Air	Water	
Particles					
α	+2	3 to 9 MeV	2 to 8 cm	20 to 40 μm	2500
β⁻	−1	0 to 3 MeV	0 to 10 m	0 to 1 mm	100
α⁺	+1	0 to 3 MeV	0 to 10 m	0 to 1 mm	100
Electromagnetic					
X rays	None	1 eV to 100 keV	1 mm to 10 m	1 μm to 1 cm	10
Gamma rays	None	10 keV to 10 MeV	1 cm to 100 m	1 mm to 10 cm	1

The number of ion pairs produced per unit path length relative to that of gamma rays.

Excitation occurs when orbital electrons are perturbed from their normal arrangement by absorbing energy from the incident radiation. Ionization occurs when the energy absorbed is sufficient to cause an orbital electron to be ejected from its orbit, creating an ion pair (a free electron and a positively charged atom or molecule). This ionizing ability of radiation is best expressed by the number of ion pairs produced per unit path length, that is, the **specific ionization**. Properties of various forms of radiation are presented in Table 9-3.

Particulate radiation. Because of their relatively large mass and double charge, alpha particles produce a great deal of ionization, which causes them to lose their energy quickly in a short distance (high specific ionization; see Table 9-3). Therefore, alpha particles are weakly penetrating and can be stopped completely by very thin layers of solid materials. For this reason, they are less hazardous externally. However, if they get into the body, they will irradiate the tissues around them intensely, causing a serious health hazard. Alpha-emitting nuclides are seldom used in medicine.

Beta particles may be negatively or positively charged. There is no known difference between the negatron particle and the electron, except for their origin. Positrons are anti-particles of electrons. The energetic negatron and positron particles also lose their energy by excitation and ionization of molecules, but because of their smaller mass and charge, their specific ionization is not as high as that of alpha particles (see Table 9-3). As described previously, the beta decay is always accompanied by the release of a neutrino and the energy released in the decay process is shared between the beta particle and the neutrino in the form of kinetic energy. Therefore, beta particles have a continuous energy ranging from zero to a maximum of E_{max}, depending on the distribution of the decay energy between the beta particle and the neutrino, and have an average energy approximately equivalent to one third of E_{max}. E_{max} is equivalent to the total energy available from the nuclear decay and is characteristic of each radionuclide. Fig. 9-3 shows the beta-particle energy spectrum of ^{14}C.

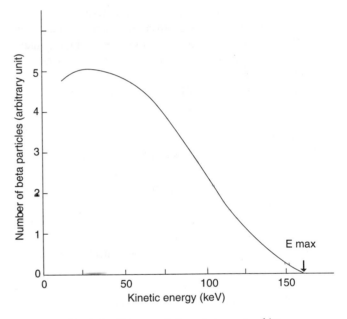

Fig. 9-3 Beta-particle spectrum for ^{14}C.

Electromagnetic radiation. Electromagnetic radiations usually encountered in the field of medicine include gamma radiation and x radiation. Except for possible differences in energy, these photons are indistinguishable and engage in the same type of interactions with matter. Because photons have no mass, are uncharged, and travel with the velocity of light, they might travel through matter for a considerable distance without any interaction and then lose all or most of their energy in a single interaction. Photons can interact with matter in several different ways, depending on their energies and the properties of the material with which they interact.

Photoelectric effect is especially important for photons with low energy (below 0.5 MeV). The photon interacts directly with one of the orbital electrons in matter (a photon-electron interaction), and the entire photon energy is transferred to the electron. Some transferred energy is used to overcome the binding energy of the electron, and the remaining energy is carried by the electron as kinetic energy. The ejected electron (photoelectron) in turn transfers its kinetic energy to many other electrons in its path. The photoelectric effect is especially pronounced if the atomic number of the absorbing material is high.

Compton effect, or *Compton scattering,* occurs primarily with photons of medium energy (0.5 to 1 MeV). In this process a collision between a photon and an electron results in the transfer of only a portion of the photon energy to the electron. The scattered photon with reduced energy emerges from the site of interaction in a new direction. The ejected electron (Compton electron) and the scattered photon lose more energy by subsequent interactions.

MEASUREMENT OF NUCLEAR RADIATION

Radioactivity measurements depend on the ability of radionuclides to produce ionized or excited atoms within the detector. Two basic types of radiation detectors are in common use: gas ionization and scintillation. The latter is capable of detecting both negatron and gamma radiation and providing information on the type and energy of the radiation and hence is currently the most commonly used detector in the field of medicine. Therefore, the following discussion is devoted primarily to scintillation detectors; other detectors are described only briefly.

Gas-Filled Detectors

The Geiger-Müller counter and the ionization chamber are examples of gas ionization detectors. In the Geiger-Müller counter the radiation is detected through ionization produced within a suitable gas. Because the ions produced are accelerated by the relatively high voltage applied between the electrodes of the detector, considerable secondary ionization occurs, leading to a large output pulse (electron multiplication). The major advantage of this type of detector, as compared with ionization chambers, is its ability to detect low levels of radiation. The ionization chamber functions on a similar principle. However, because a lower voltage is used, electron multiplication does not occur in the ionization chamber, and the output signal is relatively small. Both detectors are widely used in survey meters for measuring exposure of personnel and locating a spilled radionuclide.

Scintillation Detectors

Scintillation counting is based on the principle that a charged particle (alpha or beta) entering the detector, or an electron excited in the detector after an interaction with an incoming photon (gamma ray), will dissipate its energy within the scintillator contained in the detector by various processes of interaction mentioned previously. A portion of the energy absorbed by the scintillator is emitted as photons in the visible or near-ultraviolet region of the electromagnetic spectrum. Scintillators, or fluors, are substances capable of converting the kinetic energy of an incoming charged particle or photon into flashes of light (scintillation).

Crystal scintillation detectors. The most commonly used fluor for detecting gamma radiation by scintillation is a single crystal of sodium iodide containing small amounts of thallium (about 1%) as the activator. Fig. 9-4 is a block diagram of the common types of thallium-activated sodium iodide crystal scintillation detectors. The crystal is usually in the shape of a well, and the sample to be counted is allowed to sit in the well. The sodium iodide crystal is very hygroscopic. It is encapsulated in a can made of metal (such as aluminum) to prevent it from absorbing atmospheric moisture, except for one face (usually the bottom face) of the crystal well, which is covered by a transparent material such as Lucite and is optically coupled to the transparent face of a photomultiplier tube.

A gamma ray emitted from the sample placed in the crystal well is highly penetrating and therefore can pass through the glass or plastic wall of the test tube containing the radioactive sample and enter the crystal. As the gamma ray passes into the crystal, it produces excitation or ionization, and light photons are emitted. About 20 to 30 light photons are produced for each electron volt of energy absorbed. The photons pass through the transparent crystal and strike the photocathode of the photomultiplier tube, causing a release of electrons from the cathode. The energy required to release one photoelectron from the photocathode is about 300 to 2000 eV.

In addition to the conversion of the light photons emitted by the fluor into a pulse of detectable electrons, the photomultiplier also amplifies the minute amount of current produced from the photocathode to a level that can be effectively handled in conventional electronic amplifier circuits. This is achieved by a process of electron multiplication. As illustrated in Fig. 9-4, a series of metal plates, termed *dynodes*, are spaced along the length of the photomultiplier tube. The dynode surface is coated with a material capable of emitting secondary electrons when struck by an accelerated electron. Each dynode is maintained at a potential voltage higher than the preceding one. The initial photoelectrons are accelerated toward the first dynode and strike it to produce secondary electrons, which are then accelerated toward a second dynode. For each striking electron, the dynode releases about three or four electrons. This process is repeated until an amplification of about 10^8 is achieved.

The current output of the photomultiplier tube is amplified, and the resulting voltage pulse is shaped for optimal counting by conventional electronic circuitry such as that shown in Fig. 9-4. The preamplifier reduces the distortion of the electrical signal produced by the photomultiplier tube. The preamplifier output is further amplified by the amplifier to give a voltage of up to 10 V.

The function of the pulse-height analyzer is to sort out the pulses according to their pulse height and to allow those pulses within a restricted range (the photopeak) to reach the rate meter for counting. This is accomplished by means of **discriminators**. A lower discriminator sets the lower limit, and an upper discriminator sets the upper limit of the energy range to be counted. The lower discriminator excludes all voltage pulses below the lower limit; the upper discriminator

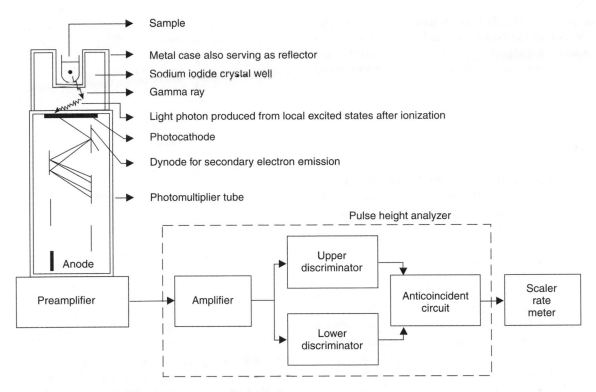

Sample

Metal case also serving as reflector

Sodium iodide crystal well

Gamma ray

Light photon produced from local excited states after ionization

Photocathode

Dynode for secondary electron emission

Photomultiplier tube

Anode

Pulse height analyzer

Preamplifier

Amplifier

Upper discriminator

Lower discriminator

Anticoincident circuit

Scaler rate meter

Fig. 9-4   Block diagram showing principal components of typical crystal scintillation counter.

excludes voltage pulses above the upper limit. The energy interval represented by the difference between the two discrimination levels is called the *window width*. Only the pulses with energy in the preset discriminator **window** pass through the **anticoincident circuit** and are counted because the anticoincident circuit will transmit a pulse arriving at its input from the lower discriminator only if there is no pulse arriving from the upper discriminator at the same time.

It is important to note that the magnitude (height) of the output pulse of the photomultiplier tube is proportional to the intensity of light photons produced in the crystal by a gamma ray and hence to the gamma ray energy deposited in the crystal, whereas the number of voltage pulses per unit time is related to the activity of radioactive samples being analyzed. Each radionuclide has a characteristic spectrum of energies (pulse height), as noted earlier.

Unlike beta particles which give a continuous energy spectrum (see Fig. 9-3), photons produced by gamma decay have a discrete and specific energy value (see Table 9-2). This specific energy value would appear in the gamma ray energy spectrum as a single vertical line at that energy level corresponding to the energy of the emitted gamma ray if the crystal scintillation detector used were perfect. In reality, however, the intensity of light produced in the crystal and transmitted to the photocathode and the number of electrons collected at the anode for each total absorption interaction in the crystal detector are slightly different. These differences produce a bell-shaped curve (photopeak) instead of a single vertical line (Fig. 9-5).

All gamma ray–emitting nuclides have their own characteristic photopeaks in their energy spectra that are very

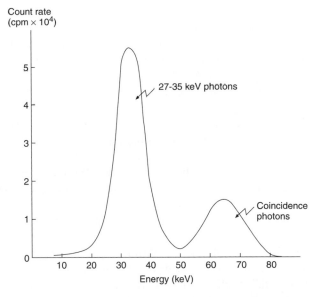

Count rate (cpm × 10^4)

27-35 keV photons

Coincidence photons

Energy (keV)

Fig. 9-5   Spectrum of ^{125}I showing the dominant peak of the x-ray photons (27 to 35 keV) and the apparent energy recorded in the detector when two photons happen to cause a scintillation simultaneously (coincidence photons). *(From Thorell JI, Larson SM:* Radioimmunoassay and related techniques: methodology and clinical applications, *St Louis, 1978, Mosby.)*

useful in the identification of such radionuclides. Fig. 9-5 shows an energy spectrum of ^{125}I. As described previously, the nuclide ^{125}I decays into ^{125}Te by electron capture with the emission of 35 keV gamma rays by the ^{125}Te daughter nuclide in the excited state and 27 and 31 keV Te x rays. The photopeak at about 28.5 keV is attributable to the single-photon detection of the two x rays and the 35 keV gamma rays, whereas the photopeak at about 56.8 keV is attributable to the coincident summing of the two x rays or one x ray and the 35 keV gamma ray. The 56.8 keV photopeak is called the *coincident photopeak* and is the result of emission of a coincidence pair of photons during the ^{125}I decay process, that is, the emission of two photons within the resolving time of the detector. Both photons of the pair are detected by a high-efficiency sodium iodide crystal detector and are recorded as a single event with a pulse height equivalent to the sum of the energies of the two photons. This unique energy spectrum is used to determine the counting efficiency for ^{125}I of some solid scintillation analyzers without the use of a standard of known disintegration rate.

A scintillation detector equipped with two or more pulse-height analyzers (multichannel analyzers) can be used to count two or more radionuclides simultaneously, either in the same sample or in different samples, provided that there is sufficient energy difference between them so that a certain portion of the energy of one radionuclide can be detected free from the second radionuclide. For example, the major photopeak of ^{125}I occurs at 27 keV and that of ^{131}I at 364 keV. In addition to the 364 keV photopeak, a minor ^{131}I photopeak occurs at 32 keV. For counting a mixture of these two isotopes, one analyzer channel (A) is centered at 27 keV and the other channel (B) at 364 keV, with the window width of about 20 to 40 keV. Channel B gives the true count for ^{131}I because ^{125}I does not contribute counts to channel B. Counts from channel A, however, represent the sum of the true counts for ^{125}I and the ^{131}I spillover. The extent of the ^{131}I spillover can be estimated by counting the pure ^{131}I standard in both channels.

Clinical laboratories performing radioimmunoassays frequently use crystal scintillation counters equipped with multiple detectors, because these assays involve counting of a large number of radioactive samples. With the use of a multidetector instrument, the total counting time can be reduced considerably. However, it is absolutely necessary to make sure that all detectors in such counters perform in an equivalent fashion.

Liquid scintillation detectors. Liquid scintillation detectors are primarily used for counting beta particle–emitting radionuclides such as ^3H, ^{14}C, and ^{32}P. Unlike that of gamma photons, the penetration of negatron particles is so short that they cannot penetrate the wall of the sample container for interaction with crystal scintillators. In liquid scintillation counting, the sample is dissolved or suspended in a solution, or "cocktail," consisting of a solvent such as toluene, a primary scintillator such as 2,5-diphenyloxazole (PPO), and a secondary scintillator such as 1,4-bis-2(5-phenyloxazolyl)benzene (POPOP) (Fig. 9-6). The beta particles from the radioactive sample dissolved in the scintillation cocktail ionize and excite the molecules of the solvent. The excitation energy is transferred to the primary scintillator, which emits light photons when the excited electrons return to the ground energy level. The wavelength

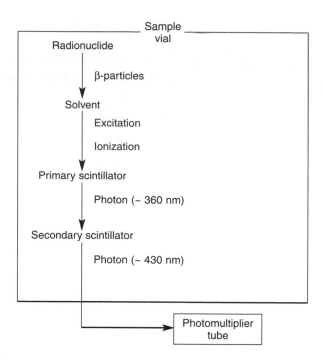

Fig. 9-6 Initial scintillation processes in a liquid scintillation analyzer. *(From Thorell JI, Larson SM: Radioimmunoassay and related techniques: methodology and clinical applications, St Louis, 1978, Mosby.)*

of light emitted by the primary scintillator is frequently too short (about 350 to 400 nm) for efficient detection by the photocathodes of photomultiplier tubes. The secondary scintillator absorbs the photons emitted by the primary scintillator and reemits them at a longer wavelength (about 430 nm). Thus the secondary scintillator is also termed a **wavelength shifter.** However, the modern photomultiplier tubes are sensitive to the wavelength of the primary scintillator. Today, the secondary scintillators are used primarily for more effective transmission of the energy from the beta particle to produce light flashes, especially when a large amount of color-quenched sample is placed in the scintillation solution. Problems related to quenching are discussed later in this chapter.

The operating principles of solid crystal scintillation analyzers and liquid scintillation analyzers are basically the same, except for the difference in scintillation detection. A typical arrangement of the principal components of a liquid scintillation counter is shown in Fig. 9-7. The light photons produced in the sample vial are detected and amplified by the photomultiplier tubes in the same manner as for the crystal scintillation counter. In the liquid scintillation detector, however, a second photomultiplier tube, a **coincident circuit**, and a **summation circuit** are incorporated to eliminate the electronic noise associated with the photomultiplier tube and to improve counting efficiency for low-energy beta-particle emitters.

Noise pulses are random events, and the probability of two photomultiplier tubes producing noise pulses simultaneously is relatively small. In contrast, the beta particle produces a

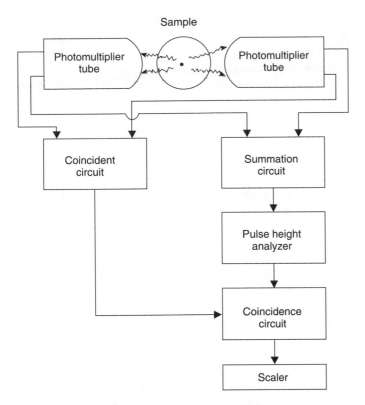

Fig. 9-7 Schema of liquid scintillation counter.

burst of photons, and two photomultiplier tubes will receive photons almost simultaneously. The output pulses from each photomultiplier tube are fed into a coincident circuit to check whether a pulse from one photomultiplier tube is accompanied by a corresponding pulse from the other within the allowed time interval (termed the **coincidence resolving time**, usually about 20×10^{-8} seconds). Pulses within the resolving time produce a coincident signal that is electrically sent to the coincident gate. Most noise pulses do not meet the requirement of the coincidence resolving time and are excluded. The summation circuit is incorporated to sum all coincident pulses to obtain the true pulse height. The summed coincident pulses are amplified, sorted, and counted in a manner similar to that for the crystal scintillation counter.

In liquid scintillation counting, proper energy transfer cannot occur unless the sample is in contact with the scintillation solution to give a colorless, transparent, homogeneous solution. Some radioactive samples are not soluble in the scintillation solution, so it may be necessary to add one or more substances to obtain a homogeneous scintillation mixture. Solubilizers such as methylbenzethonium chloride (Hyamine 10X) are used to facilitate dissolution of the sample in the scintillation solution, or jelling agents such as aluminum stearate are used to enhance the counting efficiency by stabilizing the sample suspension in liquid scintillators. Many commercial liquid scintillation cocktails of nonpolar mediums (toluene or xylene) contain some type of surfactant such as the Tritons (polyoxyethylene ethers and other surface-active compounds) to maintain aqueous

samples in colloidal suspensions so that the aqueous samples can be counted at high efficiency. Nonvolatile, radioactive materials are also counted on solid supports such as filter paper disks or glass fibers immersed in a scintillation solution. The disadvantage of this counting method is the relatively low counting efficiency because of impurity quenching.

Quenching is basically a process that results in the reduction of the overall photon output of the sample. Impurities present in the radioactive sample may compete with the scintillators for energy transfer; that is, the energy is lost to a non–light-producing process. This phenomenon is termed *impurity quenching*. Water in aqueous samples or a support medium such as a filter disk may cause impurity quenching. Colored substances such as hemoglobin may absorb the light photons produced by the scintillation process before they can be detected by the photomultiplier tubes, or these substances may change the wavelength of the light photons to a value not suitable for efficient detection by the photocathodes of photomultiplier tubes. Quenching in liquid scintillation counting is detected and corrected by efficiency determination. The efficiency of the measurement is defined as the ratio of the observed counts per minute (cpm) to the absolute units of disintegrations per minute (dpm):

$$\text{Efficiency} = \frac{\text{cpm}}{\text{dpm}}$$

Since the quenching characteristics of each sample are different, the efficiency must be determined for each sample. By knowing the counting rate (cpm) and the counting efficiency of a sample, you can calculate the absolute radioactivity (dpm) of the sample. Several methods for efficiency determination have been developed, but only those most frequently used are discussed.

Internal standardization. When properly carried out, internal standardization, one of the oldest methods, is the most accurate for efficiency determination. In this method the sample is counted before and after the introduction of a calibrated standard of the measured radionuclide. The difference between the count rates before and after the spike, divided by the calibrated activity of the spike in disintegrations per unit time, is termed the *counting efficiency*. The disadvantages of this method are the time-consuming manipulation of the sample and the loss of sample for recount after the introduction of the spike.

Sample-channels ratio. The sample-channels ratio method is based on a downward shift of the pulse-height spectrum of the photon as a result of the quenching-induced decrease in the pulse height of many energetic decays (Fig. 9-8). The degree of the shift is related to the extent of quenching or counting efficiency and is expressed by the change in the ratio of the sample counts obtained from two different discriminator window settings (channels). As shown in Fig. 9-8, one channel is usually set to measure the entire isotope spectrum (L_1 to L_3), and the second channel is restricted to only a portion of the spectrum (L_1 to L_2). In this method, channel ratios (L_1 to L_2) to (L_1 to L_3) of a set of

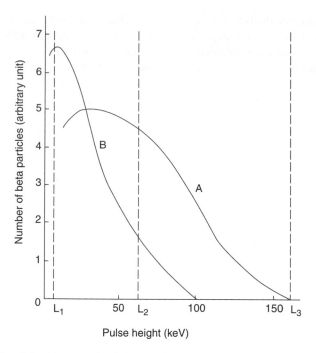

Fig. 9-8 Unquenched (*A*) and quenched (*B*) pulse-height spectra of ^{14}C. L_1 to L_3 denote discrimination levels.

artificially quenched standards of known efficiencies are determined and plotted against counting efficiency to obtain a quench curve. The efficiency of any unknown sample can be determined from its channel ratio and the quench curve. Unlike internal standardization, this method requires no additional sample manipulation and is suitable for handling a large number of samples through automation. However, this method may result in large errors in highly quenched samples or samples with low count rates.

External standards. Unlike the internal standard method, the known activity in the external standard method is provided by an external source of gamma radiation, such as ^{226}Ra, placed at a fixed position adjacent to the sample vial. The external gamma-ray source generates electrons through the Compton collision process in the scintillation solution. The Compton electrons transfer energy to the solution and cause scintillation in the same way as beta particles do in the scintillation medium. The energy spectrum produced by Compton electrons is also affected by the presence of quenching materials, as in a typical beta-particle spectrum. The sample is counted twice, once in the absence of and once in the presence of an external standard. As in the sample-channels ratio method, a set of quenched standards of known efficiencies is used to obtain a correlation curve between the sample-counting efficiency and the count rate of the external standard. The counting efficiency of a sample can be determined from the count rate of the external standard counted with the sample and from the correlation curve. The external standard method has become an integral part of almost all modern liquid scintillation detectors.

Another problem encountered in liquid scintillation counting is **chemiluminescence**, the production of light

photons by a chemical reaction between the sample material and the solute or solubilizer added to the scintillation solution. Chemiluminescence gives rise to single photons and can be excluded by the coincident circuit of the liquid scintillation counter. However, when chemiluminescence reactions are of sufficient intensity, non–beta particle coincident pulses may be generated that interfere with the beta-particle scintillation counting. The chemiluminescent effect will eventually disappear, but this may take several hours or longer, especially at low temperatures. Chemiluminescence can be monitored by repeated counting of the sample. Some modern instruments are capable of automatically monitoring and correcting for the chemiluminescent effects.

As with crystal scintillation counting, mixed-isotope counting is possible with a liquid scintillation counter with multichannel analyzers. A common example of dual-label counting involves a mixture of tritium, with a maximum beta-particle decay of 18.6 keV, and ^{14}C, with a maximum beta-particle decay of 156 keV.

Counting statistics. Since radioactive decay is essentially a random process, it is unlikely that successive measurements on a given sample will result in the same number of counts. However, radioactive decay obeys a *Poisson distribution*. The Poisson distribution density formula can be applied in the calculation of the precision of measurement at a given count rate. If a single measurement of total counts, *N,* is made, precision of this measurement in terms of the percent coefficient of variation (%CV) can be estimated to be as follows:

$$\%CV = \frac{\sqrt{N}}{N} \times 100\%$$

For example, at a total count of 100, CV = 10%; at 1000, CV = 3.2%; at 10,000, CV = 1%. This approximation is applicable only when the background count is negligible compared with the sample count. When significant background counts are present, the formula for the standard deviation of a difference must be used:

$$\%CV = \frac{\sqrt{N + B}}{S} \times 100\%$$

where *B* is the background count and *S* is the sample count (*N* − *B*). Thus a total count of 100 in the presence of a background count of 10 gives the following:

$$\%CV = \frac{\sqrt{100 + 10}}{100 - 10} \times 100\% = 11.7\%$$

Prolonging the counting time can increase precision, but a 1% CV (i.e., 10,000 counts) is satisfactory in most applications.

RADIATION HEALTH SAFETY

Although the quantity of radioactivity handled in the clinical chemistry laboratory is usually very small, every laboratory worker who has frequent contact with radioactive substances needs to have a basic knowledge of radiation safety, because the biological effects of long-term exposure to very low doses of ionizing radiation are still largely unknown and may prove to be hazardous to health.

Radionuclides commonly used in the clinical laboratory are either beta-particle emitters, such as ^{14}C and ^3H, or gamma-ray emitters, such as ^{125}I and ^{57}Co. Both forms of radiation produce their biological effects by producing ionization and excitation along their paths in the tissue. However, beta radiation is less penetrating than gamma radiation; thus beta-particle emitters are considered to be more hazardous in terms of internal radiation and less hazardous in terms of external radiation than gamma-ray emitters. Therefore, the primary concern with beta-particle emitters is to prevent the entry of radioactive materials into the body through inhalation, ingestion, or absorption by the skin. With gamma-ray emitters, radiation safety involves the consideration of other factors, such as shielding, exposure time, and exposure distance

Monitoring

Regular monitoring of both personnel and work areas is an important radiation safety procedure. It is necessary to measure periodically the radiation exposure doses of personnel to ensure that radiation doses received are below the recommended limits. The following three basic units are used to measure radiation exposure and dose.

The **roentgen (R)** is a unit of x rays or gamma rays and measures the quantity of ionization produced by photon radiation in a given sample of air. One roentgen equals that quantity of photon radiation capable of producing one electrostatic unit of either sign in 0.001293 g of air.

The **radiation absorbed dose (rad)** is a measure of local energy deposition per unit mass of material irradiated by any ionizing radiation. One rad is equal to 100 ergs of absorbed energy per gram of absorber.

The **roentgen equivalent, man (rem)** is that dose of ionizing radiation causing the same amount of biological injury to human tissue as 1 rad of x, gamma, or beta radiation. In the case of alpha radiation, the dose in rem equals the dose in rad multiplied by 20, because only 0.05 rad of alpha radiation is needed to produce the same biological effect as 1 rad of x, gamma, or beta radiation. The recommended maximum permissible dose to the whole body is 0.5 rem per year for the general public and 5 rem per year for radiation workers.

Film badges are probably the most commonly used and cost-effective way of monitoring personnel. The photographic film becomes progressively optically dense when exposed to ionizing radiation and thus may be used to monitor the radiation dose received by the wearer. Since most clinical laboratory personnel working with radioimmunoassays routinely handle ^{125}I-labeled compounds, it is advisable to monitor possible accumulation of radioactive iodine in the thyroid glands. Arrangements should be made to have the radioactive content of each worker's thyroid measured at least twice each year or after each radioiodination experiment. Records of radiation exposure of all workers

handling radioactive materials must be kept for at least 5 years. Each laboratory should have a portable radiation detector, such as a portable Geiger-Müller survey meter, to monitor radioactivity in an area in which radioactive materials are routinely handled. Monitoring of beta radiation usually requires taking samples of the work area with swabs and using a liquid scintillation counter to determine the presence of radioactivity.

Contamination Control

Internal radiation exposure is controlled only by prevention of the entry of radioactive materials into the body. This requires strict adherence to the general rules for radiation safety. No smoking, eating, drinking, applying of cosmetics, or storing of food is allowed in work areas. Mouth pipetting of radioactive materials should never be done. All persons working in radioactive areas must wear the designated protective clothing (a standard laboratory coat is satisfactory in a clinical laboratory involved in radioimmunoassays) and disposable gloves. Such protective clothing should be removed when one is leaving the laboratory and should not be taken home for washing or for any other reason. Radioactive materials must be properly labeled and stored and used only at specially designated areas. Work involving the possible generation of volatile, radioactive substances, such as radioiodination, should be performed in an exhaust hood. The working surface should be covered by a layer of disposable absorbent material. In addition to the proper operating technique, cleanliness and good housekeeping are essential to prevent and minimize the spread and buildup of contamination.

External radiation exposure is of minor concern in radioimmunoassay laboratories because the amount of radioactivity handled in any given time is very small (less than 1 µCi) and because the radiation energy of the most commonly used gamma ray–emitting radionuclide ^{125}I has weak energies ranging from 27 to 35 keV. Nevertheless, it is always a good practice to minimize the time spent in a radiation field, to maximize the distance from the source of radiation, and to use shielding between you and the source of radiation, especially for those involved in radioiodination.

Persons contaminated by radioactive materials should be quickly decontaminated to prevent the possible transfer of radioactivity to internal organs by absorption through the skin. Facilities for decontamination, such as a shower and an eyewash station, should be available in each laboratory. Use absorbent materials to remove spilled radioactive material; then scrub the contaminated area with soap and water. It is a good practice to cover the contaminated area immediately with a piece of paper to prevent spreading of the radioactivity to other parts of the laboratory.

Waste Disposal

The radioactivity level of the radioactive waste materials generated in clinical laboratories involved in radioimmunoassays is usually very low, but such radioactive waste material should still be disposed of according to the guidelines established by the Nuclear Regulatory Commission (NRC) of the United States. Some states are approved by the NRC (NRC agreement states) to regulate the use, safety, and disposal of radioactive material in the state, provided that the regulations are more restrictive than the NRC regulations. Therefore, it is important for radiation workers to be familiar with the state regulations on radioactive materials if the laboratory in which they work is located in an NRC agreement state.

Bibliography

Bernier DR et al: *Nuclear medicine technology and techniques*, ed 2, St Louis, 1989, Mosby.

Heal AV: Safety and disposal changes that affect regulations in radioassay labs, *Lab World* 50–53, Dec 1981.

L'Annunziata MF: *Radionuclide tracers,* New York, 1987, Academic Press.

L'Annunziata MF, editor: *Handbook of radioactivity analysis*, New York, 1998, Academic Press.

Radiation protection for medical and allied health personnel, Recommendations of the National Council on Radiation Protection and Measurements, NCRP report No. 105, Bethesda, MD, Oct 1989, NCRP.

Internet Sites

www.webelements.com/webelements/elements/text/periodic-table/radio.html—Links to radioisotope data

http://www.ncrp.com/—National Council on Radiation Protection and Measurements

www.ehs.ucdavis.edu/hp/shi/shi_ndex.html—UC Davis Safe Handling of Radioisotopes

http://www.stanford.edu/dept/EHS/prod/researchlab/radlaser/manual/appendices/reports.htm—Stanford University's Radiation Safety Manual

http://ntri.tamuk.edu/bio/radiation/radiation.html—Radioisotopes

www.niehs.nih.gov/odhsb/biosafe/bio.htm—Safety (In "General" section, find links to current forms used by the Health and Safety Branch)

http://research.utk.edu/ora/sections/compliances/radsaf/toc.html—Basic radiation safety

www.ehs.ucdavis.edu/hp/shi/shi_ndex.html—UC Davis Safe Handling of Radioisotopes

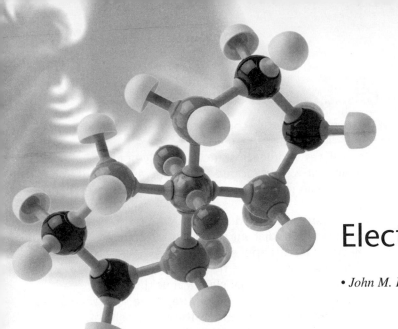

CHAPTER 10

Electrophoresis

• *John M. Brewer*

Objectives

- State the charge properties of amphoteric substances at acidic, isoelectric, and basic pH. Explain the significance of these properties in electrophoresis.
- Outline the principle of electrophoresis and summarize how electrophoretic separations of molecules are affected by the following:
  Enhanced resolution techniques
  Molecular size
  Molecular size and charge
  Thickness of support
- Describe the commonly encountered problems associated with electrophoresis and explain probable causes and corrective actions.

- Describe the principal advantages and limitations of capillary electrophoresis.
- List three common support media for electrophoresis and classify commonly used visualization stains according to the substance being separated. Describe the physical or chemical reactions that allow the use of a stain to visualize a specific substance.
- Describe the effect or effects on electrophoretic separations of the following variables:
  Ionic strength of buffer
  pH of buffer
  Electro-osmosis
  Heating

Key Terms

ampholyte   A trade name for a mixture of substances with a range of isoelectric points that have high buffering capacities at their isoelectric points.

amphoteric   A substance that can have a positive, zero, or negative charge, depending on conditions.

anion   Negatively charged particle or ion.

boundary   Edge of a zone, as of a macromolecule solution next to the solvent.

buffer   A mixture of proton-donating and proton-accepting substances the function of which is to keep the proton concentration (the pH) constant or nearly so. An example is a mixture of acetic acid and sodium acetate.

cation   Positively charged particle or ion.

coion   An ion of the same charge as the one under consideration; generally a much smaller ion.

conductivity   The readiness of a substance to carry a current. In an ionic solution, the sum of the products of the charge concentrations and charge mobilities.

convection   Mass or bulk movement of one part of a solution relative to the rest, usually because of density differences.

counterion   An ion of charge opposite to the one under consideration; generally a smaller ion.

densitometry   Measurement of the absorbance of analytes along the length of a support.

discontinuous solvent   A solution consisting of at least two separate regions that have different ions in them.

disk electrophoresis   A stacking or isotachophoretic step followed by zone electrophoresis, usually on a polyacrylamide gel.

effective mobility   The actual mobility of a substance under certain conditions; generally less than the mobility because of a lower charge or resistance by a supporting medium.

electrical field   An influence measured in volts (or volts per centimeter) that is manifested by the behavior of a charged particle in it.

electrical neutrality   A condition in which total positive charges equal total negative charges.

electroblot   Substances separated on supporting medium by electrophoresis are transferred onto a facing sheet of material using an electrical field perpendicular to the original separating field. The material on the facing sheet adsorbs and immobilizes the substances in the same pattern as the original separation.

electrochromatography   Analyte movement through a chromatographic matrix produced by an electrical field rather than hydrostatic pressure.

electrodes   Substances in contact with a conductor.

The substances are connected to a source of an electrical field.

electrolytes   Ionic substances, usually of low molecular weight, added to provide as constant and uniform an ionic environment for electrophoresis as possible.

electro-osmosis   Tendency of a solution to move relative to an adjacent stationary substance when an electrical field is applied.

electrophoresis   Movement of charged particles because of an external electrical field.

frictional coefficient   A measure of the resistance a particle offers to movement through a solvent.

gel   A network of interacting fibers, or a polymer that is solid but traps large amounts of solvent in pores or channels inside.

ionic strength   The sum of the concentrations of all ions in a solution, weighted by the squares of their charges.

isoelectric   Condition of zero net charge on an amphoteric substance.

isoelectric focusing   The ordering and concentration of substances according to their isoelectric points.

isoelectric point   The pH at which a substance has a zero net charge.

isotachophoresis   The ordering and concentration of substances of intermediate effective mobilities between an ion of high effective mobility and one of much lower effective mobility, followed by their migration at a uniform velocity.

Joule heating   Heating of a conductor by the passage of an electrical current.

micellar electrokinetic chromatography   Ionic detergents form micelles that migrate in an electrical field and analytes, even uncharged ones, which partition between the external solvent and the hydrophobic interior of the micelles will migrate depending on the extent of the partitioning. See Chapter 5 for a review of partitioning theory.

mobility   The velocity a particle or ion attains for a given applied voltage. A relative measure of how quickly an ion moves in an electrical field.

molecular sieving   Separation of molecules on the basis of their effective sizes.

polyacrylamide   Polymer of acrylamide and usually some cross-linking derivative.

polyelectrolyte   Substance with many charged or potentially charged groups.

resolving power   Ability to separate closely migrating substances.

sodium dodecyl sulfate (SDS)   A detergent and an especially effective protein denaturant.

Southern blot   A kind of *electroblot*, in which the

substances separated and transferred are nucleic acids.

stacking   Ordering or arranging and concentrating macromolecules according to their effective mobilities; compare to isotachophoresis.

Western blot   A kind of *electroblot*, in which the substances separated and transferred are proteins.

zeta potential   The potential produced by the effective charge of a macromolecule, usually taken at the boundary between what is moving with the macromolecule and the rest of the solution.

zone   A particular region or space within a larger one, generally distinguished by some property, such as its occupancy by a protein.

Movement of charged particles because of an *external electrical field* is called **electrophoresis**.[1] Because charged molecules can be made to move, different molecules can be separated if they have different velocities in an electrical field. Therefore electrophoresis is a separation technique, just as chromatography and ultracentrifugation are, and there are similarities among these techniques.

The movement of a charged species in aqueous solution is affected by the species' interaction with water molecules, that is, hydration (Fig. 10-1). The more polar a molecule is, the greater is the cluster of water molecules about it.[2]

The electrical field is applied to a solution through oppositely charged **electrodes** placed in the solution (Fig. 10-2). A particular ion then travels through the solution toward the electrode of opposite charge. Thus positively charged particles (**cations**) move to the negatively charged electrode (cathode), and negatively charged particles (**anions**) migrate to the positively charged electrode (anode).

APPLICATION OF ELECTRICAL FIELD TO A SOLUTION CONTAINING A CHARGED PARTICLE
Forces on a Particle

The force exerted on a charged particle depends on the electrical field, V (in volts or volts per centimeter), and the charge on the particle, Q. The force on the charged particle is the product:

$$F_{elec} = QV \qquad\qquad \textit{Eq. 10-1}$$

This electrical force, F_{elec}, when exerted on the particle, will cause it to move. However, a particle moving in a solvent will experience resistance because of the viscosity of the solvent.[1,3] The resistance, which is itself a force, is proportional to the velocity[3]:

$$F_{resistance} = fv \qquad\qquad \textit{Eq. 10-2}$$

The proportionality constant, f, is called the *frictional coefficient*.

The frictional coefficient depends on the viscosity of the solvent and the size and shape of the particle. The greater the viscosity, the slower is the movement. The bigger or more asymmetrical the particle, the slower is its movement through the solvent. The frictional coefficient of a large particle such as a protein is a characteristic property of the particle.

Mobility of a Particle

When an electrical field is applied to a charged particle, the particle begins to migrate. The electrophoretic and frictional forces oppose each other, and the particle's velocity increases until the forces are equal ($F_{resistance} = F_{elec}$). The velocity, v, a particle attains for a given electric field, V, is determined by two properties of the particle—its charge and its frictional coefficient. Consequently the value of v/V is also a characteristic property of the particle and is important enough to be given its own name. It is called the *mobility* of the particle.

Effect of pH on Mobility

Each ion has a particular charge and mobility. However, when a solution contains a substance the pK of which is near the pH of the solution, that substance exists in both a charged and an uncharged form in the solution. The fraction of species with a charge depends on the pK of the substance and the pH of the solution. When the pH is equal to the pK_a of a weak acid, only 50% of the particles are charged. At one pH unit below the pK_a, 90% are uncharged. At one pH unit above

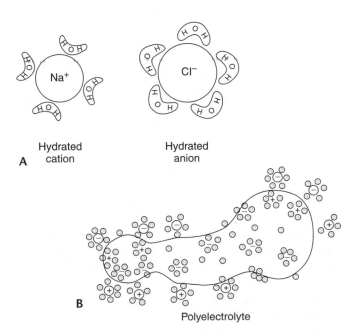

Fig. 10-1   State of charged particles in water solution. **A,** Small ions (Na⁺ and Cl⁻) with associated water molecules. **B,** Macromolecule with water molecules (*stippled smaller circles*) associated with charged and polar groups. Hydrated **coions** and **counterions** are also shown as larger circles around plus or minus signs.

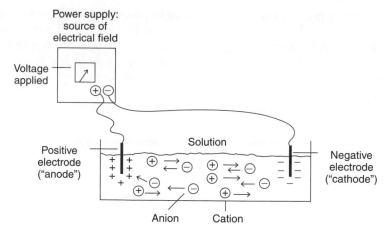

Fig. 10-2   Application of electrical field to solution of ions makes ions move.

the pK_a, 90% are in the charged state. Because the effective (average) charge of a substance varies with the pH, its ***effective mobility*** also varies with the pH.

This is particularly true for substances such as proteins. Proteins are clearly ***amphoteric*** substances; that is, they contain acidic and basic groups. Their overall (net) charge is highly positive at low pH values, zero (**isoelectric**) at a particular higher pH, and negative at still more alkaline pH values. Because mobility is directly proportional to the magnitude of the charge, the effective mobility of a protein is very much a function of the pH.

The most important practical consequence of this is that electrophoretic solutions must be buffered to maintain a constant pH. The ***buffer*** pH is chosen to give an optimum net charge for maximum separation. For proteins, pH values in the 7 to 9 range are generally used. The buffer is used to maintain this pH and thus the net protein charge throughout the electrophoretic process. Buffers are ionic substances themselves and so take part in any electrophoretic process, a fact that must also be considered.

Electrolytes

In electrophoresis, a substance such as a protein is put in one limited region, or ***zone***, of the system and is made to move into another region, or zone. Therefore much of the solution does not have protein in it at any particular time. If the protein and its associated counterions are not present to carry the current in a particular region, other ions must be present to carry the current. For this reason it is a common practice to add an excess, usually about 0.1 M, of low-molecular-weight buffer to the solution through which the protein must travel. The buffer and salt ions (**electrolytes**) provide a constant electrical environment so that the overall movement of the protein is as constant as possible and will be minimally influenced by other protein molecules.

Ion Movement and Conductivity

In any electrical system, the current produced is proportional to the voltage applied:

$$V = \text{Resistance} \times \text{Current} \qquad \textit{Eq. 10-3}$$

or

$$V = \frac{\text{Current}}{\text{Conductivity}} \qquad \textit{Eq. 10-4}$$

In electrophoresis, the current is the flow of ions (in both directions). The **conductivity** is the sum of the concentrations times the effective mobilities of all ions present. An ion with a higher effective mobility carries a larger fraction of the current[2] than one at the same concentration that has a lower effective mobility. The voltage, conductivity, and current thus are all related (equation 10-4). If the conductivity is increased by an increase in the salt concentration while the current is kept constant, the voltage must decrease. Such a decrease in voltage reduces the electrical force, F_{elec}, on charged particles, slowing the movement of the macromolecules. This increases the time needed for a given separation, and the resolution decreases because of increased diffusion. If the conductivity is increased at a fixed voltage, the current must increase, thus increasing the electrical heat (**Joule heating**) generated by the system, because heating is proportional to the square of the current. Excessive heating produces convective disturbances in the solutions, which distort the electrophoretic patterns and may also denature macromolecules. The heat generated in any electrophoretic separation is the ultimate factor in how fast the separation can be done. Because increasing the conductivity at either a fixed voltage or current has deleterious effects, optimum results are achieved when the concentration of ions and therefore the conductivity are kept at moderate values.

FACTORS AFFECTING MOBILITIES OF MACROMOLECULES
Charge and Conformation

The clinical laboratory usually deals with **polyelectrolytes**, substances with many charged or potentially charged groups on them. The net charge of a polyelectrolyte is determined by the total number of charged groups within the polyelectrolyte and its conformation. The folding, or *conformation*, of a

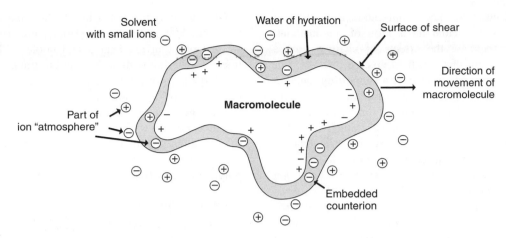

Fig. 10-3   Zeta potential of macromolecule is average effective electrical field strength (potential) produced by charges on macromolecule and any charged particles embedded in solvent carried along (water of hydration) with macromolecule. *Gray area,* water of hydration. Zeta potential is measured at surface of shear: the boundary between water of hydration and rest of solvent. Note that the small ions are hydrated also (see Fig. 10-1).

protein produces binding sites for many small molecules. In some cases electrolyte ions bind strongly and specifically to the macromolecule. For example, bovine serum albumin can bind several chloride ions. This changes the net charge of the macromolecule and therefore its mobility.

Ionic Atmosphere and Zeta Potential

Counterions, ions of opposite charge, naturally tend to hover in the vicinity of the charged groups of macromolecules.[4] However, they do not actually neutralize the charges on the macromolecule but are instead located at a range of distances from the charged groups of the macromolecule, forming a double layer of charge about the macromolecule called an *ionic atmosphere.*

The macromolecule moves with its entourage of hydration and hydrated counterions (Fig. 10-3). These reduce the effective charge of the macromolecule to a level given by the **zeta potential**. The zeta potential is the potential (voltage) produced by the effective charge of the macromolecule at the *surface of shear*. The surface of shear is the **boundary** between the entire macromolecular complex in solution (hydration layer and embedded counterions) and the material that is staying behind (the solvent).

Relaxation Effect

Because of random thermal motion, electrophoresing macromolecules move irregularly, in jumps, rather than in a continuous straight line. At each jump, the counterion atmosphere is left somewhat behind. The counterions (or their replacements from other parts of the solution) then move to catch up or reposition themselves, but this takes a little time. This is called a *relaxation effect*. It also tends to lower the mobility of the macromolecule, because the retarded or misplaced counterions momentarily produce a field that acts in a direction opposite to that of the applied field.

Electrophoretic Effect

Because ions in water solution are hydrated, the counterions of the electrolyte moving in the opposite direction carry solvent along with them. The macromolecule is thus moving against a *flow* of solvent, and its mobility is reduced by this factor also.

SUPPORT MEDIA

The goal of electrophoresis is to separate a mixture of substances, such as macromolecules, into completely separate zones. The narrower (thinner) the original zone of a mixture of macromolecules is, the smaller the migration distance necessary to achieve separation will be. Use of narrower zones means that complete separation can be effected in less time. Blurring or remixing of the separated zones as a result of diffusion is also reduced.

The major technical difficulty in using narrow (thin) zones of relatively concentrated macromolecules is a mechanical one. Such zones are considerably more dense than the solvent; thus the zones "fall" through the solvent faster than the macromolecules electrophorese. This is called *bulk flow*, or **convection**. The conventional solution to this problem is to use a supporting medium.

Functional Basis

The supporting medium must allow as free a penetration of the material to be separated as possible and yet cut off bulk flow (convection). Most media do this by offering a restricted pore size for electrophoretic movement of the macromolecules. A capillary tube has the same effect. This is the basis of *capillary zone electrophoresis*. The capillary tubes are as little as 25 to 50 μm (0.025 to 0.05 mm) across.

Electro-Osmosis

Normally the supporting medium should not interact with the molecules, because this might inhibit or stop migration (but see later discussion). The usual interaction problem encountered is not the actual adsorption of the material. More commonly seen are the effects of charged groups attached to the medium that result in **electro-osmosis**. For example, agar, which is often used as a supporting medium in electrophoresis, is a mixture of agarose and agaropectin. The agaropectin has a relatively large number of carboxyl groups in it, which at neutral pH have counterions. If a voltage is applied, the counterions move, but the carboxyl groups attached to the polysaccharide matrix do not. The counterions carry enough solvent with them to produce a *net* flow of solvent in *one* direction. This is the electro-osmosis effect, sometimes called *endosmosis*. However, electro-osmosis is a very general effect.[2] It is more pronounced when charged groups are present in the supporting medium, but it always occurs to some extent.

In capillary electrophoresis, capillaries made of fused silica, which is transparent in the ultraviolet (UV), are almost always used.[5] The surfaces of these consist of silanol groups that have a pK_a of 6.5, so capillary surfaces always bear some negative charge unless derivatized or coated with an agent such as cellulose or a plastic. These processes are performed to reduce or eliminate electro-osmosis and such effects as actual adsorption of proteins to uncoated surfaces.

Types of Supporting Media

The supporting medium can be a solution such as a sucrose density gradient, but, in general, insoluble materials are used. Some are self-supporting, whereas the apparatus mechanically supports others. Paper or sheets of plastic such as cellulose acetate have enough mechanical strength to allow electrophoresis on sheets hung or stretched over rods.

Support media can also be classified as particulate or continuous. Particulate support media include glass beads, agarose gel-permeation media (see p. 123, Chapter 5, and below) such as Sephadex, and cellulose fibers. Continuous support media include **polyacrylamide**, starch, and agarose gels.

Gels are jellylike solids in which considerable solvent is included. Starch gels, for example, are made from starch suspensions that are heated and cooled. The starch fibers interact, tangling with each other but trapping the solvent so that large gaps or pores exist between the fibers. These gaps or pores are available for macromolecular movement. Similar gels can be made from agar, agarose, and some chemical polymers. Gels can also be made by polymerization of acrylamide with a small percentage of a bifunctional acrylamide derivative that cross-links the acrylamide polymers (Fig. 10-4).

Molecular Sieving

The porosity, or average pore size, of some media is fixed, but the porosities of other media can be controlled. For example, by changing the gel concentrations of starch or agar, the pore size can be varied. If the average pore size is near the average diameter of the macromolecules that are being electrophoresed, the supporting medium will produce **molecular sieving** effects.

Sequencing of deoxyribonucleic acid (DNA) is done by electrophoresis of a mixture of radiolabeled DNA molecules that vary in length from a few nucleotides to many hundreds of nucleotides. These are separated by electrophoresis on a 6% polyacrylamide gel containing 8 M urea and so efficiently that adjacent zones of separated polynucleotide differ in length by only one nucleotide. Up to several hundred base lengths can be separated (and "read") on one such gel. Note that oligonucleotides in general have one negative charge per nucleotide at neutral pH values, a constant "charge-to-mass ratio" in other words, and usually have the same shape and so are separated exclusively on the basis of their molecular weight.

The average pore size of polyacrylamide gels cast at 5% to 10% concentrations is also comparable to the effective diameters of many globular (relatively compact) proteins of 15,000 to 250,000 D. These gels will filter such solutions, separating proteins on the basis of *both* size and mobility.[6,7]

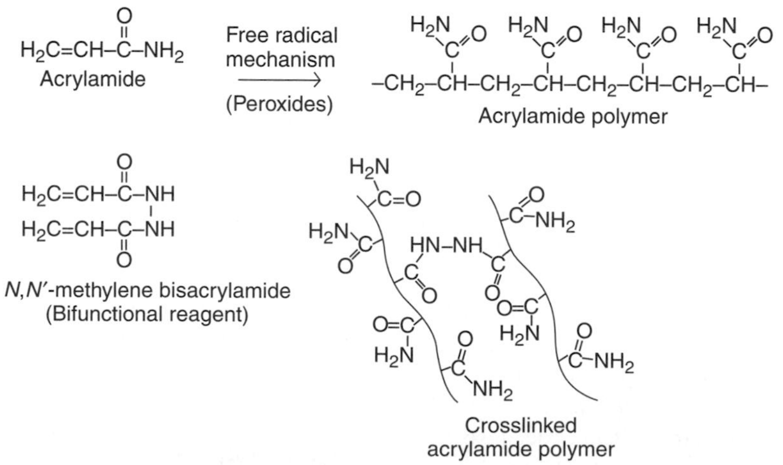

Fig. 10-4 Polyacrylamide gels are produced by polymerizing a mixture of acrylamide and a bifunctional (crosslinking) acrylamide derivative. Derivative shown is that in common use.

The molecular sieving effects can produce enhanced resolution, that is, narrower zones of macromolecules, as well.

ENHANCED-RESOLUTION TECHNIQUES
Discontinuous Buffers

Several electrophoretic techniques employ a system in which different buffer cations or anions are placed along the electrophoretic path on either side of the protein zone. The mobilities are different for each ion. If the ionic species placed before and the species placed after a mixture of high-molecular-weight substances, proteins, for example, have suitable mobilities, the proteins become *stacked* between the two ions. If a series of proteins are electrophoresed in this discontinuous buffer system, they will arrange themselves according to their effective mobilities and become concentrated, resulting in a much greater (enhanced) resolution. Simply diluting the analyte with water or an organic solvent such as acetonitrile can produce **stacking**.[5]

There are three major applications of the use of **discontinuous solvent** systems to produce enhanced resolution: **isotachophoresis, disk electrophoresis,** and **isoelectric focusing.** These techniques, briefly described in Table 10-1, are used frequently to analyze proteins.

Separations Based on Molecular Size

By enabling separations on the basis of molecular size and molecular charge, the techniques briefly described in Table 10-2 provide enhanced separation ability. They usually employ polyacrylamide or agarose to prepare gels of known pore size. Molecules of smaller molecular size electrophorese faster than larger molecules carrying similar charges. Sieving effects are also produced using linear (uncrosslinked) polyacrylamide; linear polyacrylamide is used in DNA sequencing by capillary electrophoresis.[5]

Electrophoresis of such substances is sometimes used analytically to estimate molecular weights from how far a given substance moves, compared to how far substances of known molecular weight ("standards") move under the same conditions.

SELECTION OF METHODS AND CONDITIONS

Knowledge of the **isoelectric point** and the molecular weight of the compound to be examined can help determine the optimum conditions for an electrophoretic separation. A buffer should be chosen with a pH that will provide the maximum separation without destroying the properties of the sample. Very acidic or basic conditions pose problems for

TABLE 10-1   ENHANCED-RESOLUTION TECHNIQUES

Technique	Physical Basis	Mechanism	Effect	Limitations	Advantages and Uses
Isotachophoresis	**Electrical neutrality**; current in series circuit is constant.[8,9] Lower conductivity solution after higher conductivity solution must move at same velocity and carry same current, and so the two solutions experience different voltages and adjust in concentraton.	Solution of lower conductivity containing ion of lower mobility running behind solution of higher conductivity containing higher mobility ion (e.g., chloride); ion of intermediate mobility (e.g., protein) sandwiched between; concentration of protein increases to carry same current as lower and higher mobility ions.	Intermediate-mobility ions (e.g., proteins) stack in thin concentrated zones and move in discrete zones.	Ions not separated; resolution not as good as disk electrophoresis.	No widespread clinical applications currently.
Disk Electrophoresis	Effective mobilities of some ions are pH dependent; it is often used with polyacrylamide gels.[10]	As above, then stacked proteins overrun by following ion because of pH change; change in pH produced using counterion.	Proteins, now in thin zones, migrate independently.	Ion systems and pH values limited; technically more exacting than ordinary electrophoresis	High sensitivity and resolving power; used extensively to separate proteins, mostly as research tool.
Isoelectric Focusing[11,12]	Migration of ions must occur in both directions; amphoteric ions (with both basic and acid groups) have zero effective mobility and zero net charge at their isoelectric point.	Ion movement stops because of zero counterion concentration, leaving all ions stacked in pH gradient; leading and trailing ions are an acid and a base.	Proteins in zones at isoelectric (isoionic) points; pH gradient is buffered by carrier **ampholytes**.	More complicated and exacting than ordinary electrophoresis.	High capacity and resolution to 0.001 pH unit possible;[12] primarily a research tool.

TABLE 10-2   USE OF SUPPORTING MEDIA IN SEPARATION

Method	Principle	Effect	Limitations	Advantages and Uses
Separation Based on Molecular Size				
Gradient gels[7,11]	Gels cast with increasing gel concentrations going from origin to end of gel have gradient of pore sizes.	Larger macromolecules move more slowly as they encounter higher gel concentrations; can measure relative sizes and charges.	Difficult to reproduce gels	Research tool
Gels containing denaturants[6,7,11]	Gels cast with denaturants (e.g., urea or SDS) so that macromolecules migrate in denatured forms; SDS binds uniformly and in large amounts to most proteins.	Proteins in SDS and oligonucleotides migrate inversely to subunit molecular weights or number of nucleotides.	Exacting technique; disulfide bonds in proteins must be broken; not all proteins behave normally	Research tool
Separations Based on Molecular Size and Charge				
Gel electrophoresis[6,7,11]	Pore size is small enough to restrict diffusion.	Higher resolution.	Reproducibility	Better resolution than cellulose acetate; agarose gels widely used; mostly research tool
Immunoelectrophoretic methods (see Chapter 12)	Antigen and antibody are brought together using electrophoresis to form precipitate.	Can identify and quantitate specific antigen or antibody.	Sensitivity somewhat low	Limited (e.g., *rocket immunoelectrophoresis*) clinical use
Two-dimensional electrophoresis[6,7,11]	Separation occurs according to one parameter (e.g., isoelectric point) in one dimension (direction) and then according to a second parameter (e.g., size) at right angles.	Mixture of proteins spread over a surface; information proportional to square of length of side of surface.[7,13]	Exacting technique; difficult to reproduce patterns	High information content; widely used in clinical research

SDS, *Sodium dodecyl sulfate.*

TABLE 10-3   COMMON EFFECTS OF ELECTROPHORETIC VARIABLES ON SEPARATION

Variable	Effect on Electrophoresis
pH	Changes charge of analyte and hence effective mobility; can affect structure of analyte, such as denaturing or dissociating a protein.
Ionic strength	Changes voltage or current; increased ionic strength usually reduces migration velocity and increases heating.
Ions present	Can change migration velocity if interaction is strong; can cause tailing of bands.
Current	Too high a current causes overheating.
Voltage	Migration velocity is proportional to voltage.
Temperature	Temperature gradients in support mediums cause bowed bands. Overheating can denature (precipate) proteins. Lower temperatures reduce diffusion but also reduce migration velocity; there is no effect on resolution.
Time	Separation of bands (resolution) increases linearly with time, but dilution of bands (diffusion) increases with the square root of time.
Medium	Major factors are endosmosis and pore-size effects, which affect migration velocities.

any system, because an increasing fraction of the current is carried by protons or hydroxyl ions, resulting in poorer separation. A summary of the effects of the various variables on electrophoresis is provided in Table 10-3.

Support Media

The choice of a supporting medium is based on many considerations. Slabs or sheets are useful when comparing different samples, and routine clinical electrophoresis is done using sheet supports. Thin-layer methods provide greater sensitivity (see later discussion). Gel cylinders are sometimes used in isoelectric focusing.

Paper and cellulose acetate. Paper is especially favored for separation of low-molecular-weight substances in specialized biochemical laboratories. The main advantages of these materials are their thinness and mechanical strength. A thinner support means greater sensitivity because less material is needed to produce a detectable spot or zone. In a thicker support, the same amount of sample in a zone is distributed in a greater volume and so is more dilute and hence harder to detect. Otherwise, more sample must be applied to a thicker support for equal ease of detection. Use of thinner supports means smaller samples and less material is electrophoresed. This is advantageous if little sample is available, although this is not usually the situation in clinical laboratories.

Cellulose acetate is prepared by treating cellulose with acetic anhydride. This puts acetyl groups on the sugar hydroxyl groups. The resulting material is pressed into sheets that are somewhat stronger than paper and a good deal more chemically uniform. Adsorption of material to groups in paper leads to losses of material and to *tailing* of zones. Cellulose acetate is more inert in this respect, and because of its uniformity and ease of preparation (the strips are merely soaked in electrophoresis buffer so that no air is trapped), it is very widely used in routine clinical work.

Cellulose acetate sheets can be purchased in relatively uniform batches so that results of different electrophoresis experiments are more consistent. After electrophoresis, the strips can be sliced into bands containing stained or radioactive materials. These slices can be dissolved in a solvent such as acetone for easy quantitation.

On the other hand, resolution with cellulose acetate is not as good as with polyacrylamide. (see later discussion). Eight or nine serum protein fractions can be resolved using cellulose acetate, but up to 30 fractions can be detected using disk electrophoresis on polyacrylamide gels.[11] So cellulose acetate is used because it lends itself to fast, easy, reproducible measurements, though of comparatively low resolution.

Gels. Gels can be cast with varying thicknesses to increase or decrease capacity (the amount of sample). Gels also offer the possibility of molecular sieving effects because their porosity can be controlled by changing their composition. On the other hand, their mechanical strength tends to be low.

Starch and agar. Starch gels are not as extensively used as agarose, acrylamide, or even Sephadex. The starch solution must be heated to 100° C, degassed, an awkward process, and then cast. The starch gels tend to provide greater resolution than agar or agarose does. However, the inconvenience of preparing starch gels has limited their use.

Agar and agarose (agar without the agaropectin) are easier to handle. Because agarose demonstrates a lower electro-osmotic effect and exhibits fewer problems with adsorption, it is preferred over agar. The pore size of agarose is much greater than that of polyacrylamide. This is the reason why agar or agarose is used in most immunoelectrophoretic techniques, because antigen and antibody must be able to migrate freely through the gel. Another advantage of agarose is that it may be poured after reheating to only about 50° C; thus some proteins, such as antibodies, can be mixed in without denaturing. Even so, the same disadvantages encountered when preparing starch gels are encountered when preparing agar and agarose gels. Precast agarose gels for a variety of separations are available commercially. These gels are used for separation of isoenzymes, hemoglobins, glycoproteins, and so on.

Polyacrylamide. Polyacrylamide gels are less frequently used in clinical laboratories but are a common research tool. They are clear, fairly easy to prepare, and exhibit reasonable mechanical strength over the acrylamide concentration range normally employed for proteins. In addition, they show a low endosmosis effect and have a pore size well suited for the separation of average proteins, ribonucleic acid (RNA) molecules, and smaller restriction fragments of DNA. A major clinical use of polyacrylamide gels is the separation of alkaline phosphatase isoenzymes. However, polyacrylamide gel preparation and casting are somewhat more exacting and time consuming, and reproducibility of gel preparation is difficult to achieve. It is now possible to buy commercially prepared polyacrylamide sheets from several firms.

Use of acrylamide substituted with ionizable groups that buffer at or near the isoelectric points of proteins to be separated greatly enhances the **resolving power** of isoelectric focusing. These substituted acrylamides produce what are called "immobilized pH gradient" gels.[12]

Capillary electrophoresis. Considerable attention is directed toward developing capillary electrophoresis techniques for clinical work. The actual or potential advantages of these techniques are the low volumes of buffers required, very low amounts of analyte (nanoliters) used, ease of changing conditions (buffer, pH, technique) and low cost, because the techniques tend to be easy to set up and fast. The greater speed of capillary electrophoresis separations derives from more efficient cooling of capillary tubes, enabling much greater voltages to be applied; some polymerase chain reaction (PCR)–amplified DNA fragments have been separated in seconds.[5] Even uncharged substances can be separated by electrophoresing micelles of charged detergents. The uncharged analytes partition into the interiors of the moving micelles to varying extents. This technique is called *micellar electrokinetic chromatography.*

Capillary electrophoresis must be done serially, one sample at a time. However, multicapillary instruments (currently up to 96 capillaries) are now available, so much higher sample throughput can be achieved. The major limitation is still sensitivity, because of both the very low amounts of analyte electrophoresed and the very short (0.003 to 0.006 cm) optical path lengths across 50- or 100-μm diameter capillaries. Direct observations of analytes as they migrate past an absorbance detector are possible if the analytes of interest have high extinction coefficients; otherwise a variety of techniques, some quite ingenious, for increasing sensitivity are employed. These techniques include the use of fluorescence analysis or electrospray ionization mass spectrometry (MS), prior concentration of samples using stacking, ultrafiltration, or adsorbents, and so on.[5]

Currently capillary electrophoresis in multicapillary devices is the method of choice for DNA sequencing, replacing slab gel electrophoresis. Several fold increases in sample throughput owing to shorter electrophoresis times are achieved. As of July 2001, the FDA had approved the Bio-Rad Bio-Focus 2000 and the Beckman-Coulter Paragon CZE 2000 capillary electrophoresis apparatuses for serum protein separations. The Paragon has seven capillaries, and is also approved for analysis of proteins in urine and analysis of serum proteins for monoclonal antibodies using an immunofixation method. The immunofixation method is described in reference 5.

Electroblotting. An exception to the requirement that a supporting medium not interact with the material being separated is the **Western blot** technique, a kind of **electro-blot**.[14] In this technique a gel slab containing separated proteins is electrophoresed perpendicularly to the slab, with transferal of some or all of the separated proteins onto a facing sheet of material, often nitrocellulose, which adsorbs the proteins (see Fig. 12-4). The sheet may be stained for protein or enzyme activity (see later discussion). Usually, however, the sheet is washed with some neutral protein, such as milk protein or bovine serum albumin, to block unoccupied adsorption sites. Then the locations of specific transferred adsorbed proteins are determined, usually by immunochemical assays. The resulting pattern may be compared with the original slab that is stained or examined by autoradiography for all proteins or all labeled proteins.

A major virtue of Western blots is their sensitivity. (The adsorption *concentrates* the proteins.) Adsorption of antigens or antibodies takes place at concentrations of antigen and antibody that are far too low for a precipitate to form. As little as 10^{-12} g/mm^2 of protein can be detected and hence identified.[7,14] Consequently, antigens (and antibodies) in serum that are present at very low concentrations can be detected and even quantitated. This technique is used for detecting the antigens and antibodies in patients infected with the human immunodeficiency virus (HIV).[15]

Electrochromatography. Originally, interactions between support media and analytes were minimized. However, because the aim is to produce separations of analytes, and because interactions with the support media can sometimes assist separation, increasing attention has been directed to purposefully producing and using support media in which analyte-media interactions are important. This field is called **electrochromatography**, and differs from conventional chromatography in that analyte movement through the chromatographic matrix is produced by an electrical field rather than by hydrostatic pressure.

Conditions

Horizontal versus vertical position. Electrophoresis can be performed horizontally or vertically; there is no theoretical reason for preferring one or the other procedure. Horizontal electrophoresis places less mechanical stress on the support, whereas vertical electrophoresis supporting media are often supported between glass plates.

If horizontal electrophoresis is used and the surface of the medium is open to air, evaporation of the solvent can cause problems. As a result of evaporation, salt concentrations rise, usually unevenly along the support, leading to nonuniform current flow and heating. This can lead to problems of uneven migration, especially at the sides of a horizontal, flat electrophoresis bed. "Submarine" electrophoresis is horizontal electrophoresis in which the support is covered with buffer solution so that there is no evaporation from the support. The sample is inserted into slots or holes in the support and electrophoresed through the support. If one buffer reservoir is higher than the other, convective flow of the buffer through the supporting medium may occur. Therefore the electrophoresis apparatus should always be level.

Sample application. Sometimes samples are simply applied to the surface of the supporting medium and allowed to soak in. Sometimes special slots or holes are cast or cut in a gel. Often the sample is layered onto the surface of a gel. The sample is then usually made denser than the solvent by the addition of sucrose or glycerol. Occasionally the sample may be polymerized into the gel or cast with the gel. Injection of the sample is rarely used, except with isotachophoresis. In capillary zone electrophoresis, a very small quantity (a few microliters) of the sample may be electrophoresed into the capillary tube. Commercial sample applicators can simultaneously apply a desired number of 1 or 2 μL samples of, for example, blood serum to the support surfaces; such devices help ensure greater uniformity of the initial sample zone shapes and sizes, improving reproducibility of results in clinical laboratories. If electrophoresis takes place in stages (as in two-dimensional electrophoresis), the gel containing part or all of the sample may be cut out and reattached, sometimes with an agarose "glue," to another gel for the next stage in the separation. All the above techniques are equally valid when combined with the appropriate type of assay.

Current and voltage considerations. Electrophoresis can be carried out at constant voltage, constant current, or constant power. Selection of any of these modes often depends on the power supply available. Because diffusion increases with the square root of time, it is best to complete the electrophoresis as quickly as possible. This requires use of the maximum voltage. However, the maximum voltage is always limited by the efficiency of cooling of the apparatus. Some workers claim that temperature gradients of more than 0.1° C across a gel or other support lead to noticeable distortions of macromolecule zones. For some current clinical applications, temperature control does not appear to be necessary, and separations are carried out at ambient temperatures.

Use of thinner supports (or capillaries) is now widespread because the temperature gradients that form are smaller because of the more efficient heat dissipation possible from thinner supports. This means higher voltages can be applied, producing faster separations and consequently less diffusion and clearer, sharper separation patterns. Also, more samples can be electrophoresed in a given time, an important consideration in routine clinical work. DNA-sequencing gels are about 1 mm thick. Such thin supports are very fragile and so require very careful handling. Plastic sheets are used as backing for commercial agarose or polyacrylamide supports to enable them to be used in routine clinical work.

Several commercial electrophoresis systems employ a very efficient cooling system and very thin, preformed agarose gels to perform high-voltage electrophoresis. By using 1000 to 2000 V instead of 100 V, the electrophoresis can be completed in 2 to 3 minutes instead of 20 minutes. This approach maximizes the efficiency of the electrophoretic system in time and resolution. Capillary zone electrophoresis employs voltages of 300 to 400 V/cm, resulting in electrophoresis times of often less than 10 minutes.

The conductivity of any electrophoretic system changes with time because of heating and because the ionic composition changes as a result of movement (electrophoresis) of the sample along the system. Such changes are minimal in continuous systems, such as high-voltage paper electrophoresis, and application of constant voltage is satisfactory for these systems. For disc electrophoresis and isotachophoresis, a constant velocity of zone migration is desired, and a constant current is used. For isoelectric focusing, heating is usually the limiting factor (see earlier discussion), and so constant power (wattage) should be used.[6] Pulsed power supplies provide for routine separations.[16]

Separation time. In the case of isotachophoresis, the electrophoresis is stopped when the trailing ion emerges. Isoelectric focusing is complete after the gradient is formed and the current has dropped to a stable value. The time to stop a disk or ordinary zone electrophoretic separation is usually indicated by the position of the *tracking dye,* usually when the dye band reaches a predetermined position in the stationary support (typically the end of the support). Dyes that have high mobilities, such as bromophenol blue, are employed. They are usually added to the sample. Because some proteins bind such dyes, their apparent mobilities may be changed.

LOCATING THE ANALYTE
Direct Observation

Direct observation of analytes is often employed in capillary electrophoresis. Commercial capillary zone electrophoresis apparatuses use microfocused optics to enable direct measurement of separated substances inside the capillary tube as they migrate past the light beam. With direct measurement, the patterns of separated substances must be obtained one at a time. Direct observation may be done when separating DNA molecules in gels in the presence of a fluorescent intercalating agent such as ethidium bromide. Otherwise, the practice is to physically remove the support from the apparatus after completion of the separation to determine the distribution of the analyte(s) on the support.

This can be accomplished by measurement of a physical property of a molecule, such as light absorption or refractive index, or by use of a chemical reaction such as staining. Measurements of physical properties may lack specificity, sensitivity, or resolution. For example, not all proteins absorb strongly at 280 nm.

Use of shorter wavelengths (such as 200 nm), at which most compounds absorb more strongly, improves the sensitivity of direct measurement at the cost of possible interference from other absorbing substances.

Staining

Staining of the support is routinely employed, because it often achieves the desired goals of resolution, sensitivity, specificity, and speed (Table 10-4). Because the zones of material broaden by diffusion after electrophoresis is stopped, the first step in the analytical procedure is to eliminate diffusion. This can be done in paper electrophoresis by drying the paper or in autoradiography by drying or freezing the gels. In routine clinical electrophoresis, supports are usually dried in an oven before measurement.

Proteins

Protein in gels is often denatured (i.e., precipitated in the gel matrix) by soaking the gels in dilute acetic acid or more effectively in trichloroacetic acid. Addition of sulfosalicylic acid further improves the denaturing ability of the staining solution. In the Western blot procedure, the proteins are immobilized by adsorption.

Sometimes heat must also be applied to make the proteins insoluble. However, some resist denaturation by all these conventional procedures and remain soluble in the stain. If detergents such as **sodium dodecyl sulfate (SDS)** or other soluble agents are present, they will interfere with precipitation. Inclusion of methanol in the acid solutions helps remove such substances before staining.

Choice of Stain

Many types of stains are employed, depending on the need. Sometimes it is desirable to stain everything, such as all proteins. A dye called *Stains-All* is suitable.[17] A *silver stain*, which reacts with both proteins and nucleic acids, is an alternative.[18] Proteins, after electrophoresis on cellulose acetate, are most often stained with Ponceau S.[7]

Stains and staining procedures are often specific for one chemical group. The ninhydrin (triketohydrindene hydrate) stain for amino groups, often used after paper electrophoresis of peptides or amino acids, is an example of this. Glycoproteins can be treated with periodic acid (for oxidation) and

TABLE 10-4 COMMONLY USED STAINS FOR VARIOUS SUBSTANCES

Substance	Stain	Comments
Proteins	Ponceau S.[7]	About one tenth as sensitive as Coomassie, but more specific for proteins; the most widely used stain; reversible
	Bromophenol blue[19]	About one fifth the sensitivity of Coomassie, but can be used with ampholyte gels
	Light green SF[19]	
	Coomassie brilliant blue R250[7]	Can detect less than 0.2 µg of protein; can be used with ampholyte gels
	Silver stain (silver reduced onto oxidized macromolecules)[18]	50 to 100 times more sensitive than Coomassie; different proteins give different colors, for unknown reasons
	Stains-All (a cationic carbocyanine dye)[17]	General sensitivity, including phosphoproteins
	Amino black 10B ("buffalo black")[7]	About one-fifth as sensitive as Coomassie
	India ink[7]	About 20-fold more sensitive than Coomassie; slow
	Colloidal gold[7]	About 500 fold more sensitive than Coomassie, most sensitive stain currently available; used with Western blots;[14] slow
Lipoproteins	Sudan black B[20]	
	Oil red O[20]	
	Coomassie brilliant blue R250[7]	Used with SDS (sodium dodecyl sulfate) gels
Glycoproteins	PAS (periodic acid-Schiff)[21]	Best for neutral glycoproteins; 40 ng of carbohydrate detectable using dansyl hydrazine (fluorescence)
	Stains-All[17]	Best for sialic acid-rich glycoproteins, and mucopolysaccharides
Nucleic acids	Stains-All[17]	Best for RNA, DNA
	Silver stain[17,18]	2 to 5 times more sensitive than ethidium bromide
	Ethidium bromide[22]	Fluorescent bands with DNA; less than 10 ng detectable
	TOTO-1[22]	Fluorescent bands with DNA; 4 pg detectable; binds to ssDNA and RNA
Enzymes		
Dehydrogenases	NADH (fluorescence)[23]	
	Nitroblue tetrazolium chloride[23]	
Esterases	β-naphthyl esters and tetrazotized o-dianisidine[23]	
Cholinesterases		
Phosphatases	1-Naphthyl phosphate and fast blue B[23]	

Note: The sensitivity factors given are averages, different proteins will stain with different intensities with any stain.

color developed with a dye (fuchsin) in the presence of a reducing agent (sulfite). This periodic acid-Schiff stain treatment oxidizes carbohydrate groups to aldehydes, which react with the dye to form a Schiff base. The sulfite reduces the Schiff base, making the stain permanent. There is also a specific stain for phosphoproteins. [17] (See Table 10-4 for a list of commonly used stains.)

Once the stain has been introduced, usually by soaking the support in the stain solution, excess stain must be removed. This can be done electrophoretically or, most commonly, by diffusion. Electrophoretic removal is fast but can result in distortion of the stained zones. Diffusion involves changing the solvent or using a destainer to remove free stain.

Many enzymes are identified by the use of colored or fluorescent substrates or products (zymograms), even in gels or other support media. For example, alkaline phosphatase hydrolyzes *p*-nitrophenylphosphate to *p*-nitrophenol, which has a yellow color at pH 8. Soaking a gel in such assay solutions produces colored bands where the enzymes are. If the product of enzymatic activity is of low molecular weight, rapid diffusion of the product may broaden the zone, making location of the enzyme or identification of the isozyme

difficult. Products that form polymers or insoluble substances are better, but if this is not possible, a contact print method may be used.[11] A sheet of paper or other material is impregnated with a chromophoric substrate and pressed against the support containing the separated enzyme or enzymes. Often the support is cut into slices, and the slices are incubated in assay solution. A list of such zymograms is given in the article by Heeb and Gabriel[23]; see also reference 22.

Other Localization Techniques

A common technique for localization of proteins and nucleic acids employs radioactive labels, such as iodine-125 or carbon-14, incorporated into the macromolecules. After electrophoresis, a piece of x-ray film is placed in contact with the stationary support in the dark for 12 to 24 hours. After the film is developed, a dark area corresponding to the position of the radioactively labeled macromolecule will be present. This technique, autoradiography, is commonly employed in the Western blot technique for proteins and also is used in the **Southern blot** technique for nucleic acids (see Chapter 48).

TABLE 10-5   COMMONLY ENCOUNTERED PROBLEMS IN ELECTROPHORESIS

Problem	Likely Cause	Corrective Action
No migration	Instrument not connected	Check electrical circuits.
	Wrong pH; electrodes connected backwards	Check isoelectric point of protein and pH of buffer; check electrode polarity.
Bowed electrophoretic pattern on edges of support	Overheating or drying out of support	Humidity chamber; check buffer ionic strength; reduce wattage.
Tailing of bands	Chemical reaction: subunit dissociation or adsorption to support; precipitate in sample	Use different support; try different pH; centrifuge or filter sample first.
	Salt in sample	Check sample for salt; dialyze sample against electrophoresis buffer.
	Buffer coion effect	Use different buffer coion.
Holes in staining pattern	Analyte present in too high a concentration	Apply less concentrated sample.
Very thin, sharp bands	Molecular weight of sample very high for support pore size	Use support with larger pore size.
	Sulfhydryl oxidation and aggregation	Run sample with sulfhydryl reducing compound or at lower pH.
Very slow migration	High molecular weight	Use support with larger pore size.
	Low charge	Change pH so that charge increases.
	Ionic strength too high	Check conductivity; dilute buffer.
	Voltage too low	Increase voltage.
Sample precipitates in support	pH too high or low	Run at different pH.
	Too much heating	Use lower wattage or external cooling.

Some commonly encountered problems in electrophoresis, their most likely causes, and suggested corrective action are listed in Table 10-5.

CLINICAL APPLICATIONS

For clinical research, high sensitivity of detection of analyte, high resolution of adjacent zones of analyte, and high reproducibility of separations are required. For routine clinical work, some resolution and sensitivity of detection are sacrificed for speed or throughput; reproducibility remains important but is ensured by frequent use of comparison samples from healthy people.

The most common uses of electrophoretic techniques in the laboratory today are the following:

1. Specific protein electrophoresis
2. Quantitative analysis of specific serum protein classes, such as gamma globulins and albumin (see Chapters 49 and 27, respectively)
3. Identification and quantitation of hemoglobin and its subclasses (see Chapter 36)
4. Identification of monoclonal proteins in either serum or urine (see Chapter 49)
5. Separation and quantitation of major lipoprotein and lipid classes (see Chapters 33 and 53)
6. Isoenzyme analysis: separation and quantitation of enzymes such as creatine kinase, lactate dehydrogenase, and alkaline phosphatase into their respective molecular subtypes (see Chapters 31 and 55)
7. Immunoelectrophoresis: most often used to determine qualitatively the elevation or deficiency of specific classes of immunoglobulins; also can be used to semiquantitate serum proteins, such as transferrin and complement component C3 (see Chapter 12)
8. Western blot technique to identify a specific protein: used to confirm the presence of antibodies to human immunodeficiency virus (HIV) (see Chapter 12)
9. Southern blot techniques to identify specific nucleic acid sequences (DNA or RNA) (see Chapter 48): used for prenatal diagnosis of inborn errors, diagnosis of viral infections, and identification of risk factors for cancer (see Chapter 49)

Two-dimensional techniques may replace some of the preceding procedures, but at this time more attention is directed to capillary electrophoresis. All the procedures involve measurement of alterations in an electrophoretic pattern compared with a normal control. These procedures can often be used to diagnose specific diseases[5,24] (Fig. 10-5). Nephrotic syndrome, for example, may be accompanied by a decrease of more than 25% in alpha$_2$ globulin levels and a decrease of up to 25% in gamma globulin levels because of the loss of lower molecular weight proteins in the urine. The pattern of decrease or increase in

TABLE 10-6 COMPOUNDS COMMONLY SEPARATED BY ELECTROPHORESIS

Class of Compound	Stain	Support Medium
Amino acid	Ninhydrin	Paper, cellulose acetate
Serum protein	Ponceau S	Cellulose acetate
	Coomassie blue R250	Polyacrylamide (with or without isoelectric focusing)
Lipoproteins	Oil red O	Agarose
Glycoproteins	Periodic acid-Schiff	Agarose
Nucleic acids	Ethidium bromide (fluorescent)	Agarose
Hemoglobins	Silver stain	
	o-Dianisidine	Cellulose acetate, agar
	Ferricyanide	
	Peroxide	
Isoenzymes		
Lactate dehydrogenase	Fluorescent NADH or tetrazolium	Agarose
Creatine kinase	Fluorescent NADH or tetrazolium	Agarose
Alkaline phosphatase	1-Naphthylphosphate + Fast blue B or 5-bromo-4-chloroindolyl phosphate	Polyacrylamide, cellulose acetate
Immunoglobulins	Coomassie blue R250	Agarose
Specific antigens by immunological electrophoretic techniques (such as Laurell rocket)	Amido black 10B	Agarose

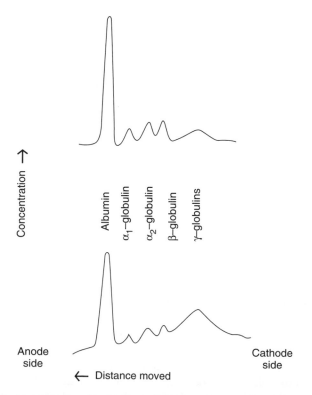

Fig. 10-5 Example of effect of disease, hepatic cirrhosis, on serum protein electrophoretic pattern. *Upper profile,* distribution characteristic of healthy people.

several disease conditions is fairly characteristic, and hence quantitation of stained cellulose acetate strips is useful in diagnosis.

The stained support may be either put through a strip scanner if the support is a strip or put through a modified spectrophotometer (*densitometer*) if it is not. Cellulose acetate supports must sometimes be "cleared," made more transparent, before analysis by **densitometry**. This result is achieved by soaking the support in a solvent. With due care, the dye absorbance on the support is a good measure of the amount of protein. With cellulose acetate electrophoresis, normal serum is electrophoresed next to the serum to be tested. The plots of absorbance (color) versus distance obtained from a strip scanner (see Fig. 10-5) allow immediate comparison of relative amounts of each class of separated proteins. Routine clinical electrophoresis such as of serum samples can be done by use of highly automated instruments. Several companies sell such equipment, such as Beckman, Ciba-Corning, and Helena Laboratories.

Use of electrophoretic techniques that provide higher resolution will increase diagnostic capabilities, but physicians will have to be trained to interpret the increased information.

Electrophoresis is sometimes used in assays of genetic defects. The two-dimensional techniques now being developed have tremendous potential in that area. Table 10-6 lists compounds normally separated by electrophoresis.

References

1. Van Holde KE: *Physical biochemistry,* ed 2, Englewood Cliffs, NJ, 1985, Prentice-Hall.
2. Moore WJ: *Physical chemistry,* ed 4, Englewood Cliffs, NJ, 1970, Prentice-Hall.
3. Tanford C: *Physical chemistry of macromolecules,* New York, 1961, Academic Press.
4. Mosher RA, Saville DA, Thormann W: *The dynamics of electrophoresis,* Weinheim, Germany, 1992, VCH.
5. Peterson JR, Mohammad AA: *Clinical and forensic applications of capillary electrophoresis,* Totowa, NJ, 2001, Humana Press.
6. Hawcroft DM: *Electrophoresis: the basics,* Oxford, UK, 1997, Oxford University Press.
7. Dunn MJ: *Gel electrophoresis: proteins,* Oxford, UK, 1993, Bios Scientific.
8. Ornstein L: Disc electrophoresis, *Ann NY Acad Sci* 121:321, 1964.
9. Brewer JM, Ashworth RB: Disc electrophoresis, *J Chem Educ* 46:41, 1969.
10. Chrambach A, Jovin TM: Selected buffer systems for moving boundary electrophoresis on gels at various pH values, presented in simplified manner, *Electrophoresis* 4:190, 1983.
11. Andrews AT: *Electrophoresis: theory, techniques, and biochemical and clinical applications,* ed 2, New York, 1986, Oxford University Press.
12. Righetti PG: *Immobilized pH gradients, theory and methodology,* Amsterdam, 1990, Elsevier.
13. Adams LD, Gallagher S: *Two-dimensional gel electrophoresis using the O'Farrell system.* In Ausubel et al, editors: *Current protocols in molecular biology, Unit 10.4,* New York, 1991, Greene Publishing and Wiley Interscience.
14. Sasse J, Gallagher SR: *Detection of proteins on blot transfer membranes.* In Ausubel et al, editors: *Current protocols in molecular biology, Unit 10.7,* New York, 1991 Greene Publishing and Wiley Interscience.
15. Gallagher S et al: *Immunoblotting and immunodetection.* In Ausubel et al, editors: *Current protocols in molecular biology, Unit 10.8,* New York, 1991, Greene Publishing and Wiley Interscience.
16. Allington RW, Nelson JW, Aron GG: *ISCO applications research bulletin,* no 18, Lincoln, NE, 1975, Instrumentation Specialties (ISCO).
17. Cutting JA: Gel protein stains: phosphoproteins, *Methods Enzymol* 104:451, 1984.
18. Merril CR: Gel-staining techniques, *Methods Enzymol* 182:477, 1990.
19. Righetti PG: *Isoelectric focusing: theory, methodology and application,* Amsterdam, 1983, Elsevier.
20. Mills GL, Lane PA, Weech PK: *A guidebook to lipoprotein techniques,* Amsterdam, 1984, Elsevier.
21. Gander JE: Gel protein stains: glycoproteins, *Methods Enzymol* 104:447, 1984.
22. Haughland RP: *Handbook of fluorescent probes and research chemicals,* Eugene, OR, 1996, Molecular Probes.
23. Heeb MJ, Gabriel O: Enzyme localization in gels, *Methods Enzymol* 104:416, 1984.
24. Annino JS, Giese RW: *Clinical chemistry, principles and procedures,* ed 4, Boston, 1976, Little, Brown.

Internet Sites

www.aesociety.org—The Electrophoresis Society
ntri.tamuk.edu/ce/ce.html—Capillary electrophoresis
www.chemsoc.org/chembytes/ezine/2000/altria_nov00.htm—Chemsoc website
www.ceandcec.com—Capillary electrophoresis and capillary electro-chromatography
web.ncifcrf.gov/events/ce_conference/program.asp
www-lecb.ncifcrf.gov/EP/Epemail.html—Two-dimensional gel electrophoresis databases
www.life.uiuc.edu/molbio/geldigest/electro.html—Gel electrophoresis of DNA
www.uct.ac.za/microbiology/sdspage.html—SDS polyacrylamide gel electrophoresis (SDS-PAGE)

www.nal.usda.gov/pgdic/Probe/v2n3/puls.html—Pulsed field electrophoresis for separation of large DNA
http://ntri.tamuk.edu/electrophoresis/home.html
http://www.ehs.berkeley.edu/pubs/helpsheets/04electro.html—Guidelines for the Safe Use of Electrophoresis Equipment, The Office of Environment, Health & Safety (EH&S), University of California Berkeley
http://www.bertholf.net/rlb/Lectures/index.htm
http://www.bertholf.net/rlb/Lectures/Lectures/Proteins%20and%20Electrophoresis.pps—PowerPoint lecture by Robert L. Bertholf, PhD, Associate Professor of Pathology, Chief of Clinical Chemistry and Toxicology

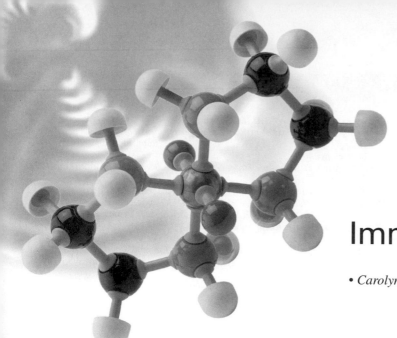

CHAPTER 11

Immunological Reactions

• *Carolyn S. Feldkamp*

Objectives

- Define antigen and antibody.
- List and explain eight factors affecting antigenicity.
- Describe the composition and structural differences of antibodies. Name five human immunoglobulins and describe the physiological role of each.
- List and explain the forces involved in antigen-antibody reactions and the factors that influence the specificity of immunochemical reactions.
- Outline the mechanism of the following antigen-antibody gel-precipitation reactions and state the principle of each: double immunodiffusion, radial immunodiffusion.

Key Terms

antibodies Proteins that combine specifically with antigens.

antibody affinity Measure of the binding strength of the antibody-antigen reaction.

antigenic determinant The portion of an antigen that reacts with antibody.

antigens Substances that induce an immune response.

avidity Measure of the binding strength of antibodies to multiple antigenic determinants on natural antigens.

B lymphocytes Lymphocytes that transform into plasma cells and produce antibodies.

constant region   C-terminus of light and heavy chains of antibodies, highly conserved. Not part of the antibody combining site.

cross-reactivity   Binding of an antibody to an antigen other than the one initiating the immune response.

Fab fragment   Portion of immunoglobulin molecule made by papain degradation and containing the antibody-combining site; composed of the light chain and a portion of the heavy chain.

Fc fragment   Portion of immunoglobulin molecule produced by papain degradation and containing most of the heavy chain (including the complement-binding site).

flocculation   A precipitation reaction producing large, loose precipitates.

hapten   Low-molecular-weight substance that can induce an immune response only when coupled to high-molecular-weight immunogenic molecules.

heavy (H) chain   Portion of immunoglobulin molecule consisting of a polypeptide chain of about 50,000 daltons.

hypervariable regions   Amino acid sequences in the variable region that have an increased likelihood of variation.

idiotype   Portion of immunoglobulin molecule conferring unique character, most often including its binding site.

immunodiffusion   Movement of antibody or antigen or both in a support medium from a region of high concentration to one of low concentration.

immunoelectrophoresis   An immunoprecipitation technique in which antigens are separated from each other by migration in an electric field, followed by reaction with antibody by immunodiffusion.

immunoglobulins (Ig)   Proteins with antibody activity.

joining (J) chain   Portion of IgM molecule possibly holding structure together.

lattice   The cross-linked, three-dimensional structure formed by the reaction of multivalent antigens with antibody.

light (L) chain   Portion of an immunoglobulin molecule composed of a polypeptide chain of about 22,000 daltons.

Ouchterlony technique   A version of the original gel diffusion technique invented by Oudin in which antigen and antibody in separate wells are allowed to spread (diffuse) toward each other.

plasma cells   Immunoglobulin-producing cells that are the end stage of B-cell differentiation.

precipitin reaction, or **precipitin line**   Also called an *immunoprecipitin*, this refers to the precipitation of antigens and antibodies in gels. Precipitin line is an insoluble complex formed by proteins; for antigens and antibodies, it occurs when their relative concentrations are approximately equivalent or optimal for lattice formation.

radial immunodiffusion (Mancini technique) Measurement of antigen concentration by allowing antigen to spread (by diffusion) into agarose containing the desired monospecific antibody. The area of the immunoprecipitin ring is proportional to antigen concentration.

rocket (Laurell) immunoelectrophoresis   Assay system in which the antigen, under the influence of an electric field, migrates into agarose-containing antibody, with a resultant immunoprecipitation reaction. The precipitin lines appear rocket-shaped.

secretory piece   Polypeptide chain attached to IgA (may participate in secretion into mucosal spaces).

valency   The effective number of antigenic determinants on an antigen molecule. Also sometimes used to describe the number of antibody-binding sites.

variable region   N-terminal portion of immunoglobulin light and heavy chains whose amino acid sequence can change; this region includes the antigen-combining site.

zone of equivalence   Region of antibody-antigen precipitin reaction in which concentrations of both reactants are equal.

Immunological reactions can occur between two types of substances, **antigens** and **antibodies.** This chapter examines these substances and the interactions between them.

ANTIGENS

Antigens, or **immunogens**, are defined as substances that induce an immune response. The immune response produced may be an antibody (humoral) response or the production of sensitized cells (cellular response). Usually both humoral and cellular responses are stimulated.

Factors Affecting Antigenicity

Many factors determine the antigenicity of a molecule. The nature and dosage of an antigen, the route of administration, the organism immunized, and the sensitivity of the detection method are important factors in the evaluation of antigenicity. Many other conditions must be satisfied for a molecule to be immunogenic. These conditions are discussed below.

Chemical nature. The first antigens investigated were bacteria and red blood cells that are complex macromolecular structures composed of many different proteins, carbohydrates, and lipids. Subsequent investigations have proved that immunogens are found in several chemical classes, including proteins, polysaccharides, glycolipids, nucleic acids, and polynucleotides.

Size. There is no absolute size requirement, but size is of considerable importance in determining the antigenicity of a molecule. The most potent immunogens are macromolecules with molecular weights greater than 100,000 daltons. The A and B polypeptide chains of insulin (2500 daltons) and of glucagon (3600 daltons) are immunogenic in guinea pigs. Nevertheless, most molecules with molecular weights less than 10,000 daltons are weakly immunogenic, if at all.

Haptens. Substances with low molecular weights can induce an immune response when coupled to higher-molecular-weight immunogenic carrier molecules. Such incomplete antigens, or **haptens**, do not elicit an immune response by themselves but do react with antibody. Many low-molecular-weight compounds have been shown to act as haptens, including monosaccharides, lipids, peptides, hormones such as adrenocorticotropic hormone and prostaglandins, toxins such as arsphenamide, and drugs such as barbiturates and sulfonamides.

Complexity. A molecule must exhibit a certain degree of chemical complexity to be antigenic. Synthetic amino acid homopolymers, composed of repeating units of a single amino acid, have been shown to be poor immunogens; copolymers of two or three amino acids are much better immunogens. Increasing immunogenicity follows increasing complexity. For example, the addition of aromatic amino acid residues such as tyrosine to synthetic amino acid copolymers increases their immunogenicity.

Antigenic determinants. The portion of an antigen involved in the reaction with an antibody is called an **antigenic determinant**, or *epitope.* An antigen may contain more than one type of antigenic determinant; the number of antigenic determinants per antigen varies with the size and complexity of the molecule (Fig. 11-1). The effective number of antigenic determinants on an antigen is its **valency.** This is the number of antibody molecules that can be bound to an antigen at the same time (see Fig. 11-1). Antibodies recognize the three-dimensional shape of an antigenic determinant (conformational antigenic determinant), as well as the basic amino acid structure (sequential antigenic determinant). An antigenic determinant sometimes comprises as few as four amino acid residues. The combining site of an antibody molecule reacts with an antigenic determinant in the complementary **lock-and-key** manner of protein-enzyme interactions. The affinity of an antibody for an antigenic determinant is directly proportional to the closeness of fit.

Conformation and accessibility. The tertiary structure or spatial folding of molecules is a significant factor in their immunogenicity. Antibodies to native proteins do not react with denatured molecules. They are directed primarily to conformational rather than sequential antigenic determinants.

In addition, accessibility or exposure to the environment is an important factor in determining immunogenicity. The terminal side chains of polysaccharides, the portions of a polysaccharide molecule that stick out from the main part of the molecule, are the most immunopotent regions of polysaccharide antigens. Accessibility of an antigen to the environment is related to the solubility of an antigen in aqueous medium. The more soluble an antigen is, the greater the probability that it will interact with an antibody. The influence of charge on immunogenicity may be a manifestation of accessibility. Charged or hydrophilic residues are more in contact with the environment than

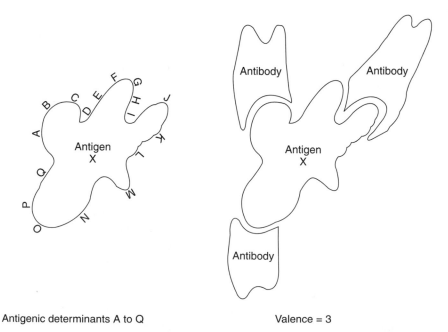

Antigenic determinants A to Q

Valence = 3

Fig. 11-1   Antigen X contains many different antigenic determinants, designated *A* to *Q* in this schematic representation. Antibody molecules when combined with antigen X bind to different sites. Maximum number of molecules of antibodies bound in this figure is 3; therefore, valence is 3.

hydrophobic residues, which tend to be sequestered in the interior of molecules.

Foreignness. The immune system is capable of distinguishing *self* from *nonself* in such a way that, under normal circumstances, a vigorous immune response is produced only to substances recognized as foreign. The more distant the evolutionary relationship between antigen and host, the more immunogenic the molecule. Thus guinea pig albumin will not evoke an immune response when injected into another guinea pig. The same guinea pig albumin will evoke a strong immune response, however, when injected into a different or more complex (higher) vertebrate, such as a rabbit or a monkey.

Genetics. It has recently been shown that the ability to recognize an antigen and the strength of the immune response produced may be under strict genetic control. Some strains of mice injected with synthetic polypeptides are capable of producing a vigorous immune response. Other mice, with closely related but nonidentical genetic backgrounds, may be poor responders or nonresponders.

In summary, many factors influence the immunogenicity of an antigen: chemical nature, size, molecular complexity, conformation, accessibility, foreignness, and genetics.

ANTIBODIES

The proteins that combine specifically with antigens are termed **antibodies.** Antibodies are produced by a subset of lymphocytes, called **B lymphocytes,** and by their progeny, **plasma cells.** B lymphocytes, through their production of antibodies, are responsible for the phenomenon of humoral immunity. Proteins with antibody activity are also called **immunoglobulins.** Immunoglobulins are an extremely heterogeneous group of molecules that constitute approximately 20% of the plasma proteins. Immunoglobulins are heterogeneous in their antigen-specificity, amino acid sequence, migration within an electrical field, and functions. There may be as many as 10,000 different molecules circulating in the human body that can be classified as immunoglobulins.

Structure

An important advance in the study of immunoglobulin structure came with the discovery that electrophoretically homogeneous proteins found in the serum of patients with multiple myeloma were structurally homogeneous and very closely related to normal immunoglobulin. Such myeloma proteins could be isolated in large quantities and chemically characterized. These studies produced an understanding of the precise structure of the antibody molecule.

H and L chains. Antibodies are glycoproteins composed of 82% to 96% polypeptide and 4% to 18% carbohydrate. All immunoglobulin molecules have a common structure of four polypeptide chains. Two identical large chains, or **heavy (H) chains,** and two identical small chains, or **light (L) chains,** are held together by noncovalent forces and covalent interchain disulfide bonds (Fig. 11-2).

The carbohydrate portion of the immunoglobulin molecule is covalently bound to amino acids in the polypeptide chains. The carbohydrates are usually found bound to the C-terminal half (Fc) of the molecule. Their function is poorly understood. They may be involved in transporting the molecule or protecting it from metabolic degradation.

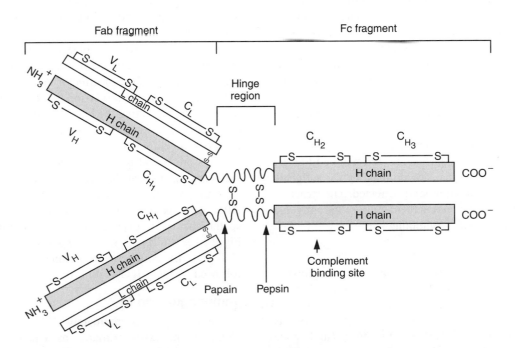

Fig. 11-2 Diagram of IgG molecule (immunoglobulin monomer). *H,* Heavy; *L,* light; *V,* variable region; *C,* constant region; *S—S,* disulfide bonds. *Arrows,* Papain and pepsin cleavage sites. *NH$_3^+$* indicates N-terminus, and *COO$^-$* indicates C-terminus of immunoglobulin.

Fab and Fc Fragments

Enzymatic digestion of immunoglobulin molecules has provided further evidence of their structure (see Fig. 11-2). Digestion with papain splits the molecule on the N-terminal side of the disulfide bonds, yielding three fragments of approximately equal size. Two of these fragments are identical and retain the antigen-binding capacity associated with an intact immunoglobulin molecule. The fragments with the antibody-combining site (**Fab fragments**) are each composed of an entire light chain and a portion of the heavy chain. The third fragment has no antigen-binding activity and is crystallizable (**Fc fragment).** The Fc fragment retains the other biological activities associated with immunoglobulin molecules: interaction with the complement system and binding to tissue. The Fc fragment is composed of the C-terminal half of the heavy chain.

Digestion with pepsin cleaves the antibody molecule on the C-terminal side of the disulfide bonds. This digestion results in the $F(ab')_2$ fragment composed of the two Fab fragments linked by disulfide bonds. The remainder of the molecule undergoes extensive degradation.

V and C Regions

Each polypeptide chain is composed of **domains**, or peptide sequences of uniform size (100 to 110 amino acid residues), that contain intrachain disulfide bonds. The domain of the N-terminal or antibody-combining site is more variable in its amino acid sequence than the rest of the polypeptide chain and is called the **variable region** (V region). The sequence and the spatial folding of the polypeptide chain are responsible for antibody specificity and affinity. The remainder of the polypeptide chain is composed of domains that are similar among immunoglobulin molecules of the same and other species. These domains are termed **constant regions** (C regions). Light chains are composed of one variable and one constant region (V_L and C_L). Heavy chains are composed of one variable and three or four constant regions (V_H and C_{H1-4}) (see Fig. 11-2).

The specific amino acid sequences of the variable regions of the light and heavy chains of an antibody molecule confer a unique three-dimensional structure to the antigen-binding potential antibody. These sequences are termed the **idiotype** of the molecule. The idiotype is determined by the antigenic determinant to which the antibody is directed. The structure of the idiotype permits the complementary fit of the antigenic determinant to the antibody-combining site.

Light-Chain Types

There are two types of light chains found in immunoglobulin molecules, kappa (κ) and lambda (λ). Kappa and lambda light chains differ in the amino acid sequence of their constant regions. A given antibody molecule always has two identical kappa light chains or two identical lambda light chains. An antibody molecule can never have both a kappa and a lambda light chain together. In human serum the ratio of kappa to lambda antibody molecules is approximately 2:1.

Heavy-Chain Types

Five types of heavy chains are distinguished in humans, based on structural differences in the constant regions of the chains. These structural differences permit functional differences. The heavy-chain types are designated gamma (γ), alpha (α), mu (μ), delta (δ), and epsilon (ε). The heavy-chain types vary in molecular weight. The gamma, alpha, and delta heavy chains are composed of three constant regions. The mu and epsilon heavy chains have four constant regions. The heavy-chain type determines the class of immunoglobulin. In humans there are five immunoglobulin classes, corresponding to the five heavy-chain types: immunoglobulin G (IgG), immunoglobulin A (IgA), immunoglobulin M (IgM), immunoglobulin D (IgD), and immunoglobulin E (IgE) (Table 11-1).

Some immunoglobulin classes have subclasses based on additional amino acid differences in their constant regions. IgG has four subclasses, and IgA and IgM each have two subclasses. The biological properties and concentrations of the subclasses may differ.

Immunoglobulin G

IgG molecules are monomers of the basic immunoglobulin subunit. They are composed of two kappa or two lambda light chains and two gamma heavy chains. IgG molecules may therefore be represented as $\gamma_2\lambda_2$ or $\gamma_2\kappa_2$. Approximately 75% of serum immunoglobulin is IgG. The frequency of IgG subclasses varies as follows: IgG_1, 60% to 70%; IgG_2, 14% to 20%; IgG_3, 4% to 8%; and IgG_4, 2% to 6%. There is evidence that antibodies to certain antigens may be restricted in their subclasses. Polysaccharide antigens tend to produce IgG_2 and IgG_4 antibodies. Antiviral and antinucleoprotein antibodies are found primarily in the IgG_1 and IgG_3 subclasses.

IgG molecules cross the placenta and are responsible for the immunological defense of the newborn. IgG molecules also fix to the surface of effector cells (T cells), which are then capable of antibody-mediated cytotoxic reactions important in protecting the host. IgG molecules bind or "fix" complement, a complex of serum proteins that assists in the lysis or elimination of foreign particles. Complement proteins are bound to the IgG molecule in the midpoint of the heavy chain, near the disulfide bond in the CH_2 domain. This area of increased flexibility is called the **hinge region.** After reaction with large antigens, this region undergoes spatial changes to expose the complement-binding site (see Fig. 11-2). Molecules in the IgG subclasses differ in their ability to fix complement proteins. IgG_3 is most active, followed by IgG_1, IgG_2, and IgG_4.

Immunoglobulin M

IgM constitutes approximately 10% of serum immunoglobulins and exists primarily as a pentamer of the basic immunoglobulin structure. The five immunoglobulin monomers are held in a circle by disulfide bonds between H chains of the subunits. In addition, the IgM molecule contains a polypeptide chain, called the **joining (J) chain,**

TABLE 11-1   PROPERTIES OF HUMAN IMMUNOGLOBULIN CLASSES

Properties	IgG	IgA	IgM	IgD	IgE
Heavy chain	γ	α	μ	δ	ϵ
Subclasses	1 to 4	1 and 2	1 and 2	None	None
Light chain	κ and λ	κ and λ	κ and λ	κ and λ	κ and λ
Form	Monomer	Monomer and dimer	Pentamer (some monomer may circulate)	Monomer	Monomer
Formula	$\gamma_2\kappa_2$ or $\gamma_2\lambda_2$	$\alpha_2\kappa_2$ or $\alpha_2\lambda_2$	$\mu_{10}\kappa_{10}$ or $\mu_{10}\lambda_{10}$	$\delta_2\kappa_2$ or $\delta_2\lambda_2$	$\epsilon_2\kappa_2$ or $\epsilon_2\lambda_2$
J chain	No	On dimer	On pentamer	No	No
Molecular weight in daltons (approximate)	150,000	Monomer 160,000 Dimer 400,000	900,000	180,000	190,000
Complement fixation (classical pathway)	$G_3 > G_1 > G_2$	No	M_1 and M_2	No	No
Crosses placenta	Yes	No	No	No	No
Concentration in serum	8 to 16 mg/mL	1.4 to 3.5 mg/mL	0.5 to 2 mg/mL	Up to 0.14 mg/mL	≤ 300 ng/mL

that may help in maintaining its structure. The J chain is a small glycoprotein (15,000 daltons) that is covalently bound to the H chains of the molecule.

IgM is the predominant immunoglobulin in the initial immune response to an antigen. It is the most efficient immunoglobulin in fixing complement. This efficiency is a result of its pentameric structure. The presence of 10 Fab units conveys on the IgM pentamer molecule a theoretical valency of 10. This means that an IgM molecule should be able to bind 10 antigen molecules simultaneously. Although this value has been computed in some experimental systems, it is not normally observed. Steric hindrance may be responsible for this disparity.

Immunoglobulin A

IgA constitutes approximately 15% of the serum immunoglobulin, but it is the predominant immunoglobulin in body secretions such as saliva, tears, sweat, human milk, and colostrum. In serum, IgA exists in both monomeric and polymeric forms. Polymeric serum IgA possesses the J chain. Secretory IgA exists as a dimer of the basic immunoglobulin unit combined with a J chain and an additional polypeptide chain called the **secretory piece.** The secretory piece is bound to dimeric secretory IgA by strong noncovalent linkages. It is important in secretory transport of the molecule and in its protection from proteolytic digestion in the gut. Secretory IgA provides the first line of defense against local infections and is important in the processing of food antigens in the gut.

Immunoglobulin D

IgD is a monomer of the basic immunoglobulin unit and is present in human serum in trace amounts. In addition, it is expressed on lymphocyte cell surface membranes. The main function of IgD is unknown. It may be involved in lymphocyte differentiation.

Immunoglobulin E

IgE is also a monomeric immunoglobulin. It is present in human serum in very low concentrations. IgE, which binds to cells by means of its Fc portion, is responsible for the physiological manifestations of allergy (see p. 473-474, Chapter 25).

ANTIGEN-ANTIBODY REACTIONS

Antigen-antibody reactions were first recognized by bacteriologists who also surmised that such reactions exhibited specificity. These bacteriologists noted that the serum of patients recovering from infectious diseases could agglutinate the organism responsible for their disease but not unrelated organisms. Serum from persons not exposed to the disease or from patients before they contracted the disease could not agglutinate the same organisms. From such evidence, scientists proposed the existence of antibody molecules, the specificity of their interactions with antigens, and the importance of such interactions in host defense.

The following sections consider the forces involved in antigen-antibody binding, the specificity of the reaction, and the mechanism of the reaction.

Binding Forces

The strength of the binding of an antigen to an antibody depends on the complementarity of fit of the antigenic determinant to the antibody idiotype and the resultant electrostatic attraction. It also depends on the sum of weak, noncovalent, intermolecular forces, such as hydrogen bonding, van der Waals forces, and hydrophobic interactions (see Table 53-2). Weak, short-range forces can operate between antigen and antibody if their closeness of fit brings them into proximity with one another.

In solution at physiological pH, charged polar groups on the amino acid residues of proteins can be strongly attracted to one another. These electrostatic forces are the strongest and most important contributors to noncovalent attraction between antigen and antibody. Hydrogen bonding between the amino and carboxy groups of peptide bonds also contributes to the attractive forces. Hydrogen bonds are weaker than electrostatic forces, but their numbers make them an important factor.

Van der Waals forces are the weakest forces involved. They can function only within a very small radius because of their low power. The increasing approximation of antigenic determinant to idiotype induces charge fluctuations within the atoms of the molecules. At very close distances the nucleus of one atom can be attracted to the external orbit electrons of a second atom. These van der Waals forces contribute to binding strength.

The final component of the attractive forces involves hydrophobic bonding between apolar groups in solution. Hydrophobic bonding functions by the exclusion of polar water molecules to bring hydrophobic molecules together. Such interactions also serve to attract polar water molecules to hydrophilic amino acid residues on protein molecules. Antibody molecules have increased numbers of hydrophobic amino acid residues such as alanine, leucine, tyrosine, tryptophan, and methionine in their antibody-combining sites, where they enhance bonding to hydrophobic residues in antigenic determinants.

Antibody Affinity

The strength of the binding of a single antigenic determinant to an antibody is a function of the closeness of fit and is called **antibody affinity.** Antibody affinity is an expression of the attraction between molecules of antibody and antigen. It is a function of the sum of the short-range, noncovalent, intermolecular forces.

Binding of antigen to antibody is a reversible reaction. The equilibrium of the reaction favors antigen-antibody association if the fit between molecules is good and the forces binding the molecules together are relatively strong and stable. The strength of the association between antigen and antibody is represented by the association constant, which may be derived as follows:

$$Ag + Ab \underset{k_2}{\overset{k_1}{\rightleftharpoons}} Ag \cdot Ab \qquad \textit{Eq. 11-1}$$

$$\frac{[Ag \cdot Ab]}{[Ag][Ab]} = K_\text{a} \text{ (Association constant)} \qquad \textit{Eq. 11-2}$$

To study these reactions, one places solutions of a small antigen, or hapten, on either side of a semipermeable membrane. As the hapten diffuses across the membrane, the reaction proceeds to the right of Eq. 11-1; that is, hapten and antibody associate to form complexes. Eventually, equilibrium is reached. At equilibrium, the rate of the forward reaction and the rate of the reverse reaction are constant. One rate constant, k_1, expresses the tendency of the reaction to move toward the right, or the tendency for association. The other rate constant, k_2, expresses the

tendency of the reaction to move to the left, or the tendency for dissociation. These reaction-rate constants differ for each antigen and antibody pair. The concentrations of antigen, antibody, and complex at equilibrium are described by Eq. 11-2. The equilibrium constant, K_a, expresses the tendency of the reaction to favor association between antigen and antibody.

Heterogeneity of Immune Response

Analysis of the binding of a simple hapten containing a single antigenic determinant shows variation in binding strength of antibody molecules. Immunization with a single antigenic determinant produces a variety of antibodies with different antibody-combining sites and with a range of antibody affinities. This is termed the **heterogeneity** of the immune response. Because haptens are three-dimensional, the immune system produces antibodies that have different areas of contact (Fig. 11-3). The antibody presents differing distributions of charged and hydrophobic residues, resulting in varying closeness of fit of hapten with each different antibody.

Antibody Avidity

In natural situations *in vivo* a variety of antibody molecules are generated in response to a large number of multivalent antigenic stimuli. Thus there are two areas of complexity: (1) multiple antibodies generated to different conformations on a single antigenic determinant and (2) multiple antigenic determinants on a single natural antigen. Both of these generate the *diversity* of the immune response. The measure of binding strength of antibodies to multiple antigenic determinants on natural antigens is termed **avidity.** Avidity is a measure of the stability of the antigen-antibody complex and is partially dependent on the affinity of each antibody for its complementary antigenic determinant. There is an enhanced effect, however, with multivalent antigens. The sum of the binding is greater than its individual parts because of the reversible nature of antigen-antibody bonds and because of the divalent nature of IgG molecules or the multivalent nature of IgM molecules. If the single bond between antigen and antibody dissociates, the antigen escapes. If an antigen has two antigenic determinants, each of which is bound by antibody, the antigen is kept in place until the broken bond re-forms (Fig. 11-4). Thus avidity is a measure of the stability of the multivalent antigen-multivalent antibody complex.

Cross-Reactivity

Cross-reactivity of antigen and antibody is a by-product of the heterogeneity of the immune response. As stated previously, immunization with a simple hapten produces a variety of antibodies of differing affinities. Some of these antibodies will combine with chemically related and structurally similar haptens. The reactivity of an antibody to a different antigen may also indicate that the two antigens in question share a previously unknown but common antigenic determinant. Thus cross-reactivity may result from similar or

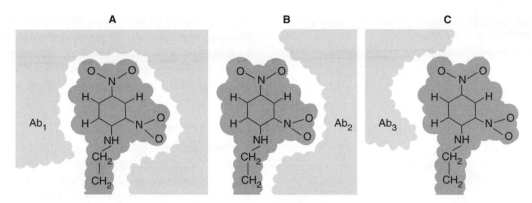

Fig. 11-3 Binding of antibodies (*Ab*) present in the same antiserum with different affinities to same hapten (dinitrobenzene linked to amino group of lysine). **A**, Ab_1 fits with nearly whole hapten and is thus of high affinity. **B**, Ab_2 fits with less of molecule and not so closely and has a moderate binding affinity, whereas **C**, low-affinity Ab_3, is complementary in shape to such a small portion of hapten surface that its binding energy is very little above that occurring between completely unrelated proteins. Only a portion of antibody-combining site is shown. *(From Roitt IM:* Essential immunology, *ed 4, Oxford, England, 1980, Blackwell Scientific Publications.)*

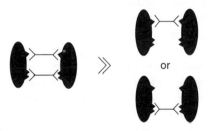

Fig. 11-4 Multivalent bonding of antigen-antibody increases bonding strength. A single bond created by divalent antibody molecules between a single antigenic determinant on two adjacent antigens is much weaker than binding created by two divalent antibodies bound simultaneously to two unique antigenic determinants on two adjacent antigens. Strength and complexity of this multivalent bonding are described by the term *avidity.*

identical antigenic determinants in different antigens. Such cross-reactivity is often observed with antibodies produced to such drugs as penicillin. The reactivity of an antibody with penicillin may be very high, but metabolic derivatives containing the basic drug structure may also react with an antibody produced to the complete drug.

In cases of prolonged antigenic challenge, such as that occurring in natural infection, the initial response is with low-affinity, low-specificity molecules, which may react with other closely related antigens. With time, animals exhibit a natural selection for clones of plasma cells producing high-affinity antibodies. As the heterogeneity of the antibody response narrows, the specificity of antigen-antibody reactions increases. This adaptation of the immune response promotes effective protection of the host against infection.

Genetic Basis of Antibody Diversity

The heterogeneity of the immune response or the variety of antibodies produced to a single antigen is known to be genetically determined. The variable (V) regions of light and heavy chains of the antibody molecule encode for antibody specificity. Some positions in the amino acid sequence of the V region have an even more increased likelihood of amino acid variation. These **hypervariable regions**, scattered throughout the amino acid sequence of the V region, are brought into proximity to one another by the natural folding (tertiary structure) of the antibody molecule. The amino acid sequence dictates possible attraction between polar amino acid residues, as well as the possibility of intrachain disulfide bonds. Folding of the protein so that the hypervariable regions are spatially close to each other forms the antibody-combining site.

ANTIGEN-ANTIBODY PRECIPITATION REACTIONS

The primary reaction of antigen with antibody is usually detected by secondary manifestations of the reaction. The nature of the secondary manifestations depends on experimental conditions, the class of antibody involved in the reaction, the number of antigenic determinants on the antigen, and the size and solubility of the antigen. The reaction of antibody with soluble molecules possessing multiple antigenic determinants that permit cross-linking is detected by precipitation of the complex out of solution. The term **flocculation** may be used to describe a precipitation reaction that produces a large, loosely bound precipitate. The reaction of antibodies with large, particulate, multivalent antigens is detected by **agglutination** of the antigen. These reactions are considered separately.

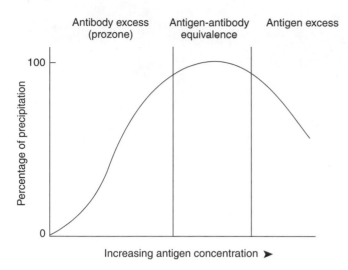

Fig. 11-5 Quantitative precipitin curve in which amount of antibody-antigen complex that precipitates is plotted as function of antigen concentration.

Precipitation Curve

When a known quantity of antibody is present in solution in a series of tubes to which increasing amounts of antigen are added, precipitation occurs in some of the test tubes. When the amount of precipitate is measured and correlated with the amount of antigen present, one obtains a curve similar to that shown in Fig. 11-5.

In the first phase of the reaction, called the *antibody-excess phase*, no free antigen (an antigen without bound antibody) can be detected in the fluid and essentially no precipitate can be found. Free (unbound) antibody can be detected, however. As greater amounts of antigen are added, the amount of precipitate increases until a point of maximum precipitation is reached. At this point, no free antigen or free antibody can be detected in the fluid. This is called the **zone**

of equivalence. As the amount of added antigen continues to increase, the amount of precipitate detected diminishes. Examination of the fluid phase of the reaction at this time shows no free antibody but increasing amounts of free antigen. This area of the curve is called the *antigen-excess phase.*

Lattice Theory

Antigen-antibody complexes precipitate out of solution because of the multivalent nature of both molecules. The reaction of antigens possessing multiple antigenic determinants and antibodies with two (as in IgG) or more (as in IgM) antibody-combining sites produces a **lattice** of interlocking molecules. Antibody molecules can cross-link antigenic sites on the same or different molecules of antigen. As the size and complexity of the lattice increase, the lattice becomes insoluble and precipitates out of solution (Fig. 11-6).

In the antibody-excess zone, a single molecule of antigen binds to each antibody molecule. The excess of antibody ensures that each molecule of antigen can encounter a free antibody molecule. The absence of cross-linking produces small soluble complexes. As the antigen concentration increases and the zone of equivalence is reached, complexes of increasing size with increasing levels of cross-linking are formed. Such large, complex lattices precipitate out of solution.

As the antigen concentration continues to increase, the zone of antigen excess is reached. In this portion of the curve, smaller complexes are again seen. The size of the lattice decreases because there is sufficient antigen to permit binding of a free antigen molecule to each antibody-combining site. At high concentrations of antigen, lack of precipitation can result in false-negative results. Obviously, detection of antigen by antibody precipitation requires optimum concentration of both reactants. Formation of

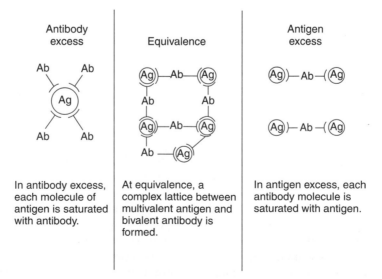

Fig. 11-6 Representation of sizes of molecular complexes formed at varying ratios of antigen and antibody.

lattices best suited for precipitation occurs at an equal equivalent concentration of antigen and antibody or at a slight antigen excess.

Other Factors Affecting Precipitation

The precipitation of antigen-antibody complexes out of solution can be affected by factors other than the ratio of antigen concentration to antibody concentration. Different antibody molecules can precipitate the same antigen to varying degrees. The efficiency of the antibody depends on its affinity and specificity. The charge and shape of the antigen-antibody complex are also important. Highly charged complexes are difficult to precipitate. The best precipitates are observed with protein antigens of molecular weights from 40,000 to 160,000 daltons. Proteins in this range are easily cross-linked by multivalent antibody molecules. Polysaccharide antigens, denatured proteins, and viruses produce broader precipitation curves. Their large size sterically hinders cross-linking. Precipitation can also be affected by temperature, pH, and ionic concentration. Such factors influence antigen-antibody interactions on a molecular level.

Precipitation Reactions in Gel

Precipitation reactions are frequently carried out in a gel-support matrix composed of agar or the more purified polysaccharide, agarose. The agar prevents convective mixing of antigen and antibody and thereby ensures establishment of concentration gradients of the two reactants. Precipitation in agar is only a moderately sensitive technique when compared with newer advances, such as chemiluminescent immunometric assays, but it is employed because of its ease and versatility. In addition, precipitation reactions in gels can be modified to permit the study of antigenic relationships among different compounds. The following section discusses two gel-precipitation reactions, double **immunodiffusion** and **radial immunodiffusion**.

Double Immunodiffusion

In double-immunodiffusion reactions, or **Ouchterlony technique**, agar or agarose is poured onto a solid support, such as a glass slide or Petri dish. Wells are then cut into the agar, and antigen and antibody solutions are placed into separate wells. The solutions then diffuse toward one another in the gel in a radial fashion during room-temperature incubation (Fig. 11-7). With diffusion into the agar, the solutions establish concentration gradients that diminish with distance from the well. At the point of antigen-antibody equivalence at the interface of the diffusing fronts, a **precipitin line** is formed (see Fig. 11-7). The positioning and shape of the line are dictated by the concentration of the reactants and the size of the molecules. The line will be closer to the well containing the reactant of lower concentration because the distance traveled is directly proportional to concentration. The rate of diffusion is also inversely proportional to molecular size. High-molecular-weight compounds, such as IgM, diffuse more slowly than lower–

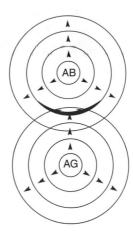

Fig. 11-7 Depiction of radial protein gradients in Ouchterlony immunodiffusion. Concentric circles represent decreasing protein concentrations. Both antigen (*AG*) and antibody (*AB*) diffuse radially from application wells. Precipitation, *heavy black arc*, occurs at point of antigen-antibody equivalence. Precipitin line is closer to well of lower concentration and concave toward reagent of higher molecular weight.

molecular-weight substances, such as IgG. The precipitation line that is formed at the interface of the two-concentration gradients will be concave to the higher-molecular-weight compound, whose diffusion rate is slower. Because precipitation occurs at a range of antigen-antibody equivalence to slight antigen excess, an inappropriate ratio of antigen to antibody will result in failure to form a precipitate.

Radial Immunodiffusion

Because of its simplicity and accuracy, radial immunodiffusion can be easily used for the quantification of antigens. Radial immunodiffusion, the **Mancini technique**, is a precipitation reaction achieved by applying an antigen solution to a gel impregnated with a monospecific antibody solution that permits quantitation of antigen. Wells are cut into the antibody-containing agar and dilutions of antigen are placed in the wells. Radial diffusion of antigen into the agar produces a concentration gradient that is inversely proportional to the distance from the well. At the point where antigen and antibody concentrations are equivalent, precipitation occurs. Because diffusion from the well is radial, the precipitation appears as a ring around the well. The precipitation reaction is dynamic rather than static; the ring first forms close to the well at the initial point of antigen-antibody equivalence. As antigen continues to diffuse from the well, antigen excess causes the precipitate to form soluble complexes that continue to diffuse outward. A new ring is formed at a new point of antigen-antibody equivalence. The square of the diameter of the ring (mm^2) is directly proportional to antigen concentration. The thickness of the ring is a function of the final concentration of antigen-antibody complexes at the equivalence point (Fig. 11-8).

When constant sample volume, temperature, pH, incubation time, and antibody concentration are maintained,

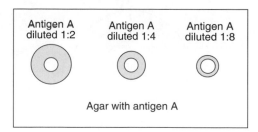

Fig. 11-8 Radial immunodiffusion patterns. Band of precipitation, *gray area*, extends as a disk from center of each circular well. Area of precipitation is proportional to concentration.

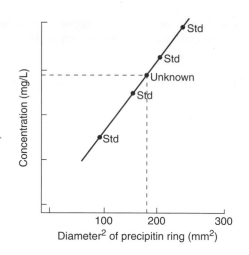

Fig. 11-9 Graph of concentration of antigen expressed as mg/L versus square of diameter of precipitin ring. *Std*, Standard.

an unknown antigen concentration can be determined. This is accomplished by comparing the area of the precipitation ring of the unknown antigen with those obtained for several dilutions of a standard antigen solution. When the concentrations of the diluted standard are plotted against ring area (or diameter squared, d^2), the concentration of the unknown can be easily determined (Fig. 11-9).

The assay is valid only over a rather narrow range of antigen concentrations. In part, this is dictated by the antibody concentration in the gel and by the ease of diffusion of the antigen into the gel. For some antigens, several dilutions are necessary to achieve the optimum concentration range. Urine and cerebrospinal fluid generally must be concentrated before they can be quantified by this technique. Excess salt must be removed from these specimens if they have been concentrated by lyophilization.

Monospecific antibody to the desired antigen is the only crucial reagent. If the antiserum binds more than one antigen, a double ring may be seen. Temperature should be kept constant. If the antigen is too large or aggregated, the resulting diffusion pattern will not be quantitative. This method is slow relative to other methods of antigen quantitation and has largely been replaced in the routine clinical laboratory.

Test sensitivity depends on antigen size; the greater the size, the poorer the diffusion. For most serum proteins, the assay is sensitive to 50 µg/mL.

Other Quantitative Methods

There are several methods for detecting or measuring antigens using adaptations and combinations of electrophoresis and precipitation reactions in gels. These include **immunoelectrophoresis** (immunoprecipitation after electrophoresis), counterelectrophoresis (movement of antigen and antibody into each other by electrophoresis), **rocket (Laurell) immunoelectrophoresis** (electrophoresis of antigen into an antibody-containing gel). Although these methods have been replaced by faster and more sensitive techniques in the contemporary clinical laboratories, they may still be used for research or for special applications. For details please refer to earlier editions of this textbook.

Bibliography

Butt WR, editor: *Practical immunoassay*, New York, 1984, Marcel Dekker.
Gosling JP, Reen DJ: *Immunotechnology*, London, 1993, Portland Press.
Keren DF: *High resolution electrophoresis and immunofixation*, ed 2, Boston, 1994, Butterworth.

Roitt IM, Brostoff J, Male DK: *Immunology*, ed 2, London, 1989, Gower Medical.
Weir DM et al, editors: *Weir's handbook of experimental immunology*, ed 5, Oxford, England, 1997, Blackwell Scientific Publications.

Internet Sites

http://www.kcom.edu/faculty/chamberlain/Website/MSTUART/lect4.htm
www.whfreeman.com/immunology/CH06/kuby06.htm
http://www.cvm.missouri.edu/vmdl/ramos/ihc/Review%20of%20IHC/html/Immunoglobulins.htm
http://www.cig.salk.edu/the_specificity_of_IR.pdf—The Salk Institute, the Specificity of Immunologic Reactions
http://www.asehaqld.org.au/pblctns.htm—Allergy, Sensitivity & Environmental Health Association

http://allergy.mcg.edu/home.html—American College of Allergy, Asthma & Immunology, Arlington Heights, IL
http://www.aaaai.org/—Professional medical organization of specialists in allergy, asthma, and immunology
http://www.niaid.nih.gov/default.htm—The National Institute of Allergy and Infectious Diseases (NIAID)

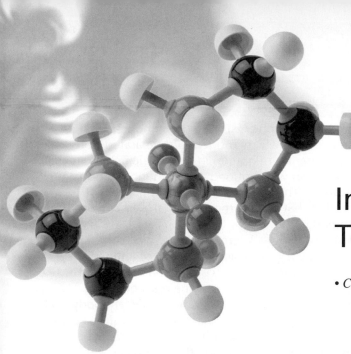

CHAPTER 12

Immunochemical Techniques

• Carolyn S. Feldkamp

Objectives

- For each of the following techniques, state the principle of the immunoreaction, describe sample requirements and preparation, list common pitfalls, and explain the interpretation of results:
  Electrophoresis
  Immunonephelometry
  Agglutination
  Complement fixation
  Western blot
  Immunofixation

- Define agglutination and differentiate between direct agglutination, indirect agglutination, and agglutination-inhibition reactions.
- Describe the principles of solid-phase, "sandwich" assays, distinguishing between those that measure antigen and those that measure antibody.
- List the labels used for "sandwich" assays, comparing their sensitivity and their ability to be used in heterogeneous and homogeneous assays.

Key Terms

agglutination Clumping or aggregating together by specific antibody of particles, such as red blood cells or latex beads, to which the specific antigenic determinant is attached.

agglutinin Specific antibody that causes agglutination.

antiantibody An antibody with specificity for immunoglobulins.

antibody absorption The process of removing or blocking nonspecific or undesired antibody in an antiserum reagent by allowing it to react with nonspecific antigens before using it as reagent.

antibody reagent A high-titer, high-affinity, IgG-class antibody prepared in animals for use in immunoassays.

antigen reagent A stabilized solution containing a known amount of an antigen that is used as a standard.

cold agglutinin An agglutinin that reacts better at temperatures less than body temperature; best reaction is usually at 4° C.

complement A group of serum proteins activated as a result of an antibody-antigen reaction. When the reaction is on the surface of a red blood cell, the activated complement can lyse the cell.

complement fixation A term applied to a set of assays in which complement is activated or "fixed" by a test reaction system.

Coombs' test A type of agglutination reaction. A direct Coombs' test measures the presence of antibody on cells; an indirect test measures its presence in serum.

cryoglobulin Protein that precipitates at temperatures less than body temperature; precipitates maximally at 4° C.

fluoroimmunoassay Any immunoprocedure that uses a fluorescent molecule as the indicator label.

hemolysin Anti–sheep-red-blood-cell antibody.

heterogeneous immunoassay Any technique that uses two phases, usually liquid and solid, to separate reacted from unreacted components.

immunodiffusion Random, spreading movement of antibody or antigen or both in a support medium.

immunoelectrophoresis An immunoprecipitation technique in which antigens are separated from each other by migration in an electric field, followed by reaction with antibody by immunodiffusion.

indicator The portion of an immunochemical reaction that can be measured; labeled antigen or antibody.

inhibition assay A term for those types of immunoassays in which an excess of antigens prevents or inhibits the completion of either the initial or indicator phase of the reaction.

monoclonal antibody A monospecific antibody that is produced by a single plasma cell or a single clone of plasma cells of a lymphocyte myeloma hybrid.

monospecific An antibody that will react with only one type of antigen molecule.

nephelometric assay Measurement of antigen or antibody by determination of the amount of light scattered as the result of the amount or rate of antibody-antigen aggregation.

nephelometric inhibition immunoassay (NINIA) Measurement of haptens by inhibition of formation of an antibody-antigen lattice.

nephelometry Measurement of light-scattering properties of large particles (such as antigen-antibody complexes) in solution.

polyclonal antiserum Serum from an immunized animal forming heterogeneous antibodies with diverse affinities toward an antigen that are produced by a large number of plasma cell clones.

prozone phenomenon Apparently lower reactivity or nonreactivity caused by a relative antigen excess.

sandwich assay A term applied to a solid-phase two-site immunometric assay in which the first layer is immobilized antibody, the second is antigen, and the third is labeled antibody.

specificity Property of an antibody molecule that restricts its reactivity to a defined molecule or group of molecules.

titer Maximum dilution of a specific antibody that gives a measurable reaction with a specific antigen; usually expressed as the reciprocal of that dilution.

Chapter 11 describes the molecular nature of antigens and antibodies and the general characteristics of the antigen-antibody reaction. This chapter deals with many techniques that use the antigen-antibody reaction as the basis to detect, characterize, or quantitate constituents in blood and other body fluids submitted to the laboratory for analysis. These constituents can range from low-molecular-weight drugs and their metabolites to high-molecular-weight proteins, such as IgM and alpha$_2$-macroglobulin. In most immunoassay formats the patient's sample contains the antigen (analyte), and antibody is added as a reagent to detect or measure the antigen. On the other hand, in cases of infectious disease, serological determinations, allergy testing (see Chapter 25, p. 474), and autoimmune antibody testing, it is the antibody measurement in the patient's sample that is clinically important. For these antibody determinations, antigen of known composition is used. The antigen may be soluble or tissue based. This chapter concentrates on the procedures that detect antigen in the patient's sample.

REAGENTS
Antibody as Reagent

Reagent antibodies are usually prepared in animals, such as rabbits or goats, by the repeated exposure of the animal to foreign substances. A group of B lymphocytes is stimulated to respond by producing antibodies. Specific areas of the molecules, or epitopes, of the immunizing material are major antigenic determinants of the antigen molecule and stimulate the production of the largest amount of antibodies; minor determinants also stimulate antibody production. Because there are many different antibodies attributable to the expansion of many clones of antibody-producing cells, the antiserum thus produced is termed *polyclonal* reagent **antiserum**. For example, an antiserum against the protein human serum albumin (anti-HSA) is a reagent that has multiple antibodies to antigenic determinants or specific molecular configurations that are characteristic and specific for the surface of HSA. This is also termed a **monospecific** antibody.

If this anti-HSA is to be used as a reagent in the clinical laboratory, its **specificity** (i.e., its reactivity with only HSA) must be verified in the same immunological test system used to generate patient results. For every reagent antibody, the specificity of its immunochemical reactivity is the single most important factor in the success or failure of any immunological technique used in the clinical laboratory.

Monoclonal antibodies. Monoclonal antibodies are formed by a technology that hybridizes individual antibody-producing cells (plasma cells) with an immortal cell line. After screening many hundreds of these hybrids, each selected cell line produces a unique antibody. Monoclonal antibodies have a single homogeneous primary structure and a unique antigen-binding site. These antibodies provide a reproducible reagent of known specificity and affinity. Monoclonal antibodies are used in competitive and noncompetitive binding assays and in tissue assays to identify specific antigens. Fig. 12-1 is a schema of how monoclonal antibodies are produced.

Selection. Selection of antibody as a reagent in an immunological procedure requires information about its characteristics such as the amount of specific antibody present (**titer**), affinity, and specificity. Because not all of the immunoglobulin in an antiserum is reactive for a specific antigen, the amount of antibody that is available for reactivity in a specific immunological method is termed the *titer of the antibody*. The titer is the reciprocal of the maximum dilution of the antibody that gives a detectable reaction for a specific method. The titer of the reagent antibody is often different for each immunological procedure for which it is to be used. For example, anti-HSA may react in an immunoprecipitation technique at a maximum dilution

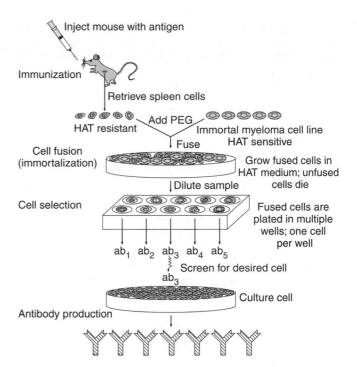

Fig. 12-1 Monoclonal antibody production. Antibody production is initiated by immunization of an animal with antigen. After the immune response, spleen cells are isolated, each of which produces a single, unique antibody. These cells are fused with an immortal myeloma cell line by exposure to polyethylene glycol (PEG). In the culture medium containing HAT (a mixture of hypoxanthine, aminopterin, and thymidine), unfused myeloma cells, which cannot bypass the metabolic block caused by aminopterin, die. Unfused spleen cells also die naturally after 1 to 2 weeks. Fused cells survive, having the immortality of the myeloma cells and HAT resistance of the spleen cells. Fused cells are then cultured at high dilution and selected by screening for secretion of antibodies with the desired characteristics. Eventually a culture of antibody-secreting cells derived from a single spleen cell produces reagent amounts of monoclonal antibody.

of 1:32, but the same antiserum may react at a maximum dilution of 1:6400 in a radioimmunoassay (RIA) procedure. Occasionally the amount of reagent antibody present may be expressed in weight, that is, milligrams per milliliter. This expression of antibody amount is determined by precipitation techniques and is often helpful in determining the amount of reagent needed. For monoclonal antibodies that are virtually pure, the indicated amount describes the total reactive proteins.

Affinity. Reagent antibodies generally fall into two categories, those of high affinity and those of low affinity. Polyclonal antibodies in the reagent may be a mixture of both, but reagents in which high-affinity antibodies are predominant should be used. This results in a strong union with the antigen that is not readily reversible and that will not be influenced greatly by alteration of the reaction conditions. Low-affinity antibodies do not bind well with the antigen and can be influenced by temperature, pH, and ionic strength with consequent changes in the reaction, resulting in dissociation of the antibody-antigen complex. Most commercial reagent antibodies are of the high-affinity type. However, if reagents are prepared in the laboratory they should be tested to be certain they are of the appropriate, preferably high, affinity.

Specificity. Specificity refers to the ability of the antibody to restrict its reaction to a defined group of molecules. Because polyclonal antibody reagents are really a collection of antibodies, they are directed to multiple antigenic determinants on a single antigen and thus could have multiple reactivities. In some cases, other reagent antibodies may react with antigenic determinants that are common to several molecular forms of plasma proteins. For example, a reagent directed to the IgG molecule should recognize only the IgG molecule, but there may be antibody in the reagent that would also react with light chains of that IgG molecule. Because light chains are common to all the immunoglobulin classes (i.e., IgA, IgM, and IgD) the reagent antibody would then react with all immunoglobulin molecules. It would not be appropriate to say that it was recognizing only the IgG molecule. The problem of cross-reactivity with other serum proteins can usually be controlled by a technique termed **antibody absorption,** by which that population of antibody reacting inappropriately with other molecules of the test solution is bound or removed from the reagent. Absorption is necessary for virtually all **antibody reagents** of the polyclonal type. It is often accomplished by addition of the undesired reacting antigen or by preparation of pure antibody by affinity columns.

Specificity of the reagent antibody is also extremely important in the enzyme immunoassays (EIA) and RIA that are frequently used to measure the presence of small molecules such as drugs and hormones. However, often there is a residual reaction between the reagent antibody and a closely related compound. This reaction between antibody and the undesired antigen is termed *cross-reactivity*.

There are times, however, when the cross-reactivity with very similar antigenic determinants cannot be avoided. For example, antibody directed to the small molecule trinitrophenol cross-reacts with dinitrophenol. To the antibody, these low-molecular-weight entities appear very similar. The only way to establish the specificity of the antibody is to determine the relative affinity of the reagent antibody to presumptive cross-reacting molecules at concentrations likely to occur in patients. Often, particularly in the case of antibody reagents used in therapeutic drug monitoring, the manufacturer gives the degree of cross-reactivity with the metabolites of the drug and with other drugs.

Because reagent antibody is protein, all precautions to prevent denaturation and degradation should be taken. The reagent should be kept free of bacterial contamination and should be stored in the refrigerator (4° C) if it is to be used within several days. Long-term storage at -20° C is usually adequate.

EXAMPLES OF MOLECULES IN BIOLOGICAL FLUIDS FREQUENTLY MEASURED BY IMMUNOLOGICAL TECHNIQUES

Large Molecules
Immunoglobulins (IgG, IgA, IgM, IgD, IgE)
Complement components (C3, C4, factor B)
Coagulation factors (factor VIII, fibrinogen)
Lipoproteins
Protein hormones
Acute-phase proteins (α_1-antitrypsin, C-reactive protein)
Albumin
Selected urine and cerebrospinal fluid proteins
Viral antigens

Small Molecules
Digoxin and digitonin
Antibiotics
Cytotoxic drugs
Prostaglandins
Hormones (steroids, thyroid hormones)
Theophylline
Anticonvulsant drugs
Antiarrhythmic drugs
Drugs of abuse

Antigen as Analyte

Range of analytes. Numerous naturally occurring molecules or antigens that are proteins, glycoproteins, or lipoproteins can be detected and measured easily in biological fluids if specific reagent antibodies are available. In addition, many small molecules such as drugs and hormones can be measured. The box above lists examples of the large and small molecules that are frequently measured by immunological techniques.

Sample types and stability. The biological fluids most commonly available to the laboratory for analysis are serum, urine, and cerebrospinal fluid. Antigens present in each of these fluids are subject to degradation depending on (1) the nature of the antigen, (2) its concentration, (3) its susceptibility to various enzymes in the body fluids, and (4) its relative stability at various storage temperatures (e.g., room temperature, 4° C, -20° C, and -70° C). Each specimen must be stored and handled properly to ensure that the antigen molecule is unaltered and the reagent antibody can react with the appropriate antigenic determinants on the molecule. **Cryoglobulins** are immunoglobulins that precipitate from serum or plasma as the temperature decreases from 37° C. Stability of antigens must be established for each biological fluid. For example, the C4 component of **complement** of serum is stable and can be measured accurately up to a week after receipt of the serum if the specimen is stored at 4° C before analysis. However, the C4 component in cerebrospinal fluid is very labile and is usually present at very low concentrations. If this kind of sample is stored more than 8 hours at 4° C before analysis, the C4 will have been degraded and will be unmeasurable. Thus spinal fluid must be frozen and stored at -70° C to ensure that the C4 will not be degraded before measurement. Another example is that of antigen denaturation in urine specimens. Because most urine specimens are acidic, immunological measurement of various proteins may be inaccurate. Proteins are degraded in an acid pH, and many antigenic determinants on these proteins are lost. β_2-Microglobulin is a protein found in both urine and plasma. In urine it is used to estimate renal tubular dysfunction. It is rapidly destroyed if the pH of urine is less than 6.0. Quantitation of specific proteins in urine samples requires immediate neutralization of the acid pH at the time of collection. In contrast, the protein in serum is stable for a week when stored at 4° C. The problems associated with specific protein measurement and antigen degradation may not be as acute when small molecules such as drugs are measured. Nevertheless, it is always good laboratory practice to store biological fluids at 4° C if the analysis is to be performed on the same day and in a frozen state if the analysis is to be performed much later.

It should be emphasized that the immunological reactivity of a molecule may not be related to its biological activity. The importance of this distinction is illustrated by the immunological measurement of α_1-antitrypsin and parathyroid hormone (PTH).

α_1-Antitrypsin is a potent inhibitor of the proteolytic enzyme trypsin, and its production is under genetic control. In certain individuals there occur genetic variations in which the molecule is estimated to be present at normal levels when measured by immunochemical techniques, but the molecule's enzyme-inhibiting capability is greatly impaired. Immunochemically the genetic variants react as well as the normally functioning molecule does; however, there is a great biological difference.

Immunological versus biological quantitation. PTH breaks down quickly in plasma and the PTH molecule may not be present as an intact molecule. In patients with end-stage renal disease, these degradation products accumulate in plasma. When levels of PTH are obtained by immunological methods, they can appear to be normal or increased when in fact there is a low level of the complete molecule. This discrepancy is attributable to the reaction of antibody with the breakdown products of PTH, which retain the appropriate antigenic determinants. Examples of immunological reactivity without biological activity occur frequently and demonstrate that normal levels of molecules assayed by immunological methods do not necessarily predict normal functional activity.

Reference materials. Qualitative and quantitative measurements of antigen in biological fluids require the use of a highly specific reagent antibody and a known reference standard of **antigen reagent.** The reactivity of the antibody with the antigen in the patient's biological fluid is compared to the reactivity of the antibody with the standard antigen. For the most part, standards are supplied in immunological test kits. If the Food and Drug Administration (FDA) approves a test kit, the technologist is reasonably assured that the reagent antibody is detecting the antigen, as stated by

the manufacturer. However, it is good practice when using immunological methods to evaluate the test system with reference antigen obtained from other sources when possible. The World Health Organization (WHO) supplies reference antigen for many of the serum proteins as primary standards. Secondary standards have been developed by the College of American Pathologists (CAP) in collaboration with the Centers for Disease Control and Prevention (CDC) and are easily available. Federal regulations established in the Clinical Laboratories Improvement Act of 1988 (CLIA '88) define laboratory requirements to validate accuracy and precision of clinical assays. Manufacturers' data may be used for kits used with no modification. Otherwise, thorough documentation of accuracy, precision, linearity, sensitivity, and normal ranges must be maintained. Periodic calibration verification and quality control (QC) programs are also required by CLIA '88.

QUANTITATION OF ANTIGENS AND ANTIBODIES BY IMMUNOLOGICAL REACTIONS IN GELS

Several techniques were developed to measure antibodies and protein antigens by immunological reactions in gels laid onto a solid support. Antigen or antibody mixtures were separated in the gel by rate of diffusion, or electrophoresis. As antigen-antibody complexes were formed at concentrations of "equivalence," the resulting precipitated complex could be visualized by eye. Quantitative relationships between distance traveled in the gel and concentration of reactants allowed quantitation. **Immunodiffusion, immunoelectrophoresis,** counterelectrophoresis, radial immunodiffusion, and Laurell ("rocket") immunoelectrophoresis have been replaced in clinical practice by nephelometric techniques and quantitative competitive binding and immunometric techniques using labeled **indicators.** The latter techniques are sensitive and are amenable to quantitation and automation. Reactions of antigens and antibodies in gels are still used in research to test antisera and antigen mixtures for cross-reacting substances. Immunofixation is still used to qualitatively identify proteins and establish light- and heavy-chain types for monoclonal proteins. **Agglutination** and techniques using antigen migration and precipitation of immune complexes are also frequently used in point-of-care devices (POC). For details of the techniques using immunological reactions in gels, please refer to earlier editions of this textbook.

IMMUNOFIXATION (WESTERN BLOT)

The immunoblotting technique known as the Western blot method is often used in clinical applications to confirm the presence of antibody (e.g., human immunodeficiency virus, [HIV], antibody) to specific antigens. The technique is also used for the detection of specific proteins, such as apoE isoforms.

Principles

The method of immunoblotting is a three-stage procedure that uses electrophoresis to separate and transfer analytes. An

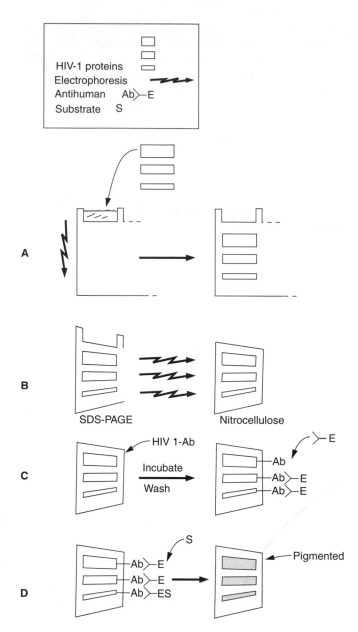

Fig. 12-2 Diagram of enzyme-linked immunoelectrotransfer blot technique (Western blot). **A**, HIV-1 proteins are layered onto an SDS-PAGE, subjected to electrophoresis, and separated according to their molecular weight. **B**, The discrete proteins are then electrophoresed (blotted) to a nitrocellulose matrix and incubated, first with a specimen containing HIV-1 antibody (Ab), which binds to the discrete HIV-1 Ag bands. **C**, Tagged antihuman Ab is then added. The excess is washed away, and substrate is added. **D**, HIV-1 Ab directed toward discrete HIV-1 antigen bands is present; the discrete bands can be visualized as pigmented bands. *(Reprinted from* American clinical laboratory, *vol 6, p 11, 1987. Copyright 1987 by International Scientific Communications, Inc.)*

antigen mixture is first electrophoresed in an appropriate support medium, such as polyacrylamide, neutral agarose, or paper strips, to separate the components by charge-to-weight differences. The agarose film is then overlaid with a sheet of nitrocellulose-based filter paper. In a second electrophoretic step, the protein is transferred from the support to the nitrocellulose. The nitrocellulose has the property of effectively irreversibly binding the transferred protein. The nitrocellulose sheet is then treated with a protein solution, which reacts with all remaining binding sites, minimizing nonspecific binding in the next step. Next, an antibody solution, usually serum from a patient, is allowed to react with the nitrocellulose sheet. Excess antibody is then removed by washing. The nitrocellulose sheet is incubated with a second labeled antibody that has specificity for the first antibody. The label allows detection of the original antigen-antibody reaction. If the label is an enzyme, such as peroxidase, the reaction is detected by substrate precipitation of, for example, a benzidine dye. A diagram is presented in Fig. 12-2.

Reagents

The reagent antibody label must have a high specificity and specific activity so that it can detect only the desired antibody or test protein, and so that the sensitivity of the assay will be great enough to determine the presence of the reaction.

Common Pitfalls

The assays commonly use peroxidase dye reactions to detect the presence of antibody or antigen. The assays often require skilled individuals to read the patterns.

Test Sensitivity and Interpretation of Results

This technique is nearly as sensitive as the enzyme immunoassay technique. However, whereas enzyme immunoassays are employed as quantitative assays, Western blots and other immunofixation methods are used primarily as qualitative techniques; that is, they are used to determine the presence or absence of a particular protein or antibody. A widely used purpose of the technique is confirmation of the results of HIV screening. The sensitivity of the technique can be the detection of less than 1 ng/mL of test protein.

IMMUNONEPHELOMETRY
Nephelometry

For a detailed discussion of **nephelometry**, see Chapter 4, pp. 101-103.

Principles. When an antibody and an antigen bind in solution, small aggregates that can scatter light form quickly, giving a turbid appearance to the solution. These aggregates then slowly associate to form a larger matrix, which eventually gives rise to the precipitate seen in immuno-precipitation assays such as double diffusion (Ouchterlony) or radial immunodiffusion (Mancini).

Development of a clinically useful assay for some plasma proteins was made possible by the observation that the intensity of scattered light was a measure of the amount of precipitate formed, as long as the reaction was carried out in antibody excess. Nephelometers used for these assays typically use a laser as a light source and measure either end-point complexes formed or rate of complex formation.

Fast (seconds to minutes) and precise methods for the specific measurement of plasma proteins, such as albumin, immunoglobulins, complement components, and acute-phase reactants, are now available. The method has also been adapted for application to small molecules such as hormones and therapeutic drugs.

In Chapter 11, the structure of the aggregates created by early lattice formation of immune complexes is shown. These aggregates from primary reactions occur within seconds to minutes, whereas the secondary interactions leading to precipitation occur over a period of hours.

Nephelometric or light-scattering assays measure this early second-order reaction, presumably between antigen and high-affinity antibody, in which there is formed a micelle of protein large enough to scatter light but not large enough to precipitate. Although the initial reaction of antigen with antibody is fast, the accumulation of small light-scattering complexes takes time. This aggregate formation can be greatly enhanced with the addition of the water-soluble polymer polyethylene glycol (6000 D) at concentrations of 2% to 4%. The polymer causes a several-fold increase in light scatter while decreasing the reaction time tenfold.

Sample requirements and preparation. Proteins in serum, cerebrospinal fluids, and urine may be measured.

Common Pitfalls

1. Antibody is not in excess. In these circumstances, the amount of precipitate formation will be recorded as a falsely low value.
2. Background scatter is too high. Rate nephelometric determinations are preferred to end-point determinations because they minimize the contribution of background. For example, it is possible to detect a 5% increase in scattering over background using a rate measurement. In contrast, such a difference may not be measurable as an end-point change. Lipidemia causes high background scatter.
3. Interference is caused by colored solution. End-point methods are most influenced by colored solutions. These absorb the scattered light, tending to yield lower values. However, even kinetic measurements are lower in highly colored solutions.
4. Mixing is insufficient. Because the rate method requires constant agitation to make uniform particles, the mixing efficacy must be constantly monitored.
5. Preformed immune complexes in the patient serum may cause false-high or false-low values, depending on whether the rate of reaction is measured and how the background correction is done.

Limitations. For most assays, quantitation is valid only when the reagent antibody is in excess. Although each instrument manufacturer has devised ways of recognizing antigen excess, the foolproof method requires the technician to carry out the measurements at two different dilutions, or to

have available a serum protein electrophoresis of the sample for comparison. The method is limited to measurements of antigens that form enough lattice to scatter light, such as proteins. Special steps are required for small molecules (see the following text).

Nephelometric Inhibition Immunoassay (NINIA)

Principles. If a small molecule such as a drug is co-valently linked to a large carrier protein such as bovine serum albumin, the resulting conjugate acts as a large light-scattering antigen when reacted with antibody to the small molecule, or hapten. In this case the complex formation can be inhibited by the addition of the specific hapten. The inhibition is dose dependent, and a quantitative assay for the small molecule results. With appropriate manipulation of the variables, the number of haptenic groups can be adjusted for adequate precipitation while allowing maximum sensitivity for inhibition by free hapten (Fig. 12-3).

Nephelometric inhibition immunoassay (NINIA) methods have been developed for rapid analysis of drugs occurring in milligram/liter amounts, such as phenytoin, phenobarbital, and theophylline.

Additional Assay Modifications

Particle-enhanced light scattering. Because the amount of light scatter is dependent on the size, amount, and refractive index of the scattering species, an increase in any of these variables should result in greater sensitivity. This potential is realized when either antigens or antibodies are coupled to various inert carrier particles. Because of availability and better control of coupling conditions, polystyrene latex beads have become the particles of choice. This type of assay is essentially a type of agglutinating procedure (see later discussion of agglutination assays). The method also offers faster signal generation and greater economy of reagents. The latex-fixation test for detection of rheumatoid factor is the classic example of this type of assay, although it depends on visual observation of agglutination and is thus only semiquantitative. More recently, several particle-enhanced methods have been developed for both direct and **inhibition assays**, and a wide variety of light-scatter detection techniques have been employed.

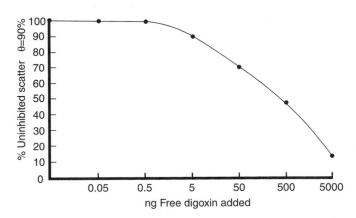

Fig. 12-3 Digoxin standard curve using nephelometric-inhibition immunoassay.

Monoclonal antibody reagents. The performance of light-scattering assays depends greatly on the quality of the antiserum used. With conventional polyclonal reagents there is a continual need to monitor and adjust antiserum titer, specificity, and affinity.

Such variability is often overcome with the use of a monoclonal antibody. However, unless the antigen has many identical antigenic sites, a single monoclonal antibody cannot cause matrix formation and will cause little or no light scatter. If an appropriate mixture of monoclonal antibodies can be made, complexes will form, causing measurable light scatter. This blending of monoclonal antibodies or the use of monoclonals in particle-enhanced light-scatter assays ensures constancy of reagent production and gives these assays further stability and specificity.

AGGLUTINATION ASSAYS

Agglutination is the clumping and sedimentation of antigen after reaction with antibody. It was first noted when the reaction of bacteria incubated with serum from an infected patient was observed. Observation of the agglutination of red blood cells after incubation with serum led to the discovery of ABO blood groups. Agglutination has been extensively used as a detection system because of its ease and versatility. It is, however, only semiquantitative, showing reproducibility only within fourfold dilutions. Agglutinating antibodies (**agglutinins**) may be directed against naturally occurring antigens on the surface of cells (active or direct agglutination) or against substances that have been applied to the surface of cells or inert particles (passive or indirect agglutination).

Principles

Agglutination reactions depend on the formation of antibody bridges by bivalent (IgG) or multivalent (IgM) antibody between antigen particles with multiple antigenic determinants. Large particles, such as red blood cells or bacteria, contain many different antigens, as well as antigens that appear hundreds of times on the cell or particle surface. Thus it is possible for antibody molecules to bind to more than one site on a single particle or to bind to equivalent sites on different particles. Such binding is called *cross-linking*. Antigens with a single antigenic determinant do not permit cross-linking and therefore do not agglutinate. Cross-linking may create a high-molecular-weight lattice that clumps together and precipitates. Because of its size and multivalency, IgM is said to be 750 times more efficient at agglutination than IgG. Agglutination reactions are generally used to detect antibody directed to particulate antigens; quantitation is by serial dilution of serum. Reverse agglutination can be used to detect soluble antigen by using antibody adsorbed onto cell or particle surfaces. Agglutination reactions are read by the naked eye or with the aid of magnification. The extent of agglutination is scored 1+ to 4+ by estimation. The titer of the serum is the reciprocal of the highest dilution giving visible (1+) agglutination.

Factors Influencing Agglutination Reaction

Factors influencing agglutination include particle charge, antibody type, electrolyte concentration, viscosity of the medium, reactant concentrations, location and concentration of antigenic determinants, and time and temperature of incubation.

Particle charge. Red blood cells, bacteria, and inert particles such as latex have a net negative surface charge called the *zeta potential*. These charges must be overcome to permit the cross-linking that results in agglutination.

Antibody type. IgM antibodies are more efficient at agglutination because of their multivalency and because their size permits more effective bridging of the gap between cells caused by charge repulsion.

Electrolyte concentration and viscosity. The ionic strength of the medium used for the agglutination reaction can assist in reducing the negative surface charge of particles. This can be accomplished by addition of charged molecules, such as albumin, to the medium. The pH of the medium should be near that present in physiological conditions. At neutral pH, high electrolyte concentrations act to neutralize the net negative charge of particles. Increasing the viscosity of the medium with polymerized molecules, such as dextran, also assists in bringing the charged particles together.

Antigenic determinants. As stated earlier, antigens with multiple antigenic determinants are necessary for agglutination. A monovalent antigen does not permit cross-linking. The placement of the antigenic determinants on the particle can also affect agglutinability. Antigenic determinants that are sparsely distributed are not as easily cross-linked as antigenic determinants that are densely distributed. Antigenic determinants can also be inaccessible to antibody binding because they are buried within cell membranes.

Concentration, temperature, and time of incubation. Concentration of reactants can therefore influence reaction time. At higher antigen concentrations, the reaction with antibody is more rapid. Agitation of the antigen suspension with antibody solution increases the reaction rate by increasing the surface area exposed to the antibody. At lower antigen concentrations, the reaction time can be shortened by centrifugation, which increases contact between the antigenic particles and the antibody. The temperature of incubation is also an important variable. Some antigens, including microbes, are bound most readily by antibody at 37° C. Some antigens react optimally with antibody at 4° C. These **cold agglutinins** include antibody to the i antigen of fetal and infant red blood cells. Optimum temperature for the agglutination reaction varies with different antigen-antibody systems. Temperature also affects the behavior of antibodies in vitro.

Direct Agglutination

Direct agglutination tests are frequently used in the immunological diagnosis of microbial infections. The titer of the serum reflects the concentration of the predominant antibody in the serum. Early detection of a high titer and documentation of a significant rise in titer are important tools in diagnosis. Antibodies to *Brucella* (brucellosis), *Salmonella* (typhoid fever), and *Proteus* (Rocky Mountain spotted fever) organisms are detected in this way. Direct agglutination tests are also used in the typing of human red blood cells in the blood bank.

Different bacterial antigens may give different patterns of agglutination. Antibodies to bacterial flagella cause cross-linking of the flagella themselves. These antibodies cause formation of a loose, rapidly formed agglutinate. Antibodies to antigens in the body of the bacterium cause cross-linking of the organisms themselves. This results in a granular, compact precipitate that develops more slowly.

Indirect Agglutination

Indirect agglutination involves reaction of antibody with antigens that have been passively transferred onto the surface of particles (Fig. 12-4). Red blood cells, usually from humans, sheep, or turkeys, are employed. Inert particles such as latex (0.81 µm in diameter) and bentonite (clay) are also used. Polysaccharide and some protein antigens, such as albumin and purified protein derivative are easily adsorbed onto the particle surface. Other antigens require pretreatment of particles with tannic acid or chromium chloride, which modifies the cell surface. Antigen can be covalently bound to the cell surface by bifunctional molecules, such as bisdiazobenzidine or glutaraldehyde. Indirect agglutination is used in the diagnosis of syphilis. The Venereal Disease Research Laboratory (VDRL) test employs cholesterol crystals coated with cardiolipin antigen. Detection of rheumatoid factor, useful in the diagnosis of rheumatoid arthritis, uses agglutination of latex particles coated with human IgG. For the quantitation of rheumatoid factor, agglutination methods have been largely replaced by immunonephelometry.

Agglutination Inhibition

Agglutination inhibition is an adaptation of the agglutination reaction that permits detection and quantitation of soluble antigen. The concentrations of antibody and particles are carefully controlled to prevent antibody excess. Antibody is incubated with the test antigen solution, and antigen is bound to available antibody combining sites. The antibody is then added to particulate antigen suspensions. The failure to agglutinate indicates that enough antibody combining sites have been saturated with a soluble form of the same antigen so that insufficient antibody binding sites are available for binding and cross-linking of the particulate antigen. Quantitation of the soluble antigen can be accomplished by assessment of the degree of inhibition in serial dilutions of the antigen solution (Fig. 12-5).

ANTIGLOBULIN TESTING

Antiglobulin testing is a modification of the agglutination reaction to permit detection of certain immunoglobulins (incomplete antibody [IgG]) that may not produce agglutination even after binding to the particle surface. IgG is less effective at agglutination than IgM because its smaller size is less effective at bridging antigen particles. If an anti-immunoglobulin, or Coombs' reagent, is added to the un-agglutinated IgG-coated particles, the Coombs' reagent will bridge the gap between particles by bivalent binding (Fig. 12-6). This enables cross-linking to achieve agglutination. The direct **Coombs' test** is used in blood banks to determine the presence of IgG antibodies to red blood cells.

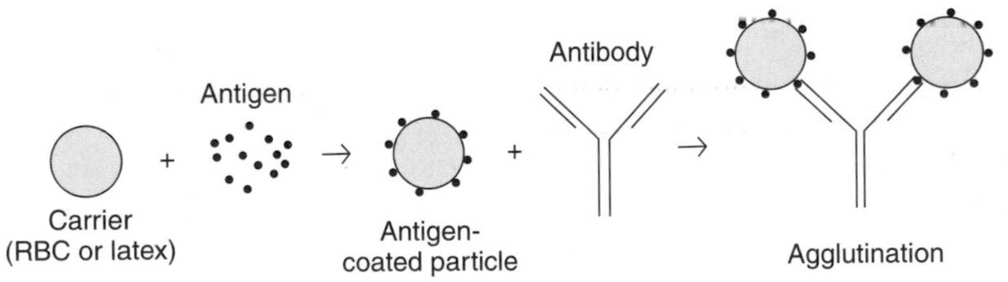

Fig. 12-4 Passive (indirect) agglutination reaction. Antigen is adsorbed onto surface of carrier particle, which is then agglutinated by antigen-specific antibody.

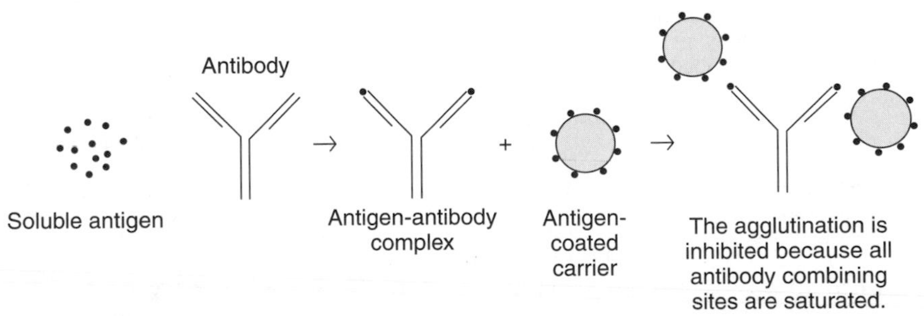

Fig. 12-5 Agglutination-inhibition reaction. Same reaction as that shown in Fig. 12-4, but inhibited by soluble antigen.

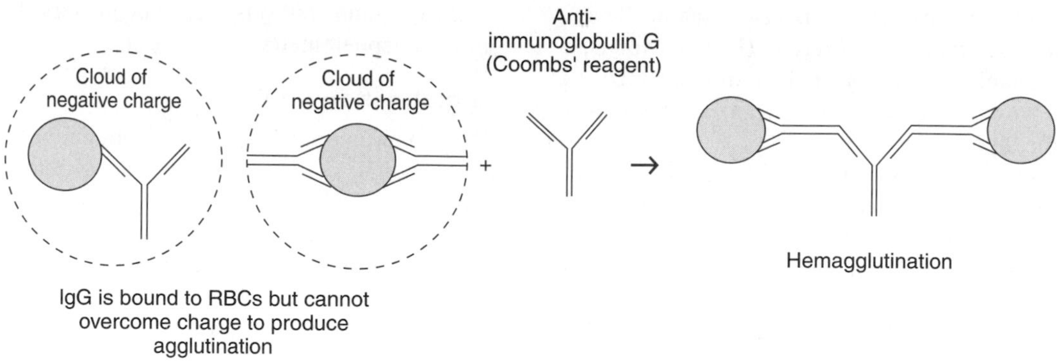

Fig. 12-6 Direct Coombs' test for antibody to red blood cells.

The indirect Coombs' test is a variation of the antiglobulin test and is used to detect free antibody to red blood cells in patient serum (Fig. 12-7). Serum is screened against a panel of red blood cells of known and varied antigenicity. Agglutination of cells to which patient serum and anti-globulin reagent have been added indicates the presence of antibody in patient serum to an antigen present on the agglutinated cells.

Sample Requirements

Agglutination reactions can be used to measure components of plasma, serum, or cerebrospinal fluid. Urine must be buffered because of its usual acidity. Because serum complement may affect agglutination, inactivation or dilution to minimize complement may be necessary.

Reagents

Similarly to red blood cell agglutination techniques, the factors influencing the reactions are particle charge, type of antibody, electrolyte concentration, and viscosity. Red blood cells, when used fresh, have a shelf life of about 2 weeks. Therefore many manufacturers have developed fixed red blood cells (usually stabilized by tannic acid or glutaraldehyde) or latex beads to overcome the need to prepare the reagents every few weeks.

Instrumentation

The great advantage of this technique is the simplicity of instrumentation. Results can be detected by eye or with the aid of a mirror or magnifying glass.

Common Pitfalls

Antigen excess often results in a **prozone phenomenon** with false-negative results. Use of expired red blood cells or other reagents can result in lack of agglutination.

Limitations

The technique is only semiquantitative and thus allows estimates of the true value within a dilution factor of two.

COMPLEMENT-FIXATION ASSAYS

The complement-fixation tests are probably the most sensitive of the immunological procedures that were developed early in the history of immunology. Tests more sensitive than **complement fixation,** such as RIA and EIA, have now been developed, but complement-fixation tests are still important, especially in the diagnosis of fungal, viral, and parasitic infections and in the quantitation of functional complement levels (total hemolytic complement) and complement components.

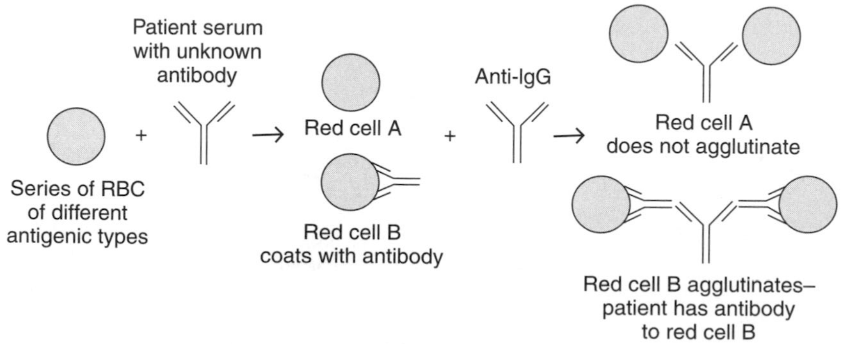

Fig. 12-7 Indirect Coombs' test for antibody.

Complement Proteins

The term *complement* is used to denote a series of plasma proteins that are activated in sequence after antigen-antibody reactions. Not all classes and subclasses of immunoglobulins are capable of activating complement or can activate it to the same degree (see Table 11-1, p. 221). The antigen-antibody complex used in complement-fixation tests therefore must involve an antibody that is capable of activating, or fixing, complement. As with agglutination reactions, pentameric IgM is 1000 times more efficient in fixing complement than IgG is.

The first protein in the complement sequence is bound to the second constant domain of the heavy chain (C_{H2}), which is inaccessible on an unreacted or unbound antibody. After interaction and binding with antigen, conformational changes in the immunoglobulin molecule cause the hinge region to open and the complement-binding site to be exposed. Subsequent complement proteins are then activated and can bind to the membrane of the cell to which the antigen-antibody complex is bound. Binding of the complete sequence of nine complement proteins results in small defects in the membranes of the cells. Cytoplasmic cell contents are lost through these holes, and extracellular fluid is admitted. This results in hypotonic swelling of the cell and ends in cell lysis. If the cells used in the test are red blood cells, cell lysis results in release of hemoglobin into the medium. The amount of hemoglobin is directly proportional to the amount of complement fixed to the surface of the cells.

One-Stage Testing

To assess total complement levels (complement activity that reflects all nine major complement proteins) or to assess individually the nine major complement proteins, a one-stage test system is used. A constant volume of red blood cells, usually sheep, is added to a constant amount of anti–sheep red blood cell, or hemolysin. A source of complement is added. For total complement measurements, dilutions of the unknown serum are used. For measurement of complement components, serum with an added excess of every complement component except the component to be measured is used. The degree of hemolysis is measured in a spectrophotometer and is directly proportional to the amount of complement available for fixation in the test serum (Fig. 12-8).

Some immunologically mediated diseases cause a decrease in total serum complement levels or in the levels of individual complement components. In addition, hereditary deficiencies of certain components of the complement system have been described.

Two-Stage Testing

Two-stage complement-fixation testing is used to measure antigen or antibody. In the first reaction, antigen and antibody are incubated with a known amount of complement. In the second stage, the residual complement activity in the solution is determined by an indicator system, such as sheep red blood cells that are coated with hemolysin. The degree of hemolysis of the indicator cells is inversely proportional to the amount of complement fixed in the first reaction (Fig. 12-9).

To determine antigen levels, a constant volume of antibody is used. To determine antibody levels, a constant amount of antigen is used.

Sample Requirements and Preparation

Plasma collected in ethylenediaminetetraacetic acid (EDTA) preservative, serum, and cerebrospinal fluid may be analyzed, but certain precautions are necessary. The samples cannot be hemolyzed. The endogenous complement of the sample must be inactivated, usually by heating of the specimen for 15 to 30 minutes at 56° C.

Reagents

Exogenous complement must be prepared daily and cannot be stored. The complement activity varies significantly from batch to batch and must be standardized daily.

Limitations

Complement-fixation tests are sensitive to many variables. They are inhibited by anticomplement activity (factors that inactivate or interfere with any of the complement proteins) in serum, including factors such as circulating immune (antigen-antibody) complexes, lipemic sera, aggregated immunoglobulins, and heparin.

It is critical to keep all components in the test constant except the one that is to be measured. Red blood cell number, concentration of complement, and concentration of antigen should be rigorously defined for antibody determinations.

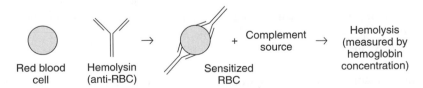

Fig. 12-8 Complement fixation one-stage testing. For measurement of total hemolytic complement, test serum is added as source of complement. For measurement of complement components as complement source, test serums to which purified complement components are added are used; for example, to measure complement component 3, all components are added, except C3, in excess to test serum. Therefore reaction is limited only by concentration of C3 in test serum.

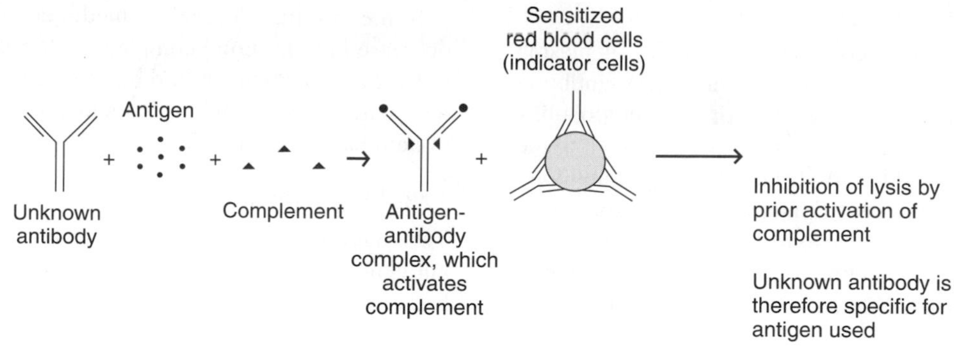

Fig. 12-9　Complement-fixation two-stage testing. Antigen or antibody can be measured by holding constant all but the variable to be tested, in this case unknown antibody.

The instability of some complement proteins, variability in red blood cells, variation between lots of hemolysin, and the narrow range of optimum reactivity for many reagents influence test results. The need for fresh reagents and the great variability make this assay one of the most difficult performed by a laboratory.

The CDC evaluates complement-fixation reagents and has developed standardized procedures for complement-fixation tests.

INDICATOR-LABELED IMMUNOASSAYS

The immunoassays described earlier all use direct measurement of a physical property of the antigen-antibody complex or aggregates formed secondarily to the initial binding step (such as precipitation or light scatter). By introducing a labeled indicator antigen or antibody to trace the initial binding reaction, an enhanced analytical sensitivity can be achieved. These indicator-labeled immunoassays use as a detection system the sensitive measurement of some property of the indicator molecule. The indicators, or labels, commonly used include enzymes, fluorescent or chemiluminescent molecules, and radioactive compounds.

Indicator-labeled assays are suitable for both qualitative and quantitative measurements. Their increasing popularity is due to the fact that they are sensitive, reproducible, use minimal reagents, and are suitable for automation. The nonisotopic immunoassays have the additional advantage over RIA in that they do not require the special precautions and waste-disposal procedures necessary for handling radioisotopes.

Quantitative immunoassays of this type usually use IgG as the reagent antibody. Although they are quite specific by virtue of the antibody specificity, the binding reactions are sensitive to the usual variations in temperature, pH, ionic strength, and sample or standard matrix. Analytical sensitivity to nanogram/milliliter range or even lower allows this type of assay to be used for analytes that are present in low concentrations, such as hormones, vitamins, and drugs.

Qualitative indicator-labeled immunoassays frequently are less sensitive but are convenient and very popular in the serology laboratory for the detection of antibodies to infectious organisms and for the characterization of autoimmune antibodies such as antinuclear antibody and antithyroid antibodies.

Indicator-labeled immunoassays may be generally classified as *competitive* or *noncompetitive* and as *heterogeneous* or *homogeneous*. Competitive reactions usually use labeled antigen and are carried out in the presence of excess antigen. The analyte and labeled analyte compete for binding sites on the antibody. Radioimmunoassay (RIA) is the prototype of the heterogeneous type of competitive immunoassay, and enzyme-multiplied immunoassay technique (EMIT) is an example of the homogeneous type (see Chapter 13). Noncompetitive assays usually employ a labeled antibody and are carried out in the presence of excess antibody. Frequently these assays are heterogeneous, using a capture antibody bound to a solid phase such as a plastic bead or test tube and a second phase consisting of the labeled antibody in solution. This latter type of assay is synonymous with the terms *immunometric* or *sandwich assay*.

Labels

A label that is suitable for use as an immunochemical reagent must have certain qualities. The label must have high specific reactivity, that is, many detectable events per indicator molecule per unit of time. The specific activity must not be reduced, or quenched, by the conjugation of the indicator to the antigen or antibody. Enzyme labels should not be normally present in the sample in high enough concentrations to interfere with the measurement. This is crucial for homogeneous assays in which the sample matrix containing interfering substances remains in the reaction mixture during the measurement step. Several enzymes, metal chelates, radioisotopes, chemiluminescent dyes, and fluorophores fulfill most of these requirements and have been successfully used as labels in immunoassays. Examples of enzymes commonly used are horseradish peroxidase, alkaline phosphatase, glucose oxidase, and β-galactosidase. Selection of the enzyme for use as a label for the immunochemical reagents is often empirical, and each enzyme has distinct advantages and disadvantages. (For the properties of enzymes, see Chapter 54.) Radioisotopes can be used to label

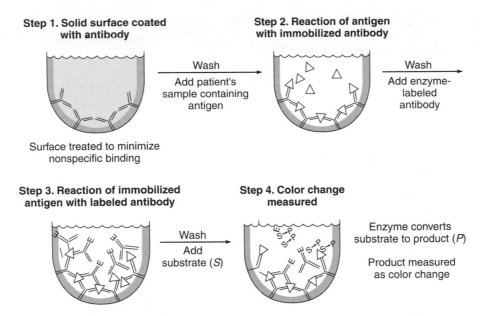

Step 1. Solid surface coated with antibody

Wash
Add patient's sample containing antigen

Surface treated to minimize nonspecific binding

Step 2. Reaction of antigen with immobilized antibody

Wash
Add enzyme-labeled antibody

Step 3. Reaction of immobilized antigen with labeled antibody

Wash
Add substrate (*S*)

Step 4. Color change measured

Enzyme converts substrate to product (*P*)

Product measured as color change

Fig. 12-10   Enzyme immunoassay. Sandwich technique with antibody label.

either antigens or antibodies. The most commonly used radioisotope is iodine-125, which has a high specific activity and a decay energy suitable for safe use in clinical laboratories (see Chapter 9).

In fluorometric immunoassays, either antigen or antibody can be conjugated, or covalently linked, with a fluorochrome molecule. The fluorochrome is a chemical that can absorb the electromagnetic energy of short-wavelength light (200 to 400 nm) and then emit light at a longer wavelength in the visible spectrum (400 to 700 nm) (see p. 98). Intensity of the emitted light is the measurable indicator in fluorometric immunoassays. The most popular fluorochrome is fluorescein isothiocyanate, often abbreviated FITC, which can be easily conjugated to free amino groups; other fluorophores include rare-earth chelates. Chemiluminescent dyes are used in a similar manner. In this case, the conjugate is activated by a chemical reaction and subsequently emits light that can be measured. The chemiluminescent molecule may be directly conjugated to the label or a chemiluminescent substrate can be used with an enzyme label such as alkaline phosphatase.

IMMUNOMETRIC ASSAYS
Principles

Heterogeneous, noncompetitive, labeled antibody (immunometric technique). A popular format for this type of immunoassay is the **heterogeneous immunoassay** using a solid phase coated with antibody for the first step of the assay. The first antibody reacts with the antigen being tested. The extent of this reaction is assessed by subsequent reaction with a second, labeled antibody. This forms the "sandwich" with the antigen between two different antibodies. The sandwich technique can be used to measure either antigens or antibodies (in which case the solid phase is coated with antigen). Antibodies have been immobilized

to polystyrene (microtiter plates), latex, or ferromagnetic particles.

For the antigen-measuring system, two different molecules of antibody must bind to the antigen. Thus this type of immunoassay can measure only large antigens, such as proteins with multiple epitopes (Fig. 12-10). Antibody of the desired specificity is immobilized to a solid surface, which may be the wells in a microtiter plate or a plastic test tube. The solid surface is washed to remove all unreacted materials and may then be coated with other material (protein) to minimize nonspecific reactions, with subsequent possible false-positive results. In the second step, the fluid containing the antigen is reacted with the immobilized antibody. All nonreacting material is then washed away. In the third step, the labeled antibody reacts with the antigen that has now been immobilized by the antibody onto the solid phase. All unreacted labeled antibody is then washed away. If enzyme is used as the label, substrate with appropriate cofactors is added. Color, fluorescence, or light is then used to measure the amount of product. Either end-point or kinetic measurements may be used. The intensity of the measured product is directly proportional to the amount of antigen bound to the solid phase. If a radioisotope was used as the label, the solid phase can be counted.

For an antibody-measuring system, the antigen of interest must be first immobilized on an insoluble matrix, such as a plastic surface or bead. Most often microtiter plates are used. Fig. 12-11 depicts this assay type. Immobilization with retention of antigenic reactivity is the first step of this procedure. In the second step, the biological fluid containing presumptive antibody toward the immobilized antigen is allowed to react. Any antibody present is bound to the antigen immobilized on the solid phase. After separation of the unreacted components by washing of the support surface,

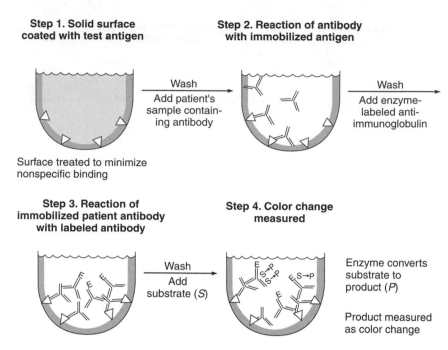

Fig. 12-11 Enzyme immunoassay. Detection of IgE specific for an allergen.

the presence of antibody is detected and quantitated by addition of labeled **antiantibody** that is directed toward the class specificity of the antibody being measured. Finally, the label is quantitated. This format is used to measure serum IgE that is specific for a particular allergen (the RAST test).

For both types of sandwich assays, the antibody or antigen coating the solid phase must be in excess over the analyte being measured. If the amount of antigen present exceeds the binding capacity of the capture molecule immobilized on the solid phase, the assay will not be quantitative, producing the so-called high dose hook effect. The labeled antibody must also be present in excess over the bound analyte to achieve a linear response and a quantitative assay.

Heterogeneous, competitive-binding assays. The simplest competitive-binding assay uses labeled antigen (Fig. 12-12) and a thorough treatment is given in Chapter 13. For the case of enzyme immunoassay, the enzyme-labeled antigen is mixed with the test solution, which contains an unknown amount of the antigen. The solution containing the labeled and unlabeled antigen is allowed to react with a limited amount of antibody that is bound to a solid matrix. Unbound antigen (both labeled and unlabeled) is removed by washing, and the amount of labeled antigen is measured by determination of the amount of enzyme bound to the solid surface. This assay is always performed in antigen excess. The test solution contains the enzyme substrate and cofactors, and the enzymatic reaction, producing a colored product, proceeds continuously. The intensity of color is inversely proportional, but not linear, to the concentration of the antigen present in the test sample. This format of immunoassay can be used to detect small molecular antigens

or hapten groups, including drugs and hormones such as steroids and thyroid hormones, in biological fluids.

Sample Requirements and Preparation

Many hormones, protein analytes, and antibodies in serum are stable for several days at refrigerator temperatures. For long-term storage, freezing is preferable.

Reagents

Solid phase. The plastic, latex, or magnetic bead should be chosen such that the bound ("capture") reagent is not removed by the wash solution under the assay conditions. Several manufacturers have developed plastic microtiter plates and test tubes specifically for enzyme immunoassays.

Substrate. In the case of enzyme labels, the appropriate pure substrate specific for the enzyme is selected to maximize the catalytic activity of the enzyme. As in any enzyme assay, care should be taken to add sufficient substrate so that it will not be depleted during the standard reaction time even if a large amount of enzyme label is bound to the solid phase.

Instrumentation

A spectrophotometer is usually used to measure the color changes that are a result of enzyme activity. With contemporary instruments, this process can be automated and kinetic measurements are possible. When the reaction occurs in microtiter plates with reaction volumes of 100 to 200 μL, special spectrophotometers called *microtiter readers,* or *microELISA readers,* are used. A drawback to the microtiter plate readers, however, is that they are frequently not as

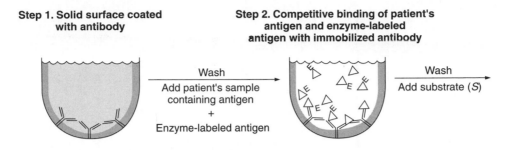

Step 1. Solid surface coated with antibody

Wash
Add patient's sample containing antigen
+
Enzyme-labeled antigen

Step 2. Competitive binding of patient's antigen and enzyme-labeled antigen with immobilized antibody

Wash
Add substrate (*S*)

Step 3. Color change measured

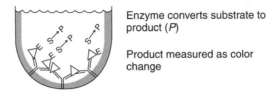

Enzyme converts substrate to product (*P*)

Product measured as color change

Fig. 12-12   Enzyme immunoassay. Competitive binding.

sensitive as a standard spectrophotometer. In addition, they are usually end-point readers. However, many have the ability to record the results of a standard 96-well microtiter plate in 1 to 2 minutes.

Instrumentation required for the measurement of radio-isotopes is presented in Chapter 9. Iodine-125, the radio-isotope most commonly used, requires a gamma counter. Specialized instrumentation is also required for the measurement of fluorescent labels. If metal chelates are employed, techniques such as time-resolved fluorescence may be used (see Chapter 4). Both the indirect and direct **fluoroimmunoassays** require a fluorometer or spectrophoto-fluorometer to obtain accurate reading of the fluorochrome-labeled antibody. Luminometers, or photon counters, measure light flashes or the "glow" emitted in chemilu-minescent assays (see Chapter 4).

Interfering Substances

Substances in the sample matrix may interfere with the antigen-antibody binding reaction or the detection of the label, or they may simulate the specific binding by increasing nonspecific binding or by cross-linking the label with the solid phase.

Nonspecific binding of labeled antigen or antibody should be tested at the time of assay development by incubating the solid support or capture phase with tracer in the absence of reagent antibody.

Any component in the sample that can link the solid phase antibody with the label will be measured as analyte. Sandwich assays using animal antibodies may show a positive interference if a patient has *heterologous (anti-species) antibodies* in his serum. This type of interference has been reported with increased frequency with the introduction of systems using mouse monoclonal antibodies as reagents. One example of heterologous, antimouse antibodies is seen in patients who have been treated with

mouse monoclonal antibodies for imaging or therapy and have subsequently developed human antimouse antibodies (*HAMA*). If HAMA interferences are suspected, they can be reduced or eliminated by preincubating with or including in the reaction mixture, additional nonimmune globulins from the same species that will bind up the antimouse, or antispecies, antibodies without interfering with the specific analytical reaction. Blocking reagents, which contain a lyophilized mixture of animal sera, are commercially available for this purpose. Rheumatoid factor, which is anti-IgG, may also interfere nonspecifically by linking solid phase antibody with labeled antibody.

In addition, the sample may contain substances that have enzyme activity or that fluoresce under assay conditions. Care must be taken to avoid contact with compounds that interfere with the detection of the enzyme label, such as inhibitors or oxidizing reagents.

Common Pitfalls

Common problems with these assays include the following:

1. Inappropriate plastic used for the microtiter plates or test tubes. This is not a common problem when using kits but is a consideration when developing new assays. Lot changes, even from the same supplier, occasionally result in poor performance because of changes in the properties of the plastic support.
2. Improper pH and ionic strengths of buffer.
3. Nonspecific adsorption of reactants to plastic surface. This nonspecific adsorption can be minimized by incubation of the solid phase with proteinaceous material, such as gelatin or bovine serum albumin, after initial adsorption of the capture reagent to the solid phase.
4. Inadequate control of experimental conditions. Precision in enzyme immunoassays depends on strict control of

TABLE 12-1   SUMMARY OF IMMUNOLOGICAL TECHNIQUES

Technique	Assay End Point	Assay Sensitivity	Time Needed for Assay Results	Common Analytes	Comments
Immunodiffusion (Ouchterlony)	Precipitation (qualitative)	45 μg/mL	8 to 72 hours	Bacterial, viral, or fungal antigens	Most frequently used to screen for presence of antigen
Immunoelectrophoresis	Precipitation (qualitative)	500 μg/mL	12 to 24 hours	Serum, urine, and cerebrospinal fluid protein	Used to assay complex mixture of analytes in biological fluids
Counterimmunoelectrophoresis	Precipitation (qualitative)	3 μg/mL	2 to 3 hours	Bacterial, viral, or fungal antigens	Commonly used to screen for antigens associated with infectious agents; more rapid than immunodiffusion
Two-dimensional immunoelectrophoresis	Precipitation (qualitative)	500 μg/mL	8 to 10 hours	Serum proteins	Research, used to examine subtle differences in proteins
Radial immunodiffusion (Mancini)	Precipitation (quantitative), CV 10% to 15%	50 μg/mL	12 to 24 hours	Serum and CSF proteins	Most commonly used immunological technique to measure serum and CSF proteins
Laurell (rocket) immunoelectrophoresis	Precipitation (quantitative), CV 8% to 12%	50 μg/mL	4 to 8 hours	Serum and CSF proteins	More rapid than radial immunodiffusion
Turbidimetry	Light-scattering of aggregates of antigen-antibody complexes (quantitative), CV ~8%	50 μg/mL	15 minutes	Serum and CSF proteins	More rapid than radial immunodiffusion
Direct and indirect agglutination	Agglutination of bacteria or red blood cell–containing antigen (semiquantitative)	15 μg/mL	1 to 5 minutes	Antibodies to bacterial antigens (such as febrile agglutinins) and red blood cell antigens	Techniques commonly used by serology laboratory and blood bank; not often used in chemistry laboratory
Agglutination inhibition	Inhibition of agglutination (semiquantitative)	15 μg/mL	2 to 5 minutes	Detect antigens such as pregnancy hormones (hCG)	Rapid test procedure often used to screen urine of pregnant women for hCG

Technique	Principle	Sensitivity	Time	Antigens/Uses	Comments
Immunofixation	Reaction of enzyme-labeled Ab with antigens fixed after electrophoresis	10 µg/mL	1 to 4 hours	Serum proteins including immunoglobulins	Used to study gammopathies and as Western blot to find antibodies to HIV
Complement fixation	Lysis of red blood cells or inhibition of red blood cell lysis (semiquantitative)	10 µg/mL	24 hours	Detect complement-fixing antibodies to bacterial, viral, or fungal antigens	Worldwide, commonly used serological procedure; sensitivity of assay approaches radioimmunoassay; assay difficult to perform
Immunonephelometry	Light-scattering of aggregates of antigen-antibody complexes (quantitative), CV 3% to 8%	1 µg/mL	1/2 to 1 hour	*Direct mode:* Serum, urine, and CSF proteins *Inhibition mode:* Drugs, such as theophylline and phenytoin	Popularly accepted technique to quantitate protein in many laboratories, this technique has replaced radial immunodiffusion
Enzyme immunoassay (ELISA, sandwich)	Color reaction between enzyme and substrate (quantitative), CV 8% to 15%	<1 ng/mL	1 to 24 hours	Serum proteins (such as IgE) Bacterial, viral, and fungal antigens Antibodies to infectious agents	Excellent assay for small amounts of antigen or antibody
Radioimmuno assay (RIA) (competitive binding)	Measurement of radioactivity	<1 ng/mL	2 to 24 hours	Capable of measuring most molecules large and small	Traditional assay, less popular because of radioisotope concerns
Enzyme immunoassay (competitive binding)	Color reaction between enzyme and substrate (quantitative), CV 8% to 15%	<1 ng/mL	2 to 24 hours	Small amounts of antigen (such as hormones, drugs, viral antigens)	Excellent assay for measuring ligands
Immunoradiometric	Radioisotope decay emission	<1 ng/mL	1 to 24 hours	Same as ELISA above	Excellent assay for quantitative measurement of low levels of antigens or antibodies; problem with radioactive wastes
Immunofluorometric	Fluorescence of dye	<1 ng/mL	1 to 24 hours	Same as ELISA and RIA above	Same as for immunoradiometric but no waste problem
Chemiluminescent	Chemiluminescence of dye	<1 ng/mL	15 to 60 minutes	Same as ELISA and RIA above	Very sensitive for quantitative measurement of low levels of antigens

CSF, *Cerebrospinal fluid;* CV, *coefficient of variation;* hCG, *human chorionic gonadotrophin hormone.*

temperature, pH, ionic strength of buffers, and concentrations of the various cofactors necessary for the enzymatic conversion of substrate into product. Finally, because enzymes are proteins and are subject to rapid denaturation under improper incubation conditions, close attention must be paid to preserve the enzyme activity during analysis.

5. Substrate depletion. If a large quantity of enzyme-labeled reagent is captured on the solid matrix, substrate can be depleted very rapidly. Sufficient substrate must be included in the reaction mixture so that a suitable working range is available, and the upper limits of linearity should be carefully defined.

Test Sensitivity and Precision

Numerous formats have been described for the performance of indicator-labeled immunoassays. The sensitivity and precision of each of these immunoassays depend on the format selected and the instrumentation used to measure the label. EIA and RIA are generally considered to be sensitive in the nanogram-to-picogram/mL range. Most currently available EIA and RIA techniques have a between-run coefficient of variation (CV) of less than 10% throughout the working range of the assay. Fluoroimmunoassays may have less sensitivity (about 100 to 200 µg/mL), but newer formats, including time-resolved fluoroimmunoassays and electrochemiluminescent assays, are as sensitive as most EIA or RIA. The variation observed within the same run is typically 3% to 6%.

Immunoassay sensitivity depends on high specific activity labels, low nonspecific binding, and excellent precision. Immunoassay *analytical sensitivity* is conventionally defined as the concentration that has a measured response at two standard deviations from the response of the zero standard. *Functional sensitivity* is defined as the lowest concentration that has a precision of 20% CV or lower. This determination is typically made from a *precision profile*, a graph of CV versus analyte concentration.

SUMMARY

The spectrum of immunological techniques is described and summarized in Table 12-1. Each of these procedures was developed to meet a specific need to identify or quantitate an antigen present in a patient's sample. The immunoprecipitation techniques are the least sensitive but have high specificity in determining the presence of an antigen within the working range of the assay. Immunonephelometry is the most sensitive of the quantitative assays using precipitation as an end point and is fast becoming the most popular form of assay to quantitate many serum and cerebrospinal fluid proteins. Recent advances in instrumentation have made this technique the most precise of the direct immunological techniques, and it has replaced radial immunodiffusion and rocket immunoelectrophoresis. Immunofixation and Western blot techniques are strictly qualitative tools. The former is commonly employed to identify an antigen present in a patient's sample, such as polyclonal IgG versus a monoclonal protein, or C3 breakdown versus C3 in native form. The Western blot technique is commonly used for the verification of the presence of antibody to a specific antigen, such as HIV. The agglutination and complement-fixation techniques are procedures used primarily in serology and blood bank laboratories.

Indicator-labeled immunoassays predominate in the clinical laboratory as quantitative tools because they extend the sensitivity and specificity of antigen detection. Nonisotopic immunoassays are the most frequently used immunoassays because of their sensitivity, specificity, and suitability for automation.

Selection of the appropriate immunological technique for detection of an antigen in the laboratory depends on many variables: technologist's skills, instrumentation, test volume and desired turnaround time, availability of test in kit form, quality control sample availability, ease of the technique, and cost to perform the assay. Whatever assay format is selected, the crucial factors that must be considered are the specificity of the reagent antibody, the antigen structure, and sample preservation.

Reference

1. Kricka LJ: Human anti-animal antibody interferences in immunological assays, *Clin Chem* 45:942, 1999.

Bibliography

General

Diamandis EP, Christopoulos TK, editors: *Immunoassay*, New York, 1996, Academic Press.

Gosling JP: A decade of development in immunoassay methodology, *Clin Chem* 36(8):1408, 1990.

Nakamura RM, Kasahara Y, Rechnitz GA, editors: *Immunochemical assays and biosensor technology for the 1990s*, Washington, DC, 1992, American Society for Microbiology.

Roitt IM: *Essential immunology*, ed 6, Oxford, England, 1988, Blackwell Scientific.

Roitt IM, Brostoff J, Male DK: *Immunology*, London, 1985, Gower Medical Publishing.

Rose NR et al, editors: *Manual of clinical laboratory immunology*, ed 5, New York, 1997, American Society for Microbiology.

Stites DP, Stobo JD, Wells JV, editors: *Basic and clinical immunology*, ed 6, Norwalk, CT, 1987, Appleton & Lange.

Weir DM, editor: *Handbook of experimental immunology*, ed 4, Oxford, England, 1986, Blackwell Scientific.

Electrophoresis and Immunofixation

Keren DF: *High resolution electrophoresis and immunofixation,* ed 2, Boston, 1994, Butterworth.

Nephelometry

Ritchie RF: The maturation of light-scattering immunoassay. In Nakamura RM, Kasahara Y, Rechnitz GA, editors: *Immunochemical assays and biosensor technology for the 1990s,* Washington, DC, 1992, American Society for Microbiology.

Whitcher JT, Perry DE: Nephelometric methods. In Nakamura RM, Kasahara Y, Rechnitz GA, editors: *Immunochemical assays and biosensor technology for the 1990s,* Washington, DC, 1992, American Society for Microbiology.

Immunonephelometry

Nishikawa T, Kubo H, Saito M: Competitive nephelometric immunoassay methods for antiepileptic drugs in patient blood, *J Immunol Methods* 29:85, 1979.

Price CP, Spencer K, Whitcher JT: Light scattering immunoassays of specific proteins: a review, *Ann Clin Biochem* 20:1, 1983.

Agglutination

Bell CA, editor: *A seminar on antigen-antibody reaction revisited,* Washington, DC, 1982, American Association of Blood Banks.

Kasahara Y: Principles and applications of particle immunoassay. In Nakamura RM, Kasahara Y, Rechnitz GA, editors: *Immunochemical assays and biosensor technology for the 1990s,* Washington, DC, 1992, American Society for Microbiology.

Lennette EH et al, editors: *Manual of clinical microbiology,* ed 3, New York, 1980, American Society for Microbiology.

Williams CA, Chase MW: *Methods in immunology and immunochemistry;* vol 3, *Reactions of antibodies with soluble antigens;* vol 4, *Agglutination, complement, neutralization and inhibition,* New York, 1977, Academic Press.

Complement Fixation

Stansfield WD: *Serology and immunology,* New York, 1981, McMillan.

Fluoroimmunoassays

Hemmil Ada L: Fluoroimmunoassays and immunofluorometric assays, *Clin Chem* 31:359, 1985.

Enzyme Immunoassays

Avrameas S et al, editors: 25 years of enzyme immunoassay, *J Immunol Methods* 150:1, 1992.

Engvall E, Perlmann P: Enzyme-linked immunosorbent assays (ELISA): quantitative assay of immunoglobulin G, *Immunochem* 8:871, 1971.

Kemeny DM, Chaldacombe SJ: *ELISA and other solid phase immunoassays,* New York, 1988, Wiley & Sons.

Precision Profile and Functional Sensitivity

Ekins R: The "precision profile": its use in RIA assessment and design, *The Ligand Quarterly* 4:33, 1981.

Sadler A et al: A method for direct estimation of imprecision profiles, with reference to immunoassay data, *Clin Chem* 35:1188, 1988.

Spenser C: Clinical utility and cost-effectiveness of sensitive thyrotropin assays in ambulatory and hospitalized patients, *Mayo Clin Proc* 63:1214, 1988.

Internet Sites

General

http://www.indstate.edu/thcme/micro/imm-tech.html—Indiana State University

www.uct.ac.za/microbiology/ababs.htm—Immunoassay techniques

www.xs4all.nl/~ednieuw/IgGsubclasses/subkl5.htm

http://www.bertholf.net/rlb/lectures/Lectures/Immunochemical%20Methods.pps—PowerPoint lecture by Robert L Bertholf, PhD, Associate Professor of Pathology, Chief of Clinical Chemistry and Toxicology

Immunoelectrophoresis

http://dpalm.med.uth.tmc.edu/Interps/Main.html—University of Texas-Houston, Immunology Page

http://www.path.queensu.ca/present/collier/monoclonal/—Kingston General Hospital (Canada)

Nephelometry and Immunonephelometry

http://swnt240.swmed.edu/medlabsci/hoypdf/nephelometry.pdf

Agglutination and Complement Fixation

http://brie.medlabscience.med.ualberta.ca/de/immunology/70imm-second.html—University of Alberta

http://www.tdh.state.tx.us/lab/serology_agg.htm—Texas Department of Health

http://www.cehs.siu.edu/fix/medmicro/cfix.htm

http://imc.gsm.com/demos/imdemo/ch2/fixation.htm

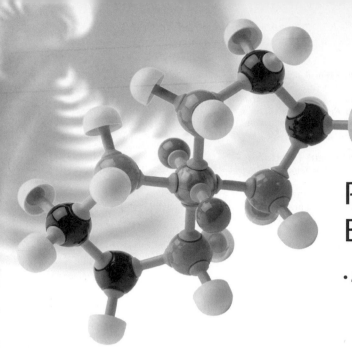

CHAPTER 13

Principles for Competitive-Binding Assays

• *Stephan G. Thompson*

Chapter Outline

Protein binding and the law of mass action
Behavior of competitive-binding assays
Competitive-binding assay formats
  Heterogeneous assays
  Homogeneous immunoassays
Labeled ligands
  Types of labels
  Factors determining choice of label
  Other labels
Detection limits (sensitivity)
Cross-reactivity (specificity)
Data reduction

Examples of competitive-binding assays
  Radioimmunoassay (RIA)
  Enzyme-linked immunosorbent assay
  Time-resolved fluorescence
  Rapid assays
Homogeneous assay techniques
  Homogeneous enzyme immunoassay
  Fluorescence polarization immunoassay
  Electrochemiluminescence
  Microparticle-based light-scattering immunoassays
Attributes and limitations of different approaches to
  competitive-binding assays

Key Terms

capture phase Ligand or specific binding protein attached to a solid surface or matrix to help separate bound from free label in a heterogeneous assay.

cloned-enzyme donor immunoassay (CEDIA) A homogeneous immunoassay in which a low–molecular-weight ligand is labeled with a genetically cloned fragment (enzyme donor) of β-galactosidase. The remaining portion of the molecule, complementary enzyme acceptor, is inactive unless the two components can combine to generate an active enzyme. In the assay, this combination is inhibited by antibody to the ligand-enzyme donor complex. The inhibition is relieved in a dose-response manner when the test ligand is present in the solution.

competitive-binding assay An analytical procedure based on the reversible binding of a ligand to a binding protein. The ligand competes in proportion to its concentration with a labeled derivative for

binding to the limited number of binding sites.

conjugate Usually refers to the labeled reagent in which either the ligand (antigen) or antibody is covalently attached to the label.

detection limit The smallest concentration of a ligand that can be statistically distinguished from a zero level in an assay. The detection limit is also referred to as the sensitivity of an assay.

electrochemiluminescence Light emission resulting from the oxidation of a reactive label at the surface of an electrode upon the application of electric potential.

enzyme-linked immunosorbent assay (ELISA) A heterogeneous immunoassay that in one configuration employs an enzyme-labeled ligand and antibody immobilized on a solid phase.

enzyme-multiplied immunoassay technique (EMIT) A homogeneous enzyme immunoassay in which a low-molecular-weight ligand is attached to an enzyme that is inhibited when the conjugate is bound by a specific antibody. Competitive binding of unlabeled ligand to the antibody relieves the inhibition in proportion to the ligand concentration.

fluorogen   A nonfluorescent molecule that becomes fluorescent when modified by a chemical or enzymatic process.

heterogeneous assay   A competitive-binding assay in which it is necessary to separate mechanically the protein-bound, labeled ligand from the unbound ligand before measurement of the signal generated by the label.

homogeneous assay   Competitive-binding assay in which it is not necessary to separate protein-bound and free ligand fractions because the signal of the label is modulated by protein binding.

immunoassay   Any binding assay in which the binding protein is an antibody.

immunogen   A substance that stimulates an antibody response when administered to an appropriate animal. Immunogens include macromolecular antigens and otherwise nonantigenic haptens coupled to a macromolecular carrier.

immunometric assay   Competitive and noncompetitive protein-binding assays in which the antibody rather than the ligand is labeled with a radioisotope or other suitable label.

label   An atom or molecule attached to either the ligand or binding protein, capable of generating a signal for monitoring the binding reaction.

ligand   A molecule or part of a molecule that is reversibly bound by the binding protein in a competitive-binding assay. It usually is the analyte but can also be a cross-reactant.

luminogenic substrates   Enzyme substrates that emit light upon hydrolysis. Light emission is either a rapid (5- to 10-second) "flash" or a long-lived "glow" where the emission is measured up to 2 hours after the reaction is started.

rapid assays   Semiquantitative immunoassays performed in a small hand-held device. Bound label is most often separated from the free label by "lateral flow" membrane chromatography.

sensitivity   The degree of response to a change in the ligand concentration in an assay. Sensitivity often refers to the detection limit.

specificity   The degree to which a binding protein binds its particular ligand while not binding structurally similar compounds.

time-resolved fluorescence   Long-lasting fluorescence emitted from the chelates of lanthanide metals such as europium and terbium. Also characterized by its high quantum yield and enormous Stokes shift.

PROTEIN BINDING AND THE LAW OF MASS ACTION

Competitive-binding assays are based on the noncovalent, reversible binding of a **ligand** to a specific binding protein. The binding assay is most often described by the following reaction:

$$\text{Ligand} + \text{Binding protein} \rightleftharpoons \text{Binding protein:ligand} \quad \textit{Eq. 13-1}$$

where the binding protein has a measurable affinity for the ligand that interacts with it. In general, only one binding protein can bind a small molecule. This reaction can be considered simply as one molecule of ligand reacting with one protein binding site. The important molecular feature of binding proteins that enables them to be used in quantitative assays is their ability to bind compounds with a high specificity and affinity (see Chapters 11 and 12). Examples of specific binding proteins are listed in Table 13-1.

Nearly all competitive binding methods use antibodies as the binding protein for small molecules. These are usually gamma immunoglobulins (IgG) directly produced in animals by a cellular response to immunization with the ligand or produced by monoclonal antibody hybridoma techniques with cells derived from an original antibody-secreting cell. These methods are discussed in great detail in Chapters 11 and 12, as well as other sources listed in the bibliography at the end of this chapter.

Small molecules by themselves normally do not provoke an immune response but do elicit antibodies when coupled with larger molecules; such small molecules are termed *haptens*.

TABLE 13-1 SPECIFIC BINDING PROTEINS PRESENT IN BLOOD OR OTHER TISSUES	
Binding Protein	**Ligand**
Antibodies	Varied antigens
Corticosteroid binding globulin (CBG)	Cortisol, corticosterone
Estrogen receptor	Estrogen
Intrinsic factor	Vitamin B_{12}
Thyroid binding globulin (TBG)	Thyroxine (T_4) Triiodothyronine (T_3)
Vitamin D receptor	1-α,25-Dihydroxyvitamin D_3

Because such small molecules participate in competitive-binding assays where the binding protein is an antibody, the ligand may be referred to as a *hapten*.

The ligand in equation 13-1 is the analyte to be quantified. Often ligands are drugs (digoxin, theophylline), hormones (cortisol, T_4), or vitamins (B_{12}). For most competitive-binding reactions, the ligand refers to both the analyte and a **labeled** derivative of the analyte. Both must bind to the specific binding protein for the analyte to be measured. The final complex of binding protein and ligand is usually stable and dissociates only very slowly under favorable circumstances.

The binding reaction described in equation 13-1 is more complex for larger ligands such as proteins because macromolecules have many different binding sites (antigenic determinants) on their surface. A protein can therefore have more than one antibody simultaneously attached to it. Such binding determinants can be structurally quite different from one another, and so the population of antibodies generated in an immune response to large molecules is heterogeneous (polyclonal antiserum). The antigenic determinants of high-molecular-weight **immunogens** and low-molecular-weight haptens are similar when one considers the behavior of antibody-binding reactions. Although macromolecules can be measured by competitive protein binding assays, noncompetitive methods are employed more often. These are discussed in Chapter 12.

The law of mass action describes some aspects of the phenomenon that occurs when molecules bind to one another. This is best illustrated by examining the concentration of an antibody **(Ab)** and its ligand **(L)** or specific binding partner under equilibrium conditions. The bimolecular reaction

$$Ab + L \underset{k_{-1}}{\overset{k_1}{\rightleftharpoons}} Ab{:}L \qquad \textit{Eq. 13-2}$$

can be rearranged for calculation of the equilibrium association constant

$$K_a = \frac{k_1}{k_{-1}} = \frac{[Ab{:}L]}{[Ab][L]} \qquad \textit{Eq. 13-3}$$

where k_1 and k_{-1} are the respective rate constants for association and dissociation of the bound complex; [Ab] is the concentration of the unbound or free antibody at equilibrium; [L] is the equilibrium concentration of unbound ligand (a term denoting the antigen, hapten, or other substance); and [Ab:L] is the equilibrium concentration of the ligand-antibody complex. K_a, also referred to as the *affinity constant*, is defined in reciprocal molar concentrations (M^{-1}) or liters per mole (L/mol). This is the volume into which a mole of the binding protein can be diluted to yield 50% binding of the ligand. The larger the K_a, the greater the affinity of the antibody for the ligand. It follows that for a constant amount of antibody in the reaction, less ligand is required for a high-affinity antibody to bind 50% of the ligand than is required for 50% binding by a low-affinity antibody. Antiserum produced by an animal that has been immunized with a high-molecular-weight immunogen usually contains a mixture of different populations of antibody (polyclonal antisera) to that antigen. These different populations of antibody vary in their ability to bind the ligand (affinity) and in their ability to recognize different sites on the protein's surface.

Only one uniform population of binding sites exists for a ligand when the binding protein or antibody is homogeneous, as in the case of monoclonal antibodies, which have a uniform binding affinity (K_a) and specificity for the antigen.

Low-affinity binding proteins and antibodies typically have association affinity constants in the order of 10^5 to 10^7 L/mol, whereas binders suitable for **immunoassays** and other competitive-binding assays have association constants between 10^8 and 10^{11} L/mol. A higher association constant makes it possible to design assays with sensitivities as low as 10^{-12} M, or lower, provided that the label itself is detectable at these low concentrations.

BEHAVIOR OF COMPETITIVE-BINDING ASSAYS

The competitive-binding assay can be imagined as the addition of increasing amounts of unlabeled ligand to reaction mixtures containing known, constant amounts of labeled ligand and a specific binding protein. In this case, labeled ligand, L*, and antibody, Ab, are added together in equimolar amounts. If one presumes that all the L* is bound, the reaction becomes

$$L^* + Ab \rightleftharpoons Ab{:}L^*$$

Two things happen with the addition of increasing amounts of unlabeled ligand (L): (1) unlabeled ligand competes with the labeled ligand for antibody-binding sites, and (2) there is an excess of the total ligand (L and L*) in solution compared with the number of binding sites. The concentration of antibody-binding sites is therefore limiting with respect to total ligand, thus modifying the preceding reaction as follows:

$$L + AbL^* \rightleftharpoons AbL + AbL^* + L^* + L$$

Less L* is antibody-bound (as Ab:L*); thus more L* is free as the amount of L increases. The amount or percentage of L* in the bound form can be calculated from the amount of L and L* present.

When the percentage of labeled ligand bound is plotted as a function of the concentration of the unlabeled ligand, it yields the dose-response curve shown in Fig. 13-1. The term *dose-response curve* applies to a plot of binding versus increasing amounts of ligand. The curvature of the dose-response plot in Fig. 13-1 is attributable to the logarithmic

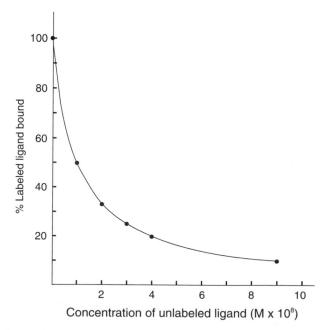

Fig. 13-1 Linear dose-response curve for a competitive protein-binding assay. Concentration (*M*) has been multiplied by 10^8.

increase in the percentage of L that is bound when the concentration of L (dose) in the assay increases arithmetically. Thus the decrease in bound L* is also logarithmic. Conversion of the concentration of L to a logarithm makes the relationship become more linear.

COMPETITIVE-BINDING ASSAY FORMATS

Fig. 13-1 shows that to derive a dose-response curve, one must know the amount of labeled ligand that is antibody-bound as a function of the amount of unlabeled ligand added. A variety of techniques have been developed to measure either the bound or free forms of the labeled ligand in a competitive-binding format.

Some of these techniques require that the antibody-bound labeled ligand be physically separated from the free labeled ligand. These assays are called **heterogeneous assays**. Immunoassay approaches that do not require physical separation of bound and free labeled ligand are called **homogeneous assays**. The activity of the label in a homogeneous assay is altered when the labeled ligand is bound to the specific binding protein; thus the bound and free labeled ligands can be directly distinguished from one another.

Heterogeneous Assays

Table 13-2 lists some of the methods commonly used to separate the protein-bound from free labeled ligand. In one example, the ligand or antibody is covalently attached or adsorbed to the hydrophobic plastic surfaces of microtiter plate reaction wells, providing a universally applied support for the **capture phases** of many different heterogeneous assays. The capture phase binds the labeled reactant in a competitive-binding heterogeneous assay, whether the latter is labeled ligand or labeled antibody. Another system, the microparticle-based capture phase, is widely used for two reasons: (1) suspended microparticle capture phases approach solution-like kinetics in that diffusion distances are very short compared with the surface of a microtiter plate well or a coated polystyrene tube, and (2) microparticles in comparison also provide a far greater surface area. For example, 1 mg of 1 μm diameter particles have 60 cm^2 of surface area for immobilization of antibody or ligand compared with the 1.0 to 1.5 cm^2 of surface area in a microtiter well. Both of these attributes shorten the assay time and potentially increase its sensitivity.

Latex and paramagnetic microparticles are used in similar heterogeneous assay formats; both can be used to readily separate the bound label from the unbound, one by filtration through a porous filter and the other by magnetic attraction.

Other methods for separating bound from free labeled ligand are listed in Table 13-2. Both the nonspecific adsorbent technique and the double antibody technique have been used with isotopic labels.

In some instances, competitive methods incorporate an indirect capture approach, in which an unrelated binding protein-ligand pair is used to bring the solid phase together with the capture antibody or ligand. In a classical example, immobilized streptavidin binds biotin that has been cova-

TABLE 13-2   TECHNIQUES TO SEPARATE PROTEIN-BOUND FROM FREE LABELED LIGAND

Technique	Principle
Adsorbents	
Nonspecific	Low–molecular-weight ligands are adsorbed by particles such as charcoal and removed by centrifugation.
Specific	Antibodies to the ligand or to the ligand-binding antibody are immobilized on the surface of a solid matrix such as glass fibers, latex microparticles, magnetic microparticles, membranes, or plastic. The immobilized antibody-ligand complex is separated from the unbound ligand by decantation, washing, filtration, diffusion, or centrifugation.
Chromatography	The protein-bound ligand moves at a rate through the chromatographic medium different from that of the free ligand. A similar behavior can occur with multilayer films.
Precipitation by ammonium sulfate	The antibody-bound ligand is precipitated by ammonium sulfate (Farr technique).
Double antibody	The antibody-bound ligand is precipitated by the addition of a second antibody specific for the antibody in the antibody-ligand or antibody-antigen complex.

lently attached to an antibody or to the ligand. Advantages to this approach are discussed below. Automation of some of the methods described in Table 13-2 has been accomplished, resulting in improved precision (see Chapter 16, pp. 297 to 301).

Homogeneous Immunoassays

By definition, the activity of the label in a homogeneous assay is modulated when bound to the specific binding protein; an exception to this generalized definition for homogeneous immunoassays is based on the scattering of light by microparticles. Instead of an antibody modulating the signal per se, changes in light scattering are produced by the formation of antibody:ligand:particle complexes, where either the antibody or ligand (or both) are multivalently attached to latex particles; the corresponding binding partner is also multivalent, thus enabling the components to form larger agglutinated complexes. An example is described later in this chapter.

LABELED LIGANDS
Types of Labels

Common types of markers used to label ligands include radioisotopes, enzymes, and fluorophores. These can be used in both homogeneous and heterogeneous competitive-binding assays. The type of label, assay, and detection system are presented in Table 13-3.

TABLE 13-3 SOME LABELS FOR COMPETITIVE-BINDING ASSAYS

Label	Detector
Enzymes	
Chromogenic substrates	Spectrophotometer
Fluorogenic substrates	Fluorometer
Luminogenic substrates	Luminometer
Enzyme fragments	Spectrophotometer, fluorometer
Enzyme substrates	Spectrophotometer, fluorometer, luminometer
Fluorophores, fluorogens	Fluorometer
Luminogens	Luminometer
Electrochemiluminescence	
Microparticles	Spectrophotometer, nephelometer
Radioactive isotopes*	Radioactivity counter

Usable only in heterogeneous assays.

TABLE 13-4 RADIOISOTOPES USED IN COMPETITIVE-BINDING ASSAYS

Isotope	Emission	Maximum Specific Activity* (Ci/g)	Half-Life	Counter[†]
^3H	Beta	9.6×10^3	12.3 years	LS
^{14}C	Beta	4.5	5730 years	LS
^{32}P	Beta	2.85×10^5	14.2 days	LS
^{125}I	Gamma	1.74×10^4	60 days	Crystal
^{57}Co	Gamma	8.48×10^3	270 days	Crystal

The curie (Ci) is a unit of radioactivity equal to 3.7×10^{10} disintegrations per second.
[†]*Beta-particle emitters are counted in liquid scintillation (LS) counters by the release of photons from organic phosphors in solution. Gamma-ray emitters are counted in detectors with a sodium iodide crystal that contains fluor from which photons are released.*

Factors Determining Choice of Label

Radioisotopes. Radioisotopic labels are used only with heterogeneous immunoassays because binding by antibody does not change the radioactive decay. In general, the desired sensitivity of the assay limits the choice of radioactive labels to certain specific isotopes that have high specific activity, high energy output, manageable half-lives, and ready availability. The radioisotope must be readily incorporated into or coupled to the ligand (or antibody) molecule, and its emission must be easily detected. Isotopes that meet these requirements are listed in Table 13-4. Consideration of all the factors, especially high specific activity, ease of incorporation, and reasonably short half-life, has made ^{125}I the label of choice for most radioassays.

Enzymes. Enzymes as labels differ from radioisotopes in that the binding reaction can modify their activity. Again, the enzymes must have high specific activity (i.e., conversion of many moles of substrate to product per minute per mole of

enzyme) and must also be easily attached to the ligand or antibody without losing significant activity. Enzymes that are commonly used include alkaline phosphatase, β-galactosidase, glucose oxidase, glucose-6-phosphate dehydrogenase, and peroxidase.

Some homogeneous enzyme immunoassays are based on the use of an inactive component of an enzyme molecule as the label. For example, in the **cloned-enzyme donor immunoassay (CEDIA)**, the reactant label is a polypeptide fragment of β-galactosidase that complexes with remainder of the enzyme. CEDIA is discussed in greater detail later.

Substrates. Substrates for enzyme labels also help define the means for detection and in some cases the format for how the assay will be performed. Examples are shown in Table 13-3. Until recently, the most commonly used substrates were either chromogenic or **fluorogenic**, with the enzyme-catalyzed product being colored or fluorescent, respectively. Luminogenic enzyme substrates that emit light upon enzyme catalysis have also been adopted for routine applications, particularly for the immunoassay of ligands that require greater sensitivity for detection and quantitation.

Although one can usually measure a thousand-fold lower concentration of a fluorophore by fluorescence techniques than by colorimetric methods, the gain in assay sensitivity with fluorogenic substrates for enzyme labels is at best only tenfold to a few hundredfold. Sensitivity greater than that seen with either fluorescence or colorimetry is generally achieved with **luminogenic substrates**. Since enzyme labels amplify the ligand or antibody molecules participating in the binding reaction, greater sensitivity can be achieved by longer incubation times for the conversion of substrate to product. This is an undesirable characteristic of some chromogenic substrates, particularly when more rapid assays are available that use either fluorogenic or luminogenic substrates. Two types of luminogenic substrates exist. When a "flash" reaction occurs, the emitted light is measured within 5 to 10 seconds after the reaction is initiated, whereas the dioxetane substrates "glow" upon hydrolysis so that the light measurement can be made from 2 minutes up to 2 hours after the reaction is started. The intensity of light and the duration of the emitted light in some flash reactions catalyzed by peroxidase are increased several orders of magnitude by the addition of phenolic enhancer molecules. Also, the emission becomes a stable glow that can be measured any time between 2 and 30 minutes after initiating the reaction.

Fluorophores. Fluorophores chosen as labels still fluoresce with a high degree of efficiency when attached to the ligand or antibody. The absorption (excitation) and emission wavelengths are well separated (Stokes shift) so that light scatter does not contribute to the fluorescence seen at the emission wavelength. Examples of fluorophores used as labels for competitive-binding assays and their properties are shown in Table 13-5. Of these, fluorescein and europium chelates are commonly used. Chelates of the rare-earth lanthanide metals europium and terbium strongly absorb light and fluoresce with properties that depend on the chelating ligand. The quantum yield (photon output/photon input) is very

TABLE 13-5   FLUOROPHORES USED AS LABELS IN COMPETITIVE-BINDING ASSAYS

Fluorophore	Excitation Wavelength (nm)	Emission Wavelength (nm)	ϵ*	Fluorescence Quantum Yield[†]
Europium chelate[‡]	340	613	90,000	>0.95
Fluorescein	490	520	72,000	0.85
β-Phycoerythrin[§]	488	576	2,400,000	0.98
Rhodamine	550	585	50,000	0.70
Umbelliferone	380	450	20,000	0.50

*ϵ is the absorbance of a 1 M solution through a 1-cm light path.
[†]The fluorescence quantum yield is relative to the quantum yield of acridine, which is 1.0.
[‡]Europium: β-diketone chelate.
[§]β-Phycoerythrin is a 240,000 dalton phycobiliprotein.

high, and the excitation and emission wavelengths are well separated. Europium and fluorescein have high extinction coefficients and quantum yields, but europium has the greatest separation between the excitation and emission wavelengths (273 nm).

Luminogens. In addition to being enzyme substrates, luminogenic molecules are also used as direct labels for immunoassays. For example, both luminol and acridinium esters emit light upon chemical oxidation and hydrolysis by hydrogen peroxide under basic conditions. The light is emitted in a "flash" over a 2- to 4-second interval. The intensity of the total light emission is measured over 5 or more seconds.

Electrochemiuminescence (ECL). Immunoassays based on ECL detection are composed of a label that emits light upon oxidation at the surface of an electrode when voltage is applied to it. The luminogenic label is a coordination complex of ruthenium, ruthenium (II) tris(bipyridyl) or $Ru(bpy)_3^{+2}$. Both $Ru(bpy)_3^{+2}$ and tripropylamine (TPA) are oxidized by the electrode to $Ru(bpy)_3^{+3}$ and the cationic radical, $TPA^{+}_{\bullet}$. Both oxidized species then react to form the excited label $Ru(bpy)_3^{+2}$*, which emits light upon returning to its ground state, ready for another excitation/emission cycle. Labels not at the surface of the electrode are not oxidized and therefore do not emit light. A description of competitive binding formats using ECL as the detection technology is presented later in this chapter.

Microparticles. When a microparticle multivalently coated with either antibody or ligand forms aggregated complexes upon binding to its specific binding partner, the increased particle size changes the amount and direction in which the light is scattered (see p. 101, Chapter 4). To minimize background signal, the measured particle should be smaller in diameter than the detection wavelength; thus optimal unaggregated particles are less than 1 μm in diameter. Both turbidimetry and nephelometry are commonly used to measure the binding reactions for microparticle-based competitive light-scattering reactions. Turbidimetry measures the decrease of incident light as a function of light scatter as the size of the aggregated particles increases. Thus these changes are detected as increases in absorbance at a particular wavelength. Nephelometry directly measures the scattered light at an angle greater than 90 degrees to the incident light (forward

light scatter). Since turbidimetry can be performed with a spectrophotometer, it has greater applicability to different analytical or clinical systems. Nephelometry, like fluorescence and luminescence, requires special optical instrumentation.

Other Labels

Two other labels that provide the basis for different homogeneous competitive protein-binding technologies are prosthetic group labels and substrate labels, respectively. Ligand labeled with an enzyme prosthetic group combines with the apoenzyme for activity. A specific antiligand antibody inhibits this interaction. Fluorogenic and luminogenic substrates have been used as reactant labels for the competitive-binding assays in which the unbound label is hydrolyzed by a specific enzyme.

DETECTION LIMITS (SENSITIVITY)

The sensitivity of a binding-reaction assay is a function of the affinity of the binding protein for its ligand. Consequently, for 50% binding to occur, a ligand present at a concentration of 1×10^{-7} M would require an antibody with a K_a of 10^7 L/mol, whereas a ligand present at a concentration of 1×10^{-10} M would need an antibody with a K_a of 1×10^{10} L/mol.

Ideally the binding protein in a competitive-binding assay would have the same affinity for both the labeled and unlabeled ligands; however, this is usually not the case. In some instances the label or the labeling procedure will alter the immunochemical properties of the ligand to the extent that antibody does not bind it as well as it does the unlabeled compound. In other instances, the converse is also true: antibodies made against haptens can include affinity for the chemical bridge used to couple the ligand to the protein carrier. Such antibodies may have a higher affinity for the labeled ligand with the chemical bridge than they do for the unmodified ligand.

The sensitivity of a competitive-binding assay is often improved if the ligand has sufficient time to bind to the antibody before the addition of the labeled ligand **conjugate**. This *sequentially* competitive-binding assay is particularly helpful when the antibody has greater affinity for the hapten conjugate than for the hapten alone compared with a *simultaneous* competitive format, in which the sample ligand

and the ligand conjugate have equal access to the antibody. The response to the presence of sample ligand is usually greater in a sequential format, since the ligand has more opportunity to occupy the available antibody-binding sites than it would in a simultaneous format.

Besides the relationship to the affinity of the binding reaction, the **detection limit**, or sensitivity of a competitive-binding assay, is also dependent on the relative detectability of the labeled species. For example, a fluorophore should provide greater sensitivity than a chromophore; the fluorescent or luminescent product of enzyme-label catalysis will place the detection limit 1 to 2 orders of magnitude below that usually observed with chromogens as substrates; europium chelates can provide greater sensitivity than ^{125}I because of their greater label density compared with ^{125}I, which is limited (to avoid damage to the radioactivity-labeled reagent).

Detection limit can be defined as the lowest concentration of a ligand that can be accurately and precisely distinguished from zero (ligand). Therefore, by definition, any nonspecific interaction that contributes to the signal in the absence of ligand compromises the detection limit by lowering the signal-to-noise ratio (S/N), thus making it more difficult to distinguish the signal derived from the specific binding reaction from that attributable to nonspecific binding (NSB) and other nonspecific interferences. Although other types of interference are prevalent in both homogeneous and heterogeneous assays, NSB is a common problem in the latter, where either a ligand-labeled conjugate or antibody-labeled conjugate nonspecifically adheres to the solid phase. This phenomenon can be attributable to sites on the solid phase available for hydrophobic or ionic adsorption, because binding sites on the solid-phase surface are not saturated or because of surface changes after coating or chemical modification. Reduction of the NSB is often achieved by inclusion of blocking proteins or detergents in the reactions.

CROSS-REACTIVITY (SPECIFICITY)

The specificity of a binding protein for its ligand is measured by its ability to bind only the ligand in contrast to other substances. Cross-reacting molecules are structurally so similar to the ligand that they are also bound by the antibody. The greater the chemical difference between the ligand and a potential cross-reactant, the less likely it is that the cross-reactant will be bound. Examples of potential cross-reactants are drug analogs and metabolites for drug assays and low-molecular-weight hormones that are similar in structure, such as T_3 and T_4 for their respective assays. Differences in antibody binding of ligand and cross-reacting substances are a function of differences in affinity. These differences are reflected by responses to cross-reactants in competitive-binding assays. Table 13-6 gives two examples of the relationship between the K_a of the antibody for its ligand, two cross-reactants, and the concentration of each that is required in the assay to deliver the same binding response. The concentration of cross-reactant$_a$ required for 50% binding to antibody$_1$ is 10 times the concentration necessary to bind 50% of ligand$_1$. Similarly, 10,000-fold less ligand$_2$ is

TABLE 13-6 CROSS-REACTANT BINDING AS A FUNCTION OF ANTIBODY AFFINITY

Antibody	Bound Species	K_a	Concentration (M) Required for 50% Binding*
1	Ligand$_1$	1×10^8	2×10^{-8}
	Cross-reactant$_a$	1×10^7	2×10^{-7}
	Cross-reactant$_b$	5×10^7	1×10^{-6}
2	Ligand$_2$	1×10^{10}	2×10^{-10}
	Cross-reactant$_c$	2×10^8	4×10^{-8}
	Cross-reactant$_d$	1×10^6	2×10^{-6}

*When 50% of the ligand or cross-reactant is bound, B/F = 1. Since $K_a = \frac{B}{F[Ab]}$; when B/F = 1 then $K_a = \frac{1}{[Ab]}$.

TABLE 13-7 CAFFEINE CROSS-REACTIVITY WITH POLYCLONAL OR MONOCLONAL ANTIBODIES TO THEOPHYLLINE

	CONCENTRATION (M) WHEN 50% OF LABEL IS BOUND		
	Theophylline	*Caffeine*	*% Cross-Reactivity*
Polyclonal	1.29×10^{-7}	1.05×10^{-6}	12.3
Monoclonal	6.15×10^{-8}	5.09×10^{-6}	1.2

required to achieve 50% binding to antibody$_2$ than is necessary to bind 50% of cross-reactant$_d$. Table 13-6 shows that with a lower K_a more antibody is required to bind 50% of the ligand or cross-reactant, further illustrating the relationship between sensitivity and K_a. The degree to which each cross-reactant in Table 13-6 interferes with the analysis of each ligand depends on the relative concentrations of ligand and cross-reactant in actual samples. For example, cross-reactants c and d would probably *not* interfere in the assay of ligand$_2$ *unless* they were present at concentrations 100 or 10,000 times higher, respectively, than that of ligand$_2$.

Ideally, antibodies or other binding proteins that participate in competitive-binding reactions are very specific for the ligand, with essentially no cross-reactivity with closely related molecules. In reality, the antibodies present in a heterogeneous antiserum bind the ligand with different affinities and orientations and are therefore also likely to bind structurally similar molecules. One of the advantages of monoclonal antibodies is the potential for selecting very specific antibodies that have essentially no cross-reactivity with other compounds. Examples of the cross-reactivity of antiserums and a monoclonal antibody are shown in Figs. 13-2 and 13-3. The dose-response curves seen with antiserum (Fig. 13-2) show that caffeine, which is structurally similar to the antiasthmatic drug theophylline, effectively competes only at much higher concentrations with the label for theophylline-binding sites. The degree of caffeine cross-reactivity, deter-

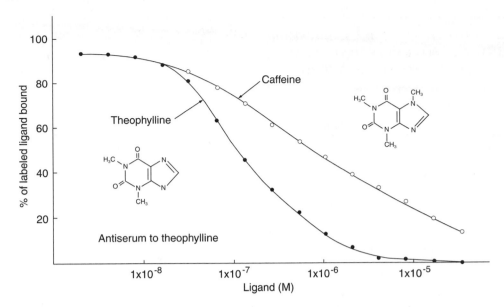

Fig. 13-2 Cross-reactivity of caffeine with a polyclonal antibody to theophylline in a homogeneous fluorescent immunoassay. Cross-reactivity is determined at concentrations of theophylline and caffeine required for 50% of the dose response. This is equivalent to 46.5% of the bound label. Refer to Table 13-7 for cross-reactivity data.

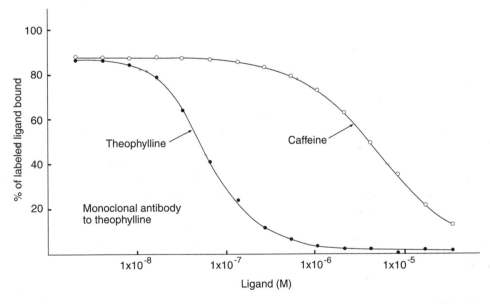

Fig. 13-3 Cross-reactivity of caffeine with a monoclonal antibody to theophylline in the same immunoassay. Cross-reactivity is determined at 43.2% of bound label.

mined by the "classical" approach, is calculated by dividing the concentration of ligand (in this case theophylline) at 50% of the maximum binding (indicated in Fig. 13-2) by the concentration of cross-reactant (caffeine), which also displaces 50% of the label according to the following equation:

$$\frac{[\text{Ligand}] \text{ at } 50\% \text{ binding}}{[\text{Cross-reactant}] \text{ at } 50\% \text{ binding}}(100) = \% \text{ cross-reactivity}$$

Eq. 13-4

Caffeine cross-reactivity for the antiserum is 12.3% in Fig. 13-2, whereas only 1.2% cross-reactivity occurs with the theophylline monoclonal antibody, as shown in Fig. 13-3.

Table 13-7 summarizes these results. A competitive-binding assay that uses the monoclonal antibody to theophylline is more specific than one that uses the antiserum; consequently, based on this analysis, the former assay would be less prone to caffeine interference.

Although the classical approach to determining cross-reactivity is useful for evaluating the comparative assay response of ligand and cross-reactant, the "functional" approach is more meaningful because it determines the contribution of a potential cross-reactant to the competitive-binding assay response in the presence of the ligand. For example, both the

TABLE 13-8 FUNCTIONAL AND CLASSICAL CROSS-REACTIVITY DETERMINATIONS FOR AN ANTITHEOPHYLLINE MONOCLONAL ANTIBODY

	CLASSICAL*		FUNCTIONAL†	
Cross-Reactant	µg/mL	%	µg/mL	%
1,3,7-trimethylxanthine (caffeine)	>10,000	<0.2	400	0.8
3,7-dimethylxanthine (theobromine)	760	2.8	390	0.8
1,3-dimethyluric acid	2900	1.0	580	0.5
3-methylxanthine	760	2.8	280	1.1

*Classical cross-reactivity determined as described by Eq. 13-4. Theophylline concentration at 50% binding was 21.3 µg/mL.
†Functional cross-reactivity is defined by the concentration of cross-reactant that increases the observed concentration of 15 µg of theophylline/mL control by 20%. Therefore, functional cross-reactivity is calculated as follows:

$$\% \text{ Cross-reactivity} = (100)\frac{3 \text{ µg theophylline/mL}}{\text{µg cross-reactant/mL at 20\% bias}}$$

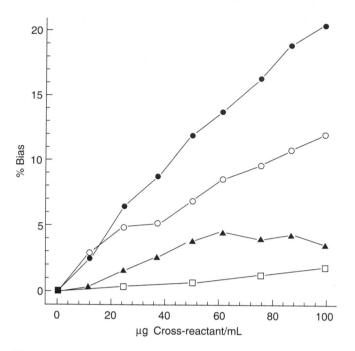

Fig. 13-4 Functional determination of cross-reactivity in a homogeneous turbidimetric inhibition assay. The observed increase in apparent concentration to a midrange control is measured in the presence of increasing concentrations of 1,3-dimethyluric acid, ●; 1-methylxanthine, ▲; 3-methylxanthine, ○; and caffeine, □.

ligand and the cross-reactant are competing with each other and with the ligand-label conjugate for antibody-binding sites. Consequently, it is not surprising when a cross-reactant with cross-reactivity of 1% to 2% in the classical method increases the known concentration of a ligand by 10% to 20%. One approach to evaluate functional cross-reactivity is to determine the assay response to increasing concentrations of cross-reactant at different concentrations of ligand. Table 13-8 summarizes the cross-reactivity of caffeine, theobromine, and various theophylline metabolites at a midlevel theophylline concentration compared with that observed using the classical approach, whereas Fig. 13-4 illustrates the response of various cross-reactants in a functional assay.

Now that the monoclonal antibodies produced from immortal cell lines can be readily screened for very high affinity ($K_a = 10^{11} - 10^{12} \, \text{M}^{-1}$) with almost absolute specificity, these binding proteins are preferred to polyclonal antibodies, which are often inconsistent in quality and availability.

DATA REDUCTION

Earlier in this chapter the displacement reaction was described by the equation

$$L + AbL^* \rightleftharpoons AbL + AbL^* + L^* + L$$

where Ab is the antibody or another binding protein providing a limited number of ligand-binding sites. The concentration of the labeled ligand, L^*, is constant and in excess of the binding-site concentration. The ligand, L, will compete with L^* for the available binding sites. As shown in Fig. 13-1, the amount of L^* bound by the antibody is inversely proportional to the concentration of L in the assay. The dose response is a measure of either the bound L^* or the free L^* that has been displaced by L. Radioimmunoassay (RIA) will serve to illustrate the common methods for generating dose-response curves and quantifying concentrations of analytes.

The data shown in Table 13-9 were generated with a double-antibody RIA for the aminoglycoside antibiotic amikacin, where ^{125}I-amikacin was the labeled ligand. The primary antibody was rabbit antiserum to amikacin. Goat antiserum to rabbit antibodies is included in the assay to precipitate the antibody-bound labeled ligand. The precipitate is collected by centrifugation, and the pellet in the bottom of the tube is counted for radioactivity after the supernatant has been removed. The *quantity nonspecifically bound (NSB) counts per minute* refers to the radioactivity nonspecifically bound to the bottom of the tube in the absence of antibody to amikacin.

Table 13-9 shows how the amikacin RIA data are processed to generate two common dose-response curves. In addition to the total bound counts per minute (TB), the y-axis can be drawn as %B, or logit B/B_0. The logit transformation is the following:

$$\text{logit } (B/B_0) = \ln \frac{B/B_0}{1 - B/B_0} \qquad \textit{Eq. 13-5}$$

The bound counts per minute and %B can be plotted as a function of the arithmetic dose of the ligand concentration even though the resulting curves are nonlinear (see Fig. 13-1), or they can be plotted versus the log of the concentration to yield the slightly sigmoid dose-response curve seen in Fig. 13-5. The graph of log dose versus the logit B/B_0 (also shown in Fig. 13-5) has been the most accepted empirical method for linearizing competitive protein-binding dose-response curves, particularly for RIA. Automatic data reduction

TABLE 13-9 DATA FOR AMIKACIN RIA RADIOACTIVITY*

Dose of Amikacin ($M \times 10^{-8}$)	Total Bound cpm (TB)	Specifically Bound cpm (B)[†]	%B[‡]	B/F[§]	B/B_0[‖]	Logit B/B_0
0	14019	13588(B_0)	64.0	1.78	1.00	—
1.07	10694	10264	48.4	0.94	0.76	1.13
2.14	9235	8805	41.5	0.71	0.65	0.61
4.28	7184	6754	31.8	0.47	0.50	−0.01
8.56	5360	4930	23.2	0.30	0.36	−0.56
17.12	3925	3495	16.5	0.20	0.26	−1.06
Unknown 1	8912	8482	40.0	0.67	0.62	0.51
Unknown 2	6910	6480	30.5	0.44	0.48	−0.09
Unknown 3	4340	3910	18.4	0.23	0.29	−0.91

*Total counts per minute (cpm), T, of ^{125}I-amikacin in each reaction are 21,225; nonspecifically bound (NSB) counts per minute are 430.
[†]Specifically bound cpm = B = Total bound cpm − NSB.
[‡]% bound = (B/T)100.
[§]$B/F = \dfrac{B}{TB - B}$.
[‖]B_0 = B at zero dose of drug.

and processing of the log-logit transformation are easily performed with computerized instruments that offer various axis transforms with polynomial and four-parameter curve-fitting equations that are well suited for curvilinear calibration lines.

EXAMPLES OF COMPETITIVE-BINDING ASSAYS
Radioimmunoassay (RIA)

In radioimmunoassay, the ligand and a constant amount of radioactively labeled ligand compete for a limited number of antibody-binding sites. The concentration of antibody is usually sufficient to bind between 30% and 80% of the labeled material. In the above example, the antibody to amikacin bound 64% of the ^{125}I-amikacin in the absence of unlabeled ligand. An addition of unlabeled ligand to the reaction yields a net increase in the total ligand (labeled plus unlabeled), but because of competition for antibody-binding sites, a decrease results in the proportion of labeled ligand that will be bound by the antibody. If you count the radioactivity bound to the antibody after the separation step, the dose-response curve will have a negative slope similar to that shown in Fig. 13-1. As the concentration of unlabeled ligand increases and the antibody-binding sites approach saturation, the slope levels off. When the unbound radioactively labeled ligand is monitored, the dose-response curve has a positive slope but with the same shape.

Radioimmunoassay is applicable to the measurement of both low- and high-molecular-weight ligands, provided that the labeling procedure or the labeled ligand conjugate itself does not adversely affect the immunoreactivity of the ligand. These problems are overcome by labeling the antibody rather than the ligand because the major structural differences between IgG molecules are substantially less than the differences between ligands. Losses in immunoreactivity are less likely to occur when the antibody is labeled.

Assays based on the use of a labeled antibody are called **immunometric assays**. One that uses a radiolabeled antibody is known as an *immunoradiometric assay (IRMA)*.

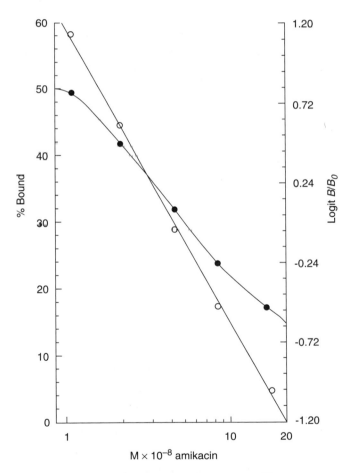

Fig. 13-5 Amikacin radioimmunoassay dose-response curves with the percentage of bound ^{125}I-amikacin, ●; and logit (B/B_0), ○; plotted as a function of the log of the amikacin concentration. To facilitate plot, concentration (*M*) has been multiplied by 10^{-8}.

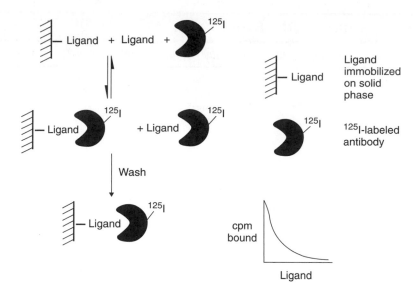

Fig. 13-6 Principle of the competitive immunoradiometric assay (IRMA) and a typical dose-response curve.

The ligand in the sample competes with the ligand attached to a solid surface for the binding sites of the labeled antibody (Fig. 13-6). The amount of labeled antibody bound to the solid surface is determined after excess label and sample have been removed. A representative dose-response curve is also shown in Fig. 13-6. The immunometric format is considered again in the discussion of ELISA techniques.

Enzyme-Linked Immunosorbent Assay

The **enzyme-linked immunosorbent assays (ELISA)** are heterogeneous nonisotopic assays that usually have an antibody immobilized onto a solid support (see Table 13-2), whereas the ligand is labeled with an enzyme. Table 13-10 lists some enzymes used for ELISA (or other enzyme immunoassays). These enzymes are useful as labels because they satisfy the following criteria:

1. *High specific activity*. The signal amplification obtained with an enzyme label corresponds to the amount of substrate converted to product during the time of incubation. Enzymes with the highest specific activities yield the greatest amplification. Assays using such enzymes have excellent sensitivity and are able to measure very low concentrations of ligand.
2. *Easily coupled to ligand*. The enzymes have sufficient acidic and basic amino acids, thiol groups, or carbohydrate to be coupled easily to the ligand without losing substantial enzymatic activity.
3. *Stability*. The enzyme labels are stable during the assay and under refrigerated storage conditions.
4. *Absent in fluid or tissue*. The enzymes are not usually present in the biological fluid or tissue sample that is to be analyzed.
5. *Retention of activity*. The enzymes retain most of their activity when attached to the ligand or antibody.

Alkaline phosphatase and horseradish peroxidase are inexpensively available in highly purified form. For this reason and those listed above, these two enzymes are most often used as labels for ELISA. Some of the enzymes listed in Table 13-10 can use chromogens, fluorogens, or luminogens as substrates. One advantage of a chromogenic substrate is that its product can be detected visually. Fluorescent and luminescent products can be detected at 100 to 1000 times lower concentrations than those of chromophores, and the incubation time can also be reduced.

Many configurations for ELISA have been devised. Some are based on competitive reactions, whereas others are direct immunometric "sandwich" assays. The sandwich ELISA is discussed in Chapter 12. The two basic formats for the competitive assays and the shape of the respective typical dose-response curves that describe the signal remaining on the solid phase are shown in Figs. 13-7 and 13-8.

TABLE 13-10 ENZYME LABELS FOR IMMUNOASSAYS

			ACTIVITY	
Enzyme	*Source*	*Molecular Weight*	*Turnover Rate**	*°C*
Alkaline phosphatase	Calf intestine	140,000	420,000	37
β-Galactosidase	*Escherichia coli*	540,000	324,000	37
Glucose oxidase	*Aspergillus niger*	186,000	53,700	25
Glucose-6-phosphate dehydrogenase	*Leuconostoc mesenteroides*	130,000	93,600	30
Peroxidase	Horseradish	40,000	220,000	25
Urease	Jack bean	540,000	450,000	25

*The turnover rate is the number of moles of product released per minute per mole of enzyme at the designated temperature.

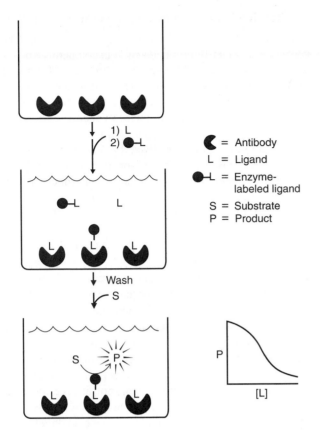

Fig. 13-7 Principle of the competitive enzyme-linked immunosorbent assay (ELISA) with the ligand labeled with an enzyme and a typical dose-response curve.

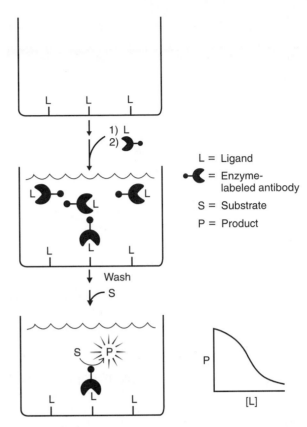

Fig. 13-8 Principle of the competitive ELISA where the antibody is labeled with an enzyme. This is an immunometric assay.

Of the two formats, the configuration in which the antibody has been immobilized onto the solid surface (see Fig. 13-7) has been described more frequently. This format is analogous to the configuration in an RIA because the ligand in the sample competes with the enzyme-labeled ligand for the limited amount of antibody-binding sites fixed to the solid phase. After the binding reaction has taken place, the solid phase is washed with buffer to remove the unbound labeled ligand so that it does not contribute to the signal. The amount of enzyme bound to the solid phase is proportional to the absorbance, fluorescence, or luminescence of the product formed after the addition of substrate, and it is inversely proportional to the concentration of unlabeled ligand. This method is applicable to both low- and high-molecular-weight analytes.

Instead of antibody, the ligand can be attached to the solid phase, as shown in Fig. 13-8. Only those antibody-enzyme binding sites not occupied by the sample ligand will bind to the immobilized ligand. The solid-phase ligand:antibody-enzyme complex is washed with buffer before addition of the substrate. Immunometric ELISAs have some of the same advantages as IRMAs when compared with an enzyme-labeled ligand ELISA.

Although both ELISA formats illustrated in Figs. 13-7 and 13-8 measure the amount of labeled conjugate bound to the solid phase, the activity remaining in solution after the binding reaction has taken place can also be measured.

In the earlier description of heterogeneous assays, some of the useful capture phases for separating antibody bound from unbound labeled ligand—namely, microtiter plates, latex, and various types of microparticles—were also described. Paramagnetic microparticles are applicable to those systems that employ magnets, whereas latex microparticles are trapped by glass-fiber filters or membranes either before or after the binding reaction takes place but always before the washing steps and addition of the enzyme substrates. Similarly, antibody has been adsorbed to glass-fiber filters with the aid of a lattice formed with secondary antibodies, or it has been adsorbed to membranes. Both glass-fiber and membrane filter capture phase supports are components of flow-through cassettes for automatic instruments, as well as the capture-support and reading area for the rapid assay devices used so frequently for pregnancy, ovulation, and infectious disease testing.

One of the drawbacks to adsorbing antibodies to solid surfaces such as the polystyrene of microtiter plates or the membranes of rapid-assay devices is that both monoclonal and polyclonal antibodies can undergo a substantial loss in antigen-binding capacity because of conformational changes upon adsorption to such surfaces. Instances in which less than 5% of the adsorbed monoclonals remained functional have been described. Major losses (~50%) are also seen where the antibodies have been covalently attached to the solid support. Indirect capture phases were developed to standardize assays and overcome losses in antigen-binding

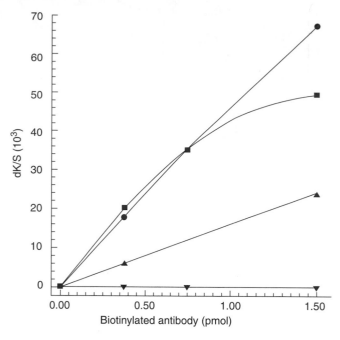

Fig. 13-9 Capture of biotinylated antipeptide antibody as a function of the biotin density in an indirect capture assay, where dK/S is a measurement of reflected light. Streptavidin immobilized to biotinylated latex microparticles is simultaneously incubated with an increasing amount of biotinylated antibody containing 1.2, ▼; 4.3, ▲; 6.0, ■; or 10.7, ●, biotins per molecule of antibody, respectively, and a constant concentration of peptide–alkaline phosphatase conjugate. The complex was retained on a glass-fiber filter and washed before the addition of substrate.

capacity. The avidin-biotin system is an example. Avidin (or streptavidin) binds biotin with very high affinity ($K_a = 10^{15}$ M⁻) and seems to retain its four binding sites upon attachment to a solid phase. The completed capture phase is formed when the immobilized avidin binds a biotinylated antibody or ligand so that the immunobinding events occur with maximal antibody-ligand binding capacity. Fig. 13-9 illustrates increased capture capacity of a biotinylated antipeptide antibody bound to streptavidin immobilized to biotinylated latex particles. The figure demonstrates increased capacity as a function of the antibody biotin density.

In addition to the biotin-avidin system, antifluorescein-fluorescein and antidigoxigenin-digoxigenin binding pairs have been used to form indirect capture phases. Aside from overcoming diminished antibody-capturing capacity, their use also has a more practical advantage: the capture phase can be a universal reagent component for a family of different heterogeneous competitive-binding assays. For example, the same antifluorescein-coupled magnetic particles are used to capture fluoresceinated antiligand antibodies in competitive-binding assays for different steroid hormones.

Cascades or amplification schemes have also been devised for ELISAs, and theoretically these schemes should enhance their sensitivity.

Time-Resolved Fluorescence (see also Chapter 4, p. 99)

Lanthanide metal chelates have strong advantages as labels compared with other fluorophores used in competitive-binding assays. For example, the fluorescence lifetimes of europium chelates are extremely long—100 µsec and greater than other fluorophores (5 nsec for fluorescein). With the appropriate instrumentation, one is able to measure such fluorescence 1 µsec or more after a pulse of excitation light and distinguish the fluorescence from short-lived background fluorescent interferences. This is the basis for time-resolved fluoro-immunoassays, heterogeneous assays with inherently low background capable of sensitivity as much as a thousandfold greater than that of other non-ELISA-based fluorescence methods.

Fluorescence of europium chelates is at wavelengths characteristic of the europium metal after light absorption by the chelator ligand with efficient energy transfer to the metal. The europium chelate complex is stable enough to withstand the washing conditions typical of heterogeneous assays. In the first time-resolved fluorescence immunoassays, highly fluorescent metal chelate complexes were insoluble in an aqueous environment, hence europium chelated by a poor energy-transferring ligand as the label was extracted and then recomplexed with a ligand appropriate for forming a highly fluorescent complex. Ligands have also been synthesized to function as highly fluorescent labels when complexed with the metal, thereby eliminating the extraction step. Carrier proteins with a multiplicity (150) of europium chelate labels attached to antibodies by means of a biotin:streptavidin bridge have been shown to increase the signal up to 7000 times in some amplification configurations. The dose-response curves for time-resolvable fluorescence assays are similar to those of other heterogeneous competitive immunoassays.

Rapid Assays

Immunoassays have been configured in small hand-held devices for qualitative and semiquantitative determinations. Similar to many home use pregnancy tests, these competitive assays have been made in flow-through and immunochromatographic (lateral flow) test formats. Labels for detection include enzymes, colored latex particles, and gold sols. Such devices do not require instrumentation, because the results can be visually read. Consequently, they are ideal for screening. One example of such a device is used to screen for various combinations of drugs of abuse. A urine sample is first incubated with a high affinity Mab and a ligand gold sol conjugate until the competitive binding reactions reach equilibrium. The antibody binds all of the conjugate and drug below a threshold concentration. The threshold drug concentrations are unique to different drugs, so it is necessary to manipulate the concentration of conjugate and antibody for each analyte to achieve the appropriate threshold. After incubation, the entire reaction mixture is applied to a solid phase in which a series of specific anti-conjugate antibodies are immobilized in different zones on a nylon membrane. When a drug threshold has been exceeded, unbound gold sol-

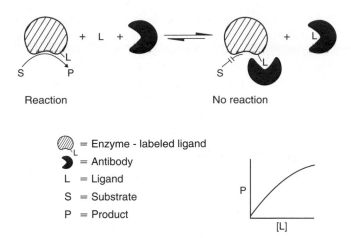

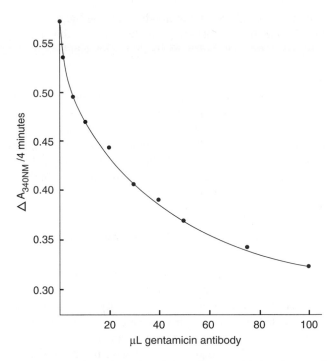

Fig. 13-10 Principle of the homogeneous enzyme immunoassay (enzyme-multiplied immunoassay technique, EMIT) and a typical dose-response curve.

ligand conjugate is bound by the solid phase antibodies in proportion to the drug concentration in the sample, creating a colored band in a particular drug zone.

HOMOGENEOUS ASSAY TECHNIQUES
Homogeneous Enzyme Immunoassay

The first reported homogeneous immunoassay was an enzyme immunoassay for low-molecular-weight ligands commonly known as the **enzyme-multiplied immunoassay technique (EMIT)**. Binding of a specific antibody to the enzyme-labeled ligand changes the enzymatic activity of the label so that the antibody-bound enzyme can be distinguished from unbound labeled ligand.

In most instances, binding of antibody to the enzyme-ligand conjugate sterically inhibits the enzyme by limiting the enzyme substrate's access to the catalytic site (Fig. 13-10). A typical enzyme-inhibition profile is shown in Fig. 13-11. Increasing the amount of gentamicin monoclonal antibody inhibits the activity of the enzyme label glucose-6-phosphate dehydrogenase (Fig. 13-11). A dose-response curve for the competitive homogeneous enzyme immunoassay is shown in Fig. 13-12. The unlabeled ligand competes with enzyme-labeled gentamicin for the limited numbers of antibody-binding sites, and as more unlabeled gentamicin is bound by the antibody, the enzymatic activity increases. Usually this response is reflected by a change in the rate of enzyme activity when two absorbance readings of the reaction are taken 30 seconds apart. The change in absorbance (ΔA) is used to calculate the dose response.

Another homogeneous enzyme immunoassay that, like EMIT, is also particularly well suited for automated high throughput immunoassay or chemistry systems is the CEDIA. The fundamental components of the method include an enzyme acceptor (EA), an inactive fragment of β-galactosidase that lacks the complementary enzyme donor (ED) fragment necessary for enzymic activity. The 10,000-dalton ED, when covalently conjugated to the haptenic ligand, is the labeled ligand for this competitive immunoassay for low–molecular-

Fig. 13-11 Inhibition of activity of gentamicin–glucose-6-phosphate dehydrogenase conjugate by monoclonal antibody to gentamicin.

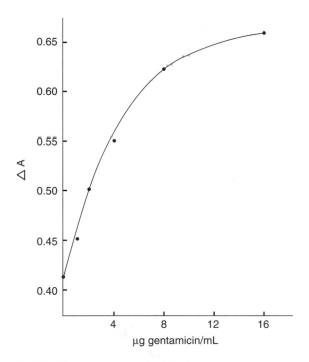

Fig. 13-12 Dose-response curve for the homogeneous gentamicin enzyme immunoassay.

weight analytes. Both β-galactosidase fragments are bioengineered by recombinant DNA techniques with the ligand attachment site to the ED so that it does interfere with the interaction of EA and ED. Reconstituted β-galactosidase activity approaches that seen with native enzyme.

When a ligand-specific antibody binds the ligand-ED, the complementation events are partially inhibited, thus making it possible to distinguish antibody-bound label from that which is free for interaction with EA. A time course for complementation-reconstituted β-galactosidase activity in the presence and absence of digoxin is shown in Fig. 13-13. The figure illustrates that although this technique is one of the more sensitive homogeneous methods, the activity in the absence of analyte ligand is only partially blocked by the antiligand-antibody complex, even though the size of the antiligand antibody is increased by addition of a second antispecies antibody to improve the steric hindrance of antibody-bound ligand-ED in generating an active enzyme.

Fluorescence Polarization Immunoassay (see Chapter 4, p. 100–101)

Fluorescence polarization immunoassay is based on the amount of polarized fluorescent light detected when the fluorophore label is excited with polarized light. The degree of polarization of the emitted fluorescent light depends on the rate of rotation of the fluorophore-ligand conjugate in solution. Small molecules rotate freely, and consequently the fluorescent light emitted by the molecule is depolarized, whereas large molecules, such as proteins, rotate more slowly and emit polarized fluorescent light. When an antibody binds a low-molecular-weight ligand labeled with a fluorophore, the fluorescence polarization of the labeled ligand is increased because rotation of the labeled ligand-antibody complex is much slower than that of labeled ligands alone. Unlabeled ligand will compete with the labeled ligand for antibody-binding sites, and so the amount of polarized fluorescent light resulting from a competitive-binding reaction is inversely proportional to the concentration of unlabeled ligand in the reaction. The principle of the fluorescence polarization immunoassay and a typical dose-response curve are shown in Fig. 13-14.

Fluorescence polarization immunoassays have been developed for all routinely monitored therapeutic drugs and are commercially available for these drugs as well as drugs of abuse and other small molecules.

Electrochemiluminescence

Electrochemiluminescent competitive binding assays for haptens and higher molecular weight ligands are quasi-homogeneous assays in that they do not necessarily require a wash step to remove the unbound label. In assays in which the hapten is labeled, a significant difference in ECL exists between the bound and free label as a result of decreased diffusion and steric hindrance of the antibody-bound label. Such assays are truly homogeneous since antibody binding modulates the activity of the ruthenium complex label. However, these assays usually incorporate a paramagnetic particle to capture and concentrate bound label on the surface of the electrode.

Both hapten-labeled and antibody-labeled approaches are used. For example, in a forward sequential competitive format for the hormone estradiol, the sample is first incubated with biotinylated antibody, then with $Ru(bpy)_3^{+2}$-labeled estradiol, and finally with streptavidin-coated paramagnetic particles. A magnet then concentrates the particle capture phase on the electrode prior to voltage application and subsequent ECL (see p. 100). Alternatively, in a simultaneous competitive immunoassay for the hormone thyroxine (T_4), sample T_4 competes with a T_4 ligand-biotin conjugate for $Ru(bpy)_3^{+2}$-labeled anti-T_4 antibody. Antibody-bound ligand-biotin conjugate is then captured by streptavidin-coated particles and magnetically concentrated on the

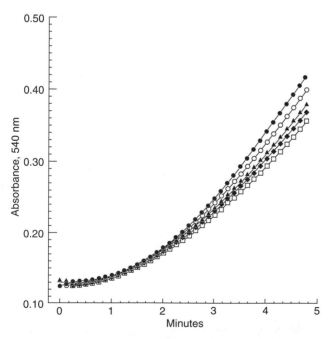

Fig. 13-13 Reaction time course for the cloned-enzyme donor immunoassay digoxin assay method. Response is in the absence, □, and presence of 1.0, ◆; 2.0, ▲; 3.0, ○; and 4.0 ng, ●, of digoxin per milliliter of sample.

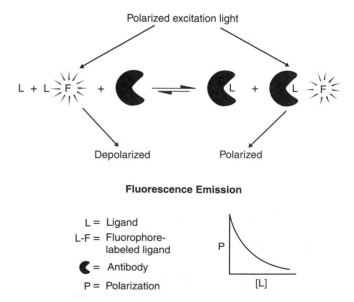

Fig. 13-14 Principle of the fluorescence polarization immunoassay (FPIA) and a typical dose-response curve.

electrode. Both of these examples introduce a separation step by removing the bound label from solution so that only it participates in the electrochemiluminescent reaction. In this sense ECL methods are a hybrid between homogeneous and heterogeneous formats in that there is a separation step without wash steps. Of course, wash steps can be introduced to lower the background and improve sensitivity.

Microparticle-Based Light-Scattering Inhibition Immunoassays

The competitive nephelometric and turbidimetric inhibition immunoassays differ only in how the scattered light is detected, as discussed earlier. These methods consist of an agglutinator, usually a water-soluble polymeric carrier substance, to which a multiple of haptenic ligands is coupled. Examples of carriers include dextran, polysucrose, and albumin. The antibody reagent is composed of antiligand antibodies adsorbed or covalently coupled to submicrometer-sized latex microparticles. For greater sensitivity, the ligand is also coupled to even smaller latex particles in a two-particle inhibition assay. The agglutination complex formed when the agglutinator and antibody reagent are combined can be measured kinetically or at a single time point. The presence of the ligand in the assay inhibits the rate of agglutination by competing for the antibody-binding sites. The course for agglutination at different ligand concentrations in a turbidimetric inhibition assay is presented in Fig. 13-15. The density of both ligand on the agglutinator and antibody on the latex microparticles is optimized to obtain maximum kinetics in the absence of ligand with appropriate inhibition

in its presence. Measuring the rate of agglutination early in the reaction provides for the greatest sensitivity, whereas the rate or fixed time point can be taken at any time during the reaction for those assays that do not require low detection limits. Fig. 13-16 presents two dose-response curves derived from the reactions course shown in Fig. 13-15.

ATTRIBUTES AND LIMITATIONS OF DIFFERENT APPROACHES TO COMPETITIVE-BINDING ASSAYS

Before describing some advantages and limitations of the competitive-binding assays described earlier, it is useful to discuss factors to be considered when one designs or chooses a particular assay format. Convenience, cost-effectiveness, and performance for an assay must be addressed.

Convenience factors include:

1. Number of pipetting steps
2. Incubation time
3. Rate or end-point assay
4. Need for additional equipment such as incubators, centrifuges, or specialized detectors
5. Automation and throughput
6. Sample volume requirement
7. Sample pretreatment (dilution, extraction, and so on)
8. Temperature-control requirements
9. Cost
10. Operator time
11. Radioactive waste disposal

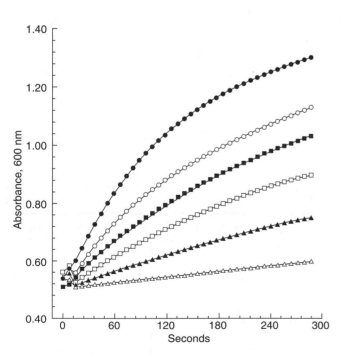

Fig. 13-15 Reaction time courses for a theophylline turbidimetric inhibition immunoassay in the absence, ● and presence of 2.5, ○; 5.0, ■; 10.0, □; 20.0, ▲; and 40.0, △, μg of theophylline per milliliter of sample.

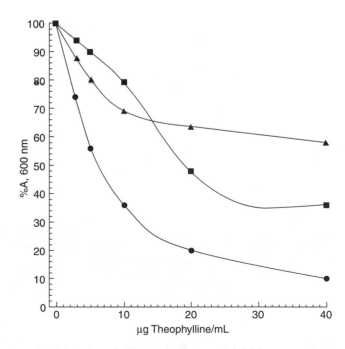

Fig. 13-16 Theophylline turbidimetric inhibition assay dose-response curves derived from the kinetic responses shown in Fig. 13-15. Rates were taken between 30 and 45 seconds, ●, and between 270 and 285 seconds, ■, and the dose response for a fixed time point at 285 seconds, ▲, is also shown. The respective responses were normalized to 100% at zero concentration for scaling purposes.

12. Applicability to a variety of analytes
13. Stability of reagents and storage temperatures
14. Stability of the calibration curve

Obviously, the ideal assay would require very little sample with no pretreatment, a very short incubation time at ambient temperature, no pipetting steps, and no additional equipment other than the detector or an automated instrument. The ideal assay would be able to be performed quickly and cheaply, with very little operator hands-on time, with walk-away capability, and with a rapid data-reduction capability. The reagents would be stable for at least a year at room temperature or on board an automated system for at least 30 days. Finally, the calibration curve would be stable so that the assay would need to be recalibrated only when the reagents had been changed or replaced.

Some of the most important performance factors are as follows:

1. Good assay response over the range of the standard curve.
2. A low background signal, that signal caused by either nonspecific interactions of the reagents in the assay or contributed by other substances in the samples. The background must be kept to a minimum to maximize the S/N, detection limits, slope, and dynamic range.
3. High antibody affinity increases the slope of the dose-response curve and contributes to the sensitivity and detection limit of an assay. Sensitivity is related to the slope of the dose-response curve, to the experimental error (accuracy and precision of the assay), and to the activity and detectability of the label.
4. Good precision and accuracy depend on the accuracy of the values used for the concentrations of standards or calibrators and on the correct interpolation of the true shape of the dose-response curve between the standards.
5. Specificity is determined by the ability of the antibody to discriminate between the ligand and similarly structured substances. In most cases, the screening and selection process for suitable antiserums or monoclonal antibodies plays a very important part in determining antibody specificity. This is true for both native ligands (such as

proteins) and the synthetic immunogens prepared to produce antibodies to low-molecular-weight substances.
6. Although some immunoassay interferences are related to antibody specificity, others that are contributed by the patient sample can affect either homogeneous or heterogeneous competitive-binding assays, or both.

For example, homogeneous assays may be influenced by endogenous enzyme activity that is the same as the enzyme label, or by substances that would interfere in the immunoreaction or detection step. These may be removed by washing (heterogeneous method). Both types of immunoassay formats are subject to "heterophilic" antibody interferences from the patient sample. Heterophilic or endogenous antispecies antibodies can bind the assay antibody so that the signal is compromised. For example, human anti-mouse antibody (HAMA) will bind to the mouse immunoglobulin coating the latex microparticle in a turbidimetric inhibition assay, with agglutination independent of the agglutinator resulting in a falsely elevated signal. HAMA is commonly neutralized by the inclusion of excessive mouse immunoglobulin in the assay.

Table 13-11 compares some characteristics of previously described competitive-binding assays, and Table 13-12 lists some of the interferences. The heterogeneous assays have the greatest potential for sensitivity, with picomolar or lower detection limits. In addition to the high specific activities of the radiolabels or enzyme labels, high-sensitivity fluorescent and luminescent labels are routinely used. Interferences originating either from substances in the sample or from impurities in the reagents are removed by the separation or wash steps. By reducing the background signal, the heterogeneous procedure also makes it possible to increase the volume of sample, which increases the sensitivity of the assay.

The short half-life of the radioactive labels used in the clinical laboratory (such as ^{125}I) limits the use of RIA reagents to between 6 and 12 weeks after their receipt. This is a short period compared with reagents for the nonisotope labeled assays, which are stable for a year or longer. In addition, radioisotopes are presumed to be hazardous and are subject to governmental regulation in their use and disposal.

TABLE 13-11   CHARACTERISTICS OF SOME COMPETITIVE-BINDING ASSAYS

Immunoassay	Homogeneous or Heterogeneous	Detection Limit (M)	Amplification	Low or High MW Ligands
CEDIA	Homogeneous	10^{-10}	Yes	Low
Chemiluminescence	Heterogeneous	10^{-13}	No	Both
ECL	Both	10^{-14}	Yes	Both
ELISA	Heterogeneous	10^{-11} to 10^{-15}	Yes	Both
EMIT	Homogeneous	5×10^{-10}	Yes	Low
FPIA	Homogeneous	5×10^{-9}	No	Low
Light scattering	Homogeneous	10^{-10}	No	Low
RIA	Heterogeneous	10^{-12} to 10^{-14}	No	Both
TRFI	Heterogeneous	10^{-12}	No	Both

CEDIA, cloned-enzyme donor immunoassay; ECL, electrochemiluminescence; ELISA, enzyme-linked immunosorbent assay; EMIT, enzyme-multiplied immunoassay technique; FPIA, fluorescence polarization immunoassay; MW, molecular weight; RIA, radioimmunoassay TRFI, time-resolved fluorescence immunoassay.

ELISA and the other nonisotopic immunoassays have many advantages, including the avoidance of radioisotope use. Because enzymes are biochemical amplifiers, the systems that employ enzyme labels are capable of producing a greatly amplified signal, depending on the specific activity of the enzyme and the incubation time for conversion of substrate to product. The use of fluorogenic or luminogenic substrates instead of chromogens can enhance the sensitivity of these assays 100 to 1000 times. Disadvantages of ELISA include the inconvenience of required washing steps compared with homogeneous assays, although available instruments automate these washing steps. Other factors are listed in Table 13-12.

The homogeneous enzyme immunoassay (enzyme-multiplied immunoassay technique, EMIT), though limited by the absorbance of the product, is still sensitive to subnanomolar levels of ligand. EMIT and other methods that use absorbance are subject to possible interferences by hemolyzed, lipemic, and icteric samples. Because a rate measurement is used for EMIT, this method is difficult to perform manually but is quickly and easily accomplished with automated equipment. However, the assay is not suitable for high-molecular-weight ligands because antibody binding of the macromolecular enzyme conjugate does not provide sufficient enzyme inhibition for unlabeled ligand to elicit a response.

Fluorescence and luminescence assays are sensitive to subpicomolar concentrations of ligand with the chemiluminescent labels providing the greatest sensitivity. The homogeneous fluorescence assays avoid errors that can be introduced by the separation steps of heterogeneous systems. With the possible exception of the time-resolved fluoroimmunoassay, which is a heterogeneous assay, fluorescence assays are prone to interferences by hemolyzed, lipemic, and icteric samples. Possible sample interferences in homogeneous fluorescence immunoassays include light scattering from lipids and particulates, fluorescence quenching, and background fluorescence from the presence of endogenous fluorophores. The fluorescence polarization immunoassay is sensitive to the depolarized scattered light of particulates in the assay and requires sophisticated instrumentation. Endogenous proteins may nonspecifically bind some fluorescein-labeled ligands, resulting in an increased polarization background.

CEDIA amplifies the signal because an active enzyme is generated in the assay. Unlike EMIT, antibody binds a ligand-label conjugate required to generate an active enzyme, rather than binding a ligand coupled to an enzyme that is already active. CEDIA, which has very high activity because of the generation of a high-turnover β-galactosidase label, would be more sensitive and require a shorter incubation time if the antiligand antibody complex was a more effective

---

TABLE 13-12 SOME POTENTIAL IMMUNOASSAY LIMITATIONS AND INTERFERENCES

Assay Type	Interferences/Limitations	Effect on Assay Response
Heterogeneous	Antibody or antigen deformation or steric hindrance at solid phase	Loss of binding affinity and capacity; reduces sensitivity
	Nonspecific binding of labeled conjugate to solid surfaces	Reduces S/N, sensitivity, detection limit
	Desorption of adsorbed binder	Loss of binding capacity over time; enhanced competitive response
	Conjugation of ligand or antibody to enzyme lowers its activity	Reduced signal that is compensated for by longer incubation times
	Increased enzyme labeling increases NSB	Lower S/N, sensitivity, detection limit
	Europium contamination with time-resolved fluorescence-labeled chelates	Increased background, lower S/N
Homogeneous	Increased sample background because of endogenous: • Fluorescence • Enzyme activity • Spectral interferences • Label-like materials	Lower S/N alleviated by dilution (which also lowers sensitivity) or by kinetic measurements (if appropriate)
	• Antibodies to label	Reduction in signal, could interfere with ligand-conjugate antibody binding
	Imprecision	Overall noise increases, thereby lowering S/N
General	Exogenous substances • Anticoagulants	Inhibit enzyme activity
	Endogenous substances • Cross-reactants, metabolites	Increased signal response
	• Heterophilic antibodies, HAMA, rheumatoid factor	Bind antiligand antibody to simulate or interfere with normal response

HAMA, Human anti-mouse antibody; NSB, nonspecifically bound; S/N, signal-to-noise ratio.

inhibitor of the donor-acceptor complementation for generating active enzymes. In addition, both fluorogenic and luminogenic substrates are available for β-galactosidase, making this method readily adaptable to most automatic instrumentation.

The immunoassays based on **electrochemiluminescence** detection are versatile in that wash steps need to be included in the format only if the assay sensitivity requires a separation step. ECL is capable of detecting subpicomolar levels of the label. In the noncompetitive immunometric formats, the dynamic range can cover greater than six orders of magnitude.

The ruthenium complex labels are very stable, with shelf lives of over a year at room temperature. Finally, the assay can be rapidly performed on an automated system.

Although the nephelometric inhibition immunoassay requires a special instrument, the turbidimetric inhibition method is applicable to most immunoassay and clinical automatic instrumentation. Although perhaps not so potentially sensitive as CEDIA and the homogeneous electrochemiluminescence immunoassay formats, in practice this method is being used to quantitate lower-level analytes such as T_4 and digoxin.

Bibliography

Immunoassays (Under a Variety of Formats)
Diamandis EP: Detection techniques for immunoassay and DNA protein applications, *Clin Biochem* 23:437, 1990.
Gosling JP: A decade of development in immunoassay methodology, *Clin Chem* 36:1408, 1990.
Price C, Newman D, editors: *Principles and Practices of Immunassays*, ed 2, New York, 1997, Stockton Press.
Self CH, Dessi JL, Winger LA: Ultra-specific immunoassays for small molecules: roles of wash steps and multiple binding formats, *Clin Chem* 42:1527, 1996.

Enzyme Immunoassay
Portsmann T, Kiessig ST: Enzyme immunoassay techniques: an overview, *J Immunol Methods* 150:5, 1992.
Tijssen P: Practice and theory of enzyme immunoassays. In Burdon RH, van Knippenberg PH, editors: *Laboratory techniques in biochemistry and molecular biology*, vol 15, New York, 1985, Elsevier Science Publishing.

Enzyme-Linked Immunosorbent Assay (ELISA)
Avrameas S: Amplification systems in immunoenzymatic techniques, *J Immunol Methods* 150:23, 1992.
Butler JE, et al: The immunochemistry of solid phase sandwich enzyme linked immunosorbent assays, *Fed Proc* 46:2548, 1987.
Pesce AJ, Michael JG: Artifacts and limitations of enzyme immunoassay, *J Immunol Methods* 150:111, 1992.

Homogeneous Enzyme Immunoassay
Henderson DR, et al: CEDIA, a new homogeneous immunoassay system, *Clin Chem* 32:1637, 1986.
Jenkins SG: Homogeneous enzyme immunoassay, *J Immunol Methods* 150:91, 1992.

Immunoassay Interference
Kricka LJ: Interference in immunoassay—still a threat, *Clin Chem* 46:1037, 2000.
Levinson SS: The nature of heterophilic antibodies and their role in immunoassay interference, *J Clin Immunoassay* 15:108, 1992.
Pesce AJ, Michael JG: Artifacts and limitations of enzyme immunoassay, *J Immunol Methods* 150:111, 1992.
Valdes R, Jr, Miller TI: Increasing the specificity of immunoassays, *J Clin Immunoassay* 15:87, 1992.

Time-Resolved Fluorescence Immunoassay
Diamandis EP: Multiple labeling and time-resolvable fluorophores, *Clin Chem* 37:1486, 1991.
Papanastasiou-Diamandis A, Christopoulos TK, Diamandis EP: Ultrasensitive thyrotropin immunoassay based on enzymatically amplified time-resolved fluorescence with a terbium chelate, *Clin Chem* 38:545, 1992.

Light-Scattering Assays
Newman DJ, Henneberry H, Price CP: Particle enhanced light scattering immunoassay, *Ann Clin Biochem* 29:22, 1992.

Luminescence Immunoassay
Blackburn GF, et al: Electrochemiluminescence detection by development of immunoassays and DNA probe assays for clinical diagnostics, *Clin Chem* 37:1534, 1991.
Kricka LT: Chemiluminescent and bioluminescent techniques, *Clin Chem* 37:1472, 1991.

Rapid Assays
Buechler KF et al: Simultaneous detection of seven drugs of abuse by the Triage' Panel for Drugs of Abuse, *Clin Chem* 38:1676, 1992.

Internet Sites

http://www.med.unc.edu/wrkunits/2depts/pharm/receptor/side5.htm—Theory and Practice of Receptor Characterization and Drug Analysis, by Richard B. Mailman, PhD, and Jose Boyer, PhD, North Carolina State University

www.curvefit.com/how_to_fit.htm—How to fit standard curves
www.m.ehime-u.ac.jp/~yasuhito/Elisa.html
www.biology.arizona.edu/immunology/activities/elisa/main.html

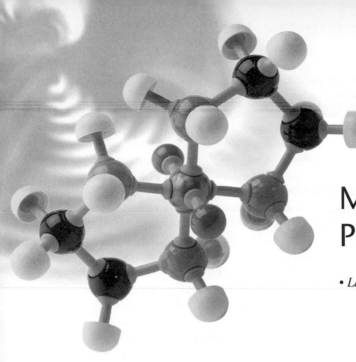

CHAPTER 14

Measurement of Colligative Properties

• *Lawrence A. Kaplan*

Objectives

- Identify the relationships among osmosis, osmotic pressure, osmolality, and osmometry.
- List four measurements that depend on colligative properties and describe what happens to each property during sample concentration.
- State the relationship between freezing-point depression and moles of particles dissolved per kilogram of water and calculate the osmolality from a given freezing point of a solution.

- Describe the techniques of freezing-point depression and vapor-pressure depression for osmolality determinations.
- State the clinical utility of performing plasma osmolality and urine osmolality determinations.
- State the clinical situations in which the measurement of the osmolal gap is useful.

Key Terms

"acetone" bodies The acetone and other ketones that are present in the serum of patients with diabetic ketoacidosis.

boiling-point elevation A phenomenon in which addition of solute molecules raises the temperature at which the solution will boil. For water, this is 1.86° C per mole of solute per kilogram of solvent.

colligative property A characteristic to which all the molecules of a solution contribute, regardless of their individual composition or nature.

colloid A large molecule, usually in aqueous solution. Normally the term is applied to protein solutions.

colloid osmotic pressure (COP) The osmotic pressure generated by that portion of a solution with high molecular weight (greater than 30,000 daltons).

crystalloids The uncharged solute molecules of a solution.

dew point The temperature at which condensation of water from the vapor phase occurs.

diffusion　Mixing or movement of molecules as a result of their random motion.

Donnan effect　The distribution of ions caused by having a high-molecular-weight ion on one side of a semipermeable membrane.

freezing-point depression　A phenomenon in which the addition of solute molecules to a solution lowers the temperature at which the solution will freeze.

molality　The number of moles of solute per kilogram of water or solvent.

oncotic pressure　Another term for colloid osmotic pressure.

osmolal gap　The difference between the observed and calculated serum osmolalities. The calculated osmolar values include sodium concentration multiplied by 2, plus glucose and blood urea nitrogen.

osmolality　The measurement of the number of moles of particles per kilogram of water.

osmometry　The measurement of a colligative property of a solution in which the number of moles of a solute per unit volume (concentration) are determined.

osmosis　Water flow across a semipermeable membrane.

osmotic pressure　The hydrostatic pressure required to prevent a change in volume when two solutions of different concentrations are placed on opposite sides of a semipermeable membrane.

plasma expander　Usually a high-molecular-weight dextran that is administered intravenously to increase the oncotic pressure of a patient.

Seebeck effect　Voltage difference seen when two ends of a specially made wire are at two different temperatures.

semipermeable membrane　A barrier that allows one type of molecule, such as water, to pass but does not allow another type of molecule, such as protein, to pass.

thermistor　A temperature measuring device in which the change of resistance is temperature dependent. It is derived from the words *thermal resistor*.

thermocouple　A device that generates a voltage (Seebeck effect) when the two ends of a wire are at different temperatures.

ultrafiltrate　The solution remaining after passage through a semipermeable membrane. Usually it contains only low-molecular-weight solutes.

vapor-pressure depression　The phenomenon in which the addition of a solute molecule to a solvent decreases the amount of solvent in equilibrium between the vapor phase and the liquid phase.

COLLIGATIVE PROPERTIES
Osmosis

Osmosis is neither simply a mixing of two fluids nor simply a diffusion. Diffusion is the mixing of molecules as a result of random motion caused by thermal kinetic energy (brownian motion). For example, if an albumin solution is carefully overlaid with water, the albumin molecules will randomly move back and forth across the original interface boundary. Because there are more albumin molecules in the albumin solution, the odds are great that an albumin molecule will cross into the water side. Thus albumin will diffuse into the water layer until the solutions become homogeneous, that is, until the odds are equal that an albumin molecule will diffuse one way or the other across the original boundary because the concentration is equal on both sides.

The term **osmosis** specifically applies to water flow across a **semipermeable membrane** such as a cell wall. Although osmosis can occur with any fluid, water is the most important fluid for this discussion. A semipermeable membrane allows some particles (molecules, ions, or aggregates of molecules) to pass through it, but it inhibits the passage of others; hence it is *semi*permeable. The simplest example of a semipermeable membrane is a dialysis membrane, which is usually made of cellophane. It has very small pores through which water and some small molecules and ions pass (often termed an **ultrafiltrate**). However, large molecules, such as proteins, cannot pass through the membrane. To demonstrate, place an albumin solution in a section of dialysis tubing and tie the ends of the tubing. If the tubing is placed in a beaker of water, the albumin molecules cannot move out of the membrane, but water molecules will move in and affect dilution of the albumin. As a result, the tubing will swell as water flows into the albumin solution inside the tubing, increasing the pressure inside the membrane. If the tubing does not burst from this pressure, an equilibrium will be maintained between the water flowing in and the water being forced out by the internal pressure. The hydrostatic pressure built up and maintained by this process is called **osmotic pressure**.

Perhaps the most graphic example of osmosis is lysis of red blood cells by water. So much water flows into the more concentrated intracellular fluid that the cell swells and bursts. Cells can also shrink if exposed to a fluid of high **osmolality**. In this case the water in the cell flows out of the cell into the concentrated solution outside. In the laboratory this process affects the measurement of mean corpuscular volume (MCV). If the diluent is not isotonic, that is, of equal osmotic pressure, the cells will swell or shrink, giving erroneous MCV and hematocrit values because the latter is calculated from the MCV.

Osmolality

The term *molarity* is used to characterize concentration, that is, the number of moles of solute per liter of water. **Molality** is the number of moles of solute per kilogram of water. Because a liter of water has a mass of 1 kg, the difference between these two expressions of concentration is usually small. Only for concentrated solutions is the difference appreciable. In practice it is the difference between adding material to a liter of water (molality) and adding water to material to make a liter of solution (molarity).

Molality is the term best suited to **osmometry** because it gives a simpler theoretical formula for osmotic pressure than molarity does. The term *osmolality* is used to identify the number of moles of particles per kilogram of water.

Because the osmolality of a solution does not depend on the kind of particles but only on the number of particles, it is called a **colligative property**. A solution that is 1 millimolal in sodium chloride is 2 milliosmolal because sodium chloride separates into sodium and chloride ions. Each kind of ion represents a particle that contributes to the osmolality. Furthermore, a 1 millimolal calcium chloride solution is 3 milliosmolal because each molecule ionizes to give one calcium ion and two chloride ions.

Osmometry

Osmometry is the measurement of the concentration, not of a particular molecule, but of molecules and ions in general. In this chapter the clinical importance and use of osmometry are discussed, the techniques for measuring osmolality are reviewed, and examples of instrumentation are provided.

Osmolal Gap

There are just a few substances in plasma that contribute significantly to the osmolality, and they are mostly small molecules and ions. For example, plasma usually contains 40 g of albumin per liter, but the number of moles of albumin is very small (only about 50 mmol). In contrast, plasma contains about 150 mmol of sodium ion and 100 mmol of a corresponding anion such as chloride. This is only 5.8 g of sodium chloride per liter. Thus sodium chloride contributes 3000 times more to osmolality than a similar mass of albumin does.

Many formulas have been used to calculate the approximate osmolality of serum or plasma. Most formulas attempt to combine accuracy with simplicity in calculation. A formula that requires measurement of many substances is not very useful clinically. The calculated osmolality can be compared with the measured osmolality; the difference is called the **osmolal gap**. An abnormal osmolal gap is an important indication of abnormal concentrations of unmeasured substances in the blood. Because the formula predicts the plasma osmolality so well, there is little new information to be gained from *routine* measurements of the osmolality. However, in certain special situations described in the next section, the measurement is informative and worthwhile.

The formulas shown below for the calculation of serum osmolality are approximations because they include only the most important contributors to osmolality:

Historical units

$$\text{Calculated osmolality (mOsm/kg)} = 2 \cdot \text{Na}^+ \text{ (mEq/L)} + \frac{\text{Glucose (mg/dL)}}{18} + \frac{\text{BUN (mg/dL)}}{2.8} \qquad \textit{Eq. 14-1}$$

SI*units

$$\text{Calculated osmolality (mOsm/kg)} =$$
$$2 \cdot \text{Na}^+ \text{ (mmol/L)} + \text{Glucose (mmol/L)} + \text{BUN (mmol/L)} \qquad \textit{Eq. 14-2}$$

The SI units formula is very straightforward. The factor 2 in both equations counts the cation (sodium) once and the corresponding anion once. Glucose and blood urea nitrogen (BUN) are undissociated molecules and are counted once each. All other components are ignored. In the historical units formula the dividing factors represent the respective molecular weights and conversion from deciliters to liters. The calculated osmolality is not corrected for the actual water content of plasma (lipids and protein take up some of the volume) because this correction does not improve the clinical utility of the osmolal gap or of osmolality in general.

Notice that these formulas use molarity rather than molality. This approximation fortuitously compensates for some of the serum components and theoretical corrections that were ignored.

The osmolal gap is defined as:

$$\text{Osmolal gap, Osm/kg} =$$
$$\text{Measured Osm/kg} - \text{Calculated Osm/kg} \qquad \textit{Eq. 14-3}$$

The average osmolal gap is near zero.

CLINICAL USE OF OSMOMETRY

There are several clinical uses of osmometry. Serum osmolality can be used to screen for the ingestion of toxic substances and to monitor mannitol therapy. In addition, osmolality measurements of urine are used to assess renal concentrating ability. Measurements of stool osmolality can be useful in differentiating various causes of diarrheic stools.

Plasma Osmolality

Screening for toxin ingestion. Only a few exogenous substances can be ingested in amounts sufficient to affect the plasma osmolality. Table 14-1 lists the substances and the concentrations necessary to increase the osmolal gap to 10 or more milliosmoles per kilogram. The most common substances are alcohols. If the measured concentration of ethanol (mmol/L) does not correspond within 10 mOsm to the calculated osmolal gap, an *excess osmolal gap* is present. An excess osmolal gap would be suggestive that another of the substances listed in Table 14-1 is also present. When calculating the osmolal gap, confidence that methodological and calculation errors have been avoided is necessary.[1] Table 14-1 shows that trichloroethane can be at near-lethal levels in the blood without being readily detected by osmometry.

Although osmometry has long been recommended as a means to detect alcohol, it should be noted that vapor-pressure osmometers are not useful for the detection of alcohol because

TABLE 14-1   TOXIC SUBSTANCES AFFECTING PLASMA OSMOLALITY

Substances	TOXIC OR LETHAL CONCENTRATIONS		Corresponding Increase in Osmolality (mOsm/kg)
	Historical Units (mg/dL)	SI Units (mmol/L)	
Ethanol	350	80	80
Isopropanol	340	60	60
Methanol	80	24	24
Ethyl ether	180	24	24
Trichloroethane	100	9	9
Acetone (including other ketones or ketone metabolites)	55	10	10

dissolved alcohol is also volatile and thus contributes to the solution's vapor pressure.

An increase in the osmolal gap will also reflect an increase in the anion gap in patients with metabolic imbalance. These changes are caused by the presence of ketone (**acetone**) "bodies" (see Chapter 32).

Screening for mannitol toxicity. Mannitol is often used as an osmotic diuretic to treat cases of edema, especially cerebral edema, by reducing the amount of intracellular water. Although mannitol is a relatively nontoxic substance, it can cause renal damage at levels greater than 50 mmol/L. Measurement of the osmolality gap for patients undergoing mannitol therapy can be useful in estimating the serum levels of mannitol. If the osmolal gap is greater than 10 mOsm/L but less than 50 mOsm/L, it is likely that mannitol is present at a therapeutic, nontoxic level.

Urine Osmolality

Renal concentrating ability is a sensitive measure of kidney function. The urine that is delivered to the bladder is typically one to three times more concentrated than the plasma. A random urine specimen is sufficient to demonstrate the kidney's ability to concentrate urine if the osmolality of the random urine specimen is greater than 600 mOsm/kg. However, if the random urine specimen is dilute, no conclusion about concentrating ability can be made. A definitive follow-up test involves overnight water restriction. After the morning void, at least one urine specimen should exceed 850 mOsm/kg. Patients who are compulsive water drinkers may need continuous observation to ensure that no water has been ingested.

The specific gravity as estimated by the refractive index can also be used to measure urine concentration. However, osmometry is less affected by the presence of protein or radiocontrast dyes.

Stool Osmolality

The measurement of the osmolality of watery (diarrheic) stools can be used to diagnose the cause of chronic diarrhea. Diarrheic stools can be caused by maldigestion of foods; the undigested nutrients cause an osmotic diuresis in the intestines, producing a stool with a high osmolality (see Chapter 30). Watery stools can also result from excessive intestinal excretion of fluids and electrolytes; this produces a stool with a low osmolality.

These two types of chronic diarrheic disorders can often be differentiated by the calculation of the *stool osmolal gap*. The stool osmolal gap is the difference between the measured stool osmolality and twice the sum of the measured stool sodium and potassium.

$$\text{Stool osmolal gap} = \text{Measured osmolality}_{stool} - 2([Na+] + [K+])_{stool}$$
Eq. 14-4

If the stool osmolal gap is less than 50 mOsm/L, the patient most likely has a secretional diarrhea.[2] A stool osmolal gap greater than 50 mOsm/L is suggestive of the presence of unabsorbed, osmotic materials such as food. A large gap may also be seen in cases of excessive use of laxatives, some of which, such as the magnesium-containing laxatives, can be detected in stool water by the measurement of magnesium.

The osmolality of fresh liquid stool is approximately equal to that of serum. A hypo-osmolar watery stool (approximately less than 280 mOsm/L) might be suggestive of a factitious diarrhea, that is, one created by the patient, such as by adding water to the stool (Munchausen syndrome).[3]

Intestinal bacteria present in the stool can very rapidly convert stool carbohydrates into osmotically active fragments, raising the stool water osmolality. Thus stool osmolality measurements should be performed within 30 minutes of the collection of the stool sample.

Serum or Plasma Osmolality

Sample-collection technique is important to obtain a valid specimen for measurement of osmolality. For example, stasis during phlebotomy should be avoided. In addition, the patient's position, supine or upright, affects the osmolality. Thus a sample from a fasting, hospitalized patient gives the most uniform results, not because lipemia or other effects are avoided but because it is more likely that the patient was supine at the time of the morning phlebotomy rounds.

Serum and heparinized plasma have similar osmolality values. The contribution to the osmolality by fibrinogen in plasma is small, and it is important only in the measurement of

colloid osmotic pressure (COP). Freezing-point depression techniques can use whole blood and are not affected by lipemia or hemolysis. Anticoagulants other than heparin increase the measured osmolality. Table 14-2 shows the estimated effect of four anticoagulants. On occasion, the kind of anticoagulant used can be verified by measurement of the osmolality of the plasma.

PRINCIPLES OF MEASUREMENT

Osmolality is a colligative property; thus any of four measurements that depend on colligative properties may be used to measure osmolality. The measurements are (1) osmotic pressure, (2) **boiling-point elevation**, (3) freezing-point depression, and (4) **vapor-pressure depression**. Osmotic-pressure measurement has been used only in a special form of osmometry called *colloid osmotic pressure (COP)* and is discussed separately in a later section of this chapter. Boiling-point elevation is not useful for clinical samples because proteins will coagulate, causing gross changes in the sample composition. Of the remaining two, freezing-point depression is the most frequently used technique. Vapor-pressure depression as measured by the **dew point** is more commonly used in pediatric laboratories.

Freezing-Point Depression

The use of salt to melt ice and snow is a well-known practice. This is an example of freezing-point depression; that is, dissolved salt increases the osmolality, thereby lowering the freezing point of the solution compared to that of the pure solvent (ice or snow). The temperature at which ice and the water solution are in equilibrium is a function of the salt concentration. More precisely, the temperature at equilibrium is a function of the number of particles in solution. The freezing-point temperature is depressed 1.86° C for each mole of particles dissolved per kilogram of water. Because the osmolality of blood is about 0.285 Osm/kg (285 mOsm/kg), the freezing point is -0.53° C. Precise measurement of this temperature requires a sensitive thermometer. A **thermistor** (thermal resistor) is made from a mixture of oxides of transition metals such as manganese, cobalt, and nickel. These materials are semiconductors, and the number of electrons in the conduction band (valence electrons of the metal lattice capable of conducting a current) depends on the temperature. They become better conductors as the temperature rises. The conductance or resistance of the metals can be related to the temperature and hence to the osmolality.

Freezing-point depression is measured as follows:

1. The sample is either cooled by a bath containing an antifreeze solution that is maintained at about -5° C by a conventional refrigerator or by a thermoelectric cooler.
2. The sample is supercooled; that is, its temperature falls below the equilibrium freezing point. This occurs because pure ice crystals are slow to form.
3. Vigorous stirring induces the crystallization process. Once ice crystals begin to form, additional water molecules are rapidly added to the ice crystals. However, heat is released in the freezing process just as it is absorbed in the melting process. The heat that is released from the formation of the ice crystals raises the temperature of the sample until the rapid freezing stops and an equilibrium temperature is established.
4. The temperature is measured at the plateau, that is, at the temperature at which the heat removed by the cooling bath is matched by the heat released by the freezing process. The temperature at this equilibrium is the freezing point of the solution and is inversely related to osmolality. The plateau's temperature is measured electronically by the thermistor, and the temperature reading is converted to milliosmoles per kilogram and displayed. At this time, before complete freezing can cause mechanical damage to the thermistor probe, the thermistor is removed from the sample.

Because 1 osmol of solute lowers the freezing point by 1.86° C, osmolality can be calculated directly by the formula:

$$\text{Osmolality (mOsmol/kg)} = \frac{\text{Freezing-point depression}}{1.86° \text{ C}} \times \text{mOsmol/kg} \qquad \textit{Eq. 14-5}$$

However, it is more practical to calibrate the osmometer using saline solutions. Calibration also corrects for systematic or procedural effects, such as the increase in concentration of the sample because of the removal of pure water (as ice) before measurement of the temperature.

Several factors must be controlled to achieve high precision in freezing-point depression osmometry. These include the bath temperature, fluid composition, and amount of fluid. The fluid composition and volume change as moisture condenses from the room air. The thickness of the sample container and the amount of sample must be standardized. The probe must be rinsed and wiped to minimize carryover from one sample to the next. This is especially important between samples of widely differing osmolality, such as standards and urine samples. Samples can be remeasured, but great care must be taken to warm the sample (e.g., by holding the sample cup in the hand) until all the ice is melted; otherwise the sample will freeze prematurely. Any sample droplets on the side of the

---

TABLE 14-2　ESTIMATED EFFECT OF ANTICOAGULANTS ON OSMOLALITY (COMPARED WITH SERUM)

Anticoagulant	Full Tube (mOsm/kg)	Half-Full Tube (mOsm/kg)
Heparin	+0	+0
EDTA (disodium salt)	+15	+30
Fluoride-oxalate (sodium fluoride–potassium oxalate)*	+150	+300
Iodoacetic acid (lithium salt)	+5	+10

*This hyperosmolal state accounts for the hemolysis usually observed in the plasma of these samples.

cup should be joined with the sample by tipping the cup to coalesce the droplets.

The most common freezing-point osmometers are listed in Table 14-3, along with several key characteristics.

Vapor-Pressure Depression

Solvent molecules on the surface of a liquid are in constant thermal motion; some of these molecules escape from the surface into the atmosphere above the surface, forming a gaseous vapor phase in equilibrium with the liquid phase. This process is called *evaporation*. If the liquid contains dissolved solute, some of these solute molecules will occupy the surface layer of the liquid. Generally a solute molecule will not evaporate but will, by its presence, prevent a solvent molecule from evaporating. As the number of solute molecules increases, the chance that a solvent molecule will evaporate decreases, reducing the vapor phase in equilibrium above the liquid. Thus there is an inverse relationship between the concentration of dissolved solute particles (osmolality) and the vapor pressure above a solution. In vapor-pressure osmometry, the vapor-pressure depression of a solution is compared with that of a standard to determine the osmolality of a solution.

The temperature at which the atmosphere is saturated with solvent can be measured by a **thermocouple**. A thermocouple generates a voltage (**Seebeck effect**) between the ends of a wire. The voltage difference between the ends depends on the difference in temperature of the ends.

Thermocouples also exhibit the Peltier effect, which is the opposite of the Seebeck effect. An electrical current through the thermocouple transfers heat from one junction to the other. One junction cools while the other heats. The vapor-pressure osmometer passes an electrical current through the thermocouple in the measurement chamber, causing it to cool. When its temperature falls low enough, water (solvent) begins to condense on it. The electrical current is discontinued, and the thermocouple comes to an equilibrium temperature at which the water condensing on it is matched by the water evaporating from it. This equilibrium temperature is measured by the Seebeck voltage, which is linearly related to the osmolality.

Vapor-pressure depression is measured as follows:

1. The sample is sealed in a chamber. The air quickly changes humidity until its humidity is in equilibrium with the sample.
2. The thermocouple cools until its temperature is below the dew point. The electrical current is turned off, and the junction temperature rises as vapor condenses on it.
3. The plateau temperature (the temperature at which an equilibrium exists between condensation and evaporation) is measured.
4. The vapor pressure of the sample is directly proportional to the thermocouple voltage. Again, it is more practical to calibrate this type of osmometer than to apply theoretical factors. Systematic or procedural effects that must be controlled include the sample volume, the size and composition of the sample absorbent disk, the time delay between sample application and sealing of the chamber, cleanliness of the chamber, and changes in room temperature.

Table 14-3 provides information on the only available clinical vapor pressure osmometer.

COLLOID OSMOTIC PRESSURE
Definitions

Osmotic pressure is a colligative property and hence reflects osmolality. This is strictly true for a semipermeable membrane that is permeable to water only. The difficulty in finding such a membrane has kept the measurement of osmotic pressure from being used as a technique in the assessment of osmolality in clinical samples. However, measurement of the osmolal contribution of a group of molecules responsible for the colloid osmotic pressure (COP) is practical and useful. This property is measured by use of membranes that are permeable to small molecules. Small molecules, less than 30,000 D molecular weight, are called **crystalloids** if they are uncharged and *ions* if they are charged. Large molecules are called *colloids*. Hence COP measures only the contribution made to osmolality by large, essentially only protein, molecules. An alternative term is the **oncotic pressure**.

TABLE 14-3 CHARACTERISTICS OF CLINICAL OSMOMETERS

Manufacturer	Model*	Technique†	Routine Sample Size (µL)	Precision (%)‡	Measurment Time (sec)
Advanced Instrument, Inc.	3D3	FP	200	1.4	120 to 180
(Needham Heights, Mass.)	3M0 Plus	FP§	20		60
Fiske Associates, Inc.	One-Ten	FP§	15	1.6	60
(Needham Heights, Mass.)					
Precision Systems, Inc.	5002	FP	200	1.6	180
(Natick, Mass.)	µOsmette	FP§	50		
Wescor, Inc. (Logan, Utah)	5500	VP	10	2.8	60 to 90
	4420	COP	450	6.7	90 to 120

*All models are manually loaded with sample and have automated measurement and reporting. Variations in sample size, automated sampling, and printing are available.
†COP, Colloid osmotic pressure; FP, freezing-point depression; VP, vapor pressure.
‡From College of American Pathologists' survey for osmolalities in normal range.
§Does not use liquid cooling bath; uses electronic cooling.

Clinical Use of Colloid Osmotic Pressure

The major use for the measurement of the COP is detection of conditions leading to pulmonary edema. In this condition, there is an accumulation of water in the lungs, which interferes with oxygen and carbon dioxide exchange. The actual diagnosis can be obtained from x-ray measurements. Two measurements are needed to predict pulmonary edema: left ventricular heart pressure and COP. As long as the COP is greater than the pulmonary blood pressure (as measured by the "pulmonary artery wedge pressure"), pulmonary edema is unlikely. If heart failure is not present, that is, if the pulmonary blood pressure is normal, COP measurements alone allow prediction of the probability of pulmonary edema.

Knowledge of the albumin or total protein content of the plasma permits the calculation of the COP. However, the formula is inaccurate when used for acutely ill patients (especially patients with heart failure) and for patients who have received dextrans, or **plasma expanders**. For these groups of patients, measurement of COP is very useful.

Measurement of Colloid Osmotic Pressure

The COP is measured with a microporous filter or membrane that contains pores or channels whose diameters are carefully controlled to be impermeable to large molecules (proteins). Physiological saline is placed in a sealed chamber on one side of the membrane, and the sample is placed on the other.

Saline flows into the sample until the back-pressure stops further flow. This back-pressure, or negative pressure, is sensed by a pressure gauge. In addition to the osmotic pressure, an additional pressure is created by the **Donnan effect**. This effect arises because at physiological pH most proteins are negatively charged. Because the sample is electrically neutral, there are positive charges equal in number to the negative charges on the proteins. These positive charges are mostly in the form of sodium ions. Charged sodium ions diffuse through the membrane, whereas the corresponding negatively charged proteins do not. This leads to a separation of electrical charges. Because of the charge separation, additional small, negatively charged molecules are attracted across the membrane. As a result, the number of particles that diffuse is larger than that resulting from simple osmosis, and the pressure across the membrane is larger. Because the net charge on proteins changes with pH, the measured COP also changes with pH.

Customarily, COP is reported in millimeters of mercury (mm Hg). In practice a maximum pressure occurs 30 to 90 sec after the sample is placed into the instrument. This value is chosen because the pressure decays with time as a result of imperfections in the membrane that slowly allow large molecules to diffuse to the saline side, thus reducing the true pressure. Characteristics of a commercially available colloid osmometer are listed in Table 14-3.

References

1. Demedts P et al: Excess serum osmolality gap after ingestion of methanol: a methodology associated phenomenon? *Clin Chem* 40:1587, 1994.
2. Binder HJ: The gastroenterologist's osmotic gap: fact or fiction? *Gastroenterology* 103:702, 1992.
3. Topazian M, Binder HJ: Brief report: factitious diarrhea detected by measurement of stool osmolality, *N Engl J Med* 330:1418, 1994.

Bibliography

Dorman HR, Sondheimer JH, Cadnapaphornchai P: Mannitol-induced acute renal failure, *Medicine* 69:153, 1990.
Dorwart VW, Chalmers L: Comparison of methods for calculating serum osmolality from chemical concentrations and the prognostic value of such calculations, *Clin Chem* 21:190, 1975.

Epstein FB: Osmolality, *Emerg Med Clin North Am* 4:253, 1986.
Geheb MA: Clinical approach to the hyperosmolar patient, *Crit Care Clin* 3:797, 1987.

Internet Sites

http://www.chem.uidaho.edu/~honors/collig.html—Description of colligative properties, University of Idaho Honors Chemistry
http://dbhs.wvusd.k12.ca.us/ColligProp/ColligativeProp.html—Description of colligative properties, Diamond Bar High School, Diamond Bar, CA

http://www.columbia.edu/cu/chemistry/edison/gallery/Lab3/collig_prop.html—College course, Chemistry 1500, Department of Chemistry, Columbia University, New York, NY
http://www.science.uts.edu.au/subjects/91326/Section11/—Osmometry

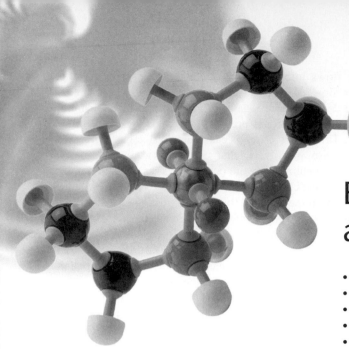

CHAPTER 15

Electrochemistry: Principles and Measurements

- *William R. Heineman*
- *Jon R. Kirchhoff*
- *John F. Wheeler*
- *Craig E. Lunte*
- *Sarah H. Jenkins*

Chapter Outline

Potentiometric methods
  Reference electrodes
  Indicator electrodes
  Care and methodology
  Experimental considerations and interferences
Voltammetric methods
  Voltammetry electrodes

  Oxygen electrode
  Glucose electrode
  Liquid chromatography with electrochemical detection
  Anodic stripping voltammetry
Coulometric methods
  Titration of chloride

Objectives

- Understand the fundamental differences between potentiometric and voltammetric techniques and understand how each technique is used for clinical measurements.

- Understand the process by which ion-selective electrodes respond to the presence of an analyte.
- Develop a knowledge of the methodology and possible interferences associated with using electrochemistry in the clinical laboratory.

Key Terms

activity (a)   The effective concentration of a solution species that accounts for interactions with other solution species.

activity coefficient (γ)   Activity divided by molar concentration. A measure of the degree with which a species interacts with other solution species.

amperometry   A controlled-potential technique in which current is measured at a fixed applied potential.

anode   The electrode at which oxidation occurs.

auxiliary electrode   The electrode in a three-electrode electrochemical cell that carries the current to maintain electrolysis at the working electrode.

cathode   The electrode at which reduction occurs.

cell potential (E_{cell})   The quantitative measure of the energy of an electrochemical cell; the difference in electron energy between two electrodes.

charge (Q)   A quantity of electricity that reflects the total current during a given time: $Q = \int_0^t i\,dt$ or $Q = it$ for constant i.

coulometry   A technique that measures the charge required to electrolyze a sample completely.

current (i)   The rate of charge flow (1 ampere = 1 coulomb/second).

electrolysis   A nonspontaneous electrochemical reaction that results from the application of potential to an electrochemical cell.

electrolyte solution   A solution of ions that provides a conducting medium for electrochemistry.

half-cell potential   The quantitative measure of the energy of a half-cell reaction relative to a reference electrode.

half-cell reaction   An electrochemical reaction that represents either an oxidation or a reduction at one of the electrodes in an electrochemical cell.

hydrodynamic voltammogram   A graphical representation of current versus applied potential for a particular electrochemical reaction that occurs in a stirred or flowing solution.

indicator electrode   An electrode whose half-cell or membrane potential varies as the concentration of reactants and products change in solution. This potential is governed by the Nernst equation.

ionophore   A neutral carrier molecule incorporated into an ion-selective electrode to detect a specific ion.

ion-selective electrode (ISE)   An indicator electrode used in potentiometry to respond to specific ions in solution.

limiting current (i_l)   The portion of a hydrodynamic voltammogram where electrolysis is occurring and the current remains constant as a function of increased applied potential.

liquid junction potential (E_{lj})   A potential that develops at the interface between two nonidentical solutions.

Nernst equation   The expression that relates the cell potential to the standard cell potential and the activities of reactants and products in an electrochemical cell.

oxidation   The process whereby a chemical species loses one or more electrons.

polarography   Voltammetry performed at a dropping mercury working electrode.

potentiometry   The technique in which the potential difference between two electrodes is measured under equilibrium conditions.

potentiostat   An instrument that controls the potential of an electrochemical cell.

reduction   The process whereby a chemical species gains one or more electrons.

reference electrode   An electrode with a stable half-cell potential that is used to measure and control the relative potential of the working electrode.

salt bridge   A device that allows ionic movement between compartments of an electrochemical cell to maintain electrical contact and at the same time prevent mixing of the separate solutions.

standard half-cell potential (E)   The electrochemical cell potential measured under standard state conditions.

stripping voltammetry   A voltammetric technique that allows sample preconcentration at the electrode before voltammetric analysis.

voltammetry   A technique whereby current is measured as a function of applied potential.

Electrochemistry involves the measurement of electrical signals associated with chemical systems that are incorporated into an electrochemical cell. The cell consists of two or more electrodes that interface a chemical system and an electrical system. The electrical system measures or controls the electrical parameters of voltage and **current (i)**, which are characteristic of a particular chemical system.

Electroanalytical chemistry makes use of electrochemistry for the purpose of analysis. In this application the magnitude of a voltage or current signal originating from an electrochemical cell is related to the activity or concentration of a particular chemical species in the cell. Excellent detection limits coupled with a wide dynamic range are exhibited by many electroanalytical techniques, with an operating range of 10^{-8} to 10^{-1} M. Measurements can generally be made on very small volumes of sample, that is, in the microliter range and below. The combination of low detection limits and microliter volume samples allows picomole amounts of analyte to be measured routinely in some instances. Furthermore, electroanalysis lends itself to measurements made in vivo. For example, miniature electrochemical sensors are used to measure pH and Po_2 in the bloodstream of patients with indwelling catheters.

In the clinical laboratory, electroanalysis is routinely used for the determination of many ions, drugs, hormones, metals, and gases. Methods are available for the rapid determination of analytes present at relatively high concentrations, such as blood electrolytes (Na^+, Cl^-, HCO_3^-), and analytes present at very low concentrations, such as heavy metals and drug metabolites in blood and urine samples.

The purpose of this chapter is to provide a fundamental background for understanding the electroanalytical techniques found in the clinical laboratory and to illustrate some of the practical applications of electroanalysis. These fundamental electrochemical techniques are divided into three basic categories: potentiometric, voltammetric, and coulometric. **Potentiometry** is the most widely used clinical application of electrochemistry and involves the measurement of a **cell potential (E_{cell})** under equilibrium conditions. **Voltammetry** and **coulometry** are considered dynamic techniques and are based on measurements made on a cell in which **electrolysis** is occurring. Many common definitions, symbols, and electrochemical nomenclature used in potentiometry, voltammetry, and coulometry are listed in Table 15-1.

POTENTIOMETRIC METHODS

Potentiometric methods are based on the measurement of a potential (voltage) difference between two electrodes immersed in solution under the condition of essentially zero

TABLE 15-1 ELECTROCHEMICAL TERMS, UNITS, CONSTANTS, SYMBOLS, AND CONVERSIONS

Term	Symbol	Unit or Constant	Symbol	Conversion or Value
Potential	E	Volt	V	V = J/C
Standard potential	(E^0)			E = i·R
Formal potential	$(E^{0\prime})$			
Current	i	Ampere	A	A = C/s
				$1A = 1.05 \times 10^{-5}$ mol of electrons per second
Charge	Q	Coulomb	C	C = A·s
				$1C = 1.05 \times 10^{-5}$ mol of electrons
Energy	H	Joule	J	
Resistance	R	Ohm	Ω	
Time	t	Second	s	
Temperature	T	Kelvin	K	
Activity	a	Moles per liter	mol/L	
Concentration	C	Moles per liter	mol/L	
		or moles per cubic centimeter	mol/cm^3	
Area	A	Square centimeters	cm^2	
Diffusion coefficient	D	Square centimeters per second	cm^2/s	
		Gas constant	R	8.31441 J/mol·K
		Faraday constant	F	9.64846×10^4 C/mol
		Number of electrons in electrode or redox reaction	n	

current. The electrodes and the solution constitute an *electrochemical cell*. Each electrode in the electrochemical cell is characterized by a **half-cell reaction** with a corresponding **half-cell potential**. Since essentially no current passes through the cell while the potential is measured, no net electrochemical reaction is occurring; thus a potentiometric technique is an equilibrium method. Potentiometric techniques are important because they can provide accurate measurements of activities, concentrations, or activity coefficients of many solution species. In general, a solution of ions or molecules is characterized by its molar concentration. However, these species can interact with other ions, molecules, or solvent. Depending on the type of interactions that occur, the *effective concentration* of the species may be less than, equal to, or greater than the actual molar concentration of species. The effective concentration is referred to as the **activity (a)** of the species and is related to the molar concentration by an **activity coefficient** as shown in the equation

$$a_i = \gamma C_i$$

where a_i is the activity of an ionic species, γ is the activity coefficient, and C_i is the molar concentration of that species.

A typical apparatus for potentiometry is shown in Fig. 15-1. The potential difference between the two electrodes is usually measured with a pH-millivolt meter. One electrode, the **indicator electrode**, is chosen so that its half-cell potential responds to changes in the activity of the particular species in solution to be measured. The other electrode is a **reference electrode** whose half-cell potential does not

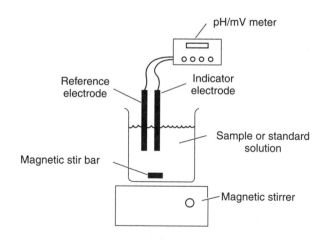

Fig. 15-1 Schema of apparatus for potentiometry.

change. It is important to understand that one does *not* measure an individual half-cell potential, but only the potential *difference* between one half-cell and a reference electrode. The most commonly used reference electrodes for potentiometry are the saturated calomel electrode and the silver/silver chloride electrode. The potential of the potentiometric electrochemical cell, E_{cell}, is given by:

$$E_{cell} = E_{ind} - E_{ref} + E_{lj} \qquad \textit{Eq. 15-1}$$

where E_{ind} is the half-cell potential of the indicator electrode, E_{ref} is the half-cell potential of the reference electrode, and E_{lj} is the **liquid junction potential**. The liquid junction

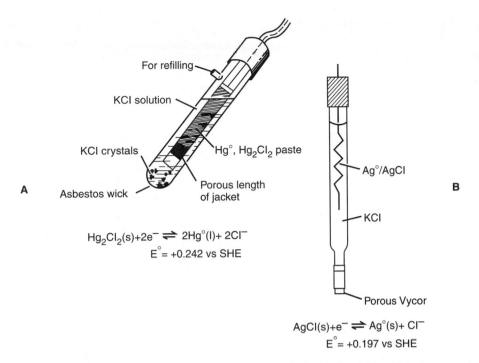

For refilling

KCl solution

KCl crystals

Asbestos wick

Hg°, Hg₂Cl₂ paste

Porous length of jacket

A

Ag°/AgCl

KCl

B

Porous Vycor

$$Hg_2Cl_2(s) + 2e^- \rightleftharpoons 2Hg°(l) + 2Cl^-$$
$$E° = +0.242 \text{ vs SHE}$$

$$AgCl(s) + e^- \rightleftharpoons Ag°(s) + Cl^-$$
$$E° = +0.197 \text{ vs SHE}$$

Fig. 15-2 Reference electrodes. **A**, Saturated calomel electrode, *SCE*, with asbestos wick for **salt bridge** function. **B**, Silver/silver chloride electrode, Ag/AgCl, with porous Vycor for salt bridge function.

potential is the electrical potential that develops at the interface between two liquids as a result of differences in the rates with which ions move from one liquid to the other. For example, the liquid junction potential arises in Fig. 15-1 at the point where the tip of the reference electrode meets the solution. Thus, E_{lj} is a potential that results from differences in **charge (Q)** rather than from an electrochemical reaction at an electrode.

Reference Electrodes

Since every electrochemical measurement must be made with respect to a reference half-cell potential, further discussion is needed with regard to the properties and types of reference electrodes. A reference electrode is an electrochemical half-cell that is used as a fixed reference for the measurement of cell potentials. Ideally, a reference electrode should possess the following characteristics: a stable, easily reproducible half-cell potential; a reversible half-cell reaction; chemical stability of its components; and ease of fabrication and use. Three reference electrodes are discussed below; one is of fundamental significance, and two are of practical importance.

The *standard hydrogen electrode (SHE)* has been chosen as the reference half-cell electrode on which tables of standard electrode potentials are based. In this half-cell, hydrogen gas at a pressure of 1 atmosphere is bubbled over a platinum electrode immersed in acid solution for which the activity of H⁺ is unity. The potential of the SHE is defined as 0.0 V at all temperatures, and the potentials of other half-cell couples are referenced to this value. The potentials of other

half-cells are either negative or positive of 0.0 V. Since other reference electrodes are easier to construct and use, the SHE is rarely used in practical applications of electrochemistry.

A commonly used reference electrode is the *saturated calomel electrode (SCE)*. A schema of a common type of SCE, its half-cell reaction, and standard half-cell potential are shown in Fig. 15-2, *A*. The electrode consists of elemental mercury covered with a thin coating of calomel (Hg_2Cl_2) that is in contact with an aqueous solution saturated with KCl. The potential of the half-cell will be constant so long as the activity of Cl⁻ does not change. The easiest verifiable way to set the activity of Cl⁻ to a fixed value is to saturate the solution with a chloride salt such as KCl. So long as crystals of KCl are present, the experimenter knows that the solution is saturated and that the activity of Cl⁻ is constant. Notice that the other participants in the electrochemical reaction (Hg_2Cl_2 and Hg) are solid and liquid components and consequently exhibit unit activity regardless of the amounts present in the cell. Thus the SCE offers the extraordinary convenience of being easily fabricated without the need for accurate preparation of the activities of any of the components.

Another commonly used reference electrode is the *silver/silver chloride electrode* (Ag/AgCl). A representative Ag/AgCl reference electrode is shown in Fig. 15-2, *B*. The electrode is prepared by coating a silver wire with a thin film of AgCl and immersing it in a solution of constant chloride concentration, which fixes the half-cell potential. The Ag/AgCl reference electrode is used routinely, especially as the inner reference electrode in potentiometric membrane electrodes.

The SCE and Ag/AgCl electrodes are commercially available or conveniently constructed.

Indicator Electrodes

The indicator electrode (or sensor) is the essence of potentiometric analysis. This electrode should interact with the analyte of interest so that the E_{ind} reflects the activity of this species in solution and not of other compounds in the sample that might interfere. The relative response of an electrode to one species and not to another species is defined as the *selectivity* of the electrode. The importance of having indicator electrodes that selectively respond to species of analytical significance has stimulated the development of many types of these electrodes.

Ion-selective electrodes. The most common indicator electrode used in clinical chemistry is the **ion-selective electrode (ISE)**. The ISE is based on the measurement of a potential that develops across a selective membrane. The response of the electrochemical cell is therefore based on an interaction between the membrane and the analyte that alters the potential across the membrane. The selectivity of the potential response to an analyte depends on the specificity of the membrane interaction for the analyte.

A representative ISE is shown schematically in Fig. 15-3. The electrode consists of a membrane, an internal reference electrolyte of fixed activity, $(a_i)_{internal}$, and an internal reference electrode. The ISE is immersed in a sample solution that contains analyte of some activity, $(a_i)_{sample}$. An external reference electrode is also immersed in this solution. The internal and external reference electrodes constitute the two half-cells of the electrochemical cell. The potential measured by the pH/mV meter (E_{cell}) is equal to the difference in potential between the external ($E_{ref,ext}$) and the internal ($E_{ref,int}$) reference electrodes, plus the membrane potential (E_{memb}), plus the liquid junction potential (E_{lj}) that exists at the junction between the external reference electrode and the sample solution.

$$E_{cell} = E_{ref,ext} - E_{ref,int} + E_{memb} + E_{lj} \qquad \textit{Eq. 15-2}$$

If the membrane is permeable to a particular ion [i], a potential develops across the membrane that depends on the ratio of activities of the ion on either side of the membrane. The half-cell potentials of the two reference electrodes are constant, sample solution conditions can be controlled so that E_{lj} is effectively constant, and the composition of the internal solution can be maintained so that $(a_i)_{internal}$ is fixed. Consequently, E_{cell} is described by the **Nernst equation:**

$$E_{cell} = K + 2.3 \frac{RT}{zF} \log (a_i)_{sample} \qquad \textit{Eq. 15-3}$$

where K represents the constant terms and z is the charge on the analyte ion (cations: +1, +2, +3, and so on; anions: −1, −2, −3, and so on). This logarithmic relationship between cell potential and analyte activity is the basis of the ISE as an analytical device. A plot of E_{cell} versus log a_i for a series of standard solutions should be linear over the working range of the electrode and have a slope of 2.3 RT/zF or 0.0591/z for measurements made at 25° C. Since membranes respond to a certain degree to ions other than the analyte (i.e., interferents), a more general expression than equation 15-3 is needed:

$$E_{cell} = K + 2.3 \frac{RT}{zF} \log [(a_i)_{sample} + k_{ij}a^{z/x}_j] \qquad \textit{Eq. 15-4}$$

where a_j is the activity of the interferent ion [j], x is the charge of the interferent ion, and k_{ij} is the selectivity constant. Small values of k_{ij} are characteristic of electrodes with good selectivity for the analyte, i.

The development of successful ISEs has hinged on the search for membranes that exhibit both sensitivity and selectivity for the analyte of interest. Of the two properties, selectivity is by far the more difficult to achieve. ISEs with selectivity for cations and anions have been developed with three basic types of membranes: liquid and polymer, solid state, and glass. All of these membranes function by selectively incorporating the analyte ion into the membrane, thereby establishing a membrane potential that depends on the activity of that ion. An ISE membrane must exhibit low solubility in the analyte medium to provide a durable electrode with a stable response. This requirement imposes a severe restriction on the material that can be used for membranes. Also, the membrane must exhibit some electrical conductivity to function in an electrochemical cell.

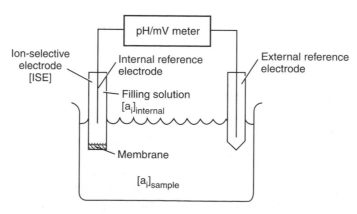

Fig. 15-3 Schema of an ion-selective electrode (ISE), external reference electrode, and pH/mV meter.

The scope of ISEs has been expanded to include the measurement of gases and neutral organic compounds by combining ISEs with gas-permeable membranes and layers of enzymes, bacteria, and tissues. These general categories of electrodes and specific ISEs are considered in the following sections.

Liquid and polymer membrane electrodes. A selective liquid membrane is the basis for many excellent ISEs. The liquid consists of a water-insoluble, viscous solvent in which is dissolved an **ionophore**, a hydrophobic organic ion-exchanger or a neutral carrier molecule that reacts selectively with the ion of interest. The liquid is typically soaked into a thin, porous solid membrane such as cellulose acetate, which is then incorporated into the ISE.

Fig. 15-4 shows the schema of the membrane portion of a liquid membrane ISE and the mechanism whereby an electrode responds to M^+ activity. The liquid membrane is in contact with internal and sample aqueous solutions of analyte M^+. The neutral carrier ionophore (R) reacts with M^+ at each membrane-solution interface and extracts M^+ into the membrane as MR^+. The extraction of M^+ into the membrane generates a positive membrane potential at each interface as a result of the charge difference that occurs when M^+ is extracted into the membrane in the form of MR^+ and the counter anion X^- that remains in the aqueous solution. As the activity of M^+ in solution is increased, the activity of MR^+ in the membrane increases and the membrane potential increases. This reaction exists at both the outer membrane surface, which is exposed to the sample, and the inner membrane surface, which contacts the inner filling solution of the ISE. The potential of the inner surface of the membrane, $E_{memb(internal)}$, is kept constant by maintenance of a constant activity of M^+ in the internal solution. Thus the only potential change measured in the circuit is the potential of the membrane surface contacting the sample, $E_{memb(sample)}$.

The availability of liquid and polymer membrane electrodes for a variety of ions is the result of the development of different neutral carrier ionophores and liquid ion exchangers that react selectively with particular ions. In the surface equilibria shown in Fig. 15-4, any ionic species other than M^+ that react to an appreciable degree with R will also generate a membrane potential and thereby cause an interference. The selectivity of the electrode for M^+ is therefore determined by the relative affinity between R and M^+ and between R and the various interferent ions in the sample.

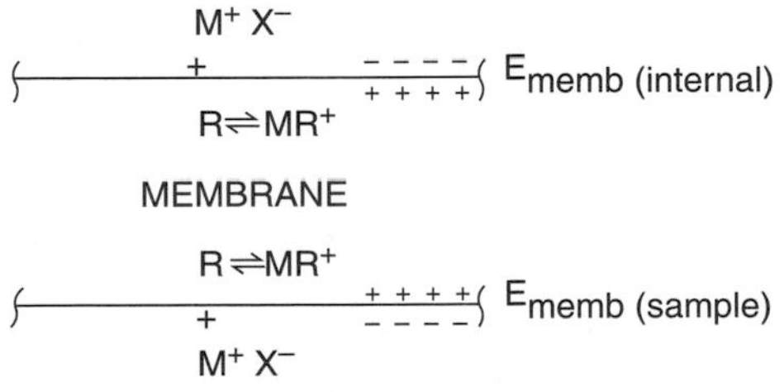

Several ionophores that selectively bind cations to nonaqueous membranes have been found. When a cation reacts with an ionophore, it is essentially inserted in a cavity within the ionophore that allows the cation to exist within a nonaqueous membrane medium. Selectivity for a particular cationic species is controlled by provision of an optimum environment in terms of number and position of binding atoms. An excellent example is the antibiotic valinomycin, which exhibits selectivity for K^+. Fig. 15-5 illustrates the K^+ complex of valinomycin. The K^+ cation fits into a snug cavity surrounded by oxygen atoms. The electrode exhibits excellent selectivity for K^+ against Na^+ because the smaller Na^+ ion is bound less tightly in the valinomycin cavity. This feature is of considerable practical importance in the clinical determination of K^+ in serum, which contains higher concentrations of Na^+ than of K^+. Ionophores for the selective determination of NH_4^+, Ca^{2+}, Na^+, Li^+, and Mg^{2+} have also been incorporated into ISEs. The selective incorporation of these cations occurs by the same principle described for the K^+ electrode. The development of liquid and polymer membrane ISEs has allowed the measurement of ions in samples of diverse origin. The electrodes have been especially successful in clinical laboratories and are now used routinely for measuring Ca^{2+}, K^+, Na^+, and Cl^- in biological fluids. The response characteristics for liquid and polymer membrane ISE systems commonly used in biomedical investigations are shown in Table 15-2.

Electrodes based on ion-pairing reactions have been developed for numerous organic compounds. These electrodes are based on insoluble ion pairs between an ionic form of the organic compound and an ion-pairing reagent. An example is

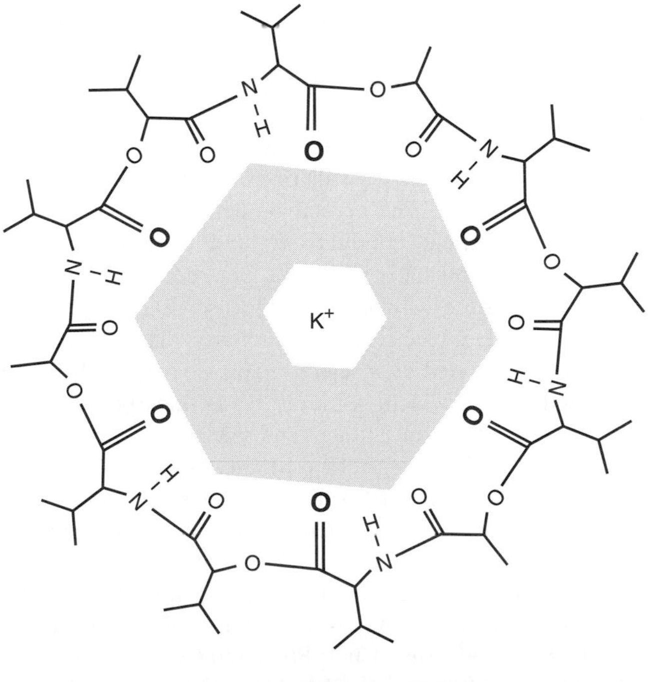

Fig. 15-4 Schema of liquid membrane ISE, where M^+ represents analyte cation, and R represents neutral carrier ionophore.

Fig. 15-5 Model of K^+ complex of valinomycin. Gray region represents K^+ ion. Bold oxygens are binding atoms.

TABLE 15-2 ION-SELECTIVE ELECTRODES (ISEs) USED IN CLINICAL CHEMISTRY

	Analyte	Membrane Composition	Linear Response Range (mol/L)	Possible Interferences
Glass	H^+	72.17% SiO_2, 6.44% CaO, 21.39% Na_2O (mol %)	10^{-12} to 10^{-2}	Na^+
	Na^+	11% Na_2O, 18% Al_2O_3, 71% SiO_2	10^{-6} to 10^{-1}	K^+, Ag^+
Solid state	F^-	LaF_3 crystal	10^{-6} to sat'd	OH^-
	Cl^-	$Ag_2S/AgCl$	5×10^{-5} to 1	Br^-, CN^-, S^{2-}
Liquid or polymer membrane	Na^+	Na^+ ionophore (ETH 227) 2-nitrophenyloctyl ether, sodium tetraphenylborate	10^{-3} to 10^{-1}	Li^+, K^+, Ca^{++}
	Cl^-	Tri-*n*-ocylpropylammonium chloride, decanol	10^{-3} to 10^{-1}	OH^-, Br^-, F^-
	K^+	Valinomycin, dioctyladipate, PVC	3×10^{-5} to 1	NH_4^+
	Li^+	Li^+ ionophores, such as crown ethers	10^{-4} to 10^{-2}	Ca^{++}, Na^+
	Ca^{++}	Ca^{++} ionophore (ETH 1001), 2-nitrophenyloctyl ether, sodium tetraphenylborate	10^{-7} to 10^{-2}	—
	Ca^{++}	Calcium di(*n*-decyl)phosphate, di(*n*-octylphenyl)phosphonate, PVC	3×10^{-5} to 1	Mg^{++}
Gas sensors	CO_2	Combination glass pH electrode, 0.01-0.1 M $NahCO_3$-NaCl filling solution; behind silicone rubber membrane	10^{-4} to 10^{-1}	Organic acids
	NH_3	Combination glass pH electrode, 0.1 M NH_4Cl filling solution; behind porous Teflon gas-permeable membrane	10^{-5} to 5×10^{-2}	Volatile amines

Modified from Meyerhoff ME, Opdycke WN: Adv Clin Chem 25:1, 1986.

an electrode for the antiepileptic drug phenytoin (5,5-diphenylhydantoin) based on the ion-pair complex between the 5,5-diphenylhydantoinate anion and the quaternary ammonium cation, tricaprylmethyl ammonium, which is immobilized in poly(vinyl chloride). The electrode measures phenytoin over the range of 10^{-1} to 10^{-4} mol/L and has a detection limit of 1.5×10^{-5} mol/L. This electrode can be used to determine phenytoin in tablets and capsules. New ion exchangers and neutral carriers are continually being evaluated in an effort to improve selectivity of existing electrodes and to develop electrodes for other ions and molecules.

Solid-state membrane electrodes. Solid-state membranes consist of single crystals or pressed pellets of salts of the ions of interest. The crystal or pellet must have some degree of electrical conductivity and exhibit very low solubility in the solvent in which the electrode is to be used—usually water. An excellent ISE for F^- uses LaF_3 doped with Eu^{2+} to provide electrical conductivity. The membrane potential is generated by a selective surface reaction between LaF_3 and F^- in which solution F^- is incorporated into vacancies in the crystal lattice. The selectivity is very good because other anions do not fit well into the crystal structure. The properties of the F^- ISE are shown in Table 15-2. Another clinically important solid-state membrane electrode for determination of Cl^- is based on pressed-pellet membranes of the ionic conductor, Ag_2S, and AgCl. Similar electrodes have also been developed for the detection of Br^-, CN^-, I^-, SCN^-, S^{2-}, Ag^+, Cu^{2+}, Pb^{2+}, and Cd^{2+}.

Glass membrane electrodes. The first and most widely used ISE is the glass membrane electrode for pH measurements. Glasses of certain compositions respond to pH when a membrane potential develops as a result of an ion-exchange mechanism with H^+ that occurs in the thin, hydrated outer layer of the glass membrane that has been soaked in solution. The outstanding properties of the glass pH electrode are attributable to the remarkable selectivity of this surface reaction for H^+.

The basic design of the glass electrode for pH is shown in Fig. 15-6. The electrode consists of a glass or plastic tube with a thin, pH-sensitive glass membrane sealed in the tip. Ordinarily the membrane is only about 50 μm thick and hence is very fragile. The bulb at the end contains an internal solution composed of 0.1 M HCl into which is dipped a silver wire coated with AgCl, which provides an internal Ag/AgCl reference electrode. This solution also maintains a fixed activity of H^+ to which the internal surface of the membrane is exposed. A shielded cable makes electrical contact between the internal Ag wire and the external pH meter.

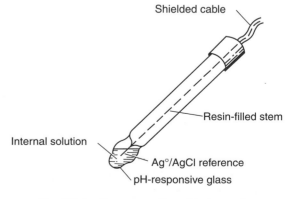

Fig. 15-6 Representative pH electrode.

The pH response of the glass membrane is determined by the composition of the glass. The glass consists of Na_2O, CaO, and SiO_2. Pure SiO_2 is essentially an insulator that is unresponsive to pH. The addition of Na_2O to the glass formulation disrupts the neutral SiO_2 structure so that negatively charged oxide sites (SiO^-) are paired with Na^+. The mobility of Na^+ in the glass renders the glass membrane slightly conductive to electrical charge. The negative oxide sites serve as ion-exchange sites in aqueous solution and provide the basis for pH response. The potential response to pH is extraordinarily accurate over a pH range of 0 to 14. At pH values above about 9 to 10 the electrode exhibits significant response to other monovalent cations such as Na^+ and K^+. This response to alkali cations at high pH is termed the *alkaline error*. This error can be minimized by replacement of Na_2O and CaO to a certain extent in the glass with Li_2O and BaO.

The membrane response to H^+ is attributed to an ion-exchange process that occurs in the vicinity of the membrane solution interface. On immersion of a dry glass membrane in an aqueous solution, the membrane surface becomes hydrated during the course of a few hours. This uptake of water leads to a gradual dissolving of the glass; this process generally determines the useful lifetime of an electrode. However, surface hydration is essential for electrode function; new electrodes immersed in solution respond poorly until adequately soaked. Soaking establishes a hydrated layer that is only 10^{-1} μm or less in thickness. This hydrated layer then functions as a cation-exchange layer in which negatively charged oxygen sites are linked to the glass matrix but in which Na^+ is mobile. Soaking the electrode in acid, for example, results in the replacement of Na^+ with H^+. The membrane response to H^+ can be understood in terms of a surface potential that results from the ion exchange of Na^+ with H^+ in the hydrated gel. Immersion of the electrode membrane in alkaline solution results in exchange of H^+ in the membrane with Na^+ as membrane H^+ moves into solution. The inner membrane potential is held constant by exposure to a fixed activity of H^+ in the internal solution. Glass electrodes for Na^+, Ag^+, and NH_4^+ have been developed by varying the composition of the glass.

Gas-sensing electrodes. Gas-sensing electrodes consist of an ISE in contact with a thin layer of aqueous electrolyte confined to the electrode surface by an outer membrane, as shown schematically for a CO_2 electrode in Fig. 15-7. The outer membrane is very thin and is chosen so that it is permeable to the gas of interest; for CO_2, the membrane is made of silicone rubber. This membrane allows CO_2 gas in the sample to pass through. Dissolution of the CO_2 in the thin layer of electrolyte causes a change in pH because of a shift in the equilibrium position of the chemical reaction shown in Fig. 15-7. The change in pH sensed by the internal ion-selective pH electrode is in proportion to the P_{CO_2} of the sample. One of the most important applications of the CO_2 electrode is the measurement of blood P_{CO_2}.

The NH_3 electrode in principle is identical to the CO_2 electrode; here the filling solution is aqueous ammonium chloride. The internal pH electrode senses the change in pH

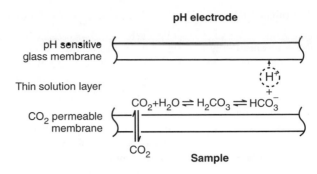

Fig. 15-7 Schema of gas-sensing electrode for CO_2.

from the ammonium/ammonia (NH_4^+/NH_3) acid-base equilibrium. The pH change is thus proportional to P_{NH_3} of the sample.

Gas electrodes have been used for other bioanalytical applications such as the measurement of CO_2 in general assays of decarboxylating enzyme activities and the measurement of NH_3 in tissue and serum. Characteristics of the CO_2 and NH_3 electrodes are shown in Table 15-2.

Care and Methodology

The care of ISEs is essentially similar for every ion type. Since the sensing tip of the electrodes is made from fragile and sensitive materials, care must be taken to prevent breakage and to maintain the tip in a moist environment. Most commercially available electrodes are supplied with protective coverings to help prevent careless damage to them while they are not in use. Each electrode is also accompanied by manufacturer's recommendations for specific cleaning and storage requirements. Storage conditions depend on the frequency of use, the type of electrode, and the application. For example, cleaning procedures are different for a pH electrode used in a protein solution and for one used in a solution of inorganic ions. Protein layers are removed by rinsing the electrode with pepsin, bleach, or 0.1 M HCl, whereas an inorganic deposit can be removed with ethylenediaminetetraacetic acid (EDTA) or acids. After each cleaning procedure, the electrode tip is thoroughly rinsed with distilled water, and the electrode is returned to the storage container.

pH measurements are easily made in the clinical laboratory with a two-point calibration procedure. Standard buffer solutions, which are commercially available, are chosen to bracket the pH of the sample solution. Electrode calibration is always initiated with a pH 7 standard buffer. The meter is adjusted to read 7.00 after the temperature control has been set to the temperature of the buffer. Depending on the sample to be measured, either an acidic or alkaline buffer is used to complete the calibration. Samples can then be measured. Multiple calibrations may be necessary for a large number of samples.

For non–H^+ sensing electrodes a calibration curve that relates the potential difference in millivolts to concentration is often used. Although ISEs measure analyte activity, the concentration can be related to millivolts as long as the ionic strength is constant between standards and samples. This is accomplished by addition of a small amount of a solution of high ionic strength to the calibrating standards. This solution must not contain any interfering ions. A potential reading is determined for each standard solution, beginning with the lowest concentration. A plot of log $(C_i)_{standard}$ versus potential is linear for a properly responding ISE. Ion concentrations in samples are then obtained by measurement of the response in millivolts of the sample and use of the calibration curve. The sample ion concentrations are valid as long as the matrix of the standard solutions is made to closely mimic the samples. Most laboratory electrodes and instruments routinely use a two-point standardization procedure to ensure similar response from analysis to analysis. Other standardization and analysis methods have been developed for various electrodes and applications.

In the clinical laboratory, the analysis of large numbers of samples is often a necessity. Thus many ISEs are incorporated into automatic analyzers in a flow-through configuration. This arrangement takes advantage of the rapid response of ISEs by placing them into multi-ion analyzers with large sample throughput capabilities. Calibrants, samples, and rinsing solutions are pumped across the electrode surfaces of the ISEs, which are placed in series. A single reference electrode is used for all ISEs in a system with the exception of the CO_2 sensor, which has its own reference electrode behind the gas-permeable membrane. Calibrants have constant ionic strength that closely matches that of physiological samples to minimize errors that result from differences in liquid junction potentials between samples and standards. It cannot be emphasized enough that the proper care and use of the ISEs in these instruments are essential to ensure accurate and reproducible analyses. This requires a constant monitoring of the performance of both the individual electrodes and the instrument as a whole. The following section is a discussion of some of the common errors and interferences that can occur with ISE measurements.

Experimental Considerations and Interferences

Errors in ISE measurement can result for any ion determination if standards and samples are not run at approximately the same temperature, since the Nernst equation is temperature-dependent. Perhaps the most important source of error is the response of an ISE to a nonanalyte or interferent ion in the sample. It is therefore important to know the selectivity properties of the electrode being used and to ensure that nonanalyte ions to which the electrode responds are not present in high enough concentrations to constitute an interference. Components in certain samples can also change the sensitivity of an electrode by adsorbing on its surface, thereby blocking access of the analyte to the surface. Such contamination is a problem in samples containing surface-adsorbing species such as proteins. For single electrode determinations in whole blood or serum, techniques that isolate the ISE from direct contact with the sample are available. However, the demand for multiple sample and ion analyses has made single electrode measurements impractical. Modern multi-ion analyzers incorporate a small size-exclusion membrane that protects the ion-selective membrane from the high–

molecular-weight components of biological fluids but allows analyte molecules access to the electrodes.

Although many ISEs are very selective, under certain conditions some ions may interfere and yield erroneous results. Specific examples are listed in Table 15-2 and are briefly discussed below. Detailed descriptions of clinical analyses for many ions can also be found in the CD-ROM.

pH measurements have few specific interferences associated with them. The linear response range is from pH 2 to 12. Sensitivity of the glass pH electrode may be reduced at pH values above 10 because of the interference of monovalent cations, especially Na^+. Although monovalent cations can enter and slowly move through the hydrated layer, multivalent cations of 2+ or 3+ charge do not interfere. In solutions of pH less than 1, low water activities also give rise to measurement error.

Na⁺ ions are determined by either a glass electrode or a polymer type of liquid membrane electrode. Interferences are minimal because of the high concentration of sodium in biological fluids, especially in blood. Because of this fact, the glass electrode exhibits excellent selectivity over K^+ and H^+. Highly acidic urine samples are an exception. The polymer-based ISE, however, can be subject to an interference from Li^+ if a patient is being treated with a lithium compound.

K⁺ is usually measured by the valinomycin/polymer electrode described above. Good results are obtained for measurements in blood; however, in undiluted urine samples a negative error may result because of the partitioning of a negatively charged lipophilic component of the urine that is permeable to the polymer. This component can be excluded by use of an ISE with a silicone-rubber membrane instead of the polymer. Alternatively, accurate measurements can be obtained by sample dilution.

Determination of Na^+ and K^+ levels in undiluted blood and urine samples requires special attention. Measurements made by the nondilutional ISE method may differ from results obtained by dilutional ISE methods, which determines the concentration of ions in the total sample volume. In contrast, the nondilutional ISE method measures the activity of the ions directly in the sample. Since the activity can be influenced by the sample environment (such as protein and water content), deviations may occur between these methods. Agreement between these methods is usually realized by calibration adjustment. Methodological differences may be greater in the case of Na^+ determinations because of the higher relative concentration of Na^+ in biological fluids. The influence of physiological effects on Na^+ and K^+ determinations in biological fluids is discussed in further detail under "Sodium and Potassium" in the CD-ROM.

Special care must also be taken in the determination of Ca^{2+}, which exists in both the bound form (with proteins or other biological molecules) and the unbound, ionized Ca^{2+} form. The Ca^{2+} ISE is one of the easiest ways to measure ionized Ca^{2+}, since it responds to only the ionized form, which is believed to be the physiologically important form.

The determination of Cl^- in biological fluids by an ISE is frequently compromised by fouling of the surface by proteins present in the sample. This problem can be minimized by using the semipermeable membrane described above to exclude the large molecules from the electrode surface. A liquid membrane electrode made of polymer that exhibits selectivity for chloride has been developed for use in electrolyte analyzers for biomedical use. The chloride ISE is subject to interference from Br^-, I^-, F^-, CN^-, OH^-, and S^{2-}, but, except for Br^-, these ions are usually not present in physiological samples at a level high enough to interfere. The F^- ISE exhibits excellent selectivity and suffers only from interference of OH^- at high pH.

ISEs for the measurement of CO_2 are relatively easy to use and are interference-free. Undiluted blood can be used directly as the sample, and calibration is typically accomplished with 5% and 10% mixtures of CO_2 in an inert gas. Total CO_2 measurements require acidification to convert CO_3^{2-} and HCO_3^- to CO_2. In this case, calibration is performed with standard $NaHCO_3$ solutions. Response times for total CO_2 measurements are generally longer because of the necessity of establishing equilibrium conditions. CO_3^{2-}-selective membranes are available in some instruments for total CO_2 measurements. Interferents are mainly organic acids to which the gas membrane is also permeable. The carbonate-selective membranes are subject to interferences from anions such as salicylate, but placement of the ISE behind the silicone-rubber membrane alleviates this problem.

The NH_3 ISE responds selectively and rapidly to the ammonia concentration in solution; the major drawback is the questionable stability of the membrane and the electrode. Interference can result from nonpolar volatile amines present in the sample. With both the CO_2 and NH_3 electrodes it is important to have a rapidly responding electrode. A decrease in the response time signifies a loss in electrode performance and may require the replacement of the membrane.

VOLTAMMETRIC METHODS

Electrochemical techniques in which a potential is applied to an electrochemical cell and the resulting current from an electrochemical reaction is measured are generally categorized as *voltammetric* methods. Electrochemical cells for voltammetry use a three-electrode configuration. The cell consists of a *working electrode, a reference electrode*, and an **auxiliary electrode**. The potential is applied between the working and reference electrode by a **potentiostat**; this applied potential can force changes to occur to any electroactive species at the working electrode surface by electrolysis. Electrolysis can occur by a **reduction**, a gain of one or more electrons, or an **oxidation**, a loss of one or more electrons. The current required to sustain the electrolysis at the working electrode and maintain electroneutrality in the cell is provided by the auxiliary electrode. This arrangement prevents the reference electrode from being subjected to large currents that could change its potential. Some voltammetry instrumentation is based on the two-electrode system. Here the auxiliary electrode is absent, and the reference electrode is subjected to the entire cell current.

The basic concept of applying a potential to an electrochemical cell and measuring the current that results from

electrolysis can be implemented in numerous ways. Several different techniques have been developed by varying how the potential is applied or how the current is measured. Although the resultant output and the practical applications of these techniques are varied, they all share the common basis of applying a potential, E, and measuring a current, i, or charge, Q. In addition, the solution may be moving or stationary with respect to the working electrode. Voltammetry in an unstirred solution is referred to as *stationary* solution voltammetry. *Hydrodynamic* voltammetry involves the forced movement of solution either through stirring the solution or flowing the solution over the electrode as in *liquid chromatography with electrochemical detection* (LCEC, see Chapter 6).

The result of a voltammetric technique is called a *voltammogram* (i.e., a current-potential curve). Voltammograms give useful quantitative and qualitative information about the electrochemical reaction. A typical **hydrodynamic voltammogram** is shown in Fig. 15-8 for the reduction of species *Ox* by one electron to species *Red*. As the potential is scanned in the negative direction, the voltammogram can be described by three distinct regions. In region A, the potential applied at the working electrode is insufficient to cause electrolysis to occur; therefore no current is observed. The onset of electrolysis is signaled by the rise in current in region B. The current continues to rise until a maximum value is reached. This takes place in region C, where electrolysis is occurring at the maximum rate possible. The maximum current in region C is defined as the **limiting current (i_l)**, and is defined by Eq. 15-5:

$$i_l = \frac{nFAD_0C_0}{\delta} \qquad \textbf{\textit{Eq. 15-5}}$$

where A is the electrode area, D_0 is the diffusion coefficient of *Ox*, C_0 is the concentration of *Ox*, and δ is the diffusion distance. As is illustrated by Eq. 15-5, the magnitude of i_l is directly proportional to the concentration of the electrochemically active analyte. Thus voltammetry can be used to quantitatively measure analyte concentration. The practical unit for current is the ampere (A), which is the transfer of one coulomb of charge per second. This corresponds to the passage of 1.05×10^{-5} moles of electrons per second. Since

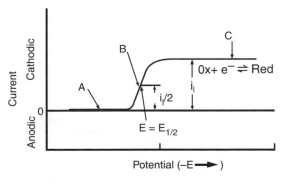

Fig. 15-8 Generalized hydrodynamic voltammogram for reduction of *Ox* to *Red*. Potential scanned negatively left to right. i_l is limiting current, and $E_{1/2}$ is half-wave potential.

the current involved in most electroanalytical techniques is very small, milliamperes (mA), microamperes (μA), and nanoamperes (nA) are commonly used units.

The *half-wave potential* ($E_{1/2}$) is defined as the potential at one half the limiting current. $E_{1/2}$ is uniquely characteristic of the species undergoing electrolysis (just as the half-cell potential is for the reference electrode), and it can be used for qualitative identification. By convention a reduction is described by a positive, or *cathodic*, current, whereas an oxidation is described by a negative, or *anodic*, current. The principles for an oxidation are similar and can be applied for a positive potential scan.

One specific type of voltammetry that is clinically useful is **amperometry**. Amperometric sensors are devices that measure the current generated at a fixed potential by an electroactive analyte in solution. The potential is set to a value of E where i_l occurs (Fig. 15-8, region C), and i_l is then measured for each sample. The current measured is directly proportional to the concentration of species present. Three clinically important amperometric sensors discussed below are the oxygen electrode, the glucose electrode, and LCEC.

Voltammetry Electrodes

Working electrodes. Working electrodes have certain properties in common. Good electrical conductance is of foremost importance; consequently, working electrodes are generally metals or semiconductors. Chemical and electrochemical inertness is important in applications for which the electrode should function simply to transfer electrons to and from species dissolved in solution. This inertness gives a wide potential region with minimum background contributions from electrode and solvent redox properties in which the electrochemistry of the analyte or analytes can be easily monitored.

Platinum, gold, mercury, and glassy carbon are commonly used materials for voltammetric electrodes. When used for voltammetry, mercury can be in the form of a *hanging mercury drop electrode*. To provide the working electrode

surface, extrude a reproducible mercury drop through a narrow glass capillary by means of a commercially available micrometer syringe. A new drop is formed by simply dislodging the old one and extruding more mercury. The *dropping mercury electrode* is the working electrode for **polarography**. In this technique, mercury is forced by gravity through a very fine capillary to provide a continuous stream of identical droplets. Each droplet expands, becomes too heavy to be suspended, and breaks loose from the capillary.

Auxiliary electrodes. Auxiliary electrodes are made from any conductive material, typically a piece of platinum wire.

Reference electrodes. The commonly used reference electrodes for voltammetry are the SCE and Ag/AgCl electrodes, which have been previously described in detail.

Oxygen Electrode

The oxygen electrode is designed as a complete electrochemical cell. The basic design, which is shown in Fig. 15-9, incorporates a platinum disk as the **cathode** and an Ag/AgCl electrode as the **anode** in a buffered **electrolyte solution**. The electrochemical cell is isolated from the sample by an oxygen-permeable membrane. Oxygen diffuses through the membrane and is reduced electrochemically at the platinum electrode, which is held at a potential that quantitatively reduces oxygen (–0.5 to –0.6 V versus Ag/AgCl).

$$O_2 + 2H^+ + 2e^- \rightarrow H_2O_2 \qquad \textit{Eq. 15-6}$$

The current generated at the platinum electrode is directly proportional to the concentration (partial pressure) of oxygen dissolved in the sample. As with potentiometric indicator electrodes, the membrane inhibits electrode fouling from serum proteins in blood and also prevents other electroactive substances from being reduced at the electrode. Calibration of the electrode system is performed with standard solutions or gases containing known concentrations of oxygen.

Few interferences are associated with the use of the oxygen electrode. Poor response times and variable results

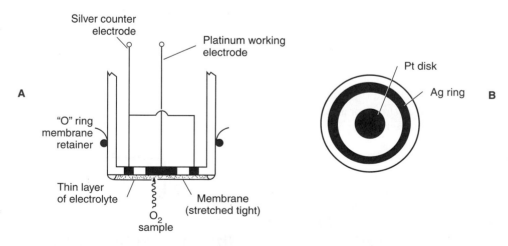

Fig. 15-9   Schema of oxygen electrode. **A,** Cross-sectional view showing diffusion of O_2 sample through membrane. **B,** View of electrode assembly from bottom.

may indicate that degradation of the membrane or a change in pH of the buffer solution has occurred. Silver metal may deposit on the platinum cathode and also affect the electrode response. Polishing the electrode with electrode polishing compound regenerates the platinum surface.

The oxygen electrode is incorporated into a blood gas analyzer, which measures oxygen, CO_2, and pH on samples of less than 250 μL of whole blood. Miniaturized O_2 electrodes have been developed for transcutaneous measurements, eliminating the need for drawing blood samples. However, the accuracy and response time of these electrodes depend on the physical characteristics of the patient's skin tissue. The oxygen electrode has been used to monitor reactions that involve consumption of O_2 to measure glucose (glucose oxidase), lactic acid (lactate oxidase), cholesterol (cholesterol oxidase), and uric acid (uricase).

Glucose Electrode

Glucose is another important constituent of serum and plasma that can be measured by an amperometric sensor. A diagram of a typical glucose electrode is shown in Fig. 15-10. The basic design of this electrode uses the enzyme glucose oxidase, immobilized between two membranes. Glucose oxidase reacts with the glucose in the sample to generate hydrogen peroxide (H_2O_2) and gluconic acid. The inner membrane is permeable to H_2O_2, which is determined amperometrically by the underlying platinum electrode held at a positive potential sufficient to oxidize H_2O_2 to O_2 (the reverse of the reaction shown in equation 15-6). The current measured from the H_2O_2 oxidation is directly proportional to the glucose concentration; glucose concentrations have been reported to be quantified in the range of 10^{-7} to 10^{-3} M. Few interferences are noted for this electrode. The inner membrane is impermeable to ascorbic acid, uric acid, and acetaminophen, which are electroactive at positive potentials and may be present in clinical samples. The design for this glucose electrode has been developed by the Yellow Springs Instrument Company (Yellow Springs, Ohio). The glucose electrode is often referred to as a **biosensor** because it incorporates a biological compound, glucose oxidase, as a key component in its

operation. Glucose, lactic acid, and urea electrodes are now common features of multi-analyte blood-gas analyzers.

Electrochemical test strips are commercially available as a personal monitoring device for patients with diabetes to measure blood glucose. The disposable test strip typically consists of thin electrodes coated on a small strip of plastic. One electrode is converted to a glucose electrode by addition of glucose oxidase; the other is made into an Ag/AgCl reference electrode. Glucose is rapidly determined by adding a drop of blood to the exposed area of the test strip and measuring the current for oxidation of glucose with a small, portable instrument.

Advances in microfabrication methodology have stimulated the commercialization of sensor arrays for whole-blood diagnostics. These are based on miniaturized potentiometric and amperometric sensors of the type already discussed. For example, a hand-held blood analyzer for Na^+, K^+, Cl^-, BUN, glucose, and hematocrit is commercially available for point-of-care testing (see Chapter 17).

Liquid Chromatography with Electrochemical Detection

LCEC is a hybrid technique that combines chromatography with electrochemistry. As discussed in Chapters 5 and 6, high-performance liquid chromatography provides a means of separating various components of solutions by making use of their chemical affinities to column-packing materials. In LCEC, electroactive materials are detected sequentially as they elute from a chromatographic column and flow across or through the working electrode. Very low detection limits (approximately 1.0 pmol) may be obtained with relatively simple instrumentation. As a result of these features, LCEC has become recognized as a powerful tool for the trace determinations of many clinically important bio-molecules, including several metabolites of the central nervous system that are easily oxidized or reduced at an electrode surface.

To optimize an LCEC determination, you must consider both chromatographic and electrochemical requirements simultaneously. A primary requirement for electrochemical detection is a mobile phase that has a relatively high conductivity. Because of this, buffered mobile phases of moderate ionic strength (0.01 to 0.1 M) are typically used. Most LCEC applications use reverse-phase, ion-exchange, or ion-pair chromatographic columns for separation (see Chapter 6). Significant amounts (up to 90% v/v) of organic modifiers, such as methanol, acetonitrile, and propanol, can be added to the aqueous mobile phase to shorten chromatographic retention. Of great advantage in LCEC is the inherent specificity of electrochemical detection, in which only compounds electroactive at the applied potential are detected. In this way many interferences that have similar chromatographic retention times are eliminated. For this reason, sample preparation may be quite simple in comparison with other detection methods available for high-performance liquid chromatography.

Most LCEC applications use a single working electrode in a conventional three-electrode system (see Chapter 6). The choice of working electrode material is an important

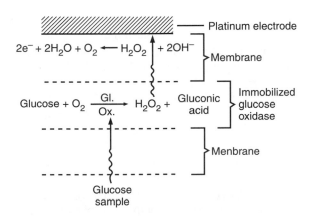

Fig. 15-10 Schema of glucose electrode.

TABLE 15-3 APPLICATION OF LCEC TO DRUG ANALYSIS

Class	Compound
Analgesic	Acetaminophen, codeine, naproxen, phenacetin, salicylic acid, ketobemidone, morphine
Tranquilizer	Diazepam
Anticonvulsant	Nitrazepam
Antibacterial	Amoxicillin
Adrenergic blockers	Labetalol, mepindolol
Antineoplastic	Methotrexate, procarbazine hydrochloride
Muscle relaxant	Theophylline
Antihypertensive	Sulfinalol hydrochloride
Antitubercular	Rifampin
Antipsychotic	Chlorpromazine
Antiarthritic	Penicillamine

Modified from Lunte CE, Heineman WR: Electrochemical techniques in bioanalysis, Top Curr Chem 143:1, 1988.

TABLE 15-4 APPROXIMATE OXIDATION POTENTIALS OF NEUROCHEMICALLY IMPORTANT COMPOUNDS

Compound	Oxidation Potential
Dopamine	0.3 V
Epinephrine	0.3 V
5-Hydroxyindoleacetic acid (5-HIAA)	0.3 V
Norepinephrine	0.3 V
Ascorbic acid	0.3 V
Vanillylmandelic acid (VMA)	0.6 V
Metanephrine	0.6 V
Normetanephrine	0.6 V
3-Methoxy-4-hydroxyphenylglycol (MHPG)	0.7 V
Homovanillic acid (HVA)	0.7 V

Modified from Lunte CE, Heineman WR: Electrochemical techniques in bioanalysis, Top Curr Chem 143:1, 1988.

consideration for LCEC. Carbon paste, a mixture of graphite powder and a coagulant such as paraffin oil, exhibits low background currents at positive potentials and is well suited to oxidative applications. Unfortunately, carbon paste electrodes are incompatible with mobile phases containing significant amounts of organic modifier. Glassy carbon electrodes are compatible with modifiers and may be used at negative potentials. Mercury or mercury-gold amalgam electrodes have the best characteristics when operated at negative potentials, and they are used principally for reductive LCEC. Any of these types of electrode surfaces can become fouled and inefficient when one is detecting high concentrations of some compounds. Additionally, high concentrations of proteins or other large biomolecules can lead to electrode fouling, which results in irreproducible data. Physical and chemical cleaning procedures have been developed to alleviate the permanent loss of electrode performance.

To obtain the best detector sensitivity and detection limits, you must determine the minimum potential that needs to be applied to the working electrode for the desired electrochemical reaction to occur. The most common method of accomplishing this is by obtaining a hydrodynamic voltammogram (Fig. 15-8) of each component being detected. Such a voltammogram is generated by making multiple injections at various applied detector potentials and then plotting the resulting current as a function of potential. To achieve maximum sensitivity, select the applied potential so that the observed oxidations or reductions are at the limiting current for all compounds to be detected.

LCEC has become a widely used analytical technique for biomedical analysis. Although space does not permit a complete review of all biochemical applications, it is important to consider many general classes of compounds detectable by both oxidative and reductive techniques. Table 15-3 lists

several compounds of pharmaceutical origin that may be determined using LCEC. Table 15-4 provides the approximate oxidation potentials obtained from hydrodynamic voltammograms used to detect some neurochemically important compounds by LCEC.

Oxidative applications. Most phenols are readily oxidized at carbon electrodes. The first and still most common LCEC application is the determination of catecholamines in biological samples. A second major use of LCEC is in the determination of the hydroxyindole metabolites of tryptophan. More recently, an electrochemical enzyme immunoassay has been developed in which phenols are detected as the electroactive product of the enzyme reaction. Aromatic amines are likewise easily oxidized at carbon electrodes and may be studied by LCEC.

Many compounds of biomedical interest are heterocyclic in structure and electroactive at potentials easily attained using LCEC. Methods for the determination of such heterocycles as ascorbic acid, uric acid, reduced nicotinamide adenine dinucleotide (NADH), biotin, and the folates have been developed. Although most amino acids are not electroactive at analytically usable potentials with reduced carbon electrodes, derivatization methods have been developed to produce electroactive products. These methods provide excellent determination of amino acids. Thiols may also be determined at a gold-mercury amalgam electrode.

Reductive applications. Wide-scale reductive LCEC applications have not been as well established in the clinical laboratory because of the difficulties presented by oxygen and trace metal-ion interferences at negative potentials. These problems can be overcome with established mobile-phase deoxygenation procedures and the use of high-purity salts, leading to more clinical applications of reductive LCEC.

Aromatic nitro and nitroso compounds are easily reduced at carbon or mercury electrodes. Other nitro compounds, such as nitrate esters, nitroamines, and nitrosamines, are also easily reduced. Additionally, several heterocycles of clinical interest may be detected by reductive LCEC, including the K vitamins, the pterins, and several pharmaceuticals.

Anodic Stripping Voltammetry

Anodic stripping voltammetry is a voltammetric technique useful in clinical chemistry for the determination of heavy metals. An example of its use is the determination of Pb^{2+} in biological fluids of patients suspected of having lead poisoning. **Stripping voltammetry** has the lowest detection limit of the commonly used electroanalytical techniques; analyte concentrations as low as 10^{-10} M have been determined. The technique consists of two steps. In the first step, analyte is deposited at a mercury electrode by the application of a potential sufficient to reduce the species of interest at the working electrode. This step serves to preconcentrate the analyte by electrochemically extracting it into a mercury electrode. It is this preconcentration feature that enables such low concentrations to be reached by stripping voltammetry. In the second step, the deposited analyte is removed, or "stripped," from the electrode by application of increasingly positive potentials; the resulting current signal is a measure of the concentration of analyte in solution. Since the stripping step gives anodic current (i.e., the species is oxidized), the technique is termed *anodic stripping voltammetry*.

In anodic stripping voltammetry only a fraction of the total analyte is deposited into the mercury electrode by electrolysis during the preconcentration step. Complete deposition of all of the analyte into the electrode is time-consuming and generally unnecessary, since adequate amounts can usually be deposited into the electrode to give a satisfactory stripping signal in much shorter times. Since the deposition is not exhaustive, it is important to deposit the same fraction of analyte for each stripping voltammogram. The parameters of electrode surface area, deposition time, and stirring must be carefully duplicated for all standards and samples. Deposition times vary from 60 seconds to 30 minutes, depending on the analyte concentration, the type of working electrode, and the stripping technique.

Anodic stripping voltammetry has become a useful method in the clinical laboratory for the determination of Pb^{2+} in blood and urine since the development of automated instrumentation by Environmental Science Associates (ESA). ESA also markets a digestion reagent, Metexchange, which frees bound Pb^{2+} from biological components of blood and urine. Detailed procedures for Pb^{2+} determination in blood and urine by anodic stripping voltammetry can be found in the literature.

COULOMETRIC METHODS

Coulometry is a very useful electrochemical method for quantitative analysis. Clinical applications use one form of coulometry that involves the application of a constant current to generate a titrating agent. In principle, the time required to titrate a sample at constant current is measured and is related to the amount of analyte in a sample by Faraday's law (equation 15-7):

$$Q = it = nFN \qquad\qquad \textit{Eq. 15-7}$$

where Q is the charge passed for a finite time, t, at constant current, i; n is the number of electrons involved in the electrochemical reaction; F is Faraday's constant; and N is the number of moles of analyte in the sample. Charge is a quantity of electricity. The unit for charge is the coulomb (C) and corresponds to 1.05×10^{-5} moles of electrons. Since N is measured directly without the need for standards, coulometry is an absolute method and can be used for very precise determinations of analyte.

Titration of Chloride

Although not in wide use currently, coulometric determination of chloride is of historical importance and has been used for the determination of Cl^- in serum, plasma, urine, and other body fluids. The determination of Cl^- takes advantage of the quantitative formation and low solubility of AgCl. Ag^+ ions (the titrating agent) are electrochemically generated at the Ag anode by application of a constant current. Cl^- ions in the sample are rapidly consumed as they react with Ag^+ to form insoluble AgCl. At any point in the titration, the Ag^+ concentration is very low.

Anode reaction: $Ag \rightarrow Ag^+ + e^-$
Solution reaction: $Ag^+ + Cl^- \rightarrow AgCl(s)$

However, the end point is signaled by a sudden increase in Ag^+ concentration that follows the consumption of all of the Cl^-. A second pair of Ag^+-specific electrodes detects the rise in concentration of silver ions in solution and immediately stops the titration. The amount of Cl^- in the sample is proportional to the amount of Ag^+ ions generated at the anode.

Coulometric determination of chloride is very precise; however, other anions that form insoluble complexes with silver ion can result in Cl^- determinations that are falsely elevated. Also, poor reproducibility can be a problem at high chloride concentrations because of the large amount of precipitate.

Bibliography

General

Luppa PB, Sokoll LJ, Chan DW: Immunosensors—principles and applications to clinical chemistry, *Clin Chim Acta* 414:1, 2001.
Vassos BH, Ewing GW: *Electroanalytical chemistry*, New York, 1983, Wiley & Sons.
Wang J: *Analytical electrochemistry*, ed 2, New York, 2000, Wiley-VCH.
Wang J: *Electroanalytical techniques in clinical chemistry and laboratory medicine*, New York, 1988, VCH Publishers

Potentiometric Methods

Diamond D, Saez de Viteri FJ, Ion-selective electrodes and optodes. In Diamond D, editor: *Principles of chemical and biological sensors*, New York, 1998, Wiley & Sons.
Koryta J, editor: *Medical and biological applications of electrochemical devices*, New York, 1980, Wiley & Sons.
Meyerhoff ME, Opdyke WN: Ion-selective electrodes, *Adv Clin Chem* 25:1, 1986.

Simon W et al: Ion-selective electrodes in biology and medicine. In Laidler KJ, editor: *Frontiers of chemistry*, New York, 1982, Pergamon Press.

Solsky RL: Ion-selective electrodes in biomedical analysis, *CRC Crit Rev Anal Chem* 14:1, 1982.

Voltammetric Methods

Bard AJ, Faulkner LR: *Electrochemical methods*, ed 2, New York, 2001, Wiley & Sons.

Kissinger PT, Heineman WR, editors: *Laboratory techniques in electroanalytical chemistry*, ed 2, New York, 1996, Marcel Dekker.

Lunte CE, Heineman WR: Electrochemical techniques in bioanalysis, *Top Curr Chem* 143:1, 1988.

Sawyer DT, Sobkowiak A, Roberts JL, Jr: *Electrochemistry for chemists*, ed 2, New York, 1995, Wiley-Interscience.

Phenytoin Electrode

Cosofret W, Buck RP: A poly(vinyl chloride) membrane electrode for determination of phenytoin in Pharmaceutical formulations, *J Pharm Biomed Anal* 4:45, 1986.

Biosensors

Blum LJ, Coulet PR, editors: *Biosensor principles and applications*, New York, 1991, Marcel Dekker.

Cunningham AJ: *Introduction to bioanalytical sensors*, New York, 1998, Wiley-Interscience.

Eggins B: *Biosensors: an introduction*, New York, 1996, Wiley & Sons.

Kessler M et al, editors: *Ion and enzyme electrodes in biology and medicine*, Baltimore, 1976, University Park Press.

Ramsey G, editor: *Commercial biosensors*, New York, 1998, Wiley & Sons.

Turner AFP, Karube I, Wilson GS: *Biosensors: fundamentals and applications*, Oxford, England, 1987, Oxford University Press.

Internet Sites

http://electrochem.cwru.edu/ed/dict.htm—Electrochemistry dictionary

www.bath.ac.uk/~chsacf/solartron/electro/html/int.htm

http://jcbmac.chem.brown.edu/baird/Chem22l/lectures/Electrochemistry/ElectroChem.html—Electrochemistry via Adobe Acrobat

http://learn.chem.vt.edu/tutorials/electrochem/—Electrochemistry help file by the Chemistry Learning Center at the Virginia Tech Chemistry Department

www.cranfield.ac.uk/biotech/chinap.htm

http://www.bertholf.net/rlb/Lectures/index.htm—PowerPoint lecture by Robert L. Bertholf, PhD, Associate Professor of Pathology, Chief of Clinical Chemistry and Toxicology

http://www.funsci.com/fun3_en/electro/electro.htm

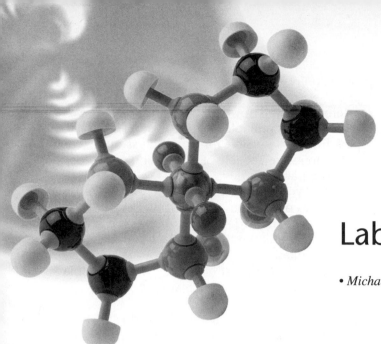

CHAPTER 16

Laboratory Automation

• *Michael A. Pesce*

Objectives

- Outline the steps in sample processing.
- Describe and compare the functions of systems for total laboratory automation, modular systems, front-end specimen processing, and specimen archiving.
- Outline the steps in analysis and describe how they may be adapted to automation.

- Describe the proportioning of samples to reagents.
- Define sample carryover, identifying systems in which it is commonly seen and suggest at least two ways by which it can be minimized.
- Outline the processes of mixing, incubation, and sensing.
- List the benefits of laboratory automation.

Key Terms

analog A measurement derived directly from an instrument's continuous signal (such as voltage) and usually presented in graphic form.

automation Use of a machine designed to follow repeatedly and automatically a predetermined sequence of individual operations.

autoverification Automatic reporting of test results without technologist review if they fall within a predetermined set of parameters.

bar code label A computer-driven sample-recognition system that identifies both the specimen and the analyses to be performed and relays this information to the automated analyzer.

bulk reagents Those that must be measured before being added to a reaction mixture to attain the desired proportion. Usually a reservoir contains the reagents for more than one analysis.

carryover Contamination of a specimen by the previous one.

computation Calculation of a desired result from the signal or readout of an instrument; it can be electronically automated by use of either digital or analog conversion.

continuous flow Process in instruments that constantly pump reagent and sample through tubing and coils, forming a continuous stream.

dead volume The volume in a sampling container that must be present for proper sample aliquot measurement but is not consumed.

digital Relating to data available in the form of discrete units or the calculations using such data.

discrete Term applied to instruments that compartmentalize each sample reaction.

dwell time The minimum time required for an instrument to obtain a result, calculated from the initial sampling of the specimen.

flow injection Placement of a sample into the stream of a continuous-flow analyzer.

incubation time The time allowed for a chemical reaction or process to proceed to completion.

mixing Process by which individual components of a chemical assay are formed into a homogeneous solution.

proportioning Addition of individual components of a chemical assay in proper ratios or amounts.

random access instrument An instrument capable of performing multiple tests on a sample. Instead of performing all possible tests on each sample, these instruments are capable of performing only those tests programmed.

readout Written or computer display of the result of an analysis performed on an instrument.

sensor A system or device that monitors changes in the reaction mixture that are related to analyte concentration.

test menu The number of different tests available at one time without changing reagents or components.

test repertoire All the different tests that are available on an instrument, including those that can be made available by changing reagents or instrument components.

throughput The maximum number of individual samples or test analyses that can be practically performed per hour by an assay system, with the required dwell time being taken into account.

total laboratory automation Automating all the steps involved in laboratory testing from specimen processing to storage and disposal of specimens.

unit reagents Premeasured reaction chemicals packaged so that only one package (unit) is used per sample test.

In this chapter, the reasons for laboratory **automation** and the ways to achieve it are considered. Examples of the major automated instrument categories are examined.

In the 1990s, healthcare costs became an important issue for hospitals. The changes in the reimbursement rates by the government and the proliferation of managed care contracts have resulted in a significant change in the laboratory environment. Cost containment or reduction has become a primary goal for the laboratory. The laboratory is now considered a cost center rather than a source of revenue. At the same time, the laboratory was asked to improve the turnaround time for reporting of test results, and to provide a more comprehensive service. For example, immunosuppressant drug monitoring for transplant patients, testing for neural tube defects and Down syndrome, maternal human immunodeficiency virus (HIV) testing, tumor marker analysis, and homocysteine and ultrasensitive C-reactive protein (CRP) measurements for assessment of patients who may be at cardiac risk must be performed as quickly as possible for physicians to treat patients in a timely fashion. Laboratories had to come up with a plan to do more with less. Laboratories had to reduce

cost, improve turnaround time, expand the **test menu**, and reduce laboratory errors. To meet these demands, the laboratory has to be on the cutting edge of technology, and automation is the key to achieve these goals.

LABORATORY PROCESSES

Automation in a hospital must be viewed as a global process. The entire sequence begins when a physician examines a patient and a decision is made to obtain specific laboratory information. The overall process is shown in Fig. 16-1, and can be broken down into the following components: test ordering, sample acquisition (phlebotomy), sample transport, front-end sample processing, sample analysis, result acquisition, result reporting, archiving, and disposal of samples. Laboratorians must be aware of each step in this process and what can cause a breakdown in these steps, resulting in longer turnaround times or in misplaced samples. In general, laboratory automation has focused on the analysis of the specimen in the laboratory and the transfer of information back to the requesting physician. There is, however, increasing interest in automating the process of transferring the sample to the laboratory and in sample processing.

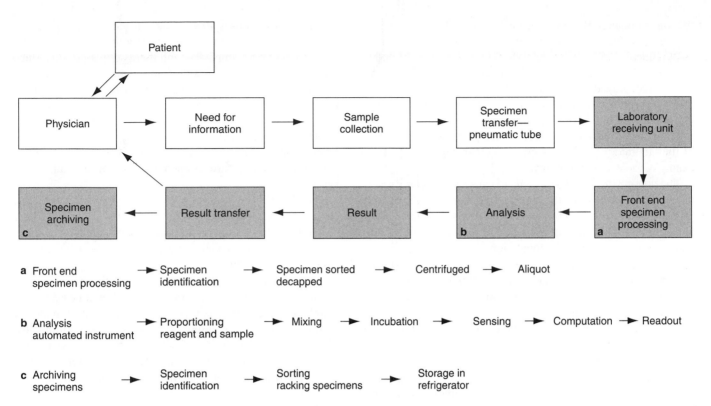

Fig. 16-1 Diagram illustrating specimen and information flow between physician and laboratory. *Shaded area* is that portion of the system usually considered part of the laboratory. Lower portion amplifies steps in sample processing and analysis.

Automating the transfer of samples to the laboratory can reduce some of the preanalytical errors associated with this step (see Chapter 3) and reduce the overall time required to produce a test result. Automation of sample transfer is usually accomplished by means of a vacuum tube system. Phlebotomy tubes are placed in a cushioned holder that is introduced into a sending station. The sending station can be programmed to send the holder to a specific receiving station. Vacuum tube systems can rapidly (in less than 5 minutes) transport samples with insignificant physiological changes to the samples (e.g., hemolysis and gas cavitation in blood-gas samples), obviating the need for slower, less reliable human transporters.

Sophisticated analytical instrumentation automates much of the analytical testing of the chemistry, immunochemistry, and hematology sections of the laboratory. Recent systems have comprehensive test menus, which have resulted in workstation consolidation. For example, instead of requiring several immunochemistry analyzers from different vendors to measure hormones, tumor markers, and cardiac markers, these analytes can now be measured with one system from a single vendor. As a result, there is less handling of specimens within the laboratory, which reduces laboratory error, and the economics of scale provide for better pricing of reagents and supplies, which reduces laboratory cost. Many hospitals have a "core" laboratory that centralizes all the automated chemistry, immunochemistry, hematology, and coagulation testing in one workspace. The core laboratory concept is a useful adjunct to the other steps of laboratory automation.

Although most automated analyzers usually operate very efficiently, the introduction of the sample to the analytical system often remains a manual process, one that accounts for a large part of the turnaround time and is responsible for the majority of laboratory cost and errors. As shown in Fig. 16-1, most of the time spent in laboratory testing is in sample handling. As laboratories seek to reduce cost and improve laboratory efficiency, increasingly they look to automate all the manual processes involved in laboratory testing. Therefore, many laboratories are concentrating on automating the last significant areas of manual work, that is, specimen processing and the archival and disposal of samples.

Goals of Laboratory Automation

The goals of laboratory automation include (1) reduction of costs, (2) expansion of laboratory testing to generate more revenue, (3) reduction of turnaround time, (4) reduction of laboratory errors, and (5) improvement of laboratory safety. The primary driving force for automation is still the reduction of costs; laboratories that have consolidated workstations have seen a reduction in their labor costs and reagent and supply budgets. This is because labor accounts for the majority of the costs in laboratory testing and successful justification for automation is usually based on staff reductions. However, a careful cost analysis must be developed because the time it takes to recover the capital investment ("payback time") for the automated equipment depends on many factors. Comparing the payback time with other laboratories can be misleading because it depends on the baseline value, which is different for each laboratory. For example, if the laboratory is not very efficient and has high staff salaries, the payback period will be more rapid and the savings greater than for a laboratory with lower salaries.

A reduction in staff because of automation usually does not mean that these workers become unemployed. They are usually redeployed for other laboratory functions, such as the measurement of new, often esoteric, tests that had been sent to commercial laboratories. Alternatively, they can use their expertise as medical technologists in the point-of-care section of the laboratory or be transferred to other departments, for example, molecular pathology.

The volume of work performed also has a significant effect on cost and must be accurately determined to optimize the type of automation needed to process the current workload and to allow for future increases in volume. The volume of work must be determined both from a global viewpoint, that is, the total number of samples or analyses in a day or week, and from a local viewpoint, that is, the number of samples at peak workflow. The laboratory also must have an estimate of the clinicians' expectation for turnaround time. The laboratory must work with the vendor to develop a realistic financial and equipment plan. A usual result of laboratory automation is a reduction in the turnaround time for reporting test results as the number of steps in the testing process is reduced. This is especially true if the front-end sample handling process becomes automated.

The majority of laboratory errors occur during front-end processing of the samples. The most common errors are mislabeling the sample, incorrectly preparing aliquot samples (pouring from the wrong sample), mislabeling the aliquot tube, and misplacing samples in the laboratory. Automation of sample processing will eliminate most of these errors.

Laboratory safety is an important issue. The staff that handles specimens is subject to exposure to potentially infectious biological fluids as the result of spills, aerosols, breakage of tubes, and when removing the stoppers from primary tubes to either prepare aliquots or for analysis. Automation of sample processing will help protect the staff from these hazards. With proper planning by the hospital administrators and laboratory staff, improved safety goals can be achieved.

AUTOMATED LABORATORY SYSTEMS
General Considerations

Although there are several approaches to maximizing the degree of automation in a laboratory, there are a number of general, nontechnical issues that should be considered before

---

GENERAL CONSIDERATIONS FOR LABORATORY AUTOMATION

Union issues
Power and cooling requirements
Cross-training of staff
LIS interface needs
Autoverification
Peak volume testing
Staff involvement
Centralized customer service area

---

the laboratory chooses an automated system. These are listed in the box at the bottom of the left column.

Union issues are important and if not addressed can reduce potential labor savings and improvements in laboratory efficiency. For example, policies that affect seniority, overtime, time off, and job responsibilities can significantly affect laboratory operations. In addition, a significant increase in efficiency may reduce the need for manpower; a critical union concern. These issues must be discussed and resolved with the union before implementation of an automated system.

The air-conditioning system must have enough capacity to cool the laboratory with present and future equipment. There should be sufficient emergency power outlets in the laboratory and enough emergency lighting to operate the laboratory in case of a power failure.

Cross-training of the staff (e.g., in both chemistry and hematology) is important if maximum laboratory efficiency is to be achieved because it provides the laboratory manager with flexibility in scheduling of the staff. Cross-training also benefits the staff because technologists that are cross-trained in chemistry and hematology usually receive higher salaries and are more marketable if they need to look for another position.

The laboratory information system (LIS) should interface with all components of the automated system. If the LIS is not compatible there could be significant delays in implementation.

Autoverification of sample results is an essential part of laboratory automation and is the automatic reporting of test results without review by the technologist. This process allows the LIS to verify laboratory results if they fall within a predetermined set of parameters (see result reporting section, p. 295, for a detailed discussion of autoverification).

In a hospital laboratory, specimens arrive throughout the day, but peak volumes usually occur in midmorning to late morning, late afternoon, and early evening. The laboratory must carefully calculate the peak volume. The automated system should be able to handle at least twice the peak load to anticipate future growth.

Staff involvement is an important part of any automation project. Committees that include laboratory staff and hospital administrators should be established for all aspects of the process, such as site coordination, stat testing , instrumentation selection, and specimen processing. For example, tube standardization is important because some automated systems only use one tube size. If a different size tube comes into the laboratory it has to be manually processed, which reduces laboratory efficiency and can result in processing errors. The staff must be convinced that automation improves patient care, makes the staff's work more efficient, and that there is some job security.

A centralized customer service area must be established to receive calls regarding laboratory testing. This should be staffed on the day and evening shifts and be located close to the laboratory. The customer service area handles, for example, calls for add-on tests, type of tube needed for specimen drawing, and reference ranges. Any technical or clinical information that is requested should be directed to the appropriate individual.

Whatever automated system is chosen, there must be careful planning for all steps. Hospital administrators, laboratory directors, laboratory managers, and staff must be convinced that the automated system will meet the needs of the laboratory. Success or failure usually depends on the cooperation of all the individuals involved in the laboratory automation process.

Laboratory Automation

The different types of laboratory automated solutions that are available are (1) **total laboratory automation** (TLA), (2) modular integrated automation, and (3) modular or stand-alone systems for front-end sample processing and archiving and sample retrieval.

Total laboratory automation. TLA employs an integrated track system that links all the laboratory's workstations (front-end processing, instrumentation, and archiving systems) together to create a continuous, comprehensive network that automates almost all the steps involved in clinical laboratory testing. TLA systems usually automate the chemistry, immunochemistry, hematology, and coagulation sections of the laboratory. TLA systems first introduced in Japan in the 1980s and now extensively used in that country are becoming important choices for laboratory automation for larger laboratories because of the potential for substantial cost savings.

TLA systems are usually turnkey systems that contain the components for each step in the process, including sample sorters, aliquoters, centrifuges, and analyzers that are interconnected by the track system. Bar code–labeled specimens are brought to an inlet station where the bar-code reader scans the bar code to check its integrity and to query the host computer for test selection. Specimens that have an unreadable bar code or have the label facing the wrong direction are placed in an exception rack for manual processing. Specimens with an acceptable **bar code label** are sorted into racks, and transported to the hematology workstation for analysis, or to a centrifuge station. After centrifugation, specimens are uncapped, sorted, placed in racks, and transported to the chemistry or coagulation workstations. If aliquots are required, the sample is sent to the aliquoting workstation, which can usually create up to five bar code–labeled aliquot tubes per specimen. At this station sample clots are detected and a liquid level sensor identifies samples with insufficient quantity of sample for the tests that have been ordered; these are also sent for manual processing. The aliquot tubes are sent to the appropriate workstations. After the analysis is completed, the specimens are recapped, transported to the archiving workstation where they are placed in racks, and sent to a refrigerator for storage or retrieval if necessary. Some TLA systems also dispose of the samples.

The major drawbacks of the TLA systems include the substantial financial investment and the considerable amount of open space required for these systems. For example, the cost of some TLA systems can range from one to three million dollars. To justify this investment a careful financial assessment must be performed. The major cost savings from automation is a reduction in labor. However, the volume of testing performed also has a significant impact on cost and a large test volume is required to justify TLA. In one analysis it was estimated that the laboratory needed to process more than 2500 tubes per day and assay more than 2,000,000 tests per year to justify TLA. In many cases, when laboratories calculate the return on investments based on current and future workloads, the anticipated increase in testing never comes to fruition. This results in an increase in time for the laboratory to recoup its initial investment and a laboratory with large amounts of unused testing capacity.

Laboratory space is an important issue when considering TLA systems. TLA requires a considerable amount of open space, which is at a premium in most hospitals; a typical TLA system requires anywhere from 3000 to 5000 square feet. Some TLA systems can use the existing space in the laboratory or be set up in another area of the hospital, or placed in a centralized laboratory off-site but relatively close to the sending hospitals. However, because of the large amounts of instrumentation and components and the additional structural support to bear the weight of the systems, installation of a TLA system usually requires extensive renovations. In some cases, TLA involves obtaining building permits, which usually delays construction. If the TLA system is to be put into the same area of the existing laboratory it usually involves removing counters and walls, and in general causing havoc in the laboratory. If possible, TLA systems should be configured into a new area within the hospital.

Other factors besides cost and space must be considered before obtaining a TLA system. Because of the complex nature of TLA, it may be necessary to have an on-site biomedical engineer to troubleshoot the system and a dedicated supervisor to ensure the day-to-day operation of the TLA system. TLA also requires standardization of the sample tubes, usually into one size. Plastic tubes are usually preferred over glass because they are less apt to break and shatter.

TLA systems, available from Roche Diagnostics and Beckman-Coulter, have been placed in large hospitals and some commercial laboratories.[1-6] TLA systems have been shown to decrease labeling errors by 27%, reduce turnaround time by 19%, and reduce full time equivalents (FTEs) by 15%.[6,7]

Modular Integrated Systems

Modular integrated systems offer an alternative to TLA. Modular systems link together multiple laboratory disciplines into a single testing platform that is interconnected by a track. This approach allows for configuration of different modules such as chemistry and immunochemistry, and consolidates into a single area sample loading and unloading, and reagent loading and unloading. Modular systems have a two-lane track system to facilitate rapid processing of stat specimens and samples that require repeat or reflex testing. The second lane allows these samples to be sent directly to the analyzer without disrupting the high volume routine testing. Front-end specimen processing systems can also be interconnected to the chemistry-immunochemistry module. Modular systems automate part of what TLA offers, but provide flexibility because different types of modules can be readily added depending on workflow or a change in test patterns.

Compared with TLA systems, the modular approach is significantly lower in cost, requires less laboratory space, is quicker to install, and is easier to interface with the LIS. A limitation of this approach is that when a front-end sample processing system is linked to a workstation, it can only process specimens for that workstation. Studies have shown that modular automated systems can decrease turnaround time by 2 to 3 hours, reduce staff, and result in a 30% increase in productivity.[8,9] Modular automated systems are available from Roche, Beckman-Coulter, Johnson and Johnson, and Bayer.

Stand-Alone Systems: Sample Processing and Archiving

Another approach to laboratory automation is to automate specific sections of the process that are still manual operations. These sections include specimen processing and sample archiving.

Sample processing. Until recently, little automation was available to automate the specimen handling that occurs before sample analysis. Front-end sample processing is usually a manual procedure in which samples are sorted, centrifuged, uncapped, and divided into aliquots if tests for more than one workstation have been requested. It is usually the rate-limiting step in providing rapid and accurate test results. In some laboratories, front-end sample processing accounts for about 60% of the testing cost caused by labor-related issues. Manual sample processing is responsible for about 40% of the turnaround time and for most of the laboratory errors and lost specimens.[4,10-12] Therefore automating this process has become a major focus of clinical laboratories.

Various approaches have been employed to automate the manual steps of front-end sample processing. There are modular systems that automate the entire process and stand-alone systems that automate one portion of front-end processing. A modular system consists of a sorting station, a centrifuge, and aliquot station all linked with a track system. Bar code–labeled primary tubes are placed on the system and the host computer queried for test selection. Tubes are sorted by test and placed into racks. If no further processing is required, for example, assays that use whole blood (complete blood count [CBC], hemoglobin A_{1c}), the tubes are manually carried to the appropriate workstation. Tests that require serum or plasma are sent to the centrifuge. The tubes are weighed and selectively loaded into the bucket to balance the centrifuge. The centrifuge should have the capacity to handle the peak load of samples that come into the laboratory, be able to accommodate more than one tube size, and be refrigerated. After centrifugation, the primary tubes are uncapped and placed into racks. Samples with unreadable bar codes are placed in an exception rack for manual intervention. If no further processing is required, samples are brought to the appropriate workstations. If an aliquot is needed the tube is sent to the aliquot workstation, where the host computer is queried

for test and sample volume requirements. The aliquoting station should have the capability of producing at least five aliquot tubes and generating the appropriate bar code labels for each tube. Disposable pipette tips should be used to eliminate **carryover** and the system should have clot detection and liquid level sensing capabilities. Samples found to have clots and inadequate sample volumes are sorted in a separate rack for manual handling. The samples are then recapped and brought to the appropriate workstation. The rate-limiting step in front-end sample **throughput** is usually the capacity of the centrifuge or aliquoting system. These modular systems provide some flexibility and may have the capability of adding another centrifuge. Some modular systems can also store and retrieve specimens.

Stand-alone systems can be used to automate part of the front-end sample processing and to archive specimens.[13] Stand-alone systems automate the sample sorting, sample uncapping, and aliquot functions of the front-end sample processing. A centrifuge is not included in the stand-alone systems, and for tests that require serum or plasma, the sample must be manually brought to the centrifuge. Table 16-1 compares the operational parameters for some of the front-end specimen processing and archiving systems.

Archiving. Archiving and retrieval of specimens is a labor-intensive process. Sample retrieval occurs when a test needs to be repeated, for reflex testing, or when the physician requests that additional tests be performed. Specimen retrieval is a very time-consuming and frustrating process, because the technologist has to manually sort through a large number of specimen racks to find the required specimen. With automated sample archiving systems, bar-coded specimens are scanned and placed in numbered positions in numbered racks. Retrieval of specimens is initiated by entering the patient's sample accession number or medical record number in the archival system database, which then displays the rack number and identifies the row and column where the specimen was placed in the rack. With this system, technologists can retrieve specimens in minutes. In addition, some archiving systems provide for refrigerated storage of samples and for automatic disposal of samples at predetermined times established by the laboratory. The ability of laboratory personnel to quickly retrieve primary and aliquot tubes automates a tedious function and reduces the time and stress associated with locating specimens within the laboratory.

Stand-alone systems have a relatively small footprint (i.e., floor or counter space) and provide maximum flexibility in placing the units in the laboratory. They are less costly and easier to set up than the modular front-end processing systems.

Studies have shown that automating front-end specimen processing decreased sample processing time by 2 to 6 hours, reduced labor cost by 30% to 40%, decreased daily phone calls from physicians waiting for stat results from 28 to less than 5 per day, reduced specimen pour-off and labeling errors by almost 98%, and reduced specimen sorting and routing errors by almost 95%.[4,10,14-15] Using stand-alone archiving systems, the time needed for specimen retrieval decreased by 67%; a potential saving of 0.4 to 0.6 FTEs.[16,17]

TABLE 16-1   AUTOMATED FEATURES OF SOME SPECIMEN PROCESSING AND ARCHIVING SYSTEMS

Automated Features	MODULAR SYSTEMS				STAND-ALONE SYSTEMS			
	Tecan Fe 500	Dade-Behring StreamLab	Beckman Power Processor	Lab-Interlink	Roche	Roche PSD 1 (Sorter, Archiver)	VA 11 (Aliquoter)	Olympus OLA 1500 (Sorter, Archiver)
Sorting*	500	300	500	400	500	900	340	1500
Centrifuge*	300	300	300	500	250	NA	NA	NA
Decapping	500	300	600	250	400	900	NA	1500
Aliquoting*	200	480	500	75	500	NA	340	NA
Recapping*	NA	NA	500	750	500	NA	NA	NA
Specimen storage/retrieval†	NA	300	300	300	NA	1200	340	1500

*Specimens processed per hour.
†Specimen capacity.
NA, Not available.

AUTOMATION OF CHEMICAL ANALYSIS

To understand how patient samples are processed by automated procedures, the process of analysis must be divided into a series of stages or steps as might be performed in a manual assay. Commonly the following steps are performed during the course of an analysis: (1) **mixing** an aliquot of the sample with a series of reagents in an ordered sequence with defined amounts, (2) incubating the reaction mixture at a specified temperature for a specified amount of time, (3) monitoring or sensing the result of the reaction, (4) quantitating the extent of the reaction, and (5) providing an appropriate **readout** of the permanent record. The automation of each one of these steps is now discussed in some detail.

Reagent Preparation

Although **bulk reagents** can be manually prepared, almost all laboratories use ready-to-use liquid reagents or lyophilates. Reconstitution of the lyophilized reagent may be automatically performed on board the instrument; however, a few instruments may require mixing of reagent with diluent before placing the reagent on the instrument. This simple step can lead to analytical errors because of improper processing. **Unit test reagent** preparation, in which sufficient reagent is present for the performance of a single test, has been automated in two ways. The first is the dry-film or impregnated-paper technique. The dry-chemical techniques use either paper or a series of thin films impregnated with the desired reagent. The analytical reactions take place when the sample is placed on the dry reagent. In this type of reagent, preparation consists in wetting the reagent with water, buffer, or sample. The second kind of unit test reagent is a container or test tube containing premeasured liquids or powders to which water, buffer, or sample is added. Unit test reagents tend to be more consistent on a long-term, within-lot basis. However, unit test reagents also tend to be more expensive than bulk reagents, a consideration that can be important for many laboratories.

Proportioning of Samples and Reagents

Most chemical reactions require the combining of reagent and sample in exact amounts to yield specific final concentrations of analyte and reagents. Because the reagents, as just described, are prepared in predetermined amounts, the ratio, or proportion, of reagent to sample must be kept constant to achieve reproducible and accurate final reagent concentrations. Thus the addition of sample to reagent is termed **proportioning**. The case of unit test reagents is considered first. In these systems the reagents are already proportioned in the required amounts; therefore only the sample must be proportioned. The dry-film reagent may have the sample added volumetrically or by saturation addition. The latter technique requires some explanation. The film is exposed to an excess of the sample, and the pores of the film allow only a fixed amount of the sample to be absorbed. This fixed amount of sample required to wet the film represents the proportioning mechanism. In some cases of saturation addition, the rate of diffusion of the sample into the film may also affect the proportioning step. In the case of bulk reagents, proportioning is always accomplished by volumetric addition.

There are three automated volumetric dispensing methods in common use. Syringes or volumetric overflow devices are used in random access test analyzers in which sample and reagents are volumetrically added to a test tube or container. The second mechanism is the **continuous-flow** technique, in which sample and reagents are proportioned by their relative flow rates. Typically, peristaltic pumps are used to move the reagents through tubing, and the cross-sectional area (diameter) of the pump tubing controls the flow rate. Usually the sample and reagent streams are allowed to flow continuously through the tubing where mixing and incubation are also accomplished. The third type uses electrical valves to control the time reagents can flow. The flow rate is controlled by the air pressure applied to the reagent container and the flow resistance in the tubing that is connected to the reaction vessel. In almost all systems the sample is introduced into the analyzer with a thin, stainless steel probe. This probe passes into a sample either by direct penetration of a stopper or after the stopper is removed from the specimen tube, aspirates a defined quantity of sample, and moves from the sample to dispense the aliquot into an appropriate vessel. A potential problem with these probes is the risk of clots; this risk is directly related to sample size. As the amount of sample pipetted decreases, the diameter of the probe decreases and the risk of clots increases. Some sample probes are designed to detect clots specifically and to reject clotted samples. Many sample probes have an associated level-sensing device that permits the tip of the probe to go a specified distance below the level of the sample to detect short samples. Because the same probe is used repeatedly for sequential samples, there is the potential for contamination of a specimen by a preceding one. This is called *sample carryover*. Various techniques have been used to minimize the interaction between samples. These include (1) aspiration of a wash liquid (such as saline solution or water) between sample aspirations, and (2) a back flush of the probe. In the latter technique, the wash liquid flows through the probe in a direction opposite to that of the aspiration, into a waste container. This procedure has the advantage of minimizing the risk of pulling a small clot further into the system.

The degree of sample carryover can be determined by assaying four identical high-level samples immediately followed by four identical low-level samples. Carryover is calculated by use of the following equation:

$$\text{Percent carryover} = \frac{L1 - (L3 + L4)/2 \times 100}{\dfrac{(H3 + H2)}{2} - \dfrac{(L3 + L4)}{2}}$$

in which *L1*, *L2*, *L3*, and *L4* are the consecutive low samples and *H1*, *H2*, *H3*, and *H4* are the consecutive high samples.

Carryover affects the test results by contaminating the current sample with a proportional part of the previous sample. The amount of contamination attributable to carryover that is permitted affects the instrument's throughput. If less carryover is permitted, a longer time must be allowed for the previous sample to be flushed out, reducing the number of samples that are processed per hour.

Mixing

Those instruments using the dry-film technique mix sample and reagents by the diffusion of sample into the reagents. Most dry-film reagents are premixed during manufacturing, though some are mixed by diffusion, which becomes possible only when the film is wet. The **random access instruments** can mix the reagent and sample by (1) motion of a test tube or container, (2) stirring by paddle or stick, (3) agitation by air bubbles or ultrasonic waves, or (4) convection resulting from forceful addition of sample into the container.

Incubation

Automated incubation is merely a delay station where the test mixture is allowed to react. This is performed, in most cases,

under conditions of a specified, constant temperature, which is most frequently achieved by the use of heating blocks or air or water baths. These constant temperature devices are monitored electronically by thermocouples. Random access analyzers accomplish incubation by allowing the reaction mixture to dwell in a chamber (test tube or cuvette) for a specified time. A similar approach is used for the dry-film analyzers. It should be noted that many test methods require an addition of a second reagent, possibly followed by an additional **incubation time**. The automated means for doing this are similar to those just discussed.

Sensing

The techniques of automation do not depend on the method of sensing, whether optical, thermal, or electrical. There are two major approaches to automated sensing: in situ and external. The term *in situ* refers to measurement in the vessel where the reaction has taken place, for example, in the reaction cuvette. The term *external* is applied to systems of measurement in which the sample is transferred from its original incubation position in the reaction vessel to the sensing device. The dry-film tests are measured in situ by reflectance photometry (see Chapter 4) or by means of integral electrodes (electrometric, see Chapter 15). Random access instruments use both in situ and external sensing mechanisms. External sensing generally exposes the sensing chamber to many samples, and so care must be taken to eliminate carryover from one sample to the next. Optical or electrode surfaces may also be contaminated by components from the samples. On the other hand, in situ sensing makes special demands on the test chamber or requires an elaborate, automated washing procedure. If the test container is disposable, it is impractical to calibrate it for optical or electrical characteristics. Such containers, therefore, must be manufactured with very good reproducibility. However, disposable containers are meant to eliminate the mechanical complexity required to wash and recertify the sensing chamber. Most sensing is done in situ because this approach decreases the mechanical complexity of the instrument. Chemical reactions can be monitored either at one time point or at many. Commonly, single-point monitoring is used for end-point analyses in which the reaction has gone to completion. Multiple-point monitoring is used for kinetic analyses. Random access analyzers are easily adapted for multiple time-point monitoring.

Spectrophotometric instruments often have the capability of automatically sensing the presence of common interferents, such as icterus, hemolysis, and lipemia. A rough "index" of the presence of these interferents is printed with test results. This helps to automate the technologist's review of results and to alert the technologist that a result may not be accurate.

Computation

Automated **computation** has taken two forms: **analog** and **digital**. Analog computations use the electrical signal such as a voltage or current from a **sensor** (such as a phototube) and quantify the signal by comparing it to a reference signal. For example, a "blank" reaction mixture will give a 100% T (blank transmittance), resulting in a certain electronic signal. A test standard will give a lower percentage of T and thus a decreased electronic signal. The analog computer compares the two signals and takes the logarithm of the result. The final result is related to the quantitation of the reaction.

Some reaction signals by their very nature are in the form of **discrete** numbers. Two examples are individual photon-counting events and counting of radioactive decay. These signals, consisting of a number of individual events, can be monitored by a digital computer that can process the signal. Digital processing is restricted to certain arithmetical functions (such as subtraction or addition) unless the computer is programmable.

For a digital computer to process signals from many types of sensing devices in automated instruments (such as the spectrophotometer and ion-selective electrodes), an analog-to-digital converter is necessary. This converts the voltage or current signal into a digital form, which can be processed by the digital computer.

There are no straightforward rules as to which is the best form of computation. The decision is usually based on economics. However, if any part of the signal processing is done digitally, virtually all the processing is done digitally. Perhaps the major exception is the analog conversion of transmittance to absorbance, which is performed to improve analytical performance.

Readouts and Result Reporting

The simplest method that can be used to visualize an instrument readout is the use of light-emitting diodes (LED) or a television monitor (cathode-ray tube) to report the data in a numerical form. These devices allow the technologist to review the data before accepting the results. The instrument readout is usually converted to a hard copy, such as a paper printout. The data must then be transferred to laboratory slips or other permanent records. If this step is performed manually, transcription errors may occur. More sophisticated automated computer systems are usually used to collate all the test results for each patient and print the results directly on the report form. When the results are transferred into a laboratory computer, the instrument readout can be directly interfaced, or connected, to the computer. Although analog connections are possible, most connections are digital. Chapter 18 discusses the use of computer interfaces for the automation of the process of reporting results.

However, in laboratories with very large workloads it is not practical for technologists to carefully review data for each patient. LIS have the capability for data *autoverification*, which is defined as the process in which the computer performs the initial review and verification of test results. Data that fall within a set of parameters or rules established by the laboratory are automatically verified in the LIS and the patient's files. The technologist must review all the data that fall outside of the set of parameters or rules established by the laboratory. Criteria for automatic data verification can include results falling within a specified range (typically, the reference range), the absence of common interferences, and delta checks. This process speeds up the result-verification process for routine results and permits

the technologist to perform a more careful review of results with potential problems.

There is usually a delay between the time when a result is entered into the LIS and becomes available to a physician and the time when a physician actually sees the result. This delay occurs because a physician never knows exactly when a result will be available and must either waste time looking for a result that is not yet in the LIS or delay looking for that result. This delay is often a very large component of the overall turnaround time for a sample result. There are available improved hospital paging systems that permit the laboratory, using the LIS, to send a result directly to a physician's pager. As soon as a technologist verifies the result in the LIS, the result is transmitted to the pager. Patient identification and the test result, as well as small amounts of text, can be displayed on the pager's screen. Automated data transfer directly to physicians decreases turnaround time, which is especially important for critical values.

Troubleshooting and Training

Medical technologists intervene to correct problems encountered when an instrument fails (see p. 394). A technologist's training and the availability of in-laboratory resources such as instrument manuals limit this process, called *troubleshooting*. These resources have been greatly expanded by the application of electronic technology, such as on-line modems and CD-ROMs.

Modems allow electronic information to be rapidly transferred over normal telephone lines. Sophisticated computers that are part of new laboratory instruments can detect an instrument problem, often before a technologist has become aware of it, and automatically transmit data about that problem to the instrument manufacturer. The manufacturer's technicians can provide the laboratory technologist with detailed instructions for resolving the problem.

On-board CD-ROMs can provide the same service within the laboratory. Multimedia CD-ROMs can contain sophisticated electronic troubleshooting manuals. Once the computer has detected a problem, the computer alerts the technologist and informs the technologist where the information to correct the problem can be found. If additional help is needed, videotapes of how to repair a problem may be available within the CD-ROM database. The electronic troubleshooting guide and its accompanying video guides can also be used to train technologists to use instruments.

CONCEPTS OF AUTOMATION: DEFINITIONS
Test Repertoire

Economic priorities require that instruments perform more than one kind of test. Once an investment has been made in an automated instrument, increasing the number of tests performed on each sample reduces the cost and labor required to produce each result. Following this logic to an extreme would require that an instrument be capable of performing every conceivable kind of test. This has not been possible. However, 6 chemistry tests account for 50% of the workload in the average chemistry laboratory, and 14 tests account for another 40% of the total workload. Thus automated instruments have been designed to perform the most frequently ordered tests. Automation, though usually not essential, is desirable for rarely ordered tests as well.

The automation of tests may also be done on the basis of type of analysis rather than test volume (number of samples); that is, an automated immunoassay instrument will perform immunoassays for many different analytes, regardless of the numbers of specimens per analysis.

The *immediate* **test repertoire** of an instrument can therefore be defined as the number of tests that can be performed by that instrument at any one time. The *total test repertoire* includes the total number of different tests that can possibly be performed on the instrument (i.e., by changing reagents and a few components). Improvements in techniques and changes in economic priorities have led to a new phenomenon called *workstation consolidation*. This phenomenon involves increasing the immediate test repertoire of random access analyzers (see later discussion) and having many high-volume tests on the least number of instruments. The automation of immunoassays on traditional chemistry analyzers has further stimulated this movement.

Random Access

Instruments that are capable of performing multiple tests are random access if the particular tests to be performed on an individual sample can be specified and if no sample and no reagent are consumed by tests that are not requested. For example, the SMAC was not a random access instrument because all tests in the immediate repertoire were performed on each sample, regardless of the exact tests requested. Random access analyzers process different test combinations for individual specimens.

Discrete

Instruments that compartmentalize each sample reaction are discrete analyzers. Typically the sample aliquot and reagent are contained in a single cuvette that is physically separated from all other cuvettes.

Continuous Flow

Instruments that continuously pump reagent through tubing and coils to form a flowing stream and continuously inject (flow injection) samples into that stream are called *continuous flow analyzers*. The proportioning of sample and reagents is accomplished by control of the respective volumetric flow rates. Such instruments are no longer very commonly used.

Batch Analyzer

Instruments that perform the same test simultaneously on all samples presented to it are termed *batch analyzers*. The type of test can vary widely, but usually only a limited number of samples are processed per analysis.

Dwell Time

The **dwell time** is the minimum time required to obtain a result after the initial sampling of the specimen. Some instruments can give results in as little as 15 sec for single tests such as glucose. Commonly, instruments that perform multiple tests on a single sample have longer dwell times, ranging from 60 sec to 15 minutes. Certain test procedures, such as kinetic analyses for enzyme activity or radioimmunoassays, that require long incubations have longer dwell times. Dwell time is extremely important when significant or life-threatening physiological changes can take place rapidly. Thus blood-gas determinations (pH, Pco_2, and Po_2) need instruments with dwell times on the order of seconds. On the other hand, a dwell time of several days for a vitamin assay is clinically acceptable.

Throughput

The throughput is the maximum number of samples or tests that can be processed in an hour. For similar analyzers the total test throughput can be calculated by multiplying the number of samples processed per hour by the number of tests performed on each specimen. For discrete analyzers, the sample throughput obviously depends on the number of different tests requested on each sample. In addition, the time required per test can vary widely (i.e., from less than 30 sec to more than 10 minutes). In general, the more tests ordered per sample, the slower is the sample throughput on a discrete analyzer. Thus it is more difficult to give a simple, accurate value for the sample throughput for a discrete analyzer. The calculation for throughput does take into account the dwell time; that is, the fact that no results are produced until the dwell time has elapsed. The desired throughput of an instrument is usually matched to the number of samples that need to be processed in a given period. For example, a higher throughput (and more costly) instrument may be required to process samples from a clinic so that results can be made available before the patient's return home. In general, an automated analyzer is chosen on the basis of its ability to process the bulk of the routine workload in time for routine clinical decision making.

Stat. Testing

The word *stat.* is an abbreviation of the Latin word *statim* meaning "immediately." Stat. tests account for a large portion (up to 30% to 50% in many laboratories) of the laboratory workload. Stat. tests must be analyzed before the less urgent test samples, resulting in the interruption of the normal workflow of the laboratory. Unfortunately, many stat requests are ordered for reasons other than a medical emergency.

The acceptable within-laboratory turnaround time (TAT, beginning when the sample is received in the laboratory and ending when the result is reported) must be defined for each stat. test, usually after consultation with the appropriate clinical staff. The Clinical Laboratory Improvement Amendments of 1988 (CLIA '88) require that the laboratory's ability to achieve the target TATs be routinely monitored. TATs are usually kept well within 60 minutes for most stat. tests but may be greater for tests that are needed quickly but not immediately (see p. 61). Point-of-care instruments are also available for the performance of stat. tests at the patient's bedside. These devices improve turnaround time in critical areas of the hospital (see Chapter

17). A test result that is needed in less than 10 minutes can be obtained by use of whole blood samples for measurement of blood gases, glucose, urea nitrogen, hematocrit, electrolytes, hemoglobin, and prothrombin time.

Instruments that are to be used for stat. testing need not necessarily have a high throughput but should have a short dwell time. Many stat. instruments are dedicated instruments that analyze no more than a half dozen high-frequency tests simultaneously.

Cost

The resources consumed in producing a patient's test result represent the cost of that test. The total cost consists of a labor cost, a cost associated with the use of the instrument, and a capital cost. The labor cost is the monetary value of the time spent by technologists processing and analyzing the sample and reporting the result. The cost associated with the use of the instrument includes the costs of instrument maintenance, service contracts, reagents (calculated from the cost of the chemicals used for the test and a proportionate part of those required for instrument start-up), calibration and quality control, and consumables (constituting the cost of sample containers and paper). The capital cost includes the proportionate amount of the life of the instrument consumed and hospital overhead including the cost of items such as laboratory slips and maintenance. See p. 57 for a more in-depth discussion of calculating costs.

AUTOMATED CLINICAL CHEMISTRY INSTRUMENTS

This section summarizes the data for a number of instruments that are either used for routine chemistry testing in the hospital laboratory or that illustrate a category of instrument type. The demand for analyzers with a high throughput and a comprehensive test menu has led to the development of systems that can perform both chemistry and immunochemistry testing. Hormones, specific proteins, and the traditional chemistry analytes can now be measured using a single platform, making workstation consolidation a reality in the clinical laboratory. Many chemistry instruments can automatically review the analysis to determine the degree of hemolysis, lipemia, and icterus present and "flag" the results to indicate the possibility of interference with chemical assays. A comparison of operational parameters for some automated instruments is shown in Table 16-2. Obviously this table is not meant to be all-inclusive but rather to demonstrate the features available for common types of instruments.

AUTOMATED IMMUNOCHEMISTRY INSTRUMENTS

During the past several years the number of immunochemistry systems available for use in the clinical laboratory has increased greatly, and the laboratory director is able to select the optimal systems for the laboratory. The immunochemistry system that best fits into a laboratory depends on the number and type of analytes to be measured, and the size and workflow of the laboratory. Requirements for turnaround time, throughput, degree of automation, data management system, and cost must all be considered when choosing an immunochemistry system. Many of the immunochemistry systems employ chemiluminescent assays, which improves analytical sensitivity and extends the dynamic range of the assay. Some immunochemistry systems (Roche, Vitros, Centaur) use disposable tips to pipet each sample, thus eliminating carryover, which can be a problem for tumor markers assays. Immunochemistry systems usually have liquid level sensing, clot detection capabilities, and an extensive test menu, which promotes workstation consolidation. A comparison of some of the operational features for some immunochemistry systems is shown in Table 16-3.

TRENDS IN AUTOMATION

The ideal scenario for the clinical laboratory is the automation of all the steps that are involved in processing and analyzing the specimen and reporting of laboratory results. In this scenario, phlebotomy information (time/place/patient) can be entered into the LIS at the time of blood draw. Order entry is performed at that time by the phlebotomist or at the nurses' station and bar-coded labels, encoded with patient demographics and test-request information, are immediately printed and placed on the tube. After the blood is drawn, the specimens are placed in a pneumatic tube that transfers the specimens to the laboratory or to a central processing area, significantly decreasing the amount of time it takes for specimens to reach the laboratory. The samples' arrival time in the laboratory is automatically recorded by means of the bar-coded labels.

For those areas that require the most rapid turnaround time two options are available. Whole blood can be used as the sample because some analyzers can perform analyses on whole blood, thus obviating the need for sample processing and greatly reducing turnaround time. Alternatively, point-of-care instruments can be used at the bedside (see Chapter 17).

Once the specimen arrives in the laboratory or in the central processing area all the steps that are required for processing and analyzing the sample should be automated. By 2003, small and large hospitals will use some type of automated front-end specimen processing systems in their laboratories. Many hospitals will use the core laboratory concept, in which all automated laboratory analyses, including chemistry (routine, immunochemistry, therapeutic drug monitoring [TDM], drugs of abuse [DAU]), hematology, urinalysis, microbiology, and coagulation, are performed in one workspace. Tests that are time-critical for patient care and are required 24 hours a day (stat testing) will also be performed here. Tests that are manual, not highly automated, or performed infrequently will be run in workspaces that are peripheral to the core laboratory. Closed tube sampling, which eliminates splashing of biological fluids when the tube is uncapped, will be used for tests that require a single workstation for analysis.

Critical to the core laboratory concept is *workstation consolidation*, which is also essential for the efficient operation of any clinical laboratory. The ideal situation is to use instrumentation from one vendor for all testing. At the present time, this is not possible. However, there are chemistry analyzers that have a comprehensive menu that includes

Text continued on p. 302.

TABLE 16-2 COMPARISON OF OPERATIONAL FEATURES FOR SOME CHEMISTRY ANALYZERS

Instrument Name	Aeroset	ADVIA 1650	Synchron Lx20	CX9 Pro	Dimension RXL	Vitros 950	AU 640	Integra
Manufacturer	Abbott	Bayer	Beckman-Coulter	Beckman-Coulter	Dade-Behring	Johnson & Johnson	Olympus	Roche
Type	Random access	Random access, batch	Random access	Random access	Batch, random access	Random access	Random access	Random access, discrete
Principle	Photometric, potentiometric	Potentiometric, photometric	Photometric, potentiometric, turbidimetric	Photometric, potentiometric, turbidimetric	Photometric, potentiometric, EIA, turbidimetric	Reflectance, potentiometric	Photometric, potentiometric	Photometric, potentiometric, fluorescence polarization, turbidimetric
Calibration frequency	8 hr – 28 days	Average 14 days	1-90 days	1-90 days	30-90 days	1-30 days	1-30 days	5 hr – 140 days
Sample volume (µL)*	2-12	2-30	3-40	3-23	2-60	10-11	1-50	2-97
Dead volume (µL)†	50	50	40-175	60-175	20-50	50	70	50-100
Sample ID‡	Bar code	Bar code	Bar code	Bar code	Bar code	Bar code	Bar code	Bar code
Reagent	Liquid	Liquid	Liquid	Liquid	Liquid or reconstitutes on board	Liquid	Liquid	Liquid or reconstitutes on board
Mixing	Probe vibrating	Rotational and reciprocating mixer assemblies	Mixing paddle	Mixing paddle	Probe mixing	Diffusion	Probe mixing	Vibrating
Optical characteristics lamp	Tungsten halogen	Tungsten halogen liquid cooled	Pulse xenon	Pulse xenon	Tungsten halogen	Tungsten halogen	Tungsten halogen	Tungsten halogen

	14 wavelengths 340-660	14 wavelengths 340-884	14 wavelengths 340-910	10 wavelengths 340-700	10 wavelengths 293-700	340-670	13 wavelengths 340-800	10 wavelengths 340-659
Wavelength, nm								
Test menu	General chemistries, specific proteins, limited TDM	General chemistries, specific proteins	General chemistries, TDM, DAU, specific proteins, limited thyroid testing	General chemistries, TDM, DAU, specific proteins, limited thyroid	Hormones, tumor markers, TDM, DAU, cardiac test, specific proteins, general chemistry tests	General chemistries, TDM	General chemistries, TDM, DAU, specific proteins, limited hormones	General chemistries, TDM, DAU
Test repertoire[§]	56	49	41	33	48	48	51	72
Total repertoire[‖]	62	38	72	72	70	48	122	127
Stat. capability	Yes	Yes	Yes	Yes	Yes	Yes	Yes	Yes
Dwell time (min)[¶]	10	10	40 sec-9 min	52 sec-10 min	50 sec-16 min	5	8	10
Throughput (tests/hr)[#]	1200	1650	1440	940	160 immunoassays, 500 tests photometric, 240 electrolytes	900	800	600

DAU, drugs of abuse; TDM, therapeutic drug monitoring.
*Sample volume needed to perform a test or simultaneous profile.
†Dead volume in sample cup.
‡Means of identifying sample for final printout.
§The number of tests available at one time, without a change of reagents or instrument module.
‖Total number of analytes for which reagents are commercially available.
¶Approximate time between sampling and availability of test.
#Calculated by multiplication of maximum number of tests per sample available times number of samples capable of being processed per hour.

TABLE 16-3   COMPARISON OF OPERATIONAL FEATURES FOR SOME IMMUNOCHEMICAL ANALYZERS

	Architect 1 2000	AXSYM	ACS: 180 System	ADVIA Centaur System	Immuno 1 System	IMMAGE	ACCESS	VIDAS	BN-II	IMMULITE 2000	Vitros ECI	ELECSYS 2010
Manufacturer	Abbott	Abbott	Bayer	Bayer	Bayer	Beckman-Coulter	Beckman-Coulter	BioMerieux	Dade-Behring	DPC	Johnson & Johnson	Roche
Type	Random access	Random access	Random access	Random access	Random access	Random access	Random access	Batch	Random access	Random access	Random access	Random access
Principle	Chemiluminescence	FPIA, MEIA	Chemiluminescence	Chemiluminescence	Magnetic particle enzyme immunoassay	Rate nephelometry, rate inhibition nephelometry/ near infrared particle immunoassay	Chemiluminescence	Fluorescence	Rate nephelometry	Enzyme enhanced chemiluminescence	Enhance chemiluminescence	Electro-chemiluminescence
Calibration frequency	30 days	30 days	2-30 days	2-30 days	30-60 days	14-30 days	28 days	14 days	30 days	7-28 days	28 days	30 days
Sample volume (µL)*	150-200	100-250	50	10-200	2.4	3.5-21	5-200	100	30-40	5-100	10-80	10-50
Dead volume (µL)*	50	50-500	50	50	30-75	40-250	100	100	200	50	70	100
Sample ID‡	Bar code	Bar code	Bar code	Bar code	Bar code	Bar code	Bar code	Bar code	Bar code	Bar code	Bar code	Bar code
Reagent	Liquid	Liquid	Liquid	Liquid	Liquid	Liquid	Liquid	Unit dose ready to use	Liquid/ lyophilized	Liquid	Liquid	Liquid

Mixing	Vortex mixing	Automated vibrational forced turbulence	On-board rotation of reagents	On-board rocker with specially designed ready-pack	Mixing of magnetic particles on-board	Mixing paddle	Ultrasonic spin	Kinetic action	Vibration	Mixing in incubator/shaking	Probe mixing	Rotation, stirring
Test menu	Hormones, tumor markers	Hormones, tumor markers, TDM, DAU, limited infectious disease markers, cardiac markers	Hormones, tumor markers, cardiac markers, TDM, anemia profile	Hormones, tumor markers, cardiac anemia profile, allergy profile, limited infectious disease markers	Hormones, tumor markers, cardiac markers, TDM, infectious disease markers, anemia profile	Specific proteins, TDM	Hormone, tumor markers, cardiac markers, anemia profile, some TDM, infectious disease markers	Infectious disease markers, hormones, some TDM, D-dimer	Specific proteins	Hormones, tumor markers, some TDM, cardiac markers, infectious disease markers, anemia profile	Hormones, cardiac markers, hepatitis	Hormones, tumor markers, cardiac markers, anemia profile, hepatitis markers
Test repertoire§	25	20	13	30	22	24	24	30	35	24	20	15
Total repertoire||	12	52	42	46 + approximately 200 allergy	48	40	41	37	50	64	27	37
Stat. capability	Yes	Yes	Yes	Yes	Yes	Yes	Yes	No	Yes	Yes	Yes	Yes
Dwell time (min)¶	28	13	15	18	38	8	15-75	30	6-12	35 and 65	24	10-20
Throughput (tests/hr)#	200	80-120	180	240	120	180	50-100	20	180	200	90	86

Anemia profile (vitamin B_{12}, folate, and ferritin); DAU, drugs of abuse; TDM, therapeutic drug monitoring.

*Sample volume needed to perform a test or simultaneous profile. Varies by test.

†Dead volume in sample cup, that is, the minimum value that must remain in the sample cup for proper sampling.

‡Means of identifying sample for final printout.

§The number of tests available at one time, without a change of reagents or instrument module.

||Total number of analytes for which reagents are commercially available.

¶Approximate time between sampling and availability of test result.

#Calculated by multiplication of the maximum number of tests per sample available times, the number of samples capable of being processed per hour.

TDM, DAU, specific proteins, and some hormones. In the next 2 years, routine immunochemistry analyzers will be able to perform, in addition to analysis of the usual menu of hormones, tumor markers, and cardiac markers, a complete hepatitis panel, antibody screening for HIV, rapid plasma reagin (RPR) test, chlamydia, Torch (*T*oxoplasmosis, *O*ther, *R*ubella, *C*ytomegalovirus, and *H*erpes) panel, Epstein-Barr virus (EBV), and Lyme testing.

Implementing these concepts of automated specimen processing and archiving of specimens, workstation consolidation, and automating as many of the laboratory tests as possible using the least number of instruments, will be the top priority of laboratories if they are to survive and prosper as independent, economically viable institutions.

References

1. Seaberg RS, Stallone RO, Statland BE: The role of total laboratory automation in a consolidated laboratory network, *Clin Chem* 46:751, 2000.
2. Bauer S, Teplitz C: Total laboratory automation: a view of the 21st century, *Med Lab Observ* 27(7):22, 1995.
3. Skjei E: Lab's quest for efficiency culminates in CLAS, *CAP Today* 11(8):30, 1997.
4. Yablonsky Stat T: Laboratory automation-boon or bust? *Lab Med* 31:369, 2000.
5. Skjei E: One lab's plunge into front-end automation, *CAP Today* 11(4):24, 1997.
6. Bissell MG: The impact of total laboratory automation (TLA) on a university medical center clinical laboratory, *Clin Chem* 47:A115, 2001 (abstract).
7. Lamb DA et al: Operational effects of total laboratory automation, *Clin Leadership Manage Rev* 14:173, 2000.
8. Foreback C: Making modular automation pay, *Adv Admin Lab* 9(9):70, 2000.
9. Demiris CH: U. Chicago takes a modular approach to automation, *Clin Lab Products* 29:12, 2000.
10. Demers M, Mowry RR, Goas SG: Pre-analytical automation, an evaluation of the TECAN Genesis FE 500, *Clin Chem* 47:A123, 2001 (abstract).
11. Mooney B: Front-end automation in the mid-sized clinical lab, *Adv Admin Lab* 13(11):18, 2001.
12. Campanelli M, Mitchell DS: ADVIA LabCell provides a modular system to manage the workflow of samples in clinical laboratories, *J Assoc Lab Automation* 3:3, 1998.
13. Orsulak PJ: Stand-alone automated solutions can enhance laboratory operations, *Clin Chem* 46:778, 2000.
14. Pawlick GF, Smith C, Smith C: A task-targeted automation system: a case study, *Clin Lab Manage Rev* 13:351, 1999.
15. Holman JW et al: Evaluation of an automated preanalytical robotic workstation at two academic health centers, *Clin Chem* 48(3):540, 2002.
16. Stauffer J, Pearlman ES, Bilello L: Automating preanalytics: total laboratory automation, preanalytical line, or task targeted? *Am Clin Lab* 19:7, Aug 2000.
17. Zibrat SJ, Berg LA, McLawhon RW: Evaluation and comparison of the Roche PSD1 task-targeted automation system to manual postanalytical methods for specimen archiving and retrievals, *Clin Chem* 47:A122, 2001 (abstract).

Bibliography

Boyd JC, Felder RA, Savory J: Robotics and the changing face of the clinical laboratory, *Clin Chem* 42:1901, 1996.

NCCLS: *Laboratory automation: systems operational requirements, characteristics, and information elements, approved standard*, AUTO4-A, 21:4, Wayne, PA, 2001, NCCLS.

Internet Sites

http://labautomation.org/—Association for Laboratory Automation (ALA)
http://marc.med.virginia.edu/library.html—Medical Automation Research Center

http://medizin.li/_mt_index/_ja/ja_000035382.html—Japanese Association for Clinical Laboratory Automation (JACLA)

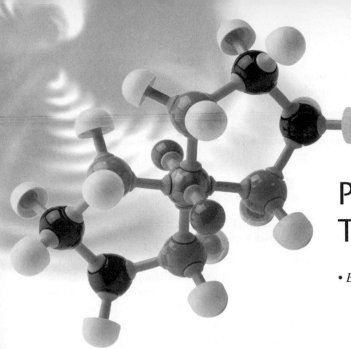

CHAPTER 17

Point-of-Care (Near-Patient) Testing

• *Ellis Jacobs*

Chapter Outline

Objectives

- Describe what is meant by near-patient testing.
- Describe the perceived medical management benefits of point-of-care testing, distinguishing between true and perceived management benefits.
- Be able to list the regulations and describe the interdepartmental coordination required for point-of-care testing.
- List the tests most frequently measured by point-of-care testing.

- Describe some of the technology used in point-of-care testing devices, including reagents and instruments.
- Describe the philosophical differences in approach to quality control between point-of-care testing and the testing performed in a central laboratory.

Key Terms

alternative site testing Laboratory testing performed under hospital jurisdiction but outside the central laboratory environment.

diagnostic test An examination of materials derived from the human body for the purpose of providing information for the diagnosis, prevention, or treatment of a disease or impairment or for the assessment of the health of human beings.

ex vivo test A diagnostic test performed on a specimen that is temporarily removed from a living organism for analysis and then returned to the organism.

in vivo test A diagnostic test in which the analyte is measured in fluids that are still within the body.

point-of-care testing (POCT) Diagnostic testing performed near or at the site of patient care. If performed within a hospital, it may also be called *alternate site testing*.

total quality management (TQM)   A management philosophy that encompasses an expansion of continuous quality management. TQM emphasizes team or institutional performance rather than individual or departmental performance.

Point-of-care testing (POCT) can be defined most simply as laboratory procedures performed near the patient. Based on advances in science and technology that have provided significant improvements in the accuracy and precision of testing procedures, near-patient testing is being used increasingly, with the same, if not improved, reliability as laboratory-based analysis.

This style of testing is referred to by numerous names (Box 17-1). The College of American Pathologists (CAP) changed the title of its inspection checklist (Section 30) from *Ancillary Testing* to *Point-of-Care Testing*. The Joint Commission on Accreditation of Healthcare Organizations (JCAHO) replaced the term *decentralized testing* with *waived tests* in their accreditation requirements to describe **diagnostic testing** that is not performed within a "traditional" laboratory setting. Regardless of the name, point-of-care testing is a form of diagnostic testing that is predominately performed by nonlaboratorians. Currently, because **in vivo** and externally attached patient-dedicated monitoring devices (such as intraarterial blood-gas catheters and pulse oximeters, respectively), do not involve a specimen being withdrawn from the body, use of these devices is not subject to federal, CAP, or JCAHO regulations even though they are forms of diagnostic testing.

Despite the fact that the technical capability exists for performing highly reliable analysis at the patient's bedside, it is not always prudent to do so. Before the decision is made to proceed with POCT, the true costs and benefits of this modality of testing must be carefully analyzed. Is there a significant improvement in patient care and/or outcome? What is the *total* financial impact, not simply the cost of equipment and supplies, of the various options for the provision of expedient diagnostic services? Additional considerations have to be made regarding integration of the data into the medical record and the proper control and supervision as mandated by professional standards and regulatory agencies.

USE OF NEAR-PATIENT TESTING
Driving Forces and Potential Benefits

Driving forces behind the use of POCT differ distinctly depending on the setting. In the ambulatory care setting, the predominant motivators for POCT are timeliness of results during the visit and convenience for the patient and physician. However, in most inpatient settings, the desire for POCT is based on other factors. These factors exist primarily in the critical care areas, including intensive care units (ICU), operating rooms (OR), and emergency departments (ED), which have expectations for the faster delivery of results that will affect immediate medical management. In addition, certain POC tests, such as fecal occult blood or urine dipsticks, can be used conveniently and easily in the nursing units. Bedside glucose testing programs have been established in most hospitals primarily to accommodate intensive insulin therapy for patients who have diabetes and the concomitant requirement for preprandial glucose determinations four times a day.

HMO-based customer-oriented economic forces are driving the health care industry; these concerns are refocusing thoughts on how laboratory services should be delivered. Anything that improves patient medical management and reduces the length of stay (LOS) of a patient in either an ICU or the general hospital is desirable. If faster laboratory services, provided by POCT, can improve patient management and reduce LOS, use of this testing will continue to increase. In certain settings, the rise of POCT is due to the perceived "failure" of the traditional, central laboratory to meet some of the current clinical needs. With proper modernization of facilities and services, the central laboratory may be able to compete with bedside testing on both a cost and a turnaround time basis.

In the hospital setting, POCT provides potential benefits for all parties involved (Table 17-1). Most of the benefits for physicians, nurses, patients, and administrative staff are based on the concept that "faster is better"; thus there is an anticipated improvement in medical care, which should translate into decreased use of hospital resources, such as supplies, rooms, and personnel. Other advantages resulting from POCT use include the patient's sense of involvement in his or her own medical care, as well as the benefit of minimal sample size (less blood withdrawn or the ability to use fingerstick samples); the use of small specimen volume with some of the bedside systems minimizes iatrogenic blood loss. For the laboratory, benefits of POCT are based on improvements in the pre- and postanalytical phases of the test cycle. Improvements in the preanalytical phase include the reduction of problems with

---

BOX 17-1

NAMES FOR POINT-OF-CARE TESTING

Alternate site testing
Ancillary testing
Bedside testing
Decentralized testing
Distributed testing
Near-patient testing
Patient-focused testing
Value-added testing
Waived testing

TABLE 17-1 POTENTIAL BENEFITS OF POINT-OF-CARE TESTING	
To physicians:	Improved turnaround time for lab results
	Better and more immediate patient care
To patients:	Patient-focused system
	Less traumatic (for fingerstick systems)
	Improved convenience
	Less blood withdrawn
To laboratory:	Decreased preanalytical errors
	Improved visibility
	Decreased manpower needs
	Collaboration with clinicians
	Direct patient involvement
	Team management system
To administration:	Shorter intensive care unit (ICU) stays
	Decreased overall length of stays
	Financial savings
	TQM (CQI) program

TABLE 17-2 CRITICAL CARE PROFILES

Physiological Function	Diagnostic Measures
Energy	Glucose, hemoglobin, hematocrit, pO_2, O_2 saturation
Conduction	K^+, Na^+, Mg^{++}, Ca^{++}
Contraction	Mg^{++}, Ca^{++}
Perfusion	Lactate
Acid-base	pH, pCO_2, TCO_2, HCO_3^-
Osmolality	Calculated as 1.86 ([Na]+[K]) + gluc/18
Hemostasis	PT, PTT, platelets, hematocrit, ACT, platelet function
Homeostasis	Phosphorus, chloride, creatinine, BUN, WBC
Cardiac ischemia	Myoglobin, CK-MB, troponin T or I

sample identification (ID), lost specimens, and changes in concentration due to time delay between sampling and testing. With a decrease in both the amount of specimen handling and time-dependent specimen degradation, POCT should considerably reduce preanalytical variance.

Immediate Medical Management Benefits

The most significant potential benefit of POCT in the hospital setting is more rapid and, ideally, more effective assessment and management of critically ill patients. Based on these criteria, although more than 40 different analytes have been evaluated as potential POC tests, only blood-gases, electrolytes (Na^+, K^+, Ca^{++}, Mg^{++}), prothrombin time (PT), partial thromboplastin time (PTT) or activated clotting time (ACT), hematocrit or hemoglobin, and glucose should be considered for analysis at the point of care. Cardiac surgery has demonstrated unique POCT benefits because of requirements for close heparin management and assessment of coagulation status, such as heparin titration, platelet counts, and platelet function assays. Cardiac markers may be performed as POCT in the emergency department or in the chest pain evaluation unit as a means to provide the recommended total (vein-to-brain) turnaround time of 1 hour or less, although their clinical efficacy has yet to be proven by suitable studies.

Other tests may be performed at the point of care for reasons of convenience or as components of critical care diagnostic profiles (Table 17-2). These profiles are groups of physiological indicators or diagnostic pivots for various vital functions. It has been suggested, but again, not proven, that use of these diagnostic clusters will improve patient care.

The notion that POCT improves patient morbidity and mortality in the critical care setting, by allowing faster response to the patient's medical needs and thus increased diagnostic and therapeutic efficiency, has been validated in the peer-reviewed literature for only a few tests. Intraoperative monitoring of potassium during cardiac surgery is associated with a 50% reduction in arrhythmias and a decreased use of antiarrhythmic pharmacological agents. Use of activated clotting time (ACT) is essential for monitoring high-dose heparin anticoagulation during cardiopulmonary bypass, vascular surgery, and angiographic/catheterization procedures. Studies have demonstrated that POC testing for coagulation studies (platelets, PT, APT, platelet function), along with the use of a treatment algorithm, decreases microvascular bleeding during surgery and reduces the consumption of blood products. POC PT and APT testing improves the management of anticoagulation therapy following thrombolytic therapy. For many other tests, there has been no demonstrable clinical benefit for POC testing.

Contraindications

The negative aspects of POCT will be covered more thoroughly in later sections of this chapter. The major drawback is cost. POCT analyzers tend to have higher disposable and reagent costs than traditional lab systems; thus POCT systems are more expensive to operate. Other areas of concern include the following: (1) maintenance of quality control and quality assurance, (2) control of diagnostic testing, and (3) proper integration of data into the patient's medical record. Despite a projected reduction in preanalytical variance due to decreased specimen handling and time delay between sampling and analysis, other preanalytical causes of variance arise in POCT. When microliter samples are obtained by fingerstick, if the site is not properly prepared, significant specimen contamination by alcohol or other disinfectant can occur. Furthermore, the physiological status of the patient has a more significant influence on the results obtained with fingerstick and noninvasive testing than it does on the analysis of arterial or venous specimens. For example, for patients with poor peripheral circulation because of shock or hypovolemia, fingerstick samples are difficult to obtain and are often contaminated with interstitial fluids. Additionally, results of POCT may not correlate with results from the central laboratory because of physiological differences between specimen source (arterial, venous, capillary, or forearm) and/or type (whole blood, plasma, serum).

The rapid availability of results with POCT creates a quality assurance dilemma. Data can be seen and acted upon before any quality control checks or other external mechanisms of ensuring test result reliability can be applied to the systems. Therefore it is critical that these POCT devices have built-in quality control/quality assurance (QC/QA) systems (see Chapter 21). These automatic functions keep improperly validated instruments from being used and prevent erroneous data being given to the health care provider.

IMPLEMENTATION AND MONITORING OF POCT
Regulations

Despite its relative simplicity, the implementation and use and point-of-care testing is subject to the various regulations associated with clinical laboratory testing. The Clinical Laboratory Improvement Amendment of 1988 (CLIA '88) subjects virtually all clinical laboratory testing to federal regulation and inspection. CLIA '88 is considered "site neutral," meaning that all laboratory testing must meet the same quality standards regardless of where it is performed. State and city governments may enact regulations which are more, but not less, stringent than federal regulations. Furthermore, these government agencies may apply for "deemed" status, by which their laboratory inspections and accreditation are accepted by the federal government. Similarly, nonprofit accrediting organizations, such as the Joint Commission for Accreditation of Healthcare Organizations (JCAHO) and College of American Pathologists (CAP), may apply for deemed status. (JCAHO and CAP have applied for, and were granted, such status.)

Test procedures are grouped into one of four categories: waived test, provider-performed microscopy test, moderate-complexity test, or high-complexity test (see Chapter 2). Test complexity is determined by seven criteria that assess knowledge, training, reagent and material preparation, operational technique, quality assurance/quality control characteristics, maintenance and troubleshooting, and interpretation and judgment. Originally there were only nine waived tests, but many more tests and devices have been added to the waived category (Box 17-2). Any analytical system approved by the Food and Drug Administration to be sold as an over-the-counter test, that is, in a store or pharmacy without the need for a prescription, is automatically placed into the waived category. Federal regulations and inspections of laboratories that perform only waived tests are minimal. However, if these tests are performed in a JCAHO and/or CAP accredited institution, they are regulated in essentially the same manner as laboratory-based testing. Also, nine provider-performed microscopy tests (Box 17-3) have been waived from accreditation requirements. Point-of-care tests fall within either the waived or moderate-complexity category, with one exception: gram stains are sometimes performed as a POC test and are classified as high-complexity testing.

Laboratories performing moderate-complexity POC tests may also perform waived tests and must fulfill all the require-

ments for personnel credentials, proficiency testing, QC, patient test management, quality assurance and inspections. Personnel standards for the performance of waived tests are minimal. However in several states, for example, California and Florida, medical technologist training and/or licensure is required, even for performance of tests in the waived category. When personnel requirements for diagnostic testing are reviewed, regardless of testing category and location, the following criteria must be satisfied:

- Those responsible for testing, direction, and supervision are identified.
- Adequate specific training and orientation of individuals to perform the test is provided.
- Testing personnel receive regular in-service training.
- Competency to perform test is checked at least annually.

A laboratory's ability to meet these requirements should be documented. As part of patient test management, written policies and procedures must be established to encompass every aspect of POCT (see box below).

State regulations in several states, including New York, New Jersey, and Pennsylvania, dictate that the central laboratory must supervise POC testing and that the laboratory director is responsible for the standards of performance in all areas, including QC, QA, and cost-effective test utilization.

Each laboratory or testing site performing waived tests must establish written policies regarding QA. An ongoing system must be in place to monitor and evaluate QC and proficiency testing data. Quality control specimens at two or three different analyte concentrations must be analyzed on a daily basis. Records of actions taken to correct out-of-range QC results must be maintained. Linearity studies, assessing the analytical range of the system, are performed before devices are initially put in use, and then every 6 months after. Split sample correlation studies with other testing systems are performed before each POCT device is initially placed into use, and then every 6 months after. Some states may require a more frequent interval. Federal standards require triannual proficiency testing only for the primary method of patient testing; however, this may be required on all testing systems by state and CAP regulations.

An integral component of both patient test management and a laboratory QA system is proper record keeping. The following information must be recorded in various logs and records:

POLICIES AND PROCEDURES NEEDED FOR POCT

Procedure for patient preparation
Procedure for specimen collection and preservation
Instructions for instrument calibration
Policies for quality control and remedial actions
Equipment performance evaluations
Procedures for test performance, result reporting, and recording

BOX 17-2

CLIA '88 WAIVED TESTS*

General Chemistry
Alanine aminotransferase
Cholesterol, total
HDL cholesterol
Creatinine
Fecal occult blood*
Fructosamine
Gastric occult blood
Glucose
Blood glucose (FDA approved for home use)*
Hemoglobin A_{1c}
Ketones
Lactate
Microalbumin
pH—body fluids—nitrazine paper
Triglycerides
Vaginal alkali volatile amines
Vaginal pH

Endocrinology
Collagen type 1 crosslink, N-teleopeptides
Estrone-3 glucuronide
Follicle-stimulating hormone
Urine pregnancy tests (hCG) (visual comparison of color)*
Urine pregnancy tests (hCG) (instrument-read)
Ovulation tests (LH) (visual comparison of color)*

Toxicology
Alcohol, saliva
Amphetamine
Cannabinoids
Cocaine metabolites
Ethanol
Methamphetamine
Methamphetamine/amphetamine
Nicotine and/or metabolites
Opiates
Phencyclidine

Urinalysis
Dipstick or tablet reagent urinalysis for bilirubin, glucose, hemoglobin, ketones, leukocytes, nitrites, pH, protein, specific gravity, and urobilinogen (nonautomated)*
Dipstick or tablet reagent urinalysis for bilirubin, glucose, hemoglobin, ketones, leukocytes, nitrites, pH, protein, specific gravity, and urobilinogen (automated)

Hematology
Erythrocyte sedimentation rate*
Hematocrit
Hematocrit, spun*
Hemoglobin
Hemoglobin (copper sulfate)*
Automated hemoglobin using single-analyte instruments with a self-contained specimen-reagent interaction and direct measurement and readout*
Prothrombin time
Semen

General Immunology
Bladder–tumor-associated antigen
Helicobacter pylori antibodies
Infectious mononucleosis antibodies
Lyme disease (*Borrelia burgdorferi*) antibodies
Rapid Strep A antigen

Bacteriology
Catalase, urine
Helicobacter pylori
Streptococcus, group A (direct from throat swab)

Virology
Influenza A/B

This list based on data as of December 2, 2001.
*Nine originally waived tests.

- Time and date of patient and QC testing
- Patient results and operator ID
- Records for quality control and patient testing
- Maintenance
- Actions taken to correct out-of-range QC results
- Initial training and recertification of personnel

Training

Point of care testing may or may not be performed by laboratory personnel. Nurses, physicians, respiratory therapists, operating room technologists, physician assistants, and medical office assistants are among those who may be involved in the performance of POCT. Qualifications for performing bedside

testing are defined by state/local and federal requirements, as well as by the laboratory director. The minimum educational and experience requirement for personnel performing POCT ranges from a high school degree with no experience to a BS with 2 years of experience. In specific cases other health care professionals may qualify by state-defined scopes of practice to perform select testing; for example, a respiratory therapist performing blood-gas analysis. In addition, all POCT personnel must have well-documented training and yearly recertification.

The degree of training depends on the background of the individuals involved, as well as the type of analytical system being used, that is, the amount of technique complexity of

BOX 17-3

CLIA '88 PROVIDER-PERFORMED MICROSCOPY

Wet-mount preparations of vaginal, cervical, or skin specimens
Semen analysis, limited to presence or absence of sperm and motility
Urine sediment examination
Potassium hydroxide preparations
Fern testing
Postcoital direct, qualitative examinations of specimens from vagina or cervix
Pinworm preps
Nasal smears for eosinophils
Fecal leukocyte examination

BOX 17-4

POC TRAINING PROGRAM AGENDA

Theory of instrument/device
Specimen collection/preservation
Instrument maintenance
Quality control procedures
Testing procedure
Sources and degree of preanalytical errors
Clinical significance

BOX 17-5

POC TESTING AS A TOTAL QUALITY MANAGEMENT PROJECT

Multidisciplinary team approach
Focus on entire system, rather than individual performance
Ongoing evaluation and refinement (CQI)
Improvement in delivery of critical care laboratory services
Cost savings

the testing system. The seven main subjects that should be included in the training program are listed in Box 17-4. In addition to teaching the specific steps for performing the test, trainers must address QC and QA issues. The greatest source of error in POCT is preanalytical error. Poor correlations or erroneous results most often derive from a poor specimen; factors that may result in a poor specimen include collection problems (interstitial fluid contamination, skin surface contamination), circulating interference (drugs, uremia, lipemia, icterus, hematocrit), specimen source (arterial, venous, fingerstick, arm, leg), and the patient's physiological status (hyper- and/or hypovolemia, poor peripheral circulation). Since sample collection is the most significant source of problems in

any POCT program, it is essential that these factors be thoroughly addressed in the training program. The training program should include pre- and postcourse written tests, as well as demonstration of acceptable performance of specimen collection and analysis. Required annual recertification of all testing personnel should include a written test and demonstration of test performance. A mechanism must be in place by which authorization for POC test performance is withdrawn from either an individual or a testing site in the case of poor technical performance or failure to follow policy. Authorization should be reinstituted only after retraining and demonstration of competency.

Coordination of Central and POC Testing

The decentralization of testing away from traditional laboratories increases the direct involvement between the laboratory and other members of the patient's health care team. One of the goals of POCT is to provide a testing system that will improve the delivery of critical laboratory results. However, to achieve this goal, the health care provider needs to view POCT as part of a larger system for cost-effective improvement of medical care, requiring the implementation of POCT as a **total quality management (TQM)** project (Box 17-5). The quality improvement issues surrounding POCT are complex; this is compounded by the fact that POCT implementation crosses many boundaries within a hospital, requiring an interdepartmental approach to the establishment, compliance review, and future direction-setting of the program(s).

Interdisciplinary committee. An interdisciplinary POCT committee must be established with representation from all participating areas, including medicine, nursing, laboratory, respiratory therapy, infection control, materials management, information systems, and administration. Laboratory leadership is the key to a successful committee; laboratorians can contribute their technical expertise, scientific perspective, and familiarity with the demands of laboratory regulatory compliance issues. In addition, the clinical laboratory staff can help assess new technology, design training programs, and help in identifying potential pitfalls in the use of new systems. Working in partnership with other health care providers, who bring their own understanding of end-user needs and priorities, the committee can forge a dynamic relationship that enhances the clinical effectiveness of POCT. The function of the committee (Table 17-3) is to determine institutional policies, define levels of service provided, evaluate and select equipment, and to assign work assignments that will help meet the various regulatory requirements. The committee reviews all requests for additional POC programs and, if approved, defines the program operationally (i.e., specifies the analytical system to be used, who will operate it, etc.) Five questions should be addressed in the request for POCT: (1) What is the medical and/or financial justification for the testing? (2) What is the anticipated frequency and volume of testing? (3) Why are current laboratory services insufficient? (4) Who, and how many individuals, will perform the testing? and (5) Who will be the key person at the testing site for ensuring QC/QA requirements?

TABLE 17-3 POINT-OF-CARE TESTING COMMITTEE RESPONSIBILITIES

Implementation Phase	Oversight Phase
Define basic system	Review QC/QA
Define what record keeping is required	Monitor compliance
Select methodology	Utilization review
Assign responsibility for test performance	Approve expansion/contraction of programs
	Assess impact/outcomes

End-use committee. Another critical component of a POCT program is an end-user committee, which is different from the interdisciplinary committee that establishes and overviews all POCT programs. An end-user committee should be established for *each* POCT program and should meet at a reasonable frequency to discuss the various compliance reports, as well as ongoing issues and problems with the program. Recommendations for change should be forwarded to the interdisciplinary committee for consideration. The interdisciplinary committee should meet on a bimonthly basis, or sooner if circumstances demand it, to review requests for changes in POCT (either additions or deletions), to consider any recommendations from the user committees, to review and discuss the overall program, and to set future directions.

POCT personnel. Ultimate responsibility and control of POCT reside within a CLIA certified laboratory and require a minimum of one laboratorian to be responsible for each POC program. This individual coordinates evaluations of all test devices before they are placed into service, including linearity and correlation studies on all devices, coordinates proficiency testing, ensures compliance with documentation and procedural requirements, reviews and performs preliminary analysis of QC data, assists in training, and provides technical guidance and troubleshooting.

If there is more than one POCT program, a laboratorian should be appointed as POCT coordinator to overview and coordinate the entire POC system. This individual has the following responsibilities:

- Ensure that all POCT systems are in compliance with accreditation requirements.
- Review and analyze QC data.
- Submit monthly QA reports for individual units as well as overall institutional performance.
- Coordinate and supervise the POCT personnel.
- Develop and coordinate training programs for individuals involved in POCT.

QUALITY ASSURANCE MONITORING

There are three ways to manage the sources of errors in POCT. The first is for the manufacturer to design the product so that errors are difficult to occur or so that it is easy to detect the error. This can be accomplished by automation of calibration function; encoding (via bar code or microchip) of crucial quality control and QA information on unit dose packages; real-time process monitoring; inclusion of calibration solution in unit-use electrode-based systems; and lockout functions for failures of any of the previous features. Second, errors in POCT can be detected with the use of matrix QC material or electronic/optical function checks. The third way to manage sources of error is to warn the end-users of likely errors by use of product labeling and training programs; for example, errors resulting from various patient conditions (such as hypovolemia or poor peripheral circulation due to shock) or analytical interferences (such as lipemia or drugs). The purpose of QA is to control errors that are not designed out of the system and to monitor the testing process in a cost-effective way. Therefore total-system POCT QA is carried out through a combination of QC testing, appropriate training of all individuals involved in POCT, proficiency testing and competency assessment, and finally, a mechanism to perform systems validation.

All POCT systems experience noncompliance problems with various QA requirements, such as record keeping, QC performance, and appropriate interpretation of results. The degree of noncompliance is directly related to the size and complexity of the program. Many of these problems result because users do not understand the regulatory requirements regarding record keeping, do not understand what quality control testing really means, or do not understand the causes of erroneous results. Additionally, external factors such as work pressures in a busy ICU or emergency department may lead to noncompliance.

Addressing compliance issues requires close coordination of all aspects of monitoring and controlling POCT, with overall responsibility residing in the laboratory (Table 17-4). Nursing or unit supervisors are responsible for work performance and compliance with policies and procedures on a daily basis, with laboratory POCT personnel providing troubleshooting and guidance as needed. Weekly and monthly reviews of system operations by POCT personnel and supervisors are important to ensure a high degree of continuous compliance with existing policies and procedures. Once a month, the POCT coordinator should generate a QC report, review the records, and then generate a report on each unit's degree of compliance with various quality indicators. The report should review QC performance, reagent storage, maintenance performance, proficiency testing, patient identification, and critical value confirmations, as well as QA indicators that are unique for each testing system. The QC report should include both a statistical and narrative analysis of individual units and system-wide QC testing and test volumes. When compliance is below established thresholds, the unit nurse managers are requested to investigate and define a follow-up action plan. The individual in charge of the program, either the lab director or POCT coordinator, and a representative from upper nursing/medicine management should perform monthly QA audit rounds. In addition to being a second level of review, these rounds focus on the proper entry of patient data in both the medical record and

TABLE 17-4 QUALITY ASSURANCE MONITORING OF POINT-OF-CARE TESTING	
Frequency	Task
Daily	Work performance and compliance is observed. POC testing personnel provides troubleshooting and guidance.
Monthly	Quality control/quality assurance reports are generated and distributed. Individual in charge of program makes quality assurance round of test sites.
Bimonthly	End-users committee meets. Interdisciplinary committee meeting is held.

TABLE 17-5 POINT-OF-CARE TESTING QUALITY MANAGEMENT STANDARDS	
Code	Description
ISO 22870	Clinical Laboratory Testing—Quality Management of Point-of-Care Testing (POCT)
ISO 15197	Requirements for In Vitro Blood Glucose Monitoring Systems for Self-Testing in Managing Diabetes Mellitus
ISO 17593	Determination of Performance Criteria for Measurement Systems for Self-Testing of Oral Anticoagulation Therapy
NCCLS C30-A	Ancillary (Bedside) Blood Glucose Testing in Acute and Chronic Care Facilities, Sept 1994
NCCLS AST2-A	Guidelines on Point-of-Care In Vivo Diagnostic Testing, June 1999
NCCLS AST4-A	Blood Glucose Testing in Settings Without Laboratory Support, June 1999
NCCLS EP18-P	Quality Management for Unit Use Testing; Proposed Guideline, Nov 1999
NCCLS POCT1-A	Point-of-Care Connectivity; Approved Standard, November 2001

ISO, International Organization for Standardization; NCCLS, National Committee for Clinical Laboratory Standards.

laboratory computer system, as well as in the workstation logs. Furthermore, these rounds open up another feedback channel for the program and send a clear signal to the system operators of the program's importance and the institution's commitment to quality.

Several management standards (Table 17-5) have been developed at both the national and international level to help improve the quality of POCT. These standards encourage a total systems approach to improve information management and data integration, increase reliance on internal QC/QA functions and electronic QC (function tests), and develop a "quality system" concept that moves away from traditional QC concepts.

COST ASSESSMENT OF POCT

A cost/benefit evaluation of POCT is difficult to perform at this time because of limited patient outcome data for POCT systems. The cost associated with POCT depends on the services that have been provided. A proper cost/benefit analysis may determine that POCT might not be the appropriate approach in every clinical setting. Stat testing in the central laboratory, a separate stat laboratory, or dedicated satellite laboratories might be considered as cost-effective alternatives to POCT. It is necessary to look at all aspects of a service delivery model, as well as the unique characteristics of each setting, to determine which testing system best services the financial and clinical needs of the institution.

An assessment of the financial impact of POCT requires consideration not only of the specific costs of test performance, but also of any cost savings associated with an improved level or quality of work. These saving may include reduced repeat testing, decreased preanalytical errors, improved patient management of service, and reduced costs derived from decreased time spent in intensive care units and in the hospital. Bedside testing systems will tend to have greater variable expenses (i.e., reagents, disposables, flexible staffing) than traditional laboratory methodologies. However, fixed expenses, such as equipment costs, instrument maintenance and QC, step-downed space allocation costs, and base staffing, may be significantly lower.

Either a cost-centered (microeconomic) or defect-rate inclusive (macroeconomic) approach can be used to determine the costs of POCT. The cost-centered approach takes into account all the fixed and variable expenses related to POCT within the affected cost center, such as the laboratory, nursing units, or operating room. It is very important that all labor associated with testing be taken into account, because even though each POCT takes only a couple of minutes to perform, those times add up. At The Mount Sinai Medical Center the nursing staff performs over 22,000 fingerstick glucose tests each month. At approximately 5 minutes per test for sample collection, analysis, and paper work, this translates into more than 22,000 nursing hours per annum, not including time for quality control testing and other functions, such as training and supervision. One institution, after performing a total cost analysis before and after restructuring laboratory services and implementing a distributed POCT system, demonstrated a total cost of $8.03 per POC test panel versus $15.33 when the testing was performed in a traditional laboratory setting.

The defect-rate inclusive approach, a subset of total cost management, is a means by which all the costs associated with the quality of a system are assessed, including preventive costs, appraisal costs, and costs of internal and external failure. Preventive costs are those associated with the various mechanisms incorporated to protect against process errors. These include QC testing, personnel training and continuing education, and preventive maintenance. The costs of ascertaining the degree to which a system meets its service requirements are known as appraisal costs. Appraisal

"IDEAL" POC TESTING SYSTEM CHARACTERISTICS

Is self-contained and portable
Has a flexible test menu
Requires minimal training; is simple to operate
Uses whole blood or urine
Demonstrates accuracy and precision comparable to main laboratory systems
Requires minimal routine and preventive maintenance
Has bar codes for test packs, controls, and specimens
Keeps reagents stable at ambient temperature storage
Generates result printouts
Is interfaceable with LIS
Provides quality assurance software for automatic calibrations, system lockouts, and data management

costs include proficiency testing, inspections and accreditation, and internal quality assurance audits. Internal failure costs are costs within the actual testing cycle that result from poor laboratory performance, including specimen re-collections, results considered useless because of the lack of timely reporting (test wastage), and repeat testing or confirmation by a second methodology because of questionable first-time results. External failure costs are costs of poor performance that result outside the testing cycle and are incurred by the receiver of testing results. These include inappropriate clinical decisions based on inaccurate or untimely results, excessive duplicate testing, and excessive use of expensive stat testing.

The defect-rate inclusion approach was applied to evaluate The Mount Sinai Medical Center's Home Health Deep Vein Thrombosis Treatment program. Prothrombin time testing performed by home health care nurses during their visits is an essential component of this program. A total cost analysis demonstrated an estimated $1,645 reduction in total health care costs per patient without any changes in the clinical outcomes.

TECHNOLOGY USED IN POCT

The environment in which POCT is performed differs from that of the traditional laboratory setting because of different workflow and workload characteristics. Furthermore, the personnel involved with POCT are more oriented to obtaining results rapidly for immediate use for patient care and may not, as laboratorians, fully understand the need to comply with all the procedures associated with laboratory medicine, such as QC, analytical procedures, record keeping, and regulatory requirements. Therefore the desirable characteristics of POC diagnostic systems (Box 17-6) are similar to, but also distinct from, laboratory-based diagnostic systems. Significant differences include the desire for POC systems that are easy and convenient to use (i.e., no venipuncture or precise pipetting required), systems that are as technique-independent as possible, and systems that have

automated record keeping functions that fulfill regulatory requirements.

Non–Instrument-Based Systems

The predominant forms of POCT are non–instrument-based systems that use competitive and noncompetitive immunoassays, enzymatic assays, or chemical reactions with a visually read end-point (Table 17-6). A variety of specimen types, such as whole blood, serum or plasma, urine, amniotic fluid, saliva, and feces, can be analyzed with non–instrument-based POCT systems. Qualitative assays with a visually read positive or negative indicator are the predominant form of non–instrument-based POCT. Systems based on either competitive or noncompetitive immunoassays are used for detecting a variety of analytes, including human chorionic gonadotropin, drugs of abuse, fetal lung maturity, cardiac markers, and markers for infectious diseases. Other major qualitative assays are occult fecal blood testing (which employs chemically impregnated paper and a color developer) and visually read blood glucose reagent strips (which use coupled enzyme reactions to form a colored product). The glucose concentration can be semiquantified by visual comparison of the color development on the glucose reagent strips with a color chart or by reflectance colorimetry. Urine dipstick systems are also semiquantitative and use chemical and enzymatic reactions to generate a colored product. There are a few non–instrument-based quantitative POC test systems that employ chemical or enzymatic reactions and immunochromatographic techniques to determine concentrations of lipids, cardiac markers, and therapeutic drugs.

Instrument-Based Systems

Instrument-based POCT systems are becoming very sophisticated. They are highly automated, using a small sample size, requiring minimal routine and preventive maintenance, and eliminating or automating calibration functions. These improvements in functionality have been facilitated by advances in reagent stabilization; in the development and miniaturization of electrodes and biosensors; in the ability to produce relatively inexpensive, precise, disposable devices; and in the development of microcomputers and microelectronics. These advances in engineering and technology have allowed reformulation of currently used reagents into different testing formats, the incorporation of real-time process control and monitoring of the analytical process, and the encoding (through microchips and bar codes) of information (such as calibration data, lot number, and test name) into the system. Through the application of these technologies and processes, the responsibility for the quality of the analytical result moves significantly toward the manufacturer.

Most but not all characteristics of the ideal POCT device are found in the various instruments on the market today. These instruments require a minimal amount of technical support because they are relatively maintenance-free. The devices are easy to operate and retain accuracy and precision with, when necessary, automatic periodic calibration. In addition to calibration functions, automation is important to

TABLE 17-6   NON-INSTRUMENTAL TECHNOLOGY EMPLOYED IN POC TESTING

Types of Assay	Assay Principle	Format	Specimen	Analytes
Qualitative	Chemical reactions	Impregnated paper strips	Feces	Occult blood
	Immunoconcentration	Dry reagent cartridges—single use	Urine and serum	hCG, Strep A
	Microparticle capture immunoassay	Dry reagent cartridges—single use	Urine	Drugs of abuse
	Latex agglutination	Dry reagent cartridges—single use	Amniotic fluid Blood	Fetal lung maturity Therapeutic drugs Myoglobin
	Latex agglutination inhibition slides	Dry reagent cartridges—single use	Urine	Drug of abuse
	Immunochromatographic	Dry reagent cartridges—single use	Blood, plasma, and serum Urine	CK-MB, Troponin I, Troponin T, myoglobin
		Dry reagent cartridges—single use	Urine	hCG
		Dry reagent cartridges—single use	Swabs	*Chlamydia*, Strep A, herpes
	Optical immunoassay	Dry reagent cartridges—single use	Swabs	Strep A, Strep B, influenza
Semi quantitative	Chemical/enzymatic reactions	Impregnated paper strips	Urine	Urinalysis
		Impregnated paper strips	Blood	Glucose
		Dry reagent cartridges—single use	Saliva	Ethanol
	Latex agglutination	Dry reagent cartridges—single use	Serum	Myoglobin
Quantitative	Chemical/enzymatic reactions	Dry reagent cartridges—single use	Blood	Lipids
	Immunochromatography	Dry reagent cartridges—single use	Blood, serum, and plasma	Therapeutic drugs CK-MB

various quality assurance functions. The ideal POCT QA/QC software includes all the characteristics listed in Box 17-7. Automatic record keeping of patient result logs, QC/QA logs, and maintenance logs with attached comments and operator ID is a feature of several systems. Quality assurance software that allows for automatic lockouts of users who are either not authorized or who do not adhere to QC/QA procedures is available in some analyzers. System lockouts can occur if QC has not been performed or is out of range, if a valid operator ID is not entered, or if patient ID is not entered. However, not all systems on the market today have the capability of interfacing with a laboratory information system. Integration of the data generated with POCT into the medical record is important.

Most POC instruments require only a few microliters of whole blood or urine, and either the analytes are tested for directly in the whole blood sample or the system internally separates the red cells by size filtration or centrifugation and analyzes the plasma obtained. Table 17-7 identifies the current technologies that are used in instrument-based POCT systems. The most common instrument systems used today are those based on either reflectance photometry or biosensors. Representative systems for the various technology/format combinations are listed, along with some of the other characteristics of these testing systems. Some of these systems employ new analytical concepts, such as optodes, paramagnetism, optical immunoassays, and centrifugal separation with optical signa-

BOX 17-7

IDEAL POCT ANALYZER QA/QA SOFTWARE

System Lockouts for the Following Problems:
  QC not performed
  QC out of range
  Patient ID not entered—override for emergency department
    (ED)
  Valid operator ID not entered
Calibration
  Automatic
  Slope/offset adjustments
Differential levels of security access
Demographic/location verification
User-definable reportable/reference and QC ranges
Alert value flagging
Delta checking
Data entry
  Bar code scanners
  Touchscreens
  Magnetic card readers
Data management
  Patient result logs
  QC/QA logs
  Maintenance logs

TABLE 17-7   CURRENT TECHNOLOGY EMPLOYED IN INSTRUMENT-BASED POC TESTING

Technology	Format	Sample Type	Precise Pipetting	Sample Volume (μL)	Representative Systems	Testing
Photometry, reflectance	Dry reagent strip—single test	Whole blood Serum/plasma	No Yes	10-45 10	Glucose meter Ektachem (Johnson and Johnson)	Glucose, chemistry, and TDM
Photometry, transmittance	Wet reagent cartridges—single test	Whole blood Serum/plasma	No	~20	Vision (Abbott)	Chemistry and drugs
	Dry reagent cartridges—single test	Whole blood	No No	10 ~20	HemoCue (Hemocue) Careside (Careside)	Glucose and hemoglobin
	Dry reagent rotors—multiple tests	Whole blood Serum/plasma	No	~90	Picolo (Abaxis)	Chemistry
Fluorometry	Dry reagent cartridges—multiple tests	Serum	No	20	IOS (Biocircuits)	Hormones
	Wet reagent cartridges—multiple tests	Whole blood Serum	No	3 mL draw tube	Alpha Dx (Sigma) Stratus CS (Dade)	CK-MB, myoglobin, cTnI
Optodes	Dry reagent cartridges—multiple tests	Whole blood	No	80 95	AVL Opti (Roche) NPT7 (Radiometer)	Blood gases/ electrolytes
	Dry reagent cartridges—multiple tests, multiple use	Whole blood	No	80	AVL OptiR (Roche)	Blood gases/ electrolytes
Potentiometry/ electrochemistry	Biosensor strips—single test	Whole blood	No	10	Precision PCX (Medisence) AccuChek (Roche)	Glucose
	Biosensor chips—multiple tests	Whole blood	No	~70 125	PCA (i-Stat) IRMA (Diametrics)	Chemistry/ blood gases
	Miniature electrodes—multiple tests, multiple use	Whole blood	No	150 180	Gem Premier (Instrumentation Labs) ABL 77 (Radiometer)	Chemistry/blood gases
Immunochromatography	Dry reagent cartridges—single test	Whole blood	Yes	140 150	Triage (Biosite) CardiacT Quant (Roche)	CK-MB, myoglobin, cTnI, BNP
Turbidimetry—latex agglutination inhibition	Dry coated latex particles cartridges—single use	Whole blood	No	10	DCA2000 (Bayer)	Hemoglobin A_{1c}
Optical motion detection	Dry paramagnetic particles motion reagent card—single use	Whole blood	No	1 large drop	Rapidpoint (Bayer) CoaguChek (Roche)	ACT, PT, PTT Heparin, protamine
	Dry sample motion cartridges—single use	Whole blood	No No	1 large drop	Biotrack (Roche) Hemochron Jr (International Technidyne)	(International Technidyne) ACT, PT, PTT
	Dry reagent tubes—single use	Whole blood	No	2 mL	Hemochron Response (International Technidyne) Hepcon (Medtronics)	ACT, PT, PTT Heparin, protamine

Continued

TABLE 17-7 CURRENT TECHNOLOGY EMPLOYED IN INSTRUMENT-BASED POC TESTING—CONT'D

Technology	Format	Sample Type	Precise Pipetting	Sample Volume (µL)	Representative Systems	Testing
Luminescence/fiber optic	Intra-arterial catheter	Not applicable	Not applicable	Not applicable	PB3300 (Puritan Bennett) Paratrend Sensor (Agilent Technologies)	Blood gases
Centrifugal separation—optical signature analysis	Single use capillary tube	Whole blood	No	250	QBC Autoread (Becton Dickinson)	Hct, HgB, platelets, granulocytes, lymphocytes/monocytes

ture analysis. Some POC instruments are miniaturized versions of traditional laboratory analyzers, often using the same chemistries and incorporating ingenious techniques to internally generate plasma for analysis.

The ability to perform analytical processes on only a few microliters of whole blood, versus having to obtain 3 to 7 mL of blood by venipuncture, helps prevent iatrogenic blood loss, a significant benefit of POCT. The only way to eliminate all blood loss associated with diagnostic testing is to use **ex vivo** and **in vivo test devices**. Ex vivo devices remove blood from the body, analyze it, and then reinfuse it. There are two main approaches to ex vivo monitoring system: (1) flow-through sensors in the extracorporeal loop on a heart-lung bypass pump (for example, CD400-3M Health Care; pH and blood-gases) and (2) withdrawal, in which blood is removed from the body, analyzed, and then reinfused (for example, VIA-Via Medical; pH, blood-gases, electrolytes, hematocrit, and glucose). Two major systems approaches to in vivo monitoring have been developed: intravascular and subcutaneous. With in vivo blood-gas and pH monitors, all three sensors (pO_2, pCO_2, and pH) are located on or near the tip of a single fiberoptic probe that is inserted through a catheter, typically into the radial artery. Probe placement is essential for proper functioning, requiring sufficient space between it and the arterial wall so as not to impede blood flow. A subcutaneous sensor has been developed that measures glucose in interstitial fluid.

Noninvasive/Minimally Invasive Technology

Minimally invasive POCT and noninvasive POCT reduce or eliminate the need for any specimen withdrawal. Most of the minimally invasive technologies have focused on glucose measurements. With these systems either microdrops of blood are tested or interstitial fluid analysis is performed (Table 17-8). By requiring only 0.3 to 1.5 µL of whole blood, sampling can be done at sites other than the fingerstick (for example, the forearm), where there are less pain receptors, helping to ensure better diabetic patient compliance with glucose self-monitoring. Interstitial fluid (ISF) analysis is

TABLE 17-8 MINIMALLY INVASIVE TECHNOLOGY

System	Sample Size
Microdrop Systems	
AtLast Blood (Almira)	1.5 µL
FreeStyle (TheraSense)	0.3 µL
Interstitial Fluid Systems	
CGMS (MiniMed)	NA
LifeGuide System (Integ, Inc.)	1.2 L
SpectRx	NA
GlucoWatch (Cygnus, Inc.)	NA
SonoPrep (Sontra Medical, Inc.)	NA
TD (Technical Chemical and Products, Inc.)	NA

another mechanism for providing minimally invasive glucose monitoring. However, before ISF glucose analysis will be routinely accepted, several issues need to be resolved or clarified. For example, what is the time delay for the concentration equilibrium to reestablish itself between blood and ISF when there is a change in blood glucose concentration? The delay may be acceptable when the patient's values are relatively stable but not when there are rapid changes that need to be assessed (e.g., for a brittle diabetic). Also, what is the correlation between blood glucose and continuously drawn and measured ISF glucose? Finally, based on the analytical systems being used, how long can "continuous" ISF glucose measurements be made, how easy is it to calibrate the systems, and how long do the calibrations hold? Most of the systems mentioned require one or more fingerstick glucose tests for the calibration process, which holds for 12 to 24 hours.

With all but three of the ISF methods, the specimen is obtained in a minimally invasive mechanism. Three of the systems, GlucoWatch (Cygnus, Inc.), SonoPrep (Sontra Medical), and TD Glucose Monitoring System (Technical Chemical and Products), use reverse ionotropheris, sonopheris, or chemical phoresis to extract the interstitial fluid for analysis. The GlucoWatch uses a disposable autosensor pack that is good for 12 hours. A single fingerstick glucose value is used to calibrate the sensor pack and the system generates three readings per hour. With the SpectrRx system a cluster of five microholes are burned in the forearm by laser and a patch containing the glucose biosensor is placed over the holes. By application of a vacuum, interstitial fluid flow is established for up to 4 days and continuous glucose monitoring is performed. As mentioned earlier regarding in vivo testing, the MiniMed Continuous Glucose monitor has a sensor approximately the diameter of a dime with a small interstitial fluid sampling stylet that is inserted under the skin. This system measures glucose continuously in the interstitial fluid. Calibration is performed with multiple fingerstick glucose tests upon initial placement of the sensor, and a one-point calibration adjustment is performed daily. This device will record the interstitial fluid glucose concentrations every 5 minutes for up to 14 days.

There are only a few noninvasive systems currently available: pulse oximeters for O_2 saturation, end-tidal CO_2 measurements for pCO_2, transcutaneous and conjunctival pO_2/pCO_2 measurements, and transcutaneous bilirubin measurements (used only for premature infants). Furthermore, since these systems do not provide exact measurements, they are used as trend indicators, providing continuous monitoring of analyte level and the ability to recognize a change in status. Other advantages of noninvasive systems are fewer infection control problems and better compliance rates with self-monitoring through the elimination of the inconvenience and discomfort of multiple fingersticks. Various noninvasive systems are in development for glucose measurements that employ infrared spectroscopy, near-infrared spectroscopy with signature analysis, and photo-acoustic technology.

Quality Control of Single-Use Devices

Quality control has traditionally been accomplished by running multiple levels of stabilized, matrix-matched specimens (QC material) within each analytical run. After various statistical rules are applied to the results, a determination is made of whether the run is "in-control" and whether the patient results can be released. As defined by the National Committee for Clinical Laboratory Standards (NCCLS) and incorporated into the CLIA '88 regulations, an analytical run for the purposes of quality control "is an interval within which the accuracy and precision of the measuring system is expected to be stable." Furthermore, because of older technological limits for the maintenance of accuracy and precision, maximum run length was set at 24 hours. However, the concept of run length does not exist with single-use diagnostic testing devices where, strictly speaking, each test is a run itself. With instrument-based systems, every time a new cartridge, pack, strip, etc., is inserted into the base instrument, a quasi new test system is created. Therefore quality control must take a different form in POCT devices.

How can this new system be tested to ensure the continued quality of the results generated? With non–instrument-based devices, QC has been integrated directly into the device by the application of visual indicators for positive and negative reaction zones, as well as for the adequacy of specimen flow. With these devices, external QC material should be analyzed upon initial receipt of a shipment and then, depending on the system, on a periodic basis. Quality control has been integrated into various POCT instruments by incorporating one or more of the following functions:

- Automation of calibration function
- Encoding (via bar code or microchip) of crucial quality control and quality assurance information on the unit dose packages
- Real-time process monitoring
- Inclusion of calibration solution in unit-use electrode-based systems

By these functions, the company ensures the reliability of test results as long as the disposable test devices are stored properly and are used before a stated expiration date. Thus part of the laboratory quality control with these POCT systems is dependent on the ability of the company to manufacture its consumable product reliably and reproducibly. Some POCT systems, such as First Medical, have incorporated liquid QC testing into each disposable unit.

An analytical instrument can be divided into three main sections: mechanical/electronic, analytical, and reagent/calibrants. The mechanical/electronic component consists of various parts such as pumps, levers, gears, chains, memory chips, logic circuits, and software. The analytical components are those parts of the system that come in contact with the sample being analyzed or that produce the signal for the electronics to convert into results; for example, ion-selective electrodes, pH electrodes, biosensors, reaction cups, optics. Traditional QC test programs validate the entire system. However, with compartmentalization of these various subsystems, it is possible to isolate and test some of the subsystems independently of the others. In this manner it may be possible to devise a more cost-effective QC program than the traditional one used for instrument-based POCT systems.

With instrument-based POCT systems, the mechanical/electronic and analytical components have been completely separated from the reagent/calibrant component. In some systems, the analytical components are individually packaged with the reagents and calibrants. With these latter devices, the only consistent part from test to test is the mechanical/electronic component. All biosensors, electrodes, reagents, and calibrants are replaced with every analysis. By separating the QC testing of these two subsystems, an effective QC system can be developed for a POCT program that uses multiple instruments. The functionality of the mechanical/electronic component of each analytical device in operation should be tested once every 24 hours. Reflectance standard strips with established ranges for acceptable values are used with some of the reflectance photometry systems to validate optical performance. Electronic test modules are available for some POCT systems. The electronic test module is inserted into the analyzer and simulates the analytical output of a test cartridge at one or more specimen concentrations. Additionally, the electronic test module may perform a series of mechanical and electronic tests on the base unit. After comparison of the various results to predefined limits, a determination is made whether or not to verify the core system as working properly and in control. Furthermore, with some systems, the electronic test module is not a passive testing system but rather requires operator intervention to further simulate sample analysis, providing additional validation of some operator techniques.

Now that the mechanical/electronic component has been validated, the analytical reliability of the test cartridges, that is, the analytical/reagent/calibrant component, has to be verified. This is done by analyzing matrix-matched (as close as possible) QC material with the test cartridges. With the operational characteristic of all the base units being verified with the electronic test module, it is necessary only to verify the analytical performance of one test cartridge per lot with one base unit. By using the electronic test module and liquid QC material in this manner, the user is properly assured that all is in control, with a minimal use of test cartridges. Since the stability and reliability of the test cartridges is contingent on proper storage conditions (temperature, humidity, light), every testing site that stores its own stock of reagents must perform QC testing on each lot in storage.

Process control incorporated into some POCT systems can identify deteriorating reagent reactivity and inappropriate biosensor response. In the PCA device, the controlling software monitors reagent rehydration, calibration, and analytical response curves from the individual biosensors. If any of the monitored biosensor parameters fall outside acceptable ranges, the output of that sensor is automatically suppressed. The Picolo analyzer has an enzyme reagent in the rotor that is sensitive to temperature, humidity, and light. If the enzyme activity does not meet expected limits, it is assumed that the environment has affected the rotor and the run is aborted. With the expansion of the application of real-time process controls in POC testing devices, the need for external QC testing will diminish. Furthermore, the definition of a "run" for quality control purposes must be changed to allow for time periods greater than 24 hours, if not eliminated completely, for systems that incorporate onboard process control. As mentioned earlier in the chapter, one of the best ways to control error in a POCT system is to manufacture better-design devices that remove the cause of error or automate error detection. By accomplishing automatic error detection, these systems are becoming a part of the total systems approach to QA. This concept of a quality system that encompasses all the aspects of a POCT system is the basis of the NCCLS document entitled Quality Management for Unit Use Testing (Proposed Guideline, November 1999).

DATA INTEGRATION AND CONNECTIVITY

Proper management of data and patient results obtained by POCT is vital for ensuring proper device function; quality processing of specimens; appropriate distribution, charting, and archiving of laboratory results; and compliance with regulatory requirements. A variety of issues are associated with managing laboratory test devices and the transmission of data generated from POCT sites that are remote from the central laboratory.

Information Flow

Fig. 17-1 shows the general flow of laboratory data at The Mount Sinai Hospital, from the time of determination of need for testing to the time the health care provider has the result. After determining the need for data, the health care provider places an order that initiates the flow of events. Ultimately, the lab results are reported back to the individual, at which time clinical decisions need to be made. The sample either is sent to a laboratory for testing or is tested in the unit with a POC device. In the latter case, the physician may have the result soon after analysis is completed. However, despite specimen transit and result reporting times being minimized with POCT, problems may still occur with recording the data in the patient's chart, especially the electronic record (see Chapter 18). Many POCT devices do not have the necessary hardware or software for connecting to the hospital information system (HIS).

POC Connectivity

There are various forms of data output used with POC testing systems: visual readings, display screens, printers, and various means of electronic transmission by RS232 ports, ethernet ports, infrared beams, radio signals, or modems. These different mechanisms provide a variety of means by which test results can be entered into the medical information system. Because handheld and small battery-powered portable systems are designed for flexibility of use, they require some degree of manual operations to get the data into the laboratory information system (LIS). This is in contrast to the analytical systems used in core and satellite laboratories and to those POCT systems with fixed location, which can be hardwired into the LIS.

Manual entry of data into the medical record is the only mechanism available for non–instrument-based POCT systems. The decision of where the data is manually entered, that is, into a computer terminal (LIS, HIS) or medical chart, depends on the institution and how the various information systems are networked. If a hospital has implemented electronic ordering of test requests on the units, and if a POC test requires an answer upon ordering, these results can be entered into the information system from the nursing station on the floor. In this case, when the health care professional places a test order in the system, there is automatically an immediate request for the result to be entered.

If POCT systems are located in a dedicated space and not moved, the best interface is a direct linkage into the LIS. Otherwise, an intermittent linkage is necessary to accommodate the flexibility and mobility needs of most POCT devices. Similar to the central laboratory's equipment, POCT systems can be hardwired into the communication network. Each instrument can be directly linked into the LIS, or multiple units can be linked to a central (network) computer that, in turn, is connected to the LIS. In the latter case, the network PC can, via an autoscripting program, log on to the LIS and

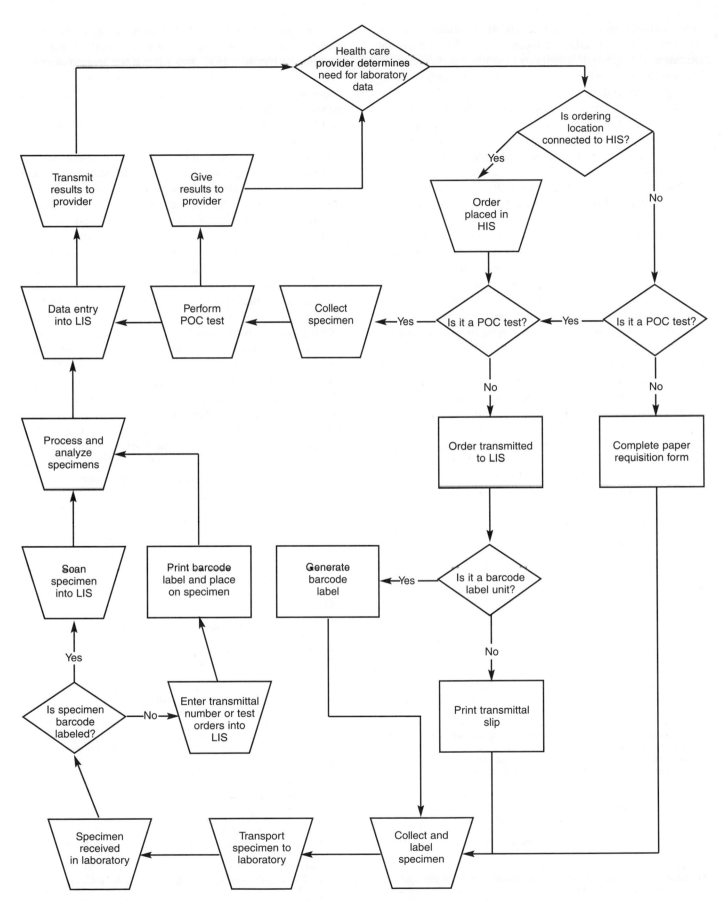

Fig. 17-1 Testing information flow—The Mount Sinai Hospital.

order, transmit, and verify test results. An alternative is to use infrared or radio signals to transmit the results to a central receiving station, which is then subsequently linked to the LIS. Infrared signal use is limited by the fact that it is usable only for short distances and must follow a line of sight. Although radio signals overcome the line of site and distance limitations of infrared data transmission, concerns exist regarding interferences within or near specific areas of a medical center, such as near telemetry units and magnetic resonance imaging installations.

Despite the various mechanisms available to transfer POC testing data into the electronic medical record, currently a majority of the data is never found there. In a recent survey by Enterprise Analysis Corp (1998) of over 500 hospitals in the United States performing POCT, it was determined that only a third of the data generated by instrument based POC systems was entered into the electronic chart. Furthermore, of the data found in the electronic record, only 45% were electronically transmitted, with the remainder being entered manually. A number of possibilities exist for why only 15% of all POC data are being downloaded into the LIS/HIS. The primary reason is that not all POCT instruments have the hardware or software to permit connection to the LIS/HIS. Furthermore, each system that does have a LIS/HIS interface currently requires a unique personal computer-based data manager for that testing. It is burdensome for the laboratory to have multiple data managers because of the space and infrastructure requirements for multiple computers and printers and because of the need of POCT personnel to learn to operate and maintain multiple software/hardware packages.

Another problem with POCT connectivity is that few laboratory information systems have an interface with the capability of handling POC data when a test request does not exist in the LIS. This is important because, in contrast to laboratory-based testing, most POC tests may not have been ordered by the time data is ready for transmission and the LIS will have to create the order at the time of result transmission.

A consortium of instrument manufacturers, information technology companies, and end-users has addressed this problem and developed three standards for POC connectivity. The first two standards govern the communication between the POCT devices and the central data manager. Protocols address both the format of the data stream and the hardware that is required to connect a POCT device to the data manager. These standards allow one data manager to handle the output from a variety of POCT devices. The third standard governs the actual interface between the central data manager and the LIS/HIS. This last standard does not overcome the obstacle of current LIS/HIS systems being unable to create an order as a result is transmitted, but it does standardize, in terms of content and format, the basic communication between a POCT data manager and the LIS/HIS. These standards, based on a robust communications structure using an HL7-type message stream, are becoming widely accepted and should correct many of the POCT communication problems noted previously. The standards have been adopted by the National Committee for Clinical Laboratory Standards as POCT1-A: Point of Care Connectivity; Approved Standards, for maintenance and further development.

Bibliography

Bailey TM et al: Laboratory process improvement through point-of-care testing, *J Qual Improv* 23:362, 1997.

Becker RC et al: A randomized, multicenter trial of weight-adjusted intravenous heparin dose titration and point-of-care coagulation monitoring in hospitalized patients with active thromboembolic disease, *Am Heart J* 137:59, 1999.

Chernow B: The bedside laboratory: a critical step forward in ICU care, *Chest* 97S:183S, 1990.

Chiquette E, Amato MG, Bussy HI: Comparison of an anticoagulation clinic with usual medical care: anticoagulation control, patient outcomes, and health care costs, *Arch Intern Med* 158:1641, 1998.

Claremont DJ: Biosensors: clinical requirements and scientific promise, *J Med Eng Technol* 11:51, 1987.

Department of Health and Human Service, Health Care Financing Administration: Clinical laboratory improvement amendments of 1988, final rule, *Fed Regist* 7:7002, 1992.

Despotis GJ et al: Prospective evaluation and clinical utility of on-site coagulation monitoring in cardiac surgical patients, *J Thorac Cardiovasc Surg* 107:271, 1994.

Dunn AS et al: Outpatient treatment of deep vein thrombosis in a diverse inner-city population, *Am J Med* 110:458, 2001.

Fleisher M, Schwartz MK: Strategies of organization and service for the critical-care laboratory, *Clin Chem* 36:1557B, 1990.

Fraser CG, Hylotft Petersen P: Desirable performance standards for imprecision and bias in alternate sites, *Arch Pathol Lab Med* 119:909, 1995.

Friedman BA, Mitchell W: Integrating information from decentralized laboratory testing sites, *Am J Clin Pathol* 99:637, 1993.

Handorf CR: POC testing: must quality cost more? *MLO* 25(9S):28, 1993.

Handorf CR: Quality control and quality management of alternate-site testing, *Clin Lab Med* 14:539, 1994.

Jacobs E, Sarkozi L, Coleman N: A centralized critical care (STAT) laboratory: The Mount Sinai experience, *Crit Care Report* 2:397, 1991.

Jacobs E et al: Analytical evaluation of i-STAT portable clinical analyzer and use by non-laboratory healthcare professional, *Clin Chem* 39:1069, 1993.

Jacobs E: Total quality management and point-of-care testing, *MLO* 25(9S):2, 1993.

Jacobs E: Bedside glucose testing: sources of variation, *ASCP Check Sample-Core Analytes* 10:1, 1994.

Jacobs E: Information integration for point-of-care and satellite testing. In Kost GJ, editor: *Clinical laboratory automation, robotics, and optimization*, New York, 1996, Wiley-Interscience.

Jacobs E: Analysis of economic models used to justify point-of-care testing. In D'Orazio P, editor: *Preparing for critical care analysis in the twenty-first century*, vol 16: proceedings of an international symposium. Medfield, MA: Electrolyte/Blood Gas Div, p 126, 1996, AACC.

Jacobs E: The laboratory as a leader of point-of-care programs, *MLO* 30(9S):6, 1998.

Jacobs E et al: Implementation and management of point-of-care testing in an academic health care setting, *Clin Chem Acta* 307:49, 2001.

Korpman RA: Health care information systems—patient centered integration is the key, *Clin Lab Med* 11:203, 1991.

Kost GJ et al: Monitoring of ionized calcium during human hepatic transplantation: critical values and their relevance to cardiac and hemodynamic management, *Am J Clin Pathol* 86:61, 1986.

Kost GJ: The hybrid laboratory: shifting the focus to the point of care, *MLO* 24(9S):17, 1992.

Kost GJ: Point-of-care testing in intensive care. In Tobin MJ, editor: *Principles and practice of intensive care monitoring*, New York, 1998, McGraw-Hill, pp 1267-1296.

Lee-Lewandrowski E et al: Utilization and cost analysis of bedside capillary glucose testing: implications for managing point of care testing, *Am J Med* 97:222, 1994.

Nanji AA, Poon R, Hinberg I: Near-patient testing: quality of laboratory test results obtained by non-technical personnel in a decentralized setting, *Am J Clin Pathol* 89:797, 1988.

National Academy of Clinical Biochemistry: Recommendations for the use of cardiac markers in coronary artery diseases. In Wu AHB, Apple FS, Warshaw MM, editors: *Standards of laboratory practice*, Washington, 1999, NACB.

NCCLS Approved Guideline AST2-A: *Guidelines on point-of-care in vivo diagnostic testing*, Villanova, PA, 1999, National Committee for Clinical Laboratory Standards.

NCCLS Approved Guideline C30-A: *Ancillary (bedside) testing in acute and chronic care facilities*, Villanova, PA, 1994, National Committee for Clinical Laboratory Standards.

NCCLS Approved Guideline POCT1-A: *Point-of-care connectivity*, Villanova, PA, 2001, National Committee for Clinical Laboratory Standards.

NCCLS Proposed Guideline EP18-P: *Quality management for unit use testing*, Villanova, PA, 1999, National Committee for Clinical Laboratory Standards.

Nuttall G et al: Efficacy of a simple intraoperative transfusion algorithm for nonerythrocyte component utilization after cardiopulmonary bypass, *Anesthesiology* 94:7731, 2001.

Parvin CC et al: Impact of point-of-care testing on patient's length of stay in a large emergency department, *Clin Chem* 42:711, 1996.

Robinson MR et al: Noninvasive glucose monitoring in diabetic patients: a preliminary evaluation, *Clin Chem* 38:1618, 1992.

Salem M et al: Bedside diagnostic testing: its accuracy, rapidity and utility in blood conservation, *JAMA* 266:382, 1991.

Santrach PJ: Point of care coagulation testing: a targeted approach, *J Clin Lig Assay* 25, 2002.

Strickland RA, Hill TR, Zaluga GP: Rapid bedside analysis of arterial blood gases and electrolytes improve patient care during and after cardiac surgery, *Anesthesiology* A257:69, 1988.

Suver JD, Nuemann BR, Boles EE: Accounting for the costs of quality, *Heathc Financ Manage* 9:29, 1992.

Winkelman JW, Wybenga DR, Tanasijevic MJ: The fiscal consequences of central versus distributed testing of glucose, *Clin Chem* 40:1628, 1994.

Zabel KM et al: Use of bedside activated partial thromboplastin time monitor to adjust heparin dosing after thrombolysis for acute myocardial infarction: results of GUSTO-I, *Am Heart J* 136:868, 1998.

Internet Sites

http://www.aacc.org/divisions/poct/default.stm—AACC Division of point-of-care testing

http://www.aacc.org/divisions/poct/latest_news.stm—Online newsletter sponsored by the AACC for point-of-care testing

http://www.cpsa.ab.ca/qoc/Point-of-Care%20Testing.doc—Accreditation survey document for laboratories by the College of Physicians and Surgeons of Alberta

http://www.springnet.com/articles/Testing1.pdf—SpringNet online newsletter (directed to nurses) sponsored by Lippincott, Williams and Wilkins

www.ascls.org/position/point.htm—ASCLS, Position on point-of-care testing

www.pointofcare.net

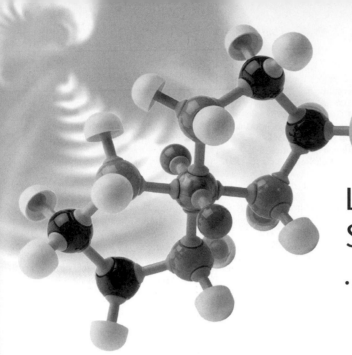

CHAPTER 18

Laboratory Information Systems

• David Chou

Objectives

- Describe the functions, operational characteristics, and workflow of a laboratory information system (LIS) in a clinical laboratory.
- Describe the problems with, importance of, and needs for instrument interfaces, computer interfaces, and data information interchange

between computers.
- Describe the basic computer terminology and the technology associated with LIS.
- Examine changes expected to occur in the laboratory, healthcare environment, and computer technology and their effects on the LIS.

Key Terms

ADT (admissions/discharge/transfer)
Administrative and demographic patient information provided by a central computer covering patient admissions, transfers, and discharges.

applications programs   Programs written to support specific end-user functions. The computer interactions visible to most users are interactions with applications programs.

archived data   Patient data that have been placed in a form not immediately accessible by the user without intervention upon the part of a computer operator.

backup   A procedure, usually performed daily, in which operational data on disks are transferred to a secondary medium, usually magnetic tape. Normally, data on these tapes will be restored to disk only in the event that the disk fails.

bar code A series of parallel lines or squares of varying thickness, printed in a fashion to represent numbers, or numbers and letters, and which can be read by automated equipment.

bidirectional interface A program that allows electronic communications between an instrument and an LIS, permitting the interchange of information in both directions.

central processing unit (CPU) The part of the computer responsible for the execution of programs and making decisions (i.e., the brains of the computer).

client A locally networked computer accessing data from other remotely networked computers, called *servers*. Data on the client may also be sent to the server for processing and/or storage.

cumulative report A report designed to display results over a period of time for a single patient in a tabular fashion.

database manager A program designed to manage the storage and retrieval of data to and from computer storage media such as disks and/or tapes.

data structure The organization of the data as they are stored in the computer.

delta check A method of quality control in which the current patient result is compared to a previous patient result.

file maintenance A program that is executed regularly for managing and reorganizing data, usually on disk, for optimal storage and retrieval.

firewall A term used for an electronic device that controls the type of information that can either enter or leave a local area network. Most often, firewalls are designed to prevent unwanted intrusions into a computer system.

hardware The physical parts of a computer. After manufacturing, updates and changes to hardware occur much less frequently than to software.

hierarchical database A database design that treats data in a hierarchical or treelike relationship.

HIPPA (The Health Insurance Portability and Accountability Act of 1996) A federal law that addresses health insurance reform, mandates the use of standardized electronic data interfaces, and sets standards for the privacy of medical records and data security.

incomplete list An LIS report listing specimens that have not yet been processed. Different incomplete lists may be printed for each task performed in the laboratory.

informatics Informatics studies the representation, processing/transformation, and communication of information in natural and artificial systems by organisms or artifacts such as computers.

interpretive reports Reports generated to provide information to the clinician that differ depending on the results and describe possible treatment or diagnostic possibilities for the given set of results.

local area network (LAN) A digital computer network that serves a localized area, usually limited to less than 2 miles in distance.

modem A device that converts digital signals from a computer to signals suitable for analog media, such as audio over a dial-up telephone line (e.g., a V.90 modem) or video for cable television (e.g., a cable modem).

network or digital computer network The use of cable television, microwave, fiber optic, or telephone lines to permit communications between a group of computers.

on-line Data that are kept in a computer in a manner that allows immediate access.

operating system Software designed to supervise the orderly execution of programs and provide support for basic functions used by most programs.

order entry The action of entering test orders into a computer system. This order process may occur on the LIS or a remote computer linked to the LIS.

patient demographics Pertinent clinical and administrative patient information collected at the time of patient admission. These include the patient number, name, sex, age, birth date, and other information relating to the patient.

personal computer A small desktop computer designed to be used by a single user in the office or home environment and costing between $500 and $5000.

privacy The need to ensure that data are accessed only by authorized individuals and parties.

program A series of instructions directing computer hardware to perform specified actions.

programming languages A structured set of instructions designed to be translated into detailed instructions for the computer hardware. Most languages are Englishlike and are designed to make writing instructions for the computer easier.

relational database A database design defined by E.F. Codd based on set theory. The operations allowable in a relational database are similar to those for sets.

run As defined by the Clinical Laboratory Improvement Amendments of 1988 (CLIA '88), a run is an interval within which the accuracy and precision of a testing system are expected to be stable but cannot be greater than 24 hours.

security The action of protecting data from being unintentionally accessed, altered, or destroyed. This includes the physical protection of computer and computer media, as well as protection of data and software against attacks.

server A networked computer, which may be remote, that acts as a data storage or data processing agent for data generated by clients (see client).

software   Collectively, the programs that operate the computer.

software maintenance   Changes in software intended to fix problems, to improve functionality, or to provide new capabilities.

specimen number   A number assigned by the LIS to a sample for identification purposes. The number may be reused periodically and must not duplicate any specimen still being processed.

unidirectional interface   A program that permits electronic communication between an LIS and instrument, permitting the instrument to send or upload information to the LIS.

uniform resource locator (URL)   A unique name assigned to an Internet resource that is translated to a single numeric address identifying a computer. URLs make it convenient for users to gain access to computers (e.g., websites).

validation   The process whereby a technologist reviews one or more analyses and releases the results to the patient file for reporting.

virus   A software program, often destructive, designed to embed itself into the operating system or other commonly available software.

wide area network (WAN)   A digital computer network that serves an area larger than 1 to 2 miles in distance. WANs are usually networks that provide intercity services.

worklist   A list of specimen numbers for pending analyses generated by a technologist before performing a specified task, such as an analytical run or a specimen collection.

The *laboratory information system*, or *LIS*, can be defined as one or more applications software packages along with the associated **operating systems**, other **software**, and the **hardware** needed to run **programs** that specifically support the operational and management needs of a clinical laboratory. Because of the variation in laboratories, the software, hardware, and the spectrum of services required from and provided by an LIS can significantly differ from one laboratory to another. Most successful information systems structure routine tasks and assist in the integration of diversified processes. As a secondary benefit, the LIS provides data management and imposes management controls. An LIS, therefore, must be closely tuned to the operating needs of each laboratory and its organization. The computer can be a powerful tool for improving both productivity and quality, and unlike an automated instrument, which may only affect the technologists using it, the LIS directly affects almost everyone within the laboratory and many users outside the laboratory. For example, physicians often request changes to an LIS to gain more information.

Most LIS vendors, like most software developers, depend on the technologies provided by many other vendors. Each vendor in the technology chain builds upon products and systems developed by other vendors. At the highest level of development are the **applications programs**, such as the end product known by clinical users as the LIS. The vendor developing a modern LIS writes applications programs using software development tools such as the **database manager**, the **programming language(s)**, and the *operating system*. Finally, a vendor provides the *hardware*, which is the physical computer itself. A single vendor may provide several components required by an LIS vendor or use products from other vendors. This technology chain presents complications and benefits. For example, a problem with an LIS program may be secondary to a defect in the operating system developed by another vendor, who is unable to correct the problem. On the other hand, the vendor of the applications software can rapidly develop software using the operating system vendor's tools and depends on that vendor for the expertise to make changes as new hardware appears. Although computer hardware has advanced rapidly, with price decreases often approaching 30% to 40% annually, similar advances have not occurred with software. Productivity improvements depend much on being able to build upon advances developed by others. Properly developed applications software then can take advantage of newer hardware with minimal or no changes.

LIS CHARACTERISTICS
Overall Functions

Most LIS support similar functions and allow a laboratory to control and monitor the execution of critical actions (Box 18-1). These functions include specimen collection, order entry, manual results entry, results reporting, and interfaces to automated instrumentation and other computer systems. Additionally, an LIS usually generates management reports and other ad hoc reports. LIS for hospitals support phlebotomy by providing blood-drawing lists and specimen labels; systems for independent laboratories usually include specimen tracking and financial and billing functions.

Most vendors separate the LIS into separate modules for marketing and functional reasons. Typically these modules include a general laboratory module, such as those supporting the high-volume hematology and chemistry areas that mostly provide numeric results; a microbiology module, a blood bank module; and an anatomical pathology module. Larger institutions may use two or more LIS vendors. In such cases, one vendor provides general laboratory functions and another vendor supports one or more other areas, such as blood bank, anatomical pathology, or customer billing. LIS vendors may also interface to third-party blood bank software to reduce Food and Drug Administration (FDA) regulatory require-

---

BOX 18-1

LIS FUNCTIONS

Preanalytical
Test ordering
Phlebotomy draw lists
Phlebotomy (labels, collection times)
Specimen accessioning and aliquoting
Specimen tracking
Incomplete list

Analytical
Manual worklist
Instrument worklist
Manual results entry
Automated results entry through interfaces
Patient delta check
Quality control
Results validation
Interfaces to laboratory automation systems

Postanalytical
Noncumulative patient chart reports
Patient cumulative chart reports
Immediate remote report printing
Electronic results inquiry
Historical patient archiving
Workload recording
Results correction
Billing
Results interfaces to other systems

DATA ACQUIRED DURING ORDER-ENTRY PROCESS

1. A patient identifier, such as a patient number and a patient name
2. One or more ordering physicians
3. One or more physicians receiving reports with their reporting locations
4. Test request time and date
5. Time the specimen was collected or will be collected
6. Person entering the request
7. Tests to be performed
8. Priority of the test request (such as stat, now, routine)
9. Any special comments or instructions pertaining to the request

---

ments. The following sections cover the features of an LIS that supports the general laboratory areas.

Patient Demographics

Before any test requesting can occur, the patient must first be defined in the system with an identifying number and other patient-specific information, called **patient demographics**. Most hospitals assign a permanent patient identification number for this purpose. Systems serving reference laboratories or outreach programs may define patients under the auspices of the client sending the test. A clerk can manually enter the demographic information into the LIS. Alternatively, an interface between an LIS and an **ADT (Admissions/Discharge/Transfer)** administrative computer system allows the information to be transmitted to the LIS when needed during test request processing, upon admission of the patient to the hospital, or when a patient is scheduled for an outpatient visit. Automated ADT interfaces can significantly reduce errors associated with data entry, as well as reduce data entry time. Demographic information entered at this time includes (1) the patient number, (2) patient name, (3) sex, (4) age or birth date, (5) referring or attending physician to receive reports by default, and (6) admitting diagnosis. Most systems also capture some patient information such as height and weight, as well as billing and accounting information. If a patient

number cannot be determined, such as when handling an unconscious accident patient treated in an emergency room, the laboratory may assign a pseudo number and pseudo name. These pseudo data must be changed later and merged into a record with the proper patient information.

Order Entry

Following the admission of the patient, the next LIS interaction is usually the processing of a test request, also known as **order entry**. Orders may be received by the LIS through a computer-to-computer interface, for example, with a hospital information system (HIS), from which nursing personnel or physicians can directly perform the test request. Alternatively, the laboratory receives a paper requisition from a clinical area, and laboratory personnel enter the test request into the LIS. Typically, order entry requires the entry of, or the acquisition of, the information listed in the box above.

Numerous checks are performed by the LIS as a part of the data entry process. Most systems maintain internal tables that contain lists of valid test entry personnel, physicians, patient locations, available laboratory tests, and even reasonable dates. These tables prevent the entry of erroneous information but also require updates, also referred to as *table maintenance*. Most institutions also incorporate a *check-digit* with patient numbers or any other number requiring some form of self-validation. This is often a single digit included as a part of the patient number that is computed during data entry from digits in the patient number. If the computed number does not match the check-digit the data entry is rejected. For example, if the patient number is 12345676 and the last digit is the check-digit, one way to generate a check-digit calculation is to use the formula:

$$\text{check-digit} = [2*C_1+3*C_2+4*C_3+5*C_4+6*C_5+7*C_6+2*C_7]\text{modulo }10$$

in which the modulo function is the remainder after dividing the result by 10. Therefore the calculated result is:

$$\text{check-digit} = [2*(1)+3*(2)+4*(3)+5*(4)+6*(5)+7*(6)+2*(7)] \text{ modulo }10$$
$$= 6$$

If the clerk types 22345676, the check-digit calculation will result in a 7. Because 6 is expected, the computer rejects the patient number. Check-digits do not guarantee accuracy, but when properly designed, help reduce errors without requiring the computer to look up details on the patient.

Test requesting in the order entry process appears deceptively simple, but numerous details complicate the process.[1] Even checking for duplicate orders by computer can be complicated, because a check for a single test must include situations in which it is ordered as a single test or as a component of ordering groups, such as a test panel. The allowable interval between duplicate test orders also depends on a number of factors, such as the ordering physician, the patient's location, the test, and the cost of performing the test. For example, a repeat electrolyte panel in an intensive care unit (ICU) might occur in less than an hour, but would not occur in less than a day for an outpatient. A daily testosterone level, however, is rarely needed as an inpatient or as an outpatient. For most tests, determining the appropriateness of a test order requires knowledge of the clinical situation. Unless ordering is performed by the physician caring for the patient, such information is rarely available at the time tests are ordered. Determination of the appropriate duplicate test interval through the consensus of all ordering clinicians or through a detailed review of their practices is a formidable task, and limitations with current computerized order entry generally make it time-consuming for physicians doing their own test ordering. Most LIS can check for duplicate orders to resolve operational problems, such as to prevent the same test from being accidentally ordered twice at the same phlebotomy draw. However, ordering rules are difficult to implement on most computer systems, and order checking is relatively ineffective in changing ordering behavior or for reducing the frequency of test ordering.

The order entry process itself can be a source of substantial errors. One study of nearly 115,000 requisitions reported that 4.8% had at least one error associated with the process and 10% of institutions reported that 18% or more of requisitions had errors.[2] Errors may be a result of clerical errors in the laboratory or nursing units. Direct entry of orders by physicians can substantially reduce clerical errors.[3] Unfortunately, most current computer systems require substantially more physician time to enter orders than paper systems. Although some improvements have been made in speeding physician order entry, physician time has been the greatest barrier to acceptance.

Phlebotomy

When the specimen is collected, laboratory personnel log it into the LIS as received. With automated equipment linked to the LIS this step can be automated (see Chapter 16). Otherwise the computer places the test requisition onto a collection list for future collection. In either case, the LIS then creates a specimen label containing collection information, such as the patient name, patient number, patient location, sex, age or birth date, tests ordered, and collection tube type (Fig. 18-1). Most specimen labels also include a *specimen*, or *accession*, *number* which is a tracking number that allows the computer to reference that sample back to a specific test request and patient. **Specimen numbers** may be assigned for each phlebotomy

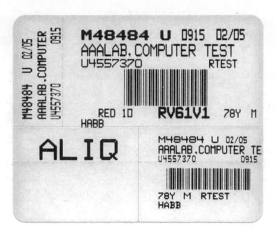

Fig. 18-1 An example of a bar-coded specimen label. The specimen number (M48484) is bar coded. The patient number, patient demographics, time/date, and test are written in human-readable form. The label is perforated so that it can be applied to both the primary specimen tube and its aliquoted samples.

transaction or, less commonly, for each orderable test. Another approach, used by larger laboratories, requires separate specimen numbers for different processing areas or for many of the larger laboratory automation systems (see Chapter 16). To keep numbers short, some LIS recycle specimen numbers. Systems reusing specimen numbers must check to see if a number is inactive before reassignment. Some systems assign a permanent specimen number by combining a date code with a number. Although this offers advantages of a permanent specimen number, the larger number adds to the work associated with manual data entry. In most cases the LIS assigns a specimen number at the time of test requisition, but for tests ordered in the future, this assignment may occur later. Some systems allow users to reserve specimen numbers for manual assignment. Although this is convenient under conditions such as computer failure, manual assignment of specimen numbers greatly increases errors, especially if the same specimen number is accidentally assigned to multiple patients.

Bar Codes

Bar codes consist of a series of lines or squares of varying widths representing numbers, or letters and numbers, and are readable by automated equipment. A number of bar code formats exist. Most bar codes used in the laboratory are linear, constructed from parallel lines. The most common of these formats are Code 39 and Code 128. The older Codabar format has been used for labeling blood bank products and is limited to representing numbers. Code 39 can represent numbers and upper case alphabets. Code 128 can represent numbers, upper/lower case alphabets, and some special symbols. Two-dimensional bar codes consist of squares of varying sizes ordered in rows and can store much more information, such as calibration data for reagents. Because of complexities of scanning a two-dimensional bar code, they are infrequently used for specimen containers where high-speed automation is likely to be used. Most bar code readers and printers can read and print multiple formats. Bar code readers may be self-scanning, such as laser-based units found in grocery stores, or user scanned with a penlike device. Self-scanning bar code readers are more expensive than pens, but are easier to use.

Specimen label bar coding decreases errors in handling and increases productivity.[4] For maximum benefit, specimen bar coding must be coordinated with automated instrumentation; preferably the instrument will have the ability to automatically read bar codes applied to the tube. Misapplication of the specimen label can cause instruments to misread bar codes. Mechanical limitations of instruments and the use of small venipuncture tubes (for pediatric purposes) may impose limitations on the use of bar codes. Larger bar codes read more reliably, but compete for label space containing valuable human-readable information. The patient number is usually not included in the specimen bar code because it is not unique to a given test request. Only the specimen number or a part of the specimen number is typically bar coded. Standards have been developed for bar codes used in specimen containers used in instruments.[5]

For samples to be collected on future scheduled phlebotomy collections, the computer prints up a collection list and specimen collection labels (Fig. 18-2). The specimen labels can also serve as the collection list. After specimen collection, the phlebotomist or a clerk verifies collected samples and deletes or reschedules uncollected requests in the LIS. Hand-held computers with built-in bar code readers can allow phlebotomists to verify collection at the bedside and download the collection status to the host computer upon return to the laboratory, reducing time for phlebotomy verification and increasing the accuracy of the draw time. To increase accuracy, bar coding of the patient identification band allows a phlebotomist with a hand-held unit to match specimen requests to the proper patient.

Following collection, the specimen must be prepared for transport or analysis. The LIS often prints additional labels for aliquots or other purposes, either as part of the initial test request or on demand. If processing occurs at a satellite, the LIS can track the sample, schedule required transportation, determine specimen location, and help locate lost specimens. Automated specimen tracking can provide laborsaving benefits in a larger laboratory, where clinicians frequently add additional tests to samples presumed to be in the laboratory. In such cases, the technologist must locate a sample, enter the add-on test into the LIS, and print a new specimen label. If a sample cannot be found, a test request must be entered into the LIS for recollection by a phlebotomist or nurse. The complexity of the process for handling add-on testing frequently results in errors. For the purposes of identifying lost specimens and to complete the process, the laboratory can print an *incomplete list*, a report listing specimens that were or should have been collected, but failed to be processed.

Instrumentation, Instrument Interfaces, and Total Laboratory Automation Interfaces

Because automated instruments perform most high-volume testing, interfacing these instruments to an LIS greatly improves productivity and decreases errors. Before an instrument can

Fig. 18-2 A draw list using bar-coded specimen labels. The bottom label bar codes the patient number. The remaining labels bar code the specimen number, one for each collection tube type. Aliquot labels are available on the left of the bar-coded specimen label.

be interfaced, however, two conditions must be satisfied. First, the LIS and the instrument must be linked by a compatible physical connection. Most clinical laboratory instruments use the Electronic Industries Association RS-232C standard,[6] a standard connecting the instrument directly to the LIS (i.e., a point-to-point connection). Because of the higher data handling rates between the LIS and newer instruments and the design of newer computers, a point-to-point Ethernet connection over a **local area network (LAN)** may be used. Second, interface software must be available on the LIS to allow it to receive data from and transmit data to the instrument. The American Society for Testing and Materials (ASTM) and the National Committee for Clinical Laboratory Standards (NCCLS) have developed standards to facilitate the interfacing of instruments to a LIS.[7,8] Standards do not always guarantee easy compatibility, but they can significantly decrease problems with incompatibilities. Most instrument manufacturers provide LIS vendors with interface specifications before instruments are introduced into the marketplace to allow time for interface software development. Interfaces, however, are often customized for each instrument, and different interfaces may be needed for different versions of the same instrument.

In an interfaced instrument, each specimen must be linked to its specific test request; typically through a bar-coded specimen number. The instrument reads the bar-coded specimen label and transmits the number to the LIS along with the analytical results. With a **unidirectional interface**, the instrument only transmits or *uploads* results to the LIS computer; a **bidirectional interface** allows the LIS to simultaneously transmit or *download* information to and receive uploaded information from the instrument. The most common information downloaded to an instrument from the LIS is the tests that have been requested for the specimen. In a bidirectionally interfaced instrument, the instrument first transmits the specimen number to the LIS, the LIS then returns the information of which tests have been ordered, and finally the instrument sends the results to the LIS. The communications and interactions between the host LIS computer and the instrument can be complex. Adding to this complexity is the requirement of some instruments for an immediate response from the LIS upon reading the bar-coded specimen number. The software required for a unidirectional interface, therefore, is considerably simpler than that for a bidirectional interface.

If the instrument does not have the ability to identify the specimen automatically through the interface, the operator must manually link the sample at the instrument to the specimen number in the computer. The order in which the LIS processes specimens for a specified instrument is called a **worklist** or a *loadlist*. At least three ways are used to create the worklist. One method is to have the instrument operator manually create ("build") a worklist on the LIS by entering specimen numbers and the instrument position. For example, position 1 on the instrument contains specimen A, position 2 contains specimen B, and so on. Alternatively, only the specimen number can be entered and the order implicitly

provided without a physical cup or tray position. This method requires that results be released from the instrument in the order that specimens are processed. The third approach is to have the computer automatically build a worklist, typically in the order that specimens are received or in sample number order, and to have the operator load the instrument in that order. This frees the operator from entering the information needed for the worklist but requires him or her to locate specimens and load them in the specified order. For the smaller laboratory, the computer-generated worklist is more efficient because the receiving area can often place the specimens in the computer-specified order. In the larger laboratory, multiple receiving areas complicate the specimen receipt order, making it easier for the operator to specify explicitly the worklist with one of the first two approaches rather than searching for a specific specimen.

Some instruments, particularly those for blood-gas analyses, process samples on a one-at-a-time basis. Test ordering frequently occurs at the time of analysis rather than in advance. For such instruments, the interaction between the analyzer, the LIS, and the operator will be greater and more labor intensive than that for other instruments. The test request, resulting, and validation processes are similar to instruments mentioned earlier but occur serially and manually for each sample. Some older hematology analyzers also operate in this fashion.

Automation (Refer to Chapter 16 for a detailed discussion of laboratory automation.)

Total laboratory automation (TLA) refers to a highly automated laboratory environment where robotics, conveyors, other mechanical devices, and computer systems significantly decrease the human handling of samples. A *front-end automation* device usually performs many steps associated with preanalytical sample handling such as centrifugation, uncapping, aliquoting, and sorting. Specimen handlers, conveyors, and robotic arms transfer specimens to and from parts of the laboratory, the automation devices, and instrumentation. Once analysis has been performed, specimens are sorted and routed to storage and refrigeration, if needed, where they can be retrieved.

TLA requires most LIS to be significantly modified, and these modifications have been designated as a third-generation design.[9] For example, whereas many LIS generate a single specimen number for each patient contact, which may include several collection tubes, most TLA systems require that *each* tube possess a unique specimen number so that it can be properly routed. A TLA system may also have a separate *laboratory automation system* (LAS), a computer system specially designed for managing the automation devices and directing specimens. The LIS may treat the TLA system as an automated instrument.

The LIS usually interacts with the analytical instruments in a TLA system in a conventional manner. LIS validation of results is also likely to be similar to that of conventional automated instruments in which an operator reviews results before they are released for general use. In most TLA systems and with most high-volume instruments, manual verification may be replaced or supplemented with some form of *autoverification* algorithm to increase the accuracy and efficiency of verifying results.

Autoverification is an approach in which an LIS uses a defined set of parameters, such as the reference interval, for automatically releasing results without technologist review. Most LIS also have another parameter, called the *release range*, which is defined separately for the purposes of autoverification. The availability of the release range offers greater flexibility by allowing the user to block or automatically release results above or below the reference range. Other common capabilities in autoverification algorithms include the blocking of one or more results performed in a given sample if another parameter is out of autoverification range. For example, it is desirable to block autorelease of both the creatinine and blood urea nitrogen (BUN) results if only the creatinine value is out of autoverification range. A more complex algorithm is to block the release of the white blood cell (WBC) differential if the WBC count is below 1000. Effective autoverification may also review instrument "flags." For example, if the instrument detects that there was insufficient sample volume, reagents have been exhausted, or excessive hemolysis is present the LIS autoverification program should block all results for that sample (insufficient sample, gross hemolysis) or for that and all subsequent samples (insufficient reagent). Autoverification algorithms may also take into consideration clinical parameters. A platelet count of 20,000 may be acceptable for an oncology ward, for example, but would be unacceptable for a primary care clinic.

Integrating Off-Site Testing

Changes in microchip technology have lead to improved LIS-interfacing of *point-of-care testing* (*POCT*) devices (see Chapter 17). This is very important because users of these devices may fail to document the testing event or the test results in the patient's chart, especially the electronic record, which are both legally required. Increasingly, point-of-care (POC) instruments support the electronic uploading of results into an LIS. In such cases, the laboratory is typically responsible for this uploading.

In an attempt to address the problems of documenting results from off-site testing, POCT vendors have developed interface standards.[10] POCT devices, such as glucose meters, sell for less than $100. Because most LIS instrument interfaces cost 10 to 100 times that amount, LIS, POCT vendors, and users have all avoided interfacing LIS and POCT instruments. To make interfacing costs acceptable, a POC data manager, usually a personal computer with special software, acts as an intermediary receiving data from one or more portable devices through a plug-in cradle transmitting through preexisting wires or through an infrared transmitter. Once the data have been uploaded into the data manager, this intermediary makes an LIS test request or finds an existing one, uploads the result through a conventional ASTM-like laboratory instrument interface along with other pertinent patient information, documents and checks devices for proper maintenance, and ensures proper operational procedures. Because both the

LIS–data manager interface and the POCT instrument–data manager interfaces are standardized, it is possible for a single data manager to serve many POCT instruments.

Results Entry

Automated. The interaction between a technologist and automated instrumentation has been partially discussed previously. For a bidirectionally interfaced instrument, the results entry process proceeds automatically, usually after the specimen has been received by the laboratory. Most LIS place the results in a pending area, waiting for the technologist to manually review and validate the entered results (see previous section). This holding area limits results access only to those in the laboratory. Upon validation, results are released for reporting to external users. A number of LIS features may be available to help the technologist during the review process. Typically these include the display of flags signifying results outside reference ranges, life-threatening results (critical or "panic" values), results outside technical ranges, or those failing **delta checks** (see Chapter 3). Most LIS can also display previous results for the same tests, allowing the operator to do a check for sample misidentification.

Manual. The laboratory must perform manual results entry for specimens analyzed manually or for tests performed on instruments that are not interfaced. Many instruments are not interfaced for economic reasons. An interface may require highly complex and idiosyncratic software, forcing the LIS vendor to price it prohibitively high for most users. Alternatively a user may have such a low volume that an interface would not pay for itself when compared with manually entering results. Manual results entry may also be used when interfaces have failed or under special conditions such as abnormal tests being repeated on a different instrument. For batched tests, the operator first generates a manual worklist, similar to that described for an instrument, and prints a worksheet. The printed worksheet usually contains a list of specimen numbers with patient demographics and blank spaces for a user to write results. This worksheet is a guide for the specimen-processing order and provides a place to manually transcribe results so that they can be later entered with a terminal.

As the technologist manually enters results into the computer terminal, most systems check the data for technical credibility, life-threatening conditions, abnormal limits, and other conditions specified by the site, similar to checks for automated systems. Most systems compare the patient's current result with his or her previous result and alert the technologists to large changes (the *delta check*). In addition, the LIS alerts the technologist to a value outside of a specified range. To assist in the data entry process, software can perform automatic calculations, and terminals can be set up so that keyboards perform special functions. For example, programs can convert the numeric pad on a data entry terminal to a differential counter. To support the urinalysis area the computer can translate the single keystroke *m* into the word *many*. After results are entered, a validation report similar to that for an automated instrument is printed. This report is similar to the initial worklist with test results replacing blank lines. Normally, the technologist performing the test also validates the worklist in a manner similar to that for automated instruments. In some areas, a second technologist may be required to validate critical results in addition to, or in lieu of the first technologist. Even with computer assistance, manual data entry can be tedious and error prone, particularly if worklists are much longer than 100 to 150 tests. For efficiency, manual data entry occurs at the end of the workday or at the end of a run. This may also delay results reporting if completed results are held for data entry.

Data verification. Whether results are generated by an interfaced instrument or entered manually, the operator reviews and approves, or *validates*, test results before they are released for patient reporting. An exception occurs if an autoverification program (see earlier discussion) releases results. Usually **validation** is performed using a worklist. This validation process usually starts with review of a printed *validation report*, followed by the technologist excluding results (for additional investigations), and then batch validating the entire worklist on a terminal. Alternatively, validation can occur one specimen at a time on a terminal without a validation report. Batch validation may be more efficient for the instrument operator but delays reporting. For most systems, the validation review occurs in the specimen order the worksheet was created or in the numeric order of specimen numbers. If results exceed predetermined parameters, the operator must perform specified activities, such as a dilution or a repeat analysis. Frequently, the LIS displays both the initial and reanalyzed results and allows the operator to validate or reject one or both results.

Results Reporting

The end product of any clinical laboratory is its results, often in the form of paper reports. Although paper reports continue to be required for the patient chart and remain an important method for communication of laboratory results, increasingly, electronic transmittal via printers and computer terminals provides a more efficient alternative. Remote terminals allow users to retrieve both current and historical data. Depending on location and user expertise, either or both of these options may be used. Computers have reduced delays associated with test result availability to seconds, even though physical charting of reports may take hours to days. Computer reporting and retrieval of laboratory results have virtually replaced the paper report, greatly reducing personnel time and errors associated with telephone and manual transmission of results.

Paper reports continue to be important for reporting test results not required immediately and placing data in the medical chart. For outpatients, the LIS often prints a nightly report with all new test results and often lists pending tests. Duplicate copies may also be sent to ordering physicians or other clinical personnel. Most outpatient reports record the result in a straightforward manner containing (1) patient demographics (see earlier discussion), (2) time of report generation, (3) name of laboratory reporting and performing the test, if all the results are not from the same laboratory, (4) test name or names, (5) collection date and time for test(s), (6) result with

abnormal flags as needed, (7) reference range, (8) result and order comments, and (9) ordering physician(s). Where electronic reporting of results is available, paper reports serve little purpose because they are less timely and are more difficult to use. Regulations and common sense dictate that LIS have the capability to reprint reports easily on demand. Printer jams and, more commonly, lost reports occur frequently with paper reports.

For inpatients, chart reports are usually in a *cumulative* format (Fig. 18-3), in which current and past results are collected and printed in a tabular format. Most commonly, tests appear as a column on the page with test result dates displayed in rows horizontally. An alternative format is to have the dates appear in columns and tests in rows. With this tabular format, a very high density of results can appear on a page. Upon admission, any results reported within the last 3 to 5 days may be included in the **cumulative report**. Typically, the report accumulates results for an entire inpatient stay or some other predetermined interval. Temporary reports are printed until the end of this interval (as on patient discharge), at which time a final permanent report is printed. The cumulative format is almost always used for inpatients, but rarely for outpatients. For these patients, *noncumulative* reports typically contain one or more lines for a single test result (Fig. 18-4). The main reason for not using cumulative reports on outpatients is the difficulty in charting reports and in determining the next time tests will be ordered.

Printer technology continues to change, resulting in changing appearances of patient reports. With impact printers, the uniformity of the typefaces in reports makes them difficult to read and prohibits graphics. With laser printers, varying print sizes and typefaces help emphasize significant findings and make reports more readable but at higher costs for printer consumables. Many LIS allow the inclusion of **interpretive reports** to assist clinicians. These reports contain comments to explain one or more result patterns (Fig. 18-5). Such reports, though welcomed by primary care practitioners, are likely to be ignored by specialists, and the laboratory must use them selectively. Most commercial LIS systems still limit the use of graphical images in reports because images require significant resources.

Quality Control

Refer to Chapter 21 for a more complete discussion of quality control.

The LIS can also contribute greatly to improved efficiency of technologists and laboratory managers by supporting quality control (QC) and quality assurance (QA) procedures (see later discussion). These activities include maintaining desired precision and accuracy of results and monitoring critical laboratory functions, such as turnaround time. QA and QC procedures tend to be consistent among most laboratories, because regulatory requirements under CLIA '88[11] require strict adherence to specified guidelines (see Chapter 2). These regulations require laboratories to retain QC information associated with any released test result, and most LIS capture these data and automatically or manually link QC results to patient data.

08/23/2001
16:54

UNIVERSITY OF WASHINGTON MEDICAL CENTER
INCLUDING LABORATORIES AT UWMC, HMC AND SCCA

CUMULATIVE SUMMARY
PAGE 1

Name: AAALAB, COMPUTER TEST
Pt #:   U4557370

Age: 25Y   Sex: F
Loc: TEST   Room: RTEST

*** BLOOD ELECTROLYTES AND COMMON CHEMISTRIES ***

TEST:	NA	K	CL	CO2	ANION GAP	GLU	WHOLE BLOOD GLU	BUN	CREAT
UNITS:	mEq/L	mEq/L	mEq/L	mEq/L		mg/dL	mg/dL	mg/dL	mg/dL
LO-HI:	136-145	3.7-5.2	98-108	22-32	5-20	62-125	62-125	8-21	0.3-1.2
01/21/01									
1130	135*	4.3	103	22	15	156*		23*	1.3*
1140	143	3.5*	105	20*	10	156*		23*	1.4*
RCV1712		3.5*							
02/01/01									
RCV0834	139	4.3	109*	19*	11	83		54*	2.1*
RCV0924	145	4.0	105	20*	NOT DONE				
04/05/01									
RCV1039						100			

= = = = = = = = = = = = = = = = = = = BLOOD ELECTROLYTES AND COMMON CHEMISTRIES =

TEST:	ALB
UNITS:	g/dL
LO-HI:	3.5-5.2
01/21/01	
1005	3.5
1145	2.3*
RCV1247	2.4*
1303	2.3*
01/23/01	
1300	2.3*

*** CALCIUM METABOLISM ***

TEST:	SERUM CALCIUM	CALCIUM SERUM IONIZED	SERUM PO4	SERUM MG	PTH
UNITS:	mg/dL	mmol/L	mg/dL	mg/dL	pg/mL
LO-HI:	8.9-10.2	1.18-1.38	3.0-4.5	1.8-2.4	10-65
01/21/01					
1005	8.8*		4.5	1.3*	
1145	7.0*		8.5*	2.0	
RCV1247	7.5*		6.0*	1.3*	
1303	8.1*		2.3*	1.3*	
01/23/01					
1300	8.8*		1.5*	1.2*	
04/04/01					
0800	10.8*			<1* NREF8	

- - - FOOTNOTES - - -
NREF8   Note new reference range effective 8/3/99

AAALAB, COMPUTER TEST
4-55-73-70

PAGE 1
INPATIENT CUMULATIVE SUMMARY
08/23/2001

Fig. 18-3   A cumulative patient report. *(Courtesy University of Washington Medical Center.)*

Name: AAALAB, COMPUTER TEST   Age: 25Y   Sex: F   *** PATIENT   ***
Pt #:   U4557370   Loc: TEST   Room: RTEST   *** DISCHARGED ***

X54 783   COLL: 01/21/2001 10:05 REC: 01/21/2001   12:10

Chemistry Panel 2
   Albumin   3.5   [3.5-5.2]   g/dL
   Magnesium   *1.3   [1.8-2.4]   mg/dL
   Calcium   *8.8   [8.9-10.2]   mg/dL
   Phosphate   4.5   [3.0-4.5]   mg/dL

X54052   COLL: 01/21/2001 11:30 REC: 01/21/2001   12:23

Chemistry Panel 1
   Sodium   *135   [136-145]   mEq/L
   Potassium   4.3   [3.7-5.2]   mEq/L
   Chloride   103   [98-108]   mEq/L
   Carbon Dioxide   22   [22-32]   mEq/L
   Ion Gap   15   [5-20]
   Glucose   *156   [62-125]   mg/dL
   Urea Nitrogen   * 23   [8-21]   mg/dL
   Creatinine   * 1.3   [0.3-1.2]   mg/dL

[   ] = Reference Range
AAALAB, COMPUTER TEST   END OF REPORT   PAGE 1

Fig. 18-4   A noncumulative patient report. *(Courtesy University of Washington Medical Center.)*

Name: AAALAB, COMPUTER TEST   Age: 25Y   Sex: F
Pt #:   U4557370   Loc: TEST   Room: RTEST

** GENETIC DNA WORKUPS **

04/26/01
0930   Hemochromatosis DNA Screen

       Hemochromatosis Results   Two mutations detected (H63D, H63D)

       Hemochromatosis Interp   This genotype may very slightly increase the risk of developing iron overload, but the DNA test
                                     results alone cannot make a diagnosis of hereditary hemochromatosis. Although this genotype
                                     occurs in 1-2% of patients with hereditary hemochromatosis, it is also very common (3–4%) in the
                                     general Caucasian population. Periodic monitoring of iron status to determine if progressive iron
                                     accumulation is occurring may be appropriate in some cases. Method: The C282Y and H63D
                                     mutations in the HFE gene were detected by melting curve analysis of amplified gene products
                                     (for details, call the Laboratory). Karen Stephens, Ph.D., Jonathan Tait, M.D., Ph.D., Laboratory
                                     Directors.

                                     This test is used for clinical purposes and should not be regarded as investigational or for research
                                     use only. This test was developed and its performance characteristics determined by the Dept. of
                                     Laboratory Medicine at UW. This laboratory is certified under CLIA-88 and is qualified to perform
                                     high complexity clinical testing.

                                     This test has not been cleared or approved by the U.S. Food and Drug Administration. The FDA
                                     has determined that such clearance or approval is not necessary.

AAALAB, COMPUTER TEST   PAGE 1
4-55-73-70   INPATIENT CUMULATIVE SUMMARY
                                                                                                08/23/2001

Fig. 18-5   An interpretive patient report. The results are analyzed in the Interp section. *(Courtesy University of Washington Medical Center.)*

CLIA '88 defines a **run** as an interval for which the accuracy and precision of a testing system is expected to be stable, but no longer than 24 hours. Most LIS allow users to define a run that matches a physical sample tray or to perform continuous analyses between controls. These runs, however, may not meet CLIA requirements if they do not have proper control samples. Most LIS evaluate the status of controls in real-time and provide the instrument operator with immediate feedback if the QC results are out of the expected range. Most instruments have built-in computers, and it is uncommon for an LIS to support the derivation of standard curves from calibration samples. Although the LIS can restrict release of results for runs by reviewing control data, calibration data, and performing other checks, such as running averages and Westgard rules, most systems leave such decisions to the operator.

Numerous QC calculations are easily and commonly performed by an LIS. These include routine checking for controls that deviate more than a specified number of standard deviations from an expected mean or that deviate from expected values determined by established rules.[12] Delta checking a patient value with his or her own previous result can also assist in identifying a QC or specimen identification problem.[13,14] In larger laboratories interinstrument, intermethod, and test-level comparisons of controls and calibrations help ensure result consistency. Most LIS systems can typically provide such QC information both in summary format and as the analysis is performed. Levy-Jennings plots are popular for following and displaying such information. Typically, LIS collect control statistics by instrument, by methodology, and by analyte and allow comparisons of controls at multiple levels.

Quality Assurance (Refer to Chapters 2, 3, and 21 for further discussions of quality assurance.)

The LIS can collect and provide much QA information as a part of its daily activities. QA differs from QC in that it monitors more global and less quantifiable parameters about the quality of the work produced by the laboratory rather than only the accuracy and precision of the testing. The ability of the LIS to perform 100% sampling with little effort encourages a level of laboratory monitoring not possible with a manual system. Several examples follow.

First, turnaround time has become an important indicator of the overall average quality of service for high acuity areas of the hospital. Coupled with specimen tracking, such information assists the manager in identifying operational bottlenecks by looking at samples exceeding predetermined parameters and by looking at the overall average service quality. This helps to properly staff areas and identify peak work periods.

Second, management reports can also assist in identifying sources of error. Errors can occur during the preanalytical processing, during test analysis, or after analysis. The most frequent error in the preanalytical process is misidentification of the patient or the specimen. Preanalytically and postanalytically, manual data entry can have as much as a 1% to 3% error rate, most of which is unlikely to be detected even with sophisticated tools such as delta checking, supervisor validation, or other tools. One way of evaluating errors is to compare

the data entered into the computer automatically with the data expected to be entered manually. Although this comparison can be tedious, it can identify systematic problems associated with data entry of results or requisitions. The computer can provide information regarding the test results that have been corrected. Summarizing this information assists in identifying causes. Proper handling of errors is a difficult, but necessary action. Most systems provide a way to change results after they have been validated. Depending on the laboratory, the responsibility for correcting results may be limited to a few or many individuals. Possibly the most difficult aspect about changing results lies in the impact on patient reports. Although reports may be reprinted, older reports remain in the chart and are potentially confusing. Most federal and other regulatory agencies require that corrected results be indicated as such on patient reports.

Third, the laboratory can monitor the quality of patient care by combining data from other hospital computer systems, such as a pharmacy system. Adverse effects associated with gentamicin, for example, can be reduced by coupling drug dispensation records with drug levels, renal function tests, and antimicrobial sensitivity patterns. This information can then be used to warn a clinician of drug toxicity or ineffective dosing. Fourth, a report of patients with grossly abnormal results provides interesting teaching cases and helps detect possible problems.

Most LIS perform significant QA reporting through epidemiology and cytology subsystems to meet Joint Commission on Accreditation of Healthcare Organizations (JCAHO) and CLIA regulations. Although these activities can be performed on other computers, the level of detail contained in most LIS in these areas allows more accurate reporting. Many other examples exist, and unfortunately, most information systems are capable of generating far more data than can be reviewed. Often, requesters of QA data also fail to realize the human resources and computer time needed to generate useful reports. For example, a programmer may be asked to retrieve historical patient data that has been stored haphazardly and inconsistently, requiring repeated searches of patient records. Such situations translate to intensive computer searches lasting weeks followed by manual examination of the collated data. Because few sites have spare computers to perform such data analyses, these searches can interfere with daily laboratory activities by slowing down response time and by consuming labor.

Management Reporting

Although some view management reports as a byproduct of implementing a computer system, others view them as a principal benefit of a computer. At the organizational level, the management information provided by information systems may not prove useful until trends have been established after several years. Much of the information collected for QC and QA mentioned earlier may also be used for managing operations. In addition to those reports, several others are most frequently used for management purposes. One of the more commonly used reports from any LIS is a list of tests and their ordering frequency. This information may be used from an operational perspective for projecting the need for instrumentation, personnel, and other resources. Another common report is a list of billing transactions, usually generated nightly. Using computer statistics, standard methods for monitoring workload provide information regarding appropriate personnel staffing and help to reschedule employees as test ordering patterns change.[15] Workload information also helps to identify inefficient work areas or individuals.

All laboratory computer systems can provide data on physician test ordering patterns. Unfortunately, these data are frequently difficult to interpret, because requisitions may contain missing ordering physicians or the order may have been performed by a medical student using an attending physician's name. The politics of managing test ordering are also difficult. With the advent of cost containment in healthcare, however, such data are being used more frequently to focus on and to eliminate unnecessary testing.

LIS TECHNOLOGY

Hardware refers to the physical parts of a computer, which are typically mass-produced. *Software* collectively refers to a series of instructions, called *programs*, which direct the behavior of a computer. Software may be mass-produced or customized for a specialized application. Both hardware and software are often updated after delivery. Because of this, the initial purchase price for an LIS may represent less than half of its total cost over its lifetime. Programming is an intellectual activity and requires large amounts of time and effort. Increasing software complexity has driven costs up dramatically. In 1970, software contributed approximately 10% of the total cost of an LIS, and by 2000 software often exceeded 90% of LIS cost. Software in an LIS includes the applications programs, database managers, interpreters, and operating systems.

Hardware

Computer technology advances even after more than 30 years of continuous improvement. New disk and microchip technology, competition, and production techniques have greatly reduced computer costs. In 1993, the total installed number of personal computers exceeded 140 million. Manufacturers predicted that 130 million worldwide and 38 million U.S. personal computers would be shipped in 2001.[16] As silicon microchip technology has advanced, distinctions between the various classes of computers have largely been lost because larger and more powerful computers are often clusters or aggregates of smaller computers. Typically, larger computers are used and are cost effective only if shared, either with other applications (such as a financial system), or if serving multiple hospitals.

At the heart of any computer lies the **central processing unit** or **CPU**. A CPU is responsible for making logical decisions, performing computations, and translating program instructions into actions. Typically, the CPU consists of one or more silicon chips and their closely associated circuitry. A CPU requires *RAM*, or *random access memory*, which is analogous to short-term memory in humans. The CPU can put data into or retrieve data from the RAM. Data requiring longer-term storage are moved to *disks* and *tapes*. Disks store data in either magnetic or optical form on a rotating medium. Optical media have higher density, that is, they can store more data in a given area. Optical media are frequently used for historical data and in CD-ROM format can be used for data distribution. Old data may be moved to magnetic tape, but the linear format of tape makes some types of data retrieval slower than from optical disk. Because writing to magnetic tape is rapid, it is often used to **backup** disks. Disk *backups* of LIS data must be performed regularly so that data can be recovered after a disk failure, or *disk crash*. Another way to protect against disk crashes is through *disk shadowing*, in which two or more disks duplicate each other.

Software

An *operating system* is a program supervising the orderly execution of programs and supporting the basic functions commonly used by all programs. Some of these functions include management of disks and disk files, support for terminals and printers, and computer networking (see following section). Microsoft Windows is an operating system for the IBM-PC. Unix and its variant Linux are common operating systems. For applications such as the laboratory, *real-time* capability is necessary. This term refers to the need to capture input data and process them immediately. For example, a high-volume instrument requires that an LIS respond with the tests to be performed within 5 seconds after being sent a specimen number.

Computers are synonymous with data management and data processing. Programs generally operate on *data* included within the program itself or on data acquired from sources external to the program, such as patient data. In either case, such data and their organization are called the **data structure**. Data stored on disks, tapes, and other devices external to the main memory, or the CPU, are organized and grouped into *files*. Although files and data structures may contain explicit information about the purpose and type of data stored, some data may be implicit. For example, an accounting system may omit the dollar sign ($) and the decimal point so that $15.25 appears as 1525. Because the possibilities for the data structure are limitless, implicit information holds significant importance.

The purpose of any database design is to store data in such a fashion as to permit their retrieval in a sufficiently fast manner. Although it is possible to store data unorganized and attempt their retrieval sequentially, computers will reach practical limits despite their speed. To make retrieval practical, data are usually stored in a manner reflecting the way they will be used. Data structures are critical to the design of programs. Stored patient data in an LIS consumes most of the disk and memory storage. In an LIS, the amount of laboratory data easily exceeds the programs needed to run a system by several orders of magnitude. The design of the data structure may impose limitations on the stored information. To describe the structure of databases, the *hierarchical* and *relational* database models have been developed. Although most databases do

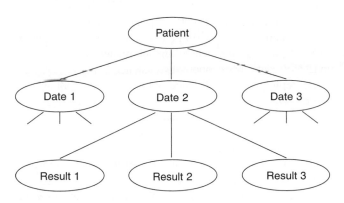

Fig. 18-6   A database with a hierarchical data relationship. The data are organized so that using the patient as the main starting index retrieves them.

not use any single model in a pure fashion, these models provide insights to some of the complications and tradeoffs associated with implementing data management systems.

The simplest and most often used model in laboratory systems is the **hierarchical database**. In this model, all data are treated as an inverted treelike structure with all data elements descending from a root. In an LIS, the root element is usually a unique patient identifier such as the patient name or a patient number (Fig. 18-6). For routine retrievals of patient care data, this data model usually works very well and can efficiently use computer resources. For selected abnormal laboratory results, however, this model fails, because it forces the computer to search all results on all patients. If such cases are frequently encountered, another tree must be built for storing the data again to gain satisfactory performance. Multiple copies of data introduce other problems, particularly if data are changed. Despite the performance of modern hardware, efficiency is still important when working with very large data sets. The M programming language, for example, directly supports a hierarchical database.

LIS vendors build their products around a *database manager*, software responsible for handling the physical storage and retrieval of data. A database manager may be viewed as a programming language. Most database managers are

constructed around the **relational database** model.[17] The relational database model is designed so that the data appear as tables and database operations become operations on tables (Fig. 18-7). This flexibility has earned relational databases a strong role in situations in which data are manipulated frequently, as in a research setting. A side effect of this flexibility is that relational databases use computer resources less efficiently than simpler models do, and this may present problems with very large data sets. Some examples of relational databases are IBM's DB2, Oracle, and Sybase. Relational databases for high-volume data transactions challenge the real-time requirements of an LIS, especially from a performance and cost perspective.

Computer Networks and the Internet

A *computer* **network** is any interconnection between computer systems, or between a computer terminal and a computer system, that supports the interchange of data. In the simplest and earliest networks in the late 1960s, computers connected to telephone lines with *modems*, devices that converted digital signals from computers to audio signals compatible with telephone lines. By the 1970s the Defense Advanced Research Projects Agency (ARPA) sponsored the research and development of a nationwide network. The ARPAnet became the precursor of the Internet. This technology was primitive compared to current **digital computer networks** that use high-speed fiber optic cables, digital subscriber lines (DSL), cable television lines, and cellular telephones. Fiber optic cables are most often used as a backbone to interconnect major parts of a network, DSL, cable television lines, and cellular telephone technologies typically connect the end user to the backbone. If the network is physically located within a limited locale, such as 1 to 2 miles, it is called a *local area network* or *LAN*. Interconnected LANs form a **wide area network** or **WAN** and the Internet is the global interconnection of many WANs. High-speed LAN technology is inexpensive (less than $10 to $20 per computer) and often user installed. Most computers found in businesses include Ethernet as an integral part of the hardware, and such systems require networks to communicate

For a data relationship that follows the structure:

{patient–1, date–1, sodium–1, potassium–1, calcium–1, TSH–1}

{patient–2, date–2, sodium–2, potassium–2, calcium–2, TSH–2}

{patient–3, date–3, sodium–3, potassium–3, calcium–3, TSH–3}

⋮
⋮

The data appear as a table:

Patient	Date	Sodium	Potassium	Calcium	TSH
James Smith	10/3/01	144 mEq/L	4.5 mEq/L	10.1 mg/dL	none
James Smith	10/20/01	138 mEq/L	none	none	3.4 µU/mL
John Jones	11/30/01	154 mEq/L	none	none	none

Fig. 18-7   Structure and data elements in a relational database. Data can be retrieved either by any single or by combinations of columns and rows.

with other computers, such as for ADT and billing functions. Interchanging data between different computers requires software to support a common protocol, or an agreed way to interchange data. On a network, computer systems interact with each other as either a **client** or as a **server**. The server computer stores the data from which the desktop client computer retrieves and processes data. In a large system hundreds of clients can access a single server computer. A single client may access one or more servers. Typically a client serves one user at a time.

The Internet has gained prominence with the introduction of the Internet browser.[18] This development integrated a number of existing network protocols into a user-friendly interface with graphics capabilities. Internet browsers, such as Netscape Navigator or Microsoft Internet Explorer, are clients supporting the hypertext transport protocol (HTTP) and the hypertext markup language (HTML) and interact with Internet web servers to enable users to perform the familiar "web surfing" activities. These browsers may also interact with traditional information systems modified to support the HTML and HTTP protocols. Internet browsers, because of their prevalence and ease of use, are frequently used as a user interface into LIS and other information systems. Internet computers often register a unique name or **uniform resource locator (URL)** so that users for e-mail, a browser, or other services can conveniently reference them. Most users connect to the Internet, through an *Internet service provider* or *ISP*. Service bureaus may also provide access to a patient information database, LIS, or billing system through the Internet. Such providers are called *application service providers* or *ASP*. Useful web sites on the Internet containing information for medical **informatics** and clinical chemistry and their URLs are listed at the end of the chapter.

Microwave satellite, cellular telephone, and other radio frequency systems are supporting mobile computing activities. For example, some vendors are providing hand-held portable units for phlebotomists to more accurately report collection times and to provide better patient identification. These systems may also be used to interconnect computer systems when cables cannot be used or are inconvenient. Most of these mobile technologies are substantially more expensive than cable-based systems. The effect of all these network technologies has been to allow the integration of information from physically diverse locations. Networks are critical for supporting laboratory facilities, by allowing remote locations to have access to patient data, and allowing the creation of a regional healthcare delivery system.[19,20] Such satellite operations become increasingly important as laboratories expand as a part of healthcare alliances.

Maintenance

Following the installation of a computer system, the user must perform numerous routine activities, often referred to as *maintenance*. *System maintenance* refers to routine housekeeping activities performed by the LIS. These activities are necessary to sustain proper functions and to allow for data recovery in case of failures. *Backup*, or making a copy of files, is one such activity. Computers also require regular **file maintenance**, during which the computer reorganizes and updates its data. Most operating systems and databases allow housekeeping activities to occur with the system still available to users. Disk space is frequently limited by design or physical limitations. As a result, inactive patient data must be *archived*, or transferred to storage tapes or optical disks periodically and *purged* from the active disk. Programs are usually available that restore the **archived data** for reprinting of reports or other purposes, or allow the processing of archived data directly. Users wishing to access archived data may incur delays while waiting for an operator to load the appropriate tape or optical disk. Magnetic tape and disks are not permanent because data may "fade" in 5 to 10 years. Optical disks, however, appear to have greater permanence and will likely satisfy legal definitions for archiving.

Software maintenance refers to the processes associated with updating software after installation. Updates may include repair of software defects or design problems, enhancements, support for new hardware or operating systems, and changes in the user environment. Because updates occur as often as several times a year, software updates usually cause more downtime than unanticipated failures. Users are often tempted to skip updates in an LIS that is operating satisfactorily, but these deferrals must be balanced by other considerations. Vendors refuse support for older software, and new software may not operate properly with older software. Maintenance charges remain a significant source of revenue for software vendors, often amounting to 1% to 1.5% per month of the original purchase price. Conversely, maintenance charges are a significant expense for users. Skilled users may terminate software support to save expenses, especially when they perceive that they are getting little benefit. Vendors often entice users to continue software support by offering enhancements. Maintenance also includes updates dictated by local changes, such as the introduction of new automated instrumentation or the replacement of a financial system with which the LIS interfaces. Locally mandated changes can easily add another 25% to maintenance costs.

Privacy and Data Security

Privacy is defined as those activities designed to protect information from being accessed by unauthorized individuals or parties. **Security** refers to activities designed to ensure that data are not altered unintentionally. Balancing privacy, data security, and access to medical information challenges computer systems, especially as computerized databases increase in use and systems are exposed to external, Internet activities. The LIS holds information directly accessible throughout the laboratory, and in many cases, throughout the hospital. As the technology for the electronic medical record improves, the availability of prepaid medical care increases, and national healthcare progresses; privacy, security, and the need for information come into even greater conflict by creating demands for greater information.[21,22] Computers can both provide ready access to information and control ordering, but can achieve this only at the risk of reducing privacy and possibly security. Federal legislation (HIPPA, see below), finalized in 2001,[23] sets standards and imposes significant penalties for violations of patient privacy and data security for healthcare providers.

Early LIS focused on laboratory activities and minimally addressed privacy issues. Access codes identified the technologist and the functions allowed to each user. Expansion of LIS access to clinicians benefited both laboratories and clinicians, but complicated privacy. Privacy remained relatively unimportant, because most data were not particularly sensitive and the number of external users was limited. As systems increased the amount of patient data being stored in electronic medical records, the likelihood of exposing sensitive information increased. Most systems today are not designed to resist systematic and determined attacks to gain access.

To control access into the LIS, most current systems require the use of a username, followed by a password. Passwords should be of sufficient length and complexity to prevent guessing. Even long passwords based on common dictionary words can be guessed by systematic attacks at an LIS. Systems or laboratory procedures should force the changing of passwords at regular intervals. Most systems limit access to system functions and test results by user codes. For example, physicians might have access only for test results inquiry, laboratory technologists might have access to ordering, resulting, and inquiry functions, whereas order entry clerks have access only to test ordering functions. A special access privilege might be needed for accessing data such as HIV results. Systems should automatically disconnect inactive terminals to prevent inappropriate access. Managing access rights in a large institution can be an extraordinarily difficult problem because residents, interns, and students change services frequently and information regarding their role can be difficult to obtain. Personal information implied by data such as home address, patient location, appointments, and billing transactions also affects privacy, but is difficult to block because of the large number of people requiring access to such data.[24]

Many new technologies have introduced substantial challenges for both privacy and security. First, most computers are connected to data networks, and many networks are connected to the Internet. Networks allow access to confidential information from physically remote sites, and make setting up physical restrictions for accessing the data difficult. Infrequently, malicious intruders destroy or alter data. Technical complexity and resource limitations prevent vendors and users from responding successfully. For example, data encryption on networks is seldom used, making interception of data easy. Second, national healthcare and healthcare costs have resulted in increased use of databases. Private insurance carriers also routinely collect and store patient information. Interchange and dissemination of such information, both for patient and provider benefits, further compromises privacy and security. Lastly, the common use of networks and microcomputers in LIS products has exposed many systems to destructive computer **viruses**, which are computer programs that embed themselves into the operating system

programs. Many viruses remain dormant for periods of time and are not destructive. Some, however, perform destructive actions, such as the alteration or destruction of data. Security and privacy require that LIS vendors deal with conflicting laws and diversified medical practices without inhibiting the convenient access to data. Users must be educated and encouraged to take steps to guard privacy. For example, networks and computers must be designed with data security considerations as forethought rather than as afterthought. Patient care computers should be isolated from outside network access, either physically or by use of **firewalls**, electronic devices designed to control traffic into and out of a network. Properly used firewalls can reduce unwanted intrusions into a computer. Messages sent over a public network should be *encrypted*, or scrambled, so that only their intended recipients can unscramble them. Messages sent over the Internet can also be encapsulated through a *virtual private network*, or *VPN*, in which all conversations between computers are encrypted by special hardware devices. Internet web sites and software using web-based software operating over the Internet are particularly vulnerable to malicious exploits because (1) the web server and the user client operate on a network open to the public, (2) because the browser and server software are inherently less secure than proprietary protocols, and (3) because the software is widely distributed. The tight integration of popular desktop software (word processors, spreadsheets, and presentation graphics) with web browsers and e-mail systems offers even more opportunities for exploits because a virus can link itself to web pages, e-mail messages, and files and propagate to other networked computers.

Regulatory Requirements

Federal regulations and accreditation agencies have greatly affected the design and functionality of LIS from both a vendor and user perspective. The most significant effects are those covering laboratory and information systems requirements under CLIA '88[11]; the FDA's ruling on LIS, especially blood bank systems as a medical device; and regulations on billing, patient privacy, and data security mandated under the **Health Insurance Portability and Accountability Act of 1996 (HIPPA)**. Lesser impacts on the LIS, but not necessarily on the laboratory, include requirements for the laboratory to collect diagnosis codes from the ordering provider on outpatient testing reimbursed by Medicare, a requirement under the Balanced Budget Act of 1997.

CLIA '88 has lead to major changes in clinical laboratory operations. Information systems are the most appropriate tool for managing record keeping and workload provisions required by this law. Areas covered by the law include the capture of quality control data, technologist workload, technologist proficiencies, and the proper operation of information systems. The major impact of CLIA '88 on the LIS lies in data-retention requirements. Records of test requests and results must be retained in a conveniently retrievable manner for 10 years for anatomical pathology and cytology results, 5 years for blood bank and immunohematology (HLA typing) results, and 2 years for all other results. Although it may be possible to retain data **on-line** in computer systems for this period of time, most laboratories archive the data to microfiche or optical disks for greater permanence.

In 1988, the FDA ruled that blood bank laboratory information systems are medical devices[25] requiring validation procedures similar to other medical devices, such as patient monitors.[26] Because such software affects the quality of blood products produced by a blood center, it is a part of the manufacturing process and is therefore subject to FDA review. LIS serving other laboratory areas are exempted from detailed validation because LIS data are reviewed by a clinician before use. Validation requires extensive testing, verification, and documentation by both the vendor and user.[27] Such procedures reduce software errors and user problems, but can greatly increase costs.

Voluntary accreditation agencies, such as the College of American Pathologists (CAP) and the JCAHO, often act as initial reviewers for compliance with federal and state regulations. Typical testing requirements for data processing include user procedures for documenting and validating software, documentation of software and hardware maintenance, and documentation of standard operating procedures.[28] CAP laboratory inspection checklists have added requirements for review of computerized verification of results, security, and privacy procedures.

MISCELLANEOUS

Role of the LIS with Other Hospital Computers

LIS often interact with other computers for receiving or transmitting of critical information. In a hospital setting, an administrative computer typically maintains patient information through interactions with other systems. These interactions include maintaining patient demographic information; verifying patient identification numbers and patient accounting information, and updating patient locations through an ADT system; receiving test requests through an order entry system; and sending results to an HIS. After performing the analysis, the LIS may send a transaction to a financial system to inform it of services that have been performed by the laboratory. The financial system then performs any needed billing and accounting, usually translating the LIS transactions into charges, common procedure terminology (CPT) codes, and other information required by most insurance carriers. If the LIS performs its own billing and accounting, it must send similar information to an insurance carrier either through an electronic data interchange (EDI) or through paper forms. Unfortunately, these complex interchanges between computers remain problematical and require constant maintenance because regulations constantly change (e.g., HIPPA has changed the procedures for EDI). Updates of test definitions in the laboratory require coordination with financial computer systems. Patient locations, test definitions, and other information must be coordinated with HIS and other clinical systems.

In most institutions, the LIS participates as one member in a complex quilt of unrelated and interconnected computerized information systems (Fig. 18-8). Depending on the institution, these computers may be operated at the departmental level, by a centralized information systems group, or a combination of both. Smaller institutions often share a centralized data processing service, which provides services for several institutions. Most often, central administrative groups operate large financial, order entry, and nursing care systems. Systems supporting ancillary services, such as pharmacy, radiology, and the laboratory, may function at either the departmental or centralized level. Typically, ancillary departments operate these systems in larger institutions whereas a centralized group supports them in small to medium-sized institutions. Some organizations attempt to improve information integration through administratively centralizing information systems and purchasing all software or hardware from a single vendor. Vendors have responded by acquiring smaller companies to broaden their services. Larger companies, however, may have bureaucracies slowing responsiveness to market changes, thus offsetting the benefits of integration. Integration of information increases in importance as hospitals face economic pressures to reduce costs.

Sharing laboratory data with other patient information systems is critical. Medical informaticians often distinguish *data*, the laboratory result by itself, from *information*, which is data aggregated and applied in a context for making decisions. For example, the report of a drug level, data, to a physician becomes information when it is coupled with other data associated with adverse drug reactions, dosing, and drug toxicity. Similarly, a surgical pathologist makes decisions regarding liver biopsies using data from liver function tests. In a broader context, the integration of ancillary and nursing data allows a hospital to make decisions to decrease costs of patient care. Ultimately, *knowledge* results when information is accumulated and organized.

The LIS therefore plays a key role in a large matrix of computer systems designed to support the delivery of patient care rather than operates as a stand-alone system. Coordinating the information in such an environment with many different systems, each with different requirements, can be a complex process. To address the high cost of software development and the lack of coordination among the various information systems, the healthcare computer industry (LIS and HIS users) and the federal government have created voluntary groups to set standards, particularly for the interconnection between information systems and between an information system and computerized equipment. For the clinical laboratory, standards address the interchange of data (1) with bedside monitoring systems, (2) with administrative systems including those associated with payers and government agencies, and (3) between laboratory systems. Of particular importance are those functions covering the interchange of laboratory test requests and results. The voluntary groups responsible for standards in the laboratory informatics arena include the NCCLS, ASTM, American National Standards Institute (ANSI), and Health Level Seven (HL7).

The HL7 protocol has become the basis for interchanging laboratory data between different systems,[7,29] such

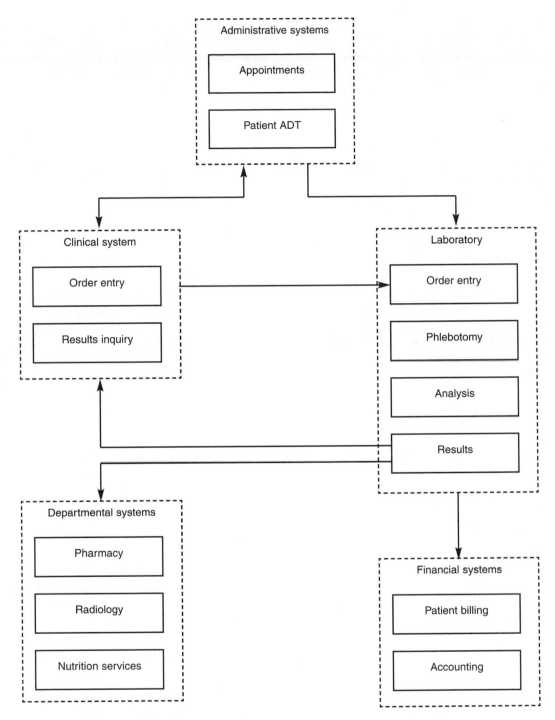

Fig. 18-8 The interchange of information between computer systems in a hospital environment. Most laboratory computer systems today are expected to interact with hospital administrative, financial, nursing, and other departmental systems.

as a reference laboratory system with a hospital laboratory system. Interfaces between an HIS and an LIS usually use HL7 or its older subset (NCCLS LIS5-A/ASTM E1238).[7,30] Intersystem interfaces provide large benefits for the laboratory. For example, significant savings result when physicians directly perform electronic order entry and results retrieval. Wide acceptance of standards has improved access to computerized medical information. Interface standards,

however, do not address differences between test definitions, ordering groups, and terminology occurring between institutions. The ultimate goal of these interfaces is the migration toward a reduction in paper use and toward the electronic patient chart. This will be difficult until medical terminology becomes more consistent. European groups have addressed the standardization of medical terminology.[31] Regenstreif Institute's Logical Observation Identifier Names and Codes

(LOINC) project has standardized test names and nomenclature used in the clinical laboratory.[32] LOINC test codes are particularly useful for interfaces between hospital LIS and reference laboratories by allowing the sending and the receiving sites to independently map LOINC to local test codes.

Future Directions

Computerizing patient records is the most effective way to decrease medical costs.[33,34] The electronic medical record (EMR), according to its proponents, would more readily transfer information between users of the chart in a more cost-effective fashion.[35] Coupled with order entry and medical practice guidelines, it can structure patient care for maximum benefits and reduce errors.[3] Unfortunately, the lack of a common medical terminology, the politics associated with large and complex projects, the difficulty of entering critical data associated with nursing care, and the high cost and technical challenge of developing complex software make this goal formidable.[36] Finally, people with combined skills in medicine and complex programming methodologies are required but are difficult to find. Creating an effective EMR continues to be a major challenge, as well as a solution, to many difficult medical care problems.[37]

Possibly the greatest potential for changing the human-computer interaction comes from computer technology already introduced, but not yet available widely in healthcare. This technology includes voice recognition devices, voice response units, handheld computers, and wireless networks. Voice recognition products have met with only moderate success because of performance limitations. Most voice recognition devices with moderate to large vocabularies require some individual user training and handle continuous speech only in limited situations. Units with vocabularies under 100 sounds can be speaker independent and are used for telephone answering systems. However, the widespread availability of inexpensive terminals and personal computers and the awkwardness of telephone menu systems have resulted in limited implementation of voice response products. Handwriting recognition in both portable computers and optical handwriting scanners has low accuracy without user training. Both technologies have the advantage of being potentially easier to use than the keyboard, but reliability of these devices must increase before they become widely used in the clinical laboratory. Wireless networks and handheld computers will permit access to information systems at the bedside rather than at the nursing station, making access to information systems more compatible with hospital workflow. These new technologies and the expansion of existing technologies hold the promise for better information systems and their impact on improving healthcare.

References

1. Sittig DF, Stead WW: Computer-based physician order entry: the state of the art, *J Am Med Inform Assoc* 1:108, 1994.
2. Valenstein P, Meier F: Outpatient order accuracy. A College of American Pathologists Q-Probes study of requisition order entry accuracy in 660 institutions, *Arch Pathol Lab Med* 123:1145, 1999.
3. Kohn LT, Corrigan JM, Donaldson MS, editors: *To err is human: building a safer health system*, Washington, DC, 2000, National Academy Press.
4. Weilert M, Tilzer LL: Putting bar codes to work for improved patient care, *Clin Lab Med* 11:227, 1991.
5. Chou D et al: *Laboratory automation: bar codes for specimen container identification*, vol 20, no 19 (Auto2-A), Wayne, PA, 2000, NCCLS.
6. EIA standard RS-232-C, Washington, DC, 1969, Electronic Industries Association.
7. LIS5-A (E1238-97), standard specification for transferring laboratory data messages between independent computer systems; LIS1-A (E1381-02), specification for low-level protocol to transfer messages between clinical laboratory instruments and computer systems; LIS2-A (E1394-97), standard specification for transferring information between clinical instruments and computer systems, Wayne, PA, 2003, NCCLS.
8. NCCLS Laboratory Automation Standards: Auto1-A *(Specimen container/specimen carrier)*, Auto2-A *(Bar codes for specimen container identification)*, Auto3-A , Auto4*(Communications with automated clinical laboratory systems, instruments, devices, and information systems)*-A *(Systems operational requirements, characteristics, and information elements)*, and Auto5-A *(Electromechanical interfaces)*, Wayne, PA, 2001, NCCLS.
9. Hoffman GE: Concepts for third generation of laboratory systems, *Clin Chem Acta* 278:203, 1998.
10. DuBois JA et al: Auto6-A: *Point of care connectivity*, approved standard, vol 21, Wayne, PA, 2001, NCCLS.
11. Department of Health and Human Services, Health Care Financing Organization, Department of Health and Human Services, 42 CFR part 405 et al, Clinical Laboratory Improvement Amendments of 1988, Final Rule, *Fed Register* 57:7001, 1992.
12. Westgard JO et al: A multi-rule Shewhart chart for quality control in clinical chemistry, *Clin Chem* 27:493, 1981.
13. Ladensen JH: Patients as their own controls: use of the computer to identify "laboratory error," *Clin Chem* 21:1648, 1975.
14. Lezotte D, Grams RR: Determining clinical significance in repeated laboratory measurements—the "clinical delta range," *J Med Sys* 3:175, 1979.
15. Koss W, Sodeman T: The workload recording method: a laboratory management tool, *Clin Lab Med* 12:337, 1991.
16. Williams G: Computer trouble: as more buyers suffer from upgrade fatigue, PC sales are falling, *Wall Street Journal* 238:A1, August 24, 2001.
17. Codd EF: A relational model for large shared data banks, *Comm ACM* 13:377, 1970.
18. Schatz BR, Hardin JB: NCSA mosaic and the world wide web: global hypermedia protocols for the Internet, *Science* 265:895, 1994.
19. Aller RD: Creating integrated regional laboratory networks, *Clin Lab Med* 19:299, 1999.
20. Connelly DP: Integrating integrated laboratory information into health care delivery systems, *Clin Lab Med* 19:277, 1999.
21. Gostin LO et al: Privacy and security of personal information in a new health care system, *JAMA* 20:2487, 1993.
22. Huston T: Security issues for implementation of e-medical records, *Communications ACM* 44:89, 2001.
23. Standards for Privacy of Individually Identifiable Health Information, 45 CFR parts 160, 164 [HIPPA], Final Rule, *Fed Register* 65:82461, 2000.
24. Essin DJ: Prying questions about privacy in a nosy world, *Clin Lab Med* 19:351, 1999.
25. Parkman PD: FDA letter to registered blood banks on recommendations for implementation of computerization in blood establishments, April 6, 1988.
26. *Application of the medical device GMPS to computerized devices and manufacturing processes: medical device GMP guidance for FDA investigators*, first draft. Office of Compliance and Surveillance, Division of Compliance Programs, Food and Drug Administration, Public Health Service, Department of Health and Human Services, Rockville MD, Nov, 1990.
27. Cowan DF, Gray RZ, Campbell B: Validation of the laboratory information system, *Arch Pathol Lab Med* 122:239, 1998.

28. Commission on Laboratory Accreditation: *Inspection checklist*, Section 1, Laboratory general—computer services, Northfield, IL, 2000, College of American Pathologists.

29. HL7 v2.4: An application protocol for electronic data interchange in health care environments, 2000, Health Level Seven, 3300 Washtenaw Ave, Ann Arbor, MI 48104.

30. McDonald CJ, Hammond WE: Standards formats for electronic transfer of data, *Ann Int Med* 110:333, 1989.

31. deMoor GJE: Standardization in medical informatics. In Bemmel JH, McCray AT, editors: *1993 Yearbook of medical informatics, sharing knowledge and information*, Stuttgart, Germany, 1993, Schattauer.

32. Huff SM et al: Development of the Logical Observation Identifier Names and Codes (LOINC) vocabulary, *J Am Med Inform Assoc* 5:276, 1998.

33. Dick RS, Steen EB, Detmer DE, editors: *The computer-based patient record: an essential technology for health care, revised edition*, Washington, DC, 1997, National Academy Press.

34. Korpman R: Health care information systems: patient-centered integration is the key, *Clin Lab Med* 11:203, 1991.

35. Barnett GO, Jenders RA, Cheuh HC: The computer-based clinical record—where do we stand? *Ann Int Med* 119:1046, 1993.

36. Brooks F: *The mythical man-month, essays on software engineering, anniversary edition*, Reading, MA, 1995, Addison-Wesley.

37. Jones J, Steindel S, Chou D, editors: *Connecting the laboratory to the electronic medical record*, National Academy of Clinical Biochemistry Symposium, Cincinnati, 2001, Pesce A, Kaplan L.

Internet Sites

www.aacc.org—American Association for Clinical Chemistry
http://www.informatics-review.com—Informatics Review: an online journal
www.imia.org—International Medical Informatics Association

www.amia.org—American Medical Informatics Association
www.nacb.org—National Academy of Clinical Biochemistry

CHAPTER 19

Laboratory Statistics*

• *Stephen E. Kahn*
• *Mark A. Jandreski*

Chapter Outline

Population distributions
- *Populations and samples*
- *Frequency distributions*

Basic distribution statistics
- *Measures of central tendencies*
- *Measures of variation*
- *Confidence intervals*
- *Measures of accuracy and precision*

Parametric comparisons of populations
- *The null hypothesis and statistical significance*
- *Two hypotheses*
- *Comparison of random variation (precision)—the F-test*

Comparison of means (accuracy or bias) —the t-test
One-way analysis of variance (ANOVA)
Testing a sample for outliers using the gap test

Nonparametric comparisons of populations
- *Nonparametric distribution statistics*
- *Sign test*
- *Mann-Whitney rank sum test*
- *χ^2 (chi-square) analysis*

Linear regression and correlation
- *Basic statistics of simple linear regression and correlation*
- *Testing for outliers using residual analysis*
- *Limitations of simple linear-regression analysis*

Objectives

- Given the appropriate data, construct frequency and relative frequency histograms.
- List three measures of central tendency and describe their utility when applied to normal and nonnormal distributions.
- List three measures of variation, calculate values for each given appropriate data, and describe their utility when applied to normal and nonnormal distributions.
- State the percentage of the values falling within the ±1s, ±2s, and ±3s confidence intervals in a normally distributed population.

- Describe three parametric techniques for comparison of populations and their utility when applied to normal distributions.
- Describe three nonparametric techniques for comparisons of populations and their utility when applied to normal and nonnormal distributions.
- Explain the use of ANOVA.
- Describe the uses and limitations of regression analysis for comparing sets of data.

Key Terms

accuracy   Estimate of nonrandom, systematic bias between samples of data or between a sample of data and the true population value.

ANOVA   Statistical method for comparison of three or more means.

central tendency   The value about which a population is centered. The mean, the median, and

---

*With acknowledgment to the previous authors, Carl C. Garber and R. Neill Carey.

the mode are all used to describe the central tendency of a population.

chi-square (χ^2)   A test statistic that measures the difference between the observed and expected frequencies of occurrences in two or more populations.

coefficient of variation (CV)   A relative standard deviation in which the standard deviation is divided by the mean and multiplied by 100%.

confidence interval   A range around an experimentally determined statistic that has a known probability of including the true parameter.

correlation coefficient   A statistic that measures the distribution of data about the estimated linear-regression line.

degrees of freedom (df)   The number of independent observations in a data set. It is the number of observations minus the number of restrictions for a set of data.

F-test   A statistical test used to determine whether there are differences between two variances.

gaussian distribution   See **normal distribution**.

histogram   A graphic display of data in which the frequency of a certain value (or range of values) is plotted against a scale of all values.

Mann-Whitney test   A nonparametric statistical test based on the ranks of data and used to test the null hypothesis that the central tendencies of two independent populations are identical.

mean   Arithmetic average of a set of data.

median   A value or interval of a population occurring in the middle of a population, of which half falls above and half falls below the median.

mode   The value or interval of a population occurring with the greatest frequency.

nonparametric statistics   Statistics employed when the assumption of a normal or symmetric (i.e., gaussian) distribution of data is not valid.

normal distribution   A population of data that has a tendency to cluster symmetrically around a central value such that the mean, median, and mode of the data are the same; also known as a *gaussian distribution*.

null hypothesis   The working hypothesis of a statistical test stating that there is no difference between the statistics of two different populations.

outlier   A result or data point that lies far outside the range of all other results or data points. The outlier is not considered to be from the population that has been sampled.

parametric statistics   Statistics employed when the assumption that a population has a symmetric distribution of data (such as gaussian or log-normal) is valid.

precision   A descriptor of the random variation in a population of data.

random error   Error that affects reproducibility of a method (precision).

range   The difference between the highest and lowest values in a population.

sign test   A nonparametric statistical test used to assess differences between population medians.

standard deviation   Square root of a variance.

standard error   A descriptor of the variability that results from sampling data from a population.

statistic   A number that describes a property of a set of data or other numbers.

statistics   The plural of *statistic*; also the science that deals with the use and classification of numbers or data.

systematic error   Nonrandom error that affects the mean of a population of data and defines the bias between the means of two populations (see **accuracy**).

t-test   A statistical test used to determine whether there are differences between two means or between a target value and a calculated mean in populations having a normal distribution.

variance   A statistic used to describe the distribution or spread of data in a population.

Generating test results, using effective quality control procedures, monitoring the performance of existing methods, and assessing the utility of new test methods are routine analytical activities performed in the clinical laboratory. All analytical techniques and methods are subject to several types of errors, or variation, that create a degree of uncertainty in the quantitative test results that a laboratory produces. The clinical laboratorian must be able to apply basic statistical techniques in order to evaluate the validity of test results. Statistics, therefore, are an important laboratory tool.

Webster[1] defines **statistics** as "(1) a branch of mathematics dealing with the collection, analysis, interpretation, and presentation of masses of numerical data, and (2) a collection of quantitative data."

A **statistic** (singular) is a number that describes some property of a set of other numbers. In the clinical laboratory, statistical descriptions of data sets can be useful in many ways:

1. To identify how a population of data is distributed
2. To assess random variation in a population of data
3. To compare the amounts of random variation within populations of data
4. To analyze which parameters are significant components of variance
5. To test for a systematic difference between populations of data
6. To assess the degree of correlation between populations of data

This chapter describes each of these uses of statistics and illustrates how each can be effectively applied in laboratory situations.

A basic and theoretical knowledge of appropriate statistical methods is critically important in the clinical chemistry laboratory. Equally important, however, is the correct application of statistical methods to relevant laboratory problems. Students are encouraged to refer to basic statistics textbooks (see, for example, references 2 to 9, as well as the Internet Sites) for an understanding of statistics beyond that presented in this chapter.

POPULATION DISTRIBUTIONS
Populations and Samples

The term *population* usually refers to a number of animate creatures or people, such as the inhabitants of the United States. However, in statistics, *population* may also refer to a collection of objects, events, procedures, or observations. For example, all the serum glucose values for all the people living in Chicago on a given day could be considered a population of glucose values. As a second example, if the glucose concentration of a single blood specimen were measured 10,000 times, a population of slightly different glucose results would be obtained, since no chemical measurement is exact because of the random variation inherent in all laboratory measurements.

The number of observations in these glucose examples is too large to study conveniently; therefore, a representative sample must be drawn from the population for an investigation. Before the sample is drawn, the population from which it comes must be carefully described. Once the attributes of the population are known, sample criteria for such variables as age, sex, occupation, family history, disease state, or any other parameter that might be relevant to the study can be applied. For example, if a serum glucose reference range analysis were carried out, serum samples from diabetic patients could not be used. The number of individual data points needed must be defined as well. If the number is too large, the study may be too difficult to carry out. If the number is too small, the sample may not be a statistically significant representation of the population. The sample must be chosen such that true inferences can be made about the population under study from results obtained from the sample. Most of the concepts and applications discussed in this chapter focus on statistical evaluations of samples of data obtained from a population.

Frequency Distributions

Conceptually, perhaps the simplest way to describe a population of data is to construct a **histogram**, also called a *frequency distribution diagram*. A histogram shows the frequency, or the number of times, a particular value or range of values is obtained versus the scale of all values. Fig. 19-1, *A*, is a histogram of 20 glucose results obtained by the repeated measurement of an individual blood specimen. The horizontal axis is glucose concentration divided into small convenient ranges, or *bins*. The vertical axis is the frequency (or relative frequency) with which results from each bin are obtained,

such as the number of patients having a given range of glucose values. When relative frequencies are used, each bin frequency is presented as a percentage of the total number of samples. The histogram's horizontal axis can also represent cumulative percentiles (cumulative percentage of the population up to and including each bin), as well as concentration units. When the number of observations, N, is small and the bins are relatively wide, the histogram has a choppy appearance (see Fig. 19-1, *A*). As N increases and the bins are made narrower, the shape of the histogram becomes smoother and the histogram becomes more truly representative of the population (Fig. 19-1, *B*). As N increases further, the histogram takes on the appearance of a continuous function (Fig. 19-1, *C*). In the histogram of hypothetical glucose data in Fig. 19-1, *C*, one can see that the population is centered around 1000 mg/L with few observations less than 920 mg/L and few greater than 1080 mg/L. The general spread of the data can also be assessed.

If enough data are represented in the histogram and the data are truly random (i.e., each result was affected by random processes alone), the histogram can be used to predict the probability of obtaining future results above or below a certain value. Fig. 19-1, *C*, shows that there is about a 2.3% chance that a future glucose result from this population will be less than 920 mg/L, and a 2.3% chance that a future glucose result will be greater than 1080 mg/L.

The curve approximated by the glucose histogram in Fig. 19-1, *C*, is a smooth "bell-shaped" curve called a *gaussian*, or *normal*, distribution, which is depicted in Fig. 19-2. This symmetric curve was first described by the French mathematician Abraham de Moivre in 1733 and further developed by the astronomer-mathematician Karl Friedrich Gauss during the 1800s. The portion of the curve on the right is usually referred to as the *upper tail*, and the portion on the left is called the *lower tail*. Many random variables of interest in medicine and health care, such as reference ranges, have distributions similar to **normal distributions**.

The *parametric* statistical tests discussed in this chapter are used under the assumption that the population being tested is distributed in a gaussian fashion. Before we proceed with parametric statistical comparisons, it is important to establish whether the population is normally distributed. A graphical analysis using *normal probability paper* can be used to test for a normal distribution. However, this method requires a visual evaluation of the sample data for deviation from a straight line and can therefore be very subjective. The graph is constructed by plotting the bin values, such as glucose concentration, along a linear *x*-axis and the cumulative frequency of the distribution on a nonlinear *y*-axis, the mathematical function of which is based on a normal distribution. Fig. 19-1, *D*, shows a normal probability plot for 600 glucose values drawn from a group of normal healthy volunteers.

The *Kolmogorov-Smirnov test* can be used to test for normally distributed data. This analysis measures the vertical distances between the cumulative distribution and the straight line on normal probability paper. Critical values for the statistically significant difference are obtained from a statistical table.

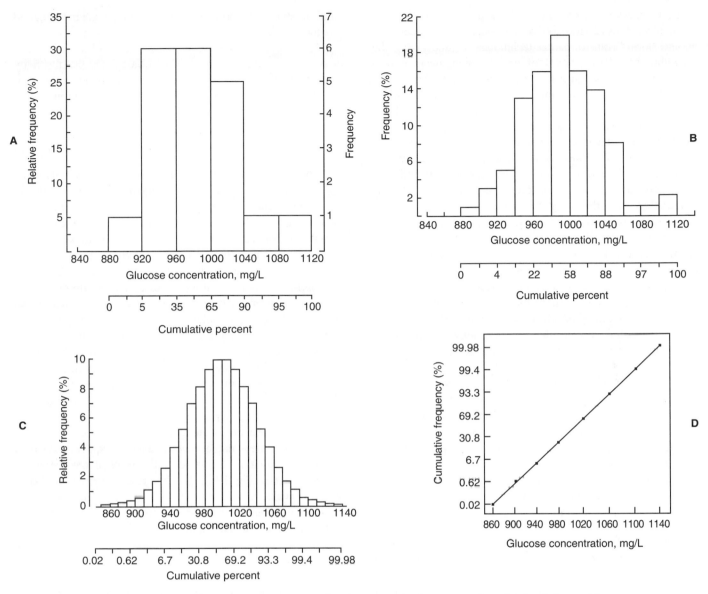

Fig. 19-1 **A,** Histogram (frequency distribution) of glucose results obtained from 20 repetitive measurements of the same specimen using bin width 40 mg/L. **B,** With N = 100 and bin width = 20 mg/L. **C,** With infinite N and bin width = 10 mg/L. **D,** Normal probability plot of glucose results obtained as described in **C.**

Another way to measure how well data fit a normal distribution is to calculate skewness and kurtosis coefficients. Skewness measures the asymmetry of the data distribution. Values greater than zero indicate that the upper tail of the curve is longer than the lower tail. Negative values indicate that the lower tail is longer. Kurtosis measures how steep or flat the distribution is with respect to a true normal distribution. Kurtosis coefficients greater than zero indicate that the curve is steep in the center and that the tails are relatively long. Values less than zero indicate that the curve is flat in the center and that the tails are short. For data that follow a reasonably **gaussian distribution**, the skewness and kurtosis coefficients should be between 1 and −1. Different types of coefficients called *standard skewness* and *kurtosis coefficients* test for significant deviations from the normal distribution and,

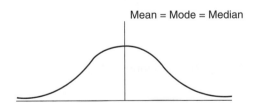

Fig. 19-2 Normal (gaussian) distribution, symmetric about mean.

analogous to standard deviation, should be between 2 and −2 for normally distributed data.[6] These calculations are usually done with computer software.

When a nonsymmetric or nongaussian distribution is observed, one option is to *transform* the nongaussian distribution into one that is more normally distributed. This can be accomplished by conversion of the population values into another form. Transformation techniques include taking the logarithm (base 10, or natural) of the data, taking the reciprocal of the data, and raising the numbers exponentially. After using one of these methods, the resulting data set is often distributed in a gaussian fashion. If the data are still not normally distributed, *nonparametric* statistical tests are used to analyze the data. In the medical and health care fields, nonparametric distributions are usually either *skewed* or *bimodal*. As alluded to previously, a skewed distribution is one where either the upper or lower tail of the distribution is longer than the other (Fig. 19-3). Serum gamma-glutamyl transferase reference interval data obtained from healthy individuals are usually skewed to the right (higher values). A bimodal distribution is seen when data are composed of two related populations (Fig. 19-4). Combined serum uric acid reference interval data obtained from healthy males and females typically demonstrate the appearance of a bimodal distribution when plotted appropriately. This type of distribution often indicates that separate, sex-based reference ranges should be established for the analyte under study.

BASIC DISTRIBUTION STATISTICS

In the previous section, plotting a histogram or frequency distribution was identified as a simple method for visually describing a population of data to assess, at least initially, whether the data set is distributed in a gaussian or a nongaussian fashion. There are two general categories of statistics that can also be used to describe the distribution of data. These two categories are measures of central tendencies and measures of variation.

Measures of Central Tendencies

Measures of central tendencies are statistics that represent some central value around which the data are distributed. Three measures of central tendencies that are often calculated for

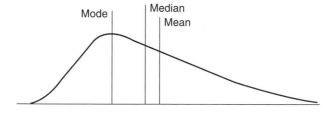

Fig. 19-3   Nonnormal distribution.

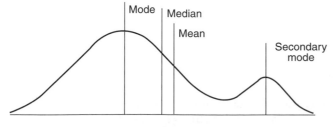

Fig. 19-4   Bimodal distribution.

clinical laboratory applications are the mean, the median, and the mode.

The **mean** is probably the most widely used statistic and is a simple *arithmetic average*. One calculates the mean by adding up all the observations and dividing by the number of observations, *N*. For a sample of data, calculation of the mean, designated as *x*, is illustrated by Eq. 19-1, where x_i is an individual observation:

$$\bar{x} = \frac{\sum x_i}{N}$$ *Eq. 19-1*

If the entire population of data is used to calculate the mean, the calculated mean is the actual mean of the population, indicated by the symbol "μ." For clinical laboratory applications, it is usually impossible to have collected the entire population of data (i.e., one can always make another measurement unless the population is restrictively defined). For these applications, use of the symbol for the sample mean, $\bar{x}$, is appropriate. This convention indicates that a subset of data from the population was used to calculate $\bar{x}$, which is an estimate of the true population mean.

If the sample data are distributed symmetrically about the mean, the arithmetic mean is actually representative of the **central tendency** of the sample. This feature is illustrated in Fig. 19-2, which depicts a *normal*, or *gaussian*, distribution. But any sample of data from a population would have a mean value, whether the distribution was gaussian or nongaussian.

A second measure of central tendency is the **mode**. The mode of a sample of data is that value most frequently observed in the sample. It is the value at the peak of the frequency distribution (see Fig. 19-3). If a frequency distribution of data has two peaks, the distribution is *bimodal*. An example of a bimodal distribution is illustrated in Fig. 19-4. For practical applications in the laboratory, every frequency distribution has a minimum of one mode (i.e., the distribution is at least unimodal).

A third measure of the central tendency is the **median**. The median is the middle value in a sample of data when all the values in the distribution are ranked individually from lowest to highest (or vice versa). Unlike the mean and mode, the median value describes a true central tendency for all types of distributions, since half of the observations are greater than the median and half of the observations are less than the median.

One characteristic of a perfect normal distribution is that the arithmetic average is the value observed most frequently and is also the middle value observed in the sample when values are ranked from lowest to highest. As illustrated in Fig. 19-2, this fact results in the mean, median, and mode all being the same value. All three of these statistics are true measures of central tendency in a true gaussian, or normal, distribution.

In contrast, in a nonnormal distribution, such as that depicted in Fig. 19-3, the mean, median, and mode are all different values. The mean does not accurately describe the center of the distribution (though it is still an arithmetic average of the data). It is also apparent that the mode of this distribution does not describe a true central tendency of the sample of data. The median is the only value that can be considered a true measure of this distribution's central tendency. For those nonnormal distributions where the mean and median might be considerably different, it may be more appropriate to use both values, or the median alone, to describe central tendencies of the distribution.

There is a significant and often overlooked limitation to using mean values to describe samples of data, even those samples that are normally distributed. Means can be strongly influenced by values in the data that lie at the extremes of the data range. This feature indicates that when calculating a mean value for a sample of data, one should be critical in evaluating which values may not be representative of the data set, that is, which values are outliers that should be excluded by the use of appropriate techniques (see below). The median is less affected than the mean by extreme values in the data set.

Measures of Variation

In addition to measures of central tendencies, other kinds of statistical data are required to characterize effectively a sample of data or a distribution. Measures of central tendencies do not provide sufficient information on how close together or far apart the values in a sample of data are. Statistics that indicate the degree to which observed values vary, or the spread of the distribution, are measures of variation. Three measures of variation that are often calculated for clinical laboratory applications are range, variance, and standard deviation.

The **range** is simply the difference between the largest and smallest values in the sample of data. The range is useful for indicating the spread of data when N is small, but when one is using the range, no assumptions can be made concerning the shape of the distribution. But a limitation of the range as a measure of variation is the fact that it is based on only two values in the sample of data.

More useful measures of variation are the **variance** and **standard deviation**. Variance is calculated by first determining the mean of the sample of data and then subtracting the mean from each value to get N differences. The squares of the differences between the individual values (x_i) and the mean are added. The sum of the squared differences is divided by $N - 1$, which yields the variance (Eq. 19-2, A):

$$\text{Variance} = s^2 = \frac{\sum (x_i - \bar{x})^2}{N - 1} \qquad \textit{Eq. 19-2, A}$$

The *standard deviation (s)* is the square root of the variance and is often represented as *SD*. The denominator of equation 19-2, A is $N - 1$ rather than N because there are only $N - 1$ **degrees of freedom (df)** for the variance once $\bar{x}$ has been used to calculate the variance. The concept of degrees of freedom is explained more fully later in this chapter.

Although s is normally calculated by use of the results of single analyses, one frequently needs to know the imprecision of replicate analyses. To calculate this estimate of variation, use the following equation:

$$s_{rep} = \left(\frac{\sum d^2}{N} \right)^{1/2} \qquad \textit{Eq. 19-2, B}$$

where d is the difference between the replicate measurements. This calculation can be useful for determining whether

duplicate analyses can help to achieve a desired level of within-run imprecision for an assay.

Another statistic that is often calculated in laboratory applications is the **coefficient of variation (CV)**. The CV indicates what percentage of the mean is represented by the standard deviation, as illustrated in Eq. 19-3:

$$\%CV = \frac{100\% \ s}{\bar{x}} \qquad \textit{Eq. 19-3}$$

One advantage in using the CV to express the variation of analytical methods is that the variation is reported in units that are independent of the particular analytical method. Keep in mind, however, that the magnitude of the CV of an analytical method is not completely independent of concentration. In certain instances, routine statistics on two levels of quality control materials may indicate a larger CV at the lower level simply because the numerator of the CV calculation, the mean, is a smaller number than the mean of the higher level of control material. Example 1 depicts the calculation of basic measures of central tendencies and basic measures of variation using data from a single level of quality control material.

Example 1. Calculation of basic statistics using a sample of data from repeated cholesterol measurements on one level of quality control material.

Calculate the mean, mode, median, variance, standard deviation, and coefficient of variation.

Sample

x_i (mg/L)	$x_i - \bar{x}$	$(x_i - \bar{x})^2$
2080	−1.4	1.96
2090	8.6	73.96
2110	28.6	817.96
2100	18.6	345.96
2010	−71.4	5097.96
2090	8.6	73.96
2040	−41.4	1713.96
2140	58.6	3433.96
2070	−11.4	129.96
2070	−11.4	129.96
2100	18.6	345.96
2110	28.6	817.96
2030	−51.4	2641.96
2090	8.6	73.96
2080	−1.4	1.96
2060	−21.4	457.96
2170	88.6	7849.96
2060	−21.4	457.96
2130	48.6	2361.96
2090	8.6	73.96
2080	−1.4	1.96
2100	18.6	345.96
2000	−81.4	6625.96
2090	8.6	73.96
2040	−41.4	1713.96
2070	−11.4	129.96
2100	18.6	345.96
2080	−1.4	1.96

$\sum x_i = 58280$ $\sum (x_i - \bar{x})^2 = 36142.88$

Mean

$$= \bar{x} = \frac{\sum x_i}{N} = 2081.4 \text{ mg/L}$$

Median*

$$= 2085 \text{ mg/L}$$

Mode

$$= 2090 \text{ mg/L}$$

Measures of Variance

$$s^2 = \frac{\sum (x_i - \bar{x})^2}{N - 1}$$
$$= 36142.88/27 = 1338.6 \text{ mg/L}$$
$$s = 36.5 \text{ mg/L}$$
$$\%CV = 100\% \ s/\bar{x}$$
$$= \frac{36.5 \text{ mg/L} (100\%)}{2081.4 \text{ mg/L}}$$
$$= 1.75\%$$

---

*When even-numbered samples of data are collected, the two middle values are averaged to obtain the median.[6] For an N of 28, the two middle values are the 14th and 15th values, 2090 mg/L and 2080 mg/L, respectively.

Confidence Intervals

Use of the mean and standard deviation values for the purposes of assessing quality control results and the determination of reference ranges are important laboratory applications. To use these statistics for these applications, the data in the sample must be normally distributed. In a normal distribution, the standard deviation and mean (which are in the same units) can be used to describe the proportion of the values falling in a given area under the normal curve.

The total area under the normal curve theoretically represents all the values in the given population. As illustrated in Fig. 19-5, the area under the perfect normal distribution from $+1s$ to $-1s$ represents 68.3% of the values, from $+2s$ to $-2s$ represents 95.4% of the values, and from $+3s$ to $-3s$ represents 99.7% of the values. These intervals that contain a stated percentage of the data are called **confidence intervals**. For samples of data that are normally distributed, confidence intervals calculated using the mean and standard deviation

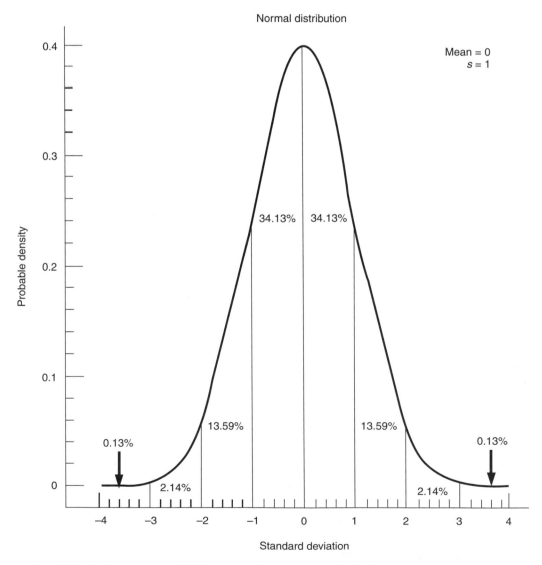

Normal distribution

Mean = 0
s = 1

Fig. 19-5 Perfect normal distribution, with a mean = 0, indicating the percentage of results that are in each standard deviation interval between –4 and +4 standard deviations.

can form the basis of statistical quality control rules for acceptance and rejection decisions concerning specific analytical runs (see Chapter 21).

If the results from analyzing the quality control material discussed in Example 1 were perfectly distributed, it would be expected that the range between the mean plus $2s$ and the mean minus $2s$ (2008.4 to 2154.4 mg/L) would exclude 4.6% of the data. In reality, this range excludes 7.1% of the data (2 of 28 values, 2000 mg/L and 2170 mg/L, are outside the $2s$ range). For this sample of data, the $2s$ range should not be expected to include exactly 95.4% of the values. It was known that the distribution was not perfectly normal once different results for the mean, median, and mode were obtained.

The measurement of cholesterol levels in Example 1 is characterized by a certain degree of imprecision (the %CV is 1.75%). Since the error of the mean measurement of the set of values is smaller than that of a single measurement, the more times a measurement is made, the more certain you can be of its true value. If several means are calculated from different groups of measurements of this quality control specimen, the individual means are distributed about the actual population mean. The random variation in this group of means is described by the **standard error** of the mean $(S_{\bar{x}})$ in Eq. 19-4:

$$s_{\bar{x}} = \frac{s}{\sqrt{N}} \qquad \textit{Eq. 19-4}$$

Suppose that for the cholesterol QC measurements discussed in Example 1, you wished to determine the $s_{\bar{x}}$ and the likelihood that the population mean is within a certain range. Putting the appropriate values into Eq. 19-4:

$$s_{\bar{x}} = \frac{36.5 \text{ mg/L}}{\sqrt{28}} = 6.9 \text{ mg/L}$$

It would then be expected that 68.3% of the various sample means (with Ns of 28) would be within 1×6.9 mg/L of the population mean (2074.5 to 2088.3 mg/L), 95.4% of the means would be within 2×6.9 mg/L of the population mean (2067.6 to 2095.2 mg/L), and 99.7% of the means would be within 3×6.9 mg/L of the true population mean (2060.7 to 2102.1 mg/L). Therefore it can be assumed with a 95% confidence that the *true* population mean lies within the range of 2067.6 to 2095.2 mg/L. This is termed the 95% *confidence interval*.

The true mean cholesterol concentration of the quality control material in Example 1 cannot be exactly determined unless an infinite number of measurements are made. In practice, the population is sampled by obtaining groups of quality control values such as those shown in Example 1. The mean obtained is therefore not the true mean but an estimate of the true mean. The standard error of the experimentally derived mean, x, can be used to develop a more exact *confidence interval* that has a known probability of including the true population mean, μ. This interval is described in Eq. 19-5:

$$\mu = \bar{x} \pm t \cdot s_{\bar{x}} \qquad \textit{Eq. 19-5}$$

The t value is obtained from a t table (Table 19-1). The t value depends on the number of degrees of freedom $(N-1)$ and the desired probability, p, that the true mean is outside the confidence interval because of chance alone. A prob-

TABLE 19-1 CRITICAL VALUES OF t FOR SELECTED PROBABILITIES, p, AND DEGREES OF FREEDOM, df			
	TWO-SIDED INTERVALS OR TESTS		
	$p = 0.10$	$p = 0.05$	$p = 0.01$
	ONE-SIDED LIMITS OR TESTS		
df	$p = 0.05$	$p = 0.025$	$p = 0.005$
1	6.31	12.70	63.70
2	2.92	4.30	9.92
3	2.35	3.18	5.84
4	2.13	2.78	4.60
5	2.01	2.57	4.03
6	1.94	2.45	3.71
7	1.89	2.36	3.50
8	1.86	2.31	3.36
9	1.83	2.26	3.25
10	1.81	2.23	3.17
12	1.78	2.18	3.05
14	1.76	2.14	2.98
16	1.75	2.12	2.92
18	1.73	2.10	2.88
20	1.72	2.09	2.85
30	1.70	2.04	2.75
40	1.68	2.02	2.70
60	1.67	2.00	2.66
120	1.66	1.98	2.62
∞	1.64	1.96	2.58

Condensed from Davies OL, Goldsmith PL: Statistical methods in research and production, *ed 4, New York, 1972, Longman.*

ability of $p = 0.05$ implies a 95% confidence $[100 \times (1 - p)\%]$ that the interval includes the true mean.

The t values describe the same probability distribution depicted in Fig. 19-5, but use of the distribution in Fig. 19-5 should be made under the assumption that the true population mean and standard deviation are known. Use of the t table makes allowances for decreasing confidence in the estimated values of specific parameters as N decreases. Therefore an appropriate use of t values is to calculate more accurate confidence intervals for statistics obtained from small samples. An illustration of this is given in Example 2. To construct a confidence interval that includes a true mean, one should be sure that the 0.05 probability of the true mean being beyond the calculated limits is spread over both ends or tails of the distribution, as shown in Fig. 19-6. For these purposes, a two-sided, $p = 0.05$, t value is used. To state that the true mean is greater than some single limit, use a one-sided t value. Notice that the t value for a two-sided interval for a $p = 0.05$ is the same as the t value for a one-sided limit of $p = 0.025$. The practical application of confidence limits is demonstrated on pp. 422-424.

Example 2. Calculating 95% confidence intervals for the mean of a small sample.

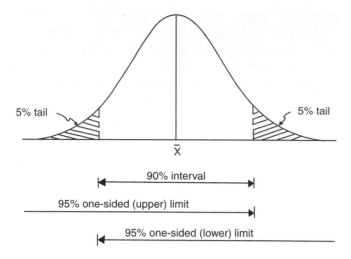

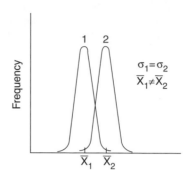

Fig. 19-6 One-sided versus two-sided *t*-values. *t*-values to calculate 90% interval and 95% one-sided limits are the same.

Fig. 19-8 Frequency distribution for replicate analysis by two different methods, *1* and *2*. Both methods are equally precise ($\sigma_1 = \sigma_2$) but are biased in relationship to each other ($\bar{x}_1$ does not equal $\bar{x}_2$).

Upper limit of confidence interval: $325 + (2.14)(5.42) =$ 336.6 IU/L

There is a 95% probability that the mean LD activity of this sample of quality control measurements is between 313.4 and 336.6 IU/L.

Measures of Accuracy and Precision

In previous sections, the mean and standard deviations of a normally distributed population were described. When a new analytical method is evaluated by the laboratory, these parameters are used to describe the accuracy and precision of the method (see Chapter 22). **Accuracy** describes the ability of an analytical method to obtain the "true" or correct result after a number of replicate analyses. The closer the mean of *N* replicate analyses of a sample comes to the "true" or known value of that sample, the more accurate the method. **Precision** describes the reproducibility of a method. The narrower the distribution of results, that is, the smaller the standard deviation, after a number of replicate analyses, the better the precision of a method.

Fig. 19-7 shows the results of replicate analyses of the same sample by three different methods. All three methods have a similar mean and thus similar accuracy. However, the distributions or standard deviations of the results are different for each method. Method *1* has the narrowest distribution or smallest standard deviation and hence has the best precision of the three methods. Method *3* has the widest distribution or largest standard deviation and thus has the poorest precision.

Fig. 19-8 shows the results of replicate analyses of the same sample by two different methods. The two methods have a similar distribution of data or similar standard deviations; therefore their precision is about the same. The means, however, are not equal, and the relative accuracies for the two methods are not the same, which indicates a nonrandom bias between the methods. Determining which method has the better accuracy will depend on which mean is closer to the "true" value of the analyte examined in the sample.

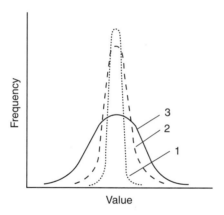

Fig. 19-7 Frequency distributions for three methods having same means, but different distributions. *1* has narrowest distribution, whereas distribution of *3* is wider than that of *2*.

Calculate the 95% confidence interval for the mean value of the lactate dehydrogenase (LD) activity of a stable control material after performing only 15 daily determinations.

Sample: All LD values are in IU/L: 324, 337, 350, 295, 284, 322, 339, 350, 309, 322, 348, 320, 298, 345, 335.

The calculated mean and standard deviation of the sample are 325 and 21 IU/L, respectively.

The standard error of the mean (SEM) is calculated:

$$s_{\bar{x}} = s/\sqrt{N} = 21/\sqrt{25} = 5.42 \text{ IU/L}$$

Using the *t* table in Table 19-1, find the two-sided *t* value for $p = 0.05$ and $N - 1$ degrees of freedom ($df = 14$). The *t* value of 2.14 is the factor used to adjust the SEM so that the correct lower and upper limits of the 95% confidence interval for the mean can be determined for this small sample. Using Eq. 19-5:

$$\mu = \bar{x} \pm t \cdot s_{\bar{x}}$$

Lower limit of confidence interval: $325 - (2.14)(5.42) =$ 313.4 IU/L

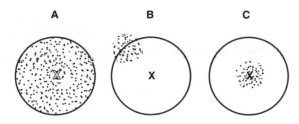

Fig. 19-9 Xs on these targets each denote the true value for a sample. The dots shown on each of the circles **A** to **C** denote the results of three replicate analyses by three different methods: **A**, imprecise but accurate; **B**, precise but inaccurate; **C**, accurate and precise.

Although the terms are sometimes used interchangeably, accuracy and precision are two distinctly different concepts and must never be interchanged with each other. This is shown in Fig. 19-9. Repeated attempts to hit the middle of the target, the true value, are indicated by dots. A method can be accurate but not very precise, as shown in Fig. 19-9, *A*. Inaccuracy but good precision is shown in Fig. 19-9, *B*, where the values fall close together but are grouped far from the middle, or "true," value. Fig. 19-9, *C*, shows the goal of all good analytical methods—excellent accuracy *and* precision.

PARAMETRIC COMPARISONS OF POPULATIONS
The Null Hypothesis and Statistical Significance

When a comparison is made between two samples from two populations, invariably a difference between the means ($\bar{x}$) and standard deviations (s) is observed. These observed differences may or may not reflect a true difference between the populations. Therefore, it is necessary to test the **null hypothesis**, which states that there is no difference between the true means (μ) or the true standard deviations (σ) of the two populations. The corresponding calculated values, $\bar{x}$ or s, are used for this purpose.

Two Hypotheses

$$s_1^2 = s_2^2 \quad \text{or} \quad \bar{x}_1 = \bar{x}_2 \qquad \text{Null hypothesis}$$

$$s_1^2 \neq s_2^2 \quad \text{or} \quad \bar{x}_1 \neq \bar{x}_2 \qquad \text{Alternative hypothesis}$$

Many different statistical tests can be used to generate a test *statistic* that indicates whether to accept or reject the null hypothesis. If the statistical test result indicates that the null hypothesis should be accepted, the possibility exists that the calculated test statistic that forms the basis for the test results does not reflect the truth and the null hypothesis may be incorrectly accepted. The level of significance or chance of this occurring is defined by the value p, where $100\% \, (1 - p)$ is the percentage of confidence that the test results are statistically significant. A minimum value of $p = 0.05$ is customarily used to test for significance. This value means that there is a 95% chance that the results of a statistical test are significant or, conversely, that there is a 5% chance that accepting the statistical test result is the wrong decision.

For many applications in clinical chemistry, a difference that is only statistically different may still be acceptable for routine applications. It is of course important to identify differences that *are* medically significant or that do not meet regulatory requirements (see Chapters 21 and 22).

Degrees of freedom. The term *degrees of freedom* is usually defined as the number of ways in which a group of numbers can vary independently. This is often a difficult idea to explain or define. It is calculated by subtraction of the number of estimated parameters from the sample size. For example, consider 20 bilirubin measurements; the sample size is 20, and for this series the number of degrees of freedom is 20. Any one of these 20 values can be altered, and the change will not affect the value of any of the other measurements in the series. However, if the mean of the 20 values is calculated, the mean has only 19, or $n - 1$, degrees of freedom. It is possible to change 19 values without changing the mean, but the 20th value will need to be a specific number so that the mean remains the same. Therefore, for the calculation of the mean, the degrees of freedom are calculated as $n - 1$. The number of degrees of freedom is an important parameter used in the calculation of many statistical tests, for example, the *t*-test.

Comparison of Random Variation (Precision)—the *F*-Test

The **t-test** is often used to compare the means ($\bar{x}$) of two groups of observations in order for one to test whether there is a significant difference between the two group means (see p. 350). Two assumptions are made with the *t*-test: that the groups are *normally* distributed and that there is no significant difference between the group variances. It is not possible to tell simply by observation of the data how different the variances in the two groups must be before the *t*-test cannot be used. However, the null hypothesis that there is no significant difference between the variances can be tested by use of the **F-test**.

The *F*-test, or variance ratio test, is used to determine whether an observed difference between the standard deviations (s) of two sets of data is statistically significant. One calculates the *F*-test statistic by dividing the larger variance (s_1^2) by the smaller variance (s_2^2), as shown in Eq. 19-6:

$$F = \frac{s_1^2}{s_2^2} \qquad\qquad \textit{Eq. 19-6}$$

The calculated *F*-value is compared with a critical *F*-value obtained from an *F*-table (Table 19-2) by using the numbers of degrees of freedom from each group at a specified level of p, such as $p = 0.05$. If the calculated *F*-value is less than the critical value, the null hypothesis is accepted as true. If the calculated *F*-value is greater than the critical value, the alternative hypothesis is accepted as true.

Example 3. *F*-test.

A comparison between folate levels in two groups is needed, but the standard deviations look considerably different. The data below show folate levels from 21 laboratory workers and 16 individuals suspected of having dietary anemia.

Serum folate (μg/L)

Workers ($n = 21$)	Patients ($n = 16$)
13	5
18	15
14	2
16	21
19	6
15	7
12	16
17	4
13	3
16	5
15	18
17	2
18	6
20	1
17	4
13	16
21	
15	
16	
19	
16	

Average	16.2	8.2
Standard deviation	2.44	6.59

$$F = \frac{(6.59)^2}{(2.44)^2} = \frac{43.43}{5.95} = 7.30$$

Use the F-table (Table 19-2) to find a critical F-value. Scan across the F-table to the column that corresponds to $n - 1$ degrees of freedom in the numerator (15) and down to the row that corresponds to $n - 1$ degrees of freedom in the denominator (20) and note a critical value of 2.20. Since the calculated value exceeds this value, the difference in precision is significant with $p < 0.05$.

The results of this test indicate that the t-test should not be used to compare the two means. The **Mann-Whitney test** may be a better alternative; this test is discussed later in this chapter.

Comparison of Means (Accuracy or Bias)—the t-Test

The t-test is used to check for statistically significant differences between two experimental means or between an experimental mean and a stated value.

Hypothesis testing. Testing the difference between an experimental mean and a stated or known value involves testing to see whether the stated value is included in the confidence interval around the experimental mean. If it is not, the null hypothesis is rejected, and there appears to be a difference between the stated value and the experimental mean value. In this case, Eqs. 19-7 and 19-8 are used to calculate the paired t-statistic, which is used to determine whether the null hypothesis will be accepted or rejected.

$$t = \frac{\text{Sample mean} - \text{Hypothesized mean}}{\text{Standard error of sample mean}} \qquad \textit{Eq. 19-7}$$

$$t = \frac{\bar{x} - \mu}{s/\sqrt{n}} \qquad \textit{Eq. 19-8}$$

For example, assume that the glucose concentration in a quality control specimen obtained from the National Institute of Standards and Technology is stated to be 1120 mg/L. This material is used as a quality control sample for 30 consecutive days.

For these data, the mean is 1110 mg/L and the s_d is 25 mg/L. Is the mean of the data significantly different from the stated value?

$$t = \frac{1110 - 1120}{\frac{25}{\sqrt{30}}} = -2.19$$

TABLE 19-2 CRITICAL VALUES OF F FOR $p = 0.05$ AND SELECTED DEGREES OF FREEDOM, df

	DEGREES OF FREEDOM FOR NUMERATOR						
df for Denominator	*5*	*10*	*15*	*20*	*30*	*60*	*∞*
1	230.00	242.00	246.00	248.00	250.00	252.00	254.00
2	19.30	19.40	19.40	19.40	19.50	19.50	19.50
3	9.01	8.79	8.70	8.66	8.62	8.57	8.53
4	6.26	5.96	5.86	5.80	5.75	5.69	5.63
5	5.05	4.74	4.62	4.56	4.50	4.43	4.36
6	4.39	4.06	3.94	3.87	3.81	3.74	3.67
7	3.97	3.64	3.51	3.44	3.38	3.30	3.23
8	3.69	3.35	3.22	3.15	3.08	3.01	2.93
9	3.48	3.14	3.01	2.94	2.86	2.79	2.71
10	3.33	2.98	2.85	2.77	2.70	2.62	2.54
15	2.90	2.54	2.40	2.33	2.25	2.16	2.07
20	2.71	2.35	2.20	2.12	2.04	1.95	1.84
30	2.53	2.16	2.01	1.93	1.84	1.74	1.62
60	2.37	1.99	1.84	1.75	1.65	1.53	1.39
∞	2.21	1.83	1.67	1.57	1.46	1.32	1.00

Modified from Barnett RN: Clinical laboratory statistics, ed 2, Boston, 1979, Little, Brown & Co.

The critical t-value for $p = 0.05$ and 29 df (rounded to 30 in Table 19-1) is 2.04. Thus this month's mean of 1110 mg/L is significantly different from the assigned glucose concentration of 1120 mg/L. See also p. 415 for an application of the t-test to assess bias in a methods-comparison experiment.

Testing the statistical significance between two measured means using the t-test involves testing the degree of overlap of their respective probability distributions. If there is little or no overlap, the populations are considered to be different. If significant overlap exists, you cannot be sure that there is any difference. A t-value is calculated from the data and compared with a critical t-value. Table 19-1 gives many of the critical values from the t-distributions. If the absolute value of the calculated t-value does not exceed the critical t-value, the null hypothesis is accepted, and such acceptance indicates that a statistically significant difference between the two distributions does not exist; that is, the means are the same.

Two different t-tests are available for comparing the means of different sample populations: the *unpaired t-test* and the *paired t-test*.

Unpaired t-test. The unpaired t-test is used when the difference between the means of two independent populations is being analyzed. One example is the comparison of the means of patients' glucose values from two different hospitals. When the unpaired t-test is used, it is assumed that the variances of the two populations are equal, and this must first be verified with the F-test. If there is no statistically significant difference between the variances, it is proper to proceed with the t-test. The *pooled sample variance* (s_p^2) is first calculated as shown in Eq. 19-9:

$$s_p^2 = \frac{(n_1 - 1)s_1^2 + (n_2 - 1)s_2^2}{n_1 + n_2 - 2} \qquad \textbf{\textit{Eq. 19-9}}$$

where s_1 and s_2 are the standard deviations of the two groups of sizes n_1 and n_2. Using $\bar{x}_1$ and $\bar{x}_2$ for the means of the two groups, the *unpaired t-statistic* is calculated as shown in Eq. 19-10:

$$t = \frac{\bar{x}_1 - \bar{x}_2}{s_p \sqrt{1/n_1 + 1/n_2}} \qquad \textbf{\textit{Eq. 19-10}}$$

where s_p is the pooled standard deviation. Each group contributes to the degrees of freedom associated with s_p, so that the calculated unpaired t-statistic has $(n_1 - 1) + (n_2 - 1)$ or $n_1 + n_2 - 2$ degrees of freedom. The critical t-value is found from a t-table using the calculated degrees of freedom and comparing with the calculated t-value.

Example 4. Equal variance unpaired t-test.

A reference laboratory begins using a new method for serum immunoglobulin A. Samples are received from two regions of the country. Random samples from healthy patients from each region are tested to find out whether the reference range for these two regions is the same.

	Region A	Region B
Mean ($\bar{x}$) (mg/L)	2260	2650
Standard deviation (s) (mg/L)	584	473
Number of samples (n)	33	29

The unpaired t-test is used to determine whether the observed differences between the two means are significant.

The F-test is first performed to ensure that the variances are statistically the same.

$$F = \frac{(584)^2}{(473)^2} = \frac{341056}{223729} = 1.52$$

Use the F-table (see Table 19-2) to find a critical F-value. Scan across the F-table to the column that corresponds to $n - 1$ degrees of freedom in the numerator (32) and down to the row that corresponds to $n - 1$ degrees of freedom in the denominator (28) and note a critical value of 1.84. (You can interpolate the table to obtain the exact value for $n_1 = 32$ and $n_2 = 28$ or round off to 30, as shown in this example.) Since the calculated value is less than the critical value, the difference in precision is insignificant with $p < 0.05$. The result of this test indicates that the t-test can be used to compare the two mean values.

To calculate the t-statistic, first calculate s_p:

$$s_p^2 = \frac{(33 - 1)(584)^2 + (29 - 1)(473)^2}{33 + 29 - 2}$$
$$s_p^2 = 286303$$
$$s_p = \sqrt{286303} = 535$$

Then calculate the t-statistic:

$$t = \frac{2260 - 2650}{535 \times \sqrt{1/33 + 1/29}} = -2.86$$

Use the t-table (see Table 19-1) to find a critical t-value. Scan down the t-table to the column that corresponds to $n_A + n_B - 2$, or 60 degrees of freedom, and note a critical value of 2.00. Since the absolute value of the calculated t-value $|-2.86| = 2.86$, and this is greater than 2.00, the difference in the means is significant with $p < 0.05$. Thus the sample distributions for the two regions do not overlap enough to declare them the same. The laboratory would need separate regional reference ranges for the samples it is testing.

Suppose that $s_1 \neq s_2$, but you are reasonably certain that the two populations are normally distributed. In this case, the pooled estimate of the variance, s_p^2, cannot be used. However, another form of the unpaired t-test sometimes called the separate-variance t-test can be utilized. The formula in Eq. 19-11 approximates a student's t-distribution for normally distributed response variables and does not require that the population variances be equal:

$$t = \frac{\bar{x}_1 - \bar{x}_2}{(s_1^2/n_1 + s_2^2/n_2)^{1/2}} \qquad \textbf{\textit{Eq. 19-11}}$$

The number of degrees of freedom can be found by use of the formula shown in Eq. 19-12. The answer is rounded down to the next lowest integer. For example, 7.6 becomes 7 degrees of freedom.

$$df = \frac{(w_1 + w_2)^2}{w_1^2/(n_1 - 1) + w_2^2/(n_2 - 1)} \qquad \textbf{\textit{Eq. 19-12}}$$

where df = degrees of freedom and $w_1 = s_1^2/n_1$ and $w_2 = s_2^2/n_2$.

Example 5. Separate variance unpaired t-test.

In a study of chronic hepatitis, serum alkaline phosphatase levels were reported for 9 patients with inactive disease and

25 patients with active disease. Use the unpaired *t*-test to test the hypothesis that there is a difference between the alkaline phosphatase means for the active-disease and the inactive-disease populations.

Serum alkaline phosphatase (IU/L)

Inactive	Active
65	103
72	210
84	92
68	225
89	110
110	286
77	96
95	216
81	94
	150
	195
	208
	95
	163
	184
	89
	238
	99
	116
	224
	124
	135
	201
	92
	176

$\bar{x}$	82	157
s	14.2	58.5
n	9	25

The *F*-statistic for the sample variances is $(58.5)^2/(14.2)^2$ = 16.74, which is much greater than the critical value of 3.12 (see Table 19-2). Since the variances are very different, the separate-variance *t*-test is used.

$$t = \frac{82 - 157}{[(14.2)^2/9 + (58.5)^2/25]^{1/2}}$$

$$t = -75/12.6 = -5.95$$

The degrees of freedom are:

$$w_1 = (14.2)^2/9 = 22.4$$

$$w_2 = (58.5)^2/25 = 136.9$$

$$df = \frac{(w_1 + w_2)^2}{w_1^2/(n_1 - 1) + w_2^2/(n_2 - 1)}$$

$$df = \frac{(22.4 + 136.9)^2}{(22.4)^2/(9 - 1) + (136.9)^2/(25 - 1)}$$

$$df = 25376/843 = 30.1 \approx 30.$$

For 30 degrees of freedom from Table 19-1, the critical *t*-value at $p = 0.05$ is 2.04.

Since the absolute value of the calculated *t*-value $|-5.95|$ = 5.95, and this is greater than 2.04, the difference in the means is significant with $p < 0.05$. Thus the sample distributions for the two disease groups do not overlap enough to declare them the same.

Paired *t*-test. A special case of comparison of means is the paired-sample *t*-test. Paired-sample testing (also called "split" sample testing) is used to minimize the effects of sample variations, which can lead to ambiguous results. For example, if you were comparing the blood-gas Po_2 method x with the blood-gas Po_2 method y and specimens were drawn from different random patient populations for each method, extraneous variations in the populations could mask true methodological differences. To eliminate this variance, analyze the same specimens by both methods (see Example 6). The equation used to calculate the paired *t*-statistic is:

$$t = \frac{\bar{x}_1 - \bar{x}_2}{s_d/\sqrt{n}} \qquad \text{Eq. 19-13}$$

where $\bar{x}_1$ and $\bar{x}_2$ are the means of the two paired populations, s_d is the standard deviation of the *difference* between the populations, and n is the number of samples. There are $n - 1$ degrees of freedom. To calculate s_d, find the standard deviation of the differences between each pair of results or between each result and a known or stated value. Example 6 shows the calculation of a paired *t*-test between two groups of data.

Example 6. Paired *t*-test.

A laboratory examines a new method for Po_2 by running 40 samples in a paired fashion on the old and new instruments. Using a paired *t*-test, compare the data to determine whether any bias exists between the methods.

Po_2 (mm Hg)

Old	New	Difference
88	88	0
118	121	−3
115	119	−4
189	198	−9
36	36	0
123	123	0
123	118	5
200	203	−3
60	62	−2
86	86	0
61	62	−1
81	87	−6
33	31	2
223	232	−9
47	48	−1
38	36	2
140	142	−2
67	67	0
87	90	−3
218	225	−7
79	80	−1
56	56	0
228	224	4
65	67	−2
86	88	−2
327	334	−7
59	62	−3
36	36	0

Continued

Po$_2$ (mm Hg), cont'd		
Old	New	Difference
100	101	−1
146	140	6
112	106	6
218	212	6
95	94	1
67	68	−1
71	72	−1
102	100	2
92	91	1
106	105	1
64	60	4
105	114	−9
Avg 108.7	109.6	−0.93
s 64.1	65.3	3.86

First the variances must be checked by using the F-test to verify that there is no significant difference between the methods. The F-statistic for the sample variances is: $(65.3)^2/(64.1)^2 = 1.04$, which is less than the critical F-value of 1.69 (see Table 19-2) for $p = 0.05$ at 39 degrees of freedom. Since the variances are not significantly different, the t-test can be used.

$$t = \frac{\bar{x}_1 - \bar{x}_2}{s/\sqrt{n}}$$

$$t = \frac{-0.93}{3.86/\sqrt{40}}$$

$$t = -1.52$$

The critical t value for $p = 0.05$ at 39 degrees of freedom is 2.02. Since the absolute calculated t value $|-1.52| = 1.52$, which according to Table 19-1 is less than the critical value, 2.02, the means are not significantly different. The methods are yielding results that are not statistically biased from each other.

One-Way Analysis of Variance (ANOVA)

ANOVA is a method for testing the hypothesis that several different groups (three or more), the distributions of which are normal, all have the same mean. A logical approach to this problem might be to perform a t-test on each difference, beginning with the largest, until the null hypothesis is rejected for one test. For example, if three population means were compared by testing of the hypothesis that all three population means are equal, it would be necessary to carry out three t-tests: a test of the hypothesis that $\bar{x}_1 = \bar{x}_2$, a test of the hypothesis that $\bar{x}_1 = \bar{x}_3$, and a test of the hypothesis that $\bar{x}_2 = \bar{x}_3$. However, this approach would become increasingly inefficient as the number of populations increased. Also, when many comparisons are being performed, some may fail because of chance alone.

In ANOVA, k means (where $k \geq 3$) are compared by testing with the null hypothesis that $\bar{x}_1 = \bar{x}_2 = \bar{x}_3 = \ldots \bar{x}_k$. An F-statistic is calculated, and if this statistic is less than a specified value, the null hypothesis is accepted and the means for all groups are not significantly different from one another. The alternative hypothesis is always that at least one sample mean does not equal another sample mean. If the null hypothesis is rejected, it cannot be stated that all the sample means are different. It can only be concluded that one of the sample means does not equal one other sample mean. Since ANOVA analysis cannot tell which of the means is significantly different from the others, alternative methods, such as the Bonferroni method for multiple comparisons,[6] are used to determine which of the means are different.

A major advantage of ANOVA compared with the use of individual t-tests is that ANOVA deals with the larger overall sample population. By using as many data as possible, ANOVA is essentially calculating the best estimate of the true population variance. Differences among the group means are then tested with reference to this best estimate of the population variance. This decreases the possibility that random differences in the variances within individual groups will obscure true findings. In the clinical chemistry laboratory, ANOVA can be a useful statistical tool.

Testing a Sample for Outliers Using the Gap Test
(See also p. 369)

When results or data points are distributed in gaussian fashion, graphing a frequency plot of the data allows them to be visually assessed. It is possible that during this assessment the investigator may identify an **outlier**, which is a result or data point that is so far outside the range of all other results or data points that it is considered unlikely that the result is from the population which has been sampled. Unfortunately, although the experienced investigator might feel comfortable with this assessment, a visual inspection of a frequency distribution or histogram is subjective in nature.

Certain samples of data can be evaluated for the presence of outliers using more rigorous criteria established by the investigator, for example, exclusion of data points that exceed a given percentage of the mean or median value. A statistical technique that allows the investigator to test a sample for outliers is the *gap test*.[8,9]

Use of the gap test provides valid statistical evidence that justifies the exclusion of an outlier from a particular sample. To use the gap test on a sample, you must arrange the series of results in order, from the lowest to the highest value. Then assign the results particular values of x in one of the following two ways:

$$x_1 < x_2 < \ldots < x_n \text{ when testing an extreme high value}$$

$$x_n < x_{n-1} < \ldots < x_1 \text{ when testing an extreme low value}$$

In the first case, the smallest value is designated as x_1; whereas in the second, the largest value is x_1. Particular sample test quotients are then selected from standard statistical tables comparing different values of n and varying levels of significance.[9] A sample test quotient is a ratio of two different equations that describe the relationship of x to the overall range of data. Once the sample test quotient is calculated, it is possible to determine whether there is a statistically unacceptable "gap" between this x and the rest of the data. If so, the x can be justifiably discarded from the data set as an outlier. Since there are different levels of significance and different values of *n*, there are different sample test quotients that can be used. Texts that provide these tables indicate which sample test quotient should be used given the value of *n*, the level of significance selected, and the value (extreme high or extreme low value) that is to be tested. Tests of an extreme high value require the use of a table different from that used for the test of extreme low values.

Use of the sample test quotient allows for calculation of a gap using specific data points in the ordered list. As an example, the sample test quotient used for an *n* of 15 when testing an extremely high value would require a gap calculation based on the ordered results designated as:

$$\frac{x_n - x_{n-2}}{x_n - x_3}$$

The recommended gap is then calculated based on the *n* of the sample and compared with the value listed in the statistical table in the significance column of choice (for example, $p < 0.05$). If the calculated gap is greater than the value listed in the table (at the desired probability level and *n* value), the investigator is justified in discarding this value as an outlier with the significance limit selected in the table.

NONPARAMETRIC COMPARISONS OF POPULATIONS
Nonparametric Distribution Statistics

The statistical tests described above are termed **parametric statistics** because they assume a gaussian, or normal, distribution of the data. Many populations do not meet this criterion, and the analyst needs techniques for describing and comparing these populations statistically. **Nonparametric statistics** require no assumptions about the distribution and thus can be considered more general than parametric statistics.

The simplest nonparametric procedure is to rank the data in order from the lowest (value = 1) to the highest (value = *n*). The range of the data set is the difference between the lowest and highest value, and the median value indicates the central tendency of the data set. The ranked data can be used, for example, to determine the limits of reference intervals for those analytes whose distributions are not gaussian. The lower 2.5 percentile and upper 97.5 percentile of the ranked data are usually selected as the lower and upper limits of a reference interval. The central 95% of the data are within the reference interval limits (see p. 347).

Sign Test

One of the simplest nonparametric tests for the comparison of two nongaussian populations is the **sign test**, which is analogous to the *t*-test. The sign test essentially uses the median rather than the mean of a data set. In one application, all the data in a single data set can be compared with some stated (critical) value. Data points higher than the stated value are assigned a plus value (+), lower points are assigned a minus value (−), and zeros are assigned to those values equal to the critical value. The sign test can also be used to compare the results of two methods (A with B) using paired samples. If the B value is higher than A for a given sample,

the sample is assigned a plus value. If the B value is less than A, it is assigned a minus value, and zeros are assigned to those samples in which A = B. A hypothesis is assumed that there is no difference between the median of the sample data set and the critical value or between the two samples in each pair, depending on how the test is used. If this hypothesis is correct, the median difference (A − B) should be zero and there should be approximately equal numbers of positive and negative differences.

The investigator performs the test by designating the difference between each data pair as negative, positive, or zero, with the actual numerical difference being unimportant, and then tabulating the results. The number of negative results is then compared with a critical range from a table of "exact" confidence limits for *Np* (Table 19-3), entering the table at the level of the number of nonzero differences observed between the two populations. *Np* is a short-term designation for the sample size, *N*, and the significance level of probability, *p*. So, Table 19-3 can be said to describe exact confidence limits for a given sample size at a given probability. If the negative difference value (the number of negative results) is outside the critical range, the difference between the median values of the two populations is considered significant. Example 7 demonstrates the use of the sign test.

Example 7. Sign test.

To determine whether there is a significant difference between plasma and serum potassium concentrations (mmol/L), investigators obtain for analysis both types of samples from 18 volunteers.

Plasma	Serum	Difference
4.0	4.2	−
3.8	3.8	0
3.6	3.7	−
3.9	3.8	+
4.4	4.5	−
4.6	4.4	+
4.8	4.9	−
4.5	4.7	−
4.3	4.5	−
4.0	3.9	+
4.1	4.1	0
4.0	4.1	−
3.5	3.6	−
3.7	3.7	0
3.6	3.7	−
4.2	4.2	0
4.1	4.0	+
4.5	4.5	0

The null hypothesis assumes that there is no difference between the medians of the two samples, and if this hypothesis is correct, the difference between the median of the plasma samples and the median of the serum samples should be zero. There should be approximately equal numbers of positive and negative differences.

Negatives 9

Positives 4

Zeros 5

TABLE 19-3   EXACT CONFIDENCE LIMITS FOR *Np* (BINOMIAL DISTRIBUTION), *P* = 0.05; *N* = 0 TO 99

N	0	1	2	3	4	5	6	7	8	9
0	—	—	—	—	—	—	0-6	0-7	0-8	1-8
10	1-9	1-10	2-10	2-11	2-12	3-12	3-13	4-13	4-14	4-15
20	5-15	5-16	5-17	6-17	6-18	7-18	7-19	7-20	8-20	8-21
30	9-21	9-22	9-23	10-23	10-24	11-24	11-25	12-25	12-26	12-27
40	13-27	13-28	14-28	14-29	15-29	15-30	15-31	16-31	16-32	17-32
50	17-33	18-33	18-34	18-35	19-35	19-36	20-36	20-37	21-37	21-38
60	21-39	22-39	22-40	23-40	23-41	24-41	21-42	25-42	25-43	25-44
70	26-44	26-45	27-45	27-46	28-46	28-47	28-48	29-48	29-49	30-49
80	30-50	31-50	31-51	32-51	32-52	32-53	33-53	33-54	34-54	34-55
90	35-55	35-56	36-56	36-57	37-57	37-58	37-59	38-59	38-60	39-60

Condensed from Lenter C: Geigy scientific tables, vol 2, Introduction to statistics, statistical tables, mathematical formulae, *ed 8, Allschwil, Switzerland, 1982, Ciba-Geigy.*

Take the number of negative differences to a table of "exact" confidence limits for *Np*. Enter the table at *N* = (total number of data pairs) – (number of zero differences). (See Table 19-3.)

$$N = 18 - 5 = 13$$

The critical range for an adjusted sample size of 13 is 2 – 11. Since the observed number of negative differences, 9, does not fall outside this range, the median difference between the paired plasma and serum samples is not significantly different from zero at the 5% level.

Mann-Whitney Rank Sum Test (See Example 8)

Another alternative to the t-test is the *rank sum test*. There are two forms of this test, one by Wilcoxon, the other by Mann and Whitney. The test is commonly called the *Mann-Whitney test* to avoid confusion with the paired test also developed by Wilcoxon.

The test is performed by taking the sample data from the two populations being compared, ranking them as if the data belonged to one population, and then calculating the sum of the ranks of each group. The sum of the smaller *N* is designated *T* and is used in a table of *acceptance regions for the rank sum T* (Table 19-4); the larger *N* is designated in the table as N_2. If the *T-value* is outside the acceptance range for the number of values in each sample, the difference in the median values of the two populations is taken to be significant at a chosen *p* value.

If the populations were identical, an even distribution among the ranks of the two samples would be expected. An

TABLE 19-4   ACCEPTANCE REGION FOR THE RANK SUM *T* (MANN-WHITNEY-WILCOXON 2 SAMPLE TEST), *P* = 0.05

N_1	1	2	3	4	5	6	7	8	9	10	11	12	13	14	15
N_2															
1	—	—	—	—	—	—	—	—	—	—	—	—	—	—	—
2	—	—	—	—	—	—	—	36-52	45-63	55-75	66-88	79-101	92-116	106-132	121-149
3	—	—	—	—	15-30	22-38	29-48	38-58	47-70	58-82	69-96	82-110	95-126	110-142	125-160
4	—	—	—	10-26	16-34	23-43	31-53	40-64	49-77	60-90	72-104	85-119	99-135	114-152	130-170
5	—	—	6-21	11-29	17-38	24-48	33-58	42-70	52-83	63-97	75-112	89-127	103-144	118-162	134-181
6	—	—	7-23	12-32	18-42	26-52	34-64	44-76	55-89	64-104	79-119	92-136	107-153	122-172	139-191
7	—	—	7-26	13-35	20-45	27-57	36-69	46-82	57-96	69-111	82-127	96-144	111-162	127-181	144-201
8	—	3-19	8-28	14-38	21-49	29-61	38-74	49-87	60-102	72-118	85-135	100-152	115-171	131-191	149-211
9	—	3-21	8-31	14-42	22-53	31-65	40-79	51-93	62-109	75-125	89-142	104-160	119-180	136-200	154-221
10	—	3-23	9-33	15-45	23-57	32-70	42-84	53-99	65-115	78-132	92-150	107-169	124-188	141-209	159-231
11	—	3-25	9-36	16-48	24-61	34-74	44-89	55-105	68-121	81-139	96-157	111-177	128-197	145-219	164-241
12	—	4-26	10-38	17-51	26-64	35-79	46-94	58-110	71-127	84-146	99-165	115-185	132-206	150-228	169-251
13	—	4-28	10-41	18-54	27-68	37-83	48-99	60-116	73-134	88-152	103-172	119-193	136-215	155-237	174-261
14	—	4-30	11-43	19-57	28-72	38-88	50-104	62-122	76-140	91-159	106-180	123-201	141-223	160-246	179-271
15	—	4-32	11-46	20-60	29-76	40-92	52-109	65-127	79-146	94-166	110-187	127-209	145-232	164-256	184-281

Condensed from Lenter C: Geigy scientific tables, vol 2, Introduction to statistics, statistical tables, mathematical formulae, *ed 8, Allschwil, Switzerland, 1982, Ciba-Geigy.*

extremely large or extremely small rank sum in one of the samples should not be observed when the populations are the same. The rank sum table gives the limits for these extremes, and if these limits are exceeded, it makes sense to reject the null hypothesis of equality between the two populations.

Example 8. Mann-Whitney rank sum test.

A comparison is conducted to determine whether there is any difference between the blood urea nitrogen (BUN) concentrations in renal transplant recipients with stable graft function and a group of patients with urinary tract infections (UTI). The following results in milligrams per liter are observed in the two groups:

UTI ($n_1 = 14$)		Transplant ($n_2 = 12$)	
Rank	BUN	Rank	BUN
1	150		
2	170		
3	180		
*4.5	190		
		*4.5	190
**7	200		
**7	200		
		**7	200
9.5	210		
		9.5	210
12	220		
		12	220
		12	220
14	230		
16.5	240		
16.5	240		
		16.5	240
		16.5	240
		19	250
20.5	260		
		20.5	260
		22	270
23	280		
24	290		
		25	310
		26	320
Sum =	160.5	Sum =	190.5

$$*4.5 = \frac{4 + 5}{2}$$

$$**7 = \frac{6 + 7 + 8}{3}$$

The smaller of the two sums ($T = 160.5$) is taken to a table of acceptance ranges for the rank sum T (see Table 19-4) at a level of $p = 0.05$ for $n_1 = 14$, $n_2 = 12$. The range of acceptance is 150 to 228. The calculated T-value falls within this range, and the difference in the median values of BUN between these two populations is not considered significant at the 5% level.

χ^2 (Chi-Square) Analysis

When populations contain a continuum of numbers, regression analysis and **correlation coefficients** can usually be used to measure their association. However, when the

values of two populations are discrete, with few possible values, such as yes/no, or positive/negative, **chi-square (χ^2)** analysis is used to test whether the populations are related. The analysis is based on the difference between the observed frequency of the values in a population and the expected frequency of the values of a population.

Often, the results obtained with real samples do not agree exactly with the theoretical results expected according to the rules of probability. For example, if a fair coin is tossed 100 times, 50 heads and 50 tails would be the expected result. However, these exact results are rarely obtained. A statistical method would be needed to determine whether the observed frequencies, say 47 heads and 53 tails, differ significantly from the expected frequencies (50 heads and 50 tails). The χ^2 statistical method provides a measure of the chance discrepancy that may exist between the observed and expected frequencies of the results of an analysis. The formula for the calculation of χ^2 is shown in Eq. 19-14:

$$\chi^2 = \frac{(o_1 - e_1)^2}{e_1} + \frac{(o_2 - e_2)^2}{e_2} + \ldots \frac{(o_k - e_k)^2}{e_k} \qquad \textit{Eq. 19-14}$$

where o = the observed frequency result and e = the expected frequency result. If $\chi^2 = 0$, the observed and expected frequencies agree, whereas if $\chi^2 > 0$, they do not agree exactly. The larger the value for χ^2, the greater is the discrepancy between the observed and the expected frequencies.

In medical and healthcare research, chi-square analysis is often used to answer questions about the relationship between sex, age, race, or hormonal status, and some laboratory test result or physical condition of a patient (such as diabetes or hypertension).

Example 9. χ^2 (chi-square analysis).

In a study designed to determine whether there was a significant difference in estrogen receptor positivity between breast tumors resected from premenopausal and postmenopausal women, the following frequency of positive results were observed:

Premenopausal women:	ER+	308/581
Postmenopausal women:	ER+	648/1079

Is the observed difference in ER (estrogen receptor) positivity between the two groups significant?

	Pos	Neg	Total
Observed			
Pre	308	273	581
Post	648	431	1079
Total	956	704	1660
Expected			
Pre	335	246	581
Post	621	458	1079
Total	956	704	1660

$$\chi^2 = \frac{(308 - 335)^2}{335} + \frac{(648 - 621)^2}{621} +$$

$$\frac{(273 - 246)^2}{246} + \frac{(431 - 458)^2}{458}$$

$$\chi^2 = 7.90$$

TABLE 19-5 CRITICAL VALUES FOR CHI-SQUARE

Level	0.10	0.05	0.01
df			
1	2.706	3.841	6.635
2	4.605	5.991	9.210
3	6.251	7.815	11.345
4	7.779	9.488	13.277
5	9.236	11.070	15.086
6	10.654	12.592	16.812
7	12.017	14.067	18.475
8	13.362	15.507	20.090
9	14.684	16.919	21.666
10	15.987	18.307	23.209

Condensed from Lenter C: Geigy scientific tables, *vol 2*, Introduction to statistics, statistical tables, mathematical formulae, *ed 8, Allschul, Switzerland, 1982*, Ciba-Geigy.

The critical value $\chi^2_{0.05}$ for 1 degree of freedom is 3.84 (Table 19-5). Since $7.90 > 3.84$, the hypothesis that there is no difference between the groups is rejected, and the hypothesis that there is a significantly higher estrogen receptor rate of positivity in breast tumors resected from postmenopausal women is accepted.

When a comparison is made between one sample and another, as in this estrogen receptor sample, an easy rule for the degrees of freedom is that they equal:

(Number of variables in columns − 1) ×

(Number of variables in rows − 1)

Sample: (Pos + Neg −1) × (Pre + Post − 1) = 1

Example 10. A continuation of χ^2 (chi-square analysis). The numbers in the previous chi-square table are represented by variables in the chart below. The expected values are calculated under the assumption that the percentage of distribution between the positive and negative values should be equal for both the premenopausal and postmenopausal populations. This is true with any 2×2 chi-square table.

	Pos	Neg	Total
Observed			
Pre	a_1	a_2	N_a
Post	b_1	b_2	N_b
Total	N_1	N_2	N_T
Expected			
Pre	$N_1(N_a/N_T)$	$N_2(N_a/N_T)$	N_a
Post	$N_1(N_b/N_T)$	$N_2(N_b/N_T)$	N_b
Total	N_1	N_2	N_T

There are simple formulas for computing χ^2 that use only the observed frequencies. The following give results for the 2×2 contingency table used in the previous estrogen receptor example.

$$\chi^2 = \frac{N(a_1b_2 - a_2b_1)^2}{(a_1+b_1)(a_2+b_2)(a_1+a_2)(b_1+b_2)} = \frac{N\Delta^2}{N_1N_2N_aN_b}$$

$$\chi^2 = \frac{1660(132,748 - 176,904)^2}{956 \times 704 \times 581 \times 1079} = 7.67$$

LINEAR REGRESSION AND CORRELATION

For a wide variety of clinical laboratory applications, it is useful to determine the relationship between two variables, x and y. If x can be considered a "fixed," or an *independent*, variable and y can be considered a "not fixed," or a *dependent*, variable, then it is mathematically valid to describe y as a *function* of x. A widely used, and sometimes misused, statistical procedure for assessing this relationship or describing this function is regression analysis.

Simple "linear" regression analysis can be used when the relationship between the independent x and dependent y variables is a linear one. This type of regression analysis is termed "simple" because there is one independent variable. The simplest model for a relationship between two variables would be a straight line. Linear-regression analysis can be graphed on a rectilinear x,y plot where each pair of values is a point on the graph. Once all the x,y pairs are plotted, a straight line of "best fit" can be manually drawn through the points. If the straight-line model appears to be a valid depiction of the relationship between x and y, the line is termed the *regression line*, and its calculation is referred to as "regressing y on x."

Simple linear-regression analysis is used to answer this question: If you know what one variable (x) is, can you calculate what the other variable (y) would be under certain conditions? Here is another way to ask this question: Can changes in x be used to predict changes in y? In consideration of this question, the x variable can also be termed the "predictor" variable and the y variable can be called the "response" variable.

In simple linear-regression analysis, the equation that describes the linear relationship between x and y also can be said to describe y as a function of x, that is, $y = f(x)$. This function is described in Eq. 19-15:

$$y = \alpha + \beta x + \epsilon \qquad \textit{Eq. 19-15}$$

where α is the true value of the intercept of the regression line and β is the true value of the slope of the regression line. Using this function, x can be used to make a prediction of y.

In practice, the values of α and β in Eq. 19-15 are unknown and must be estimated as a and b respectively. It is also expected that the majority of the data points will not fall precisely on the regression line. The term ϵ is included in Eq. 19-15 to describe the distance between any observed value of y and the corresponding value of y that would be predicted or expected for y, which is denoted as $\hat{y}$. This value of ϵ is also termed the residual and exists because there is variability expected in y for any fixed, accurately known value of x. This basic assumption for using simple regression analysis is that for every known value of x, there is a corresponding normal distribution of y values. This assumption is graphically illustrated in Fig. 19-10, *A*. Notice

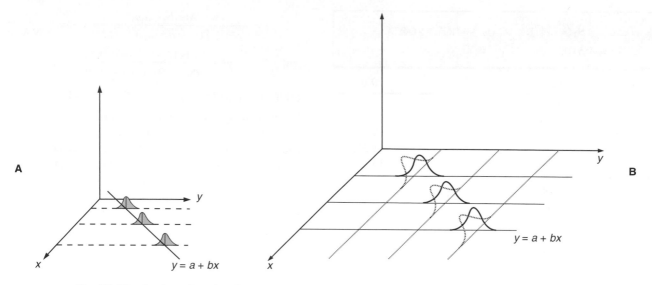

Fig. 19-10 **A,** Gaussian distributions of *y* values around simple linear-regression line. **B,** Gaussian distribution around Deming regression.

that the regression line passes through the means of the distributions.

Use of the simple linear-regression model for appropriate applications requires that the two variables *x* and *y* satisfy several conditions.

1. The x values are considered fixed, and any **random error** in the measurement of *x* can be considered "negligible."
2. For every value of *x*, there is a normal distribution of *y* values as illustrated in Fig. 19-10, A.
3. The distribution of *y* values for every value of *x* has the same variance; that is, the variance around the line is independent of the value of *x*.
4. The expected values of *y* for each *x* generally fit the straight-line model.
5. The straight-line model that is estimated is not horizontal (i.e., β does not equal 0). If the straight line were horizontal, the values of *y* on the regression line would not be a better predictor of *y* than the mean *y* value, or $\bar{y}$.

If these conditions are met, use of the simple linear-regression model will allow the correct estimates of expected *y* values for each fixed value of *x* to be inferred.

The above conditions for simple linear regression should be satisfied for the majority of clinical laboratory applications. But in certain instances, the *x* values cannot be considered "fixed" or "invariable" as defined in condition 1. The most common misuse of simple linear-regression analysis involves the false assumption that values of *x* are fixed or that *x* is an independent variable when, in fact, it is not. For example, in a typical comparison of two methods, the results of one method will be considered to be the "*x*," independent variable (see pp. 415–417). Although this may be the current method, each "*x*" result cannot be considered "fixed" but is reported with a certain error. In this instance, it is appropriate to consider using a different type of regression analysis. Although several types of regression techniques are

described in the literature, the technique that may be most appropriate to apply when variability exists in the values of x and in the values of y is the Deming regression technique (Fig. 19-10, *B*).[10,11]

In a simple linear-regression analysis, an investigator could attempt to determine values for *a* and *b* using the manual plot of the data and the "best-fit" regression line (see p. 357). Conventionally, however, the method used to determine the correct regression parameters is the *method of least squares*. Using this method, the analyst mathematically minimizes the sum of the squares of the residuals of all the *y* values. Predicting expected *y* values based on the actual *x,y* data points by this method and calculating the subsequent regression statistics, for either the simple or Deming's model, are most easily accomplished with the use of a calculator or software program that can generate the appropriate statistics automatically.

The method of least squares is valid if the residuals are random (i.e., independent of values of *x* and *y*) and have a gaussian distribution with a mean of 0 and a standard deviation, $S_{y,x}$.[11] The standard deviation of the residuals, or *standard error of the estimate*, should be constant at every *x* value (see p. 359). It has been reported that within the range of measurement commonly encountered in most clinical laboratory applications, the method of least squares also correctly calculates a regression line when $S_{y,x}$ is proportional to *x*.[11]

Appropriate clinical laboratory applications for simple linear-regression analysis, when *x* can legitimately be considered a fixed or independent variable, are:

1. Comparison of results from a new procedure to results from an established procedure.
2. Comparison of a technique to a reference method (see Chapter 22 for these two applications).
3. Comparison of paired results for the same test or analyte

collected from two different analytical systems in current use. This application could be used to validate test systems secondarily with a test system that has been validated by external proficiency testing. This application would satisfy the Clinical Laboratory Improvement Amendments of 1988 regulations for proficiency testing.

4. Comparison of results from the same analytical system collected during two different analytical runs.

In either simple linear or Deming regression analysis, a relationship exists between the *x* and *y* variables, though the mathematical description of this relationship would be somewhat different for each type of regression technique. When a linear relationship exists between two variables, these variables can be considered to have a *correlation* with each other. If increasing values of *x* are related in a linear fashion to increasing values of *y*, there is a *positive correlation* between these variables. If increasing values of *x* are related in a linear fashion to decreasing values of *y*, there is a *negative correlation* between these variables (see p. 360).

It is, of course, possible that the relationship between two variables is a nonlinear relationship. If this is the case, the computation of basic linear-regression parameters may reflect this relationship. For example, determination of the correlation coefficient, *r*, may indicate a value much closer to 0 than either 1 or –1. It is also likely that a nonlinear relationship would be reflected in an increased value $s_{y,x}$. If this were the case, the application of either simple linear regression or Deming regression analysis would be inappropriate and other regression techniques would be utilized.[4-8] Of course, it is also true that a nonlinear relationship or an increased amount of scatter may be apparent upon visual inspection of the regression plot.

Basic Statistics of Simple Linear Regression and Correlation

With the two methods of linear regression described above, the line of best fit would be determined by either the method of least squares or the method of Deming. In either case, once the correct line to fit the appropriate model is identified, this line can then be described by Eq. 19-16:

$$y = bx + a \qquad \textit{Eq. 19-16}$$

where *b* is the estimated slope of the regression line and *a* is the estimated intercept of the regression line on the *y*-axis.

Although the "best fit" of the regression line may appear obvious by visual examination of the graphed scatterplot, this method is not recommended. More appropriately, calculation of the regression parameters, *a* and *b*, with the use of a calculator or software program allows for an exact prediction of any additional value of *y* once the *x* value is known. Automatic calculation of the regression parameters and the subsequent determination of two predicted *y* values from two different *x* values would then allow for the correct graphical placement of the regression line, since two points determine the location of a straight line.

In simple linear regression, the statistical parameters, *a* and *b*, the *y*-intercept, and the slope of the regression line

respectively can be calculated by use of Eqs. 19-17 and 19-18:

$$a = \bar{y} - b\bar{x} \qquad \textit{Eq. 19-17}$$

$$b = \frac{\sum(x - \bar{x})(y - \bar{y})}{\sum(x - \bar{x})^2} \qquad \textit{Eq. 19-18}$$

To measure the variability of the data points about the regression line, the investigator must determine the standard deviation about the regression line of the differences between the observed and the predicted values of *y* (i.e., the residuals). This variability, termed the *standard error of the estimate*, is calculated by use of Eq. 19-19:

$$S_{y,x} = \left(\frac{\sum(y - \bar{y})^2}{N - 2}\right)^{1/2} \qquad \textit{Eq. 19-19}$$

Use of $(N - 2)$ degrees of freedom in the denominator is appropriate because two regression coefficients, *a* and *b*, had to be determined from the data in order to calculate the predicted values of *y*. That is, two restrictions are placed on the N observations.

The variability of the estimated slope, *b*, of the simple linear-regression line is determined by first calculating the standard deviation of the slope, s_b, using Eq. 19-20:

$$s_b = s_{y,x} / [\Sigma(x_i - \bar{x})^2]^{1/2} \qquad \textit{Eq. 19-20}$$

and then determining a $100(1 - p)\%$ confidence interval for the true slope, β, using Eq. 19-21:

$$\beta = b \pm t \cdot s_b \qquad \textit{Eq. 19-21}$$

where *t* is obtained from a two-sided *t*-table for $N - 2$ degrees of freedom and the desired level of significance.

The variability of the estimated intercept, *a*, of the simple linear-regression line is determined in a similar manner. The estimated standard deviation of *a*, s_a, is calculated by use of Eq. 19-22:

$$s_a = s_{y,x}[\Sigma x_i^2 / N\Sigma(x_i - \bar{x})^2]^{1/2} \qquad \textit{Eq. 19-22}$$

and then by determination of a $100(1 - p)\%$ confidence interval for the true intercept, *a*, by use of Eq. 19-23:

$$\alpha = a \pm t \cdot s_a \qquad \textit{Eq. 19-23}$$

where *t* is, again, obtained from a two-sided *t*-table for $N - 2$ degrees of freedom and the desired level of significance.

The statistic that provides a measure of how closely the data points lie to the regression line is *r*, or the Pearson correlation coefficient. This correlation coefficient, *r*, is a measure of the degree to which two variables are linearly related. The calculation of *r* is illustrated in Eq. 19-24:

$$r = \frac{\sum(x_i - \bar{x})(y_i - \bar{y})}{\{\sum[(x_i - \bar{x})^2][\sum(y_i - \bar{y})^2]\}^{1/2}} \qquad \textit{Eq. 19-24}$$

Essentially, *r* describes the strength of correlation between the *x* and *y* variables.

The correlation coefficient, *r*, can range in value from –1 to 1. If *r* is equal to 1, there is a perfect positive correlation between the variables. If *r* is equal to –1, there is a perfect negative correlation between the variables. The further the correlation coefficient is from 0, the stronger the correlation is, positive or negative, between the variables. If the correlation coefficient is equal to 0, there is no *linear* relationship between the variables. This should not be interpreted to mean that there is no relationship between the two variables; it is possible that these two uncorrelated variables are strongly related in *nonlinear* fashion (this would be apparent from a visual inspection of the *x,y* scatterplot).

At what value of *r* can one assume there is not a linear relationship between the *x* and *y* variables? From an empirical perspective, an *r* value between –0.7 and 0.7 would indicate that the probability of the relationship between *x* and *y* being linear is less than 50%. As *r* approaches zero, this probability also approaches zero. If the data collected for analysis by linear regression is from routine laboratory methods, a practical consideration is that a low *r* value can be caused by very poor precision in the method used to obtain *x* values, *y* values, or both variables.

An example of the use of equations 19-17 to 19-24 for calculation of basic statistics of simple linear-regression analysis is illustrated in Example 11. This example illustrates the use of simple linear-regression analysis and Deming regression analysis for the comparison of two potassium methods. Equations for the calculated Deming regression statistics are given elsewhere.[10]

Example 11. Linear-regression analysis.

In an initial method comparison study, 42 pairs of potassium measurements are obtained from an established method (old) and an experimental method (new). Calculate regression statistics, first assuming there is negligible variability in the old method (use simple linear-regression analysis) and then assuming there is variability in the established method (using Deming regression equations, as cited in references 10 and 11).

Assuming there is negligible variability in the established method, calculate the standard error of the estimate, variability of the estimated slope and intercept, and the 95% confidence intervals for the actual slope and intercept for the population.

All *x,y* (old,new) potassium results are in millimoles per liter:

3.9, 3.9	3.9, 3.9	3.4, 3.4	5.4, 5.2	4.0, 4.0
4.6, 4.5	4.2, 4.2	4.3, 4.1	4.3, 4.3	4.8, 4.7
3.7, 3.6	4.4, 4.3	4.4, 4.4	4.5, 4.4	3.9, 3.9
4.3, 4.3	3.8, 3.7	3.8, 3.7	3.9, 3.8	4.0, 3.9
4.6, 4.5	3.4, 3.4	4.2, 4.1	3.8, 3.8	3.6, 3.6
4.3, 4.3	4.1, 4.0	3.5, 3.4	4.6, 4.8	4.1, 4.2
3.7, 3.1	4.1, 4.1	4.8, 4.7	3.3, 3.2	5.4, 5.4
4.0, 3.9	4.5, 4.4	3.5, 3.6	3.7, 3.7	4.1, 4.1
3.6, 3.5	3.0, 3.1			

	Simple linear-regression analysis	Deming regression
Slope (*b*)	0.99	0.98
Intercept (*a*)	–0.03	0.22
$S_{y,x}$	0.12	0.09
r	0.97	0.98

For 95% confidence intervals and $N - 2$ degrees of freedom (40), *t*-value from a two-sided table = 2.021.

Variability of estimated slope:
Standard deviation of estimated slope (*b*) =
$$s_b = s_x / [\Sigma(x_i - \bar{x})^2]^{1/2} = 0.12/3.24 = 0.04$$
Confidence interval for the true slope (*β*) =
$$\beta = b \pm t \cdot s_b = 0.99 \pm 2.021 \,(0.04) = 0.99 \pm 0.07$$

Variability of estimated intercept:
Standard deviation of estimated intercept (*a*) =
$$s_a = s_{y,x}[\Sigma x_i^2 / N\Sigma (x_i - \bar{x})^2]^{1/2} = 0.12(1.28) = 0.15$$
Confidence interval for the true intercept (*α*) =
$$\alpha = a \pm t \cdot s_a = -0.03 \pm 2.021 \,(0.15) = -0.03 \pm 0.30$$

Testing for Outliers Using Residual Analysis

Simple linear-regression analysis can be used to identify outliers, or extreme paired values, in the *x,y* data points. This procedure involves the plotting of the residuals, or ∈, against the independent variable *x*.[8] It may then be appropriate to exclude any data points that generate residuals greater than $4\,s_{y,x}$. The plot of residuals can be evaluated against the independent variable *x* for assessment of the equality of variances. If the variances are equal, the plotted residuals will be seen as a horizontal band of points independent of *x* (one of the conditions necessary to apply simple linear regression to a pair of variables).

Additional information can be obtained by plotting the residuals against the predicted values of *y*. If there is truly a linear relationship between the *x* and *y* variables, the residuals would be randomly scattered, in horizontal fashion, around zero.

Limitations of Simple Linear-Regression Analysis

When paired data spanning a limited range are analyzed by the simple linear-regression method, an acceptable level of random error can still result in inaccurate estimates of the slope and intercept of the regression line. This problem is magnified if the *x* variable should really not be considered fixed or independent. In this instance, an unacceptably large standard error of the slope and intercept, as well as an unacceptably low correlation coefficient, may also be calculated, and it is appropriate to use Deming regression analysis instead of simple linear-regression analysis.

Other considerations may suggest that Deming regression should be used instead of simple linear-regression analysis. An initial assessment of this question can be made by plotting one variable on the *x*-axis in a first *x,y* plot and generating regression statistics. The procedure is then, repeated with the second variable plotted on the *x*-axis. If the two least-squares regression lines are substantially different from each other, the Deming regression should be used. The Deming method will yield one regression line between *x* and *y* that takes into account the error in measuring both variables. A characteristic of the Deming regression technique is that switching the variables and recalculating regression statistics will give identical statistics to the initial calculation.

Finally, it must be noted that the value of *r* in simple linear-regression analysis is sensitive to both the scatter of the data points and the range of data points. The scatter of the data points is a characteristic of the dependent method being evaluated. But it is possible to increase the value of r by simply extending the range of data. Extension of the range of data by one single point farther away from the majority of data points where this single point coincidentally happens to demonstrate close agreement between x and y will dramatically increase the value of r. This characteristic is described in Eq. 19-25:

$$r = (1/s_x)\,(s_x^2 + s_{y,x}^2)^{1/2} \qquad \textit{Eq. 19-25}$$

where s_x is the standard deviation of the x population, an indication of the spread in the x data. As s_x becomes very large relative to $s_{y,x}$, r approaches 1.0. Because of this characteristic, it is always wise to evaluate an x,y plot, visually examining the simple linear-regression line generated from the data. It may be obvious that a point lying far above or below the regression line is an outlier. But a more insidious outlier might be the point that lies exactly on the regression line but is considerably removed from the range of the remaining data points used to generate the regression statistics.

References

1. *Webster's Ninth New Collegiate Dictionary*, Springfield, MA, 1988, Merriam-Webster, Inc.
2. Sheskin DJ: *Handbook of parametric and nonparametric statistical procedures*, Boca Raton, FL, 1996, CRC Press.
3. Jones RG and Bayne RB: *Clinical investigation and statistics in laboratory medicine*, London, 1997, ACB Ventures Publications.
4. Freedman D, Pisani R, Purves R: *Statistics*, ed 3, New York, 1998, W.W. Norton & Company.
5. Strike PW: *Measurement in laboratory medicine—a primer on control and interpretation*, Oxford, England, 1996, Butterworth-Heinemann.
6. Shott S: *Statistics for health professionals*, Philadelphia, 1990, Saunders.
7. Fisher LD and Van Belle G: *Biostatistics: a methodology for the health sciences*, New York, 1993, Wiley Press.
8. Lenter C: *Geigy scientific tables, vol 2, Introduction to statistics, statistical tables, mathematical formulae*, ed 8, Allschwil, Switzerland, 1982, Ciba-Geigy.
9. Hollander M, Wolfe DA: *Nonparametric statistical methods*, ed 2, New York, 1999, Wiley-Interscience.
10. Wallers PJM, et al: Applications of statistics in clinical chemistry—a critical evaluation of regression lines, *Clin Chem Acta* 64:173, 1975.
11. Cornbleet PJ, Gochman N: Incorrect least-squares regression coefficients in method-comparison analysis, *Clin Chem* 25(3):432, 1979.

Internet Sites

http://www.math.uah.edu/stat/index.html—University of Alabama at Huntsville, Mathematics Department

http://www.math.yorku.ca/SCS/StatResource.html—University of York, Mathematics Department, with a statistical resource link in their Statistical Consulting Service area

http://nimitz.mcs.kent.edu/~blewis/stat/scon.html—Department of Mathematics and Computer Science, Kent State University, guide to elementary inferential statistical methods

http://www.ruf.rice.edu/~lane/rvls.html—Rice Virtual Lab in Statistics

http://www.statistics.com—A general web page detailing a myriad of statistical resources

http://www.bertholf.net/rlb/Lectures/Statistics.pps—PowerPoint lecture by Robert L. Bertholf, PhD, Associate Professor of Pathology, Chief of Clinical Chemistry and Toxicology

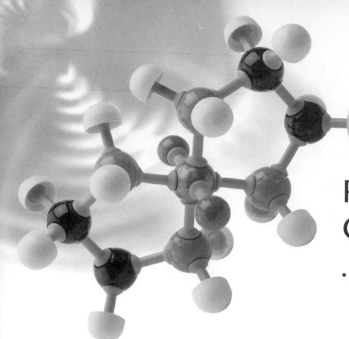

CHAPTER 20

Reference Intervals and Clinical Decision Limits*

• *Edward A. Sasse*

Objectives

• State the purpose of reference intervals and identify primary considerations of the sampling process when establishing a reference interval.

• Suggest a statistical approach for establishing the reference interval for nongaussian distributions.

Key Terms

abnormal   Test results outside of reference intervals observed in people with disease or in less than good health.

cutoff values   Those limits above or below which the patient is abnormal or positive for a condition such as substance abuse.

decision analysis   Strategy comparing risks and benefits of predicting the true diagnosis or outcome.

gaussian   A particular symmetrical statistical distribution; also called the *normal distribution.*

healthy   A relative term that must be defined for each reference population.

log normal   A symmetrical gaussian population distribution obtained by a plot of the logarithm of the data.

log normal distribution   A sample of values with a long tail to the right can often be made to act as a gaussian distribution when the logarithms of values are used.

medical decision limits   The values or changes in values that result in immediate medical intervention or change in medical management.

---

*The editors wish to acknowledge Paul Horn as a reviewer of this chapter.

negative predictive value   The probability that a laboratory result falling within the reference interval reflects the true absence of disease; defined as true negatives divided by the sum of true negatives and false negatives, or as the predictive value of a negative result.

normal   A term with many meanings, including those persons in the nondiseased population and an equivalent term for a gaussian distribution (see later discussion).

observed value   The quantitative value (test result) obtained for a test subject (such as a patient) to be compared with reference values, reference distributions, reference limits, or reference intervals.

outlier   An observation that arises from a population different from the reference population. The outlier can be an erroneous result or an observation on a subject that does not conform to the characteristics of a reference individual.

partitioning of reference values   The process of separating reference intervals of subjects based on criteria of age, sex, and race, as well as statistical analysis showing significant differences between the populations.

positive predictive value   The probability that a laboratory result outside the reference interval actually reflects the presence of disease; defined as true positives divided by the sum of true positives and false positives.

predictive value   Probability that a laboratory result accurately reflects the true presence or absence of disease. It is dependent on the actual prevalence of the disease.

prevalence   The number of persons who have a disease in a given population at any one point in time, or more often the rate of such disease, which is also called *disease frequency.*

receiver-operating characteristic (ROC) curve   A graphical presentation of discrimination of disease from nondisease by plotting sensitivity.

reference distribution   The distribution of reference values. Hypotheses regarding the distribution of reference values of a reference population may be tested statistically.

reference individual   An individual selected on the basis of well-defined criteria. It is usually important to define the individual's health, age, sex, and race.

reference interval (Listed in the Clinical Laboratory Improvement Amendments of 1988, CLIA '88, as a reference range.)   The interval between and including two reference limits. It is designed as the central interval of values bounded by the lower reference limit and upper reference limit at certain designated percentiles. For example, for fasting glucose the central 95th percentile reference interval is 65 to 110 mg/dL (3.6 to 6.1 mmol/L), that is, 95% of the apparently healthy population will have a fasting glucose value of 65 to 110 mg/dL.

reference limit   A numeric value or values derived from the reference distribution and used for descriptive purposes. It is common practice to define a reference limit so that a stated fraction of the reference values will be less than or equal to, or more than or equal to, the respective upper or lower limit.

reference population   A group consisting of all the reference individuals. The reference population usually has an unknown number of members and therefore is a hypothetical entity.

reference range   The entire range (actual minimal to maximal measured values) of laboratory values of people without disease.

reference sample group   An adequate number of reference individuals selected to represent the reference population.

reference value   The value (test result) obtained by the observation or measurement of a particular analyte for a reference individual. Reference values are obtained from a reference sample group.

sensitivity   A term used to describe the probability that a laboratory test is positive (i.e., outside of the reference interval) in the presence of disease; defined as true positives divided by the sum of true negatives and false positives.

specificity   Used to describe the probability that a laboratory test will be negative (i.e., within the reference interval) in the absence of disease; defined as true negatives divided by the sum of true negatives and false positives.

standard deviation   A measure of variability. In the gaussian distribution, two standard deviations above and below the mean encompass the central 95% of the population data, and one standard deviation above and below encompasses 68.3% of the data.

DEFINITION OF REFERENCE INTERVAL

The medical interpretation of clinical laboratory data is a comparative decision-making process in which a laboratory test result for an individual is compared with a **reference interval** derived from **reference values.** Therefore, reliable reference values are required for all tests in the clinical laboratory and must be provided by clinical laboratories and diagnostic test manufacturers. The reference intervals most commonly used (often known as *normal values*, and sometimes *expected values*) are often poorly defined.

Reference intervals should be determined in a systematic and scientific manner that provides an acceptable degree of confidence for the clinical decision-making process, which includes a consideration of the significant factors and variables introduced by the specific individual's reference sample or by the analytical process itself. Understanding the process used to establish a reference interval yields a better understanding of the limitations of the defined reference interval.

To facilitate the generation of reliable reference intervals, the National Committee for Clinical Laboratory Standards (NCCLS) has recently published a document entitled *How to Define and Determine Reference Intervals in the Clinical Laboratory; Approved Guideline* (NCCLS Document C28-A2),[1] which establishes guidelines and procedures for determining valid reference values and reference intervals for quantitative clinical laboratory tests. The NCCLS document catalogs the significant factors and variables that may affect the reference interval and is based on the recommendations of the Expert Panel on Theory of Reference Values (EPTRV) of the International Federation of Clinical Chemistry (IFCC).[2-7] The recommendations given in the NCCLS guideline are intended to comprise a standard protocol for determining reference intervals that meet the minimum, mandatory requirements for reliability.

Consequently, reference interval determination should follow the guidelines of the NCCLS protocol. However, there are instances, particularly for geriatric and pediatric populations, when it is difficult to collect data from the recommended number of **reference individuals.** In these instances, the proper and well-defined selection of reference individuals becomes preeminent. These reference values, with their limitations, are still useful to the practice of medicine in these particular patient categories.

Reference values may be associated with good health or with specific physiological or pathological conditions and may be used for different reasons. For example, to establish the **sensitivity** and **specificity** of a laboratory test, the laboratory must carefully define the population. In all cases, the reference values allow comparison of observed data to reference data for a defined population of subjects. This comparison then becomes part of the decision-making process.

TERMINOLOGY

Specific definitions for terms permit relatively unambiguous description and discussion of the subject of reference values. The definitions listed in the key terms have been proposed by the EPTRV of the IFCC[2] and International Council for Standardization in Hematology and have been endorsed by the World Health Organization (WHO) and other organizations worldwide.

The scheme[2] at the top of the right column demonstrates the relationship between the defined terms.

The **reference limits** and associated reference interval are usually estimated by a statistical method. Reference limits

(1) REFERENCE INDIVIDUALS
comprise a
↓

(2) REFERENCE POPULATION
from which is selected a
↓

(3) REFERENCE SAMPLE GROUP
on which are determined
↓

(4) REFERENCE VALUES
on which is observed a
↓

(8) OBSERVED VALUE
in an individual may
be compared with (5)

(5) REFERENCE DISTRIBUTION
from which are calculated
↓

(6) REFERENCE LIMITS
that may define
↓

(7) REFERENCE INTERVALS

serve only to describe the **reference sample group** or **reference population** and are strictly a function of the characteristics of the designated population.

The term **reference range** has commonly been used as a substitute for *reference interval;* however, such a term should be avoided. *Range* should be reserved for describing a set of values defined by the actual minimal and maximal measured values, that is, the entire range of values of the measured set.

The reference intervals most commonly used to describe **healthy** individuals have been known as *normal values,* referring to reference values that have been observed in **normal,** or healthy, people. Test results outside of these reference intervals may, therefore, be observed in people with disease or in states of less than good health and have consequently been termed as **abnormal.** However, there is often an overlap of *normal* and *abnormal* values in disease because most disease processes and associated biological analytes change in a continuing fashion. Consequently, *normal* values do not always indicate a lack of disease (Figs. 20-1 to 20-3), nor does a value exceeding a defined limit always indicate disease. The use of the term *normal* in this context is now considered to be ambiguous.

The word *normal* has several different connotations in laboratory medicine that can cause confusion. Values are often described as normal if their observed distribution

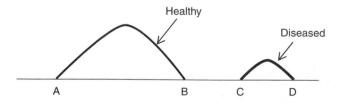

Fig. 20-1 Perfectly separated test result distributions of healthy and diseased populations. This clear separation rarely occurs in reality.

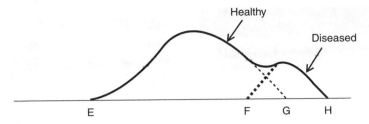

Fig. 20-2 Usual test result distributions of healthy and diseased populations in which an overlap between the two occurs.

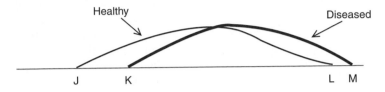

Fig. 20-3 Degree of test result overlap does not permit differentiation between healthy and diseased populations.

seems to follow the theoretical **gaussian** ("normal") distribution. However, biological data from a reference sample group are often not gaussian, and the use of *normal* may be misleading by implying that the data are symmetrical or bell-shaped in distribution. Other meanings of *normal* are *common, frequent, usual,* and *typical,* which also may be used in statements referring to biological or clinical values. Therefore it is more precise and less confusing to avoid the terminology *normal values* and replace it with *reference values* (or *reference interval*) *obtained from healthy individuals, health-associated reference values* (or *reference intervals*), or colloquially, *healthy reference values* (*intervals*). As previously mentioned, reference intervals can also be established for physiological conditions other than good health.

PROTOCOL OUTLINE FOR OBTAINING REFERENCE VALUES AND ESTABLISHING HEALTH-ASSOCIATED REFERENCE INTERVALS[1]

The collection or verification of reference values from healthy subjects and the subsequent estimation of the reference interval for a given analyte is a requirement of CLIA '88 regulations (§493.1213), *Federal Register* 57(40) Feb 28, 1992, and must be carried out in accordance with a well-defined protocol. This involves following the sequence of operations listed in the box.

It is sometimes acceptable to transfer a previously established reference interval that is based on a valid reference value study from a donor laboratory or manufacturer to a receiving laboratory without performing a new, full-scale study. Such a transfer is acceptable only if the test subject population and the entire methodology, from preparation of the test individual to the analytical measurement in the receiving laboratory, are the same as or appropriately comparable to those of the donor laboratory (see following text). The comparability of the analytical measuring system

PROTOCOL OUTLINE FOR OBTAINING REFERENCE VALUES AND REFERENCE INTERVALS

The procedure manual must include the following, when applicable to the test procedure:
1. Consult the medical and scientific literature and list possible biological variations and analytical interferences. (In the case of a totally new analyte, a laboratory may need to perform its own studies.)
2. Establish selection (or exclusion) and partition criteria and an appropriate questionnaire designed to reveal these criteria in the potential reference individuals.
3. Categorize the potential reference individuals based on the questionnaire findings and the results of other appropriate health assessments.
4. Exclude individuals from the reference sample group, based on the exclusion criteria or other assessments indicating a lack of good health.
5. Select the appropriate reference individuals.
6. Prepare the reference individuals properly and consistently for specimen collection following the specific requirements for the analyte and consistent with routine practice for patients.
7. Collect and process the biological specimens properly and uniformly and consistent with the routine practice for patient specimens.
8. Determine the reference values by analyzing the specimens according to the respective analytical methodology under well-defined conditions.
9. Inspect the reference value data and prepare a histogram.
10. Identify data errors and values that are outliers.
11. Analyze the reference values, that is, select a statistical method of estimation and estimate reference limits and the reference interval (include partitioning into subclasses for separate reference intervals, if appropriate).
12. Document all the above steps and procedures.

BOX 20-1

EXAMPLES OF POSSIBLE EXCLUSION CRITERIA

Alcohol consumption
Recent illness
Abnormal blood pressure
Lactation
Blood donor, frequent
Obesity
Drug abuse
Occupation
Prescription drugs
Oral contraceptives
Over-the-counter drugs
Pregnancy
Environment
Recent surgery
Fasting or nonfasting
Tobacco use
Genetic factors
Recent transfusion
Current/recent hospitalization
Vitamin abuse

From National Committee for Clinical Laboratory Standards: How to define, determine and utilize reference intervals in the clinical laboratory: proposed guideline, ed 2, NCCLS Document C28-A2, Villanova, PA, 2000, NCCLS.

BOX 20-2

EXAMPLES OF POSSIBLE PARTITIONING FACTORS

Age
Posture when sampled
Blood group
Race
Circadian variation
Sex
Diet
Stage of menstrual cycle
Ethnic background
Stage of pregnancy
Exercise
Time of day when sampled
Fasting or nonfasting
Tobacco use
Geographical location

From National Committee for Clinical Laboratory Standards: How to define, determine, and utilize reference intervals in the clinical laboratory: proposed guideline, ed 2, NCCLS Document C28-A2, Villanova, PA, 2000, NCCLS.

can be validated using the techniques discussed in NCCLS Document EP9-A, *Method Comparison and Bias Estimate Guideline.*[8] It may be necessary to carry out an abbreviated reference value study, as described later, to validate the transferred reference interval.

SELECTION OF REFERENCE INDIVIDUALS

Health is a relative condition lacking a universal definition. Defining what is to be considered healthy becomes the initial problem in any study, and establishing the criteria used to exclude nonhealthy subjects from the reference sample is the first step in selecting reference individuals. Frequently, it can only be determined that a particular individual is apparently "disease free," that is, does not have a specific medical condition that might affect the reference interval study. In some cases, individuals with minor illnesses or "unrelated" conditions may be used as reference individuals. However, it is often difficult to estimate the potential physiological and pharmacological influences in these subjects, and appropriate caution is required.

The selection of reference individuals for a reference value study is important and should be systematic.[1,3,9] Each institution or investigator may have different criteria for health; these criteria should be defined *before* selection proceeds. As a minimum it is recommended that the investigator establish lists of selection, exclusion, and potential partition criteria (examples are shown in Boxes 20-1 and 20-2) and use a questionnaire to evaluate these criteria in the potential reference individuals. The use of designed questionnaires is one of the best ways to consistently implement the exclusion and partitioning criteria. Forms should be simple and nonintimidating, requiring only *yes* or *no* responses to questions. The questionnaire may be used with simple measurements, such as blood pressure, height, and weight, and with an interview during which it is appropriate to ask individuals if they consider themselves to be in good health. Name, address, and phone number and any additional information, such as a patient identification number, should be included to facilitate contacting the reference individual when abnormal results are obtained. Certainly there is an obligation to notify the individual or the individual's physician in such cases. In some situations anonymous questionnaires may be a better vehicle for obtaining the required information. In these instances a numbering system can be used. (The reference individual is then responsible for contacting the laboratory to determine if the testing showed any problems that require follow-up study.) In all cases, the usual policy for patient confidentiality must be enforced.

Informed consent should be obtained from reference individuals for specimen collection and testing. In some cases, protocol review and approval by an institutional research committee (human use committee) may be necessary. A sample questionnaire is provided in the NCCLS C28-A2 document.[1] Determination of the health status of the individuals by medical examinations and laboratory testing is not considered to be essential. However, if these assessments are performed, they will, of course, strengthen the reliability of the reference interval determination. All criteria and assessments used should be documented so that others can evaluate the health status of the reference sample group.

Reference individuals used for the determination of a health-associated reference interval do not have to be young healthy adults but should closely resemble the patient population in the specific hospital or practice that will be using the results. However, for some particular analytes a "standard" population of young healthy adults may be appropriate. For others, age-related sets of reference intervals may be more appropriate. In the elderly population, it may be particularly important to rule out disease by use of additional diagnostic assessments. Patient populations should not be used as disease-free reference individuals unless it is absolutely essential, as in certain instances for pediatric or geriatric populations.

It is necessary to determine for each analyte whether there are age-related differences, whether these differences are clinically important, and whether the use of age sub-groups for reference intervals will be clinically appropriate. For certain biological constituents, age-related differences are consistent with good health and are part of a normal process of growth or maturation, such as alkaline phosphatase levels in children versus those in adults. However, for levels of other substances, such as cholesterol or possibly growth hormone in the elderly, the use of different levels to reflect age differences may not be medically suitable when developing health-associated reference intervals. Consequently, determination of the need for separate reference intervals for age subgroups at specified age-group intervals is a rather complex medical decision. Review of the literature can be very helpful in making this evaluation.

The terms *a priori* and *a posteriori* are used to describe two general methods of selecting reference individuals from the reference population. *A priori* sampling is a method that is best used for well-studied, established laboratory procedures. Well-defined exclusion and partitioning criteria are established before the selection of the reference individuals. For established methods, a thorough search of the literature should allow identification of known sources of biological variation, enabling the researchers to establish exclusion and partitioning criteria and to develop an appropriate questionnaire. Reference individuals are then selected and partitioned into subclasses, if necessary. This process should take place *before* any blood samples are collected. The number of reference individuals selected for analysis must closely match the number required to be statistically valid.

The *a posteriori* approach is especially appropriate for new or poorly studied laboratory procedures for which the literature contains little information. In *a posteriori* sampling the process of exclusion and partitioning takes place after sampling and analyte testing rather than before. Because the factors defining a subclass are not usually known, the questionnaire for this approach should be more detailed than the one designed for the *a priori* sampling process. Generally the *a posteriori* approach requires large numbers of subjects and substantial computing power to be implemented effectively.

PREANALYTICAL AND ANALYTICAL VARIABLES

Analytical results from reference populations are affected by preanalytical and analytical variables. Therefore, all these variables must be considered and controlled consistently when reference intervals are determined.[10-15] In addition, it is important that reference subjects and samples be handled in an approved manner[16-22] and in exactly the same manner as patients and patient samples will be handled in the actual clinical analysis situation. All the preanalytical variables discussed in detail in Chapter 3 and reviewed in Box 20-3 must be carefully considered, controlled if necessary, and documented.

ANALYTICAL METHOD CHARACTERISTICS

The validity of information provided by the laboratory is critical; thus the methods chosen for specimen analysis must be described in detail, clearly stating accuracy, precision, minimum detection limit, linearity, recovery, and interference characteristics.[10-12] Other factors that affect analytical performance also require control and documentation. These include equipment or instrumentation, reagents (including water), calibration standards, and calculation methods.

BOX 20-3

EXAMPLES OF PREANALYTICAL VARIABLES

Subject Preparation
Prior diet
Fasting versus nonfasting
Abstinence from pharmacological agents
Drug regimen
Synchronization in analysis
Relation to biological rhythms
Physical activity
Rest period before collection
Stress

Specimen Collection
Environmental conditions during collection
Time
Body posture
Specimen type
Collection site analysis
Site preparation
Blood flow promotion
Equipment
Technique

Specimen Handling
Transport
Clotting
Separation of serum/plasma
Storage
Preparation for analysis

From National Committee for Clinical Laboratory Standards: How to define and determine reference intervals in the clinical laboratory: approved guideline, ed 2, NCCLS Document C28-A2, Villanova, PA, 2000, NCCLS.

Reagent lot-to-lot and technologist variability, as well as instrument-to-instrument variability (if the test will be performed on more than one instrument), must be determined. Thus the use of more than one technologist and more than one lot of reagent should be incorporated in the study protocol.

It is important to document the validity of the data generated during the reference interval study. Therefore, during the determination of reference intervals, quality control materials are routinely analyzed in the same format used for patient samples. This not only monitors the analytical protocol used during the process, but also ensures equivalence of results over the long term.[13] Ideally, data will be gathered by analyzing specimens over several days, resulting in values that reflect average run-to-run variation (see Chapter 21). In addition, an assessment of the interference from naturally occurring constituents is essential.

ANALYSIS OF REFERENCE VALUES[1]
Statistical Methods

The reference interval is defined here as the interval between and including two numbers, an upper and lower reference limit. These two numbers are estimated to enclose a specified percentage (usually 95%) of the values for a population from which the reference subjects have been drawn. For most analytes, the lower and upper reference limits are assumed to demarcate the estimated 2.5th and 97.5th percentiles, respectively, of the underlying distribution of values. In some cases, only one reference limit is of medical importance, usually an upper limit, say, the 97.5th percentile.

Two general statistical methods for determining such limits are the nonparametric and the parametric procedures (see Chapter 19). Detailed presentations of these procedures have been published by Solberg.[6,9] The nonparametric method of estimation makes no specific assumption concerning the mathematical form of the probability distribution represented by the observed reference values. The parametric method, as applied in practice, is used under the assumption that the **observed values**, or some mathematical transformation of those values, follow a gaussian (i.e., "normal") probability curve. Because the reference values of many analytes do not follow the gaussian form, use of the parametric method requires that they be transformed to some other measurement scale that will "normalize" them. This requires selecting the most suitable transform (such as log, power, or some other function of the original scale) and then testing whether, on this new scale, the reference values do indeed appear to conform to a gaussian distribution. When the log function is used to transform the data to gaussian, the data are considered to have a log normal distribution. The chi-squared goodness-of-fit test and the Kolmogorov-Smirnov nonparametric test of the cumulative distribution may be used to determine if the reference values have a gaussian distribution. This may involve some moderately complex statistical theory and corresponding computer programs.

The NCCLS Guideline document[1] recommends that the reference interval be estimated by the nonparametric method

TABLE 20-1 FREQUENCY DISTRIBUTIONS OF CALCIUM LEVELS IN 240 MEDICAL STUDENTS, BY SEX			
	FREQUENCY		
Analyte (mg/L)	Women	Men	Combined
88	1	0	1
89	2●	0	2
90	1	0	1
91	3	2	5●
92	11	1●	12
93	11	8	19
94	8	6	14
95	16	11	27
96	16	12	28
97	26	13	39
98	8	16	24
99	7	14	21
100	3	7	10
101	2	10	12
102	3◆	11	14
103	2	7◆	9◆
104	0	1	1
106	0	1	1
Total	120	120	240

From National Committee for Clinical Laboratory Standards: How to define and determine reference intervals in the clinical laboratory: approved guideline, ed 2, NCCLS Document C28-A2, Villanova, PA, 2000, NCCLS.
●*Indicates the 2.5th percentile.*
◆*Indicates the 97.5th percentile.*

and that a minimum of 120 reference values be used for the reference interval determination. The nonparametric method is simple, depending only on the ranks of reference data arrayed in order of increasing values. As an example, the frequency distribution for calcium reference values is shown in Table 20-1. The rank of the percentile observation is the percentile times ($n + 1$) the number of degrees of freedom. Thus for 120 values, the rank of the 2.5th percentile observation is 3, that is, $0.025 \times 121 = 3.025$; and the rank for the 97.5th percentile observation is 118, that is, $0.975 \times 121 = 117.975$. These are indicated in Table 20-1 by ● and ◆, respectively. Using these rank values to estimate upper and lower reference limits, we obtain the following 95% reference intervals: 89 to 102 mg/L for women and 92 to 103 mg/L for men, or 91 to 103 mg/L for the combined population.

Using the nonparametric method, it is impossible to distinguish between two percentiles of a distribution unless the number of observations, n, equals $(100/P) - 1$, in which P is the difference between the two percentiles. Consequently, the nonparametric method requires an absolute minimum of 39 measurements to distinguish the 2.5th percentile from the 5th percentile or the 95th percentile from the 97.5th percentile, $n = (100/2.5) - 1 = 39$. Reed, Henry, and Mason[23] have suggested that a minimum of 120 observations be secured, one from each reference group, allowing 90% confidence limits to be computed nonparametrically for each reference limit at the 2.5th and 97.5th percentiles. To estimate the reference limits for these same percentiles with 95% confidence, 153 reference values are needed; for 99% confidence, 198 reference values are needed. Recently Lott et al,[24] using a Monte Carlo simulation technique and large numbers of samplings of a medical student population, found that increasing the size of the sample had a stabilizing effect on the 2.5th and 97.5th percentiles. At about 200 individuals, the lower and upper reference limits for seven tests (Na, K, Cl, glucose, hemoglobin, erythrocytes, hematocrit), as determined by the nonparametric method, became stable. This experimental finding agrees with the 198 subjects required by strictly statistical criteria to define the same limits with a 99% confidence level. Linnet[25] has proposed that up to 700 observations should be obtained for highly skewed distributions. Clearly, a greater number of observations will improve the statistical accuracy of the estimation.

The minimum number of 120 samples is made under the assumption that no observations have been deleted from the reference set. If aberrant or outlying observations have been deleted, additional subjects should be selected until at least 120 acceptable reference values have been obtained for each determination of a reference interval. Moreover, if separate intervals are needed for different subclasses (for sex or age class, for example), each such interval should be determined using the recommended number (at least 120) of reference observations.

Confidence Intervals

The reference limits computed from a sample of selected subjects are estimates of the corresponding percentiles in the population of individuals studied. Confidence intervals are useful for two reasons. First, they remind the investigator of the variability of estimates and provide a quantitative measure of this variability. Second, confidence intervals narrow as the size of the sampling increases. Therefore the investigator can get an idea of the improved precision in an estimated 95% reference interval that would be obtained from a larger sampling of reference individuals.

Table 20-2 demonstrates the 90% confidence intervals for the lower and upper 95% reference limits for calcium.

TREATMENT OF OUTLYING OBSERVATIONS

An important implicit assumption in the estimation of reference limits is that the set of measured reference values represents a "homogeneous" collection of observations. This means that all values come from the same underlying probability distribution.

It may be that this condition is satisfied by almost all the reference values but that one or two arise from a probability distribution different from that of their fellows. When such values fall within the expected distribution, they are practically impossible to identify unless the individual performing the biochemical analysis happens to know that these observations represent atypical analytical conditions or

TABLE 20-2 90% Confidence Intervals for Lower and Upper 95% Reference Limits		
Analyte	Lower Reference Limit	Upper Reference Limit
Calcium (mg/L)		
Women (*n* = 120)	88 to 91	101 to 103
Men (*n* = 120)	91 to 93	103 to 106
Combined (*n* = 240)	88 to 91	103 to 106

From National Committee for Clinical Laboratory Standards: How to define and determine reference intervals in the clinical laboratory: approved guideline, ed 2, NCCLS Document C28-A2, Villanova, PA, 2000, NCCLS.

are the result of some arithmetic or procedural mistake. Often, however, such "aberrant" values lie outside the range of the remaining measurements and often can be identified as **outliers** requiring special attention.

Unless outliers are known to be aberrant observations, that is, the result of a mistake in the analysis or a lapse in the preanalytical controls applied to the remaining subjects, the emphasis should be on retaining rather than deleting them. Nonparametrically estimated reference limits based on at least 120 observations would be only slightly changed, or not changed at all, if an extreme value were deleted. There are many statistical techniques available for testing the atypicality of outlying observations.[26] A test proposed by Dixon[27] uses the ratio *D/R*, in which *D* is the absolute difference between an extreme observation (large or small) and the next largest (or smallest) observation, and *R* is the range of all observations including extremes, to evaluate outlying observations. Reed, Henry, and Mason[23] have suggested the use of 1/3 as a **cutoff value** for the ratio *D/R*; that is, if the observed value of *D* is equal to or greater than one third of the range *R*, the extreme observation is deleted. For sample sizes as large as 120, this criterion is rather conservative[23]; that is, it would often fail to reject outliers that are really not part of the distribution. However, in the absence of evidence that an outlier is indeed an aberrant observation and given that the underlying distribution will often not be exactly gaussian in form, the one-third rule for the ratio *D/R* seems appropriate, especially when reference intervals are determined by the nonparametric method. Therefore the NCCLS guideline supports the use of this test and the cutoff value of one third suggested by Reed, Henry, and Mason when looking for statistically significant outliers in a set of observed reference values.

When two or three outliers are present on the same side of the distribution (i.e., all are extremely large or extremely small), the one-third rule (or any similar *D/R* rule) can fail to label the most extreme outlier as statistically significant and thereby mask the presence of the other outliers just slightly less extreme. Common sense indicates that, in such a case, the one-third rule should be applied to the least extreme outlier as if it were the only outlier. If the rule leads to rejection of this outlier, the more extreme observations should naturally be rejected as well. If the rule does not reject the least extreme value, either all the extreme values should be accepted or, alternatively, a test that considers all the outliers together should be applied. Such a test is called a *block procedure;* examples are given by Barnett and Lewis.[26] When any outlier is rejected, it is appropriate to test the remaining data for an additional outlier or outliers.

PARTITIONING OF REFERENCE VALUES

The possibility that separate reference intervals will be required for subclasses of subjects should be considered before the process of securing and analyzing subject specimens is begun. However, the use of separate reference intervals for men and women or for different age groups, for example, may not be justified unless these separate intervals will be clinically useful or are well grounded physiologically. When necessary, at least 120 subjects of each sex or age or other subclass should be sampled. The information necessary to decide whether **partitioning of reference values** is needed may not be available in advance for a new analyte.

It has been generally assumed that when the difference between the observed means of two subclass populations is statistically significant (at the 5% or 1% probability level), each subclass warrants its own reference interval. However, any observed difference, no matter how unimportant clinically, will become statistically significant if the sample sizes are large enough. It is important to consult with an appropriate clinician to define what a *clinically* significant difference is. If the difference between subgroups is *not clinically significant*, the reference values should not be partitioned, even if there is a statistically significant difference between the means (as determined by a *t*-test).

Recent research by Harris and Boyd[28] has shown that differences between subclass means or differences in the **standard deviations (SD)** of the subclasses, even when the means are identical, can lead to deviations in the sensitivity and specificity for disease detection. They found that at times there is a statistical need for separate reference intervals, which, if ignored, could potentially hamper the interpretation of laboratory results as part of the diagnostic process. An approach suggested by Harris and Boyd[1,28] tests the *statistical* significance of the difference between subclass means by the standard normal deviate test (*z*-test), beginning with a pilot sample of 60 subjects in each subclass. If the calculated statistic *z* exceeds a "critical" *z* value (see Chapter 19), separate reference intervals should be calculated for each subclass. In addition, if the larger SD of the two subclasses exceeds 1.5 times the smaller SD regardless of the *z* value, separate reference intervals should be calculated.

For two subclasses, such as men and women or two age groups, the statistical significance of the difference between subclass means should be tested by the standard normal deviate test:

$$z = \frac{[\bar{x}_1 - \bar{x}_2]}{[(s_1^2/n_1) + (s_2^2/n_2)]^{1/2}} \qquad \text{Eq. 20-1}$$

in which $\bar{x}_1$ and $\bar{x}_2$ are the observed means of the two subgroups, s_1^2 and s_2^2 are the observed variances, and n_1 and n_2 are the number of reference values in each subclass, respectively. If at least 60 subjects are assumed in each subclass, the *z*-test is essentially a nonparametric test and may be applied to the original data whether or not the values represent a gaussian distribution. The calculated statistic *z* should be compared with a "critical" value *z**:

$$z^* = 3\,(n_{\text{average}}/120)^{1/2} = 3[(n_1 + n_2)/240]^{1/2} \qquad \text{Eq. 20-2}$$

In addition, the larger standard deviation, for example s_2, should be checked to see whether it exceeds $1.5s_1$, or, equivalently, whether $s_2/(s_2 - s_1)$ is less than 3 (see box).

For example, suppose that at the end of the first stage of sampling the average number of reference values in each subclass is 60. Then, if the calculated *z* exceeds a *z**, that is, $3(60/120)^{1/2} = 2.12$, or if the larger standard deviation exceeds 1.5 times the smaller standard deviation, sampling should be continued to obtain at least 120 subjects in each subclass. The *z*-test and standard deviation comparisons should be repeated. If the average number of subjects in each subclass is now 120, $z^* = 3$.

At this point, if the calculated *z* value exceeds *z**, or if the larger standard deviation exceeds 1.5 times the smaller, regardless of the *z* value, separate reference intervals should be calculated for each subclass, under the assumption that the difference between the two reference intervals is likely to be of importance in medical practice. If these conditions do not hold, a single reference interval for the combined group of reference subjects should be calculated for general use. The box below gives an example of this calculation.

When more than two subclasses are being compared, the problem is more complicated. A statistically significant

---

CALCULATION OF A *z* STATISTIC TO TEST FOR SUBCLASS DIFFERENCE

Example: To test for subclass difference between the calcium reference values for men and women, the means and standard deviations of each group are needed:

Calcium (mg/L), $n_1 = n_2$

$\bar{x}$, men	$\bar{x}$, women	SD, men	SD, women
98.0	95.7	3.1	2.9

Inserting these statistics into the formula given above for *z*, the results are:

Calcium:
$$z = \frac{|98.0 - 95.7|}{\left[\frac{(3.1)^2}{120} + \frac{(2.9)^2}{120}\right]^{1/2}} = 5.94$$

The *z* value exceeds the critical value $z^* = 3$ for $n = 120$, indicating that separate reference intervals for men and women should be considered. The SD of the male population is not greater than 1.5× the SD of the female group and thus does not indicate a subclass difference on this basis.

difference found when the means of all subclasses are compared may, in fact, be attributable only to a difference between two means, such as the mean of one subclass versus the mean of the other subgroups combined. For three or more subclasses, the common statistical analysis of results would be the analysis of variance, if it is assumed that all subclasses have equal standard deviations. In this case, a critical F-statistic comparable to the z^* value defined earlier (and therefore dependent on the sample sizes in each subclass) would have to be defined. It is suggested that in this situation the aid of a statistical consultant should be sought.[29]

The statistical tests and criteria recommended earlier may also be applied to the question of whether reference intervals determined in one laboratory should be transferred without change for use in another laboratory (see the discussion of transference).

In the preceding examples, the differences in calcium values between men and women, although statistically significant, are small and may not be clinically significant. The z-test in this case is certainly sensitive. Considering the imprecision of the assay and the 90% confidence intervals calculated previously for calcium, a laboratory may choose to provide only a single reference range of 91 to 103 mg/L for both men and women in this age group. The final decision may be made based on the clinical relevance of the statistically significant difference.

TRANSFERENCE

Because the determination of reliable reference intervals can be a major and costly task, it is cost-effective to transfer a reference interval from one laboratory to another by a convenient process of validation. As new tests and methods are introduced in laboratories, it is unrealistic to expect each laboratory, large or small, to develop its own reference intervals. Consequently, clinical laboratories rely on other laboratories or on manufacturers of diagnostic tests to provide adequate reference value data that can be transferred. To transfer reference values properly, certain conditions must be fulfilled. For example, the original reference value study must meet the minimum requirements of a valid study as outlined by NCCLS C28-A2. The preanalytical and the analytical procedural details, analytical performance, the complete set of reference values, and the method of estimating the reference interval must be stated.

If it is assumed that the original reference value study was properly performed, the transference of a reference interval from one testing agency to another involves two problems: the comparability of the two analytical systems and the comparability of the two test subject populations. If both testing agencies do not use the same closed analytical system, the comparability of the two systems can be assessed as outlined by the NCCLS Approved Guideline EP9-A.[8] In addition, all preanalytical procedures used during the reference value study, such as preparation of the test subjects and specimen collection and handling procedures, must also be the same as those used by the receiving laboratory. The factors that must be considered before a reference interval is

---

> ### FACTORS TO CONSIDER FOR TRANSFERENCE OF REFERENCE INTERVALS
>
> 1. Appropriateness of donor laboratory reference interval (i.e., selection of reference individuals, exclusions and partitions, number of reference values, method of estimation, and valid reference interval determination according to NCCLS C28-A2 requirements).
> 2. Comparability of preanalytical factors (i.e., subject preparation and specimen collection and handling and other items listed in Box 20-3).
> 3. Comparability of analytical method (i.e., same [closed method] or different [use NCCLS EP9-A] method).
> 4. Comparability of test subjects in terms of factors listed in Box 20-2.
> 5. Validation study, if necessary.

---

transferred are reviewed in the box above. If, in the judgment of the laboratorian, these factors are consistent with the receiving laboratory's operation and test subject population, the reference interval may be transferred.

The NCCLS approved guideline[1] has two alternative procedures for the transference protocol that use either $n = 20$ or $n = 60$. Both shorter protocols require the same considerations as the larger protocol does (see the box on p. 370).

PRESENTATION OF REFERENCE INTERVALS

Every quantitative clinical result should be accompanied by an appropriately presented *reference interval*. The reference intervals should reflect the subclass partitions that have been determined to be significant for that laboratory's particular reference population. Reports that include the results of many tests should clearly highlight those results that are not within the reference interval. It is helpful to indicate the relationship of a patient's results to those of the reference interval. Printing *high* or *low* adjacent to a result is an acceptable option.

When forms with preprinted reference intervals are used, reference intervals for all appropriate subclasses should be included. This can result in a confusing report. A better approach is for the computer or instrument to print the reference interval appropriate for the particular patient. In most cases, the age and sex of the patient will determine the subclass reference intervals. Any report that uses subclass reference intervals should have the patient's partitioning factors included in the heading or in the demographics portion of the report.

Ideally, detailed information describing the reference population and the details of the reference interval study should be available to all users of a laboratory service. This information should be updated any time a change is made in the laboratory that affects the reference intervals in use. A memo addressing changes in a reference interval should be sent to all users of the laboratory.

INTRAINDIVIDUAL REFERENCE INTERVALS

The National Institutes of Health (NIH) has shown that even healthy individuals studied over several weeks under standardized conditions exhibited a range of values for numerous analytes.[30,31] (See Table 3-1, Chapter 3, for examples of intraindividual variations.) For the same analyte, some individuals had analyte values that fell within a narrow range, whereas for others the variability was quite large. The larger component of variability in some analytes was the preanalytical and analytical variation, whereas in others it was biological variability. In the NIH study, the spread of results obtained in any one individual was consistently less than the population-based reference interval. Thus an intraindividual abnormal result for a particular individual could fall within the so-called healthy population–based reference interval. The variability of results also means that a healthy individual might occasionally have test results that fall outside a reference interval derived from a central 95% population–based interval and therefore be falsely categorized as having abnormal test results. Another individual might have a result that is abnormal for his or her specific range but falls within the population-based reference interval; this individual would therefore have a falsely normal result.

These studies showed that it is clearly impossible to develop a reference interval from 120 healthy individuals that is appropriate for every individual. They also showed that it is impractical to develop a series of reference intervals that consider each and every possible variable that might affect the concentration of an analyte. Consequently, laboratorians are left with the compromise of the population-based reference interval developed under those conditions that can be controlled and that is reasonably consistent with the patient testing conditions. D.S. Young[32] discusses this in detail.

TABLE **20-3** Purposes for Which Laboratory Tests are Ordered and Importance of Reference Intervals in Interpretation of Their Results

Purpose	*Reference Interval*
Diagnosis of disease	++
Screening for disease	+++
Determination of severity of disease	+
Monitoring progress of disease	+
Monitoring response to therapy	+
Monitoring therapy	+++
Monitoring drug toxicity	++
Predicting response to treatment	+
Predicting prognosis	+
Reassurance of patient	++

From Young DS: Determination and validation of reference intervals, Arch Pathol Lab Med *116:704, 1992.*
+, Minor importance; ++, moderate importance; +++, great importance.

Many clinicians are unaware of the preanalytical and analytical factors that may affect the interpretation of test results. It is important for all clinicians to understand that all results within the reference interval are not always considered healthy, nor are all results outside the reference interval considered abnormal. Thus it is essential that clinical laboratories interact with the clinicians who use their services to ensure the proper interpretation of test values in patients.

CLINICAL DECISION LIMITS
Predictive Value Theory

Clinical decision limits are different from reference intervals because they are based on medical information related to a specific medical condition. They may be "critical values," describing limits of analyte concentrations that demand immediate medical intervention or change in management, they may be diagnostic cutoff values with a high association for a disease or clinical condition, or they may be therapeutic window limits for pharmaceutical agents (Table 20-3).

Decision analysis is a practical strategy for considering the risks and benefits of decision-making based on the quantitative probability of predicting the true diagnosis or outcome. The respective quantitative approaches used by the laboratorian or clinician in evaluating clinical laboratory measurements and data have been well described[33,34] and have been generally accepted. The concepts of sensitivity, specificity, and **predictive values** of test results are fundamentally important to these probabilistic approaches. These concepts are now being applied more frequently in the clinical laboratory, not only to establish clinical decision limits but also to assist in determining the relative clinical merits of a given test (Fig. 20-4).[32]

The *diagnostic sensitivity* of a test is the probability of obtaining a positive result for a patient with a given disease, that is, the percentage of individuals with the disease who test positive. In contrast, the *diagnostic specificity* of a test is the probability of obtaining a negative result for a patient without the disease, that is, the percentage of individuals without the disease who test negative. The true positives (TP) are the individuals with the disease who are correctly classified by the test, that is, individuals with the disease who have positive test results. The false positives (FP) are the individuals without the disease who are incorrectly classified by the test, that is, healthy individuals who have positive test results. The false negatives (FN) are the individuals with the disease who are incorrectly classified by a negative test result. The true negatives (TN) are the individuals without the disease that correctly test negative. Because sensitivity is the true-positive rate, the complement, 100% minus sensitivity, is the false-negative rate. For example, if the sensitivity is 75%, the false-negative rate will be 25%. Accordingly, because specificity is the true-negative rate, 100% minus specificity is the false-positive rate.

The *predictive value of a positive test* is the probability that the patient with a positive test result has the given disease, that is, the fraction obtained when the number of true-positive results is divided by the total number of positive

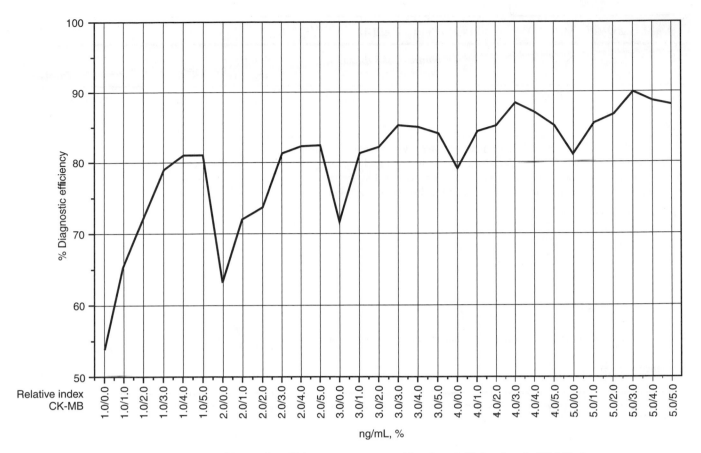

Fig. 20-4   Percent diagnostic efficiency versus combined cutoff levels of CK-MB in nanograms per milliliter (lower set of values on *x*-axis) and percent relative index, expressed as (CK-MB/total CK) × 100. Combining these two tests at different respective cutoff levels produced the highest diagnostic efficiency, 90%, at a cutoff of 5 ng/mL for CK-MB and 3% for the relative index. *(Courtesy D. Obzansky, Du Pont Co., Wilmington, Delaware.)*

test results. The *predictive value of a negative result* is the probability that the patient with a negative result does not have the disease, that is, the fraction obtained when the number of true-negative results is divided by the total number of negative test results. The *efficiency* of the test is the fraction of all the tested individuals who were correctly classified as either having or not having the disease. These probabilities are often converted to and discussed as percentages.

Predictive values and diagnostic efficiency are greatly influenced by the false-positive and false-negative rates and the **prevalence** of the disease in the population being tested (Table 20-4). The importance of prevalence in determining the predictive value (expressed as a percentage) can be seen by rearrangement and substitution of the terms for the predictive value of a positive result (PV+) to give the following equivalent equation:

$$\text{PV+} = \frac{[\text{Prevalence} \cdot \text{Sensitivity}] \times 100\%}{[\text{Prevalence} \cdot \text{Sensitivity}] + [(1 - \text{Prevalence})(1 - \text{Specificity})]} \qquad \textit{Eq. 20-3}$$

Thus, for a test with a diagnostic sensitivity of 95% and a diagnostic specificity of 95%, the predictive value for a

positive result in a population with a prevalence of the disease of 50% is 95%. However, if the prevalence is 5%, the PV+ is 50%, or for a prevalence of 1%, the PV+ is only 16.1%. When the PV+ is 50%, the predictive value of the test is no better than chance; thus a coin may be tossed to decide if a patient with a positive test result actually has the disease.

It is clear that although a test has high sensitivity and specificity and is a good diagnostic test in a defined population of patients, it will perform less well in another population where the prevalence is very low. For example, a positive creatine kinase-MB (CK-MB) result is more significant (has a higher PV+) in a population of patients in a cardiac care unit (with prevalence of myocardial infarction at 30% to 50%) than in an emergency unit (with prevalence of myocardial infarction at ~5%).

The sensitivity of a specific laboratory test can vary as the disease progresses through various stages in the continuum of disease development over a relatively long term. This variability is seen, for example, with atherosclerosis, cancer, and diabetes. Thus a tumor marker test may have low sensitivity for very early cancer, but a much higher sensitivity for detecting advanced stages of the same cancer. On the other hand, certain tests can be so sensitive as to detect or predict

TABLE 20-4 SENSITIVITY, SPECIFICITY, PREDICTIVE VALUE*

	Number of Subjects with Positive Test Result	Number of Subjects with Negative Test Result	Total
Number of subjects with disease	TP	FN	TP + FN
Number of subjects without disease	FP	TN	FP + TN
TOTALS	TP + FP	FN + TN	TP + FP + TN + FN

TP, True positives, or number of diseased patients correctly classified by the test.
FP, False positives, or number of patients without the disease misclassified by the test.
FN, False negatives, or number of diseased patients misclassified by the test.
TN, True negatives, or number of patients without the disease correctly classified by the test.

$$\text{Diagnostic sensitivity} = \frac{TP}{TP + FN}$$

$$\text{Diagnostic specificity} = \frac{TN}{FP + TN}$$

$$\text{Predictive value of positive test, PV+} = \frac{TP}{TP + FP}$$

$$\text{Predictive value of negative test, PV–} = \frac{TN}{TN + FN}$$

$$\text{Efficiency of the test (number fraction of patients correctly classified), that is,} \ \frac{TP + TN}{TP + FP + TN + FN}$$

$$\text{Prevalence} = \frac{TP + FN}{TP + FP + TN + FN}$$

*From Statland BE et al: Quantitative approaches used in evaluating laboratory measurements and other clinical data. In Henry JB, editor: Clinical diagnosis and management by laboratory methods, Philadelphia, 1979, Saunders.

disease before there are symptoms. The predictive value of the test in a population will then also be, in part, dependent on the relative proportion of patients with disease that has advanced to a detectable level.

As a general rule, tests that are used for the screening of occult disease in the general population (low disease prevalence) should have as high a diagnostic sensitivity as possible, consistent with an acceptable level of false-positive results (specificity). Generally, both maximal sensitivity and specificity are desired. In the example above of a test with 95% sensitivity and specificity, if the test is used to screen for a disease present in a population with a 1% prevalence, 83.9% of the people who have a positive test result will *not* have the disease. If this rate of false-positive values is unacceptable, the specificity of the test will have to be increased at the expense of the sensitivity. Alternatively, if the diagnostic sensitivity and positive predictive value are not mutually acceptable, the test should not be used for screening but should be applied only to populations with a higher prevalence of the disease.

Galen and Gambino[34] have suggested the following guidelines for deciding whether a test should have the highest sensitivity, the highest specificity, the highest **positive predictive value**, or the highest efficiency. Please note that it is *not* possible to have all these attributes at the same time.

The highest sensitivity (preferably 100%) is desired in the following diagnostic situations:

1. The disease is serious and should not be missed, and

2. The disease is treatable, and
3. False-positive results do not lead to serious physical, psychological, or economic trauma to the patient.

Example. Pheochromocytoma. This disease can be fatal if missed, but if diagnosed, it is nearly 100% curable. Other examples include phenylketonuria, venereal disease, and other treatable infections.

The highest specificity (preferably 100%) is desired in the following diagnostic situations:

1. The disease is serious but is not treatable or curable, and
2. The knowledge that the disease is absent has psychological or public health value, and
3. False-positive results can lead to serious psychological or economic trauma to the patient.

Example. Multiple sclerosis and most occult cancers. These diseases are serious but not generally treatable or curable.

A high predictive value for a positive result is essential in the following diagnostic situation:

1. Treatment of a false-positive individual might have serious consequences.

Example. Occult cancer of the lung, in which the treatment of lobectomy or radiation has significant morbidity.

The highest efficiency is desired in the following diagnostic situations:

1. The disease is serious but treatable, and
2. False-positive results and false-negative results are essentially equally serious or damaging.

Example. Myocardial infarction. The disease may be fatal but is treatable. Other examples include lupus erythematosus, some forms of leukemia and lymphoma, and diabetes mellitus.

It is apparent that the predictive value or efficiency estimation for a given test is highly dependent on the population of patients tested. Comparisons of the predictive value or efficiency of different tests or different methodologies are valid only if the populations studied are the same. Unless the patient populations studied are carefully defined, sufficiently large, and very similar, predictive values from different studies may be misleading if the relative merits of the tests are judged. For example, as suggested earlier, a study of the predictive value or efficiency of a CK-MB assay for diagnosing myocardial injury will most certainly give different results when the patient population consists of patients in the cardiac intensive care unit from the results it would give for a population of patients with chest pain in the emergency room. Caution must even be used in comparing predictive values between different studies of critical care unit patients from different institutions because the institutions may treat different patient populations and may use different specific criteria for admission to the unit or for making a final diagnosis.

Medical Decision Limits

Another important use of the concepts of sensitivity, specificity, and predictive value is in the determination of an optimal cutoff value or **medical decision limit** for a clinical laboratory test. The diagnostic sensitivity and specificity are dependent on the cutoff value selected. When a relatively low medical decision limit is used for CK-MB, the diagnostic sensitivity of the test may approach 100% for the diagnosis of myocardial injury (few or no false-negative results); however, the diagnostic specificity may decrease to a range of 50% to 60% (a large number of false-positive results). When a higher cutoff value is used, the specificity will improve but the sensitivity will decrease. Whenever a medical decision limit is changed, there is a tradeoff between the diagnostic sensitivity and the specificity of the test. The perfect test, if it were to exist, at a perfect cutoff value would have both a sensitivity and a specificity of 100% and a diagnostic efficiency of 100%.

Certainly, laboratories and clinicians have to collaborate and agree on the balance of false positives versus false negatives for each diagnostic situation. Some knowledge of the distributions of test results for diseased versus nondiseased populations can be very helpful when medical decision limits (Figs. 20-1, 20-2, and 20-3) are chosen. As illustrated in Figs. 20-2 and 20-3, test result distributions of healthy and diseased populations commonly overlap. For some diseases and certain tests, not all individuals with a particular disease will ever have a test result for a particular

test outside the healthy reference interval. Also the test results may be affected by more than one disease. In addition, the test results distribution can reflect the continuum from good health to the diseased condition or the stage of a given disease. For example, knowledge of the distribution of prostate-specific antigen (PSA) levels in men with benign prostate hypertrophy (BPH), in men with prostate cancer, and in men with normal prostates has led to the adoption of four decision limits: 0 to 4 ng/mL associated with normal prostates; 4 to 10 ng/mL normally associated with BPH but rarely with prostate cancer; 10 to 20 ng/mL often associated with prostate cancer; and >20 ng/mL associated almost always with prostate cancer. Thus, as the concentration of PSA increases, the likelihood of disease increases, and the specificity of the assay increases. Most experienced clinicians have a practical feel for such medical decision limits, using a relative high (or low) analyte level as an inclusion level to conclude confidently that a patient is in the population with the disease, or vice versa, to exclude the patient from the population with the disease. The medical decision limit helps the clinician make choices regarding diagnosis, follow-up care, or the need for adjunct diagnostic testing.

The intended clinical use of a test will also be a factor in selecting the best cutoff value. In a given clinical setting the consequences of a false-negative result may be far more serious than those of a false-positive result. False negatives are entirely unacceptable when testing for human immunodeficiency virus (HIV) infection among blood donors and organ transplant donors. Alternatively, less harm may be caused by classifying a patient as having myocardial injury by a CK-MB test when the patient in fact did not have a myocardial infarction (MI) (a false positive) than by classifying a patient with an MI as negative (a false negative). Clearly, discharging a patient with an MI from the emergency department or clinic could be catastrophic for that patient. On the other hand, needlessly subjecting a patient with a falsely positive test result to other diagnostic procedures or interventions associated with a certain amount of risk is also not desirable. In addition, it could be prohibitively expensive to admit too many patients who have not had an MI to the cardiac intensive care unit. Galen and Gambino[34] have suggested that the best cutoff value to use for classifying a patient as having had an MI is the value that produces the highest diagnostic efficiency.

There is no simple way to select the optimum combination of sensitivity and specificity. The choice, as discussed earlier, depends on the nature of the disease, the clinical population, and the relative cost of a false-positive or false-negative result. Additional sequential, supplemental, or confirmation testing can often compensate for a test with a high rate of false-positive results and minimize the associated undesirable consequences.

Receiver-Operating Characteristic Curve

The ability of a test, using a specific analyte concentration, to discriminate disease from nondisease can be graphically portrayed by use of **receiver-operating characteristic**

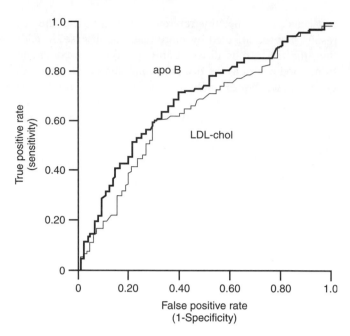

Fig. 20-5 Receiver-operating characteristic (ROC) curves showing discrimination between subjects with and without any coronary artery disease as measured by cardiac catheterization for two different biochemical indicators. *(From Zweig MH, Broste SK, Reinhart RA: ROC curve analysis: an example showing the relationships among serum lipid and apolipoprotein concentrations in identifying patients with coronary artery disease,* Clin Chem *38:1425, 1992.)*

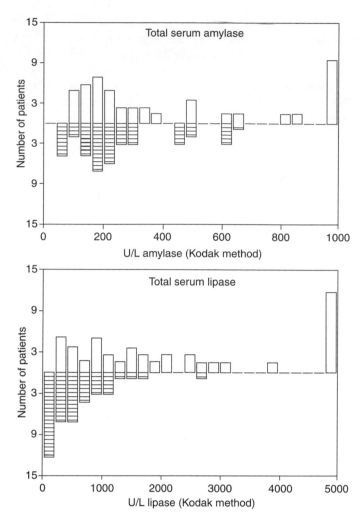

Fig. 20-6 Modified Gerhardt plots for serum amylase, lipase, and in the diagnosis of acute pancreatitis. *(From Gerhardt W: The Bayes approach: systematic graphic evaluation of diagnostic tests. In Keller H, Trendelenburg CH, editors:* Data presentation, interpretation, *New York, 1989, Walter de Gruyter.)*

(ROC) curve analysis. Plotting several ROC curves on the same graph, the laboratory staff can compare the merits of two different tests or the performance of one test under different conditions such as different cutoff values or different patient populations. An example of such curves is shown in Fig. 20-5 showing the discrimination between subjects with and without coronary artery disease at different decision levels for apolipoprotein B and low-density lipoprotein (LDL) cholesterol. Refer to the article by Zweig, Broste, and Reinhart[35] and the review by Zweig and Campbell[36] for a good discussion of the use of ROC curves.

An ROC curve is derived by plotting the sensitivity (the true-positive rate) of the test versus 1.0 minus specificity (the false-positive rate). The multiple points on a curve represent the true-positive rate and false-positive rate using different cutoff values for the diagnosis or differentiation of illness versus nonillness. The point on the curve that is the closest to the upper left-hand corner of the plot represents the cutoff value or decision limit that provides the greatest diagnostic accuracy, that is, the efficiency of the test. The area under the curve represents the overall accuracy of the test.

There are other useful ways of representing and examining the relative diagnostic value of different cutoff values. One example is the modified Gerhardt plot,[37] as used in a study of the relative utility of serum total amylase, total lipase, pancreatic amylase isoenzyme, and a lipase isoform in the diagnosis of acute pancreatitis.[38] These four tests were used

on the same population of 81 patients with suspected acute pancreatitis. In this population, 41 of the patients did have pancreatitis and 40 did not. In Fig. 20-6, the open bars in the plots above the zero line represent patients with pancreatitis, and the striped bars, below the line, represent patients without pancreatitis. Using these graphs, the investigators could judge the best discrimination or cutoff point to maximize the sensitivity or specificity of each test. They also concluded that, at least in this set of patients studied, total amylase was a poor test for evaluating patients with an "acute abdomen," and a better test choice would be total lipase.

Other representations of cutoff values are also useful, such as those shown in Figs. 20-4 and 20-7, for a hypothetical immunochemical CK-MB assay for use in the diagnosis of myocardial injury.[39] When diagnostic efficiency is the goal, a simple plot of the percent efficiency versus the diagnostic cutoff values is helpful. The highest efficiency at the lowest cutoff is the most appropriate, because increasing the cutoff value produces more false-negative results. Fig. 20-4 is interesting in that the diagnostic efficiency is plotted as a function of the combination of two cutoff values, the CK-MB in nanograms per milliliter and the percent relative index of CK-MB to total CK. The maximum diagnostic efficiency for this studied and defined patient population for these specific CK-MB and CK assays appears to be 90% at a CK-MB cutoff of 5 ng/mL and a relative index of 3%:

$$\text{relative index} = \frac{\text{CK-MB } (\mu g/L)}{\text{CK-MB } (U/L)} \times 100$$

The decision analysis involving multiple testing or combination testing may be similar to the concepts presented here for the measurement of a single variant value and is discussed in Galen and Gambino's text.[34] It can also be quite complex regarding the sequential or simultaneous assessment of multiple variate values according to the Bayes theorem as discussed by Statland et al.[33]

ACKNOWLEDGMENT

The author wishes to acknowledge the efforts of the members of the NCCLS Subcommittee on Reference Intervals who prepared the C28-P Guideline: Edward A. Sasse (Chairman), Kaiser J. Aziz, Eugene K. Harris, Sandy Krishnamurthy, Henry T. Lee, Jr., Andy Ruland, and Bette Seamonds. The C28-P was revised to C28-A, 1995.

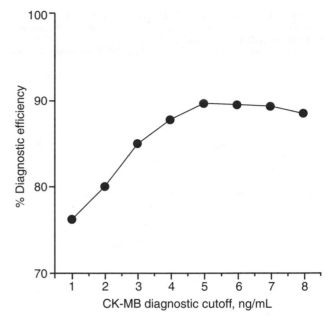

Fig. 20-7 Percent diagnostic efficiency plotted versus different diagnostic cutoff levels in nanograms per milliliter for a hypothetical immunochemical serum CK-MB assay. The highest diagnostic efficiency, 90%, at the lowest cutoff, 5 ng/mL, for CK-MB is the optimal decision level. *(Courtesy D. Obzansky, Du Pont Co., Wilmington, Delaware.)*

References

1. National Committee for Clinical Laboratory Standards: *How to define and determine reference intervals in the clinical laboratory: approved guideline*, ed 2, NCCLS document C28-A2, Villanova, PA, 2000, NCCLS.
2. Solberg HE: Approved recommendation (1986) on the theory of reference values. Part 1. The concept of reference values, *Clin Chem Acta* 167:111, 1987; *J Clin Chem Clin Biochem* 25:337, 1987; *Ann Biol Clin* 45:237, 1987; *Labmedica* 4:27, 1987.
3. PetitClerc C, Solberg HEL: Approved recommendation (1987) on the theory of reference values. Part 2. Selection of individuals for the production of reference values, *J Clin Chem Clin Biochem* 25:639, 1987; *Clin Chem Acta* 170:S1, 1987.
4. Solberg HE, PetitClerc C: Approved recommendation (1988) on the theory of reference values. Part 3. Preparation of individuals and collection of specimens for the production of reference values, *Clin Chem Acta* 177:S1, 1988.
5. Solberg HE, Stamm D: Approved recommendation on the theory of reference values. Part 4. Control of analytical variation in the production, transfer and application of reference values, *Eur J Clin Chem Clin Biochem* 29:531, 1991.
6. Solberg HE: Approved recommendations (1987) on the theory of reference values. Part 5. Statistical treatment of collected reference values: determination of reference limits, *J Clin Chem Clin Biochem* 25:645, 1987; *Clin Chem Acta* 170:S13, 1987.
7. Dybkaer R, Solberg HE: Approved recommendations (1987) on the theory of reference values. Part 6. Presentation of observed values related to reference values, *J Clin Chem Clin Biochem* 25:657, 1987; *Clin Chem Acta* 170:S33, 1987; *Labmedica* 5:27, 1988.
8. National Committee for Clinical Laboratory Standards: *Method comparison and bias estimate using patient samples: approved guideline*, NCCLS document EP9-A, Villanova, PA, 1995, NCCLS.
9. Solberg HE: Establishment and use of reference values. In Burtis CA, Ashwood ER, editors: *Tietz textbook of clinical chemistry*, ed 2, Philadelphia, 1994, Saunders.
10. Schultz EK: Analytical goals and clinical relevance of laboratory procedures. In Tietz NW, editor: *Textbook of clinical chemistry*, Philadelphia, 1986, Saunders.
11. Koch DD, Peters T, Jr: Selection and evaluation of methods. In Burtis CA, Ashwood ER, editors: *Tietz textbook of clinical chemistry*, ed 2, Philadelphia, 1994, Saunders.
12. Stamm D: Control of analytical variation in the production of reference values. In Grasbeck R, Alstrom T, editors: *Reference values in laboratory medicine*, New York, 1981, Wiley & Sons.
13. National Committee for Clinical Laboratory Standards: *Internal quality control testing: principles and definitions: approved guideline*, ed 2, NCCLS document C24-A2, Villanova, PA, 1999, NCCLS.
14. Statland BE, Winkel P: Selected preanalytical sources of variation in reference values. In Grasbeck R, Alstrom T, editors: *Reference values in laboratory medicine*, New York, 1981, Wiley & Sons.
15. Hjelm M: Preparing reference individuals for blood collection. In Grasbeck R, Alstrom T, editors: *Reference values in laboratory medicine*, New York, 1981, Wiley & Sons.
16. National Committee for Clinical Laboratory Standards: *Procedures for the collection of diagnostic blood specimens by venipuncture: approved standard*, ed 4, NCCLS document H3-A4, Villanova, PA, 1998, NCCLS.
17. National Committee for Clinical Laboratory Standards: *Procedures for the collection of diagnostic blood specimens by skin puncture: approved standard*, ed 4, NCCLS document H4-A4, Villanova, PA, 1999, NCCLS.
18. National Committee for Clinical Laboratory Standards: *Percutaneous collection of arterial blood for laboratory analysis: approved standard*, NCCLS document H11-A3, ed 3, Villanova, PA, 1999, NCCLS.
19. National Committee for Clinical Laboratory Standards: *Collection, transport, and preparation of blood specimens for coagulation testing and performance of coagulation assays: approved guideline*, ed 3, NCCLS document H21-A3, Villanova, PA, 1998, NCCLS.

20. National Committee for Clinical Laboratory Standards: *Collection and transportation of single-collection urine specimens: proposed guideline*, NCCLS document GP8-P, Villanova, PA, 1985, NCCLS.

21. National Committee for Clinical Laboratory Standards: *Collection, transportation, and preservation of timed urine specimens: approved guideline*, ed 2, NCCLS document GP16-A2, Villanova, PA, 2001, NCCLS.

22. National Committee for Clinical Laboratory Standards: *Procedures for the handling and processing of blood specimens: approved guideline*, ed 2, NCCLS document H18-A2, Villanova, PA, 1999, NCCLS.

23. Reed AH, Henry RJ, Mason WB: Influence of statistical method used on the resulting estimate of normal range, *Clin Chem* 17:275, 1971.

24. Lott JA et al: Estimation of reference ranges: how many subjects are needed, *Clin Chem* 38:648, 1992.

25. Linnet K: Two-stage transformation systems for normalization of reference distributions evaluated, *Clin Chem* 33:381, 1987.

26. Barnett V, Lewis T: *Outliers in statistical data*, New York, 1978, Wiley & Sons.

27. Dixon WJ: Processing data for outliers, *Biometrics* 9:74, 1953.

28. Harris EK, Boyd JC: On dividing reference data into subgroups to produce separate reference ranges, *Clin Chem* 36:265, 1990.

29. Harris EK: Personal communication.

30. Cotlove E, Harris EK, Williams GZ: Biological and analytical components of variation in long-term studies of serum constituents in normal subjects, III: physiological and medical implications, *Clin Chem* 16:1028, 1970.

31. Young DS, Harris EK, Cotlove E: Biological and analytical components of variation in long-term studies of serum constituents in normal subjects, IV: results of a study designed to eliminate long-term analytic deviations, *Clin Chem* 17:403, 1971.

32. Young DS: Determination and validation of reference intervals, *Arch Pathol Lab Med* 116:704, 1992.

33. Statland BE et al: Quantitative approaches used in evaluating laboratory measurements and other clinical data. In Henry JB, editor: *Clinical diagnosis and management by laboratory methods*, Philadelphia, 1979, Saunders.

34. Galen RS, Gambino SR: *Beyond normality: the predictive value and efficacy of medical diagnoses*, New York, 1975, Wiley & Sons.

35. Zweig MH, Broste SK, Reinhart RA: ROC curve analysis: an example showing the relationships among serum lipid and apolipoprotein concentrations in identifying patients with coronary artery disease, *Clin Chem* 38:1425, 1992.

36. Zweig MH, Campbell G: Receiver-operating characteristic (ROC) plots: a fundamental evaluation tool in clinical medicine, *Clin Chem* 39:561, 1993.

37. Gerhardt W: The Bayes approach: systematic graphic evaluation of diagnostic tests. In Keller H, Trendelenburg CH, editors: *Data presentation, interpretation*, New York, 1989, Walter de Gruyter.

38. Lott JA, Lu CJ: Lipase isoforms and amylase isoenzymes: assays and application in the diagnosis of acute pancreatitis, *Clin Chem* 37:361, 1991.

39. Obzansky D: Personal communication, Wilmington, Del.

Internet Sites

http://130.189.200.66/Flow%20Lab%20manual/1.%20Policy%20statements/refrange.html—Reference intervals by Marc Langweiler, Flow Cytometry Laboratory at Mary Hitchcock Memorial Hospital, Hitchcock Medical Center, Dartmouth, New Hampshire

http://www.analyse-it.com/products/clinical/diagnostic-testing.htm—Trial software that works with Microsoft Excel, Analyse-It Software, Leeds, United Kingdom

http://www.cche.net/usersguides/decision.asp—Centres for Health Evidence: How to use a clinical decision analysis

http://www.westgard.com/essay8.htm—Medical decision limits by Westgard

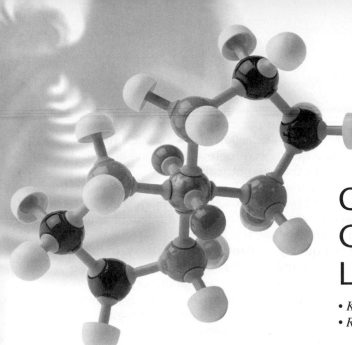

CHAPTER 21

Quality Control for the Clinical Chemistry Laboratory

• *Kenneth E. Blick*
• *Richard B. Passey*

Chapter Outline

Objectives

- Provide a practical approach to quality control.
- Establish a method to evaluate performance specifications during the process of controlling quality.
- Furnish practical methods for carrying out quality control.

- Develop criteria for judging the out-of-control condition.
- Provide a practical approach to solving an out-of-control condition.
- Provide a link between the costs of quality control to instrument features and performance.

Key Terms

action limits   Ranges set for quality control pools that, if exceeded, signal a possible deterioration of the quality of the testing system and require an investigation by a technologist. (See **out of control**.)

autoverification   Verification and release of patient results using software-based algorithms with decision-making logic on the laboratory information system.

CMS   Center for Medicare and Medicaid Services; formerly named Health Care Finance Administration (HCFA).

certified reference material (CRM)   "A reference material that has one or more property values certified by a technically valid procedure and is accompanied by, or traceable to, a certificate or another document issued by a certifying body."[1] The material has high purity for the specified compound. Certified reference materials are used in preparing calibrators or specimens of known concentration.

CLIA compliance   The term used to describe the laboratory program and plan to ensure that all aspects of the CLIA regulations are followed.

control limits   Numerical limits (expressed in test units) within which the assay values of control samples must fall for the assay to be considered valid or in control.

definitive method   An analytical method that has been subjected to thorough investigation and evaluation for sources of inaccuracy, including analytical nonspecificity. The magnitude of the definitive method's final imprecision and bias, as expressed in the uncertainty statement, is compatible with the definitive method's stated end purpose. The assay value obtained by a definitive method is taken as the true value.[2]

electronic quality control   Type of quality control available on selected point-of-care instruments provided that manufacturer's claims are verified and the system is tested periodically with liquid QC materials.

error budget   A testing system's total allowable error, which must be determined by each laboratory on the basis of medical or regulatory requirements. The error expenditure comprises all sources of error including imprecision, bias, interferences, and other errors.

external quality control   A program in which an external agency provides unknown samples for analysis. (See **survey or proficiency testing specimen**.) The results are returned to the participant with an evaluation of "acceptable" or "not acceptable" performance. Under CLIA '88 this process is called *proficiency testing*.

false rejection   Rejection of an analytical run because quality control results indicate analytical problems that are not really present.

inherent variability   Repeated measurements on the same material vary around an average value. The standard deviation measures the magnitude of this variability.

internal quality control   An analysis program, using quality control samples, that is used to verify the acceptability and stability of laboratory results.

Levey-Jennings plot   A visual tool for evaluating quality control data in the context of previous QC results where data are plotted relative to the mean +/− 2 SD on the vertical (y) axis versus days on the horizontal (x) axis.

method   The methodological principles used in the performance of a laboratory test; must include the chemical or physical basis of the test.

monthly average   Daily quality control values averaged over the period of 1 month.

monthly standard deviation   Standard deviation calculated using the daily quality control values over the period of 1 month.

out of control   A circumstance when a testing system has been shown, by quality control results or other indicators, to be unusable for patient care. This circumstance must be formally declared by the laboratory director or technical supervisor, since this decision implies that specified actions need to be taken under CLIA '88 regulations (see §493.1219, Remedial Actions, and §493.1705, Quality Assurance of Quality Control). Routine responses to quality control results that exceed set limits should be documented; see **action limits**.

peer group   A term that, when used in proficiency testing programs, indicates a group of laboratories that use the same or similar methods. Commercial quality control suppliers also provide monthly peer group comparisons.

performance specifications   Numerical limits established by each laboratory for each analyte and each testing system to delineate acceptable performance. Performance specifications for accreditation and good laboratory practice often include accuracy, precision, analytical sensitivity (minimum reportable amount), analytical specificity (interfering substances), the reportable range of patient test results, and the reference intervals or normal values.

power curves   Plots of the magnitude of the error detected by a control system versus the probability of detecting that size error under various control rules.

primary standard   Chemicals of the highest known purity that can be used to produce calibrators for analytical systems.

procedure   A set of instructions for using a particular method that, when followed, will produce an analytical test value.

proficiency testing   See **external quality control**.

proficiency testing specimen   A sample that is prepared by an independent agency and submitted to a laboratory that is participating in an external quality control program.

quality control pool   A quantity of stable material (such as serum, plasma, or urine) that is used in an **internal quality control** program to evaluate the acceptability and stability of a testing system.

reference method   "A thoroughly investigated method in which exact and clear descriptions of the necessary conditions and procedures are given for the accurate determination of one or more property values; the documented accuracy and precision of the method are commensurate with the method's use for assessing the accuracy of other methods, for measuring the same property values, or for assigning reference method values to reference materials."[3]

regional quality control   A group of laboratories that jointly purchase a large amount of quality control material so that target values and data can be shared.

results verification   The final step of the testing process whereby an analyst with both clinical and analytical expertise verifies and releases patient results for clinical use purposes.

run   "An interval within which the accuracy and precision of a testing system are expected to be stable but cannot be greater than 24 hours." (CLIA '88 §493.1218[b])

shift   An abrupt and sustained change (in one direction) in control values. A shift usually indicates a problem (or change) with the analytical system or the control material.

significant difference   A difference that is statistically shown to be outside the expected variability limit; *medically* it is a difference that is large enough to influence a medical decision; *operationally* it is a statistically significant difference that testing personnel and supervisors believe to be large enough to require investigation.

systemic bias   Systemic bias can be constant or proportional. *Constant systemic bias* denotes a constant difference between the true value and the observed value regardless of the concentration level. *Proportional systemic bias* denotes a difference between the true value and the observed value, which changes proportionally as the concentration level changes.

target value   The established mean value for an analyte in a quality control pool. Target values for both method and instrument types are often used for peer group comparison purposes.

testing system   The combination of the following: an analytical method; a procedure for using the method; reagents, calibrators, and supplies; and an instrument for measurements.

trend   A gradual change in the test results obtained from control material that is suggestive of a progressive problem with the testing system or control material; also termed *drift*.

true rejection   The rejection of an analytical run because the control specimens indicate that a problem truly exists.

usual standard deviation (USD)   The average of 3- to 6-month average standard deviation values based on consecutive quality control values. This estimates the usual precision that a laboratory's testing system is capable of achieving.

Westgard Multirule System   Warning and rejection rules developed by James Westgard to evaluate quality control data more effectively. These rules are used on many computerized quality control programs found on LIS and laboratory instruments.

This discussion of quality control, as practiced in clinical laboratories, is designed to provide a practical guide for establishing and maintaining quality in laboratory practice. We will present quality control as it is handled manually in laboratories with the knowledge that computerized quality control is now commonplace in many clinical laboratories. Breitenberg[4] identified 10 quality ensuring items from the International Organization for Standardization series 9000 standards that are common to all quality control systems: (1) effective quality system; (2) ensuring valid and timely measurements; (3) using calibrated measuring and testing equipment; (4) using appropriate statistical techniques; (5) developing a product identification and traceability system; (6) maintaining adequate record-keeping systems; (7) ensuring adequate product handling, storage, packaging, and delivery systems; (8) maintaining an adequate inspection and **testing system**; (9) establishing processes for dealing with nonconforming items; and (10) ensuring adequate personnel training and experience. It should be the goal of quality control procedures to meet all 10 of these standards. Careful examination of the rules delineated by Clinical Laboratory Improvement Amendment of 1988 (CLIA '88) shows that all these items must be included by law in a laboratory's quality control system.

The primary analytical goals of a clinical laboratory's quality control program should be:

1. Establishing and maintaining accurate **methods**.
2. Determining the level of precision needed by the laboratory and maintaining that level of reproducibility.
3. Ensuring that analytical systems are stable and operating according to **performance specifications**. This increases the reliability of both short- and long-term medical decisions.
4. Ensuring that all regulatory requirements relative to **CLIA compliance** are followed.
5. Providing objective analytical benchmarks for methods and instruments so that continuous improvement of existing methods is achievable.

To achieve these analytical goals, a laboratory must meet the 10 quality-assuring goals, institute policies that govern patient preparation, reduce preanalytical errors (see Chapter 3), and maximize the effective use of the laboratory's personnel and physical facilities. A laboratory's quality control program is designed to evaluate how well these analytical goals are being met.

GOALS FOR A QUALITY CONTROL PROGRAM
Setting Goals

The first step in establishing a laboratory quality control program is to develop criteria for acceptable laboratory performance. How accurate and precise *should* the laboratory be? How precise and accurate *must* it be? These considerations include the determination of what constitutes acceptable analytical error based on the use of the test result in clinical care.[5,6] Control beyond that required for medical purposes can waste time and materials; hence it is important to evaluate whether error reduction improves medical diagnosis, treatment, or prognosis.

Several bases exist upon which performance criteria can be formulated. The first is the body of regulatory standards; for example, the precision and accuracy demanded by CLIA '88 regulations. Second are the precision and accuracy that appear to be attainable performance by most laboratories. This information can be obtained by communication with other laboratory professionals or from data derived from proficiency surveys, such as that of the College of American Pathology (CAP). Third and probably most important, it is essential to determine the precision and accuracy required by the clinical staff, the users of data produced by the laboratory. In general, a testing system's analytical error should be much smaller than the allowable error in the regulatory requirements. Otherwise, the laboratory may not meet its regulatory and perhaps medical requirements. The following section will review the medical criteria used to establish and evaluate performance.

Total Allowable Error

The total allowable error of a testing system is composed of individual components. In general, each component of a testing system can be a source of imprecision or bias. If the total error can be likened to an **error budget**, the individual components of the total allowable error make up the total error expenditure of that budget. When the error budget is exceeded, more error than can be tolerated exists in the testing system. The more completely one can identify the components of error, the better one can adjust the testing system to reduce these errors. Medical and CLIA '88 requirements are not based on whether the error is introduced by imprecision or bias; rather it is the combination that determines the effect of the total error. Therefore, the laboratory staff must know what roles imprecision and systemic bias play in the error expenditure because the resolution processes for these errors are often different. The systemic bias between testing systems can be constant or proportional, depending on whether the error is constant with changes in analyte concentration or varies proportionally with changes in concentration (see Chapter 22).

Total error[7] is estimated from imprecision and bias by:

$$\text{Total error} = \text{Sum of bias errors} + 1.96 \times \text{SD (standard deviation)} \qquad \textit{Eq. 21-1}$$

Notice that 1.96 is the 95% confidence limit (often rounded to 2.0 for convenience) for a normally distributed set of results (see Chapter 19).

Example. If your medical requirements for glucose require that the total error be less than 60 mg/L at a concentration of 1200 mg/L and you know that your imprecision is ± 20 mg/L, the maximum bias that your method can have is calculated as follows:

$$60 \text{ mg/L} = x \text{ mg/L} + 1.96 \times 20 \text{ mg/L}$$
$$\text{Maximum bias} = x = 60 - (1.96 \times 20) = 20.8 \text{ mg/L}$$

If the bias of the assay is too large, it can often be reduced by more accurate calibration **procedures** and materials. Imprecision is often increased by poor mechanical and electronic components in the analyzer or measurement device. Thus the state of instrument calibration and maintenance can affect both bias and imprecision. An accuracy-based quality control system can provide information on both accuracy and precision.

Table 21-1 contains analytical data from the Oklahoma Medical Center showing the total error for each listed test. The total errors are large because they include error contributions from all the instruments used to report the test values. Accurate error budgeting must include the bias introduced by the use of multiple testing systems. The problem of bias between different testing systems is one that can affect the medical use of test results because a test is often performed by more than one testing system.

Performance Required for Proficiency Testing

The federal government has set allowable error criteria for 154 tests in 13 laboratory disciplines plus cytology (**proficiency testing** rules of CLIA '88 *Federal Register,* February 28, 1990, pp. 7152-7162). The CLIA criteria for chemistry tests are listed in Table 21-2. These allowable error criteria define the total amounts of error a proficiency testing value can have. The **target value** used to determine bias is

TABLE 21-1 Performance Specifications for Total Error (%)*

Test	Analytical†	Medical‡	CLIA '88§
Albumin	13 to 15	—	10
Alkaline phosphatase	10 to 15	—	30
Aspartate aminotransferase (AST)	5 to 20	14 to 26	20
Bilirubin, total	12 to 16	5 to 28	20% or 4 mg/L
Blood urea nitrogen (BUN)	18 to 33	12 to 25	9% or 20 mg/L
Calcium	5.5 to 6.4	5 to 7	10 mg/L
Chloride	5	—	5
Cholesterol	11 to 14	9‖	10
Cholesterol, high-density lipoprotein	5	—	30
Creatine kinase (CK)	8 to 10	—	30
Creatinine	15 to 47	10 to 20	15% or 3 mg/L
Glucose	5 to 11	11 to 16	10% or 60 mg/L
Iron	—	17	20
Lactate dehydrogenase (LD)	7 to 8	—	20
Phosphorus	4 to 10	14 to 17	NA
Potassium	10 to 12	5 to 10	0.5 mmol/L
Protein, total	7 to 8	8	10
Sodium	5 to 6	2 to 3	4 mmol/L
Triglycerides	10 to 16	16	25

NA, *Not applicable.*
Total analytical error calculated by: T.E. = Bias + 1.96 × standard deviation.
†*Data from Oklahoma Medical Center, University of Oklahoma. Tested systems include Beckman CX3 and Kodak 700XRC; bias differences between these two systems are important sources of the high total error. The difference between the systems is part of the error for a patient's results when different systems are used interchangeably.*
‡*Rounded to the nearest whole percentage. (From Skendzel LP, Barnett RN, Platt R:* Am J Clin Pathol *83:200, 1985.)*
§*Tests and acceptable performance are from the* Federal Register, *p 7158, Feb. 28, 1990.*
‖*Cholesterol medical goals are now set at 3% bias and 3% imprecision. (From NCEP: NIH Pub. No. 90-2964, 199025).*

defined by the proficiency testing service using either the overall mean, a **peer group** mean, or the value established by a definitive or **reference method**. It is noteworthy that CLIA '88 error windows (budgets) are too large for routine quality **control limits** because imprecision errors this large will cause frequent proficiency testing failure.[8]

Compare the total errors listed in Table 21-1 to the suggested allowable medical errors and the maximum error windows specified by CLIA '88. Notice that several tests in Table 21-2 show potential problems with proficiency testing because of unacceptably high total errors when the analysis is performed by more than one testing system. This would be the case if proficiency testing truly mimicked laboratory practice. However as currently practiced, proficiency testing usually compares testing systems only with instrument peer grouping.

Medical Decision Limits

For true control of quality it is necessary to evaluate, from the customer's perspective, the performance required for each aspect of the clinical laboratory's operation.[8-11] The elements of a good quality control program include establishment of analytical accuracy and precision performance criteria based on medical usefulness requirements.[7,12-17]

In Table 21-1, the total analytical error for several analytical instruments is compared with the allowable error

suggested by medical requirements and with the CLIA '88 mandated allowable error. An example of medically defined criteria for precision and accuracy are the guidelines formulated by the National Institutes of Health (NIH) for cholesterol analysis.[18,19] To minimize the errors in diagnosing hyperlipidemias, the NIH established a target of 3% for the limits of imprecision and 3% for an acceptable degree of bias (inaccuracy). Documents from professional organizations can provide estimates based on review of accepted practice (e.g., National Academy of Clinical Biochemistry, www.nacb.org). Each laboratory should consult the appropriate users or clinicians to obtain their estimate of allowable error based on their particular medical practice.[20-23] If their suggestions are reasonable and would not place the laboratory in conflict with regulatory requirements, the laboratory should try to attain these limits of error. If no information is available about the precision and accuracy targets needed for medical decision making, one can then estimate a theoretical error based on the degree of intraindividual and interindividual variation for each analyte.[24,25] Page 406 of Chapter 22 lists the equations relating total analytical imprecision with these biological variabilities. Table 3-1 lists some examples of the intrapersonal variability of certain analytes. Once the allowable total error based on medical requirements has been decided, the methods and testing systems chosen must be capable of producing values that consistently meet those

TABLE 21-2 CLIA REQUIRED PERFORMANCE ON PROFICIENCY TESTING (FEDERAL REGISTER, FEB. 28, 1992)

Analyte or Test	Criteria for Acceptable Performance
Immunology Tests	
Alpha$_1$-antitrypsin	Target value ± 3 SD
Alpha-fetoprotein (tumor marker)	Target value ± 3 SD
Antinuclear antibody	Target value ± 2 dilutions or positive or negative
Antistreptolysin 0	Target value ± 2 dilutions or positive or negative
Antihuman immunodeficiency virus	Reactive or nonreactive
Complement C3	Target value ± 3 SD
Complement C4	Target value ± 3 SD
Hepatitis (HBsAg, anti-HBc, HBeAg)	Reactive (positive) or nonreactive (negative)
IgA	Target value ± 3 SD
IgE	Target value ± 3 SD
IgG	Target value ± 25%
IgM	Target value ± 3 SD
Infectious mononucleosis	Target value ± 2 dilutions or positive or negative
Rheumatoid factor	Target value ± 2 dilutions or positive or negative
Rubella	Target value ± 2 dilutions or immune or nonimmune or positive or negative
Chemistry Tests	
Alanine aminotransferase (ALT/SGPT)	Target value ± 20%
Albumin	Target value ± 10%
Alkaline phosphatase	Target value ± 30%
Amylase	Target value ± 30%
Aspartate aminotransferase (AST/SGOT)	Target value ± 20%
Bilirubin, total	Target value ± 4 mg/L or ± 20% (greater)
Blood-gas Po$_2$	Target value ± 3 SD
Pco$_2$	Target value ± 5 mm Hg or ± 8% (greater)
pH	Target value ± 0.04
Calcium, total	Target value ± 10 mg/L
Chloride	Target value ± 5%
Cholesterol, total	Target value ± 10%
Cholesterol, high-density lipoprotein	Target value ± 30%
Creatine kinase	Target value ± 30%
Creatine kinase isoenzymes	MB elevated (presence or absence) or target value ± 3 SD
Creatinine	Target value ± 3 mg/L or ± 15% (greater)
Glucose (excluding glucose performed on monitoring devices cleared by FDA for home use)	Target value ± 60 mg/L or ± 10% (greater)
Iron, total	Target value ± 20%
Lactate dehydrogenase (LD)	Target value ± 20%
LD isoenzymes	LD$_1$/LD$_2$ (+ or −), or target value ± 30%
Magnesium	Target value ± 25%
Potassium	Target value ± 0.5 mmol/L
Sodium	Target value ± 4 mmol/L
Total protein	Target value ± 10%
Triglycerides	Target value ± 25%
Urea nitrogen	Target value ± 20 mg/L or ± 9% (greater)
Uric acid	Target value ± 17%
Endocrinology	
Cortisol	Target value ± 25%
Free thyroxine	Target value ± 3 SD
Human chorionic gonadotropin	Target value ± 3 SD positive or negative
Triiodothyronine uptake	Target value ± 3 SD
Triiodothyronine	Target value ± 3 SD
Thyroid-stimulating hormone	Target value ± 3 SD
Thyroxine	Target value ± 20% or 10 µg/L (greater)

TABLE 21-2   CLIA REQUIRED PERFORMANCE ON PROFICIENCY TESTING (FEDERAL REGISTER, FEB. 28, 1992)—CONT'D

Analyte or Test	Criteria for Acceptable Performance
Toxicology	
Alcohol, blood	Target value ± 25%
Blood lead	Target value ± 10% or 40 µg/L (greater)
Carbamazepine	Target value ± 25%
Digoxin	Target value ± 20% or ± 0.2 ng/mL (greater)
Ethosuximide	Target value ± 20%
Gentamicin	Target value ± 25%
Lithium	Target value ± 0.3 mmol/L or ± 20% (greater)
Phenobarbital	Target value ± 20%
Phenytoin	Target value ± 25%
Primidone	Target value ± 25%
Procainamide (and metabolite)	Target value ± 25%
Quinidine	Target value ± 25%
Tobramycin	Target value ± 25%
Theophylline	Target value ± 25%
Valproic acid	Target value ± 25%
Hematology	
Cell identification	90% or greater consensus on identification
White blood cell differential	Target ± 3 SD based on the percentage of different types of white blood cells in the samples
Erythrocyte count	Target ± 6%
Hematocrit (excluding spun hematocrits)	Target ± 6%
Hemoglobin	Target ± 7%
Leukocyte count	Target ± 15%
Platelet count	Target ± 25%
Fibrinogen	Target ± 20%
Partial thromboplastin time	Target ± 15%
Prothrombin time	Target ± 15%

requirements. In addition, the quality control program must be designed to ensure that the testing system maintains these limits.

Reference intervals for laboratory tests describe the expected values for carefully selected groups of individuals determined by testing systems that are assumed to be performing appropriately (see Chapter 20). Increased bias will cause a **shift** in test values and will thus invalidate the medical usefulness of the established reference intervals and may in fact lead to inappropriate patient care.

Meeting Medical Usefulness Criteria by Calculating the Significant Change Limit

The day-to-day medical usefulness of clinical laboratory tests depends on maintaining the accuracy and precision of the testing system. Physicians make many clinical decisions on the basis of the day-to-day differences in patient test values, assuming that the day-to-day accuracy and precision are maintained at the same level from month to month and year to year. Thus the actual accuracy and precision of the measurement procedure directly influence the medical interpretation of these day-to-day changes in test values. One

key element in interpreting the medical usefulness of a test result is an estimate of the magnitude of an analytically significant change in concentration. This estimate is called the *significant change limit (SCL)*.

The significant change limit is a decision-making tool that helps physicians distinguish day-to-day changes in results that are caused by the **inherent variability** of the analytical procedure from changes that are caused by modifications in the patient's physiology and pathology. The significant change limit is based on the assumption that the **usual standard deviation (USD)** represents day-to-day method variability. The theoretical standard deviation of the difference (SD_{diff}) between two separate analyses of the same material on different days is related to the usual standard deviation (USD) of the procedure by the following formula:

$$SD_{diff} = \sqrt{2(USD)^2} = 1.4 \, USD \qquad \textit{Eq. 21-2}$$

The SCL is then the 95% confidence limits (or ± 2 SD_{diff}) that define the extent of the inherent method variability:

$$SCL = \text{Mean value} \pm 2 \, SD_{diff} = \text{Mean value} \pm 2.8 \, USD$$

$$\textit{Eq. 21-3}$$

As an approximation, the significant change limit is three times the usual standard deviation (Table 21-3). Changes greater than the significant change limit are likely to represent a real change in the patient. For example, if the usual standard deviation for cholesterol is 50 mg/L, the significant change limit is 2.8 times 50, or 140 mg/L. A change from 2000 to 2200 mg/L would exceed the significant change limit and would represent a real change in the patient. A change from 2000 to 1900 mg/L would not exceed the SCL and could be the result of the method's imprecision. Clearly, in order to facilitate consistent decision making by the attending physician, it is important to maintain a consistent level of precision from month to month and year to year.

CONTROL OF QUALITY (PROCESS CONTROL) AND ERROR DETECTION

Once a laboratory's performance criteria are established, a process control system must be put into place. The purpose of this system is to allow continuous monitoring of the testing process (including preanalytical and postanalytical testing) to ensure that either the performance goals are met or that steps are taken to achieve the goals. It is important to recognize the key role of laboratory personnel in the quality process.

Levels of Activity in the Control Process

The control process that we call quality control (QC) is designed to detect error in the measurement system. There

---

TABLE 21-3   CALCULATION OF QUALITY CONTROL PARAMETERS

Test/method: Potassium by ion-selective electrode
Analyst: RBP
Start/finish date: 3/15/02-3/26/02
Control source and level: Superior control-elevated
Manufacturer's target value: 6.02 mEq/L
How determined: By NRSCL definitive method
Manufacturer's typical standard deviation for users: 0.15 mEq/L

| Day | VIAL 1 | | VIAL 2 | |
	Sample A	Sample B	Sample A	Sample B
1	6.1	6.1	6.2	5.9
2	6.2	6.2	6.0	6.0
3	5.7	5.8	6.0	6.0
4	5.9	5.8	5.9	5.8
5	6.0	6.0	6.0	6.0
6	5.9	6.0	6.0	6.0
7	5.9	6.0	6.0	6.0
8	5.9	5.8	6.0	5.9
9	6.0	6.1	6.1	6.2
10	6.0	6.1	6.1	6.1

Grand total (sum of all observations) = 239.7; n = 40 observations.
Average initial target value = 239.7/40 = 5.99 mEq/L.
Temporary standard deviation = 0.12 mEq/L.

Calculation of average final target and usual standard deviation (USD) values

Initial Target Value	Average Target Value	Standard Deviation
Data	5.990	0.12 mEq/L
1 April	6.070	0.13 mEq/L
2 May	6.020	0.11 mEq/L
3 June	6.010	0.13 mEq/L

Average final target = 6.02 (average of 5.99, 6.07, 6.02, and 6.01)
Usual standard deviation (USD) = 0.12 mEq/L (average of 0.12, 0.13, 0.11, and 0.13)
Medically allowable error = 0.3 mEq/L (set by the medical staff Jan. 14, 2002)
Number of USDs in the medically allowable error = 0.3/0.12 = 2.5
Significant change value = 2.8 × USD = 2.8 × 0.12 = 0.34 mEq/L
Chosen control range is the average final target value ± 2.5 USD, or 6.02 ± 2.5(0.12) = 6.02 ± 0.3 mEq/L, or 5.72 to 6.32 mEq/L.

If the chosen control range is the average final target value ± 3 USD, range = 6.02 ± 3(0.12) = 6.02 ± 0.36, or 5.66 to 6.38 mEq/L (larger than the medical requirements).

Also be careful when less than 2.5 SD is contained in the medically allowable error because the imprecision may be too large to show medically required changes in test results.

are at least three levels in this process, each the responsibility of different individuals. For the control process to be most effective, active communication among the individuals within each level of responsibility is crucial.

The first level of the process is the responsibility of the bench medical technologist and the supervisors. At this level, the control process includes the daily analysis of quality control specimens (discussed in this section) and the review and verification of patient results (results verification) and reports. The technologist is responsible for performing quality control analyses at the appropriate intervals and for determining that, during any given run, there is no significant systematic error in that run. Both the technologists and the supervisor are responsible for reviewing patient data to ensure that no random error exists.

The second level of control ensures that minimal systematic bias enters into the system over a relatively short period of weeks to months. The responsibility for this level of error control is usually shared by supervisors and the laboratory director, though technologists often contribute greatly. The control process at this level requires timely review of the quality control data and proficiency testing that have accumulated over that period of time.

The third level of the control process ensures that the analytical systems are as precise and accurate as possible. This is the responsibility of the laboratory director or technical consultant. The control process at this level requires review of proficiency testing results, knowledge of the levels of precision and accuracy achievable by other laboratories, and, when applicable, the use of accuracy-based standards to verify or correct errors. This level of quality control review occurs over a longer period of time, from months to years. Discussion of proficiency testing is provided in a later section.

Quality control of the *entire* testing system (i.e., from the physician order to phlebotomy to generating a patient report) requires additional process control measures. Many of these measures include regulatory-mandated monitors of individual steps in the process, which are reviewed in Chapter 2. One important factor that is rarely formally recognized is the complaints of physicians about perceived problems. Physicians' complaints are very often based on real deficiencies in one part of the testing system. These errors may not be known to the laboratory until revealed by the laboratory staff's investigation of a complaint. Monitoring physicians' complaints and their resolutions is thus an important monitor to help control the overall quality of the testing system. Accreditation standards such as ISO9001:1987 and ISO9001:1994 for error and incident detection in the testing process have also been implemented by some clinical laboratories.

Testing Quality Control Specimens—Daily Decision Making

The daily preparation and analysis of quality control samples is a regular responsibility of the analyst. The **quality control pools** are analyzed as "known" controls during analysis of patient samples. The values are considered "known" because some attempt has been made to determine the actual levels of each constituent using the procedures employed for routine analysis. The laboratory can estimate the target values of the control samples by repeated analysis (the "true value" being estimated as the mean), use the manufacturer's estimates of the values, or ideally, determine the values by definitive or reference methods (see below, p. 397). The frequency of analysis of the QC material is established by each laboratory for each method. CLIA '88 requires the analysis of at least two controls of different values for each **run** (defined as up to 24 hours of stable operation) as do other accrediting bodies with deemed status from CLIA.

Most laboratories use two different pools, one normal and one abnormal. A normal pool contains constituents at concentrations within the nondiseased reference interval, whereas an abnormal pool contains the analytes at concentrations outside the reference interval. Some laboratories may employ three pools—low abnormal, normal, and high abnormal—especially when medically significant decisions are made at each level. CLIA allows each laboratory to set its own protocols for chemistry testing assay control samples as long as at least two control samples of different concentrations are assayed every 24 hours. Some states mandate three pools for certain tests. CLIA mandates special rules for blood-gases, requiring as a minimum the analysis of one QC sample every 8 hours of testing and the use of a combination of QC samples and calibrators that includes samples with both high and low concentrations each day of testing. The Clinical Laboratory Improvement Amendment also requires the use of one calibrator or control each time a patient sample is analyzed, unless the blood-gas instrument is calibrated at least every 30 minutes (§493.1243). Because of this complexity of blood-gas quality control, some manufacturers have included QC reagents as part of the reagents resident on blood-gas analyzers and have thus assumed a more active role in the QC process. More commonly, however, the manufacturer of a testing system recommends the testing frequency that should be used as a basis for a laboratory's quality control policy.

Testing personnel must use the data from each quality control analysis to make a decision about the validity of patients' test data. Generally, if the results for a quality control sample are within the accepted target range, technologists may assume that the patients' results obtained during the same run are equally valid and can "accept" the run. On the other hand, if the results for the quality control pool are unacceptable, the run is not acceptable (see pp. 390 and 392). The decision to accept or reject an analytical run should be documented and include the decision (either *accept* or *reject*), the analyst's name (or code number), and the date on a work sheet, in a separate log book, on a data sheet, or in the laboratory information system (LIS) (see Chapter 18). Usually, the process of verification of patient data in the LIS by technologists is regarded as implied acceptance of the associated quality control data included in the run. Although the term *run* implies a batch process, current laboratory practice usually has the measurements continuously performed in real-time on automated analyzers. That is, the run is more generally associated with the 8-hour work shift.

Although daily bench-level quality control testing is most useful for detecting systematic errors, it can also be used to detect increases in imprecision. However, random errors, which occur unpredictably, are not usually detectable by a quality control system. Random errors can be detected only by review of reported problems and patients' results (see pp. 392–394).

Quality Control Mechanics

How to choose a quality control pool. Quality control material should have a matrix that closely matches that of the specimens in the analytical run. This means that if the run includes cerebrospinal fluid, serum, and urine, then controls composed of cerebrospinal fluid (CSF), serum, and urine should also be included in the analytical run.

Because the quality control material is analyzed in every run along with patients' specimens, large amounts of control material are needed each year. Several sources currently exist from which a laboratory can obtain sufficient quantities of quality control material: (1) commercial lyophilized pool material; (2) commercial stabilized liquid pools; and (3) frozen, pooled, patient specimens. Patient serum is more frequently used than plasma because it is more readily available and is less likely to include precipitated material. Frozen liquid or pools that have been clarified (with materials that reduce turbidity) generally show smaller standard deviations than do lyophilized pools.[26] The smaller imprecision errors of the liquid pools derive, in part, from the absence of the errors involved with the lyophilization and reconstitution processes. However, the liquid pools may experience greater instability errors associated with shipping batches of a lot to the customer. Some characteristics of three sources of quality control material are listed in Table 21-4. It is important to select a pool with a matrix that interacts least with the methods employed in the laboratory. Certain characteristics of a control pool, including turbidity or chemical constituents, can render it unusable.

Notice that control pools prepared in the laboratory from pooled patient samples (serum, plasma, urine, and CSF) can be contaminated with viruses; thus it is essential to test each specimen or group of specimens and the final pool for harmful viruses. Therefore, the following statements apply to *all* specimen pools used for quality control. First, all pooled human material should be monitored for the human immunodeficiency virus and the hepatitis B virus. No pools should be used if there is evidence of either virus. Second, all control material requires refrigerator or freezer space for storage of a 1- to 2-year supply. Alternatively, commercial distributors may supply quantities from a single lot number of stored material on a monthly or quarterly basis so that the laboratory can use the same lot number over 1 to 2 years. This helps bring long-term stability to the quality control process, though the possibility of shipment-to-shipment variations within the lot must be considered.

Some professional groups and manufacturers offer participation in **regional quality control** programs in which laboratories use the same batch of pooled serum. This offers both scientific advantages and cost benefits. The comparison between laboratories can help predict how similar testing systems (peer groups) will perform in proficiency testing. This comparison becomes more valuable when the accuracy of the quality control pool is established by reference or **definitive methods** (see p. 397, below).[1-3, 27-29]

Preliminary Considerations for Estimating Limits for Quality Control Pools

Unless the true value of a pool is established by definitive or reference methods, the target values are only averages of repeated measurements of the pool. The average temporary or average final target values of the quality control pool are the estimated concentrations of each analyte within the pool. Each laboratory usually establishes its own average target values for the analytes by performing the laboratory's test procedures on each pool. CLIA '88 allows the pool's manufacturer to establish target values, with the laboratory confirming that each target value is applicable to its testing system.

TABLE 21-4 COMPARISON OF QUALITY CONTROL MATERIALS

Criteria	Frozen	Lyophilized	Low-Temperature Liquid
Cost	Low, if not manipulated* Medium, if manipulated	High	Highest
Clarity	Clear, if carefully collected	Turbid	Clear
Stability	12 months	18 to 24 months	18 to 24 months
Validation	Compare with accurately measured materials (NIST and CAP†)	Regional and manufacturer's peer group analysis available, or by NIST and CAP	Regional and manufacturer's peer group analysis available
Lyophilization error	Absent	Present	Absent

*That is, if additional analyte is added.
†NIST, National Institute of Standards and Technology; CAP, College of American Pathologists.

Laboratories must resolve a dilemma regarding target limits that result from CLIA's rules. On one hand, the need exists to optimize a testing system's calibration according to the manufacturer's instructions, but on the other hand, there is the need to meet proficiency testing requirements. The Center for Medicare and Medicaid Services (**CMS**, formerly the Health Care Financing Administration) allows each proficiency testing provider to determine how the program will establish the target values that will be used to judge acceptable performance. If the target value is calculated from peer group means for each testing system, it is better to establish the laboratory's QC system target values by use of the manufacturer's recommendations for both calibration and QC. However, if the target values for proficiency testing are set by the mean of all participants or by the true target values established by definitive methods, optimizing assays to the manufacturer's specifications may result in problems with the proficiency testing results if a bias is present as a result of those specifications.

Part of the problem with establishing a quality control program using manufacturers' recommendations is the effect of lyophilization (which causes matrix changes) on various constituents, resulting in method-specific interferences or bias, for example, as a result of the turbidity of these specimens. The dilemma, then, arises from the fact that if a laboratory adheres to the requirement of CLIA '88 and follows the manufacturer's instructions, failure in proficiency testing may result. However, a laboratory can, by the rules of CLIA '88, modify the manufacturer's instructions if the laboratory has data validating a method based on these changes.

When new target values are established for a new lot of quality control material, it is important to be sure that, during the data collection period, the analytical systems perform according to normal performance specifications. The new lot of quality control material should be tested in parallel with the current lot of quality control material. If the analytical data from the current quality control material indicate satisfactory performance of the methods, the data for the new lot can be assumed to be valid. When a quality control system is being set up for the first time, the current methodology is accepted as valid if the method meets performance specifications. As mentioned earlier, the choice of the laboratory's testing method (or testing system) is based on experience with medical usefulness, significant change limits, **external quality control** and accuracy comparisons, and quality control performance.

Three approaches can be used to establish the limits of acceptable values for a control pool. One method is to use the medically allowable error for choosing the range. Another, more usual, approach is to estimate the target value and usual standard deviation (SD) for the method and use some number of SDs to establish the range. The third technique is to employ the more statistically accurate method of **power curves**. These approaches are described in the following pages.

A Simple Method for Establishing Average Temporary Target Values for Quality Control Pools

1. Procure a minimum of a 1-year supply of quality control test material.
2. If possible, plan a 6-week lead time before changing control pools to allow for (a) comparative analyses of old and new lots of control materials (3 weeks); (b) data reduction and calculation and evaluation of control limits (1 week); and (c) a buffer of 2 additional weeks because not all planning is perfect. It is also advisable to retain 20 or 30 vials of each expiring pool for evaluating problems resulting from system changes. Clearly identify the expiring pool to ensure that it is not used beyond its expiration date and that it is not mistaken for the current lot of control materials. CLIA prohibits a laboratory from using out-of-date reagents, solutions, controls, calibrators, or culture media (§493.1205[e][1]). Any exception must be specifically granted by the Food and Drug Administration (FDA).
3. Always reconstitute the lyophilized material carefully, following the label's directions. Mixing too quickly or too vigorously may interfere with the solubilization of the lyophilized material or denature its protein constituents. Denatured enzymes have reduced activity. The date, time, and technologist's initials should be recorded on each vial of control material after reconstitution. If a frozen liquid pool is used, after thawing, mix the sample six times by inversion because the protein and other compounds become concentrated at the bottom of the vial during freezing.
4. Test duplicate samples from two separate vials (20 vials, 40 measurements) each day for 10 days. An alternative procedure is to reconstitute one vial per day and perform the tests in duplicate on each of 20 consecutive days (20 vials, 40 measurements). See Table 21-3 for an example of these calculations.
5. Determine temporary target values for each constituent by calculating the mean of these 40 analytical values ($n = 40$). This temporary target value is replaced after 2 months with a final average target value (see #7 following text).
6. Calculate the standard deviation of the 40 values. Note that this calculated standard deviation is a hybrid between within-run and total imprecision because the tests are done both in single runs and over several days. Set the range of allowable control values around the average temporary target by using the newly calculated standard deviation multiplied by the laboratory's control limit, expressed as the number of standard deviations (such as 2.5 or 3.0). The number of standard deviations for the control range can also be set according to the size of the USD and the test's allowable error (see following text and Table 21-3). If the allowable error for glucose at 1200 mg/L is ± 60 mg/L, the control range should fit within these boundaries. In other words, the testing system's full control range (such as ± 3 standard deviations) should fit within the allowable ± 60 mg/L. For this example, a single standard deviation can be as large as

20 mg/L. Alternatively, if the usual standard deviation is 15 mg/L, then ± 4 standard deviations can fit within the allowable window. For the next 2 months, use the temporary average target and range of allowable control values for routine quality control in the laboratory.

7. After the second month use three values to calculate the average final target value: the temporary target value and two **monthly averages** (Table 21-3). If the control material is slightly unstable over time (e.g., alkaline phosphatase activity often changes over time), the process used to change the target value must include evidence that the test value of the control material changed while the testing system remained constant. Such evidence can be provided by the use of additional stable materials with known values (such as a different control, excess proficiency testing material, or additional calibrator materials). The decision process for changing the target value must be well documented. It is best to avoid unstable control material.

Calculation of the Usual Standard Deviation

Every method has a characteristic inherent variability termed the *usual standard deviation*. The USD is calculated from a series of three to six consecutive **monthly standard deviations** that are obtained during a time when the testing instrument is assumed to be stable. The USD is a valid estimate of the usual day-to-day variability of individual measurements. The USD can eventually be used instead of the temporary SD to establish the daily control limits around the average final target value. Table 21-3 shows how the USD can be used to calculate the allowable number of standard deviations for control values that will still maintain the medical usefulness of the testing system. The medically allowable error is divided by the USD to calculate the number of USDs in the medically allowable error. This calculation assumes no significant bias. If significant bias is present, first subtract the bias from the total medically allowable error and then divide the result by the USD. This calculated number of standard deviations should be equal to or more than the number of standard deviations used for the laboratory's control range. Otherwise the test will either be persistently out of control or its medical usefulness will be compromised.

The USD can also be used to establish the statistical significance of the difference between two values from the same patient. The latter is often referred to as the *significant change limit* (see p. 385).

Setting the Action Control Limits for Each Level of Control Pool

The limits of acceptable results are used to determine the **action limits** of the control range. Historically, a QC result that exceeded the set limits was known as an *out-of-control* value. However, CLIA regulations now specifically define the term **out of control** as a situation in which a testing system cannot be used for reporting patients' results. Thus the term *exceeding action limits* is now used to designate

the less serious condition in which the result of a routine QC analysis exceeds the set limits. The documented response of a medical technologist to a QC result that exceeds action limits (see following text) does not include shutting the procedure down. This occurs only when the laboratory director formally declares that a testing system is *out of control* and the laboratory begins a formal remedial process to correct this more serious situation (see following text). A laboratory will be best served by designating in their laboratory manual the conditions that will define these two situations.

Historically the ranges were ± 2 standard deviations and covered 95% of expected control values. However, this means that 5% of results for control pools are expected to exceed action limits even when the method is working perfectly. A **false rejection** of a run results in excessive rerunning of samples and necessitates performing the documentation required under CLIA regulations. Therefore, limits other than ± 2 SDs have been suggested for establishing control limits. Currently many laboratories use 2.5 or 3 standard deviations for the acceptable limits in an attempt to reduce false-run rejection time and unnecessary retesting.

However, the use of 2.5 or 3 standard deviations to set error limits may not result in error detection that is sufficient for medical and CLIA requirements.[8,10,15] Thus a second approach is to establish daily quality control ranges based on the considerations discussed earlier. The target range must be equal to or less than the total allowable error (see p. 382), which in turn is equal to or less than the allowable medical and legal (CLIA) error. The target control limits will therefore be some multiples of the USD or temporary SD that will fulfill these requirements. The number of multiples chosen will be based on the need to detect true cases of inaccurate measurements and yet minimize false rejections of acceptable runs (see following text).

Another approach is to set the allowable range based only on medical usefulness criteria. The range is expressed as plus or minus the medically allowable error window around the target value. This process does not require that the laboratory use ± 2 or more standard deviations. The control window is as wide as medical use will allow. An "action limit" situation is demonstrated when the test value of the control material exceeds the error limits. One should determine that this approach will not place the laboratory at risk for failure of proficiency testing. For all these approaches, the final control range must not be so large that the testing system will fail to detect true instances of failure of the method.

Setting Quality Control Limits by Power Curves

Among the main questions in quality control are the following: "How much quality control testing is enough?" "Am I sure that I am detecting appropriately small errors?" and "Is my error detection sensitive enough to show whether the testing system is appropriate for the medical needs?" If a laboratory has adequately set allowable errors for medical needs, the second question is of academic interest only, because the detection of the smallest errors is costly and time-consuming.

A more scientific approach to answering these questions uses power curves to determine how many controls should be run, how frequently controls should be run, and what control rules should be used. Power curves are plots of the size of the error detected by a control system versus the probability of detecting that size error by various control rules. The power curve rules can calculate the probability of falsely rejecting a valid test run, the probability of **true rejection** (the detection of a significant error in the run), the probability of error detection, and the average number of control observations required to identify a given error.[7, 30-36] The design of specific control rules for a laboratory requires a five-step process[35] that includes (1) defining total allowable analytical error, (2) estimating the method's actual standard deviation and bias at the medical decision concentrations, (3) determining the systematic and random error that must be detected by the control system, (4) determining the probability level used for error detection (i.e., do you want to detect 90%, 95%, or 99% of errors?), and (5) plotting and inspecting the power curves to determine the number of control specimens that should be tested per run. In general, the most difficult part of these evaluations is determining how much error is allowable.

Westgard[37] (www.westgard.com) used these power curves to develop a series of specific control guidelines, popularly called the "Westgard rules." The rules, which are used to determine whether an analytical run is out of control, are written in shorthand as follows: (1) 1_{2s}, $1_{2.5s}$, and 1_{3s} mean one control value exceeding two, two and one half, or three standard deviations, (2) 2_{2s} means two control values exceeding two standard deviations, and (3) R_{4s} means the range of two control specimens exceeds four standard deviations. For many testing situations the sequential application of the $1_{3s}/2_{2s}/R_{4s}$ set of control rules allows two control specimens to give sufficient error detection for a single run.[38] These rules mean that the run is rejected (action limits are exceeded) if *any* of the following happen: (1) 1_{3s}, if one control value differs by more than three standard deviations from the mean value, (2) 2_{2s}, if two control values differ by more than two standard deviations from the mean value, and (3) R_{4s}, if the range between two controls in the same run exceeds a combination of four standard deviations (i.e., one control $\geq$1.5 SD from mean and the other >-2.5 SD from mean). The first two rules will detect excessive bias, whereas the last rejects the run because of excessive imprecision. With use of these rules, the data in Fig. 21-1 for one control show values that exceed the action limits on days

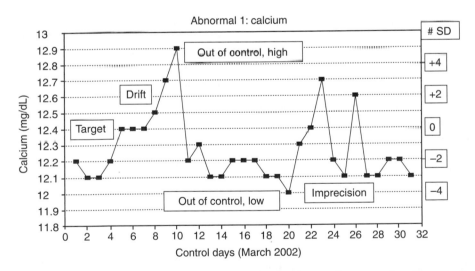

Fig. 21-1 Levey-Jennings plot of quality control values. *Quality control actions (testing personnel documentation of how all out-of-control values were resolved)*: Days 5-7 represent a shift from the target value (monitor carefully). Days 6-10 demonstrate a gradual trend toward higher values. Day 10 patients' results were not reported, an unresolved problem (one control >3 SD), probably need new bottle of calibrator. On day 11 recalibrated using new bottle of calibrator. Control values are now in control range; the patients' specimens from day 9 were retested. Day 13 begins a shift to lower values. This shift was investigated on day 20 when one control was low by more than 3 SD. Recalibration on day 21 resolved the problem because values were nearer to the target value (RBP). Days 23 through 26 show increased imprecision. On day 27 cleaning the flow cell resolved the problem; however, the low bias is still present. *General note*: When this method shows acceptable imprecision, the values are below the target. It was subsequently determined that the manufacturer's target value for this QC pool was inaccurate. Proficiency results from testing performed on March 16 were within 0.01 mg/dL from the all participants' target value. After this documentation, the laboratory director approved a new target value for this QC pool.

10 (1_{3s}) and 20 (1_{3s}). Notice that, for rejection, the control value should exceed the control limit, not just be equal to that value. For many chemistry tests, power curves allow cost-effective detection of significant total errors (based on clinical usefulness) when two controls are used and the limits are set somewhere between 2.5 to 3.5 standard deviations.[7] For this reason, many use 3.0 usual standard deviations as a generalized control limit. For best implementation of Westgard rules, the LIS or the analyzer must have the proper software present to support this level of quality control checks. A more sophisticated approach to quality control will minimize run rejection and, at the same time, ensure the quality of patient results. Accordingly, some version of the Westgard approach are a useful feature on most LIS QC applications.

DETECTION AND RESOLUTION OF QUALITY PROBLEMS
The Out-of-Control Decision

A testing system is designated as "out of control" when the validity of the results is not considered to be appropriate. Grossly out-of-control testing systems are usually unsuitable for medical purposes. This determination is made by the director or technical supervisor.

The conditions for an out-of-control determination should be set by each laboratory; as a minimum, the criteria for an out-of-control decision include the following elements:

1. Control values exceed predetermined out-of-control limits within a specified period. Technologists must be directed to document their response to every control value that exceeds the established limits.
2. A method is determined to have an inappropriate reference interval; if the range is not immediately correctable, the method is "out of control."
3. A method demonstrates unacceptable imprecision, non-linearity, or interferences. Interferences usually are limited to specific specimen types or substances.
4. A pattern of inappropriate patient results with large numbers of abnormal values is observed or individual patient results exceed "delta" checking against previous results.
5. The laboratory director, section director, or technical supervisor declares the method out of control for other reasons.

Techniques for detecting and resolving out-of-control situations are discussed in the following text.

Detection of Quality Problems

Computer assistance. The target values and limits for acceptable results that are established for each control pool are used in daily practice to detect analytical problems. A control result can be reviewed in a variety of ways by a technologist to evaluate acceptability. The technologist can simply compare the result with the posted range. This limits the technologist's ability to employ the Westgard rules or to evaluate the **trend** of previous results. More complex

selection rules are now available as part of some computer programs, either on the instrument or as part of the laboratory's information system (LIS, see Chapter 18). Computer assistance allows real-time review of control results, early detection of QC problems, and better documentation of the quality control process.

Levey-Jennings plots.[39,40] Current quality control data are best interpreted in the context of previous QC results as described above. In order to facilitate this goal, the data obtained from daily analysis of quality control pools can be plotted to give a visual presentation of the data. The most common visual analysis is the **Levey-Jennings plot**. The expected analyte concentrations, the established target value, and the desired number of standard deviations are drawn on the *y*-axis and the days of the month (typically 31) are indicated on the *x*-axis (Fig. 21-1). A large piece of graph paper can be used to show the data for several months. Thus cumulative information from quality control results can be observed at one time. Levey-Jennings plots are usually available on the LIS (see Chapter 18) or on the instrument performing the assays, obviating the need to plot these QC results manually.

Fig. 21-1 shows an example of a Levey-Jennings plot. The sudden change in control values (days 1 to 4 versus days 5 to 7) from one average to a new average is called a *shift*. The increasing deviation from the target value, seen from day 8 to day 10, is called a *trend*. Changes in the precision of the testing system are shown on days 21 to 26, that is, a greater dispersion of data points than that shown for days 13 to 19. This system was judged as unacceptable for the reasons documented at the bottom of Fig. 21-1. On day 32, the laboratory director reevaluated the target value and concluded that it had been set too high. A lower value was set, and QC results for the next month were closely monitored to assess this change.

All positive or negative trends (or drifts) or shifts from the target value represent biases that should be evaluated. Levey-Jennings plots should be routinely evaluated by technologists and supervisory personnel looking for trends or shifts in the data that could indicate problems in the testing system. Normally a trend or a shift is noticed within 6 to 10 days after it begins. A shift or trend that exists over this period is usually a nonrandom, permanent change in the assay system.

Using Patients' Data in Decision Making

Pattern of patients' results. The results of most patients' sample analyses fall within reference (healthy) intervals established for each analyte.[41] Thus, for an analytical run of patients' samples, the results fall into a familiar pattern; that is, most results are within the nondiseased patient reference interval and a few results are abnormal. The distribution of abnormal results, that is, the percentage of high or low results, will vary from test to test and even from hospital to hospital. Deviations from the usual pattern of cumulative patient results should alert the testing personnel that a shift in the system's performance may be occurring and that the patient analyses may be invalid. For example, a series of patient results for potassium greater than 5 should alert a technologist to a possible bias problem (Table 21-5). The example in Table 21-5 shows a typical set of potassium values (patient set A) and a clearly abnormal series (patient set B). The technologist should, of course, evaluate special circumstances. For example, a work load that includes a larger number than usual of patients' specimens from renal dialysis or cancer chemotherapy clinics will abnormally skew the otherwise typical pattern of test results. Clearly, the verification of patient results by the technologist serves as a critical final check of quality control and especially so when results are reviewed as part of a batch of results from the same run.

The delta check. Another important quality control check is the pattern of consecutive results for an individual patient. For most analyses, it is unlikely that a consecutive series of two or three test values from one patient will show large differences unless a major medical change has occurred. Unexpected changes from a single patient's serial specimens are called *delta changes,* meaning that a value for a single patient changed from the previous results more than the laboratory's delta limit allows. Delta limits are set primarily to detect misidentified specimens or other errors (see p. 80 in Chapter 3). When these types of changes are noted, the analyst must determine whether the change is real or whether problems exist that are not identified by analysis of quality control specimens. Delta checks are usually part of an **autoverification** program (pp. 326–327 in Chapter 18).

Actions To Bring a Testing System Back into Control

When analytic problems are found, it is best to have a plan of action that is executed sequentially until the problem is resolved. For CLIA '88 it is necessary to document the problem, the investigation, the problem resolution, and any data that indicate that the problem is actually resolved (so called corrective action). In a manual QC system, this documentation is kept in a separate "action limits" or "out-of-control" log book. A good LIS system also allows the analyst to point and click on a specific QC point on a displayed Levey-Jennings plot and list comments regarding the point including associated corrective action. A list of actions follows that are among the sequential actions that might be taken to identify a problem. After each step is taken, the routine QC pools are analyzed; if the results are now within limits, it is assumed that the problem has been resolved, and patient results can be released. If the QC results are still not satisfactory, the next step is taken.

1. Repeat assays on control specimens using fresh aliquots of QC pools.
2. Repeat assays on control specimens using a separate or newly reconstituted set of controls. A set of controls can be mishandled, resulting in changed analyte concentrations because of possible enzyme deterioration, evaporation, precipitation, or other causes.
3. Look for obvious problems: clots, reagent levels, mechanical fault.
4. Recalibrate the instrument for the out-of-control analyte, then reassay all the controls.
5. Install a new bottle or new lot number for one or all of the reagents, recalibrate, and reassay all the controls.
6. Perform periodic maintenance, recalibrate, and reassay all the controls.

If any of these responses results in acceptable QC data, results for patients' results can be released if and *only* if at least three (or the entire run, whichever is less) patients' specimens taken from the last run are reassayed and the differences between previous and new results are within the performance specification for precision (see p. 390). If the differences exceed the performance specifications, further action must be taken (see example below). This requirement is established by CLIA, which states (§493.1219[b]) that "all patient test results obtained in the unacceptable test run or since the last acceptable test run must be evaluated to determine if patient test results have been adversely affected and the laboratory must take the remedial action necessary to ensure the reporting of accurate and reliable patient test results."

Technologists should be encouraged to perform all the above steps by themselves before requesting help from a supervisor. However, in a critical testing area, time limits for instrument downtime should be set. For an instrument in a stat. area, probably no more than 15 to 20 minutes should be spent in problem solving before supervisors are notified.

Example. At the start of the day, the laboratory's method for potassium produced results for controls that were elevated by over 5 standard deviations. The change coincided with a change in the potassium ion-selective electrode (ISE). A new potassium ISE was installed, the instrument was

---

TABLE 21-5   USE OF PATIENT DATA IN DAILY QUALITY CONTROL

Sample Number	Patient Set A	Patient Set B
Control I	4.4—in control	4.4—in control
Control II	6.9—in control	6.8—in control
1	3.8	4.1
2	4.6	3.9
3	5.0	5.7
4	4.3	6.1
5	4.2	6.5
6	3.6	5.8
7	4.7	6.4
8	4.0	6.2
9	4.6	5.1
10	3.9	4.7
Control I	4.3—in control	4.6—in control (at +2 SD)
Control II	6.8—in control	7.0—in control (at +2 SD)

Would you wait until the quality control samples after the tenth sample to make a judgment about the system? No. After about the third or fourth patient sample with an extremely high or low value, quality control could be moved ahead and trouble detection should begin. Keep in mind that occasionally, by chance, a series of specimens from very ill patients may fall in consecutive order. Repeated testing will usually solve the problem.

recalibrated, and the controls were retested; they were then back in control. Three patient samples from the last run were retested to see if the problem affected the reported values. The potassium results reported for the previous runs were 3.9, 4.6, and 5.3 mmol/L and, when repeated, the results were 4.1, 4.5, and 5.3 mmol/L. The method's performance specification for potassium precision is 1 SD = 0.11 mmol/L. The patients' potassium results each changed by <0.22 mmol/L. This is less than a 2 SD change; therefore, the old report does not have to be changed. This reevaluation of a patient's results should continue until either a **significant difference** is seen or the previously accepted quality control sample is reached.

When reevaluation of previous patients' results shows unacceptable differences, *all* the patients' specimens that were tested after the last in-control QC sample must be reassayed. If problems persist, the test may need to be performed on an alternative system or sent to a reference laboratory. If there is insufficient quantity (or quantity not sufficient, QNS) of a patient's specimen to reevaluate, the laboratory should request that another specimen be collected. It is inappropriate to report a result when the assay quality is in question.

7. Assay a different control of similar known concentration to determine if the original control material is at fault. In such situations, it is good policy to have some alternative control materials that are different from the QC materials routinely used, possibly with previously established, reliable assay values. The determination of a shift in the control material's assay value (which requires resetting the target value) is to be made only by the director or technical supervisor. If the values for a routine QC pool have changed slightly, assuming a new, stable pattern, but the test system appears stable (as judged by values from separate QC materials), then the target values of the routine QC pool may be changed. The laboratory director, with concomitant documentation of the decision process, must authorize such changes. If only one of the controls is showing the slight shift while a material of similar concentration continues to give a stable value and the test system shows stable performance, the initial estimation of the control material's target value was probably incorrectly set. In this case the target value should be modified. If both controls and additional controls show similar shifts or trends, the problem is probably in the testing system.

8. Call the manufacturer to help determine the cause of the problem. Follow the manufacturer's instructions and then reassay all the controls.

9. Have the instrument serviced by the manufacturer, recalibrate, and reassay all the controls, if necessary to resolve the problem.

10. Use commercial accuracy-based materials to evaluate the quality of the analytical system, checking linearity (reportable range), accuracy, bias, precision, analytical sensitivity, and minimal detectable change (smallest concentration change that is significant). Careful evalua-

tion of these data should help reveal the cause of the control problem. Performing parallel testing on patient samples on a second instrument can also be very helpful at this point.

11. Determine whether the testing system has changed by reevaluating the reference interval. You can do this by obtaining data on the last 100 patients who have near-normal chemistry profiles with two or fewer slight abnormalities (acceptable patients are determined by the director or technical supervisor). Estimate the reference interval by excluding the 2.5% of the values from the tails of the distribution. This interval should agree (within ± 1 SD) with the laboratory's established reference interval. This procedure will only demonstrate gross changes in the system. The director or technical supervisor should determine if there has been a significant shift in the reference interval.

12. Reestablish the method's linearity using either the National Committee for Clinical Laboratory Standards (NCCLS) protocols EP-6 to P2 (2001). If the method is linear over the reporting range and the reference interval has not changed, the method is probably usable with adjustments to the appropriate target values for the control specimens.

13. Consult the director or technical supervisor to declare the method out of control if the above steps fail.

14. A final action is replacement of the method or instrument with one that will allow the laboratory to meet its medical and proficiency testing goals.

Every quality control decision should be recorded in a permanent record. To meet CLIA '88's requirements, the quality control records should state acceptable limits and include written documentation of the actions taken in response to out-of-range values. These responses must include date, analyte, complete testing system (i.e., source of reagents, instrument, calibrators, and controls), description of the problem, problem resolution, and names of the persons performing the test and approving the final actions. It may be convenient to prepare check-off forms or graphs for each control and analyte (Fig. 21-2). These records are also useful for predicting the need for maintenance, repair, or replacement of deteriorating reagents and instrument components as indicated by the circled check marks in Fig. 21-2. Computerized records can greatly simplify and speed the documentation process.

Actions To Be Taken When a Method Is Out of Control

1. The decision that a testing system is out of control and must be suspended is communicated to all laboratory personnel, including the director, technical consultant, technical supervisor, clinical consultant, general supervisor, and all appropriate testing personnel. As stated above, the time frame for making this problem known will vary from section to section and should be stated in the laboratory's manual.

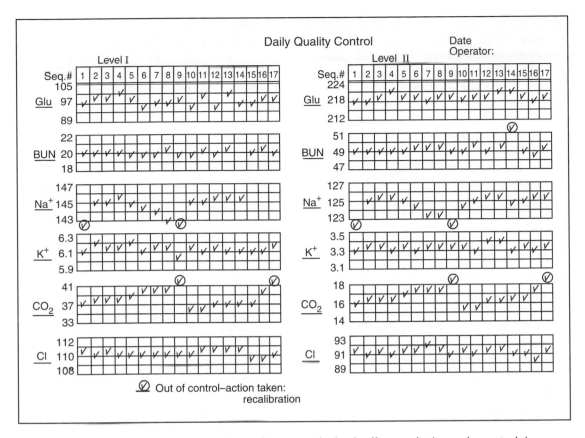

Fig. 21-2 Multiple analyte daily quality control check-off record. As each control is reported, it is quickly logged on a data sheet. Notes of out-of-control values and action taken are included. A daily value for quality control calculation is selected by use of a random-number table basis. *(Form developed by Rosvoll RV: In Copeland BE, Rosvoll RV, Casella JM: Quality control workshop manual, Chicago, 1978, American Society of Clinical Pathologists Commission on Continuing Education.)*

2. Suspension of a testing system means that no further patient test results are to be released until the out-of-control condition is corrected and the director or technical supervisor approves resumption of the testing.

3. Steps must be taken to have the test performed either by an alternative method or by a reference laboratory. The alternative procedure must be listed in the laboratory manual. Notify the appropriate clinicians if the alternative method will have any adverse influence on test results or turnaround times.

4. An out-of-control condition that cannot be dealt with by use of alternative methods or testing systems must be communicated within a reasonable time to the medical staff and any other authorized persons (such as senior administrative staff).

5. Supervisory personnel may define, for medical or analytical reasons, out-of-control conditions that differ from those stated in the general policy. These special conditions must be documented in the procedure as well as in the method's file.

6. Bringing a suspended test back into production requires the following actions as a minimum. The method must be recalibrated, or a calibration verification must be performed. Two levels of controls and at least one other material, such as proficiency testing materials of known or established value, must be used. The method can be used when the results of the known specimens are within the expected mean ± 2 times the appropriate usual standard deviation (established at a concentration close to the control value that was out of control). The method's reuse must be authorized by the technical supervisor or director. This authorization must be entered into the laboratory's problem log and formally signed and dated.

Procedures To Follow during a Testing System Failure

An out-of-control condition that is not immediately correctable can constitute a laboratory emergency. These emergencies can be managed by (1) using a suitable backup method, (2) sending the test to a reference laboratory, or (3) temporarily discontinuing the test. A laboratory must list an alternative or backup method of analysis in the procedure manual. Laboratory policy should define how much time the technologist can spend troubleshooting a method before using the alternative system. Other factors that affect the decision include the medical requirements of the test (stat.

versus routine), laboratory staffing, and the laboratory's work load. For example, a stat. potassium analysis would be treated very differently from a 72-hour fecal fat determination. In the case of a potassium test, a delay of more than 30 minutes in providing a backup result may affect a critical medical decision, whereas several days' delay in the fecal fat analysis may not be crucial to patient care. Decisions about processing patient samples during a testing system failure should be made in consultation with the laboratory technical supervisor/consultant and the laboratory director, as specified by laboratory policy.

CALIBRATION AND QUALITY CONTROL
Use of Calibrators

Controls may not be used as calibrators. Controls and calibrators must be different because each has a separate and important function. Calibrators set the reported values accurately, whereas controls verify the stability and accuracy of the calibration and the testing system. However, for those tests that do not have suitable controls available, CLIA '88 allows calibration materials to be used as controls. For evaluation of the system's stability, in these cases it is best to find calibrator materials other than those used for calibration of the testing system.

A commercially available calibrator has an assigned value that the manufacturer establishes by using a definitive or reference method or by using reference materials (traceable to **primary standards**). The calibrator is then used to set the value reported by the laboratory's method or instrument. This process establishes correspondence of the instrument output signal with known concentrations. Differences between an aqueous and serum matrix can affect the transfer of known concentrations to a reported patient result. These matrix differences include turbidity, surface tension, which can affect sample pipetting, interactions between analytes and proteins, and the effect of the volume fraction occupied by protein or other large molecules (especially lipoproteins) on the actual concentration of the analytes.

Calibrators are usually purchased in lots large enough to last 12 or more months. It is recommended that a new lot of calibrator material be tested 6 weeks before it is used. This time delay allows the laboratory to detect any systematic bias between the values of the current and the new calibrator. Bias in a new lot of calibrator is detected when changes are seen in the mean value of quality control pools or patients' test results. Some testing systems do not allow calibrators (especially calibrators from other systems) to be run as an unknown because of matrix mismatch. Often a calibrator will have assigned values that don't represent actual analyte values. These assigned-value calibrators are designed to calibrate testing systems to produce accurate test values when patients' samples are used. Although the FDA requires manufacturers to use reference methods to assign calibrator values, there are frequently significant differences between calibrator lots. Because of matrix effects, errors can be introduced into the calibration process when calibrators are used that are not specifically designed for the analytic system.

Under CLIA '88 any modification of the manufacturer's instructions for the analytical portion of an FDA-cleared procedure requires documentation of the validity of the change. A laboratory that wishes to change a manufacturer's calibration set point must document that the change does not adversely affect the method's performance specifications. Some of the newer analyzers employ a two-dimensional bar code with a specific calibration associated with the particular lot of reagents. In this case, the manufacturer provides one or two point "adjusters" or calibrator-like reagents to refine the calibration curve prior to placing the reagents into use. Of course, controls are subsequently run to verify the accuracy of such factory calibrations.

A Practical System for New Calibrator Verification

1. Use a 10-day verification period.
2. If the manufacturer allows the assay of calibrators as unknowns, each day insert two aliquots from one vial of new calibrator as an unknown into the regular daily run (n = 10 vials; 20 values). Calculate the average for each analyte. Compare each average with the value assigned by the manufacturer. Any difference between the assigned and measured values will allow you to predict the average change expected in the quality control pool's target value (and also in patients' test values) when the new calibrator is introduced. A change in the quality control pool's target value greater than 1.0 usual standard deviation is statistically significant, and a decision must be made as to which calibrator value is truly accurate. This decision must include consideration of CLIA's requirements (especially those that concern proficiency testing) and consultation with the manufacturer.

CLIA '88 requires that, when control values demonstrate significant changes (defined by each laboratory), the laboratory must establish, through calibration verification, that calibration has not been changed. Calibration verification requires that three specimens with high, low, and normal analyte concentrations be run to verify the quality of the test results. These specimens can be controls, calibrators, or other specimens with known values. If the manufacturer has specified a calibration verification protocol, you may follow it (§493.1217). The CLIA rules do not set the quantity of allowable error except as judged by proficiency testing. By setting an allowable error that is too large, however, a laboratory increases the danger of failing proficiency testing and may compromise patients' test values. Performance specifications can be used to judge excessive change (see Table 21-3).

Quality Control of Reagent Changes and Instrument Maintenance

Each lot of reagent or separate shipment must be evaluated for quality before it is put into use. The laboratory can show that new lots or shipments of reagents (including calibrators and quality control pools) are acceptable if, after their use, the control values do not change significantly. It is also a good practice, after any maintenance is performed, to test a set of controls and run several patient samples from a previous batch before testing is resumed. Maintenance problems can lead to an "action-limits" situation because operating parameters may be changed. A chronological record of all reagent changes, instrument repairs, and maintenance procedures along with any calibration-verification tests must be kept.

EXTERNAL QUALITY CONTROL PROGRAMS AND OTHER TOOLS FOR ACCURACY CONTROL
Accuracy Control Is Required by CLIA '88

CLIA '88 requires that all laboratories holding a certificate that allows testing of moderately or highly complex tests must participate successfully in proficiency testing. Proficiency testing (PT) specimens are used to evaluate the adequacy of laboratory performance in all laboratory specialties. The analyst must test these specimens in the same manner as patients' specimens. Historically, PT has been part of a volunteer peer review and educational process. Proficiency testing is now regulatory, and failure on PT has serious penalties. However, the value of proficiency testing is the provision of independent validation of the internal quality control programs. Some of the providers of proficiency testing programs approved by the CMS are listed in Table 21-6. Because the analyst does not know the target value of the PT sample, it is difficult for the operator to influence the results. These programs, if properly used, can give an estimation of the inherent accuracy of a system, at least as compared with a peer group or to the overall mean.[19]

TABLE 21-6 PARTIAL LIST OF CMS (HCFA)-APPROVED PROVIDERS OF PROFICIENCY TESTING PROGRAMS FOR CLIA '88

Provider	Telephone Number
Accutest	800-356-6788
American Academy of Family Physicians	800-274-2237
American Association for Bioanalysts	800-234-5315
American Association of Pediatrics	800-433-9016
American Osteopathic Association	800-621-1773
American Proficiency Institute	800-333-0958
American Society of Internal Medicine	800-338-2746
American Thoracic Society	212-315-8789
California Thoracic Society	714-730-1944
College of American Pathologists/Excel	800-323-4040
College of American Pathologists/Surveys	800-323-4040
State of Idaho	208-334-2235
State of New York	518-485-5378
State of Ohio	614-466-2278
Wisconsin State Laboratory of Hygiene	800-462-5261

CMS (HCFA), *Center for Medicare and Medicaid Services (formerly Health Care Financing Administration).*
From the American Association for Clinical Chemistry, Clinical Laboratories Improvement Act, Fax No. 800-254-2329.

Continued or significant deviations from the PT target levels, even if there is no failure, should alert the laboratory to a possible accuracy problem. If a method's USD is not significantly smaller than the comparative group's SD, that method is at increased risk for PT failure.

An *estimation* of a system's bias can also be made from proficiency testing performance. To do this, evaluate the specific test method's observed values against a comparison value, which is either the mean value reported for all similar methods (peer group mean), the mean value for all methods, or the definitive method value. Bias is calculated by subtracting the comparison value from your method's value. The algebraic sign shows whether your method's value is higher (positive bias) or lower (negative bias) than the group mean. Notice that comparison to a peer group mean or even to the mean of all participants doesn't establish accuracy. These comparisons show bias only from the comparison value. Accuracy is determined only when the comparison value is the true value. Certainly repeated bias on proficiency tests must raise the suspicion of a true bias and will require that additional steps be taken to either prove or disprove a real bias.

Definitive and Reference Methods

Definitive and reference methods are established by the National Reference System for the Clinical Laboratory (NRSCL) through applications by groups of interested persons representing different disciplines and organizations from professional societies or practitioners, industrial companies, and governmental agencies. The NRSCL is a part of the NCCLS. Definitive and reference methods are used to establish accuracy-based reference materials (see below).

A *definitive method*[2, 42-43] is the most accurate way to measure a particular chemical substance. Analysis by definitive methods usually involves instrumentation of the most sophisticated type and a separation procedure to purify the analyte before its concentration is measured. These methods are available in institutions such as the National Institute of Standards and Technology (NIST), the Centers for Disease Control and Prevention (CDC), and large reference laboratories. Table 21-7 lists the seven definitive and 18 reference methods defined by the NRSCL.

A *reference method*[3] is less rigorously proved than a definitive method, but it is well accepted because there is considerable evidence of its analytical ability. Thus the reference method has a demonstrated record of transferability of accuracy. The equipment and methodology are such that these methods are usually available in a university hospital-level laboratory. If a definitive method is not available for comparison, the reference method is established by consensus among authorities in the field. Reference methods credentialed by the NRSCL are listed in Table 21-7. There are other reference methods that will become NRSCL-credentialed in the near future. The NRSCL is currently designing specifications for designated comparison methods that could be readily used by many laboratories.

A *field method* is one that is in common use. It is not classified as a reference or definitive method. It has been

TABLE 21-7 NRSCL DEFINITIVE AND REFERENCE METHODS

Document Number	Analyte
Definitive Methods	
NCCLS RS1-A	Glucose
NCCLS RS3-A	Cholesterol
NCCLS RS7-P	Sodium
NCCLS RS8-P	Potassium
NCCLS RS9-P	Calcium
NCCLS RS10-P	Chloride
NCCLS RS11-P	Urea
Reference Methods	
NCCLS RS1-A	Glucose
NCCLS RS2-A	Aspartate aminotransferase (AST)
NCCLS RS3-A	Cholesterol
NCCLS RS4-A	Alanine aminotransferase (ALT)
NCCLS RS5-A	Total protein
NCCLS RS6-A	Total bilirubin
NCCLS RS7-P	Sodium
NCCLS RS8-P	Potassium
NCCLS RS9-P	Calcium
NCCLS RS10-P	Chloride
NCCLS RS11-P	Urea
NCCLS RS12-P	Creatinine*
NCCLS RS13-P	Rubella antibody*
NCCLS RS14-P	Creatine kinase
NCCLS RS15-P	Hemoglobin*
NCCLS RS16	Antimicrobial susceptibility testing
NCCLS RS17	Gamma-glutamyl transferase
NCCLS RS18	Uric acid*

NRSCL, *National Reference System for the Clinical Laboratory.*
A, *Approved;* P, *proposed.*
*In development.

this material have levels measured by reference and definitive methods.

There are other materials (similar to quality control materials) that have consensus values established by thousands of laboratories. These values are reported as overall average values or average values of methods performed by a specific testing system. The College of American Pathologists (CAP) produces survey-validated sera that have values established by thousands of individual assays from laboratories participating in proficiency testing.[44] Some systems will show matrix effects caused by the lyophilization process or the presence of interfering compounds, and so one must be careful when using these materials as the sole judge of a testing system's bias.

Primary standards are always required for definitive and reference methods. The NIST provides a number of standard reference materials (SRMs) that may be used to prepare primary liquid standards. These include albumin, angiotensin, anticonvulsant drugs, aspartate aminotransferase, bilirubin, blood-gases, calcium, chloride, cholesterol, cortisol, creatinine, electrolytes for ion-selective electrodes, fat-soluble vitamins, glucose, hydrogen ion, inorganic ions in bovine serum, iron, lead, lithium, magnesium, potassium, phosphorus, sodium, trace metals in serum, tripalmate, urea, and uric acid. Aqueous materials in sealed vials prepared from these NIST primary standards are available from CAP. When NIST reference materials are used for calibration, a method's accuracy may be said to be "traceable to NIST reference materials." It is essential that the matrix of the prepared calibrator is consistent with the requirements of the testing system. Some testing systems require protein or other constituents in the calibrator before it will behave appropriately in the testing system. A catalog of reference materials (NIST Special Publication 260) can be obtained from NIST at 1-301-975-6776.

compared to a reference method and has been shown to give comparable results acceptable to the user. Information on these method comparisons and evaluations is available in the medical literature and often from the manufacturer of a testing system.

Reference Materials

Commercially available aqueous and protein-based materials may be used as calibrators or controls to determine or monitor the accuracy of assays. Each of these reference materials is useful for investigating the accuracy of a method. True target concentrations are assigned by use of definitive or reference methods, and can be certified by a certifying body to produce certified reference materials (CRM). Alternatively, the reference material is prepared with a specific concentration by use of known amounts of high-purity analytes. These true target values are the most accurate values obtainable by state-of-the-art technology and thus are preferable when they are available. An example of such a reference material is the lyophilized human serum product, SRM909, produced by the NIST. A number of constituents in

Selection of a Reference Laboratory for Assistance in Accuracy Control

One procedure that a laboratory can use to confirm the accuracy of a method is to send aliquots of patients' samples to a reliable reference laboratory. It is important, however, to be completely confident of the quality of the reference laboratory's analytical work. Always obtain information on the accuracy and precision of their analytical methods. The laboratory should request a list of the methods and performance specifications used by the reference laboratory as well as the results of their proficiency testing. The laboratory should evaluate all data carefully to determine whether the methods are appropriate for its needs. The laboratory's method is considered accurate if its results are not significantly different from those of the reference laboratory.

Manufacturer's Responsibility in the Control of Testing Systems

The responsibility for solving systematic and random bias problems does not belong solely to the user but should also be shared by the manufacturer of equipment and reagents.

Manufacturers should provide performance specifications so that the laboratory can determine whether the system can be used appropriately to meet its medical and CLIA requirements. After the laboratory chooses a testing system, the technical supervisor must determine (often with the manufacturer) that the performance specifications are met by laboratory operation. Careful perusal of national proficiency surveys quickly reveals instrument systems and reagent systems that show the presence of significant systematic bias in the analysis of proficiency testing specimens. Proficiency testing specimens are the same or very similar to the specimens used for quality control evaluation. However, some bias may be shown only because of the difference in the matrix of the control materials.[45] These matrix-specific biases are not seen when fresh patients' specimens are tested. The presence of matrix bias is shown by testing of fresh human specimens and control materials by the laboratory's test method and a different method that doesn't show the matrix bias. Any differences found between the methods may be the result of the matrix effect. Analytical problems that cannot be resolved after consultation with the manufacturer should be reported through the FDA's reporting system, administered by the U.S. Pharmacopeia, at 1-800-638-6725.

Automated Quality Control Initiatives

Manufacturers are playing an ever-increasing role in the quality control of new instruments and, in some cases, taking over some of the traditional roles of the analyst. This is especially true for point-of-care testing (or decentralized testing, see Chapter 17)[37,46] where in many cases the operator of the testing device is much less knowledgeable about issues of quality control than the technologists and scientists in the central laboratory. New blood-gas instruments for example have included quality control material in test packs and allow the user to program when quality control is to be performed. A one-point calibration in some blood-gas instruments is performed automatically after each patient sample, while some manufacturers have included plans to automatically generate maintenance procedure and other corrective actions based on out-of-control results. Such automated QC systems use expert software tools and automatically document QC and maintenance activities in computer files for CLIA requirements (42 CFR 492.801.01.3000). The concept of a reagent lot-specific factory calibration stored on two-dimensional barcodes with "adjusters" to refine the factory calibration on site is becoming more common in the laboratory industry. With the Federal Drug Administration (FDA) becoming more involved in their traditional oversight of medical devices, one might regard built-in, automated quality control features on laboratory instruments as a requirement to ensure accuracy and reliability of generated test results. In this regard, it is not surprising that many newer chemistry analyzers have features allowing for quality control materials to be stored on the system and run periodically without operator intervention. Many vendors of chemistry analyzers provide continuous monitoring of their customers' instrument functions and quality control using Web initiatives and modem communications. Using modem access, this allows the vendor to assume remote control of the instrument for testing and troubleshooting without having to go onsite, greatly speeding the response time needed to correct a testing problem. In addition, one manufacturer of quality control materials is providing real-time evaluation of quality control results generated at customer sites, again using modem and Web communication tools. As automated instruments improve in terms of reliability, stability, redundancy of components, remote QC and QA monitoring, and self-diagnostics/expert software tools, defects in the analytical system will frequently be detected prior to any observable change in testing accuracy and precision. In addition, as vendors obtain real-time access to QC results, they will be empowered to possibly identify problems with field-installed instruments prior to requests from the local analyst.

Frequency of Calibration, Reagent Systems, and QC

Clearly, one goal of the laboratory must be to minimize the number of assays required to produce a patient result. Manual calibration *in lieu* of factory calibration, frequent recalibration resulting from out-of-control QC, frequent re-analysis of QC and patient are characteristics of older, poorly designed analyzers and QC programs. New analyzers tend to be much more stable with reagents stored "onboard" in temperature-controlled, refrigerated compartments and calibrations lasting for at least 30 to 60 days. If a method is entirely in control over this period of time, then theoretically one can compute the costs of performing quality control. The example of such a computation, shown in Table 21-8, assumes that calibration is part of quality control expense and that the only controls that would be repeated would be outliers or those 5% beyond the ± 2 SD limits. The theoretical achievable test performed to reportable test ratio (TRR)[47] for a hypothetical laboratory test would be in the 1.02 to 1.46 range, or 2% to 46% QC overhead cost. Of course, dilutions on patient assays beyond linear range would increase the TRR slightly, however new analyzers have expanded the linear range on most of their assays to minimize this occurrence. Extending the shelf-life of reagents minimizes waste and tends to lower the TRR; vendors have accomplished this, as described above. All of the design features now available on new analyzers have markedly increased the overall efficiency and cost-effectiveness of the laboratory as demonstrated by TRRs in the 1.2 to 1.3 range on some well-designed instruments. On the other hand, analyzers for immunoassay are still being manufactured that operate with TRRs in the 2 to 3 range. Note that these are instruments where reagents must be manually calibrated (6 calibrators or more in duplicate), frequently recalibrated because of reagent or calibration instability, packaging of as little as 50 assays per calibration, and daily controls at two to three levels with frequent repeats. Also, as seen in Table 21-8, higher TRRs and thus higher QC costs will be seen in lower

**TABLE 21-8   THEORETICAL TEST TO REPORTABLE RATIOS ON AN AUTOMATED CHEMISTRY/
IMMUNOCHEMISTRY ANALYZER BASED ON 31-DAY ONBOARD REAGENT AND CALIBRATION
STABILITY***

Patient Assays per Day	Control Assays per Month (2/Day) +5% Outlier Repeats	Factory Calibration Verification Assays	Theoretical Test to Reportable Ratio (TRR)	Theoretically Achievable QC Overhead
100	65	6	1.02	2%
10	65	6	1.23	23%
5	65	6	1.46	46%

*Assumptions: A totally in-control, stable method for 31 days with no recalibrations required, manufacturer's factory calibration with two "verifiers" run in triplicate, no patient dilution reruns due to expanded linear range on the assay, and no reagent or control lot number changes during the 31-day period.

volume esoteric assays like PSA and troponin-I, which may be performed only once or twice daily in a smaller hospital laboratory. Clearly, instruments with high TRRs are much more expensive to operate. These days, instrument vendors are highly motivated to achieve the lowest TRRs possible in the US market because many of them are paid on a per reportable patient result system (CRR, Cost per Reportable Result), with the vendor supplying the required instrument, reagents, calibrators, and expendable supplies. A high TRR will therefore be expensive to the manufacturer as well as to the hospital.

Electronic Quality Control (See also p. 315, Chapter 17)

For most of the quality control discussion above, we have assumed that laboratory testing is being performed in the traditional manner, that is, in the central laboratory (or core laboratory) and that QC has been performed on liquid

materials similar to the patient sample. However, as computer chip and biosensor technology allow for more testing to be conveniently and cost-effectively performed at the patient's bedside, one can anticipate the need for a more sophisticated approach to quality control. Handheld testing devices that employ **electronic quality control** have already demonstrated a high level of success in the marketplace. Indeed, CLIA rules accept the concept of electronic controls with the provision that verification of the manufacturer's claims is performed, as well as periodic assessment with liquid control materials, as required by the Joint Commission on Accreditation of Healthcare Organizations (JCAHO) and the College of American Pathologists (CAP).

ACKNOWLEDGMENT

Special thanks to Bradley E. Copeland, M.D., for his previous authorship of this chapter, much of which is retained.

References

1. National Committee for Clinical Laboratory Standards: *Development of certified reference materials for the National Reference System for the Clinical Laboratory, approved guideline*, NCCLS publication NRSCL3-A (ISBN 1-56238-106-7), Villanova, PA, 1991, NCCLS.
2. National Committee for Clinical Laboratory Standards: *Development of definitive methods for the National Reference System for the Clinical Laboratory, approved guideline*, NCCLS publication NRSCL1-A (ISBN 1-56238-104-0), Villanova, PA, 1991, NCCLS.
3. National Committee for Clinical Laboratory Standards: *Development of Reference Methods for the National Reference System for the Clinical Laboratory, approved guideline*, NCCLS publication NRSCL2-A (ISBN 1-56238-105-9), Villanova, PA, 1991, NCCLS.
4. Breitenberg M: *Questions and answers on quality, the ISO 9000 standard series, quality systems registration, and related issues*, U.S. Department of Commerce, National Institute of Standards and Technology Publication NISTIR 4721, Gaithersburg, MD, 1991, USDC.
5. Dorsey DB: Evolving concepts of quality in laboratory practice: a historical overview of quality assurance in clinical laboratories, *Arch Pathol Lab Med* 113:1329, 1989.
6. Harris EK: Statistical principles underlying analytic goal-setting in clinical chemistry, *Am J Clin Pathol* 72:374, 1979.
7. Koch DD et al: Selection of medically useful quality-control procedures for individual tests done in a multitest analytical system, *Clin Chem* 36:230, 1990.
8. Ehrmeyer SS et al: 1990 Medicare/CLIA final rules for proficiency testing: minimum intralaboratory performance characteristics (CV and bias) needed to pass, *Clin Chem* 36:1736, 1990.
9. Barnett RN: Analytic goals in clinical chemistry: the pathologist's viewpoint. In *Analytical goals in clinical chemistry*, Northfield, IL, 1977, College of American Pathologists.
10. Ehrmeyer SS, Laessig RH: The relationship of intralaboratory bias and imprecision on laboratories' ability to meet medical usefulness limits, *Am J Clin Pathol* 89:14, 1988.
11. Tonks DB: A study of the accuracy and precision of clinical chemistry determination in 170 Canadian laboratories, *Clin Chem* 9:217, 1963.
12. Barnett RN: *Clinical laboratory statistics*, ed 2, Boston, 1979, Little, Brown & Co.
13. Douville P, Cembrowski GS: An approach to the use of clinical limits for quality control, *Lab Med* 406, June 1989.
14. Gilbert RK: Progress and analytic goals in clinical chemistry, *Am J Clin Pathol* 63:960, 1975.
15. Ross JW et al: Goals for allowable analytical error better based on medical usefulness criteria, *Am J Clin Pathol* 85:391, 1986.
16. Skendzel LP, Barnett RN, Platt R: Medically useful criteria for analytic performance of laboratory tests, *Am J Clin Pathol* 83:200, 1985.
17. Turcotte G et al: Analytic clinical chemistry precision and medical needs: the Canadian interlab program (CID), *Am J Clin Pathol* 74:336, 1980.

18. National Cholesterol Education Program: *Recommendations for improving cholesterol measurements,* NIH Publication No. 90-2964, Bethesda, MD, 1990, U.S. Department of Health and Human Services, National Institutes of Health.
19. Oxley DK: Cholesterol measurements: quality assurance and medical usefulness interrelationships, *Arch Pathol Lab Med* 112:387, 1988.
20. Cotlove E, Harris EK, Williams GZ: Biological and analytic components of variation in long-term studies of serum constituents in normal subjects: III. Physiological and medical implications, *Clin Chem* 16:1028, 1970.
21. Elion-Gerritzen WE: Analytic precision in clinical chemistry and medical decisions, *Am J Clin Pathol* 73:183, 1980.
22. Linnet K: Choosing quality-control systems to detect maximum clinically allowable analytical errors, *Clin Chem* 35:284, 1989.
23. Kaplan LA: Determination and application of desirable analytical performance goals: the ISO/TC 2121 approach, *Scand J Clin Lab Invest* 59:479, 1999.
24. Fraser CG: The application of theoretical goals based on biological variation data in proficiency testing, *Arch Pathol Lab Med* 112:404, 1988.
25. Ricós C et al: Current databases on biological variation: pros, cons, progress, *Scand J Clin Lab Invest* 59:491, 1999.
26. Hardin E et al: The use of "clear" enzyme control materials, *Am J Med Technol* 45:183, 1979.
27. Bowers GN Jr: Clinical chemistry analyte reference systems based on true value, *Clin Chem* 37:1665, 1991.
28. CastaZeda-MJndez K, Chemometrics: measurement reliability, *Clin Chem* 34:2494, 1988.
29. Lasky FD: Proficiency testing linked to the National Reference System for the Clinical Laboratory: a proposal for achieving accuracy, *Clin Chem* 38:1260, 1992.
30. Carey RN: Implementation of multi-rule quality control procedures, *Lab Med,* 393, June 1989.
31. Groth T, Falk H, Westgard JO: An interactive computer simulation program for the design of statistical control procedures in clinical chemistry, *Comput Programs Biomed* 13:73, 1981.
32. Parvin CA: Comparing the power of quality-control rules to detect persistent systematic error, *Clin Chem* 38:358, 1992.
33. Parvin CA: Comparing the power of quality-control rules to detect persistent increases in random error, *Clin Chem* 38:364, 1992.
34. Westgard JO et al: Performance characteristics of rules for internal quality control: probabilities for false rejection and error detection, *Clin Chem* 23:1857, 1977.
35. Westgard JO, Groth T: Power functions for statistical control rules, *Clin Chem* 25:863, 1979.
36. Westgard JO, Oryall JJ, Koch DD: Predicting effects of quality-control practices on the cost-effective operation of a stable multitest analytical system, *Clin Chem* 36:1760, 1990.
37. Westgard J, Qia E, Barry T: Basic QC practices—training in statistical quality control for healthcare laboratories, Westgard Quality Corp., 1998; www.westgard.com.
38. Westgard JO, Barry PL, Hunt MR, Groth T: A multi-rule Shewhart chart for quality control in clinical chemistry, *Clin Chem* 27:493, 1981.
39. Levey S, Jennings ER: The use of control charts in the clinical laboratory, *Am J Clin Pathol* 20:1059, 1950.
40. Shewhart WA: *Economic control of quality of the manufactured product,* New York, 1931, Van Nostrand Co.
41. Ladenson JH: Patients as their own controls: use of the computer to identify "laboratory error," *Clin Chem* 21:1648, 1975.
42. Gilbert RK: Accuracy of clinical laboratories studied by comparison with definitive methods, *Am J Clin Pathol* 70:450, 1978.
43. Velapoldi RA et al: *A reference method for the determination of potassium in serum,* NBS Spec. Pub. No. 260-63, Washington, D.C., 1979, National Measurement Laboratory, National Bureau of Standards.
44. Hartmann AE et al: Accuracy of participant results utilized as target values in the CAP Chemistry Survey Program, *Arch Pathol Lab Med* 109:894, 1985.
45. Uldall A: Quality assurance within clinical chemistry—a brief review emphasizing "good laboratory practice," *Scand J Clin Lab Invest* 47(suppl 187):507, 1987.
46. Ehrmeyer SS: U.S. legislation for decentralized testing, *Blood Gas News* 8:20, 1999. 42 CFR Part 493, *CLIA Laboratory Requirements,* Federal Register, October 1, 1997.
47. Blick KE: Cost effective workstation consolidation using the Chiron ACS:180 and valuanalysis *J Clin Ligand Assay* 43:908, 1997.

Bibliography

CLAS 19th National Meeting, Complying with CLIA '88 (Spring 1993), Clinical Ligand Assay Society, Wayne, MI 48184.
CLIA '88 final rules (1992) College of American Pathologists, Northfield, IL 60093,
Evaluation of matrix effects, approved guideline (March 2001), EP14-A, NCCLS, 940 West Valley Road, Suite 1400, Wayne, PA 19087-1898. (Website: www.nccls.org; 610-688-0100).
Method comparisons and bias estimation using patient samples, approved guideline (1995), EP9-A, NCCLS, 940 West Valley Road, Suite 1400, Wayne, PA 19087-1898.

Preliminary evaluation of quantitative clinical laboratory methods; approved guideline (1998), EP10-A, NCCLS, 940 West Valley Road, Suite 1400, Wayne, PA 19087-1898.
Quality management for unit-use testing; proposed guideline (1999), EP18-P, NCCLS, 940 West Valley Road, Suite 1400, Wayne, PA 19087-1898.
Statistical quality control for quantitative measurements: principles and definitions, approved guideline—second edition (1999), C24-A2, NCCLS, 940 West Valley Road, Suite 1400, Wayne, PA 19087-1898.
User demonstration of performance for precision and accuracy, approved guideline (2001), EP15-A, NCCLS, 940 West Valley Road, Suite 1400, Wayne, PA 19087-1898.

Internet Sites

www.nccls.org—National Committee for Clinical Laboratory Standards
http://www.vh.org/Providers/CME/CLIA/CLIAHP.html—NIST
www.iso.ch/—International Organization for Standardization
www.nccls.org/nrscl.htm—National Reference System for the Clinical Laboratory (NRSCL)
www.cap.org—College of American Pathologists (CAP)

www.jcaho.org—Joint Commission on Accreditation of Healthcare Organizations (JCAHO)
www.hcfa.gov/—Centers for Medicare and Medicaid Services (formerly HCFA)
http://www.multiqc.com/—Multivariate QC in clinical laboratories

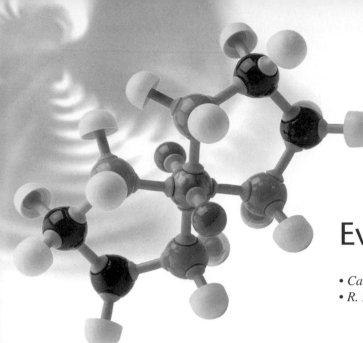

CHAPTER 22

Evaluation of Methods

- *Carl C. Garber*
- *R. Neill Carey*

Chapter Outline

Objectives

- List three purposes of a method evaluation.
- List aspects to consider when selecting a method to evaluate for use in a clinical chemistry laboratory.

- Differentiate among random, constant, proportional, and total error.

Key Terms

accuracy The agreement between the mean estimate of a quantity and its true value.[1]

allowable error (E_A) The amount of error that can be tolerated without invalidating the medical usefulness of the analytical result or the maximum

amount of error defined for successful performance in proficiency testing.[2]

assigned value The value assigned either arbitrarily (as by convention) or from preliminary evidence (as in the absence of a recognized reference method).[1]

bias   A systematic component of analytical error, estimated from a comparison-of-methods experiment.[3] Also known as the difference between two quantities. A measure of inaccuracy.

coefficient of variation (CV)   The standard deviation expressed as a percentage of the mean.

comparative method   The analytical method to which the test method is compared in the comparison-of-methods experiment. This term makes no inference about the quality of the comparative method.[4]

comparison-of-methods experiment   An evaluation experiment in which a series of patient samples are analyzed by both the test method and comparative method. The results are assessed to determine whether differences exist between the two methods.[3,4]

confidence interval   The numerical interval that contains the population parameter with a specified probability.

constant systematic error (CE)   An error that is always in the same direction and of the same magnitude, even as the concentration of analytes changes.[4]

demonstration   A minimum evaluation needed for a laboratory to show that it is able to obtain expected results by following the manufacturer's instructions. This is appropriate for test systems whose performance characteristics have been well studied and documented.[5]

error   The difference between a single estimate of a quantity and its true value. If a good estimate of the true value is not available, the difference may have to be expressed as the deviation from an assigned value.[1]

evaluation   Determination of the analytical performance characteristics of a new method.

ideal value   The value of a parameter under conditions of zero error.

imprecision   The standard deviation or coefficient of variation of the results in a set of replicate measurements. The mean value and number of replicates must be stated as well as the particular type of imprecision, such as between-laboratory, within-day, or between-day imprecision.[1]

inaccuracy   The systematic error estimated by the difference between the mean of a set of data and the true value known or estimated from other approaches.

interference   The effect of any component of the sample on the accuracy of measurement of the desired analyte.[1]

interference experiment   An evaluation experiment that is used to estimate the systematic error in a method, resulting from interference or lack of specificity.[4,6]

limit of absence   The lowest concentration of analyte that a method can differentiate from zero.

limit of detection (LOD)   The minimum concentration of analyte whose presence can be *qualitatively* detected under defined conditions.

limit of quantification (LOQ) or **functional sensitivity**   The minimum concentration of analyte whose presence can be *quantitatively* measured reliably under defined conditions. For example, a functional sensitivity has been defined as the lowest concentration with an imprecision of 20%.

linear regression   An approach that is used to choose a single line through a data set that "best" describes the relation between two subsets or two methods. This approach is used assuming there are no errors in the data by the X (comparative) method. (Also see Chapter 19.)

medical decision level (X_c)   A concentration of analyte at which some medical action is indicated for proper patient care. There may be several medical decision levels for a given analyte. (Also see Chapter 20.)

parameter   A number that describes a feature of a population. This is in contrast to a statistic, which is an estimate of a parameter derived from a sample of the population.

precision   The agreement among replicate measurements.[1]

proficiency testing   A program in which specimens are periodically sent to laboratories for analysis for the purpose of assessing overall analytical performance. Participation in proficiency testing is required under CLIA '88.[2] (Also see Chapter 21.)

proportional systematic error (PE)   An error that is always in one direction and the magnitude of which is a percentage of the concentration of the analyte being measured.[4]

random analytical error (RE)   An error, either positive or negative, the direction and exact magnitude of which cannot be predicted; imprecision.[4]

recovery experiment   An evaluation experiment that estimates proportional systematic error.[4] The determination of recovery is based on the measurement of added analyte. Percent recovery is the ratio of the measured amount to the added amount. Deviation of percent recovery from 100% is one example of proportional systematic error.

replication experiment   An evaluation experiment that estimates random analytical error.[4,7] Measurements are made on aliquots of a stable sample over specified periods, as within a run, within a day, or over a period of days.

reportable range   The concentration range of a method over which the analytical performance (i.e., imprecision and inaccuracy) has been determined and judged to meet medical application requirements.

sample The appropriately representative part of a specimen used in the analysis. This sample should be called a *test sample* when it is necessary to avoid confusion with the statistical term *random sample from a population*.[1]

standard deviation (SD) Square root of the variance. A measure of imprecision (see Chapter 19).

standard deviation of differences The standard deviation of the differences (s_d) between the observed *y* values and corresponding *x* values for a group of samples where each sample is measured by the *x* method and the *y* method. This is a measure of the dispersion of differences around the average difference.

standard error of the estimate The standard deviation of the differences ($s_{y,x}$) between the observed *y* values and the *y* values predicted by the regression line for a given *x*. This statistic measures the dispersion or spread of the data around the regression line.

systematic analytical error (SE) An error that is always in one direction; inaccuracy.[4]

test method In this chapter, the method that is chosen for experimental testing or study by means of method evaluation.[4]

total error (TE) A combination of the random and systematic analytical errors; an estimate of the magnitude of error that might occur in a single measurement.

true value A term considered to have self-evident meaning requiring no definition. In practice the true value is closely approximated by the definitive (method) value and somewhat less closely by the reference (method) value.[1] (Also see Chapter 21.)

validation Confirmation by examination and provision of objective evidence that the particular requirements for a specific intended use of an analytical procedure can be consistently fulfilled (21 CFR Section 820.3 Definitions).[8]

variance A statistic used to describe the distribution or spread of data in a population (see Chapter 19).

verification Confirmation by examination of objective evidence that specified requirements have been fulfilled (21 CFR Section 820.3 Definitions).[8]

Over the past several decades the quantitative analytical methods used in clinical laboratories have become more reliable and more standardized. Commercial manufacturers supply most analytical procedures. The emphasis of the hospital clinical chemist has shifted away from methods development to the selection and evaluation of those commercially available methods that suit a particular laboratory situation best. Since implementation of the Clinical Laboratory Improvement Amendments of 1988[2] (CLIA '88), this selection and evaluation process has taken on more significance because these regulations require, among other things, successful performance in **proficiency testing** for any laboratory to continue to perform tests in that specialty, subspecialty, or test procedure.

The process of method evaluation has been evolving.[9] It is critical to recognize that a method's performance can be objectively judged as acceptable only if its **errors** are small enough to be acceptable for medical use and to pass proficiency testing. The protocols developed by Westgard et al[4] and the National Committee for Clinical Laboratory Standards (NCCLS)[3,5-7,10,11] measure error in terms of analyte concentration units, but present different criteria for assessment of error. Westgard and associates take a quality management approach and include an error budget for the operation of the quality control (QC) procedure when they compare derived estimates of error to medically allowable error. NCCLS protocols provide procedures for comparing observed errors either to manufacturers' claims or to an allowable error specified in terms of a statistical **parameter** (such as allowable **standard deviation** or allowable **bias**).

This chapter describes both the Westgard and NCCLS approaches.

PURPOSE OF METHOD EVALUATION
Laboratory Requirements

New analytical methods are usually developed to improve **accuracy** or **precision** over existing methods, to allow automation, to reduce reagent or labor cost, or to measure a new analyte. In any case the method's analytical performance in a clinical laboratory setting must be verified experimentally, even if the new method is believed to be an improvement over all previous methods. Beyond the scientific and medical reasons for performing an evaluation, there are regulatory (CLIA '88) and accreditation requirements to evaluate new methods.

The process of evaluating a method is different from the process of routine QC of a method after it has been introduced into daily use. Routine (daily) QC (see Chapter 21) is a process established to detect increases in the analytical errors of a method to avoid the release of incorrect patient data. Routine QC detects errors only when they exceed the error that was present in the method when the control ranges were established. The use of routine QC does not enable the investigator to determine the magnitude of the inherent errors of the method or to decide whether they are acceptable. Method-evaluation experiments are required to assess the inherent analytical errors of the method and relate them to medical or regulatory requirements, and to select effective QC procedures.

The scope of a method evaluation depends on who is doing the evaluation, and what is already known about the

SCOPES OF METHOD EVALUATION STUDIES

Evaluation is the determination of the analytical performance characteristics of a new method.

Validation is confirmation by examination and provision of objective evidence that the particular requirements for a specific intended use can be consistently fulfilled (21 CFR Section 820.3 Definitions).[8]

Verification is confirmation by examination of objective evidence that specified requirements have been fulfilled (21 CFR Section 820.3 Definitions).[8]

Demonstration is a minimum evaluation for a laboratory to use to show that it is able to obtain expected results by following the manufacturer's instructions. This is appropriate for test systems whose performance characteristics have been well studied and documented.

analytical performance of the method. In order of decreasing amounts of effort, the scope of different evaluations can be described by the terms in the box above. These are also described in several NCCLS documents, such as NCCLS Guideline EP15-A: User Demonstration of Precision and Accuracy.[5]

Manufacturer Requirements

When a manufacturer develops a new method and prepares to market it, the manufacturer is required by the Food and Drug Administration (FDA) to make claims about the analytical performance of the method, specifically about its precision and accuracy.[8,12] In addition, the final rule of CLIA '88 requires that the FDA assess whether the manufacturer's claims meet the CLIA '88 requirements for general quality control.[13] All claims must be supported by experimental method-evaluation data. It is essential that these claims be realistic and conservative. The level of performance of the method in most laboratories must be consistent with that claimed by the manufacturer. Extensive experimental data are required for the manufacturer to develop defensible claims. The protocols proposed by NCCLS have been modified for manufacturers to enable them to produce defensible performance claims that can be verified by the laboratory.

Laboratory personnel in hospital and commercial laboratories perform most method evaluations. These evaluations are performed to determine whether the performance of a method meets, primarily, the requirements for the medical applications intended by the user and, secondly, the quality goals specified by CLIA '88 for successful performance in proficiency testing. The method may be a commercial method, a "home-grown" method, a method using Analyte Specific Reagents (ASR),[14] or a method the user has seen in the literature and is setting up in his or her own laboratory. The user needs to perform the evaluation as efficiently as possible and to determine with a minimum of experimental work whether the method's performance is acceptable as each experiment is completed. If performance is not acceptable at any stage of the evaluation, the user can "repair" or reject the method without performing all the time-consuming studies required for acceptance.

Medical Requirements

The decision to accept or reject a candidate laboratory method should be based on the ability of the method to meet the requirements of the final user, the physician who is using the results of a laboratory test for patient care (see Chapter 21). The error of the test result is excessive if it causes a misdiagnosis. The greatest chance for misdiagnosis caused by an analytical error in a test result occurs at the concentration at which a medical diagnosis is made; this concentration is termed the **medical decision level (X_C)** concentration. For example, a fasting glucose concentration below 500 mg/L may be diagnostic of hypoglycemia.[15] For each decision-level concentration, a performance standard consisting of the decision-level concentration, X_C, and the **allowable error**, E_A, may be formulated. Allowable error is stated in concentration units so that errors of the **test method** may be judged by comparison with clinically allowable error. The method-evaluation data are interpreted by using the data to estimate the error of the method at the medical decision level of concentration and then comparing this estimate with the allowable error. If the method's error exceeds allowable error, performance is not acceptable. If the error is less than the allowable error, performance is acceptable.

The amount of error present in the single measurement of an analyte is different each time the analyte is measured because a portion of the error is purely random. Thus the magnitude of error for a measurement on a given patient specimen cannot be known exactly, and the absolute maximum error a method could ever make on the analysis of a single patient specimen cannot be predicted. However, an estimate of the upper limit of the error can be calculated such that there is only a 5% or 1% chance that the actual error would exceed the upper limit and possibly cause a misdiagnosis.

Exact performance standards for allowable error based on medical criteria have not been defined for most analytes. Performance standards have been proposed for those analytes that are measured most often, but generally, professional judgment and input from clinicians must be used to establish the performance standard for a particular analyte. Barnett[16,17] presented a summary of medically allowable standard deviations. Tonks[18] proposed that allowable error be either one fourth of the reference range or 10%, whichever is less. For enzymes, the limit is expanded to 20%.[19] Cotlove, Harris, and Williams[20] recommended a "tolerable analytical variation" based on one half the combined individual and group biological variation. The 1976 Aspen Conference[21] sponsored by the College of American Pathologists (CAP) also recommended the use of intraindividual and interindividual biological variations for determining the goals for the precision of a method used for group testing. The analytical **coefficient of variation (CV)** is denoted as CV_A:

$$CV_A = \tfrac{1}{2}\sqrt{CV^2_{Intra} + CV^2_{Inter}} \qquad \textit{Eq. 22-1}$$

in which CV_{Intra} is the biological variation observed within an individual and CV_{Inter} is the biological variation observed between individuals. To enable the physician to monitor intraindividual changes, the method must be even more precise:

$$CV_A = \tfrac{1}{2}\sqrt{CV^2_{Intra}} \qquad \textit{Eq. 22-2}$$

Fraser and associates[22-25] and Ricos et al[26] have reviewed and summarized various approaches that have been used to establish quality goals, concluding that biological variation should be a key consideration for establishing allowable error for most analytes. For therapeutic drugs, quality goals were based on pharmacokinetic theory. Professional organizations have made recommendations; such as the National Academy of Clinical Biochemistry for cardiac markers,[27] and the National Glycohemoglobin Standardization Program for hemoglobin A_{1c}.[28]

Other factors, such as turnaround time, may affect the medically allowable error. Clinicians may sometimes accept increased error if turnaround time is small.

Performance Standards Based on Proficiency Testing

The government specifies allowable error for proficiency testing for many analytes, the most notable of which are contained in the CLIA '88 regulations.[2] The Occupational Safety and Health Administration (OSHA) has specified allowable errors for monitoring of heavy metals.[29] CAP has specified allowable errors for many nonregulated analytes[30] (see the participant summary of a recent CAP survey for current allowable errors). A laboratory must select, evaluate, and then monitor (by statistical QC, see Chapters 19 and 21) the test method so that when it is in routine use the laboratory will have confidence that the method will meet proficiency testing requirements. These requirements are given as (1) fixed limits, such as an absolute limit of the amount of variability or a limit expressed in terms of a fixed percentage of concentration or activity, or (2) as three–standard deviation limits based on the overall or peer-groups standard deviation, or (3) as plus or minus two dilutions for assays reported in units of titers. Ehrmeyer et al[31] showed that if the internal laboratory standard deviation (SD) for a procedure is less than one third of the fixed-limit criteria and the assay's bias is "small," the likelihood for passing proficiency testing is greater than 99%. Westgard and Burnett,[32] using error budget analysis, found that the assay's "bias + 4 × SD" should be less than the specified limit. In practice, this indicates that the internal SD should be less than 25% of the limit. Table 22-1 lists the CLIA '88 proficiency testing requirements. The fifth column shows the maximum allowable within-laboratory SD (using the 4 × SD criterion and zero bias). For comparison, in the recommendations based on biological variation,[22-26] maximum internal SD are listed. Note that for some analytes the SD derived from

---

TABLE 22-1 **COMPARISON OF ALLOWABLE ERROR AS SPECIFIED BY CLIA '88 TO THAT RECOMMENDED BY FRASER ET AL BASED ON BIOLOGICAL VARIABILITY**

Analyte	Acceptable Performance Criteria, CLIA '88	Decision Level (X_c*)	Allowable Error (CLIA '88[†])	Maximum SD (CLIA '88[‡])	Medically Based Maximum SD (Fraser[§])
Routine Chemistry					
Albumin	±10%	3.5 g/dL	0.35	0.09	0.05
Bilirubin	±0.4 mg/dL or ±20%	1.0 mg/dL	0.40	0.10	0.11
		20 mg/dL	4.0	1.0	2.2
Calcium	±1.0 mg/dL	7.0 mg/dL	1.0	0.25	0.08
		10.8 mg/dL	1.0	0.25	0.10
		13.0 mg/dL	1.0	0.25	0.12
Chloride	±5%	90 mmol/L	4.5	1.1	0.63
		110 mmol/L	5.5	1.4	0.77
Cholesterol	±10%	200 mg/dL	20	5.0	5.4
Creatinine	±0.3 mg/dL or ±15%	1.0 mg/dL	0.30	0.08	0.02
		3.0 mg/dL	0.45	0.11	0.07
Glucose	±6 mg/dL or ±10%	50 mg/dL	6.0	1.5	1.1
		126 mg/dL	12.6	3.2	2.8
		200 mg/dL	20	5.0	4.4
Hemoglobin A_{tc}		7.0%	0.35%[‖]	0.14%	
Iron	±20%	150 mg/dL	30	7.5	24
Magnesium	±25%	2.0 mg/dL	0.50	0.12	0.02

*Medical decision levels, most of which are based on Barnett.[16,17]
[†]Allowable error based on CLIA '88 performance requirements at the respective medical decision level.[2] SD limits are based on peer group data.
[‡]Maximum internal SD based on criteria that 4 SD is less than the allowable error[32] (see column 3 for units).
[§]Maximum internal SD based on biovariability criteria (Fraser et al[22-24]) (see column 3 for units).
[‖]No CLIA criterion. Maximum allowable SD calculated from National Diabetes Data Group recommendation.[27]

> **TABLE 22-1** COMPARISON OF ALLOWABLE ERROR AS SPECIFIED BY CLIA '88 TO THAT RECOMMENDED BY FRASER ET AL BASED ON BIOLOGICAL VARIABILITY—CONT'D

Analyte	Acceptable Performance Criteria, CLIA '88	Decision Level (X_c*)	Allowable Error (CLIA '88[†])	Maximum SD (CLIA '88[‡])	Medically Based Maximum SD (Fraser[§])
pH	±0.04	7.35	0.04	0.01	0.01
P_{CO_2}	±5 mm Hg or ±8%	35 mm Hg	5.0	1.2	0.84
		50 mm Hg	5.0	1.2	1.2
P_{O_2}	±3 SD	30 mm Hg	3 SD	0.75 SD	
		80 mm Hg	3 SD	0.75 SD	
Potassium	±0.5 mmol/L	3.0 mmol/L	0.50	0.12	0.07
		6.0 mmol/L	0.50	0.12	0.14
Protein, total	±10%	7.0 g/dL	0.70	0.18	0.10
Sodium	±4 mmol/L	130 mmol/L	4.0	1.0	0.38
		150 mmol/L	4.0	1.0	0.44
Triglycerides	±25%	160 mg/dL	40	10	18
Urea nitrogen	±2 mg/dL or ±9%	27.0 mg/dL	2.4	0.6	1.7
Uric acid	±17%	6.0 mg/dL	1.0	0.25	0.25
Enzymes					
Alkaline phosphatase	±30%	150 U/L	45	11	5.1
ALT	±20%	50 U/L	10	2.5	6.8
Amylase	±30%	100 U/L	30	7.5	3.7
AST	±20%	30 U/L	6.0	1.5	2.2
		70 U/L	14	3.5	5.0
CK	±30%	200 U/L	60	15	40
LD	±20%	300 U/L	60	15	12
Endocrinology					
Cortisol	±25%	5 µg/dL	1.25	0.3	
		30 µg/dL	7.5	1.8	
Free thyroxine	±3 SD	2.3 ng/dL	3 SD	0.75 SD	0.1
hCG	±3 SD positive/negative	25 IU/L	3 SD	0.75 SD	
T_3 uptake	±3 SD	25%	3 SD	0.75 SD	
Triiodothyronine	±3 SD	100 ng/dL	3 SD	0.75 SD	4.0
		200 ng/dL	3 SD	0.75 SD	8.0
TSH	±3 SD	0.1 mlU/L	3 SD	0.75 SD	0.025
		5.0 mlU/L	3 SD	0.75 SD	0.4
Thyroxine	±1.0 µg/dL or ±20%	3 µg/dL	1.0	0.25	0.1
		13 µg/dL	2.6	0.65	0.45
Toxicology					
Alcohol, blood	±25%	0.10 g/dL	0.025	0.006	
β-2-microglobulin, urine		300 µg/L	45.0	11.25[#]	
		750 µg/L	112.5	28.1[#]	
		1500 µg/L	225.0	56.2[#]	
Cadmium, blood		5 µg/L	1.0	0.25[#]	
		10 µg/L	1.5	0.375[#]	
		15 µg/L	2.2	0.505[#]	
Cadmium, urine		3 µg/L	0.45	0.11[#]	
		7 µg/L	1.05	0.26[#]	
		10 µg/L	1.5	0.375[#]	
Blood lead	±4 µg/dL or ±10%	10 µg/dL	4.0	1.0	
		40 µg/dL	4.0	1.0	
Carbamazepine	±25%	8 mg/L	2.0	0.5	0.8
		12 mg/L	3.0	0.8	1.2
Digoxin	±0.2 µg/L or ±20%	0.8 µg/L	0.2	0.05	0.04
		2.0 µg/L	0.4	0.10	0.10
Ethosuximide	±20%	40 mg/L	8.0	2.0	2.0
		100 mg/L	20.0	5.0	4.9

ALT, Alanine aminotransferase; *AST*, aspartate aminotransferase; *CK*, creatine kinase; *CLIA*, CLinical Laboratories Improvement Amendments; *hCG*, human chorionic gonadotropin; *IU*, international units; *LD*, lactate dehydrogenase; *SD*, standard deviation; T_3, triiodothyronine; *TSH*, thyroid-stimulating hormone; *U*, units; X_c, concentration of x analyte to indicate medical intervention.
[#]No CLIA criterion. Allowable error is from OSHA regulations on cadmium monitoring.[28] Actual medical decision levels for cadmium in urine is in terms of µg Cd/g creatinine. Similarly for β-2-microglobulin (µg/g creatinine). However, for the purposes of this table, we assumed a urinary creatinine elimination rate of 1 g/L.

Continued

TABLE 22-1 COMPARISON OF ALLOWABLE ERROR AS SPECIFIED BY CLIA '88 TO THAT RECOMMENDED BY FRASER ET AL BASED ON BIOLOGICAL VARIABILITY—CONT'D

Analyte	Acceptable Performance Criteria, CLIA '88	Decision Level (X_c*)	Allowable Error (CLIA '88[†])	Maximum SD (CLIA '88[‡])	Medically Based Maximum SD (Fraser[§])
Gentamicin	±25%	10 mg/L	2.5	0.6	
Lead, blood	±4 µg/dL or ±10%	10 µg/dL	4.0	1.0	
		40 µg/dL	4.0	1.0	
Lithium	±0.3 mmol/L or ±20%	0.5 mmol/L	0.3	0.08	0.06
		1.5 mmol/L	0.3	0.08	0.18
Phenobarbital	±20%	15 mg/L	3.0	0.75	1.3
		40 mg/L	8.0	2.0	3.6
Phenytoin	±25%	10 mg/L	2.5	0.6	0.7
		20 mg/L	5.0	1.2	1.3
Primidone	±25%	5 mg/L	1.2	0.3	0.56
		12 mg/L	3.0	0.75	1.36
Procainamide	±25%	4 mg/L	1.0	0.25	
		20 mg/L	5.0	1.25	
Quinidine	±25%	7 mg/L	1.8	0.45	
Theophylline	±25%	10 mg/L	2.5	0.6	0.7
		20 mg/L	5.0	1.2	1.4
Valproic acid	±25%	50 mg/L	12	3.0	3.3
		100 mg/L	25	6.2	6.7

proficiency testing and from biological variation are quite similar, whereas they are different for others. A laboratory method must be able to pass proficiency testing and provide medically useful test results.

More recently, Westgard[33] has related laboratory performance to the Six Sigma model as defined by Motorola in the 1980s and subsequently adopted by many manufacturing and service industries.[34] This model states that if the process SD is less than one sixth of the allowable **total error (TE)**, the process is said to be *six sigma capable* with a potential defect rate of 3.4 defects per million tests, when a defect is a result that has an error that exceeds the allowable TE.

SELECTION OF METHODS
Evaluation of Need

The quality of service achievable by a laboratory is determined by selection of personnel, equipment, and analytical methods. The many considerations involved in the process of method selection are shown in Fig. 22-1. Unless this process is well organized, method selection can be a traumatic and costly experience. The box on the right provides a logical sequence to follow in method selection.

Often the decision to set up a new method or instrument is based on a medical or economic requirement for the laboratory to provide a new test on site. Advances in laboratory practice may also dictate a change in the methodology of a presently offered test. For example, many laboratories have converted their immunoassays from radiolabeled to non-isotopic-labeled reagents to enable automation, reduce or eliminate the special procedures required for managing radioactive materials, and to take advantage of the longer shelf lives of newer reagents. The need for a new method or

STEPS IN THE SELECTION PROCESS

Determine need
Define requirements
    Application
    Methodological
    Performance
Review literature
Select candidate methods

device may also be dictated by the age and lack of operational reliability of the present method.

Application Characteristics

After the need for a new method or analyzer has been determined, all the practical features required of the method are defined. These are termed *application characteristics* (see box on p. 409). Emphasis may be placed on **sample** size for pediatric applications, on turnaround time and interrupt features for stat applications, and on the sample throughput rate for high-volume screening applications. It is essential that a candidate method meet these fundamental requirements before it is considered any further.

Cost per test is an important application characteristic, because cost can also be considered separately in light of the present emphasis on reducing medical costs. The factors that affect direct cost should be considered when comparing candidate methods. These include the depreciated capital cost (see example in Chapter 2), reagent (including water for many analyzers) and supplies cost, service and repair cost, computer interface cost, and labor cost. Much of this

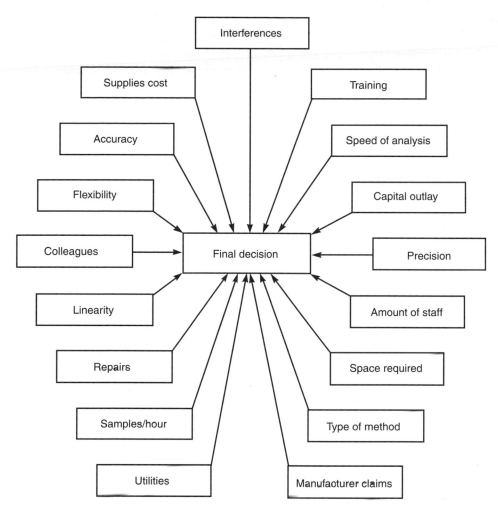

Fig. 22-1   Factors in method selection.

APPLICATION CHARACTERISTICS

Sample size
Turnaround time
Sample throughput rate
Specimen type
Automated calibration
On-line quality control review
Self-diagnostics
Laboratory space required
Reagent storage facilities required
Availability and skill of laboratory staff
Time available for training
Cost per test
Safety and environmental hazards

information is available from the manufacturer including initial equipment cost, estimated reagent and supplies consumption and cost, estimated productivity, and service cost (by contract or per visit). Other information, such as the expected workload and anticipated modifications in the productivity based on the internal QC procedures, is

available from within the laboratory. Users must adjust this information to their own laboratory situations. The example in the box on p. 410 illustrates how this information may be combined to arrive at a total direct cost per test. By far the largest cost component is labor at 88% of the total. If the laboratory wishes to add new tests in a way that minimizes added overall cost, the new tests that have the smallest labor component should be selected.

Method Characteristics

The next step in the selection process is the definition of ideal methodological characteristics that will enable the selected method to have a good chance for success in the user's laboratory. These characteristics include preferred methodology, which will potentially have the necessary chemical specificity (freedom from **interferences**) and chemical sensitivity (ability to detect small quantities or changes in the analyte's concentration). The ability to use primary aqueous standards for calibration (freedom from matrix effects) is also important. The reagents, temperature, reaction time, measurement time, and measurement approach (such as end-point, two-point, or multipoint kinetic methods) are all characteristics of a method and should be defined. A source

ESTIMATION OF DIRECT COSTS

Laboratory information
    8000 patient tests (samples) per year
    50% estimated test yield (sample, quality control, repeats, dilutions, troubleshooting)
    16,000 total number of assays
    4 minutes labor per test, estimated
    64,000 total minutes of labor, estimated
    5-year depreciation of capital
    $750 setup costs (change laboratory bench)
Manufacturer information
    $11,000: cost of equipment
    $1200: cost of reagents and supplies (for 16,000 assays)
    $1100: service contract (two visits)
    $500: replacement parts
Calculate equipment costs
    Capital and setup: $11,750 \div 5$ yr $= \$2350/yr \div 8000 =$
    $0.294/sample
    Service and repair: $1100 + $500 = \$1600/yr \div 8000 =$
    $0.20/sample
    Subtotal = $0.494/sample
Calculate labor costs (assume $35.00/hour, including benefits)
[(64,000 minutes of labor $\div$ 60 minutes/hour) $\times$ $35.00/hour] $\div$
8000 samples = $4.667/sample
Calculate reagent costs
    $1200 \div 8000$ samples = $0.15/sample
Total direct costs = $5.311/sample

---

of recommended principles for clinical chemistry methods has been developed by the National Reference System for the Clinical Laboratory (NRSCL).[35]

Analytical Performance Characteristics

The method should also be defined in terms of its analytical performance capabilities. Overall goals for analytical performance have been discussed in terms of allowable error based on the medical application of the test and on proficiency testing requirements. Other aspects of performance that must be defined are working range of the method (reportable range, which may or may not be the same as the linear range), stability of the reagents and calibration materials, ability of the analyzer to detect reagent depletion in the case of enzyme substrates, expected reference range, amount of error caused by interfering substances, precision (within-run, between-run, between-day, and total), and accuracy of the method (determined by comparison of results to those obtained by a reference or standard method). Although the manufacturer is required to provide information about precision and accuracy, the selected method must be evaluated experimentally to determine if the method's actual performance in the user's laboratory is good enough to meet the medical application needs in the user's institution. The manufacturer's claimed performance should be considered as a starting point for determining the actual performance in the user's laboratory setting.

Next, the technical and professional literature and proficiency testing data should be reviewed to determine what methods are available and to obtain some information about their application and methodological and performance characteristics. It is also very useful to confer with colleagues about their experience and recommendations.

The final step in the selection process involves putting all the information together to arrive at a final choice. The use of a rating scheme enables a more objective overall ranking of the candidate methods.[36,37] The rating scheme can be customized by use of appropriate weighting factors for the characteristics that are more important. The final choice may include several candidate methods that meet the desired criteria. These methods can then be subjected to the evaluation process described later to choose the method with the best analytical performance characteristics.

LABORATORY EVALUATION OF A METHOD

Usually a method-evaluation study is not performed to test all methods to determine the method with the smallest error but to determine whether the selected method has acceptably small analytical errors. The process of method evaluation involves estimation of the magnitude of analytical error for a single patient specimen. The laboratory experiments performed to obtain data for estimating the errors are chosen because they give quantitative estimates of random and systematic errors with a minimum of experimental work. The error estimates obtained may be invalid, however, if certain underlying assumptions are not true. These assumptions include operator familiarity with the method's procedure; stability of calibrators, controls, and reagents; and linearity of response throughout the working range.

Familiarization

It is essential that the operators of the method become thoroughly familiar with the details of the method and instrument operation before the collection of any data that will be used to characterize the method's performance. This familiarization period has been addressed by NCCLS[3,6,7,10] and may include training by the manufacturer. It should be of sufficient duration that, at its completion, the operators can perform all aspects of the method or instrument operation comfortably. Obviously the length of time for device familiarization varies with the complexity of the method or analyzer.

Stability

Verification of the stability of reagents, calibrators, and control materials, especially those prepared in house, can be a lengthy procedure. The matter is simplified considerably for commercially prepared materials. The manufacturer's expiration date can be used during the method evaluation because serious stability problems will be detectable through unacceptable analytical performance of the method. For in-house preparations it is necessary to document these characteristics. Preliminary studies should be performed with crossover analyses comparing the results of patient samples analyzed using both fresh calibrators and old calibrators and fresh reagents to test the stability of calibrators. This should be done several times, and the differences for each specific age of calibrator should be averaged to reduce the effects of different preparations. Similarly, the stability of reagents can be tested by periodically (daily, weekly, or monthly, depending on the anticipated decay rate) preparing new reagents and testing them against the older reagents by analyzing patient samples under both configurations of reagents. The older reagents should be stored under specified conditions for the subsequent measurements. The observed differences between the old and new reagents can be tested by use of a *t*-test (see pp. 350 and 415).

Linearity

The International Federation of Clinical Chemistry has defined the analytical range in a qualitative sense, stating that it is "the range of concentration or other quantity in the specimen over which the method is applicable without modification."[1] CLIA '88 regulations do not explicitly require that a "linearity" experiment be performed but instead discuss "verification" of the **reportable range**,[2] which is the range defined by a minimum (or zero) value and a maximum-value calibration material. When the limits of linearity are studied experimentally, the range of concentrations included should at least encompass the limits claimed by the manufacturer. The absolute minimum number of different concentrations that must be measured for linearity verification is three. Replicate measurements, at least in duplicate, should be made on each concentration sample.

Random and Systematic Error

In general, errors that affect the performance of analytical procedures are classified as either random or systematic. Factors contributing to **random analytical error (RE)** are those that affect the reproducibility of the measurement. These include (1) instability of the instrument, (2) variations in the temperature, (3) variations in the reagents and calibrators (and calibration-curve stability), (4) variability in handling techniques such as pipetting, mixing, and timing, and (5) variability in operators. These factors superimpose their effects on each other at different times. Some cause rapid fluctuations, and others occur over a longer time. Thus RE has different components of variation that are related to the actual laboratory setting. The *within-run* component of variation (σ_{wr}) is caused by specific steps in the procedure, such as sampling and pipetting precision, and short-term variations in the temperature and stability of the instrument. Within-day, *between-run* variation (σ_{br}) is caused by instability of the calibration curve or by differences in recalibration that occur throughout the day, longer term variations in the instrument, small changes in the condition of the calibrator and reagents, changes in the condition of the laboratory during the day, and fatigue of the laboratory staff. The *between-day* component of variation (σ_{bd}) is caused by variations in the instrument that occur over days, changes in calibrators and reagents (especially if new vials are opened each day), and changes in staff from day to day. Although not

a true random component of variation, any drift in the stability of the calibration curve over time greatly affects the between-day component of variation as well. These components can be combined in such a way as to produce an estimate of the total **variance** of a method (σ_t^2).

$$\sigma_t^2 = \sigma_{wr}^2 + \sigma_{br}^2 + \sigma_{bd}^2 \qquad \textit{Eq. 22-3}$$

Terms used to indicate RE include *precision*, **imprecision**, *reproducibility*, and *repeatability*. In each case they refer to the random dispersion of results or measurements around some point of central tendency.

Systematic analytical error (SE) describes error that is consistently low or high. If the error is consistently low or high by the same amount, regardless of the concentration, it is called **constant systematic error (CE)** (Fig. 22-2). If the error is consistently low or high by an amount proportional to the concentration of the analyte, it is called **proportional systematic error (PE)**.

Factors that contribute to CE are independent of the analyte concentration, and the magnitude of this error is constant throughout the concentration range of the analyte. CE is caused by an interfering substance in all samples or in reagents that gives rise to a false signal. The error can be positive or negative. A reaction between an interfering substance and the reagents, caused by a lack of specificity, is an example of a CE. Another cause of systematic error is an interfering substance that interferes in the reaction between the analyte and the reagents. This type of error is seen in enzymatic methods using oxidase-peroxidase–coupled reactions in which the hydrogen peroxide intermediate is destroyed by endogenous reducing agents, such as ascorbic acid. An

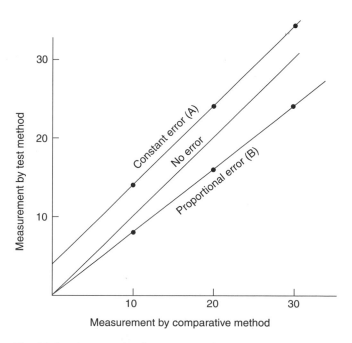

Fig. 22-2 Constant and proportional errors. *(From Westgard JO et al: Concepts and practices in the evaluation of laboratory methods. I. Background and approach,* Am J Med Technol *44:290, 1978.)*

interfering substance may also inhibit or destroy the reagent, causing it to remain in suboptimal amounts for the reaction with the analyte. A nonchemical source of CE is the error caused by improper blanking of the sample or the reagents.

PE is most often caused by incorrect assignment of the amount of substance in the calibrator. If the calibrator has more analyte than is labeled, all the unknown determinations will be low; less analyte than is labeled will result in a positive error. The error will be proportional to the original calibration error. PE may also be caused by a side reaction of the analyte. The percentage of analyte that undergoes a side reaction will be the percentage of error in the method.

EXPERIMENTS TO ESTIMATE MAGNITUDE OF SPECIFIC ERRORS

In designing experiments that will be used to determine the analytical errors of a method, it is imperative that the experiments be carefully conceived to avoid ambiguous conclusions. The aim of this section is to describe specific experiments that will enable estimation of the magnitude of a specific error. The size of the error can then be compared to the allowable error to determine the acceptability of the method. This approach is used for all the types of errors described previously. Each type of error is considered individually before combinations of errors are considered. Fig. 22-3 presents an organization of experiments to be performed for specific error determinations, arranged in such a way that the easy experiments can be done first. The more extensive (and expensive) final studies are performed only if the errors estimated by these preliminary experiments are acceptable.

Random Error Estimated from Replication Studies

The within-run **replication experiment** is the simplest type of study and should be one of the first performed to assess the performance of a new method. Because it allows assessment of precision over a very short time, the results cannot be extrapolated to indicate long-term performance. The short-term performance must be judged acceptable before the long-term performance of the method is studied.

The replication study should be performed with samples whose matrix is as similar as possible to that of the intended patient samples. The concentrations to be studied should be at or near the medical-decision concentrations for the analyte. This is where the laboratory data will be interpreted most critically; thus the method's performance at these concentrations must be ensured.

An estimate of RE is developed by consideration of repeated analyses of the same specimen. Sixty-eight percent of the results are within ±1.0 SD of the test mean, and 95% of the results are within 1.96 SD of the mean (see p. 346). Using the error budget approach recommended by Westgard and Burnett,[32] we define the RE as four times the SD. If the estimate of RE is less than the allowable error, RE is acceptable. An example of the calculation of RE is shown on p. 422.

Constant Error Estimated from Interference Studies

The **interference experiment** measures the CE caused by the presence of a substance suspected of interfering with the test method. To perform the study, a sample that is spiked with the interferent is used. The volume of this addition should be small, less than 10% of the sample volume, so that the disruption of the matrix is minimal. To compensate for the dilution of the spiked sample, a baseline sample should be prepared by addition of an equal amount of the solvent that was used for the interferent to another aliquot of the sample. The two samples should then be analyzed, at least in duplicate. The difference between the results in the two samples is attributable to an interference caused by the added substance.

A scheme for studying the effects of hemolysis involves taking two blood samples. One is centrifuged and analyzed directly (baseline sample), and the red blood cells in the other blood tube are physically traumatized to rupture the cell membranes to yield an elevated amount of serum hemoglobin. After centrifugation, this hemolyzed sample is analyzed. The difference between the two samples is attributable to the effects of hemolysis. Mild, moderate, or severe hemolysis may be simulated, depending on the volume of red blood cells traumatized. This approach is more consistent with the actual problems encountered in the laboratory than the approach in which pure hemoglobin is added to a sample. However, this procedure is not valid if red blood cells contain the analyte.

Type of Analytic Error	Evaluation Experiments	
	Preliminary	Final
Random error	Replication within-run Pure materials Real samples	Replication run-to-run Real samples
Constant error	Interference	Comparison with comparative method
Proportional error	Recovery	
Other systematic errors	Linearity Limit of detection	

Fig. 22-3 Specific evaluation experiments for estimating specific types of analytical error. *(From Westgard JO et al: Concepts and practices in the evaluation of laboratory methods. I. Background and approach,* Am J Med Technol 44:290, 1978.)

The effects of lipemia may be studied by dividing a lipemic sample into two portions and analyzing one directly while centrifuging the other with an ultrahigh-speed centrifuge to remove the lipoproteins before analysis. The difference in results is attributable to the effects of lipemia. Alternatively, turbid specimens may be prepared for each decision-level concentration by adding small amounts of lipid-containing materials (e.g., IntraLipid [KabiVitrum, Inc.] or Lyposin [Abbott Laboratories]) to nonlipemic specimens of appropriate analyte concentrations to obtain slightly, moderately, and grossly lipemic samples. Baseline concentrations are prepared by addition of equal volumes of water to the original specimens.

Pools with increased amounts of unconjugated bilirubin are produced from a stock solution of bilirubin prepared by dissolving pure bilirubin in dimethylsulfoxide to 2500 mg/L. Clear, nonicteric patient sera are spiked to the desired bilirubin concentration. Baseline specimens are prepared as already described. This technique does not test the effect of the more water-soluble conjugated bilirubin on the analysis.

The choice of substances to be tested is almost infinite. For all spectrophotometric methods, the effects of hemolysis, icterus, and lipemia should be determined. Other substances that have been reported to affect methods similar to the one under review should be tested (see NCCLS guideline EP7-P).[6] Pipetting should be (1) precise so that the baseline and spiked samples reflect the same extent of dilution and (2) accurate so that a known amount of interfering substance is added. Again, it is important that the concentration of the analyte in the sample be near the medical-decision levels. A substance that is a possible interferent should be added so that its final concentration is at the maximum physiologically expected concentration. If no errors are caused at this high concentration, it can be assumed that lower concentrations will not adversely affect the performance of the method. If an error is too large at the maximum concentration of interfering substance, it is appropriate to test the interference at lower concentrations. A slightly icteric sample may be acceptable, but a grossly icteric one may not. It is recommended that these interference studies be conducted on the **comparative method** (see later discussion) at the same time, as a check on the experimental technique.

An example of the calculation of CE from data obtained from an interference experiment is shown on p. 422. The overall average difference (bias) is called a *constant error* because it is independent of the analyte concentration. This CE is compared directly to the E_A for the appropriate decision level. If the CE is less than E_A, the CE caused by the interference is judged acceptable. This decision is based on clinical limits instead of a statistical test of significance (see pp. 406 and 407). The SD of the interference values is a measure of the uncertainty of the estimated CE.

Proportional Error Estimated from a Recovery Experiment

Another preliminary study is the **recovery experiment.** This procedure involves the addition of a known amount of analyte to an aliquot of sample. As in the interference experi-

ment, the sample is divided into two aliquots. One aliquot is spiked with a stock solution that contains the analyte. An equal volume of diluent is added to the second; this is the baseline sample. The two samples are then analyzed. The baseline sample provides the original amount of analyte. The difference between the results of the analyses of the spiked sample and the baseline sample indicates the amount of added analyte "recovered." The amount of analyte added to the sample is calculated from the concentration of the stock solution of the analyte and the volume added. The volume of analyte added to the sample should be less than 10% to avoid major disruption of the sample matrix. Pipetting accuracy is critical because the amount of added analyte is calculated from the volume. The concentration of the sample and the amount added should be such that they test the performance of the method near the medical-decision levels of the analyte. In some instances a very small amount of analyte is added to the sample, and the amount recovered is lost in the randomness of the method. Thus it is advisable to make two to four measurements on each sample to reduce the effects of the imprecision of the method. Analysis of these samples with the comparison method is recommended as a check on the experimental technique.

The calculation of recovery is illustrated with an example on p. 423. Recovery is defined as the ratio of the amount of analyte recovered to the amount added and is given as a percentage. The difference between the calculated percentage of recovery and 100% recovery is the percentage of PE. The SD of the percentage of recovery is a measure of the uncertainty of the percentage of PE. The percentage of PE cannot be directly compared to E_A to decide acceptability because the percentage of PE is not in concentration units. PE can be converted to concentration units at the medical-decision level, as shown on pp. 406 and 407. If the PE is less than the E_A, the PE is acceptable. Again, the decision is based on medical requirements rather than statistical tests of significance.

Error Caused by Nonlinearity

An initial linearity study could use aqueous standards to identify the capabilities of the method in an ideal specimen matrix. This should be followed by the analysis of the analyte in a dilution series of samples containing the biological matrix,[10] such as serum or urine, that will be used for patient tests. The aqueous and matrix samples will provide important information about the influence of the biological matrix on the method.

It may be difficult to prepare specimens in a biological matrix with a range of analyte concentrations from zero to the limit of linearity. For analytes not normally present in the matrix, such as drugs, the analyte is simply added to an analyte-free specimen to obtain the desired maximum concentration, and a dilution series is prepared using analyte-free serum or urine. Diluting stock aqueous pools of analyte with human serum albumin, enzyme-inactivated serum, or Plasmonate (Miles, Inc., Elkhart, Indiana) can also approximate serum matrices. A patient specimen containing the analyte at a concentration known to exceed the linearity of the method can also be used and then a dilution series constructed using analyte-free materials. The accuracy of the volumetric dilutions is very important, and serial dilutions are not recommended because errors are propagated through the subsequent samples. Rather, each sample should be prepared by direct dilution from the original high sample or pool. For commonly measured analytes, linearity materials are available from commercial sources and proficiency testing providers.

Finally, all the data points should be plotted for visual inspection of linear performance. The actual result of the analysis of each dilution is plotted against the percentage of high pool present in each dilution (or against known concentrations). The straight portion of the resulting curve represents the linear portion of the assay. In the case of methods with curvilinear response, such as radioimmuno-assay procedures, the results obtained from the recommended curve-straightening algorithms should be plotted to show linearity of final results. If linearity is not certain on visual inspection, the significance of the degree of nonlinearity can be tested statistically.[10,38]

Sensitivity (Limit of Detection)

Several terms describe the different aspects of the minimum analytical sensitivity of a method.[39] These terms are demonstrated graphically in Fig. 22-4. The **limit of absence** is the lowest concentration of analyte that the method can differentiate from zero. Typically a specimen with zero concentration, or blank, is tested repeatedly, and the limit of absence is taken as an upper confidence limit of the resulting population of blank values. It is calculated from the mean and SD of the blank values.

$$\text{Limit of Absence} = \overline{Y}_{blank} + z \cdot SD_{blank} \qquad \textbf{\textit{Eq. 22-4}}$$

When the limit of absence is calculated using typical z values of 2 or 3, it represents the upper 97.5% or 99.7% confidence limit of the blank. If the method under evaluation reports negative results as zero, it may be necessary to collect data in terms of raw signal units and convert into concentration units before performing this calculation. Note, this threshold can be viewed as a qualitative definition of analytical sensitivity, providing an indication as to whether analyte is *absent* or *present* (a no/yes response based on the result compared to this value).

The **limit of detection (LOD)** is the minimum concentration of analyte whose presence can be qualitatively detected under defined conditions. It is the mean of the population in the center of Fig. 22-2. It is calculated as the upper confidence limit of the blank (limit of absence) plus two or three times the SD of a spiked sample.

$$\text{Limit of Detection} = \overline{Y}_{blank} + z \cdot SD_{blank} + z \cdot SD_{spike} \qquad \textbf{\textit{Eq. 22-5}}$$

Defined in this manner, limit of detection is 4 to 6 SD_{blank} above the average value for a zero sample.

The **functional sensitivity** or **limit of quantification (LOQ)** is the minimum concentration of analyte whose presence can be quantitatively measured reliably under defined conditions. It is the concentration at which the CV is a stated amount, usually 20%. The desired CV may be analyte specific, and set by a consensus group. Determining the functional sensitivity is somewhat empirical, and involves testing method precision at several low concentrations until the concentration with the desired CV is determined.

FINAL-EVALUATION EXPERIMENTS

The final-evaluation experiments take the most time to perform and potentially yield the most information about the test method's day-to-day performance on real patient specimens.

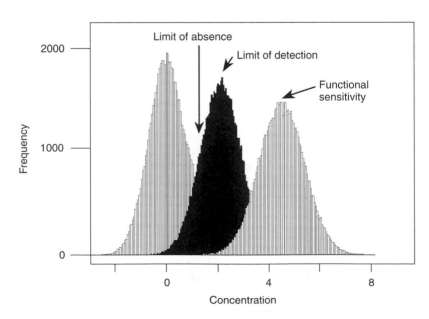

Fig. 22-4   Illustration of different aspects of analytical sensitivity or detection limits.

Between-Day Replication Experiment

The between-day replication experiment is an expansion of the within-run experiment over many days, usually 20, This period must be long enough to allow the random effects occurring over several days to influence the long-term estimate of RE. This experiment and the comparison-of-methods experiment described next are usually combined for better efficiency in the study.

A material known to be stable for the time of the experiment is used, usually a frozen serum or plasma pool or a lyophilized control product. Aliquot-to-aliquot variation of the material must be minimal because it will appear to be day-to-day variance of the test method.

RE is estimated as four times the total SD and compared to E_A, as described previously for the within-run study.

Comparison-of-Methods Experiment

The comparison-of-methods experiment determines the systematic error of the test method, using real patient specimens. A group of patient specimens are analyzed by both the test method and a comparative method, a method known to be accurate and precise. Systematic differences between the two methods are interpreted as errors of the test method if the results of the comparison method are known to have little or no error (negligible random and systematic errors). Thus the comparative method should be of the highest quality possible so that errors will not be erroneously assigned to the test method. Methods may be classified in terms of the quality of their performance as definitive, reference, or routine methods. See Chapter 21 for a description of definitive and reference methods.

In practice the comparative method is often the method in routine use in the laboratory and not a method of reference quality. It is useful to see how results from the test method compare with those of the routine method, but differences between the two methods should be interpreted cautiously unless the quality of the comparative method is known to be high.

At least 40 and preferably 100 or more patient specimens should be analyzed. They should include the variety of disease states that will be encountered by the test in routine use. Analyte concentrations of the specimens should be evenly distributed throughout the analytical range; otherwise regression analysis of the comparison data will be inaccurate. However, even distributions are not always practical. The NCCLS guideline for comparison of methods[3] has suggested some alternative distributions. Hemolyzed, lipemic, and icteric specimens should be included if they are not proscribed by the manufacturer of the test method and if they do not cause errors by the comparative method. If included in the study, they should be identified. Specimens must be carefully selected from the routine workload to be an efficient representation of the patient mix; preanalysis by the routine method is usually necessary.

Specimens are analyzed in duplicate by each method. Results should be examined carefully and plotted daily. Any specimen with large differences between results either for duplicate pairs within a method or paired results between methods should be reanalyzed in duplicate by both methods in the next run. A large difference (outlier) is defined as being greater than four times the average difference (using the within-assay difference or between-assay difference as appropriate).[3] If the large between-method difference is confirmed for a given specimen, the patient should be investigated for disease or diseases present and the specimen for other analytes (possible interferents) to determine the cause of the large difference. An immediate follow-up examination is essential to avoid unanswerable questions about outliers later.

The test and comparative methods should be run at the same time, or as close in time to each other as possible. If this is not possible, specimens must be stored in a manner that guarantees analyte stability.

The comparison-of-methods experiment is usually combined with the between-day replication experiment. Patient specimens should be evenly spread over at least five runs and preferably all 20 runs, to ensure that day-to-day effects have a chance to influence the data and to ensure that day-to-day effects are "fully confounded" (in statistical parlance). Both methods must be maintained in acceptable QC during the period.

***t*-Test statistics: bias, S_d.** The systematic differences between the test and comparative methods are most easily estimated from the comparison-of-methods data by the bias. The bias is the difference between the average result by the test method and the average result by the comparative method. Bias can indicate the magnitude of the systematic error between the two methods. (Each patient specimen must be analyzed by both methods for bias to be valid.) Bias is calculated by equation 22-6, in which y_i and x_i are the analyte concentrations of the individual specimens by the test method and comparative method, respectively and N is the number of paired results compared.

$$\text{Bias} = \frac{\sum (y_i - x_i)}{N} \qquad \textit{Eq. 22-6}$$

The standard deviation about the bias, called the *standard deviation of the differences*, s_d, is calculated in a manner analogous to that used to calculate the SD in the replication experiment. The s_d may be viewed as an indicator of the RE between the two methods.

$$s_d = \sqrt{\frac{\sum (y_i - x_i - \text{Bias})^2}{(N-1)}} \qquad \textit{Eq. 22-7}$$

The statistical significance of the bias, that is, whether it really differs from zero, or no bias, is determined by use of the *t*-test. A *t* value is calculated according to the formula

$$t = \frac{\text{Bias} \sqrt{N}}{s_d} \qquad \textit{Eq. 22-8}$$

This is the same *t* statistic described in equation 19-13. The *t* value is the ratio of a systematic-error term (bias) to a random-error term (s_d). If the bias increases relative to the standard deviation of differences, there is less of a probability that the observed bias is caused by random variations and more of a probability that there really is a systematic difference between the test and comparative method mean values. For example, in a comparison of glucose methods there were 101 specimens, the bias was 30 mg/L, and the *t* value was 2.11. The critical *t* value for *p* = 0.05 and for 100 degrees of freedom (obtainable from a statistics textbook) is 1.99. (The two-sided critical *t* value is used because the bias could be either positive or negative.) The calculated *t* value exceeds the critical *t* value; therefore a statistically real bias exists between the two methods (see also p. 350).

The acceptability of the systematic error, as estimated by the bias, is judged by comparison with E_A. If bias is less than E_A, the systematic error is acceptable. If bias exceeds E_A, the systematic error is not acceptable. Decisions about acceptability should never be based on the *t* value alone. A large bias and large s_d may combine to give an insignificant *t* value, even though the bias is unacceptably large. Also from this equation, it can be seen that if *N* is very large, the value of *t* can become statistically significant for some ratio of bias to s_d, indicating a statistically significant bias even though that bias may be medically unimportant.

Westgard and Hunt[40] have shown that bias can give inaccurate estimates of systematic error if a PE is present, because both proportional and constant errors are combined in the bias. PE also increases s_d. Bias should not be used as an estimator of systematic error unless PE is absent, or unless the mean analyte concentration as measured by the comparative method is very near the decision-level concentration (X_C) and the data are well distributed around X_C. Otherwise the bias will be weighted toward the side of X_C that has the most samples with large individual biases.

Correlation coefficient. The statistic most frequently cited in reports of comparison-of-methods experiments is the correlation coefficient (*r*). An *r*-value of zero indicates that there is no correlation between the methods. A value of +1 indicates perfect positive correlation. See Chapter 19 for a more extensive discussion of the calculation of **linear-regression** statistics and their interpretation.

The correlation coefficient is frequently misused in method evaluation reports. Westgard and Hunt[40] demonstrated that the correlation coefficient is extremely sensitive to the range of analyte concentrations of the patient specimens in the comparison-of-methods experiment. In a comparison of bilirubin methods over a range of 0 to 45 mg/L, a correlation coefficient of 0.950 was obtained. When data pairs with bilirubin concentrations above 15 mg/L were eliminated, the correlation coefficient dropped to 0.773. This is shown in Fig. 22-5.

The correlation coefficient is simply a means to look for a correlation, not agreement, between pairs. Thus, if the values for one population were twice that of the other, as one population's value doubled, the other population's value would double as well. The correlation between the two methods would be excellent (high *r*). Thus decisions about the acceptability of the analytical performance of a method should never be based on the value of the correlation coefficient alone.

Linear-regression statistics. If the test method and comparative method do correlate with each other, an *x:y* plot of results resembles a straight line, which can be described by the linear-regression expression

$$Y_i = a + bx_i \qquad \textit{Eq. 22-9}$$

in which Y_i is the calculated value on the straight line corresponding to the actual comparative method result, x_i. The proportionality between the methods is given by the slope, *b*, the **ideal value** of which (no proportional error) is 1. CE is indicated by the *y* intercept, *a*. RE between the methods is indicated by the standard error of the regression, $s_{y,x}$, also called the **standard error of the estimate**, or the *standard deviation of the residuals*.

Statistic	Range of Concentrations Studied		
	0 to 1.5 mg/dL	0 to 2.5 mg/dL	0 to 4.5 mg/dL
r	0.773	0.878	0.950
bias	0.17	0.17	0.17
s_d	0.30	0.29	0.31
$S_{y/x}$	0.29	0.29	0.31
a	0.17	0.17	0.20
b	1.025	1.007	0.966

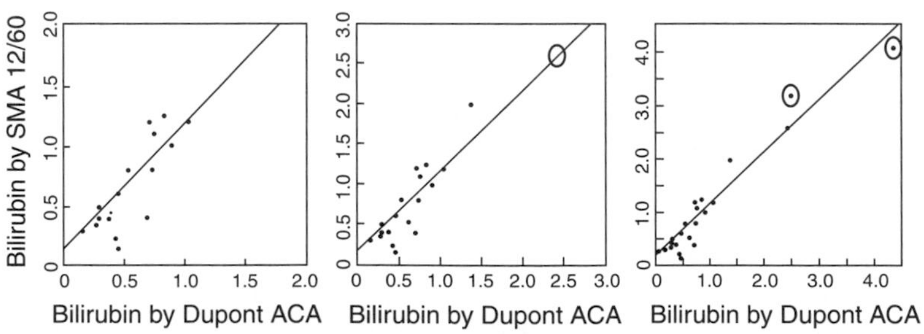

Fig. 22-5 Effect of range of data on correlation coefficient, *r. (From Westgard JO et al: Concepts and practices in the evaluation of laboratory methods. III. Statistics,* Am J Med Technol *44:552, 1978.)*

An estimate of systematic error at X_C, the decision-level concentration, may be obtained from the linear-regression statistics by substitution of X_C for x_i in Eq. 22-9, to calculate Y_C, the concentration the test method would measure for a specimen whose true analyte concentration is designated as X_C. The systematic error, SE, is calculated by subtraction of X_C from this Y_C:

$$SE = |Y_c - X_c| = |a + bX_c - X_c| \qquad \textit{Eq. 22-10}$$

This estimate of error will be valid only if the following limitations of linear regression are observed.

The data used to calculate the regression equation (Eq. 22-9) must first be plotted and carefully examined for nonlinearity, and the data used for the final calculation must be limited to the data in the linear range. Nonlinearity at higher concentrations will lower the slope, increase the y intercept, and increase $s_{y,x}$.

The importance of daily examination and plotting of comparison-of-methods data cannot be overemphasized, and the data must be carefully examined for outliers. A commonly used definition of an outlier from a regression line is a specimen for which $|y_i - Y_i| > 4 \cdot s_{y,x}$, (see Chapter 19). As stated before, outlier specimens must be detected immediately and reanalyzed by both methods so that the data can correct or confirm the outlier. The linear regression line is "pulled" toward the outlier, with the greatest effects caused by outliers at the extreme ranges of the data. Confirmed outliers should be investigated for their causes. A confirmed outlier really is representative of the true analytical performance of the method. The SE of the test method should be calculated both with the outlier included in the data set and with it excluded. If errors are acceptable with the outlier excluded and excessive with it included, extreme caution should be exercised. There are other statistical tests for removal of an outlier,[41] but no more than one outlier should be excluded in a set of 40 patient comparisons. If the outlier discrepancy is less than the E_A, do not exclude it even though

it may be a statistically significant outlier. If more than one clinically significant outlier is present per 40 patient comparison samples, the test method should be rejected until a cause for the outliers can be found and corrected.

The range of analytical concentrations must be wide. The effects of a narrow range of data on the least-squares statistics are seen in Fig. 22-6. Methods-comparison data often fail to meet one additional assumption of linear-regression calculations. This assumption requires that the x data (comparison) be known without error. Actually, in a methods-comparison experiment, random errors do affect the results of the comparison method. When the range of the data is sufficiently large, the effect of the failure to know the x values without error becomes negligible.[42,43]

Waakers et al[42] have suggested that the correlation coefficient be used to decide whether the range of data is sufficient for using traditional least-squares calculation. If the correlation coefficient is greater than 0.99, calculation by the traditional least-squares approach will produce a slope whose mathematical error will be less than 1%. If the correlation coefficient is less than 0.99, the slope will be falsely low and the y intercept will be too high. Cornbleet and Gochman[43] have suggested another decision limit. If the ratio of the analytic SD of the comparative (x) method, S_{CM}, to the SD of the x-method population, S_x, is less than 0.2, the least-squares calculation will be appropriate. If these tests on the data fail, another "debiased" regression approach should be used to calculate regression coefficients, such as those discussed by Cornbleet and Gochman[43] (see also Chapter 19).

One debiased regression method is Deming's regression,[42,43] which is based upon minimizing the sum of squares of residuals determined perpendicularly from the line (as opposed to only in the y direction by the traditional least-squares method). The Deming approach is much more robust and provides a good estimate of the slope, even when the data are not precise, or when the data are limited to a narrow range (see also pp. 358-360). Another approach, the method

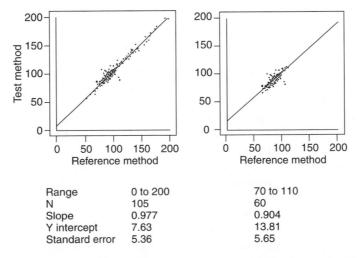

Range	0 to 200	70 to 110
N	105	60
Slope	0.977	0.904
Y intercept	7.63	13.81
Standard error	5.36	5.65

Fig. 22-6 Effect of range of data on linear-regression statistics. *(From Westgard JO, Hunt MR: Use and interpretation of statistics in method-comparison studies,* Clin Chem *19:49, 1973.)*

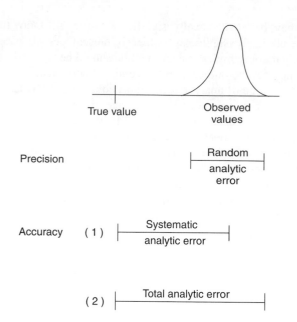

Fig. 22-7 Total analytical error. *(From Westgard JO, Carey RN, Wold S: Criteria for judging precision and accuracy in method development and evaluation,* Clin Chem *20:825, 1974.)*

of Passing-Bablock,[44] involves drawing a straight line between each pair of data points and then ranking the slopes and selecting the median slope as the best nonparametric estimate of the slope. This approach makes no assumption about the distribution of the data.

Calculation of SE by use of linear-regression statistics is demonstrated on p. 424.

ESTIMATION OF TOTAL ERROR

Estimates of RE and SE are combined to estimate the total error (TE) of the test method. This is the most severe criterion for the test method to meet. The rationale for the TE concept is shown in Fig. 22-7. The horizontal line is error in concentration units, and the vertical line is located at the true-value concentration, the medical decision-level concentration, or zero error. The vertical distance from the horizontal line represents the probability of obtaining a test-method result at any given amount of error (difference from X_C). The bell-shaped curve shows the distribution of test-method data obtained from repeated analyses of a patient specimen whose true analyte concentration is designated as X_C. The distance from the mean of that curve to the **true value** is the SE. The dispersion around the mean of the data is the RE, which is defined as four times the SD. There will be (1) instances in which the combined error will be exactly equal to the SE, (2) other times when the combined error for a given result will be less than the average SE by some amount because of the RE of the method, and (3) other times when the combined error will be greater than the SE, again by some amount caused by the RE of the method. The physician has no way of knowing what the various components of error are or when they will cause a larger error. Therefore it is essential to consider the worst-case combination and to define this as total error, TE:

TABLE 22-2 POINT-ESTIMATE CRITERIA FOR ACCEPTABLE PERFORMANCE

Type of Error	Criteria
Random (RE)	$4 \times s_{TM} < E_A$
Constant (CE)	Bias $< E_A$
Proportional (PE)	$\dfrac{|\bar{R} - 100|}{100} \times X_C < E_A$
Systematic (SE)	If $\bar{X} = X_C$, $|\bar{Y} - \bar{X}| < E_A$
	or $|Y_C - X_C| = |a + bX_C - X_C| < E_C$
Total (TE)	RE + SE = $4 \times s_{TM} + |a + bX_C - X_C| < E_A$

$$TE = RE + SE \qquad \text{Eq. 22-11}$$

If TE is less than E_A, the method's overall performance is acceptable. Calculation of TE is demonstrated on p. 424.

Equations for estimating the magnitudes of the various errors and the criteria for judging their acceptability are summarized in Table 22-2.

Medical Decision Charts

A graphic aid can best illustrate the relationship between method performance (determined in the method evaluation studies) and QC. If a method's inherent errors are small relative to allowable error, large deviations from the method's usual performance are required for total error to exceed allowable error. Relatively insensitive QC procedures will be able to detect errors before they are large enough to exceed E_A. If a method's inherent errors are larger, smaller deviations from routine performance cause TE to exceed E_A, and more sensitive QC procedures are necessary to ensure adequate error detection. When a method's inherent errors are so large that they exceed E_A frequently (for example, over 5% of the time), no QC procedure can maintain acceptable performance.

The Medical Decision Chart (also called OpSpecs QC chart) developed by Westgard,[45] shows the interrelationship between SD, bias, and E_A (Fig. 22-8). Fig. 22-8 shows that the combination of RE (some multiple of SD) and SE (bias) must be less than the allowable (total) error defined for the assay. The chart is divided into regions according to the magnitude of the SD. From right to left on the chart, they are *Unacceptable*, *Marginal*, *Fair*, *Good*, and *Six Sigma*, according to the complexity of QC procedure required to maintain the method's errors below the E_A. The lines on the chart are defined by the following equations:

- TE = 2 SD + bias (crosses y axis where SD = 0, or bias = E_A and crosses x axis where bias = 0, hence, 2 SD = E_A, or SD = 50% E_A)
- TE = 3 SD + bias (crosses y axis where SD = 0, or bias = E_A and crosses x axis where bias = 0, hence, 3 SD = E_A, or SD = 33.3% E_A)
- TE = 4 SD + bias (crosses y axis where SD = 0, or bias = E_A and crosses x axis where bias = 0, hence, 4 SD = E_A, or SD = 25% E_A)

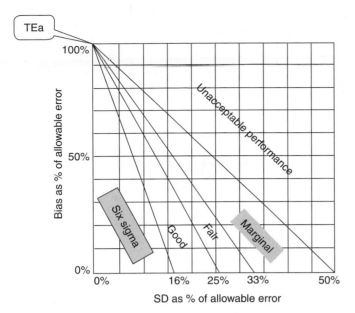

Fig. 22-8 Medical Decision Chart. In the *unacceptable performance* region, the SD exceeds 50% of E_A, and precision errors alone will exceed E_A more than 5% of the time regardless of bias and QC procedure. In the *marginal* performance region, the SD is so large (between 33% and 50% of E_A) that the method's total error is very close to E_A. Only QC procedures with unacceptably high rates of false rejection could maintain errors below E_A. This means many rejected runs. In the *fair* performance region, QC procedures must be carefully developed to maintain errors below E_A. This can be done with four to six QC measurements per run. In the *good* performance region, ordinary multirule QC procedures will detect unacceptable method performance. This will involve two to three QC measurements per run. In the *six Sigma* region, relatively weak QC procedures will be sufficient to detect errors that might exceed the EA. Only one or two QC measurements per run are required. See Chapter 21 for a discussion of QC procedures. *(From Westgard JO: Six sigma quality design and control, Madison, WI, 2001, Westgard QC.)*

- TE = 6 SD + bias (crosses *y* axis where SD = 0, or bias = E_A and crosses *x* axis where bias = 0, hence, 6 SD = E_A, or SD = 16.7% E_A)

CONFIDENCE-INTERVAL CRITERIA FOR JUDGING ANALYTICAL PERFORMANCE

To this point it has been assumed that the error estimated by each of the previous equations is absolutely accurate. However, if the same experiment were repeated in as identical a manner as possible, a slightly different estimate of error would probably be obtained. Exact measurements of random and systematic error cannot be obtained from the limited numbers of specimens analyzed in the procedures recommended above.

In the approach developed by Westgard, Carey, and Wold,[46] 95% upper and lower limits of error are calculated. If the 95% upper limit of an error is smaller than the E_A, there

TABLE 22-3 FACTORS FOR COMPUTING ONE-SIDED CONFIDENCE LIMITS FOR STANDARD DEVIATION

Degrees of Freedom (N – 1)	$A_{.05}$	$A_{.95}$
1	.5103	15.947
5	.6721	2.089
10	.7391	1.593
15	.7747	1.437
20	.7979	1.358
25	.8149	1.308
30	.8279	1.274
40	.8470	1.228
50	.8606	1.199
60	.8710	1.179
70	.8793	1.163
80	.8861	1.151
90	.8919	1.141
100	.8968	1.133

From Natrella MG: Experimental statistics, National Bureau of Standards Handbook 91, Washington, DC; 1963, US Government Printing Office.[47]

is at least a 95% certainty that estimated error is acceptable. If the 95% lower limit is greater than the E_A, there is at least a 95% certainty that the error, and thus the method's performance, is not acceptable, and no further testing is indicated. The method should be rejected or modified to improve its analytical performance. When the lower 95% limit is less than E_A and the 95% upper limit of error exceeds E_A, no decision can be made about whether the method is unacceptable or acceptable, and more data are required to make a definitive decision.

Calculations of confidence-interval estimates of each type of error are demonstrated on pp. 422-424. For additional discussion of confidence limits, see pp. 346-348.

Confidence-Interval Criterion for Random Error

In the calculation of RE, the true value of the SD is not known. The upper and lower confidence limits of the SD can be estimated by multiplying the observed SD by the appropriate one-sided 95% factors. These factors (Table 22-3) are referenced to $N – 1$ degrees of freedom.

$$s_{TM_u} = s_{TM} \cdot A_u \qquad \textit{Eq. 22-12, A}$$

and

$$s_{TM_l} = s_{TM} \cdot A_l \qquad \textit{Eq. 22-12, B}$$

in which A_u and A_l are the factors for computing the upper and lower one-sided limits of the SD.[47] The upper confidence limit of RE is four times the upper confidence limit of the SD, and the lower confidence limit of RE is four times the lower confidence limit of the SD.

$$RE_u = 4 \cdot s_{TM_u} \qquad \textit{Eq. 22-13, A}$$

and

$$RE_l = 4 \cdot s_{TM_l} \qquad \textit{Eq. 22-13, B}$$

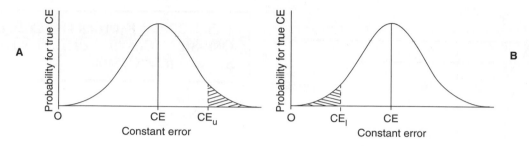

Fig. 22-9 **A,** One-sided 95% upper limit of constant error, CE$_u$. **B,** One-sided 95% lower limit of constant error, CE$_l$.

Confidence-Interval Criterion for Constant Error and for Proportional Error

Upper (E$_u$) and lower (E$_l$) confidence limits for constant and proportional error can be derived from the point estimates ($\bar{E}$) of constant and proportional error calculated above, and their SD, using the general equation:

$$E_u = \bar{E} + \frac{t \cdot s}{\sqrt{N}}$$ *Eq. 22-14, A*

and

$$E_l = \bar{E} - \frac{t \cdot s}{\sqrt{N}}$$ *Eq. 22-14, B*

Fig. 22-9, A, shows the upper 95% limit of constant error, leaving only a 5% chance that the error exceeds this upper limit, CE$_u$. Similarly, Fig. 22-9, B, shows the lower 95% limit of constant error, CE$_l$. A one-sided t-value is used only when there is interest in an upper limit on the error without regard to how small the error is, and vice versa for a lower limit. (A two-sided t is used to answer the question, "Is there a difference?" without regard to whether the difference is positive or negative, as in the *t*-test used in the comparison-of-methods experiment.)

Confidence-Interval Criterion for Systematic Error

Fig. 22-10 shows the profile of a **confidence interval** around a least-squares regression line. The expression for the limits, w, of this interval is given as

$$w = t \cdot s_{y,x} \sqrt{\frac{1}{N} + \frac{(X_c - \bar{X})^2}{\Sigma(x_i - \bar{X})^2}}$$ *Eq. 22-15*

This equation is similar to those used to calculate the limits for constant and proportional error in terms of the component $t \cdot s_{y,x}$. The component under the square-root sign becomes $1/N$ if X_C equals the mean of the patient data by the comparative method. As X_C moves away from the mean, the right term begins to contribute to the widening of the limits. The denominator of this second term can be calculated from the SD of the patient population by the comparative method (s_x) as follows:

$$\Sigma(x_i - \bar{X})^2 = s_x^2 (N - 1)$$ *Eq. 22-16*

In this situation, what the regression line is cannot be known exactly, and for a given X_C, the corresponding Y_C could be as large as ($Y_C + w$) or as small as ($Y_C - w$). The

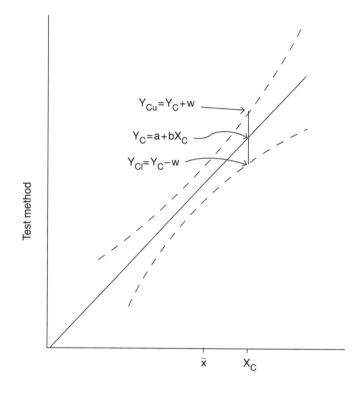

Fig. 22-10 Confidence interval around regression line. *(From Westgard JO et al: Concepts and practices in the evaluation of laboratory methods. IV. Decisions on acceptability, Am J Med Technol 44:727, 1978.)*

limit that is farther from the ideal value is used to estimate the upper limit of SE, and the limit closer to the ideal value is used to estimate the lower limit of SE:

$$SE_u = |(Y_c \pm w) - X_c|_u$$ *Eq. 22-17, A*

and

$$SE_l = |(Y_c \pm w) - X_c|_l$$ *Eq. 22-17, B*

Eq. 22-15 may not provide a valid estimate of the confidence limits of the linear-regression line if the precision of the test method is not reasonably constant throughout the concentration range of the patient specimens included in the comparison-of-methods experiment.

TABLE 22-4 POINT-ESTIMATE CRITERIA FOR ACCEPTABLE PERFORMANCE

Error	Acceptable Performance	Unacceptable Performance
Random (RE)	$4 \times s_{TM_u} < E_A$	$4 \times s_{TM_l} > E_A$
Constant (CE)	$\|Bias\| + \dfrac{t \cdot s}{\sqrt{N}} < E_A$	$\|Bias\| - \dfrac{t \cdot s}{\sqrt{N}} > E_A*$
Proportional (PE)	$\dfrac{\|\overline{R}_u \text{ or } \overline{R}_l - 100\|_u}{100} \cdot X_C < E_A$	$\dfrac{\|\overline{R}_l \text{ or } \overline{R}_u - 100\|_l}{100} \cdot X_C > E_A*$
Systematic (SE)	$\|(a + bX_c \pm w) - X_c\|_u < E_A$	$\|(a + bX_c \pm w) - X_c\|_u > E_A*$
Total error (TE)	$\sqrt{RE_u^2 + w^2} + SE < E_A$	$\sqrt{RE_l^2 + w^2} + SE > E_A*$

* If the idea value is between the two limits, it is possible that there is no error, and thus the lower limit of error might be zero. In these cases, therefore, CE_l is defined as zero, or PE_l is redefined as zero, or SE_l is redefined as zero, whatever the case might be. If $SE_l = 0$, TE_l becomes RE_l.

Confidence-Interval Criterion for Total Error

As described before, TE is the worst-case combination of the random and systematic errors. Because both the random and systematic errors have variances included in the equations used to calculate them, they must be combined vectorially. Their variances are combined as shown:

$$TE_u = \sqrt{RE_u^2 + w^2} + SE \qquad \textit{Eq. 22-18, A}$$

and

$$TE_l = \sqrt{RE_l^2 + w^2} + SE \qquad \textit{Eq. 22-18, B}$$

If the upper 95% limit of the TE is less than the E_A, there is a 95% certainty that the method performs acceptably. If the lower 95% limit of the TE exceeds E_A, there is a 95% certainty that the method does not perform acceptably and should be modified or rejected.

It should be noted that whenever the ideal value (zero error condition) is between the upper and lower limits of the estimated error there is a chance that the true error might be zero. Thus in these situations the lower limit of error is simply zero. The upper limit of error remains as just calculated. This situation can arise for the constant, proportional, or systematic error estimates but not of course for RE. If the lower limit of SE is zero, the lower limit of the estimate of TE is equal to the lower limit of the estimate of RE because there may not be a SE present. Equations for calculating confidence intervals of the various errors and criteria for judging their acceptabilities are summarized in Table 22-4.

Confidence limits for the calculated SD and SE (bias) can be used with the method decision chart to define the confidence interval of the operating point. Appropriate QC procedures should be used that take into account the worst case limits for SD and for bias when the method is put into routine use. See the example on pp. 424-425.

OTHER EVALUATION PROTOCOLS

The NCCLS has proposed a series of evaluation protocols. The first, EP5-A, is for evaluation of precision and verification of manufacturer's precision claims.[7] It requires duplicate measurements on sample pools that contain at least two different levels of the analyte in a run, two runs per day, for 20 days. An analysis of variance calculation is used to determine within-run, within-day, and day-to-day components of variance. These are combined to estimate the total SD.

Guideline EP6-P2 addresses both experimental procedure and data analysis for evaluating the linearity of an assay.[10] Statistical procedures are presented for determining the limit of linearity and for estimating errors caused by nonlinearity at a particular concentration.

Another NCCLS guideline, EP7-P, presents two approaches for interference testing in the clinical chemistry laboratory.[6] The first approach is similar to that already discussed on pp. 412-413. The second approach describes the determination of interferences with increasing concentrations of interferent (dose-response method). This guideline also presents extensive lists of exogenous and endogenous interferents and recommended testing concentrations.

The NCCLS guideline EP9-A[3] addresses key issues in method-comparison studies. The protocol requires that duplicate results be obtained for each procedure to facilitate tests for outliers. A minimum of 40 specimens distributed over the reportable range are to be tested. Various approaches to estimate the bias between the two methods and its confidence interval are described for use, depending on the nature of the data as determined in the preliminary review.

A protocol for user demonstration of precision and accuracy is described in EP15-A.[5] This protocol assumes that the method's performance is already well documented and the user believes it will perform acceptably in his laboratory. Its purpose is for the user to demonstrate that he can obtain performance similar to that claimed by the manufacturer, as required by CLIA.[2] Precision is estimated in a replication experiment of 5 days or less. Accuracy is estimated by either a comparison-of-methods experiment with 20 patient specimens, or analysis of materials with known analyte concentration such as proficiency testing specimens or materials recommended by the manufacturer.

Multifactor experimental designs have been proposed to study several method characteristics at one time.[48] A special example of this approach is given in NCCLS guideline EP10-A, *Preliminary Evaluation of Quantitative Clinical*

Laboratory Methods.[11] This protocol enables the estimation of imprecision, **inaccuracy**, nonlinearity, carryover, and drift in one series of studies over 5 days, using three levels of analyte. Samples must be measured in a specific sequence for a total of three readings each day as well as two "primer" samples of the midlevel sample, for a total of 11 analyses per day, or 55 for the whole study. If unusual effects are observed, each effect should be investigated more thoroughly with a specific study performed for each factor separately, as described in this chapter.

DISCUSSION

There are situations, as in the study of different enzyme methods, in which suitably close agreement is not expected or possible because of different reaction conditions or different definitions of enzyme units. In these cases, rather than conclude that the method is unacceptable, a new clinical baseline of information is necessary, and a new reference interval is needed (see Chapter 20). Specific disease-related data should be obtained to provide new clinical information for interpretation of test-method results.

Evaluation of a method for a "new" analyte previously not measured in the user's laboratory is an analogous situation. Because there is no comparative method on site, accurate estimates of SE are harder to obtain. Reliance on published evaluation reports increases. The conclusions of these reports must be reviewed cautiously after the analysis of a laboratory's own experimental data is completed. If an analyte is not usually measured, the emphasis of the laboratory should shift to experiments to estimate specific errors. Accurate recovery studies are essential. The interference studies are expanded to include a broader range of chemicals that could interfere with the measurement reactions. Patient specimens that have been analyzed in another laboratory may be analyzed for comparison purposes, but specimen instability and lack of user control of the other laboratory's procedure may decrease the reliability of the SE estimate. However, if the other laboratory is the reference laboratory to which the user has previously referred specimens for measurement of this analyte, the comparison is really being made to present practice.

Smaller laboratories often do not have the resources for exhaustive method-evaluation studies, but fortunately these are usually not among the first to evaluate a new method. Usually some evaluation reports have been published. Even when a method's performance is well documented by published evaluation studies, the user should still evaluate RE and perform the comparison-of-methods experiment to verify acceptable performance in his or her own laboratory. A reference interval study should be performed (see Chapter 20).

Using the decision-making approaches and tools that have been described in this chapter, it is possible to perform evaluations of methods efficiently and objectively. Conducting a method evaluation enables the laboratory scientist to understand the capabilities and quality of an assay before its routine use for patient testing, regardless of whether an evaluation is required by government regulation.

AN EXAMPLE PERFORMANCE EVALUATION FOR GLUCOSE

1. **Estimation of RE from replication data**
   a. **Statistics calculations.** (y_i = Results from the method being tested)

   Mean:

   $$\bar{y} = \frac{\Sigma y_i}{N}$$

   SD:

   $$s_{TM} = \sqrt{\frac{\Sigma(y_i - \bar{y})^2}{N - 1}}$$

   or

   $$s_{TM} = \sqrt{\frac{\Sigma y_i^2 - (\Sigma y_i)^2/N}{N - 1}}$$

   Coefficient of variation:

   $$CV = \frac{s_{TM}}{\bar{y}} \cdot 100\%$$

   Example. For glucose

   $$N = 20, \Sigma y_i = 25,652, \Sigma y_i^2 = 32,905,141$$
   $$\bar{y} = 1283 \text{ mg/L}$$
   $$s_{TM} = 14.3 \text{ mg/L}$$
   $$CV = 1.1\%$$

   b. **Point estimate of RE**

   $$RE = 4 \cdot s_{TM}$$

   If $RE < E_A$, performance is acceptable.
   Example.
   For glucose, E_A = 126 mg/L at Y_C = 1260 mg/L
   $$\bar{y} = 1283 \text{ mg/L}$$
   $$s_{TM} = 14.3 \text{ mg/L}$$

   $RE = 4 \cdot 14.3 = 57.2$ mg/L; RE is acceptable.

   c. **Confidence-interval estimate of random error (RE_u, RE_l)**

   $$s_{TM_u} = s_{TM} \cdot (A_{0.95}) \ldots \text{(see Table 22-3)}$$
   $$s_{TM_u} = 14.3 \cdot 1.358 = 19.4 \text{ mg/L}$$
   $$s_{TM_l} = s_{TM} \cdot (A_{0.05})$$
   $$s_{TM_l} = 14.3 \cdot 0.7979 = 11.4 \text{ mg/L}$$
   $$RE_u = 4 \cdot s_{TM_u} = 4 \cdot 19.4 \text{ mg/L} = 78 \text{ mg/L}$$
   $$RE_l = 4 \cdot s_{TM_l} = 4 \cdot 11.4 \text{ mg/L} = 45 \text{ mg/L}$$

   Because $RE_u < E_A$, it is 95% certain that RE is acceptable.

2. **Estimation of CE from an interference study for a glucose method**
   a. **Sample preparation**
      (1) 1.00 mL of serum A + 0.10 mL of water
      (2) 1.00 mL of serum A + 0.10 mL of 1000 mg/L of creatinine standard
      (3) 1.00 mL of serum A + 0.10 mL of 3000 mg/L of creatinine standard

b. Results

	Creatinine added (mg/L)	Glucose measured (mg/L)	Interference (mg/L)	Average interference (CE) (mg/L)
(1)	—	1200, 1220, 1190	—	—
(2)	91	1240, 1240, 1230	+40, +20, +40	+33
(3)	273	1310, 1340, 1290	+110, +120, +100	+110

c. Formulas for calculations

Concentration added =

$$\text{Concentration of standard} \cdot \frac{\text{Volume standard}}{\text{Total volume}}$$

Interference = Concentration (test) − Concentration (baseline)

d. Point estimate of constant error (CE)

CE = Interference

If CE < E_A, performance is acceptable.

Example. For glucose, E_A = 126 mg/L at X_C = 1260 mg/L. In the presence of 91 mg/L of creatinine, CE = 33 mg/L; CE is acceptable.

In the presence of 273 mg/L of creatinine, CE = 110 mg/L; CE is acceptable, but doesn't allow for much imprecision.

e. Confidence-interval estimate of constant error (CE_u, CE_l)

(1) In the presence of 91 mg/L of creatinine, CE = 33 mg/L, s = 11.5 mg/L, N = 3, and t for ($N-1$), or 2 degrees of freedom; 95% one-sided limit is 2.92 (see p. 3).

$$CE_u = CE + \frac{t \cdot s}{\sqrt{N}}$$

$$CE_u = 33 + \frac{2.92 \cdot 11.3}{\sqrt{3}} = 52 \text{ mg/L}$$

$$CE_l = CE - \frac{t \cdot s}{\sqrt{N}}$$

$$CE_l = 33 - \frac{2.92 \cdot 11.3}{\sqrt{3}} = 14 \text{ mg/L}$$

Because $CE_u < E_A$ (52 mg/L < 126 mg/L), the CE caused by creatinine of 91 mg/L is acceptably small.

(2) In the presence of 273 mg/L of creatinine, CE = 110, s = 10 mg/L, N = 3.

$$CE_u = 110 + \frac{2.92 \cdot 10}{\sqrt{3}} = 127 \text{ mg/L}$$

$$CE_l = 110 = \frac{2.92 \cdot 10}{\sqrt{3}} = 93 \text{ mg/L}$$

Because $CE_l < E_A < CE_u$, we cannot be 95% sure the method is acceptable or 95% sure the method is not acceptable for glucose analysis in the presence of 273 mg/L of creatinine. More data should be obtained to narrow the confidence limits to one side of E_A or the other.

3. Estimation of PE from a recovery study for a glucose method

a. Sample preparation

(1) 2.0 mL of serum A + 0.1 mL of water
(2) 2.0 mL of serum A + 0.1 mL of 10,000 mg/L of glucose standard
(3) 2.0 mL of serum B + 0.1 mL of water
(4) 2.0 mL of serum B + 0.1 mL of 10,000 mg/L of glucose standard

b. Results (mg/L)

Sample	Glucose added	Glucose measured	Glucose recovered (test— baseline)	Percentage recovery*
(1) Baseline	—	510, 530, 540	—	—
(2) Spike	476	970, 1000, 980	460, 470, 440	96.6%, 98.7%, 92.4%
(3) Baseline	—	1240, 1200, 1210	—	—
(4) Spike	476	1690, 1660, 1640	450, 460, 430	94.5%, 96.6%, 90.3%

*Average recovery ($\bar{R}$) = 94.8%; SD of recovery (s_R) = 3.09%; SD of average recovery = 1.26%.

c. Formulas for calculations

Concentration added =

$$\text{Concentration of standard} \cdot \frac{\text{Volume standard}}{\text{Total volume}}$$

Concentration recovered =

Concentration (test) − Concentration (baseline)

$$\% \text{ Recovery} = \frac{\text{Concentration recovered}}{\text{Concentration added}} \cdot 100$$

d. Point estimate of PE

$$PE(\%) = |\bar{R} - 100|$$

$$PE \text{ (concentration units)} = \left| \frac{|\bar{R} - 100|}{100} \right| \cdot X_C$$

If PE < E_A, performance is acceptable.

Example: For glucose, E_A = 126 mg/L at X_C = 1260 mg/L

$$\bar{R} = 94.8\%$$

$$PE(\%) = |94.8\% - 100| = 5.2\%$$

or

$$PE = \left| \frac{|94.8 - 100|}{100} \right| \cdot 1260 \text{ mg/L} = 66 \text{ mg/L}$$

PE is acceptable.

e. Confidence-interval estimate of proportional error (PE_u, PE_l)

$\bar{R}$ = 94.8%, s = 3.09%, N = 6, and t for ($N-1$), or 5 degrees of freedom, and the 95% one-sided limit is 2.02.

$$\bar{R}_u = \bar{R} + \frac{t \cdot s}{\sqrt{N}}$$

$$\bar{R}_u = 94.8\% + \frac{2.02 \cdot 3.09}{\sqrt{6}} = 97.4\%$$

$$\bar{R}_l = \bar{R} - \frac{t \cdot s}{\sqrt{N}}$$

$$\bar{R}_l = 94.8\% - \frac{2.02 \cdot 3.09}{\sqrt{6}} = 92.3\%$$

The limit that deviates more from the ideal recovery of 100% is used to estimate the upper limit of proportional error, $PE_u\%$.

$$PE_u\% = |92.3 - 100| = 7.7\%$$

and for the lower limit

$$PE_l\% = |97.3 - 100| = 2.7\%$$

To relate $PE_u\%$ or $PE_l\%$ to E_A, convert them to concentration units at X_C.

$$PE_u = \frac{PE_u}{100} \cdot X_C$$

$$= \frac{7.7\%}{100} \cdot 1260 \text{ mg/L} = 97 \text{ mg/L}$$

$$PE_l = \frac{PE_l}{100} \cdot X_C$$

$$= \frac{2.7\%}{100} \cdot 1260 \text{ mg/L} = 34 \text{ mg/L}$$

Because $PE_u < E_A$, it is 95% certain PE is acceptably small for this glucose method.

4. Estimation of SE from a comparison-of-methods study for glucose

a. In the comparison of an automated glucose oxidase method (*y*) versus the manual glucose national reference method (*x*), the following statistics were obtained by linear-regression analysis: $y = 0.973 \cdot x - 6$ mg/L, $s_{y,x} = 37$ mg/L, $N = 82$, $\bar{x} = 1723$, $\bar{y} = 1670$, $s_x = 571$ mg/L (in which s_x is the SD of the *x* values for the 82 samples), and $r = 0.9941$.

b. Point estimate of SE

Consider bias:

$$\text{Bias} = |\bar{y} - \bar{x}| = 53 \text{ mg/L}$$

The bias provides an estimate of SE at the mean of the data. However, if is not equal to the X_C of interest, there must be no PE between methods for the bias to provide an accurate estimate of SE at these other concentrations. If PE is present, use linear-regression statistics or calculate the bias using only those samples whose analyte concentrations are close to X_C.

Consider linear regression:

$$SE = |Y_C - X_C|$$

in which $Y_C = a + b \cdot X_C$

For

$$X_C = 1260 \text{ mg/L glucose,}$$

Then

$$Y_C = 0.973 \cdot 1260 - 6 \text{ mg/L}$$
$$Y_C = 1220 \text{ mg/L}$$

and

$$SE = |1220 - 1260| = 40 \text{ mg/L}$$

Because $SE < E_A$, the SE is acceptable.

c. Confidence-interval estimate of systematic error (SE_u, SE_l)

$$Y_{C_u} = Y_C + w$$

and

$$Y_{C_l} = Y_C - w$$

in which

$$w = t \cdot s_{y,x} \sqrt{\frac{1}{N} + \frac{(X_c - \bar{X})^2}{\Sigma(x_i - \bar{X})^2}}$$

in which

$$\Sigma (x_i - \bar{X})^2 = s_x^2 (N - 1)$$

in which *w* is the width of the confidence interval around the regression line (Fig. 22-10). The value for *t*, obtained from a 95% one-sided *t* table and $N - 2$ degrees of freedom, has the value of 1.66.

$$w = 1.66 \cdot 37 \sqrt{\frac{1}{82} + \frac{(1260 - 1162)^2}{571^2 \cdot 81}} = 7 \text{ mg/L}$$

thus

$$Y_{C_u} = 1220 + 7 = 1227 \text{ mg/L}$$
$$Y_{C_l} = 1220 - 7 = 1213 \text{ mg/L}$$

The limit that deviates more from the ideal value for Y_C (ideally, $Y_C = X_C$) will be used to estimate the upper limit of SE.

$$SE_u = |(Y_C \pm w - X_C|_u$$
$$SE_u = |1213 - 1260| = 47 \text{ mg/L}$$

and

$$SE_l = |(Y_C \pm w - X_C|_l$$
$$SE_l = |1227 - 1260| = 33 \text{ mg/L}$$

Because $SE_u < E_A$, we can be 95% sure that the SE between these methods is acceptable.

5. Estimation of TE

a. Point estimate of TE

$$TE = RE + SE \text{ (see Fig. 22-7)}$$
$$TE = 4 \cdot s_{TM} + |Y_C - X_C|$$
$$TE = 57 \text{ mg/L} + 40 \text{ mg/L} = 97 \text{ mg/L}$$

Because $TE < E_A$, the TE of the new glucose method is acceptable.

b. Confidence-interval estimate of total error (TE_u, TE_l)

$$TE_u = \sqrt{RE_u + w^2} + SE$$

and

$$TE_l = \sqrt{RE_l + w^2} + SE$$

Notice that the variance of the uncertainty in repetitive measurements and the uncertainty of the regression line are added, and the square root of the sum is taken to estimate the overall uncertainty, which is then combined with the point estimate of SE to yield the appropriate limit for TE. Thus

$$TE_u = \sqrt{78^2 + 7^2} + 40 = 118 \text{ mg/L}$$

and

$$TE_l = \sqrt{46^2 + 7^2} + 40 = 87 \text{ mg/L}$$

Because $TE_u < E_A$ we can be 95% sure the TE is acceptable.

6. **Method decision chart analysis of point estimates of precision and bias**
   a. **Express SD as percentage of E_A.**
   b. **At $X_C = 1260$ mg/L, $s_{TM} = 14.3$ mg/L, $E_A = 126$ mg/L, or SD = 11.3% of E_A.**
   c. **Express bias as percentage of E_A.**
   d. **At $X_C = 1260$ mg/L, SE = 40 mg/L, $E_A = 126$ mg/L, or SE = 31.7% of E_A.**
   e. **Plot percent bias and SD on the medical decision chart.**

   The operating point is in the region of *Good* performance.

   f. **Calculate the upper and lower confidence limits of SD as percentages of E_A.**

   $$s_{TM_u} = 19.4 \text{ mg/L} = 15.4\% \text{ of } E_A.$$
   $$s_{TM_l} = 11.4 \text{ mg/L} = 9.0\% \text{ of } E_A.$$

   g. **Calculate the upper and lower confidence limits of bias (SE by regression) as percentages of E_A.**

   $$SE_u = 47 \text{ mg/L} = 37.0\% \text{ of } E_A.$$
   $$SE_l = 33 \text{ mg/L} = 26.2\% \text{ of } E_A.$$

   h. **Plot confidence limits of percent bias and percent SD on medical decision chart ("+" marks the confidence limits).**

The uncertainty limits indicate that the method's performance could be either *Fair* or *Good*.

The QC Rules that are selected for this assay should accommodate the worst case SD of 15.4% of E_A and inaccuracy of 37.0% of E_A. For example, a simple, single rule QC procedure could be the $1_{2.5s}$ rule with three controls in the run. This would give a probability for error detection (P_{ed}) of 80% and a probability for a false rejection (P_{fr}) of 3%. (For more discussion on probability of error detection and probability for false rejection, and QC rules, see Chapter 21).

If the inaccuracy were reduced to near zero (method is in the Six Sigma zone), the $1_{2.5s}$ rule could be used with only one control per run. This would give a P_{ed} of >94% and P_{fr} of 1%.

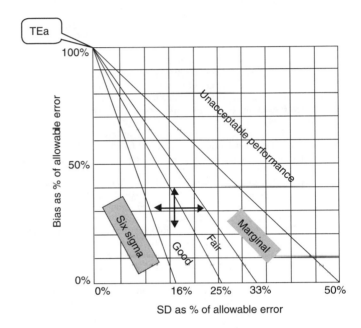

References

1. Buttner R et al: Approved recommendation (1978) on quality control in clinical chemistry. Part 1. General principles and terminology, *Clin Chem Acta* 98:129F, 1979.
2. Health Care Financing Administration (42 CFR Part 493, et al), the Public Health Service, U.S. Department of Health and Human Services: Clinical Laboratory Improvement Amendments of 1988, Final Rule, *Fed Reg* 57:7003, 1992. For latest updates go to the Government Printing Office Internet site (www.access.gpo.gov) and proceed as follows:
   1) Select "GPO access"
   2) Select "Regulatory"
   3) Select "Code of Federal Regulations (CFR), April 1996 and forward"
   4) Select "Attention new CFR browse feature"
   5) Scroll down to "Title 42" and select latest year indicated (note Title 42 is updated every October 1)
   6) Select parts "430-end"
   7) Select part "493"
   8) Select section of interest. For example, Quality Control begins with section 1201. These can be downloaded as text files or PDF files.
3. *NCCLS approved guideline EP9-A User comparison of quantitative clinical laboratory methods using patient samples*, Wayne, PA, 1999, Evaluation Protocols Area Committee.
4. Westgard JO et al: Concepts and practices in the selection and evaluation of methods, *Am J Med Technol*: Part I, Background and approach, 44:290, 1978; Part II, Experimental procedures, 44:420, 1978; Part III, Statistics, 44:552, 1978; Part IV, Decision on acceptability, 44:727, 1978; Part V, Applications, 44:803, 1978.
5. *NCCLS proposed guideline EP15-A, User demonstration of precision and accuracy of quantitative clinical methods*, Wayne, PA, 2001, Evaluation Protocols Area Committee.
6. *NCCLS proposed guideline EP7-P, Interference testing in clinical chemistry*, Wayne, PA, 1986, Evaluation Protocols Area Committee.
7. *NCCLS approved guideline EP5-A, Guidelines for user evaluation of precision performance of clinical chemistry devices*, Wayne, PA, 1999, Evaluation Protocols Area Committee.
8. 21 Code of Federal Regulations (CFR) Section 820.3 Definitions.
9. Westgard JO: Precision and accuracy: concepts and assessment by method evaluation testing, *CRC Crit Rev Clin Lab Sci* 13:283, 1981.
10. *NCCLS proposed guideline EP6-P2, Evaluation of the linearity of quantitative analytical methods*, Wayne, PA, 2001, Evaluation Protocols Area Committee.
11. *NCCLS approved guideline EP10-A, Preliminary evaluation of quantitative clinical methods*, ed 2, Wayne, PA, 1993, Evaluation Protocols Area Committee.

12. Labeling requirements and standards development for in-vitro diagnostic products, 21 CFR 809.10, 1974. For latest updates, go to www.access.gpo.gov and follow the instructions cited in Reference 2, selecting Title 21, section 809, and parts of that section as desired.

13. Draft guidance to manufacturers of in vitro analytical test systems for preparation of premarket submissions implementing CLIA '88, *Fed Reg*, p 3592, Jan 12, 1993.

14. Analyte Specific Reagents. 21 CFR 809.30 (November 21, 1997) and 21 CFR 864.4020 (November 21, 1997). For latest updates, go to www.access.gpo.gov and follow the instructions in Reference 2 to locate Title 21 and sections 809 and 864.

15. Berkow R, editor: *The Merck manual of diagnosis and therapy*, ed 16, Rahway, NJ, 1992, Merck Sharp & Dohme Research Laboratories.

16. Barnett RN: Medical significance of laboratory results, *Am J Clin Pathol* 50:671, 1968.

17. Barnett RN: Analytic goals in clinical chemistry: the pathologist's viewpoint. In Elevitch FR, editor: *Proceedings of the 1976 Aspen conference on analytic goals in clinical chemistry*, Skokie, IL, 1977, College of American Pathologists.

18. Tonks D: A study of the accuracy and precision of clinical chemistry determinations in 170 Canadian laboratories, *Clin Chem* 9:217, 1963.

19. Tonks D: A quality control program for quantitative clinical chemistry estimations, *Can J Med Technol* 30:38, 1968.

20. Cotlove E, Harris E, Williams G: Biological and analytic components of variation in long-term studies of serum constituents in normal subjects. III. Physiological and medical implications, *Clin Chem* 16:1028, 1970.

21. Elevitch FR, editor: *CAP Aspen Conference 1976: analytical goals in clinical chemistry*, Skokie, IL, 1977, College of American Pathologists.

22. Fraser CG: The application of theoretical goals based upon biological variation in proficiency testing, *Arch Pathol Lab Med* 112:404, 1988.

23. Fraser CG: Desirable standards of performance for therapeutic drug monitoring, *Clin Chem* 33:387, 1987.

24. Fraser CG et al: Quality specifications. In Haeckel R, editor: *Evaluation methods in laboratory medicine*, New York, 1993, VCH.

25. Fraser CG: *Biological variation: from principles to practice*, Washington, DC, 2001, AACC Press.

26. Ricos C et al: Current databases on biological variation: pros, cons, and progress, *Scand J Clin Lab Invest* 59:491, 1999.

27. Dufour DR et al: Diagnosis and monitoring of hepatic injury. I. Performance characteristics of laboratory tests, *Clin Chem* 46:2027, 2000.

28. Nation glycohemoglobin standardization program. Internet site: http://web.missouri.edu/~diabetes/ngsp.html. Please go to this Internet site for current information.

29. OSHA regulations on cadmium surveillance (29CFR 1910.1027), *Fed Regist* 58:21778ff, Appendix F, April 23, 1993.

30. Ross JW: A theoretical basis for clinically relevant proficiency testing evaluation limits. Sensitivity analysis of the effect of inherent test variability on acceptable method error, *Arch Pathol Lab Med* 112:421, 1988.

31. Ehrmeyer SS et al: 1990 Medicare/CLIA final rules for proficiency testing: minimum intralaboratory performance characteristics (CV and bias) needed to pass, *Clin Chem* 36:1736, 1990.

32. Westgard JO, Burnett RW: Precision requirements for cost-effective operation of analytical processes, *Clin Chem* 36:1629, 1990.

33. Westgard JO: *Six sigma quality design and control*, Madison, WI, 2001, Westgard QC.

34. Pande PS, Neuman RP, Cavanaugh RR: *The six sigma way: how GE, Motorola, and other top companies are honing their performance*, New York, 2000, McGraw/Hill.

35. National Reference System for the Clinical Laboratory, *NRSCL6-T, Development of methodological principles documents for analytes in the clinical laboratory: tentative guideline*, Villanova, PA, 1989, NRSCL.

36. Tremblay MM: Evaluation of instruments in biochemistry, *Can J Med Technol* 41:65, 1979.

37. Shaikh AH: A systematic procedure for selection of automated instruments in the clinical laboratory, *Am J Med Technol* 45:710, 1979.

38. Kroll MH, Emancipator K: A theoretical evaluation of linearity, *Clin Chem* 39:405, 1993.

39. Miller JC, Miller JN: *Statistics for analytical chemistry*, Chichester, UK, 1984, Ellis Horwood Limited.

40. Westgard JO, Hunt MR: Use and interpretation of common statistical tests in method-comparison studies, *Clin Chem* 19:49, 1973.

41. American Society for Testing and Materials: *ASTM Standard E178-68: standard recommended practice for dealing with outlying observations*, Philadelphia, 1968, ASTM.

42. Waakers PJM et al: Applications of statistics in clinical chemistry: a critical evaluation of regression lines, *Clin Chem Acta* 64:173, 1975.

43. Cornbleet PJ, Gochman N: Incorrect least-squares regression coefficients in method-comparison analysis, *Clin Chem* 25:432, 1979.

44. Passing H, Bablock W: Comparison of several regression procedures for method comparison studies and determination of sample sizes, *J Clin Chem Clin Biochem* 22:431, 1984.

45. Westgard JO: *Six sigma quality design and control*, Madison, WI, 2001, Westgard QC.

46. Westgard JO, Carey RN, Wold S: Criteria for judging precision and accuracy in method development and evaluation, *Clin Chem* 20:825, 1974.

47. Natrella MG: *Experimental statistics*, National Bureau of Standards Handbook 91, Washington, DC, 1963, US Government Printing Office; also published by Wiley & Sons, 1966.

48. Krouwer J: A multifactor experimental design for evaluating random access analyzers, *Clin Chem* 34:1984, 1988.

Internet Sites

www.westgard.com
www.dgrhoads.com
www.krouwerconsulting.com
www.asq.org
www.nccls.org

www.access.gpo.gov—Use this site for the latest updates to Code of Federal Regulations (CFR) information
www.fda.gov
www.cms.gov

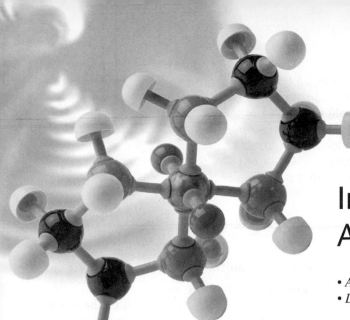

CHAPTER 23

Interferences in Chemical Analysis

• *Amadeo J. Pesce*
• *Lawrence A. Kaplan*

Chapter Outline

Limitations of detectors
  Absorption spectrophotometer
  Fluorescence spectrophotometer
In vitro interferences
  Spectral interferences
  Correction of spectral interferences
  Chemical interferences
  Correction of chemical interferences

  Chromatographic interferences
  Immunochemical interferences
In vivo interferences
  Drugs
Source-reference material
  Evaluation of analytical interference
  Allowable interference

Objectives

• To understand how the accuracy of analytical results are minimized by reducing errors from interferents in instrumentation, methodology, and sample.

• To be aware of limitations to analytical accuracy.
• To be able to determine and recognize allowable levels of laboratory data inaccuracy.

Key Terms

Allen correction Multichromatic analysis of a reaction to correct for background absorbance. Two wavelengths, in addition to the A_{max} (maximum absorption) of the chromophore, are monitored to subtract average background absorbance.

bichromatic analysis Spectrophotometric monitoring of a reaction at two wavelengths. Used to correct for background color.

chemical interferent A compound that either produces an endogenous color or interferes directly in the reaction or process being monitored.

DLIF Digoxin-like immunoreactive factor. An endogenous substance that cross-reacts with antibody to digoxin.

end-point analysis Monitoring of a reaction after it has been essentially completed.

HAMA Human antimouse antibody found in serum of individuals.

hemolysis Breakage of red blood cells, either in vitro or in vivo. Hemolysis will give a plasma specimen a red color.

icteria Pertaining to the orange color imparted to a sample because of the presence of bilirubin.

interferent Any chemical or physical phenomenon that can interfere in or disrupt a reaction or process.

in vitro interferent An interferent that is not caused by any in situ physiological process. Also called *exogenous interferent.*

in vivo interferent An interfering process resulting from physiological processes within the body. Also called *endogenous interferent.*

kinetic analysis Analysis in which the *change* of the

monitored parameter with time is related to concentration, such as change of absorbance per minute. Measurements are made very early in the reaction period.

lipemia   Presence of lipid particles (usually very-low-density lipoprotein) in a sample, which gives the sample a turbid appearance.

reagent blank   Reaction mixture *minus* the sample;

used to subtract endogenous reagent color from the absorbance of the complete reaction (plus sample).

sample blank   Sample plus diluent; used to correct absorbance of complete reaction mixture for endogenous sample color.

turbidity   Scatter of light in a liquid containing suspended particles.

A chemistry laboratory uses many techniques for measuring the concentration of specific biochemicals. All these techniques are subject to interferences from a variety of sources. Specific interferences that affect one technique may not be important for another. There are, however, general concepts that, when understood, help to control and minimize the effects of interferences on method accuracy and precision.

Four basic types of interferences may occur in laboratory analysis: (1) those that arise from limitations of detectors; (2) chemical substances in the sample that directly interfere with the analytical method; (3) disease states or exogenous agents that modify certain physiological processes, thus changing the concentrations of an analyte in vivo; and (4) those that occur as a result of sample (blood) processing.

LIMITATIONS OF DETECTORS

Methods yielding quantitative answers usually employ a detector, such as a spectrophotometer. It is then possible to obtain a relationship between the detector response and the concentrations of analytes in various samples. In the case of absorption spectrophotometry, there is a complex logarithmic relationship between concentration and detector response (see Chapter 4). When fluorescence is used, a linear relationship exists between concentration and the fluorescence signal. Similarly, when other optical properties, such as refractive index, or electrochemical properties, such as ion current from oxidation, are used by detectors, the response is also linear. Knowledge of the type of relationship that exists between concentration and detector response is important.

The first section describes errors in absorption spectrophotometry. Because this is the technique by which the clinical chemistry laboratory quantifies most of its analytes, it is extremely important to understand the interference problems associated with this mode of measurement. As the nature and sophistication of the laboratory change, other types of interferences will become important to consider when performing a laboratory analysis.

Absorption Spectrophotometer

Two interrelated types of error may occur in spectrophotometric measurement. The first is caused by the nature of the mathematical relationship between absorbency and percentage of transmittance, and the second is related to limitations of the instrument.

Absorbance variance. As discussed in Chapter 4, there is a logarithmic relationship between the percentage of transmittance (%T), which is the quantity actually measured, and the absorbance (A), which is calculated. Fig. 23-1 shows the relationship between the linear percentage of transmittance and the log absorbance scales. At very low percentages of transmittances, small changes in the percentage of transmittance result in large changes in absorbance. For example, a change in percentage of transmittance of 60% to 50% T produces only a small absorbance change of approximately 0.08 A. A change in percent transmittance from 15% to 5%, however, results in a change of absorbance of 0.65 A. Thus small changes of percent T at very low transmittances will result in disproportionately large changes in the calculated absorbance at this part of the scale and will lead to an increased error of analysis.

One can consider the error of a spectrophotometric measurement as a function of the total or full-scale deflection of the detection meter or its electronics. When the absorbance scale is set at 0.000 or the transmittance scale is adjusted to 100%, the maximum electronic signal is obtained. For error analysis, the variation in this measurement is presumed to be constant throughout all readings on the scale. Because percent T directly reflects the electrical signal, some simple calculations using percent T can be done. At full-scale deflection (100% T), a 1% variation in percent T means an error of ±1% T. At half scale, a 1% variation of the 50% T value means a 2% absolute error (1/50), and at 10% T, this becomes a 10% error (1/10). However, it is not percent T that is directly proportional to concentration; it is absorbance. One can convert these percent T values into absorbance and calculate the error (Table 23-1).

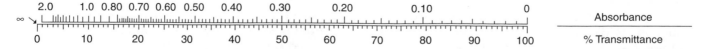

Fig. 23-1   Absorbance and percentage of transmittance scales juxtaposed.

TABLE 23-1 ABSORBANCE ERROR AS A FUNCTION OF PERCENTAGE OF TRANSMITTANCE

%T and Error	Absorbance	Variation in Absorbance	Percent Error of Absorbance Measurement
4 ± 1	1.398	0.22	15.8
10 ± 1	1.000	0.041	8.60
25 ± 1	0.602	0.035	5.79
35 ± 1	0.456	0.025	5.44
50 ± 1	0.301	0.017	5.78
70 ± 1	0.155	0.012	8.03
90 ± 1	0.046	0.0097	21.2

Because the conversion of percent T to absorbance is a logarithmic function, both ends of the scale, 0.000 absorbance and high absorbance (more than 1.0), have the greatest error. In simple terms, when the solution has little color, it is difficult to tell the difference between no color and some color. The relative error can be huge because this difference is so small. At high absorbances, it is not easy to record accurately a small amount of light passing through the solution. Thus differences between the two values are minute compared with the total incident light used to calibrate 100% T, and it is difficult to measure these small changes.

The relative error of spectrophotometric measurements versus percentage of transmittance and absorbance is shown in Fig. 23-2. One should make most spectrophotometric measurements at absorbances between 0.1 and 1.1 to minimize this type of error.

Instrument limitations. Consider how a spectrophotometer functions. At 100% T, or zero absorbance, the entire light signal is converted to an electronic signal. Assume that this signal measures 1000 nanoamps (nA). If the absorbance changes by 0.010, there is a decrease to 990 nA, and the instrument must measure accurately 10/1000 nA, or a 1% change in signal. To do this accurately (1%), the instrument must measure the signal to ±0.10 nA (1% of 10). Thus at zero absorbance there is the difficulty of accurate measurement of one part in 10^4 of signal. In contrast, if the absorbance is 2.0, the signal to the photomultiplier is only 10 nA because only 1% of the light reaches the photodetector. To achieve the same degree of accuracy between a value of absorbance of 2.00 and 2.02, the instrument must measure the difference between 10 and 9.9 nA, or 0.1 nA.; the signal must be measured accurately to within 0.001 nA (1% of 0.1). Thus at high absorbances the limitations are caused by the inability of the detection system to measure small differences between high levels of absorbance accurately.

Thus in analyses with relatively high levels of absorbing compound or **interferent**, a large spectrophotometric error occurs. An initial dilution to lower total absorption *in addition to* a **sample blank** may be needed to eliminate this

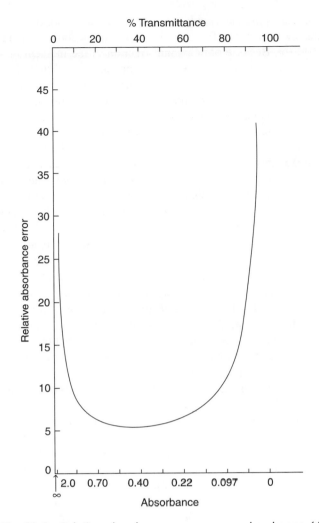

Fig. 23-2 Relative absorbance error versus absorbance (*A*) and percentage transmittance (%*T*) for a ±1% error in measurement of transmitted light. Relative error is minimum at 36.8% T, and A is 0.434.

problem (see the discussion of **turbidity** on pp. 430-431 for an example).

Fluorescence Spectrophotometer

Fluorescence measurements are different from those of transmission spectrophotometry in that the intensity of the fluorescence signal is linearly related to concentration. A doubling of the fluorescence signal is indicative of a twofold increase in concentration. However, this is true only if there is very little light absorbed by the sample. If a significant portion of the light passing through a fluorescence sample is absorbed, the relationship is no longer linear; it becomes a more complex mathematical function. Thus, to minimize error, fluorescence analysis should be performed with relatively dilute solutions, the absorbance of which is less than 0.1.

Scattering of light or the presence of stray light has pronounced effects on fluorescence measurements. If the sample scatters light, some may be observed by the detector as fluorescence. Similarly, if there is *stray light* (i.e., the light used to excite the sample was not pure, that is, not of a very narrow color band), this also may be recorded by the detector. Because only a small fraction of the incident light (less than 1% and often less than one part in a million of the total light input into the instrument) is detected as fluorescence, these extraneous signals have a disproportionate effect on the reading and thus on the error.

Fluorescence measurements, like absorption measurements, can be inaccurate or invalid because of high signals. Unlike absorption spectrophotometry, this usually occurs because of the blanking system. If the fluorometer is adjusted to read zero for the blank, the entire detector sensitivity is adjusted for this zero reading. Assume that there is a blank solution which the instrument records as 10 units on its most sensitive scale. The instrument is now set to read zero fluorescence units. If the instrument can record accurately this zero unit to ±1 unit and if it can also measure a full scale of 100 units in the same way, it can accurately measure a signal of 100 ±1 units. If a different blank solution is used and this is recorded as 100 units, this value can be set at zero by use of an electronic manipulation (subtraction of the signal). At this new full-scale deflection of 100, the detector is really recording 200, of which 100 is subtracted as the blank. Because the instrument is accurate to 1%, it is now accurate to 1% of the new full scale of 200 units. The inaccuracy of measurement is now ±2 units. The accuracy is therefore twice as poor as that for the first example. Similarly, if a blank records as 1000, the accuracy is one tenth as great. Therefore the blank limits the accuracy of fluorescence measurements.

This same line of argument applies to other linear measurements, such as in electrochemical analysis. The background can be blanked, but this must be considered in relation to the total signal.

IN VITRO INTERFERENCES

In vitro interferences arise from the fact that biochemical analyses are performed in the complex matrices that make up biological fluids (serum, plasma, urine, cerebrospinal fluid, and so on). These fluids contain hundreds of compounds that have chemical groups capable either of reacting to some extent with the test reagents or mimicking the physical, chromatographic, or spectral properties of the desired analyte. This situation is further complicated because the chemical composition of body fluids can vary with the nature and extent of disease processes. This variability is increased by the possible presence of a large number of drugs. Each of these factors, alone or in combination, can result in a possible interference.

The **in vitro interferents** can be subclassified into those of a spectral nature and those caused by competing chemical reactions. The most commonly observed interferences are **hemolysis**, **icteria**, and **lipemia**. From one fourth to one third of samples obtained from clinic patients[1] or hospitalized patients[2] are lipemic, icteric, or hemolyzed. A compendium listing the degree of interference by hemolysis, icterus, and lipemia on the analysis of 21 analytes on 22 different instruments is available.[3]

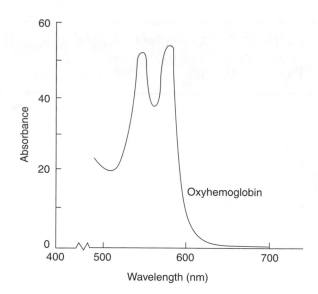

Fig. 23-3　Partial spectrum of oxyhemoglobin (HbO_2).

Spectral Interferences

Absorbance. Spectral interferences are observed when a compound causes a response in the spectrophotometer similar to that of the analyte of interest, though the interferents themselves do not necessarily undergo any chemical change during the analytical reaction. The simplest and most common example is the effect of hemoglobin (Hb) on many analytical procedures. A partial spectrum of HbO_2 (Fig. 23-3) shows significant absorption in the 500 to 600 nm portion of the visible spectrum. If the reaction of a colorimetric procedure in this region of the visible spectrum were being monitored, a significant positive interference would occur whenever Hb contaminated the specimen. Other molecules, such as bilirubin, cause a similar interference.

An example of hemoglobin interference can be seen when a serum total protein (TP) concentration is determined by monitoring the biuret reaction at 540 nm. A standard curve for this reaction is depicted in Fig. 23-4. If a significant concentration of hemoglobin is added to a sample, the absorption at 540 nm is increased, thus giving a falsely high total protein reading. In this example, the A_{540} of a 50 g/L standard is 0.550. If small amounts of hemoglobin are added to this standard, the A_{540} is 0.650. When this solution is read from the standard curve, a higher apparent concentration of protein is calculated (*dotted line*). Most spectral interferences give falsely elevated results in this manner.

Turbidity. A common type of spectral interference is caused by the turbidity of the sample. Turbidity is caused by large lipoprotein molecules called very-low-density lipoproteins (VLDL), which are suspended in serum. When a turbid specimen is analyzed in a colorimetric reaction, the lipoproteins cause the incident light to scatter, much as in nephelometry (see Chapter 4).

Because spectrophotometric analysis normally measures transmitted light at 180 degrees to the incident light, any light scattering tends to decrease the transmitted light and

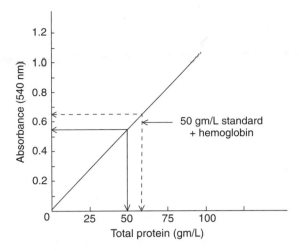

Fig. 23-4 Standard curve for measurement of total protein by the biuret reaction: A_{540} versus concentrations: *Solid arrow*, A_{540} for 50 gm/L standard; *dotted arrow*, A_{540} for same standard containing hemoglobin.

therefore to increase the apparent absorbance of the specimen. This, of course, results in falsely elevated results. Sample blanks normally work poorly here, just as two-point **kinetic analysis** does (see below), because of the error resulting from the very high absorbances often encountered. The best method for eliminating the interference caused by turbidity is dilution of the specimen. The extent to which the sample can be diluted to minimize turbidimetric interference is limited by the ability of the analytic procedure to measure the diluted analyte. If possible, several dilutions should be analyzed simultaneously to determine the best response. An example of the effect and elimination of turbidometric interference is presented in the analysis of equal amounts of lactate dehydrogenase (LD) activity in a turbid and a nonturbid specimen (Table 23-2). When the nonturbid specimen is diluted, all the corrected LD activities calculate out to the same approximate value. This indicates linearity of dilution. In contrast, when the turbid specimen is diluted, the calculated LD activity changes with dilution. Only at higher dilutions containing minimum turbidity do the calculated LD

activities converge with the true values of the nonturbid specimen.

Fluorescence. Turbidity affects fluorescence measurements in a similar fashion. Here, some scattered light will reach the detector set at 90 degrees to the incident light, thus giving an apparent increase in fluorescence and falsely elevated concentrations. Reducing problems of turbidity in fluorescence measurements is more difficult than for absorption spectroscopy. The best approach is the elimination of the source of light scattering by filtration or centrifugation.

Correction of Spectral Interferences

Sample blank. One can minimize spectral interferences by measuring the absorbance of the assay against a sample blank. The simplest sample blank is obtained by a mixture of the sample and diluent (instead of reagent). The correction for spectral interference is made by subtracting the absorbance value of the blank from the absorbance of the complete reaction mixture. Any significant color inherent to the sample is eliminated by this calculation. In the example of the biuret reaction discussed previously, the absorbance of the sample and the hemoglobin diluted with saline is 0.100. If this is subtracted from the absorbance of the complete reaction mixture (0.650), the true absorbance of the standard (0.550) is obtained. Such a sample blank can usually work unless there are gross amounts of the interferent present. In these cases, the very large total absorption ($A_{interferent}$ + $A_{reaction}$) results in large spectrophotometric and calculation errors. Random access analyses (see Chapter 16) easily permit the measurement of sample blank absorbances before the addition of reagent. **Reagent blanks** (reagent plus diluent) are used in a similar fashion to correct for high absorbance of the reagent. In the case of fluorescence, the sample blank allows for the correction of nonspecific fluorescence; however, the fluorescence of this blank cannot be a great portion of the total fluorescence signal (see preceding text).

Kinetic measurements. One frequently used method for the correction of spectral interference is the measurement of a typical end-point reaction as a two-point kinetic reaction. If the absorbance of a noninstantaneous, colori-

TABLE 23-2   EFFECT OF TURBIDITY ON MEASUREMENT OF LD ACTIVITY (U/L)

Dilution (with Saline)	LD ACTIVITY (U/L)			
	NONTURBID SAMPLE		TURBID SAMPLE	
	Uncorrected	*Corrected*	*Uncorrected*	*Corrected*
Undiluted	440	—	28	—
1:2	245	450	32	64
1:4	136	444	30	120
1:8	62	496	26	208
1:16	30	480	25	400
1:32	14	450	13	416

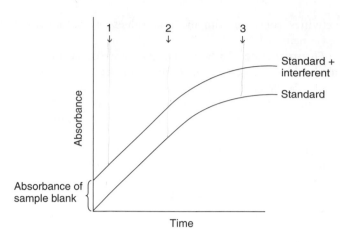

Fig. 23-5 Absorbance changes versus time for colorimetric reaction, with and without interferent present. *Arrows 1 and 2,* time frame for kinetic analysis; *arrow 3,* end-point reading.

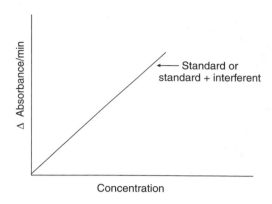

Fig. 23-6 Kinetic analysis of both reactions shown in Fig. 23-5. Change in absorbance per minute versus concentration during linear portion of curve of absorbance versus time between arrows 1 and 2 in Fig. 23-5.

metric reaction is monitored versus time, a reaction curve as shown in Fig. 23-5 will be observed. An **end-point analytical** reaction is monitored at a single time point when the reaction is mostly completed (Fig. 23-5, arrow 3). If no spectral interferences are present, the reaction curve should pass through the origin. If such interferences are present, the curve will be *parallel* to the original curve but biased high because of the endogenous color in the sample. If a sample blank was used to subtract endogenous color, a line identical to the sample containing no interferences would be obtained.

In a two-point kinetic assay, the absorbance is measured at *two* different time points (Fig. 23-5, arrows 1 and 2) when (1) the final color development has not occurred and in fact may be small and (2) the response of absorbance versus time response is still linear.

The initial absorbance reading (Fig. 23-5, arrow 1) is actually taken when almost no color formation has occurred. Thus any absorbance at this time is primarily caused by endogenous spectral interferents. A second reading is taken a short time later, when only a small amount of color has formed and the response of absorbance versus time is still linear (Fig. 23-5, arrow 2). This absorbance therefore includes both the original endogenous color and the color formed because of the specific analytical reaction. By subtraction of the first reading from the second, the calculated *delta absorbance* (ΔA) is caused only by the specific color formed by the analytical reaction. Standard curves based on kinetic analysis have the change in absorbance (ΔA) plotted versus concentration (Fig. 23-6). In this standard curve the presence of a *nonreacting,* endogenous, colored interferent has no effect. Thus no separate sample blank measurement is necessary; a two-point kinetic reaction is self-blanking when there is no change in the nature of the interferent during the reaction. This technique plays an important part in performing automated chemical analysis on large numbers of specimens.

Biochromatic analysis.[4] Many currently used instruments employ a spectral interferent correction technique that

involves measurement of the absorbance of the reaction mixture simultaneously at two different wavelengths. These are the primary wavelength (λ_1) and one other wavelength (λ_2) close by. As shown in Fig. 23-7, λ_1 is the wavelength at which the chromogen maximally absorbs. At λ_2 there is minimum absorbance of the chromogen. Because the reaction is monitored simultaneously at two wavelengths, this is known as *bichromatic analysis.* This technique is based on the premise that although a compound may give a spectral interference, the absorbance maxima of the interferent will differ from that of the actual analytical reaction. In addition, this analysis is made under the assumption that the absorption caused by the interfering compound is approximately the same at λ_1 as at λ_2. Although the measured absorbance at λ_1 will be caused by both the analytical reaction and the interferent, the absorbance at the second wavelength (λ_2) will be caused by only the interferent. This technique can also correct for instrument problems such as dirt on the cell, which causes light scattering or reflectance. Standard curves are then based on either $A_1 - A_2$ or the ratio of the two absorbances (A_1/A_2). Use of this procedure also allows each sample to serve as its own blank for endogenous color.

Another similar method for the correction of background interference is the measurement of absorbance at the primary wavelength A_{max} and at two additional wavelengths, usually equidistant from the peak, A_1 and A_2. The absorbance readings at these last two wavelengths are averaged to give the average background absorbance in the specimen. This technique for the correction of background absorbance from interfering substances is known as the **Allen correction.**[5]

The Allen correction is valid only if the background absorbance is approximately linear with wavelength over the region in which the measurements are being taken. Thus the shape of the absorption curve for both the analyte and the interferent (*solid line*) and the interferent or interferents (*dotted line*) must be obtained as shown in Fig. 23-8. Use of the Allen correction in this example, when the wavelengths

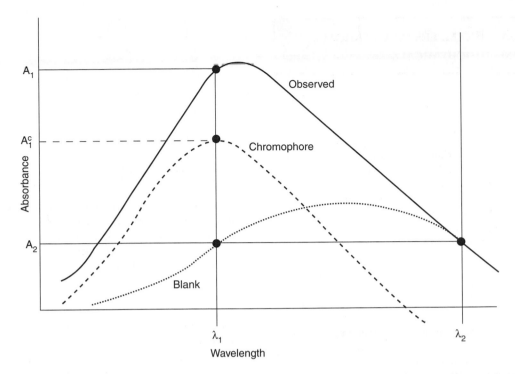

Fig. 23-7   Spectral curves for chromophore and nonreactive blank, where blank absorbance is equal at λ_1 and λ_2.

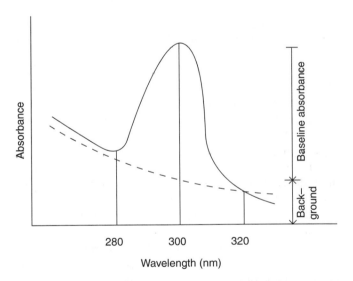

Fig. 23-8   Spectral curves of chromophore and interferent, *solid line*, and background interferents, *dotted line*. Average of A_{280} and A_{320} represents background absorbance at A_{max} for chromophore (300 nm).

used to correct for background are equidistant from the absorbance maxima, would result in the following equation:

$$A_{300} \text{ corrected} = A_{300} - \frac{A_{320} + A_{280}}{2} \qquad \textit{Eq. 23-1}$$

The "A_{300} corrected" has the average background absorbance subtracted from the absorbance maximum to give the actual absorbance above base-line value. The Allen correction is widely used, but improper use of the Allen correction, that is, with nonlinear background interference, can lead to even larger errors. Because the final corrected absorbance is based on three measurements, there is a decrease in the precision of the assay.

Dilution. As discussed for turbidity, dilution of a sample containing a spectral interferent can sometimes reduce the problem. One must be careful not to overdilute the desired analyte or chromogen to a concentration below the minimum detectable level for a given assay. Several dilutions should be assayed simultaneously to determine the most effective dilution.

Instrument indices. A number of automated chemistry analyzers have replaced visual inspection of patent samples for spectral interferences with automated semiquantitative spectral analysis. This method gives three indices, one each for hemoglobin, bilirubin, and turbidity.[6] The operator is alerted to the extent of each interferent and may choose to dilute the sample or inform the physician about the problem.

Chemical Interferences

All the interferences discussed so far have been spectral interferences caused by compounds that do not react in the analytical chemical reaction. However, many interferents do react with the chemicals of the analytical reaction. The reaction products of these interferences usually result in positive interferences, though negative interferences are observed.

The types of nonspecific, chemically reacting interferents can vary greatly, as seen in the examples in Table 23-3. Uric acid produces a positive interference, and bilirubin and ascorbic acid yield negative interferences in the glucose

TABLE 23-3 EXAMPLES OF CHEMICALLY INTERFERING BIOCHEMICALS

Analyte	Method	Interferences
Glucose	Reducing sugar	Uric acid (+), creatinine (+), protein (+), glutathione (+)
	Glucose oxidase— horseradish peroxidase	Uric acid (+), ascorbic acid (−), bilirubin (−)
	Glucose oxidase— O_2 consumption	Hemoglobin (−), ascorbic acid (+)
	Hexokinase	Fructose
Creatinine	Alkaline picrate	Ascorbic acid (+), glucose (+), protein (+), ketones (+)
Vanillylmandelic acid	Pisano	Certain foods (such as bananas), vanilla, aspirin (+)
	High-performance liquid chromatography	Certain drugs and their metabolites (+)

+, Positive interference; −, negative interference.

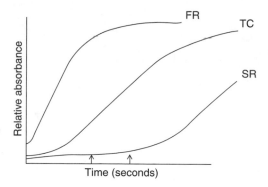

Fig. 23-9 Relative absorbance versus time curves for alkaline picrate reaction, for creatinine (*TC*), slow-reacting interferents (*SR*), and fast-reacting interferents (*FR*). *Arrows*, time during which absorbance, over time, primarily reflects change attributable to the TC reaction.

oxidase methods used for glucose measurement. The alkaline picrate reaction for the measurement of creatinine is known to have both positive (ketones, protein) and negative (bilirubin) interferences. Remember that these types of interference are functions of the concentration of the interferent, which itself is dependent on the extent of the pathophysiological process. Thus, testing for interference using healthy serum will often render far different results compared with using sera from a patient with liver failure.

Correction of Chemical Interferences

Elimination of many nonspecific **chemical interferents** is often achieved by one or more of the following techniques:

1. Diluting the interferent
2. Increasing the specificity of the reaction
3. Removing the interferent
4. Monitoring an assay by kinetic measurement
5. Monitoring an assay by bichromatic measurement

Dilution of the sample is an effective method in the case of interferents that do not react at the same rate or produce the same color intensity as the analyte. Interference by protein is minimized in many automated analyzers by a large specimen dilution.

Increased specificity of an analytic reaction is often achieved by use of specific enzymes as reagents. Examples of this approach include the measurement of glucose by hexokinase or glucose oxidase, uric acid by uricase, and urea by urease. Immunochemical-based reactions are also used to increase the specificity of the analysis. An example would be the measurement of theophylline by enzyme immunoassay

versus the older methods, which employed ultraviolet absorbance.

Separation of an interferent from the analyte may be achieved by the use of (1) a protein-free sample, (2) liquid-liquid extraction, or (3) adsorption or partition chromatography. Protein-free samples were originally prepared by precipitation of serum proteins and separation of the protein-free sample by filtration or centrifugation. Agents used to precipitate proteins include tungstic acid (Folin-Wu procedure) and heavy-metal salts (such as barium and zinc; Somogyi-Nelson procedure). Protein-free specimens obtained by the dialysis technique were the basis of many Technicon Auto-Analyzer procedures.

Liquid-liquid extractions are used when the analyte and interferent or interferents can be separated into different liquid phases. Similarly, in adsorption and partition chromatography, the analyte and interferent are separated by their differential affinity for the stationary phase (see Chapters 5 to 7).

The basis for the elimination of nonspecific chemical reactants by use of a two-point kinetic reaction is the fact that many interferents react at a rate different from the one at which the specific analyte of interest reacts. This is observed in the example of the Jaffe reaction with creatinine.[7]

Creatinine reacts with alkaline picrate at a finite rate (curve TC, true creatinine) (Fig. 23-9). Many of the nonspecific interferents (such as acetone) react at a faster kinetic rate (FR), whereas some (such as protein) react at a slower rate (SR), giving a complex change of absorbance with time for the reaction of a mixture of all three species (Fig. 23-10). Therefore, by properly choosing an optimal window of time for the two absorbance readings for the kinetic analysis (*arrows*, Fig. 23-9), you can minimize the effect of the fast-reacting and slow-reacting nonspecific interferents and isolate the absorbance change caused primarily by creatinine. During the window of time, the reaction of the FR interferents is essentially complete, whereas that of the SR interferents is not yet occurring (Fig. 23-10). The ΔA during

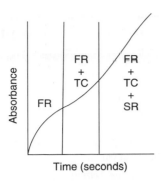

Fig. 23-10 Complex reaction of mixture containing fast-reacting (*FR*) and slow-reacting (*SR*) interferents plus creatinine (*TC*). Only by measurement of the change in absorbance over time can TC reaction be isolated and SR and FR interferences minimized.

this time is caused by the analyte, that is, creatinine. This concept has also been used for the glucose oxidase reaction and is, in fact, a popular technique for increasing the specificity of reactions in many instruments.

Chromatographic Interferences

The third type of common in vitro, or methodological, interference is chromatographic interference. This often occurs when an interfering compound cochromatographs with the compound of interest to give falsely elevated results.

Currently, many analytical procedures use chromatography to separate the analyte to be measured from interfering compounds. A chromatographic method is made under the assumption that the desired analyte is completely isolated from other compounds that may be recorded by the detection system. However, no single set of chromatography conditions can possibly prevent interferences from cochromatographing or closely chromatographing compounds, especially when the patient may be receiving several potentially interfering drugs.

An example of this type of interference and its correction can be seen in the high-performance liquid chromatographic (HPLC) separation of catecholamines and the drug methyldopa (Aldomet), which is used in the treatment of hypertension. In some HPLC assays, methyldopa is eluted from the column just before norepinephrine. Because the pharmacological dose of Aldomet is much greater than the physiological concentrations of norepinephrine, it will obliterate or be confused with the norepinephrine peak. The only way to eliminate this type of interference is to remove the source of exogenous interferent. In the case of methyldopa, removal of the drug from the patient for 2 to 10 days is required. Drug or diet restrictions before biochemical analysis are often a necessity for many compounds.

Two primary modes are used to minimize chromatographic interferents: (1) increasing the specificity of the detector and (2) removing the interferent from the analyte. Detectors can measure compounds based on a variety of principles. If the interferent has physical or chemical properties different from those of the analyte, it is possible to select a detector that will not respond significantly to a potential interferent. In liquid chromatography, refractive index detectors can detect almost any compound in the eluant; thus they are very nonspecific. Fluorescence detectors have much higher specificities because not all compounds fluoresce. By appropriate setting of excitation and emission wavelengths, the detector becomes even more specific. Electrochemical detectors also have high specificities because not all compounds are electrochemically active. The specificity can be further increased by selection of an electrode voltage at which the interferent will not react.

As discussed earlier, separation of the analytes from potentially interfering compounds is achieved by several techniques, based on differences in solubility or chromatographic behavior between the analyte and interferents. The techniques commonly used are single liquid-liquid extractions, multiple extractions including back-extractions, and adsorption and ion-exchange chromatography. The complexity of the procedure used depends on the nature of the interference and required sensitivity. HPLC methods for serum theophylline, present in relatively large amounts, usually employ only a simple liquid-liquid extraction. In contrast, the HPLC analysis of the tricyclic antidepressants present in nanogram quantities requires several extraction steps, including back-extractions. Chapter 5 discusses these types of procedures in more detail.

A technique for detecting contaminating or cochromatographing compounds is dual-detection analysis, which uses two different types of detectors or parameters, such as multiple wavelengths, to monitor the column eluate. The response of the two different detectors (D_1 and D_2) is determined for a standard, and the ratio of the responses is calculated (D_1 standard/D_2 standard). The probability that another compound would have a similar characteristic ratio is quite small. Thus significant deviations of the ratio found in patient analyses are strongly suggestive that the analyte peak contains a contaminating, coeluting compound.

Often the presence of a cochromatographing interferent is recognized because of the abnormal shape of the peak. The presence of a contaminant often causes a normally symmetric peak to be skewed. In these cases, rerunning the chromatogram at lower flow rates will sometimes separate or partially separate the analyte from the interfering compound, allowing quantitation.

Immunochemical Interferences

Immunochemical methods are subject to the usual causes of exogenous interference (see box at top left of p. 436).[8] In addition, however, they are subject to matrix effects of the reaction solution and, in some cases, the surface where the reaction is occurring. Hyperlipidemia can greatly affect immunochemical reactions that use turbiditometric or nephelometric measurements because of the increased sample turbidity. The most difficult interference to detect is that in which the patient has antibodies to the test reagent antibodies (heterophile antibodies) or to the actual test

INTERFERENCES COMMON TO IMMUNOASSAYS

Exogenous Interferences
- Sample collection and preparation, including anticoagulants, sample storage, drugs, and serum-separating gels
- Calibration matrix
- Changes in solid-phase surface binding caused by coating molecule
- Incomplete saturation of solid-phase binding sites for antigen or antibody

Endogenous Interferences
- Hyperlipidemia—turbidity
- Heterophilic anti-immunoglobulin antibodies (HAMAs)
- Iatrogenic antibodies, such as Digabind [see Methods on CD-ROM]
- Rheumatoid factor
- Autoantibodies against analyte
- Complement
- Cross-reacting substance, such as DLIF
- Competing immunospecific antibodies to analyte

DLIF, Digoxin-like immunoreactive factor; HAMAs, human antimouse antibodies. Modified from Pesce AJ, Michael JG: Artifacts and limitations of enzyme immunoassay, J Immunol Methods *150:111, 1992.*

INTERFERENCES FOR ENZYME IMMUNOASSAYS

Exogenous Interference
- Enzyme inhibitor

Endogenous Interferences
- Endogenous enzyme
- Endogenous substrate
- Spectral: lipids, hemoglobin
- Drugs that inhibit enzyme activity

Measurement of Enzyme Activity
- Temperature
- Substrate reaction on solid phase
- Nonlinear kinetics
- Limited sensitivity
- Substrate depletion

Modified from Pesce AJ, Michael JG: Artifacts and limitations of enzyme immunoassay, J Immunol Methods *150:111, 1992.*

antigen. The most frequently encountered heterophile antibodies, those against mouse antibodies (**HAMA**s), can cause interference in assays using mouse monoclonal antibodies. Methods for reducing these interferents include adding specific animal sera, such as mouse serum, to the test reagent to combine with the heterophile antibodies and neutralize them.[9] Often the only indication that the patient has antibodies to the test analyte is the patient history, which can indicate that the test results are not consistent with the clinical findings. An interesting example of the problem of endogenous antibodies can be seen in the measurement of digoxin. In acute digoxin overdoses, the patient may be treated with Digibind, an Fc fragment of IgG antibodies to digoxin that binds digoxin, minimizes toxicity, and increases clearance. Digabind will also react with labeled digoxin in an immunoassay and cause apparently highly elevated digoxin levels.

For enzyme immunoassays, some of the interferences are the same as those observed in ordinary enzyme assays, as shown in the box at right.

IN VIVO INTERFERENCES

Factors such as age and sex, time of day, diet, pregnancy and menses, as well as sample-processing errors can affect the test result. These **in vivo interferents** are discussed in Chapter 3. The presence of drugs in the patient is a common source of interference.

Drugs

Virtually every drug affects some laboratory procedure, and any laboratory procedure may be affected by one or more drugs. The interference may be either in vivo or in vitro. An example of a commonly encountered drug is alcohol, whose ingestion may affect glucose, lactate, urate, bicarbonate, γ-glutaryltransferase, and creatine phosphokinase levels.[10] Smoking may alter catecholamine, cortisol, and blood-gas results. Reference to source material is needed to determine the effect of any one of the vast number of drugs on a specific test.

SOURCE-REFERENCE MATERIAL

This chapter provides only a brief description of the wide variety and types of interferences in chemistry laboratory testing. Many common interfering substances are well documented, and an alert laboratory staff can often eliminate these as a source of interference. For example, the development of the interferogram[2] allows the laboratory to estimate the effect of hemolysis, icterus, and lipemia on the analyses performed on frequently used instruments. Newer automated chemistry analyzers can be calibrated to detect increased levels of hemolysis, lipemia, and icterus.

However, as the number of drugs produced by pharmaceutical companies and consumed by the public increases, the laboratory must determine both the in vivo and in vitro effects exerted by each of these drugs on clinical laboratory analysis.

A list of the known effects of drugs and other interferences on chemical analysis has been compiled by Donald Young and the American Association for Clinical Chemistry.[11] Because of the constant introduction of new drugs and the lag time for observations of their reported interference effects, this work is not complete; however it remains the best and only single listing of drug effects on laboratory tests. The first of the two major sections of Young's study provides a listing of analytes. Under each analyte is a listing of drugs that may effect its measurement because of analytical or physiological causes. In the second section these effects are cross-indexed by the effect of the drug on the test. Fig. 23-11 shows a section of Young's study in which glucose is the listed test. The figure is a partial listing of the drugs that can cause an increase in serum glucose because of their effect on the analytical method. After each test is the indication of how the tested interferent affects the laboratory test and the concentration at which this effect is observed.

Laboratory Test Listings

Glucose *(continued)*

Serum Increase Analytical

Acetaminophen At 1 mmol/L affects Technicon SMA 12/60 method *5576* At concentrations of 125 µmol/L and above had significant effect on the methods on Bayer Glucometer Elite and BMC Accu-chek Advantage *904* In YSI glucose analyzer with potentiometric measurement of hydrogen peroxide produced. Effect can be quite marked *5042* At concentrations up to 1.30 mmol/L caused significant increase of up to 0.38 mmol/L in whole blood glucose concentration as measured by Medisense Exatech analyzer *5904*

Acetylsalicylic Acid Increase by 11% with 8326 µmol/L on glucose-peroxidase method with 2,4-Dichlorophenol. Increase by 3% with 8326 µmol/L on glucose-peroxidase method with ABTS *2920*

Aminosalicylic Acid At 1 mmol/L affects Technicon SMA 12/60 method *5576* At concentrations above 100 mg/L raised concentration as measured by Kodak Ektachem® method *5704*

Ascorbic Acid At 1 mmol/L affects Technicon SMA 12/60 method *5576* 17.9% increase in absorbance with 1 mmol/L and 11.4% increase with 0.5 mmol/L on glucokinase based assay of Scott *5414* At concentrations above 60 mg/L (maximum serum concentration 34 mg/L) raised concentration as measured by glucose dehydrogenase method *5704* Increases sensitivity of o-toluidine procedures: 1 g/dL equivalent to 3.3 mmol/L with alkaline ferricyanide *3531*

Cefotaxime Statistically significant effect of metabolite on American Monitor Parallel method *320*

Cefuroxime False positive reaction may be given ferricyanide procedures *1693*

Dextran 10 g/dL equivalent to 0.3 mmol/L in alkaline ferricyanide. 10 g/dL equivalent to 0.7 mmol/L in p-HBAH procedure *3531* 10 g/dL equivalent to 6.7 mmol/L with o-toluidine procedure. 10 g/dL equivalent to 0.3 mmol/L with glucose oxidase procedures *3531*

Dextran 40 At concentrations above 10,000 mg/L raised concentration as measured by Kodak Ektachem® method *5704*

Fig. 23-11 Example of format used in *Effects of Drugs on Clinical Laboratory Tests*. (Modified with permission from Young DS, editor: Effects of drugs on clinical laboratory tests, vol 1, ed 5, 2000, AACC Press.)

The complexity and extent of Young's work highlight the awareness laboratory personnel must have concerning interferences with clinical laboratory tests. A complementary volume lists the effects of disease on clinical laboratory tests.[12] The format for this volume is similar to the one just described. The first section lists each analyte and those disease states in which changes in the concentration of that analyte have been noted. The second section lists diseases and those analytes that change during the course of the disease. A third volume in this compilation lists the effects of preanalytical variables on tests.[13]

Evaluation of Analytical Interference

Because virtually all clinical chemistry analytical procedures can experience interference by the factors of preanalytical variation and the patient specimen itself (see Chapter 3), many protocols for evaluating the extent of the potential interference have been proposed.[14-16] Often the testing of spectral interference involves the addition of a lipid substance Intralipid (Kabi Vitrum, Alameda, California), a hemolysate, or bilirubin.[3] A series of graphical representations of these interferences has been compiled by Glick et al.[17] In some cases the test method is compared with a reference or definitive method that is not subject to the interference being evaluated. These techniques include isotope dilution mass spectroscopy, neutron activation, atomic absorption, and other specialized techniques.

Allowable Interference

Because some interference is potentially present for every assay, clinical chemists must determine how much interference is allowable. A statistically significant interferent

may not be a clinically significant one. One approach is to use the medical decision limit.[18] The concept of clinically important errors is reviewed in Chapter 21, and examples of its application are found in Chapter 22. The size of allowable error is determined from consultations with the clinicians who are using the results of the testing and from discussions of allowable error in the literature.

The total analytical error, E_A, of a method is the sum of its imprecision, which equals the sum of twice the standard deviation (2SD), its analytical bias (E_B), and the error resulting from interferents (E_I):

$$E_A = 2SD + E_B + E_I \qquad \textit{Eq. 23-2}$$

For an assay to be clinically useful, the total analytical error, E_A, must be less than the total allowable error at the medical decision level, E_{MDL}, for each analyte. If the laboratory knows the errors SD + E_B and can estimate E_{MDL}, the allowable contribution from an interferent, E_I, can be calculated:

$$E_I = E_{MDL} - 2SD - E_B \qquad \textit{Eq. 23-3}$$

This discussion is made under the assumption that the total allowable error based on medical decision making needs is greater than the total allowable error permitted for CLIA '88 regulated analytes. These calculations can be used to determine the analytical errors permissible under these regulations (see Chapter 21).

In summary, for precise assays with small standard deviations and large changes before the medical decision value is reached, larger errors caused by interferences can be tolerated. In contrast, some measurements, such as creatinine in transplant patients, have a small allowable error (often less than 20%), which must include bias, method variability, and interference. Thus, in these methods there is less tolerance to interference.

References

1. Glick MR: *Ohio Valley Section Meeting on "Interferences,"* Cincinnati, Ohio, Feb 27, 1988.
2. Kaplan LA: *Ohio Valley Section Meeting on "Interferences,"* Cincinnati, Ohio, Feb 27, 1988.
3. Glick MR, Ryder KW: *Interferographs: user's guide to interferences in clinical chemistry instruments*, Indianapolis, 1987, Science Enterprises, Inc.
4. Hahn B et al: Polychromatic analysis: new applications of an old technique, *Clin Chem* 25:951, 1979.
5. Allen E, Rieman W: Determining only one compound in a mixture, short spectrophotometric method, *Anal Chem* 25:1325, 1953.
6. *Boehringer Mannheim Reference Guide Hitachi 917 System*, Indianapolis, 1998, Hitachi.
7. Soldin SJ, Henderson L, Hill JG: The effect of bilirubin and ketones on reaction rate methods for the measurement of creatinine, *Clin Biochem* 11:82, 1978.
8. Pesce AJ, Michael JG: Artifacts and limitations of enzyme immunoassay, *J Immunol Methods* 150:111, 1992.
9. Bjerner J et al: Immunometric assay interferences: incidence and prevention, *Clin Chem* 48:613, 2002.
10. Freer DE, Statland BE: The effect of ethanol (0.75 g/kg body weight) on the activities of selected enzymes in sera of healthy young adults. I. Intermediate-term effect, *Clin Chem* 23:830, 1977.
11. Young DS: *Effects of drugs on clinical laboratory tests*, ed 5, Washington, DC, 2000, American Association for Clinical Chemistry.
12. Young DS, Friedman KB: *Effect of diseases on clinical laboratory tests*, ed 4, Washington, DC, 2001, American Association for Clinical Chemistry.
13. Young DS: *Effects of preanalytic variables on clinical laboratory tests*, ed 2, Washington, DC, 1997, American Association for Clinical Chemistry.
14. Buttner R et al: International Federation of Clinical Chemistry expert panel on nomenclature and principles of quality control in clinical chemistry: approved recommendation (1978). II. Assessment of analytical methods for routine use, *Clin Chim Acta* 98:129F, 1979.
15. Galteaux MM, Siest G: IFCC. Drug effects in clinical chemistry. II. Guidelines for evaluation of an analytical interference, *J Clin Chem Clin Biochem* 22:275, 1984.
16. *Interference testing in clinical chemistry: proposed guideline*, NCCLS Publication EP7-P, Villanova, PA, 1986, National Committee on Clinical Laboratory Standards.
17. Glick MR, Ryder KW, Jackson SA: Graphical comparison of interferences in clinical chemistry instrumentation, *Clin Chem* 32:470, 1986.
18. Castano-Vidriales JL: Interferences in clinical chemistry, *J Int Fed Clin Chem* 6:7, 1994.

Internet Sites

http://www.edie.net/Library/Features/IEI9825.html
http://bashful.ehem.washington.edu/abstracts/Stand-abst.htm

http://courses.chem.ukans.edu/Fall2000/516/LectureNotes/Overview%20Of%20Chemical%20Analysis.htm
http://www.caeal.ca/Simplified%20Uncertainty.pdf

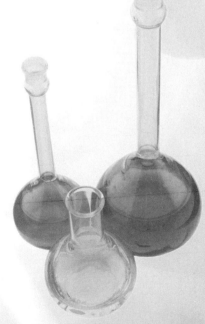

PART II

Pathophysiology

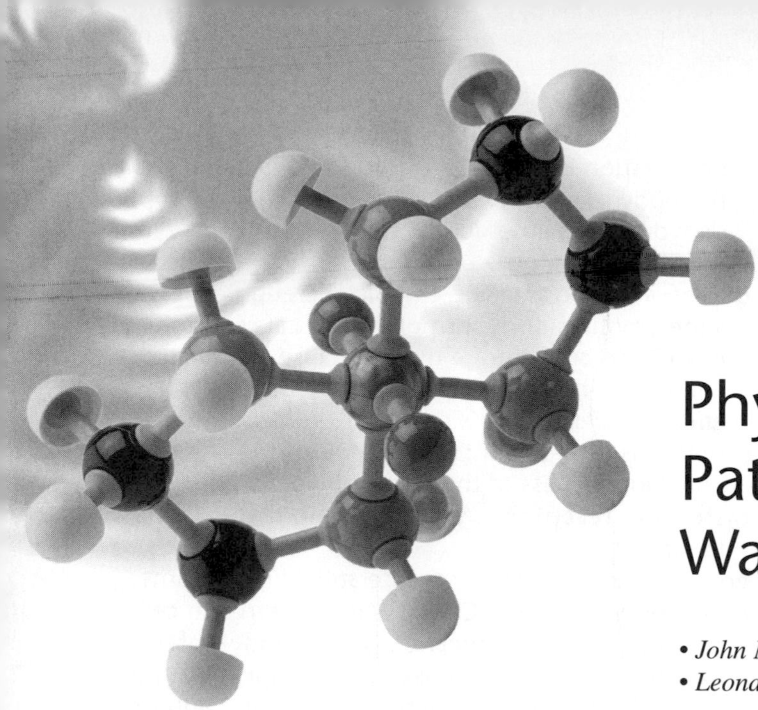

CHAPTER 24

Physiology and Pathophysiology of Body Water and Electrolytes

- *John M. Lorenz*
- *Leonard I. Kleinman*

Chapter Outline

Body water compartments
  Volume of body water compartments
  Maturational changes in body water compartment
    volumes
  Composition of body water compartments
  Osmotic pressure and osmolarity of body fluids
Regulation of body fluid compartment osmolarity and
  volume
  Extracellular compartment
  Plasma and interstitial fluid compartments
  Intracellular compartment
Water metabolism
  Water balance
  Disorders of water imbalance
  Dehydration
  Overhydration

Sodium metabolism
  Sodium balance
  Disorders of sodium balance
  Abnormalities of plasma sodium concentration
Potassium metabolism
  Potassium balance
  Disorders of potassium balance
  Abnormalities of plasma potassium concentration
Chloride metabolism
  Chloride balance
  Disorders of chloride balance
  Abnormalities of plasma chloride concentration
  Urine chloride concentration

Objectives

- List the electrolyte composition of the two main compartments of total body water.
- Define anion gap and state its clinical significance; calculate and interpret anion gap results from given data.
- Outline the homeostatic regulation of sodium, potassium, chloride, and body water.

- Define the various states of decreased or increased plasma electrolyte concentrations in terms of an excess or deficit of water or electrolyte.
- List and briefly describe the symptoms and at least two causes or clinical conditions associated with increased and decreased amounts of electrolytes and body water.

Key Terms

acidosis Abnormally low body fluid pH. **Respiratory acidosis** is caused by an abnormally high Pco_2; **metabolic acidosis** is caused by an abnormally low bicarbonate concentration.

active transport The passage of ions or molecules across a cell membrane by an energy-consuming process. This energy is generated by cellular metabolism.

aldosterone   A mineralocorticoid hormone secreted by the adrenal cortex that influences sodium and potassium metabolism.

alkalosis   Abnormally high body fluid pH. *Respiratory* alkalosis is caused by an abnormally low P_{CO_2}; **metabolic alkalosis** is caused by an abnormally high bicarbonate concentration.

angiotensin   A vasoconstrictive polypeptide produced by the enzymatic action of renin on angiotensinogen. A converting enzyme from the lung removes two C-terminal amino acids from the inactive decapeptide angiotensin I to form the biologically active octapeptide angiotensin II.

angiotensinogen   A serum globulin produced in the liver that is the precursor of angiotensin.

anion   An ion that carries a negative charge.

anorexia   Diminished appetite for food.

antidiuretic hormone   A peptide hormone of the neurohypophysis that acts on the collecting tubule of the kidneys to allow increased water reabsorption and therefore decreased free water excretion by the kidney. Also known as *vasopressin*.

arrhythmia   Irregularity of the heartbeat.

ascites   The accumulation of fluid in the peritoneal cavity.

asphyxia   Interference with oxygen delivery to and carbon dioxide removal from the tissue.

atrial natriuretic peptide (ANP)   A natriuretic peptide hormone secreted primarily by the cardiac atria.

baroreceptor   A nerve ending that responds to change in pressure.

brain natriuretic peptide (BNP)   A natriuretic peptide hormone secreted primarily by the cardiac ventricles.

cation   An ion that carries a positive charge.

cirrhosis   Progressive disease of the liver characterized by damage to hepatic parenchymal cells.

colloid   As used in this chapter, this term applies to the large molecules in the body to which the capillary endothelium and cell membrane are impermeable.

colloid osmotic pressure   The effective osmotic pressure of plasma and interstitial fluid across the capillary endothelium, largely the result of the presence of protein.

C-type natriuretic peptide (CNP)   A natriuretic peptide produced locally in the brain and vascular endothelium.

dehydration   Abnormal decrease in total body water (see Table 24-4). **Hypernatremic** dehydration is a net loss of sodium and water from the body, with net water loss exceeding net sodium loss. **Hyponatremic** dehydration is a net loss of sodium and water from the body, with net sodium loss exceeding net water loss. **Normonatremic**

dehydration is a net loss of sodium and water from the body in equal extracellular proportions. **Simple** dehydration is a net loss of body water alone with no net sodium loss.

diabetes insipidus   The chronic excretion of very large amounts of hyposmotic urine caused by inability to concentrate urine because of the lack of antidiuretic hormone (ADH) production, secretion, or effect. *Pituitary* form is caused by inadequate ADH synthesis or secretion; *nephrogenic* form is caused by unresponsiveness of the renal tubules to ADH.

distension receptor   A nerve ending that responds to stretch.

edema   An increase in the interstitial fluid volume.

extracellular water (ECW)   Water external to cell membranes. **Anatomical ECW** is all body water external to cell membranes; **physiological ECW** is plasma and body water into which small solutes can freely diffuse; excludes the transcellular portion of the anatomical extracellular water; includes the plasma and interstitial fluid (Fig. 24-1).

free water   Water containing no solute.

Gibbs-Donnan equilibrium   The steady-state distribution of permeable ions and transmembrane potential that results across a semipermeable membrane when an impermeant ion exists in unequal amounts on either side of the membrane and solvent movement across the semipermeable membrane is exactly opposed (see Fig. 24-9).

hyperaldosteronism   A disorder caused by excessive secretion of aldosterone and characterized by hypokalemic alkalosis, muscular weakness, hypertension, polyuria, polydipsia, and normal or elevated plasma sodium concentration.

hyperchloremia   An abnormally high plasma chloride concentration.

hyperkalemia   An abnormally high plasma potassium concentration.

hypernatremia   An abnormally high plasma sodium concentration.

hyperosmotic   Denoting an effective osmotic pressure higher than that of plasma.

hypertonic   Denoting a theoretical osmotic pressure higher than that of plasma.

hypochloremia   An abnormally low plasma chloride concentration.

hypokalemia   An abnormally low plasma potassium concentration.

hyponatremia   An abnormally low plasma sodium concentration. **Dilutional hyponatremia** is caused by an excess of water (relative to sodium) in the extracellular compartment.

hyposmotic   Denoting an effective osmotic pressure lower than that of plasma.

hypothalamus   Portion of brain beneath the thalamus and connected to the pituitary gland (see Chapter 43).

hypotonic   Denoting a theoretical osmotic pressure lower than that of plasma.

hypovolemia   An abnormally low blood volume.

insensible water loss   Evaporation of water through the skin or from the respiratory tract.

interstitial fluid (ISF)   Extravascular, extracellular water (see Fig. 24-2).

intracellular water (ICW)   Water inside the cells of the body; water within cell membranes.

juxtaglomerular cells   Smooth muscle cells that synthesize and store renin and release it in response to decreased renal perfusion pressure, increased sympathetic nerve stimulation of the kidneys, or decreased sodium concentration in fluid in the distal tubule.

macromolecule   A molecule of colloidal size, notably proteins, nucleic acids, and polysaccharides.

natriuretic peptides   A family of peptides secreted in response to intravascular volume expansion that reduce blood pressure and plasma volume through coordinated actions on the brain, vasculature, adrenal glands, and kidneys.

osmolarity   Osmotic concentration expressed as **osmoles** or milliosmoles of solute per liter of solvent (see Chapter 14).

osmole   The total number of moles of a solute in solution after dissociation.

osmotic pressure   The force necessary to exactly oppose the movement of water across a semipermeable membrane from a solution with low solute particle concentration to a solution with high solute particle concentration.

paresthesia   An abnormal spontaneous sensation, such as burning, pricking, numbness, and so on.

plasma   The extracellular, intravascular fluid of the body (see Fig. 24-2).

polyanionic   Possessing multiple negative charges.

polydipsia   Excessive fluid intake secondary to extreme thirst. **Psychogenic polydipsia** is secondary to a psychiatric disorder, without a demonstrable organic lesion.

polyuria   Excessive urine output, that is, more than 1 to 2 L/day in the adult.

pseudohyperkalemia   Abnormally high plasma potassium concentration in a sample obtained from a patient in the absence of true elevation of plasma potassium concentration in that patient.

renin   An enzyme produced, stored, and secreted by the juxtaglomerular cells of the kidney, which acts on circulating angiotensinogen to form angiotensin I.

semipermeable   Permeable to certain molecules but not to others; usually permeable to water.

syndrome of inappropriate antidiuretic hormone secretion (SIADH)   A grouping of findings, including hypotonicity of the plasma, hyponatremia, and hypertonicity of the urine with continued sodium excretion, that is produced by excessive ADH secretion and that improves with water restriction.

total body water (TBW)   All water within the body, both inside and outside the cells, including that contained in the gastrointestinal and genitourinary systems.

transcellular water   That portion of extracellular water that is enclosed by an epithelial membrane, the volume and composition of which are determined by the cellular activity of that membrane.

urodilatin   A natriuretic peptide similar in structure to ANP that is peptide produced locally in the kidneys.

water intoxication An increase in free water in the body; results in dilutional hyponatremia.

Methods on CD-ROM

Anion gap
Chloride

Osmolality
Sodium and potassium

Water is the most abundant constituent of the human body, accounting for approximately 60% of the body mass in a normal adult. Water is important not only because of its abundance but also because it is the medium in which body solutes, both organic and inorganic, are dissolved and metabolic reactions take place. The discussion in this chapter focuses on (1) description of the dynamic steady-state compartmentalization of body fluid and its inorganic solutes, (2) physiological mechanisms involved in the maintenance of this compartmentalization, and (3) pathophysiological events that occur during certain clinical states that alter the composition of body fluids.

BODY WATER COMPARTMENTS

Total body water (TBW) includes water both inside and outside of cells and water normally present in the gastrointestinal and genitourinary systems (Fig. 24-1). TBW can be theoretically divided into two main compartments. The **anatomical extracellular water (ECW)** includes all water external to cell membranes and constitutes the medium

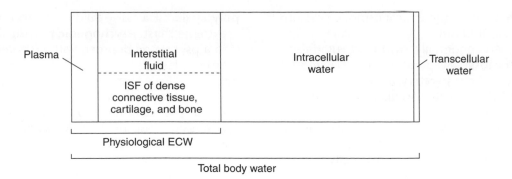

Fig. 24-1   Body water compartments. Notice that anatomical extracellular water (*ECW*) includes physiological extracellular water and transcellular water. *ISF*, Interstitial fluid.

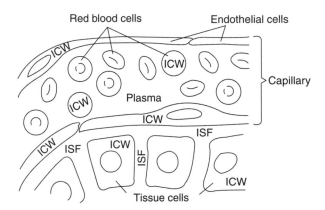

Fig. 24-2   Diagram of plasma, interstitial fluid (*ISF*), and intracellular water (*ICW*), in tissue at the microscopic level.

through which all metabolic exchange occurs. **Intracellular water (ICW)** includes all water within cell membranes and constitutes the medium in which chemical reactions of cell metabolism occur (Fig. 24-2). This compartment is heterogeneous and discontinuous; the interior of each cell is separated from the ECW and from the interior of every other cell by the **semipermeable** cell membrane.

The anatomical ECW is functionally subdivided into **physiological extracellular water** and **transcellular water**. The physiological ECW is the portion of the anatomical ECW whose volume is accessible to direct measurement; it includes **plasma** (intravascular water) and **interstitial fluid (ISF)**. The ISF, which includes extravascular, extracellular water into which ions and small molecules diffuse freely from plasma, is the fluid that directly bathes the cells of the body. In addition, there are potential spaces in the body (pericardial, pleural, peritoneal, and synovial) that are normally empty except for a few milliliters of viscous lubricating fluid and are considered to be part of the ISF compartment. Transcellular water includes water in extracellular compartments enclosed by an epithelial membrane, the volume and composition of which are determined by the cellular activity of that membrane. These heterogeneous compartments include the aqueous humor in the eye, the cerebrospinal fluid, and water within the gastrointestinal, genitourinary, and nasorespiratory systems. The volume of the transcellular water portion of the anatomical ECW is not included in conventional measurements of extracellular water (see Chapter 41).

Volume of Body Water Compartments

TBW is 65% of body weight in average adult men and 55% of body weight in women (Table 24-1). This difference between men and women is largely the result of differences in body fat. As a percentage of total body weight, TBW varies inversely with body fat content, from approximately 70% in very thin persons to 50% in very obese persons.

Physiological ECW volume is approximately 20% of body weight and one third of TBW in the average adult. Unlike TBW, neither physiological nor anatomical ECW volumes can be accurately measured. Plasma volume can be accurately measured and is approximately 5% of body weight. ISF volume is calculated as the difference between the ECW and plasma volumes. It is approximately 15% of body weight and one fourth of TBW. ICW is calculated as the difference between the TBW and ECW volumes. It is equal to 40% of body weight and two thirds of TBW in the average adult. ICW volume calculated in this manner includes transcellular water, which has been estimated to be 1% to 3% of body weight.

TABLE 24-1	COMPARTMENT VOLUMES		
	Percentage of Body Weight	*Percentage of Total Body Water*	*Volume in 70 kg Man*
Total body water	60		42 L
Extracellular water	20	33	14 L
Plasma	5	8	3.5 L
Interstitial fluid	15	25	10.5 L
Intracellular water	40	67	28 L

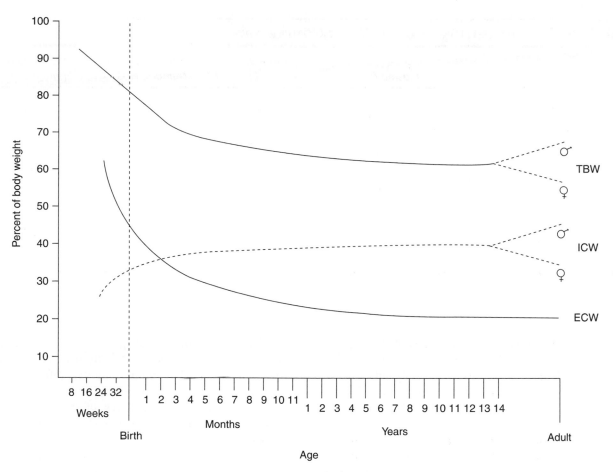

Fig. 24-3 Changes in body water compartments (expressed as a percentage of body weight) with age. *TBW*, Total body water; *ICW*, intracellular water; *ECW*, extracellular water. *(Modified from data of Friis-Hansen B: Changes in body water compartments during growth, Acta Paediatr Scand 46[suppl 110]:1, 1957.)*

Maturational Changes in Body Water Compartment Volumes

The fraction of body weight that is water and the proportions of TBW that are ECW and ICW do not remain constant during growth (Fig. 24-3). When expressed as a percentage of body weight, TBW gradually decreases during intra-uterine gestation and early childhood, reaching a value approximating that in the adult by about 3 years of age. During this time ECW (expressed as a percentage of body weight) decreases and ICW (expressed as a percentage of body weight) increases. Thus, ECW becomes a lesser and ICW a greater proportion of TBW. Plasma volume remains constant at 4% to 5% of body weight throughout life. Of course, the absolute volumes of TBW, ECW, ICW, and plasma all increase with growth.

Composition of Body Water Compartments

Plasma compartment. The plasma compartment is the only compartment the composition of which is directly measurable. Notice that the concentration of ions in the plasma is lower than that in plasma water (Table 24-2). The reason is that plasma is composed of water, ions, and **macromolecules**. Ions are present only in the water phase.

The term *plasma water* is used to indicate this aqueous fraction in distinction to the remainder, which is composed of protein, lipid, and other macromolecules. The concentration of ions in plasma is lower than that in plasma water because plasma contains both the plasma water (in which plasma ions are dissolved) and the macromolecule fraction (in which no ions are dissolved). Plasma water represents only 93% of total plasma volume. Consequently the concentration of ions in plasma is 93% of that in plasma water (see p. 446). It should be emphasized that although the concentration of ions in plasma is that portion conventionally measured and reported, it is the concentration of ions in plasma water that affects the distribution of ions across the capillary endothelium. If there is an abnormally increased amount of macromolecules in the plasma (such as lipids), the measured plasma concentration of ions will be low even though the concentration of ions in plasma water and the resultant chemical activities of these ions may be normal. In addition to protein, plasma contains high concentrations of sodium and chloride, moderate concentrations of bicarbonate, and low concentrations of calcium, magnesium, phosphate, sulfate, and organic acids.

The sum of all the charges of positively charged ions **(cations)** must be equal to the sum of all the charges of

TABLE 24-2 COMPOSITION OF BODY WATER COMPARTMENTS

	Plasma (mmol/L)	Plasma Water (mmol/L)	Interstitial Fluid (mmol/L H₂O)	Intracellular Water (mmol/L H₂O)
Cations	153	164.6	153	195
Na⁺	142	152.7	145	10
K⁺	4	4.3	4	156
Ca⁺⁺	5	5.4	(2 to 3)	3.2
Mg⁺⁺	2	2.2	(1 to 2)	26
Anions	153	164.6	153	195
Cl⁻	103	110.8	116	2
HCO₃⁻	28	30.1	31	8
Protein	17	18.3	—	55
Others	5	5.4	(6)	130
Osmolarity (mOsm/L)		296	294.6	294.6
Theoretical osmotic pressure (mm Hg)		5712.8	5685.8	5685.8

negatively charged ions (**anions**) to maintain electrical neutrality in the plasma. Most often in clinical medicine, however, the plasma concentrations only of sodium, potassium, chloride, and bicarbonate are measured. The sum of these *measured* cations exceeds that of the *measured* anions. Therefore the sum of unmeasured plasma anions must be greater than that of the unmeasured cations. The difference between the sum of measured cations and the sum of measured anions is known as the *anion gap* and is calculated either as $[Na^+] + [K^+] - [Cl^-] - [HCO_3^-]$ or as $[Na^+] - [Cl^-] - [HCO_3^-]$ (see Anion gap in Methods on CD-ROM). The latter is frequently used because the plasma potassium concentration is relatively constant and may be spuriously elevated because of hemolysis (see p. 73). Because total plasma cation concentration must equal total plasma anion concentration and decreases in unmeasured cations have little effect in the calculation, an increased anion gap is usually indicative of an increase in the concentration of one or more of the unmeasured anions (Fig. 24-4). A decrease in the anion gap is suggestive of the opposite possibility. The most frequent use of the anion gap clinically is in the differential diagnosis of **metabolic acidosis** (see Chapter 25).

Interstitial fluid compartment. The ISF cannot normally be sampled in amounts sufficient for chemical analysis. The major difference between the ISF and plasma is the presence of protein in the plasma and its relative absence in the ISF. Although the concentrations of freely diffusible solute in ISF might be expected to be equal to those in plasma water, this is true only for uncharged solutes. The presence of **polyanionic** protein molecules in plasma, which cannot cross semipermeable membranes, leads to the **Gibbs-Donnan equilibrium** (see p. 450). This equilibrium results in plasma water cation concentrations slightly greater than those in ISF and plasma water anion concentrations slightly less than those in ISF. Values for ISF ion concentrations given in Table 24-2 are theoretical approximations based on Gibbs-Donnan equilibrium calculations.

Intracellular water compartment. Solute concentrations in cell water cannot be directly determined. The ICW compartment is heterogeneous; important differences exist in intracellular solute concentrations between different cell types. However, certain features of most cell fluids are quantitatively similar and distinguish ICW from ECW. The major cations of ICW are potassium and magnesium, and the concentration of sodium is always low; the major anions of cell fluids are protein, organic phosphates, and sulfates, whereas chloride and bicarbonate concentrations are low. The profile presented in Table 24-2 is for muscle cells.

Osmotic Pressure and Osmolarity of Body Fluids

Osmotic pressure is an important factor determining the distribution of water among the body water compartments. (See Chapter 14 for a description of colligative properties that determine osmotic pressure.) The *theoretical* osmotic pressure (and water attractability) of a solution is proportional to its **osmolarity**. The theoretical osmotic pressure of a solution at body temperature is calculated as follows:

$$\text{Theoretical osmotic pressure (mm Hg)} = 19.3 \text{ (mm Hg/mOsm/L)} \times \text{Osmolarity (mOsm/L)} \qquad \textit{Eq. 24-1}$$

Notice that the solute permeability of specific biological membranes is not considered in this calculation. The osmolarity and theoretical osmotic pressure of each of the body water compartments are listed in Table 24-2.

Osmotic pressure can be simply seen as the force that tends to move water from dilute solutions to concentrated solutions. When a membrane is permeable to a solute, the solute exerts no osmotic pressure across the membrane—it does not contribute to the effective osmotic pressure of the solution. The effective osmotic pressure of a solution thus depends on the total number of solute particles in solution *and* the permeability characteristics of the particular membrane in question. The higher the permeability of a membrane to a solute, the lower the effective osmotic pressure of a

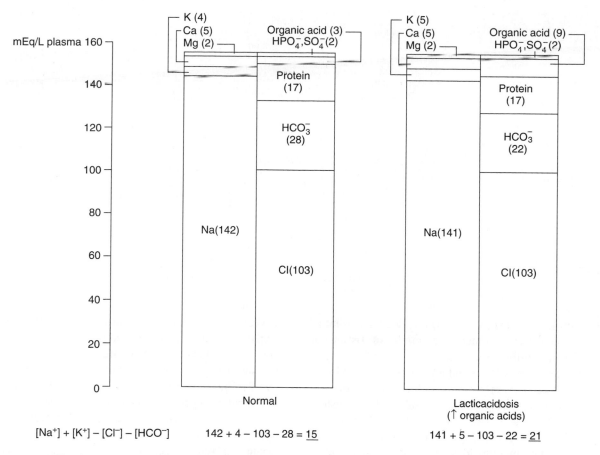

$$[Na^+] + [K^+] - [Cl^-] - [HCO^-] \qquad 142 + 4 - 103 - 28 = \underline{15} \qquad\qquad 141 + 5 - 103 - 22 = \underline{21}$$

Fig. 24-4 Increased anion gap because of an increase in unmeasured anions. *Numbers in parentheses*, concentration of ions in units of mEq/L plasma. Notice that the sum of cations (left-hand side of each bar graph) is always equal to the sum of anions (right-hand side of each bar graph), both under normal conditions and in the presence of lactic acidosis. The sum of concentrations of unmeasured anions (organic acids, HPO_4^{2-}, SO_4^{2-}, and proteins) is larger than the sum of concentrations of unmeasured cations (Ca^{2+} and Mg^{2+}). During lactic acidosis, the difference between unmeasured anions and cations becomes greater because production of lactic acid increases the concentration of organic acids.

solution of that solute at any given osmolarity. For example, cell membranes are much more permeable to urea than to sodium and chloride. Therefore the effective osmotic pressure of a solution of urea across the cell membrane would be much less than that of a solution of NaCl of the same osmolarity. Measurement of the osmolarity of body compartment water is a measure only of its *theoretical*, not effective, osmotic pressure.

A solution with an *effective* osmotic pressure greater than that of plasma is said to be **hyperosmotic** with respect to plasma. A solution with a *theoretical* osmotic pressure greater than plasma is said to be **hypertonic**. **Hyposmotic** and **hypotonic** solutions are those with effective and theoretical osmotic pressures, respectively, less than those of plasma.

The effective osmotic pressure of plasma and ISF across the capillary endothelium by which they are separated is referred to as their **colloid osmotic pressure**. The capillary endothelium is freely permeable to most solutes in plasma and ISF. Therefore these solutes contribute to theoretical but not to effective osmotic pressure. The capillary endothelium is impermeable to large protein molecules (**colloids**) under usual circumstances. It is these colloids that are responsible for the effective osmotic pressure of plasma and ISF.

REGULATION OF BODY FLUID COMPARTMENT OSMOLARITY AND VOLUME
Extracellular Compartment

Regulation of the ECW osmolarity and volume depends on the independent control of each of these variables by the **hypothalamus**, the **renin-angiotensin-aldosterone** system, atrial natriuretic factor, and the kidney.

Water metabolism and hypothalamus. The regulatory centers for water intake and water output are located in separate areas of the hypothalamus in the brain (Fig. 24-5). Neurons in each of these areas respond to increases in ECW osmolarity, to decreases in intravascular volume, and to angiotensin II. Increased ECW osmolarity stimulates these neurons directly by causing them to shrink (increased osmolarity of ISF bathing any cell will cause water to move

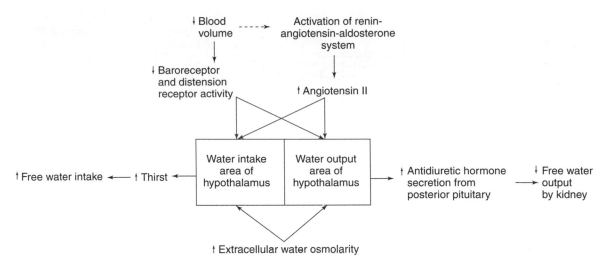

Fig. 24-5   Hypothalamic regulation of water balance.

out of the cell into the ISF; see p. 451). A decrease in intravascular volume causes a reduction in activity of **distension receptors** located in the atria of the heart, the inferior vena cava, and the pulmonary veins and a reduction in activity of blood pressure receptors in the aorta and the carotid arteries. Relay of this information to the central nervous system stimulates neurons in the water-intake and water-output areas of the hypothalamus. Circulating angiotensin II seems to act directly to stimulate neurons located in these water-control areas of the hypothalamus. Stimulation of neurons located in the water-intake area produces the conscious sensation of thirst and thereby stimulates water intake. Stimulation of neurons located in the water-output area results in the release of **antidiuretic hormone** (ADH) from the posterior pituitary gland. Antidiuretic hormone stimulates water reabsorption in the collecting ducts of the kidney, which results in the formation of hypertonic urine and decreased output of **free water** (water without solute). The integration of all these control mechanisms governing water intake and output ensures maintenance of appropriate water balance.

Water and sodium metabolism and renin-angiotensin-aldosterone system. The renin-angiotensin-aldosterone system (Fig. 24-6) functions as a neurohormonal regulating mechanism for body sodium and water content, arterial blood pressure, and potassium balance. Renin is a proteolytic enzyme synthesized, stored, and secreted by cells in the **juxtaglomerular cells** of the kidney. Renin secretion is increased by decreased renal perfusion pressure, stimulation of sympathetic nerves to the kidneys, and decreased sodium concentration in the fluid of the distal tubule. Renin converts **angiotensinogen** (a polypeptide synthesized in the liver) to angiotensin I. Angiotensin I is converted to angiotensin II in the lung and kidney. Angiotensin II is a potent vasoconstrictor. In addition, angiotensin II stimulates aldosterone secretion by the adrenal cortex, thirsting behavior, and ADH secretion. Aldosterone stimulates sodium reabsorption in the distal nephron. As a consequence of this sodium reabsorption, the body retains water.

Water and sodium metabolism and the natriuretic peptides. Natriuretic peptides (Fig. 24-7) are a family of peptides that have reciprocal effects to the renin-angiotensin-aldosterone system. They include **atrial natriuretic peptide (ANP), brain natriuretic peptide (BNP),** and **C-type natriuretic peptide (CNP).** Each is tissue specific and independently regulated. Increased secretion of these natriuretic peptides in response to intravascular volume expansion reduces blood pressure and plasma volume through coordinated actions on the brain, vasculature, adrenal glands, and kidneys. Natriuretic peptides are important in defending against salt-induced hypertension and in mitigating congestive heart failure.

ANP is a hormone produced primarily in the cardiac atria, which is released in response to an increase in transmural atrial pressure. It relaxes venous capacitance of blood vessels by suppressing sympathetic nervous system activity. This reduces the increase in venous pressure that occurs with a given increase in blood volume. ANP also increases vascular permeability and promotes natriuresis and diuresis. The latter are the result of direct effects on renal hemodynamics (which increase glomerular filtration rate [GFR]), suppression of the renin-angiotensin-aldosterone system (which inhibits tubular sodium reabsorption), and antagonization of the effect of ADH in the collecting ducts (which inhibits water reabsorption). In the brain, ANP inhibits salt appetite, water intake, and secretion of ADH and corticotrophin.

BNP is a hormone produced primarily in the cardiac ventricles in response to increases in ventricular wall tension resulting from increased volume expansion and pressure overload. The main circulating form of BNP is a 17–amino acid residue ring structure, formed by a disulfide bridge between two cysteine amino acid residues, and a 9-residue and a 6-residue N-terminal and C-terminal extension, respectively. It has cardiovascular, natriuretic, and diuretic effects similar to ANP.

CNP is produced in the brain, vascular endothelial cells, and renal tubules. Little, if any, is found circulating in the

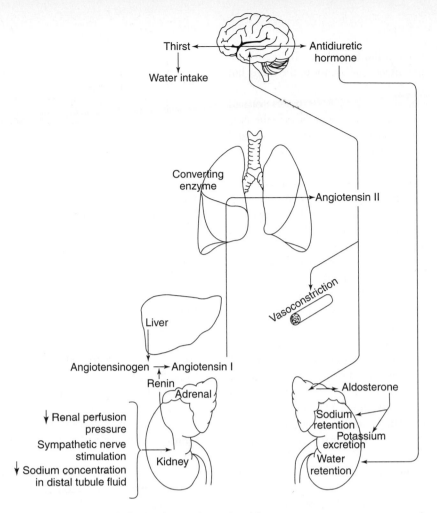

Fig. 24-6   Renin-angiotensin-aldosterone system.

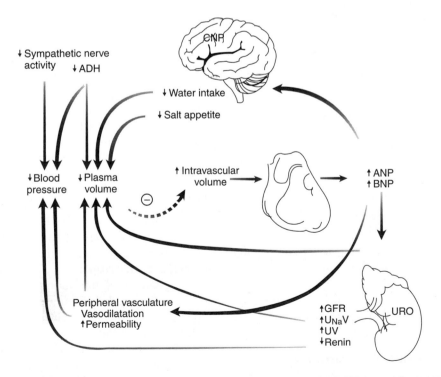

Fig. 24-7   Natriuretic peptide effects in response to increase in intravascular volume. *ANP,* atrial natriuretic peptide; *BNP,* brain natriuretic peptide; *CNP,* C-type natriuretic peptide; *URO,* urodilatin; *GFR,* glomerular filtration rate; $U_{Na}V$, urinary sodium excretion; *UV,* urinary water excretion. *(Modified from Levi ER, Gardner DG, Samson WK: Natriuretic peptides,* New Engl J Med *339:321, 1998. Copyright 1998, Massachusetts Medical Society. All rights reserved.)*

plasma. Thus it seems to act at the local level. Its regulation is unclear. It is the most potent venous dilator of the three, but has no natriuretic effects.

Urodilatin is similar in structure to ANP, but is formed directly in the kidney from the same precursor protein as is ANP in the atria. Its regulation is unclear. Its diuretic and natriuretic effects are more potent than those of ANP.

Measurement of circulating natriuretic peptide concentrations to classify and predict mortality in patients with congestive heart failure might reduce the need for more expensive and invasive evaluations (see Chapter 31). However, several analytical problems must be resolved before these assays can be used routinely.

Control of extracellular water osmolarity. ECW *osmolarity* is regulated by the hypothalamic control of water intake (regulatory thirst) and renal excretion of free water (Fig. 24-5). Increased ECW osmolarity stimulates water intake and ADH secretion. ADH secretion decreases renal water excretion. Increased water intake and decreased renal water excretion result in a positive water balance, that is, water gain in excess of water loss. Positive water balance decreases ECW osmolarity to normal. The opposite occurs with decreased ECW osmolarity: thirst and ADH secretion are inhibited. Negative water balance (water loss in excess of water gain) results, and ECW osmolarity is restored to normal.

Control of extracellular water volume. Control of ECW *volume* depends on the integrated control of water and sodium balance by the water intake and output areas of the hypothalamus, the renin-angiotensin-aldosterone system, atrial natriuretic factor, and the kidney.

When water and sodium output exceed intake (water and sodium balance are negative), the ECW volume contracts. The associated decrease in plasma volume results in decrease in venous blood return to the heart and decrease in cardiac output. These cardiovascular changes produce the following effects:

1. Stimulation of the water-intake area of the hypothalamus and thirst center (Fig. 24-5)
2. Stimulation of the water-output area of the hypothalamus and ADH secretion (Fig. 24-5)
3. Stimulation of the renin-angiotensin-aldosterone system and increase in angiotensin II (Fig. 24-6)
4. Inhibition of release of atrial natriuretic factor
5. Retention of sodium and water by the kidney

The net result of these effects is that water and sodium balance become positive, and ECW volume is restored to normal.

Expansion of the ECW volume results in the opposite sequence of events, with net loss of water and sodium and restoration of ECW balance to normal.

Plasma and Interstitial Fluid Compartments

Water and solute distribution between the plasma and ISF compartments depends on an intact capillary endothelial surface and is controlled passively by the interaction of

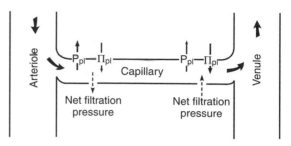

Fig. 24-8 Starling's hypothesis of water distribution between plasma and interstitial fluid compartments. Thickness of *arrows* representing plasma hydrostatic pressure, P_{pl}, and plasma oncotic pressure, Π_{pl}, indicate their relative magnitudes. *Dashed arrows*, direction of net filtration pressure.

hydrostatic, osmotic, and electrochemical forces. The capillary endothelium functions as a continuous tube, with numerous intercellular channels 4 to 5 nm in diameter. It is freely permeable to water and small solutes and relatively impermeable to protein.

Water distribution. Water distribution across the capillary endothelial surface is controlled by the balance of forces that tend to move water from the plasma to the ISF (filtration forces) and forces that tend to move water from the ISF into the plasma (reabsorption forces). The major filtration force is plasma hydrostatic pressure in the capillary. A much weaker filtration force is the ISF colloid osmotic pressure. Because the protein concentration in ISF is negligible, colloid osmotic pressure is low. Another weak filtration force is a small *negative* ISF hydrostatic pressure. The major reabsorption force is the colloid osmotic pressure exerted across the capillary endothelium by plasma proteins. As a broad generalization, plasma hydrostatic pressure (which tends to drive water out of the capillary) exceeds plasma colloid osmotic pressure (which tends to draw water into the capillary) at the arteriolar end of the capillary so that net filtration occurs. As plasma moves along the capillary and filtration occurs, plasma hydrostatic pressure decreases and plasma protein concentration (and therefore plasma colloid osmotic pressure) increases along the course of the capillary so that net reabsorption occurs toward the venous end of the capillary. This is depicted schematically in Fig. 24-8. Overall, filtration exceeds reabsorption; therefore water must be returned to the plasma from the ISF compartment by way of the lymphatic system to prevent **edema** (defined as an abnormal increase in ISF volume).

Solute distribution. The small differences in the concentrations of the various extracellular solutes across the capillary endothelium are the result of the presence of polyanionic protein molecules (i.e., having multiple negative charges) in plasma to which the capillary endothelium is relatively impermeable. This results in the Gibbs-Donnan equilibrium (Fig. 24-9): the presence of impermeant polyanionic macromolecules restricted to one side of a membrane permeable to solvent and small ions establishes a characteristic distribution of the permeable ions. At electrochemical

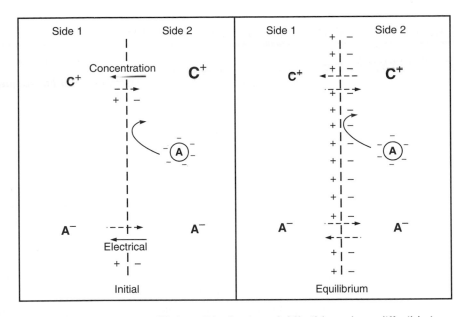

Fig. 24-9 Gibbs-Donnan equilibrium. Distribution of diffusible and nondiffusible ions and development of an electrical potential gradient across a membrane when a nondiffusible, polyvalent anion ($^-\widehat{A}^-$) with a diffusible cation (C^+) is added to one side of membrane in solution of diffusible cation (C^+) and anion (A^-). Initially, a diffusible cation moves down its concentration gradient from side 2 to side 1. This movement generates an electrical potential gradient across the membrane (side 2 negative with respect to side 1). The diffusible anion moves down this electrical potential gradient from side 2 to side 1. At equilibrium, the concentration of diffusible cation will be greater on side 2 than side 1 (as indicated by size of symbols), whereas the concentration of diffusible anion will be greater on side 1 than on side 2. No *net* movement of diffusible ions occurs across the membrane because no net electrochemical gradients exist. The concentration gradient for each ion is balanced by an equal but oppositely directed electrical gradient.

equilibrium, the concentrations of *diffusible cations* are slightly *higher* and the concentrations of *diffusible anions* slightly *lower* in the compartment containing the impermeant polyanionic macromolecule.

In the cases of calcium and magnesium, the larger differences between plasma water and ISF concentrations result from the fact that approximately 45% of plasma calcium and 25% of plasma magnesium is protein bound and therefore is nondiffusible.

Intracellular Compartment

Water and solute distribution across the cell membrane between the ISF and ICW depends on the integrity of the cell membrane and on osmotic and electrochemical forces; all these factors are sustained by cell metabolism. The cell membrane behaves as though it were an oil film with numerous 0.7 nm-diameter pores. This membrane is highly permeable to water but differentially permeable to solutes. The permeability of the cell membrane to a solute is directly related to the lipid solubility of the solute and inversely related to its hydrophilicity (water attractability) and molecular size. Other factors being constant, membrane permeability is greater to anions than to cations.

Cell volume. Cell volume is controlled by ISF osmolarity. Osmolarity inside the cell must equal osmolarity outside

the cell because the cell membrane is highly permeable to water and no hydrostatic pressure gradient can be maintained across animal cell membranes. The osmotic content of the intracellular compartment is maintained relatively constant by cell metabolism. Therefore osmotic equilibrium across the cell membrane can be maintained in the face of changes in ISF osmolarity only by the movement of water between the intracellular compartment and interstitial space. A decrease in ISF osmolarity causes movement of water into cells and an increase in intracellular volume. Conversely, an increase in ISF osmolarity causes movement of water out of cells and a decrease in intracellular volume.

Cell solute content. The ionic composition of the intracellular fluid is shown in Table 24-2. This composition is largely the result of an energy-dependent ion-transport pump (Na^+,K^+-ATPase) found in the cell membrane that extrudes sodium from the cell in exchange for potassium. In addition, the intracellular solute composition depends on the intracellular production of nonpermeable polyanionic macromolecules. The cellular content of the other, permeable ions results from (1) electrochemical gradients produced by Na-K exchange and nonpermeable intracellular polyanionic macromolecules (Gibbs-Donnan effect) (Fig. 24-9), (2) the specific permeability characteristics of the cell membrane to the various ions, and (3) other energy-dependent ion-specific

TABLE 24-3	WATER BALANCE IN AVERAGE ADULT UNDER VARIOUS CONDITIONS							
	INTAKE (mL/DAY)				**OUTPUT (mL/DAY)**			
	Normal	*Hot Environment*	*Strenuous Work*			*Normal*	*Hot Environment*	*Strenuous Work*
Drinking water	1200	2200	3400	Urine		1400	1200	500
Water from food	1000	1000	1150	Insensible water				
Water of oxidation	300	300	450	Skin		400	400	400
				Lung		400	300	600
				Sweat		100	1400	3300
				Stool		200	200	200
TOTAL	2500	3500	5000			2500	3500	5000

transport pumps. The latter two factors vary from cell type to cell type and are responsible for the differences in ionic content among various cell types.

All factors influencing cell solute content depend on normal cellular metabolism. When cellular metabolism is disrupted, as during **asphyxia**, solute and water enter the cell, causing it to swell.

WATER METABOLISM
Water Balance

Extracellular water osmolarity is maintained constant at 285 to 298 mOsm/L as a consequence of the dynamic balance between water intake and water excretion, which is controlled by the mechanisms discussed previously. Average daily water turnover in the adult is approximately 2500 mL; however, the range of water turnover possible is great and depends on intake, environment, and activity (Table 24-3).

Under normal conditions approximately one half to two thirds of water intake is in the form of oral fluid intake, and approximately one half to one third is in the form of oral intake of water in food. In addition, a small amount of water (150 to 350 mL/day) is produced by oxidative metabolism. Oral fluid intake is the only source of water that is regulated in response to changes in ECW volume and osmolarity.

Routes of water excretion include urinary water loss, **insensible water loss**, sensible perspiration (sweating), and gastrointestinal water loss. The kidney is the principal organ regulating the volume and composition of the body fluids. Urine volume varies over a wide range in response to changes in ECW volume and osmolarity. Solute excretion is regulated independently.

Loss of water by diffusion through the skin and through the respiratory tract is known as *insensible water loss* because it is not apparent. It is the only route by which water is lost without solute. Normally, half of insensible water loss occurs through the skin and half through the respiratory tract. The magnitude of cutaneous insensible water loss is a function of body surface area; therefore it is disproportionately greater in infants and children in relation to their weight. Insensible water loss varies directly with ambient temperature, body temperature, and activity, and inversely with ambient humidity.

Sensible perspiration is negligible in a cool environment but may be quite substantial with increases in ambient temperature, body temperature, or physical activity. Sodium and chloride are the major ionic components of sweat, but sweat is almost invariably hypotonic to plasma. An increase in ECW osmolarity causes a decrease in the rate of sensible perspiration.

Net water loss from the gastrointestinal tract is normally small, approximately 150 mL/day. However, the *flux* of water and electrolytes between the gastrointestinal tract and ECW compartment is quite large. Therefore, if reabsorption is impaired, water and electrolyte losses from the gastrointestinal tract can be great, as with diarrhea. Except for saliva, which is hypotonic, the total solute concentration of most gastrointestinal secretions is similar to ISF.

Disorders of Water Imbalance

Disorders of water balance (**dehydration** and overhydration) result from an imbalance of water intake and output or sodium intake and output (Table 24-4).

Dehydration

Deficit of water. Simple dehydration, defined as a decrease in total body water with relatively normal total body sodium, may result from failure to replace obligatory water losses or failure of the regulatory or effector mechanisms that promote conservation of water by the kidney (see box, p. 453). Simple dehydration is by definition associated with **hypernatremia** and hyperosmolarity because water balance is negative and sodium balance is normal. The increase in ECW osmolarity as water is lost from the body results in movement of water out of the ICW compartment. Therefore simple dehydration results in contraction of both the ECW and ICW compartments (Table 24-4).

Deficit of water and sodium. More often dehydration results from a net negative balance of both water and sodium. In this case water balance may be more negative than, equal to, or less negative than sodium balance (Table 24-4). If water balance is more negative than sodium balance, the result is **hypernatremic** or *hyperosmolar* dehydration; if it is equally negative, **normonatremic** or *isomolar* dehydration results; and if it is less negative, **hyponatremic** or *hyposmolar* dehydration results. Hypernatremic dehydration is

TABLE 24-4   Changes in Total Body Water Volume and Distribution, Total Body Sodium Content, and Plasma Sodium Concentration with Dehydration and Overhydration

	Total Body Water	Extracellular Water	Intracellular Water	Total Body Sodium	Plasma Sodium Concentration
Dehydration					
Hypernatremic	↓	sl ↓	↓	nl or sl ↓	↑
Normonatremic	↓	↓	nl	↓	nl
Hyponatremic	↓	↓↓	↑	↓↓	↓
Overhydration					
Water intoxication	↑	↑	↑	nl	↓
Extracellular water volume expansion					
Normonatremic	↑	↑	nl	↑	nl
Hyponatremic	↑	↑	↑	sl ↑	↓

nl, *Normal*; sl, *slightly*.

CAUSES OF DEHYDRATION (WATER AND SODIUM DEFICITS)

Hypernatremic Dehydration
Water and food deprivation
Excessive sweating*
Osmotic diuresis (with glucosuria)
Diuretic therapy*

Normonatremic Dehydration
Vomiting, diarrhea
Replacement of losses in the above conditions with
　low-sodium liquids

Hyponatremic Dehydration
Diuretic therapy†
Excessive sweating
Salt-wasting renal disease
Adrenocortical insufficiency

*If free water intake is inadequate.
†If free water intake is excessive.

most common. Some causes of water and sodium deficits are listed in the box above.

The degree of extracellular volume contraction for a given sodium deficit and the associated change in intracellular volume is different for each of these types of dehydration (Table 24-4). The degree of extracellular volume contraction is least with hypernatremic dehydration because the increase in ECW osmolarity causes water to move out of the cell; contraction of ICW volume occurs. Thus the total body water deficit is "shared" by the extracellular and intracellular compartments. The degree of extracellular volume contraction is intermediate with normonatremic dehydration, because no water moves out of or into cells because there is no change in ECW osmolarity. There is also no change in ICW volume. The degree of ECW volume depletion is largest with hyponatremic dehydration because the decrease

in ECW osmolarity causes water to move into cells. Intracellular water volume is actually increased.

Symptoms of dehydration. The signs and symptoms of dehydration include thirst, dry mucous membranes, decreased skin turgor, decreased urine output and increased urine osmolarity (except when caused by failure of the kidney to conserve free water), increased blood urea nitrogen, and increased hematocrit. With increasing severity, weakness, lethargy, hypotension, and shock may occur.

Overhydration

Excessive water. Water intoxication is defined as an increase in TBW with normal total body sodium. It rarely results from excessive water consumption (**polydipsia**). More often water intoxication results from impaired renal free water excretion as the result of ADH secretion in excess of that required to maintain normal ECW osmolarity (**syndrome of inappropriate ADH secretion, SIADH;** see box on p. 454).

With water intoxication the **dilutional hyponatremia** and hyposmolarity of the ECW result in water movement into the cells. Therefore water intoxication produces expansion of the ECW and ICW compartments (Table 24-4).

The symptoms of water intoxication are related to the degree and rate of fall in sodium. With an acute fall in serum sodium to 120 to 125 mmol/L, nausea, vomiting, seizures, and coma can occur.

Excessive water and sodium. *Expansion of the extracellular compartment* usually results from retention of sodium and water. This occurs with oliguric renal failure, nephrotic syndrome, congestive heart failure, **cirrhosis**, and primary **hyperaldosteronism**. In these conditions TBW excess is associated with normal or low serum sodium and osmolarity (Table 24-4). Hypernatremia is rare with water excess. If the serum sodium is normal, the increase in TBW will be limited to the ECW. With **hyponatremia** the increase of TBW will be shared by the ECW and ICW compartments.

CAUSES OF WATER INTOXICATION

Polydipsia

Psychogenic—secondary to a psychiatric disturbance
Organic—secondary to an anterior thalamic lesion

SIADH

Increased secretion of ADH by hypothalamus secondary to
   decreased venous return to heart with no decrease in total
   blood volume
   Asthma
   Pneumothorax
   Bacterial or viral pneumonia
   Positive pressure ventilation
   Chronic obstructive pulmonary disease
   Right-sided heart failure
   Disease of spinal cord or peripheral nerves (Guillain-Barré
      syndrome, poliomyelitis)
Increased secretion of ADH by hypothalamus in absence of
   appropriate osmolar or volume stimuli
   Central nervous system disorders (intracranial hemorrhage,
      hydrocephalus, skull fracture, severe asphyxia, brain
      tumors, cerebrovascular thrombosis, meningitis,
      encephalitis, seizures, acute psychoses, and cerebral
      atrophy)
   Hypothyroidism
   Pain, fear
   Anesthesia or surgical stress
   Drugs such as morphine, barbiturates, cyclophosphamide,
      vincristine, and carbamazepine

Ectopic, Autonomous Secretion of ADH

Bronchogenic carcinoma
Adenosarcoma of pancreas
Lymphosarcoma
Duodenal adenocarcinoma
Pulmonary tuberculosis
Pulmonary abscess

SODIUM METABOLISM
Sodium Balance

In a normal adult the total body sodium is about 55 mmol/kg of body weight; about 30% is tightly bound in the crystalline structure of bone and thus is nonexchangeable. Thus, only 40 mmol/kg is exchangeable among the various compartments and accessible to measurement. The exchangeable sodium is distributed primarily in the extracellular space (Fig. 24-10). About 97% to 98% of the exchangeable sodium is found in the ECW space and only 2% to 3% in the ICW space. Approximately 16% of exchangeable sodium is in plasma, 41% is in ISF that is readily accessible to the plasma compartment, 17% is in ISF of dense connective tissue and cartilage, 20% is in ISF of bone, and 3% to 4% in the transcellular water compartment. Total bone sodium (exchangeable and nonexchangeable) accounts for 40% to 45% of the total body sodium. The concentrations of sodium in the various fluid compartments are displayed in Table 24-2. As discussed previously, the difference in sodium concentration between plasma and ISF is the result of the Gibbs-Donnan equilibrium. The difference in sodium concentration between ISF and ICW is the result of the **active transport** of sodium out of the cell in exchange for potassium.

The amount of sodium in the body is a reflection of the balance between sodium intake and output. Sodium intake depends on the quantity and type of food intake. Under normal conditions the average adult takes in about 50 to 200 mmol of sodium/day. Sodium output occurs through three primary routes: the gastrointestinal tract, the skin, and the urine.

Under normal circumstances loss of sodium through the gastrointestinal tract is very small. Fecal water excretion is only 100 to 200 mL/day for a normal adult, and fecal sodium excretion only 1 to 2 mmol/day. However, it should be borne in mind that although fecal losses of water and electrolytes

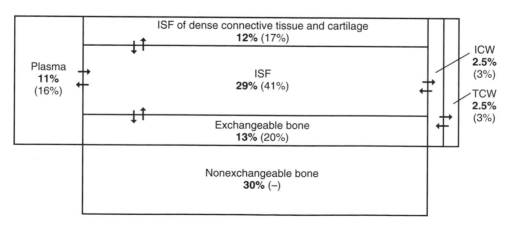

Fig. 24-10　Distribution of sodium among body compartments. *Bold numbers,* percentages of *total body* sodium in various compartments; *numbers in parentheses,* percentages of *exchangeable* sodium in various compartments; *ICW,* intracellular water; *ISF,* interstitial fluid; *TCW,* transcellular water.

are normally small, the total volume of gastrointestinal fluid secreted is large, averaging about 8 L/day. Almost all this volume is normally reabsorbed. However, with impaired gastrointestinal reabsorption, losses of water and electrolytes are large. The volume and electrolyte content of various gastrointestinal secretions are shown in Table 24-5. Notice that most of the secretions have sodium contents much higher than that of the feces. Thus, with severe diarrhea or with gastric or intestinal drainage tubes, sodium losses through the gastrointestinal tract may exceed 100 mmol/day.

The sodium content of sweat averages about 50 mmol/L but is somewhat variable. The sweat sodium concentration is decreased by aldosterone and increased in cystic fibrosis. The rate of sweat production is highly variable, increasing in hot environments, during exercise, and with fever. Under extreme conditions sweat production can exceed 5 L/day, accounting for a loss of more than 250 mmol of sodium. Under normal conditions, in a cool environment, sodium losses from the skin are small. With extensive burns or exudative skin lesions there is great loss of sodium and water.

The major route of sodium excretion is through the kidney. Furthermore, the urinary excretion of sodium is carefully regulated to maintain body sodium homeostasis, which in turn is critical to control of extracellular volume. The details of the mechanisms and regulation of renal sodium excretion are discussed in Chapter 26.

Sodium is freely filtered by the glomerulus. Approximately 70% of the filtered sodium is reabsorbed by the proximal tubule, about 15% by the loop of Henle, about 5% by the distal convoluted tubule, 5% by the cortical collecting tubule, and another 5% by the medullary collecting duct; thus normally less than 1% of the filtered sodium is excreted.

Disorders of Sodium Balance

Sodium excess. Sodium accumulates in the body when sodium intake exceeds sodium output because of some abnormality of sodium homeostatic mechanisms. Some major clinical causes of sodium retention appear in the box.

CLINICAL CONDITIONS RESULTING IN EXCESS BODY SODIUM

Cardiac failure
Liver disease
Renal disease—nephrotic syndrome
Hyperaldosteronism
Pregnancy

Because sodium is distributed in the extracellular space, an increase in total body sodium is usually accompanied by an increase in ECW volume. An abnormal increase in ECW volume, particularly an increase in the interstitial space, produces tissue swelling known as *edema*. Thus those clinical conditions associated with sodium retention are frequently characterized by the presence of edema. Clinically, edema is characterized by swelling and puffiness of the body.

Congestive heart failure. When the heart begins to fail as a pump, a series of pathophysiological mechanisms occur leading to retention of sodium. The failing heart does not pump as much blood to the kidney, resulting in less sodium filtration, greater reabsorption, and consequently less excretion. The greater venous back pressure generated from the failing heart causes fluid to move from the vascular space to the interstitial space, decreasing the effective plasma volume and cardiac output. These factors stimulate the secretion of angiotensin II, aldosterone, and ADH and decrease release of atrial natriuretic factor. These hormone responses further enhance salt and water retention.

Liver disease. In some liver diseases there is venous obstruction, which results in increased sinusoidal and portal venous pressure. These in turn lead to leakage of fluid out of the vascular space into the peritoneal space (**ascites**), which lowers the effective plasma volume. The lowered plasma volume leads to salt and water retention by mechanisms similar to those described for heart failure.

TABLE 24-5   ELECTROLYTE COMPOSITION AND VOLUME OF VARIOUS GASTROINTESTINAL SECRETIONS IN A NORMAL ADULT

Fluid	Volume Secreted (mL/Day)	ELECTROLYTE CONCENTRATION (mmol/L)			
		Na⁺	K⁺	Cl⁻	HCO₃⁻
Gastric juice*	2500	8 to 120	1 to 30	8 to 100	0 to 20
Bile	700 to 1000	134 to 156	4 to 6	83 to 110	38
Pancreatic juice	>1000	113 to 153	2 to 7	54 to 95	110
Small bowel	3000	72 to 120	3.5 to 7	69 to 127	30
Ileostomy	100 to 4000	112 to 142	4.5 to 14	43 to 122	30
Cecostomy	100 to 300	480 to 116	11 to 28	35 to 70	15
Feces	100	<10	<10	<15	<15

Electrolyte composition of gastric juice varies, depending on acidity. The higher the acidity, the lower the sodium concentration, the higher the chloride concentration, and the lower the bicarbonate concentration. The average sodium concentration is approximately 100 mmol/L. (From Lockwood JS, Randall HT: Bull NY Acad Med 25:228–243, 1949.)

Renal disease. If the kidneys are damaged to such a degree that the GFR is greatly reduced and sodium excretion is thereby compromised, sodium retention will occur (see Chapter 26). Sodium retention occurs by another mechanism in the nephrotic syndrome. This syndrome is characterized by proteinuria and decreased serum albumin levels, which result in low plasma colloid osmotic pressure and therefore a shift of fluid from the vascular space to the ISF space. This in turn results in **hypovolemia** with consequent salt and water retention, as previously discussed.

Pregnancy. The reasons for sodium accumulation during pregnancy are still unclear, but there is no question that most women accumulate between 500 and 800 mmol of sodium during a normal pregnancy. Some suggest that the sodium accumulation may be a resetting of the normal homeostatic mechanism regulating body sodium and water.

Sodium depletion. Sodium depletion occurs when the output of sodium exceeds the intake (see the box below). As discussed previously, only small amounts of sodium are lost in the feces under normal conditions. However, under conditions of severe diarrhea or drainage of gastrointestinal secretions, gastrointestinal sodium excretion can be quite large. If this is not replaced by increased intake, sodium depletion will result. Moreover, because the gastrointestinal route may not be available, the intravenous replacement of water and electrolytes may be necessary. Similarly, losses of sodium through the skin are normally relatively small. However, when the volume of sweat becomes large, when the concentration of sodium in sweat is abnormally high (as with cystic fibrosis), or when there is abnormal exudation of fluid and electrolytes from the surface of the body (as occurs with extensive burns), the amount of sodium lost from the skin may be substantial and sodium depletion may occur.

When the tubules of the kidney are unable to reabsorb sodium because of disease or hormonal abnormalities, sodium loss can be excessive. For example, aldosterone deficiency, caused by disease of the adrenal gland or abnormalities in the aldosterone-regulating system, leads to decreased reabsorption of sodium in the distal nephron and total body sodium depletion. Inhibition of tubular sodium reabsorption by a diuretic also may lead to body sodium depletion.

In SIADH (see p. 453) there is water retention and hypotonic expansion of the ECW and ICW spaces. This in turn inhibits sodium reabsorption in the proximal nephron and also perhaps the distal nephron, leading to body salt depletion.

Abnormalities of Plasma Sodium Concentration

Changes in total body sodium are not necessarily associated with similar changes in plasma sodium concentration. That is, with salt retention, plasma sodium concentration is not necessarily increased. In fact, plasma sodium is frequently decreased in sodium-retentive states. Similarly, salt depletion is not necessarily associated with decreased plasma sodium concentrations. Plasma sodium concentration reflects the relative balances of extracellular sodium and water.

Hyponatremia (low plasma sodium) occurs when there is a greater excess of extracellular water than of sodium or a greater deficit of sodium than of water. Some causes of hyponatremia are listed in the box below. Notice that in many cases there is an excess of total body sodium.

The symptoms of hyponatremia depend on the cause, magnitude, and rate of fall in serum sodium. With acute, pronounced hyponatremia caused by water intoxication, nausea, vomiting, seizures, and coma occur. Symptoms are less fulminant with chronic hyponatremia caused by salt depletion in excess of water depletion. With progressively

---

CLINICAL CONDITIONS THAT CAN RESULT IN DEFICITS OF BODY SODIUM

Gastrointestinal losses—vomiting, diarrhea, fistulas, drainage tubes
Excessive sweating—exercise, fever, hot environment
Renal disease
Adrenal insufficiency—hypoaldosteronism
Diuretic therapy
Osmotic diuresis—diabetes mellitus
Burns
SIADH

CLINICAL CONDITIONS ASSOCIATED WITH HYPONATREMIA

Water excess greater than sodium excess*
    Inappropriate ADH secretion
    Glucocorticoid deficiency
    Hypothyroidism
    Psychogenic polydipsia (excessive water intake)
    Heart failure[†]
    Liver disease[†]
    Renal failure[†]
    Nephrotic syndrome[†]
Sodium deficit greater than water deficit
    Certain gastrointestinal losses—vomiting, diarrhea, fistulas,
        and intestinal obstruction
    Burns
    Diuretic therapy
    Adrenal insufficiency—hypoaldosteronism
    Salt-losing nephropathy
    Renal tubular acidosis
    Osmotic diuresis
    Bicarbonaturia, ketonuria
Movement of sodium from the extracellular to intracellular
    water space
    Adrenal insufficiency—hypoaldosteronism
    Sick cell syndrome—shock
Pseudohyponatremia—hyperglycemia, hyperlipidemia,
    hyperglobulinemia

*Hyponatremia is dilutional, that is, secondary to excessive water retention.
†Total body sodium is increased.

severe degrees of chronic hyponatremia, constant thirst, muscle cramps, nausea, vomiting, abdominal cramps, weakness, lethargy, and finally delirium and impaired consciousness occur.

Hypernatremia (high plasma sodium) occurs when there is greater deficit of extracellular water than of sodium. Greater excess of sodium than of water rarely occurs. Causes of hypernatremia are listed in the box below. Notice that in many cases there is actually a deficit of total body sodium.

Hypernatremia usually occurs as a chronic process secondary to loss of water in excess of sodium. Symptoms are therefore those of dehydration.

Measurement of urine sodium and urine osmolarity can be useful in the diagnosis of abnormalities of serum sodium concentration (Tables 24-6 and 24-7). However, it is critical to interpret these values in light of the clinical picture, particularly assessment of ECW volume. Interpretation of these measurements may be misleading in the case of coexisting abnormalities. Failure to find the expected values when the clinical picture is otherwise consistent with given clinical condition should lead to consideration that one or more abnormalities coexists.

POTASSIUM METABOLISM
Potassium Balance

Approximately 98% of the total body potassium is found in the ICW space, reaching a concentration there of about 150 to 160 mmol/L. In the ECW space, the concentration of potassium is only 3.5 to 5 mmol/L. Total body potassium in an adult male is about 50 mmol/kg of body weight and is influenced by age, sex, and, very importantly, muscle mass, because most of the body's potassium is contained in muscle.

The concentrations of potassium in the various fluid compartments are listed in Table 24-2. The difference in potassium concentration between plasma and ISF is attributable to the Gibbs-Donnan equilibrium. The difference

in potassium concentration in ISF and intracellular fluid is the result of the active transport of potassium into the cell in exchange for sodium. Factors that enhance potassium transport into the cell and thereby increase the ratio of intracellular to extracellular potassium are insulin, aldosterone, **alkalosis**, and β-adrenergic stimulation. Factors that decrease potassium transport into the cell or enhance leakage out of the cell include **acidosis**, α-adrenergic stimulation, and tissue hypoxia.

The amount of potassium in the body is a reflection of the balance between potassium intake and output. Potassium

---

CLINICAL CONDITIONS ASSOCIATED WITH HYPERNATREMIA

Sodium excess greater than water excess:
    Ingestion of large amounts of sodium
    Administration of hypertonic NaCl or NaHCO$_3$
    Primary hyperaldosteronism
Water deficiency greater than sodium deficiency:
    Excessive sweating*—exercise, fever, hot environment
    Burns*
    Hyperventilation
    Diabetes insipidus
        Pituitary—ADH deficiency
        Nephrogenic—kidney unresponsive to ADH
    Osmotic diuresis*—diabetes, mannitol infusion
    Diminished fluid input—diminished thirst
    Essential hypernatremia—reset "osmostat"
    Certain diarrheal states and vomiting*

Total body sodium is decreased. Serum sodium concentration is increased because the magnitude of water loss exceeds the magnitude of sodium loss.

TABLE 24-6 URINE SODIUM CONCENTRATION AND OSMOLARITY IN THE DIFFERENTIAL DIAGNOSIS OF HYPONATREMIA

Urine Osm (mOsm/L)	Urine [Na] (mmol/L)	Etiology
Greater than serum Osm	>20	SIADH Glucocorticoid deficiency Hypothyroidism
<200	Variable	Psychogenic polydipsia
Greater than serum Osm	<10	Heart failure Liver failure Nephrotic syndrome
Greater than serum Osm	<15	Gastrointestinal losses Burns
≈300	>20	Renal failure
Greater than serum Osm	>20	Diuretic therapy Adrenal insufficiency Salt-losing nephropathy Renal tubular acidosis Osmotic diuresis Bicarbonaturia, ketonuria

---

TABLE 24-7 URINE SODIUM CONCENTRATION AND OSMOLARITY IN THE DIFFERENTIAL DIAGNOSIS OF HYPERNATREMIA

Urine Osm (mOsm/L)	Urine [Na] (mmol/L)	Etiology
>400	>20	Excessive sodium intake Primary hypoaldosteronism
>400	<10	Burns Excessive sweating Diarrhea in children
>400	Variable	Hyperventilation Thirst deficit
<300	Low	ADH deficiency
≈300	Low	Nephrogenic diabetes insipidus

CAUSES OF POTASSIUM RETENTION

Increased potassium intake:
    High-potassium diet
    Oral potassium supplementation
    Intravenous potassium administration
    Potassium penicillin in high doses
    Transfusion of aged blood
Decreased potassium excretion:
    Renal failure
    Hypoaldosteronism—adrenal failure
    Diuretics that block distal tubular potassium secretion:
        triamterene, amiloride, spironolactone
    Primary defects in renal tubular potassium secretion

CAUSES OF POTASSIUM DEPLETION

Decreased potassium intake:
    Low-potassium diet
    Alcoholism
    Anorexia nervosa
Increased gastrointestinal losses:
    Vomiting
    Diarrhea
    Fistulas
    Gastrointestinal drainage tube
    Malabsorption
    Laxative or enema abuse
Increased urinary losses:
    Increased aldosterone
        Primary aldosteronism
        Adrenal hyperplasia
        Bartter's syndrome
    Adrenogenital syndrome
    Renal disease
        Renal tubular acidosis
        Fanconi syndrome
    Diuretics
        Thiazides
        Loop diuretics—ethacrynic acid, furosemide
        Carbonic anhydrase inhibitors—acetazolamide
Alkalosis

intake depends on the quantity and type of food intake. Under normal conditions the average adult takes in about 50 to 100 mmol of potassium/day, about the same amount as sodium. Potassium output occurs through three primary routes: the gastrointestinal tract, the skin, and the urine.

Under normal conditions loss of potassium through the gastrointestinal tract is very small, amounting to less than 5 mmol/day for an adult. The concentration of potassium in the sweat is less than that of sodium; therefore potassium losses through the skin are usually quite small.

The major means of potassium excretion is by the kidney. The kidney is capable of regulating the excretion of potassium to maintain body potassium homeostasis. The details of the mechanisms of renal potassium excretion are discussed in Chapter 26.

Disorders of Potassium Balance

Potassium excess. Potassium accumulates in the body when the intake of potassium exceeds output because of some abnormality of the potassium homeostatic mechanisms. Some major conditions causing potassium retention are presented in the box above. It should be noted that under most conditions the normal kidney is capable of excreting a great deal of potassium, and a high potassium intake leads to potassium retention only when kidney function is compromised.

Potassium depletion. Potassium depletion occurs when potassium output exceeds intake. As discussed previously, only small amounts of potassium are lost in the feces under normal conditions. As is the case for water and sodium, however, gastrointestinal potassium loss during diarrhea or drainage of gastrointestinal secretions can be quite large (Table 24-5). Some major clinical conditions causing potassium depletion are presented in the box at right.

Note that alkalosis results in total body potassium depletion. With alkalosis, potassium moves from the extracellular to the intracellular space. In the cells of the distal nephron of the kidney, this increase in intracellular potassium stimulates potassium secretion and therefore increases renal excretion of potassium.

Abnormalities of Plasma Potassium Concentration

Abnormalities in plasma potassium concentration can occur, not only because of abnormalities in total body potassium, but also because of shifts of potassium between the extracellular and intracellular compartments. Although similar shifts may occur with sodium, the effect of intracellular to extracellular shifting on plasma concentration is more pronounced for potassium, because 98% of the total potassium is intracellular. For example, if only 2% of the intracellular potassium were to shift to the extracellular space, plasma potassium concentration would double. Fortunately, the plasma potassium concentration is held fairly constant despite large fluctuations in potassium intake. This homeostatic mechanism is depicted in Fig. 24-11 for increased potassium intake. The opposite effect occurs with decreased potassium intake.

Hyperkalemia. Clinical conditions associated with elevated plasma potassium are listed in the box on the top left of p. 459. Actual plasma potassium may be normal, but measured plasma potassium may be elevated (**pseudohyperkalemia**) if the blood sample is hemolyzed or if there is leakage of potassium from white blood cells when there is leukocytosis (elevated white blood cell number). In addition, vigorous arm exercise, tight application of the tourniquet, or squeezing of the area around the venipuncture site may result in cellular potassium release and spurious elevation of plasma potassium concentration.

True **hyperkalemia** can result from movement of potassium out of the cell into the extracellular water space,

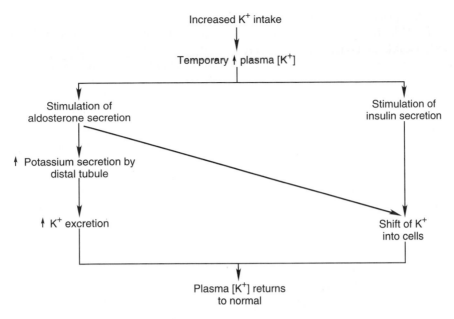

Fig. 24-11   Control of plasma potassium concentration.

Causes of Hyperkalemia

Pseudohyperkalemia:
   Hemolysis
   Leukocytosis
Intracellular to extracellular shift:
   Acidosis*
   Crush injuries
   Tissue hypoxia*
   Insulin deficiency*
   Digitalis overdose*
High potassium intake (see top left box, p. 458)
Decreased potassium excretion (see top left box, p. 458)

*May be associated with total body potassium depletion.

Causes of Hypokalemia

Extracellular to intracellular potassium shift:
   Alkalosis
   Increased plasma insulin*
   Diuretic administration
Decreased potassium intake
Increased gastrointestinal losses (see top right box, p. 458)
Increased urinary losses

*May be associated with total body potassium excess.

increased intake, or decreased output. Hyperkalemia caused by potassium shifts may in fact be associated with total body potassium depletion. This is the case in diabetic ketoacidosis. Hyperkalemia caused by increased intake or decreased output is associated with total body potassium excess.

The clinical signs and symptoms of hyperkalemia include changes in the electrocardiogram, cardiac **arrhythmia**, muscular weakness, and **paresthesias**. The greatest danger of hyperkalemia is life-threatening cardiac arrhythmia or arrest.

Hypokalemia. Low plasma potassium concentration (**hypokalemia**) can be caused by movement of potassium into the cell from the extracellular water space, increased output, or decreased intake (see box at right). Hypokalemia caused by potassium shifts may in fact be associated with increased total body potassium. Hypokalemia caused by increased excretion or decreased intake is associated with total body potassium depletion.

Signs and symptoms of hypokalemia are numerous and include **anorexia**, nausea, vomiting, abdominal distension,

muscle cramps or tenderness, paresthesias, electrocardiographic changes, arrhythmias, inability to concentrate the urine with resultant **polyuria** and polydipsia, lethargy, and confusion. For methods of analysis see sodium and potassium described previously and Sodium and Potassium Methods on CD-ROM.

Urine potassium concentration. Urine potassium concentration can be useful in the differential diagnosis of hypokalemia. As with urine sodium concentration, it is important to interpret these values in light of the clinical picture. A urine potassium concentration <20 mmol/L with hypokalemia is consistent with inadequate intake of potassium or nonurinary losses; a urine potassium level >20 mmol/L is consistent with urinary loss. On the other hand, urine potassium is of little help in the differential diagnosis of hyperkalemia.

CHLORIDE METABOLISM
Chloride Balance

Chloride is the major anion in the ECW space. In a normal adult the total body chloride is about 30 mmol/kg of body weight. Approximately 88% of chloride is found in the ECW space and 12% in the ICW space. Approximately 14% of total body chloride is in the plasma, 27% in ISF that is readily accessible to plasma, 17% in ISF of dense connective tissue and cartilage, 15% in ISF of bone, and 5% in the transcellular space. The concentrations of chloride in the various fluid compartments are listed in Table 24-2. Notice that the concentration of chloride in ISF is greater than that in plasma water, whereas the concentrations of sodium and potassium in ISF are less than that in plasma water. These differences between plasma and ISF are caused by the Gibbs-Donnan equilibrium. Chloride is passively distributed across the cell membrane. The difference in chloride concentration between ISF and ICW is caused by the electrical potential difference across the cell membrane. Because the inside of the cell is negative compared to the outside, the concentration of chloride outside the cell will be higher than that inside.

The amount of chloride in the body is a reflection of the balance between chloride intake and output. Chloride intake depends on the quantity and type of food intake. The chloride content of most foods parallels that of sodium. Under normal conditions the average adult takes in about 50 to 200 mmol of chloride/day. Chloride output occurs by way of three primary routes: the gastrointestinal tract, the skin, and the urinary tract.

Under normal circumstances loss of chloride through the gastrointestinal tract is very small. Fecal chloride excretion for a normal adult is only 1 to 2 mmol/day. The concentrations of chloride in gastrointestinal secretions are shown in Table 24-5. With severe diarrhea or with gastric or intestinal drainage tubes, chloride loss through the gastrointestinal tract may exceed 100 mmol/day.

The chloride composition of sweat averages about 40 mEq/L but is somewhat variable. As in the case of sodium, the concentration of chloride in sweat is decreased by aldosterone and increased in cystic fibrosis. Under conditions of excessive sweating, chloride losses through the skin can exceed 200 mmol/day. However, under normal conditions chloride losses through the skin are small.

The major route of chloride excretion is through the kidney. Details of the mechanisms of renal chloride excretion are discussed in Chapter 26.

Disorders of Chloride Balance

Chloride excess. Chloride accumulates in the body when the intake of chloride exceeds output because of some abnormality of a chloride homeostasis mechanism. For the most part, the causes of chloride retention mainly are the

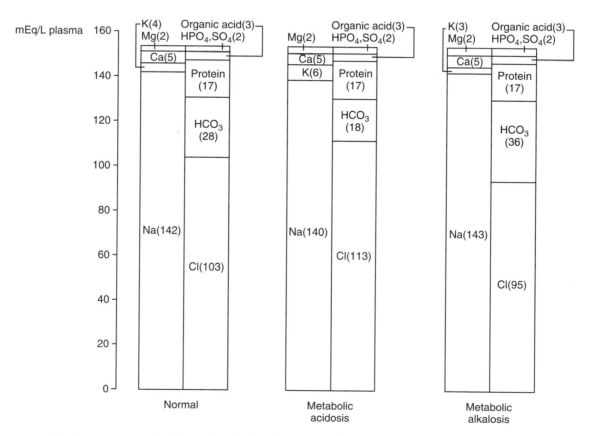

Fig. 24-12 Concentration of electrolytes in plasma (mEq/L) with metabolic acidosis and metabolic alkalosis compared with normal. In the example of metabolic acidosis shown, there is no increase in organic acids, only loss of bicarbonate. Metabolic acidosis may be attributable to an increase in organic acids (see Fig. 24-4). In these cases chloride may not be increased. Notice that the extracellular potassium concentration is elevated in metabolic acidosis and lowered in metabolic alkalosis. Under all conditions the concentration of anions equals concentration of cations.

same as those of sodium retention. Therefore the pathophysiology of chloride excess is in most cases similar to that of sodium excess (see box, p. 453). However, there is one clinical condition in which chloride excess may not be associated with sodium excess: certain types of metabolic acidosis. The two major extracellular anions are chloride and bicarbonate. Extracellular bicarbonate is consumed by the reaction with hydrogen ions produced in metabolic acidosis. If no organic anions are produced with the H^+, chloride ions are needed to replace the consumed bicarbonate ions to maintain electrical neutrality. The increase in chloride concentration is caused by the reabsorption of a relatively greater proportion of sodium with chloride than with bicarbonate by the tubules of the kidney.

Chloride depletion. Chloride depletion occurs when the output of chloride exceeds intake. For the most part, the causes of chloride depletion are the same as those of sodium depletion (see box, p. 456). However, in one clinical condition, hypochloremic **metabolic alkalosis**, there may be chloride depletion without sodium depletion. Hypochloremic metabolic alkalosis may result from loss of chloride in excess of sodium loss, usually from abnormal loss of gastric fluid. Bicarbonate must be retained to maintain electrical neutrality. **Hypochloremia** may also be associated with other disorders that involve bicarbonate retention, such as renal compensation for chronic **respiratory acidosis** (see Chapter 25).

Abnormalities of Plasma Chloride Concentration

As for sodium, changes in total body chloride are not necessarily associated with similar changes in plasma chloride concentration. That is, with body chloride retention the plasma chloride concentration will remain normal if there is a proportional increase in ECW and will decrease if there is a relatively greater increase in ECW. Similarly, plasma chloride concentration may remain normal or even increase with chloride depletion, depending on the concomitant change in ECW.

In most cases the causes of hypochloremia and **hyperchloremia** are the same as those of hyponatremia and hypernatremia (see pp. 456-457). The major clinical exceptions to the usual parallel changes in plasma sodium and chloride concentrations occur during chronic metabolic acidosis and alkalosis. With metabolic acidosis, hyperchloremia may not be associated with hypernatremia; with metabolic alkalosis, hypochloremia may not be associated with hyponatremia. The reasons for this are those previously discussed for chloride excess and depletion.

Symptoms are not directly attributable to hypochloremia or hyperchloremia. Rather, symptoms that occur in patients with an abnormal serum chloride concentration are caused by the associated abnormality in serum sodium or pH. A summary of the plasma electrolyte changes in metabolic acidosis and alkalosis is presented in Fig. 24-12.

Urine Chloride Concentration

The concentration of chloride in the urine is important in the differential diagnosis of metabolic alkalosis (see Chapter 25). Metabolic alkalosis as the result of contraction of the ECW volume will be associated with a urine chloride concentration of less than 15 mmol/L. The metabolic alkalosis can be corrected with saline administration. Metabolic alkalosis with a normal ECW volume will be associated with a urine chloride concentration of greater than 15 mmol/L and be resistant to saline administration.

Bibliography

Abraham WT, Schrier RW: Body fluid volume regulation in health and disease, *Adv Intern Med* 39:23, 1994.

Adrogué HJ, Madias NE: Hypernatremia, *New Engl J Med* 342:1493, 2000.

Adrogué HJ, Madias NE: Hyponatremia, *New Engl J Med* 342:1581, 2000.

Badrick T, Hickman PE: The anion gap. A reappraisal, *Am J Clin Pathol* 98:763, 1992.

Fulop M: Algorithms for diagnosing some electrolyte disorders, *Am J Emerg Med* 16:76, 1998.

Halperin ML, Kamel KS: Potassium, *Lancet* 352:135, 1998.

Ishihara K, Szerlip HM: Anion gap acidosis, *Sem Nephrol* 18:83, 1998.

Koch SM, Taylor RW: Chloride ion in intensive care medicine, *Crit Care Med* 20:227, 1992.

Kumar S, Berl T: Sodium, *Lancet* 352:220, 1998.

Levin ER, Gardner DG, Samson WK: Natriuretic peptides, *New Engl J Med* 339:321, 1998.

Lumbers ER: Angiotensin and aldosterone, *Regul Peptides* 80:91, 1999.

Mandal AK: Hypokalemia and hyperkalemia, *Med Clin N Amer* 81:611, 1997.

Maxwell MH, Kleeman CR, Narins RG, editors: *Clinical disorders of fluid and electrolyte metabolism*, ed 5, New York, 1994, McGraw-Hill.

Oiso Y, Iwasaki Y: Vasopressin and related disorders, *Intern Med* 37:213, 1998.

Internet Sites

http://www.ut.edu.co/fcs/

http://family.georgetown.edu/welchjj/netscut/fen/fluids_intro.html

http://www.cord.edu/faculty/blarson/Water.ppt

http://blue.temple.edu/~pathphys/surgery/fluids.html

http://www.virtual-anaesthesia-textbook.com/vat/acidbase.html—The Virtual Anaesthesia Textbook: Water, Electrolytes, Renal, and Acid-Base

http://www.rrca.org/publicat/wat.htm—Road Runners Club of America (RRCA)

http://www.canr.uconn.edu/nusci/hpg/Water.pdf—University of Connecticut Department of Nutritional Science

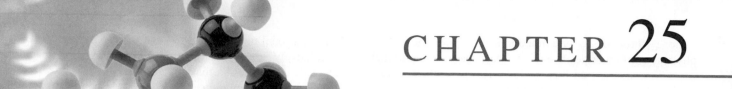

CHAPTER 25

Acid-Base Control and Acid-Base Disorders

• *John E. Sherwin*

Chapter Outline

Objectives

- Outline the blood-buffering mechanism of the bicarbonate and hemoglobin buffering systems.
- Explain acid-base balance regulation by the kidney with respect to the following:
  Hydrogen ion excretion
  Bicarbonate ion reaction
  Sodium-hydrogen exchange
  Ammonium secretion
- State the Henderson-Hasselbalch equation, identifying the respiratory and metabolic components; relate the equation to acid-base disorders; and calculate the pH, given appropriate data.
- For each of the following pathological states,

identify the expected pH, P_{O_2}, and P_{CO_2} values as normal, increased, or decreased, and state the physiological response to the following disease states:
Drug-induced hyperventilation
Acute hyperglycemic ketoacidosis
Hypochloremia resulting from persistent vomiting
Chronic emphysema
- Define oxygen saturation and P_{50}, and describe the effect of the following on dissociation of oxygen from hemoglobin:
2,3-DPG
pH
P_{CO_2}

Key Terms

acidemia A condition of decreased pH of the blood.
acidosis A pathological condition resulting from accumulation of acid in the blood or loss of base from the blood.

alkalemia A condition of increased pH of the blood.
alkalosis A pathological condition resulting from accumulation of base or loss of acid from the body.
alveoli Small outpouchings of walls of alveolar space

through which gas exchange takes place between alveolar air and pulmonary capillary blood.

anlon gap   The concentration of undetermined anions, calculated as the difference between the measured cations and the measured anions.

apnea   Cessation of breathing.

base excess   Elevated HCO_3^-/H_2CO_3 ratio caused by a decrease in P_{CO_2}. As in the relative base deficit, the HCO_3^- (base) is elevated relative to the P_{CO_2}.

base excess or deficit   The difference between the titratable acids and bases of a blood sample and a normal blood sample at a pH of 7.4, a P_{CO_2} of 40 mm Hg, and a temperature of 37° C.

bradycardia   Slowing of the heartbeat to less than 60 beats per minute.

carbamino group   A stable, protein-bound form of CO_2 resulting from the covalent chemical reaction between CO_2 and the primary amino group ($—NH_2$) of a protein.

carbonic anhydrase   An enzyme that catalyzes the reaction between CO_2 and water to form carbonic acid (H_2CO_3).

chloride shift   Exchange of Cl^- in serum for HCO_3^- in red blood cells in peripheral tissues as a response to the P_{CO_2} of the blood. The shift reverses in the lungs.

conjugate base   Unprotonated anionic form of a corresponding weak acid.

Henderson-Hasselbalch equation   Describes the relationship among pH, the pK_a of a buffer system, and the ratio of the conjugate base to a weak acid.

hypercapnia   A condition of excess carbon dioxide in the blood.

hypochloremic alkalosis   A metabolic alkalosis resulting from increased blood bicarbonate secondary to loss of chloride from the body.

hypoxia   A condition of low oxygen content in tissues.

isohydric shift   The series of reactions in red blood cells in which CO_2 is taken up and oxygen is released without the production of excess hydrogen ions.

metabolic acidosis   Pathological loss of base in the body.

metabolic alkalosis   Pathological accumulation of base in the body.

metabolic component   The bicarbonate concentration of plasma.

oxygen saturation   The fraction of total hemoglobin (Hb) in the form of HbO_2 at a defined P_{O_2}. Percentage of saturation = $100(HbO_2)/(HbO_2 + Hb)$.

P_{50}   The partial pressure of oxygen at which hemoglobin is half-saturated with bound oxygen.

partial pressure   The pressure exerted by a gas, whether it is alone or mixed with other gases. The partial pressure of a gas is denoted by the letter P preceding the symbol for that gas (usually in small capital letters); for example, the partial pressure of CO_2 is P_{CO_2}.

pH   The negative logarithm of the hydrogen-ion concentration.

relative base deficit   Lowered HCO_3^-/H_2CO_3 ratio caused by an increase in P_{CO_2}. The HCO_3^- (base) is low relative to the P_{CO_2}.

respiratory acidosis   Pathological retention of CO_2 in the body caused by respiratory change.

respiratory alkalosis   Pathological decrease in CO_2 caused by respiratory change.

respiratory component   The "αP_{CO_2}" or acid component, which is immediately modified by respiratory status; "α" is the solubility (or Bunsen) coefficient of CO_2.

surfactant   An agent that decreases surface tension. Applies to agents that coat pulmonary alveolar surfaces.

ventilation   The exchange of gases between the lungs and ambient air.

Methods on CD-ROM

Blood gas analysis and oxygen saturation
Carbon dioxide
Henderson-Hasselbalch calculating algorithm

Ketones
Lactic acid
Pyruvic acid

ACID-BASE CONTROL
Acids and Bases (see also p. 39)

Definitions. Using the simplest definition, an acid is a substance that releases protons or hydrogen ions (H^+), whereas a base is simply defined as a substance that accepts protons or H^+. Both acids and bases are further defined by their degree of affinity for H^+. A strong acid has little affinity for H^+ and so readily dissociates H^+, whereas a weak acid has

some affinity for H^+ and thus less readily dissociates H^+. A strong base has a high affinity for H^+; a weak base has low affinity for H^+. If one molecule differs from another by only a proton, the two are called a *conjugate acid-base pair*. Physiological examples of a weak acid and its **conjugate base** are carbonic acid (H_2CO_3) and bicarbonate (HCO_3^-). The equilibrium reaction is as follows:

$$H_2CO_3 \rightleftharpoons H^+ + HCO_3^-$$ *Eq. 25-1*

Dietary and metabolic sources of acids and bases.

Two types of acids are dealt with in physiological states: fixed acids and volatile acids. Fixed acids are nongaseous acids such as phosphate (HPO_4^{2-}) and sulfate (SO_4^-) ions or organic acids such as lactic acid, acetoacetic acid, and beta-hydroxybutyric acid. The physiologically important volatile acid is carbonic acid (H_2CO_3). The volatility of carbonic acid arises from its ability to dissociate into water and carbon dioxide (CO_2), which can be released as a gas. The reaction scheme for carbonic acid is as follows:

$$CO_2 \text{ (gas)} \rightleftharpoons CO_2 \text{ (dissolved)} \underset{-H_2O}{\overset{+H_2O}{\rightleftharpoons}} H_2CO_3 \rightleftharpoons H^+ + HCO_3^-$$

Eq. 25-2

At one end of the equilibrium is carbon dioxide, which can be considered the anhydrous form of H_2CO_3, and at the other end is HCO_3^-, the conjugate base of H_2CO_3. Although the reaction of CO_2 and water to form H_2CO_3 will occur spontaneously, the enzyme **carbonic anhydrase** facilitates this reaction in vivo.

Carbohydrates, lipids, and proteins are metabolized by oxidation reactions that generate acids which must be neutralized in order to maintain constant cellular pH. Under anaerobic conditions such as those produced by respiratory distress or strenuous exercise, carbohydrates are metabolized to lactic and pyruvic acids, which accumulate until normal oxygenation is achieved. These acids can be further metabolized to the ultimate oxidation product, carbon dioxide, when aerobic metabolism is resumed. Triglycerides are metabolized to fatty acids, which can be further metabolized to ketone bodies (acetoacetic acid and β-hydroxybutyric acid) under anaerobic conditions. Ultimately these lipid metabolites are further oxidized to carbon dioxide. Proteins are hydrolyzed to amino acids, which are then converted to carbon dioxide. Those proteins composed of sulfur-containing amino acids are catabolized in part to the salt of sulfuric acid. Nucleic acids and some lipids contain phosphorus and are metabolized to salts of phosphoric acid.

pH, hydrogen ion, and buffers. Please review the discussion of pH and buffer calculations in Chapter 1. Remember, the accepted convention is to describe the concentration of H^+ in terms of **pH** (the negative logarithm of the concentration of H^+) rather than in moles per liter (M).

Physiological buffers. Normal human whole blood is buffered at a slightly alkaline pH in a range of 7.35 to 7.45, which corresponds to an H^+ concentration of 4.5×10^{-8} M to 3.5 to 10^{-8} M. Buffering capacity depends on the concentration of the buffer and the relationship between the pK_a of the buffer and the desired pH. A buffer is considered most effective within ±2 pH units of its pK_a. It has maximum buffering capacity when its pK_a equals the pH. For maximum blood buffering, the pK_a of the buffers should therefore be near physiological pH, that is, pH 7.4. The physiologically important buffers that maintain this narrow pH range observed in the body are hemoglobin, bicarbonate, phosphate, and proteins. Table 25-1 lists the pK_a and concentrations of these buffer systems and their relative buffering capacities.

TABLE 25-1   PHYSIOLOGICALLY IMPORTANT BUFFERS AND THEIR CONCENTRATION, pK_a, AND BUFFERING CAPACITY

Buffer	pK_a	Concentration (mmol/L)	Relative Buffering Capacity (mEq/L)
Bicarbonate	6.33	25	1
Hemoglobin	7.2	53	40
Phosphate	6.8	1.2	0.3
Protein	—	—	8

Bicarbonate buffer system. The **Henderson-Hasselbalch equation** for the bicarbonate-carbonic acid buffer system is as follows:

$$pH = pK_a + \log \frac{[HCO_3^-]}{[H_2CO_3]}$$

Eq. 25-3

The measured pK_a is 6.33 at 37° C. Instead of being at the maximum buffer capacity with a 1:1 ratio of HCO_3^- to H_2CO_3, the bicarbonate-carbonic acid buffer system at the blood pH of 7.4 is at a ratio of 20:1.

$$pH = pK_a + \log \frac{[HCO_3^-]}{[H_2CO_3]} = 6.33 + \log 20 = 7.4$$

Eq. 25-4

This 20:1 ratio is maintained primarily by the lungs, which expel CO_2 produced during the metabolism of nutrients.

In Eq. 25-3 there are three unknowns: pH, $[HCO_3^-]$, and $[H_2CO_3]$. Although pH is measurable, there is no direct measure of $[HCO_3^-]$ or $[H_2CO_3]$. To use this equation, replace the term H_2CO_3 with an analyte that is measurable. The concentration of H_2CO_3 is proportional to the amount of dissolved CO_2 (Eq. 25-2). Thus, you can replace $[H_2CO_3]$ with the term αP_{CO_2} where α (the Bunson coefficient) is the solubility coefficient of CO_2. The pK_a term in the Henderson-Hasselbalch equation is modified to reflect the equilibrium between CO_2 (dissolved) and HCO_3^-. The modified Henderson-Hasselbalch equation describing the equilibrium in Eq. 25-2 is as follows:

$$pH = pK_a' + \log \frac{[HCO_3^-]}{\alpha P_{CO_2}}$$

Eq. 25-5

The apparent pK_a' in human plasma is 6.1 at 37° C. The solubility coefficient for CO_2 in plasma at 37° C is 0.031 mmol $\times$ L^{-1} $\times$ mm Hg^{-1}. The concentration of base greatly exceeds that of acid in this plasma buffer system, reflecting the demands put on the body by metabolism, which primarily produces acids. This buffer system is designed to process the primary metabolic waste product, CO_2. The CO_2 component of the buffer system is eliminated by the lungs.

The total CO_2 content (T_{CO_2}) of plasma is described as

$$T_{CO_2} = CO_2 \text{ (dissolved)} + [HCO_3^-] + [H_2CO_3]$$

Eq. 25-6, A

The $[H_2CO_3]$ term can be disregarded because it is so small (one twentieth the $[HCO_3^-]$) and CO_2 (dissolved) can be replaced with the term αPco_2. Thus the equation can be reduced to

$$Tco_2 = \alpha Pco_2 + [HCO_3^-] \qquad \textit{Eq. 25-6, B}$$

Two of the three unknowns are readily determined, allowing calculation of the third (see pp. 39 and 472).

Hemoglobin. The major buffer of blood is hemoglobin, which is localized in the red blood cells. Hemoglobin (Hb) takes up free H^+ so that the following reaction proceeds to the right:

$$CO_2 + H_2O \rightleftharpoons H_2CO_3 \rightleftharpoons HCO_3^- + H^+$$
$$\searrow \; HHb^+ + O_2$$
$$HbO_2 \qquad \textit{Eq. 25-7}$$

Hemoglobin and serum proteins have high concentrations of histidine residues. The imidazole group of histidine (Fig. 25-1) has a pK_a of approximately 7.3. It is this combination of high concentration and appropriate pK_a that makes hemoglobin the dominant buffering agent of blood at physiological pH. The bulk of the CO_2 formed in peripheral tissues is transported in the plasma portion of blood as HCO_3^- with the H^+ bound to hemoglobin within the erythrocyte (Fig. 25-2). The CO_2 of carbonic acid accounts for about 2 mmol/L of CO_2 in venous blood but accounts for only about 1 mmol/L in arterial blood.

Significant amounts of CO_2 are transported as a protein-bound moiety. CO_2 reacts nonenzymatically with the accessible amino groups of proteins to form a **carbamino group**:

$$\underset{\text{C}}{\overset{\text{O} \;\; \text{O}}{\diagdown\diagup}} + \; \underset{\overset{|}{\text{H}}}{\overset{\overset{\text{H}}{|}}{\text{N}}} - \text{Protein} \;\rightarrow\; {}^-\text{O-C-N-Protein} \; + \; H^+$$
$$\textbf{Carbamino}$$
$$\textbf{group} \qquad \textit{Eq. 25-8}$$

Approximately 0.5 mmol/L of CO_2 is transported in this fashion.

The observed arteriovenous difference in total CO_2 content is almost entirely the result of formation of bicarbonate in the red blood cell. In the lungs, as deoxygenated hemoglobin becomes oxygenated and the CO_2 is expelled, the H^+ is released from hemoglobin because oxygenated hemoglobin (HbO_2) is a stronger acid than deoxyhemoglobin (HbH). In the lungs, then, the reaction in Eq. 25-7 proceeds to the left. H^+ is released and reacts with the transported HCO_3^- to form CO_2, which the lungs can now release (Fig. 25-2). The overall equation linking the oxygenation process to buffering is

$$H^+ + HbO_2 \rightleftharpoons HHb^+ + O_2 \qquad \textit{Eq. 25-9}$$

The forward reaction occurs in tissues in which there is a relatively high H^+ and a relatively low O_2 concentration, whereas the reverse reaction occurs in the lungs, where the O_2 concentration is relatively high.

Phosphate and proteins. Phosphate is a minor buffering component of the blood, with the following equilibrium reaction occurring:

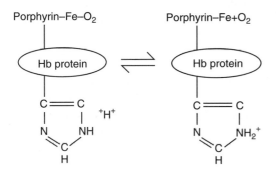

Fig. 25-1 Effect of hemoglobin oxygenation on buffering action of imidazole group of histidine. Oxygen binding affects the pK_a of the imidazole ring, making the ring more acidic with release of an H^+.

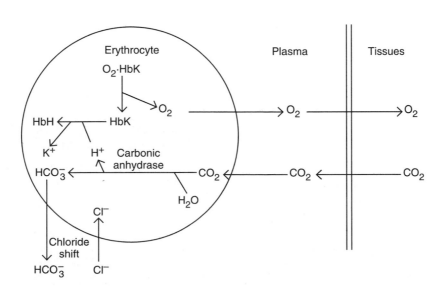

Fig. 25-2 Hemoglobin buffering action in peripheral tissues. *HbK*, potassium salt of hemoglobin; *HbH*, protonated form of hemoglobin.

$$H_2PO_4^- \rightleftharpoons H^+ + HPO_4^{2-} \qquad Eq.\ 25\text{-}10$$

The pK_a of this reaction is 6.8. Phosphate buffer is an important buffer in urine, which has relatively little protein, hemoglobin, or bicarbonate. The phosphate buffers in the blood are inorganic phosphates, but both inorganic and organic phosphates act as intracellular buffers.

Plasma proteins also act as buffers in the blood, although their buffering effect is minor compared with that of the bicarbonate system or hemoglobin system (see Table 25-1).

Oxygen and Carbon Dioxide Homeostasis

Partial pressure. Blood-gas analysis is performed to determine the **partial pressures** of oxygen and carbon dioxide (Po_2 and Pco_2, respectively). Historically, the units of Po_2 and Pco_2 have been millimeters of mercury (mm Hg), or torr, and these units are still used by a majority of laboratories in the United States. The international unit for partial pressure is the *pascal*, or Pa (1 mm Hg = 133.3224 Pa).

Table 25-2 shows the composition of atmospheric air, alveolar air (air inside the lung), and expired air. Humidity makes a substantial contribution to the composition of air in the lungs, thus altering the partial pressures of the other gases. A correction for the gas-volume contributed by water vapor is therefore essential; at 37° C, the P_{H_2O} of blood is approximately 47 mm Hg.

Two terms used in discussing the oxygen content of blood are **oxygen saturation** and **P$_{50}$**. Oxygen saturation is the percentage of the total hemoglobin present as oxygenated hemoglobin. P_{50} denotes that partial pressure of oxygen at which the hemoglobin is 50% saturated with oxygen.

Ventilation. **Ventilation** is differentiated from respiration in that *ventilation* is the mechanical process of moving air in and out of the lungs, and *respiration* is the exchange of gases between the atmosphere and the body. The exchange of gases between air and the capillaries of the pulmonary circulation occurs in the **alveoli**. The normal respiration rate is 13 to 16 times per minute.

The walls of the lung contain elastic connective tissues that would collapse the lung were it not for the surface tension between the wall of the lung and the wall of the thoracic cavity. The surface tension of the inner walls of the alveoli, in contrast, has a tendency to collapse the alveoli after expiration, when the alveoli are deflated. This surface tension is reduced by the presence of a phospholipid-lipoprotein complex, a **surfactant** that lines the alveolar walls in a thin film and allows the alveolar walls to be easily reinflated. Premature babies without sufficient surfactant lining the alveolar walls can have respiratory difficulties because of the tendency of alveoli to collapse. It is for this reason that the levels of surfactant (e.g., lecithin/sphingomyelin ratio) in amniotic fluid are determined to assess fetal lung development (see Chapter 40).

Gas exchange. Gas transfer in the alveoli is a concentration-dependent phenomenon. Inspired (room) air has a relatively high Po_2 (158 mm Hg) and a low Pco_2 (0.3 mm Hg). Pressures of oxygen and carbon dioxide in capillary blood in the lungs are 50 and 40 mm Hg, respectively. Because the Po_2 of blood is lower than that of inspired air and the Pco_2 of blood is higher than the Pco_2 of room air, the gases diffuse from higher to lower concentration areas. That is, CO_2 gas moves from the capillaries to the alveolar air space, whereas O_2 moves from the alveoli to the capillaries. Reference values for adult blood-gas parameters in arterial and venous blood are summarized in Table 25-3. Because of its greater water solubility, CO_2 exchanges more rapidly and more efficiently than O_2 does. In **respiratory acidosis**, this phenomenon of differential gas diffusibility can result in low blood Po_2 but relatively normal Pco_2.

Control of ventilation. Ventilatory control regulates the carbonate-bicarbonate buffer system but is in turn regulated by the resulting pH of cerebrospinal fluid and plasma. Control of ventilation is localized in a respiratory center of the brain where chemoreceptors are influenced by the pH of the cerebrospinal fluid. Other chemoreceptors influenced by the changes in pH of arterial blood are located in the carotid and aortic vessels. A rise in Pco_2 of arterial blood will result in a fall in pH. This will in turn stimulate the chemoreceptors, initiating a rise in the respiration rate that will result in the release of more CO_2 from the blood in the lungs.

Acid-Base Balance

The maintenance of a constant pH is important because changes in pH will alter the functioning of enzymes, the cellular uptake and use of metabolites and minerals, the

---

TABLE 25-2 COMPARISON OF AIR (PARTIAL PRESSURE EXPRESSED IN MM HG)

Air	N$_2$	O$_2$	CO$_2$	H$_2$O	Total Pressure
Atmospheric air	598.0	158.0	0.3	3.7	760
Alveolar air	573.0	100.0	40.0	47.0	760
Expired air	566.0	115.0	32.0	47.0	760

TABLE 25-3 REFERENCE VALUES FOR ADULT BLOOD-GAS PARAMETERS IN ARTERIAL AND VENOUS BLOOD

Parameters	Arterial	Venous
pH	7.35 to 7.45	7.33 to 7.43
Pco$_2$	35 to 45 mm Hg	38 to 50 mm Hg
Po$_2$	80 to 100 mm Hg	30 to 50 mm Hg
HCO$_3^-$	22 to 26 mmol/L	23 to 27 mmol/L
Total CO$_2$	23 to 27 mmol/L	24 to 28 mmol/L
O$_2$ saturation	94% to 100%	60% to 85%
Venous anion gap	5 to 14 mmol/L	5 to 14 mmol/L
Base excess	−2 to +2 mEq/L	−2 to +2 mEq/L

conformation of biological structural components, and the uptake and release of oxygen.

In the body, physiological buffers act to maintain a constant pH in the following manner. Fixed acids enter the blood and are immediately neutralized by the bicarbonate buffering system.

$$H^+A^- \text{ (fixed acid)} + HCO_3^- \rightleftharpoons H_2CO_3 + A^- \text{ (unmeasured anions)}$$
$$\Updownarrow$$
$$H_2O + CO_2 \qquad \textit{Eq. 25-11}$$

However, the volatile acid, CO_2, is neutralized by the hemoglobin buffering system, because all the buffering systems are at equilibrium with one another. It is this overall equilibrium that gives the blood the relative buffering capacities described in Table 25-1.

Thus one of the important buffer systems required to maintain the pH of the blood is the carbonic acid-bicarbonate buffer system. Although this system has relatively low buffering capacity (see Table 25-1), it plays a large role in maintaining blood pH because it acts as the immediate buffer when fixed acids enter the blood.

Changes in respiration rate will alter the bicarbonate-carbonic acid ratio and pH. To understand this process, one must reconsider Eqs. 25-2 and 25-5. A decrease in the ventilation rate will cause a decrease in release of CO_2 from the blood in the lungs. The increased blood CO_2 will result in the formation of more bicarbonate (shifting Eq. 25-2 to the right), though the increase in bicarbonate will be less than the increase in PCO_2. Thus there will be a decrease in the bicarbonate-carbonate ratio and a decrease in the pH (see Eq. 25-5). If the ventilation rate were to remain constant and the metabolic release of fixed acid were to increase, the same effect would be observed. In this case H^+ reacts with HCO_3^- to form CO_2, which is released in the lungs. There is an immediate decrease in the concentration of bicarbonate with essentially no change in PCO_2, resulting in a decreased bicarbonate/αPCO_2 ratio and a decreased pH. If the ventila-

tion rate increases, more CO_2 is released from the blood at the lungs and the bicarbonate-carbonic acid ratio and pH increase. The ventilation rate can range from zero to 15 times the normal, allowing a significant degree of regulation of the bicarbonate-carbonic acid ratio. Thus when the rate of ventilation is increased, excess acid in the form of CO_2 is quickly removed. Similarly, when the rate of ventilation is decreased, acid (CO_2) is added to neutralize excess alkali (HCO_3^-).

The other important blood buffer, hemoglobin, which is vital for the regulation of blood pH, buffers the CO_2 produced by the tissues. The major function of hemoglobin is the transport of oxygen through the blood to the cells of the body. There is a complex relationship between the degree of oxygenation of hemoglobin and the pH, PCO_2, and total CO_2 (TCO_2) of blood. Oxygenated hemoglobin is a stronger acid than deoxygenated hemoglobin, and therefore in the lungs hemoglobin will release H^+ as it becomes oxygenated (Eqs. 25-7 and 25-12), decreasing the bicarbonate level and increasing the levels of carbonic acid and its anhydrous form CO_2, and thus increasing the PCO_2 of the blood. The rate at which this reaction proceeds is enormously increased by the presence in the red blood cells of the enzyme carbonic anhydrase. It is the action of this enzyme that allows the rapid transfer of CO_2 into and out of red blood cells, with consequent buffering by hemoglobin. This process is summarized by the following series of reactions and by Fig. 25-3.

$$\text{Carbonic anhydrase}$$
$$\downarrow$$
$$\text{Gas exchange in the lungs } CO_2 \rightleftharpoons dCO_2 \rightleftharpoons$$
$$\text{(gas)} \qquad \text{(dissolved)}$$
$$H_2CO_3 \rightleftharpoons H^+ + HCO_3^-$$

$$TCO_2 = dCO_2 + HCO_3^- \text{ or } TCO_2 = \alpha PCO_2 + HCO_3^- \qquad \textit{Eq. 25-12}$$

In the lungs ventilation will eliminate this increased PCO_2 by releasing the CO_2 from the blood and thereby return the ratio of bicarbonate to carbonic acid to 20.

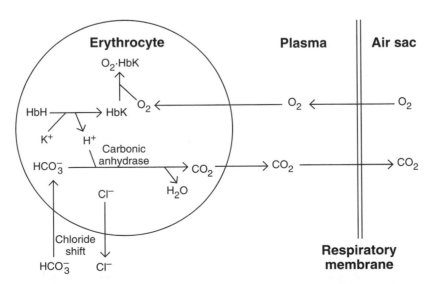

Fig. 25-3 Transfer of CO_2 in lungs from erythrocytes to air sacs. *HbK*, potassium salt of hemoglobin; *HbH*, protonated form of hemoglobin.

Oxygenated hemoglobin is transported in the blood to cells that have relatively low Po_2 tension and are releasing metabolic products such as CO_2 and organic acids into the blood, thus raising the Pco_2 and Tco_2 and lowering the pH. The relatively low Po_2 causes the dissociation of O_2 from HbO_2 and the consequent delivery of O_2 to the cells. The high CO_2 pressure in the cells drives the CO_2 along a concentration gradient into the red blood cells. Carbonic anhydrase rapidly converts the CO_2 into H^+ and HCO_3^- (see Fig. 25-2). Deoxygenated hemoglobin is a weaker acid than oxygenated hemoglobin. It neutralizes the H^+ to raise the pH and causes the dissociation reaction of carbonic acid to proceed to the right to increase the level of bicarbonate and decrease the Pco_2.

The dissociation of oxygen from hemoglobin as a function of the Pco_2 is shown in Fig. 25-4, which is a graph of the percentage of O_2 saturation of hemoglobin versus Po_2. The sigmoidal shape of the curve indicates that at critical levels of Po_2 near the P_{50} there is a strong increase or decrease in the percentage of O_2 saturation, with a minimal shift in Po_2. In an area of the body in which there is a drop in Po_2 below that of P_{50} on the sigmoid curve, the hemoglobin will release a larger portion of O_2 than at a Po_2 level above the P_{50}. Similarly, in areas of high O_2, such as the lungs, the hemoglobin will be essentially saturated with O_2.

Another factor that has an effect on the position of the oxygen dissociation curve is 2,3-diphosphoglycerate (2,3-DPG), an intermediate in glycolysis. By interacting with the N-terminal amino groups of the hemoglobin molecule itself, 2,3-DPG induces the release of oxygen from hemoglobin. This is reflected in the shift to the right of the O_2 dissociation curve (Fig. 25-4). With a shift to the right, the critical Po_2 level that causes 50% saturation of hemoglobin by oxygen is

increased so that areas of active metabolism, which contain increased 2,3-DPG levels, do not require Po_2 levels as low as those required in areas without increased 2,3-DPG for significant O_2 release from hemoglobin. See Chapter 36 for additional details on factors affecting oxygen binding by hemoglobin.

As more oxygen is released in response to increased levels of Pco_2 and H^+, more deoxyhemoglobin, which acts as a buffer, is formed. Increased Pco_2 leads to formation of bicarbonate (HCO_3^-). Most H^+ ions are bound by the deoxygenated hemoglobin, and the rest are buffered by the proteins and phosphate buffer in the plasma. Because all the H^+ formed is buffered, there is essentially no change in the pH. This buffering phenomenon is referred to as the **isohydric shift**. The HCO_3^- formed in the red blood cells as a result of uptake of H^+ by the hemoglobin diffuses out of the cells into the plasma. To preserve the electrical neutrality of the red blood cell, as HCO_3^- diffuses out of the cell, Cl^- diffuses into the erythrocytes from the plasma. This increase in the erythrocyte Cl^- is termed the **chloride shift**. Thus the plasma chloride concentration of venous blood (where HCO_3^- is formed in red blood cells) is *lower* than that of arterial blood. When CO_2 is expelled from the lungs, Cl^- again shifts out of red blood cells into plasma (see Figs. 25-2 and 25-3). As the anion charges on the polyvalent hemoglobin molecule are replaced by the diffusing monovalent chloride anions, the osmolality of the erythrocyte increases, leading to diffusion of water into the erythrocyte, slightly increasing the mean volume of venous red blood cells over the mean cell volume (MCV) in arterial blood.

Although the intact respiratory system acts as an immediate regulator of the $HCO_3^-/\alpha Pco_2$ system, long-term control is exerted by renal mechanisms (see Chapter 26 for

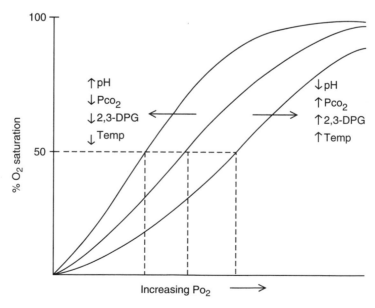

Fig. 25-4   Hemoglobin-oxygen dissociation curves and factors that shift the curve right and left. A shift of curve right or left changes the level of Po_2 at which hemoglobin is 50% saturated (P_{50}).

details). The kidneys excrete nonvolatile acids such as sulfuric, hydrochloric, phosphoric, and some organic acids into the urine. Hydrogen ions are excreted by the kidneys into the urine and are buffered by HPO_4^{2-} and ammonia, which is derived from deamidation of the amino acid glutamine. Sodium is the cation exchanged for excreted hydrogen ions by the kidney. The kidney also affects the bicarbonate-carbonic acid buffer system by regulating the excretion of bicarbonate (Fig. 25-5). The kidney reabsorbs almost all filtered bicarbonate at plasma bicarbonate concentrations below 25 mEq/L. Only when bicarbonate levels become elevated above 25 mEq/L will bicarbonate be excreted into the urine. The reabsorbed bicarbonate is electrically neutralized by the reabsorbed sodium ions, which have been exchanged for the hydrogen ions excreted in the urine (Fig. 25-5).

ACID-BASE DISORDERS
Definitions

Acid-base disorders are most readily classified in terms of their immediate cause. Thus acidoses and alkaloses are described as being of either respiratory or metabolic origin.

These classifications should always be considered in terms of the modified Henderson-Hasselbalch equation:

$$pH = pK_a' + \log \frac{[HCO_3^-]}{\alpha P CO_2} \qquad \textit{Eq. 25-13}$$

The term $\alpha P CO_2$ represents the acid component that is directly and immediately modified by respiratory status. Thus the term $\alpha P CO_2$ is called the **respiratory component**. The concentration of bicarbonate is most immediately affected by changes in the hydrogen-ion concentration caused by production of metabolic acids other than CO_2 (i.e., fixed acids) and by physiological processes that directly change the concentration of serum bicarbonate. Thus the bicarbonate concentration of plasma is called the **metabolic component** of acid-base status. Acid-base homeostasis is accomplished when one or both of these components is

controlled. Keep in mind that the pH of plasma depends on the *ratio* of the concentration of bicarbonate to $\alpha P CO_2$ rather than on the absolute concentration of these components (see Eq. 25-13).

Base excess. Base excess is a calculated parameter used to assess the metabolic component of the patient's acid-base disturbance. The term *base excess* is used to describe clinical situations in which there is an excess of bicarbonate (positive base excess) or a deficit of bicarbonate (negative base excess). We use the term *base deficit* for a negative base excess because this is a more accurate description of the physiological condition. Base excess in the blood at a pH of 7.40, $P CO_2$ of 40 mm Hg, a hemoglobin concentration of 150 g/L, and a temperature of 37° C is zero. The hemoglobin concentration is important because the blood-buffering capacity is greatly dependent on this quantity. The addition of a base, such as bicarbonate, raises the buffer content of the blood and results in a positive base excess. The loss of base, as occurs in diarrhea or with the addition of acids, lowers the blood buffer content and results in a base deficit. The calculation of the **base excess or deficit** is useful in the management of patients with acid-base disturbances because it permits estimation of the number of milliequivalents of sodium bicarbonate or ammonium chloride that should be administered to correct the patient's pH to normal. In practice the base excess is only a crude estimate because as the patient's condition improves, changes in respiration and metabolism will invalidate the original calculation. It is for this reason that blood-gas status is closely monitored by the analysis of sequential blood specimens.

$$\text{Base excess} = (1.0 - 0.0143\ \text{Hgb})\ (HCO_3^-) - (9.5 + 1.63\ \text{Hgb})\ (7.4\ \text{pH}) - 24 \quad \textit{Eq. 25-14}$$

where Hgb is the hemoglobin concentration in g/dL.

Oxygen saturation. Oxygen saturation indicates the amount of oxygen bound to hemoglobin and is used to determine the effectiveness of respiration or oxygen therapy. Oxygen saturation is calculated by use of the measured

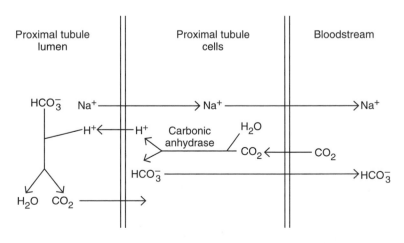

Fig. 25-5 Kidney reabsorption of bicarbonate with excretion of H^+.

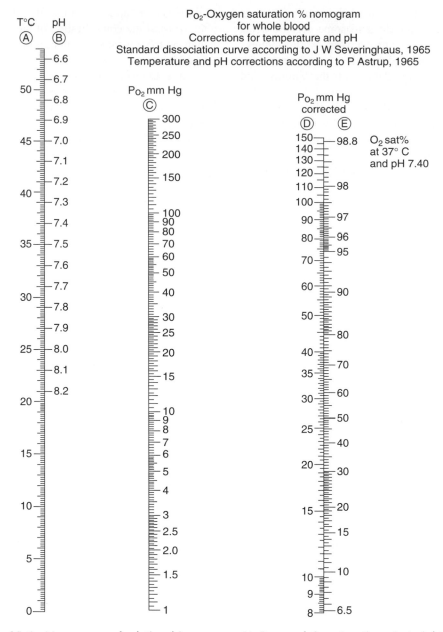

Fig. 25-6   Nomogram of relationship among pH, Po_2, and O_2 saturation. A straight line through a value of pH and of Po_2 will connect with a calculated value of O_2 saturation at 37° C. *(Courtesy Radiometer Corp., Copenhagen, Denmark.)*

parameters of pH and Po_2 and the equation for a normal oxygen dissociation curve. A nomogram to derive O_2 saturation from pH and Po_2 values is presented in Fig. 25-6. Oxygen saturation is also measured directly by use of the difference in the wavelengths of maximum absorbance for oxyhemoglobin and deoxyhemoglobin. This measurement is performed with a co-oximeter. Table 25-3 contains reference values for the calculated blood-gas parameters.

Anion gap. If the total measured cations are subtracted from the total measured anions, the difference is the **anion gap,** or the amount of unmeasured anions present, as shown by the following equation:

$$\text{Anion gap} = [Na^+] + [K^+] - [Cl^-] - [HCO_3^-] \qquad \textit{Eq. 25-15}$$

Usually the only electrolytes measured are sodium, potassium, chloride, and bicarbonate (as total CO_2). However, other anions exist in blood, such as phosphates, ketones, lactic acid, proteins, and sulfates. These other anions are not measured, whereas their counterions are, resulting in an apparent excess, or gap, of measured cations over measured anions. Increases in the amounts of these unmeasured anions and of the accompanying Na^+ ions will increase the apparent gap. Usually the anion gap averages 12 mEq/L. The anion gap increases with production of organic acids. Diabetic ketoacidosis is the most common cause of an elevated anion gap. If diabetes is ruled out, other causes of the acidosis must be sought, such as lactic acidosis, dehydration, renal tubular acidosis, sepsis, and toxic acidosis.

Base-Deficient Disorders

Any condition associated with a lower-than-normal blood pH (**acidemia**) is referred to as an **acidosis**.

Metabolic acidosis. In base-deficient disorders the pH is below the reference interval. Such disorders occur if metabolic processes result in the accumulation of abnormal amounts of organic acids other than carbonic acid. Examples of acids that accumulate are lactic acid, β-hydroxybutyric acid, and acetoacetic acid. Metabolic organic acids entering plasma react with plasma bicarbonate to form H_2CO_3; this is immediately converted to CO_2 gas, which in turn is rapidly eliminated from the body by the lungs. The net result is an immediate decrease in bicarbonate concentration with essentially no loss of PCO_2. This leads to a lowered bicarbonate/αPCO_2 ratio and a lowered pH, or metabolic acidosis.

In contrast to this accumulation of acids is the pathological loss of base from the body. In severe diarrhea, bicarbonate ion is lost as part of the watery stool, resulting in a base deficit ($\downarrow[HCO_3^-]$, $\downarrow$ bicarbonate/αPCO_2 ratio). These types of disorders are termed **metabolic acidoses**.

Respiratory acidosis. A relative base-deficient disorder can result from a decrease in the bicarbonate-carbonic acid ratio as a result of an increase in carbonic acid. This occurs if the lungs are not able to expel CO_2 from the blood. This disorder is termed *respiratory acidosis*. The increase in PCO_2 results in an increase in the concentration of bicarbonate as the CO_2 is buffered by hemoglobin. However, the rise in bicarbonate is less than the increase in PCO_2, resulting in a **relative base deficit** and a decrease in the bicarbonate/αPCO_2 ratio, which results in a blood pH below the reference interval.

Base-Excess Disorders

Any condition associated with a blood pH above the reference interval (**alkalemia**) is called an **alkalosis**.

Metabolic alkalosis. In base-excess disorders, the pH is above the reference interval. If the disorder is caused by an increase in bicarbonate, with little or no change in carbonic acid, the disorder is termed **metabolic alkalosis**. Such a disorder occurs when excess amounts of bicarbonate of soda are ingested or administered or when there is an increased renal reabsorption of bicarbonate, as in **hypochloremic alkalosis**.

Respiratory alkalosis. If the disorder is caused by a decrease in carbonic acid, as when respiration is overly stimulated, the disorder is termed **respiratory alkalosis**. In this condition, rapid ventilation greatly decreases the PCO_2 of blood, with minimal change in bicarbonate concentration. This results in a relative excess of bicarbonate so that the bicarbonate/αPCO_2 ratio increases. This increased ratio yields a higher plasma pH.

Instrumentation (see also pp. 313-315 and CD-ROM)

The traditional laboratory blood-gas analyzer includes a pH electrode, a PO_2 electrode, and a PCO_2 electrode. As point-of-care testing has gained acceptance, the use of noninvasive electrodes has expanded. Current technology permits reliable assessment of both PO_2 and PCO_2 using noninvasive techniques but *not* blood pH. The noninvasive devices use essentially the same electrodes as the traditional blood-gas analyzer. They are widely used in neonatal intensive care units because they do not require blood collection from these small infants. It is common practice to verify the performance of these noninvasive instruments by performing a traditional blood-gas analysis periodically.

With the development of disposable microelectrodes and fully automated analyzers that are reliable, blood-gas analysis is now being done in the surgery suite and other nonlaboratory settings, resulting in shortened turnaround times for results and permitting more rapid medical intervention.

The central laboratory is usually responsible for maintaining the devices, whereas the operator, physician, or respiratory therapist is responsible for performing quality control. Documentation of operator training is required.

Calculated parameters. The remainder of the blood acid-base parameters are not measured but are instead calculated using Eqs. 25-6, *B*, and 25-13. One of the parameters is bicarbonate, which is calculated by use of the measured parameters pH and PCO_2 in the Henderson-Hasselbalch equation:

$$HCO_3^- = [\alpha PCO_2] \text{ antilog } [pH - pK_a']\qquad \textit{Eq. 25-16}$$

Nomograms have also been developed to derive bicarbonate levels from pH and PCO_2 measurements (Fig. 25-7 and the Henderson-Hasselbalch calculating algorithm on the CD-ROM). Bicarbonate levels are useful in the assessment of the degree to which metabolic and renal control are involved in the acid-base status of the patient.

ACIDOSIS

Metabolic Acidosis

Etiology. Increased organic acid production resulting in metabolic acidosis can have many causes. Uncontrolled diabetes results in accumulation of acetoacetic and hydroxybutyric acids, which are produced by the excessive oxidation of fatty acids (see Chapter 32). Fasting or fad diets also lead to increased levels of these acids.

Lactic acid increases as a result of increases in anaerobic metabolism caused by strenuous muscular exercise or systemic infections. Lactic acidosis also results from local tissue **hypoxia** (low tissue PO_2), which is caused by dehydration, poor perfusion as a result of circulatory collapse, or cardiac failure.

Renal tubular acidosis results from a failure of the kidney to acidify the urine by exchanging H^+ for Na^+. This renal insufficiency may be acquired as a result of infection or may be congenital, as in cases of severe de Toni-Fanconi syndrome. Liver disease that impairs the formation of urea and ammonia also results in a metabolic acidosis because of retention of H^+.

Siggaard-Andersen alignment nomogram

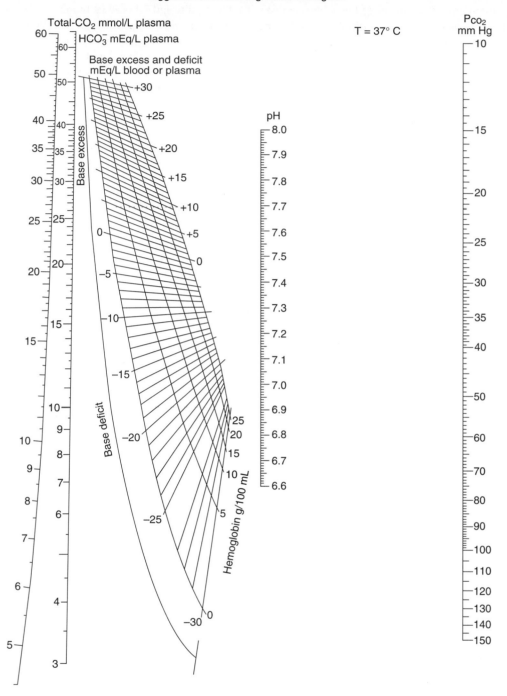

Fig. 25-7 Nomogram of relationship among P_{CO_2}, pH, base excess, hemoglobin, bicarbonate, and total CO_2. A straight line through a value of pH and of P_{CO_2} will connect with a calculated value of HCO_3^- and total CO_2. Base excess or deficit can be derived from that straight line if the hemoglobin level is known. *(Modified from Radiometer Corp., Copenhagen, Denmark.)*

Salicylate intoxication initially induces respiratory alkalosis because of hyperventilation, which is a result of a stimulatory effect of the drug on the respiratory center. The ingested drug is converted to an acid before excretion, and the large quantities of acid formed ultimately result in metabolic acidosis. Other poisons ingested as acids or as compounds will lead to acid metabolites; for example, methanol (converted to formic acid), ethylene glycol (converted to oxalic acid), paraldehyde, and ammonium chloride. These compounds initially cause respiratory alkalosis, followed by metabolic acidosis. Infusion of large quantities of isotonic sodium chloride results in a metabolic acidosis because the

> **TABLE 25-4 CLASSES OF ACID-BASE DISORDERS WITH CORRESPONDING EFFECTS ON SELECTED BLOOD-GAS PARAMETERS**
>
> | Disorder | pH | PCO_2 | HCO_3^- | Base Excess |
> |---|---|---|---|---|
> | Metabolic acidosis | ↓ | ↓N | ↓ | ↓ |
> | Respiratory acidosis | ↓ | ↑ | ↑N | ↑N |
> | Metabolic alkalosis | ↑ | ↑N | ↑ | ↑ |
> | Respiratory alkalosis | ↑ | ↓ | ↓N | ↓N |
>
> N, *initially normal (within the reference interval).*

high sodium load competes with hydrogen ions for renal excretion. Metabolic acidosis is also caused by the ingestion of carbonic anhydrase inhibitors, such as acetazolamide or sulfonamides, which interfere with the formation of bicarbonate in the erythrocyte and the renal tubule cells (see Figs. 25-2, 25-3, and 25-5).

Metabolic acidosis may also be caused by a decreased bicarbonate concentration. Diarrhea and colitis lead to losses of intestinal fluids, which contain high concentrations of bicarbonate. The resultant reduction of the HCO_3^-/H_2CO_3 ratio causes acidemia.

Physiological response. The acidoses just described usually result from the presentation to the body of an acid load that is compensated for, at least in part, by retention of bicarbonate. When acidemia occurs as a result of acute metabolic acidosis, the body attempts to correct this acidemia by hyperventilation. Hyperventilation lowers the PCO_2 (and to a smaller extent the HCO_3) and at least partially increases the ratio of HCO_3^-/H_2CO_3, thereby returning the pH toward normal. This mechanism of correcting the pH during acidosis is known as *compensatory respiratory alkalosis*. The result is a decrease in the PCO_2 and HCO_3^- concentration and a pH value closer to the reference interval.

In a metabolic acidosis that does not involve renal dysfunction, the kidney will excrete organic acids and exchange H^+ for Na^+ in the distal region of the tubule, resulting in a more acidic urine. This renal compensatory mechanism becomes effective over a period of time and will eventually correct both the blood pH and the bicarbonate toward the reference interval. This correction can take place only when the underlying cause of the acidosis has been eliminated. Part of the renal response to chronic acidosis is the excretion of ammonia by the renal tubular cells. This excretion of ammonia into the presumptive urine allows additional H^+ to be excreted and thus reduces the H^+ load in blood.

Laboratory findings. The findings seen in metabolic acidosis, summarized in Table 25-4, include a decrease in both pH and HCO_3^-. Initially the PCO_2 may be within the reference interval but it will decrease as a result of the respiratory response to the acidemia. A base deficit (negative base excess) will also be present.

The laboratory findings in lactic acidosis are those of a metabolic acidosis with a decreased pH, an initially normal PCO_2 and PO_2, a decreased O_2 saturation (the hemoglobin saturation curve is shifted to the right), a decreased bicarbonate and total CO_2, an increased anion gap, a negative base excess, and increased potassium and lactic acid concentrations. As the body attempts to correct the metabolic acidosis, the PCO_2 decreases.

In cases of toxic drug ingestion, such as methanol, ethylene glycol, or paraldehyde poisoning, the patient develops a metabolic acidosis. Laboratory findings include a decreased pH; an initially normal PCO_2 and PO_2; a decreased O_2 saturation, bicarbonate, and total CO_2; an increased anion gap (caused by the ingested poisons or their metabolites); and a negative base excess. As the body attempts to compensate for the acidosis, the PCO_2 decreases initially and the bicarbonate slowly increases toward normal as the kidney reabsorbs increasing amounts of bicarbonate.

Treatment. Initially, if possible, the cause of the acidemia is corrected, for example, by insulin treatment of diabetes. If the pH falls below 7.2, there is sometimes a deleterious effect on the cardiovascular system, and the base deficit may have to be corrected immediately. This is frequently accomplished by administration of bicarbonate, which corrects the base deficit by raising the HCO_3^-/H_2CO_3 ratio. In all cases the cause of the metabolic acidosis must ultimately be corrected.

Respiratory Acidosis

Etiology. Respiratory acidoses are caused by disorders that interfere with the usual ability of the lungs to expel CO_2. These disorders include pulmonary edema, bronchoconstriction, pneumonia, asthma, emphysema, **apnea**, and **bradycardia**. Morphine injection and barbiturate poisoning cause an immediate respiratory depression, resulting in respiratory acidosis.

Respiratory distress syndrome (RDS), which is common in premature infants, results in a respiratory acidosis because the infants lack sufficient levels of surfactant in their lungs to allow the alveoli to expand in their usual manner. Gas exchange is thus inhibited. Respiratory distress is also seen in some adults who experience systemic shock or oxygen toxicity (adult respiratory distress syndrome, ARDS). Initially, the observed blood-gas parameters are decreased pH, increased PCO_2, decreased PO_2, and decreased oxygen saturation. Base excess, bicarbonate, and anion gap are initially within normal limits.

Asthma is a chronic respiratory condition that affects more than 10 million Americans and is one of the leading causes of absence from school and work. Asthma attacks are associated with episodes of airflow obstruction in the bronchial tubes; respiratory symptoms of asthma are listed in the box on the upper left of p. 474. As in other cases of physical obstruction of the air pathway, asthmatic attacks tend to result in respiratory acidosis and often require hospitalization.

Although asthma affects both adults and children, more than half the cases are found in children between the ages of 2 and 17. A wide variety of agents may initiate an episode of

SYMPTOMS ASSOCIATED WITH ALLERGY

Respiratory
Asthma
Runny nose or eyes
Frequent colds
Coughs, frequent sore throats
Wheezing and shortness of breath
Swelling (lips, eyes)
Bouts of sneezing
Bronchitis
Nasal or chest congestion
Sinus headaches, postnasal drip
Recurrent ear infections
Respiratory acidosis

Gastrointestinal
Abdominal cramps
Diarrhea
Vomiting
Nausea

Dermatological
Eczema
Itching
Hives (urticaria)

COMMON ALLERGENS

Plant pollen (tree, grass, and weed)
Household animal dander (dog, cat)
Cockroaches
Mouse or rat
House dust mites
Molds
Latex (see p. 33)
Foods
Tobacco smoke

asthma. The most common causes are allergens, physical irritants, viral respiratory infections, and physical exertion. Allergens are substances to which susceptible individuals may become allergic. A partial list of common allergens is listed in the box on the upper right.

Inner-city children have very high rates of asthma and are especially susceptible to a number of common indoor allergens, including cockroaches, dust mites, and cats.

Normally the body produces an immune response, in this case IgE (see p. 240), to allergens in the respiratory and gastrointestinal tracts or allergens on the skin. An allergic response is an abnormal reaction, or overreaction, of the body to one or more substances from the outside environment to which a person has become sensitized. The IgE stimulates a response from mast cells, which results in the production of histamine and other inflammatory response chemicals to produce many of the symptoms (see below) associated with an allergic response. Laboratory assays (RAST, RadioAllergo Sorbent Test; see p. 240) are available to detect the presence of IgE specific for an allergen that may be the cause of allergy.

Physiological response. The physiological response to respiratory acidosis includes the increased renal excretion of acids, the retention of sodium and bicarbonate, and if possible, hyperventilation. If a response compensates for the respiratory acidosis and results in its correction, the acidosis is referred to as *compensated respiratory acidosis*. This response may be viewed as the development of a metabolic alkalosis that compensates for the respiratory acidosis. In chronic respiratory acidosis, the pH becomes essentially normal but a base excess remains. When the respiratory disorder is corrected, the usual respiratory response to the

acidosis removes the excess CO_2, and a transient metabolic alkalosis may result. Generally this alkalosis does not require treatment.

Laboratory findings. Respiratory disorders frequently lead to an increase in plasma CO_2 concentration with a smaller increase in HCO_3^- and a concurrent decrease in the ratio of HCO_3^-/H_2CO_3, which results in respiratory acidosis. However, as a result of the low oxygen levels in the tissue, a coexisting metabolic lactic acidosis can develop. This metabolic acidosis results in an increased anion gap, and the decrease in bicarbonate results in a negative base excess. Table 25-4 is a review of these findings.

As a result of the renal compensatory response, very elevated concentrations of HCO_3^- with almost normal pH are often seen. In chronic respiratory disease, the concentration of HCO_3^- and pH are near normal, though the P_{O_2} may be somewhat depressed.

Medical treatment. Medical treatment is primarily aimed at correction of the respiratory disorder and ventilation of the patient with gases containing higher P_{O_2} and lower P_{CO_2} by use of mechanical respirators. However, initial correction of the acidemia may be achieved by injection of sodium bicarbonate.

ALKALOSIS
Metabolic Alkalosis

Etiology. Occasionally, excessive chronic ingestion of bicarbonate of soda for gastrointestinal distress results in an increased concentration of blood bicarbonate and a resultant metabolic alkalosis. Similarly, treatment of peptic ulcers with ingestion of large quantities of alkali antacids will also produce metabolic alkalosis. More commonly, metabolic alkalosis arises from the loss of chloride. Prolonged vomiting or aspiration of gastric fluids leads to loss of gastric hydrochloric acid. This in turn raises the pH of the blood, because the loss of the chloride anion results in increased renal retention of bicarbonate to counter the sodium reabsorbed by the proximal tubule. This condition is known as *hypochloremic alkalosis*. Corticosteroid administration and diseases such as hyperaldosteronism and Cushing's syndrome, which affect the ability of the kidney to regulate electrolyte balance, will also raise the blood pH. In the distal tubule, Na^+ is retained at the expense of K^+ and H^+. The resultant hypokalemia causes a release of K^+ by cells into the blood and a concurrent balanced movement of H^+ from blood into the cells, thereby leading to a rise in the pH of the blood.

Physiological response. To compensate for the increase in the HCO_3^-/H_2CO_3 ratio during metabolic alkalosis, the respiratory system slows, raising the Pco_2 and the bicarbonate concentration of the blood. The Pco_2 rises more rapidly than the HCO_3^-, thereby decreasing the pH. This mechanism of readjusting the pH during metabolic alkalosis is termed *compensatory respiratory acidosis*. The result is a pH closer to the reference interval in the presence of an elevated concentration of HCO_3^-.

If the alkalosis persists, the body will attempt to correct the condition by increasing the renal excretion of the excess bicarbonate unless the proximal tubule of the kidney actually increases the reabsorption of bicarbonate, as in hypokalemia, dehydration, or hypochloremia.

Laboratory findings. During metabolic alkalosis, the ratio of HCO_3^-/H_2CO_3 increases as a result of a rise in the concentration of blood bicarbonate. Because of the physiological response to the alkalemia, additional laboratory findings are an increased Pco_2 and an alkaline urine containing titratable bicarbonate (see Table 25-4).

Treatment. Treatment of metabolic alkalosis involves administration of NaCl or KCl, depending on the degree of hypokalemia, and perhaps also administration of NH_4Cl if the alkalosis is severe and persistent. The Cl^- anion of NH_4Cl compensates for the chloride deficit, which may have led to excessive retention of bicarbonate initially. This permits the kidney to begin to excrete the excess bicarbonate and correct the alkalosis.

Respiratory Alkalosis

Etiology. Hyperventilation causes respiratory alkalosis. The conditions resulting in hyperventilation include hysteria, excessive crying, pregnancy, salicylate intoxication, impairment of the central nervous system's control of the respiratory system, asthma, fever, pulmonary embolism, and excessive use of a mechanical respirator.

Physiological response. The kidneys respond to the alkalosis by excreting increased amounts of bicarbonate under the conditions of lower Pco_2 that occur during respiratory alkalosis. In response to the alkalosis, the proximal tubules of the kidney decrease the reabsorption of bicarbonate. This renal response to respiratory alkalosis is termed *compensatory metabolic acidosis*.

Laboratory findings. Hyperventilation leads to increased loss of CO_2 from the blood at the alveolar surface, which causes the HCO_3^-/H_2CO_3 ratio to increase as carbonic acid is lost. Because of the physiological response to the alkalemia, additional laboratory findings include decreased Pco_2 and an alkaline urine containing titratable bicarbonate (see Table 25-3).

Treatment. Respiratory alkalosis is corrected by lowering the respiration rate with drugs, such as sedatives, or by having the patient breathe air with a higher CO_2 content. This can be easily accomplished by having the patient breathe in a restricted environment, for example, as into a paper bag, which raises the Pco_2 of the air and the blood. The increased Pco_2 returns the HCO_3^-/H_2CO_3 ratio to within the reference interval and corrects the respiratory alkalosis. Table 25-4 summarizes the changes in blood-gas parameters seen in several diseases.

CHANGE OF ANALYTE IN DISEASE (Table 25-5)

Diabetic ketoacidosis in patients with uncontrolled diabetes is an example of metabolic acidosis. Laboratory findings include a decreased pH, acidemia, a decreased Pco_2, a normal Po_2, a decreased O_2 saturation (see CD-ROM for blood-gas methods), a decreased bicarbonate and total CO_2 (see CD-ROM, Tco_2), an increased anion gap, a negative base excess, and increased serum potassium, ketones (see CD-ROM), and lactic and pyruvic acids (see CD-ROM) caused by the disturbed carbohydrate and fat metabolism.

Emphysema is a disease of impaired respiration that frequently results in respiratory acidosis. Laboratory findings include a decreased pH and Po_2, an increased Pco_2 and potassium, and a decreased oxygen saturation. Initially the anion gap, base excess, bicarbonate, and Tco_2 are within the reference interval. As the body compensates for the acidosis, the bicarbonate and Tco_2 rise. As in respiratory distress syndrome (RDS), the low Po_2 may result in a metabolic acidosis caused by a rise in blood lactate because of increased anaerobic metabolism.

TABLE 25-5   COMMON DISORDERS OF ACID-BASE BALANCE AND EFFECTS ON SELECTED BLOOD-GAS PARAMETERS

Disorders	pH	Pco_2	Po_2	HCO_3^-	Base Excess	Anion Gap	O_2 Saturation
Respiratory distress syndrome	↓	↑	↓	N	N	N	↓
Lactic acidosis	↓	N*	N, ↓	↓	↓	↑	↓
Diabetic ketosis	↓	N*	N	↓	↓	↑	↓
Emphysema	↓	↑	↓	N*	N	N	↓
Methanol poisoning	↓	N*	N	↓	↓	↑	↓
Renal failure	↓	N*	N	↓	↓	↑	↓

N*, *initially normal;* N, *always normal (within the reference interval).*

Hemoglobinopathies, such as sickle cell anemia, can lead to unusual oxygen-saturation kinetics caused by the abnormal hemoglobin molecule. Some laboratory findings associated with hemoglobinopathies are decreased oxygen saturation and P_{O_2} levels, which result in increased anaerobic metabolism and thereby metabolic acidosis. Persistence of the hypoxemia results in decreased bicarbonate and total CO_2, an increased anion gap (see CD-ROM) and blood lactate, and a negative base excess. The respiratory response to this acidosis is hyperventilation, which decreases the P_{CO_2}. The renal response to this acidosis is an increase in the reabsorption of bicarbonate, which tends to return the HCO_3^-/H_2CO_3 ratio to normal.

Renal failure leads to metabolic acidosis with the associated laboratory findings of a decreased pH, initially normal P_{CO_2} and P_{O_2}, decreased oxygen saturation, increased potassium level, and decreased bicarbonate level and T_{CO_2}. As the anion gap increases because of organic acid production and retention, the base excess becomes negative. The respiratory compensation for the metabolic acidosis will lead eventually to a decrease in P_{CO_2}.

Bibliography

Abg blood gas interpretation on a CD-ROM for Microsoft Windows, SymBioSis, 1997.

Arieff AI, DeFronzo RA: *Fluid, electrolyte and acid-base disorders*, ed 2, New York, 1995, Churchill Livingstone.

Busse WW, Lemanske RF: Asthma: a review, *N Eng J Med* 344:350, 2001.

Cohen JJ, Kassirer JP: *Acid-base*, Boston, 1982, Little, Brown & Co.

Davenport HW: *The ABC of acid-base chemistry*, ed 6, Chicago, 1974, University of Chicago Press.

Haber RJ: A practical approach to acid-base disorders, *West J Med* 155(2): 146, 1991.

Rosenstreich DL, Eggleston P, Kattan MM: The role of cockroach allergy and exposure to cockroach allergen in causing morbidity among inner-city children with asthma (The National Cooperative Inner-City Asthma Study), *N Engl J Med* 336:1356, 1997.

Scanlan CL, Wilkins RL, Stoller JK: *Egan's fundamentals of respiratory care*, ed 7, St Louis, 1999, Mosby.

Soloway HB: How the body maintains acid-base balance, *Diagn Med* 32-41, Feb 1979.

Internet Sites

Asthma
www.niaid.nih.gov
www.foodallergy.org
www.aaaai.org
http://www.asthmainamerica.com/

General
www.acid-base.com—Acid-base balance
www.science.ubc.ca/~chem/tutorials/pH—pH tutorial

www.madsci.com/manu/indexgas.htm—Blood gases manual
www.int-med.uiowa.edu/education/abg.htm—Introduction to interpreting arterial blood gases
www.mtsinai.org/pulmonary/books/abg/preface.html—All you really need to know to interpret arterial blood gases
http://www.home.eznet.net/~webtent/acidbase.html
http://umed.med.utah.edu/ms2/renal/Word%20files/h)%20Acid_Base%20Physiology.htm
http://cnserver0.nkf.med.ualberta.ca/cn/Schrier/Volume1/chap6/ADK1_06_4-6.pdf

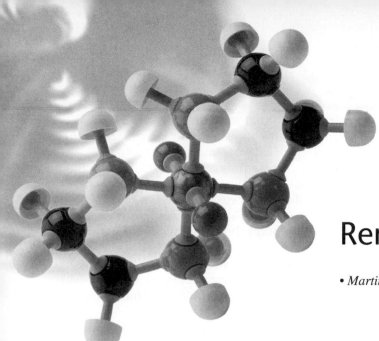

CHAPTER 26

Renal Function

• *Martin Roy First*

Objectives

• List the five main functions of the kidney and outline the formation of urine, including the function of the following:
Glomerulus
Proximal tubule
Loop of Henle
Distal convoluted tubule
Collecting duct
• Outline the mechanism by which the kidney conserves protein and describe the metabolic production and renal control of blood urea nitrogen, serum creatinine, and uric acid.

• Given pathological conditions associated with the kidney, state the expected abnormal laboratory results.
• State the purpose of performing a renal clearance test and the reasons why creatinine is most frequently used for renal clearance testing. State the advantages and disadvantages of using inulin or urea for clearance testing.
• Outline two types of studies used to evaluate renal tubular function.

Key Terms

albuminuria   The presence of albumin in urine.

aldosterone   A steroid hormone produced in the adrenal cortex that acts on the distal tubules to stimulate sodium reabsorption and potassium and hydrogen excretion.

antidiuretic hormone (ADH)   Also called *vasopressin*; a pituitary hormone that acts at the collecting duct to increase absorption of water, resulting in the formation of a more concentrated urine.

anuria   A condition in which no urine is formed.

ascending limb   The straight portion of the loop of Henle in which the presumptive urine flows up toward the convoluted distal tubule. Osmolality of urine decreases because of loss of chloride (plus Na$^+$).

bladder   A sac used to collect formed urine before voiding.

Bowman's capsule   A structure consisting of glomeruli and extended opening of the proximal tubule.

carbonic anhydrase   The enzyme at the brush border of the proximal tubule that catalyzes the reaction $H_2O + CO_2 \rightarrow H_2CO_3$.

casts   Protein aggregates, outlined in the shape of renal tubules, secreted into the urine.

clearance   A theoretical concept expressing that volume of plasma filtered at the glomeruli per unit of time from which an analyte would be completely removed and placed in final urine. It is usually expressed as milliliters of plasma per minute.

collecting tubule   The last portion of the nephron, connecting the distal convoluted tubule and the larger collecting ducts, which in turn empty into the ureter. The final concentrating processes under the influence of ADH occur here.

countercurrent mechanism   The process by which two streams flowing in opposite directions exchange material. In the kidney, urine and blood form opposing flows, and this mechanism allows reabsorption of substances.

creatinine clearance   An estimate of the glomerular filtration rate obtained by measurement of the amount of creatinine in the plasma and its rate of excretion into the urine.

descending limb   The straight portion of the loop of Henle in which forming urine flows down from the convoluted proximal tubule. This portion of the loop of Henle is freely permeable to water, which leaves the presumptive urine.

distal convoluted tubule   The convoluted tubule connecting the ascending loop of Henle with the collecting tubule. It has secretory and reabsorptive functions as part of the final urine formation and acidification process.

diuretic   A drug that promotes the increased excretion of salt and water, thus increasing the flow of urine.

filtered load   The amount of a substance presented to the tubules for reabsorption.

glomerular filtration rate (GFR)   The rate in milliliters per minute at which plasma substances are filtered through the glomeruli into the proximal tubule.

glomerulus   Cluster of small blood vessels in the kidney that projects into the expanded end (capsule) of the proximal tubule and functions as a filtering mechanism of the nephron.

hematuria   The presence of blood or red blood cells in the urine.

loop of Henle   A U-shaped tubule connecting the proximal and distal convoluted tubules. It reduces the volume of tubule fluid.

microalbuminuria   Low-grade, dipstick-negative increase in urine albumin excretion.

micturition   Urination.

nephron   The functional unit of the kidney containing Bowman's capsule, the proximal and distal convoluted tubules, the ascending and descending limbs of the loop of Henle, and the collecting tubules.

oliguria   The formation of small amounts of urine.

proteinuria   The presence of protein in urine.

proximal tubule   The convoluted tubule beginning at the glomeruli and connecting to the descending loop of Henle. It has secretory and reabsorptive functions as part of the mechanism for urine formation.

pyuria   The presence of pus (an inflammation fluid with leukocytes and dead cells) in the urine.

reabsorption (active and passive)   The process of uptake of substance into tissues or cells. Active absorption requires the expenditure of energy to move substances against a concentration gradient, whereas, in the case of passive absorption, substances move from higher to lower concentrations.

renal cortex   The outer part of the kidney that contains mostly glomeruli and convoluted tubules.

renal medulla   The inner part of the kidney that contains mostly collecting ducts and the loops of Henle.

renal threshold   The plasma concentration of a substance above which it will be present in urine.

renin   An enzyme formed by the juxtaglomerular apparatus in the kidney. It converts plasma angiotensinogen to angiotensin I.

specific gravity   The ratio of the weight in grams per milliliter of a body fluid compared with water.

titratable acid The combination of hydrogen ion with phosphate present in final urine.

urethra A membranous tube through which urine passes from the bladder to the exterior of the body.

urine The aqueous liquid and dissolved substances excreted by the kidney.

Methods on CD-ROM

Creatinine
Albumin
Anion gap
Creatinine clearance algorithm
Electrolytes (sodium, potassium, calcium, magnesium, phosphate), serum and urine

Urea
Uric acid
Urinalysis infobase
Urine protein, total

ANATOMY OF KIDNEY

Gross Anatomy

The kidneys are paired organs located in the posterior part of the abdomen on either side of the vertebral column. Underneath the capsule of fibrous tissue that encloses the kidney lies the **renal cortex**, which contains the **glomeruli**. The inner portion of the kidney, the **renal medulla**, contains the collecting ducts. A vertical section through the kidney is shown on the left-hand side of Fig. 26-1.

The urinary system is illustrated on the right-hand side of Fig. 26-1. The renal pelvis rapidly diminishes in caliber and merges into the ureter. Each ureter descends in the abdomen alongside the vertebral column to join the **bladder**. The bladder provides temporary storage for **urine**, which is eventually voided through the **urethra** to the exterior.

Microscopic Anatomy

Each kidney is made up of approximately 1 million functional units, or **nephrons**. The component parts of the nephron are illustrated in Fig. 26-2. The nephron begins with the glomerulus, which is a tuft of capillaries that is formed from the afferent (incoming) arteriole and drained by a smaller efferent (outgoing) arteriole. The glomerulus is surrounded by **Bowman's capsule**, which is formed by the blind, dilated end of the renal tubule. The proximal convoluted tubule runs a tortuous course through the cortex, entering the medulla and forming first the **descending limb** of the **loop of Henle** and then the **ascending limb** of the loop of Henle. The thick section of the ascending limb of the loop of Henle reenters the cortex, forming the distal convoluted tubule. The merging of two or more distal tubules marks the beginning of a collecting duct. As the collecting duct descends through the cortex and medulla, it receives the effluent from a dozen or more distal tubules. The collecting ducts join and increase in size as they pass down the medulla. The ducts of each pyramid coalesce to form a central duct, which empties through the papilla into a minor calyx, eventually draining into the renal pelvis.

RENAL PHYSIOLOGY

The kidney is the chief regulator of all body fluids and is primarily responsible for maintaining homeostasis, or equilibrium of fluid and electrolytes in the body. The kidney has six main functions, as follows:

1. Urine formation
2. Regulation of fluid and electrolyte balance
3. Regulation of acid-base balance
4. Excretion of waste products of protein metabolism
5. Hormonal function
6. Protein conservation

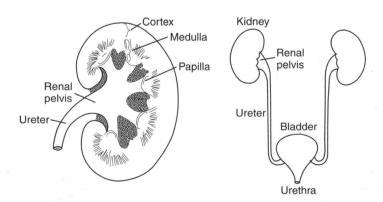

Fig. 26-1 Gross anatomy of kidney and urinary system.

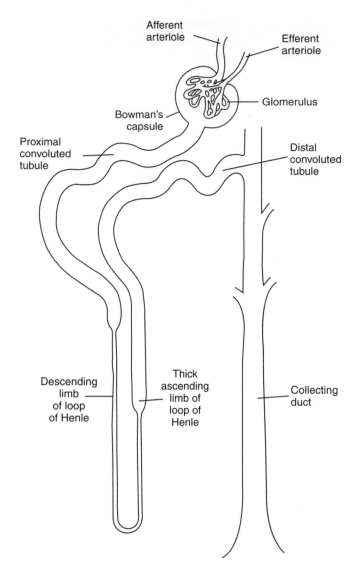

Fig. 26-2 Components of the nephron.

Afferent
arteriole

Efferent
arteriole

Glomerulus

Bowman's
capsule

Proximal
convoluted
tubule

Distal
convoluted
tubule

Descending
limb
of loop
of Henle

Thick
ascending
limb of
loop of
Henle

Collecting
duct

The kidney is able to carry out these complex functions because approximately 25% of the volume of blood pumped by the heart into the systemic circulation is circulated through the kidneys; therefore the kidneys, which constitute about 0.5% of total body weight, receive one fourth of the cardiac output.

Urine Formation

The removal of potentially toxic waste products is a major function of the kidneys and is accomplished through the formation of urine. The basic processes involved in the formation of urine are *filtration, reabsorption,* and *secretion.* The kidneys filter large volumes of plasma, reabsorb most of what is filtered, and leave behind for elimination from the body a concentrated solution of metabolic wastes called *urine.* In healthy individuals the kidneys, highly sensitive to fluctuations in diet and fluid and electrolyte intake, compensate for any changes by varying the volume and consistency of the urine.

Glomerular filtration. Each minute 1000 to 1500 mL of blood pass through the kidneys. The glomerulus has a semipermeable basement membrane that allows free passage of water and electrolytes but is relatively impermeable to larger molecules. The architecture of the human glomerular capillary wall is illustrated in Fig. 26-3. In the process of transfer from capillary lumen (CL) to Bowman's space, or urinary space (US), water, solutes, and macromolecules must traverse three layers: (1) the endothelial wall cytoplasm (En), containing numerous fenestra with a mean diameter of 70 nm; (2) the basement membranes (B) with a mean thickness of 320 nm; and (3) the layer of foot process (F), which are separated 25 to 60 nm from each other by slit pores. The cytoplasm (EpCy) and nucleus (EpN) of an epithelial cell are also shown. In glomerular capillaries the hydrostatic pressure is approximately three times greater than the pressure in other capillaries. As a result of this high pressure, substances are filtered through the semipermeable membrane into Bowman's capsule at a rate of approximately 130 mL/min; this is known as the **glomerular filtration rate (GFR)**. Cells and the large plasma proteins are unable to pass through the semipermeable membrane. Therefore the glomerular filtrate is essentially plasma without the proteins. The GFR is an extremely important parameter in both the study of kidney physiology and the clinical assessment of renal function. In the average healthy person, more than 187,000 mL of filtrate are formed per day. Normal urine output is around 1500 mL per day, which is only about 1% of the amount of filtrate formed; therefore the other 99% must be reabsorbed.

Proximal tubule. The proximal tubular cells perform a variety of physiological tasks. Approximately 80% of salt and water are reabsorbed from the glomerular filtrate in the proximal tubule. All the filtered glucose and most of the filtered amino acids are normally reabsorbed here. Low-molecular-weight proteins, urea, uric acid, bicarbonate, phosphate, chloride, potassium, magnesium, and calcium are reabsorbed to varying extents. A variety of organic acids and bases, as well as hydrogen ions and ammonia, are secreted into the tubular fluid by tubular cells. Under normal conditions, no glucose is excreted in the urine; all that is filtered is reabsorbed. As the plasma concentration of glucose is increased above some critical level, termed the *renal plasma threshold,* the tubular maximum for glucose is exceeded, and glucose appears in the urine. The higher the plasma concentration of glucose, the greater is the quantity excreted in the urine. Renal plasma thresholds also exist for phosphate and bicarbonate ions.

Most of the metabolic energy consumed by the kidney is used to promote **active reabsorption**. Active reabsorption can produce net movement of a substance against a concentration or electrical gradient and therefore requires energy expenditure by the transporting cells. Active reabsorption of glucose, amino acids, low-molecular-weight proteins, uric acid, sodium, potassium, magnesium, calcium, chloride, and bicarbonate is regulated by the kidney according to the levels of these substances in the blood and the body's needs. **Passive reabsorption** occurs when a substance moves by

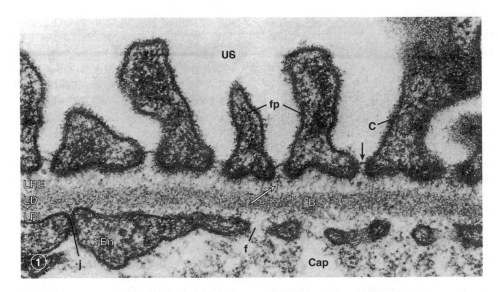

Fig. 26-3 Portion of a glomerulus showing a peripheral region of a capillary loop cut into a healthy section. The filtration surface consists of the endothelium (*En*) with its open fenestrae (*f*) lacking diaphragms, the glomerular basement membrane (*B*), and the epithelial foot processes (*fp*) between which are the filtration slits, bridged at their base by slit membranes (*short arrow*). Notice that the glomerular basement membrane (GBM) consists of three layers—a central dense layer, the lamina densa (*LD*), and two adjoining layers of lower density, the lamina rara interna (*LRI*) and externa (*LRE*). A thick cell coat (*C*) is visible on the membrane of the foot processes. The lamina densa is composed of a fine (~3 nm) filamentous meshwork, and wispy filaments are seen extending from the lamina densa to the endothelial and epithelial (*long arrow*) membranes on either side. *Cap,* Capillary lumen; *j,* junction between two endothelial cells; *US,* urinary spaces; 80,000 ×. *(From Farquhar MG, Kanwan YS: In Cummings NB, Michael AF, Wilson CB, editors:* Immune mechanisms in renal disease, *New York, 1983, Plenum Medical Books.)*

simple diffusion as the result of an electrical or chemical concentration gradient, and no cellular energy is involved in the process. Water, urea, and chloride are reabsorbed in this way.

Tubular secretion, which transports substances into the tubular lumen (i.e., in the direction opposite to tubular reabsorption), may also be an active or passive process. Substances that are transported from the blood to the tubules and excreted in the urine include potassium, hydrogen ions, ammonia, uric acid, and certain drugs, such as penicillin. Table 26-1 gives an idea of the magnitude and importance of these reabsorptive mechanisms.

Loop of Henle. The descending limb of the loop of Henle is highly permeable to water. In the medulla, the loop of Henle descends into an environment that is increasingly hypertonic as the papilla is approached. Passive reabsorption of water occurs in response to this osmotic gradient, leaving the presumptive urine highly concentrated at the bottom of the loop. The ascending limb is relatively impermeable to the passage of water but actively reabsorbs sodium and chloride. This segment of the nephron is often called the *diluting segment* because the removal of salt with little water from the tubular contents lowers the salt and osmotic concentration, in effect diluting the tubular fluid. The ascending thick limb of

TABLE 26-1 FILTRATION, REABSORPTION, AND EXCRETION BY KIDNEY

Component	Amount Filtered per Day	Amount Excreted per Day	Percentage Reabsorbed
Water	180 L	1.5 L	99.2
Sodium	24,000 mEq	100 mEq	99.6
Chloride	20,000 mEq	100 mEq	99.5
Bicarbonate	5000 mEq	2 mEq	99.9
Potassium	700 mEq	50 mEq	92.9
Glucose	180 g	0	100
Albumin	360 mg	18 mg	95

the loop of Henle transfers sodium chloride actively from its lumen into the interstitial fluid (ISF). The tubular fluid in its lumen becomes hypotonic, and the ISF becomes hypertonic. This phenomenon is known as the **countercurrent mechanism**. A series of successive steps results in sodium chloride being trapped in the ISF of the medulla. As the isotonic fluid in the descending limb reaches the area into which the ascending limb is pumping out sodium, it becomes slightly hypertonic because of the movement of water into the hypertonic interstitium. The first step repeats itself, and again, as more sodium and chloride are added to the interstitium by the ascending limb, more water is drawn out of the descending limb.

Distal convoluted tubule. A small fraction of the filtered sodium, chloride, and water is reabsorbed in the **distal convoluted tubule**. The distal tubule responds to the **antidiuretic hormone (ADH)**, and so its water permeability is high in the presence of the hormone and low in its absence. Potassium can be reabsorbed or secreted in the distal tubule. **Aldosterone** stimulates both sodium reabsorption and potassium secretion in the distal tubule. Hydrogen, ammonia, and uric acid secretion and bicarbonate reabsorption occur, but there is little transport of organic substances. This segment of the nephron has a low permeability to urea.

Collecting duct. ADH controls the water permeability of the **collecting tubule** throughout its length. In the presence of the hormone, the hypotonic tubular fluid entering the duct loses water. Sodium and chloride are reabsorbed by the collecting tubule, with the transport of sodium stimulated by aldosterone. The collecting duct also reabsorbs potassium, hydrogen, and ammonia. When ADH is present, the rate of water reabsorption exceeds the rate of solute reabsorption, and the concentration of sodium and chloride in the presumptive urine rises. The collecting duct is relatively impermeable to urea.

Regulation of Fluid and Electrolyte Balance

Water. Water is the most abundant component of the human body, constituting approximately 60% of body weight. Body water, and therefore body weight, remains fairly constant from day to day in normal persons, despite wide fluctuations in fluid and salt intake.[1,2] One of the most remarkable properties of the human kidney is its ability to elaborate urine that is either more concentrated or more dilute than the plasma from which it is derived. When the human body needs to conserve water, as in dehydration, the concentrating mechanism operates maximally, and urine osmolality increases to about 1200 mOsm/kg. Conversely, when there is excess water in the body, urine flow increases, and the diluting mechanism reduces urine osmolality to as low as 50 mOsm/kg. The capacity of the kidney to form urine of greatly varying osmolality enables it to regulate the solute concentration and hence the osmolality of body fluids within narrow physiological limits, despite wide fluctuations in intake of salt and water.[1,2] Water balance is controlled primarily through voluntary intake (which is regulated through the thirst center in the hypothalamus) and urinary

loss of water. The control of urinary water loss is the major automatic mechanism by which body water is regulated. In dehydrated states the urine is concentrated when the kidney reabsorbs water without solute. Conversely, urine is diluted when the kidney reabsorbs solute without water.

Sodium. Sodium is the main cation found in extracellular fluid. Sodium is freely filtered through the glomerulus and actively reabsorbed by the tubules. Sodium reabsorption is very important because it affects the regulation of several other electrolytes. Active reabsorption of the sodium ion in the proximal tubule results in passive transport of chloride and bicarbonate as counterions and in passive reabsorption of water. In normal persons, daily urinary sodium excretion fluctuates widely according to the dietary intake, thereby keeping the body sodium content remarkably constant. In the normal person, the kidneys reabsorb more than 99% of the **filtered load** of sodium. The sodium reabsorption by the nephron is controlled by the renin-angiotensin-aldosterone system (see Chapters 24 and 46).[3,4]

Chloride. The concentration of chloride in the extracellular fluid parallels that of sodium and is influenced by the same factors. However, chloride reabsorption is passive in the proximal tubule and probably active in the distal tubule and collecting duct.

Potassium. Potassium is the chief cation of the intracellular fluid. Maintenance of a normal potassium level is essential to the life of the cells. The distribution of potassium is such that 90% of total body potassium is intracellular and only 2% is extracellular. The high intracellular-to-extracellular potassium ratio is maintained by the Na^+,K^+-ATPase pump.[5] The normal person maintains potassium balance by excreting daily an amount of potassium equal to the amount ingested minus the small amount eliminated in the feces and sweat. Renal function is the major mechanism by which the body potassium is regulated. Potassium is freely filtered at the glomerulus, and active tubular reabsorption occurs throughout the nephron, except in the descending loop of Henle. Only about 10% of the filtered potassium enters the distal tubule. The distal tubule and collecting ducts are able to both secrete and reabsorb potassium, thus regulating potassium excretion.[6] The hormone aldosterone, which stimulates tubular sodium reabsorption, simultaneously enhances potassium secretion in the distal tubule.[6,7]

Calcium. Calcium reabsorption in the proximal tubule parallels that of sodium and water. The maintenance of calcium homeostasis depends on the balance between calcium intake and calcium loss. The body loses calcium in the urine, through the gastrointestinal tract, and in sweat. Calcium balance is achieved largely by the control of calcium **absorption** rather than by the regulation of calcium excretion. The percentage of ingested calcium absorbed decreases as the dietary calcium content increases, and so the amount absorbed can remain relatively constant. The slight increase in absorption that occurs on a high-calcium diet is reflected in an increased renal excretion.[8]

Phosphorus. Over a wide range of dietary intakes, roughly two thirds of ingested phosphorus is absorbed into the bloodstream. The maintenance of the phosphorus balance is achieved largely through renal excretion.[9] Proximal tubular reabsorption of inorganic phosphate is normally about 90% of the filtered load. Parathyroid hormone depresses the renal tubular reabsorption of inorganic phosphate. In progressive chronic renal failure, there is a progressive increase in the serum phosphorus level.[10]

Magnesium. The filtration of magnesium at the glomerulus and its reabsorption from the proximal tubules parallels that of calcium and is also under the influence of parathyroid hormone. A moderate elevation of the plasma magnesium concentration occurs in patients with advanced chronic renal failure.[11]

Acid-Base Balance

Each day acid waste products are produced in the body. If they were not disposed of efficiently, they would accumulate and cause cellular damage. Body pH is controlled by three systems: acid-base buffers, the lungs, and the kidneys (see Chapter 25).

Excretion of hydrogen ions. In subjects on a normal diet, about 50 to 100 mEq of hydrogen ions are generated each day. To prevent a progressive metabolic acidosis, these hydrogen ions are excreted in the urine.[12] Hydrogen ions are generated in the cells of the proximal and distal tubule and the collecting duct as a result of the formation of carbonic acid by the enzyme **carbonic anhydrase** (CA). The cells secrete these hydrogen ions into the lumen[13]:

$$H_2O + CO_2 \xrightleftharpoons[]{CA} H_2CO_3 \xrightleftharpoons[]{} H^+ + HCO_3^- \qquad \textit{Eq. 26-1}$$

The kidneys' role in the maintenance of the acid-base balance centers on the generation of bicarbonate. The hydrogen ions are excreted into the urine while newly generated bicarbonate ions pass from the tubular cells into the blood at the same rate as bicarbonate is consumed by the metabolic processes.[13] Four mechanisms exist to handle the hydrogen ions that have been secreted into the tubular fluid.

Reaction with filtered bicarbonate ions. Bicarbonate is completely filterable at the glomerulus. In the tubular lumen, the excreted hydrogen ion combines with the filtered bicarbonate to form carbonic acid, which decomposes to water and carbon dioxide, the latter then diffusing into the cell, where it can be converted by CA to carbonic acid to generate another hydrogen ion. One bicarbonate ion is regenerated for every hydrogen ion that is secreted into the tubular lumen. The bicarbonate ion is reabsorbed into the blood as sodium bicarbonate, thus conserving most of the filtered bicarbonate. The **renal threshold** for bicarbonate is 28 mM; at a plasma level below this, all filtered bicarbonate is reabsorbed.

Reaction with filtered buffers to form titratable acids. Inorganic monohydrogen phosphate is present in the tubular lumen as the disodium salt. The secreted hydrogen ions react with the filtered phosphate, releasing sodium that combines with the bicarbonate; the sodium bicarbonate is reabsorbed, and dihydrogen phosphate is excreted:

$$Na_2HPO_4 + H^+ \rightarrow NaH_2PO_4 + Na^+$$
$$Na^+ + HCO_3^- \rightarrow NaHCO_3 \text{ (reabsorbed)} \qquad \textit{Eq. 26-2}$$

Hydrogen ions combine with phosphate to form **titratable acid**. The rate of excretion of titratable acid is limited by the filtered load of buffer and cannot increase greatly in acidosis. The lowest possible pH of urine is 4.4.

Reaction with secreted ammonia to form ammonium ion. The glomerular filtrate does not contain ammonia. This compound is synthesized in renal tubular cells by deamination of glutamine in the presence of glutaminase.[13] The ammonia diffuses into the tubular fluid, where it reacts with a secreted hydrogen ion to form an ammonium ion. Once again this results in the addition of new bicarbonate to the blood. The most important renal adaptation to acidosis is the increased excretion of ammonium ions[13]:

$$\text{Glutamine} \xrightarrow{\text{Glutaminase}} \text{Glutamic acid} + NH_3$$
$$NH_3 + H^+ \rightarrow NH_4^+ \qquad \textit{Eq. 26-3}$$

Excretion as free hydrogen ions. Only negligible quantities of hydrogen ions are handled in this way by the kidneys.

Nitrogenous Waste Excretion

One of the major functions of the kidney is the elimination of nitrogenous products of protein catabolism. The enormous reserves of the kidney for excretion of the products of protein catabolism are indicated by the fact that the blood concentrations of these products are not elevated in renal failure until renal function is reduced to less than one half of normal.[14]

Urea. As amino acids are deaminated, ammonia is produced. The development of toxic levels of ammonia in the blood is prevented by the conversion of ammonia to urea. This takes place in the liver. Urea in the blood is reported as the blood urea nitrogen (BUN). Urea production and the BUN are increased when more amino acids are metabolized in the liver.[15] This can occur with a high-protein diet, tissue breakdown, or decreased protein synthesis. In contrast, urea production and the BUN are reduced in the presence of a low-protein intake and severe liver disease. Urea production exceeds renal urea excretion in normal persons. The remaining urea is degraded to ammonium ions by intestinal bacteria. Urea is readily filtered, but approximately 40% to 50% of the filtered urea is normally reabsorbed by the proximal tubules. Because many factors may influence the BUN level while the GFR remains constant, BUN is a less specific indicator of renal function and should not be relied on for that purpose.

Creatinine. Serum creatinine levels and urinary creatinine excretion are a function of muscle mass in normal persons and shows little response to dietary changes.[16] Creatinine is derived from the nonenzymatic dehydration of creatine in skeletal muscle:

$$\begin{array}{ccc}
CH_3-NCH_2-COOH & & CH_3-N-CH_2 \\
\quad | & \longrightarrow & \qquad | \qquad\quad C=O + H_2O \\
\quad C=NH & & \qquad\quad / \\
\quad | & & HN=C-NH \\
\quad NH_2 & & \\
\textbf{Creatine} & & \textbf{Creatine} \qquad \textit{Eq. 26-4}
\end{array}$$

The amount of creatine per unit of muscle mass is constant, and thus the rate of spontaneous breakdown of creatine is also constant. As a result, the plasma creatinine concentration is very stable, varying less than 10% per day in serial observations in normal subjects. Because the serum creatinine concentration is a direct reflection of muscle mass, the serum level is higher in males than in females. Creatinine is freely filtered at the glomerulus and is not reabsorbed by the tubules. A small amount of the creatinine in the final urine is derived from tubular secretion. Because of these properties of creatinine, the **creatinine clearance** can be used to estimate the GFR (see tests of glomerular function, p. 487):

Uric acid. Uric acid is derived from the oxidation of purine bases. Plasma levels of uric acid are quite variable and are higher in males than in females. Plasma urates are completely filterable, and both proximal tubular resorption and distal tubular secretion occur. With advanced chronic renal failure there is a progressive increase in the plasma uric acid level.

Hormonal Function

The kidneys have important metabolic and endocrine functions. The kidney as an endocrine organ is discussed in this section.[17]

Vitamin D metabolism. In vitamin D metabolism the kidney produces the major biologically active hormone 1,25-dihydroxycholecalciferol.[18] The enzyme responsible for the production of 1,25-dihydroxycholecalciferol is present only in the mitochondria of the renal cortex (see Chapter 28).

Renin. The kidney releases **renin** in response to a decrease in extracellular fluid volume. This results in stimulation of the renin-angiotensin-aldosterone axis, with subsequent sodium and water conservation.[4] (See Chapters 24 and 46.)

Erythropoietin. The kidneys play a major role in the production and release of erythropoietin, a hormone that stimulates red blood cell production. The central role of the kidneys in erythropoietin production explains the anemia associated with chronic renal failure.[19]

Protein Conservation

Under normal physiological conditions, the kidney helps to maintain the homeostasis of the body's proteins. In humans 180 L of plasma, each liter containing 70 g of protein, are filtered each day by the glomerulus.[20] Without an efficient conservation mechanism, body protein stores would be depleted very rapidly. Yet normal urine contains less than 200 mg of protein per day, only a minute percentage of the 12,600 g passing through the glomerulus daily.[20] Most of the filtered proteins are absorbed by the proximal tubules and returned to the circulation. Most plasma proteins, except those of very high molecular weight, have been found in the urine. Albumin excretion is less than 20 mg/day.[20] Many proteins of nonserum origin are also found in the urine. One of these, uromucoid or Tamm-Horsfall mucoprotein, is the predominant protein in normal urine, with about 40 mg excreted daily. This high-molecular-weight mucoprotein is excreted by the cells of the distal tubule and collecting ducts. Commercially available dipsticks are in widespread use and are accurate for rapid assessments of urinary protein concentration.

PATHOLOGICAL CONDITIONS OF KIDNEY

There are many syndromes that singly or in combination indicate possible renal disease. These have been elegantly described by Coe.[21]

Acute Glomerulonephritis

Acute glomerulonephritis is an acute inflammation of the glomeruli, resulting in **oliguria**, **hematuria**, increased BUN and serum creatinine levels, decreased GFR, edema formation, and hypertension. The presence of red blood cells in the urine (hematuria) alone is insufficient evidence of acute glomerulonephritis, for blood can originate from elsewhere in the kidney or from the urinary tract. The presence of red blood cell **casts** in the urine indicates glomerular inflammation and is a finding of great importance. Other abnormalities present in acute nephritis include **proteinuria** and anemia.

Nephrotic Syndrome

The nephrotic syndrome has been classically defined as a clinical entity characterized by massive proteinuria, edema, hypoalbuminemia, hyperlipidemia, and lipiduria.[20] This syndrome, which can have many causes, is characterized by increased glomerular membrane permeability that results in massive proteinuria and excretion of fat bodies. Protein excretion rates are usually greater than 2 to 3 g/day in the absence of a depressed GFR. Hematuria and oliguria may be present. The causes of the nephrotic syndrome are illustrated in the box on p. 485. As a result of the massive loss of serum proteins, primarily albumin, into urine, the plasma protein concentration is decreased, with a concomitant reduction in plasma oncotic pressure. This results in fluid movement from the vascular to interstitial space with consequent edema formation.

Tubular Disease

In some disorders of renal tubular function, the depressed renal function cannot be explained by the reduction in the GFR. Defects of tubular function may result in depressed secretion or reabsorption of specific biochemicals or impairment of urine concentration and dilution mechanisms. Renal tubular acidosis (RTA) is the most important clinical disorder of tubular function.[22] There are two main types of RTA: (1) proximal RTA, which is a result of reduced proximal tubular bicarbonate reabsorption and causes *hyperchloremic acidosis*, and (2) distal RTA, in which there is an inability of the tubular cells to create and maintain the usual pH difference between tubular fluid and blood. Failure of either the proximal or distal secretory mechanisms occurs in several disease states. Failure of the proximal tubule to reabsorb bicarbonate causes acidosis because more bicarbonate is passed on to the low-capacity distal mechanism

CAUSES OF NEPHROTIC SYNDROME

Associated with various forms of glomerulonephritis
Associated with generalized disease processes
    Amyloidosis
    Carcinoma
    Systemic lupus erythematosus
    Diabetic glomerulosclerosis
    Polyarteritis nodosa
Associated with mechanical or circulating disorders
    Renal vein thrombosis
    Constrictive pericarditis
Associated with infection
    Syphilis
    Malaria
    Subacute bacterial endocarditis
Associated with toxins and allergens
    Penicillamine
    Gold salts
    Bee sting
    Serum sickness
Miscellaneous
    Severe preeclampsia
    Transplant rejection

than it can reabsorb. The loss of alkali in the urine causes the blood to become acidotic. Defects in potassium and uric acid secretion may result in elevations of the serum potassium and uric acid levels that cannot be explained by the reduction in the GFR. Reabsorptive disorders of the proximal tubules may result in hypouricemia, hypophosphatemia, aminoaciduria, and renal glucosuria. The Fanconi syndrome is a group of renal defects resulting in glucosuria, aminoaciduria, hypophosphatemia, and renal tubular acidosis. Tubular proteinuria may occur as a result of a tubular defect in the handling of proteins. In tubular proteinuria, less than 2 g/day of protein are excreted. Disorders of urine concentration and dilution occur in all renal disease as the GFR falls appreciably, but occasionally these disorders become extreme and dominate the clinical presentation.[21]

Urinary Tract Infection

Infection of the urinary tract may occur in the bladder *(cystitis)* or may involve the kidneys *(pyelonephritis)*. The presence of a urine bacterial concentration of more than 100,000 colonies/mL is diagnostic of urinary tract infections. In a urinary tract infection there is an increased number of white blood cells in the urine. The presence of white blood cell casts indicates pyelonephritis. An increased number of red blood cells may also be present in the urine.

Vascular Diseases

Hypertension. Long-standing and severe hypertension can result in progressive renal damage and chronic renal insufficiency (hypertensive nephrosclerosis). In contrast, hypertension can be caused by the sodium and water retention that occurs in chronic renal failure, acute glomerulo-

nephritis, and the nephrotic syndrome (volume-dependent hypertension), or it can occur as a result of increased renin release from chronically damaged kidneys (renin-dependent hypertension).

Arteriolar disease. Disease of the small arteries of the kidneys (arteritis) may occur in association with generalized disease processes affecting the kidney, such as systemic lupus erythematosus, polyarteritis nodosa, and progressive systemic sclerosis (scleroderma). These diseases may result in the clinical and biochemical abnormalities seen in acute glomerulonephritis, the nephrotic syndrome, or chronic renal insufficiency.

Renal vein thrombosis. Thrombosis of the renal veins results in massive proteinuria and the nephrotic syndrome. Hypertension, edema, hematuria, and impaired renal function may accompany the proteinuria.

Diabetes Mellitus

Diabetes mellitus results in a wide variety of abnormalities in kidney function. The early phases of the disease are manifested by the presence of pronounced glucosuria, polyuria, and nocturia as a result of the osmotic diuresis caused by the glucose load. In insulin-dependent diabetes (type I diabetes mellitus), kidney disease is the leading cause of morbidity and mortality. In the juvenile diabetic, overt proteinuria develops approximately 17 years after the diagnosis has been made, hypertension develops 1 to 2 years later, and chronic renal insufficiency is seen after another year.[23] Early in the course of this disease, protein excretion, particularly **albuminuria** and IgG, is increased. A urinary albumin excretion in the range of 50 to 200 mg/24 hr is usually predictive of diabetic nephropathy.[24] The level of albumin excretion rate has been shown to be increased with age and disease duration after 10 years in patients with type I diabetes mellitus.[25] A significant link also occurred with a declining renal function and elevation of blood pressure. In recent years, attention has been focused on dipstick-negative, low-grade increase in albumin excretion, or **microalbuminuria**. This latent phase has been shown to be predictive of clinical nephropathy and eventual renal failure in patients with type I diabetes mellitus.[26,27]

Urinary Tract Obstruction

Lower urinary tract obstruction is characterized by residual urine in the bladder after **micturition** or urinary retention, whereas the presence of upper tract obstruction is established by the demonstration of a dilated collecting system above a constricting lesion.[14] Lower urinary tract obstruction is characterized by a slow urinary stream, difficulty in emptying the bladder, hesitancy in initiating micturition, and dribbling. Chronic renal damage may result from obstruction and incomplete bladder emptying, and symptoms of chronic renal insufficiency may develop. With complete obstruction, oliguria or **anuria** will occur. Symptoms of urinary tract infection may also be seen. Urinary tract obstruction may occur as a result of congenital disorders of the lower urinary tract, neoplastic lesions (benign prostatic hypertrophy, carcinoma of the prostate or bladder, or lymph nodes compressing the ureters), or acquired disorders (retroperitoneal fibrosis, renal calculi, or urethral strictures).

Renal Calculi

Renal calculi, or stones, are seen in combination with renal colic, hematuria, and symptoms of urinary tract infection or obstruction. Kidney stones may form after recurrent urinary tract infections by urease-producing organisms or when the urine is supersaturated by large quantities of calcium, uric acid, cystine, or xanthine.

Acute Renal Failure

In acute renal failure there is an abrupt deterioration in renal function. Acute renal failure can be classified as follows:

1. Prerenal (occurring before blood reaches the kidney) because of hypovolemia or poor perfusion as a result of cardiovascular failure
2. Renal (occurring in the kidney) because of acute tubular necrosis, which is the most frequently observed cause of acute renal failure, or because of other renal diseases, causing rapid deterioration in renal function, including arterial or venous obstruction
3. Postrenal (occurring after urine leaves the kidney) because of obstruction

The causes of acute renal failure are listed in the box below. Acute renal failure is usually accompanied by oliguria or anuria; in addition, nonoliguric acute tubular necrosis can occur. Acute renal failure is associated with varying degrees of proteinuria, hematuria, and the presence of red blood cell casts and other casts in the urine. Serum urea nitrogen and creatinine levels increase rapidly, and metabolic acidosis becomes evident. Depending on the cause, acute renal failure can progress to chronic renal insufficiency or failure, or can be followed by recovery of renal function. Most patients with acute tubular necrosis recover once the offending cause has been treated or removed.

CAUSES OF ACUTE RENAL FAILURE

Prerenal
Hypovolemia
Cardiovascular failure

Renal
Acute tubular necrosis
Glomerulonephritis
Vasculitis
Malignant nephrosclerosis
Vascular obstruction
    Arterial
    Venous

Postrenal
Obstruction of lower urinary tract
Rupture of bladder

Chronic Renal Failure

Chronic renal failure is a clinical syndrome resulting from the progressive loss of renal function. The symptoms of chronic renal failure result not only from simple excretory failure but also from the onset of regulatory failure, the kidney's failure to regulate certain substances, such as sodium and water; from biosynthetic failure, such as the kidney's inadequate production of erythropoietin, resulting in anemia; and from the excessive production of certain normal substances in response to the chemical derangements that occur in chronic renal failure, such as the excessive production of parathyroid hormone.[14] There are four stages in chronic, progressive renal disease. In the first stage renal function is diminished, but plasma urea and creatinine levels remain normal. At least 50% of normal function must be lost before the concentrations of these chemicals rise above the normal range. The second stage is characterized by mild renal insufficiency. The third stage is the development of frank renal failure with advancing anemia, acidosis, and other clinical and biochemical manifestations. The fourth and final stage is that of uremia, when all the consequences of renal failure become overt.[14] A classification of the causes of chronic renal failure is shown in the box below.

CLASSIFICATION OF CAUSES OF CHRONIC RENAL FAILURE

Primary Glomerular Diseases
Chronic glomerulonephritis of various types
Systemic lupus erythematosus
Polyarteritis nodosa

Renal Vascular Disease
Malignant hypertension
Renal vein thrombosis

Inflammatory Disease
Chronic pyelonephritis
Tuberculosis

Metabolic Disease with Renal Involvement
Diabetes mellitus
Gout
Amyloidosis

Nephrotoxins
Aminoglycosides
Analgesic nephropathy
Chronic heavy metal poisoning

Obstructive Hypertrophy
Calculi
Prostatic hypertrophy
Congenital anomalies of lower urinary tract

Congenital Anomalies of Kidneys
Hypoplastic kidneys
Polycystic kidney disease

Miscellaneous
Chronic radiation nephritis
Balkan nephropathy

RENAL FUNCTION TESTS

The kidney performs many physiological and excretory functions. By performing a relatively small number of tests, a physician can deduce accurately the functional state of the kidney.[28] The clinician first determines whether any significant impairment of renal function exists and then assesses a particular renal function to make a specific diagnosis. In this section, evaluation of glomerular and tubular function and urinalysis are discussed.

Tests of Glomerular Function

Glomerular function is most conveniently measured by the creatinine clearance test. **Clearance** is defined as that volume of plasma from which a measured amount of substance can be completely eliminated into the urine per unit of time. This depends on the plasma concentration of the substance and its excretory rate, which in turn depends on the GFR and renal plasma flow. The creatinine clearance is a renal function test based on the rate of excretion by the kidneys of metabolically produced creatinine. The amount of creatinine produced by endogenous creatine metabolism is relatively constant and directly proportional to the body surface area. The amount of creatinine present in the urine depends on renal excretion. Creatinine is freely filtered at the glomerulus and is not reabsorbed by the tubules. The creatinine clearance can therefore be used to estimate the GFR. Generally, a 24-hour urine collection is performed. However, shorter collection periods are acceptable. Precise timing is critical to this test. The bladder is emptied at the beginning of the test period and the urine discarded; all urine passed subsequently during the timed collection is kept in a single container. A sample of blood is drawn during the urine collection period. The creatinine clearance is calculated from the following formula:

$$\text{Creatinine clearance (mL/min)} = UV/P \qquad \textit{Eq. 26-5}$$

in which U is urinary creatinine (mg/L), V is volume of urine excreted per time (mL/min), and P is plasma creatinine (mg/L). The healthy reference interval for creatinine clearance corrected to a surface area of 1.73 m^2 is 90 to 120 mL/min (see creatinine method on CD-ROM). The creatinine clearance usually parallels true GFR. However, at low filtration rates, creatinine clearance becomes increasingly inaccurate.[16] The creatinine clearance is lower in women, the elderly, and smaller persons. Measurement of creatinine clearance by collection of a timed (24-hour) urine specimen is burdensome to the patient and frequently difficult to perform. Inaccurate results caused by incomplete bladder emptying, failure to collect the entire specimen, and wide intraindividual variation impair the usefulness of this procedure.[16] Numerous formulas and nomograms have been developed for estimating creatinine clearance from the serum creatinine concentration, thereby bypassing the need for urine collection. The simplest and most widely used is the formula described by Cockcroft and Gault.[29]

$$C_{cr} \text{ (males)} = \frac{[140 - \text{Age (years)} \times \text{Weight (kg)}]}{[7.2 \times \text{Serum creatinine (mg/L)}]}$$

$$C_{cr} \text{ (females)} = \text{Above equation result} \times 0.85 \text{ (based on}$$
$$\text{15\% lower muscle mass on average)} \qquad \textit{Eq. 26-6}$$

Inulin clearance is the method of choice when precise determination of the GFR is required.[16] The glomerular capillary wall is freely permeable to inulin, and inulin is not reabsorbed, secreted, or metabolically altered by the renal tubule. The clearance of endogenous creatinine may exceed that of inulin by up to 30% in healthy individuals. The main disadvantages in the measurement of inulin clearance are the need for its intravenous administration and the technical difficulty of the analysis.

Urea clearance may also be employed as a measure of the GFR. Urea is freely filtered at the glomerulus, and approximately 40% is reabsorbed in the tubules. Thus, urea clearance values will parallel the true GFR. The measurement of a small, endogenous nonglycosylated peptide, cystatin C (MW ~13,000 D), in serum has been proposed as an alternative way of assessing glomerular function.[30] Cystatin C is produced at a steady rate from most body tissues, and is freely filtered by the glomerulus.

From a practical point of view, creatinine clearance is used in clinical medicine as an assessment of the GFR. It is important to understand that there is a large margin of reserve in renal function; more than two thirds of the GFR may be lost in the course of chronic renal disease with few clinical symptoms and biochemical abnormalities.[28] For a person whose usual serum creatinine is 7 mg/L, an increase to 14 mg/L, which is still defined as within the reference interval for healthy individuals for serum creatinine, is indicative of a fall in the GFR to 50% of normal.

Tests of Tubular Function

Concentration-dilution studies. Assessment of the concentrating and diluting ability of the kidney can provide the most sensitive means of detecting early impairment in renal function, because the ability to concentrate urine and conserve water requires an adequate GFR, renal plasma flow, and tubular mass and healthy tubular cells that are able to pump salt against a sizable electrochemical gradient.[28] The urinary **specific gravity** and *osmolality* are used as measures of the concentrating and diluting ability of the tubules. As long as the urine does not contain appreciable amounts of protein, sugar, or exogenous material such as contrast dye, specific gravity is proportional to osmolality, and a specific gravity of 1.032 will correspond to an osmolality of 1200 mOsm/kg.[28]

Impairment of renal concentrating ability is a relatively early manifestation of chronic renal disease and becomes evident before changes in other function tests appear. However, it is a nonspecific test for reduced renal function, and any disease resulting in chronic renal failure, diabetes insipidus, or the use of **diuretics** may impair renal concentrating ability. The test is performed after 15 hours of fluid deprivation, and urine is then collected on the hour for 3 hours. Dehydration maximally stimulates endogenous ADH secretion. Under these conditions the urine osmolality should be at least three times that of plasma (286 mOsm/kg).

TABLE 26-2 ASSOCIATION OF PATHOLOGICAL CONDITIONS AFFECTING THE KIDNEY AND CLINICAL AND BIOCHEMICAL ABNORMALITIES

	AGN	NS	TD	UTI	HT	RVT	DM	UTO	RC	ARF	CRF
Hypertension	++	+	0	0	++	±	±	0	0	+	+
Edema	+	++	0	0	0	+	+	0	0	+	+
Oliguria or anuria	+	±	0	0	0	±	0	+	0	+	+
Polyuria	0	0	+	0	0	0	+	0	0	0	0
Nocturia	0	±	+	±	0	0	+	±	0	0	0
Frequency	0	0	0	+	0	0	0	±	±	0	0
Loin pain	0	0	0	+	0	+	0	+	+	0	0
Anemia	+	0	0	0	0	0	0	0	0	0	++
↑Blood urea nitrogen	+	0	0	0	±	±	±	±	0	+	+
↑Serum creatinine	+	−	−	−	±	±	±	±	0	+	+
↓GFR	+	0	0	0	±	±	±	±	0	+	+
↑Serum potassium	±	±	0	0	0	0	0	0	0	+	+
↑Serum phosphorus	±	0	0	0	0	0	0	0	0	+	+
↓Serum calcium	0	+	0	0	0	0	0	0	0	+	+
↑Serum uric acid	0	0	+	0	±	0	±	0	±	+	+
Acidosis	0	0	+	0	0	0	0	0	0	+	+
Proteinuria	+	++++	+	±	±	++	+	0	0	±	±
Hematuria	++	+	±	+	0	+	0	0	++	+	±
RBC casts	+	0	0	0	0	0	0	0	0	±	0
Pyuria	±	0	0	++	0	0	0	±	±	0	0
WBC cast	0	0	0	+	0	0	0	+	0	0	0
Glucosuria	0	0	+	0	0	0	++	0	0	0	0

AGN, *Acute glomerulonephritis;* ARF, *acute renal failure;* CRF, *chronic renal failure;* DM, *diabetes mellitus;* GFR, *glomerular filtration rate;* HT, *hypertension;* NS, *nephrotic syndrome;* RBC, *red blood cells;* RC, *renal calculi;* RVT, *renal vein thrombosis;* TD, *tubular disease;* UTI, *urinary tract infection;* UTO, *urinary tract obstruction;* WBC, *white blood cells.* 0, *Absent;* ±, *variable;* +, *present.*

A specific gravity of 1.025 or more or an osmolality of 850 mOsm/kg or above in one of the specimens is accepted as evidence of concentrating ability within the healthy reference interval. A patient within the healthy reference interval of concentrating ability is unlikely to have a serious kidney malfunction of any type.[28] As chronic renal disease progresses, tubular ability to concentrate urine slowly decreases until the urine has the same specific gravity as the plasma ultrafiltrate, 1.010. Clinically the loss of concentrating ability is manifested by nocturia and polyuria.

To test the urinary diluting capacity, the following procedure is used. The patient empties the bladder and is given 1000 to 1200 mL of water. Urine specimens are then collected every hour for the next 4 hours. Under these circumstances, the urinary specific gravity should fall to 1.005 or less or an osmolality of less than 100 mOsm/kg. In the patient with chronic renal disease who is unable to dilute the urine, there is a danger of fluid overload with this test.

In diabetes insipidus, which can arise from inadequate ADH production or from insensitivity of the renal tubules to ADH, the distal tubular walls are impervious to water. As sodium is reabsorbed, the fluid left behind may be very dilute. In this disease the baseline urine might have a specific gravity of less than 1.005 and an osmolality of 50 mOsm/kg.

Urinalysis (see Urinalysis section of CD-ROM)

Urinalysis is an indispensable tool for assessing renal disease. It may reveal disease anywhere in the urinary tract. Observations that can be made in the standard urinalysis include the appearance of the specimen, pH, specific gravity, protein semiquantitation, presence or absence of glucose and ketones, and a microscopic examination of the centrifuged urinary sediment. The importance of the urinalysis is indicated in Table 26-2. Microscopic examination of the centrifuged urinary sediment for cells, crystals, and casts should be done on a freshly voided specimen.

Casts are protein conglomerates outlining the shape of the renal tubules in which they were formed. Hyaline casts are composed almost exclusively of protein. Cellular elements may be trapped within hyaline casts, resulting in the formation of granular casts. When there is heavy proteinuria, accumulation of protein within tubular cells leads to fatty degeneration of the cells and desquamation of cells into the urine; these appear in the urine as oval fat bodies. In acute pyelonephritis, white blood cells may aggregate in the tubules to form pus casts. Red blood cell casts are important markers of glomerular inflammation and should be diligently searched for when any form of glomerular nephritis is suspected.

Microscopic examination of the urinary sediment is completed by a search for bacteria and crystals. The presence

TABLE 26-3 CHARACTERISTIC URINE MICROSCOPIC FINDINGS IN RENAL DISEASE

Condition	Protein	Red Blood Cells (per High-Power Field)	White Blood Cells (per High-Power Field)	Bacteria	Casts (per Low-Power Field)
Normal	0 to trace	0 to 3	0 to 5	0	Hyaline, occasionally
Glomerulonephritis	1 to 2+	>20	0 to 10	0	Granular red blood cells
Nephrotic syndrome	4+	0 to 10	0 to 5	0	Oval fat bodies; hyaline
Pyelonephritis	0 to 1+	0 to 10	>30	++	Granular white blood cells

of crystals in the urine may be a clue to the diagnosis of a specific type of renal calculus. The characteristic urine microscopic findings in healthy individuals and in renal disease are indicated in Table 26-3. (See Urinalysis section of CD-ROM.)

CHANGE OF ANALYTE IN DISEASE

The changes that occur in analytes are discussed in the section on pathological conditions of the kidney and summarized in Table 26-2. In this section the following question is examined from a different perspective: What does the finding of a biochemical abnormality or group of abnormalities mean in the diagnosis of the pathological condition in the kidney?

Serum Electrolytes (see also pp. 454-461)

Sodium. Sodium is the major cation in the extracellular fluid and usually has a serum concentration of 136 to 145 mmol/L. Sodium and its attendant anions are the major contributors to serum osmolality.[31]

Hyponatremia. Hyponatremia with hypo-osmolality can occur in renal disease because of an increased extracellular fluid volume resulting from the kidney's inability to excrete water. This state occurs in chronic renal insufficiency and the nephrotic syndrome. Hyponatremia, with decreased extracellular fluid, can be associated with the use of diuretic agents and the syndrome of inappropriate ADH secretion.

Hypernatremia. Hypernatremia, by definition a relative water deficit, can occur in patients with hypotonic fluid loss. Hypernatremia also occurs in diabetes insipidus whenever the oral fluid intake cannot keep pace with urinary losses.

Chloride. The concentration of chloride in extracellular fluid parallels that of sodium and is influenced by the same factors. Chloride imbalances occur concurrently with sodium imbalances. Hyperchloremia occurs in association with renal tubular acidosis.

Potassium. Potassium is the major cation of intracellular fluid.

Hypokalemia. Hypokalemia is usually associated with overt potassium depletion as a result of excessive losses of potassium-rich fluids. Potassium loss may be renal or extrarenal. Increased renal excretion of potassium occurs with diuretic agents, prolonged use of corticosteroids, primary or secondary aldosteronism, and Cushing's syndrome. Hypokalemia from extrarenal potassium losses usually occurs in

the gastrointestinal tract and is seen with prolonged vomiting, diarrhea, fistulas of the intestinal tract, and villous adenomas of the colon.

Hyperkalemia. Hyperkalemia, an acute medical emergency, is usually caused by either increased cellular breakdown exceeding the normal renal excretory capacity or impaired renal excretion.[31] Hyperkalemia may result from (1) increased intake of potassium, as occurs with dietary excess or intravenous potassium administration in the patient with compromised renal function; (2) cellular breakdown, as occurs with extensive burns or rhabdomyolysis (acute muscle necrosis); (3) decreased potassium excretion, as occurs in acute or chronic renal failure, secondary to potassium-sparing diuretics, in adrenal insufficiency, and in hypoaldosteronism; or (4) transcellular redistribution of potassium, as occurs with acute acidosis, diabetic ketoacidosis, familial hyperkalemic periodic paralysis, and certain drugs (see Chapter 24 for specific details).

Urinary Electrolytes

Sodium. Urinary sodium determinations are diagnostically useful in three clinical settings. First, in volume depletion, the measurement of urinary sodium excretion is helpful in determining the route of sodium loss. A low urinary sodium concentration (less than 10 mEq/L) indicates an extrarenal sodium loss, whereas the presence of a high concentration of sodium in the urine indicates renal salt wasting or adrenal insufficiency. Second, in the differential diagnosis of acute renal failure, the urinary sodium excretion will be less than 10 mEq/L in patients with volume depletion who have no intrinsic renal disease and usually more than 30 mEq/L in patients with acute tubular necrosis.[32] In volume depletion a urine-to-plasma osmolality ratio of more than 1.1 and a urine-to-plasma urea ratio of more than 10 is observed, compared with values of less than 1.05 and less than 10, respectively, in acute tubular necrosis.[32] Third, in hyponatremia a low urinary sodium concentration (less than 10 mEq/L) indicates avid renal sodium retention, which may be attributable to either severe volume depletion or sodium-retaining states seen in cirrhosis, the nephrotic syndrome, and congestive heart failure. When hyponatremia is associated with urinary sodium excretion that equals or exceeds the dietary sodium intake, it is likely that the syndrome of inappropriate ADH secretion is present.[31] In these three situations a random urinary sodium concentration can rapidly supply valuable diagnostic information (see Chapter 24 for additional details).

Chloride. The measurement of urinary chloride is of clinical value only in patients with persistent metabolic alkalosis who are not receiving diuretics (see Chapter 24 for additional details).[31]

Potassium. Urinary potassium levels are helpful in the evaluation of patients with unexplained hypokalemia.[31] The finding of a urinary potassium concentration of more than 10 mEq/L indicates that the kidney is responsible for the potassium loss, whereas a urinary potassium concentration of less than 10 mEq/L in the presence of hypokalemia is strongly suggestive that the gastrointestinal tract is the route of potassium loss (see Chapter 24 for additional details).

Anion Gap

An increased anion gap occurs in renal failure because of the retention of sulfate, phosphate, and organic acid anions. (See Chapters 24 and 25.)

Creatinine, Urea, and Uric Acid

With progressive renal insufficiency there is retention in the blood of urea, creatinine, and uric acid. Normally the ratio of serum urea nitrogen to serum creatinine is between 10:1 and 20:1. In the usual case of renal failure, a similar ratio is seen. Ratios higher than 20:1 occur in disease states of extrarenal origin, such as prerenal azotemia, gastrointestinal bleeding, or excessive protein intake with marginally adequate renal function. In contrast, urea production and the BUN are reduced in the presence of a low protein intake and in severe liver disease. Uric acid concentration in the blood rises in advanced chronic renal failure, but this rarely results in classical gout.

Calcium and Phosphorus

In chronic renal failure there is impaired excretion of phosphate, and progressive hyperphosphatemia occurs. This results in a fall in the plasma calcium concentration (hypocalcemia), giving rise to secondary hyperparathyroidism. The elevated parathyroid hormone level causes calcium resorption from bone, and normocalcemia or hypercalcemia may result. However, hypocalcemia is more prevalent in uremia, both as a result of the reciprocal fall in the plasma calcium concentration as the plasma phosphate level rises and because of reduced calcium absorption in the gut as a result of impaired 1,25-dihydroxycholecalciferol production.[10,18] Hypocalcemia is also present in the nephrotic syndrome, as a result of the hypoalbuminemia. However, the ionized serum calcium level remains normal in this condition.

Proteinuria

Proteinuria may be of two types. In *glomerular proteinuria*, large quantities of high-molecular-weight proteins enter the glomerular filtrate and ultimately appear in the urine. Heavy proteinuria (more than 2 g/day) results from increased glomerular permeability, and the protein loss may be great enough to result in the nephrotic syndrome.[20] In *tubular proteinuria* the amount of protein filtered by the glomeruli is not increased, but the low–molecular-weight proteins, which are normally filtered, appear in larger quantities in the final urine because tubular reabsorption is incomplete. Impaired tubular reabsorption of filtered proteins results in modest increases (1 to 3 g/day) in the urinary excretion of low–molecular-weight proteins and albumin.[20] Physiological increases in protein excretion occur during the maintenance of an upright posture, after strenuous exercise, and in normal pregnancy.[20]

The traditional method for measuring proteinuria is to collect all urine for a 24-hour period. The first voided specimen of the morning is discarded, all urine is then saved for the next 24 hours, ending at the same time on the next morning, saving the last voided urine. Quantitation of 24-hour protein and creatinine excretion is made. In any given patient whose diet, renal function, and muscle mass remains constant, 24-hour urine creatinine excretion also remains fairly constant. Because of this, creatinine excretion serves as a measure of completeness of the 24-hour collection. The average man excretes 16 to 26 mg, and the average woman excretes 12 to 24 mg of creatinine per kilogram of ideal body weight. With aging, this value drops to 8 to 15 mg/kg of ideal body weight. Because a timed 24-hour urine specimen is inconvenient to collect, and because there are often difficulties in assessing the completeness of collection, the concept of measuring the protein-to-creatinine ratio of "spot" morning urine samples has developed.[33] A value grater than 3 mg protein/mg creatinine indicates nephrotic range proteinuria. The degree of proteinuria by this method correlates with the rate of loss of renal function and is a risk factor for progression to end-stage renal disease.[33]

Enzymes in Urine

Enzymes may appear in urine because of filtration, secretion, or tissue damage.[20] Enzymes of low molecular weight, such as lysozyme and amylase, appear because they are filtered and not completely reabsorbed. High–molecular-weight enzymes, such as lactic dehydrogenase, can be excreted because of parenchymal renal damage.

Hemoglobin and Hematocrit

Anemia is a common feature of chronic renal failure, and its severity reflects the extent of renal impairment.[19] Progressive anemia usually occurs when the GFR falls below 25 mL/min. The anemia of chronic renal failure is attributable to (1) reduced erythropoietin production as renal mass decreases, (2) inhibitors of erythropoiesis present in the serum of the uremic patient, (3) reduced red blood cell survival in advanced renal failure, and (4) iron deficiency caused by blood loss as a result of the hemostatic defect characteristic of renal failure.[19]

References

1. Narins RG et al: Diagnostic strategies in disorders of fluid electrolyte and acid-base homeostasis, *Am J Med* 72:496, 1982.
2. Schrier RW: *Renal and electrolyte disorders*, ed 3, Boston, 1986, Little, Brown.
3. Hackenthal E et al: Morphology, physiology and molecular biology of renin secretion, *Physiol Rev* 70:1067, 1990.
4. Singh I et al: Coordinate regulation of renal expression of nitric oxide synthase, renin, and angiotensinogen mRNA by dietary salt, *Am J Physiol* 270: F1027, 1996.
5. MacKnight ADC: Epithelial transport of potassium, *Kidney Int* 11:391, 1977.
6. Suki WN: Disposition and regulation of body potassium: an overview, *Am J Med Sci* 272:31, 1976.
7. Giebisch G, Malnic G, Berliner RW: Renal transport and control of potassium excretion. In Brenner BM, Rector FC, editors: *The kidney*, Philadelphia, 1991, Saunders.
8. Friedman PA, Gesek FA: Cellular calcium transport in renal epithelia: measurement, mechanisms, and regulation, *Physiol Rev* 75:429, 1995.
9. Slatopolsky E et al: Hyperphosphatemia, *Clin Nephrol* 7:138, 1997.
10. Felsenfeld AJ, Llach F: Parathyroid function in chronic renal failure, *Kidney Int* 43:771, 1993.
11. Contiguglia SR et al: Total-body magnesium excess in chronic renal failure, *Lancet* 1:1300, 1972.
12. Androgue HJ, Madias NE: Management of life-threatening acid-base disorders, *N Engl J Med* 338:26, 1998.
13. Flessner MF, Knepper MA: Renal acid-base transport. In Schrier RW, Gottchalk CW, editors: *Diseases of the kidney*, Boston, 1993, Little, Brown.
14. First MR: *Chronic renal failure*, Garden City, NY, 1982, Medical Examining Publishing.
15. Walser M: Urea metabolism in chronic renal failure, *J Clin Invest* 53:1385, 1974.
16. Perrone RD, Madias NE, Levey AS: Serum creatinine as an index of renal function: new insights into old concepts, *Clin Chem* 38:1933, 1992.
17. Stein JH: Hormones and the kidney, *Hosp Pract* 14:91, 1979.
18. Brown AJ, Dusso A, Slatopolsky E: Selective vitamin D analogs and their therapeutic applications, *Semin Nephrol* 14:156, 1994.
19. Jones SS et al: Human erythropoietin receptor: cloning, expression and biological characterization, *Blood* 76:31, 1990.
20. Pesce AJ, First MR: *Proteinuria: an integrated review*, New York, 1979, Marcel Dekker.
21. Coe FL: Clinical and laboratory assessment of the patient with renal disease. In Brenner BM, Rector FC, editors: *The kidney*, vol 1, Philadelphia, 1986, Saunders.
22. Madias NE, Perrone RD: Acid-base disorders in association with renal disease. In Schrier RW, Gottschalk CW, editors: *Diseases of the kidney*, Boston, 1993, Little, Brown.
23. First MR, Pollak VE: Renal insufficiency in the diabetic patient with heart disease. In Scott RC, editor: *Clinical cardiology and diabetes*, vol 3, part 2, Mount Kisco, NY, 1981, Futura Publishing.
24. Bennett PH et al: Screening and management of microalbuminuria in patients with diabetes mellitus: recommendations to the Scientific Advisory Board of the National Kidney Foundation from an Ad Hoc Committee of the Council on Diabetes Mellitus of the National Kidney Foundation, *Am J Kidney Dis* 25:107, 1995.
25. Wiegmann TB et al: The role of disease duration and hypertension in albumin excretion of type I diabetes mellitus, *J Am Soc Nephrol* 2:1587, 1992.
26. Mathiesen ER et al: Relationship between blood pressure and urinary albumin excretion in development of microalbuminuria, *Diabetes* 39:245, 1990.
27. The Diabetes Control and Complications Trial Research Group: Effect of intensive therapy on the development and progression of diabetic nephropathy in the DCCT, *Kidney Int* 47:1703, 1995.
28. Ware F: Renal function tests: a guide to interpretation, *Hosp Med* 9:77, 1981.
29. Cockcroft DW, Gault MH: Prediction of creatinine clearance from serum creatinine, *Nephron* 16:31, 1976.
30. Coll E et al: Serum cystatin C as a new marker for noninvasive estimation of glomerular filtration rate and as a marker for renal impairment, *Am J Kidney Dis* 36:29, 2000.
31. Harrington JT: Evaluation of serum and urinary electrolytes, *Hosp Pract* 17:28, 1982.
32. Oken DE: On the differential diagnosis of acute renal failure, *Am J Med* 71:916, 1981.
33. Ruggenenti P et al: Cross-sectional longitudinal study of spot morning protein: creatinine ratio, 24-hour urine protein excretion rate, glomerular filtration rate, and end-stage renal failure in chronic renal disease in patients without diabetes, *Br Med J* 316:504, 1998.

Internet Sites

www.kidney.org—National Kidney Foundation (US)
www.kidney.ca—Canadian Kidney Foundation
www.kidney.org.au—Australian Kidney Foundation
http://www.fpnotebook.com/REN63.htm
http://www.kcl.ac.uk/teares/gktvc/vc/lt/rtg/sbdl18.pdf
www.isn-online.org—International Society of Nephrology

www.asn-online.org—American Society of Nephrology
http://www.bertholf.net/rlb/lectures/Lectures/Cardiac%20Markers%20and %20Renal%20Function.pps—Microsoft PowerPoint lecture by Robert L. Bertholf, PhD, Associate Professor of Pathology, Chief of Clinical Chemistry and Toxicology

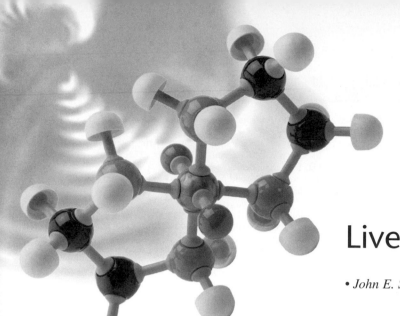

CHAPTER 27

Liver Function

• *John E. Sherwin*

Objectives

• Explain the role of the liver in carbohydrate metabolism, nitrogen metabolism, bile pigment formation, and metabolic end-product excretion and detoxification.
• Describe pathological liver conditions and the serum biochemical alterations associated with these diseases.

• Describe the processing of bilirubin by the liver, define jaundice, and describe the various pathological states associated with jaundice.
• List the serum proteins derived from the liver and describe their functions.

Key Terms

biliary canaliculi   Fine channels running between liver cells.
cirrhosis   A liver disorder characterized by loss of normal microscopic architecture with fibrosis. Cirrhosis has a variety of causes but is most commonly secondary to chronic alcohol abuse. Obstructive biliary cirrhosis may also be caused by obstruction of major intrahepatic or extrahepatic bile ducts.

Crigler-Najjar syndrome   A familial form of nonhemolytic jaundice caused by the absence of glucuronide transferase activity from the liver. Associated with increased serum unconjugated bilirubin and nervous system disorders.
cytochrome P-450   A series of cellular proteins that are one-electron carriers and whose active centers are heme groups. These proteins are involved in hydroxylation reactions of drugs and other

xenobiotics. The *450* refers to the nanometer position of the *Soret* absorption band.

detoxification The process of changing the chemical structure of a foreign substance or poison to make it less poisonous or more readily eliminated.

Dubin-Johnson syndrome A familial form of chronic, nonhemolytic jaundice caused by a defect in the hepatic excretion of conjugated bilirubin.

focal necrosis The death of cells in a small area of tissue.

Gilbert's disease A benign, hereditary form of hyperbilirubinemia and jaundice caused by a defect in the hepatic uptake of unconjugated bilirubin from serum.

gluconeogenesis The formation of glucose from lactate or amino acids by means of the Cori cycle.

glycogenesis The biochemical formation of glycogen from glucose.

glycogenolysis The biochemical degradation of glycogen to form glucose.

hepatitis Inflammation of liver produced by a variety of infections, toxins, and other causes, such as obstruction of the biliary tract in obstructive hepatitis.

hepatobiliary Relating to liver and biliary ducts.

hepatocellular disease Any disease in which the liver cells are destroyed.

hepatocyte A parenchymal liver cell that performs all the functions ascribed to the liver.

jaundice A syndrome characterized by hyperbilirubinemia and deposition of bilirubin pigment in skin and mucosal membranes, resulting in a yellow appearance to the skin (also called *icterus*).

kernicterus Literally "nuclear jaundice," resulting from deposition of unconjugated bilirubin in nuclei of brain and nerve cells, which causes cell destruction and encephalopathy.

ketone bodies Compounds with carbonyl groups; usually referring to acetoacetic acid, acetone, and beta-hydroxybutyric acid (though the last compound is chemically not a ketone).

LCAT Lecithin-cholesterol acyltransferase; esterifies cholesterol with fatty acids.

neonatal jaundice (physiological jaundice) A disorder of newborns characterized by increased serum levels of unconjugated bilirubin and caused by transient immaturity of liver.

oncofetal proteins Any protein, such as alpha-fetoprotein, produced by fetuses and tumors.

parenchymal cells A general term indicating the functional elements of an organ (see **hepatocyte**).

periportal fibrosis The deposition of fibers or fibrous material in the cells lining the portal blood vessels of the liver.

porphyrias A group of disorders caused by disturbances of porphyrin metabolism characterized by increased formation and excretion of porphyrins and their precursors.

Reye's syndrome Acute, often fatal encephalopathy and fatty degeneration of the liver, seen primarily in children.

Wilson's disease Hepatocellular degeneration, also associated with a change in the iris and lens of the eye and caused by a defect in copper metabolism.

xenobiotics Any organic compound that is foreign to the body, such as drugs and organic poisons.

Methods on CD-ROM

Alanine aminotransferase
Albumin
Alkaline phosphatase, total
Alpha$_1$-antitrypsin
Aspartate aminotransferase

Bilirubin
Gamma-glutamyl transferase
Lactate dehydrogenase and lactate dehydrogenase enzymes

ANATOMY AND NORMAL FUNCTION OF LIVER

The liver is the largest organ of the body and is responsible for producing most of the endogenous energy sources used by the body. Divided into two primary lobes, the liver is located in the abdominal cavity just below the diaphragm. The two primary cells of the liver are the **hepatocytes** and the *Kupffer cells* (Fig. 27-1). The parenchymal hepatocytes secrete metabolites into veins or the **biliary canaliculi**; the canaliculi eventually dispense wastes into the bile duct and gallbladder. The hepatocytes are responsible for the metabolic functions of the liver.[1]

The liver is the primary organ responsible for the metabolism of carbohydrates, proteins, lipids, porphyrins, and bile acids. It is responsible for synthesizing most plasma proteins except the immunoglobulins, which are produced by the lymphocytic plasma cell system. The liver is also the principal site for storage of iron, glycogen, lipids, and vitamins. Furthermore, the liver plays an important role in

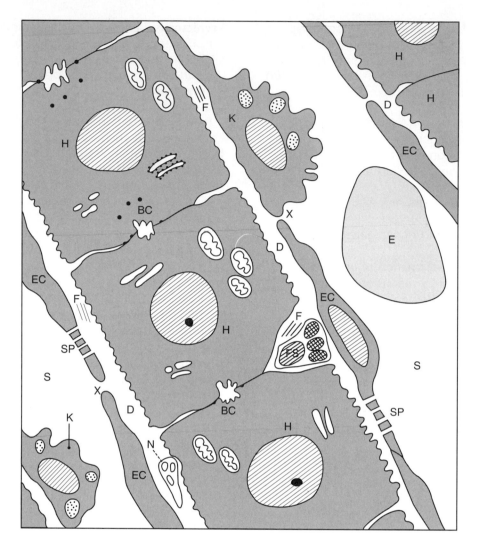

Fig. 27-1 Schema of structures within the lobule. *BC,* Bile canaliculus; *D,* space of Disse; *E,* erythrocyte; *EC,* endothelial cell; *F,* reticulum fibers; *FS,* fat-storing cell; *H,* hepatocyte; *K,* Kupffer cell; *N,* nerve fiber; *S,* sinusoid; *SP,* fenestrae of endothelial cell forming a sieve plate; *X,* intercellular gap. *(From Tanikawa K, editor:* Ultrastructural aspects of the liver and its disorders, *ed 2, Tokyo, 1979, Igaku-Shoin.)*

the **detoxification** of **xenobiotics** and excretion of metabolic end products such as bilirubin, ammonia, and urea.

Carbohydrate Metabolism and Liver Function

Polysaccharides are a form of energy storage; glycogen is the principal storage polysaccharide. The liver is capable of both producing glycogen through **glycogenesis** and degrading glycogen by **glycogenolysis**. Whether the glycogen synthetic reaction or the glycogen degradation reaction predominates depends on an individual's metabolic status. Only liver glycogen is available for maintenance of a constant blood glucose, since only the liver and kidneys contain the enzyme glucose-6-phosphatase, which converts glucose-6-phosphate to glucose. As a result of the highly branched structure of glycogen, approximately 10% of the glucose of glycogen is available for immediate enzymatic release (see Chapter 32 for details on glucose metabolism). Liver glycogen in the normal adult is not a static storage pool; instead it functions as a source of glucose for the rest of the body, except for

muscle. Under conditions of stress, increased body energy requirements must be met by increased glucose use, that is, glycogenolysis and glycolysis. Additional glucose required for the body is provided by increased secretion of glucose by the liver. This is accomplished when the rate of glycogen degradation and the rate of **gluconeogenesis** are increased. Gluconeogenesis is not simply a reversal of glycolysis, since several of the glycolytic enzymes, such as pyruvate kinase, phosphofructokinase, and hexokinase, are not reversible. Lactate and amino acids serve as the precursors for the gluconeogenic pathway. The liver's use of blood lactic acid (of muscle origin) is an important factor in the clearance of this analyte from serum. Gluconeogenesis is an important source of blood glucose when liver glycogen has been depleted. When a person begins fasting, liver glycogen depletion will occur within several hours. The net result of these metabolic pathways is to provide a constant supply of glucose to the blood for export to peripheral tissues to meet their energy requirements.

TABLE 27-1   MAJOR REPRESENTATIVE PLASMA PROTEINS AND THEIR PROPERTIES

Electrophoretic Fraction	Protein	Approximate Concentration (g/L)	Principal Function
	Transthyrethin (prealbumin)	0.1 to 0.4	Binds retinol-binding protein, T_4
	Albumin	40 to 50	Binds Ca^{2+}, T_4, bilirubin
α_1	Antitrypsin	2 to 4	Inhibits some proteolytic enzymes
	Lipoprotein, high density (HDL)	3 to 8	Transport of cholestrol from peripheral tissue to liver
	Retinol-binding	0.03 to 0.06	Transport of retinol
α_2	Thyroxine-binding globulin	0.01 to 0.02	Transport of thyroxine
	Haptoglobins (three types)	1 to 3	Transport of free hemoglobin from destroyed red blood cells
	Lipoprotein, very low density (VLDL)	1.5 to 2.0	Transport of cholesterol and triglycerides
	Ceruloplasmin	0.2 to 0.6	Transport of copper; increases use of iron as ferroxidase
	Prothrombin (bovine)	0.1	Proenzyme of thrombin
	Angiotensinogen	—	Precursor of angiotensin I
	Erythropoietin	<0.05	Erythropoietic hormone
β_1	Lipoprotein, low density (LDL)	4 to 10	Transport of cholesterol and other lipids
	Plasminogen	0.3	Profibrinolysin, precursor of fibrinolysin
	Fibrinogen	3	Coagulation factor I
$\beta_1\beta_2$	Complement (C_4)	0.5 to 1.8	Lysis of foreign cells
	Transferrin	2 to 4	Transport of iron
β_2	Glycoproteins	0.3	Unknown
γ	Blood group globulins and immunoglobulins	7 to 15	Contain various antibodies, blood globulins, complement C_1, C_2, and so on

Modified from Orten JM, Neuhaus OW: *Human biochemistry, ed 10,* St Louis, 1982, Mosby.

Protein Metabolism in Liver

Most blood proteins are synthesized in the liver, with two exceptions in the adult: immunoglobulins and hemoglobin. In the infant the liver retains the ability to synthesize hemoglobin. As in carbohydrate synthesis, liver function must be extensively impaired before a decrease in protein synthesis can be unequivocally demonstrated. The changes associated with **focal necrosis** or **periportal fibrosis** are not extensive enough to affect protein synthesis. The normal concentrations of the major electrophoretic subgroups of proteins are quite variable and depend at least in part on the person's age. Tumors of the liver may express **oncofetal proteins** such as alphafetoprotein, which can be used as both a diagnostic and a monitoring tool (see p. 501 and Chapter 49).

Many liver enzymes exhibit half-lives of several weeks, though structural proteins are stable nearly indefinitely. Plasma proteins synthesized by the liver exhibit quite varied rates of synthesis and degradation (i.e., turnover rates). Under normal conditions, the rate of synthesis of each protein equals its rate of degradation, since its concentration in plasma remains constant. Many proteins synthesized by the liver are excreted into *extravascular fluid* to carry out specific functions. These functions include nutrition, blood pressure control (oncotic pressure), and transport. Table 27-1 lists some liver proteins found in plasma and some of their properties.

One of the most important serum proteins produced in the liver is albumin. Present in concentrations of 40 to 50 g/L, albumin represents 50% to 60% by weight of all plasma protein. This molecule has an extraordinarily wide range of functions, including nutrition; maintenance of oncotic pressure; and serum transport of Ca^{++}, unconjugated bilirubin, free fatty acids, drugs, and steroids. Its multifactorial role in human physiology makes it an important analyte in the monitoring of liver disease.

The liver is also the site for the synthesis of several *acute phase reaction* proteins. When the body is stressed (as by an infectious disease), the serum levels of these proteins may become elevated. Some of these acute phase reaction proteins are used as markers for infectious disease, such as *C-reactive protein (CRP)*. Others, such as *transthyretin (prealbumin)*, are used as markers for the protein-nutritional status of an individual. When the body is protein-malnourished, serum prealbumin levels are decreased; thus measurement of prealbumin and albumin can be useful for the diagnosis and monitoring of malnutrition (see Chapter 37).

Metabolic pools of amino acids are present in the liver. From these pools amino acids are drawn for the synthesis of proteins. When a protein is degraded, the bulk of the constituent amino acids are returned to these intracellular pools. The released amino acids can also be used in gluconeogenesis, transamination, or deamination reactions or be reincorporated into new proteins. Important transamination reactions are catalyzed by the enzymes alanine amino-transferase (ALT, or formerly SGPT) and aspartate amino-transferase (AST, or formerly SGOT). In the healthy person who is in nitrogen equilibrium or positive nitrogen balance, the amino groups of excess amino acids in serum are converted to ammonia or urea for excretion.[2] Some amino acids are also excreted unchanged in the urine. Negative nitrogen balance (i.e., insufficient dietary nitrogen) leads to a diminution of amino acid pools and thus decreased urea excretion.

Urea, creatinine, ammonia, and uric acid account for 70% to 75% of the serum nonprotein nitrogen; urea accounts for 60% of the total. Most of the metabolism of nonprotein nitrogen occurs in the liver. Urea is produced in the liver because arginase, the enzyme that converts arginine to urea and ornithine, is present only in the liver. Although blood ammonia concentration is normally quite low, 500 mg/L, ammonia is an important intermediate in amino acid synthesis. Sources of ammonia include hepatic oxidation of glutamate to oxoglutarate, the transamination and oxidative deamination of amino acids and catecholamines, and bacterial breakdown of urea in the gut. Most blood ammonia is formed from the gut. The primary mechanisms for the metabolic disposal of ammonia is the synthesis of glutamate, glutamine, and carbamyl phosphate. Carbamyl phosphate may be used to synthesize orotic acid and ultimately pyrimidines for nucleic acids or to synthesize urea, which is the principal pathway for the excretion of excess nitrogen.

Lipid Biosynthesis and Transport in Liver Function

Lipids, for the sake of this discussion, include only free fatty acids, triglycerides, glycerophosphatides, sphingolipids, cholesterol, and cholesterol esters. General chemical structures for these lipids are shown in Chapter 53, and their metabolism is discussed in Chapter 33.

Lipids are synthesized in the liver in response to excess carbohydrate intake and to normal intake of dietary lipids. Excess carbohydrate is converted to acetyl coenzyme A (acetyl CoA), and a cytoplasmic enzyme system converts it to the fatty acid palmitate, using reduced nicotinamide adenine diphosphonucleotide (NADPH) and adenosine triphosphate, which are also produced from glucose metabolism.

In the liver, fatty acids are broken down to acetyl CoA, which can then be oxidized to CO_2 by the citric acid cycle. However, a small portion of acetyl CoA is converted to **ketone bodies**, such as acetoacetate, beta-hydroxybutyrate, and acetone. In normal persons, these products are present in blood to the extent of only about 30 mg/L. In the presence of excess mobilization of fatty acids, as in diabetic ketoacidosis or alcohol intoxication, limiting amounts of NAD and NADP results in an increased hepatic synthesis of the ketone bodies.

The liver repackages dietary lipids and secretes them in the form of triglyceride-rich, very–low-density lipoproteins. These are eventually converted to low-density lipoprotein for delivery of cholesterol to peripheral cells. Cholesterol is also synthesized in the liver microsomes from acetyl CoA. Approximately 70% of the total cholesterol in plasma is

esterified with fatty acids by the enzyme **lecithin-cholesterol acyltransferase (LCAT)**, which is also produced by the liver. Bile acids are produced from cholesterol by the cells lining the biliary canaliculi and ductules of the liver.[2] The bile acids are the final excretory metabolites of cholesterol. They also serve as aids in the digestion of dietary lipids (see Chapter 30). Approximately 80% of the available cholesterol is converted into the four major bile acids (Table 27-2). Cholic acid and chenodeoxycholate are the primary bile acids and are present in a fivefold to tenfold excess over the secondary bile acids, deoxycholic acid and lithocholic acid, which are produced by metabolism of the primary hepatic bile acids by intestinal bacteria.

Bile acids are collected in the biliary canaliculi and ductules and stored in the gallbladder. They are then transported to the intestinal lumen, where they emulsify ingested lipids. This emulsification of the lipids permits the intestinal mucosa to digest the lipids and absorb the liberated triglycerides and cholesterol. More than 90% of the secreted bile acids are reabsorbed and returned to the liver through the portal circulation.[2] Periportal fibrosis can alter the utilization of bile acids.

Liver as a Storage Depot

The liver is an important site for the storage of iron, glycogen, amino acids, and some lipids and vitamins. The adult liver contains about 700 mg of iron. Nutritional iron is absorbed primarily in the intestine. To be absorbed, ferric iron (Fe^{3+}) must be converted to ferrous iron (Fe^{2+}). Immediately after absorption, the Fe^{2+} is reconverted to Fe^{3+} and temporarily stored in the intestinal mucosa as the ferritin complex. The ferritin apoprotein is synthesized in the liver. The iron is then released once more as Fe^{2+} into the plasma and is rapidly oxidized into Fe^{3+} and complexed with transferrin, a hepatic synthesized α_1-globulin. In the healthy adult, transferrin is 25% to 30% saturated with Fe^{3+}. In the liver, transferrin releases iron, and a new ferritin-Fe^{3+} complex is formed. Ferritin is the primary storage form of iron; apoferritin binds iron as a colloidal hydrous ferric oxide. However, a small amount of iron is stored as hemosiderin,

TABLE 27-2 Names of Bile Acids, Their Relative Contribution to the Total Bile Acid Pool, and Normal Serum Concentrations

Name	Relative Content (%) in Bile	Normal Serum Concentration (mmol)
Cholylglycine	38	0.2 to 0.9
Deoxycholylglycine	20	0.08 to 0.7
Lithocholylglycine	4	0.07 to 0.3
Chenodeoxycholylglycine	38	0.05 to 0.2

From Shaw LM: Lab Management 20:56, 1982.

which is an insoluble cellular inclusion of Fe^{3+} complexed with ferritin. Hemosiderin granules serve as a storage form for iron when there are insufficient levels of apoferritin. The ratio of iron to protein is much greater in hemosiderin than in ferritin. Additional details of iron metabolism are found in Chapter 35.

Lipid is stored, primarily as triglyceride, in subcutaneous adipose tissue. Lipid is also stored in the liver, where it functions as an energy reservoir. Under normal circumstances the liver functions as a temporary storage site for lipids as they are synthesized in the liver or absorbed from the intestine after a meal.

Bile Pigment Formation

About 126 days after emergence from the reticuloendothelial tissue, the senescent erythrocytes are phagocytized and the hemoglobin is released. The heme portion of hemoglobin is converted to bilirubin, with the release of iron and the globin proteins. The liberated iron is bound by transferrin and returned to the iron stores of the liver or bone marrow; the globin is degraded to its constituent amino acids. The conversion of heme to bilirubin requires 2 to 3 hours (Fig. 27-2). Bilirubin, bound to albumin, is transported from the reticuloendothelial cells to the hepatocytes. In the liver, bilirubin is transported through the cellular microvilli of the sinusoids to the hepatocytes. Bilirubin is dissociated from albumin and taken up into the hepatocytes by specific proteins. Within the hepatocyte, bilirubin glucuronide is formed by reaction of bilirubin with uridine diphosphoglucuronate (UDP-glucuronate) in the presence of UDP-glucuronyl-transferase. Approximately 8 to 10 mg/L of unconjugated bilirubin is present in normal adult serum; normal adult serum contains no conjugated bilirubin. Formation of bilirubin diglucuronide represents the usual (85% to 90%) conjugation reaction, but in disease states, monoglucuronides of bilirubin form as a result of the accumulation of unconjugated bilirubin in the face of a limited supply of glucuronate. In disease states, a small fraction of unconjugated bilirubin is also covalently conjugated to albumin.

This fraction of bilirubin, termed *delta-bilirubin*, reacts like conjugated bilirubin in most chemical assays used to measure this fraction.

After formation, the bilirubin-diglucuronide is excreted by the hepatocyte into the biliary canaliculi. Any disease resulting in a decreased secretion of the conjugated bilirubin will result in an increased serum concentration of this analyte. As part of the bile, these water-soluble conjugates are secreted into the lumen of the small intestine. The bilirubin conjugates are hydrolyzed by a beta-glucuronidase, and the regenerated bilirubin is converted to *d*-urobilinogen and further reduced to *l*-urobilinogen and *l*-stercobilinogen by the anaerobic bacteria of the intestinal lumen. The urobilinogens are reabsorbed from the intestine and recirculated in the extrahepatic circulation, where they are ultimately excreted in the urine. Stercobilinogen is not reabsorbed from the intestine but is a normal constituent of the feces. These bilinogens oxidize spontaneously in air to the corresponding bilins and thereby contribute to the color of both urine and feces (Fig. 27-3). (See Chapter 35 for additional details on bilirubin metabolism.)

Metabolic End-Product Excretion and Detoxification

Humans have two mechanisms for detoxification of foreign, or xenobiotic, materials (such as drugs and poisons) and toxic metabolic products (such as ammonia and bilirubin). The first is to bind the compound reversibly to a protein so that the material is inactivated; thus bilirubin is bound to albumin and lead is bound to hemoglobin. The second mechanism is to modify the compound chemically so that it is readily excreted; thus ammonia is converted to urea and bilirubin is converted to bilirubin-glucuronide.

The inactivation and detoxification of exogenous compounds are usually accomplished by hydroxylation mediated by one of the **cytochrome P-450** enzymes or by conjugation of the parent compound or its metabolite with sulfate or carbohydrate. These reactions are localized in the microsomes of the liver. The sulfated compounds are more water-soluble than the parent compounds and are excreted directly in the urine. Carbohydrate conjugates are commonly excreted into the intestinal lumen as part of the bile.

LIVER-FUNCTION ALTERATIONS DURING DISEASE

Jaundice

Jaundice is a general condition that results from abnormal metabolism or retention of bilirubin. Jaundice causes a yellow discoloration of the skin, mucous membranes, and sclera. Jaundice can typically be seen at serum bilirubin levels of approximately 50 mg/L. The three principal types of jaundice are prehepatic, hepatic, and posthepatic.

Prehepatic jaundice is the result of acute or chronic hemolytic anemias. *Hepatic jaundice* includes disorders of bilirubin metabolism and transport defects, such as **Crigler-Najjar syndrome**, **Dubin-Johnson syndrome**, and **Gilbert's disease**, as well as neonatal physiological jaundice

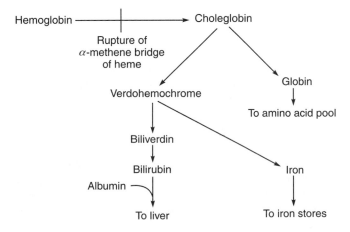

Fig. 27-2 Formation of bilirubin from hemoglobin occurs primarily in reticuloendothelial tissues.

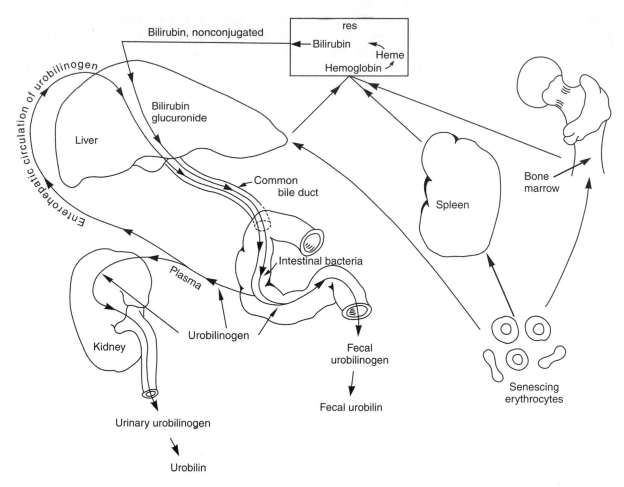

Fig. 27-3 Bilirubin metabolism. *res,* Reticuloendothelial system. *(From Bauer JD, editor: Clinical laboratory methods, ed 9, St Louis, 1982, Mosby.)*

and diseases resulting in hepatocellular injury or destruction. *Posthepatic jaundice* results from a compromised ability of the liver to excrete bilirubin.

Each of the specific diseases of bilirubin metabolism represents a defect in one of the steps in the hepatic processing of serum bilirubin (Fig. 27-4). Thus *Gilbert's disease* is caused by a defect in the transport of bilirubin from plasma albumin into the hepatocyte. Although levels of unconjugated bilirubin are elevated in this familial disorder, levels of conjugated bilirubin are not. Impairment in the conjugation step by UDP-glucuronide caused by a deficiency in the enzyme UDP-glucuronyl transferase will also lead to a large increase in unconjugated bilirubin. When this enzyme deficiency is congenital, it is known as *Crigler-Najjar disease.*

Deficiencies in glucuronyl transferase are most frequently encountered as **neonatal jaundice,** or **physiological jaundice.**[3] This enzyme activity is one of the last liver functions to be activated in prenatal life, since unconjugated bilirubin formed in the fetus is cleared by the placenta into maternal blood. However, in premature births, infants are sometimes born without the enzyme activity present. This leads to a rapid buildup of unconjugated bilirubin, which can be life-threatening. The unconjugated bilirubin, which is much more lipid-soluble than water-soluble, readily passes

into the brain and nerve cells and is deposited in the nuclei of these cells, resulting in **kernicterus.** Kernicterus often results in cell damage and death. Neonatal jaundice will persist until the glucuronyl transferase is produced by the newborn's liver.[3] The newborn's blood must be monitored frequently so that dangerously high levels of unconjugated bilirubin (about 200 mg/L) can be detected. At this point the infant is treated either with ultraviolet radiation to destroy the bilirubin as it passes through the capillaries of the skin or with exchange transfusion.[3] Monitoring serum bilirubin in premature infants is particularly important. These infants are at greater risk for bilirubin-induced encephalopathy because (1) the blood-brain barrier may be incomplete, (2) these infants often have lower concentrations of albumin than normal, (3) acidosis is present, whereby the increase in hydrogen ions can displace bilirubin from albumin, and (4) these infants are often treated with substances that may displace bilirubin from albumin, such as free fatty acids in hyperalimentation fluids or drugs such as phenytoin (Dilantin) or phenobarbital. In hospitals where babies are at risk for **hepatitis,** measurements of conjugated bilirubin may also be needed (see below).

The last step in the hepatic processing of bilirubin is the post-conjugation step of excretion of the bilirubin-glucuronide

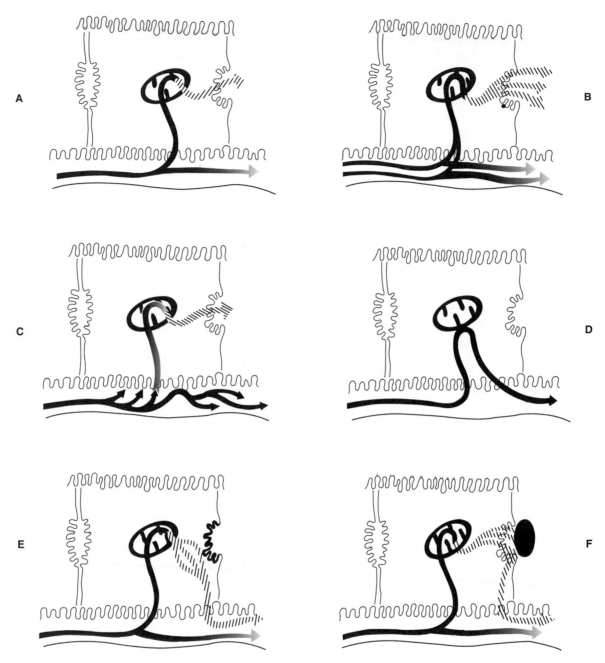

Fig. 27-4 Mechanisms of hyperbilirubinemia. **A**, Normal bilirubin metabolism with hepatocyte uptake of unconjugated bilirubin *(dark arrow)* and microsomal conjugation and excretion of conjugated bilirubin *(striped arrow)*. **B**, Hemolytic jaundice, in which increased bilirubin production results in increased excretion of conjugated bilirubin and a rise in excess (exceeding liver capacity) unconjugated bilirubin in blood. **C**, Gilbert's disease, in which decreased hepatic uptake results in a large increase in blood levels of unconjugated bilirubin. **D**, Physiological jaundice, in which microsomal conjugating system is not functional, resulting in a large increase in unconjugated bilirubin. Congenital deficiency is called *Crigler-Najjar syndrome.* **E**, Dubin-Johnson syndrome, in which there is a biochemical defect preventing secretion of conjugated bilirubin, resulting in a backflow into blood. **F**, Intrahepatic or extrahepatic obstruction in which a physical block prevents secretion of conjugated bilirubin. Hepatocellular disease results in a pattern similar to a combination of **C** and **D**. *(From Leevy CM, editor:* Evaluation of liver function, *ed 2, Indianapolis, 1974, Lilly Research Laboratories.)*

from the hepatic microsomes into the canaliculi. Impairment of this process, called the *Dubin-Johnson syndrome*, results in large increases in the conjugated bilirubin fraction of serum and a urine showing the presence of bilirubin.

The measurement of delta-bilirubin (δ-bili) has been advocated as a means of better assessing hyperbilirubinemia resulting from obstructive hepatic disease.[4] If elevated to significant concentrations, it may result in an apparent slowed decrease in the drop in serum bilirubin, giving a false impression of a lack of progress as the liver disease responds to treatment. However, this test is very rarely used.

Hepatic jaundice also encompasses the disorders characterized by hepatocellular damage or necrosis, such as hepatitis and **cirrhosis**. *Posthepatic jaundice* is generally caused by biliary obstructive disease resulting from spasms or strictures of the biliary tract, ductal occlusion by stones, or compression by neoplastic disease. Since the hepatic functions of transport and conjugation of bilirubin are normal in these diseases, the major increase in serum bilirubin involves the conjugated fraction. Unable to be properly excreted by the liver in these disorders, the conjugated bilirubin fraction increases in serum, resulting in the appearance of bilirubin in the urine. If the **hepatocellular disease** is severe enough to cause jaundice, both the conjugated and the unconjugated bilirubin fractions are increased. The reason is the general disruption of bilirubin metabolism. The laboratory findings for bilirubin and its metabolites in these diseases are summarized in Table 27-3.

Hepatitis

Hepatitis, a general term meaning "inflammation of the liver," is used to describe diseases resulting in hepatocellular damage. Hepatitis is usually caused by infections or toxic agents. Viral hepatitis is the most common cause of acute hepatocellular disease. Four types of hepatitis virus have been recognized: type A virus; type B virus; type C virus; and the delta hepatitis virus. The type C virus is now an important cause of hepatitis in the United States.[5] The delta virus is a biologically active agent but may require the hepatitis B virus (HBV) for production of disease. Certainly, coinfection by both viruses results in a more aggressive chronic liver disease than infection by HBV alone.[6] The clinical symptoms of the four types are similar, and the majority of hepatitis cases are anicteric because despite the hepatic necrosis, the liver retains sufficient residual functional capacity to handle the bilirubin load from normal hemoglobin turnover. Other viruses known to cause hepatitis include cytomegalovirus, coxsackievirus B, and Epstein-Barr virus.

Serum levels of ALT and AST rise rapidly during the early course of hepatitis because of hepatic necrosis (see NACB monograph listed in bibliography). In patients who develop jaundice, the rise in the transaminases precedes the increase in bilirubin, which persists for 2 to 8 weeks. AST is usually more elevated than ALT. Serum alkaline phosphatase and γ-glutamyltransferase (GGT) are elevated during the early cholestatic portion of the disease and remain elevated until the disease has resolved. Diagnosis of the type of viral hepatitis is accomplished by measurement of the specific viral antigen during the prodromal phase of the illness. Specific antibodies to virus antigens are detectable for several weeks after the antigen is no longer detectable. Chronic hepatitis is generally the result of a persistence of hepatitis B infection. It is associated with elevation of serum bilirubin, minimally but persistently elevated serum transaminases (with ALT now greater than AST) caused by hepatic necrosis, and occasionally, elevated alkaline phosphatase.

Drug-Induced Hepatic Damage

The most common cause of drug-induced hepatic damage is chronic excessive ingestion of alcohol. Laboratory findings associated with this damage are an elevation of GGT, a mild elevation of the transaminases, an increase in the globulin with a decrease in the albumin fractions of the serum proteins, and a decrease in sulfobromophthalein (Bromsulphalein, BSP) or indocyanine green clearance. (See Chapter 34 for a detailed review of alcoholic liver disease.)

TABLE 27-3   Concentrations and Changes in Concentration of Bilirubin and its Metabolites in Healthy Persons and Those with Jaundice

| | SERUM | | URINE | | |
Condition	Total Bilirubin	Conjugated Bilirubin	Conjugated Bilirubin	Urobilinogen	Feces Pigment
Healthy	2 to 10 mg/L	0 to 2 mg/L	Negative	0.5 to 3.4 mg/day	Brown
Prehepatic jaundice	Increased	Normal	Negative	Increased	Normal
Hepatic jaundice					
Hepatocellular disease	Increased	Increased	Positive	Decreased (normal)	Light brown
Gilbert's disease	Increased	Normal	Negative	Decreased (normal)	Normal
Crigler-Najjar syndrome	Increased	Decreased	Negative	Decreased	Light brown
Dubin-Johnson syndrome	Increased	Increased	Positive	Decreased (normal)	Light brown
Posthepatic obstructive jaundice	Increased	Increased	Positive	Decreased	Light brown

Other classes of drugs that induce hepatic damage include barbiturates, tricyclic antidepressants, antiepileptics, isoniazid, and acetaminophen. These drugs typically cause an increase in serum GGT. Acetaminophen is highly hepatotoxic. Overdoses require careful monitoring to prevent death from liver failure. Drug withdrawal permits liver regeneration. Chemotherapeutic drugs such as vincristine, vinblastine, actinomycin D, and 5-fluorouracil will typically cause an elevation of the serum transaminases and lactate dehydrogenase because of hepatic tissue damage and enzyme release.

Reye's Syndrome

Reye's syndrome typically occurs in children between 2 and 13 years of age. The liver has fatty infiltration with necrosis and cholestasis, and encephalopathy occurs because of accumulation of ammonia. Laboratory findings include an elevated blood ammonia, elevated serum transaminases, and a prolonged prothrombin time.

Congenital Deficiency Syndromes with Altered Liver Function

Porphyrias. The **porphyrias** are caused by congenital enzyme deficiencies in the pathways leading to the synthesis of the heme moiety of hemoglobin and other heme proteins, such as myoglobin and the cytochromes. Increased excretion of specific porphyrin metabolites, varying with the enzyme defect, is seen. The six types of porphyria are acute intermittent porphyria, variegate porphyria, congenital erythropoietic porphyria, coproporphyria, porphyria cutanea tarda, and erythropoietic protoporphyria. Chapter 35 summarizes porphyrin metabolism and includes a discussion of the enzyme defects.

Wilson's disease. Wilson's disease is an autosomal recessive disorder of copper metabolism. The accumulation of copper in the liver results in jaundice followed by liver cirrhosis. Wilson's disease is characterized by a low serum concentration of ceruloplasmin, glycosuria, phosphaturia, aminoaciduria, and an elevated urinary copper concentration with excretion greater than 50 mg/day. (See p. 712, in Chapter 38 for additional information.)

Hemochromatosis. Hemochromatosis is another genetic disorder of metal metabolism (see Chapter 48). In this disease, iron accumulates in the liver, and the resulting cirrhosis is similar to alcoholic cirrhosis. An elevated serum iron, a low iron-binding capacity, and an elevated serum ferritin value in the presence of normal dietary iron intake are characteristic of this disorder. (See Chapters 34 and 35 for a discussion of acquired hemochromatosis.)

Alpha₁-Antitrypsin Deficiency

Alpha$_1$-antitrypsin deficiency is an inborn error of protein metabolism that results in emphysema and liver cirrhosis. Numerous alpha$_1$-antitrypsin phenotypes have been identified and carry varying risks for disease.[7] The tissue damage seen in alpha$_1$-antitrypsin deficiencies may be caused by hydrolytic damage to structural protein by trypsin-like enzymes that have not been neutralized by alpha$_1$-antitrypsin. Since alpha$_1$-antitrypsin represents approximately 80% of the alpha$_1$ fraction of serum proteins on electrophoresis, a severe deficiency is often diagnosed by the absence of this fraction in the electrophoretogram. Phenotyping of the various alpha$_1$-antitrypsin deficiencies is best done by isoelectric focusing.

Other genetic disorders associated with liver disease include the lipid-storage diseases and the glycogen-storage diseases. These are discussed in detail in Chapter 48.

Liver Tumors and Other Hepatic Disorders

The incidence of hepatocellular cancer is increasing as the result of increased exposure to agents, such as hepatitis C, which cause chronic liver disease.[8] Congenital hepatic fibrosis, hepatic cysts, and liver abscesses are generally best diagnosed by liver biopsy. However, nonspecific changes in liver enzymes and indocyanine green retention can accompany these disorders. Liver tumors frequently alter liver function as a result of tissue compression during tumor growth and infiltration. This results in an increase in serum alkaline phosphatase, 5′-nucleotidase, and especially GGT. BSP and indocyanine green clearances are frequently prolonged. The demonstration of an elevation of serum alpha-fetoprotein is diagnostic of hepatic tumor in the presence of an abnormal liver scan.

Liver Transplantation

Liver transplantation is becoming increasingly common, and between 85% and 90% of patients survive their first transplant for at least 1 year. It is important to monitor these patients for function as well as early signs of rejection (see Chapter 52). Both cyclosporin A and FK-506 (Tacrolimmus) are used as immunosuppressive agents to aid in graft acceptance. Monitoring whole blood concentrations of these drugs is important for maintaining effective drug concentrations.

Maintenance of posttransplantation liver function can be assessed by measurement of the traditional liver-function enzymes such as ALT, lactate dehydrogenase (LD), GGT, and alkaline phosphatase in conjunction with other tests, such as prothrombin time. Findings of these tests in posttransplantation patients should be interpreted in the same manner as those in other patients.

LIVER-FUNCTION TESTS

Liver-function tests are generally used to identify liver disease in the absence of jaundice or when the jaundice is the result of hemolytic disease and the existence of complicating liver disease is suspected. Liver function is tested by injecting a dye intravascularly and observing the retention of dye in the serum. It is essential to choose a dye that is excreted into the bile rather than filtered by the kidney. Thus indocyanine green is acceptable, whereas phenolsulfonphthalein, which is excreted preferentially in the urine, is not. Indocyanine green retention depends on hepatic blood flow, biliary duct function, and liver cell function. Therefore these tests cannot distinguish between hepatocellular disease and obstructive liver disease. In the normal person the percentage of retention is less than 5% at 45 minutes. An increase in the

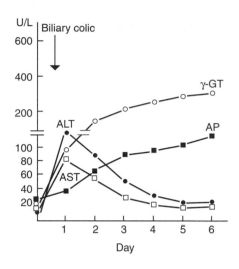

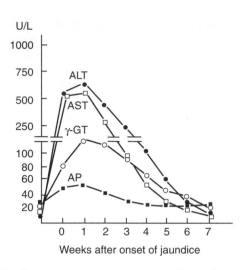

Fig. 27-5 Course of serum enzyme activities in obstructive jaundice. *(From Schmidt E, Schmidt FW: Brief guide to practical enzyme diagnosis, Houston, 1977, Boehringer Mann-heim Diagnostics.)*

Fig. 27-6 Course of serum enzyme activities in acute viral hepatitis. *(From Schmidt E, Schmidt FW: Brief guide to practical enzyme diagnosis, Houston, 1977, Boehringer Mann-heim Diagnostics.)*

TABLE 27-4   CHANGE OF SERUM ANALYTE WITH DISEASE

	Alkaline Phosphatase	GGT	5'-Nucleotidase	AST	ALT	Bile Acids	Albumin	NH₃
Acute hepatitis (viral and so on)	↑	↑	↑	↑↑↑	↑↑	↑↑	N	N, ↑
Alcoholic (drug) hepatitis	N, ↑	↑↑↑	↑	↑	↑	↑	N	N, ↑
Chronic hepatocellular disease	N, ↑	N, ↑	N, ↑	↑	↑	↑	↓	N, ↑
Cirrhosis	N, ↑	N, ↑	N, ↑	N, ↑	N, ↑	↑	↓	N, ↑
Reye's syndrome	N			↑	↑			↑↑
Hepatomas	↑↑	↑↑↑↑	↑↑	↑	↑		N, ↓	N
Cholestatic disease	↑	↑↑	↑↑↑	↑	↑	↑	N	N

N, Normal; ↑, elevated; ↓, lowered.

---

retention is consistent with liver dysfunction resulting from hepatocellular disease, biliary obstructive disease, and space-filling lesions such as tumors in the liver. It should be emphasized that BSP testing is not done routinely any longer, in part because it is known to cause anaphylaxis in some patients.

A second group of liver function tests relates changes in liver's ability to metabolize drugs to changes in serum concentration of the parent drug or its metabolite, or in the of drug metabolite excreted into urine.

CHANGE OF ANALYTE IN DISEASE

Changes of serum analyte with disease are summarized in Table 27-4.

Enzymes

In this section, six serum enzymes are described: alkaline phosphatase, GGT, AST, ALT, 5'-nucleotidase, and lactate dehydrogenase. Although numerous other enzymes useful in the evaluation of liver function have been identified, the six

enzymes discussed here are those generally used. We will also examine the value of these enzymes in the differential diagnosis of liver disease. Examples of the course of activity for several of these enzymes in hepatic disease are illustrated in Figs. 27-5 to 27-7.

Alkaline phosphatase (EC 3.1.3.1). Alkaline phosphatase is actually a group of enzymes that hydrolyze monophosphate esters at an alkaline pH. Optimal pH levels of these enzymes are generally about 10. The natural substrates for alkaline phosphatase are not known. The enzyme has been identified in most body tissues and is generally localized in the membranes of cells. Alkaline phosphatase activity is highest in the liver, bone, intestine, kidney, and placenta, and as many as 11 different isoforms of alkaline phosphatase have been identified in serum. Since alkaline phosphatase normally contains significant amounts of sialic acid, most of these multiple enzyme forms are the result of different degrees of sialation. The enzyme produced by the placenta is known to have a protein composition different from the other enzyme compositions.

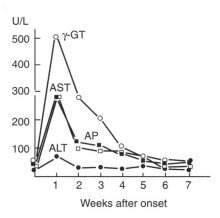

Fig. 27-7 Course of serum enzyme activities in acute alcoholic hepatitis. *(From Schmidt E, Schmidt FW:* Brief guide to practical enzyme diagnosis, *Houston, 1977, Boehringer Mannheim Diagnostics.)*

Measurement of serum alkaline phosphatase is useful in differentiating **hepatobiliary** disease from osteogenic bone disease. Alkaline phosphatase activity increases greatly (10 times) as a result of membrane-localized enzyme synthesis after extrahepatobiliary obstruction such as cholelithiasis or gallstones. Intrahepatic biliary obstruction is also accompanied by an increased serum alkaline phosphatase activity, but the degree of increase is smaller (two to three times).

Liver disease resulting in **parenchymal cell** necrosis does not elevate serum alkaline phosphatase unless the liver disease is associated with damage to the canaliculi or biliary stasis.

Interpretation of serum alkaline phosphatase measurements is complicated by the fact that enzyme activity can increase in the absence of liver disease. The most common disorders causing elevation of alkaline phosphatase are bone diseases, such as Paget's disease, rickets, and osteomalacia. Additionally, rapid bone growth during puberty elevates serum alkaline phosphatase activity, as does the release of alkaline phosphatase from the placenta during the third trimester of pregnancy (see **Methods on CD-ROM**).

Gamma-glutamyltransferase (EC 2.3.2.2). GGT (or γ-GT) is a membrane-localized enzyme that plays a major role in glutathione metabolism and resorption of amino acids from the glomerular filtrate and from the intestinal lumen. Glutathione (γ-glutamylcysteinylglycine) in the presence of GGT and an amino acid or peptide transfers glutamate to the amino acid, resulting in a peptide bond on the γ-carboxylic acid and thereby forming cysteinylglycine and the corresponding γ-glutamyl peptide (see **Methods on CD-ROM**).

Although the GGT activity is highest in renal tissue, serum GGT is generally elevated as a result of liver disease. Serum GGT is elevated earlier than other liver enzymes in diseases such as acute cholecystitis, acute pancreatitis, acute and subacute liver necrosis, and neoplasms of multiple sites at which liver metastases are present. Since GGT is a hepatic microsomal enzyme, chronic ingestion of alcohol or drugs such as barbiturates, tricyclic antidepressants, and anti-convulsants induces microsomal enzyme production. These drug-induced elevations precede any change in other liver enzymes, and if drug ingestion is stopped at this point, the liver changes are generally reversible. GGT permits differentiation of liver disease from other conditions in which serum alkaline phosphatase is elevated because serum GGT levels are usually normal in Paget's disease, rickets, and osteomalacia and in children and pregnant women without liver disease. Since the prostate contains significant GGT activity, serum activity is higher in healthy men than in women. Serum GGT is most useful in the diagnosis of cholestasis caused by chronic alcohol or drug ingestion, mechanical or viral cholestasis, liver metastases, bone disorders in which alkaline phosphatase is elevated but GGT is normal, and skeletal muscle disorders in which the transaminase AST is elevated but GGT is normal.

5′-Nucleotidase (EC 3.1.3.5). 5′-Nucleotidase (NTD) is a microsomal and cell membrane-localized enzyme that catalyzes the hydrolysis of nucleoside-5′-phosphate esters. The serum enzyme has an apparent pH optimum of 7.5:

$$\text{Nucleoside-5′-monophosphate} + H_2O \xrightarrow{\text{NTD}} \text{Nucleoside} + P_i$$

Like GTT, serum NTD is increased in hepatobiliary diseases such as gallstone obstruction of the bile duct, cholestasis, biliary cirrhosis, and obstructive disease caused by neoplastic growth. Serum NTD is not generally elevated in drug-induced liver damage.[9] Therefore, during the course of chemotherapy for patients with liver neoplasms, it is useful to measure NTD in conjunction with GGT. Since NTD is not elevated in bone disease, it (like GGT) is useful in differentiating hepatic causes of alkaline phosphatase increase from other causes, such as bone disease, pregnancy, and normal childhood growth.

Lactate dehydrogenase (EC 1.1.1.27). Lactate dehydrogenase (LD) is present in numerous tissues and catalyzes the interconversion of pyruvate and lactate (see **Methods on CD-ROM**):

$$\text{NAD} + H^+ + \text{Lactate} \underset{}{\overset{\text{LD}}{\rightleftharpoons}} \text{Pyruvate} + \text{NADH}^+$$

LD activity is highest in the kidney and heart and lowest in the lung and serum. LD is localized in the cytoplasm of cells and thus is extruded into the serum when cells are damaged or necrotic.

The measurement of total LD can be useful in cases when only a specific organ, such as the liver, is known to be involved. Total LD is increased in viral or toxic hepatitis, extrahepatic biliary obstruction, acute necrosis of the liver, and cirrhosis of the liver.

Aspartate aminotransferase (EC 2.6.1.1) and alanine aminotransferase (EC 2.6.1.2). The transaminases AST and ALT catalyze the conversion of aspartate and alanine to oxaloacetate and pyruvate, respectively. (See **Methods on CD-ROM** for discussion of the measurement of the transaminases.) These transaminases are still the most useful tests for detecting hepatic cell damage.[10] The highest ALT levels are found in the liver, whereas AST is present in nearly equal levels in the heart, skeletal muscle, and liver. Serum activity of both AST and ALT increases rapidly during the onset of viral jaundice and remains elevated for 1 to 2 weeks (see NACB monograph in Bibliography). In toxic hepatitis, ALT and AST are also elevated, but LD is elevated to an even greater extent as a result of hepatic cell necrosis. Patients with chronic active hepatitis also exhibit increased AST and ALT.

Acute liver necrosis is accompanied by significant increases in the activity of both ALT and AST. The increase in ALT activity is usually greater than the increase in AST activity. In cirrhotic liver disease, serum transaminase activities are generally not elevated above 300 U/L, regardless of the cause of the cirrhotic disease. The elevations of serum ALT and AST seen in Reye's syndrome are directly attributable to hepatic damage, and the increase in ALT is generally greater than the increase in AST. Neoplastic disease also elevates serum transaminase activity.

Measurement of ALT and AST serum levels is valuable in the diagnosis of liver disease. However, these laboratory tests are best used in conjunction with other enzyme assays, such as LD and creatine kinase, and with other measures of liver and kidney function, such as blood urea, creatinine, ammonia, and bilirubin.[11] Because ALT and AST are present in tissues other than the liver, serum activity of these enzymes may reflect organic disease in these other tissues. ALT and AST serum activities are elevated in myocardial infarction, renal infarction, progressive muscular dystrophy, and numerous diseases that affect the liver only secondarily, such as Gaucher's disease, Niemann-Pick disease, infectious mononucleosis, myelocytic leukemia, diabetic ketoacidosis, and hyperthyroidism.

Other Hepatic Analytes

Bilirubin (see Chapter 35). Serum bilirubin analysis is helpful in differentiating the cause of jaundice. *Prehepatic jaundice* results in a large increase in unconjugated bilirubin because of the increased release and metabolism of hemoglobin after hemolysis. However, because the transport of bilirubin into the liver and the formation of the glucuronide conjugate become rate-limiting in prehepatic jaundice, no increase or only a slight increase in serum conjugated bilirubin is observed. Additionally, because of the increased levels of conjugated bilirubin excreted by the liver, urinary urobilinogen and fecal urobilin concentrations are elevated, but urinary bilirubin (the freely soluble, conjugated form) is absent. In contrast, *posthepatic obstructive jaundice* is characterized by large increases in serum-conjugated bilirubin. Delta bilirubin (bilirubin covalently bound to albumin) also increases in this disorder; however, the measurement of delta bilirubin as a diagnostic tool has not achieved widespread acceptance. The accumulation of bilirubin in the serum is the result of decreased biliary excretion after the conjugation of bilirubin in the liver rather than the result of an increased bilirubin load caused by hemolysis. Hepatic excretion of bilirubin metabolites is low in posthepatic obstructive jaundice, and urinary bilirubin

can usually be demonstrated. *Hepatic jaundice* presents an intermediate pattern, wherein levels of both conjugated and unconjugated serum bilirubin are increased to the same degree and conjugated bilirubin is present in the urine. However, the fecal concentration of urobilin is generally decreased in hepatic jaundice.

Cholesterol. Serum cholesterol comprises two forms, free cholesterol and esterified cholesterol. Since this esterification takes place in the liver, intrahepatic disease or biliary obstruction is characterized by an increase in the free cholesterol and occasionally a shift in the serum free fatty acid profile, though the total cholesterol usually remains unchanged. In chronic disease associated with parenchymal cell destruction, the total cholesterol may fall below the reference range.

Bile acids. Bile acid secretion and production is altered in disease.[2,12] In the healthy adult, serum contains 1 to 2 mg/mL of bile acids. In hepatobiliary disease, serum bile acid concentrations may rise as much as a thousandfold. Other diseases that can cause a significant rise in serum bile acid concentrations are hepatitis, cirrhosis, drug-induced liver disease, and hepatoma. Serum bile acid concentrations are normal in Gilbert's disease, hemochromatosis, and polycystic liver disease. Measurement of serum bile acids is useful in the diagnosis of minimal liver dysfunction when other biochemical parameters are still unchanged and is the diagnostic test for cholestasis of pregnancy (see Chapter 40).

Triglycerides. Serum triglycerides should be measured in a fasting sample. Increases are relatively nonspecific[12]; liver dysfunctions resulting from hepatitis, extrahepatic biliary obstruction, and cirrhosis are associated with an increase in serum triglycerides, but so are such disorders as acute pancreatitis, myocardial infarction, renal failure, gout, pernicious anemia, and diabetes mellitus. Free fatty acids exhibit a similar nonspecificity. They are decreased in chronic hepatitis, chronic renal failure, and cystic fibrosis. Serum free fatty acid concentrations are elevated in Reye's syndrome, hepatic encephalopathy, and chronic active hepatitis but also in myocardial infarction, acute renal failure, hyperthyroidism, and pheochromocytoma.

Serum proteins in evaluation of liver function. A healthy functioning liver is required for the synthesis of all serum proteins, except for the immunoglobulins. The liver has the ability to increase protein output approximately twofold during diseases associated with protein loss. Therefore it is not surprising that total protein measurements are not altered until an extensive impairment of liver function has occurred.

Albumin is decreased in chronic liver disease and is generally accompanied by an increase in the beta and gamma globulins as a result of production of IgG and IgM in chronic active hepatitis and of IgM and IgA in biliary or alcoholic cirrhosis, respectively. It is important to note that these immunoglobulins are not produced by the liver but by the plasma cells of the reticuloendothelial system. Immunoelectrophoresis may facilitate the identification of these subclasses of gamma globulin. However, a decrease in serum albumin is not specific for liver disease, since decreases are also seen in malabsorption, malnutrition, renal disease, alcoholism, and malignant diseases.

The alpha$_1$-fraction of the serum protein globulin is decreased in chronic liver disease, and when this fraction is absent or nearly absent, it indicates that alpha$_1$-antitrypsin deficiency may be the cause of the liver disease. Serum alpha$_2$-globulin and beta-globulin are increased in obstructive jaundice. The increase in alpha$_2$-globulin and beta-globulin in obstructive jaundice is largely associated with interferences of normal lipoprotein metabolism. Thus a lipid disorder cannot be phenotyped accurately in the presence of liver disease. The use of high-density lipoprotein cholesterol for assessment of the risk for coronary heart disease is obviated in patients with alcoholic liver disease, biliary obstruction, and acute liver necrosis.

Coagulation factors are produced by the liver and can decrease significantly in the presence of liver disease. Plasma fibrinogen is normally present in a concentration of 2 to 4 g/L. A decrease in plasma fibrinogen is usually an indication of severe liver disease and is associated with decreased concentrations of other clotting factors, most notably prothrombin. Since prothrombin synthesis occurs in the liver and requires the fat-soluble vitamin K, prothrombin time may be increased in biliary obstructive disease, liver cirrhosis or necrosis, hepatic failure, Reye's syndrome, liver abscess, vitamin K deficiency, and hepatitis. The response of the prothrombin time to exogenous vitamin K is useful in differentiating intrahepatic disease associated with a decrease in clotting factor from extrahepatic obstructive disease with decreased absorption of vitamin K.

Urea and ammonia in evaluation of liver function.

Blood ammonia concentration is higher in infants than in adults because the development of the hepatic circulation is completed after birth. Hyperammonemia results infrequently from congenital defects of the urea cycle, most often as a result of ornithine transcarbamylase deficiency. A much more frequent cause of hyperammonemia in infants is hyperalimentation.[13] Reye's syndrome is frequently diagnosed by an elevated blood ammonia in the absence of any other demonstrable cause.

Adult patients exhibit elevated blood ammonia in the terminal stages of liver cirrhosis, hepatic failure, and acute and subacute liver necrosis. The onset of hepatic encephalopathy is presaged by an elevated blood ammonia. Urinary ammonia excretion is increased in acidosis and decreased in alkalosis, since ammonia salt formation is a significant mechanism for excretion of excess hydrogen ions. Damage to the renal distal tubules, as occurs in renal failure, glomerulonephritis, hypercorticoidism, and Addison's disease, results in decreased ammonia excretion but no changes in blood ammonia levels.

Since urea is synthesized in the liver, diseases of the liver without renal impairment result in a low serum urea nitrogen, although the urea-to-creatinine ratio may remain normal.[14] An elevated serum urea nitrogen does not necessarily imply renal damage; dehydration alone may result in a urea nitrogen as high as 600 mg/L, and infants receiving high-protein formula may exhibit urea nitrogen levels of 250 to 300 mg/L. Naturally, renal diseases such as acute glomerulonephritis, chronic nephritis, polycystic kidney, and renal necrosis result in an elevated urea nitrogen.

References

1. Johnson TR: Development of the liver. In Johnson TR, Moore WM, Jefferies SE, editors: Children are different: developmental physiology, ed 2, Columbus, OH, 1978, Ross Laboratories.
2. Demers LM: Serum bile acids in health and in hepatobiliary disease. In Demers LM, Shaw LM, editors: *Evaluation of liver function*, Baltimore, 1978, Urban & Schwarzenberg.
3. Dennery PA, Seidman DS, Stevenson DK: Neonatal hyperbilirubinemia: a review article, *N Engl J Med* 344:581, 2001
4. Doumas BT, Wu FW: The measurement of bilirubin fractions in serum, *Crit Rev Clin Lab Sci* 28:415, 1991.
5. Alter MJ et al: The natural history of community-acquired hepatitis C in the United States, *N Engl J Med* 327:1899, 1992.
6. Craig JR: Hepatitis delta virus (editorial), *Am J Clin Pathol* 98:552, 1992.
7. Jeppson JO et al: Typing of genetic variants of alpha-1-antitrypsin by electrofocusing, *Clin Chem* 28:219, 1982.
8. Tsukuma H et al: Risk factors for hepatocellular carcinoma among patients with chronic liver disease, *N Engl J Med* 328:1797, 1993.
9. Ellis G et al: Serum enzyme tests in diseases of the liver and biliary tree, *Am J Clin Pathol* 70:248, 1978.
10. Kew MC: Serum aminotransferase concentration as evidence of hepatocellular damage (editorial), *The Lancet* 355:591, 2000.
11. Friedman RB et al: Effects of diseases on clinical laboratory tests, *Clin Chem* 26:1D, 1980.
12. Lloyd-Still JD: Disorders of the liver in childhood. In Demers LM, Shaw LM, editors: *Evaluation of liver function*, Baltimore, 1978, Urban & Schwarzenberg.
13. Nanji AA, Blank D: The serum urea nitrogen/creatinine ratio and liver disease, *Clin Chem* 28:1398, 1982.

Bibliography

Bishop ML, Duben-Engelkirk JL, Fody EP, editors: *Clinical chemistry: principles, procedures, correlations*, ed 2, Philadelphia, 1992, JB Lippincott.
Dufour DR, editor: *Laboratory guidelines for screening, diagnosis, and monitoring of hepatic injury*, Washington, DC, 2000, National Academy of Clinical Biochemistry (NACB).
Feldman M et al, editors: *Sleisenger and Fordtran's gastrointestinal and liver disease: pathophysiology/diagnosis/management*, ed 6, New York, 1998, Saunders.
Gitnick G: *Hepatology*, New York, 1986, Medical Examination Publishing Co.
Halsted JA: *The laboratory in clinical chemistry: interpretation and application*, Philadelphia, 1976, Saunders.

Meites S, editor: *Pediatric clinical chemistry: reference (normal) values*, ed 3, Washington, DC, 1989, American Association of Clinical Chemists.

Orton SM, Neuhaus OW: *Human biochemistry*, ed 10, St Louis, 1982, Mosby.

Suchy LJ, Sokol RJ, Balistreri WF, editors: *Liver disease in children*, ed 2, Baltimore, 2001, Lippincott Williams & Wilkins.

Tilton RC et al, editors: *Clinical laboratory medicine*, St Louis, 1992, Mosby.

Internet Sites

www.aasld.org—American Association for the Study of Liver Disease (AASLD)

www.childliverdisease.org—Children's Liver Disease Foundation

http://cpmcnet.columbia.edu/dept/gi/—Click on "Diseases of the Liver"

www.niddk.nih.gov/health/digest/summary/pricir/pricir.htm—A look at primary biliary cirrhosis: what it is, its causes, symptoms, diagnosis, and treatment

http://www.nacb.org/lmpg/hepatic_lmpg.stm

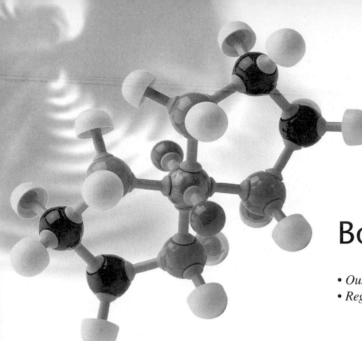

CHAPTER 28

Bone Disease

• *Oussama Itani*
• *Reginald C. Tsang*

Chapter Outline

Bone structure and function
  Bone structure
  Bone mass
  Bone function
  Biochemical markers of bone turnover
  Bone modeling
  Hormonal regulation of bone remodeling
Biochemistry and physiology
  Determinants of bone health
  Gonadal steroids
  Growth hormone and body composition
  Mineral physiology
  Hormone physiology
Bone disorders
  Osteoporosis

  Osteomalacia
  Osteitis fibrosa
  Paget's disease
  Heritable bone disease
Change of analyte in disease
  Biochemical measurements of bone turnover
  Vitamin D
  Parathyroid hormone
  Calcium
  Magnesium
  Phosphate
  Calcitonin
  Alkaline phosphatase (ALP)
  Osteocalcin
  Hydroxyproline (HP)

Objectives

• Describe the structure and function of normal bone.
• Describe effects of vitamin D metabolites, parathyroid hormone (PTH), magnesium, and phosphorus on calcium metabolism and regulation.
• Define osteopenia, osteoporosis, osteomalacia,

rickets, osteitis fibrosa, and Paget's disease.
• State expected levels of calcidiol, PTH, calcium, phosphorus, magnesium, calcitonin, alkaline phosphatase, and urinary hydroxyproline in the disease states listed above.

Key Terms

bone density Expressed as grams of mineral per area or volume of bone.
bone mass The total amount of bone material, including calcium and phosphorus, in a person.
bone quality The architecture, turnover, damage accumulation, and mineralization of bone.

bone remodeling The coupling of bone formation and bone resorption.
bone resorption Breakdown of the bone matrix.
bone sialoprotein Part of the noncollagen bone matrix.
calcidiol 25-Hydroxyvitamin D (25-OHD) is

cholecalciferol hydroxylated at the carbon-25 position in the liver.

calcitonin A hormone of 32 amino acids involved in calcium regulation.

calcitriol 1,25-Dihydroxyvitamin D (1,25-(OH)$_2$D), the active vitamin D metabolite, is cholecalciferol hydroxylated at both the carbon-1 and carbon-25 positions.

cholecalciferol The parent vitamin D compound.

cortical bone Dense compact bone that provides structural support.

diaphysis Shaft of a long bone.

epiphysis End of a long bone.

ionized calcium The unbound divalent calcium ion.

metaphysis Region in which diaphysis and epiphysis converge.

N-telopeptides Peptide fragments of the protein that links collagen fragments in bone.

osteoblasts Cells that synthesize bone matrix.

osteocalcin The major component of bone's noncollagen proteins.

osteoclasts Cells that resorb bone.

osteocytes Mature bone cells that have limited function and are encased in bone matrix, the composition of which they help to maintain.

osteoid Bone matrix.

osteolysis Process of being able to resorb bone.

osteomalacia Disorder in which bone contains normal amounts of osteoid but deficient amounts of mineral.

osteopenia The roentgenographic appearance of subnormally mineralized bone.

osteoporosis A generalized reduction in bone mass involving both mineral and osteoid.

parathyroid hormone An 84 amino acid polypeptide hormone that regulates calcium levels in blood.

peak bone mass Maximum bone material during the life of an individual.

rickets Osteomalacia in childhood.

trabecular bone Interlacing delicate spicules of bone that are predominantly involved in mineral homeostasis.

vitamin D Major hormone controlling calcium and phosphorus homeostasis and bone mineralization.

Methods on CD-ROM

Alkaline phosphatase, total
Calcium
Ionized calcium

Magnesium
Parathyroid hormone
Phosphorus

BONE STRUCTURE AND FUNCTION

More than 90% of the cells in bone are encased in calcified tissue and separated by great distances from a vascular supply. This gives the cells the appearance of inactivity. However, it is now clear that the skeletal system is a dynamic organ. The modern theory of skeletal system function proposes that bone has two interdependent roles: provision of support and maintenance of mineral homeostasis. Both functions are successfully achieved by continuous bone remodeling. Disturbances in the balance and nature of bone formation and resorption produce the common bone diseases.

Bone Structure[1]

Macroscopically, the major bones are classified as long bones or flat bones.[1] Long bones are confined to the limbs and consist of a shaft (**diaphysis**), two ends (**epiphyses**), and a region in which the two converge (**metaphysis**) (Fig. 28-1, *A*). Seen in cross section, the diaphysis is lined by dense, compact (**cortical) bone**, whereas the metaphysis contains interlacing bony spicules that resemble the structure of a sponge (**trabecular** or *cancellous* **bone**) (Fig. 28-1, *B*). Flat bones, typified by the bones of the skull, consist of two thin layers of cortical bone that enclose a layer of trabecular bone. Dense cortical bone provides strength needed for structural support, and the spicules of trabecular bone provide a large surface area for bone synthesis and resorption and provide a reservoir of minerals for the maintenance of mineral homeostasis.

Bone contains three major types of mature cells, **osteoblasts**, **osteocytes**, and **osteoclasts**.[2] *Osteoblasts*, found along surfaces of both cortical and trabecular bone, synthesize bone matrix. The plasma membrane of the osteoblast is very rich in alkaline phosphatase (ALP), the activity of which is an index of bone formation. Osteoblasts have receptors for PTH, **calcitriol** (1,25-dihydroxyvitamin D, [1,25(OH)$_2$D]) and estrogen but not for calcitonin. Stimulation by PTH, 1,25(OH)$_2$D, growth hormone, and estrogen causes osteoblasts to produce insulin-like growth factor I (IGF-I), which has a significant role in local bone regulation and modeling. As osteoblasts become embedded in bone matrix, they differentiate into mature *osteocytes*. Osteocytes synthesize small amounts of matrix continuously to maintain bone integrity, and they are able to resorb bone (osteocytic **osteolysis**) in exceptional circumstances when normal mineral homeostasis is altered.

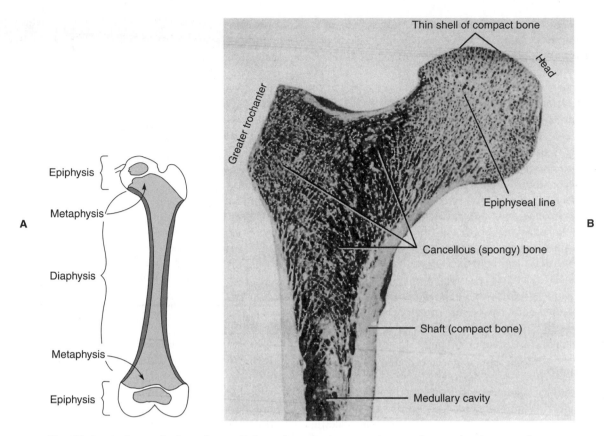

Fig. 28-1 **A**, Parts of a long bone. **B**, Long bone in cross section: notice predominance of trabecular, cancellous bone in diaphysis. *(From Copenhaver WM, Kelly DE, Wood RL, editors: Bailey's textbook of histology, ed 17, Baltimore, 1978, Williams & Wilkins.)*

Osteoclasts contain enzymes that demineralize and digest bone matrix. The process of osteoclastic bone resorption has been understood only recently. Bone resorption occurs at a special part of the osteoclast cell membrane, the "ruffled border," which comprises a sealed lysosomal compartment. Because of their acidic pH, lysosomes dissolve bone crystals, and their proteolytic enzymes digest bone matrix.[1] Although bone resorption is primarily effected by the osteoclast, other cells influenced by bone resorbing hormones can direct the osteoclasts. Both osteoblasts and osteoclasts have receptors for bone resorbing hormones and appear to play a significant role in bone resorption. The moth-eaten appearance of bone that indicates bone resorption is evident in histological sections of areas in which osteoclasts are numerous.

Only a small portion of bone is cellular; calcified matrix predominates. This matrix is primarily composed of collagen fibers (mostly type I), a glycosaminoglycans-containing ground substance, and noncollagenous proteins. Type I collagen is the major collagen produced by osteoblasts and represents more than 90% by weight of the nonmineral component of bone. **Osteocalcin** is the major component of bone's noncollagen proteins (see later discussion). Although most bone proteins are synthesized by osteoblasts, some proteins, such as α_2-HS-glycoprotein, are produced by the liver and absorbed by bone matrix. Spindle-shaped hydroxyapatite, $Ca_{10}(PO_4)_6(OH)_2$, crystals are present in the ground

substance and aligned on and within collagen fibers. Glycosaminoglycans are highly anionic complexes that may play a major role in the calcification process and the fixation of hydroxyapatite crystals to collagen fibers. Approximately one fourth of the amino acids present in collagen are either proline or hydroxyproline, neither of which is present to any great extent in other tissues. When collagen is metabolized, hydroxyproline-containing oligopeptides are excreted in the urine, and the amount present correlates with the amount of bone turnover. The mineral elements of bone consist mostly of crystals of calcium and phosphate arranged either amorphously or as hydroxyapatite. A wide range of other elements may be present, including sodium, magnesium, copper, zinc, lead, and fluoride.

Bone Mass

About 45% of the adult skeleton is built and enlarged during adolescence.[3-6] The concept of peak bone mass has become crucial in understanding **osteoporosis**, especially postmenopausal osteoporosis.[4-6] **Peak bone mass** is determined by several factors including genetics, nutrition, mechanics, and environment.[7] The genetic effect on adult bone mass may be mediated largely through effects on bone formation premenopausally and postmenopausally, rather than through effects on resorption. There is a strong positive relationship between current and past calcium intake and the peak bone mass achieved.[8] Higher calcium intake during adolescence theoretically may optimize, within genetic limits, peak bone mass. Physical activity, use of estrogenic oral contraceptives, and dietary calcium intake exert a positive effect on bone gain in young adult women. Androgens and estrogen are important determinants of peak bone density in young women. The optimal dietary calcium intake for bone growth is a debatable issue. Calcium retention requirements for growth are as follows: an average of 100 mg/day must be retained during childhood, 220 mg/day during adolescence, and probably 20 to 30 mg/day during early adulthood from 20 to 30 years of age.[1,9]

Bone strength is determined by *bone density* and *bone quality*. **Bone density** is expressed as grams of mineral per area or volume and in any given individual is determined by peak bone mass and amount of bone loss. Bone mineral density (BMD) accounts for approximately 70% of bone strength. **Bone quality** refers to architecture, turnover, damage accumulation (e.g., microfractures) and mineralization. A fracture occurs when a failure-inducing force (e.g., trauma) is applied to osteoporotic bone.

Bone Function

The large surface area and excellent blood supply of trabecular bone permit a quick response to perturbations in plasma mineral concentrations. In contrast, the abundant calcified matrix of cortical bone provides the strength to support body weight. Despite this segregation of structure and function, disturbances in both often coexist. Examples include vitamin D deficiency, which causes both hypocalcemia and easily fractured bone, and immobilization, which causes bone resorption, osteoporosis, and hypercalcemia. Under normal circumstances such disturbances do not occur because, in **bone remodeling** that occurs throughout the body, bone formation and **bone resorption** are "coupled," resulting in equal amounts of bone formation and resorption.[10] Most bone diseases result from alterations in coupling that are either new or secondary to hormonal imbalance, which produce either excessive bone formation or excessive resorption.

Biochemical Markers of Bone Turnover[11-15]

The processes of bone formation and resorption are accompanied by production of a plethora of proteins. Measurement of several of these molecules in serum and urine provides a valuable indicator of ongoing homeostatic bone processes (Box 28-1). These markers serve as noninvasive indicators of osteoblastic or osteoclastic activities. However, interpretation of their results is difficult because the concentrations depend on age, pubertal stage, growth velocity, mineral accrual, hormonal regulation, nutritional status, circadian variation, method of expression of results of urinary markers, specificity for bone tissue, and the sensitivity and specificity of different assays. In addition, studies have shown that the accuracy of these markers for osteoporosis diagnosis and monitoring is inferior to bone mineral density measurements. Furthermore, there are no pediatric reference ranges for many of the newer markers. However, measurement of these

---

BOX 28-1

BIOCHEMICAL MARKERS OF BONE TURNOVER

Bone Formation
- Serum osteocalcin
- Serum alkaline phosphatase (ALP), bone specific ALP
- Serum procollagen I extension peptides

Bone Resorption Markers
- Urine hydroxyproline
- Urine deoxypyridinoline
- Urine pyridinoline
- Type I collagen telopeptides (peptides containing crosslinks) N-terminal telopeptide to helix in urine (NTX-I), C-terminal telopeptide-1 to helix in serum (ICTP) C-terminal telopeptide-2 in urine and serum (CTX)
- Serum tartrate-resistant acid phosphatase, hydroxylysine and its glycosides

---

markers in conjunction with clinical evaluation and radiologic findings may aid in the initial investigation of osteoporosis and possibly assist in monitoring therapy. Because of their multiple limitations, bone metabolism markers should not be relied on exclusively to make important clinical decisions. Measurement of several indices at once, as well as serial measurements, may help to overcome some of these limitations.

Osteocalcin is the major noncollagenous bone protein. It is a 49–amino acid protein that is synthesized by osteoblasts. Osteocalcin can serve as a marker of osteoblastic activity and bone formation. It contains γ-carboxyglutamic acid, which is a vitamin K–dependent calcium binding amino acid. Most of synthesized osteocalcin is incorporated in bone where it constitutes 1% of the organic matrix of bone. Minute amounts of osteocalcin in the circulation are derived from new protein synthesis rather than from resorption of bone matrix. The synthesis of osteocalcin is stimulated by $1,25(OH)_2D$.

Procollagen I extension peptides. Procollagen, a precursor of collagen, undergoes cleavage to collagen and extension proteins before collagen becomes incorporated into bone matrix. These proteins serve as indicators of osteoblastic activity. For instance, serum concentration of type I procollagen is elevated in Paget's disease. However, from recent evidence it appears that assay of procollagen propeptides as an indicator of bone formation is less sensitive and specific than serum osteocalcin and bone isoenzyme of alkaline phosphatase.

Urine collagen pyridinoline cross-linking amino acids. These are the among the best available specific biomarkers of bone resorption. These compounds, which include hydroxylysylpyridinoline and lysylpyridinoline, are released upon degradation of mature collagen from skeletal tissues. The hydroxypyridinium collagen crosslinks, pyridinoline and deoxypyridinoline, are also released upon degradation of mature collagen. These compounds are present in urine either in the free, non–peptide bound (40%) state or peptide-bound (60%).

Urinary telopeptides. Urinary **N-telopeptides** are the peptide fragments of the protein that links the collagen bundles in bones. These fragments are liberated into the circulation as a result of the breakdown of collagen in the bones, and they are excreted unchanged in the urine. Urine levels of N-telopeptides therefore reflect the degree of *bone resorption.* Because there are diurnal variations in the degree of bone resorption, with the highest levels occurring during the night, the N-telopeptides are best measured either in a 24-hour urine sample or in the early morning sample. A single urine N-telopeptides level on its own is not of much use because the normal range is so wide. On the other hand, a reduction of 40% to 50% in these levels over a period of 8 to 12 weeks is suggestive that the increased rate of bone resorption has been suppressed, and that the patient is probably responding well to the prescribed therapy. Pyridinoline crosslinks and collagen telopeptides are the best indices of bone resorption.

Urinary hydroxyproline. Urinary hydroxyproline level is mainly used as an index of greatly increased rate of bone resorption. However, it is not a specific test because sources of hydroxyproline include bone, diet, connective tissues, serum proteins, and degradation of propeptides from collagen biosynthesis. This test correlates poorly with bone resorption as assessed by bone histomorphometric and calcium kinetic studies.

Bone sialoprotein (BSP). **Bone sialoprotein** (BSP) accounts for 5% to 10% of noncollagenous bone matrix. It may play a role in cell-matrix adhesion processes and organization of the extracellular matrix of mineralized tissues. Serum BSP drops following bisphosphonate therapy, suggesting that serum BSP levels reflect bone resorption activity. Usefulness of this marker is still not well studied.

Bone Modeling

Inherent to bone physiology is the physiological "coupling" of the processes of bone formation and resorption, called **remodeling.**[1] Remodeling continues throughout life and requires a balance between bone formation and resorption. At any time approximately 10% of bone mass participates in bone remodeling. Growth during infancy and adolescence is associated with predominance of bone formation over bone resorption, resulting in increased bone mass and bone deposition. In young adults, the processes of bone resorption and formation are equal. With aging, bone resorption exceeds bone formation thereby predisposing the older individual to net bone loss and osteoporosis. In bone disease states, this balance is altered. For instance, in osteoporosis the volume of bone resorbed outweighs the volume of bone formed, resulting in a net loss of bone at each remodeling site.

Hormonal Regulation of Bone Remodeling[8]

Both systemic and local regulators control the dynamic balance between bone formation and resorption. Systematic regulators of bone homeostasis include primarily the calcitropic (PTH and vitamin D) hormones. Local regulation of bone homeostasis involves prostaglandins and growth factors, such as IGF-I and IGF-II,[8] which act as autocrine or paracrine effectors of bone formation by increasing osteoblastic proliferation and bone matrix biosynthesis.

PTH and $1,25(OH)_2D$ play an important role in activating bone remodeling. PTH has a biphasic effect on bone homeostasis: on the one hand, intermittent administration of PTH stimulates bone formation, possibly through production of local growth factors IGF-I and IGF-II; on the other hand, continuous PTH administration has a catabolic effect on bone and favors bone resorption. Prostaglandins, particularly of the E series, are potent local bone resorbing agents. $1,25(OH)_2D$ and thyroid hormones also have a biphasic effect on bone homeostasis.[16] Thyrotoxicosis is a significant risk factor for osteoporosis. Growth hormone also has an anabolic effect on bone metabolism; it increases bone formation by increasing local concentrations of IGF-I.[17] Estradiol and progesterone stimulate osteoblastic activity to increase bone formation,[18] and estrogen increases production of both IGF-I and IGF-II. Several cytokines have osteoclast-activating effects and promote osteoclastic bone resorption.[1,8-10,17,19] These cytokines include interleukin-1, tumor necrosis factors a and b, and differentiation-inducing factor. Osteoclasts carry receptors for calcitonin. Calcitonin directly inhibits bone resorption by binding to specific receptors on osteoclasts to inhibit osteoclast formation, motility, and activity.[1]

BIOCHEMISTRY AND PHYSIOLOGY

Determinants of Bone Health[3-6]

Although most growth in bone size and strength occurs during childhood, bone accumulation is not completed until the third decade of life, after the cessation of linear growth. The bone mass attained early in life is perhaps the most important determinant of life-long skeletal health. Individuals with the highest peak bone mass after adolescence have the greatest protective advantage when the declines in bone density associated with increasing age, illness, and diminished sex-steroid production take their toll. Peak bone mass is influenced by *genetic, physiological, environmental,* and *lifestyle* factors. Among these are adequate nutrition and body weight, exposure to sex hormones at puberty, and physical activity.[3,7] Therefore, maximizing bone mass early in life presents a critical opportunity to reduce the impact of bone loss related to aging. Childhood is also a critical time for the development of lifestyle habits conducive to maintaining good bone health throughout life. Cigarette smoking, which usually starts in adolescence, may have a deleterious effect on achieving bone mass.

Nutrition (see Chapter 37). Good nutrition is essential for normal bone growth and health.[3,9] Supplementation of calcium and vitamin D may be necessary. Proper calcium intake is most important for attaining peak bone mass and for preventing and treating osteoporosis. Although the Institute of Medicine recommends calcium intakes of 800 mg/day for children ages 3 to 8 and 1300 mg/day for children and adolescents ages 9 to 17, only about 25% of boys and 10% of girls ages 9 to 17 are estimated to meet these recommendations. For older adults, calcium intake should be maintained at 1000 to 1500 mg/day, yet only about 50% to 60% of this population meets this recommendation.

Vitamin D is required for optimal calcium absorption and bone health (see later discussion). Most infants and young children in the United States have adequate vitamin D intake because of supplementation and fortification of milk. During adolescence, when consumption of dairy products decreases, vitamin D intake is less likely to be adequate, and this may adversely affect calcium absorption. A recommended vitamin D intake of 400 to 600 IU/day has been established for adults. High dietary protein, caffeine, phosphorus, and sodium can adversely affect calcium balance, but their effects appear not to be important in individuals with adequate calcium intakes.

Exercise. Physical activity early in life contributes to higher peak bone mass, with resistance and high-impact exercise providing the most benefit.[7] It is clear that exercise later in life, even beyond 90 years of age, can increase muscle mass and strength twofold or more in frail individuals, and have a modest effect on slowing the decline in bone mass and density (BMD).

Gonadal Steroids (see Chapter 45)

Sex steroids secreted during puberty increase BMD and peak bone mass in both women and men. In adolescent girls and women, sustained production of *estrogens* is essential for the maintenance of bone mass. Reduction in estrogen production with menopause is the major cause of loss of BMD during later life. Timing of menarche, absent or infrequent menstrual cycles, and the timing of menopause influence both the attainment of peak bone mass and the preservation of BMD. *Testosterone* production is important for achieving and maintaining maximal bone mass in adolescent boys and men; estrogens have also been implicated in the growth and maturation of the male skeleton. Delayed onset of puberty is a risk factor for diminished bone mass in men, and hypogonadism in adult men results in osteoporosis.

Growth Hormone and Body Composition

Growth hormone and insulin-like growth factor-I, which are maximally secreted during puberty, play a role in the acquisition and maintenance of bone mass and the determination of body composition into adulthood. Growth hormone deficiency is associated with a decrease in BMD. Children and youth with low body mass index (BMI) are likely to attain lower-than-average peak bone mass. Although there is a direct association between BMI and bone mass throughout the adult years, it is not known whether the association between body composition and bone mass is due to hormones, nutritional factors, higher impact during weight-bearing activities, or other factors.

Mineral Physiology

Calcium and mineral metabolism represents a delicate and complex biological process composed of many intricate and interrelated components. Normal homeostatic metabolism depends on the availability of mineral substrates and the interactions of tissues such as bone, kidney, and the gastrointestinal tract with the calcitropic hormones PTH, calcitonin (CT), and $1,25(OH)_2D$.

Calcium and phosphorus. Calcium is the fifth most abundant inorganic element in the human body. The human body contains about 1200 g of calcium in the adult and approximately 28 g in a full-term newborn. Almost all the body's calcium (99%) resides in bone. The remainder resides in body fluids and serves a crucial role in a multitude of physiological processes including muscular contraction, neurotransmission, membrane transport, enzyme reactions, hormone secretion, and blood coagulation. In the circulation, calcium exists in three forms: 45% of total serum calcium is the biologically active ionized calcium, 45% is protein-bound mainly to albumin, and 10% is complexed to anions (phosphate, lactate, citrate).

Bone contains 80% to 85% of total body phosphorus; approximately 9% is in muscle, and the remainder is in the viscera and extracellular fluid. The intracellular concentration of phosphorus (phosphates and organic phosphorus) is greater than the extracellular levels.

Metabolism. In the adult, dietary calcium is absorbed by the gut by specific calcium-binding proteins. This process is under the active control of vitamin D (see the text following for details). Most absorbed calcium is deposited in bone. The major route for excretion of body calcium is through the kidneys. Both processes, deposition and renal excretion, are under the control of PTH, as described later. Control of serum calcium homeostasis is under control of PTH and will also be discussed later.

By an active energy-dependent process, the placenta transfers calcium ions from mother to fetus against a concentration gradient. This results in relative fetal hypercalcemia and a calcium concentration higher in cord blood than in maternal blood. An intrinsic placental calcium-binding protein (CaBP, calbindin) is present only in the presence of specific receptors for $1,25(OH)_2D$, which have been demonstrated in the human placenta and human fetal gut. It is likely that calbindin may play a significant role in the active transport of calcium transplacentally to the fetus.

Magnesium. Magnesium (Mg) is the fourth most abundant cation and the second most abundant intracellular cation within the body.[20] Most of the total body Mg content (50% to 60%) is concentrated in bone tissue as an integral component of the hydroxyapatite lattice (30% to 40%) and as an exchangeable fraction (15% to 20%) adsorbed to apatite and in equilibrium with the extracellular fluid compartment. About 20% of total body Mg is concentrated in muscle and another 20% is in the intracellular compartment of blood cells and other body tissues. Changes in total body Mg content are largely reflected by changes in skeletal Mg and to a lesser extent in serum Mg concentrations. Only 1% of the body's magnesium is in blood. Magnesium serves as a cofactor for a multitude of enzymatic reactions involved in storage, transfer, and production of energy and the synthesis of nucleic acid. Further, Mg plays a significant role in calcium and bone homeostasis.

Metabolism. Magnesium is absorbed through the intestinal tract, with absorption rates ranging from 44% on an ordinary diet to 76% on a low-magnesium diet. There is an efficient conservation of magnesium in the kidney so that in magnesium deficiency extremely low magnesium excretion rates occur. PTH appears to cause increases in serum magnesium concentrations, possibly by mobilizing magnesium from bone. In acute conditions an increase in the serum magnesium concentration results in suppression of the parathyroids, thus theoretically preventing further PTH increase and completing a "feedback" loop for magnesium-parathyroid interrelationships.[20] This feedback mechanism is thus similar to that for calcium-parathyroid interrelationships (see p. 515).

Although acute lowering of serum magnesium appears to increase serum PTH concentrations, chronic magnesium deficiency results in *decreased* release of PTH. In addition to this impairment in parathyroid function, magnesium deficiency can decrease the response of target organs to PTH. Thus magnesium deficiency leads to hypoparathyroidism and, secondarily, hypocalcemia. Hypocalcemia can thus accompany magnesium deficiency because calcium release from bone is decreased. Under normal circumstances magnesium and calcium undergo an exchange in bone related to their release into the circulation. Lowered magnesium content in bone results in lowered interchange with calcium and lowered release of calcium from bone.[21]

Hormone Physiology

Vitamin D. Attention has been focused on vitamin D since its discovery in 1925 led to the elimination of the widespread problem of nutritional **rickets**. Initially considered a vitamin because rachitic patients were cured with oral supplementation of vitamin D, vitamin D is now considered to be a hormone.[18] The major source of vitamin D is not the diet, but its production in skin after exposure to sunlight.[17] Dietary vitamin D includes vitamin D_2 (derived from plant sterols) and D_3 (from animal or synthetic origin). Normally, in adults, at least 90% of vitamin D requirements are provided by endogenous photosynthesis in the skin, which may amount to 1.5 to 10 mg/day (100 to 400 IU/day). Vitamin D is then transported in the bloodstream to the liver and kidneys for activation. It subsequently localizes at sites of activity in intestine and bone because of the presence of specific cellular receptors in these organs. Finally, as in other hormone systems, the plasma level of activated vitamin D is rigidly controlled by feedback regulation. Vitamin D is regarded as one of the three major hormones controlling calcium and phosphorus homeostasis and bone mineralization.[18,19]

Biochemistry and metabolism. Under the effect of small intestinal mucosal dehydrogenase, dietary cholesterol is converted into 7-dehydrocholesterol, which is then transported to the malpighian layer of the skin (Fig. 28-2). Ultraviolet (UV) radiation (of wavelengths 290 to 320 nm) penetrates the skin to break the C9-C10 bond of 7-dehydrocholesterol (provitamin D_3) to form previtamin D_3. Previtamin D_3 undergoes several reactions: it may be photoisomerized to lumisterol and tachysterol or converted by a temperature-dependent isomerization to **cholecalciferol** (vitamin D_3). Cholecalciferol is then released in the circulation where it is bound to vitamin D–binding protein and transported to the liver.

In the liver, cholecalciferol undergoes 25-hydroxylation to yield 25-hydroxyvitamin D, or 25(OH)D (**calcidiol**) (Figs. 28-2 and 28-3), which is released into the circulation once again before reaching the kidney. In the kidney mitochondrion, 25(OH)D undergoes 1-α-hydroxylation to produce 1,25-dihydroxyvitamin D (calcitriol), or 24-hydroxylation to form 24,25-dihydroxyvitamin D (24,25-(OH)$_2$D) (Fig. 28-2). Plasma calcitriol concentrations are relatively low (approximately 30 pg/mL). Although normal plasma concentrations vary with age,[22,23] they are probably under strict feedback control.[23] The details of this control are discussed later. If plasma calcitriol concentrations are sufficient, calcidiol is hydroxylated in the kidney at the C-24 position to yield 24,25-dihydroxycholecalciferol (Fig. 28-2). Most investigators currently regard this last metabolite as a waste product of vitamin D metabolism. The role of 24,25(OH)$_2$D in mineral and vitamin D homeostasis is not very well known.

Although the human newborn has undetectable plasma vitamin D concentration, vitamin D metabolites are necessary for optimal human fetal and maternal bone mineralization. The fetus is totally dependent on maternal vitamin D.

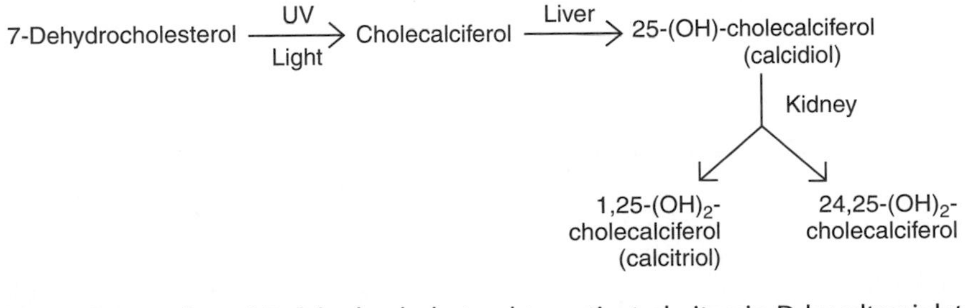

7-Dehydrocholesterol $\xrightarrow[\text{Light}]{\text{UV}}$ Cholecalciferol $\xrightarrow{\text{Liver}}$ 25-(OH)-cholecalciferol (calcidiol)

Kidney

1,25-(OH)$_2$-cholecalciferol (calcitriol)   24,25-(OH)$_2$-cholecalciferol

Fig. 28-2 Conversion of 7-dehydrocholesterol to activated vitamin D by ultraviolet *(UV)* light and by liver and kidney.

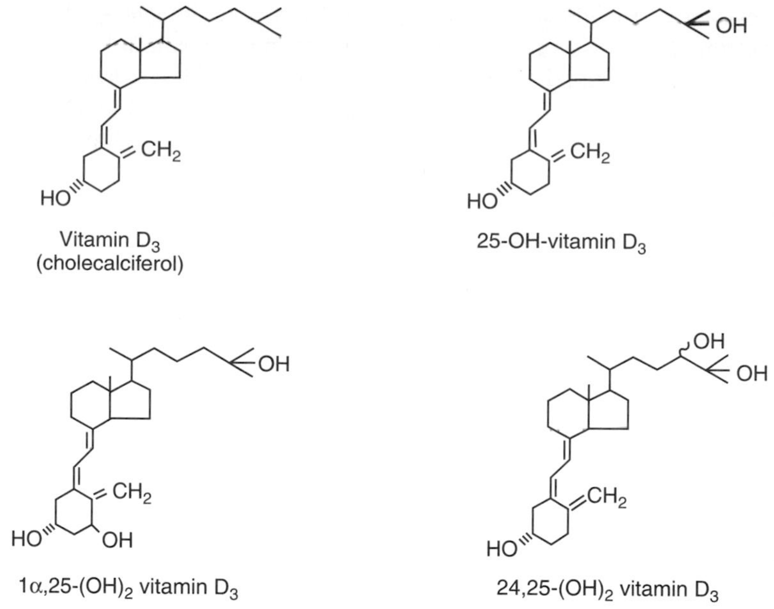

Fig. 28-3 Some common metabolites of cholecalciferol.

Cholecalciferol and its metabolites pass through the circulation attached to vitamin D–binding protein.[24] Certain tissues contain an intracellular protein that serves as a specific receptor for calcitriol. This protein, located in the cytosol of the kidney, intestine, bone, and selected other tissues, functions like other established cellular steroid hormone receptors (see Chapter 40). It facilitates entry of calcitriol into cells and transports the calcitriol to the cell nucleus, where the hormone, in theory, directs protein synthesis to achieve its desired effect.

Mechanisms of action.[18,19,24] The three major target organs of calcitriol are intestine, bone, and kidney (see the following box). Calcitriol facilitates both calcium and phosphate absorption in the intestine and induces a specific calcium-binding protein in the intestines, calbindin D. Phosphate transport accompanies calcium transport, but it is also increased by an unknown, calcium-independent mechanism. Calcitriol works cooperatively with PTH to increase bone resorption by increasing osteoclast activity. This may be considered paradoxical because vitamin D is believed to enhance bone mineralization. However, the net effect of the action of calcitriol at bone and intestine is to increase available blood calcium and phosphorus concentrations, which subsequently facilitate mineralization of newly formed bone matrix. Calcitriol increases the renal reabsorption of both calcium and phosphorus, but because 99% of filtered calcium is normally reabsorbed, the overall effect of alterations in plasma calcitriol concentrations on renal calcium reabsorption is small.

Calcitriol has a regulatory effect on PTH and CT gene transcription. In humans with secondary hyperparathyroidism, intravenous $1,25(OH)_2D$ administration leads to a sharp reduction in serum PTH concentration. Oral administration of calcitriol to children with hypophosphatemic rickets and secondary hyperparathyroidism also has an inhibitory effect on PTH secretion. Calcitriol upregulates its own receptor in the parathyroid glands; $1,25(OH)_2D$ administration increases the concentration of vitamin D receptor mRNA in the parathyroid gland.

Regulation of vitamin D metabolism. The regulation of vitamin D metabolism is easily understood once calcitriol function is known (see the following box). Although plasma calcidiol levels are poorly controlled,[23] there appears to be relatively strict control of plasma calcitriol concentrations. The activity of renal 1-α-hydroxylase is stimulated by IGF-I, PTH, and hypophosphatemia and by periods of high calcium demand such as growth, pregnancy, or low calcium intake. Activity may be inhibited by $1,25(OH)_2D$ and other vitamin D metabolites.

PTH is the major stimulus for calcitriol formation. PTH administration is now used as a clinical tool to assess the ability of the kidney to produce calcitriol.[25] PTH may stimulate renal 1-α-hydroxylase, the enzyme that hydroxylates

---

TARGET ORGANS FOR CALCITRIOL

Intestine—Increased calcium and phosphorus absorption
Bone—Enhanced PTH-induced bone resorption
Kidney—Increased reabsorption of calcium and phosphorus

PRIMARY STIMULI FOR CALCITRIOL SYNTHESIS

Decreased serum calcium concentration
Increased parathyroid hormone secretion
Decreased intracellular phosphorus concentration

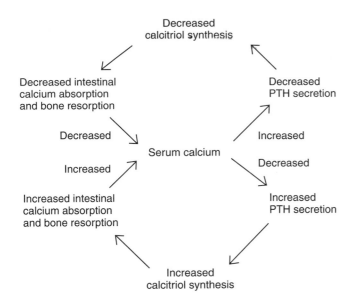

Fig. 28-4 Interrelationships of serum calcium concentrations and parathyroid hormone *(PTH)* and calcitriol.

calcidiol at the C-1 position, indirectly by lowering intracellular phosphorus concentrations. Because phosphorus depletion increases calcitriol synthesis in normal or parathyroidectomized animals, decreased intracellular phosphorus levels may be the ultimate common stimulus for calcitriol synthesis.

Understanding the metabolic control of vitamin D allows comprehension of the control of serum calcium and phosphorus concentrations (Fig. 28-4). When the serum calcium concentration falls, PTH is secreted and acutely restores normal serum calcium concentrations by stimulating osteoclasts to resorb bone. Within hours, calcitriol production is increased, which causes enhanced intestinal calcium absorption, which subsequently restores the serum calcium concentration and indirectly the PTH concentration to normal. Elevations in serum calcium concentration produce the opposite effect, that is, a reduction in both serum PTH concentrations and calcitriol synthesis.

Plasma calcitriol concentrations are altered by aging and pregnancy; they are elevated during adolescence and decline in old age.[26] Pregnancy and subsequent lactation are associated with elevated serum estrogen or prolactin concentrations; both hormones increase calcitriol synthesis.[27] It should be noted that the adolescent growth spurt, pregnancy, and lactation all increase requirements for calcium. Thus the elevated serum calcitriol concentrations represent an appropriate response to a physiological need.

Parathyroid hormone

Biochemistry and metabolism. PTH is an 84–amino acid polypeptide (at 9500 D) synthesized in the parathyroid glands. The precursor protein for PTH is *preproparathyroid hormone.* This precursor is sequentially converted in the gland, first to proparathyroid and then to PTH, which is released into the circulation. Full biological activity resides in the amino-terminal 1-34 peptide; the middle and carboxy-terminal sequences (35 to 84 amino acids) are biologically inert though immunologically highly reactive. Thus fragments of PTH bearing the amino terminal generally are active, whereas those bearing the carboxy terminal are inactive.

Mechanisms of action. PTH acts on two major target organs, bone and kidney, to produce three major effects: increase in serum calcium concentrations, decrease in serum phosphorus concentrations, and increase in the active hormonal form of vitamin D (calcitriol). In bone, PTH predominantly mobilizes calcium and phosphorus to the extracellular fluid, thus raising serum calcium and phosphorus concentrations. PTH has a synergistic effect with $1,25(OH)_2D$ in stimulating bone resorption.

At the other target organ, the kidney, PTH causes increased calcium retention, increased phosphorus excretion, stimulation of renal 1-α-hydroxylase activity (see earlier discussion), and increased conversion of 25-hydroxycholecalciferol (calcidiol) to 1,25-dihydroxycholecalciferol (calcitriol). Calcitriol, in turn, as described earlier, predominantly causes increased intestinal calcium and phosphorus absorption. The effects of PTH on the kidney are mediated through the formation of cyclic adenosine monophosphate (cAMP), and urinary levels of this substance rise when PTH production is increased. The resultant effect of PTH on the bone, kidney, and indirectly the intestine is to increase calcium concentrations in the blood. Although phosphorus concentrations may be elevated through parathyroid actions on bone and indirectly the intestine, the effect on increased renal phosphorus excretion overwhelms the other effects and, overall, results in decreased serum phosphorus concentrations (Fig. 28-5).

Serum **ionized calcium** (iCa) (the unbound divalent calcium ion) concentration is the main determinant of PTH secretion: a drop in serum iCa concentration stimulates PTH secretion, whereas a rise in serum iCa concentration suppresses it. However, other ions and hormones influence PTH secretion by the parathyroid glands: for instance, a rise in serum $1,25(OH)_2D$ decreases PTH secretion. An acute drop in serum Mg concentration stimulates PTH secretion but to a much smaller extent (tenfold less on a molar basis) compared to the effect of acute hypocalcemia.[28] Chronic hypomagnesemia impairs PTH secretion and causes blunting of PTH action at target organs.[20,29] Magnesium ions are essential for adenylate cyclase–mediated secretion of secretory granules and subsequent release of PTH from the parathyroid chief cells. Therefore, magnesium deficiency may cause secondary hypocalcemia. Hypermagnesemia also suppresses PTH secretion.[30]

Perinatal PTH homeostasis. Theoretically, because PTH does not cross the placenta, the relative fetal hypercalcemia should suppress the fetal parathyroid glands. Paradoxically, fetal PTH secretion is not suppressed. A possible explanation for the nonsuppression of PTH secretion, despite relative fetal hypercalcemia, is that the negative-feedback system regulating PTH secretion by calcium concentration operates with a higher "set point" in the fetus so that suppression of

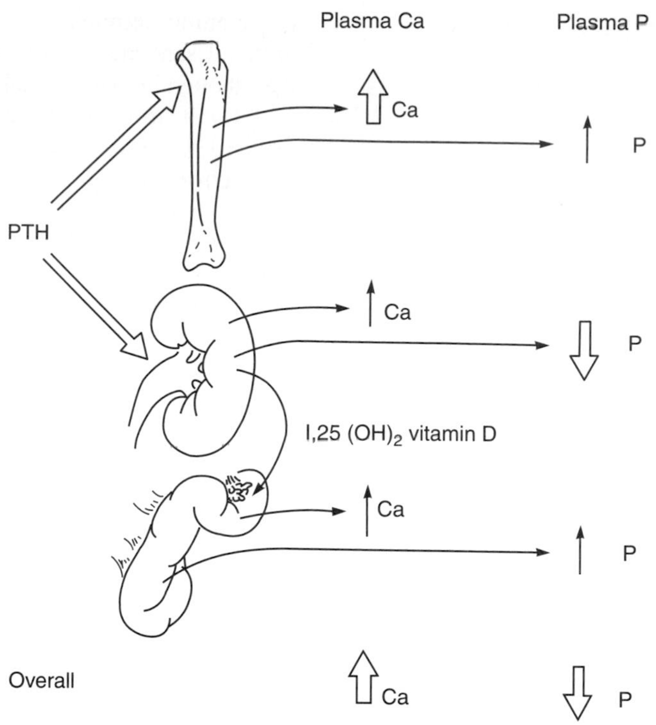

Fig. 28-5 Normal PTH physiology. PTH action increases serum calcium concentrations predominantly through its bone and kidney effects but reduces plasma phosphorus concentrations *(P)* through increasing renal phosphorus excretion. *(From Tsang RC, Noguchi A, Steichen JJ: Pediatric parathyroid disorders,* Pediatr Clin North Am *26:223, 1979.)*

PTH secretion in the fetus requires higher serum calcium concentrations than those required after birth. Both PTH and PTH-related peptide (PTHRP) may have a significant role in placental transport of calcium, and PTHRP may significantly contribute to the PTH bioactivity in fetal serum.

PTH-related peptide[31]

Biochemistry and metabolism. **PTH-related peptide** (PTHRP) and PTH genes are members of the same gene family; the amino terminal of PTHRP has a sequence homology in eight amino acids with the PTH amino terminal. PTHRP is also found to be equipotent to PTH when assessed by cytochemical bioassay and in situ biochemistry.[31] PTH synthesis is restricted to the parathyroid glands in normal subjects, but PTHRP messenger RNA is widely distributed in normal tissues, including the skin, thyroid, bone marrow, hypothalamus, pituitary, parathyroid, adrenal cortex, adrenal medulla, and stomach. Several studies suggest that PTHRP may have a significant physiological role. One of the major production sites of this peptide is lactating breast tissue, and PTHRP is present in large quantities in milk.

Mechanisms of action. In normal adults, plasma PTHRP concentrations range from less than 2 to 5 pmol/L. Infusion of PTHRP causes an elevation in serum 1,25-dihydroxy vitamin D concentration and an increase in bone formation parameters.[31] PTHRP may play a causal role in the hypercalcemia of malignancies. It is possible that PTH and PTHRP act on the same bone receptor to cause increased bone resorption and formation and hypercalcemia and hypo-

phosphatemia. PTHRP, produced in the fetal parathyroid glands, may be responsible for stimulation of placental calcium transport.

Calcitonin (CT). Calcitonin,[32] discovered in 1962, is generally regarded as one of three hormones (along with vitamin D and PTH) responsible for the control of calcium and phosphorus homeostasis. Despite great research efforts, a definitive role for CT in calcium homeostasis has not yet been clarified. Neither CT deficiency nor CT excess is clearly associated with bone disease or alteration of serum calcium homeostasis.

Localization, biochemistry, and metabolism. CT is produced by the parafollicular C-cells of the thyroid gland, though the pituitary gland, gastrointestinal tract, and liver may also produce the hormone.[32] CT is secreted in a precursor form, with a molecular weight of 15,000 D, that is cleaved into the active 32–amino acid CT polypeptide, which has a molecular weight of 3500 D.[32] Normal serum CT concentrations are less than 100 pg/mL. CT is rapidly excreted, with a half-life of 10 minutes after intravenous administration.[33] Excretion is predominantly by the kidney, and serum CT concentrations are increased in patients with renal failure.[34]

Biological effects. The best recognized physiological effect of CT is to counteract the action of PTH at several organ sites in the human body. The biological effects of CT may be divided into those related to calcium and phosphorus homeostasis and those related to gastrointestinal function. Intravenous CT administration causes a prompt decline in the serum calcium and phosphorus concentrations. This occurs because of effects of CT on both bone and kidney. CT alters cell function by increasing intracellular cAMP production.[35] Receptors specific for CT have been demonstrated on bone osteoclasts, and CT antagonizes PTH-mediated bone resorption by suppressing osteoclastic activity. Consequently, CT decreases the flux of calcium and phosphorus from bone into the circulation with urinary hydroxyproline excretion decreasing in parallel with the inhibition of bone resorption. CT also decreases the renal reabsorption of calcium, phosphorus, sodium, potassium, and magnesium.[35] CT also acts on vitamin D metabolism; it enhances $1,25(OH)_2D$ production by proximal renal tubules. These described effects on both bone and kidney have been produced with pharmacological CT concentrations.

In the human fetus, the thyroid C-cells appear to be well developed by 14 weeks of gestation. However, the role of CT in fetal mineral and bone homeostasis is not very well understood. CT does not cross the placenta, and, as with PTH, fetal CT function may be autonomous from that of the mother and may play a role in fetal bone mineralization.

Regulation of CT secretion. CT secretion is influenced by serum calcium concentrations; the gastrointestinal hormones gastrin, cholecystokinin, and glucagon; and sex steroids. CT release is affected primarily by the concentration of serum iCa and is stimulated by hypercalcemia and inhibited by hypocalcemia.[36] Vitamin D has a direct inhibitory effect on CT gene expression and CT secretion; receptors for $1,25(OH)_2D$ have been demonstrated on para-follicular C-cells. Serum CT concentrations may be higher in pregnant and lactating women than in controls. Men have higher circulating CT concentrations than women.[37]

BONE DISORDERS

Disorders of calcium, phosphorus, vitamin D, or PTH homeostasis frequently produce **osteopenia**, a general term for the x-ray appearance of a subnormal amount of mineralized bone. Many illnesses are associated with osteopenia[38] (see box at right). The bone histopathological condition of osteopenia can reveal decreased **osteoid** (bone matrix) formation, decreased osteoid mineralization, or increased bone resorption.[39] These histological categories correlate with the clinical diagnosis of *osteoporosis*, **osteomalacia**, or *osteitis fibrosa*, respectively. Osteopenia can result in the crush-fracture syndrome in adults and either fractures or growth failure in children. Trabecular bone is more frequently affected than cortical bone, and so fractures most often occur

in vertebrae, the femoral neck, and the distal ends of the long bones, where trabecular bone is abundant. Whereas specific diagnoses of osteopenic bone are best made histologically, occasionally, characteristic laboratory abnormalities will permit differentiation among osteoporosis, osteomalacia, and osteitis fibrosa (Table 28-1).

A PARTIAL DIFFERENTIAL DIAGNOSIS OF OSTEOPENIA

Osteoporosis
Primary
Premature and low birth weight infants
Aging (senile)
Postmenopausal
Juvenile

Secondary
Malnutrition and malabsorption syndromes
Immobilization
Cushing's syndrome
Hyperthyroidism
Multiple myeloma
Rheumatoid arthritis
Leukemia
Turner's syndrome
Alcoholism
Chronic liver disease
Irradiation
Drug-induced
Glucocorticoid therapy
Anticonvulsant therapy
Immunosuppressive therapy (e.g., cyclosporin)

Osteomalacia
Vitamin D deficiency
Chronic gastrointestinal disease
Anticonvulsant medication induced
Vitamin D dependency
Vitamin D resistance (hypophosphatemia)
Chronic acidosis
Fanconi's syndrome
Chronic renal failure
Phosphorus and calcium deficiency

Osteitis Fibrosa
Primary hyperparathyroidism
Chronic renal failure

Paget's Disease

TABLE 28-1	COMMON SERUM ABNORMALITIES ASSOCIATED WITH METABOLIC BONE DISEASE					
Disease	*Ca*	*P*	*PTH*	*Alk PO$_4$*	*Calcidiol*	*Calcitriol*
Osteoporosis	NL	NL	NL	NL	NL	LO
Osteomalacia	LO	LO	HI	HI	NL or LO	NL or LO
Osteitis fibrosa	HI or NL	LO or NL	HI	HI	NL	HI or NL

Alk PO$_4$, *alkaline phosphatase;* HI, *increased;* LO, *decreased;* NL, *normal;* PTH, *parathyroid hormone.*

Osteoporosis

The National Institutes of Health (NIH), in a recent consensus statement, has declared osteoporosis to be a major health threat to Americans.[4,5] The NIH believes that at least 10 million individuals have osteoporosis, and 18 million more have low bone mass, placing these individuals at increased risk for this disorder. Osteoporosis is no longer considered a disease of postmenopausal women only, and it is by no means entirely age- or gender-dependent. Prevention of osteoporosis necessitates optimizing the factors that influence bone health (see earlier discussion) throughout the life span in both males and females.[6]

Osteoporosis is characterized by a disturbed balance between bone resorption and bone formation, which results in a progressive decrease in bone mass and a decrease in the amount of normally mineralized bone; the mineral-collagen ratio is normal. The major sequelae are fragility of bone and predisposition to fractures; particularly spine-vertebral crush fracture, hip-femoral neck fracture, and distal radius fracture, which may occur either spontaneously or in response to minor trauma. The World Health Organization (WHO) associates osteoporosis with bone density 2.5 standard deviations below the mean for young white adult women. It is not clear how to apply this diagnostic criterion to men, children, and across ethnic groups. Because of the difficulty in accurate measurement and standardization between instruments and sites, controversy exists among experts regarding the continued use of this diagnostic criterion.

Osteoporosis can be further characterized as either primary or secondary.

Primary osteoporosis. Primary osteoporosis can occur in both genders at all ages but often follows menopause in women and occurs later in life in men and women (senile osteoporosis). However, osteoporosis is not always the result of bone loss, and individuals who do not reach optimal bone mass during childhood and adolescence may also develop osteoporosis without occurrence of accelerated bone loss. Hence suboptimal bone growth in childhood and adolescence is as important as bone loss to the development of osteoporosis. It occurs only rarely in childhood as an idiopathic illness and can also accompany certain systemic diseases.

Secondary osteoporosis. Secondary osteoporosis can result from medications, medical conditions (see box on p. 517 and Table 28-2), and environmental factors.[25] Medical disorders (Table 28-3) associated with osteoporosis can be organized into several categories: *genetic* disorders, *hypogonadal* states, *endocrine* disorders, *gastrointestinal* diseases, *hematologic* disorders, *connective tissue disease*, *nutritional deficiencies*, *drugs*, and a variety of chronic systemic disorders, such as congestive heart failure, end-stage renal disease, and alcoholism. Among men, 30% to 60% of osteoporosis is associated with secondary causes, with hypogonadism, glucocorticoids, and alcoholism the most common. In perimenopausal women, more than 50% of osteoporosis is most commonly associated with secondary causes, the most common of these are hypoestrogenemia, glucocorticoid therapy, thyroid hormone excess, and anticonvulsant therapy.

TABLE 28-2 TREATMENTS THAT INCREASE THE RISK OF SECONDARY OSTEOPOROSIS

Treatments	Comments
Irradiation	Direct effects on bone; decreased osteoblastic activity
	Pituitary hormone deficiencies from cranial irradiation
Chronic glucocorticoid use	Definitely with oral use and possibly with high-dose inhaled steroids
Chemotherapy	Methotrexate
	Cyclosporin A
	FK-506
Long-term anticonvulsant therapy	Vitamin D deficiency

Environmental factors that predispose to bone loss and osteoporosis include medications (Table 28-2), cigarette smoking, chronic low dietary calcium intake, a sedentary lifestyle, high-acid animal protein diet, and alcohol intake.[25] The incidence of osteoporotic fracture is increased by various risk factors (see the following box) in addition to decreased bone strength and density.

Senile osteoporosis. Progressive bone loss normally occurs during aging. This process begins at 50 years of age in women and 65 to 70 years of age in men and results in a loss of 0.5% of total bone mass per year and approximately 20% in a lifetime.[40] Patients with senile osteoporosis experience accelerated losses of 1% to 2% per year, with symptoms of osteoporosis beginning when 30% of bone mass is lost. It has been suggested that osteoporosis is a natural part of the aging process manifested earlier in those persons who have accrued less skeletal mass during early

RISK FACTORS ASSOCIATED WITH LOW BONE DENSITY AND FRACTURE

Female gender
Estrogen deficiency
Late menarche
Early menopause
Low endogenous estrogen
Increased age (both genders)
White race
Hypogonadism (males)
Low weight and body mass index (BMI)
Family history of osteoporosis
Smoking and alcohol use
Excessive caffeine-containing beverages
Chronic low dietary calcium intake
Sedentary lifestyle
High-acid animal protein diet
History of prior fracture

TABLE 28-3 DISORDERS THAT INCREASE THE RISK OF SECONDARY OSTEOPOROSIS	
Disorder	*Pathophysiology*
Celiac disease	Malabsorption of calcium and vitamin D
Inflammatory bowel disease	Glucocorticoid use
Cholestatic liver disease	
Solid organ and bone marrow transplants	Glucocorticoid use
	Immunosuppressive use
Collagen-vascular disease	Glucocorticoid use
Hypogonadism/amenorrhea	Secondary amenorrhea in female athletes
Chronic renal disease	Secondary hyperparathyroidism
	Impaired vitamin D hydroxylation
Growth hormone deficiency	Decreased osteoblastic activity
Cushing's syndrome	Increased bone resorption caused by excess adrenal hormones
Spina bifida	Lack of weight bearing
Neuromuscular disorders	Hypotonia and decreased weight bearing
Severe cerebral palsy	Effect of anticonvulsants on vitamin D
Cystic fibrosis	Malabsorption of calcium and vitamin D
	Glucocorticoid use
"Steroid-dependent" asthma	Chronic oral glucocorticoids
	High doses of inhaled glucocorticoids
Anorexia nervosa	Malnutrition
	Secondary amenorrhea
Osteogenesis imperfecta	
Hyperthyroidism	Increased bone resorption
Hyperparathyroidism	Increased bone resorption

adult life. The causes of senile osteoporosis are largely unknown. Hormonal alterations that occur during senescence undoubtedly potentiate bone loss (see box below). Decreased serum calcitriol concentrations found in elderly persons[41] probably result from a blunted synthetic response to PTH.[42] In addition, serum PTH concentrations increase[43] and serum CT concentrations decrease[44] with aging. The net effect of these hormonal alterations is diminished intestinal calcium absorption and increased bone resorption.

Residents of long-term care facilities, such as nursing homes, are at particularly high risk of fracture. Most have low BMD and a high prevalence of many of the risk factors associated with fracture, including advanced age, poor physical function, low muscle strength, decreased cognition and high rates of dementia, poor nutrition, and, often, use of multiple medications. There also appears to be a significant role for vitamin D deficiency in the cause of senile osteoporosis. Up to 60% of elderly people living in nursing homes

develop vitamin D deficiency by the end of the winter season; also a significant number of elderly subjects with hip fractures (40% of males and 30% of females) are vitamin D deficient. Evidence supports a defective renal 1-α-hydroxylase activity with aging and secondary hyperparathyroidism as a cause of vitamin D deficiency in elderly people and secondary osteoporosis.

Postmenopausal osteoporosis. Postmenopausal osteoporosis, which occurs in females at a younger age than senile osteoporosis does, is caused by estrogen deficiency.[45] Affected women have diminished intestinal calcium absorption and lower serum calcitriol concentrations than their normal age-matched peers.[46] Although serum PTH concentrations are normal when compared to controls with normal serum calcitriol concentrations, they are low when viewed in the context of calcitriol deficiency.[46] Estrogen supplementation increases intestinal calcium absorption and serum calcitriol and PTH concentrations.[47] These data have been interpreted to indicate that estrogen deficiency produces postmenopausal osteoporosis by causing bone resorption, which releases calcium into the extracellular space and which in turn suppresses PTH secretion, calcitriol synthesis, and intestinal absorption of calcium (Fig. 28-6). It has been suggested that magnesium deficiency may play a role in postmenopausal osteoporosis.

Approximately 30% of postmenopausal white women sustain at least one osteoporotic fracture. However, the true incidence of these fractures is difficult to assess because a

CALCIUM-REGULATING HORMONE ABNORMALITIES ASSOCIATED WITH AGING

Decreased serum calcitriol concentration and calcitriol secretory reserve
Increased serum PTH concentration
Decreased serum CT concentration

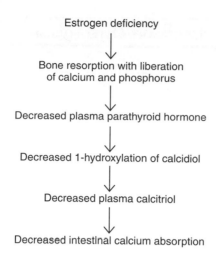

Estrogen deficiency

↓

Bone resorption with liberation
of calcium and phosphorus

↓

Decreased plasma parathyroid hormone

↓

Decreased 1-hydroxylation of calcidiol

↓

Decreased plasma calcitriol

↓

Decreased intestinal calcium absorption

Fig. 28-6 Hypothesized pathogenesis of postmenopausal osteoporosis.

large number of vertebral fractures remain asymptomatic. Osteoporotic hip fractures occur in the third and fourth decades after menopause; they are twice as common in women as in men. By 90 years of age, about 33% of women and at least 17% of men sustain a hip fracture.

Idiopathic juvenile osteoporosis. Idiopathic juvenile osteoporosis is a rare form of bone demineralization that affects prepubertal children. Clinical features manifest as fractures of long bones and vertebrae, in addition to bone pain. It is characterized by spontaneous recovery after puberty. In severe cases, characteristic metaphyseal compression fractures of the lower extremities occur because of compaction of osteoporotic newly formed bone, a pathognomonic feature of this disease. The etiology of the disease is unknown to date. Some patients have transient calcitriol deficiency, which correlates with the clinical course of the disease. Treatment of these patients with calcitriol reduces bone fracture rate and increases bone mineralization within a year. Other patients may have a negative calcium balance, low $25(OH)D$ and high $1,25(OH)_2D$, or possible CT deficiency.

Corticosteroid-induced osteoporosis.[48-50] Diseases that are treated with glucocorticoid therapy may affect more than 30 million Americans. It is estimated that up to 50% of patients on chronic glucocorticoid therapy will experience loss of bone substance and osteoporotic fractures. The mechanism of steroid-induced bone resorption is not completely known. Corticosteroids do exert direct inhibitory effects on osteoblast function, decreasing bone formation. Serum osteocalcin concentration, an indicator of bone formation, is significantly reduced in steroid-treated patients. Corticosteroid therapy reduces intestinal calcium and phosphorus absorption.

Hyperthyroidism. Both deficient and excessive circulating thyroid hormones can have deleterious sequelae on bone. The major role of thyroid hormone is to increase the number of bone-remodeling units, thereby increasing bone-remodeling activity. Thyrotoxicosis causes increased bone resorption and a decrease in bone mineral density.

Hypogonadal states. Hypogonadism, characterized by delayed menarche, oligomenorrhea, or amenorrhea, is relatively common in adolescent girls and young women. Settings in which these occur include strenuous athletic training, emotional stress, and low body weight. Failure to achieve peak bone mass, bone loss, and increased fracture rates have been shown in this group. *Anorexia nervosa*, a hypogonadic state, is further complicated by the associated profound undernutrition and nutrition-related bone demineralization. This latter point is evidenced, in part, by the failure of estrogen replacement to correct the bone loss.

Drugs. Patients with impaired renal functions are not able to excrete *aluminum* contained in antacids, dialysis fluids, foods, and nutritional supplements. Accumulation of aluminum in bone can increase the risk for fractures. *Immunosuppressant* drugs, such as cyclosporin, predispose to osteoporosis by stimulating bone resorption. *Lithium* stimulates the production of PTH and increases the rate of bone resorption; chronic lithium therapy can therefore increase the risk for osteoporosis. *Cytotoxic medications* inhibit bone turnover and predispose to osteoporosis. An excessive amount of vitamin D increases the rate of bone resorption and can increase risk for osteoporosis.

Diagnosis of osteoporosis.[4,5] The diagnosis of osteoporosis should (1) confirm the presence of osteoporosis, (2) rule out secondary causes of osteoporosis, and (3) establish a baseline against which the patient's progress can be monitored. The most commonly used measurement to diagnose osteoporosis and predict fracture risk is an assessment of BMD by *bone densitometry*, which is principally a measure of the mineral content of bone.[51-54] BMD measurements correlate strongly with load-bearing capacity of the hip and spine and with the risk of fracture. Bone density measurements are performed by dual energy x-ray densitometry (DEXA) and scored by criteria developed by WHO. Patients with evidence of osteoporosis are started on medications (alendronate (10 mg), hormonal replacement therapy, or CT), whereas patients with *osteopenia* (see later discussion) need a medication to prevent osteoporosis (alendronate (5 mg), hormonal replacement therapy, or raloxifene).[55,56]

The National Osteoporosis Foundation (NOF) recommends women have a bone density test if they meet the following criteria:

- Over 65 years old
- Postmenopausal with at least one risk factor besides menopause or with a fracture
- Considering osteoporosis therapy
- On prolonged hormone replacement therapy

Other patients who are candidates for a bone density measurement include individuals who meet the following criteria:

- On long-term (longer than 2 months) corticosteroid therapy
- Have parathyroid gland disorders
- Have had x-ray films that are suggestive of osteoporosis

SERUM TESTS TO RULE OUT SECONDARY OSTEOPOROSIS

Calcium
Alkaline phosphatase
Inorganic phosphate
Total protein
Creatinine and urea (renal function)
AST, ALT, total bilirubin (liver function)
Testosterone

Repeat DEXA scans at annual or biennial intervals allow clinicians to determine whether the patient is responding to the prescribed medication to correct a low bone density condition.

Laboratory tests to rule out secondary causes of osteoporosis. The main purpose of laboratory investigations is to rule out secondary causes of osteoporosis and to monitor the patient's response to therapy. There are as yet no laboratory tests that can be used to diagnose osteoporosis. The most frequently ordered tests are listed in the box above and discussed in more detail in the Change of Analyte with Disease section.

Treatment for osteoporosis.[4,5,57-63] Therapies available for treating osteoporosis are listed in the box below.

Adequate calcium and vitamin D intake modulates age-related increases in PTH levels and bone resorption, increasing spine BMD and reducing fractures. The maximal effective dose of vitamin D is thought to be 400 to 1000 IU/day. Optimal treatment of osteoporosis with any drug therapy also requires calcium and vitamin D intake meeting recommended levels. The consensus opinion of the North American Menopause Society (NAMS) has shed light on the role of calcium in prevention and treatment of osteoporosis in postmenopausal women. The conclusions derived from this consensus are the following:

1. Daily calcium intake should not exceed 2500 mg because it increases the risk of hypercalcemia
2. The NIH recommends the following calcium intake:
   a. 1000 mg/day for women aged 25 to 50 years and postmenopausal women younger than 65 years taking hormone replacement therapy (HRT)
   b. 1500 mg/day for menopausal women not using HRT and all women 65 years and older

THERAPY FOR OSTEOPOROSIS

Calcium	Selective estrogen receptor
Vitamin D	modulators
Physical activity	CT
Drug therapy (biphosphates)	PTH
Estrogen replacement	

Bisphosphonates. Treatment with bisphosphonates enhances the calcium content of bone.

Hormone replacement therapy (HRT).[57,58] Estrogen increases bone mass and BMD by (1) reducing bone resorption by directly inhibiting the activity of the osteoclasts and indirectly by stimulating the secretion of CT, (2) increasing collagen synthesis and osteoid formation, probably by stimulating the activity of the osteoblasts, and (3) enhancing the absorption of calcium across the intestines.[59]

Selective estrogen receptor modulators (SERMs). SERMs maximize the beneficial effect of estrogen on bone.

Calcitonin. CT is approved for the treatment of osteoporosis in women who have reached menopause more than 5 years earlier. CT has demonstrated positive effects on BMD at the lumbar spine, but this effect is less clear at the hip.

Parathyroid Hormone (PTH). Recombinant human PTH (1-34) stimulates the formation of new bone. PTH can build bone in men with osteoporosis and in women taking glucocorticoid medications.[61]

Monitoring osteoporosis and treatment. Patients with osteoporosis not only have decreased bone mass but also increased rates of *bone remodeling* (see p. 511). Monitoring patients' response to therapy for osteoporosis can be achieved by the measurement of a baseline DEXA, with repeat measurements every 1 to 3 years, depending on the expected rate of loss and the clinical situation. Alternatively surrogate markers of bone turnover in the blood or urine (N-telopeptides) assayed at baseline and then 8 to 12 weeks after specific therapy has been initiated are useful. These markers are discussed on pp. 510-511. The level of these markers may identify changes in bone remodeling within a relatively short time interval, several days to months, before changes in BMD can be detected. However, marker levels do not predict bone mass or fracture risk, are only weakly associated with changes in bone mass, and thus are of limited utility in the clinical evaluation of individual patients. Despite these limitations, these markers have been shown in research studies to correlate with changes in indices of bone remodeling and may provide insights into mechanisms of bone loss.[4,5]

Osteomalacia

Osteomalacia is diagnosed when bone contains normal quantities of osteoid that fail to mineralize. When seen in the growing child, osteomalacia is termed *rickets*. The terms *rickets* and *osteomalacia* are used interchangeably in this chapter. The major causes of osteomalacia are listed in the box on p. 517 and their associated biochemical abnormalities are summarized in Table 28-4.

Clinically the earliest rachitic features in infancy may be hypocalcemic tetany or seizures, particularly in vitamin D–unsupplemented, exclusively human milk–fed infants and in infants with congenital rickets born to vitamin D–deficient osteomalacic mothers. Acute infection may precipitate hypocalcemic tetany, possibly by mobilizing bone phosphate into the circulation and therefore decreasing serum calcium concentration. In the first 6 months of life, abnormal bones will be seen on x-ray film. The wrist and the knee are most

TABLE 28-4　Biochemical Abnormalities Associated with Rickets

	Serum Calcium	Serum Phosphorus	Parathyroid Hormone	Calcidiol	Calcitriol
Vitamin D deficiency	LO	LO	HI	LO	LO, NL, or HI
Vitamin D dependency					
I	LO	LO	HI	HI	LO
II	LO	LO	HI	HI	HI
Vitamin D resistance	NL	LO	NL	NL	NL or LO
Dietary phosphorus deficiency	NL	LO	NL	LO	HI

HI, *Increased;* LO, *decreased;* NL, *normal.*

useful in demonstrating even the earliest signs of rickets. "Rachitic lungs" indicate rib cage weakening, with secondary defective pulmonary ventilation. This feature occurs in the very young child, particularly among preterm infants. Beyond infancy, increased weight bearing aggravates rachitic changes particularly in vertebral, pelvic, and lower limb bones, resulting in spinal and pelvic deformities that cause a waddling gait and bowed legs, or "knock knees." Muscular weakness and hypotonia frequently involve proximal muscle groups in rickets and contribute to waddling gait, protuberance of the abdomen, and inefficient lung ventilation in rachitic children. The muscular weakness is believed to be caused by decreased calcium uptake by myocytes.

Vitamin D–deficient osteomalacia. Historically the most common cause of osteomalacia was *vitamin D deficiency* caused by a combination of insufficient sunlight exposure and inadequate dietary intake of vitamin D–containing foods.[64] Serum calcidiol concentrations, which reflect the adequacy of vitamin D in the body, are low in osteomalacia. Supplementation of foods with vitamin D has virtually eliminated the problem in industrialized countries, but it may still be seen in underdeveloped nations, particularly among dark-skinned people because skin pigment decreases the production of cholecalciferol, which normally occurs after UV radiation exposure. It is also encountered in exclusively human milk–fed infants and in strict vegetarian adults, even in developed countries. These individuals have limited exposure to sunshine and do not ingest vitamin D–fortified milk.

Alterations of vitamin D metabolism that can lead to rickets range from conditions of insufficient intake or production of cholecalciferol to disturbances in its activation by the liver and kidneys. Generally the biochemical response to a deficiency of calcitriol can be predicted (Fig. 28-4). The absorption of intestinal calcium will decrease and produce hypocalcemia. This will stimulate PTH release (secondary hyperparathyroidism), which will mobilize calcium from bone and increase phosphorus excretion by the kidney. Initially, serum calcium concentrations will be maintained at the expense of bone resorption, but as minerals are depleted, hypocalcemia occurs. Hypophosphatemia occurs because of increased urinary phosphorus losses. Thus the characteristic serum abnormalities associated with calcitriol deficiency are hypocalcemia, hypophosphatemia, and hyperparathyroidism

(Table 28-4). In addition, hyperphosphaturia, aminoaciduria, rachitic bone disease, and elevated serum alkaline phosphatase concentration will be observed.

Osteomalacia also results from phosphorus deficiency. In this situation, low intracellular phosphorus concentrations should stimulate calcitriol synthesis, which will increase both intestinal and renal phosphate absorption. Serum calcium and PTH concentrations should be unaffected (Table 28-4).

Osteomalacia secondary to gastrointestinal disorders. Patients with gastrointestinal disease, particularly those with hepatobiliary disease, often develop osteomalacia. Vitamin D is fat-soluble and requires bile acids for absorption (see Chapter 30). Patients with hepatobiliary disease have low serum calcidiol levels that appear to be caused in part by defective intestinal cholecalciferol or ergosterol absorption, impaired calcidiol production by the liver, and enhanced calcitriol metabolism. Osteopenia also may be seen after gastric surgery, though the pathogenesis is not understood.

Hepatic rickets.[65] Hepatobiliary disease predisposes to rickets, presumably because of decreased 25-hydroxylase activity, vitamin D malabsorption, and decreased enterohepatic circulation of 25(OH)D. Malabsorption of vitamin D is probably a major factor in the pathogenesis of hepatic rickets. Biochemically, serum 25(OH)D and 1,25(OH)$_2$D concentrations are low. Clinically, signs of rickets are superimposed on the primary hepatic disease. Infants with hepatitis and infants who require prolonged parenteral hyperalimentation may develop varying degrees of hepatic dysfunction and secondary rickets.

Osteomalacia secondary to anticonvulsant medication. Rickets may occur in up to 30% of children receiving anticonvulsant medications, such as phenytoin (Dilantin) and phenobarbital, that induce the hepatic microsomal mixed-oxidase enzyme system.[65] This enzyme system, when stimulated, converts calcidiol to polar inactive metabolites, which results in calcidiol deficiency. Other biochemical effects of the therapy can include hypocalcemia, hypophosphatemia, hypocalciuria, and elevated serum concentrations of alkaline phosphatase and PTH. In addition, anticonvulsants inhibit calcitriol-dependent intestinal calcium uptake.

Vitamin D–dependent osteomalacia (types I and II). After foods were fortified with vitamin D, it became apparent that normal antirachitic doses of analogs of vitamin D failed to heal the rickets of a small subpopulation of rachitic patients. One group of such patients had the classical signs and symptoms of vitamin D deficiency, including early infantile hypocalcemia, hypophosphatemia, and tetany, but these patients required up to 100 times the normal intake of vitamin D to heal their rickets. This group of patients with *vitamin D–dependent rickets* has recently been classified into two subgroups with distinct pathophysiological bases.

Patients with vitamin D–dependent rickets type I have the classical biochemical abnormalities of vitamin D–deficient rickets, but their serum calcidiol concentrations are normal and they lack circulating calcitriol.[65] The presumed defect is an abnormal or absent renal 1-α-hydroxylase enzyme. Clinically, the disease occurs before 2 years of age, most often in the first 6 months of life. A sporadic form of the disease has been described less often, and its onset is in late childhood and adolescence. The osteomalacia of these patients heals when physiological doses of calcitriol are administered.

Patients with vitamin D–dependent rickets type II have normal calcidiol and calcitriol levels and are resistant to physiological doses of calcitriol.[66] The cause of the disease is an end-organ resistance to the effect of 1,25(OH)$_2$D because of a defective calcitriol-receptor effector system, and mechanistically should be called *calcitriol (1,25[OH]$_2$D)– resistant rickets*.[66] Clinically, the disease manifests as rickets and osteomalacia, most commonly before 2 years of life, rarely later in life. Biochemically these patients have low serum calcium and phosphorus concentrations, normal serum 25(OH)D concentration, and elevated serum 1,25(OH)$_2$D and PTH concentrations. Both types of vitamin D–dependent rickets are inherited in an autosomal recessive pattern.

There are five classes of defective calcitriol receptors: (1) Defect in the hormone-binding domain. Calcitriol concentration is elevated but does not evoke a biochemical response. This is the most common defect. (2) Hormone-binding affinity is normal, accompanied by reduction in the number of receptors and hormone-binding sites (10% of normal). (3) Hormone-binding affinity is reduced twenty-fold to thirty-fold although the number of binding sites is normal. (4) Defective nuclear localization. In this form, calcitriol does not localize to the cell nucleus. (5) Decreased affinity of hormone-receptor complex to DNA. Intracellular defect categories 1, 2, and 5 do not respond to therapy with high vitamin D doses. In contrast, intracellular defects types 3 and 4 can be cured with high vitamin D doses. Prenatal diagnosis of this disease is now feasible and is indicated in high-risk families.

Vitamin D–resistant osteomalacia. Patients with *vitamin D–resistant rickets* lack most of the usual biochemical markers associated with rachitic patients. Serum phosphorus is severely decreased, whereas serum calcium concentrations may be normal or decreased.[67] Serum PTH concentration is either normal or increased, and serum 1,25(OH)$_2$D concentration is either normal or low. This disorder is caused by a congenital defect in phosphate resorp-tion in the proximal renal tubules, resulting in massive phosphaturia and hypophosphatemia. The defective gene responsible for this disease has been mapped to the short arm of the human X chromosome. Because low intracellular phosphorus concentrations are a major stimulus for calcitriol synthesis, serum calcitriol concentrations should be elevated in this disorder; however, when measured, serum calcitriol concentrations have been found to be low or low-normal.[65,68] This finding is suggestive of a potential second defect in this condition, that is, dysfunction of the renal 1-α-hydroxylase enzyme. Vitamin D–resistant rickets may be inherited in a sex-linked recessive or an autosomal dominant pattern. The most frequent type is the X-linked concomitant pattern and affects males. Traditionally, patients with vitamin D–resistant rickets have been treated with cholecalciferol and phosphate supplements.

Calcium-deficiency rickets. Also termed *calcipenic rickets*, this form of osteomalacia occurs when the diet is low in calcium or when the bioavailability of the calcium is reduced. Children who follow strict vegetarian or high cereal diets are at risk of developing rickets. Some of these children have clinical and biochemical features of vitamin D deficiency, attributed to vitamin D binding by dietary phytates in the intestinal lumen.

Clinically, affected children have rachitic features with "knock" knees, bow legs, or "wind-swept" deformities but no muscular weakness. Radiological features correspond to clinical findings of rachitic changes (see earlier discussion). The bone histological pattern reveals features of osteomalacia and secondary hyperparathyroidism. Biochemical features of calcipenic rickets include hypocalcemia and hypocalciuria, normal serum 25(OH)D, elevated serum alkaline phosphatase, and elevated serum calcitriol and PTH concentrations.

Hyperalimentation-induced osteopenia. Long-term parenteral alimentation (TPN) has been associated with osteopenia and bone demineralization. The main feature seen in this metabolic bone disease is hypercalciuria. Several factors have been implicated in the cause of hypercalciuria including cyclic infusion of TPN solutions, sulfur-containing acidic amino acids, hypertonic dextrose infusions, which result in hyperinsulinemia and decreased tubular resorption of calcium, acidosis, and low phosphate in infused solutions. Hypercalciuria may be ameliorated by phosphate supplementation.

Aluminum-containing parenteral hyperalimentation solutions are responsible for causing a peculiar metabolic bone disease characterized by reduced bone formation. The degree of aluminum accumulation in bone correlates with decreased bone formation.

Other causes of osteomalacia. Chronic acidosis causes osteomalacia, hypercalciuria, and hyperphosphaturia because of neutralization of acids by bone with subsequent release of bone mineral. Patients with renal Fanconi's syndrome have diminished proximal tubule reabsorption of bicarbonate (resulting in chronic acidosis), phosphorus, glucose, and amino acids. Osteomalacia may be severe because of the chronic acidosis and severe hypophosphatemia. In addition, as part of the proximal tubulopathy, there may be subnormal activity of the renal 1-α-hydroxylase enzyme.[69]

Sufficient substrate must be supplied in the diet for proper bone mineralization. Delayed bone mineralization commonly occurs in very low birth weight, premature infants who are fed normal infant formulas or breast milk,[70] both of which contain insufficient quantities of calcium and phosphorus for the rapid bone mineralization of premature infants.

Drug-induced osteomalacia. Prolonged administration of heparin has been associated with osteoporosis and decreased bone density. The incidence of heparin-induced osteopenia is unknown. It appears that an individual has to receive a dose of at least 15,000 U/day for 6 months before osteopenia occurs. The symptoms are nonspecific and basically manifest as back pain and vertebral fractures and are reversible after withdrawal of heparin. Methotrexate is a commonly used antineoplastic agent, particularly in childhood leukemias. It has been shown to decrease osteoblastic activity in animals and to increase bone resorption in humans. Consequently, prolonged use of this agent may induce osteopenia.

Osteitis Fibrosa

Osteitis fibrosa is the histopathological bone lesion produced by excessive PTH secretion. It is primarily seen in two conditions, primary hyperparathyroidism and chronic renal failure. Bone disease is of lesser significance in primary hyperparathyroidism because surgical removal of the involved parathyroid glands cures the disease. The pathophysiological condition of secondary hyperparathyroidism associated with chronic renal failure is more complex and less amenable to treatment. Thus uremic patients frequently suffer from severe bone disease.

The complex bone abnormality associated with chronic renal failure is termed *renal osteodystrophy*. Two distinct histopathological forms of renal osteodystrophy, osteomalacia and osteitis fibrosa (see box at right), frequently coexist in the same patient. Osteomalacia is probably caused by decreased synthesis of calcitriol secondary to renal parenchymal disease. Serum concentrations of calcitriol and 24,25-dihydroxyvitamin D are decreased in both children and adults with chronic renal failure, and calcidiol concentrations are normal.[71] Factors that contribute to secondary hyperparathyroidism of renal disease include (1) decreased phosphorus excretion and hyperphosphatemia, which directly decreases renal calcitriol synthesis (Figs. 28-7 and 28-8), (2) decreased renal hydroxylase activity because of renal damage, (3) a higher set point for PTH secretion in uremia possibly because of a decrease in the number of vitamin D receptors in parathyroid cells, (4) hypocalcemia, and (5) skeletal resistance to PTH.

Paget's Disease[29,72]

Paget's disease is a disorder of bone metabolism characterized by increased osteoclastic bone resorption followed by disordered bone formation. The incidence of this disease is difficult to determine because the majority of affected patients are asymptomatic. The incidence of Paget's disease varies with age and geographic location. It is more common among elderly than among middle-aged people. In an autopsy series of persons over 40 years of age, 3% of this group was affected. Family history is positive in 14% of cases. Males are more prone to have the disease than females (3:2). The disease occurs more frequently among people of European ancestry. It is uncommon among Scandinavians,

---

PATHOLOGICAL FORMS OF RENAL OSTEODYSTROPHY

Predominant osteitis fibrosa
   Normal serum calcium level—calcitriol responsive
   Pretreatment hypercalcemia—exacerbated by calcitriol
Predominant osteomalacia
   Small amount of fibrosis present—calcitriol responsive
   Pure osteomalacia—hypercalcemia with calcitriol treatment
Mixed osteitis fibrosa and osteomalacia—calcitriol responsive
Mild—calcitriol responsive

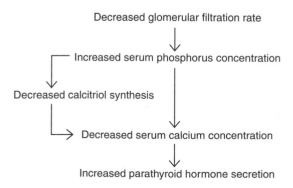

Fig. 28-7 Pathogenetic mechanism of secondary hyperparathyroidism in renal failure according to phosphate theory.

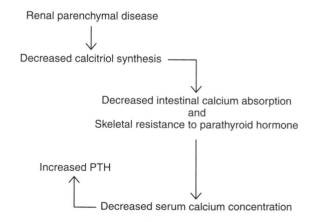

Fig. 28-8 Pathogenetic mechanism of secondary hyperparathyroidism in renal failure according to vitamin D theory.

Asians, and black Africans. The cause of the disease is unknown.

The histological pattern of patients with Paget's disease proceeds through three stages. In the early phase of the illness, resorption predominates and the bone marrow is replaced with a highly vascular fibrous connective tissue. In the second phase of the disease, bone formation predominates. The pagetic bone is coarse-fibered, dense trabecular bone. In the final phase the rate of bone resorption declines, and continued bone formation produces hard, dense bone. The largest amount of bone resorption that initially occurs produces greatly elevated urinary hydroxyproline concentrations, and the subsequent rapid rate of bone formation results in dramatically elevated serum alkaline phosphatase concentrations. Serum calcium and phosphorus concentrations are normal. However, pathological fractures occur and are treated by immobilization of the patient. Hypercalcemia frequently occurs because immobilization increases the rate of bone resorption. Paget's disease is treated successfully with CT, which inhibits osteoclastic bone resorption.[72]

Heritable Bone Disease

Hypophosphatasia. Hypophosphatasia is a rare heritable bone disease characterized by generalized reduction in alkaline phosphatase activity in liver, bone, and kidney tissues. Placental and intestinal alkaline phosphatase isoenzyme activities remain normal. The disease occurs in all races but is especially common among Mennonites in Canada, among whom the incidence is up to 1 per 100,000 live births. Clinically, the disease affects bone and dentition and ranges from a severe, lethal in utero form to an asymptomatic adult disease. Four clinical forms of the disease are known: perinatal (lethal) form, commonly associated with stillbirth and polyhydramnios; infantile form, usually seen during the first 6 months of life; childhood form; and the adult form, usually appearing in middle age.

Osteogenesis imperfecta. The condition osteogenesis imperfecta is a heritable disorder of connective tissue involving abnormal synthesis of type I collagen fibers, the most abundant protein in bone matrix. The prime clinical manifestations of this disease are pronounced bone fragility, generalized osteopenia, and recurrent fractures in response to mild trauma. Hearing loss, which occurs in about 50% of patients less than 30 years of age, is most often conductive and rarely sensorineural. The pathogenesis of the disease involves defective mutations in the genes coding for pro-α 1 and pro-α 2 chains of type I collagen, resulting in bone fragility.

Osteopetrosis. Osteopetrosis encompasses a group of diseases characterized by failure of osteoclast-mediated bone resorption. The mechanism of osteoclast malfunction is poorly understood. The disease is classified into eight types according to clinical and genetic factors. The main two forms of osteopetrosis are a more common benign type, often asymptomatic and inherited as an autosomal dominant mode, and the rare malignant form, which typically occurs in infancy and childhood and is inherited in an autosomal recessive mode. Rare forms of osteopetrosis may be associated with renal tubular acidosis, carbonic anhydrase deficiency, or neuronal storage disease.

CHANGE OF ANALYTE IN DISEASE
Biochemical Measurements of Bone Turnover

Biochemical measurements of bone turnover are helpful in the study of the pathophysiology of skeletal metabolism and growth. However, interpretation of their results is difficult because it depends on a number of physiological variables including age, pubertal stage, growth velocity, mineral accrual, hormonal regulation, nutritional status, and circadian variation. Methodological considerations, including the expression of results of urinary markers, specificity of the markers for bone tissue, and the sensitivity and specificity of assays, also affect interpretation. These limitations have minimized the widespread use of these markers.[14]

Vitamin D

Serum concentrations of vitamin D metabolites may be altered in a variety of disease states (see box below). Decreased concentrations result from deficient intake, defective metabolic regulation, or increased excretion. Serum calcidiol concentrations are low in patients who have both an insufficient exposure to sunlight and a low intake of foods that contain vitamin D. Patients who receive anticonvulsant drugs convert calcidiol into biologically inactive polar metabolites.[66] Production of calcidiol is impaired in patients with liver disease.[73] Inactive or absent renal 1-α-hydroxylase activity and secondary low serum calcitriol concentrations are associated with vitamin D–dependent rickets type I,[65] postmenopausal and senile osteoporosis,[40-47] hypoparathyroidism,[74] pseudohypoparathyroidism,[75] vitamin D–resistant rickets,[65-68] and chronic

---

DISEASES AND CONDITIONS ASSOCIATED WITH CHANGES IN SERUM CONCENTRATIONS OF VITAMIN D METABOLITES

Calcidiol (25-hydroxycholecalciferol) deficiency
    Nutritional osteomalacia
    Anticonvulsant-induced osteomalacia
    Liver disease
    Nephrotic syndrome
Calcitriol (1,25-dihydroxycholecalciferol) deficiency
    Vitamin D–dependent rickets type I
    Postmenopausal and senile osteoporosis
    Hypoparathyroidism
    Pseudohypoparathyroidism
    Vitamin D–resistant rickets
    Nephrotic syndrome
Calcidiol (25-hydroxycholecalciferol) excess
    Vitamin D intoxication
    Excessive sunlight exposure
Calcitriol (1,25-hydroxycholecalciferol) excess
    Childhood
    Pregnancy and lactation
    Sarcoidosis
    Hyperparathyroidism

renal failure.[76] Patients with nephrotic syndrome have low serum concentrations of both calcidiol and calcitriol because of urinary losses of both metabolites, as well as the serum protein (vitamin D–binding protein) to which they are attached.[30]

High serum calcidiol concentrations result from either increased exogenous intake or increased endogenous production secondary to an unusually large sunlight exposure. High serum calcitriol concentrations occur in physiological states of increased calcium requirements such as growth[77] and pregnancy and lactation.[78] High serum calcitriol concentrations are also seen in sarcoidosis, in which an extrarenal source of calcitriol production has been implicated, and in hyperparathyroidism, in which the serum concentrations of PTH, a major stimulus for calcitriol production, are elevated.

Parathyroid Hormone

Hypoparathyroidism

Primary idiopathic hypoparathyroidism. *Idiopathic hypoparathyroidism* describes the condition of a decreased production of PTH whose cause is not known. In pseudo-hypoparathyroidism, production of PTH is intact, but there is target organ resistance to PTH; in other words, PTH, though

present, does not exert its physiological actions because the target organs are not responsive. In current terminology, there may be a "receptor defect" for PTH. Another way of describing idiopathic hypoparathyroidism would be *hormone-deficient hypoparathyroidism*, and pseudohypoparathyroidism would be described as *hormone-sufficient, receptor-deficient hypoparathyroidism* (Fig. 28-9). Hypoparathyroidism classically manifests itself with hypocalcemia and hyperphosphatemia, usually in childhood.

Secondary hypoparathyroidism. Hypoparathyroidism may result from other disorders. Inadvertent surgical removal of the parathyroids may occur during thyroidectomy. Because magnesium is important for PTH secretion, magnesium deficiency may result in hypoparathyroidism. An interesting physiological hypoparathyroidism occurs in infants. In utero, calcium is transferred actively across the placenta, and serum calcium concentrations in the fetus are extremely high. These high serum calcium concentrations appear to inhibit fetal parathyroid function. Inhibited parathyroid function persists for a short interval after birth and appears to be a cause of hypocalcemia in the first 3 days of life, especially in the premature infant.[75]

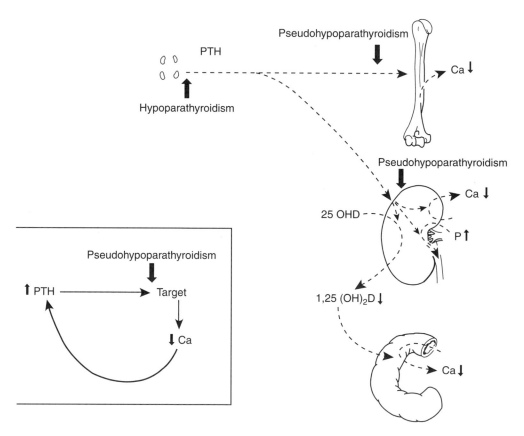

Fig. 28-9 In idiopathic hypoparathyroidism, decreased PTH results in decreased serum calcium, increased serum phosphorus, and decreased production of 1,25-dihydroxyvitamin D. In pseudohypoparathyroidism, although there is sufficient hormone, target organs are unresponsive and biochemical result is similar. *Inset,* In pseudohypoparathyroidism, resultant low serum calcium concentrations serve as a stimulus to PTH production. Because parathyroid glands are intact, in contrast to idiopathic hypoparathyroidism, serum PTH concentrations will be *elevated* in an attempt to overcome target organ resistance and rectify hypocalcemia.

The diagnosis of hypoparathyroidism is made from the clinical presentation of lowered serum calcium and elevated serum phosphorus concentrations. PTH concentrations will be low in hypoparathyroidism but elevated in pseudohypoparathyroidism. To further distinguish idiopathic hypoparathyroidism from pseudohypoparathyroidism, PTH infusion is administered. After the infusion, serum calcium and urinary phosphorus and cAMP concentrations are measured. Patients with pseudohypoparathyroidism may have varying "degrees of block" in response to PTH, at the bone site or at various "levels" in the kidney.[79] Patients with hypoparathyroidism are treated with supplements of calcium salts and calcitriol.

Hyperparathyroidism

Primary hyperparathyroidism. Primary hyperparathyroidism is often described as being related to hyperplasia or adenoma of the parathyroids. In contrast to hypoparathyroidism, which usually begins in childhood, hyperparathyroidism is usually discovered in adulthood. As expected from the physiological action of PTH, excess concentrations of the hormone result in increased serum calcium concentrations and decreased serum phosphorus concentrations. Demineralization occurs as a consequence of the bone lytic action of PTH and is associated with areas of extensive resorption (osteitis fibrosa, see p. 524). Many clinical problems are associated with the high serum calcium concentrations. The major organ systems adversely affected by hypercalcemia are the nervous system and the kidney.

Secondary hyperparathyroidism. Conditions that are associated with chronic hypocalcemia will result in chronic stimulation of the parathyroids and secondary hyperparathyroidism. The two major factors resulting in chronic hypocalcemia of nonparathyroid cause are vitamin D–metabolite deficiencies and high phosphorus loads. Any deficiency of vitamin D or its major metabolites will result in decreased intestinal absorption of calcium and hypocalcemia. The initial response to this hypocalcemia will be secondary hyperparathyroidism, which helps maintain serum calcium concentrations in the normal range. High phosphorus loads occur with infusion of phosphorus-containing fluids, ingestion of high phosphorus content milk (such as cow milk given to newborn infants), or retention of phosphorus by failing kidneys. High serum phosphorus concentrations result in a secondary decrease in serum calcium concentrations. With decreased serum calcium concentrations there is compensatory secondary hyperparathyroidism.[80]

The diagnosis of primary hyperparathyroidism is based on the findings of high serum calcium, low serum phosphorus, and high serum PTH concentrations. However, not all hyperparathyroid patients will have increased serum calcium concentrations or increased serum PTH concentrations. Ionized calcium measurements in blood may provide additional diagnostic help because the ionized calcium fraction is the physiologically active calcium.

In secondary hyperparathyroidism, serum calcium concentrations are low or normal because the parathyroid overactivity results from an initial decline in serum calcium.

Serum phosphorus concentrations are low except in situations of phosphorus overload, when they are high. Serum PTH concentrations should be elevated in secondary hyperparathyroidism.

Calcium (see Methods on CD-ROM)

Hypercalcemia. Hypercalcemia resulting from primary hyperparathyroidism has been described earlier. Other causes of hypercalcemia are listed in the box below.

Endocrine and tumor-related hypercalcemia. Hypercalcemia may occur with disorders of endocrine organs other than the parathyroids. Overproduction of thyroid hormone (thyrotoxicosis) and underproduction of corticosteroids (Addison's disease or abrupt withdrawal of steroid hormones) are associated with hypercalcemia. A wide variety of tumors appear to produce PTH-like substances with osteoclast-stimulatory activity, which results in hypercalcemia. Hypercalcemia and hyperparathyroidism are sometimes associated with *pheochromocytoma* or multiple endocrine neoplasia type II syndrome. Pancreatic *VIPoma* tumors secrete vasoactive intestinal peptide (VIP), which causes severe diarrhea. About 50% of these cases have hypercalcemia possibly because of VIP-induced bone resorption. The mechanism of hypercalcemia in malignancy may, in part, be the result of the production of PTHRP (humoral hypercalcemia of malignancy), $1,25(OH)_2D$ in lymphoma, lymphotoxin in multiple myeloma, or other substances that cause bone resorption.

Vitamin A- and vitamin D-related disorders. Excessive intake of vitamin A or vitamin D may result in hypercalcemia. Hypercalcemia may be a feature of granulomatous diseases such as *tuberculosis* and *sarcoidosis*, which are associated with abnormal vitamin D metabolism and increased serum levels of $1,25(OH)_2D$. In sarcoidosis, elevated calcitriol concentrations appear to be the cause of the hypercalcemia. Vitamin A in high doses appears to have a direct effect on bone resorption. Therapy for vitamin D–resistant rickets or hypoparathyroidism with high doses of vitamin D is a common cause of hypercalcemia. Idiopathic hypercalcemia of infants is believed to be related to disordered vitamin D metabolism, possibly increased sensitivity to vitamin D.[81]

CAUSES OF HYPERCALCEMIA

Primary hyperparathyroidism
Thyrotoxicosis
Addison's disease
Withdrawal of steroids
Tumors
Vitamin D and vitamin A intoxication
Sarcoidosis
Idiopathic hypercalcemia of infancy
Immobilization
Subcutaneous fat necrosis in infants
Thiazide diuretics
Milk-alkali syndrome
Benign familial hypercalcemia

Iatrogenic causes. Immobilization of patients, especially male adolescents, results in rapid mobilization of calcium from bone and resultant hypercalcemia. Lactation causes a transient increase in bone resorption and secondary hypercalcemia, reversed by weaning. In infants born after traumatic deliveries, a curious condition of hypercalcemia can occur related to subcutaneous fat necrosis. Use of thiazide diuretics is classically associated with hypercalcemia. *Thiazides* act directly to increase calcium release from the skeleton and promote renal tubular reabsorption of calcium. Chronic *lithium* intake may cause hyperparathyroidism and mild hypercalcemia and hypermagnesemia. Excessive ingestion of milk and alkali in the treatment of peptic ulcer (the milk-alkali syndrome) also results in hypercalcemia.

Neonatal hypercalcemia (total serum calcium concentration higher than 110 mg/L or serum ionized calcium concentration higher than 58 mg/L) can be the result of prolonged *maternal hypocalcemia* resulting from a multitude of causes. Consequently a variable degree of congenital, transient hyperparathyroidism results. Neonatal hypercalcemia in the *phosphorus-deficiency syndrome* has been reported in preterm infants fed human milk.

Familial form. There is a benign form of familial hypercalcemia that is inherited as a dominant trait. Mild hypercalcemia (less than 130 mg/L) occurs and apparently is without adverse effects.

Hypocalcemia. The causes of hypocalcemia are currently classified in relation to the major hormone or biochemical involved: vitamin D, PTH, CT, calcium, magnesium, and phosphate (see box below).

CAUSES OF HYPOCALCEMIA

Vitamin D
  Decreased solar exposure and endogenous synthesis
  Decreased intestinal intake (malabsorption, dietary deficiency)
  Altered hepatic metabolism of vitamin D (hepatic disease, anticonvulsant therapy)
  Decreased renal synthesis of calcitriol (vitamin D dependency, renal failure)
Parathyroid
  Hypoparathyroidism (primary and secondary)
  Pseudohypoparathyroidism
Calcitonin
  Calcitonin or mithramycin infusion
Calcium
  Intestinal malabsorption
  Acute pancreatitis
  Infusion of agents complexing calcium
  Alkalosis decreasing ionized calcium
Magnesium
  Magnesium deficiency (see box on right side of p. 530)
Phosphorus
  Renal failure
  Phosphate infusion
  Cow milk formulas

Vitamin D deficiency, which has been covered earlier, occurs as a result of reduced synthesis or intake of the parent vitamin D, altered hepatic metabolism of vitamin D, and decreased renal synthesis of calcitriol, the final active metabolite of vitamin D.

Hypoparathyroidism (primary and secondary) and pseudohypoparathyroidism have been discussed previously. CT or mithramycin infusions decrease calcium transport from bone to extracellular space and result in hypocalcemia. Intestinal malabsorption of calcium may lead to hypocalcemia. Acute pancreatitis is associated with fatty acid–calcium complex precipitates in the pancreas and hypocalcemia. Decreased blood ionized calcium occurs with infusion of agents complexing calcium (citrate and acid-citrated blood for transfusion, or EDTA), or alkalosis, which shifts the fraction of calcium that is ionized to that which is protein bound.

Hypomagnesemia results in hypocalcemia mostly related to the adverse effect of hypomagnesemia on parathyroid function. Conditions in which phosphorus concentrations in blood are elevated; as in renal failure (see earlier discussion), phosphate infusion, or infants receiving cow milk formulas with their high phosphate content; will result in decreased serum calcium concentrations because calcium is shifted from the extracellular space into bone and soft tissues and probably because there is a blunted bone response to the effects of PTH.[82]

Neonatal hypocalcemia is defined as a total serum calcium concentration of less than 70 mg/L for preterm infants or 80 mg/L for term infants (serum ionized calcium concentration less than 44 mg/L). Neonatal hypocalcemia is the direct result of the relatively high PTH set point (see p. 515) established in the fetus. After birth, this PTH set point is lowered, with a commensurate lowering of serum calcium. At birth, termination of the high transplacental calcium influx to the fetus can result in a transient hypocalcemia. *Prematurity* is the major cause of neonatal hypocalcemia, which may develop in a large proportion (30% to 90%) of preterm infants. The incidence of hypocalcemia correlates inversely with gestational age and birth weight. Its cause is uncertain. About 30% of infants with *birth asphyxia* may develop hypocalcemia in the neonatal period.

Parathyroid gland adenoma is the most common cause of *maternal hyperparathyroidism* and hypercalcemia. Maternal hypercalcemia suppresses the fetal parathyroid glands, resulting in transient neonatal, or congenital, hypoparathyroidism. At least 50% of infants born to hyperparathyroid mothers have hypocalcemic tetany.

Mothers with *insulin-dependent diabetes mellitus* have excessive urinary magnesium losses, especially if euglycemia is not maintained. Consequently, these mothers, and theoretically their fetuses, may be magnesium depleted. *Hypomagnesemia* impairs PTH secretion and may explain the transient neonatal hypoparathyroidism and hypocalcemia that may develop in about 50% of infants of diabetic mothers.

Hypocalcemia in infants born to mothers with gestational exposure to *anticonvulsant* therapy may be related to the

TABLE 28-5 PARATHYROID HORMONE–VITAMIN D AXIS ANALYTES IN HYPERCALCEMIA

Disorder	Serum Phosphorus	Parathyroid Hormone (PTH)	PARATHYROID HORMONE–VITAMIN D AXIS		VITAMIN D STATUS
			Nephrogenous Cyclic AMP	Calcitriol (1,25-Dihydroxycholecalciferol)	Calcidiol (25-Hydroxycholecalciferol)
Hyperparathyroidism	LO	HI	HI	HI	NL
Vitamin D disorders					
Vitamin D intoxication	NL	LO	LO	HI or NL	HI
High calcitriol in sarcoidosis	NL	LO	LO	HI	NL
Sensitivity to vitamin D: idiopathic hypercalcemia of infancy	NL	LO	LO	NL	NL
Non–parathyroid hormone, non–vitamin D disorders					
Malignancy	NL	LO	HI/LO	LO or HI	NL
Immobilization	NL	LO	LO	LO	NL
Thyrotoxicosis	NL	LO	NL	LO	NL

HI, *Increased;* LO, *decreased;* NL, *normal.*

effect of phenobarbital or phenytoin in enhancing accelerated hepatic metabolism of 25(OH)D (see p. 522). Hypocalcemia has also been described in a few infants born to hypercalcemic women with familial hypocalciuric hypercalcemia.

Changes in PTH: vitamin D–axis analytes in hypercalcemia and hypocalcemia. Changes in the serum concentrations of phosphorus, the PTH–vitamin D axis, and vitamin D status help in evaluation of the causes of hypercalcemia and hypocalcemia. If the PTH–vitamin D axis is intact, two effects are seen: (1) cAMP production by the kidney is active; renal cAMP is best determined as "nephrogenous" cAMP, which takes into account the cAMP not produced in the kidney,[83] and (2) 1,25-dihydroxycholecalciferol (calcitriol) production is also active (Tables 28-5 and 28-6).

Of the *hypercalcemic* disorders listed in Table 28-5, serum phosphorus concentrations are decreased in hyperparathyroidism because of the phosphaturic effects of PTH; in the remaining hypercalcemic disorders, little effect on serum phosphorus is evident. In hyperparathyroidism, serum PTH concentrations and the PTH–vitamin D axis analytes are increased. In hypercalcemia from other causes, serum PTH is suppressed. In turn the PTH–vitamin D axis may be suppressed, except in sarcoidosis, in which elevation of serum calcitriol concentrations appears to be a primary problem.

Vitamin D status is best assessed through measurement of serum 25-hydroxycholecalciferol (calcidiol) concentrations. Thus serum 25-hydroxycholecalciferol concentrations are elevated in vitamin D intoxication, with or without elevations in the serum 1,25-dihydroxycholecalciferol (calcitriol) concentrations.

In *hypocalcemia* (Table 28-6) related to parathyroid disorders, hypoparathyroidism or pseudohypoparathyroidism, serum phosphorus is elevated because of decreased urinary phosphorus excretion. The PTH–vitamin D axis is generally hypofunctioning, except in pseudohypoparathyroidism, in which serum PTH concentrations are elevated because of target-organ resistance to the hormone.

In the vitamin D disorders, serum phosphorus concentrations are generally low because one of the major actions of vitamin D is to raise serum phosphorus concentrations. However, in renal osteodystrophy (renal failure) serum phosphorus concentrations are elevated because of decreased renal phosphorus excretion. The PTH-cAMP axis in this circumstance may be increased because of hyperparathyroidism secondary to hypocalcemia; however, serum 1,25-dihydroxycholecalciferol concentrations will remain decreased because of deficiency of vitamin D or blocks in vitamin D metabolism. In the condition of increased resistance to 1,25-dihydroxycholecalciferol, high serum concentrations of the metabolite are found, analogous to elevated PTH concentrations in pseudohypoparathyroidism. Serum 25-hydroxycholecalciferol measurements will be low in vitamin D deficiency or when there is a block in 25-hydroxylation of vitamin D but normal in vitamin D disorders caused by metabolic blocks beyond the liver step of hydroxylation.

In the mineral disorders causing hypocalcemia, little effect on the PTH–vitamin D axis has been reported. Secondary hyperparathyroidism can be a consequence of hypocalcemia. In hypomagnesemia, however, hypoparathyroidism can occur secondary to the magnesium deficiency.

Magnesium (see Methods on CD-ROM)

Hypermagnesemia. Excess of magnesium is usually a consequence of increased medicinal intake of magnesium. Magnesium ($MgSO_4$) is used in the treatment of hypertension induced by pregnancy (preeclampsia). The mother will become hypermagnesemic (up to 110 mg/L), as will her infant. Recent clinical studies demonstrated the apparent

			PARATHYROID HORMONE–VITAMIN D AXIS		VITAMIN D STATUS
Disorder	**Serum Phosphorus**	**Parathyroid Hormone (PTH)**	**Nephrogenous Cyclic AMP**	**Calcitriol (1,25-Dihydroxycholecalciferol)**	**Calcidiol (25-Hydroxycholecalciferol)**
Parathyroid disorders					
Hypoparathyroidism	HI	LO	LO	LO	NL
Pseudohypoparathyroidism	HI	HI	LO	LO	NL
Vitamin D disorders					
Vitamin D deficiency	LO	HI	HI	HI*; NL or LO	LO
Hepatic disease and anticonvulsant therapy	LO	HI	HI	NL or LO	LO
Renal					
Vitamin D–dependent rickets	LO	HI	HI	LO	NL
Osteodystrophy	HI	HI	—	LO	NL
Resistance to 1,25-dihydroxycholecalciferol	LO	HI	HI	HI	NL
Mineral disorders					
Calcium malabsorption	NL	NL or HI	—	—	—
Hypomagnesemia	NL	LO, NL, or HI	—	—	NL
High phosphate load	HI	NL or HI	—	—	NL

TABLE 28-6 PARATHYROID HORMONE–VITAMIN D AXIS ANALYTES IN HYPOCALCEMIA

HI, Increased; LO, decreased; NL, normal.
*Especially in childhood.

benefits of maternal magnesium supplementation in reducing the incidence of preterm labor and allowing greater fetal growth. Reduced magnesium excretion may occur in severe renal failure, and the use of medicines that contain magnesium (antacids, purgatives) in this situation may result in hypermagnesemia[21] (see box below).

Hypomagnesemia and magnesium deficiency. Severe magnesium deficiency in humans is uncommon, possibly because of the body's highly developed ability to conserve magnesium. Decreased uptake of magnesium caused by gastrointestinal disorders (steatorrhea, malabsorption syndromes, gut resections) can cause magnesium deficiency. Specific intestinal malabsorption of magnesium also occurs and can cause hypomagnesemia in infancy. Protein-calorie malnutrition is often associated with magnesium depletion. Increased urinary magnesium losses may result from generalized renal disease or a specific renal defect in reabsorption of magnesium. Dialysis of patients may result in magnesium depletion if a low magnesium–content dialysate is used. High rates of production of aldosterone (hyperaldosteronism), hyperparathyroidism, and diabetes mellitus cause increased urinary magnesium losses. Alcoholism, intensive diuretic therapy, and treatment with the antibiotic gentamycin also result in increased urinary magnesium losses[20] (see box below).

Magnesium deficiency is often associated with hypocalcemia, and the signs and symptoms of magnesium deficiency normally are the signs of hypocalcemia. Although serum magnesium concentrations can be low, because magnesium is predominantly an intracellular mineral, serum measurements may not reflect intracellular concentrations. Red blood cell magnesium concentrations have been advocated as a measure of intracellular magnesium status.

CAUSES OF HYPERMAGNESEMIA

Magnesium sulfate therapy
Magnesium-containing antacids and purgatives
Renal failure

CAUSES OF HYPOMAGNESEMIA

Decreased intake of magnesium
  Steatorrhea
  Malabsorption syndromes
  Gut resections
  Specific intestinal malabsorption of magnesium
  Protein-calorie malnutrition
Increased loss of magnesium
  Renal tubular loss
  Dialysis with low magnesium dialysate
  Hyperaldosteronism
  Hyperparathyroidism
  Diabetes mellitus
  Alcoholism
  Diuretic therapy
  Aminoglycoside therapy

Phosphate (see Methods on CD-ROM)

Hyperphosphatemia. Hyperphosphatemia is most often the result of decreased renal excretion of phosphate anions as encountered in acute or chronic renal failure, particularly when the glomerular filtration rate is reduced to less than 25% of normal. Hyperphosphatemia can also result from an increased body phosphate load, which can in turn result from phosphate-containing laxatives and enemas, blood transfusions, or hyperalimentation, or as the result of massive cell destruction after cell lysis by cytotoxic therapy (the tumor lysis syndrome), or tissue injuries (hyperthermia, hypoxia, or crush injuries), which result in rhabdomyolysis and hemolysis. Increased renal tubular reabsorption of phosphate is responsible for the hyperphosphatemia seen in hypoparathyroidism, hyperthyroidism, hypogonadism, and growth hormone excess.

Hypophosphatemia. Moderate hypophosphatemia, which is defined as a serum phosphorus concentration between 10 and 25 mg/L in adults, is usually asymptomatic. In children, serum phosphorus concentrations below 40 mg/L are often considered abnormal. Hypophosphatemia may be caused by decreased intestinal absorption of phosphate or by increased urine losses of phosphate and an endogenous shift of inorganic phosphorus from extracellular to intracellular fluid compartments.

Calcitonin

Abnormal serum CT concentrations are rarely found (see box below). Serum measurements are most useful in patients suspected of having medullary thyroid carcinoma, a malignancy of the thyroid C-cells. This cancer is frequently seen in different members within families and is often associated with a tendency for other malignancies (termed *multiple endocrine neoplasia syndrome type II*).[84] Serum CT measurements are useful both in the screening of family members who are potentially at risk of developing the disease and in the follow-up examination of previously treated patients suspected of recurrent metastatic disease. Serum CT elevations are produced by a wide variety of other neoplasias, the most frequent one being bronchogenic carcinoma.[85] Because gastrin is a potent stimulus for CT secretion, serum CT concentrations are elevated in Zollinger-Ellison syndrome, a pancreatic tumor of gastrin-secreting

cells. Finally, CT excretion is decreased in patients with renal failure, and that decrease results in secondary elevation of serum concentrations of CT in these patients.

Because the thyroid gland is usually the sole source of CT production, athyroid patients lack circulating CT. CT levels are also decreased in some patients with osteoporosis. This may be caused by altered regulation of CT synthesis or release.[86]

Alkaline phosphatase (ALP) (see Methods on CD-ROM)

In clinical practice, ALP determinations measure a group of enzymes that catalyze the hydrolysis of phosphate esters in an alkaline medium.[87] Alkaline phosphatase is produced by many tissues (see the first box below), but only the portion produced by bone and liver is usually detected in serum from healthy persons. The second box below lists causes of abnormal serum bone alkaline phosphatase concentrations. Note that ALP lacks sensitivity and specificity for bone disease, particularly in patients with osteoporosis, when serum ALP is usually within reference ranges. Alkaline phosphatase is produced by osteoblasts and, as previously discussed, lowers bone pyrophosphate levels, which probably facilitates mineralization. Alkaline phosphatase synthesis is deficient in hypophosphatasia, a rare hereditary illness associated with undermineralized bones and pathological fractures, and achondroplasia, an inherited disorder of endochondral bone growth. Production is also decreased with generalized malnutrition or scurvy.

Far more common than decreased concentrations are diseases associated with elevated bone serum alkaline phos-

---

SOURCES OF ALKALINE PHOSPHATASE

Osteoblasts
Bile canalicular cells
Placenta
Leukocytes
Proximal renal tubule cells
Active mammary gland

BONE DISEASES ASSOCIATED WITH ABNORMAL SERUM ALKALINE PHOSPHATASE CONCENTRATIONS

Deficiency
  Hypophosphatasia
  Achondroplasia
  Severe malnutrition
  Scurvy
Excess
  Osteoblastic sarcoma
  Osteomalacia
  Paget's disease
  Hyperparathyroidism
  Growing children

DISEASES ASSOCIATED WITH ABNORMAL SERUM CALCITONIN CONCENTRATIONS

Deficiency
  Thyroid agenesis
  Thyroidectomy
  Osteoporosis
Excess
  Medullary thyroid carcinoma
  Bronchogenic carcinoma
  Zollinger-Ellison syndrome
  Renal failure

phatase concentrations. Such elevations signify increased osteoblastic activity, as seen in osteoblastic sarcoma, rickets, Paget's disease, and acromegaly. The elevated levels associated with hyperparathyroidism result from secondary bone mineralization rather than PTH-induced osteoclastic activity. Caution should be exercised when considering the pathological significance of alkaline phosphatase increases in childhood because growth is an important physiological cause of such elevations.[63] Liver alkaline phosphatase elevations reflect biliary obstruction and do not occur to any great extent with pure hepatocellular disease (see pp. 502-503).

Osteocalcin

Clinically, serum osteocalcin concentration is elevated in bone diseases characterized by increased osteoblastic activity including Paget's disease, osteomalacia, osteitis fibrosa, and renal osteodystrophy. Serum osteocalcin levels in these diseases correlate with other markers of bone formation, such as serum alkaline phosphatase and bone histomorphometry. Decreased serum concentrations of PTH, thyroid hormone, or growth hormone are associated with a decrease in the serum osteocalcin concentration, whereas the reverse is true; hyperparathyroidism, thyrotoxicosis, and acromegaly are associated with elevated serum osteocalcin concentrations. Puberty is associated with a rise in serum osteocalcin concentration, consistent with the increase in osteoblastic activity that accompanies the pubertal growth spurt and gonadal hormone surges. Circadian variation in serum osteocalcin concentration (peak levels at 4 AM and nadir at 5 PM) as well as in other serum markers of bone formation and resorption have been reported, but the etiology and

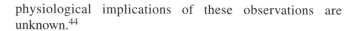

CONDITIONS ASSOCIATED WITH ELEVATED URINARY HYDROXYPROLINE CONCENTRATIONS

Paget's disease
Acromegaly
Osteomalacia
Rheumatoid arthritis
Neoplastic bone disease
Osteoporosis
Hyperthyroidism
Aseptic bone necrosis
Osteomyelitis
Chronic renal failure
Burns

physiological implications of these observations are unknown.[44]

Hydroxyproline (HP)

Collagen, which is present predominantly in bone and skin, is the sole source of the amino acid hydroxyproline, which, together with proline, makes up approximately one third of the total amino acid content of collagen. Collagen digestion, associated with either bone or skin breakdown, results in elevated urinary hydroxyproline (UHP) concentrations (see box above).[88] However, the determination of UHP concentration is not a specific test because sources of hydroxyproline include bone, diet, connective tissues, serum proteins, and degradation of propeptides from collagen biosynthesis. UHP correlates poorly with bone resorption as assessed by bone histomorphometric and calcium kinetic studies.[46]

References

1. Shipman P, Walker A, Bichell D, editors: *The human skeleton*, Cambridge, MA, 1985, Harvard University Press.
2. Ham AW, Cormack DH: *Histology*, ed 8, Philadelphia, 1979, Lippincott.
3. Chan GM: Calcium needs during childhood, *Pediatr Ann* 30:666, 2001.
4. National Osteoporosis Foundation: *Physicians guide to prevention and treatment of osteoporosis*, Belle Mead, NJ, 1999, Exerpta Medica.
5. Osteoporosis prevention, diagnosis, and therapy, *NIH Consens Statement* 17:1, 2000.
6. Steelman J, Zeitler P: Osteoporosis in pediatrics, *Pediatr Rev* 22:56, 2001.
7. Slemenda C et al: Role of physical activity in the development of skeletal mass in children, *J Bone Mineral Res* 6:1227, 1991.
8. Potts JT, Deftos LJ: Parathyroid hormone, calcitonin, vitamin D, bone and bone mineral metabolism. In Bondy PK, Rosenberg LE, editors: *Duncan's diseases of metabolism*, Philadelphia, 1974, Saunders.
9. Committee on Nutrition: Calcium requirements of infants, children, and adolescents, *Pediatrics* 104:1152, 1999.
10. Baylink DJ, Lin CC: The regulation of endosteal bone volume, *J Periodontol* 50:43, 1979.
11. Szulc P, Seeman E, Delmas PD: Biochemical measurements of bone turnover in children and adolescents, *Osteoporos Int* 11:281, 2000.
12. Looker AC et al: Clinical use of biochemical markers of bone remodeling: current states and future directions, *Osteoporos Int* 11:467, 2000.
13. Ganero P, Delmas PD: Biochemical markers of bone turnover. Applications for osteoporosis, *Endocrinol Metab Clin North Am* 27:303, 1998.
14. Seibel MJ, Lang M, Geilenkeuser: Interlaboratory variation of biochemical markers of bone turnover, *Clin Chem* 47:1143, 2001.
15. Fassbender WJ et al: Serum levels of immunoreactive bone sialoprotein in osteoporosis: positive relations to established biochemical parameters of bone turnover, *In Vivo* 14:619, 2000.
16. Avioli LV: Hormonal aspects of vitamin D metabolism and its clinical implications, *Clin Endocrinol Metab* 8:547, 1979.
17. Hollick MF et al: Photometabolism of 7-dehydrocholesterol to previtamin D_3 in skin, *Biochem Biophys Res Commun* 176:107, 1977.
18. Avioli LV, Haddad JG: Vitamin D: current concepts, *Metabolism* 22:507, 1973.
19. DeLuca HF: The kidney as an endocrine organ for production of 1,25-dihydroxyvitamin D_3, a calcium-mobilizing hormone, *N Engl J Med* 289:359, 1973.
20. Alkawa JK: *Magnesium: its biologic significance*, CRC series on cations of biological significance, Boca Raton, FL, 1981, CRC Press.
21. Tsang RC: Neonatal magnesium disturbances, *Am J Dis Child* 124:282, 1972.
22. Chesney RW et al: Serum 1,25-dihydroxyvitamin D levels in normal children and in vitamin D disorders, *Am J Dis Child* 134:135, 1980.
23. Chesney RW et al: Absence of seasonal variation in serum concentrations of 1,25-dihydroxyvitamin D despite a rise in 25-hydroxyvitamin D in summer, *J Clin Endocrinol Metab* 53:139, 1981.
24. DeLuca HF: The vitamin D system in the regulation of calcium and phosphorus metabolism, *Nutr Rev* 37:161, 1979.
25. Eisman JA et al: Modulation of plasma 1,25-dihydroxyvitamin D in man by stimulation and suppression tests, *Lancet* 2:931, 1979.

26. Gallagher JC et al: Intestinal calcium absorption and serum vitamin D metabolites in normal subjects and osteoporotic patients: effect of age and dietary calcium, *J Clin Invest* 64:729, 1979.

27. Kumar R et al: Elevated 1,25-dihydroxyvitamin D levels in normal human pregnancy and lactation, *J Clin Invest* 63:342, 1979.

28. Massry SG, Ritz E: The pathogenesis of secondary hyperparathyroidism of renal failure: is there a controversy? *Arch Intern Med* 138:853, 1978.

29. Singer FR et al: Paget's disease of bone. In Avioli LV, Krane SM, editors: *Metabolic bone disease*, vol 2, New York, 1978, Academic Press.

30. Strewler GJ: Mechanisms of disease: the physiology of parathyroid hormone-related protein, *N Engl J Med* 342:177, 2000.

31. Goldstein DA et al: Vitamin D metabolites and calcium metabolism in patients with nephrotic syndrome and normal renal function, *J Clin Endocrinol Metab* 52:116, 1981.

32. Austin LA, Heath H III: Calcitonin physiology and pathophysiology, *N Engl J Med* 304:269, 1981.

33. Huwler R et al: Plasma kinetics and urinary excretion of exogenous human and salmon calcitonin in man, *Am J Physiol* 236:15, 1979.

34. Ardaillou R: Kidney and calcitonin, *Nephron* 15:250, 1975.

35. Heersche JNM, Marcus R, Aurbach GD: Calcitonin and the formation of 3',5'-AMP in bone and kidney, *Endocrinology* 94:241, 1974.

36. Deftos LJ: Calcitonin. In Gray CH, James VHT, editors: *Hormones and blood*, New York, 1979, Academic Press.

37. Cooper CW: Recent advances with thyrocalcitonin, *Ann Clin Lab Sci* 6:119, 1976.

38. Chase L: Osteopenia, *Am J Med* 69:915, 1980.

39. Parfitt AM, Oliver I, Villanueva AR: Bone histology in metabolic bone disease: the diagnostic value of bone biopsy, *Orthop Clin North Am* 10:329, 1979.

40. Wallach S: Management of osteoporosis, *Hosp Pract* 13:91, 1978.

41. Gallagher JC et al: Intestinal calcium absorption and serum vitamin D metabolites in normal subjects and osteoporotic patients: effect of age and dietary calcium, *J Clin Invest* 64:729, 1979.

42. Slovik DM et al: Deficient production of 1,25-dihydroxyvitamin D in elderly osteoporotic subjects, *N Engl J Med* 305:372, 1981.

43. Gallagher JC et al: Effect of age on serum immunoreactive parathyroid hormone in normal and osteoporotic women, *J Lab Clin Med* 95:373, 1980.

44. Shamonki IM et al: Age-related changes of calcitonin secretion in females, *J Clin Endocrinol Metab* 50:437, 1980.

45. Ivey JL, Baylink DJ: Postmenopausal osteoporosis: proposed roles of defective coupling and estrogen deficiency, *Metab Bone Dis Rel Res* 3:3, 1981.

46. Avioli LV: Postmenopausal osteoporosis: prevention versus cure, *Fed Proc* 40:2418, 1981.

47. Gallaher JC, Riggs BL, DeLuca HF: Effect of estrogen on calcium absorption and serum vitamin D metabolites in postmenopausal osteoporosis, *J Clin Endocrinol Metab* 51:1359, 1980.

48. Lukert BP: Glucocorticoid and drug-induced osteoporosis. In Favus M, editor: *Primer on the metabolic bone diseases and disorders of mineral metabolism*, ed 3, Philadelphia, 1996, Lippincott-Raven.

49. Ziegler R, Kasperk C: Glucocorticoid-induced osteoporosis: prevention and treatment, *Steroids* 63:344, 1998.

50. Rackoff PJ, Rosen CJ: Pathogenesis and treatment of glucocorticoid-induced osteoporosis, *Drugs Aging* 12:477, 1998.

51. Lane NE, Jergas M, Genant HK: Osteoporosis and bone mineral assessment. In Koopman WJ, editor: *Arthritis and allied conditions*, ed 13, Baltimore, 1997, Williams & Wilkins.

52. Blake GM, Fogelman I: Applications of bone densitometry for osteoporosis, *Endocrinol Metab Clin North Am* 27:267, 1998.

53. Levis S, Altman R: Bone densitometry: clinical considerations, *Arthritis Theum* 41:577, 1998.

54. Prins SH et al: The role of quantitative ultrasound in the assessment of bone: a review, *Clin Physiol* 18:3, 1998.

55. Karpf DB et al: Prevention of nonvertebral fractures by alendronate. A meta-analysis. Alendronate Osteoporosis Treatment Study Groups, *JAMA* 277:1159, 1997.

56. Prostko M: Meta-analysis of prevention of nonvertebral fractures by alendronate, *JAMA* 278:631, 1997.

57. Eastell R: Treatment of postmenopausal osteoporosis, *N Neg J Med* 338:736, 1998.

58. McNagny SE: Prescribing hormone replacement therapy for menopausal symptoms, *Ann Intern Med* 131:605, 1999.

59. Chesnut CH et al: A randomized trial of nasal spray salmon calcitonin in postmenopausal women with established osteoporosis: the prevent recurrence of osteoporotic fractures study, *Am J Med* 109:267, 2000.

60. Hodsman AB et al: A randomized controlled trial to compare the efficacy of cyclical parathyroid hormone versus cyclical parathyroid hormone and sequential calcitonin to improve bone mass in postmenopausal women with osteoporosis *J Clin Endocrinol Metab* 82:620, 1997.

61. Neer RM et al: Recombinant human PTH [rhPTH(1-34)] reduces the risk of spine and non-spine fracture in postmenopausal osteoporosis. In *Endocrine Society's 82nd Annual Meeting*, Toronto, Ontario, 2000, Endocrine Society Press.

62. Bryant HU et al: Selective estrogen receptor modulators: an alternative to hormone replacement therapy, *Proc Soc Exp Biol Med* 217:45, 1998.

63. The role of calcium in peri- and postmenopausal women: consensus opinion of The North American Menopause Society, *Menopause* 8:84, 2001.

64. Avioli LV: Hormonal aspects of vitamin D metabolism and its clinical implications, *Clin Endocrinol Metab* 8:547, 1979.

65. Scriver CR et al: Serum 1,25-dihydroxyvitamin D levels in normal subjects and in patients with hereditary rickets and bone disease, *N Engl J Med* 299:976, 1978.

66. Brooks MH et al: Vitamin D–dependent rickets type II: resistance of target organs to 1,25-dihydroxyvitamin D, *N Engl J Med* 298:996, 1978.

67. Scriver C: Rickets and the pathogenesis of impaired tubular transport of phosphate and other solutes, *Am J Med* 57:43, 1974.

68. Drezner MK et al: Evaluation of a role for 1,25-dihydroxyvitamin D_3 in the pathogenesis and treatment of X-linked hypophosphatemic rickets and osteomalacia, *J Clin Invest* 66:1020, 1980.

69. Chesney RW et al: Serum 1,25-dihydroxyvitamin D levels in normal children and in vitamin D disorders, *Am J Dis Child* 134:135, 1980.

70. Steichen JJ et al: Elevated serum 1,25-dihydroxyvitamin D concentrations in rickets of very low–birth-weight infants, *J Pediatr* 99:293, 1981.

71. Chesney RW et al: Circulating vitamin D metabolite concentrations in childhood renal diseases, *Kidney Int* 21:65, 1982.

72. Singer FR: Human calcitonin treatment of Paget's disease of bone, *Clin Orthop* 127:86, 1977.

73. Kooh SW et al: Pathogenesis of rickets in chronic hepatobiliary disease in children, *J Pediatr* 94:870, 1979.

74. Drezner MK, Neelon FA, Jowsey J: Hypoparathyroidism: a possible cause of osteomalacia, *J Clin Endocrinol Metab* 45:114, 1977.

75. Drezner MK, Neelon FA, Haussler M: 1,25-Dihydroxycholecalciferol deficiency: the probable cause of hypocalcemia and metabolic bone disease in pseudohypoparathyroidism, *J Clin Endocrinol Metab* 42:621, 1976.

76. Juttmann JR et al: Serum concentrations of vitamin D in patients with chronic renal failure: consequences for the treatment with 1-α-hydroxy derivatives, *Clin Endocrinol* 14:225, 1981.

77. Chesney RW et al: Serum 1,25-dihydroxyvitamin D levels in normal children and in vitamin D disorders, *Am J Dis Child* 34:135, 1980.

78. Kumar R et al: Elevated 1,25-dihydroxyvitamin D levels in normal pregnancy and lactation, *J Clin Invest* 63:342, 1979.

79. Tsang RC, Brown DR: The parathyroids. In Kelley V, editor: *Practice of pediatrics*, vol 1, New York, 1979, Harper & Row.

80. Tsang RC, Venkataraman P: Pediatric parathyroid and vitamin D–related disorders. In Kaplan LA, editor: *Clinical pediatric and adolescent endocrinology*, Philadelphia, 1982, Saunders.

81. Taylor AB, Stern PH, Bell NH: Abnormal regulation of circulating 25-hydroxyvitamin D in the Williams syndrome, *N Engl J Med* 306:972, 1982.

82. Juan D: Hypocalcemia differential diagnosis and mechanisms, *Arch Intern Med* 139:1166, 1979.

83. Broadus AE: Nephrogenous cyclic AMP, *Recent Prog Horm Res* 37:665, 1981.

84. Grace K, Spiler IJ, Tashjian AH, Jr: Natural history of familial medullary thyroid carcinoma: effect of a program for early diagnosis, *N Engl J Med* 229:980, 1978.

85. Silva OL, Brode LE, Doppman JL: Calcitonin as a marker for bronchogenic cancer, *Cancer* 44:680, 1979.

86. McTaggert H et al: Deficient calcitonin response to calcium stimulation in post-menopausal osteoporosis, *Lancet* 1:475, 1982.

87. Kaplan M: Alkaline phosphatase, *N Engl J Med* 286:200, 1972.

88. Niejadlik DC: Hydroxyproline, *Postgrad Med* 51:214, 1972.

Bibliography

Broadus AE, Stewart AF: Parathyroid hormone-related protein: structure, processing and physiologic actions. In Bilezikian JP, editor: *Parathyroids: basic and clinical concepts*, New York, 2001, Raven Press.

Christakos S, Gabrielides C, Rhoten W: Vitamin D–dependent calcium binding proteins: chemistry, distribution, functional considerations, and molecular biology, *Endocr Rev* 10:3, 1989.

Favus M, editor: *Primer on the metabolic bone diseases and disorders of mineral metabolism*, ed 2, New York, 1993, Raven Press.

Itani O, Tsang R: Calcium, phosphorus and magnesium in the newborn: pathophysiology and management. In Hay W, editor: *Neonatal nutrition and metabolism*, St Louis, 1991, Mosby.

Itani O, Tsang RC: Calcium and mineral metabolism in the fetus. In Thorburn GD, Harding R, editors: *Textbook of fetal physiology*, Oxford, UK, 1994, Oxford University Press.

Mughal M, Tsang R: Calcium, phosphorus, and magnesium transport across the placenta. In Polin RA, Fox WW, editors: *Fetal and neonatal physiology*, vol 2, ed 2, Philadelphia, 1998, Saunders.

Schrier RS, editor: *Renal and electrolyte disorders*, ed 5, Boston, 1997, Little, Brown.

Tsang R, editor: *Calcium and magnesium metabolism in early life*, Boca Raton, FL, 1995, CRC Press.

Internet Sites

General

http://pathophysiology.uams.edu

http://www.ectsoc.org/review.htm

www.meddean.luc.edu—Loyola University Medical Education Network

Osteoporosis

www.nof.org—National Osteoporosis Foundation

www.osteo.org—NIH Osteoporosis and Bone Related Disease

www.learn-about-osteoporosis.com—Osteoporosis & Women's Health

www.nos.org.uk—National Osteoporosis Society

Osteomalacia

http://uwcme.org—University of Washington CME credits for a fee

Osteitis Fibrosa

www.nlm.nih.gov—NIH MEDLINE plus Medical Encyclopedia

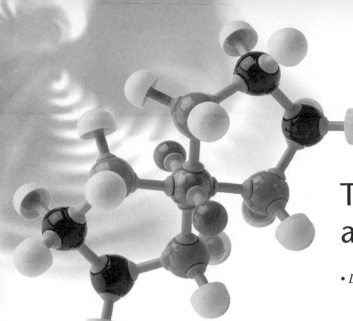

CHAPTER 29

The Pancreas: Function and Chemical Pathology*

• D. Robert Dufour

Chapter Outline

Anatomy
Endocrine physiology
Exocrine physiology
  Normal pancreatic exocrine secretions
  Normal pancreatic fluid secretions
  Control of exocrine pancreatic secretions
Pathological conditions

Endocrine pancreatic disorders
Inflammatory or necrotic pancreatic injury
Destructive disorders
Pancreatic function tests
  Tests for volumes or analytes in pancreatic fluid
  Pancreatic infections
  Pancreatic neoplasms

Objectives

- Describe the anatomy of the pancreas.
- Describe the normal endocrine (islets) and exocrine (digestive) physiology of the pancreas.
- Describe the factors controlling normal exocrine pancreatic secretions.
- List the major disease groups of the endocrine and exocrine pancreas and how they affect laboratory measurements made on body fluids.
- Discuss exocrine pancreatic insufficiency, its causes, clinical findings, and specific changes that occur in clinical laboratory tests.

- Outline the presumed causes of acute pancreatitis, the clinical findings, the factors portending a poor prognosis, and the effects on serum and urine tests.
- Discuss cystic fibrosis and the laboratory tests, especially those of pancreatic function, that aid in the diagnosis of this disease.
- Briefly discuss pancreatic adenocarcinoma, its prognosis, and tests that are used to follow disease progression.
- Outline the current knowledge of islet cell tumors and the role of the laboratory in their diagnosis.

Key Terms

acinar From the Latin word *acinus*, meaning "berry" or "grape." In anatomy, the term refers to a small sacklike dilation and is accented on the first syllable.

adenocarcinoma A malignant growth that begins in the epithelial cells; for the pancreas, it affects the cells that line the pancreatic ductules and duct. Nearly all pancreatic cancers are adenocarcinoma.

ampulla of Vater A flasklike dilation at the point where the biliary and pancreatic ducts join. The ampulla joins the duodenal papilla (a nipple-shaped structure), and its orifice is encircled by a ring of smooth muscles called the "sphincter of Oddi." Note that the ampulla and the sphincter are two distinct structures.

---

*With acknowledgment to the previous author, John A. Lott.

cachexia   A state of progressive weakness, loss of appetite, malnutrition, and weight loss that is observed in some chronic disorders, such as advanced cancer.

cholecystitis   Inflammation of the gallbladder.

cholecystokinin (CCK)   A gastrointestinal hormone that is released when the duodenum is distended after ingestion of food or alcohol. It is a powerful secretagogue for the pancreas, producing a high-volume secretion that is high in bicarbonate concentration but low in proteins and enzymes. CCK and secretin potentiate each other's actions.

endoscopic retrograde cholangiopancreatography (ERCP)   An invasive diagnostic technique whereby the pancreatic duct is cannulated and an x-ray contrast medium is injected into the duct to visualize the biliary and pancreatic ducts.

enterokinase   An enzyme produced by the mucosa of the small intestine that converts the inactive, digestive proenzymes from the pancreas into their active forms.

gastrin   A hormone produced primarily by the G-cells of the stomach that stimulates the secretion of HCl by the parietal cells in the stomach. Plasma gastrin is greatly increased in Zollinger-Ellison syndrome, usually a pancreatic neoplasm, but gastrin is not normally produced by the pancreas.

glucagon   An islet cell hormone that has multiple actions to raise plasma glucose.

hypoglycemia   A low blood glucose concentration, generally <2.8 mmol/L (<500 mg/L), causing some individuals to become symptomatic.

immunoreactive trypsin   A form of the digestive enzyme found in blood. Because of the presence of potent antiproteases in blood, the enzyme must be measured in serum as a protein. It has little or no enzymatic activity in blood.

insulin   An islet cell, anabolic hormone that controls glucose uptake, fat synthesis, and synthesis of proteins.

islets of Langerhans   Clusters of cells in the pancreas that produce the endocrine secretions of the gland. They constitute about 1% of the pancreatic mass.

laparoscopy   A technique used to view the pancreas or any other abdominal organ. A small incision is made in the abdomen to allow the insertion of the viewing instrument. It is probably the most objective and reliable method for diagnosing pancreatitis.

multiple endocrine neoplasias (MEN)   An autosomal dominant inherited disorder that has many different clinical presentations. Type I MEN disorder often involves the pancreas and other endocrine organs, particularly the pituitary and parathyroid glands.

pancreatic duct   A conduit that passes through the pancreas, collects the pancreatic exocrine secretions of enzymes, water, and electrolytes, and carries them to the ampulla of Vater.

pancreatic polypeptide   An islet cell hormone (PP) that slows the absorption of food, stimulates gastric and intestinal secretions, and inhibits intestinal mobility.

proteolytic   Having the ability to break down proteins to peptides and amino acids.

secretin   A gastrointestinal hormone that is released when the duodenum is distended after ingestion of food or alcohol. It is a powerful secretagogue for the pancreas, producing a secretion high in protein and enzymes but low in volume.

somatostatin   An islet cell hormone that has largely inhibitory effects on insulin and glucagon secretion, gastric secretions, and exocrine pancreatic secretions.

trypsin   A potent proteolytic enzyme produced in the pancreas but stored there in zymogen granules as the enzymatically inactive protrypsin form.

trypsinogen   The enzymatically inactive or zymogen form of trypsin; also called *protrypsin*.

vagus nerve   The tenth cranial nerve that carries motor, sensory, and autonomic nerve fibers to the neck, thorax, and abdomen, including the pancreas (see also Fig. 30-3). Vagal stimulation of the pancreas causes release of pancreatic fluid that is high in enzymes but low in volume and electrolytes.

vasoactive intestinal peptide (VIP)   A hormone that can be produced by pancreatic islet tumors. It stimulates production of profuse diarrhea and is associated with hypokalemia and non–anion gap metabolic acidosis.

Zollinger-Ellison syndrome   The clinical picture of a patient with a gastrinoma (frequently malignant) in the pancreas, duodenum, or both. It causes excessive acid production in the stomach, typically producing multiple peptic ulcers and diarrhea.

zymogen granules   The storage form of the digestive enzymes in the pancreatic acinar cells. Some of the enzymes, especially the **proteolytic** and lipolytic forms, are present as their zymogens or inactive precursors.

Methods on CD-ROM

Amylase
Chloride
Fat absorption

Gastric fluid analysis
Lipase

ANATOMY

The pancreas is an elongated, flattened pyramidal organ, located mostly behind the stomach; the tail points to the spleen, and the head is nestled in the duodenal loop (Fig. 29-1). This soft, easily traumatized gland lies behind the peritoneum, the serous membrane lining the abdominal cavity. Blood from the pancreas drains into the portal vein; pancreatic islet cell hormones (such as insulin and glucagon) are both active in and metabolized by the liver. The exocrine acini (Fig. 29-2) are drained by ductules that combine into a single **pancreatic duct**; in most individuals this duct joins the common bile duct at the **ampulla of Vater**. The latter opens through the duodenal papilla, the orifice of which is encircled by the

sphincter of Oddi, so that pancreatic exocrine secretions can flow into the gastrointestinal tract.[1] Except when pancreatic fluid is secreted, the sphincter is tightly closed, preventing stomach and duodenal contents from reaching the pancreas. Exocrine **acinar** cells and their associated structures account for more than 98% of the pancreatic mass.

About 1% of the pancreas consists of unique cell clusters, the **islets of Langerhans**, that produce endocrine hormones. A normal pancreas contains 1 to 2 million islets (Fig. 29-3).[2] Nerve fibers in pancreatic tissue stimulate production of **vasoactive intestinal peptide (VIP)**, substance P, somatostatin, enkephalin-related peptides, and bombesin-like peptides (see also p. 553).

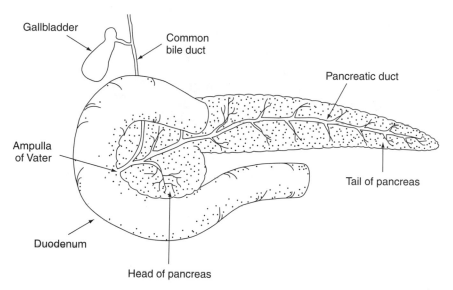

Fig. 29-1 Structure of pancreas, including nearby organs. The pancreatic duct carries the exocrine secretions to the ampulla of Vater, where it empties into the duodenum at the sphincter of Oddi. Notice that the sphincter is closed except during periods of secretion. The common bile duct usually joins the pancreatic duct before the latter reaches the duodenum.

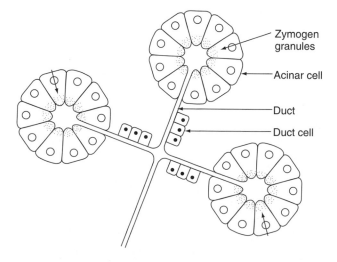

Fig. 29-2 Diagram of acinar cells and associated ductules. The exocrine acini terminate with a collection of acinar cells that contain zymogen granules; the latter contain the proenzymes and other digestive enzymes described in Fig. 29-4. Special cells line the ductules that secrete fluid and electrolytes, especially bicarbonate.

Cell type		Hormone produced	Percentage of islet cells producing hormone
Alpha	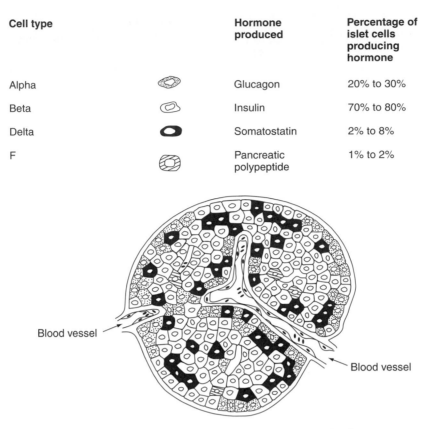	Glucagon	20% to 30%
Beta		Insulin	70% to 80%
Delta		Somatostatin	2% to 8%
F		Pancreatic polypeptide	1% to 2%

Blood vessel

Blood vessel

Fig. 29-3 Diagram of an islet of Langerhans. At least four types of cells secrete hormones into the blood. Most of the cells (beta-cells) produce insulin, while only a small fraction are F cells, which produce pancreatic polypeptide. *(Adapted from Unger RH, Orci L: Glucagon and the A cell: physiology and pathophysiology (first of two parts),* N Engl J Med *304:1518, 1981. Copyright 1981, Massachusetts Medical Society. All rights reserved.)*

ENDOCRINE PHYSIOLOGY

Pancreatic endocrine secretion from the islets of Langerhans includes the hormones glucagon from the alpha-cells, insulin from the beta-cells, somatostatin from the delta-cells, and pancreatic polypeptide from the F cells. The action and control of these hormones are summarized in Table 29-1.[3] Gastrin was once believed to be present in the normal pancreas; however, the current contention holds that, normally, gastrin originates only from the G cells in the stomach.[4]

Alpha-cells, constituting 20% to 30% of the islet cells, produce **glucagon**, a hormone that increases plasma glucose concentrations (see Chapter 32); it has a half-life in blood of 5 to 10 minutes. The release of glucagon is stimulated by the factors shown in Table 29-1.

Beta-cells (60% to 70% of islet cells) produce **proinsulin**, which consists of A and B chains and the C-peptide (see Chapter 32). **Insulin** is stored in secretory granules; when plasma glucose is high, these particles migrate to the cell wall and are released by exocytosis. Proinsulin is normally converted to insulin, C-peptide, and other proteins before release, although a small amount is normally found in plasma. Insulin has a half-life of about 10 to 25 minutes. C-peptide has no insulin-like action but can be measured in

plasma to evaluate beta-cell function, even in persons receiving insulin (which does not contain the C-peptide).

Delta-cells, constituting about 2% to 8% of islet cells, produce **somatostatin**, a hormone that inhibits the action of insulin and of gastrin, inhibits the secretion of exocrine pancreatic enzymes, and decreases the flow of bile. Somatostatin plays a role in glucose metabolism by inhibiting insulin secretion; an abnormal increase of somatostatin may lead to diabetes mellitus. Somatostatin is also produced in other sites, notably the hypothalamus, and is important in inhibiting growth hormone production. The F cells produce **pancreatic polypeptide (PP)**, a hormone that stimulates gastric and intestinal enzyme secretion and inhibits intestinal motility.

EXOCRINE PHYSIOLOGY
Normal Pancreatic Exocrine Secretions

The pancreas produces at least 22 digestive enzymes, 15 of which are proteases, that act on three major sources of energy: proteins, digested by the enzymes **trypsin**, chymotrypsin, and elastase; lipids, digested by the enzymes lipase, phospholipase A_2, and cholesterol esterase; and complex carbohydrates, digested by α-amylase.[5] The functional units of the exocrine pancreas consist of clusters of acini that store

TABLE 29-1	NORMAL PANCREATIC ISLET CELL HORMONES			
Cell of Origin	**Hormone**	**Release Stimulated By:**	**Release Inhibited By:**	**Hormone Causes:**
Alpha	Glucagon (3500*)	Low plasma glucose, sympathetic nervous system, epinephrine, any factors lowering plasma glucose	Somatostatin, glucose, secretin, insulin	Increased plasma glucose by stimulating hepatic glycogenolysis, gluconeogenesis; adipose tissue lipolysis; mobilizes amino acids
Beta	Proinsulin (11,500*) Insulin (5734*) C-peptide (3000*)	Plasma glucose above 1000 mg/L, keto acids, arginine, leucine, sympathetic and parasympathetic nervous system stimulation, gastric inhibitory polypeptide, gastrin, secretin, CCK, glucagon, cortisol, growth hormone, thyroxine, progesterone, sex hormones, sulfonylureas	Alpha-adrenergic agonists, somatostatin, insulin, thiazide diuretics, phenytoin	Glucose uptake by liver, muscle, adipose tissue; inhibition of gluconeogenesis; glycogen formation; fat synthesis and storage; inhibition of mobilization and oxidation of fats; conversion of glucose to fatty acids or cholesterol; production of acetyl CoA; synthesis of proteins; inhibition of protein breakdown; increased RNA synthesis, entry of K, phosphate, Mg into muscle and liver cells
Delta	Somatostatin (1640*)	Food intake, increased plasma glucose, arginine, leucine, CCK	Unknown	Inhibition of insulin and glucagon release, inhibition of gastric and exocrine pancreatic secretions
F	Pancreatic polypeptide (2400*)	Food intake, especially protein; fasting; exercise; hypoglycemia	Hyperglycemia	Decreased rate of food absorption, stimulation of gastric and intestinal enzyme secretion, inhibition of intestinal mobility

CCK, Cholecystokinin.
*Molecular weight in daltons.

most of the digestive enzymes in inactive forms (zymogens, in **zymogen granules**); the free enzymes are not normally present in the acinar cell cytoplasm (see Fig. 29-2). The granules are released from the acinar cells by exocytosis into the collecting ductules and finally reach the pancreatic duct. Ribonuclease, deoxyribonuclease, cholesterol esterase, amylase, lipase, and colipase are the only digestive enzymes produced in their active forms.

Fig. 29-4 illustrates the modification of exocrine digestive enzymes from zymogen granules in the acinar cells to their active forms after entry into the duodenal lumen. The potent proteolytic enzymes trypsin, chymotrypsin, carboxypeptidase A and B, and elastase constitute more than 75% of the mass of the digestive enzymes secreted. The proenzyme forms of the proteolytic enzymes contain a small amino acid chain that blocks their proteolytic site. This propitious arrangement of nature prevents the autodigestion of the zymogen granules, the acinar cells, and of course the pancreas itself.

The pancreas also secretes protease inhibitors to neutralize any prematurely activated enzymes.

Upon entering the duodenum, **enterokinase** (also called *enteropeptidase*), a duodenal peptidase that is active at acid pH, cleaves off the small amino acid chains from the proenzymes, converting protrypsin to active trypsin. Free trypsin activates the other proenzymes in a cascade or chain reaction–like fashion and, to a small degree, protrypsin itself (see Fig. 29-4).

Normal Pancreatic Fluid Secretions

A normal adult weighing 75 kg produces about 2 to 3 liters of water-clear, colorless pancreatic juice per day, containing the proenzymes and enzymes described above and 120 to 300 mmol/day of bicarbonate. Amylase and lipase, for example, are present in pancreatic juice in activities of about 500,000 to 1 million U/L,[2,6] with an approximately 10,000:1 gradient in the enzyme activities between pancreatic fluid and plasma. Damage to the pancreas can thus produce

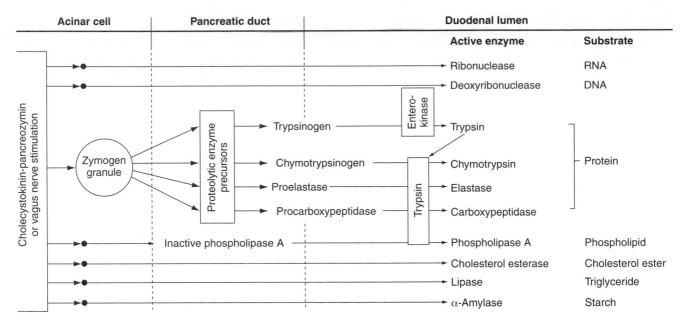

Fig. 29-4   The pancreatic enzymes and their conversion to active forms in the duodenum. The enzymes are stored in zymogen granules that reach the pancreatic duct by exocytosis. Upon reaching the duodenum, the proenzymes are converted to their active form by enterokinase and to a lesser extent by trypsin.

considerable increases in plasma activities of amylase, lipase, trypsin, and other digestive enzymes. The principal cations in pancreatic fluid, totaling about 150 mmol/L, are Na^+, K^+, Ca^{++}, and Mg^{++}. The principal anions are bicarbonate (120 mmol/L) and Cl^- (30 mmol/L).

Water and electrolytes in pancreatic fluid are secreted by the ductal and centroacinar cells. The healthy pancreas can secrete bicarbonate into the pancreatic juice and hydrogen ions into blood. There is normally more than enough pancreatic bicarbonate to neutralize the acid coming from the stomach; this is critical, since the activity of pancreatic enzymes is inhibited at acid pH.

Control of Exocrine Pancreatic Secretions

Exocrine secretions from the pancreas have both neural and hormonal controls, as summarized in Table 29-2.[4,7,8] Three upper gastrointestinal tract hormones—**cholecystokinin (CCK)**, **secretin**, and **gastrin**—affect pancreatic juice secretion; they are discussed more fully in Chapter 30. Distention of the duodenum by food or by ethanol leads to the release of all three hormones. Fat and ethanol are particularly active stimulators of secretin production. A negative-feedback loop exists; trypsin released as a consequence of CCK activity has an inhibitory action on further CCK secretion.[9] VIP is structurally similar to secretin and glucagon; this probably

TABLE 29-2   FACTORS THAT CONTROL THE NORMAL EXOCRINE PANCREATIC SECRETIONS

Event or Release of Factor	Result
Vagal nerve stimulation of pancreas	Secretion of fluid high in protein and enzymes (such as trypsin), low in bicarbonate, low in volume; release of pancreatic polypeptide
Distension of duodenum by food; alcohol ingestion	CCK and gastrin secretion by duodenum
CCK or gastrin release	Release of zymogen granules from acinar cells; secretion of fluid high in protein and enzymes, low in bicarbonate, low in volume; release of pancreatic polypeptide
Secretin release	Secretion of fluid high in bicarbonate and volume but low in enzymes
Fatty acids or acid food ingestion	CCK release
Amino acids or Ca^{++} ingestion	CCK, gastrin release
Vasoinhibitory polypeptide (VIP) release	Secretin-like effect on gland
Somatostatin release	Inhibition of basal pancreatic secretions, increased fecal fat, decreased intestinal mobility
Trypsin in duodenum	Inhibition of CCK release
Thyroid hormone release	Maintenance of normal pancreatic function and response to stimuli

CCK, Cholecystokinin.

explains the similar action of VIP on the pancreas. All pancreatic exocrine secretions and other gastrointestinal functions are inhibited by somatostatin.

PATHOLOGICAL CONDITIONS

Diseases of the pancreas can be broadly grouped into islet cell disorders such as diabetes mellitus (insulin deficiency) and glucagon excess; exocrine insufficiency, producing pancreatic insufficiency and associated malabsorption; inflammatory disorders such as acute or chronic pancreatitis; and neoplastic disorders such as **adenocarcinomas** and islet cell tumors, which may lead to bile duct obstruction if the mass occurs in the head of the pancreas. The emphasis here is on those disorders associated with chemical changes in body fluids or abnormal chemical responses to certain stimuli. Interpretation of laboratory tests is one of the major tools used in defining pancreatic diseases. A carefully obtained history and physical examination may suggest pancreatic disease; imaging techniques such as **endoscopic retrograde cholangiopancreatography** (**ERCP**), ultrasonography, computerized tomography, and magnetic resonance imaging are also of great importance. Estimating pancreatic size by imaging methods is important in suspected acute pancreatitis, because an inflamed, edematous gland is generally larger than normal. Mass lesions can usually be diagnosed only by imaging, and chronic pancreatitis is typically associated with calcification in the region of the pancreas. Laparotomy or **laparoscopy** with visual observation and palpation are useful in defining pancreatic anatomy.

Endocrine Pancreatic Disorders

Diabetes mellitus. The major endocrine disorder is diabetes mellitus (DM), discussed more fully in Chapter 32. Diabetes mellitus is usually caused by islet cell destruction (type 1) or insulin resistance (most type 2 diabetes). Chronic inflammation of the pancreas (as in chronic pancreatitis), pancreatic resection, or drugs toxic to the islets (such as pentamidine) are rare causes of DM. Laboratory findings in DM are discussed fully in Chapter 32. An abnormal serum amylase in the absence of pancreatitis is common in uncontrolled DM, especially in the presence of diabetic ketoacidosis. Typically, the increase is due to high levels of salivary amylase. Transplantation of the pancreas (often along with renal transplantation) is currently being used with excellent success for patients with DM and end-stage renal disease (see Chapter 50). With whole organ transplantation, exocrine pancreatic function is unnecessary and can cause destruction of normal tissue if the enzymes are not eliminated from the body. For this reason, the pancreatic duct in a transplanted gland is usually attached to the bladder. Measurement of urinary amylase is a good test of graft function, and can be used to monitor evidence of graft rejection (which will cause decreased urine amylase excretion). When intestinal drainage is used, measurement of serum lipase is helpful in assessing graft function.[10]

Insulinoma. One of the less common causes of **hypoglycemia** is overproduction of insulin by a tumor of the pancreatic islets, termed an *insulinoma*. Insulinomas are typically small, benign tumors that can be difficult to locate by imaging procedures. Hypoglycemia is most commonly the result of an imbalance between glucose ingestion or production and medications in patients with diabetes. Among patients who do not have diabetes, hypoglycemia often occurs in ill patients because of shock, renal failure, liver failure, and endocrine diseases such as adrenal insufficiency and hypopituitarism.[11] In otherwise healthy individuals, excess insulin production or ingestion is usually the cause of hypoglycemia and requires careful evaluation of the patient. The initial workup of hypoglycemia in such persons involves a period of fasting (24 to 72 hours), with frequent determinations of blood glucose. If the person becomes hypoglycemic (plasma glucose <400 mg/L [2.2 mmol/L]), samples should be collected for insulin and C-peptide measurement. Insulin levels are best reported as a ratio of insulin to glucose, with glucose reported in mg/dL and insulin in U/L; a ratio above 0.3 indicates inappropriate insulin production. In insulinoma, the ratio is increased along with elevated C-peptide, whereas exogenous insulin administration causes a high ratio but undetectable C-peptide. Ingestion of oral insulin secretagogues, which can produce a pattern similar to that of insulinoma, can be detected by screening for their presence in urine or serum.

Glucagonoma. Tumors that produce glucagon almost always arise in the pancreas and present with a distinctive combination of hyperglycemia, weight loss, and a peculiar skin rash that often calls attention to the presence of the tumor. Most cases occur in adults older than 40. Diagnosis depends on measurement of plasma glucagon; the upper reference limit is 200 pg/mL, but 70% to 90% of glucagonoma cases show glucagon levels greater than 1000 pg/mL. Although increased glucagon also occur in conditions such as renal failure, starvation, pancreatitis, and other endocrine diseases, glucagon levels are rarely above 500 pg/mL in these disorders (although they may be over 1000 pg/mL in cirrhosis).[12] Most glucagon-producing tumors are very large at the time of diagnosis, and the majority behave in a malignant fashion.

Somatostatinoma. Tumors of the pancreas (or, less frequently, the intestine) can produce excess somatostatin.[13] These tumors usually occur in older adults (average age of onset is about 50), and they are somewhat more common in women. The most common clinical features are nonspecific and include glucose intolerance or diabetes, gallbladder disease, and diarrhea (often with steatorrhea). However, these symptoms are much more likely to be present with intestinal tumors than with pancreatic tumors, in which these symptoms occur in a minority of cases, and an endocrine tumor is usually not suspected until the tumor is removed and examined histologically. Within the pancreas, the tumors are often large and malignant and predominantly arise in the head of the pancreas (in contrast to most other endocrine tumors), where they may produce bile duct obstruction. Because the tumors are usually malignant, plasma somatostatin levels are typically elevated even after surgery. Excess

TABLE 29-3   PROPOSED EVENTS IN THE DEVELOPMENT OF ACUTE PANCREATITIS

Event	Likely Causes
Injury to acinar cell membranes	Reflux of bile or pancreatic juice into pancreas, alcoholic irritation of duodenum or precipitation of protein plugs in gland, infection or inflammation in gallbladder spreading to pancreas, viral and other microbiological infections of pancreas, ischemia, circulatory failure, trauma, surgery
Biochemical changes in gland	Activation of proenzymes such as protrypsin, proelastase, prophospholipase A_2 to their biochemically active forms; occlusion of pancreatic ductules or duct; conversion of kallikreinogen to kallikrein
Edema, swelling of pancreatic capsule	Inflammation of gland, disturbance of gland's afferent or efferent blood flow
Tetany and cardiac arrhythmias, respiratory distress	Peripancreatic fat necrosis, Ca^{++} sequestration by fatty acids, refractory hypocalcemia, unknown toxic substance(s) (phospholipase A_2?) acting on lung and other organs
Hemorrhagic necrosis of gland, shock, circulatory collapse, profound reduction of plasma volume	Autolysis and digestion of gland with bleeding into retroperitoneal space, release of hypotensive kinins, cytotoxic effect of lysolecithin (from bile)
Death	Acute circulatory and respiratory failure, refractory hypotension

CLINICAL PROBLEMS ASSOCIATED WITH ABDOMINAL PAIN AND ELEVATED PANCREATIC ENZYMES

Pancreatitis, perforated stomach ulcer, mesenteric artery infarction, biliary tract disorders, an inflamed gallbladder, gangrenous gallbladder, inflammation or obstruction anywhere along the gastrointestinal tract or abdominal cavity, an abscess anywhere in the abdomen, peritonitis, renal failure, volvulus, dissecting aortic aneurysm, diabetic ketoacidosis, connective tissue disorders with vasculitis, ectopic pregnancy, inflammation of the fallopian tubes[7]

production of other hormones (such as insulin, calcitonin, and gastrin) is common.

PPoma. Tumors producing pancreatic polypeptide are uncommon and usually asymptomatic. As with somatostatinomas, they are usually large, malignant tumors found in the head of the pancreas, often presenting as a mass or with obstructive jaundice, with diagnosis becoming apparent only at the time of resection.[13] Elevation of PP levels and levels of other hormones such as chromogranins are usually present even after surgery; these can be used as tumor markers to follow success of therapy.

Gastrinoma, VIPoma. Tumors producing gastrin and VIP almost always arise in the pancreas. Excess production of gastrin produces **Zollinger-Ellison syndrome**, whereas excess production of VIP produces the syndrome of watery diarrhea, hypokalemia, and achlorhydria (WDHA). Since the manifestations of these tumors are primarily intestinal, they are discussed in Chapter 30.

Inflammatory or Necrotic Pancreatic Injury

Acute pancreatitis. Acute pancreatitis can be a life-threatening emergency; it must be distinguished from other disorders with a similar presentation. The box at left lists several of the leading differential diagnoses of patients with abdominal pain and generally abnormal pancreatic enzymes.[5]

Severe, knife-like pain associated with nausea and vomiting is a common presenting feature in acute pancreatitis. The disease varies from a mild, self-limiting, edematous form to full-blown necrotizing, hemorrhagic pancreatitis that is often fatal.[14] Any factors that obstruct the pancreatic afferent (incoming) or efferent (outgoing) blood supply, the pancreatic ducts, or the ampulla of Vater can precipitate pancreatitis. A proposed mechanism for the evolution of pancreatitis is shown in Table 29-3, though the precise factors leading to pancreatitis are unknown. Leading causes of pancreatitis are alcohol abuse and biliary tract diseases, especially cholelithiasis. A history of alcohol abuse or biliary tract diseases is present in about 75% of patients with pancreatitis; other important causes are listed in the box below.

Alcohol has a double effect of stimulating pancreatic secretion and at the same time irritating the duodenal

CAUSES OF ACUTE PANCREATITIS

Alcoholism, biliary tract diseases, surgery to the pancreas or nearby organs, atherosclerotic plaques in the pancreatic arteries, abdominal trauma, post-ERCP as a complication, metabolic disorders such as hypertriglyceridemia (especially with triglyceride concentrations above 10,000 mg/L), and infections

Drugs associated with or possibly causing pancreatitis include azathioprine, cimetidine, cytarabine, didanosine, estrogens, furosemide, 6-mercaptopurine, methyldopa, metronidazole, nitrofurantoin, pentamidine, sulfonamides, sulindac, tetracycline, and valproic acid.

mucosa, possibly to the point of occluding the pancreatic duct or the duodenal sphincter. There may even be alcohol-generated protein plugs in the pancreatic ductules that lead to pancreatic obstruction.

Although autopsy studies indicate that a stone or obstructing tumor in the common bile duct can lead to the reflux of bile into the pancreas, which may lead to pancreatitis, these are infrequent causes of the disorder. Rather, gallstones tend to promote the development of **cholecystitis** that spreads to and inflames the pancreas. Gallstone pancreatitis is especially common in older adult women. Routine laboratory tests can often suggest that gallstones are the etiology; whereas ALT is increased to over 150 U/L in 91% of cases of gallstone pancreatitis, it is increased to this level in only 17% of other causes of pancreatitis.[15] Patients with very high triglycerides (>10,000 mg/L) are also at increased risk for developing pancreatitis.

A number of drugs listed earlier in the box *Causes of Acute Pancreatitis* are linked to pancreatitis, occasionally causing the disorder. There are many other drugs with a less-clear association with pancreatitis.[16]

Prevalence of pancreatitis. Inflammatory diseases of the pancreas, including acute pancreatitis, pancreatic pseudocyst, and pancreatic abscess, are uncommon. In one series,[17] pancreatitis was suspected in 1800 patients because of abdominal pain or other suggestive symptoms, and serum amylase and lipase were ordered; of these, 188 patients had abnormal results reported from either or both tests, and only 25 (1.4%) had confirmed inflammatory pancreatic disease. Nevertheless, establishing a correct diagnosis of pancreatitis is important, given the potentially fatal outcome; the death rate from pancreatitis is about 1.5 per 100,000 population.

Pathogenesis of pancreatitis. A likely mechanism in the pathogenesis of acute pancreatitis is the activation of protrypsin within the gland by reflux of pancreatic fluid, pancreatic hypoxia, viral infections, endotoxins, trauma, and other factors. The release of active enzymes in the gland results in a self-digestive attack on the gland's structure and blood vessels. Lysosomal enzymes such as cathepsin B may cause intracellular coalescence of zymogen granules leading to premature acinar cell activation of protrypsin and other proenzymes. Activation and release of vasoactive substances probably produce shock, circulatory collapse, and death in some patients. Conversion of prekallikrein to kallikrein in the pancreatic islets activates kinin and the clotting and complement systems; these act to promote inflammation, thrombosis, tissue damage, and bleeding.[2] If there is sufficient damage to the pancreatic blood vessels, hemorrhagic pancreatitis can ensue. Lecithin from bile may be converted to highly toxic lysolecithin by phospholipase A_2, promoting the destruction of acinar cell membranes.

Adult respiratory distress syndrome (ARDS), a grave complication of pancreatitis, may be caused by autodigestive injury to the pulmonary capillaries by circulating activated pancreatic enzymes, such as phospholipase A_2.[2,5] If the activated enzymes enter the peritoneal space and the systemic circulation, host antiprotease defenses such as α_1-antitrypsin

and α_2-macroglobulin may be overwhelmed, and dysfunction in distant organs such as the lung, kidneys, and parathyroids may occur.

Sensitivity and specificity of tests in pancreatitis. When pancreatitis is suspected, the commonly ordered studies are amylase and lipase. A somewhat arbitrary but useful ranking of tests from least to most efficient for diagnosing pancreatitis is as follows: urinary amylase, urinary amylase/creatinine ratio, serum phospholipase A_2, serum amylase, pancreatic elastase 1, lipase, pancreatic amylase, pancreatic lipase, lipase L2 isoenzyme, **trypsinogen**, and **immunoreactive trypsin (IRT)**.[18-21]

Urine amylase is a poor test for pancreatitis because of the enormous range of values observed in healthy persons and its poor specificity. Serum phospholipase A_2, amylase, and lipase have good sensitivity but poor specificity, particularly the first of these. A single, moderately abnormal amylase or lipase is usually of no help in a patient with abdominal pain; only about 15% of such patients have pancreatitis.[17] The disorders that are often associated with secondary pancreatitis and with an increased serum amylase and lipase are listed in the box below and on p. 542. Appropriate use of the pancreatic enzymes to diagnose pancreatitis includes repeat studies during the first 24 to 48 hours after admission. In a patient with signs and symptoms suggestive of acute pancreatitis with serum amylase or lipase values greater than four to five times the assay's upper reference limit and with amylase and lipase values that move in parallel over time, a diagnosis of acute pancreatitis is highly likely.[6,17] With optimized lipase assays, serum lipase levels are usually greater than those of serum amylase. The half-life of lipase is somewhat longer than that of amylase, so lipase is more likely to be the only enzyme elevated in patients first seen several days after the onset of abdominal pain.[22]

The sensitivity and specificity of any tests used to diagnose pancreatitis, including amylase and lipase, are affected by the selection of patients for testing, the time of blood collection following onset of symptoms, and the methods used for the tests. Reported sensitivities and specificities for amylase are 70% to 100% and 33% to 89%, respectively; for lipase, 63% to 100% and 34% to 100%.[23] The general consensus is that amylase and lipase levels above the upper reference limit (URL) have good sensitivity but only fair specificity. Fig. 29-5 shows an ROC curve for total amylase, P3 isoenzyme of amylase, total lipase, and the L2 isoenzyme of lipase.[18,24] From this data, P3 amylase or total amylase are inferior to total lipase or L2 lipase. For lipase, increasing

---

DISEASES ASSOCIATED WITH SECONDARY PANCREATITIS

All types of biliary tract disorders, any inflammatory process or abscess in the abdomen, renal failure, burns, shock, sepsis, diabetic ketoacidosis, status after surgery, volvulus, gastrointestinal perforation of any kind, pancreas and kidney transplantation

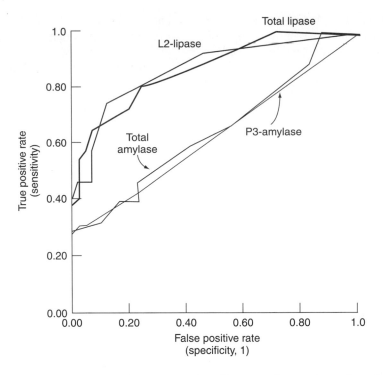

Fig. 29-5   Receiver-operating-characteristic (ROC) curves for total amylase, P3-amylase, total lipase, and L2-lipase in the diagnosis of pancreatitis. The total lipase and L2-lipase tests are significantly better than the total amylase and P3-amylase tests. The ideal test should show a sensitivity of 1 and a false positive rate of zero. The closer the curve gets to the top left corner of the figure, the better the test. *(Adapted from Zweig MH, Campbell G: Receiver-operating characteristic (ROC) plots: a fundamental evaluation tool in clinical medicine,* Clin Chem *39:561, 1993.)*

the cut-off point between normal and abnormal improves the specificity of the test with little effect on the sensitivity. The URLs for amylase and lipase do not serve well as limits to separate the healthy from the ill (see above).

Amylase has six isoenzymes, though not all are expressed in most individuals.[25] The major groupings of the amylase isoenzymes are salivary and pancreatic; they are readily separated by electrophoresis on cellulose acetate or agarose. The isoenzymes are of limited diagnostic use. The pancreatic forms cannot be used to discriminate among various types of abdominal causes of an increased total amylase or between edematous and necrotizing pancreatitis, with the possible exception of fallopian tube disorders in which salivary rather than pancreatic isoamylases predominate. Isoamylases assayed by electrophoresis are rarely performed because of the time-consuming nature of the test. Pancreatic amylase, obtained by inhibiting salivary amylase with wheat germ lectin or an antibody to salivary amylase, appears superior to total serum amylase.

Severity of pancreatitis. It is possible to give only a very rough estimate of the severity of pancreatitis from the magnitude of increase of pancreatic enzyme activities in serum. In some patients, trivial inflammation and edema can lead to large increases in the plasma activities of the pancreatic enzymes; in those with end-stage pancreatitis, plasma enzyme activities may be relatively low because of

TABLE 29-4   RANSON'S LABORATORY INDICATORS OF SEVERITY IN ACUTE PANCREATITIS

On Admission	Within 48 Hours
Glucose >2000 mg/L (7.1 mmol/L)	Hematocrit decrease >10%
LDH >350 IU/L	BUN increase >50 mg/L (1.8 mmol/L)
AST >250 IU/L	Calcium <80 mg/L (2 mmol/L)
	PO_2 <60 mm Hg

Modified from Ranson JH, Rifkind KM, Turner JW: Prognostic signs and nonoperative peritoneal lavage in acute pancreatitis, Surg Gynecol Obstet *143:109, 1976.*

preexisting gland destruction. A host of disorders other than pancreatitis increase both amylase and lipase, though many afflicted patients may have undiagnosed secondary pancreatitis. A number of routine laboratory features were determined by Ransom to have prognostic importance in patients with pancreatitis; these are summarized in Table 29-4. Although their positive predictive value for determining a poor prognosis is only about 50%, their negative predictive value in ruling out severe disease is about 90%.[26,27]

Miscellaneous causes of increased serum amylase. Diseases of the salivary gland, fallopian tubes, renal failure, some lung cancers, and macroamylasemia increase the serum amylase. Amylase has a broader tissue distribution than lipase has; organs containing amylase but not lipase include the salivary glands and fallopian tubes. The amylase activity in saliva is at least 10,000 times that in normal plasma. An increased serum amylase is common in mumps (sialoadenitis) and other inflammatory disorders of the salivary glands. The salivary form of amylase is generally increased in radiation injury of the salivary glands and in many tubal-ovarian disorders, including ectopic pregnancy. After coronary artery bypass surgery, amylase is often increased because of the entry of saliva into the lungs during intubation and surgery and absorption of salivary amylase into the bloodstream; in these cases, amylase typically returns to normal in about 48 hours.[28] In a few patients with lung cancer, an increased amylase may be observed because the tumor produces salivary amylase.[25]

In renal failure, amylase and lipase are typically both increased, as the result of decreased amylase clearance and reduced lipase metabolism in the renal tubules, a normal catabolic process for lipase.

A persistently abnormal amylase in an asymptomatic patient may be macroamylasemia, a laboratory curiosity, usually composed of amylase bound to an immunoglobulin.[29] The normal clearance mechanisms for amylase are blocked, and macroamylase accumulates. It is important to identify macroamylase when present to avoid unnecessary and costly diagnostic studies. After electrophoresis of amylase, macroamylase gives a smear of activity; normally, distinct salivary and pancreatic amylase bands are seen. In the presence of macroamylasemia, the urinary amylase is usually low, and the fractional excretion of amylase is typically much less than the normal 3% to 5% (often <0.1%).

Chronic pancreatitis. Chronic pancreatitis is often a consequence of repeated bouts of acute pancreatitis and extensive destruction of the gland; usually much of the pancreas has been replaced with scar (fibrotic) tissue.[30-32] Protein plugs in the small ductules may be present and lead to pancreatic fibrosis, calcification, loss of acinar cell function, and even destruction of the islets. DM and pancreatic insufficiency (see below) and nutritional problems may be present. Individuals with episodes of chronic pancreatitis may be in acute distress but show no or trivial laboratory abnormalities because of the loss of much of the functional pancreatic tissue. While chronic alcohol abuse is the most common cause of chronic pancreatitis, chronic pancreatitis is present in only a minority of habitual alcoholics.[6] Other causes include tropical pancreatitis and familial hereditary pancreatitis. A calorie- and protein-deficient diet appears to predispose patients to tropical pancreatitis. Attacks may also be provoked by overeating. Atherosclerosis of the pancreatic artery causing recurrent pancreatic ischemia is an uncommon cause of chronic pancreatitis.

Destructive Disorders

Cystic fibrosis. Exocrine pancreatic malfunction is a hallmark of cystic fibrosis (CF), an autosomal, recessively inherited disease primarily diagnosed in infants and children (see also Chapters 47 and 48).[33] CF is caused by a number of different mutations in the chloride transporter gene that lead to a missing or nonfunctional cell-membrane protein (CFTR), which plays a role in the selective cellular uptake of ions. In CF, pancreatic secretions (as well as those of the lungs and other organs) are viscous and of low volume. In the pancreas this leads to greatly reduced pancreatic flow, in many cases resulting in pancreatic duct obstruction and atrophy. In the early stages of pancreatic injury from cystic fibrosis, IRT is elevated, whereas in pancreatic insufficiency it is reduced.[34] Between the ages of 2 and 5 years, IRT levels are often normal in children with cystic fibrosis. Malabsorption syndromes (see below and p. 557) and malnutrition often occur in CF patients.

The diagnosis of CF is based on finding genotypic defects using polymerase chain reaction (PCR) technology (see Chapter 48),[32] an abnormal sweat chloride test, abnormal pancreatic function tests, the characteristic pulmonary disease, and a history of a blood-related family member with the disease.[35,36] The chromosome defects are multifaceted, and depending on the genetic error, CF can present in varying severity, from mild to lethal. With some mutations, there may be a discrepancy between the severity of lung and pancreatic injury.[37]

Pancreatic insufficiency. Reduction or loss of pancreatic exocrine (digestive) function leads, in its late stages, to severe gastrointestinal disturbances, such as diarrhea, constipation, and malabsorption. With advanced disease, a catabolic state leading to weight loss and **cachexia** appears. The exocrine pancreas has extensive reserve capacity; symptoms generally appear only after about 85% to 90% of the acinar tissue has been lost. The most common causes of pancreatic insufficiency differ in children and adults; in children, it is almost always due to cystic fibrosis, while in adults it is usually due to chronic pancreatitis. The causes of acinar cell loss are listed in the box below.

PANCREATIC FUNCTION TESTS

Pancreatic function tests are used to measure the ability of the pancreas to produce enzymes, proteins, and bicarbonate and to secrete an adequate volume of fluid into the duodenum. Pancreatic function tests (Table 29-5) can be classified into four groups:

CAUSES OF ACINAR CELL LOSS

- Repeated bouts of pancreatitis, especially that caused by chronic alcoholism
- Cystic fibrosis (CF)
- Atherosclerosis and subsequent pancreatic atrophy
- Any obstruction of the pancreatic ductules or duct as caused by a stone or stones or calcification of the gland, a benign or malignant tumor pressing on the pancreas, or other types of mechanical blockage

TABLE 29-5	TESTS OF PANCREATIC FUNCTION		
Test	Patient Preparation	Specimen	Normal Finding
Secretin/CCK stimulation test	Secretin or CCK (or both) given IV	Duodenal aspirate	Adequate fluid output containing bicarbonate, enzymes, proteins
Fecal fat excretion	80 to 100 g of fat/day and meat for at least 1 week	Feces, 72-hour collection	Less than 7 g of fat excretion per day; no obvious meat fibres observed microscopically on smear
Urinary amylase excretion	24-hour urine collection	Urine	Healthy amylase; greatly increased amylase in pancreas transplant recipients
Pancreatic enzymes in serum	None	Serum	Healthy IRT, trypsinogen
Fat or cholesterol labeled with ^{13}C or ^{14}C	^{13}C- or ^{14}C-labeled fats or cholesterol given by mouth in a controlled meal	Breath	Healthy $^{13}CO_2$ or $^{14}CO_2$ excretion
β-Carotene in serum	Controlled β-carotene in diet	Serum	Normal β-carotene

IRT, *Immunoreactive trypsin*; IV, *intraveneously*.

1. Tests that measure fluid volume and bicarbonate output or residual enzymatic activity in pancreatic fluid
2. Tests on feces to measure undigested fat, meat, or enzymes
3. Tests on duodenal fluid, blood, or urine to measure endogenous or exogenously administered agents
4. Tests on breath to measure $^{13}CO_2$ or $^{14}CO_2$ produced by the action of pancreatic enzymes on labeled compounds, commonly fats or other esters

Tests for Volumes or Analytes in Pancreatic Fluid

A double-lumen tube is inserted through the esophagus and stomach to a point in the duodenum below the ampulla; pancreatic secretion is then stimulated with intravenous CCK, secretin, or both. Bicarbonate, fluid volume, and (less frequently) enzymes such as amylase, lipase, trypsin, or chymotrypsin are measured in the collected duodenal fluid. The bicarbonate production and fluid volume are reasonably insensitive tests of adequate pancreatic function, and patients with significant losses of pancreatic function may show a normal bicarbonate and volume because of the large reserve capacity. Although duodenal fluid enzyme levels are the first to become decreased, reference values are not widely available for fluid enzyme content. In those with extensive exocrine pancreatic impairment, such as in patients with repeated bouts of pancreatitis or children with cystic fibrosis, tests on duodenal fluid have good sensitivity. These tests are considered the most sensitive available for detecting pancreatic exocrine insufficiency.

Tests on feces. An abnormal fecal fat test on a 72-hour collection remains the standard, noninvasive test for the initial recognition of pancreatic insufficiency. Fecal fat excretion generally becomes abnormal only after 85% to 90% of pancreatic acinar tissue loss. In general, the percentage of stool weight composed of fat is higher in pancreatic insufficiency than in intestinal disease, but there is overlap in the results between the two conditions. Tests for trypsin and chymotrypsin in feces are unreliable in early pancreatic

insufficiency, although chymotrypsin as measured by immunoassay is typically decreased when steatorrhea results from pancreatic insufficiency. (See Chapter 30 for additional information.)

Serum, urine, and breath tests. Because they lack sensitivity, serum amylase, lipase, and phospholipase A_2 are essentially useless for estimating pancreatic function; however, in the late stages of pancreatic insufficiency, serum amylase and lipase are often reduced. Immunoreactive trypsin (IRT) consists of at least two unique proteins, an anionic and a cationic form, that differ in their isoelectric point and electrophoretic mobility at pH 8.6. Cationic trypsin, anionic trypsin, or chymotrypsin measured in serum as proteins are better tests, and IRT on dried blood spots has been recommended as a screening test for cystic fibrosis in newborns.[36] The NBT-PABA (Bentiromide) test is used in a few laboratories for estimating pancreatic digestive function, but is not commercially available in the United States. NBT-PABA is *p*-aminobenzoic acid linked to a short chain of synthetic amino acids. In normal individuals, proteolytic enzymes in pancreatic fluid split the molecule, and PABA is absorbed by the small intestine and metabolized to hippurate, which is excreted in urine. Urine hippurate excretion is quantified to determine PABA release and absorption. Unfortunately, the test has poor sensitivity for early pancreatic damage and is affected not only by pancreatic enzyme secretion but also by intestinal absorption, liver function (conjugation), and renal excretion. Hippurate can be measured in serum, thereby eliminating the renal component in patients with kidney diseases.

Fats labeled with ^{131}I, ^{13}C, or ^{14}C have been advocated as pancreatic function tests. If the pancreatic enzymes hydrolyze the fat or cholesterol esters, ^{131}I can be measured in urine with a gamma counter, or alternatively, $^{13}CO_2$ or $^{14}CO_2$ is measured in the breath with a mass spectrometer or beta counter, respectively.[22] A similar strategy employs the fluorescein ester of lauric acid. Pancreatic lipase will split the ester, and the fluorescein is measured in urine or blood.

As with the NBT-PABA procedure, the test has poor sensitivity in the earlier stages of pancreatic insufficiency.

Pancreatic Infections

Infections are both a cause and a complication of pancreatitis. Causative agents are believed to include the mumps virus, echovirus, hepatitis A and B virus, Epstein-Barr virus, coxsackievirus B, HIV, *Ascaris* worms (producing ascariasis, a roundworm infection), and *Mycoplasma* bacteria.[38] Acute pancreatitis has been observed in some HIV-infected children in whom pancreatitis is normally rare. The onset of pancreatitis in a child with AIDS portends imminent death. Also, drugs such as pentamidine isethionate and didanosine given to AIDS patients tend to provoke pancreatitis.[39,40]

Pancreatic Neoplasms

Adenocarcinoma. Most pancreatic cancers are adenocarcinomas, arising from the ductal epithelial cells and carrying an ominous prognosis. Only about 1% of pancreatic cancers originate in the acinar cells. Pancreatic cancer is the fifth most lethal malignancy in the developed world after colorectal, breast, lung, and prostate cancer.[2] The death rate from pancreatic cancer in the United States is about 12 per 100,000 and is increasing. Predisposing factors are smoking, diabetes mellitus, a diet high in fat, and exposure to certain carcinogens such as coal tar, coke, benzidine, and β-naphthylamine. It may be possible to reduce the risk for pancreatic cancer by stopping cigarette smoking and reducing fat intake. Pancreatic cancer is extremely rare in vegetarians. Smokers have a two- to threefold greater incidence of pancreatic carcinoma. The earlier presumed association of coffee consumption and pancreatic cancer has not been confirmed.

Most pancreatic cancers are invasive and inoperable when clinically apparent. Death within 1 year of diagnosis is common, and the 5-year survival rate is a dismal 1%. Jaundice develops early in 60% to 70% of patients with cancer in the head of the pancreas because of tumor-caused occlusion of the bile duct. If jaundice does occur with carcinoma of the body or tail of the pancreas, it usually manifests late in the disease. Malabsorption of fats and proteins with weight loss is common. Rarely, a search for the cause of the jaundice may reveal surgically curable pancreatic cancer. Testing for the recurrence of pancreatic cancer is possible with the fetoacinar pancreatic protein; pancreatic cancer-associated antigen (CA-19-9), carcinoembryonic antigen, galactosyltransferase, CA-50, or DU PAN-2.[41] However, many acute but benign conditions (including bile duct obstruction) also lead to abnormal results for these tests.[42,43] Unfortunately, no satisfactory screening tests are available for pancreatic cancer.

Islet cell tumors. Production of hormones is very common in islet cell tumors; about 20% of islet cell tumors are biochemically silent and do not secrete. Islet cell tumors have been found that secrete one or more of the following hormones: ACTH, β-chorionic gonadotropin, C-peptide, calcitonin, gastrin, glucagon, insulin, parathormone, prostaglandins, secretin, serotonin, somatostatin, and VIP.[11-13] Islet cell tumors may occur as part of the type I **multiple endocrine neoplasia syndrome** (see Chapter 30). In nearly all cases, patients have significant endocrine disturbances (these disorders are discussed previously under **Endocrine Pancreatic Disorders**).

References

1. Bannister LH: Alimentary system. In Williams PL, editor: *Gray's anatomy*, ed 38, New York, 1995, Churchill Livingstone.
2. Crawford JM, Cotran RS: The pancreas. In Cotran RS, Kumar V, Collins T, editors: *Robbins' pathologic basis of disease*, ed 6, Philadelphia, 1999, WB Saunders.
3. The pancreas. In Guyton AC, Hall JE, editors: *Textbook of medical physiology*, ed 10, Philadelphia, 2001, WB Saunders.
4. Dockray GJ et al: The gastrins: their production and biological actions, *Ann Rev Physiol* 63:119, 2001.
5. Soergel KH: Pancreatitis. In Goldman L, Bennett JC, editors: *Cecil's textbook of medicine*, ed 21, Philadelphia, 2000, WB Saunders.
6. Lott JA et al: Assays of serum lipase: analytical and clinical considerations, *Clin Chem* 32:1290, 1986.
7. Gullo L et al: Influence of the thyroid on exocrine pancreatic function, *Gastroenterology* 100:1392, 1991.
8. Lembcke B et al: Effect of the somatostatin analogue Sandostatin (SMS 201-995) on gastrointestinal, pancreatic, and biliary function and hormone release in normal men, *Digestion* 36:108, 1987.
9. Owyang C, Louie DS, Tatum D: Feedback regulation of pancreatic enzyme secretion: suppression of cholecystokinin release by trypsin, *J Clin Invest* 77:2042, 1986.
10. Sugtiani A et al: Serum lipase as a marker for pancreatic allograft rejection, *Clin Transplant* 12:224, 1998.
11. Service FJ: Approach to the adults with hypoglycemic disorders, *Endocrinol Metab Clin North Am* 28:519, 1999.
12. Leichter SB: Clinical and metabolic aspects of glucagonoma, *Medicine* 59:100, 1980.
13. Vinik AI et al: Somatostatinomas, PPomas, neurotensinomas, *Semin Oncol* 14:263, 1987.
14. Baron TH, Morgan DE: Acute necrotizing pancreatitis, *N Engl J Med* 340:1412, 1999.
15. Kazmierczak SC, Catrou PG, Van Lente F: Enzymatic markers of gallstone-induced pancreatitis identified by ROC curve analysis, discriminant analysis, logistic regression, likelihood ratios, and information theory, *Clin Chem* 41:523, 1995.
16. Young DS: *Effects of drugs on clinical laboratory tests*, ed 5, Washington, DC, 2000, American Association for Clinical Chemistry Press.
17. Lott JA, Ellison EC, Applegate D: The importance of objective data in the diagnosis of pancreatitis, *Clin Chem Acta* 183:33, 1989.
18. Lott JA, Lu CJ: Lipase isoforms and amylase isoenzymes: assays and application in the diagnosis of acute pancreatitis, *Clin Chem* 37:361, 1991.
19. Vissers RJ, Abu-Laban RB, McHugh DF: Amylase and lipase in the emergency department evaluation of acute pancreatitis, *J Emerg Med* 17:1027, 1999.
20. Tietz NW: Support of the diagnosis of pancreatitis by enzyme tests: old problems, new techniques, *Clin Chem Acta* 257:85, 1997.
21. Kylanpaa-Back M et al: Reliable screening for acute pancreatitis with rapid urine trypsinogen-2 test strip, *Br J Surg* 87:49, 2000.
22. Eskfeldt JH et al: Serum tests for pancreatitis in patients with abdominal pain, *Arch Pathol Lab Med* 109:316, 1985.
23. Wong ECC et al: The clinical chemistry laboratory and acute pancreatitis, *Clin Chem* 39:234, 1993.
24. Zweig MH, Campbell G: Receiver-operating characteristic (ROC) plots: a fundamental evaluation tool in clinical medicine, *Clin Chem* 39:561, 1993.
25. Lott JA: Amylase. In Lott JA, Wolf PL, editors: *Clinical enzymology: a case-oriented approach*, St Louis, 1986, Mosby.

26. Malfertheiner P, Dominguiez-Munoz JE: Prognostic factors in acute pancreatitis, *Int J Pancreatol* 14:1, 1993.
27. Dervenis C et al: Diagnosis, objective assessment of severity, and management of acute pancreatitis (Santorini consensus conference), *Int J Pancreatol* 25:195, 1999.
28. Kazmierczak SC, Van Lente F: Incidence and source of hyper-amylasemia after cardiac surgery, *Clin Chem* 34:916, 1988.
29. Mifflin TE et al: Macroamylase, macro creatine kinase, and other macroenzymes, *Clin Chem* 31:1743, 1985.
30. Mergener K, Baillie J: Chronic pancreatitis, *Lancet* 350:1379, 1997.
31. Clain JE, Pearson RK: Diagnosis of chronic pancreatitis. Is a gold standard necessary? *Surg Clin North Am* 79:829, 1999.
32. Manes G et al: Chronic pancreatitis: diagnosis and staging, *Ann Ital Chir* 71:23, 2000.
33. Robinson P: Cystic fibrosis, *Thorax* 56:237, 2001.
34. Couper RT et al: Longitudinal evaluation of serum trypsinogen measurement in pancreatic-insufficient and pancreatic-sufficient patients with cystic fibrosis, *J Pediatr* 127:408, 1995.
35. Farrell PM, Koscik RE: Sweat chloride concentrations in infants homozygous or heterozygous for F508 cystic fibrosis, *Pediatrics* 97:524, 1996.
36. Ranieri E et al: Neonatal screening for cystic fibrosis using immunoreactive trypsinogen and direct gene analysis: four years' experience, *BMJ* 308:1469, 1994.
37. Mickle JE; Cutting GR: Genotype-phenotype relationships in cystic fibrosis, *Med Clin North Am* 84:597, 2000.
38. Miller TL et al: Pancreatitis in pediatric human immunodeficiency virus infection, *J Pediatr* 120:223, 1992.
39. Shelton MJ, O'Donnell AM, Morse GD: Didanosine, *Ann Pharmacother* 26:660, 1992.
40. Bonacini M: Pancreatic involvement in human immunodeficiency virus infection, *J Clin Gastroenterol* 13:58, 1991.
41. Sataka K et al: The possibility of diagnosing small pancreatic cancer (less than 4.0 cm) by measuring various serum tumor markers: a retrospective study, *Cancer* 68:149, 1991.
42. Fabris C et al: Serum CA 19-9 and alpha-fetoprotein levels in primary hepatocellular carcinoma and liver cirrhosis, *Cancer* 68:1795, 1991.
43. Akdogan M et al: Extraordinarily elevated CA 19-9 in benign conditions: a case report and review of the literature, *Tumori* 87:337, 2001.

Internet Sites

http://www.pancreasfoundation.org
http://arbl.cvmbs.colostate.edu/hbooks/pathphys/digestion/pancreas/

http://www.teaching-biomed.man.ac.uk/student_projects/2000/mnby7lc2/pancreas.htm
http://www.udel.edu/Biology/Wags/histopage/colorpage/cp/cp.htm

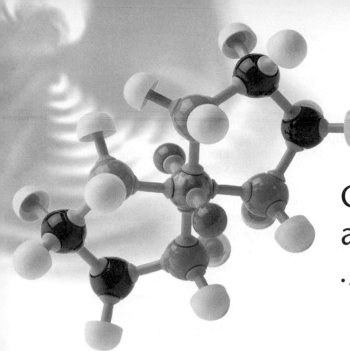

CHAPTER 30

Gastrointestinal Function and Digestive Disease

• *D. Robert Dufour*

Chapter Outline

Objectives

- Describe the anatomy of the normal digestive tract.
- Outline the digestive and absorptive functions of the normal digestive tract.
- List the major pathological conditions of the gastrointestinal tract and the causes of these conditions.
- Describe diagnostic tests used for patients with dyspepsia and/or peptic ulcer disease.
- Outline the major causes of malabsorption and list

laboratory tests helpful in its recognition and differential diagnosis.
- In general terms, define gastrointestinal hormones and describe their role in gastrointestinal function.
- Describe tests useful in the differential diagnosis of diarrhea.
- Describe the advantages and disadvantages of different methods for measurement of occult blood loss from the intestinal tract.

Key Terms

achlorhydria　Literally "without hydrochloric acid." Refers to lack of acid production by the stomach.

brain-gut axis　Similar peptides that are found in the gut, nerves, and central nervous system.

chyme　The semisolid end product of gastric action on food. Chyme consists of mucus, gastric secretions, and broken-down food.

gastrointestinal hormones　Substances that are produced by gastrointestinal cells and then travel through the bloodstream to act at a separate site. These hormones include cholecystokinin, secretin, glucagon, gastric inhibitory polypeptide, vasoactive intestinal polypeptide, bombesin, somatostatin, motilin, bulbogastrone, enterooxyntin, and pancreatic polypeptide.

gluten　A protein found in wheat and wheat products.

intubation　The procedure of introducing a tube-shaped instrument into the body, usually through an anatomical opening, such as the mouth.

pancreatic exocrine enzymes　Enzymes required for digestion. Often released in a precursor form. These enzymes include trypsinogen, chymotrypsinogen, proelastase, procarboxypeptidase, ribonuclease, deoxyribonuclease, amylase, lipase, phospholipase A, and cholesterol esterase.

pancreatic hormones　Endocrine hormones mainly concerned with carbohydrate intermediary metabolism and including glucagon, insulin, and gastrin.

Methods on CD-ROM

D-xylose
Fat absorption

Gastric fluid analysis

The gastrointestinal tract is a muscular tube lined with epithelial cells and extending 10 m from the mouth to the anus. Along its course its structure is modified to suit particular requirements for the digestion and absorption of food.

The gastrointestinal tract is an extremely elaborate organ with several structural and functional regions, serving as both a digestive and absorptive organ. In addition, the gastrointestinal tract is controlled by an elaborate hormonal and neural regulatory network, and itself produces a number of hormones that largely act locally to affect the function of the intestine and other organs (particularly the pancreas and gall bladder) involved in the digestive process. The lower digestive tract contains a large number of microorganisms that coexist with the body without causing disease; in some cases, they serve a symbiotic role in providing nutrients (such as vitamin K) to the body. Changes in the microbial flora or introduction of unusual microorganisms can lead to disease of the intestinal tract.

ANATOMY AND GENERAL FUNCTIONS

The gastrointestinal tract has seven distinct regions: mouth, esophagus, stomach, duodenum, jejunum, ileum, and large bowel (Fig. 30-1).

The mouth contains teeth, tongue, salivary glands, and an elaborate swallowing mechanism. It is responsible for

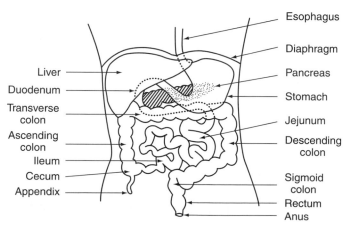

Fig. 30-1　Diagram of gastrointestinal tract.

tasting, grinding, and lubricating food, and beginning the process of digestion through the action of salivary amylase (and to a much smaller extent, lingual lipase). The swallowing mechanism propels the food down the esophagus, through the thoracic cavity, and into the stomach.

The stomach is a rough-surfaced, muscular bag coated with a protective mucous layer; it has four functional areas (Fig. 30-2). The very top part is known as the *fundus*, and the main portion is known as the *body*. The outlet of the stomach, known as the *antrum*, is segregated from the duodenum by the *pylorus*, which contains a strong, muscular sphincter. The gastric mucosa is arranged in numerous coarse folds known as *rugae*. The rugae assist in mixing and breaking down food particles during the churning action of the stomach. Hydrochloric acid and the enzyme pepsin are also secreted and continue the digestive breakdown. These actions convert food into **chyme**.

Chyme enters the duodenum, into which bile and **pancreatic exocrine enzymes** (see Chapter 29) are secreted. Further enzymatic degradation of the basic food materials takes place in the duodenum and continues as the food material enters the rest of the small intestine. Through this process, complex macromolecules in food are broken down to amino acids, simple sugars, free fatty acids, and glycerol to allow their absorption by the intestines and ultimate entry into the bloodstream.

The small intestine is 4 m long. Its microvillus substructure increases its absorptive surface area. In addition to the duodenum, the small intestine consists of two additional segments (see Fig. 30-1), the jejunum proximally and the ileum distally, the sites of final digestion and absorption. The nondigestible residual matter enters the large intestine, where a process of selective water and electrolyte absorption occurs. The digestive process terminates with the formation of feces.

The entire absorptive surface of the gastrointestinal tract is drained by the portal venous blood vessels. These convey the newly absorbed materials directly to the liver so that they may be immediately used.

The intestinal tract, from the stomach to the small bowel, also contains many endocrine cells. The peptide hormones produced by these cells are involved in the regulation of gastrointestinal function. In addition, a significant number of these peptides are present in the nerves of the gastrointestinal tract[1] and in the central nervous system, thus establishing the **brain-gut axis** for these hormones. The knowledge that gut hormones are distributed not only in endocrine cells but also in peripheral and central nerves has established the fact that these peptides function not only as hormones but also as neurotransmitters.

DIGESTION

Digestion is the chemical process of rendering food into a form that can be absorbed by the body. The digestive process begins in the mouth and is generally completed in the proximal portion of the small intestine. The digestive process for various foods is summarized in Table 30-1.

Digestive Action of the Mouth

Ingestion of food stimulates the production of saliva from the three pairs of salivary glands: parotid, mandibular, and sublingual. These glands produce viscid, water-based, mucin-containing secretions that act as a lubricant. They also secrete salivary amylase to initiate the digestion of starch and lingual lipase to initiate metabolism of complex lipids. Chewing breaks up food into smaller pieces, increasing the surface area to enhance the action of digestive enzymes.

Digestive Action of the Stomach

The gastric mucosa contains four types of cells. Mucous cells are found throughout the entire stomach and secrete mucus to protect the surface from attack by acid and enzymes. Also found in all parts of the stomach are the surface epithelial cells, which are also capable of secreting mucus but which proliferate rapidly and shed readily, producing a continually

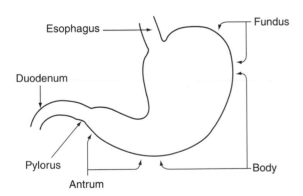

Fig. 30-2 Diagram of stomach.

TABLE 30-1	CHEMICAL PROCESSES FOR DIGESTION OF FOOD	
Food Material	**Digestive Action**	**End Product**
Starch	Pancreatic amylase	Disaccharides (mainly maltose)
Disaccharides	Mucosal disaccharidases	Monosaccharides
Monosaccharides	None	
Protein	Gastric hydrochloric acid and pepsin	Partial degradation into large polypeptides
	Pancreatic trypsin, chymotrypsin, and carboxypeptidase	Polypeptides, dipeptides, and amino acids
Long-chain triglycerides	Emulsification with bile, hydrolysis by lipase	Fatty acids and glycerol

viable surface for the stomach. Parietal cells produce hydrochloric acid and intrinsic factor. Chief cells produce the proenzyme pepsinogen. These last two cell types are found throughout the body of the stomach.

The *antral* cells secrete mainly mucus but also some pepsinogen. The hormone gastrin is synthesized and stored in the G cells of the antrum.

There are three phases of gastric activity. The first of these is the cephalic phase, which is initiated by the sight and smell of food. This sensation triggers a direct vagus nerve message from the brain to the stomach to initiate the digestive process by stimulating the production of HCl both directly and through production of gastrin, which further stimulates HCl production.

In the gastric phase of digestion, distension of the gastric antrum stimulates production of additional gastrin (Fig. 30-3). The *chief* cells contain receptors that respond to the acid en-

vironment by secreting pepsinogen, which is rapidly converted into its active form (pepsin) at pH 3. Lipase and other enzymes are also liberated, but these enzymes are of little consequence in the digestive process.

Stomach activity subsides with time, and the chyme is then permitted to pass into the duodenum.

Digestive Action of the Duodenum

As chyme enters this portion of the intestine, several **gastrointestinal hormones** are released by both neural and local stimulation (Table 30-2). These hormones enter the portal blood system and act primarily on various regions of the gastrointestinal tract, stimulating contraction of the gall bladder (releasing bile salts), pancreatic secretion of bicarbonate (to neutralize gastric acid), and release of pancreatic proenzymes into the duodenum. The action of these agents on the primary food substances is now considered.

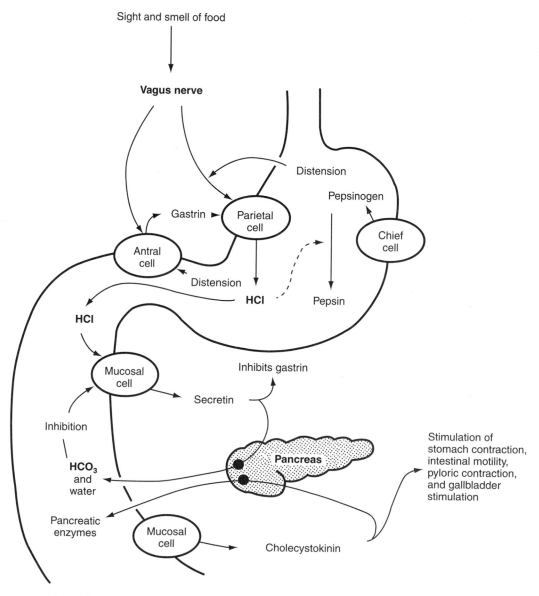

Fig. 30-3   Schema demonstrating various stimuli of stomach and duodenum.

Carbohydrate Digestion

Carbohydrates are present in the diet primarily as complex polysaccharides (starches), but also as monosaccharides and disaccharides (especially sucrose and lactose). Only the polysaccharides and disaccharides require digestion before their carbohydrate constituents can be absorbed.

Starch is the most common complex polysaccharide. It has a branching structure based on 1,4-carbohydrate or 1,6-carbohydrate linkages. Amylase is capable of hydrolyzing the 1,4 linkages in starch into oligosaccharides and ultimately into disaccharides. The dominant disaccharide produced from starch is maltose. Thus, as chyme leaves the duodenum, monosaccharides and disaccharides from the diet and disaccharides resulting from the action of amylase are passed to the jejunum and ileum, where hydrolysis of disaccharides and absorption of monosaccharides takes place.

Protein Digestion

Dietary protein is partially degraded in the stomach by hydrochloric acid and pepsin. In the duodenum, trypsin, chymotrypsin, and carboxypeptidase secreted by the pancreas (see Chapter 29) act on the partially degraded protein to yield polypeptides, dipeptides, and amino acids.

These tiny molecules then pass into the ileum and jejunum for assimilation.

Fat Digestion

Fat digestion is more complex than digestion of other basic food substances. Most dietary fats are long-chain triglycerides (palmitic, stearic, oleic, and linoleic acids). The stomach decreases the particle size of the fatty substances by its churning action. In the duodenum, fats are emulsified by the detergent action of bile salts (synthesized in the liver, see Chapter 27). Emulsification allows the pancreatic enzyme, lipase, in the presence of colipase, to attack the otherwise water-insoluble lipids. Lipase causes stepwise hydrolysis, which first forms diglycerides, monoglycerides, and finally free fatty acids and glycerol (see Chapter 33).

ABSORPTION

Absorption is the process whereby digested food substances enter the body. The intestinal mucosa is thrown into many fingerlike projections known as *villi* (Fig. 30-4). Each villus increases the absorptive surface many times. Each surface epithelial cell in the villus is covered by hairlike projections known as *microvilli*; there are 200 million microvilli per centimeter of epithelium. The villus and microvillus

TABLE 30-2 INTESTINAL HORMONES

Hormone	Number of Amino Acids	Source	Stimulating Factor	Function
Cholecystokinin	33	Mucosa of upper small intestine	Amino acids, fatty acids, hydrochloric acid, and food in duodenum	Stimulates pancreatic enzyme secretion, gallbladder contraction, contraction of stomach and pylorus, intestinal motility
Gastrin	14 to 34	Stomach, gut lumen	Protein digestion products, food in duodenum	Stimulates stomach acid secretion, gastric mobility, gastric mucosal growth
Secretin	27	Throughout gut mucosa but concentrated in duodenum	Acid in duodenum	Stimulates pancreatic secretion of water and bicarbonate, gastric pepsin secretion; relaxes pyloric sphincter
Motilin	22	Upper small intestine	High-fat meal, duodenal acidification	Stimulates motility of small intestines and duodenum
Glucagon	29	Pancreatic and intestinal mucosa	Arginine, alanine, stress	Stimulates gluconeogenesis; raises blood glucose
Gastric inhibitory polypeptide (GIP)	43	Duodenal mucosa	Glucose and fat	Cholecystokinin-like activity
Vasoactive intestinal polypeptide (VIP)	28	Wide distribution throughout gut		Vasodilation and hypotensive effects; inhibits histamine, pentagastrin acid release, and pepsin secretion; stimulates electrolyte and water secretion from pancreas; stimulates bile flow
Enteroglucagon (glucagon-like peptides)	29	Lower small intestine	Meal	Inhibits intestinal transit; enhances mucosal growth
Bombesin	14			Stimulates pancreatic secretion and gastrin release

structure gives the small intestine a massive absorptive surface area of 500 m^2.

It was once believed that enzymes were secreted by the small intestine to produce a digestive juice known as *succus entericus*. It is now known that the main enzymatic action occurs in intimate association with the epithelial surface. Rather than being a purely passive sieve through which food substances are permitted to pass, the intestinal mucosa contains a highly selective mechanism for the absorption of each nutrient.

Although there are regional differences in the ability of the intestine to absorb different food substances, these details are not considered here.

Carbohydrate Absorption

The monosaccharides (glucose, galactose, and fructose) are absorbed by specific active-transport mechanisms. Disaccharides are split into monosaccharides by the enzymatic activity of disaccharidases located on the microvilli. For example, the milk sugar, lactose, is split by lactase into glucose and galactose, whereas sucrose (table sugar) is cleaved by sucrase into glucose and fructose. Maltose, the common product of starch hydrolysis, is split by a surface maltase into two molecules of glucose. Lactase deficiency is discussed later in the text.

Protein Absorption

The digested products of protein are small polypeptides, dipeptides, and amino acids. Dipeptides are absorbed more rapidly than amino acids because of special transport mechanisms. Proteins are not absorbed directly. A very large number of specific absorptive mechanisms designed for various types of amino acids are located in the mucosal surface.

Fat Absorption (see also Chapter 33)

The successfully digested fat enters the intestine as a micelle. By diffusion the fatty acids and monoglycerides enter the intestinal epithelial cells, where they then interact with a binding protein. Long-chain fatty acids of 16 to 18 carbons are reesterified to form triglycerides and then bound to apolipoprotein B-48 to form chylomicrons. These tiny lipid droplets are released into the lymphatic system and transported to the thoracic duct before entry into the bloodstream. Medium-chain fatty acids (8 to 10 carbons) are not reesterified and rapidly enter the portal bloodstream bound to albumin.

Vitamins D, E, A, and K

Vitamins D, E, A, and K (see also Chapter 39) are not water-soluble and must therefore be absorbed with lipids.

Water and Sodium Absorption

The control over water absorption is not fully understood, but it is believed that bulk flow with sodium absorption is the mode for water transport in the intestine. Sodium is absorbed by an active-transport mechanism that is linked to the absorption of amino acids, bicarbonate, and glucose.

Calcium

Calcium transport (see also Chapter 28) is primarily under the influence of vitamin D and is regulated by a calcium-binding protein in the mucosal cells.

Iron Absorption (see also Chapter 35)

Gastric acid is required to convert iron to the absorbable ferrous form.[2] Iron then enters the mucosal cells and is transported across these cells, released into plasma after oxidation to the ferric state, and attached to transferrin for delivery to iron storage cells in the bone marrow and other

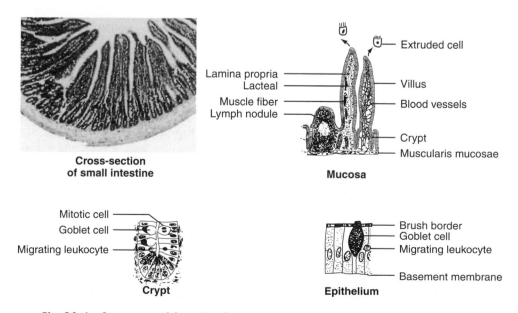

Fig. 30-4   Structures of functional components of small intestine. *(From Arey LB:* Human histology: a textbook in outline form, *ed 4, Philadelphia, 1974, Saunders.)*

organs. The *HFE* gene (defective in most cases of hereditary hemochromatosis) codes for a transmembrane protein that binds iron/transferrin/transferrin receptor complexes, signaling enterocytes to decrease iron absorption.[1,3] The exact mechanisms by which this affects iron absorption have not been determined.

Formation of Stool

Having passed through the ileum and jejunum, the residual intestinal contents enter the large bowel. Very little absorption of nutrients occurs in this region, but water, potassium, and bicarbonate are actively absorbed and returned to the circulation. Progressive dehydration of undigested food substances and the action of the bacteria that normally inhabit the colon lead to the formation of feces.

HORMONE PHYSIOLOGY
Gut Hormone Structure

The two main families of gut hormones are the gastrin and secretin families. The *gastrin* family consists primarily of gastrin and cholecystokinin, but, in addition, motilin and enkephalin share several structural similarities. The *secretin* group includes secretin, gastric inhibitory polypeptide (GIP), vasoactive intestinal polypeptide (VIP), glucagon, and bombesin. Many of these hormones are present in multiple forms of varying molecular size.

Gut hormones regulate digestion and absorption; they are released in response to nutrients in the lumen of the gastrointestinal tract and stimulate the release of acid, bicarbonate, and enzymes for the digestion of food. Once nutrients enter the blood, **pancreatic hormones** are released from the islets of Langerhans. This link has led to the term *enteroinsular axis*. Different steps of digestion, absorption, and storage can be both stimulated and inhibited by different gastroenteropancreatic peptides.

Each gastrointestinal function has several agonists and antagonists. Final control thus depends on a fine balance of numerous influences. In the case of gastric acid secretion, at least 21 different factors appear important in its normal control. Motilin, gastrin, VIP, and glucagon are the major hormones involved in the control of secretion, absorption, motility, and growth in the stomach and intestine. Secretin, cholecystokinin (CCK), VIP, and pancreatic polypeptide (PP) control exocrine pancreatic function, whereas insulin and GIP are involved in the enteroinsular axis. Insulin, glucagon, and somatostatin are primarily involved in the metabolism of carbohydrate, fats, and protein. Substance P, VIP, and the enkephalins have a major neurotransmitter involvement in the central, peripheral, and autonomic nervous systems. Only the most important of these hormones will be discussed in detail.

Gastrin[4,5]

Gastrin exists in multiple molecular forms, containing from 14 to 34 amino acids. The cellular origin of gastrin is the G cell of the gut. These cells extend into the gut lumen, where they terminate in a tuft of microvilli.

Gastrin stimulates gastric acid secretion, gastric motility, and the growth of fundic small bowel mucosa.[5] Secretion of gastrin is mediated by luminal, neural, and blood-borne stimuli. The principal luminal stimuli are the amino acid products of protein digestion. Other luminal stimuli include calcium, alcohol, and increased intragastric pH. Excess acid provides a feedback mechanism for autoregulation of gastrin release. Secretin, GIP, VIP, glucagon, calcitonin, and somatostatin are known to inhibit the release of gastrin.

Cholecystokinin[6]

The molecule is a basic peptide of 33 amino acid residues. CCK is found in the brain and in the K cells of the upper small intestinal mucosa.

The finding of CCK-like peptides in the central nervous system and in the gut indicates that these peptides may function as both neurotransmitters and hormones. The physiological role of CCK is the regulation of gallbladder and intestinal motility and pancreatic secretion.[7] Physiological actions of CCK in the pancreas include release of enzymes, potentiation of the action of secretin, and stimulation of growth of the pancreas.[8] A mixture of polypeptides and amino acids is a strong stimulus for the release of CCK. Fatty acids with chains longer than nine carbons also stimulate CCK release.[9]

Secretin[6]

Secretin is a basic peptide of 27 amino acid residues with strong similarities in sequence to glucagon. Secretin is predominantly located in the S cells of the mucosa of the duodenum and jejunum.

Secretin inhibits smooth muscle contraction, decreases gastric acid secretion, lowers the lower esophageal sphincter pressure, and stimulates pancreatic growth. In addition to these effects, it stimulates water and bicarbonate secretion from the pancreas and Brunner's glands. It is synergistic with CCK in the stimulation of gallbladder contraction and pancreatic enzyme secretion. The primary physiological role of secretin appears to be the modulation of pancreatic bicarbonate secretion.

A principal stimulus for duodenal secretin release is the presence of stomach acid, but in the adult jejunum there is seldom if ever likely to be sufficient acid to liberate secretin. Fatty acids with 10 or more carbons weakly stimulate duodenal secretin release.

Vasoactive Intestinal Polypeptide[6]

VIP has 28 amino acids and has been shown to be present in both endocrine cells and nerves of the gut and central nervous system.[10] VIP has a wide range of gastrointestinal activities, including inhibition of gastric acid secretion, stimulation of insulin release, stimulation of pancreatic water and bicarbonate secretion, and stimulation of intestinal fluid and electrolyte secretion. Recently, increasing attention has been paid to the role of VIP in immune function.[11]

Glucagon-Like Immunoreactive Peptides[6]

Several molecular forms of this family of hormones, which includes pancreatic glucagon, have been identified. Each intestinal peptide probably has a separate physiological role, though only one cell type containing glucagon-like immunoreactivity is found in the intestine.[12]

Glucagon and the glucagon-like immunoactive peptides have several biological actions, which include relaxation of smooth muscle, inhibition of pancreatic enzyme secretion, inhibition of gastric acid secretion, stimulation of intestinal fluid and electrolyte secretion, and stimulation of cardiac output. Pancreatic glucagon is secreted primarily in response to hypoglycemia and is important in the mobilization of hepatic glycogen stores and carbohydrate homeostasis (see Chapters 27 and 32).

PATHOLOGICAL CONDITIONS
Malnutrition

Malnutrition is caused by an abnormal food intake or by abnormal digestion or absorption of food. See Chapter 37 for a general review of malnutrition. Diseases of the gastrointestinal tract that may prevent nutrients from being digested or absorbed are discussed below.

Stomach Pathological Conditions

Ulcers. An ulcer results from the loss of the normal internal or external surface of the body caused by a variety of factors; in the intestinal tract, mucosal ulcers occur most commonly in the stomach and duodenum, where excess acid action (peptic ulcers) is responsible for most cases. The cause of peptic ulcer disease[2] is multifactorial, with risk factors including genetic (blood group O), local (decreased mucosal prostaglandins, damage to the mucosal lining), and infectious (*Helicobacter pylori*). *H. pylori* is now considered to be the direct cause of most cases of chronic gastritis and peptic ulcers, as well as increasing risk of development of gastric cancer and primary gastric lymphoma.[13] Eradication of *H. pylori* is associated with reduced symptoms of gastric pain (dyspepsia) and cure of ulcers.[14]

Although a definitive diagnosis of an ulcer is generally based on morphological grounds, with roentgenographic and endoscopic examinations of prime importance, an increasing emphasis is now placed on identifying patients with dyspepsia who are infected with *H. pylori* and treating the infection, rather than performing more expensive and invasive imaging procedures.[15] A number of tests are available for determination of exposure to or infection by *H. pylori*. The most widely employed have been serological tests that detect antibodies to *H. pylori*; these are relatively sensitive, but nonspecific.[16] Because *H. pylori* produces the enzyme urease, a number of tests have been developed to determine the presence of urease activity in the stomach. The most widely used is the *urea breath test*, in which the individual ingests a test meal containing carbon-13- or carbon-14-labeled urea.[17] Urease releases CO_2, and the amount of labeled CO_2 in breath is directly related to urease activity. The sensitivity and specificity of urea breath tests are around

99% in untreated patients; treatment with proton pump inhibitors such as lansoprazole markedly reduces test sensitivity.[18] More recently, a stool antigen test has become available for detection of *H. pylori*; sensitivity and specificity are similar to urea breath tests.[19,20] With successful eradication of *H. pylori*, the antigen test remains positive for a short period, but becomes negative by 4 to 6 weeks.[20]

If endoscopy is performed, a number of additional methods are available to detect *H. pylori*. Urease activity can also be determined in gastric biopsies; the most widely used method for detecting this is the CLO test, in which a small fragment of gastric tissue is incubated with urea and a pH indicator. Direct examination of histologic sections is also available. Culture and amplification techniques can also be used; culture is becoming more important in detecting antibiotic resistance in those individuals that do not respond to therapy.[10]

Cancer. The incidence of stomach cancer is declining in the United States, but it remains high in the Soviet Union and in Japan (54% of all cancers). It appears most often in the seventh and eighth decades of life, and the 5-year survival remains at 15%. Over half of all gastric cancers are found in the pylorus or antrum. Surgery in combination with radiotherapy or chemotherapy is used to treat the lesion. *H. pylori* infections of the stomach are associated with an approximately six-fold increase in the incidence of gastric cancer[13]; in a recent study, no cases of gastric cancer were found in individuals negative for *H. pylori*.[21] Although tumor markers are of no use in initial diagnosis, many gastric carcinomas produce CEA and CA 19-9, which may be useful for monitoring response to treatment.

Zollinger-Ellison syndrome. The Zollinger-Ellison syndrome is an extreme form of peptic ulcer disease, caused most commonly by a gastrin-secreting tumor of the pancreas (gastrinoma)[22] or by antral G-cell hyperplasia of the stomach. The unrelenting gastrin release stimulates hypersecretion of hydrochloric acid by the stomach. The Zollinger-Ellison syndrome is characterized by high basal acid output (BAO) (Table 30-3). The maximal acid output (MAO) is generally only 40% to 60% higher than the BAO because the stomach is close to maximal stimulation. Indeed, a BAO/MAO ratio greater than 60% is virtually pathognomonic for the Zollinger-Ellison syndrome. The typical clinical presentation (not seen in all patients) is recurrent peptic ulceration, often accompanied by diarrhea. Seventy-five percent of patients with this syndrome have ulcers in the duodenal bulb or immediate postbulbar area.

The gastrin-secreting tumors are often very small and can be difficult to identify. Sixty percent of tumors metastasize, and multiple tumors are common. Some tumors (10%) arise in the duodenal wall. The excess secretion of hydrochloric acid accounts for most of the clinical manifestations of the syndrome. The large amount of gastric acid entering the duodenum interferes with fat digestion and leads to steatorrhea. Because gastrin also inhibits salt and water absorption by the intestine, diarrhea occurs in 50% of patients. The very large volumes of gastric contents that are presented to the intestine enhance the diarrhea. The prolonged secretion of gastrin causes hypertrophy of the stomach, with parietal cell hyperplasia. Often, more distal parts of the intestine also become ulcerated. The Zollinger-Ellison syndrome is associated with hyperparathyroidism in 20% of patients. Other endocrine abnormalities that appear less commonly include pituitary, adrenal, ovarian, and thyroid tumors.[23] This cluster of endocrine adenomas and carcinomas is known as the *multiple endocrine neoplasia (MEN) syndrome I.* It may occur with autosomal dominant inheritance, as described originally by Werner, or it may occur sporadically. It is due to mutations in the MEN 1 tumor suppressor gene, located on the long arm of chromosome 11.[24] This syndrome manifests from the second decade to old age with an equal sex distribution. The areas involved in order of frequency are parathyroids (88%), pancreatic islets (81%), anterior pituitary (65%), adrenal cortex (38%), and thyroid follicular cells (19%).

A fasting serum gastrin concentration four times the upper limit of normal in the absence of **achlorhydria** or renal failure is strongly suggestive of the Zollinger-Ellison syndrome. This criterion is not met in 40% of cases. Because marked elevation of gastrin can also occur with achlorhydria (as occurs with atrophic gastritis), it is important to document that a patient actually is producing excess gastric acid before proceeding further.

Provocative testing has been used. Serum gastrin can be measured after administration of (1) intravenous secretin, 1 to 2 U/kg (as an intravenous bolus), (2) intravenous calcium gluconate, or (3) a standard meal. When secretin is administered, serum gastrin is collected at 2, 5, 10, 15, 30, and 60 minutes. A postsecretin increase of gastrin of $\geq$110 pg/mL is the most reliable criterion for Zollinger-Ellison syndrome, because secretin responses of this magnitude typically do not occur with antral G-cell hyperplasia or other causes of hypergastrinemia.[25] The sensitivity of the test is 95% and specificity virtually 100%.

Pernicious anemia and other causes of Vitamin B$_{12}$ malabsorption. Vitamin B$_{12}$ is an essential nutrient that is required for normal synthesis of myelin and nucleic acids (see Chapter 39). Vitamin B$_{12}$ is absorbed in a complex series of steps. After liberation from food in the stomach, vitamin B$_{12}$ becomes bound non-specifically to proteins termed *R-binders*. In the duodenum, pancreatic proteases degrade R-binders, but cannot digest the specific vitamin B$_{12}$ binding protein, intrinsic factor (produced by gastric parietal cells). In the terminal ileum, receptors bind the intrinsic factor-vitamin B$_{12}$ complex, leading to absorption of vitamin B$_{12}$.

Pernicious anemia is a disease that consists of gastric achlorhydria, gastric atrophy, and failure to secrete intrinsic factor. It is caused by autoimmune destruction of gastric mucosa (particularly parietal cells), often associated with antibodies to parietal cells (a nonspecific finding) and intrinsic factor blocking antibodies (specific, but seen in only 50% to 70% of cases). The intrinsic-factor deficiency prevents absorption of vitamin B$_{12}$. This leads to damage to the posterior columns of the spinal cord (causing a sensory neuropathy), and in many cases megaloblastic anemia. Pernicious anemia is covered in greater detail in Chapter 39.

The Schilling test of vitamin B$_{12}$ absorption is an elegant evaluator of both gastric and intestinal function. The Schilling test may be normal in the early stages of pernicious anemia, in which vitamin B$_{12}$ absorption may be related more to impaired degradation of R-binders, as the result of lack of acid needed to activate pancreatic enzymes, than to deficiency of intrinsic factor. Some studies have suggested that administration of labeled vitamin B$_{12}$ along with food may be a more sensitive method to detect pernicious anemia.[26] Recent studies have suggested that tests of B$_{12}$ absorption are less sensitive indicators of B$_{12}$ deficiency than measurement of methylmalonic acid, which accumulates with tissue B$_{12}$ deficiency.[27,28] The procedure for performing this test is described in the Methods section of the CD-ROM; however, in many North American institutions the Schilling test is no longer available because the company that manufactured diagnostic kits for performing the test has discontinued their production.

Malabsorption Syndromes

Malabsorption syndromes are the result of any interference with the process of digestion and absorption of food. Clinical features of malabsorption syndromes commonly include loose stools, typically containing fat that gives a greasy appearance and foul odor to the stools (steatorrhea); loss of weight or failure to gain weight (in children); and features secondary to deficiencies of fat-soluble vitamins (bone disease, prolonged clotting times, poor night vision, neuropathy).[28-30] In true malabsorption, the gastrointestinal tract is impaired so that it cannot absorb a variety of nutrients, generally the result of a disorder that causes damage to the intestinal mucosa. The other category of malabsorption syndrome should in fact be called *maldigestion*, in which the digestive process is in some way impaired.[31] This is most commonly caused by pancreatic insufficiency (see Chapter 29), but may also occur with inadequate pancreatic enzyme activation in severe achlorhydria or with excessive acid production (see ulcers and Zollinger-Ellison

TABLE **30-3** PENTAGASTRIN STIMULATION TEST		
	Basal Acid Output (BAO) (mmol/hour)	*Maximal Acid Output (MAO) (mmol/hour)*
Healthy adult men		
Under 30 years old	2.2 to 2.7	14 to 42
Over 30 years old	2.2 to 2.7	3 to 33
Healthy adult women	1 to 1.5	7 to 20
Zollinger-Ellison syndrome	10 to 100 (or more)	40% to 60% above BAO
Ulcer predisposition		
Likely		>35
Highly likely		>45
Low risk		<11

syndrome described earlier) or inadequate bile acid production or secretion. Maldigestion syndrome typically leads to fat malabsorption and steatorrhea, but protein and carbohydrate absorption may be less affected.

A variety of serum tests may be abnormal in patients with malabsorption syndromes, including decreases in serum iron, vitamin B_{12}, albumin, calcium, and phosphorus; and increases in prothrombin time. In addition, immunoglobulin determinations can be useful to rule out IgA deficiency, a condition that permits intestinal parasitic infestations to occur. In persons suspected of malabsorption syndromes, laboratory tests can be useful in confirming its presence and in distinguishing true malabsorption from maldigestion.

Steatorrhea. Steatorrhea is a clinical syndrome caused by the malabsorption of dietary fat. The undigested fat travels into the large bowel, and the stools contain an excess amount of lipid and are characteristically pale, bulky, and greasy with a repugnant odor. It is important to distinguish clinically the stools produced in steatorrhea from those produced in other causes of diarrhea. When steatorrhea is suspected, testing should be undertaken to estimate the actual amount of fat in the stool. When excess fat has been identified, the specific cause is sought. A deficiency of any factor important for lipid digestion and absorption can cause steatorrhea. Conditions producing steatorrhea include the Zollinger-Ellison syndrome, increased duodenal acid (postgastrectomy syndromes), abnormal bile output (biliary tract obstruction), pancreatic insufficiency, intestinal mucosal impairment, and disease of the large bowel that has caused an interruption of bile-salt enterohepatic circulation.

Celiac disease (celiac sprue).[32] Celiac disease is an extremely important cause of malabsorption. In this condition, persons appear to have an abnormal immunological response to the presence of **gluten** in the diet. Ingestion of gluten (found principally in wheat products) leads to inflammation of the intestine and loss of both villi and microvilli, drastically reducing the absorptive surface area and causing malabsorption. There is also an increased incidence of intestinal lymphomas in individuals affected by celiac disease, and an increased incidence of other autoimmune disorders, particularly those involving the endocrine system. Up to 90% of celiac patients have circulating antibodies to gluten, although the finding of these antibodies is nonspecific. More recently, antibodies to the endomysium of muscle (specifically those to the enzyme tissue transglutaminase), particularly those of the IgA class, have been found to be both sensitive and specific markers of celiac disaese.[33] Celiac disease may manifest in very subtle ways such as iron-deficiency anemia, and may be definitively diagnosed only by the response to a gluten-free diet; however, antibodies to both gluten and transglutaminase may become negative after several months on this diet.[34]

Lactose intolerance and other carbohydrate malabsorption disorders. The most common carbohydrate malabsorption disorder is lactose intolerance.[35] All infants have the intestinal enzyme lactase, necessary to break the milk disaccharide, lactose, into glucose and galactose,

thereby allowing their absorption. In those population groups who characteristically feed on animal milk throughout life, these enzyme mechanisms persist into adulthood. However, in those groups who are historically not milk drinkers (individuals of African and Asian ancestry), the enzyme system regresses. If persons lacking lactase ingest milk or milk products, they will fail to split the lactose; unabsorbed sugar creates an osmotic force that pulls fluid into the intestinal lumen. This causes cramping, bloating sensations, and diarrhea. Moreover, large-bowel bacteria can metabolize the sugar to produce gas. Although most people with lactose intolerance are aware of their problem and avoid milk products, there are persons with milder forms who experience discomfort in much more subtle ways. In infants, transient lactase deficiency can occur after episodes of gastroenteritis, producing similar symptoms; lactase activity typically becomes normal in less than 2 weeks. The diagnosis of lactose malabsorption can be made by use of the lactose-tolerance procedures discussed later in the chapter, but this step is usually unnecessary. Malabsorption syndromes of other disaccharides have been reported but are extremely rare. Malabsorption of monosaccharides is seen only in extreme impairment of the mucosal surface.

Carcinoid Syndrome[36]

A syndrome manifesting as vascular flushing, diarrhea, occasional tricuspid insufficiency, and, rarely, pellagra associated with an intestinal carcinoid tumor is called the *carcinoid syndrome*. Carcinoid tumors, which are the most common of small bowel tumors, are located predominantly in the distal ileum or appendix. The remainder of gastrointestinal carcinoid tumors are found in the rectum and stomach. These tumors metastasize most commonly to the regional lymph nodes, liver, and skeleton. Primary carcinoid tumors of the appendix are common but rarely metastasize, whereas those that arise from other parts of the gastrointestinal tract do metastasize. The tumors produce serotonin and kinins in vast excess, which are responsible for the characteristic clinical syndrome. The presence of the disorder can be detected by measuring serotonin or its metabolite 5-hydroxyindoleacetic acid (5-HIAA),[37] formed by the conversion of tryptophan to 5-hydroxytryptamine (serotonin), which is ultimately converted to 5-HIAA. The amount of 5-HIAA found in the urine is highly method dependent. Many screening procedures are very nonspecific and should therefore not be used to make diagnoses. An appropriate approach is the use of a screening procedure for all requests for 5-HIAA values; those that exhibit an elevated value should be subjected to a more specific test.

In healthy adults, up to 6 mg (31.2 mmol) of 5-HIAA is excreted per 24 hours. In the carcinoid syndrome, results are usually between 25 and 1000 mg (130 and 5200 mmol) per day.

False-negative results are produced by many drugs, including *p*-chlorophenylalanine, corticotropin, ethanol, imipramine, isoniazid, monoamine oxidase inhibitors, methenamine, methyldopa, and phenothiazines. Reduction of an elevated value is also seen in renal disease and in phenyl-ketonuria. False-positive results have been reported in celiac disease, intestinal obstruction, pregnancy, sleep deprivation, small cell carcinoma of the lung, and with ingestion of avo-cados, bananas, eggplants, pineapples, plums, and walnuts. Drugs that are known to cause an increase in 5-HIAA value are acetanilid, ephedrine, mephenesin, nicotine, phenacetin, phenobarbital, phentolamine, rauwolfia, reserpine, metho-carbamol, and glycerol guaiacolate cough medicines. Chromogranin, a marker of neuroendocrine cells, is elevated in a high percentage of persons with carcinoid syndrome and a number of other neuroendocrine tumors.[38,39]

Large Intestine Disease

Diarrhea. Diarrhea[40] is defined as the excessive produc-tion of feces, usually as a result of overabundance of water in the stool. Severe diarrhea causes sodium and water depletion and loss of potassium and bicarbonate. There are three main mechanisms for diarrhea: solute malabsorption, secretion of fluid into the intestine, and motility disturbance.

Solute malabsorption is caused by the ingestion of poorly absorbed substances, "dumping," or intestinal malabsorption. Secretion of fluid occurs in many conditions. Passive secretion occurs if obstruction or inflammation increases the epithelial permeability. Secretion of ions occurs through the activity of $3',5'$-cyclic adenosine monophosphate as stimulated by cholera toxin, endotoxin, prostaglandins, bile acids, and certain tumor products (such as VIP). Another secretory mechanism is the replacement of absorptive epithelium by crypt epithelium (as occurs with viral gastroenteritis).

Cathartics and irritable bowel syndrome can cause motility disturbances. These will increase the motility and decrease the transit time and therefore the absorptive efficiency.

Cancer. Malignancies of the colon and rectum account for over half the cancers of the entire gastrointestinal system. Early detection through screening is the most effective approach to curing this often fatal disorder. Digital, sigmoid-oscopic, and colonoscopic examination of the rectum is supplemented by screening for the presence of occult blood. Roentgenological studies are useful only in screening patients with a high risk of cancer. Colonoscopy is becoming the preferred method of examining high-risk patients.[41]

Blind-loop syndromes. A variety of inflammatory and anatomical disorders of the gastrointestinal tract may cause regional outpouchings to occur in the large bowel. These pockets can trap intestinal material and allow bacterial overgrowth. If this happens, the overabundant bacteria can cause excessive breakdown of bile conjugates. When these materials have been deconjugated, they cannot be reabsorbed by the body and are lost in the feces. This may be the cause of diarrhea. The bile acid breath test can be used in the diagnosis of this condition. The use of breath analysis in gastroenterology has been extensively reviewed by Newman.[42] In the carbon-14 bile acid breath test, glycine-1-$[^{14}C]$cholate is administered orally. If the patient has an intestinal blind loop or other source of bacterial overgrowth,

deconjugation of the tracer will occur, allowing the ^{14}C-labeled compound to enter the bloodstream; metabolism in the liver releases $^{14}CO_2$. Breath CO_2 is trapped in an alkaline solution, and the subsequent detection of radioactivity is a sensitive indication of the presence of bacterial overgrowth.

Inflammatory bowel disease. Two idiopathic inflam-matory disorders of the intestinal tract, ulcerative colitis and Crohn's disease, may present with signs and symptoms such as abdominal pain, diarrhea, and (in the case of Crohn's disease) malabsorption. The exact pathogenesis of these disorders is unknown, but there is evidence of familial predisposition and autoimmune phenomena in many cases. Characteristically, Crohn's disease affects the small intestine, and ulcerative colitis is limited to the large intestine, but in some cases it is not possible to distinguish these two disorders clinically or by pathologic examination of samples. Autoantibodies can be found in about half of patients with each disorder. In ulcerative colitis, atypical perinuclear anti-neutrophil cytoplasmic antibodies are present, whereas in Crohn's disease, antibodies to *Saccharomyces cerevisiae* are found. The specificity of these autoantibodies is bout 90% to 95% for each disorder.[43]

GASTROINTESTINAL FUNCTION TESTS
Tests of Gastric Acidity (see CD-ROM)

Tests of gastric acidity can be used to screen for the ability of the parietal cells to produce hydrochloric acid, but are rarely performed at present. The discovery of achlorhydria (anacidity) is strong evidence for the presence of pernicious anemia and rules out peptic ulcer disease. The presence of acid in the stomach is very strong evidence against pernicious anemia. As discussed later, acid detection must be carried out to determine the significance of increased serum gastrin.

The only suitable test for the presence of gastric acid is **intubation** and withdrawal of stomach juice. A pH measure-ment may then be made directly and should be less than 3. Anacidity is confirmed by a pH over 6.

Gastric Stimulation Tests

Gastric analysis. With the recognition that most cases of peptic ulcer are related to *H. pylori* infection, tests of gastric acid stimulation are seldom used. Gastric analysis involves collecting gastric secretions for a baseline period to deter-mine basal or unstimulated acid production. Next, a parietal cell stimulant is administered and gastric juice is collected to evaluate maximum secretory ability. Currently, pentagastrin, the active 5–amino acid portion of gastrin, is the recommended stimulant.[44,45]

The procedure involves (1) removing residual gastric fluid from a fasting patient by intermittent suction on a nasogastric tube positioned within the stomach, (2) collecting basal secre-tions for four 15-minute periods, (3) administering penta-gastrin in a dose of 5 mg/kg body weight intramuscularly, and (4) collecting gastric secretions for six consecutive 15-minute periods. All collections are then evaluated for appearance, pH, volume, millimoles of H^+ per liter, millimoles of H^+ per total volume, and millimoles of H^+ per hour for each collection.

After stimulation, pH values should fall to less than 2; failure to do so indicates inadequate parietal cell function because of pernicious anemia or other causes (gastric carcinoma, iron deficiency anemia, rheumatoid arthritis, and myxedema). BAO is determined by averaging the mmol/hr output for the three closest basal collections. The MAO is calculated as the mean of the two highest poststimulation values in mmol/hr. Healthy adult men have a BAO of 2.2 to 2.7 mmol/hr, with 5 mmol/hr being the upper reference limit. The MAO for men under 30 years of age is 14 to 42 mmol/hr, but 3 to 33 mmol/hr for men over 30 years of age. The values for women are approximately 50% of those for men. Detailed tables of reference intervals have been published[46] and are reviewed in Table 30-3.

Hollander insulin test. The Hollander insulin test[47] is used to assess whether a surgical vagotomy has successfully denervated the stomach. In this procedure, regular insulin (0.15 U/kg of body weight) is administered intravenously to render the patient hypoglycemic (plasma glucose less than 400 mg/L [2.2 mmol/L]). Vagus stimulation is a normal response to hypoglycemia. Those with an intact gastric vagus release acid in response to hypoglycemia. A successful denervation will result in MAO less than 0.05 mmol/hour, and pH will remain over 3.5. The test is not often performed because clinical evaluation is generally sufficient.

Fat Absorption Tests (see CD-ROM)

The definitive test of fat absorption is the quantitative measurement of fat in timed collections of feces obtained while the patient is maintained on a diet containing an approximately known amount of fat.[28] Because the collection is extremely difficult for the patient, a variety of alternative approaches have been promoted. Unfortunately, none of these entirely replaces the diagnostic ability of the quantitative fecal fat measurement.

Fat screening. Fat screening is carried out first by evaluation of the weight and appearance of the stool. A pale, frothy appearance is virtually diagnostic of excessive fat. More reliable than this is the application of a small amount of the fecal material onto a standard microscopic slide, followed by staining with a fat-specific stain. Trained observers are able to identify excessive fat in 80% to 90% of persons with fat malabsorption. Using quantitative microscopy (including grading size and number of fat droplets) improves sensitivity and specificity of fecal fat stains.[47] Another screening procedure is the steatocrit, in which the percentage of fat is quantified in a random stool sample; this correlates reasonably well with quantitative fecal fat determination.[48]

Serum carotene. Carotenoids are a group of related fat-soluble compounds that are found in yellow vegetables and serve as precursors of vitamin A. Unlike vitamin A, carotenoids are not stored in the body; thus, serum carotene levels reflect recent intake and absorption of fat. One particular carotenoid, β-carotene, a naturally occurring pigment found in vegetables and fruit, has found the most use as a screening test for fat malabsorption. The reference interval for serum carotene is 500 to 2500 µg/L (0.19 to 1.6 mmol/L). The concentration of carotene is determined by the balance between the degree of malabsorption and the oral carotene intake.[50] Serum carotene is decreased in low carotene diets (low vegetable diets), abetalipoproteinemia, Tangier disease, liver failure, and 86% of patients with clinically significant fat malabsorption.

Quantitative fecal fat estimation. Quantitative fecal fat estimation is performed after collection of feces for 3 consecutive days. In the 2 days preceding the collection and during the period of collection, patients must include approximately 100 g of medium-chain triglycerides in their diet. The actual amount of fat in diet can be difficult to determine, even for a dietitian; however, within the range of fat intakes from about 60 to 200 g, normal fecal fat excretion is less than 7 g per day.[28] Quantitative fecal fat measurements are unreliable in patients without diarrhea (defined as stool output >200 g per day). The nonabsorbable fat substitute Olestra is also measured as fat in quantitative measurements; individuals collecting stool fat specimens should be instructed to discontinue use of products containing this compound for 72 hours before they start a fecal fat collection.[51]

Feces can be collected in plastic bags. The plastic bags may then be closed with a tin tie and held in a preweighed, 5-gallon paint can. On arrival in the laboratory the can and contents are weighed and the weight of the collection is determined. The chemical analysis is then carried out on a thoroughly mixed aliquot of this 3-day collection. Persons consuming a 100 g fat diet will excrete no more than 5 g of fecal fat per day. More than 10 g per day is certain evidence of fat malabsorption. Failure to adhere to the diet may invalidate the results; low fat intake will mask minimum fat malabsorption, whereas grossly excessive fat intake will raise the fecal content above 5 g.

Isotope tests. A radioactively labeled, medium-chain triglyceride is administered to patients in whom fat malabsorption is suspected.[52] After a suitable time interval, blood is collected and its radioactivity determined. It is assumed that the radioactivity that finds its way into the bloodstream is a result of the successful digestion and absorption of the radioactive fat. Unfortunately, radioactive iodine tags are not suitable for this procedure because they must be linked to unsaturated fats and because the size of the iodine tag gravely distorts the triglyceride molecule, making it susceptible to incidental breakdown. Thus the absorption of the radioactive iodine from these materials might not indicate successful fat absorption.

D-Xylose Absorption Test[53] (see Methods on CD-ROM)

D-Xylose is an aldopentose that is absorbed passively in the small intestine; its successful absorption is a reflection of the integrity of the surface area of the small intestine. Once D-xylose is absorbed, at least 50% is excreted in the urine within the next 24 hours. The amount excreted over a 5-hour period is closely correlated with the amount absorbed in the gastrointestinal tract.

The patient is instructed to fast overnight but is encouraged to drink an ample amount of water during this time. Two doses have been advocated; most authors suggest that 25 g of D-xylose dissolved in approximately 300 to 500 mL of water is a suitable dose for adults, but a 5 g dose appears adequate and is less likely to cause abdominal cramps. Smaller subjects are given 1 g/kg of body weight to a maximum of 25 g. After administration, urine is collected for a 5-hour period. At least 25% of the administered dose will appear in the urine over a 5-hour period if renal function is within the reference interval. For children who cannot be relied on to collect a urinary sample or for subjects with severe renal insufficiency, blood collections at 1 and 2 hours may be substituted. Most persons demonstrate plasma levels greater than 300 mg/L in one of the samples. In children, values above 100 mg/L should be considered within the reference interval.

Low levels of urine or plasma xylose are suggestive of an absorptive defect in the jejunum. Low levels are also seen in ascites, vomiting, delayed gastric emptying, improper urine collection, and high-dose aspirin therapy and with neomycin, colchicine, indomethacin, atropine, and impaired renal function. Values within the reference interval are seen in persons who have absorptive defects occurring in a skip pattern (such as Crohn's disease). Such a disease distribution allows a sufficient amount of healthy mucosa to remain and absorb an amount of D-xylose within the usual interval.

Lactose Tolerance Test

In this test, 50 g of lactose dissolved in water is administered orally to the patient, who is observed carefully for the onset of symptoms. The standard protocol includes the collection of a baseline specimen and 5-, 10-, 30-, 60-, 90-, and 120-minute specimens for plasma glucose measurements. Glucose levels will be increased if lactose has been successfully cleaved and its components absorbed. The galactose moiety of the lactose is converted quickly into glucose by the liver. Healthy persons will demonstrate a glucose rise to greater than 2000 mg/L (11.1 mmol/L) over the baseline sample. Those with lactase deficiency will exhibit notable abdominal discomfort and will have a peak plasma glucose of less than 1000 mg/L (5.5 mmol/L).

An alternate method of determining lactose absorption is the measurement of the amount of hydrogen appearing in exhaled breath after the oral administration of lactose.[35] Lactase-deficient persons will not absorb lactose, and it will find its way into the large bowel, where bacteria will metabolize it. Hydrogen, one of the by-products of this bacterial action, passes quickly into the bloodstream and is removed in the exhaled breath. Special-purpose gas chromatographs can detect the presence of postlactose hydrogen. A healthy person allows no lactose to enter the colon and therefore has less than 10 parts per million (ppm) of hydrogen in the exhaled breath. Persons with lactase deficiency demonstrate at least 50 ppm of hydrogen. Intermediate amounts of hydrogen in the breath can be caused by large doses of lactose and are of questionable significance.

The definitive diagnosis is made by tissue enzyme assays carried out on biopsy samples of the intestinal mucosa.

CHANGE OF ANALYTE IN DISEASE (Table 30-4)
Malabsorption Testing

Screening approach. Screening for malabsorption syndromes is best done using clinical signs and symptoms associated with malabsorption and looking at populations at high risk. For example, elderly persons are at greatest risk for occult malabsorption. Laboratory screening for malabsorption is not very sensitive; however, measurement of serum albumin, calcium, vitamin B_{12}, and a peripheral smear looking for evidence of macrocytosis and iron-deficiency anemia constitute a reasonable general laboratory screen for malabsorption. If necessary, more specific tests for iron deficiency can be carried out. Persons believed to have specific malabsorption syndromes should be tested accordingly. Those with steatorrhea and suspected fat malabsorption should first have their feces examined visually. Next, a rapid slide evaluation of a stool sample should be carried out, looking for meat fibers and excess (see p. 560) fat. A carotene determination is easily performed and reflects gross abnormalities of fat absorption. A D-xylose absorption test (see earlier discussion) will indicate whether significant generalized absorptive problems are present. Protein malabsorption is difficult to assess biochemically, and only when there is serious amino acid malabsorption will the serum albumin be depressed.

Vitamin A. Vitamin A is an alcohol derived from β-carotene by hydrolytic cleavage at the midpoint of the C-18 polyene chain. Because it is chemically similar to carotene, it is also hydrophobic and must be absorbed into the body along with fat. Thus its presence in serum is also a reasonable estimate of the ability of the body to absorb fat. Serum vitamin A concentrations are less dependent on diet than serum carotene concentrations are. Reduced serum vitamin A concentrations are seen in association with fat malabsorption and liver disease.

Because the serum vitamin A determination is significantly more difficult to perform than the serum carotene and because its diagnostic ability is not significantly greater, it has never achieved popular acceptance as a screening test for fat malabsorption.

Trypsin. The measurement of trypsin in stool has been advocated as a screening test of pancreatic insufficiency.[54] Trypsin determination is much more reliable in infants and young children than in adults because there is less colonic degradation of pancreatic enzymes. The simplest test of tryptic activity is the application of a smear of fecal material to a thin film of gelatin. If trypsin is present, an enzymatic breakdown of the film will be seen. The test will be abnormal in all patients with significant pancreatic insufficiency, except in unusual cases of isolated defects of amylase and lipase. Some healthy infants, however, will fail to produce sufficient trypsin to degrade the gelatin layer. Although such tests have some validity in screening, a strong clinical suggestion of pancreatic insufficiency warrants specific testing, as outlined in Chapter 29.

Chymotrypsin. Although trypsin measurements are seldom performed, measurement of fecal immunoreactive

TABLE 30-4 CHANGE OF ANALYTE AND FUNCTION TESTS IN DISEASE

Disease	Fecal Fat	Lactose Intolerance	S-Carotene S-Vitamin A	S-Vitamin B12 S-Folate	Schilling Test	D-Xylose Absorption	Stool Occult Blood	Carcino-embryonic Antigen	5-HIAA	Pancreatic Enzyme Testing	Stool Examination
Steatorrhea	↑↑	N	↓	N,↓	AB	AB	Neg	N	N	AB	Foul smelling, greasy
Celiac disease	N,↑	N	N,↓	N	N, AB	N, AB	Neg	N	N	N	Variable
Lactose intolerance	N	AB	N	N	N	N	Neg	N	N	N	Loose in association with abdominal cramps
Carcinoid syndrome	N	N	N	N,↓	N, AB	N	Neg, pos	N,↑	↑↑	N	Loose in association with cutaneous flushing
Functional diarrhea	N	N	N	N	N	N	Neg	N	N	N	Loose
Bowel carcinoma	N	N	N	N,↓	N	N	Neg, pos	N,↑	N	N	Change in bowel habits
Inflammatory bowel	N	N	N	N,↓	N	N	Neg, pos	N,↑	N	N	Loose, bloody

AB, Abnormal; N, normal (within the reference interval); S, serum; ↑, increase; ↓, decrease.

chymotrypsin has been suggested as a better indicator of pancreatic protease production, as discussed in Chapter 29.

Evaluation of Diarrhea

In persons with acute onset of diarrhea, laboratory tests (other than culture and gram stain for fecal leukocytes) are usually not required or indicated, because most acute diarrhea will resolve with or without treatment.[55] In persons with chronic diarrhea, laboratory tests can be helpful in distinguishing secretory diarrhea from that resulting from the presence of osmotically active substances (as also occurs in those who have malabsorption).[56,57] Normally, most of stool solute is composed of the electrolytes, and normal stool osmolality is approximately 290 mosm/kg. Measurement of stool electrolytes in liquid stools (after centrifugation) can be used to calculate an osmotic gap, defined as the difference between normal stool osmolality (290) and stool electrolytes (two times the sum of Na^+ and K^+ concentrations in mmol/L).[58] Measurement of actual stool osmolality, although theoretically more accurate in calculating osmotic gap, is limited by the rise in stool osmolality that occurs because of bacterial metabolism of undigested solutes after sample collection. A normal stool osmotic gap (<50 mmol/L) indicates the presence of increased water and electrolytes in normal balance, caused by secretory diarrhea or abnormal motility. An increased osmotic gap indicates the presence of unabsorbed solutes, as can be found with malabsorption and with ingestion of nonabsorbable solutes such as magnesium salts. Alkalinization of a stool sample and inspection for the pink color of phenolphthalein can be used to detect occult ingestion of cathartics.

Vasoactive intestinal polypeptide.[59] Elevated levels of VIP are found in the plasma in some patients with watery diarrhea syndrome (Verner-Morrison syndrome). This syndrome was subsequently named *WDHA* after the initial letters of its main characteristics: *w*atery *d*iarrhea, *h*ypokalemia, and *h*ypochlorhydria or *a*chlorhydria. The syndrome is rare; about one tenth as common as Zollinger-Ellison syndrome. It is sometimes part of the multiple endocrine neoplasia syndromes (see p. 557). In patients with WDHA syndrome, a non-β islet cell tumor (VIPoma) of the pancreas is usually present (D_1 cells); about half of these tumors are malignant. Tumors that occur elsewhere (such as small cell carcinoma, or retroperitoneal neuroblastoma) may also secrete VIP. In high levels, VIP causes vasodilation with facial flushing, increases intestinal blood flow, induces watery diarrhea, and inhibits gastric secretion. The diarrhea, which is explosive and consists of up to 30 stools per day, causes profound hypokalemia (1 to 3 mmol/L).

The diagnosis is made by elimination of the common causes of watery diarrhea and hypokalemia. Gastric secretion tests often show the presence of hypochlorhydria, and the diagnosis is confirmed by measurements of elevated blood levels of immunoreactive VIP.

Tests Related to Specific Disorders

Occult blood in stool. A number of methods are available to detect trace amounts of hemoglobin in feces. Most rely on the ability of hemoglobin and its derivatives to act as peroxidases and catalyze the reaction between hydrogen peroxide and a chromogenic, organic compound. Benzidine has been used but is carcinogenic and therefore not currently available; most commercial assays employ *guaiac*. A number of immunochemical tests to detect hemoglobin directly are also available.[60] Immunochemical tests produce false-negative results if stool is exposed to toilet bowl sanitizers.[61] With peroxidase-based tests, a number of dietary substances are capable of producing false-positive results, including iron and peroxidases found in red meat and various plants. Most kit manufacturers and practice guidelines suggest putting the patient on a diet in which red meat is withheld for several days prior to collection,[62] but this may not be necessary to prevent false-positive results.[63] Allowing samples to stand for 2 to 3 days (as occurs with mailing of completed cards to the laboratory) reduces the rate of false-positives derived from plant peroxidases and may reduce the interference from other food peroxidases as well.[64] Rehydration of dried stool samples before testing reduces the rate of false-negative results,[65] but increases the rate of false-positive results as well.[62]

Carcinoembryonic antigen. Carcinoembryonic antigen (CEA), also discussed in Chapter 49, is a glycoprotein that is abundant in fetal entodermally derived tissues (gastrointestinal mucosa, pancreas, lung).[66] CEA is not a single chemical compound; numerous glycoproteins cross-react in CEA assays, including fetal sulfoglycoprotein, normal colonic antigen, and normal glycoprotein. CEA is produced in a variety of tumors, including most tumors of the GI tract but especially in colon cancer. Serum CEA levels are related to tumor mass; CEA is elevated in less than one fourth of localized tumors, preventing its use in screening for colon cancer. CEA is most useful in monitoring the course of disease in persons who have been treated for colon cancer. CEA should be measured at the time of surgery to establish a baseline level, and checked again starting at least 1 month after surgery. Persistent elevations and increases after surgery indicate residual and metastatic disease, respectively. The reference interval for CEA is typically 0 to 5 ng/mL. Higher values occur in liver disease, inflammatory bowel disease, heavy smoking, and chronic renal failure, but levels above 10 to 15 ng/mL are rare in these conditions. Immunoassays for CEA are not interchangeable; patients being followed for colon cancer should have levels checked by the old and new assays in parallel (rebaselining) before the laboratory switches to a new CEA methodology.

References

1. Parkkila S et al: Molecular aspects of iron absorption and HFE expression, *Gastroenterology* 121:1489, 2001.
2. Mirsky IA: Physiologic, psychologic, and social determinants in the etiology of duodenal ulcer, *Am J Dig Dis* 3:285, 1958.
3. Feder JN: The hereditary hemochromatosis gene (HFE): a MHC class I-like gene that functions in the regulation of iron homeostasis, *Immunol Res* 20:175, 1999.
4. Dockray GJ et al: The gastrins: their production and biological activities, *Annu Rev Physiol* 63:119, 2001.
5. Dockray GJ: Topical review. Gastrin and gastric epithelial physiology, *J Physiol* 518:315, 1999.
6. Holst JJ, Schmidt P: Gut hormones and intestinal function, *Baillieres Clin Endocrinol Metab* 8:137, 1994.
7. Owyang C: Physiological mechanisms of cholecystokinin action on pancreatic secretion, *Am J Physiol* 271:G1, 1996.
8. Shulkes A, Baldwin GS: Biology of gut cholecystokinin and gastrin receptors, *Clin Exp Pharmacol Physiol* 24:209, 1997.
9. Liddle RA: Regulation of cholecystokinin secretion by intraluminal releasing factors, *Am J Physiol* 269:G319, 1995.
10. Glupczynski Y: Microbiological and serological diagnostic tests for *Helicobacter pylori*: an overview, *Acta Gastroenterol Belg* 61:321, 1998.
11. Gozes I et al: Pharmaceutical VIP: prospects and problems, *Curr Med Chem* 6:1019, 1999.
12. Drucker DJ: Minireview: the glucagon-like peptides, *Endocrinology* 142:521, 2001.
13. The Eurogastric Study Group: An international association between *Helicobacter pylori* infection and gastric cancer, *Lancet* 341:1359, 1993.
14. Cohen H: Peptic ulcer and *Helicobacter pylori*. *Gastroenterol Clin North Am* 29:775, 2000.
15. Anderson J, Gonzalez J: *H. pylori* infection. Review of the guideline for diagnosis and treatment, *Geriatrics* 55:44, 2000.
16. Herbrink P, van Doorn LJ: Serological methods for diagnosis of *Helicobacter pylori* infection and monitoring of eradication therapy, *Eur J Clin Microbiol Infect Dis* 19:164, 2000.
17. Fallone CA, Veldhuyzen van Zanten SJ, Chiba N: The urea breath test for *Helicobacter pylori* infection: taking the wind out of the sails of endoscopy, *CMAJ* 162:371, 2000.
18. Laine L et al: Effect of proton-pump inhibitor therapy on diagnostic testing for *Helicobacter pylori*, *Ann Intern Med* 129:547, 1998.
19. Forne M et al: Accuracy of an enzyme immunoassay for the detection of *Helicobacter pylori* in stool specimens in the diagnosis of infection and posttreatment check-up, *Am J Gastroenterol* 95:2200, 2000.
20. Ishihara S et al: Diagnostic accuracy of a new non-invasive enzyme immunoassay for detecting *Helicobacter pylori* in stools after eradication therapy, *Aliment Pharmacol Ther* 14:611, 2000.
21. Uemura N et al: *Helicobacter pylori* infection and the development of gastric cancer, *N Engl J Med* 345:784, 2001.
22. Hirschowitz BI: Zollinger-Ellison syndrome: pathogenesis, diagnosis, and management, *Am J Gastroenterol* 92(4 suppl):44S, 1997.
23. Mignon M, Cadiot G: Diagnostic and therapeutic criteria in patients with Zollinger-Ellison syndrome and multiple endocrine neoplasia type 1, *J Intern Med* 243:489, 1998.
24. Phay JE, Moley JF, Lairmore TC: Multiple endocrine neoplasias, *Semin Surg Oncol* 18:324, 2000.
25. Lamers CBH et al: Comparative study of the value of the calcium, secretin, and meal stimulated increase in serum gastrin to the diagnosis of the Zollinger-Ellison syndrome, *Gut* 18:128, 1977.
26. Lindgren A et al: Schilling and protein-bound cobalamin absorption tests are poor instruments for diagnosing cobalamin malabsorption, *J Intern Med* 241:477, 1997.
27. Brigden ML: Schilling test: still useful in pernicious anemia? *Postgrad Med* 106:37, 1999.
28. Riley SA, Marsh MN: Maldigestion and malabsorption. In Feldman M, Scharschmidt BF, Sleisenger MH: *Sleisenger & Fordtran's gastrointestinal and liver disease*, ed 6, Philadelphia, 1998, Saunders.
29. Marousis CG, Cerda JJ: Malabsorption: a clinical update, *Compr Ther* 23:672, 1997.
30. Bai JC: Malabsorption syndromes, *Digestion* 59:530, 1998.
31. Ebert EC: Maldigestion and malabsorption, *Dis Mon* 47:49, 2001.
32. Collin P, Kaukinen K, Maki M: Clinical features of celiac disease today, *Dig Dis* 17:100, 1999.

33. Schuppan D: Current concepts of celiac disease pathogenesis, *Gastroenterology* 119:234, 2000.
34. Fasano A, Catassi C: Current approaches to diagnosis and treatment of celiac disease: an evolving spectrum, *Gastroenterology* 120:636, 2001.
35. Shaw AD, Davies GJ: Lactose intolerance: problems in diagnosis and treatment, *J Clin Gastroenterol* 28:208, 1999.
36. Donaldson D: Carcinoid tumors–the carcinoid syndrome and serotonin: a brief review, *J R Soc Health* 120:78, 2000.
37. Nuttall KL, Pingree SS: The incidence of elevations in urine 5-hydroxyindoleacetic acid, *Ann Clin Lab Sci* 28:167, 1998.
38. Obert K: Biochemical diagnosis of neuroendocrine GEP tumor, *Yale J Biol Med* 70:501, 1997.
39. Boomsma F et al: Sensitivity and specificity of a new ELISA method for determination of chromogranin A in the diagnosis of pheochromocytoma and neuroblastoma, *Clin Chem Acta* 239:57, 1995.
40. Schiller LR: Diarrhea, *Med Clin North Am* 84:1259, 2000.
41. Lieberman DA et al: One-time screening for colorectal cancer with combined fecal occult-blood testing and examination of the distal colon, *N Engl J Med* 345:555, 2001.
42. Newman A: Breath-analysis tests in gastroenterology, *Gut* 15:1, 1974.
43. Peeters M et al: Diagnostic value of anti-Saccharomyces cerevisiae and antineutrophil cytoplasmic autoantibodies in inflammatory bowel disease, *Am J Gastroenterol* 96:730, 2001.
44. Ward S et al: Comparison of Histalog and histamine as stimulants for maximal gastric secretions in human subjects and in dogs, *Gastroenterology* 44:620, 1963.
45. Abernethy RJ et al: Pentagastrin as a stimulant of maximal gastric acid response in man: a multicentre pilot study, *Lancet* i:291, 1967.
46. Blackman AH et al: Computed normal values for peak acid output based on age, sex and body weight, *Am J Dig Dis* 15:783, 1970.
47. McNeely MDD: Gastrointestinal function. In Sonnenwirth AC, Jarett L, editors: *Gradwohl's clinical laboratory methods and diagnosis*, ed 8, St Louis, 1980, Mosby.
48. Fine KD, Ogunji F: A new method of quantitative fecal fat microscopy and its correlation with chemically measured fecal fat output, *Am J Clin Pathol* 113:528, 2000.
49. Sugai E et al: Steatocrit: a reliable semiquantitative method for detection of steatorrhea, *J Clin Gastroenterol* 19:206, 1994.
50. Galvan-Guerra E et al: Diagnostic utility of serum beta-carotene in intestinal malabsorption syndrome, *Rev Invest Clin* 46:99, 1994.
51. Balasekaran R et al: Positive results on tests for steatorrhea in persons consuming olestra potato chips, *Ann Intern Med* 132:279, 2000.
52. Perri F, Andriulli A: "Mixed" triglyceride breath test: methodological problems and clinical applications, *Rev Med Univ Navarra* 42:99, 1998.
53. Craig RM, Ehrenpreis ED: D-Xylose testing, *J Clin Gastroenterol* 29:143, 1999.
54. Erlanger BF, Kokowsky N, Cohen W: The preparation and properties of two new chromogenic substrates of trypsin, *Arch Biochem Biophys* 95:271, 1961.
55. Aranda-Michel J, Giannella RA: Acute diarrhea: a practical review, *Am J Med* 106:670, 1999.
56. Branski D, Lerner A, Lebenthal E: Chronic diarrhea and malabsorption, *Pediatr Clin North Am* 43:307, 1996.
57. Silk DB: In-patient assessment of difficult diarrhoea, *Eur J Gastroenterol Hepatol* 12:595, 2000.
58. Castro-Rodriguez JA, Salazar-Lindo E, Leon-Barua R: Differentiation of osmotic and secretory diarrhoea by stool carbohydrate and osmolar gap measurements, *Arch Dis Child* 77:201, 1997.
59. Jensen RT: Overview of chronic diarrhea caused by functional neuroendocrine neoplasms, *Semin Gastrointest Dis* 10:156, 1999.
60. Nakama H et al: Sensitivity and specificity of several immunochemical tests for colorectal cancer, *Hepatogastroenterology* 45:1579, 1998.
61. Imafuku Y, Nagai T, Yoshida H: The effect of toilet sanitizers and detergents on immunological occult blood test, *Clin Chem Acta* 253:61, 1996.
62. American College of Physicians: Suggested technique for fecal occult blood testing and interpretation in colorectal cancer screening, *Ann Intern Med* 126:808, 1997.
63. Rozen P, Knaani J, Samuel Z: Eliminating the need for dietary restrictions when using a sensitive guaiac fecal occult blood test, *Dig Dis Sci* 44:756, 1999.

64. Sinatra MA, St John DJ, Young GP: Interference of plant peroxidases with guaiac-based fecal occult blood tests is avoidable, *Clin Chem* 45:123, 1999.

65. Simon JB: Fecal occult blood testing: clinical value and limitations, *Gastroenterologist* 6:66, 1998.

66. Gold P, Freedman SO: Specific carcinoembryonic antigens of the human digestive system, *J Exp Med* 122:467, 1965.

Internet Sites

http://www.iffgd.org/GIDisorders/GImain.html
http://www.karger.ch/journals/ddi/ddi_jh.htm
http://pages.prodigy.com/DVBL86A/drk3_hp.htm

MENS 1
http://www.pituitary.com/Articles/MEN1Article1.htm
http://www.niddk.nih.gov/health/endo/pubs/fmen1/fmen1.htm

Ulcers
www.gastro.com/ulcers
www.niddk.nih.gov/health/digest/summary/nsaids
www.digestivedisorders.org.uk/leaflets/ulcers.html
www.faseb.org/opar/pylori/pylori.html

British Society of Gastroenterology
www.bsg.org.uk/clinical_prac/guidelines/malabsorb.htm

Glucose Galactose Malabsorption
www.ncbi.nlm.nih.gov/disease/ggm.html

Celiac Disease
www.niddk.nih.gov/health/digest/pubs/celiac/

Celiac Disease Foundation
www.celiac.org

Lactose Intolerance
www.niddk.nih.gov/health/digest/pubs/lactose/lactose.htm

Carcinoid Disease
www.carcinoid.org/review.html

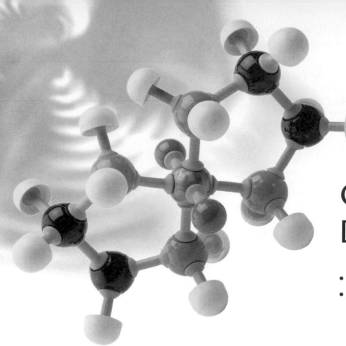

CHAPTER 31

Cardiac and Muscle Disease

• *Wendy R. Sanhai*
• *Robert H. Christenson*

Chapter Outline

Muscle anatomy and function
 Types of muscle
 Proteins involved in muscle contraction
 The neuromuscular connection
 Mechanism of contraction
Anatomy and function of the heart
Energy metabolism
Energy demands of different muscle types
 Skeletal muscle
 Cardiac muscle
 Smooth muscle

Pathological conditions
 Cardiac disorders
 Skeletal muscle disorders
Function tests
Drug therapy
 Glycosides
 Lidocaine
 Quinidine and other drugs
Change of analyte in disease
 Protein markers in myocardial cells

Objectives

• List the proteins involved in muscle contraction.
• Describe the layout of the sarcomere and the orientation of the different filaments.
• Describe the sliding filament mechanism of contraction in cardiac and skeletal muscle.
• Describe the series of events that occurs at the neuromuscular junction following a wave of depolarization.
• Define MI.

• Describe the spectrum of ACS.
• List proteins and enzymes (and their isoforms and isoenzymes) that are routinely measured in serum to assess myocardial disease, and state the time periods for the expected enzyme elevations following myocardial infarction.
• Describe the diagnostic use of cardiac troponins T and I in cardiomyopathy.
• Define CHF and describe the use of BNP in CHF.

Key Terms

actin One of the proteins involved in myocardial and arterial smooth muscle contraction.
action potential An electrical event produced by the ion flux across a membrane when its permeability is changed upon stimulation.
acute coronary syndromes The continuum of

ischemic heart disease from unstable angina (reversible injury) through myocardial infarction (irreversible injury), having the unstable coronary plaque as a common physiological feature.
adenosine-5′-triphosphate (ATP) The high-energy compound that can be hydrolyzed to adenosine-5′-

diphosphate (ADP) or adenosine-5'-monophosphate (AMP), releasing energy that can be used to drive metabolic reactions.

atherosclerosis   A process that results in gradual deposition of lipid, fibrin, and calcium in the walls of arteries. Often called "hardening of the arteries," this condition is the most common cause of death in Western countries.

atria   The chambers of the heart that collect blood from the veins and contract to expel the blood into their respective ventricles. There are two atria: the right atrium collects blood from systemic veins and fills the right ventricle; the left atrium collects blood from the pulmonary vein and expels it into the left ventricle.

cardiac failure   Failure of the heart to maintain blood circulation, which leads to inadequate perfusion of essential organs, usually resulting in accumulation of salt and water.

cardiomyopathy   A heterogeneous group of disorders that have in common a genetic component or toxic insult that affects contracting myocardial cells directly.

Embden-Meyerhof pathway   The pathway of anaerobic glycolysis that converts glucose or glycogen to lactate.

glycoside   A generic term for a group of drugs originally obtained from the foxglove plant. These drugs improve the contractility of the failing heart and slow the rate of ventricular contraction in atrial fibrillation. Digoxin is a member of this family of drugs.

infarction   A process of cell death caused by an inadequate blood supply (ischemia). Thus myocardial infarction or heart attack occurs when one of the coronary arteries is occluded and the tissue distal to the occlusion dies.

ischemia   A reduction of blood supply to tissue sufficient to prevent the tissue from functioning normally.

Krebs citric acid cycle   The pathway of intermediary metabolism that will accept metabolic products from the Embden-Meyerhof pathway and oxidize, decarboxylate, and reduce them, with the production of a relatively large amount of adenosine triphosphate.

myosin II   A protein that contains ATP- and actin-binding sites and is involved in skeletal, cardiac and smooth muscle contraction.

sarcolemma   The plasma membrane of muscle cells.

sarcoplasm   The cytoplasm of muscle cells.

sarcoplasmic reticulum   The endoplasmic reticulum of muscle cells.

syncytium   A group of cells that maintain cytoplasmic continuity and contain many nuclei.

technetium 99m (^{99m}Tc)   An isotope injected intravenously to measure left ventricular output (*m* = metastable).

thallium 201   An isotope injected intravenously to delineate either the ischemic part of the ventricular muscle mass or a scar caused by an old infarction.

titin   A giant (3mDa) protein that is a major constituent of the sarcomere in vertebrate skeletal muscle. It spans half the length of the sarcomere joining the Z-line to the M-band. Functions include thick-filament assembly, muscle elasticity, and tension generation. Also called *connectin*.

tropomyosin   A rigid, rod-shaped protein made up of two identical α-helical proteins that wind around each other in a coiled fashion. It binds along the length of the actin filaments, making them more rigid and altering their affinity for other proteins, such as myosin.

troponins   Three distinct polypeptides: troponin T, responsible for tropomyosin-binding activity; troponin I, which binds to actin and inhibits the activity of actomyosin ATPase; and troponin C, responsible for calcium-binding activity of muscle contraction. Together with tropomyosin, the troponins form a complex that regulates actin and myosin interactions and muscle contraction.

ventricles   The main right and left pumping chambers of the heart that expel blood. The right ventricle pumps blood into the pulmonary artery, and the left ventricle pumps blood to the aorta. The left ventricle is more massive and powerful than the right ventricle because the pressure in the systemic circulation, against which it must expel blood, is higher than that in the pulmonary circulation.

Methods on CD-ROM

Creatine kinase
Creatine kinase isoenzymes
Digoxin and digitoxin
Lactate dehydrogenase and lactate dehydrogenase
  isoenzymes

Myoglobin
Procainamide and *N*-acetylprocainamide
Troponin

MUSCLE ANATOMY AND FUNCTION
Types of Muscle

There are three distinct groups of muscle: skeletal, cardiac, and smooth. The *skeletal muscle* consists of unbranched, cylindrical muscle cells that are multinucleated (form a **syncytium**) and arranged in parallel bundles (Figure 31-1) as a result of the fusion of many individual progenitor cells (myoblasts) during myogenesis. The nuclei are located just under the plasma membrane (sarcolemma), and the fibers run the whole length of the muscle. They have well-defined nerve end-plates and are under voluntary control. Contractions are initiated by nerve impulses and are termed *neurogenic*. Nerve endings are attached to the outer surface of the **sarcolemma** through the motor end-plate of an axon. Within the sarcolemma-enclosed space the fibrils are bathed by the intracellular fluid of muscle, the **sarcoplasm**.

Each muscle cell contains bundles of cylindrical *myofibrils*, which make up about two-thirds of the dry mass of the cytoplasm (Fig. 31-1). Myofibrils are the contractile elements of the muscle cells and are surrounded by an extensive network of tubular channels known as the **sarcoplasmic reticulum**, which is analogous to a "net stocking" around the muscle fibers (see Fig. 31-1). The myofibrils are composed of repeating units called *sarcomeres*. The parallel arrangement of the filaments within each sarcomere gives muscle its characteristic cross-striation, a pattern of light and dark bands visible at high magnification. The darker bands are called *A bands* (anisotropic, containing both thick and

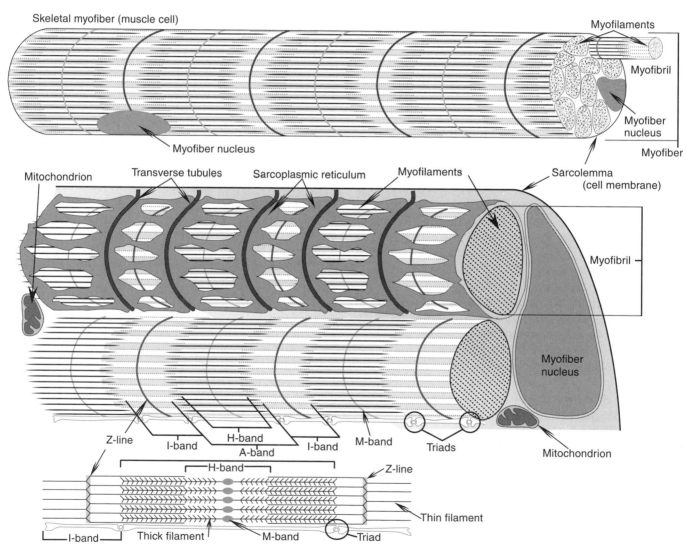

Fig. 31-1 Schematic representation of a skeletal muscle fiber with increasing magnification. Diagram illustrates the structure of the muscle cell (myofiber) and the juxtaposition of the individual myofibrils, sarcoplasmic reticulum, transverse tubules, and nucleus within the muscle cell. The structural components of the myofilaments and arrangement of the thick (myosin) and thin (actin) filaments within the A-, H- and I-bands of the sarcomere are demonstrated. *(Drawing adapted with permission from Wu A: Cardiac markers, Totowa, NJ, 1998, Humana Press.)*

thin filaments); the light bands are called *I bands* (isotropic, containing only thin filaments). In the electron microscope, each I band is bisected by a dense transverse band called the *Z line*, or *Z disc*, which separates one sarcomere from the next. Each sarcomere contains a precisely arranged assembly of partly overlapping *thick* and *thin* filaments. The thick filaments are polymers of specific isoforms of **myosin II**. Thin filaments composed of **actin** and associated proteins are attached to the Z discs at either end of the sarcomere. They extend toward the middle of the sarcomere, where they overlap with the thick filaments. The sarcoplasm is filled with long cylindrical filamentous bundles called *myofibrils*, which have a diameter of 1-2 mm and run parallel to the long axis of the muscle fiber. Myofibrils consist of an end-to-end chainlike arrangement of sarcomeres (Fig. 31-1).

Skeletal muscles can also be divided into two types, "fast-twitch" and "slow-twitch," which differ in their biochemical nature (see below, p. 572) and their motor nerve endings (see below, p. 571).

Cardiac muscle is found exclusively in the heart and, like skeletal muscle, contains actin and myosin filaments arranged in a similar banding pattern. However, cardiac muscle cells bifurcate, or branch, and contain only 1 or 2 nuclei per cell. Cardiac muscle consists of tightly knit bundles of interwoven cells, which contribute to the characteristic wave of contractions that leads to the "pumping" of blood from **atria** and **ventricles**. There are no defined end-plates in cardiac muscle, and control is involuntary; that is, no conscious effort is required to initiate and maintain contraction of cardiac muscle, which is therefore termed *myogenic*.

Smooth muscle is composed of elongated, nonstriated cells with a single, centrally located nucleus. The smooth muscle cell does not have a structurally defined end-plate and is not under voluntary control; therefore it is also called *involuntary* muscle. Found in the walls of tubes or sacs such as blood vessels, the wall of the uterus, the urinary bladder, the intestines, and the bronchioles, smooth muscle is characterized by slow contraction and can maintain tension or a given length without fatigue at low energy cost.

Proteins Involved in Muscle Contraction[1,2-4]
(see Table 31-1)

Many proteins are required for muscle contraction, including myosin II (consisting of heavy and light chains), **actin**, **troponins**, and **tropomyosin**. Muscle myosin belongs to the myosin II subfamily while myosin I is present in nonmuscle cells. Myosin II is a large filamentous molecule (540 kD) made up of six peptide chains, two heavy chains (230 kD), and four light chains (MCLs, 26 kD). The heavy chains contain two head domains and a long rod-like tail composed of two α-helical peptide chains arranged in a coiled motif as shown in Figure 31-2. When stimulated by the binding to actin filaments in skeletal muscle, the globular head, or motor domain, of myosin II binds to actin filaments and hydrolyzes **adenosine-5'-triphosphate (ATP)** to adenosine-5'-diphosphate (ADP) and inorganic phosphate (*Pi*).

Two types of myosin light chains (MLCs) bind to the head domains of the myosin heavy chains: cardiac and noncardiac. The phosphorylation of one of the two light chains by myosin light chain kinase (MLCK) causes a change in the conformation of the myosin head, exposing its actin-binding site. MLCs from cardiac and noncardiac sources can be differentiated by using antibodies specific for cardiac MLCs.[5]

Actin, a critical component of a wide range of structures in eukaryotic cells, has the same fundamental structure in all cells, and consists of long filamentous (F-actin) polymers consisting of two strands of globular (G-actin) monomers. However, the length of the filaments, their stability, and the number and geometry of attachments vary, depending on the *actin-binding proteins*, such as α-actinin and desmin. α-actinin, a major component of the Z-line, is thought to anchor the actin filaments. Specialized accessory proteins, tropomyosin and troponins, also associate with polymerized actin filaments and mediate the Ca^{2+} regulation of muscle contraction. Sarcomere shortening is caused by the myosin filaments sliding past the actin filaments with no change in the lengths of either filament.

The troponin complex is a set of three proteins that, together with Ca^{++} ions and tropomyosin, regulate

TABLE 31-1   CHARACTERISTICS OF MYOFIBRILLAR PROTEINS

Proteins	Location	Protein (as a Percentage of Total Cellular Protein)	Molecular Weight (kD)
Myosin II	A-band	60	2×260 (2 heavy and 4 light chains)
Actin	I-band	20	42
Tropomyosin	I-band	3	2×35
Troponin (TIC-triple complex)	I-band	4.5	T-component = 31 I-component = 21
C-protein	A-band	Less than 1	128
α-actinin	Z-line, I-band	Less than 1	2×100 (dimer)
Titin (also called *connectin*)	Z-line	Less than 1	3 MDa
Desmin	Z-line	Less than 1	55

Data from Politou AS, Thomas DJ, Pastore A: The folding and stability of titin immunoglobulin-like modules with implications for the mechanism of elasticity, Biophys J 69:2601, 1995; Squire JM: Architecture and function in the muscle sarcomere, Curr Opin Struct Biol 7:247, 1997; Trinick J, Tskhovrebova L: Titin: a molecular control freak, Trends Cell Biol 9:377, 1999.

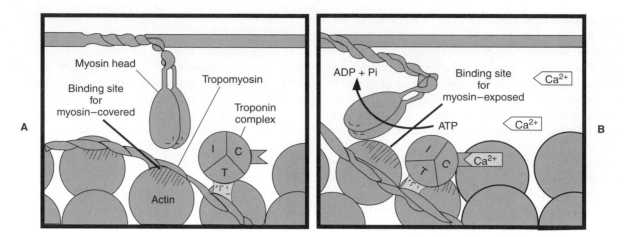

Fig. 31-2 Schematic representation of the spatial configuration of myosin, actin, tropo-myosin, and the troponin complex in the presence and absence of calcium ions. **A,** In the absence of calcium ions, the long tropomyosin molecule is bound to the myosin-binding site on the actin filament (large spheres representing actin monomers polymerize to form the actin filament). **B,** Calcium ions (Ca^{2+}), upon their release from the sarcoplasmic reticulum, bind to troponin C subunit of the troponin complex (TIC spherical complex with Ca^{2+}-binding site on the C subunit), and the subsequent conformational changes increase the affinity of the troponin T subunit for the tropomyosin molecule. The troponin-tropomyosin-Ca^{2+} complex triggers the movement of the tropomyosin molecule away from the myosin-binding site on the actin filament. ATP binds to a site on the myosin head domain and upon hydrolysis to ADP and Pi, triggers a conformational change that allows the myosin head to move along the actin filament in the direction of the Z-line (not shown). *(Drawing adapted with permission from Wu A:* Cardiac markers, *Totowa, NJ, 1998, Humana Press.)*

muscle contraction (seen as the spherical triple complex in Fig. 31-2). Localized primarily in the myofibrils (94-97%), with a smaller soluble, cytoplasmic fraction (3-6%), the troponin complex consists of three proteins: *troponin C* (the calcium-binding component), *troponin T*[2] (the tropomyosin-binding component) and *troponin I*[4] (the inhibitory component). The subunits exist in a number of different isoforms, whose distributions vary between cardiac muscle and slow- and fast-twitch skeletal muscle. Troponin C is found in human heart and skeletal muscle. However, cardiac-specific troponin T (cTnT) and cardiac-specific troponin I (cTnI) isoforms have been isolated. cTnI and cTnT have different amino acid sequences compared with the skeletal muscle isoforms and are encoded by different genes. Only one form of cTnI has been identified and it has never been shown to be expressed in normal, regenerating, or diseased skeletal muscle.

Tropomyosin is a rod-shaped molecule containing two polypeptide chains that bind within the grooves of the actin filaments (see Figure 31-2). Troponin T is bound to tropomyosin and positions the complex on the actin filament. The troponin T–tropomyosin complex, together with troponin I, which binds to actin filaments, inhibits interactions between actin filaments and the head domain of myosin II. However when **action potentials** (produced by an ion flux across membranes, resulting in increased permeability) stimulate Ca^{2+} ion release from the sarcoplasmic reticulum, troponin C

binds up to 4 Ca^{2+} ions. This binding changes the conformation of the tropomyosin-troponin complex and removes the inhibition of myosin binding to actin produced by the other two troponin components. With the myosin-binding site on the actin filament now exposed, the myosin head domain is free to bind to actin filaments, and in the presence of ATP, muscle contraction can occur.

The Neuromuscular Connection

The force-generating molecular interactions just described take place only when a signal passes to the muscle from its motor nerve. At the site of innervation, motor nerves have no myelin sheath and the exposed end sits within a trough on the muscle cell surface. This structure is called *the motor end-plate,* or *myoneural junction.* Within the axon terminal are numerous mitochondria and synaptic vesicles, the latter containing the neurotransmitter acetylcholine. When an action potential innervates the motor end-plate, acetylcholine is liberated from the axon terminal, diffuses through the synaptic cleft, and binds with receptors in the sarcolemma of the adjacent muscle cell. Binding of the transmitter makes the sarcolemma more permeable to sodium, which results in membrane depolarization. This depolarization is propagated along the length of the muscle cells and triggers the release of Ca^{2+} ions, stored in the sarcoplasmic reticulum, into the vicinity of the myofibrils. Ca^{2+} ions initiate the contraction by acting as a second messenger, activating the ATPase in the troponin complex and triggering the interaction between myosin and actin (see Fig. 31-2). When depolarization ceases, the Ca^{2+} ions are actively transported back into the sarcoplasmic reticulum and the muscle relaxes.

Motor nerve endings differ depending on the main fiber type. A single nerve fiber (axon) can innervate one muscle fiber/cell, or it may branch and innervate more than 160 muscle fibers. Slow-twitch fibers, which respond to nerve stimuli with prolonged contractions, are generally innervated by multiple nerve endings. Fast-twitch fibers are usually innervated by individual end-plates. Acetylcholine, which serves as a neurotransmitter (see Chapter 42, p. 792), is synthesized and stored in vesicles of both types of neurons.

Mechanism of Contraction

The general function of the muscles is to respond mechanically to stimulation, producing fiber shortening and force development, both of which usually occur together. Skeletal muscle function is modified by leverage, as a result of attachment to the skeleton. In cardiac muscle the force development is manifested by the development of pressure within the chambers of the heart during cardiac muscle shortening, which results in reduced chamber size and pumping. Smooth muscle shortening is seen when smooth muscle sacs or cavities are emptied, as in the expulsion of urine from the bladder or of a child from the uterus.

Muscle contraction is driven by the interaction between myosin II heads and adjacent actin filaments. The energy for muscle contraction in generated by the hydrolysis of ATP by myosin. The amount of ATP hydrolyzed in contraction is not constant but depends on the duration of contraction and on the amount of work done by the muscle. ATP hydrolysis produces an ordered set of allosteric changes in the conformation of the myosin molecule that allows it to move from its original binding site on the actin filament. With each cycle of ATP hydrolysis, the myosin molecule alters its affinity for the actin filaments and moves or "walks" along the actin filament in the direction of the Z-line (i.e., toward the positive end of the actin filament), sliding the myosin and actin filaments past one another at rates up to 15 mm/second. This sliding filament mechanism of contraction can shorten the sarcomere by as much as one-third its original length.

Relaxation of the muscle is a passive process. The interdigitated filaments slide back to a less overlapped position, thereby increasing the length of the muscle. The same basic mechanism of contraction/relaxation applies to all muscle types. In the absence of ATP, the myosin-actin complex becomes stable; this accounts for the extreme muscular rigidity (*rigor mortis*) that occurs after death.

ANATOMY AND FUNCTION OF THE HEART

The pumping action of the heart[6] is the prime factor in the maintenance of the body's circulation. The heart is a muscular organ composed of four chambers, two atria and two ventricles. The right atrium collects blood from the systemic circulation and pumps it into the right ventricle. The right ventricle pumps blood to the lungs for reoxygenation; the blood is then collected by the left atrium, which pumps the blood to the left ventricle. The left ventricle pumps blood to the rest of the body, including the heart itself. Cardiac output is determined primarily by the volume of blood pumped, by systemic blood pressure, and by the contractile force developed in the wall of the left ventricle. Cardiac muscle, which is extremely active, requires large quantities of energy (as ATP) and oxygen for metabolism. Delivery of the oxygen needed to fuel the heart requires a rich capillary bed.

ENERGY METABOLISM

Various substrates are used by muscle cells for energy production. Energy is liberated from these fuels by several pathways, including the Embden-Meyerhof glycolytic pathway, the pentose phosphate shunt, fatty acid oxidation, and the **Krebs citric acid cycle** (see Chapter 32). The energy produced by the breakdown of substrates is then transported through the electron-transport system of the mitochondria to produce ATP, the chemical form of stored energy that is used by muscle tissue to perform work. To perform their functions, muscle cells must maintain a high [ATP]/[ADP] ratio, and all muscles require an effective storage method to maintain a reserve of ATP. This is achieved through the synthesis of creatine phosphate (CP), which functions as an energy reservoir source that can be used for rapid regeneration of ATP when levels fall as a result of increased demand.

This high-energy reservoir uses the enzymes creatine kinase (CK) and myokinase (MK) to maintain an equilibrium concentration of ATP, ADP, and creatine phosphate (CP). The immediate effect of increased ADP concentrations caused by the hydrolysis of ATP during contraction is a disturbance of the equilibrium of the creatine kinase-catalyzed reaction:

Creatine phosphate + ADP $\underset{CK}{\rightleftharpoons}$ ATP + **Creatine**

The equilibrium is reestablished by the phosphorylation of ADP to ATP by this reaction, thus preserving a high [ATP]/[ADP] ratio. Another enzyme, myokinase, catalyzes the reaction:

$$2\ ADP \xrightarrow{\ MK\ } ATP + AMP$$

This reaction also ensures the reestablishment of the original high [ATP]/[ADP] ratio.

A third enzyme present in the muscle, adenosine deaminase (AD), prevents the accumulation of AMP produced by the myokinase reaction by deamination of the AMP:

$$AMP \xrightarrow{\ AD\ } IMP + NH_3^+$$

Inosine monophosphate (IMP) then either returns to the nucleoside pool as inosine or is degraded further to uric acid. For a single contraction (twitch) or for short periods of muscle activity, the only measurable change in the intracellular high-energy phosphate pool is a small change in CP concentration.

ENERGY DEMANDS OF DIFFERENT MUSCLE TYPES
Skeletal Muscle

Human skeletal muscle contains both red and white fibers, which differ in their metabolic properties. Red or slow fibers are rich in myoglobin and mitochondria. In these fibers the main metabolic pathway is oxidative phosphorylation. White or fast fibers contain little myoglobin and mitochondria, and the main route for energy metabolism is glycolysis. Rested, well-nourished muscle synthesizes and stores glycogen, which serves as a ready source of fuel that can be converted to glucose-6-phosphate for entry into the glycolytic pathway. Skeletal muscle at rest uses about 30% of the oxygen consumed by the human body. At maximal activity, skeletal muscle can increase its oxygen uptake 20-fold or more during the transition from rest to full activity to supply the oxygen needed for the oxidative process. However, its rate of ATP hydrolysis can increase by a much greater amount. Therefore, at maximal activity the skeletal muscles still are relatively oxygen-poor (anoxic), and lactate, the end product of anaerobic glucose metabolism, increases in blood.

Acidosis occurs when either metabolic or other abnormal processes result in a lower-than-normal pH of the arterial blood. Lactic acidosis, which results from an excessive production of lactic acid, can occur in normal skeletal muscles after excessive exercise. The localized acidosis in skeletal muscle contributes to fatigue and can result in muscle cramps and pain, especially when it is accompanied by excessive imbalance of sodium and potassium ions.

Cardiac Muscle

The highly aerobic metabolism of the heart allows it to use as fuel many substrates normally present in plasma, and cardiac uptake of most of these substances is proportional to their arterial concentration once certain levels are exceeded. In general terms, the heart uses free fatty acids as its predominant fuel. It also consumes significant quantities of glucose and lactate, as well as lesser amounts of pyruvate, ketone bodies, and amino acids. Most of the energy for cardiac function is obtained from the breakdown of metabolites through the citric acid cycle and oxidative phosphorylation. These enzyme pathways are found principally in the mitochondria, which make up some 35% of the total volume of cardiac muscle. Although free fatty acids are the resting heart's fuel of choice, upon the imposition of a heavy workload the heart greatly increases its rate of glucose consumption, derived mainly from its relatively limited glycogen supply.

Smooth Muscle

Compared with skeletal and cardiac muscle, the energy needs of smooth muscle contraction are very modest. An influx of Ca^{2+} ions is involved in the initiation of contraction in smooth muscle cells. Ca^{2+} complexes with the binding protein calmodulin, and the Ca^{2+}-calmodulin complex activates MLC kinase, the enzyme responsible for the ATP-dependent phosphorylation of myosin. The myosin of smooth muscle interacts with actin only when its light chain is phosphorylated. For this reason, and because troponin is absent, the contraction mechanism of smooth muscle differs from that of skeletal and cardiac muscle. Smooth muscle contraction is slow and concerted, is not subjected to voluntary control, and does not demand the high aerobic metabolism of skeletal and cardiac muscle.

PATHOLOGICAL CONDITIONS
Cardiac Disorders

Ischemic heart disease. Ischemia[6] is a condition in which an organ has an inadequate blood supply for maintaining its essential functions. Although there are many causes of myocardial ischemia, including vascular contraction and spasm, the most common cause by far is coronary **atherosclerosis**, believed by many to be an inflammatory condition of arterial vessels that generally progresses over many years, often beginning in childhood. Atherosclerosis causes the arteries supplying blood to the heart to gradually narrow (occlude) because of deposition of cholesterol and other substances in the arterial wall. The most common cause of ischemia is related to unstable lipid-filled deposits, termed *plaques* (see p. 628, Chapter 33). Unstable plaques are the common physiological feature of acute coronary syndrome, a continuum of ischemic disease ranging from unstable angina, associated with reversible myocardial cell injury, to frank myocardial **infarction** (MI) with large areas of necrosis. Another condition that can cause ischemia and cell death is coronary vasospasm, in which the arterial wall constricts in an abnormal and prolonged fashion because of hypersensitivity to normal vasoconstrictor signals. Other less common causes of myocardial ischemia are severe anemia and hypotension.

Effects of occlusion on myocardium. Cessation of blood flow produces a complex series of metabolic consequences to the cells deprived of blood flow. Severe *hypoxia* occurs because tissue oxygen concentration drops drastically; also contributing to this condition are delayed clearance of toxic cellular metabolites from ischemic tissue and the production of free radicals after reperfusion of the damaged tissues. Hypoxia prevents aerobic metabolism, and the oxygen supplies remaining in the microvasculature are readily consumed. Instead of the aerobic Krebs cycle, myocardial metabolism switches to the use of glycogen or glucose in the anaerobic **Embden-Meyerhof pathway**. The end product of anaerobic glucose metabolism, pyruvate, is reduced to lactate, which accumulates and is one of the earliest and most dramatic signs of myocardial ischemia.

As ischemia continues, accumulation of lactate and other acidic intermediates of glycolysis occurs. CP reserves are depleted, and ATP levels fall. Generally, if tissue is reperfused, it will recover in 15 to 20 minutes after an ischemic incident. However, after 15 to 20 minutes of occlusion, over

60% of the cellular ATP is depleted and the amount of lactate in myocardial tissue is 12-fold higher than its normal aerobic level. In addition, all cellular glycogen is exhausted. With the glycogen and CP reserves depleted, dramatic ultrastructural changes occur, indicating irreversible cell damage. At this point, even if the obstruction is relieved and the myocardial tissue is reperfused, the myocardial tissue is unable to tolerate the arrival of fresh blood, resulting in cell lysis, loss of muscle tone, and fibrosis.

At the point when reversible ischemic injury becomes irreversible, the cell is no longer able to maintain membrane integrity. Damage to the cell membrane results in the release of intracellular contents. Once membrane damage has occurred, the rate of appearance of intracellular proteins in the circulation depends on the clearance mechanism, rate and extent of reperfusion of the damaged myocardium, and the size of the protein molecule. The greater the reperfusion and the smaller the size, the sooner the molecule will be seen in peripheral blood. For example, myoglobin with a molecular weight of 17,800 daltons will be observed before CK and the cardiac troponins T and I, which have molecular weights in the range of 85,000 daltons. Release of these proteins can be used as markers for the evaluation and confirmation of irreversible ischemic injury. Marker release (cTnT, cTnI, or CK-MB) reflecting death to myocytes indicates that the patient has had an MI rather than a transient ischemic episode. Mitochondrial enzymes are also released, but there is usually some delay before they appear in plasma.

Acute coronary syndromes (ACS). The acute coronary syndromes represent the following continuum of events:

angina

↓

reversible tissue injury

↓

unstable angina, frequently associated with
minor myocardial damage

↓

myocardial infarction

↓

extensive tissue necrosis

Based on World Health Organization (WHO) criteria of ischemic symptoms, assessment of coronary artery disease has focused mainly on electrocardiogram changes and a rise and fall in biochemical markers. From the 1980s to mid-1990s, CK-MB was the benchmark for markers; however CK-MB is not completely specific for myocardium. The cardiac specific proteins cTnT and cTnI have emerged as sensitive and specific indicators for myocardial infarction and, more important, for risk stratification of acute coronary syndrome patients (see below). In addition to these markers of necrosis, other indicators are of potential use; for example, markers for inflammation (C-reactive protein[7] and serum amyloid A), "angry" platelets (P-selectin), ischemia (ischemia-modified albumin[8]), and the procoagulant state and thrombosis (soluble fibrin). Also, CK-MB and myo-globin have been combined with clinical indicators for monitoring reperfusion after thrombolytic therapy.

Each year 8 million patients with chest pain are evaluated in hospital emergency departments in the United States; approximately 1.1 million of these are diagnosed as having MI.[9] The cost of caring for suspected and confirmed MI patients is approximately $4 billion per year. A system of triage based on the results of cardiospecific biochemical markers obtained within 12 hours after onset of symptoms could potentially reduce the number of patients admitted to coronary care units by as much as 70%. This system would operate under the assumption that all patients with negative results, even those with unstable angina (chest pain but without ischemic injury), could be adequately cared for in a regular hospital unit.[10] The use of biochemical markers will, therefore, continue to be a cost-effective and important clinical adjunct for MI diagnosis, risk assessment, and reperfusion monitoring in the future.

Congestive heart failure (CHF). Congestive heart failure is a disease related to the decreased capability of the heart to pump blood. The prevalence in the United States is rising, and the projection is that this trend will continue. It is now recognized that CHF represents a spectrum of disease that can progress from left ventricular dysfunction (LVD), in which at least half of subjects have an absence of symptoms, to end-stage overt CHF with a markedly high morbidity and mortality. The contributing factors to CHF are increased age, hypertension, and coronary atherosclerosis. Regardless of its etiology, CHF is divided into four classes based upon symptoms by the New York Heart Association (NYHA) classification index. Class I represents ventricular dysfunction in the absence of symptoms. Class II represents minimal symptoms that may occur with exercise. Class III is classified as moderate symptoms associated with mild exercise, and Class IV represents symptoms that may occur at rest. The diagnosis of CHF is difficult because its symptoms may occur with pulmonary disease, syndromes associated with edema, and syndromes associated with fatigue.

An important therapy for CHF is treatment with angiotensin-converting enzyme (ACE) inhibitors, which is usually used throughout the spectrum of CHF from Class I through IV. An increasing role for beta-adrenergic blockers has emerged, particularly in symptomatic heart failure. Diuretics are indicated for patients with sodium retention, and digitalis is recommended for those with symptomatic heart failure to reduce the progression of disease and hospitalization. The laboratory may be used to monitor these therapeutic agents.

Brain natriuretic peptide (BNP), a protein released from the heart in response to cardiac stretch receptors, may help to differentiate between CHF and other conditions that have similar clinical presentations and to guide therapy for CHF. However, it is unclear as to what extent other conditions (such as renal disease) or medications (such as beta-blockers) might interfere with the use of BNP as a biomarker in the diagnosis of heart failure.

Cardiomyopathy.[11,12] **Cardiomyopathy** represents a diverse group of disorders, generally falling into two categories: disease originating in heart tissue and disease that is secondary to other, nonmyocardial disorders. Cardiomyopathy is characterized by inadequate muscle contraction caused by direct damage to myocardial cells and typically results in hemodynamic overload and heart failure. Although there are some specific forms of cardiomyopathy, most clinical cases are idiopathic; that is, the cause is unclear. Cardiomyopathy manifests as an enlargement of all four chambers of the heart and **cardiac failure**. The biochemical findings in most cases of cardiomyopathy are nonspecific and reflect cardiac failure, the major clinical presentation. At least two forms of this disease, *familial hypertrophic cardiomyopathy* and *viral myocarditis*, can now be diagnosed using molecular genetic techniques.[13,14]

Arrhythmias. A complex neuroregulatory system controls and coordinates the pattern of contraction for the four chambers of the heart and regulates cardiac function in relation to the changing needs of body organs. Damage to the neuroregulatory system, which can occur during and after cardiac injury (such as MI), is relatively nonspecific and is frequently related to the disease process affecting the heart muscle. Whatever the cause, damage frequently distorts the transmission of cardiac nerve impulses, producing abnormal, irregular, and self-sustaining contractile activity of the heart, termed *arrhythmia*.

In functional terms the rhythm abnormalities are classified as *bradycardias* (resulting in heartbeat rates less than 60 beats/min) or as *tachycardias* (producing heartbeat rates faster than 100 beats/min). The dysrhythmia can affect atrial or ventricular contractions and can be acute or chronic. Atrial fibrillation is a fairly common rhythm abnormality in which the atria beat in an irregular and abnormally rapid fashion. Chronic arrhythmias are controlled by medications, the serum levels of which should be routinely monitored during the initial period to determine the optimal dosing levels.

Congenital and valvular heart disease. Many congenital heart abnormalities have been described, but these are beyond the scope of this chapter. In general terms, all components of the heart can be affected by maldevelopment or infectious disease. In many cases the cause of these defects are unknown. One important exception is rubella infection of the mother during the first trimester of pregnancy. Of the acquired valvular diseases of the heart, one large group is caused by rheumatic carditis. In susceptible patients affected by the hemolytic streptococcus, the body develops an immune reaction against all myocardial tissue, but particularly the valves, which become damaged and deformed.

Skeletal Muscle Disorders

Diseases of muscle are characterized by motor dysfunction, such as muscular weakness. The three major categories of muscle disorders, according to the part of the motor unit affected, are (1) neurogenic muscular atrophies, (2) muscle fiber disorders, and (3) disturbances of the neuromuscular junction. Within each major class further distinctions are

made based on the loci, or known origins of the defects. These categories are listed below.

The *muscular atrophies* are caused by a loss of efferent innervation as a result of a degeneration of either an anterior horn cell or an axon at the level of an anterior efferent root or peripheral nerve cell. The *myopathies* are characterized by major defects at the level of the muscle fiber. Certain hereditary progressive myopathies are called, by convention, *muscular dystrophies*. *Nonhereditary myopathies* can result from inflammation or from an endocrine or metabolic abnormality.

Anterior root and peripheral nerve involvement. *Acute polyneuropathy*, or Guillain-Barré syndrome, is a parainfectious and postinfectious disease presumed to be caused by an immunological reaction with peripheral nerves. *Metabolic neuropathies* include damage to nerves resulting from metabolic diseases such as diabetes mellitus or malnutrition.

Disorders of muscle fibers: muscular dystrophies. Muscular dystrophy is a general name for a group of chronic diseases of muscle. The general characteristics are progressive weakness and degeneration of skeletal muscle with no evidence of neural degeneration. They are genetic diseases with different inheritance patterns. The age of onset, the course of disease, and the effect on the different fiber types differ among the individual diseases.

Pseudohypertrophic muscular dystrophy, or *Duchenne muscular dystrophy* (DMD), the most common of the muscular dystrophies, is an X-linked recessive disease that causes progressive muscle weakness and muscle wasting starting at 1 or 2 years of age, progressing to heart failure or weakness of the respiratory muscles; most patients are confined to wheelchairs by 10 to 12 years of age, and death typically occurs in early adulthood. Most patients with DMD have deletions that eliminate large portions of the dystrophin gene, one of the largest known genes in the human genome. This gene codes for the protein dystrophin, which is thought to stabilize the sarcolemma during muscle contraction.

Serum enzymes are greatly elevated in the disease even before symptoms develop; especially noted is the rise in CK. The CK values in heterozygous females and normal persons overlap so that the enzyme is elevated in only about 50% to 70% of heterozygous females. Diagnosis of this disease by DNA analysis and genetic counseling has significantly decreased DMD occurrence in the last 10 years. No effective treatment exists for DMD, but the disease is a prime candidate for gene therapy.

Disturbances of the neuromuscular junction. *Myasthenia gravis* is an autoimmune disorder characterized by progressive muscular weakness caused by reduction in the number of functionally active acetylcholine receptors in the sarcolemma of the myoneural junction. Circulating antibodies bind to the acetylcholine receptors in the junctional folds and inhibit normal nerve-muscle communication. As the body attempts to correct the condition, membrane segments with affected receptors are internalized, digested by lysosomes and replaced by newly formed receptors. These receptors, however, are rapidly rendered unresponsive to acetylcholine by the same antibodies, and the disease follows in its progressive course.

FUNCTION TESTS

The most important tests for assessment of cardiac function are the electrocardiogram (ECG)[15] and myocardial imaging techniques.[1] The ECG involves noninvasive recording of the electrical impulses through the heart and is an effective but not perfect means of assessing cardiac rhythm abnormalities and diagnosing a myocardial infarction. Although relatively specific for myocardial infarction, the diagnostic sensitivity of the ECG is believed to range from 43% to 65%. Data from a recent study on the diagnostic reliability of the initial ECG in the emergency department setting found the sensitivity and specificity for acute myocardial infarction to be 79% and 83%, respectively.[16] Myocardial imaging techniques (**technetium 99m [^{99m}Tc]** pyrophosphate and **thallium 201**) are used to assess cardiac output and wall-motion abnormalities and to detect nonfunctioning regions of the myocardium caused by infarction. The diagnostic sensitivity of the technetium 99m pyrophosphate scan may be as high as 84% in transmural infarctions; however, the sensitivity may be as low as 32% in patients with nontransmural infarctions. The thallium 201 scan is not typically used for initial diagnosis of infarction.[17]

DRUG THERAPY

Two groups of drugs[18,19] have a direct effect on cardiac tissue and are therefore monitored by the clinical chemistry laboratory. These are the cardiac glycosides and the antiarrhythmic drugs.

Glycosides

The **glycosides** increase contractility in the heart and are particularly useful in treating heart failure. The problem with glycosides is that the therapeutic-to-toxic ratio is very low. At toxic dosage levels, the glycosides can upset the electrical activity of the heart and induce fatal arrhythmias. Since they have long half-lives in the body, they tend to have cumulative effects, necessitating careful monitoring of blood levels to reduce the possibility of toxic side effects. These tests are often needed on a stat basis.

Lidocaine

Lidocaine is an anesthetic compound given intravenously as a bolus or infusion to suppress ventricular irregularities and to prevent the induction of life-threatening arrhythmias, such as ventricular tachycardia. Lidocaine is a particularly attractive drug because it has few side effects and because it has little or no effect on myocardial function and cardiac conduction. Requests for serum lidocaine measurements are most often associated with cardiac surgery patients.

Quinidine and Other Drugs

Many antiarrhythmic drugs have a major side effect of inducing severe arrhythmias, and for this reason, drug blood levels are usually monitored so that one may use antiarrhyth-

mic drugs as safely as possible. Infrequently monitored antiarrhythmic drugs are quinidine and procainamide and its metabolite, N-acetyl procainamide (NAPA).

CHANGE OF ANALYTE IN DISEASE
Protein Markers in Myocardial Cells

When myocytes become necrotic, they lose membrane integrity, and intracellular macromolecules diffuse into the cardiac interstitium and ultimately into the cardiac microvasculature and lymphatics. Eventually, these macromolecules are detectable in the peripheral circulation. The term currently used to collectively describe these macromolecules is *cardiac markers*. The ideal cardiac marker of MI should be abundant in myocytes and low in blood, released early after injury, and absent from nonmyocardial tissue. It should be rapidly released into the blood at the time of myocardial injury, and there should be a direct relation between the plasma level of the cardiac marker and the extent of myocardial injury. The marker should persist in blood for a sufficient length of time to allow a high rate of diagnosis. Finally, measurement of the marker should be easy, inexpensive, and rapid.[20,21]

Definition of myocardial infarction (MI). MI represents the end of the acute coronary syndrome continuum, in which ischemic injury is irreversible, leading to cell death and necrosis. Based on the ECG, two classifications of MI are possible: ST elevation MI, which tends to be larger and tends to affect the anterior location of the heart, and non-ST elevation (NSTE) MI, which tends to involve less myocardial tissue. In the past, a general consensus existed for the clinical entity designated as MI. In studies of disease prevalence by the WHO, MI was defined by a combination of at least two of three characteristics: typical symptoms (such as chest discomfort), a rise in biochemical marker levels, and a typical ECG pattern involving the development of Q waves. However, current clinical practice, health care delivery systems, epidemiologic studies, and clinical trials all require a more precise definition of MI.

In response to increased evidence gained by new cardiac markers such as troponin and the development of other technologies for assessment of the acute coronary syndromes including MI, the European Society of Cardiology (ESC) and the American College of Cardiology (ACC) held a consensus conference during July 1999 to reexamine the definition of MI.[20,21] As a result of these activities, cTnT and cTnI now represent the cornerstone for the definition of and detection of MI. It became apparent from these deliberations that the term *MI* required further qualifications. Such qualifications should refer to the amount of myocardial cell loss (infarct size), the circumstances leading to the infarct (spontaneous or in a setting of a coronary artery diagnostic or therapeutic procedure), and the timing of the myocardial necrosis relative to the time of the observation (evolving, healing, or healed MI).

Also necessitating reevaluation of established definitions of MI is the advent of sensitive and specific serologic biomarkers capable of detecting small infarcts (as little as 1.0 g of dead tissue) that may not have been considered an MI in an earlier era. If it is accepted that any amount of myocardial necrosis caused by ischemia should be labeled as an infarct (as proposed by the ASC/ACC) then individuals formally diagnosed with severe, stable or unstable angina, might be diagnosed today as having had MI. According to the ESC/ACC document, the cutoff for MI is the ninety-ninth percentile of a reference control population. Currently, adherence to this definition is difficult because of the limitations of many quantitative troponin assays. The American Association for Clinical Chemistry (AACC) and International Federation of Clinical Chemistry (IFCC) are actively working toward improvement of this situation. The increased-sensitivity criteria for MI means more cases will be identified; in contrast, the increased specificity would lessen the number of false-positive MI results. Such changes in the definition of MI will have a profound effect on the traditional monitoring of disease rates and outcomes.

Cardiac markers in MI. After the onset of symptoms in MI there is a "time window" during which elevated values for the cardiac markers released from the myocardial tissue become elevated in blood. This temporal relationship is unique for each cardiac marker and varies somewhat among persons, though a typical pattern is defined for each marker (Fig. 31-3). Usually, 4 to 6 hours are required after the onset of chest pain before CK-MB becomes elevated in the serum of patients with MI; this marker has high diagnostic sensitivity and specificity by 8 to 12 hours after presentation. This time course represents the classic temporal sequence of CK-MB changes and is often helpful in distinguishing uncomplicated MI from extension or reinfarction.

Clinical interpretation of cardiac marker data for the diagnosis of MI requires that samples be collected and analyzed at appropriate intervals. Since the temporal sequence of events is critical in the assessment of the biochemical changes, the diagnosis of an MI with cardiac markers should not be made on the basis of a single isolated specimen, particularly if the result is negative. Some studies have recommended sampling a sequence that includes samples collected on admission and at 2 to 4 hours, 6 to 8 hours, and 12 hours after an MI is suspected.[17-19] The ESC/ACC consensus report stressed the importance of serial sampling for cardiac markers, recommending sampling upon presentation, at 6 to 9 hours, and again at 12 to 24 hours if the earlier samples were negative and the clinical index of suspicion is high.[21]

Results of cardiac marker measurement should be available 24 hours a day, within 30 to 60 minutes of sample collection. Numerous cases in which elevated CK-MB levels are accompanied by normal total CK levels during the initial course of a MI have been documented.[22] In most of these cases, however, there is a distinct rise and fall of the total CK values, though none ever exceeds the upper limit of normal.

Recommendations for the use of cardiac markers in coronary disease. The ESC/ACC conference in 1999 recognized the preferred biomarker for assessment of myocardial injury as the cardiac troponins (T and I),[20, 21] because these proteins have nearly absolute myocardial tissue specificity. Because even small elevations of cTn reflect microscopic zones of myocardial necrosis, the cardiac troponins (T and I) have become surrogates of myocardial necrosis. In the event that the cardiac troponins are not

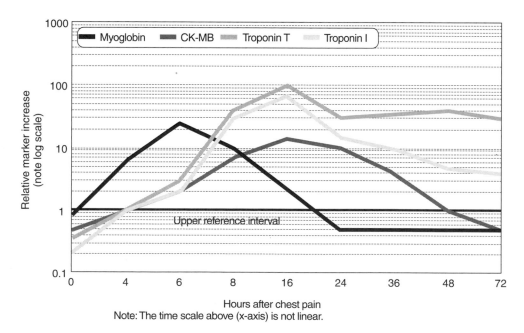

Fig. 31-3 Relative marker increase after myocardial infarction. Markers are expressed as multiples of the upper limit of the reference interval. Therefore, the relative increase varies depending on the normal reference interval used. The time scale above (x-axis) is not linear. *(Drawing adapted with permission from Wu A: Cardiac markers, Totowa, NJ, 1998, Humana Press.)*

available, the recommended alternative is CK-MB (measured by mass assay). CK-MB is less tissue-specific than cTnT and cTnI, but there is significant evidence demonstrating clinical specificity for irreversible cardiac injury. Measurement of total CK is not recommended for the routine diagnosis of MI because of the wide tissue distribution of this enzyme. Nevertheless, total CK has a long history, and some physicians may opt to continue to employ it for epidemiological or scientific purposes. In such a setting, total CK should be combined with more sensitive biomarkers, such as the cardiac troponins or CK-MB, for more accurate clinical diagnosis of MI.[21]

The following are biochemical indicators for detecting myocardial necrosis: (1) maximal concentration of cTnI or cTnI exceeding the decision limit (ninety-ninth percentile of the values for a reference control group) on at least one occasion during the first 24 hours after chest pain onset (thus in the setting of cardiac ischemia, a single positive troponin is diagnostic of MI); (2) maximal value of CK-MB (preferably CK-MB mass) exceeding the ninety-ninth percentile of the values for a reference control group on two successive samples, or maximal value exceeding twice the upper limit of normal for the specific institution on one occasion during the first hours after chest pain onset. Values for CK-MB must rise and fall; values that remain elevated without change, are almost never due to MI. In the absence of the cardiac troponins or CK-MB mass assay, total CK (greater than two times the upper reference limit) or the B fraction of CK may be employed, but these last two biomarkers are considerably less satisfactory than CK-MB.[21]

Although myoglobin is also used as a diagnostic indicator of myocardial injury, the use of LD and AST is anachronistic and is *not* recommended for routine use in the diagnosis of MI.

Diagnostic use of cardiac troponin T (cTnT) and cardiac troponin I (cTnI).

Troponin plays a vital role in the diagnosis and risk stratification of acute coronary syndromes (ACS). Several general impressions can be made regarding cTnT and cTnI. First, the release kinetics of both cTnT and cTnI are similar to those of CK-MB after MI. Second, troponin remains elevated in blood for 4 to 10 days after MI. The long temporal elevation after MI has led to replacement of LD for detection of late-presenting patients. Third, the very low troponin values in patients without cardiac disease permits use of lower discriminator values for the determination of MI based on cutoff at the ninety-ninth percentile of a reference control population. Finally, troponin's cardiac specificity helps eliminate the diagnostic uncertainty caused by increased CK-MB following skeletal muscle injury.

It must be emphasized that the use of troponin for MI diagnosis requires a setting of cardiac ischemia. The clinical interpretation of elevated troponin levels that are common in heart failure, end-stage renal disease, and other conditions is uncertain at this time. However, troponin positively suggests that these positive patients are at greater risk for adverse events. Also, troponin measurements are based on immuno-

assays, so false-positive results may occur from a variety of factors unrelated to heart disease (See Interferences, Chapter 23).

cTnI. Although cTnI has a lower molecular weight (27 kDa) than cTnT (37 kDa) and CK-MB (85 kDa), its release characteristics and use as an early indicator of MI are similar to those of cTnT and CK-MB. cTnI is similar to cTnT in most clinical applications, and its measurement offers the same advantages over CK-MB as cTnT. cTnI remains elevated 3 to 7 days after AMI. Thus cTnI and CK-MB have comparable diagnostic sensitivity for MI during the initial 48 to 72 hours after MI with improved cTnI sensitivities 72 to 96 hours after MI.

In contrast to CK-MB and total CK, cTnI is not elevated in patients with extreme skeletal muscle injury, including (1) acute skeletal muscle injury following marathon racing, (2) chronic myopathy of Duchenne muscular dystrophy, or (3) chronic renal failure requiring dialysis.

cTnT.[2-4] Although more than 10 diagnostic companies manufacture cTnI assays, only one company (Roche Diagnostics, Indianapolis, IN) manufactures cTnT for diagnostic use. Once an MI has occurred, cTnT increases in serum after 4 hours, achieving an initial peak or plateau at 1 to 6 days. A second cTnT peak is observed in some MI patients, which is thought to occur because cTnT has both cytosolic and structurally bound cTnT pools; the first peak is believed to result from release of the cytosolic pool, and the second peak may reflect the slower release of the bound fraction later in the myocardial necrosis process.

By the traditional WHO definition of MI, clinical sensitivity of cTnT is similar to that of CK-MB during the first 48 hours after the onset of chest pain. Thus cTnT is not an early marker of MI, showing clinical sensitivity of 50% to 65% from 0 to 6 hours after chest pain onset. Therefore, like CK-MB, cTnT is insufficient for effective early diagnosis. Because of cTnT's extended lifetime in serum, levels may provide important diagnostic information about an MI after serum CK-MB has achieved normal levels. In addition, cTnT may offer substantial information about the recent history of myocardial dysfunction. cTnT is useful for risk stratification of acute coronary syndrome patients and is advocated in clinical guidelines[20] for coronary intervention and for targeting therapy with low–molecular-weight heparin and platelet inhibitors in high-risk patients.

cTnI Versus cTnT. Few direct comparison studies have been conducted between cTnI and cTnT for the diagnosis of MI. However, direct comparisons of cTnI and cTnT measurements in serum from patients with chronic renal failure indicated that both were increased in patients with documented myocardial injury. However, cTnT elevations were also seen in patients without evidence of myocardial injury. Interpretation of these findings must wait for further study because patients on chronic hemodialysis having cTnT may have poorer outcomes.

There is currently no cTnI reference material available for manufacturers, and there can be as much as a 30-fold difference in values between methods. Explanation for this disparity is related not only to calibration but also to the fact that the reagent antibodies used in various assays recognize different epitopes on the troponin molecule. In addition, cTnI may be present in the circulation in three forms: (1) free, (2) bound as a two-unit complex (cTnI-cTnC), and (3) bound as a three-unit complex (cTnT-cTnI-cTnC). Issues involving calibration and antibody targets are an active area of investigation by AACC and IFCC committees.

Myoglobin. Myoglobin is present in both cardiac and skeletal muscle, limiting its diagnostic specificity. The value of myoglobin assay[15,16] in MI is its early appearance in serum after MI. Because the interval between the onset of symptoms and clinical presentation is variable, it has been suggested that multiple markers are needed to enable detection of MI in patients who present either very early or late after the onset of pain. Currently, myoglobin most effectively fits the role of an early marker. A rise in myoglobin is detectable in blood as early as 1 to 2 hours after symptoms onset and is highly sensitive for MI diagnosis and effective for rule-out in the 2- to 6-hour timeframe after onset of symptoms (see Figure 31-3). Myoglobin is not cardiac-specific, so patients with renal failure injury, trauma, or diseases involving skeletal muscle can have abnormal concentrations in the absence of MI. The presence of myoglobinuria can be used to confirm massive muscle cytolysis (trauma- or drug-induced) and as a diagnostic aid for assessing myoglobin-induced acute renal failure.

CK-isoforms[23-25] (see also Chapter 55). Because the enzyme responsible for lysine cleavage is found in blood, only the unconverted MM and MB isoforms, MM_3 and MB_2, are found within cells; for this reason, MM_3 and MB_2 are termed the *tissue isoforms*. As part of normal cell turnover, MM_3 and MB_2 are released into circulation, where normally MM_3 constitutes only 30% of the CK-MM concentration in serum and MB_2 normally constitutes 50% of total serum CK-MB. After tissue injury, however, greater amounts of MM_3 and MB_2 isoforms are released from the intracellular compartment into circulation. Because the tissue/plasma ratio of CK-MB is very high and isoform conversion is not immediate, soon after cell death the plasma levels of unconverted MB_2 are present in great proportions relative to their respective seroconverted form. Therefore, it is possible to formulate tissue to a seroconverted isoform ratio (MB_2/MB_1), and an increase in this isoform ratio is sensitive for early diagnosis of myocardial cell death. Overall, the MB_2/MB_1 ratio is relatively cardiospecific, demonstrating an excellent diagnostic sensitivity, at over 90%, within 4 to 6 hours after onset of symptoms in patients with MI.

CK and CK isoenzymes in conditions other than MI. Frequently the pattern of cardiac isoenzyme elevation in conditions other than MI does not follow a rise-and-fall pattern, but instead is chronically elevated. These potential false-positive situations emphasize the importance of documenting an acute ischemic event in the timeframe of testing and measuring multiple samples obtained at appropriate intervals. The pattern of CK isoenzymes that is

found in the developing fetus is duplicated in the adult in certain pathological states. This alteration is most commonly observed in skeletal muscle. In the adult, CK is predominantly present in the MM form. Fetal muscle, however, is predominantly BB until the 16th week of gestation, at which time the expression of the gene coding for the M subunit is significantly increased. Diseases of skeletal muscle characterized by blood-perfusion regeneration are often associated with chronically increased levels of the fetal isomeric forms of CK. Thus Duchenne muscular dystrophy, polymyositis, and some forms of rhabdomyolysis frequently show increased levels of CK-MB in serum. These increases are in proportion to the degree of muscle fiber regeneration. Because skeletal muscle contains CK-MB, levels are frequently in the range associated with MI. Since the absolute amount of CK in skeletal muscle is about 5- to 10-fold that observed in cardiac tissue, the actual elevations of total CK observed in serum in skeletal muscle abnormalities are frequently dramatically higher than those observed in MI, though the proportion that is CK-MB is typically quite low.

Caveats for diagnostic performance of cardiac markers for MI. The interpretation of cardiac markers for the diagnosis of MI becomes obscured by the causes of false-positive and false-negative results. A fundamental issue for use of cardiac markers is that the diagnosis of myocardial ischemia without cell death is extremely difficult because there is little objective data and clinically ischemia can present as many clinical signs and symptoms.[26] A proper interpretation requires an understanding of the clinical setting of ischemia for which testing will occur. The use of cardiac markers in the setting of a coronary care population, with a 50% prevalence of disease assumed, clearly increases the predictive values of cardiac markers. In a low-prevalence population such as the emergency department (3%), the usefulness of positive predictive values of cardiac markers for MI will be diminished. In all cases laboratory data must be used within the context of other clinical findings, such as history of prior cardiac disease, history of coronary pain, and ECG changes.

B-type natriuretic peptide, or brain natriuretic peptide (BNP). BNP and atrial natriuretic peptide (ANP) act as a dual natriuretic system in regulating blood pressure and fluid balance.[27] See Chapter 24 for additional details on the natriuretic peptides. The heart is the major source of circulating BNP[28]; the heart releases BNP in response to both ventricle volume expansion and pressure overload. The underlying rationale for use of BNP as a diagnostic tool for heart failure is its substantial release from the failing heart into the plasma, making it an appealing target for further development.

Albumin cobalt binding (ACB) test for ischemia. The release of currently used myocardial markers into the circulation is believed to require tissue necrosis, whereas the assessment of cardiac ischemia before or in the absence of cell death is an important component of clinical decision making in the suspected acute coronary syndrome patient.

With regard to biochemical markers of ischemia, initial data for glycogen phosphorylase-BB were encouraging, but these results have not been confirmed. Recently, a test has been developed for measurement of ischemia-modified albumin; the test is based on differences between normal albumin and ischemia-modified albumin in binding the transition metal cobalt (Ischemia Technologies, Inc., Denver, CO). Although studies are currently ongoing, other markers such as free fatty acid, nourin, and others may play an important role in the future for assessment of myocardial ischemia.

References

1. Hearse DJ: *Enzymes in cardiology: diagnosis and research*, New York, 1979, Wiley & Sons.
2. Mair J, Dienstl F, Puschendorf B: Cardiac troponin T in the diagnosis of myocardial injury, *Crit Rev Clin Lab Sci* 29:31, 1992.
3. Apple FS: Acute myocardial infarction and coronary reperfusion, *Am J Clin Pathol* 97:217, 1992.
4. Bodor GS et al: Development of monoclonal antibodies for an assay of cardiac troponin-I and preliminary results in suspected cases of myocardial infarction, *Clin Chem* 38:2203, 1992.
5. Nolan AC et al: Patterns of cellular injury in myocardial ischemia determined by monoclonal antimyosin, *Proc Natl Acad Sci* 80:6046, 1983.
6. Hurst JW et al, editors: *The heart, arteries, and veins*, ed 6, New York, 1986, McGraw-Hill.
7. de Ferrantim S, Rifai N. C-reactive protein and cardiovascular disease: a review of risk and interventions, *Clin Chim Acta* 317:1, 2002.
8. Christenson RH et al: Characteristics of an albumin cobalt binding test for assessment of acute coronary syndrome patients: a multicenter study, *Clin Chem* 47:3, 2001.
9. Storrow AB, Gibler WB. Chest pain centers: diagnosis of acute coronary syndromes, *Ann Emerg Med* 35:449, 2000.
10. Puleo PR et al. Use of a rapid assay for subforms of creatine kinase MB to diagnose or rule out myocardial infarction, *N Engl J Med* 331:561, 1994.
11. Tears RD: Asymmetrical hypertrophy of the heart in young adults, *Br Heart J* 20:1, 1958.
12. Wigle ED: Hypercardiomyopathy, *Mod Concepts Cardiovasc Dis* 57:1, 1988.
13. Elstein E, Liew CC, Sole MJ: The genetic base of hypertrophic cardiomyopathy, *J Mol Cell Cardiol* 24:1471, 1992.
14. Weiss LM et al: Detection of enteroviral RNA in idiopathic dilated cardiomyopathy and other human cardiac tissues, *J Clin Invest* 90:156, 1992.
15. Grenadier E et al: The rules of serum myoglobin, total CPK and CK-MB isoenzyme in the acute phase of myocardial infarction, *Am Heart J* 105:408, 1983.
16. Drexel H et al: Myoglobinuria in the early phase of acute myocardial infarction, *Am Heart J* 105:642, 1983.
17. Guzy PM: Creatinine phosphokinase-MB (CPK-MB) and the diagnosis of myocardial infarction, *West J Med* 127:445, 1977.
18. Lott JA, Stang JM: Serum enzymes and isoenzymes in the diagnosis and differential diagnosis of myocardial ischemia and necrosis, *Clin Chem* 26:1241, 1980.
19. Mair J et al: Equivalent early sensitivities of myoglobin, creatine kinase MB mass, creatine kinase isoform ratios, and troponin I and T for acute myocardial infarction, *Clin Chem* 41:1266, 1995.
20. ACC/AHA guidelines for the management of patients with acute myocardial infarction: a report of the American College of Cardiology/American Heart Association Task Force on Practice Guidelines (Committee on Management of Acute Myocardial Infarction), *JACC* 34:890, 1999.
21. ESC/ACC Committee: Myocardial infarction redefined—a consensus document of the joint European Society of Cardiology/American College of Cardiology Committee for the Redefinition of Myocardial Infarction, *Eur Heart J* 21:1502, 2000.
22. Irvin RG, Cobb FR, Roe CR: Acute myocardial infarction and creatine phosphokinase, *Arch Intern Med* 140:329, 1980.
23. Wu ABW: Creatine kinase isoforms in ischemic heart disease, *Clin Chem* 35:7, 1989.
24. Puleo PR et al: Early diagnosis of acute myocardial infarction based on assay for subforms of creatine kinase-MB, *Circulation* 82:759, 1990.
25. Christenson RH et al: Characteristics of creatine kinase-MB and the MB isoforms in serum after reperfusion in acute myocardial infarction, *Clin Chem* 35:2179, 1989.
26. Hamm CW et al: The prognostic value of serum troponin T in unstable angina, *N Engl J Med* 327:146, 1992.
27. Yandle T: Biochemistry of natriuretic peptides, *J Int Med* 235:561, 1994.
28. McDowell G et al: The natriuretic peptide family, *Eur J Clin Inv* 25:291, 1995.

Internet Sites

General

http://www.cardiac-disease.net/
http://www.ynhh.org/cardiac/diagnosis/
www.acc.org/—American College of Cardiology

Guidelines for MI

www.acc.org/clinical/guidelines/nov96/1999/—ACC/AHA Guidelines for the Management of Patients with Acute Myocardial Infarction
www.acc.org/clinical/consensus/mi_redefined/—Myocardial Infarction Redefined: A Consensus Document
www.escardio.org—European Society of Cardiology
http://www.fodsupport.org/cpt2.htm—Fatty oxidation disorder website

http://medlib.med.utah.edu/WebPath/TUTORIAL/MYOCARD/MYOCARD.html—University of Utah tutorial
www.nlm.nih.gov/medlineplus/ency/article/000158.htm—National Medical Library, Encyclopedia; Heart Failure
http://www.ultranet.com/~jkimball/BiologyPages/M/Muscles.html#Muscle_Diseases
http://www.bertholf.net/rlb/lectures/Lectures/Cardiac%20Markers%20and%20Renal%20Function.pps—Microsoft PowerPoint lecture by Robert L. Bertholf, PhD, Associate Professor of Pathology, Chief of Clinical Chemistry and Toxicology
http://www.nacb.org/lmpg/cardiac_lmpg.stm

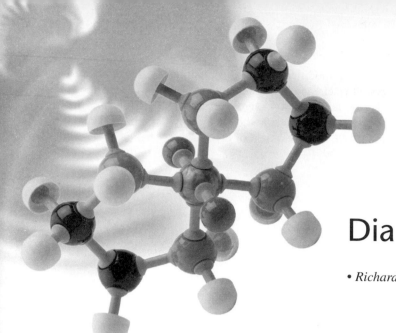

CHAPTER 32

Diabetes Mellitus

• *Richard F. Dods*

Chapter Outline

Objectives

- Describe normal glucose homeostasis.
- Differentiate between diabetes mellitus (types I and II), impaired glucose tolerance, and gestational diabetes.
- Describe common acute and chronic complications of diabetes mellitus.
- List steps in performing an oral glucose tolerance test.
- State expected levels of the following analytes in controlled diabetes mellitus I and II, ketoacidosis, and hyperosmolar coma: glucose, ketones, pH, bicarbonate, P_{CO_2}, insulin, C-peptide, sodium, potassium, glycated hemoglobin, BUN, osmolality, and triglycerides.

Key Terms

acromegaly   Growth hormone excess in adults and characterized by enlargement of features such as the head, hands, and feet.

adenosine 3′,5′-cyclic monophosphate (cAMP)   An organic molecule that is obligatory for the action of enzymes such as protein kinases.

aerobic glycolysis   Glycolysis that is linked to the tricarboxylic acid cycle by the presence of oxygen. Aerobic glycolysis produces 36 moles of ATP per mole of glucose.

anaerobic glycolysis   Glycolysis that occurs in the absence of oxygen. In this case glycolysis is not linked to the tricarboxylic acid cycle and only 2 moles of ATP are produced per mole of glucose.

angiogenesis   A complication of diabetes mellitus. Abnormal proliferation of blood vessels in a tissue such as the eye lens.

angiopathy   A complication of diabetes mellitus manifesting as damage to the basement membranes of blood vessels.

anoxia   Lack of oxygen.

basement membrane   A layer of noncellular material that underlies the epithelium.

diabetic ketoacidosis   A complication of diabetes mellitus characterized by hyperglycemia, hyperosmolarity, low pH, ketonuria and ketonemia, and lethargy or coma.

disaccharide   Two monosaccharides linked by a glycosidic bond.

electron transport chain   A series of molecules that transfers electrons from NADH and FADH$_2$ to oxygen.

gestational diabetes   Glucose intolerance that occurs in some pregnancies.

glucagon   A hormone produced by the α-cells of the pancreas. Glucagon is primarily involved in energy release.

glucagonoma   Excessive glucagon levels caused by a tumor.

gluconeogenesis   Production of glucose from pyruvic acid.

glucose   A six-carbon polyhydroxyl aldehyde;

primary source of energy in living organisms. Its metabolism produces adenosine triphosphate.

glucosuria   Excessive quantities of urinary glucose.

glycation   Reaction in which glucose binds covalently to protein.

glycogen   Highly branched, high–molecular-weight polysaccharide composed only of glucose units.

glycogenesis   Formation of glycogen from glucose-6-phosphate.

glycolysis   Metabolism of glucose-6-phosphate to pyruvic acid or lactic acid.

growth hormone   Hormone produced by the anterior part of the pituitary. Also called somatotropin. Raises blood glucose.

hexose monophosphate shunt   Metabolic pathway in which glucose-6-phosphate is metabolized to ribose and carbon dioxide.

histocompatibility antigen (human lymphocyte antigen, HLA)   Proteins responsible for rejection of tissue transplanted to an individual from another unrelated individual. Specific HLAs are present at a high frequency in persons who develop certain diseases.

hyperglycemia   High blood glucose concentrations.

hyperglycemic hyperosmolar nonketotic coma (HHNC)   A complication of diabetes mellitus characterized by hyperglycemia, hyperosmolarity, normal keto acid levels, and lethargy or coma.

islet cell antibodies (ICA)   Antibodies frequently found in type I diabetics that are suggestive of an autoimmune cause.

islets of Langerhans   Group of cells in the pancreas composed of α-cells, which secrete glucagon; β-cells, which secrete insulin; and δ-cells, which secrete somatostatin.

ketonemia   Excess of ketones and derived keto acids in the blood.

ketonuria   Excess of ketones and derived keto acids in the urine.

lactic acidosis   Acidosis (low blood pH) caused by excess lactic acid.

lipolysis Hydrolysis of triglycerides to free fatty acids and glycerol.

monosaccharide A polyhydroxyl aldehyde or ketone, such as glucose, fructose, or mannose.

nephropathy A complication of diabetes mellitus referring to damage to the glomerulus and capillaries associated with the glomerulus.

neuropathy The most common complication of diabetes mellitus. It refers to reduced motor and sensory nerve conduction velocities caused by axonal degeneration and demyelination.

oxidative phosphorylation The process linking the tricarboxylic acid cycle with ATP formation.

polydipsia Excessive thirst. A symptom of diabetes mellitus.

polyphagia Constant hunger. A symptom of diabetes mellitus.

polysaccharide A carbohydrate composed of more than two monosaccharides linked by glycosidic bonds.

polyuria Excessive urinary output. A symptom of diabetes mellitus.

preproinsulin Precursor to proinsulin.

proinsulin Precursor to insulin.

protein kinases Enzymes that phosphorylate other proteins. Some protein kinases depend on adenosine monophosphate for activity.

receptor sites Sites on or in cells where hormones are bound. Hormone binding to the receptor site is the initial step for hormone action.

retinopathy A complication of diabetes mellitus. A disorder of the retina caused in diabetics by cataract formation or proliferation of small blood vessels (angiogenesis).

somatostatin A hormone produced in the δ-cells of the pancreas. Inhibits insulin and glucagon secretion.

somatostatinoma A tumor that produces excess quantities of somatostatin, resulting in hyperglycemia.

thyroxine A hormone produced by the thyroid gland that increases blood glucose levels.

tricarboxylic acid cycle Metabolic pathway that converts glucose-6-phosphate via pyruvic acid to CO_2 and water. When coupled to oxidative phosphorylation, adenosine triphosphate is formed.

uronic acid pathway Converts glucose-6-phosphate to glucuronic acid.

Methods on CD-ROM

Albumin
Anion gap
Blood gas analysis and oxygen saturation
BUN
Glucose
Glycated hemoglobin
Insulin and C-peptide

Ketones
Lactic acid
Osmolality
Sodium and potassium
Triglycerides
Urine protein, total

According to Harris et al,[1] the prevalence of diabetes in the American population is 5.9%. Thus there are approximately 15.7 million diabetic Americans. Of this number about 34% are undiagnosed. Although rates are equal by gender, there are significant race-based differences. Mexican-Americans are 1.9 times, non-Hispanic blacks are 1.7 times, and American Indians and Alaska Natives are 2.8 times as likely to have diagnosed diabetes than whites of similar age. The prevalence of diabetes in the Asian-American and Pacific Islanders populations is unknown but one study suggests that Native Hawaiians are 2 times as likely to have diabetes than whites living in Hawaii. The cost of diabetes, both direct and indirect (disability, work loss, premature mortality), to the American economy is estimated at $98 billion.[2]

The implications of diabetes extend beyond its direct effects and long-term complications, because it has been established that diabetes is a risk factor for coronary heart disease[3] and cerebrovascular disease (stroke).[4] A diabetic has a twofold greater risk of suffering a myocardial infarction than a nondiabetic of the same age and sex.

Research has demonstrated that diabetes mellitus is not a single disease but an array of diseases that exhibit a common symptom, inability of the individual to regulate **glucose** levels (glucose intolerance).

The primary symptoms of diabetes mellitus are abnormally high blood and urine glucose levels (**hyperglycemia** and **glucosuria**, respectively), **polyuria**, excessive thirst (**polydipsia**), constant hunger (**polyphagia**), sudden weight loss, and, during acute episodes of diabetes mellitus, excessive blood and urinary ketones (**ketonemia** and **ketonuria**, respectively). All these symptoms are the result of the inability to metabolize glucose and the consequences of high glucose levels.

GLUCOSE: PROPERTIES AND METABOLISM

Definition (see also p. 1035)

Carbohydrates are defined as polyhydroxyl aldehydes (aldoses) and ketones (ketoses). Simple carbohydrates such as glucose are also called **monosaccharides**. Two monosaccharides linked by a bond called a glycosidic bond form a **disaccharide**. More than two monosaccharides linked by glycosidic bonds form a **polysaccharide**. Dietary carbohydrates consist of monosaccharides such as glucose, fructose, and galactose; disaccharides such as sucrose, lactose, and maltose; and polysaccharides such as starch. Intestinal enzymes convert disaccharides and polysaccharides to monosaccharides (see p. 553).

Function

The principal biochemical function of glucose is to provide energy for life processes. *Adenosine triphosphate* (ATP) is the universal energy source for biological reactions. Glucose oxidation by the glycolytic and tricarboxylic acid pathways is the primary source of energy for the biosynthesis of ATP.

Glucose Transport Across Cell Membranes

The initial event in glucose metabolism is facilitated transport of glucose across the plasma membrane. Five glucose transporters, called GluT-1 through GluT-5, have been identified.[5] The glucose transporters are integral components of the cell membrane and are glycoproteins with molecular weights of approximately 55,000 Daltons (D).

The glucose transporters vary with respect to tissue distribution and apparent Michaelis-Menten constant (K_m). GluT-1, GluT-3, and GluT-5 possess a low K_m of <1 to 2 mM, whereas GluT-4 has an intermediate K_m of 5 mM, and GluT-2 has a high K_m of 17 mM. There is considerable significance in the locations of the different forms of the glucose transporters. GluT-1 and GluT-3, predominantly located in glucose-sensitive, insulin-dependent cells such as brain and erythrocytes, permit cell uptake of glucose at levels below the normal fasting range despite low levels of insulin and glucose. The highest K_m glucose transporter, GluT-2, is located in cells that are directly involved in blood glucose regulation and permit these cells to increase their glucose uptake, independent of insulin, in the presence of increased blood glucose levels. Thus small intestine, renal tubule, and liver cells, and pancreatic β-cells possess GluT-2. High K_m transporters allow glucose uptake over a wide range of extracellular glucose levels. GluT-4, which has a K_m in the intermediate range, is found principally in the insulin-dependent muscle and adipose cells.

Principal Glucose-6-Phosphate Metabolic Pathways

Within the cell, glucose is rapidly converted to *glucose-6-phosphate* (G6P), a major intermediate in glucose metabolism. The enzyme catalyzing the phosphorylation of

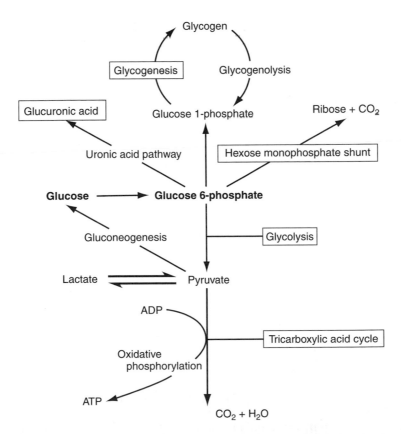

Fig. 32-1 The five principal pathways of glucose metabolism: glycolysis, tricarboxylic acid pathway, glycogenesis, hexose monophosphate shunt, and the uronic acid pathway.

glucose by ATP is hexokinase (or glucokinase in the liver and β-cells of the pancreas). Glucokinase may play a key role in the regulation of glucose homeostasis by maintaining a gradient for glucose transport in hepatocytes.[6]

As shown in Fig. 32-1, glucose-6-phosphate serves as a starting point for four metabolic pathways. Glucose-6-phosphate is converted by **glycolysis** to pyruvate, a substance that is further metabolized by the tricarboxylic acid pathway to carbon dioxide and water. Glucose-6-phosphate is also oxidized by the **hexose monophosphate shunt** to ribose and carbon

dioxide, converted by the **uronic acid pathway** to glucuronic acid, and incorporated into glycogen by **glycogenesis**.

Aerobic Glycolysis

Glycolysis. Glucose-6-phosphate metabolism by the glycolytic pathway (also called the *Embden-Meyerhof pathway*) results in the formation of ATP (Fig. 32-2). Glycolysis converts the six-carbon glucose molecule to two molecules of a three-carbon compound called pyruvic acid. This process produces 2 mol of ATP per mole of glucose. An

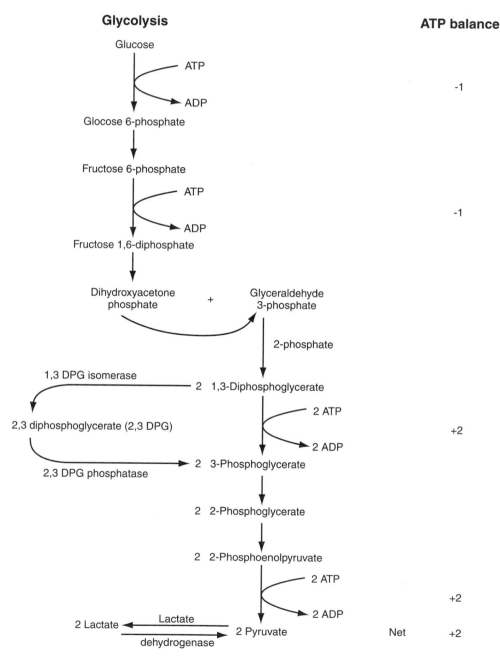

Glycolysis

ATP balance

Fig. 32-2 Two stages of glycolysis. First stage proceeds from glucose to formation of 1,3-diphosphoglycerate and consumes 2 mol of ATP. Second stage proceeds from 1,3-diphosphoglycerate to pyruvate and produces 4 mol of ATP. Glycolysis therefore results in net gain of 2 mol of ATP per mole of glucose. The synthesis of 2,3-DPG by the Rapoport-Luebring cycle is important for the regulation of oxygen transport.

important aspect of glycolysis is the formation of pyruvic acid. In **aerobic glycolysis**, pyruvate is metabolized further by means of the **tricarboxylic acid cycle**.

Tricarboxylic acid cycle. Pyruvic acid enters the tricarboxylic acid cycle (citric acid cycle, Krebs cycle) where it is metabolized to carbon dioxide and water. Fig. 32-3 shows the intermediate steps in the tricarboxylic acid cycle and the steps that are used to reduce nicotinamide adenine dinucleotide (NAD) and flavin adenine dinucleotide (FAD) to their corresponding analogs, NADH and FADH$_2$. The tricarboxylic acid cycle does not directly produce ATP, but ATP is produced by the oxidation of NADH and FADH$_2$.

Electron transport chain and oxidative phosphorylation. Electron transport is a complex process that takes place in the mitochondria and that involves electron transfer from NADH and FADH$_2$ to a series of compounds, ending with the reduction of oxygen to yield a water molecule. Oxidative phosphorylation involves the phosphorylation of ADP by inorganic phosphate to form ATP, the energy for this reaction being caused by the flow of electrons through the electron transport chain. The mechanism for this process was formulated by Peter Mitchel in 1961 and called the *chemiosmotic mechanism*. The flow of electrons causes the pumping of protons from the inner matrix through the inner membrane into intermembrane space. The intermembrane space becomes more acidic and the matrix more basic. The protons cannot migrate back. The proton gradient that is established provides the energy for the phosphorylation of ADP. Thus it is the reoxidation of NADH and FADH$_2$, compounds produced by the tricarboxylic acid cycle, that produces ATP. In contrast to glycolysis, which produces 2 mol of ATP per mole of glucose, the tricarboxylic acid cycle linked with oxidative phosphorylation produces 36 mol of ATP per mole of glucose. The oxidative and ATP synthesis processes are tightly coupled because the availability of adenosine diphosphate (ADP) controls the rate of oxidation and oxygen availability regulates phosphorylation.

Anaerobic Glycolysis

In fatigued muscle where there is a deficiency of oxygen, or **anoxia**, the above pathways cannot further metabolize glucose converted by glycolysis to pyruvic acid. Instead (Fig. 32-2) pyruvate is converted by the enzyme lactate dehydrogenase to lactate. This is called **anaerobic glycolysis**. In contrast to aerobic glycolysis, only 2 mol of ATP per mole of glucose are produced by anaerobic glycolysis. Lactic acid produced by anoxic tissue is carried by the circulation to the liver, where it is reconverted to glucose in a process called **gluconeogenesis** (see the following text).

Alternate energy sources. As indicated in Fig. 32-3, amino acids and fatty acids also enter the tricarboxylic acid cycle to produce ATP and are therefore alternative sources of energy.

Glycogenesis, Glycogenolysis, and Gluconeogenesis

Glycogen. Excess glucose is stored in the cells as the polymer **glycogen** for later energy demands. Glycogen (Fig. 32-4) is a high–molecular-weight polysaccharide composed entirely of glucose units in 1,4-glycosidic bonds with 1,6-branches occurring approximately every 10 units. Glycogen is located in the cytoplasm of liver and muscle cells in granules that contain the enzymes involved in the synthesis (**glycogenesis**) and hydrolysis (glycogenolysis) of glycogen. Refer again to Fig. 32-1 to see how glucogenesis and glycogenolysis fit into the overall scheme of glucose metabolism. Fig. 32-5 presents a simplified representation of glycogenesis and glycogenolysis.

Glycogenesis. The first step in glycogenesis is conversion of glucose-6-phosphate to glucose-1-phosphate (see Fig. 32-5). Reaction of glucose-1-phosphate with uridine-5'-triphosphate produces uridine diphosphate glucose, a substance that reacts with the preexisting glycogen molecule to form 1,4-glycosidic linkages. Synthesis of 1,4-glycosidic bonds is catalyzed by the enzyme glycogen synthetase. Glycogen synthetase exists in two forms: the phospho-

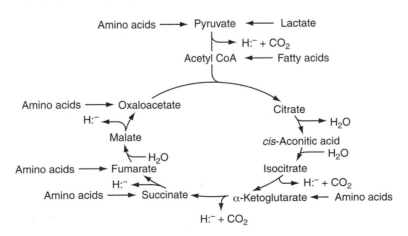

Fig. 32-3 Tricarboxylic acid cycle produces CO$_2$ and water from pyruvate, fatty acids, and amino acids, which enter the cycle at the points indicated. Hydride ions (H:$^-$) are produced and used in oxidative phosphorylation process to produce ATP from ADP and inorganic phosphate.

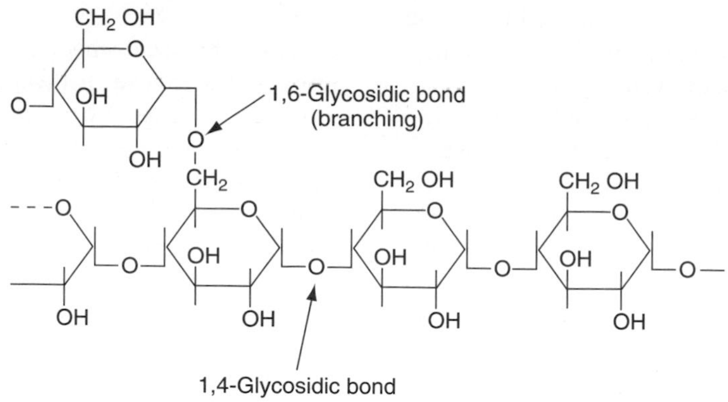

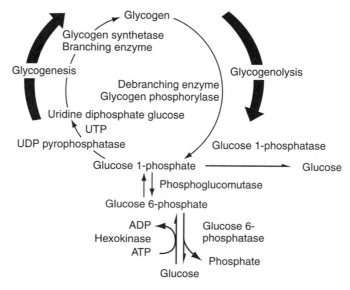

CH₂OH... (chemical structure)

1,6-Glycosidic bond
(branching)

1,4-Glycosidic bond

Fig. 32-4   Glycogen is a 1- to 4-million Dalton polysaccharide composed of glucose units in 1,4- and 1,6-glycosidic linkage. The 1,6-bonds produce branches at intervals of approximately 10 glucose units.

rylated, inactive enzyme form and the dephosphorylated, active enzyme form. Phosphorylation of the active enzyme is accomplished by any of several enzymes of the **protein kinase** class. Protein kinases are activated by low levels of **adenosine 3′,5′-cyclic monophosphate (cAMP)**. Thus glycogen synthetase activity (and thereby glycogenesis) is regulated by intracellular cAMP levels. Glycogenesis is enhanced by low cAMP levels and inhibited by high cAMP levels; cAMP levels are in turn regulated by insulin, which causes decreased cAMP levels.

Branching of glycogen is accomplished by an enzyme called a *branching enzyme*. This branching enzyme hydrolyzes the 1,4-glycosidic bond of glycogen to form five to six glucose unit fragments, which are reattached to the glycogen molecule through 1,6-glycosidic bonds.

Glycogenolysis. Although glycogenolysis (see Fig. 32-5) is the opposite of glycogenesis, it does not occur through a simple reversal of each step of glycogenesis but by a unique enzyme system. The *debranching enzyme* splits off trisaccharides from branches and reattaches them by 1,4-glycosidic bonds to the ends of the glycogen molecule. *Glycogen phosphorylase* hydrolyzes the 1,4-glycosidic bond producing glucose-1-phosphate:

$$\text{Glycogen} + P_i \rightarrow \text{Glycogen} + \text{Glucose-1-phosphate}$$
(*n* residues)   (*n* − 1 residues)   *Eq. 32-1*

Like glycogen synthetase, glycogen phosphorylase exists in two forms. The active form, called *phosphorylase a*, is a tetramer. The inactive form, phosphorylase b, is the dimer. The active tetramer is formed in three steps; phosphorylation of the dimer by a protein kinase called phosphorylase kinase followed by binding of the phosphorylated dimer with another phosphorylated dimer. The third and final step in the activation process is the binding of one molecule of

Fig. 32-5   Glycogen, storage molecule for glucose, is synthesized from glucose-1-phosphate by a process called *glycogenesis* (*left side*). *Glycogenolysis* releases glucose units from glycogen. Debranching is first step in glycogenolysis (*right side*).

pyridoxal phosphate to each subunit of the tetramer. Phosphorylase kinase is activated by cAMP. Note that high cellular cAMP levels favor glycogenolysis over glycogenesis. The activation of glycogen phosphorylase is under hormonal control (see later discussion).

Gluconeogenesis. The steps in gluconeogenesis are shown in Fig. 32-6. Gluconeogenesis produces glucose-6-phosphate from amino acids, fatty acids, glycerol, and lactate. Pyruvate is an important intermediary in gluconeogenesis (Fig. 32-6), because it can be formed directly from lactate oxidation (by lactate dehydrogenase) and from the amino acid alanine (via transamination by alanine transaminase). Glycerol, derived from hydrolysis of triglyceride **(lipolysis)**, enters the gluconeogenic pathway after pyruvate as glycerol-3-phosphate. These three substances, lactate,

alanine, and glycerol, are the primary precursors for glucose synthesis. Gluconeogenesis is not a simple reversal of glycolysis, though gluconeogenesis does share some of the enzymes of the glycolytic pathway. Glucose is formed only in the liver and kidney, which have the enzyme glucose-6-phosphatase, which hydrolyzes G6P to glucose. In fact, the liver is the major nondietary source of serum glucose of the body and is critical for maintaining blood glucose levels.

Hormone Regulation of Glucose Metabolism[7]

The system for regulating blood glucose levels is designed to achieve two ends. The first is to store glucose in excess of the body's immediate needs in a compact reservoir (glycogen), and the second is to mobilize the stored glucose to maintain the blood glucose level. The regulation of blood glucose is

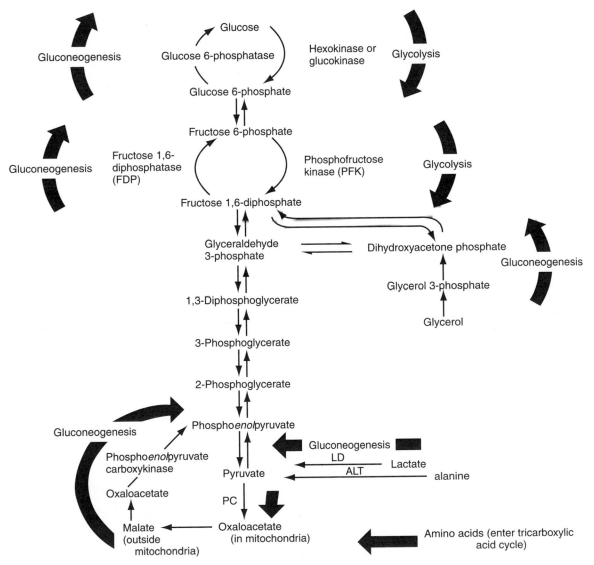

Fig. 32-6 Pathways involved in gluconeogenesis from amino acids, fatty acids, glycerol, and lactate. This pathway shares many of the enzymes of glycolytic and tricarboxylic acid pathways. Gluconeogenesis provides glucose whenever scarcity of glucose occurs and whenever lactate accumulates. *ALT,* Alanine transaminase; *LD,* lactate dehydrogenase; *PC,* pyruvate carboxylase.

essential to keep the brain, whose primary energy source is glucose, supplied with a constant amount of glucose. The role of insulin is to shift extracellular glucose to intracellular storage sites in the form of macromolecules (such as glycogen, fats, and proteins). Thus glucose is stored away in times of plenty for times of need.

In response to low blood glucose, as in periods of fasting, a series of hyperglycemic agents acts on intermediary metabolic pathways to form glucose from storage macromolecules. Thus proteins and glycogen are metabolized to form glucose-6-phosphate (gluconeogenesis), which in the liver is hydrolyzed to glucose and released into the blood to maintain blood glucose levels.

The most important hyperglycemic agents are **glucagon**, epinephrine, cortisol, **thyroxine**, **growth hormone**, and certain intestinal hormones. The behavior of each of these agents in regulating blood glucose is different; whereas insulin promotes anabolic metabolism (synthesis of macromolecules), these hormones in part induce catabolic metabolism to break down large molecules.

Insulin. Insulin is synthesized in the endocrine pancreas by the β-cells of the **islets of Langerhans** as a high–molecular-weight precursor called **preproinsulin**.[8] Preproinsulin (11,500 D) is shown in Fig. 32-7. Cleavage at the link marked by the line labeled *1* results in the formation of proinsulin (9000 D). Proinsulin has only 5% of the activity

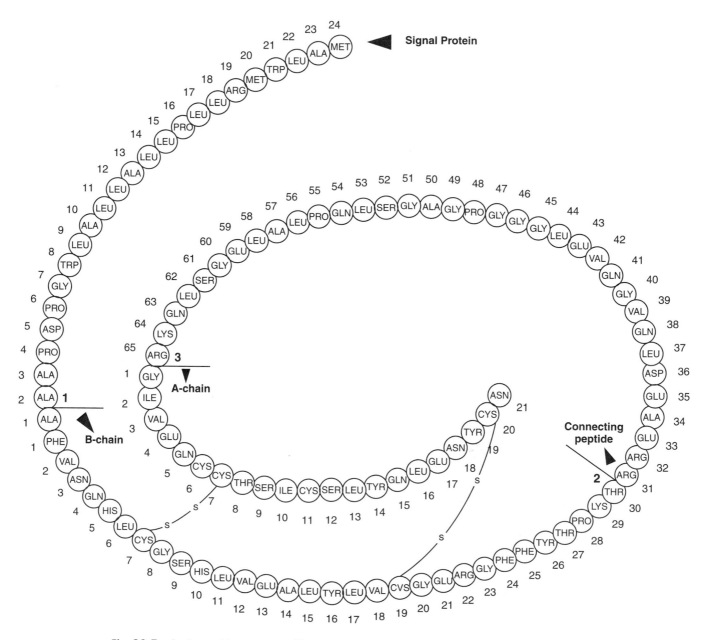

Fig. 32-7 Amino acid sequence of human preproinsulin. The series of enzymatic cleavages of preproinsulin *(site 1)* to proinsulin and of proinsulin *(sites 2 and 3)* to insulin are described in text.

of insulin. The proinsulin molecule consists of the A and B chains of insulin connected by disulfide bonds and by a connective peptide called *C-peptide*. During processing the C-peptide (3000 D) is removed from the molecule by cleavage at the links marked by lines *2* and *3*. The resulting insulin molecule (6000 D) consists of chains A and B connected by two disulfide bonds. This entire process occurs within the β-cell. The initial synthesis of preproinsulin occurs at the Golgi apparatus. The molecule is packaged in a vesicle called a β-*granule*. Cleavage first to proinsulin and next to insulin occurs within the granule. Equal quantities of C-peptide and insulin are released into the circulation when the granule is dissolved at the plasma membrane of the β-cell after neural, dietary, or hormonal stimuli. Only small quantities of proinsulin are found in the circulation.

Glucagon and cortisol. Glucagon is a 3500-D polypeptide hormone that is synthesized in the α-cells of the pancreas.[9] In diabetes mellitus, because of insulin deficiency, glucagon levels are elevated and are not suppressed by carbohydrate loading.[10] Cortisol and the other adrenal corticosteroids increase the rate of gluconeogenesis from protein and amino acids, especially in the liver.

Epinephrine. Epinephrine raises glucose levels by inhibiting insulin secretion, stimulating glucagon secretion, stimulating glycogenolysis, and inhibiting gluconeogenesis.

Other hormones. *Growth hormone* and *thyroxine* also act to raise circulating levels of glucose. **Somatostatin** is a polypeptide hormone that is synthesized primarily in the δ-cells of the pancreas. Somatostatin inhibits both insulin and glucagon release. *Gastric inhibitory polypeptide* stimulates insulin release. This hormone is located in the intestinal mucosa, and glucose and amino acids stimulate its release. Thus food ingestion results in increased levels of circulating insulin. Insulin-like growth factors are proteins with structured homology to proinsulin and somatomedin C. These factors may play a role in glucose control.

Opposite actions of insulin and glucagon. Insulin and glucagon have opposing effects. Insulin inhibits proteolysis, lipolysis, gluconeogenesis, and glycogenolysis and stimulates lipid synthesis and glycogenesis in the liver; increases protein synthesis in muscle; and accelerates triglyceride synthesis in fat cells (see table below). Insulin

acts as the body's only hypoglycemic agent. In contrast, glucagon stimulates lipolysis, ketogenesis, gluconeogenesis, and glycogenolysis. A meal rich in carbohydrates induces insulin secretion and suppresses glucagon release. Hypoglycemia stimulates the release of glucagon. Thus, in general, insulin and glucagon act oppositely to each other, with insulin promoting energy storage and glucagon promoting energy release. The net result of the hypoglycemic agent (insulin) and the hyperglycemic agents is glucose homeostasis.

Glucose Metabolism in Diabetes Mellitus

Metabolic processes in the normal individual. The hormonal regulation of blood glucose levels and metabolic processes is abnormal in diabetics and results in the classic sign of diabetes mellitus: elevated blood glucose levels.

In the postabsorptive (fasting) state of normal individuals, the blood insulin/glucagon ratio is low, causing muscle and hepatic glycogen to be degraded as a source of glucose. Additional fasting results in the breakdown of protein to amino acids in skeletal muscle, and the lipolysis of triglycerides to fatty acids in adipose tissue. The amino acid alanine and glycerol are used to synthesize glucose by means of glucagon-stimulated gluconeogenesis. In addition, free fatty acids can be used as fuel by the heart, skeletal muscles, and liver.

Just minutes after ingestion of a meal, blood insulin levels rapidly increase. Dietary glucose and amino acids, such as leucine, isoleucine, and lysine, are potent stimulants of the β-cells of the pancreas, causing them to secrete insulin. Most peripheral cells respond to the rise of blood glucose by rapidly increasing glucose transport into cells. Thus blood glucose levels increase by only 20% to 40% in nondiabetic individuals. However, approximately 80% of the glucose uptake is *not* insulin dependent, because the brain, red blood cells, liver, and intestines do not require insulin for increased glucose uptake in the presence of elevated blood glucose. Muscle is the most important insulin-dependent tissue. Increased blood insulin and glucose levels do inhibit lipolysis as well as approximately 60% of the normal hepatic release of glucose.

Metabolic processes in the diabetic.[7,11] In the diabetic, both the production and metabolism of glucose are increased. Thus, in the fasting state, hepatic glucose release is greatly elevated, causing the diagnostic, fasting hyperglycemia of diabetics.

In addition, both the release of insulin (type I diabetics) and the cellular response to insulin (insulin resistance in type II diabetics, see later discussion) are decreased in diabetics, especially relative to a given blood glucose level. The decreased insulin control causes the diabetic to be in a semistarvation state, with an increased dependence on triglycerides as a source of fuel and on protein as a source of glucose precursors. Thus, in the fasting state, the diabetic may have increased blood free fatty acids and ketones (see p. 593).

After a meal, the inhibition of hepatic glucose output is much smaller in the diabetic. Combined with both the

METABOLIC ACTION OF INSULIN			
	TISSUE		
	Liver	*Adipose*	*Muscle*
Inhibits:	Glycogenolysis Gluconeogenesis Ketogenesis	Lipolysis	Protein breakdown Amino acid release
Stimulates:	Glycogen and fatty acid synthesis	Glycerol and fatty acid synthesis	Glucose uptake and metabolism Amino acid uptake Synthesis of protein Glycogenesis

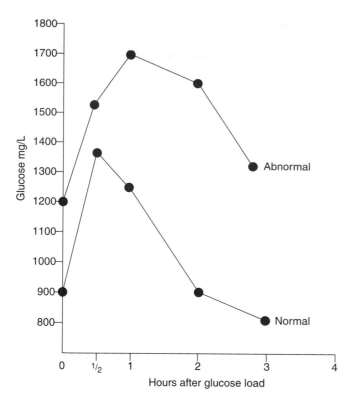

Fig. 32-8 Oral glucose tolerance test (OGTT, see p. 596). Diabetic's response to OGTT is compared to normal response. In diabetics, glucose curve is elevated and delayed. In normal response, peak is reached after 30 minutes and returns to baseline value after 2 hours. Type I diabetics produce a nearly flat insulin curve after glucose load. If there is a peak, it occurs late (later than 1 hour). In type II diabetics, insulin response is often exaggerated, peak is late, and return to baseline value is later than 3 hours.

diminished insulin output and insulin resistance, this results in an abnormal and prolonged rise in blood glucose in diabetics after a meal (Fig. 32-8).

In summary, the carbohydrate metabolism in a diabetic is strikingly similar to that of a nondiabetic in the fasting state. In both cases metabolism of fatty acids has replaced the metabolism of glucose-6-phosphate as the principal source of energy for the cell.

CLASSIFICATION OF DIABETES MELLITUS

In 1979 the National Diabetes Data Group of the National Institutes of Health (NIH) developed a classification scheme for diabetes mellitus and other types of glucose intolerance based on current knowledge of the biochemistry of this disease.[12] Table 32-1 summarizes the NIH classification system.

Type I Diabetes

Type I diabetes accounts for 5% to 10% of the diagnosed cases of diabetes. Its prevalence is 1 in 300 persons younger than 20 years of age, the time when this disease is usually diagnosed. This type of diabetes is caused by insufficient insulin secretion (insulinopenia). Insulin injections are

necessary to maintain normal glucose metabolism. Individuals with type I diabetes are especially prone to ketoacidosis. *Ketoacidosis* refers to excessive formation of keto acids and low blood pH (acidosis). This condition is discussed on p. 593. Other complications of type I diabetes include cataracts, diseases of nerves (**neuropathy**), kidney disease (**nephropathy**), and blood vessel diseases (**angiopathy**).

Type II Diabetes

The occurrence of type II diabetes has no correlation with blood insulin levels. Type II diabetes accounts for 90% to 95% of the diagnosed cases of diabetes; onset is usually after 40 years of age. The type II individual is usually not dependent on insulin injection, is less prone to ketoacidosis, and is often obese.

Secondary Diabetes

Diabetes mellitus caused by other conditions and diseases is called *secondary diabetes*. Secondary diabetes can be caused by pancreatic disease, **acromegaly** (growth hormone excess), Cushing's syndrome (elevated cortisol), pheochromocytoma (excessive catecholamines), **glucagonoma** (excessive glucagon produced by a tumor), **somatostatinoma** (excessive somatostatin produced by a tumor), primary aldosteronism, severe liver disease, and administration of certain drugs, hormones, and chemicals.

Impaired Glucose Tolerance

Impaired glucose tolerance (IGT) includes persons who have had an abnormal glucose tolerance test but no frank hyperglycemia. The oral glucose test is discussed later in this chapter. Estimates of IGT prevalence range from 4.6% to 11.2%.[2]

Gestational Diabetes

Gestational diabetes refers to diabetes that occurs temporarily during pregnancy. Gestational diabetes occurs in 2% to 5% of pregnancies in the United States resulting in 135,000 cases annually.[13] One study[14] estimates that 39% of women with gestational diabetes manifest type II diabetes mellitus 20 years after delivery. Screening of pregnant women for gestational diabetes, to prevent perinatal complications associated with maternal hyperglycemia, has become a widespread, accepted practice. Gestational diabetes is derived from a woman's inability to secrete sufficient insulin to compensate for increased nutritional needs of pregnancy, the greater numbers of adipose cells during pregnancy, and the pregnancy-associated secretion of increased quantities of hyperglycemic hormones, including human placental lactogen, cortisol, prolactin, and progesterone. This results in a nearly fourfold increase in the need for insulin secretion. When this need for additional insulin is not totally met, hyperglycemia develops in a pregnant woman. Gestational diabetes is therefore similar to type II diabetes but probably has a different etiology.[15]

The increased rates of fetal and newborn complications associated with gestational diabetes (see later discussion, p. 595 and Chapter 40) have resulted in routine screening

TABLE 32-1 CLASSIFICATION OF DIABETES AND OTHER CATEGORIES OF GLUCOSE INTOLERANCE

Class	Description

Type I diabetes mellitus	Deficiency of insulin (insulinopenia)
	Dependence on injected insulin
	Usually occurs before 40 years of age
	Prone to ketoacidosis
	Prone to diabetic complications
	  Cataracts (six times greater than in nondiabetics)
	  Neuropathy (60% to 70% show mild to severe symptoms; 10% serious)
	  Nephropathy (40% to 50% develop renal failure)
	  Angiopathy (high risk for heart attack and stroke)

Type II diabetes mellitus	Variable levels of insulin Not dependent on exogenous insulin for control of hyperglycemia; often obese individuals Usually occurs after 40 years of age Not prone to ketoacidosis Not prone to diabetic complications
Secondary diabetes mellitus	Diabetes caused by various secondary conditions such as pancreatic disease, acromegaly, Cushing's syndrome, pheochromocytoma, glucagonoma, somatostatinoma, primary aldosteronism, severe liver disease, and certain drugs, chemicals, and hormones
Impaired glucose tolerance	Persons who exhibit in their oral glucose tolerance test a 2-hour value between 1400 mg/L and 2000 mg/L
Impaired fasting glucose	Persons exhibiting a fasting plasma glucose level between 1100 mg/L and 1260 mg/L fall into this new category[18]
Gestational diabetes mellitus	Diabetes that occurs during pregnancy
Statistical risk classes; previous abnormality of glucose tolerance	Previous transient hyperglycemia that occurred either spontaneously or in response to specific stimuli but presently testing normally
Potential abnormality of glucose tolerance	Persons not presently exhibiting any indications of diabetes but at substantially increased risk to develop diabetes in the future; includes monozygotic twin of a type II diabetic; person who has parent, sibling, or offspring who is type II diabetic; obese individuals; members of certain racial or ethnic groups with a high prevalence of diabetes

for this form of diabetes. Once detected, gestational diabetes is treated aggressively, with either insulin or hypoglycemic agents.

PATHOGENESIS OF DIABETES MELLITUS[16]
Epidemiology

Epidemiologists have studied identical twins and offspring and siblings of diabetics.[16,17] These studies demonstrate clearly that diabetes mellitus develops from a complex interaction between environmental and genetic factors. If the development of diabetes were determined by hereditary factors alone, the disease should always affect both identical twins. Three different studies show that when type I diabetes occurs in one twin its subsequent appearance in the other occurs only about 50% of the time. On the other hand, development of type II diabetes in one twin presages its appearance in the other nearly 100% of the time.

Studies of offspring of type II diabetic parents show that diabetes is transmitted to offspring at a frequency of only 6% to 10%. The prevalence of type II diabetes in the general American population is estimated at about 2%. However, a propensity to diabetes exists in the offspring because 25% to 40% of them have abnormal glucose tolerance test results.

Similar results have been obtained using siblings of diabetics.

The principal conclusions derived from these studies are as follows:

1. Offspring and siblings of diabetics are more likely to develop diabetes than are those of nondiabetics.
2. The offspring of two diabetics are more likely to develop diabetes than offspring having only one diabetic parent.
3. The lower-than-expected frequencies of diabetes in identical twins and offspring and siblings of diabetics are suggestive of the importance of environmental factors in the expression of the genetic component for diabetes.
4. A second event occurring early in life is postulated to trigger type I diabetes in genetically susceptible individuals. This event is likely to be a viral infection or a disturbance in the immune system. Type II diabetes occurs without such an event though its expression is modulated by factors such as obesity.
5. Diabetes is generally transmitted true to type. For example, diabetic siblings and offspring of type I diabetics are usually type I diabetics.
6. Inheritance plays a more important role in development of type II diabetes than type I diabetes.

Human Lymphocyte Antigens and Diabetes Mellitus

Inherited susceptibility or resistance to type I diabetes mellitus is supported by studies that associate the production of specific **human lymphocyte antigens** (HLAs) to the occurrence of the disease. HLAs are dimeric proteins produced by the major histocompatibility complex on chromosome 6. The *class II* HLA loci so far identified with susceptibility to type I diabetes are DP, DQ, and DR. HLAs DR3 or DR4, or both types, occur in 90% of type I diabetics. Resistance to type I diabetes is associated with DR2.[19] Recently it was determined that susceptibility to type I diabetes was greater when DR4 protein was produced in conjunction with a protein produced by the DQ locus, called DQw3.2.

The DQw3.2 allele has a gene frequency of 35.7% in type I diabetics as contrasted to 10.1% in nondiabetics. Individuals possessing the DQw3.1 allele are less likely to acquire type I diabetes than their DQw3.2 counterparts.[20] Susceptibility to type I diabetes is further increased when the DQ β-chain lacks aspartic acid at position 57 and has arginine present at position 52 of the DQ α-chain.[21]

The autoimmune cause for type I diabetes mellitus has been suggested by observations of progressive lymphocyte infiltration of the islet cells of the pancreas with concomitant β-cell destruction and the appearance of **islet cell antibodies (ICA)** before the manifestation of overt diabetes.

Markers for the autoimmune destruction of the β-cell include autoantibodies to glutamic acid decarboxylase, β-islet cells, insulin, and tyrosine phosphatases. At least one of these autoantibodies is present in 85% to 90% of persons diagnosed with diabetes.[22,23]

An inherited susceptibility or resistance to type II diabetes is complicated by the genetic heterogeneity of the disease. Attempts to identify type II diabetes genes have led to conflicting results in different populations.[24,25] Studies have shown that even within the same ethnic group, different genes may be involved in different families.[26]

Viruses

Viral infections have long been considered to be initiating factors in the autoimmune cause of type I diabetes. Epidemiological studies report a seasonal incidence for type I diabetes[17,27] and correlate the occurrence of viral infections such as mumps and measles with subsequent development of this type of diabetes.[28,29]

Further evidence for viral infection as a cause of type I diabetes comes from studies with coxsackievirus B4. Direct evidence that this virus causes diabetes in humans is derived from the isolation of coxsackievirus B4 from the pancreas of a child who had developed diabetic ketoacidosis shortly after the onset of a viral infection.[30] The child died of the disease, and autopsy showed extensive β-cell destruction. Injection of the virus into mice produced diabetes. Since the coxsackievirus B4 reports, mumps virus, coxsackievirus B1, and rubella reovirus type 3 have been implicated in the transmission of type I diabetes.[31]

Receptor Site Defects

Insulin receptor proteins. Insulin binds reversibly to sites on cell membranes. Insulin-binding sites (called *receptor sites*) are found only on certain cell types (monocytes, adipocytes, and muscle). The insulin receptor site is composed of two glycoprotein molecules.[32] One subunit is a tyrosine-specific protein kinase.[33] Insulin binding to the receptor site triggers a chain of events resulting in an increase of cell membrane permeability to glucose and amino acids, alteration of enzyme activities, and promotion of protein biosynthesis.

Insulin resistance. In type II diabetes, hyperglycemia is often associated with hyperinsulinemia. This is in strong contrast to type I diabetes, in which hyperglycemia is always associated with insulin *deficiency*. In fact, whereas type I diabetics depend on insulin to maintain normal blood glucose, type II diabetics respond to relatively high doses of insulin with only small reductions in circulating glucose levels. Type II diabetics are said to be *insulin resistant*, that is, although the cellular uptake of glucose does increase in response to a glucose load, it is low relative to both the blood glucose and insulin levels. Most patients exhibiting this type of diabetes are obese or have a preponderance of fat distributed in the abdominal area.[34]

Recent studies show that these diabetics range from those that are insulin resistant to those who have a defect of insulin secretion in addition to insulin resistance. In individuals with the insulin secretion–insulin resistant defect, insulin levels are normal or elevated but these individuals have a hyperglycemia that would be associated with even greater insulin levels if their insulin secretion was normal.[35] When these diabetics reduce their weight, insulin resistance improves but never returns to normal.[36] For years it was thought that the insulin resistance of type II diabetes was caused by a malfunction in the insulin receptor.[37] However, except for the rare mutation, a scarcity of functioning receptor sites has failed to have been proven as the principal cause of type II diabetic resistance to insulin.[38,39] The cause of type II diabetes remains a puzzle. One of the more promising theories implicates intracellular signaling pathways that involve two related proteins, IRS-1 and IRS-2, which are activated when the insulin receptor binds insulin.[40]

Antibodies to receptor. The presence of circulating antibodies to the insulin receptor has also been reported.[32] Type II diabetes caused by such antibodies to insulin receptor sites is called *type B diabetes*. Type B diabetics usually have symptoms of autoimmune disorders such as antinuclear antibodies, arthralgia, and enlargement of the parotid gland. Type B diabetes has a lower incidence than type A.

Impaired glucose transport. Glucose transport is reduced in both type I and type II diabetics because of significantly reduced levels of the high-K_m glucose transport protein, GluT-2.[41] The underlying defect appears to be an underexpression of the mRNA for GluT-2. The effect of this transport abnormality is a reduction in the insulin response to elevated glucose levels. This further aggravates the diabetic condition.

Summary

It is likely that type I diabetes mellitus is most commonly caused by destruction of islet cells resulting from an autoimmune response to viral infection, whereas type II diabetes is probably caused by a defect in a step that occurs after insulin binds to its receptor. Other causes of diabetes described in this section are probably rare (<10%).

COMPLICATIONS OF DIABETES MELLITUS[17,42]

The principal complications of diabetes mellitus are **retinopathy**, neuropathy, angiopathy, nephropathy, susceptibility to infection, hyperlipidemia, ketoacidosis, and **hyperglycemic hyperosmolar nonketotic coma (HHNC)**. With the single exception of HHNC, these diabetic complications occur more frequently for type I diabetics than for type II diabetics.

Retinopathy

Opaque areas in the lens of the eye are called *cataracts*. Cataract formation is the principal retinopathy of diabetes. Retinopathy is also caused by **angiogenesis**, a proliferation of small blood vessels in the lens. Diabetic retinopathy is the primary cause of blindness in people 20 to 74 years old.

Neuropathy[43]

Neuropathy is the most common complication of diabetes mellitus. It is apparent in about 60% to 70% of diabetics and is recognized by a variety of symptoms that include pain, numbness, tingling or burning sensations in extremities, dizziness, and double vision. Decreased motor and sensory nerve conduction velocities caused by axonal degeneration and demyelination cause these symptoms. Secondary manifestations of neuropathy include cardiac failure, excessive sweating, and male impotence.

Angiopathy

Angiopathy refers to damage to linings **(basement membranes)** of blood vessels. Angiopathy increases the risk of coronary heart disease and stroke and can lead to retinopathy and nephropathy.

Nephropathy

Nephropathy refers to damage to the glomerulus (filtering apparatus of the nephron) and capillaries associated with the glomerulus; this damage is associated with a reduction in the filtering capability of the kidneys (see Chapter 26). Capillary damage is caused by angiopathy, a common feature of diabetes. According to a study released in 1995 approximately 25% to 30% of individuals treated for end-stage renal failure are diabetics and approximately 27% of diabetics developed end-stage renal disease. Both the prevalence and incidence of end-stage renal disease are approximately twice the rates of the early 1990s and diabetic nephropathy accounts for most of the increase.[44]

Proteinuria is often the first sign of diabetic nephropathy. The Diabetes Control and Complications Trial convincingly demonstrated that maintaining a diabetic's blood glucose levels within or near the normal range reduced the risk of developing small quantities of protein in the urine by 35% and the risk of developing substantial quantities of protein in the urine by 56%.[45] Close control of blood glucose levels in combination with new treatment modalities may well make diabetic-associated nephropathy a preventable disease.

Infection

Diabetics are highly susceptible to infection, ulceration, and gangrene (especially in the extremities). Approximately half of lower limb amputations in the United States occur in diabetics. Skin disorders are also more common in diabetics than in nondiabetics.

Hyperlipidemia and Atherosclerosis

Abnormal triglyceride, cholesterol, and very-low-density lipoprotein (VLDL) levels are often associated with type II diabetes.[46,47] High-density lipoprotein (HDL) levels have been reported to be significantly lower in diabetics than in nondiabetics. These results are consistent with the high incidence and natural history of atherosclerotic coronary heart disease in diabetics and with the higher death rates from myocardial infarction in diabetics. These incidences are two to four times higher than those of persons without diabetes (see Chapter 33).[48]

Diabetic Ketoacidosis (DKA)

Keto acid metabolism. As shown in Fig. 32-9, acetyl coenzyme A (acetyl CoA) is at the crossroads of glucose, protein, and lipid metabolism. It either enters the tricarboxylic acid cycle or is metabolized to 3-hydroxy-3-methylglutaryl coenzyme A (HMG CoA). HMG CoA can be metabolized to cholesterol, or it can be converted to acetoacetate. Acetoacetate has two possible fates, spontaneous decarboxylation to acetone (in the lungs) or enzymatic reduction to β-hydroxybutyrate. Acetoacetate and β-hydroxybutyrate are commonly called keto acids, or ketone bodies. Keto acids are normally a source of energy for the brain, kidneys, and cardiac muscle. The kidneys excrete a considerable quantity of acetoacetate and β-hydroxybutyrate with concomitant loss of sodium and potassium. Kidney excretion of sodium and potassium results in the retention of hydrogen ions.

Keto acids and insulin. In nondiabetics keto acid formation is a minor pathway. In type I diabetics insulinopenia causes fat cells to mobilize fatty acids from triglycerides. Fatty acid degradation increases as it becomes the major source of energy for the cell. Increased fatty acid catabolism produces excessive quantities of acetyl CoA. Although a significant portion of the acetyl CoA is able to enter the tricarboxylic acid cycle to produce energy, an excess quantity of acetyl CoA is metabolized to produce abnormal levels of keto acids (ketosis). Increased production of keto acids consumes bicarbonate and thereby lowers blood pH (acidosis). This same metabolic pattern occurs in starvation except that hypoglycemia is present instead of hyperglycemia.

Diagnosis of ketoacidosis. Blood gas and blood glucose levels are useful in detecting **diabetic ketoacidosis**. Low pH, normal P_{CO_2}, low bicarbonate, high anion gap, and

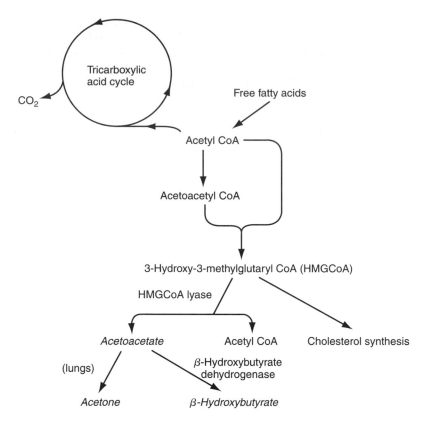

Fig. 32-9 Pathways involved in keto acid metabolism. Accumulation of keto acids, acetoacetate, and β-hydroxybutyrate is a principal feature of diabetic ketoacidosis. Metabolic pathway leading from acetyl-CoA to acetoacetate and β-hydroxybutyrate is accelerated in diabetes because of free fatty acid mobilization.

high glucose are suggestive of uncompensated ketoacidosis. Low pH, low P_{CO_2}, low bicarbonate, a high anion gap, and high glucose are suggestive of partially compensated diabetic ketoacidosis. The elevated anion gap is caused by the accumulation of keto acids (sodium salts).

Lactic acidosis. Lactic acidosis is caused by the accumulation of lactic acid resulting from tissue hypoxia (oxygen deficiency). Like the accumulation of keto acids, lactate accumulation causes increased blood hydrogen ions and therefore low pH. In the diabetic, lactic acidosis often occurs simultaneously with diabetic ketoacidosis, especially if the pH falls below 7.10, if renal insufficiency occurs, or if certain hypoglycemic agents such as phenformin (DBI) are administered.

Hyperglycemic Hyperosmolar Nonketotic Coma

Hyperglycemic hyperosmolar nonketotic coma (HHNC) has been reported with increasing frequency over the past few years. It is characterized by a blood glucose level above 6000 mg/L, normal or slightly low blood pH, serum osmolality above 350 mOsm/kg, normal keto acid levels, and lethargy or coma. Although diabetic ketoacidosis occurs primarily in type I diabetics, HHNC occurs primarily in type II diabetics. The absence of keto acids in HHNC is probably caused by the differential sensitivity of lipid and glucose metabolism to insulin. Lipolysis is inhibited by one tenth

the insulin level that is required to enhance glucose metabolism.[49] In type I diabetics, insulinopenia enhances lipolysis with resulting accumulation of keto acids and glucose utilization is blocked, resulting in hyperglycemia. In type II diabetics, although insulin resistance occurs, there is sufficient insulin activity to limit lipolysis and thus keto acid production but insufficient insulin activity to avoid hyperglycemia. HHNC is often brought on by stressful events and major illness.

Hypoglycemia

Hypoglycemia causes numerous neurogenic problems, ranging from mild to severe coma, seizures, and death. The level of blood glucose when symptoms become obvious varies but will tend to be less than 500 mg/L for adults and less than 400 mg/L for newborns. This potentially life-threatening disorder is most often the result of treatment of hyperglycemia with insulin, usually because of mismanagement. However, aggressive use of insulin treatment to maintain normoglycemia can greatly increase the risk of hypoglycemia.[50]

There are several other causes of hypoglycemia[51] that are listed in the box at the bottom of p. 595. Many of these are detected in emergency room cases as coma, treatable simply with intravenous glucose. Differential diagnosis may require measurement of blood glucose, insulin, and C-peptide. C-peptide is important in diagnosing surreptitious or overzealous insulin treatment because commercial insulin preparations contain no C-peptide.[52] In these cases, although blood insulin levels are elevated, C-peptide levels are low. Production of autoantibodies against insulin can also result in a similar pattern, though these cases are often associated with postprandial hyperglycemia.

The risk for hypoglycemia is increased for hospitalized patients. This risk is often unrelated to diabetes but is associated with advanced liver disease, renal insufficiency, and malnutrition. Such severely ill patients will have increased mortality.

Other Complications of Diabetes

The acutely ill diabetic, with ketoacidosis or hyperosmolar coma, is at risk for immediately life-threatening complications. The hypovolemia associated with these acute illnesses can result in shock and renal failure. Cerebral edema may arise in patients with ketoacidosis and hyperosmolar coma as a result of insulin and fluid administration. Loss of salts usually occurs in DKA and HHNC. Although patients' serum electrolytes may be elevated, normal, or low, they usually have a deficit of body potassium.

Effect of diabetes on the fetus (see also Chapter 40). The fetus of a pregnant diabetic is at increased risk for adverse complications directly resulting from hyperglycemia. These include spontaneous abortion, birth defects, macrosomia, hypoglycemia, hypocalcemia, polycythemia, and hyperbilirubinemia. A child who has been exposed to hyperglycemia *in utero* is at greater risk for the development of diabetes later in life.[53,54] Increased rates of cesarean section and hypertensive disorders have been reported as maternal complications. The risk for these complications is directly related to the degree of maternal hyperglycemia, and the greatest risk for intrauterine death or neonatal mortality occurs when the mother's glucose levels are greater than 1050 mg/L when fasting or greater than 1200 mg/L after a meal. The risk for perinatal morbidity and mortality is reduced to that which is seen in the general population when normal fasting and postprandial levels are maintained.

CAUSES OF FASTING HYPOGLYCEMIA

Depressed blood insulin/decreased glucose production
Liver disease
Alcoholism
Renal insufficiency
Galactosemia and glycogen storage disease
Malignancy (increases consumption of glucose or production of insulin-like growth factor)
Infection
Late pregnancy
Malnutrition
Overtreatment with insulin
   Insulinoma
   Factitious (exogenous) treatment with insulin
   Treatment with sulfonylurea drugs
   Antiinsulin antibodies

PATHOGENESIS OF DIABETIC COMPLICATIONS
Protein Glycation

Nonenzymatic protein **glycation** commonly occurs in red blood cells, glomeruli, nerve cells, and in other tissues. The extent of the glycation is proportional to extracellular glucose concentrations. Such glycation occurs by the mechanism shown for the glycation of hemoglobin (see Methods on CD-ROM). The carbonyl functional groups of glucose and other sugars react with free amino groups of proteins to form intermediates called *Schiff bases*, or *aldimines*. The amino group that reacts is either an N-terminal amino group or a lysine e-amino group. The aldimine subsequently rearranges to form a ketamine. This rearrangement is called the *Amadori rearrangement*. The aldimine is labile; it can readily hydrolyze to reform a free amino group and a carbonyl group. The ketamine is relatively stable, and its formation is not reversible.

Excessive glycation is known to produce significant alterations in a protein's physical and biochemical properties. For example, glycation of α-crystallin, a protein occurring in the lens of the eye, greatly reduces its solubility. Hyperglycemia in rats has been shown to increase α-crystallin glycation simultaneously with cataract formation.[55] Glycation of the basement membrane of blood vessels is known to cause basement membrane thickening similar to that found in most if not all diabetics.[56] Functional alterations of immunoglobulin G (IgG) by nonenzymatic glycation have been reported[57] to be associated with increased susceptibility to infection.

Based on these and other findings, a hypothesis has been proposed stating that many of the complications of diabetes are caused by glycation of specific proteins such as α-crystallin, IgG, and basement membrane protein, which impairs their function and results in disease such as diabetic nephropathy.[55-57]

Sorbitol Accumulation

The intracellular accumulation of sorbitol is the basis for another hypothesis designed to explain diabetic complications.[58] Aldose reductase reduces glucose to sorbitol, which in turn is oxidized to fructose by sorbitol dehydrogenase. Sorbitol does not easily cross cell membranes. The removal of sorbitol from the cell depends on its conversion to fructose, which does pass freely through the cell membrane. However, when glucose levels are high, the quantities of sorbitol produced outstrip the cell's ability to convert sorbitol to fructose, resulting in the intracellular accumulation of sorbitol. Intracellular accumulation of ketones, glucose, and sorbitol causes osmotic swelling and injury to cell structures. Only cells that do not depend on insulin for glucose transport across the plasma membrane are affected. These cells include nerve, ocular lens, and glomerulus cells. This osmotic effect is the cause of life-threatening cerebral edema that can occur during treatment for DKA and HHNC. The decreased blood osmolality after treatment can increase the shift of extracellular water into brain cells. Supporting this hypothesis are reports of elevations in sorbitol and fructose levels in the nerve and ocular lens cells of diabetics. The strongest support for this hypothesis is derived from studies using aldose reductase inhibitors. The aldose reductase inhibitors sorbinol and tolrestat are reported to improve nerve conduction in diabetic rats[59] and diabetic humans.

FUNCTION TESTS
Postprandial Plasma Glucose

Diabetes is more readily detected when the carbohydrate metabolic capacity is tested. This can be done by stressing the system with a defined glucose load. Measurement of the rate that the glucose load is cleared from the blood, as compared to the rate of glucose clearance in healthy persons, detects impairment in glucose metabolism. A meal high in carbohydrates is often used as the carbohydrate load, though a 75-g glucose drink is usually preferred over a meal. It is called the *postprandial test*. Two consecutive postprandial tests are recommended for diagnosis.

Blood is drawn at 2 hours after ingestion of the meal or glucose drink. Two postprandial tests with glucose levels of 2000 mg/L or higher at 2 hours are suggestive of diabetes.[60] The postprandial glucose test, though widely used for detection of diabetes, is highly inaccurate because of several variables that are difficult to control or adjust for. These variables include age, weight, previous diet, activity, illness, medications, time of day that the test is conducted, and actual size of the glucose dose. When a meal is used as the load, the effective glucose load depends on the digestion of disaccharides and polysaccharides and their subsequent absorption from the intestinal tract.

Oral Glucose Tolerance Test

The oral glucose tolerance test (OGTT) evaluates glucose clearance from the circulation after glucose loading under defined and controlled conditions. The Committee on Statistics of the American Diabetes Association has standardized the test.[61]

Standard conditions call for a minimum carbohydrate intake of 150 g/day for 3 days before the test. Daily carbohydrate intake less than this lowers carbohydrate intolerance. There should be an 8- to 16-hour fast before testing. The patient must be ambulatory, because inactivity decreases glucose tolerance. However, exercise and emotional stress should be avoided.

Illness reduces glucose tolerance. Abnormalities of such hormones as thyroxine, growth hormone, cortisol, and catecholamines interfere. Drugs and medications such as oral contraceptives, salicylates, nicotinic acid (found in cigarettes, cigars, pipe tobacco, chewing tobacco), diuretics (including caffeine), and hypoglycemic agents (insulin, sulfonylureas) interfere. Testing time affects the test. The best time to conduct the test is between 7 AM and noon. Evaluation criteria should also be adjusted for age. If adjustments for age are not made, about 80% of persons over 60 years of age will be judged diabetic.[62]

The glucose load should consist of glucose only. Some commercial preparations labeled "100 grams glucose equivalent" contain disaccharides and polysaccharides. The rate that these saccharides are hydrolyzed and absorbed from the intestinal tract varies from person to person. Such a preparation is obviously not desirable for individuals with pancreatic or malabsorptive disorders. The size of the load is 40 g of glucose per square meter of body area. For most subjects 75 g of total glucose is sufficient. The drink can be flavored if caffeine or theophylline is not used.

In accordance with the World Health Organization (WHO) recommendations, a blood glucose measurement should be made 2 hours[63] after a 75-g glucose challenge is given. A glucose value of greater than or equal to 2000 mg/L is suggestive of diabetes mellitus. This value is supported by evidence from several studies (Pima Indians in the United States, Egyptian study, Third National Health and Nutrition Examination Survey in the United States [NHANES III]) that diabetic complications such as retinopathy and nephropathy increase significantly beyond this glucose level. In addition the Paris Prospective Study demonstrated that the incidence of fatal coronary heart disease increased dramatically as the 2-hour plasma glucose value increased above 1400 mg/L.

The shape of the glucose tolerance curve is useful in evaluating the OGTT (Fig. 32-8). Healthy subjects peak at $\frac{1}{2}$ hour and return to fasting levels at 2 hours. Diabetics peak late (approximately 1 hour) or even show a plateau at 2 to 3 hours and return to baseline value after 3 hours. Insulin determinations performed along with glucose determinations are useful in evaluating the OGTT. Plasma insulin levels after a glucose load differentiate type I from type II diabetes. In nondiabetics, insulin levels peak 1 hour after a glucose load and return to fasting levels at 2 to 3 hours. Type I diabetics respond to a glucose load with little or no insulin increases above fasting levels. Type II diabetics respond to the challenge with an abnormally late and often excessive increase in insulin levels. Type I diabetics often have low fasting insulin levels. Type II diabetics have variable fasting insulin levels.

The OGTT has been criticized[64,65] because many of the variables affecting test results are difficult to control and the reproducibility of the test is poor. In fact, the OGTT is used rather infrequently.[66] The American Diabetes Association recommends a fasting plasma glucose level rather than the OGTT to detect diabetes mellitus. This has brought some criticism from some investigators[67,68] who have identified a sizable number of patients who test below the 1260 mg/L cutoff for fasting plasma glucose levels but who are diabetic by OGTT criteria. The consensus opinion is that the OGTT is best used to assess individuals who have borderline fasting glucose levels or who are at risk for the development of diabetes and to distinguish (in concert with insulin levels) type I from type II diabetes.

O'Sullivan-Mahan Glucose Challenge Test and Carpenter-Coustan OGTT for Gestational Diabetes

The O'Sullivan-Mahan glucose challenge test is frequently used to detect gestational diabetes. A 50-g load of glucose is given to a fasting patient and a blood glucose measurement is made 1 hour after dosage. A plasma glucose level above 1400 mg/L suggests gestational diabetes and a full oral glucose tolerance test is recommended for such patients.[69,70]

In 1982 Carpenter and Coustan proposed a 75-g, 2-hour OGTT for the detection of gestational diabetes.[71] The American Diabetes Association supported this alternative approach for the detection of gestational diabetes in a workshop conducted in March 1997. The new criteria[72] for the detection of gestational diabetes as proposed at that workshop are summarized as follows:

1. Women with the following characteristics need not be screened for gestational diabetes: those who are younger than 25 years of age, with normal body weight, no family occurrence of diabetes, no history of abnormal glucose tolerance, no history of poor obstetric outcome, and not of an ethnic or racial group with a high prevalence of diabetes (Hispanic, Native American, Asian, African, and Pacific Islander).
2. Women who do not fulfill all of the above criteria should be tested as soon as possible after pregnancy has been detected.
3. If glucose tolerance is found to be normal, women should be retested between 24 and 28 weeks of gestation.
4. The test should consist of a fasting plasma blood glucose or a random plasma blood glucose.
5. A fasting value of greater than 1260 mg/L or a random value of greater than 2000 mg/L suggests gestational diabetes, if subsequently confirmed.
6. If the fasting or random plasma blood glucose is normal the follow-up testing should consist of the O'Sullivan-Mahan glucose challenge or the O'Sullivan-Mahan glucose challenge (as modified by Carpenter-Coustan) or the Carpenter-Coustan OGTT.
   a. O'Sullivan-Mahan test procedure and criteria are reported earlier.
   b. O'Sullivan-Mahan test (as modified by Carpenter-Coustan) is an OGTT that uses a 100-g glucose load. Cut-off criteria for a normal response to this test are: fasting 950 mg/L, 1-hour 1800 mg/L, 2-hour 1550 mg/L, 3-hour 1400 mg/L.
   c. Carpenter-Coustan OGTT uses a 75-g glucose load. Criteria for this test are: fasting 950 mg/L, 1-hour 1800 mg/L, 2-hour 1550 mg/L.
   d. For b and c two or more of the plasma glucose values must be equaled or exceeded for a diagnosis of gestational diabetes. The test is done in the morning after a fast of 8 to 14 hours and after 3 days of unrestricted diet (greater than 150 g of carbohydrate/day) and unlimited physical activity. During the test the patient should remain seated and should not smoke.

There are two protocols recommended by the Expert Committee on the Diagnosis and Classification of Diabetes Mellitus for testing for gestational diabetes. In the one-step approach an OGTT is the initial action. In the two-step approach initial screening is performed using the O'Sullivan-Mahan glucose challenge. For those women who test abnormally in the first step a second step consisting of a diagnostic OGTT (either O'Sullivan-Mahan glucose challenge as modified by Carpenter-Coustan or the Carpenter-Cousin OGTT) is recommended to confirm the diagnosis.

Intravenous Glucose Tolerance Test

The intravenous glucose tolerance test is often used for persons with malabsorptive disorders or previous gastric or intestinal surgery. Glucose is administered intravenously over 30 minutes, using a 20% solution. A glucose load of 0.5 g/kg of body weight is used. Nondiabetics respond with a plasma glucose level of 2000 to 2500 mg/L. Discontinuation of the glucose loading leads to a decrease in plasma glucose levels with fasting levels reached at about 90 minutes. Diabetics demonstrate plasma glucose levels above 2500 mg/L during administration of the load. On discontinuation of the loading, plasma glucose levels of diabetics also return to fasting levels at about 90 minutes. An alternative procedure called the Soskin method uses 50% glucose delivered intravenously within 3 to 5 minutes. The glucose load used is 0.3 g/kg of body weight. Nondiabetics reestablish fasting levels less than 60 minutes after discontinuing the glucose infusion. In diabetics fasting levels are reestablished significantly later than 60 minutes.

CHANGE OF ANALYTE IN DISEASE

The following is a summary of analyte changes in diabetes mellitus. For each analyte, levels in controlled diabetes, diabetic ketoacidosis, and HHNC are compared.

Fasting Plasma Glucose

Fasting plasma glucose and urinary glucose levels are the most commonly used markers for diabetes mellitus. In general, repeated fasting plasma glucose levels of greater than 1260 mg/L are strongly suggestive of diabetes, provided that drugs such as glucocorticoids are not being administered and diseases and conditions such as those listed in the box are not present. Values from 1100 to 1260 mg/L are suggestive of impaired fasting glucose.

Fasting plasma glucose is directly proportional to the severity of diabetes mellitus. As with the OGTT, results greater than the upper range of normal (1260 mg/L), coincide with a dramatic increase in the incidence of retinopathy, nephropathy, and fatal coronary heart disease.[73] Blood glucose levels above 1800 mg/L may produce glucosuria. Ketoacidosis can occur at almost any level above 1400 mg/L but is more common at levels above 1800 mg/L. HHNC is associated with glucose levels above 6000 mg/L.

Diabetics who are under control exhibit wide variations in their plasma glucose concentrations. Plasma glucose levels in controlled diabetics range during a typical 24-hour period from as low as 250 mg/L to as high as 3250 mg/L. These variations are considerably wider than those of nondiabetics.[74] Wide swings in plasma glucose contribute to the development of diabetic complications. Management of insulin therapy remains a significant challenge for the physician. Excessive quantities of insulin cause insulin-induced

Conditions and Diseases that Often Cause Both Hyperglycemia and Glucosuria or Glycosuria in the Absence of Hyperglycemia

Hyperglycemia and Glucosuria
Septicemia
Hypercortisolism
Pancreatic cancer
Glucagonoma
Acute pancreatitis
Somatostatinoma
Pheochromocytoma
Primary aldosteronism
Hyperthyroidism
Acute myocardial infarction
Acromegaly
Cerebral hemorrhage

Glucosuria and Normal Plasma Glucose
Pregnancy (renal threshold is reduced)
Vitamin D–resistant rickets
Osteomalacia (proximal tubular malfunction)
Hepatolenticular degeneration

hypoglycemia, which often leads to coma. On the other hand, inadequate control of glucose levels causes diabetic complications such as those described earlier. Generally, fasting plasma glucose in diabetics is maintained at normal or slightly above normal concentrations.

Urinary Glucose

Urinary glucose is a poor marker for diabetes mellitus. The normal renal threshold for glucose is 1800 mg/L. Blood glucose levels must exceed this value before excessive glucose is apparent in the urine. Further complicating this picture is the fact that the renal threshold in diabetics is often increased to above 3000 mg/L. Some diseases and conditions that produce both hyperglycemia and glucosuria are listed in the box above. This box also lists conditions that cause glucosuria in the absence of hyperglycemia.

Self-Monitoring and Bedside Monitoring of Blood Glucose

The goal of therapy for diabetics is to maintain normal levels of glucose so as to minimize the acute and long-term complications of the disease. Aggressive therapy to achieve this goal has the primary side effect of an increased risk for hypoglycemia (see earlier discussion). However, close monitoring of blood glucose levels has been aided by the development of increasingly accurate and reliable bedside glucose monitors (see Chapter 17). In a consensus statement on blood glucose monitoring, many insulin-treated populations have been recommended for self-monitoring programs.[75] These include pregnant women; patients with unstable diabetes; patients with histories of severe ketosis or hypoglycemia, especially those who do not demonstrate warning

symptoms of hypoglycemia; patients receiving intensive insulin therapy; and patients with abnormal renal thresholds for glucose.

The consensus panel also had important recommendations on the blood-glucose monitoring devices that are widely employed in hospitals for bedside monitoring and control of blood glucose levels. The correct use of such devices should minimize the wide variations of blood glucose experienced by diabetics and, as a result, the hypoglycemic events and even the long-term complications of diabetes.

Glycated Hemoglobin and Plasma Albumin

A minor hemoglobin derivative called $Hb\ A_{1c}$ is produced by glycation, the covalent binding of glucose to hemoglobin. Because this reaction is nonenzymatic and because the red cell is completely permeable to glucose, the quantity of $Hb\ A_{1c}$ formed is directly proportional to the average plasma glucose concentration that the red blood cell is exposed to during its 120-day life span, that is, the 4 to 6 weeks before sampling. Thus, in long-term hyperglycemia, $Hb\ A_{1c}$ constitutes a higher percentage of total hemoglobin than in normoglycemia. Transient elevations in plasma glucose only mildly affect $Hb\ A_{1c}$ levels.

$Hb\ A_1$ actually consists of four principal components, called $Hb\ A_{1a1}$, $Hb\ A_{1a2}$, $Hb\ A_{1b}$, and $Hb\ A_{1c}$.[76] As seen in Table 32-2, each consists of two components, a labile component, which is actually the aldimine, and a stable component, which is actually the ketamine. For normoglycemic persons, $Hb\ A_{1a1}$, $Hb\ A_{1a2}$, and $Hb\ A_{1b}$ constitute 0.4% to 0.8% of the total hemoglobin. $Hb\ A_{1c}$ constitutes 4% to 5% of total hemoglobin. Total $Hb\ A_1$ is normally 5.0% to 7.0% (see Methods on CD-ROM). As shown in Table 32-2, diabetics have total $Hb\ A_1$ and $Hb\ A_{1c}$ percentages that are significantly elevated. The elevations are directly proportional to the long-term degree of hyperglycemia.[77]

The Report of the Expert Committee on the Diagnosis and Classification of Diabetes Mellitus[78] noted that differing assay methods[79] and reference intervals among laboratories make it difficult to establish a standard upper range of healthy for glycated hemoglobin. To allow physicians to more readily follow the Diabetes Control and Complications Trial (DCCT) guidelines for monitoring glycated hemoglobin, most laboratories now employ procedures that use a common standard, can achieve a high degree of reproducibility, and can report results, either directly measured or calculated, as $Hb\ A_{1c}$.

The DCCT[80] demonstrated that patients with type I diabetes reduced their risk of development or progression of retinopathy, nephropathy, and neuropathy by 50% to 70% by maintaining their average $Hb\ A_{1c}$ at 7.2% as compared to diabetics who maintained their values at an average of 9.0%. In addition, the reduction of the risk for these complications progressively decreased with decreased levels of $Hb\ A_{1c}$, suggesting that if normal $Hb\ A_{1c}$ were achieved, risk of complications would approach that of the nondiabetic population with a reference interval of 4.0% to 6.0%. When $Hb\ A_{1c}$ levels are kept below 8% the risk of developing an

TABLE 32-2   Comparison of Four Criteria for Evaluation of Oral Glucose Tolerance Test

Time of Blood Drawing (Hours)	PLASMA GLUCOSE LEVELS (mg/L)			
	Wilkerson Point System	Fajans-Conn System	WHO	UGDP
Fasting	>1290 (1)*	—	>1390	Sum
1	>1940 (½)*	>1840	—	Sum
1½	—	>1640	—	—
2	>1390 (½)*	>1390	1400–2000 (IGT)	Sum
			>2000 (diabetes)	
3	>1290 (½)*	—	—	Sum

UGDP, *University Group Diabetes Program;* WHO, *World Health Organization.*
Points given in Wilkerson Point system.

early sign of diabetic nephropathy, microalbuminuria (see later discussion), is greatly reduced.[81] Although measurements of glycosylated hemoglobins are recommended for the monitoring of diabetes, they are not sufficiently sensitive to effectively detect borderline cases of diabetes mellitus.[82] The American Diabetes Association recommends fasting plasma glucose of 1260 mg/L and Hb A_{1c} of less than 7% as goals for treatment.[83]

As stated earlier, serum albumin is also glucosylated to a degree proportional to plasma glucose levels. The relatively short half-life for albumin of 15 days makes it a good monitor of short-term blood plasma glucose levels.[84]

Insulin

Fasting plasma insulin levels in type I diabetics are usually low. Those of type II diabetics are low only when fasting plasma glucose levels exceed 2500 mg/L. Otherwise, they are normal.[85] A glucose challenge separates type I diabetics from type II diabetics. Glucose loading elicits no significant insulin response for type I diabetics and a delayed, often exaggerated response in type II diabetics.

Keto Acids

Significant elevations of acetoacetate and β-hydroxybutyrate cause diabetic ketoacidosis. It is important to measure both blood and urinary keto acid levels, because plasma keto acid levels can be normal even though urinary keto acid concentrations are high. This effect is caused by increased urinary keto acid excretion resulting from renal compensation to low pH. Both ketonemia and ketonuria are absent in HHNC. Controlled diabetics should have both normal plasma and normal urinary keto acid levels.

The nitroprusside test (commonly known as Acetest) is useful for the detection of acetoacetic acid (AcAc) in the blood or urine. Nitroprusside does not react with β-hydroxybutyrate (β-HBA) and reacts only weakly (20%) with acetone. In the early stages of diabetic ketoacidosis, acetoacetate levels are often normal (AcAc:β-HBA, 1:3) or only mildly elevated. In later stages of ketoacidosis β-hydroxybutyrate levels are highly elevated (AcAc:β-HBA, 1:30). Under these conditions the nitroprusside test can signi-

ficantly produce an underestimate of the severity of the ketoacidosis. As the ketoacidosis becomes controlled, the β-hydroxybutyrate is metabolized to acetoacetic acid, and the nitroprusside test can become strongly positive.

Urinary Protein

One of the earliest signs of impending glomerular nephropathy is the increased excretion of albumin in the urine, also termed *microalbuminuria*. It has been recommended[86,87] that diabetics be routinely monitored for microalbuminuria (see p. 485), so this complication of diabetes can be treated early and prevented. The determination of the urine albumin/creatinine ratio on a random urine sample is an effective screening test.[88] An albumin/creatinine ratio that is equal to or greater than 20 to 30 mg/g suggests microalbuminuria.[89]

Lactic Acid

Plasma lactic acid levels are frequently elevated (lactic acidosis) during DKA.

Hydrogen Ion (pH)

High plasma hydrogen-ion concentrations (low pH) occur in DKA, ketoacidosis with lactic acidosis, and HHNC. A pH level below 7.00 is associated with a poor prognosis.

Electrolytes

Uncontrolled diabetics can exhibit normal, low, or high plasma sodium levels. Plasma sodium levels in diabetics are influenced by three factors, described next.

Hyperglycemia causes an increase in the osmotic pressure of plasma. As a result water flows from cells to plasma. Plasma substituents are thereby diluted. Thus hyponatremia (low plasma sodium) is common in diabetes. In diabetic ketoacidosis excessive quantities of sodium are excreted in the urine, further lowering plasma sodium levels. However, complicating matters is the preferential excretion of water relative to sodium. This effect often compensates for sodium loss from high plasma glucose levels and ketosis, thus resulting in normal or even elevated plasma sodium levels.

The same factors described above affect plasma potassium levels. However, for potassium, two additional factors are operative. First, insulin causes the transport of intracellular potassium to the plasma. Thus hypokalemia (low plasma potassium) occurs in insulin deficiency (type I diabetes). Second, in acidosis, potassium moves out of cells. Thus, in DKA, significant quantities of potassium ion are shifted from cells to plasma. This produces hyperkalemia (high plasma potassium). Type II diabetics normally exhibit hypokalemia or normokalemia. However, because of urinary losses of potassium, diabetics in DKA always require potassium replacement and monitoring during therapy.

Plasma bicarbonate levels are normal in controlled diabetes. Ketoacidosis causes low plasma bicarbonate levels. The body responds to ketoacidosis by kidney retention of bicarbonate and rapid, deep respiration called *Kussmaul breathing*, which removes CO_2. Both of these compensatory mechanisms raise pH. Kussmaul breathing lowers the P_{CO_2}. Both plasma bicarbonate and P_{CO_2} are low in DKA.

Osmolality

Serum osmolality is increased in both ketoacidosis and HHNC because of the water loss that accompanies glucose excretion. Serum osmolality in HHNC is usually above 350 mOsm/kg, a hallmark of the condition.

Body Fluid Volume

Renal loss of water in DKA produces severe volume depletion, often as much as 6 to 8 L. Patients with HHNC can have fluid deficits greater than 9 L. Low fluid volume (hypovolemia) often coexists with hyponatremia. Insulin therapy restores both fluid volume and plasma sodium to normal.

Anion Gap

In ketoacidosis the anion gap is always increased because of the excessive formation of keto acids. Lactic acidosis further increases the gap because of the high lactate levels.

Blood Urea Nitrogen (BUN)

BUN levels are increased in both DKA and HHNC because of increased protein catabolism and prerenal azotemia secondary to loss of extracellular fluids. Prerenal azotemia refers to increased BUN caused by decreased renal flow. In DKA, prerenal azotemia is caused by hypovolemia.

Lipids

Elevated plasma triglyceride, cholesterol, and VLDL are commonly found in diabetics. On the other hand, HDL-cholesterol levels are usually low.

References

1. Harris MI et al: Prevalence of diabetes, impaired fasting glucose, and impaired glucose tolerance in U.S. adults, *Diabetes Care* 21:518, 1998.
2. American Diabetes Association: Economic consequences of diabetes mellitus in the U.S. in 1997, *Diabetes Care* 21:296, 1998.
3. Smith JW et al: Prognosis of patients with diabetes mellitus after myocardial infarction, *Am J Cardiol* 54:719, 1984.
4. Oppenheimer SM et al: Diabetes mellitus and early mortality from stroke, *Br Med J* 291:1014, 1985.
5. Mueckler M et al: Sequence and structure of a human glucose transporter, *Science* 229:941, 1985.
6. Froguel P et al: Familial hyperglycemia due to mutations in glucokinase, *N Engl J Med* 328:697, 1993.
7. Cryer PE, Gerich JE: Glucose counterregulation, hypoglycemia, and intensive insulin therapy in diabetes mellitus, *N Engl J Med* 131:232, 1985.
8. Chan SJ, Keim P, Steiner DF: Cell-free synthesis of rat preproinsulin: characterization and partial amino acid sequence determination, *Proc Natl Acad Sci USA* 73:1964, 1976.
9. Unger RH, Orci L: Glucagon and the A cell, *N Engl J Med* 304:1518, 1981.
10. Hartmann H et al: Inhibition of glycogenolysis and glycogen phosphorylase by insulin and proinsulin in rat hepatocyte cultures, *Diabetes* 36:551, 1987.
11. Dinneen S, Gerich J, Rizza R: Carbohydrate metabolism in non–insulin-dependent diabetes mellitus, *N Engl J Med* 327:707, 1992.
12. National Diabetes Data Group: Classification and diagnosis of diabetes mellitus and other categories of glucose intolerance, *Diabetes* 28:1039, 1979.
13. Engelgau MM et al: The epidemiology of diabetes and pregnancy in the U.S., *Diabetes Care* 18:1029, 1995.
14. O'Sullivan JB, Worshop Y: Subsequent morbidity among gestational diabetes women. In Sutherland HW, Stowers M, editors: *Carbohydrate metabolism in pregnancy and the newborn*, Edinburgh, UK, 1984, Churchill Livingstone.
15. American Diabetes Association: Clinical practice recommendations. Gestational diabetes mellitus; Position Statement, *Diabetes Care* 21(suppl 1):S60, 1998.
16. Atkinson MA, Maclaren NK: The pathogenesis of insulin-dependent diabetes mellitus, *N Engl J Med* 331:1428, 1994.
17. Krolewski AS et al: Epidemiologic approach to the etiology of type I diabetes mellitus and its complications, *N Engl J Med* 317:1390, 1987.
18. Charles MA et al: Risk factors for NIDDM in white population: Paris Prospective Study, *Diabetes* 40:796, 1991.
19. Tiwari JL, Terasaki PI: *HLA and disease*, New York, 1985, Springer-Verlag.
20. Baisch JM et al: Analysis of HLA-DQ genotypes and susceptibility in insulin-dependent diabetes mellitus, *N Engl J Med* 322:1836, 1990.
21. Khalil I et al: A combination of HLA DQ beta Asp 57-negative and HLA DQ alpha Arg 52 confers susceptibility to insulin-dependent diabetes mellitus, *J Clin Invest* 85:1315, 1990.
22. Hagopian WA et al: Glutamate decarboxylase-, insulin- and islet cell-antibodies and HLA typing to detect diabetes in a general population-based study of Swedish children, *J Clin Invest* 95:1505, 1995.
23. The Expert Committee on the Diagnosis and Classification of Diabetes Mellitus: Report of the Expert Committee on the Diagnosis and Classification of Diabetes Mellitus. In American Diabetes Association: Clinical practice recommendations 2001, *Diabetes Care* 24(suppl 1): S5, 2001.
24. Hanis CL et al: A genome-wide search non–insulin-dependent diabetes gene reveals a major susceptibility locus on chromosome 2, *Nat Genet* 13:161, 1996.
25. Horikawa Y et al: Genetic variation in the gene encoding calpain-10 is associated with diabetes mellitus, *Nat Genet* 26:163, 2000.
26. Mahtani MM et al: Mapping of a gene for diabetes associated with an insulin secretion defect by a genome scan in Finnish families, *Nat Genet* 14:90, 1996.
27. Gamble DR, Taylor KW: Seasonal incidence of diabetes mellitus, *Br Med J* 3:631, 1969.
28. Hinden E: Mumps followed by diabetes, *Lancet* 1:1381, 1962.
29. Johnson GM, Tudor RB: Diabetes mellitus and congenital rubella infection, *Am J Dis Child* 120:453, 1970.
30. Yoon JW et al: Virus induced diabetes mellitus. XI. Replication of Coxsackie B3 in human pancreatic beta cell cultures, *Diabetes* 27:778, 1978.
31. Craighead JE: Does insulin dependent diabetes mellitus have a viral etiology? *Hum Pathol* 10:267, 1979.

32. Kasuga M et al: Autoantibodies against the insulin receptor recognize the insulin binding subunits of an oligomeric receptor, *Diabetes* 30:354, 1981.

33. Roth RA, Cassell DJ: Insulin receptor: evidence that it is a protein kinase, *Science* 219:299, 1983.

34. Kissebah AH et al: Relationship of body fat distribution to metabolic complications of obesity, *J Clin Endocrinol Metab* 54:254, 1982.

35. Polonsky KS, Sturis J, Bell GI: Non–insulin-dependent diabetes mellitus: a genetically programmed failure of the beta cell to compensate for insulin resistance, *N Engl J Med* 334:777, 1996.

36. Wing RR et al: Caloric restriction per se is a significant factor in improvements in glycemic control and insulin sensitivity during weight loss in obese NIDDM patients, *Diabetes Care* 17:30, 1994.

37. Moller DE, Flier JS: Insulin resistance-mechanisms, syndromes, and implications, *N Engl J Med* 325:938, 1991.

38. Alper J: New insights into diabetes, *Science* 289:37, 2000.

39. Withers DJ, White M: Perspective: the insulin signaling system—a common link in the pathogenesis of diabetes, *Endocrinology* 141:1917, 2000.

40. Kido Y et al: Tissue-specific insulin resistance in mice with mutations in the insulin receptor, IRS-1, and IRS-2, *J Clin Invest* 105:199, 2000.

41. Shepard PR, Kahn BB: Glucose transporters and insulin action. Implications for insulin resistance and diabetes mellitus, *N Engl J Med* 341:248, 1999.

42. Nathan DM: Long-term complications of diabetes mellitus, *N Engl J Med* 328:1676, 1993.

43. Understanding diabetic neuropathy, *Lancet* 338:1496, 1991 (editorial).

44. U.S. Renal Data System: *USRDS 2001. Annual data report: atlas of end-stage renal disease in the United States*, Bethesda, MD, 2001, National Institutes of Diabetes and Digestive and Kidney Disease.

45. The Diabetes Control and Complications Trial Research Group: The effect of intensive diabetes therapy on the development and progression of nephropathy, *Kidney Int* 47:1703, 1995.

46. O'Brien T, Nguyen TT, Zimmerman BR: Hyperlipidemia and diabetes mellitus, *Mayo Clin Proc* 73:969, 1998.

47. Betteridge DJ: Diabetic dyslipidemia, *Diabetes Obes Metab* 2(suppl 1):S31, 2000.

48. Krolewski AS et al: Evolving natural history of coronary artery disease in diabetes mellitus, *Amer J Med* 90(suppl 2A):2A, 1991.

49. Zierler KL, Rabinowitz D: Effect of very small concentrations of insulin on forearm metabolism: persistence of its action on potassium and free fatty acids without its effect on glucose, *J Clin Invest* 43:950, 1964.

50. The DCCT Research Group: Epidemiology of severe hypoglycemia in the Diabetes Control and Complications Trial, *Am J Med* 90:450, 1991.

51. Polonsky KS: A practical approach to fasting hypoglycemia, *N Engl J Med* 326:1020, 1992 (editorial).

52. Fischer KF, Lees JH, Newman JH: Hypoglycemia in hospitalized patients, *N Engl J Med* 315:1245, 1986.

53. Jovanoic J: The diabetic pregnancy: a clinical challenge. Symposium of the Diabetes and Pregnancy Council: 60th Scientific Sessions of the American Diabetes Association, Day 2, June 11, 2000.

54. American Diabetes Association: Clinical practice recommendations. Gestational diabetes mellitus: Position Statement, *Diabetes Care* 21(suppl 1):S60, 1998.

55. Cerami A, Stevens VJ, Monnier VM: Role of nonenzymatic glycosylation in the development of the sequelae of diabetes mellitus, *Metabolism* 28:431, 1979.

56. Makita Z et al: Advanced glycosylation end products in patients with diabetic nephropathy, *N Engl J Med* 325:836, 1991.

57. Kaneshige H: Nonenzymatic glycosylation of serum IgG and its effect on antibody activity in patients with diabetes mellitus, *Diabetes* 36:822, 1987.

58. Gabbay KH: The sorbitol pathway and the complication of diabetes, *N Engl J Med* 288:831, 1973.

59. Notvest RR, Inserra JJ: Tolrestat, an aldose reductase inhibitor, prevents nerve dysfunction in conscious diabetic rats, *Diabetes* 36:500, 1987.

60. Report of the Expert Committee on the Diagnosis and Classification of Diabetes Mellitus, *Diabetes Care* 20:1183, 1997.

61. Report on the Committee on Statistics of the American Diabetes Association: Standardization of the oral glucose tolerance test, *Diabetes* 18:299, 1969.

62. Davidson MB: The effect of aging on carbohydrate metabolism: a review of the English literature and a practical approach to the diagnosis of diabetes mellitus in the elderly, *Metabolism* 28:688, 1979.

63. Harris MI et al: International criteria for the diagnosis of diabetes and impaired glucose tolerance, *Diabetes Care* 8:562, 1985.

64. Sherwin RS: Limitations of the oral glucose tolerance test in diagnosis of early diabetes, *Primary Care* 4:255, 1977.

65. Nelson RL: Subspecialty clinics: endocrinology: oral glucose tolerance test: indications and limitations, *Mayo Clin Proc* 63:263, 1988.

66. Stolk RP, Orchard TJ, Grobbee DE: Why use the oral glucose tolerance test? *Diabetes Care* 18:1045, 1995.

67. The DECODE Study Group on behalf of the European Diabetes Epidemiology Group: Is fasting glucose sufficient to define diabetes? Epidemiological data from 20 European studies, *Diabetologia* 42:647, 1999.

68. Shaw JE et al: Impact of new diagnostic criteria for diabetes on different populations, *Diabetes Care* 22:762, 1999.

69. American Diabetes Association: Report of the Expert Committee on the Diagnosis and Classification of Diabetes Mellitus, *Diabetes Care* 21(suppl 1):S5, 1998.

70. Metzger BE, editor: Proceedings of the Third International Workshop-Conference on Gestational Diabetes Mellitus, *Diabetes* 40(suppl 2):1, 1991.

71. Carpenter MW, Coustan DR: Criteria for screening tests for gestational diabetes, *Am J Obstet Gynecol* 144:768, 1982.

72. Metzger BE, Coustan DR: Summary and recommendations of the Fourth International Workshop-Conference on Gestational Diabetes Mellitus, *Diabetes Care* 21(suppl 2):B161, 1998.

73. Report of the Expert Committee on the Diagnosis and Classification of Diabetes Mellitus, *Diabetes Care* 20:1183, 1997.

74. Mauer AC: The therapy of diabetes, *Am Scientist* 67:422, 1979.

75. Consensus Development Panel: Consensus statement on self-monitoring of blood glucose, *Diabetes Care* 10:95, 1987.

76. Gonen B, Rochman H, Rubenstein AH: Metabolic control in diabetic patients: assessment by hemoglobin A1 values, *Metabolism* 28:448, 1979.

77. Larsen ML, Horder MN, Mogensen EF: Effect of long-term monitoring of glycosylated hemoglobin levels in insulin diabetes mellitus, *N Engl J Med* 323:1021, 1990.

78. Report of the Expert Committee on the Diagnosis and Classification of Diabetes Mellitus, *Diabetes Care* 20:1183, 1997.

79. Bry L, Chen PC, Sachs DB: Effect of hemoglobin variants and chemically modified derivatives on assays for glycohemoglobin, *Clin Chem* 47:153, 2001.

80. American Diabetes Association: Position statement: standards of medical care for patients with diabetes mellitus, *Diabetes Care* 21:S23, 1998.

81. Krolewski AS et al: Glycosylated hemoglobin and the risk of developing microalbuminuria in patients with insulin-dependent diabetes mellitus, *N Engl J Med* 332:1251, 1995.

82. Dods RF, Bolmey C: Glycosylated hemoglobin assay and oral glucose tolerance test compared for detection of diabetes mellitus, *Clin Chem* 25:764, 1979.

83. American Diabetes Association: Position statement: standards of medical care for patients with diabetes mellitus, *Diabetes Care* 24(suppl 1):S33, 2001.

84. Guthrow CE et al: Enhanced nonenzymatic glucosylation of serum albumin in diabetes mellitus, *Proc Natl Acad Sci USA* 76:4528, 1979.

85. Ward WK et al: Pathophysiology of insulin secretion in non–insulin-dependent diabetes mellitus, *Diabetes Care* 7:491, 1984.

86. Hawthorne V, Herman WH, editors: International symposium on preventing the kidney disease of diabetes mellitus: public health perspectives, *Am J Kidney Dis* 13:2, 1989.

87. American Diabetes Association: Position statement: standards of medical care for patients with diabetes mellitus, *Diabetes Care* 17:616, 1994.

88. Nelson RG et al: Assessment of risk of overt nephropathy in diabetic patients from albumin excretion in untimed urines, *Arch Intern Med* 151:1761, 1991.

89. Emancipator K: Laboratory diagnosis and monitoring of diabetes mellitus, *Am J Clin Pathol* 112:665, 1999.

Internet Sites

http://www.bsc.gwu.edu/bsc/studies/dcct.html—A brief summary of the 10-year Diabetes Control and Complications Trial and links pertaining to it

http://www.aafp.org/afp/981015ap/mayfield.html—"Diagnosis and Classification of Diabetes Mellitus: New Criteria" by J Mayfield

http://www.zoomph.net/diabetes.world/dcct.htm—American Diabetes Association Position Statement: Implications of the Diabetes Control and Complications Trial

http://www.diabetes.org—American Diabetes Association

http://www.diabetes.org/main/professional/journals/diabcs21_2_898.jsp

http://www.diabetes.org/main/community/forecast/pg112.jsp

http://www.diabetes.org/main/application/commercewf

http://www.cdc.gov/diabetes/faqs.htm

http://www.cdc.gov—Centers for Disease Control and Prevention

http://www.ohsu.edu/cliniweb/C18/C18.452.297.html

http://www.aace.com/pub/pf/index.php—Click on "Revised Diabetes Guidelines"

http://www.bsc.gwu.edu/bsc/studies/dcctbib.htm—Diabetes Control and Complications Trial (DCCT) bibliography, with links to journal abstracts

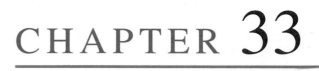

CHAPTER 33

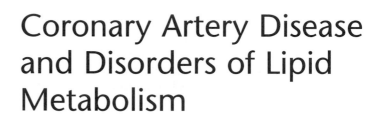

Coronary Artery Disease and Disorders of Lipid Metabolism

• *Herbert K. Naito*

Objectives

• Describe digestion, absorption, and metabolism of cholesterol and triglycerides, including the role of the liver and adipose tissue.
• List the lipoproteins and their apolipoprotein content; state the primary function of each lipoprotein.
• Describe the synthesis and catabolism of HDL, LDL, VLDL, and chylomicrons.

- Discuss each of the six types of lipoproteinemias with respect to lipid and lipoprotein levels, appearance of the specimen, and genetic etiology.

- Discuss the initiation and development of atherosclerosis.
- Discuss the risk factors for coronary atherosclerosis.
- State the clinical significance of hyperlipidemia.

Key Terms

amphipathic From *amphi-* ("on both sides") and *pathic* ("of feeling"); pertaining either to a molecule having two sides with characteristically different properties, or to a detergent that has both a polar (hydrophilic) end and a nonpolar (hydrophobic) end but is long enough so that each end demonstrates its own solubility characteristics.

apolipoprotein The protein component of lipoprotein complexes.

chylomicron Large lipid-protein complexes that are made by the gut and serve an important function in the transport of fats (mainly dietary triglycerides).

high-density lipoprotein (HDL) A lipoprotein complex is also called *alpha-lipoprotein* and is the most dense of the lipoproteins.

intermediate-density lipoprotein (IDL) A lipid-protein complex that has a density between VLDL

and LDL and has (relatively) a very short half-life. It is present in the blood in very low concentrations in a healthy person. In a person with dysbetalipoproteinemia, the IDL concentration in the blood is elevated.

low-density lipoprotein (LDL) A lipid-protein complex that is the end product of VLDL catabolism and the major carrier of serum cholesterol. Also called *beta-lipoprotein*.

lipoproteins Lipid-protein complexes consisting of discrete families of macromolecules with known physical, chemical, and physiological properties.

very–low-density lipoprotein (VLDL) A relatively large lipid-protein complex that transports mainly endogenously synthesized triglycerides. Also called *pre-beta-lipoprotein*.

Methods on CD-ROM

Cholesterol
High-density lipoprotein (HDL) cholesterol

Triglycerides

Part 1: Lipids
NORMAL PHYSIOLOGY OF LIPIDS
Lipid Composition of Foods

The fat found in food is composed mainly of triglycerides, about 98% to 99%, of which 92% to 95% is fatty acid and the remainder is glycerol. The remaining 1% to 2% of the lipids includes cholesterol, phospholipids, diglycerides, monoglycerides, fat-soluble vitamins, steroids, terpenes, and other fats. Most fats are mixtures of triglycerides containing four or five major fatty acids and many more minor or trace constituents. The individual glyceride molecules in most food fats contain both saturated and unsaturated fatty acids. Several polyunsaturated acids (linoleic, linolenic, and arachidonic acids) cannot be synthesized in the animal body and must be provided in the diet. These have been termed *essential fatty acids (EFAs)* (see Chapter 37).

The small amount of nonhydrolyzable matter in food fats consists of sterols, fatty alcohols, hydrocarbons, pigments, glycerol esters, and various other compounds. Cholesterol occurs in all animal fats. Most sterols are cholesterol, but depending on the diet, other sterols, such as phytosterols, can

make up an appreciable percentage of the total sterols, particularly in people on vegetarian diets. The phytosterols are important because they compete with cholesterol for uptake by the mucosal cell. Thus the more phytosterols consumed, the less dietary cholesterol is absorbed by the mucosal cells of the gut.

Fat Digestion, Absorption, and Metabolism of Lipids

Fat absorption occurs in three phases: the *intraluminal phase* (or digestive phase), during which the dietary fats are modified both physically and chemically before absorption; the *cellular phase* (or absorptive phase), in which the digested material enters the intestinal mucosal cells where it is reassembled into its preabsorptive form; and the *transport phase*, during which the absorbed lipids are carried from the mucosal cell to other tissues through the lymphatics and blood.[1-4]

Intraluminal phase. Most digestion of food fat is carried on in the intestine through the action of intestinal and pancreatic enzymes (lipases) and bile acids (see Chapters 29 and 30, respectively). Because of their surface-active properties, the bile salts emulsify the dietary triglyceride into very small particles with diameters of approximately 1 μm. The emulsification process thus forms particles that can be readily acted on by digestive enzymes.

In the intestinal lumen the action of pancreatic lipase on ingested fat results in the progressive digestion of triglycerides to 1,2-diglycerides and then to 2-monoglycerides and fatty acids. Only a small percentage of the fat is completely hydrolyzed to free fatty acids (FFAs) and glycerol. Cholesterol esters are hydrolyzed to free cholesterol and free fatty acid; the reaction is catalyzed by the enzyme cholesterol esterase.

Absorptive phase. After monoglycerides and fatty acids enter the endoplasmic reticulum of the mucosal cell, presumably by diffusion, the monoglycerides and fatty acids are reesterified into triglycerides by either of two pathways. The monoglyceride pathway is peculiar to the intestinal mucosa and involves the direct acylation of the absorbed monoglyceride from the lumen with activated FFA. The alpha-glycerophosphate pathway present in most tissues involves the formation of a coenzyme A (acyl-CoA) derivative of the fatty acid. This reaction, which requires adenosine triphosphate (ATP), is catalyzed by the enzyme fatty acid:CoA ligase (AMP). This enzyme has a pronounced specificity for longer-chain fatty acids. Thus long-chain fatty acids appear in thoracic duct lymph transported as triglycerides in the **chylomicrons**, whereas short- and medium-chain fatty acids are transported bound to albumin in the portal circulation.

The percentage of cholesterol absorbed from the diet is self-regulating. Increased levels of triglyceride in the diet and an expanded bile acid pool tend to promote cholesterol absorption. When the continuous intake of cholesterol is less than about 300 mg/day, more is absorbed (about 40% to 60%). If the intake is increased to 2 to 3 g/day, as little as 10% may be absorbed. In a typical American diet, about 600 mg of steroids are consumed per day, and the coefficient of absorption of dietary cholesterol is generally 25% to 40%. It should be stressed that there is a large individual variation in cholesterol absorption. This could account partially for the difference in individual responsiveness to diet-induced hypercholesterolemia.

Transport phase. Once triglycerides have been resynthesized within the intestinal mucosal cell, they are assembled in the mucosal cell endoplasmic reticulum and the Golgi apparatus into water-soluble macromolecules called *chylomicrons*. The intestinal **lipoproteins** leave the mucosal cells presumably by reverse pinocytosis. They first appear in the lymphatic vessels of the abdominal region and later in the systemic circulation. The intestinal release of chylomicrons persists for several hours after the ingestion of a fat meal. Because the chylomicrons are large enough to scatter light (up to 0.5 μm in diameter), the plasma becomes lactescent (turbid) so as to produce what is commonly called an *alimentary lipemic response*. These larger lipid-protein complexes are mixtures of triglycerides (82%), some proteins (2%, as

apoproteins), small amounts of cholesterol (9%, mainly as ester), and phospholipids (7%). Although the amount of protein is small, there is a good deal of evidence that its presence is necessary for the release of the chylomicrons. For example, in abeta-lipoproteinemia (a genetically determined disease in which apoprotein B cannot be made in the body), triglyceride is not released from the intestinal cells.

The bloodstream transports chylomicrons to all tissues in the body, including adipose tissue, which is their principal site of uptake. The large chylomicrons, heavily laden with triglyceride (Fig. 33-1), are removed rather rapidly (within minutes). Chylomicrons are normally present in only trace amounts in blood samples taken from individuals after an overnight fast.

Under normal conditions, chylomicron catabolism proceeds in two known phases. In the first, triglycerides are hydrolyzed at extrahepatic tissue sites under the influence of triglyceride (or lipoprotein) lipase. The process results in a relatively triglyceride-poor, cholesterol-rich remnant particle. In the second catabolic phase, the remnant particle, which has been implicated as a highly atherogenic lipoprotein, is removed by the liver.

The hydrolysis by lipoprotein lipase of triglyceride-rich, plasma proteins takes place at the luminal surface (bloodstream side) of the capillary endothelium. The enzyme is bound to the capillary endothelial cells in muscle and adipose tissue and can be released by intravenous administration of heparin (postheparin lipolytic activity, PHLA).

As a result of the first phase of chylomicron metabolism, unesterified fatty acids are released into the bloodstream, and the diglycerides and monoglycerides are taken up in vacuoles and transported across the capillary wall for hydrolysis.

Within tissue cells, the fatty acids derived from triglycerides in chylomicrons or very–low-density lipoproteins (VLDL) can be stored or used for energy when needed, especially by the heart. FFAs are also used for cellular phospholipid synthesis, including the synthesis of prostaglandins, the ubiquitous local hormones.

Remaining chylomicron remnant particles are cleared by the liver. Further catabolism of the VLDL remnant occurs at an extracellular site and results in the formation of low-density lipoprotein (LDL), a cholesterol-rich particle.

Role of Liver in Metabolism of Lipids

In addition to the intestines and other organs, the liver can synthesize lipoprotein particles from recently absorbed dietary constituents. In fact, the liver is the major organ that synthesizes cholesterol; about 70% of the daily cholesterol production comes from the liver. Newly synthesized hepatic triglycerides are coupled with phospholipid, cholesterol, and proteins to form VLDL. These macromolecules are then released into the circulation and transported to adipose tissue.

Hepatic triglyceride synthesis is accelerated when the diet is rich in excess calories. This results in VLDL overproduction, which may explain the hypertriglyceridemia observed when diets are particularly rich in simple sugars.

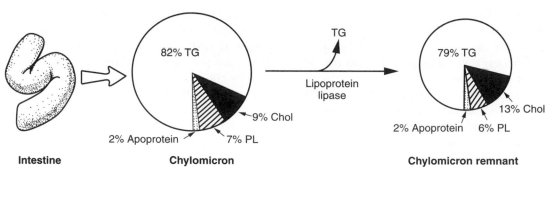

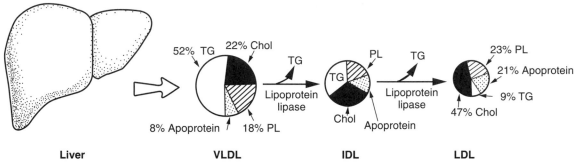

Fig. 33-1 Origin and catabolic pathway of chylomicron and very–low-density lipoprotein (VLDL). End product of chylomicron is chylomicron remnant; end product of VLDL is LDL. *Chol*, Cholesterol; *PL*, phosphatidyllecithin; *TG*, triglyceride.

Cyclopentanoperhydrophenanthrene

Fig. 33-2 Chemical structure of cyclopentanoperhydro-phenanthrene ring. This common four-ring structure is the basic structure of all steroids.

During fasting, the metabolic pathways in the liver are reversed. Blood glucose concentration falls, and insulin levels are diminished. Hepatic VLDL triglyceride synthesis is diminished during normal fasting. FFAs derived from adipose tissue are taken up by the liver, and their oxidation to ketone bodies provides energy for gluconeogenesis. FFAs of adipose tissue origin can be esterified to triglycerides, incorporated into hepatic VLDL, and then released into the bloodstream. During periods of stress and in certain metabolic conditions, such as uncontrolled diabetes, FFAs are the principal precursors of hepatic VLDL.

CHOLESTEROL METABOLISM
Biological Functions

Cholesterol is a member of a large class of biological compounds called *steroids* that have a similar four-ring structure, a cyclopentanoperhydrophenanthrene ring (Fig. 33-2).

Because of the well-established positive association between plasma cholesterol concentration and coronary heart disease (CHD), we are apt to think of cholesterol as a harmful substance. Contrary to that belief, cholesterol is essential for normal functioning of the organism because it is:

1. An essential structural component of the membranes of all animal cells and subcellular particles.
2. An obligatory precursor of bile acids.
3. A precursor of all steroid hormones, including sex and adrenal hormones.

Physiology of Cholesterol Metabolism

Tissue cholesterol is in constant exchange with plasma cholesterol; the turnover rate and the amount of tissue cholesterol that is exchangeable with the plasma cholesterol will vary from one tissue to another.

Because of loss and replacement, about 2% of the body's cholesterol is renewed each day. The main channel for outflow from the pool is the gastrointestinal tract; the absolute rate of turnover (in grams per day) as estimated by measurement of the daily fecal output is 1 to 2 g/day of cholesterol, with excretion of bile acids accounting for about half the total turnover. Fig. 33-3 illustrates that the concentration of a given cholesterol pool is under the influence of cholesterol input, output, and turnover rates. It should be stressed that because of the continuous cycling of cholesterol into and out of the bloodstream, the plasma cholesterol concentration is not a simple additive function of dietary cholesterol intake and endogenous cholesterol synthesis. Rather, it reflects the rates of synthesis of the cholesterol-carrying lipoproteins and the efficiency of the receptor mechanisms that determine their catabolism. A detailed discussion of the dynamics of lipoprotein concentration can be found in the section on lipoprotein metabolism.

Cholesterol is present in all plasma lipoproteins, but about 60% of the total cholesterol in plasma from a fasting human subject is carried in the LDL.[5] About two thirds of the plasma total cholesterol is esterified with long-chain fatty acids, with linoleic acid being the predominant fatty acid in humans. The cholesteryl esters in the plasma are in a state of constant turnover because of their continual hydrolysis and resynthesis. Hydrolysis of cholesteryl esters takes place in the liver, but synthesis occurs mainly in the plasma by transfer of a fatty acid residue from lecithin to free cholesterol (Fig. 33-4). This reaction is catalyzed by a plasma enzyme known as *lecithin:*

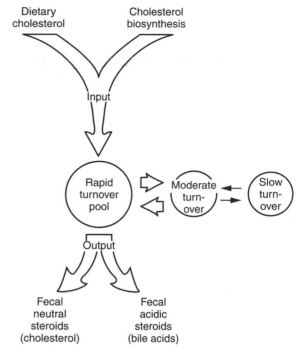

Fig. 33-3 Scheme of dynamics of cholesterol metabolism.

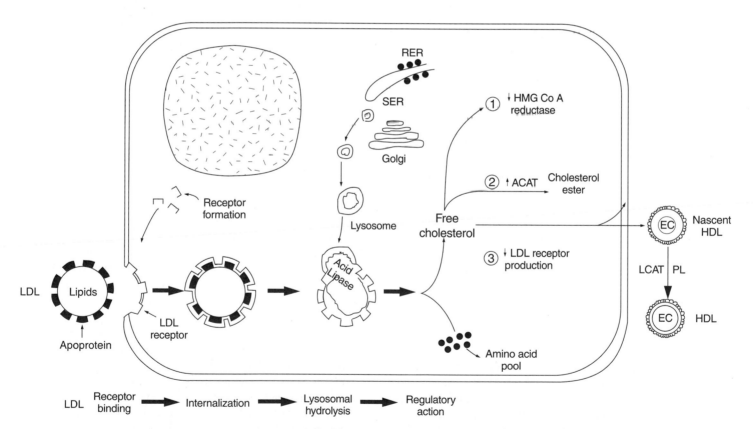

Fig. 33-4 Scheme of LDL uptake and catabolism by a cell. Mechanism not only clears LDL from circulation but also aids in regulation of cholesterol synthesis and storage. High-density lipoprotein, *HDL*, plays an integral role in removing cellular cholesterol, esterifying free cholesterol in blood and transporting cholesterol to liver for catabolism. *ACAT*, Acyl-CoA:cholesterol acyltransferase; *EC*, cholesteryl ester; *HMG-CoA reductase*, β-hydroxy-β-methylglutaryl-coenzyme A reductase; *LCAT*, lecithin:cholesterol acyltransferase; *PL*, phospholipid; *RER*, rough endoplasmic reticulum; *SER*, smooth endoplasmic reticulum.

cholesterol acyltransferase, or *LCAT*. The preferred lipoprotein substrate for human LCAT is **high-density lipoprotein (HDL)**, and it seems likely that the bulk of the esterified cholesterol in the plasma is formed on HDL.[6] The cholesteryl ester then is transferred from HDL to LDL and VLDL, partly in exchange for triglyceride.

It is believed that one of the functions of HDL is to transport cholesterol, in esterified form, from the tissues to the liver[6] by the following sequence of events. Free cholesterol from peripheral tissues is transferred to HDL; it is then esterified by LCAT, enabling HDL to take up more free cholesterol. The esterified cholesterol formed on HDL is transferred to LDL and VLDL, where it is incorporated into the nonpolar core of the lipoprotein molecules. LDL, carrying its load of cholesteryl ester to peripheral tissues, reaches the liver, where the cholesteryl esters are hydrolyzed, entering the pool of free cholesterol in the hepatocyte. The free cholesterol can leave the hepatic pool by secretion into the bile, directly or after conversion into bile acids, or by reincorporation into plasma lipoprotein (VLDL). Hepatic excretion of cholesterol via the biliary pool is one of the major mechanisms for removing cholesterol from the circulation.

Synthesis

Almost all animal tissues synthesize cholesterol from acetyl CoA. In adults the liver and intestinal wall probably supply over 90% of the plasma cholesterol of endogenous origin. Hepatic cholesterogenesis, unlike intestinal cholesterol synthesis, is inhibited by dietary cholesterol. Cholesterol production rate (absorbed cholesterol plus endogenously synthesized cholesterol) amounts to about 1 g/day. In most tissues the rate of synthesis of cholesterol is determined by the capacity of β-hydroxy-β-methylglutaryl CoA (HMG-CoA) reductase, which catalyzes a rate-limiting step in the biosynthetic sequence from acetyl CoA to cholesterol. Although this appears to be the main rate-limiting reaction, other sites of suppression are likely in the biosynthetic cholesterol pathway. Hepatic HMG-CoA reductase is subject to induction and repression by several hormones, dietary factors, and drugs. Feedback control of hepatic cholesterogenesis is also mediated by cholesterol itself and directly or indirectly by bile acids. A brief scheme of the control of hepatic cholesterogenesis is shown in Fig. 33-5.

Catabolism

In humans, increased absorption of cholesterol is followed by increased excretion of cholesterol from the exchangeable pool. Increased conversion of cholesterol into bile acids can be brought about by interruption of the enterohepatic circulation of bile salts. Bile salts returning to the liver from the intestine repress the formation of an enzyme catalyzing the rate-limiting step in the conversion of cholesterol into bile acids. When bile salts are prevented from returning to the liver, the activity of this enzyme increases and degradation of cholesterol to bile acids is stimulated. This effect may be exploited therapeutically in the treatment of hypercholes-

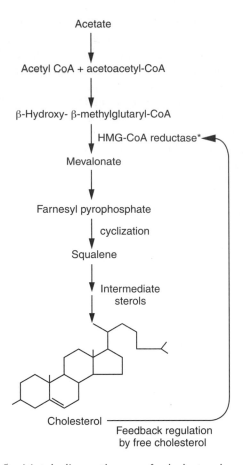

Fig. 33-5 Metabolic pathway of cholesterol synthesis, emphasizing negative feedback end-product inhibition step at β-hydroxy-β-methylglutaryl CoA step with the important enzyme HMG-CoA reductase.

terolemia by the use of unabsorbable resins, which bind bile acids in the lumen of the intestine and prevent their return to the liver.

These mechanisms for excretion of cholesterol by means of bile acids or cholesterol in the bile depend on the receptor-mediated activity in the hepatocytes. The hepatocytes have receptor sites specific for apoproteins (Apo) B and E. The major function of the liver in lipoprotein clearance is to remove lipoproteins containing Apo E (such as chylomicron remnants and VLDL remnants) and Apo B (such as LDL remnants) from plasma. However, the Apo E–containing lipoproteins are cleared with much greater efficiency than the Apo B–containing lipoproteins. For this reason chylomicron remnants and VLDL remnants (intermediate-density lipoprotein, IDL) are not normally measurable in healthy individuals (see Fig. 33-1).

The uptake of LDL by the peripheral tissues is also receptor-site–dependent (see Fig. 33-4). The binding of LDL to the receptor site followed by internalization and hydrolysis of the LDL serves to deliver free cholesterol to the cell. The intracellular free cholesterol then functions (1) as a regulator for the rate of receptor synthesis, (2) as a regulator for cholesterol synthesis by the end-product negative-feedback mechanism, or (3) as a regulator for ACAT (acyl-CoA:

cholesterol acyltransferase) activity, which determines how much cholesterol is stored in the cell as cholesteryl oleate, a cholesterol ester. It is believed that the availability of HDL is one of the determining factors for the efflux of cholesterol from the cell into the blood.[6] By this process, the cholesteryl oleate in the cell is hydrolyzed to free cholesterol and fatty acid. The liver and to some extent the gastrointestinal tract and other organs, such as the adrenal glands and gonadal tissues, take up the HDL and catabolize it to its protein and lipid constituents (including cholesterol).

Expected Cholesterol Values

Unlike many of the blood analytes that we measure in the laboratory, lipids and lipoproteins require a different approach when normal expected values are being defined.[7] A problem arises in defining what levels of plasma lipids separate persons with elevated blood fats, who have or will develop CHD, from the rest of the "normal" population. Before addressing the question of what is adequate dietary or drug therapy for the control of serum lipid and lipoprotein concentrations, we must first consider the degree to which blood lipids should be lowered. In other words, at what level should the clinician consider a sample "hyperlipidemic"? Many clinical laboratories and practicing physicians used reference intervals derived from the central 95% of values when classifying a sample as normal or abnormal. Unfortunately, because of the way we have defined "normal" in the past, many lipid and lipoprotein test results do not correlate very well with health-risk conditions on an individual basis. Thus a cholesterol value in the normal range for a given population may not represent a healthy cholesterol level. For example, a cholesterol value of 2500 to 2800 mg/L (to convert mg/L to mmol/L, divide by 387) may be within the 95th percentile of the distribution of an apparently healthy male population between 51 and 59 years of age in the United States, but about 40% to 50% of these persons eventually will develop CHD. In Japan, where CHD is less common than in the U.S., the mean total cholesterol value for the adult population is around 1850 mg/L—up about 250 mg/L from several decades ago.

Critical values for serum lipids and lipoproteins have been established that are highly predictive of disease or disease risk, irrespective of the "normal" distribution (see the discussion of the National Cholesterol Education Program, p. 631).

Because of the positive correlation between blood cholesterol concentration and the increased risk for CHD, many investigators believe that the average cholesterol concentration for the entire population should be as low as possible. According to clinical data,[8] individuals with plasma cholesterol values below 1800 mg/L experience minimum CHD mortality (about 3.3/1000). In addition, clinical trials have documented that reversal of the coronary stenosis of the blood vessels is possible when total cholesterol is reduced to less than 1800 mg/L or when LDL cholesterol is lowered to less than 1000 mg/L. On the other hand, the relative risk is increased by 25% for those with values between 1800 and

2000 mg/L. For values between 2000 and 2390 mg/L, the relative risk is increased about 80%; for values above 2400 mg/L, the relative risk rises almost two and one-half times, or 230%. For individuals with plasma cholesterol concentrations near 2600 mg/L, the relative risk is increased by 400%. In simplistic terms, concentrations below 2000 mg/L can be considered more ideal than concentrations above 2000 mg/L for the adult population. Using such a definition, this means that about 58% of adults in the United States have undesirably elevated cholesterol concentrations. The plasma concentration in young American men is essentially within the ideal range. If it did not increase with age, the risk of CHD in the United States would perhaps be much lower than it is now. Recent reports suggest that the mean cholesterol value of the U.S. population declined from 2200 to less than 2150 mg/L, and the CHD morbidity and mortality have decreased. Again, it should be remembered that the relationship between blood cholesterol concentration and CHD shows no threshold for the disease.

The newest guidelines of the National Institutes of Health (NIH) National Cholesterol Education Program Adult Treatment Panel III[9] suggest that the total cholesterol should be less than 2000 mg/L for the high-risk adult. These new guidelines place most of the emphasis on the LDL cholesterol, the major carrier for the transport of cholesterol in the blood and a causal agent for atherogenesis. Thus the newest focus for assessment of CHD risk, goal setting, and primary target of therapy is the LDL cholesterol concentration and not the total and HDL cholesterol concentrations, as in the past.[10] The new guidelines recommend that all adults 20 years or older have a fasting lipoprotein profile (total cholesterol, LDL cholesterol, HDL cholesterol, and triglycerides) every 5 years. These recommendations are listed in the following box.

The risk for coronary heart disease increases from low to very high as fasting lipid values rise from optimal to very

---

NATIONAL INSTITUTES OF HEALTH NATIONAL CHOLESTEROL EDUCATION PROGRAM ADULT TREATMENT PANEL III[9] GUIDELINES

Optimal Fasting Levels
Total cholesterol <2000 mg/L
LDL cholesterol <1000 mg/L
HDL cholesterol >400 mg/L
Triglycerides <1500 mg/L

Near or Above Optimal Fasting Levels
LDL cholesterol 1000 to 1290 mg/L

Borderline High Fasting Levels
LDL cholesterol 1300 to 1590 mg/L

High Fasting Levels
LDL cholesterol 1600 to 1890 mg/L

Very High Fasting Levels
LDL cholesterol >1900 mg/L

high. If the patient is *nonfasting*, the values for total cholesterol and HDL cholesterol will be usable. Specimens from nonfasting patients can be used for the determination of LDL cholesterol *only* if a direct measurement of LDL is employed. Calculated LDL cholesterols will not be accurate in these specimens because the VLDL cholesterol values (triglycerides divided by 5) are elevated in nonfasting conditions (see Methods on CD-ROM). In such a case, a total cholesterol of less than 2000 mg/L or an HDL cholesterol under 400 mg/L can be considered *desirable*. However, if the total cholesterol and/or HDL cholesterol values are abnormal, a follow-up fasting lipoprotein profile is necessary.

In addition to LDL cholesterol, risk determinants for CHD include the current presence or absence of CHD, other clinical forms of atherosclerotic disease, and the major risk factors other than LDL cholesterol (see Box 33-1 on p. 634). The ATP III guidelines[9] focus attention on intensive treatment of patients with CHD and on the primary prevention of CHD in persons with multiple risk factors; the latter have a relatively high risk for CHD and will benefit from more intensive LDL-lowering treatment than recommended in ATP II.[11]

It is well known that as people age, they become more susceptible to the atherosclerotic process (coronary artery disease, peripheral arterial disease, abdominal aortic aneurysm, and carotid artery disease) because of changes in lifestyle and the accumulation of CHD risk factors. The more risk factors accumulated, the greater the risk for early heart disease, including angina pectoris, myocardial infarction, or for an unfortunate 35% of the population, acute cardiac death. It has been calculated that, for an individual with a total cholesterol level of 2000 mg/L and no other risk factors, a critical degree of significant atherosclerosis (greater than 60% stenosis) may be reached by the time the person reaches the age of 70 years. If the same individual had a cholesterol value of 2500 or 3000 mg/L, this degree of coronary artery disease (CAD) would probably be attained by 60 or 50 years of age, respectively. This timetable is accelerated when multiple risk factors for CHD are involved (e.g., smoking, hypertension, obesity, physical inactivity, atherogenic diets, Lp(a), homocysteine, peripheral arterial disease, abdominal aortic aneurysm, symptomatic carotic artery disease, prothrombotic and proinflammatory factors, impaired fasting glucose). With the addition of a single CHD risk factor (smoking), the critical age is reached by 60 years of age, and with addition of a second CHD risk factor (hypertension), this age drops to 50 years. A plasma cholesterol concentration of 2500 mg/L moves the critical age back to 50 years with one risk factor and to 40 years with two risk factors. Greater than 20% of the general population can expect to develop CHD or have a recurrent CHD event within 10 years if they have multiple risk factors (two or more). Thus the number of CHD risk factors is a determinant in deciding how aggressive the patient's treatment protocol should be.

For the first time, the guidelines consider high triglycerides (or VLDL cholesterol) a risk factor that should be treated. The ATP III[9] guidelines also include individuals with *metabolic syndromes* as a high-risk group (see below). These persons have a constellation of major risk factors such as abdominal obesity, atherogenic dyslipidemia (elevated triglyceride, small LDL particles, low HDL cholesterol), raised blood pressure, insulin resistance (with or without glucose intolerance), and prothrombotic and proinflammatory states. Management of the *metabolic syndrome* has a two-fold objective: (a) to reduce the underlying causes (such as, obesity and physical inactivity) and (b) to treat associated nonlipid and lipid risk factors. The changes in the ATP III guidelines[9] include lowering the *normal plasma triglycerides* cutoff point from <2000 mg/L to <1500 mg/L. The treatment strategy for hypertriglyceridemia depends on the cause and severity of the triglyceride elevation. If a patient has borderline-high or high triglycerides, the primary aim is to achieve the target goal for LDL cholesterol. When triglycerides are *borderline high* (1500 to 1990 mg/L), emphasis should also be placed on weight reduction and increased physical activity. For *high triglycerides* (2000 to 4990 mg/L), non-HDL cholesterol becomes a secondary target of therapy. The term *non-HDL cholesterol* refers to VLDL, LDL, IDL (intermediate-density lipoprotein), and Lp(a) cholesterol. In addition to weight reduction and increased physical activity, hypolipemic medication therapy can be considered in high-risk persons to achieve the non-HDL cholesterol goal. In rare cases in which triglycerides are *very high* (>5000 mg/L), treatment may include very-low fat diets, weight reduction, increased physical activity, and triglyceride-lowering drugs. It should be emphasized that a person's serum or plasma total cholesterol concentration is under the influence of many other factors, some of which are controllable and some uncontrollable.[12]

Genetics. Genetic factors are probably the most important influence on a person's cholesterol concentration. It is estimated that about half of the variability in blood cholesterol concentrations has a genetic basis.

Age. Serum cholesterol concentration starts out around 650 mg/L at birth and steadily increases with age (about 15 mg/L per year).

Sex. Cholesterol concentration in the blood of males is generally higher than that in premenopausal females. After menopause, however, the cholesterol concentration is higher in females than in males. Serum cholesterol levels in males seem to reach a plateau by 50 to 60 years of age.

Diet. Saturated fat in the diet increases serum cholesterol levels, whereas polyunsaturated fat decreases cholesterol concentration; monounsaturated fats have some lowering effect. Trans-fatty acids are another LDL-raising fat that should be kept at a low intake. Dietary cholesterol elevates serum cholesterol levels. Plant sterols and certain types of fiber decrease serum cholesterol concentration. Fish oils seem to lower triglycerides and Lp(a) more than cholesterol. Current guidelines[9] suggest that the saturated fat intake should not exceed 7% of the total calories and total fat intake should not exceed 35% of the total calories with cholesterol intake of <200 mg/day. In addition, it is recommended that other therapeutic options for lowering LDL cholesterol can be achieved with greater dietary intake of phytosterols (plant sterols) and viscous fiber (both found in fruits and vegetables).

Obesity. Although obesity is commonly regarded as an important contributor to the development of hypertriglyceridemia, it is well established that as the percentage of individuals with obesity increases with age, so do blood cholesterol concentrations. Approximately 30% of American adults can be considered obese (see also Chapter 37). The problem is especially pronounced for Hispanic populations, low socioeconomic Caucasian populations, and African American women. It is estimated that over 65 million American adults are obese, and the problem is acute for American children. Weight reduction therapy for overweight or obese patients will enhance lowering of LDL cholesterol levels and will provide other health benefits, including modifying other lipid and nonlipid risk factors. The current ATP III guidelines[9] recommend that diet be focused on a balanced energy intake and expenditure to maintain desirable body weight and to prevent weight gain. Additional risk reduction can be achieved by simultaneously increasing physical activity.

Physical activity. Physical activity tends to lower serum total cholesterol. Much of this effect depends on the type, intensity, duration, and frequency of physical activity. Exercise also lowers total cholesterol, LDL cholesterol, triglycerides, and VLDL cholesterol, and it increases HDL cholesterol concentration. Physical activity also can lower blood pressure, reduce insulin resistance, and reduce stress. In addition, physical *inactivity* further enhances the risk for CHD by impairing cardiovascular fitness and coronary blood flow. Over 60% of American adults have a sedentary lifestyle or no regular physical activity. The prevalence is higher in women, minority groups, and older adults. It has been demonstrated that when women with diabetes exercised at least 4 hours per week (moderate to vigorous exercise), they had a 40% reduced risk for cardiovascular diseases.

Hormones. Growth hormone, thyroxine, and glucagon decrease serum cholesterol levels, whereas anabolic steroids and progestins increase cholesterol levels. The loss of estrogen in the postmenopausal women is associated with elevated blood concentrations of total cholesterol, Lp(a), and homocysteine in older women.

Primary disease states. Diabetes mellitus, thyroid dysfunction, obstructive liver disease, acute porphyria, dysgammaglobulinemias, and nephrotic syndrome all have an effect on blood cholesterol concentrations. The current guidelines[9] categorize diabetic patients as high-risk individuals who need aggressive intervention therapy. This is based on the fact that diabetes confers a high risk for new CHD within 10 years from the onset of the disease, in part because of its frequent association with multiple risk factors. Furthermore, a more intensive prevention strategy is recommended for diabetics because myocardial infarction in these patients results in an unusually high death rate, either immediately or in the long term. *Hypothyroidism* is relatively common in the geriatric population and is a common cause for secondary hypercholesterolemia. Thus appropriate screening and treatment for thyroid dysfunction in older adults is warranted (see Chapter 44).

TRIGLYCERIDE METABOLISM
Biological Functions

Triglycerides are the major form of fat found in nature, and their primary function is to provide energy for the cell. One gram of fatty acids liberates about 9 kcal. The human body stores large amounts of fatty acids in ester linkages with glycerol in the adipose tissue. This form of reserve energy storage is highly efficient because of the magnitude of the energy released when fatty acids undergo catabolism. Most of the fatty acids come from our diets, can be synthesized endogenously, and are called *nonessential fatty acids*. There are three fatty acids (linoleic, linolenic, and arachidonic acids) that cannot be made by the human body. These fatty acids are called *essential fatty acids* and are important for proper growth and development of cells, cell membrane integrity, prostaglandin synthesis, and myelinization of the central nervous system. Insufficient intake of the essential fatty acids will lead to an essential fatty acid deficiency.

Physiology

Triglycerides are by far the most abundant subclass of neutral glycerides in nature. Mammalian tissues also contain some diglycerides and monoglycerides, but these occur in trace levels when compared with triglycerides. Most triglyceride molecules in mammalian tissues are mixed glycerides.

Because of their water insolubility, triglycerides are transported in the plasma in combination with other more polar lipids (phospholipids) and proteins, as well as with cholesterol and cholesteryl esters, in the complex lipoprotein macromolecules. It appears that the essentially nonpolar triglycerides (and cholesteryl ester) are largely in the center of the lipoprotein, whereas the more polar protein and phospholipid components are at the surface, with their polar groups directed outward to stabilize the whole structure in the aqueous plasma environment.

Synthesis

The concentration of triglyceride in the plasma at any given time is a balance between the rate of entry into the plasma and the rate of removal. A change in concentration may therefore be the result of a change in either or both of these factors. Moreover, a primary change in one may result in a secondary change in the other. Thus, perhaps the main problem to be considered in any situation in which the plasma triglyceride concentration is abnormally high is whether this is attributable to a rise in the rate of entry or to a fall in the rate of removal of plasma triglycerides.

Plasma triglycerides are derived from two sources, intestinal and liver. Intestinal triglycerides are synthesized from dietary fat. The source of the fatty acids present in the triglycerides entering the blood from the liver depends greatly on the individual's nutritional state. Thus in the fasting state, fatty acids derived from adipose cell triglycerides are taken up by the liver and a portion is reexcreted as VLDL. Following a meal, dietary carbohydrates are taken up by the liver and converted to triglycerides, which are secreted as lipoproteins. It is important to realize that, except during the absorption of dietary fat, the liver is the main contributor of triglyceride to the plasma.

The size, triglyceride content, and particle density of the lipoprotein complexes formed by the intestines and liver varies according to the amount of triglyceride being released. Thus high rates of release result in large complexes with a higher triglyceride load and a correspondingly lower density. In fact, the lipoprotein complexes released from the liver under such conditions may reach a size not much smaller than that of the intestinal chylomicrons, even though they normally have a somewhat lower triglyceride content and therefore a higher density.

Catabolism

The action of clearing-factor lipase at the endothelial cell surface not only facilitates the removal of triglyceride fatty acid from the blood but also determines where it is used, and this has important consequences. For example, in a state of caloric excess, the amount of triglyceride fatty acid in the bloodstream in excess of the immediate caloric needs is taken up by adipose tissue. Most fatty acids are reconverted to intracellular triglyceride and stored. In contrast, in a state of caloric deficit (as during fasting) the tissues derive their energy primarily from the oxidation of unesterified fatty acids, which are mobilized from adipose tissue and carried to the body tissues in the blood. Triglyceride is still present in the blood in VLDL under these conditions, but instead of being taken up by adipose tissue, it is now directed away from this tissue and toward muscle to supplement the supply of energy from the mobilized fatty acids. This switch in triglyceride fatty acid uptake is achieved through changes in the activity of intracellular lipase in the tissues concerned. Thus fasting results in a decrease in the activity of the enzyme in adipose tissue and an increase in its activity in muscle.

The intracellular adipose triglyceride enzyme is distinct from the plasma enzyme and is called *hormone-sensitive lipase* because it is converted from an inactive to an active form by epinephrine, norepinephrine, adrenocorticotropin, thyroid-stimulating hormone, and glucagon. Moreover, its activity is promoted by growth hormone. On the other hand, insulin inhibits the activity of this lipase. Unlike the lipoprotein lipase of adipose tissue, hormone-sensitive lipase of other tissue exhibits increased activity during fasting, possibly because of falling insulin levels. It is believed that hormone-sensitive lipase plays an important role in fat mobilization from adipose tissue.

Expected Triglyceride Values

Rather than base triglyceride reference intervals on traditional 95th percentile ranges, the NIH ATP III guidelines recommended that the most useful triglyceride value to remember is 5,000 mg/L or greater, which represents an increased risk for acute pancreatitis.[9] (To convert triglyceride units from mg/L to mmol/L, divide by 886.) There are other

clinical presentations when a patient has marked elevations in triglycerides, such as lipaemia retinalis, eruptive xanthoma hepatomegaly, and splenomegaly. The adult upper limit of normal was once defined as 2000 mg/L for both sexes, regardless of age.[10] The new NIH ATP III guidelines[9] define the upper limits of *normal* for serum triglycerides as less than 1500 mg/L. *Borderline-high* triglyceride level is now defined as 1500 to 1990 mg/L, and *high* triglyceride level is 2000 to 4990 mg/L. *Very high* triglyceride level is defined as ≥5000 mg/L. Factors that contribute to elevated serum triglycerides are listed in the following box.

According to the NCEP III[9] guidelines, the treatment strategy for elevated triglycerides depends on the causes and severity of the elevation. For all persons with borderline-high or high triglyceride levels, the primary aim of therapy is to achieve the target goal for LDL cholesterol. Emphasis should be placed on weight reduction and increased physical activity. In many instances, the lowering of the triglycerides will normalize the below-normal HDL cholesterol levels (<400 mg/L) because of the existence of the reverse relationship between triglyceride and HDL cholesterol concentrations. However, the NCEP ATP III[9] recommendations do not specify a goal for raising HDL. Although many clinical trial results suggest that raising HDL will reduce the CHD risk, the evidence is insufficient to specify a goal for therapy, unless the patient has documented CHD.

Part 2: Lipoproteins

As discussed earlier, lipids are insoluble in aqueous media, including that of plasma.[3,4] Only when the hydrophobic lipids are bound to protein-containing "lipoproteins" do they become soluble in the bloodstream. Because lipoproteins are generally viewed as a class of macromolecules associated with lipid transport, recommendations were made in the late 1960s and early 1970s to transfer the diagnostic emphasis from hyperlipidemia to hyperlipoproteinemia.[1,2,5,13]

FACTORS THAT CONTRIBUTE TO ELEVATED SERUM TRIGLYCERIDES

Excess weight or obesity
Physical inactivity
Cigarette smoking
Excess alcohol intake
Excessively high carbohydrate diets (>60% of the caloric intake)
Primary disease states
 Type II diabetes
 Chronic renal failure
 Renal failure (such as nephrotic syndrome)
Drugs (such as corticosteroids, estrogens, retinoids, high doses of beta-adrenergic blocking agents)
Certain genetic metabolic disorders (including familial combined hyperlipidemia, familial hypertriglyceridemia, and familial dysbeta-lipoproteinemia)

A lipoprotein can be visualized most simply as a globular structure with an outer solubilizing coat of protein and phospholipid and an inner hydrophobic, neutral core of triglycerides and cholesterol (Fig. 33-6). The protein and phospholipid impart solubility to the otherwise insoluble lipids. The binding of the inner lipid to the phospholipid and protein coat is noncovalent, occurring primarily through hydrogen bonding and van der Waals forces. The protein, free of lipid, is called **apolipoprotein (Apo)**. Note that the lipids, which are weakly bound to the protein and phospholipid, are bound loosely enough to allow the ready exchange of lipid between the serum lipoproteins as well as between serum and tissue lipoproteins. On the other hand, the lipids are bound strongly enough to allow the lipid and protein moieties to be separated in the analytical systems used to isolate and classify the lipoproteins.

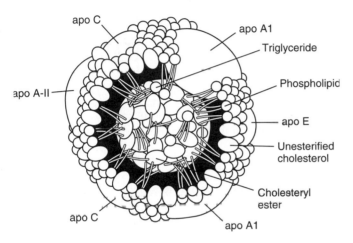

Fig. 33-6 Scheme of a lipoprotein complex showing polar outer surface and a core filled with neutral lipids. *HDL,* High-density lipoprotein.

CLASSIFICATION OF LIPOPROTEINS

The four most frequently used systems to isolate, separate, and characterize lipoproteins are based on analytical ultracentrifugation, preparative ultracentrifugation, electrophoresis, and precipitation techniques.[14] The most frequently used systems are those based on ultracentrifugation and electrophoresis (Fig. 33-7). With a paper or agarose support medium, electrophoretic patterns show that chylomicrons remain at the origin whereas pre-beta-lipoproteins and beta-lipoproteins migrate in the beta$_1$- and beta$_2$-globulin areas, respectively, and alpha-lipoproteins migrate in the alpha$_1$-globulin area. A new high-definition agarose support media (Helena Laboratories; Beaumont, TX) can identify Lp(a) as a fast-migrating pre-beta-lipoprotein, which typically migrates between the alpha- and pre-beta-lipoprotein bands. Using the conventional ultracentrifuge methods and taking advantage of the fact that lipoproteins are lighter than the other serum proteins, one can separate the lipoproteins into chylomicrons (the lightest lipoproteins, of a density less than plasma), VLDL at a density below 1.006 g/mL (after chylomicron removal), LDL of density 1.006 to 1.063 g/mL, and HDL of density 1.019 to 1.210 g/mL.[1-4,13] These lipoprotein classes correlate with electrophoretic patterns; for example, pre-beta-lipoprotein is generally synonymous with VLDL, beta-lipoprotein with LDL, and alpha-lipoprotein with HDL. Table 33-1 and Fig. 33-7 summarize the physical, chemical, and physiological characteristics of the major plasma lipoproteins.

Chylomicrons

Chylomicrons contain mainly triglyceride combined with cholesterol, small amounts of phospholipid, and specific apoproteins (Apo B-48, A-I, A-II, C-I, C-II, C-III, with small amounts of Apo B and E-II, E-III, E-IV) (see Table 33-1). Most models for chylomicron structure have been made under the assumption that the neutral lipids (triglycerides and

Feature	Chylomicrons	VLDL	IDL	LDL	HDL
Density (g/mL)	<1.006	<1.006	1.006 to 1.019	1.019 to 1.063	1.063 to 1.21
Electrophoretic mobility	Origin	Pre-beta	Beta	Beta	Alpha
Flotation rate (S$_f$)	>400	20 to 400	12 to 20	0 to 10	—
Diameter (nm)	80 to 500	40 to 80	24.5	20	7.5 to 12
Lipids (% by weight)	98	92	85	79	50
Cholesterol	9	22	35	47	19
Triglyceride	82	52	20	9	3
Phospholipid	7	18	20	23	28
Apoproteins (% of weight)	2	8	15	21	50
Major	A-I, A-II	B-100	B-100	B-100	A-I, A-II
	B-48	C-I, C-II, C-III	C-I, C-II, C-III		C-I, C-II, C-III
	C-I, C-II, C-III	E	E		
Minor	B-100	A-I, A-II	B-48	C-I, C-II, C-III	B-100
	D	B-48		E-II, E-III, E-IV	D
	E-II, E-III, E-IV				E-II, E-III, E-IV

TABLE 33-1   PHYSICAL AND CHEMICAL DESCRIPTION OF PLASMA LIPOPROTEINS IN HUMANS

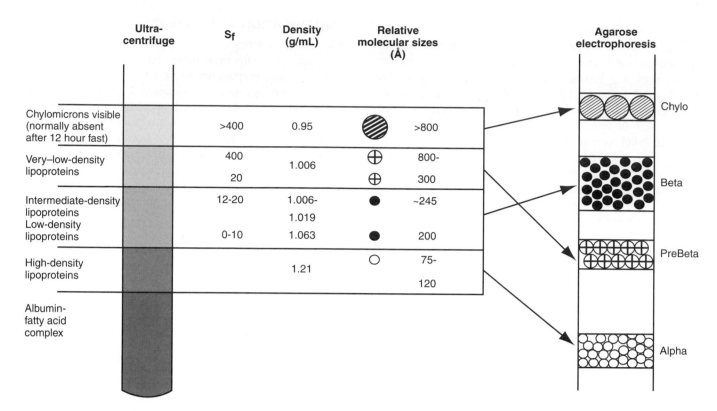

Fig. 33-7 Overview of major types of lipoproteins, showing some basic chemical and physical properties. *alpha*, Alpha-lipoprotein; *beta*, beta-lipoprotein; *chylo*, chylomicrons; *preBeta*, a very–low-density lipoprotein; S_f, Svedberg flotation rate.

cholesteryl ester) are partially surrounded by an outer shell of phospholipid, free cholesterol, and protein. Under fasting conditions (more than 10 to 12 hours after a meal), no chylomicrons are generally found in the blood of healthy persons. The presence of chylomicrons makes the serum appear turbid or milky.

Very–Low-Density Lipoprotein

An average preparation of **very–low-density lipoprotein (VLDL)** contains 52% triglyceride, 18% phospholipid, 22% cholesterol, and about 8% protein. Cholesterol and cholesteryl esters occur in a ratio of about 1:1 by weight. Sphingomyelin and phosphatidylcholine are the major phospholipids. The larger the size of a VLDL particle, the greater the proportion of triglycerides and Apo C and the smaller the proportion of phospholipid, Apo B, and other apoproteins. Apo B appears to be present in a constant absolute quantity in all VLDL fractions. Apo B-100 accounts for approximately 30% to 35%, with Apo C-I, C-II, and C-III making up over 50% of the apoprotein content in VLDL. Apo E-II, E-III, and E-IV and varying quantities of other apoproteins (A-I, A-II, B-48) may also be present. The relative quantity of each protein varies with the individual and with the degree of hyperlipidemia. Partially degraded VLDL, commonly called *remnant lipoprotein* is a triglyceride-poor lipoprotein, known to be highly atherogenic. In clinical practice, remnant lipoproteins are not easily measured. Although VLDL is not known to be atherogenic, it would be

prudent to lower VLDL cholesterol only if triglycerides are >2000 mg/L (or VLDL cholesterol >300 mg/L) and the LDL cholesterol values are abnormal.

Low-Density Lipoprotein

Low-density lipoprotein (LDL) contains, by weight, 80% lipid and 20% protein. Consistent with this increased protein content, LDL is smaller (21 to 25 nm) and is of higher hydrated density (1.006 to 1.063 g/mL) than are VLDL and chylomicrons. About 50% of LDL lipid is cholesterol. LDL constitutes 40% to 50% of the plasma lipoprotein mass in humans. Its average concentration in normal adult American males is about 4000 mg/L; in females it is 3400 mg/L. LDL is the major carrier of cholesterol and is considered an atherogenic lipoprotein. Apo B-100 is the major apoprotein of normal LDL, and LDL Apo B represents 90% to 95% of the total plasma Apo B-100. Experimental evidence suggests that the LDL Apo B in healthy humans is derived almost entirely from VLDL Apo B in plasma. LDL is frequently separated into two classes—LDL₁ (or IDL) and LDL₂—on the basis of flotation density. The lower-density fraction, IDL (1.006 to 1.109 g/mL), is more lipid-rich than LDL₂ (1.019 to 1.063 g/mL) and probably represents an intermediate in VLDL catabolism (see Fig. 33-1). Thus a comparison of IDL with LDL₂ demonstrates the gradual disappearance of triglyceride and of apoproteins more characteristic of VLDL (Apo C and Apo E) and an enrichment with Apo B-100 and cholesterol ester. Recently, it has been reported that there is a significant size heterogeneity in all the major lipoprotein classes, including that of LDL. It has been shown that small, dense LDL is metabolically more active and is more atherogenic than the conventional-size LDL. Case studies have shown that individuals with an abundance of small, dense LDL particles are at greater risk for CHD than persons with normal size LDL. The ATP III report[9] has acknowledged this as a CHD risk factor.

High-Density Lipoprotein

The HDL macromolecular complex (see Fig. 33-6) contains approximately 50% protein and 50% lipid. HDL is the smallest of the lipoproteins (9 to 12 nm) and floats at the highest density (1.063 to 1.21 g/mL) of any of the lipoprotein molecules. Quantitatively, the most important HDL lipid is phospholipid, though HDL cholesterol is of particular interest. The major phospholipid species is phosphatidylcholine (also known as *lecithin*), which accounts for 70% to 80% of the total phospholipid. Phosphatidylcholine plays an important functional role as a reactant in plasma cholesterol esterification, which is catalyzed by the enzyme lecithin:cholesterol acyltransferase (LCAT).

HDL may be further subfractionated by differential ultracentrifugation into HDL_2 (with a density of 1.063 to 1.110 g/mL) and HDL_3 (1.110 to 1.21 g/mL); the former is present in premenopausal women at about three times its concentration in men. Persons with lower HDL_2 levels are apparently more susceptible to premature CHD.

Other Lipoproteins

Floating beta-lipoprotein, or beta-migrating VLDL.

The lipoprotein fraction called *floating beta-lipoprotein* is found in persons with type III hyperlipoproteinemia, or "broad-beta disease" (derived from the broad smear from beta- to pre-beta-lipoprotein regions frequently present on whole plasma lipoprotein electrophoresis in these subjects); the condition is also called *dysbeta-lipoproteinemia*.[12] This fraction has a density of 1.006 g/mL, which is a VLDL characteristic, but has a beta-lipoprotein migration pattern. The abnormal lipid composition of VLDL in type III hyperlipoproteinemic persons is attributable to a proportionately larger amount of cholesterol in that fraction. This is considered to be a very atherogenic lipoprotein; most individuals with this lipoprotein disorder die of CHD by 20 to 30 years of age.[12]

Type III hyperlipoproteinemia is a very rare genetic disorder, affecting approximately 1 in 10,000 individuals, or less than 0.1% of the population. A hallmark clinical presentation of this disease is palmar xanthoma (also called *xanthoma striatum palmare*). Occasionally, tuberous or tuberoeruptive xanthomas occur on the arms and, less frequently, on the buttocks. In addition to premature CHD, dysbeta-lipoproteinemia causes cerebral and peripheral vascular disease. This biochemical abnormality is reflected by an increase in IDL and chylomicron remnants, a VLDL cholesterol-to-VLDL triglycerides ratio greater than 0.35, and an isoelectric focusing pattern demonstrating the presence of the E-II/E-II apolipoprotein isoform, which is presently the definitive diagnostic test.

Lp(a), or sinking pre-beta-lipoprotein.

Similarities in lipid composition, concentration, and density (1.05 to 1.10 g/mL) between Lp(a) and LDL prevented clear discrimination of these two lipoproteins until immunological tests demonstrated the uniqueness of their protein moieties. Apo B-100 makes up 65% of Lp(a) protein, but another 15% is albumin, and the remainder is an apoprotein unique to Lp(a), called *apo Lp(a)*. Lp(a) structurally resembles LDL and the apo B protein is connected to the apo Lp(a) by disulfide bridges. It is polymorphic in size and has several isomers. Despite its high frequency in the population, the functional significance of this lipoprotein is still not entirely clear. However, it is known that Lp(a) competes with plasma plasminogen for the latter's binding sites, resulting in decreased synthesis of plasmin and inhibition of fibrinolysis. Thus Lp(a) may have a role in thrombogenesis. It also plays a role in atherogenesis by causing cholesterol deposition in the arterial wall, inducing monocyte-chemotactic activity in the arterial wall subendothelial space, enhancing foam cell formation, and promoting smooth muscle cell proliferation (see below).

From a pathological standpoint, there is increasing evidence that high Lp(a) levels (i.e., greater than 300 mg/L) are associated with an elevated risk for CHD.[15] It appears that a person can have a normal LDL cholesterol but an elevated Lp(a) concentration and be at increased risk for CHD. Most perspective studies have demonstrated that Lp(a) is a primary, and independent CHD risk factor that aggravates the coronary risk exerted by elevated LDL cholesterol, low HDL cholesterol, hypertension, or the combined effects of multiple risk factors (e.g., smoking, hypertriglyceridemias, diabetes, angina pectoris, and a family history for premature MI). Persons with elevated levels of Lp(a) and a familial history of hypercholesterolemia are at very high risk for premature CHD. Although about a third of Americans have normal or low Lp(a) levels (less than 100 mg/L), about 50% have elevated levels. The elevation of Lp(a) occurs early in childhood and persists throughout adulthood. Lp(a) increases are seen in postmenopausal women and especially in African-American males. Lp(a) levels are not affected by any dietary intervention techniques and are not responsive to most lipid-lowering therapies, except for use of nicotinic acid and exercise. Estrogen, hormonal-replacement therapy, thyroxine, growth hormone, nicotinic acid, ACE inhibitors, neomycin sulfate, *N*-acetylcysteine, and fish oil appear to have the ability to decrease Lp(a) concentration.

Lipoprotein X. Although lipoprotein X has a flotation density similar to that of LDL, the lipid and protein compositions are quite different, and this abnormal lipoprotein migrates in an electrophoretically different manner from LDL. Lipoprotein X is characterized by an unusually high proportion of plasma phospholipid and unesterified cholesterol and by a low protein content consisting of Apo B, Apo C, and albumin. Electrophoretically, Lp-X migrates in the opposite direction from the conventional lipoproteins on an agar support medium. On the new high-definition agar support media, Lp-X migrates as a slow-migrating beta-lipoprotein (a lipoprotein cathodal to the beta lipoprotein band) and is found most characteristically in plasma of patients with biliary obstruction. Lp-X is not found in healthy persons but is often found in patients with a familial deficiency of the enzyme LCAT and in patients with obstructive liver disease. Lp-X has been used in Europe for differentiating cholestasis from hepatic parenchymal disease. However, it is not a useful marker for differentiating extrahepatic from intrahepatic cholestasis.

LIPOPROTEIN METABOLISM
Chylomicrons

As discussed previously, chylomicrons are made exclusively in the intestine and traverse the lymphatic system to the thoracic duct where they then enter the systemic circulation. The major function of the chylomicron is the transport of dietary or exogenous triglycerides. It is postulated that the newly synthesized and secreted chylomicrons (80 to 500 nm) from the intestinal mucosal cells ultimately pick up Apo C-II from HDL. Apo C-II then catalyzes lipoprotein triglyceride hydrolysis by lipoprotein lipase. The hydrolysis results in the liberation of FFAs and monoglycerides.

As shown in Fig. 33-1, endothelial cell lipoprotein lipase-catalyzed hydrolysis results in progressive triglyceride depletion of the chylomicron molecule, resulting in the chylomicron remnant particle. This transformation involves maintenance of lipoprotein structure by simultaneous removal of phospholipid, unesterified cholesterol, and Apo C peptides from the lipoprotein surface to plasma HDL. A reciprocal transfer of cholesteryl ester from HDL may occur; Apo D may aid in this transfer process. The chylomicron remnant particle is then released from the capillary wall and cleared from circulation through the liver, where it is metabolized. This particle, now smaller (30 to 80 nm), retains its cholesteryl ester and Apo B and Apo E, which play an important role in the uptake of these particles by a high-affinity hepatic receptor uptake mechanism (see Fig. 33-4). When binding occurs, the remnants are immediately internalized by receptor-mediated endocytosis and degraded in hepatic lysosomes.

Very–Low-Density Lipoprotein

After the postprandial rise in chylomicron triglyceride, a secondary rise in triglyceride concentration occurs 4 to 6 hours after a meal. This represents predominantly hepatic VLDL triglyceride synthesized from glucose and chylomicron triglyceride not hydrolyzed in the peripheral tissue. The relative contributions of glucose and dietary fat vary with diet composition. Consumption of a high-carbohydrate diet may lead to a phenomenon known as *carbohydrate-induced hypertriglyceridemia*. With high dietary carbohydrate, glucose influx into the hepatocyte is in excess both of energy demands and of glycogen-storage capacity. This results in the shunting of acetyl CoA into fatty acid synthesis and dihydroxyacetone phosphate into activated glycerol.

This phenomenon may not persist in healthy persons, but others may be unusually susceptible to carbohydrate induction of VLDL synthesis. This is the basis for reduction of dietary carbohydrate (simple sugars and alcohol) in the treatment of hypertriglyceridemia, but this approach is not successful if the hypertriglyceridemia has other causes, such as overproduction or a clearance defect. Normally, VLDLs represent about 10% to 15% of the total circulating lipoproteins in a normal healthy individual.

VLDL triglycerides are believed to have a fate similar to that of the lipids from chylomicrons (see Chylomicron Catabolism, p. 605, and just above). During the catabolism of VLDL, more than 90% of Apo C is transferred to HDL, whereas essentially all the Apo B remains with the original lipoprotein particle. According to this postulated catabolic pathway, breakdown of VLDL leads to the formation of the cholesterol-rich particle LDL. HDL plays an important role by serving as an acceptor macromolecule for Apo C and unesterified cholesterol and phospholipids, the excess surface materials from a saturated VLDL. Apo C may recycle from HDL to newly synthesized chylomicrons or VLDL. The half-life of VLDL is 1 to 3 hours.

Intermediate-Density Lipoprotein

Intermediate-density lipoprotein (IDL) is a transient particle (22 to 28 nm) usually present in very low concentrations in plasma from fasting persons. IDL, as discussed previously, is a lipoprotein derived from VLDL catabolism. The HDL particles interact with the plasma enzyme LCAT, which esterifies the excess HDL free cholesterol with fatty acids derived from the carbon-2 position of lecithin, the major phospholipid of plasma. The newly synthesized cholesteryl ester is transferred back to the IDL particles from HDL, apparently through the action of a plasma cholesteryl ester exchange protein (possibly Apo D). The net result of the coupled lipolysis and exchange reactions is the replacement of most of the original triglyceride core of VLDL with cholesteryl ester.

After lipolysis, the IDL particles are released from the capillary wall into the circulation. They then undergo a further conversion in which most of the remaining triglycerides are removed and all the apoproteins except Apo B are lost. The resultant particle, which contains almost pure cholesteryl ester in the core and Apo B at the surface, is LDL.

Low-Density Lipoprotein

As discussed previously, LDL formation occurs primarily from the catabolism of VLDL. In normal healthy persons, LDL cholesterol constitutes about two thirds of the total plasma cholesterol; LDL cholesterol concentration in women is slightly less than that in men (except after menopause). LDL delivers cholesterol to extrahepatic tissues (and to the liver), where it is used, deposited, or excreted.

Delivery of the LDL particles to peripheral tissue is accomplished when the LDL binds to high-affinity receptors located in regions of the plasma membrane called *coated pits*. These pits invaginate into the cell and pinch off to form endocytic vesicles that carry the LDL to the lysosomes (see Fig. 33-4). Fusion of the vesicle membrane with the lysosomal membrane exposes the LDL to a host of hydrolytic enzymes, which degrade the Apo B to amino acids. The cholesteryl esters are hydrolyzed by an acid lipase, and liberated free cholesterol leaves the lysosomes for use in cellular reactions. As a result of this uptake mechanism, extrahepatic cells have low rates of cholesterol synthesis, relying instead on LDL-derived cholesterol. The free cholesterol thus released is used for membrane synthesis and serves to regulate, that is, depress cellular cholesterol synthesis by HMG-CoA reductase. LDL internalization also regulates synthesis of the LDL receptor itself.

Excess cholesterol activates the enzyme acyl-CoA:cholesterol acyltransferase (ACAT), leading to intracellular cholesteryl ester storage. Thus the net result of LDL binding and internalization is the reciprocal inhibition and activation of enzymes synthesizing and storing cellular cholesterol and a reduction in the number of receptors available to bind LDL.

The significance of this process for regulation of plasma cholesterol levels in humans is illustrated by patients with the homozygous form of familial hypercholesterolemia. These patients are deficient in LDL receptors and have excessive LDL production and defective LDL catabolism because of an inability of tissues to bind, internalize, degrade, and thus regulate cholesterol synthesis. Except for the receptor-deficient state of familial hypercholesterolemia, however, the role of the LDL receptor in the final control of plasma cholesterol levels is uncertain and is probably only complementary to other regulatory processes. It has been recognized that the specificity of the LDL receptor extends to lipoproteins containing Apo E and Apo B as well. It appears that although extrahepatic receptors take up LDL readily, hepatic receptors take up chylomicron remnants with greater efficiency (about 20 times greater) and LDL with much less efficiency. This difference is probably attributable to the Apo E content of chylomicron remnants and IDL, which has a higher receptor affinity than that of Apo B.

In addition to its normal degradation mechanism, the high-affinity LDL receptor pathway, plasma LDL can be degraded by less efficient mechanisms that require high plasma levels to achieve significant rates of removal. One of these mechanisms occurs in scavenger cells (macrophages) of the reticuloendothelial system. When the plasma level of LDL rises, these scavenger cells degrade increasing amounts of LDL. When macrophages are overloaded with cholesteryl esters, they are converted into foam cells, which are classic components of atherosclerotic plaques (see below). In humans, estimates of the proportion of plasma LDL degraded by the LDL receptor system range from 33% to 66%. The remainder is degraded by the scavenger cell system and perhaps by other mechanisms not yet elucidated.

High-Density Lipoprotein

Nascent HDL molecules are synthesized in intestinal mucosal cells and in hepatocytes by a process analogous to that of VLDL and chylomicron synthesis. This involves microsomal lipid and protein synthesis followed by secretion. During the synthetic process, phospholipid and free cholesterol are combined with specific apoproteins to form disk-like structures that undergo extensive compositional and structural modifications after secretion. The most important of these modifications is the esterification of free cholesterol to form cholesteryl ester by an enzymatic reaction catalyzed by LCAT. In humans this is the major source of plasma ester cholesteryl. Persons with LCAT deficiency have an accumulation of these cholesteryl ester-deficient particles in plasma. This finding possibly indicates that the cholesteryl ester formed in the LCAT reaction allows the expansion of the disk-like structures to form spheres characteristic of normal plasma HDL. Cholesteryl ester thus formed may be transferred to VLDL during catabolism.

The apoprotein profile of nascent HDL is modified concomitantly with changes in lipid content. Apo E is a major component of newly secreted (nascent) HDL, unlike the plasma HDL, which is characterized by a predominance of Apo A with minor contributions by Apo C and Apo E. The functional significance of this modification is not completely understood, but Apo A-I is an activator of LCAT, and its acquisition must facilitate all LCAT reactions. In addition, HDL participates in the regulation of triglyceride catabolism and cholesteryl ester formation by providing the respective cofactors, Apo C-II for activation and Apo C-III for inhibition of lipoprotein lipase activity. Also, normal HDL may balance LDL transport by mediating cholesterol removal from peripheral sites to degradative and excretory sites. This role of HDL in reverse cholesterol transport may be the basis for the protection afforded by HDL against cardiovascular disease. Like the other lipoprotein classes, HDL is a class of lipoproteins with size polymorphism. It appears that the HDL_2 is more protective to arterial wall damage than HDL_3

The plasma half-life of HDL in normal subjects ranges from 3.3 to 5.8 days. The Apo A-I catabolism and Apo A-II catabolism within HDL are similar. HDL catabolism is enhanced in nephrotic patients but decreased in hypertriglyceridemic subjects, especially those with hyperchylomicronemia. It is also increased in subjects on high-carbohydrate diets and is greatly enhanced in patients with familial HDL deficiency (Tangier disease). It appears that changes in HDL catabolism may play a major role in regulating HDL levels in plasma.

HYPERLIPIDEMIA

By definition, hyperlipidemia is an elevated concentration of lipids in the blood. The major plasma lipids of interest are total cholesterol (free cholesterol + cholesteryl ester) and the triglycerides. When one or more of these major classes of plasma lipids is elevated, a condition referred to as *hyperlipidemia* exists.

Cholesterol and triglyceride concentrations can be used to detect hyperlipoproteinemia. Over 90% of persons with hyperlipidemia, as defined previously, have hyperlipoproteinemia. The major exceptions are individuals with excessive amounts of LDL whose plasma cholesterol is kept within normal limits by a concomitant decrease in HDL.

Just over a decade ago, the NIH suggested that treatment for hyperlipidemia in the United States should be initiated when an adult has a serum cholesterol level above 2000 mg/L.[8,11] The new ATP III guidelines[9] have lowered the upper limit for *normal* (minimal risk for CHD) to <1500 mg/L. Triglyceride levels of 1500 to 1990 mg/L are considered *borderline high*, whereas levels of 2000 to 4990 mg/L are considered *high*. Values greater than 5000 mg/L are considered *very high* levels and can be considered undesirable because of the increased risk for acute pancreatitis.[10,11] Dietary therapy, weight reduction, and increased physical activity should be initiated when these limits are exceeded in order to prevent or minimize the development of CHD. In rare cases, triglyceride-lowering drugs (fibrate or nicotinic acid) can be used. Elevated triglycerides are an independent CHD risk factor and some triglyceride-rich lipoprotein are atherogenic, particularly the partially degraded VLDL (commonly called *remnant lipoproteins*). Type 2 diabetics have what is called *diabetic dyslipidemia*, a disorder involving elevated triglycerides, low HDL cholesterol, or both. Aggressive treatment should be sought because of the atherogenic nature of this type of dyslipidemia.

HYPERLIPOPROTEINEMIA

Hyperlipoproteinemia is an elevation of serum lipoprotein concentrations. The classification of hyperlipoproteinemia begins with the determination of the type of abnormal lipoprotein profile.[1-3,8,9,11-16] However, other differentiation and analyses, such as the following, are necessary:

1. Separation of hyperlipoproteinemia into primary and secondary forms (Table 33-2). The secondary form is caused by another known disease that can result in secondary hyperlipoproteinemia manifesting itself in any of the five major types of lipoprotein profiles.
2. Differentiation of primary hyperlipoproteinemia into heritable and nonheritable forms.
3. Determination of the relative concentration of the lipoprotein fractions, that is, VLDL cholesterol, LDL cholesterol, and HDL cholesterol.

There are numerous types of hyperlipoproteinemias, but the majority of patients with heritable hyperlipidemia have one of six common abnormal lipoprotein patterns. These patterns are summarized in Fig. 33-8, which illustrates that three of the four lipoprotein families serve as determinants. These three families are (1) chylomicrons, (2) VLDL, and (3) LDL (including IDL). The original Fredrickson phenotyping system[1,2] disregarded the importance of HDL and other lipoproteins discussed in this chapter. For a current understanding of the use of lipoprotein profiling for the assessment of CHD risk, refer to the new guidelines from NCEP ATP III,[9] discussed in detail elsewhere in this chapter.

TABLE 33-2 CAUSES OF SECONDARY HYPERLIPOPROTEINEMIA	
Pattern	**Causes**
Hyperchylomicronemia	Insulinopenic diabetes mellitus
	Dysglobulinemia
	Lupus erythematosus
	Pancreatitis
Hyperbeta-lipoproteinemia	Nephrotic syndrome
	Hypothyroidism
	Obstructive liver disease
	Porphyria
	Multiple myeloma
	Portal cirrhosis
	Viral hepatitis, acute phase
	Myxedema
	Stress
	Anorexia nervosa
	Idiopathic hypercalcemia
Dysbeta-lipoproteinemia	Hypothyroidism
	Dysgammaglobulinemia
	Myxedema
	Primary biliary cirrhosis
	Diabetic acidosis
Hyperpre-beta-lipoproteinemia	Diabetes mellitus
	Nephrotic syndrome
	Pregnancy
	Hormone use (oral contraceptives)
	Glycogen-storage disease
	Alcoholism
	Gaucher's disease
	Niemann-Pick disease
	Pancreatitis
	Hypothyroidism
	Dysglobulinemia
Mixed type of lipoproteinemia	Insulinopenic diabetes mellitus
	Nephrotic syndrome
	Alcoholism
	Myeloma
	Idiopathic hypercalcemia
	Pancreatitis
	Macroglobulinemia
	Diabetes mellitus (insulin-independent)

CLASSIFICATION OF HYPERLIPOPROTEINEMIAS

Although the classification of hyperlipoproteinemia is based on identification of elevated concentration of blood lipids and abnormal lipoprotein patterns (Fig. 33-8), it must be emphasized again that each form of dyslipoproteinemia is not a homogeneous entity from a genetic, clinical, or pathological point of view.

The hyperlipoproteinemias are now described in somewhat greater detail, with emphasis on distinctive clinical, diagnostic, genetic, biochemical-pathophysiological, and therapeutic aspects.[1-4,8,9,11-16]

	Electrophoretic pattern	24 hr standing plasma (4° C)	Choles-terol	Triglyc-erides	Dietary management	Drugs
Hyperchylo-micronemia (very rare)	Chylomicrons↑↑↑ chylo β pre β α ⊢— migration —→ +	Creamy layer over clear plasma	↔↕	↑↑↑	1. Restriction of fat to about 35 g/day 2. Supplementation with medium-chain triglycerides 3. Restriction of alcohol intake	None effective at present
Hyperbeta-lipoprotein-emia (common)	LDL↑↑↑ β pre β α	Clear	↑↑↑	↔	1. Low-cholesterol diet (less than 300 mg/day) 2. Decreased intake of saturated fats (S) 3. Increased intake of polyun-saturated fats (P) 4. P/S ratio: 1.0-1.2	1. Cholestyramine, 16-24 g/day 2. Nicotinic acid, 3 g/day 3. Probucol, 1g/day 4. Colestipol, 4-6 sachets/day 5. Mevacor, 10-40 mg/day 6. Zocor, 5-40 mg/day 7. Pravachol, 10-40 mg/day 8. Lescol, 20-40 mg/day
Combined hyperlipo-proteinemia (common)	LDL↑↑↑ VLDL↑ β pre β α	Clear to slighty cloudy	↑↑↑	↑	1. Reduction to ideal body weight 2. Low-cholesterol diet (less than 300 mg/day) 3. Decreased intake of saturated fats (S) 4. Increased intake of polyun-saturated fats (P) 5. P/S ratio 1.0-1.2	1. Cholestyramine, 16-24 g/day 2. Nicotinic acid, 3 g/day 3. Lopid, 600-1200 mg/day 4. Probucol, 1g/day 5. Colestipol, 4-6 sachets/day 5. Mevacor, 10-40 mg/day 6. Zocor, 5-40 mg/day 7. Pravachol, 10-40 mg/day 8. Lescol, 20-40 mg/day
Dysbeta-lipoprotein-emia (very rare)	β-VLDL, LDL of abnormal composition β pre β α	Slighty cloudy to cloudy	↑↑	↑↑	1. Reduction to ideal body weight 2. Low-cholesterol diet (less than 300 mg/day) 3. Decreased intake of saturated fats 4. Restriction of alcohol intake	1. Clofibrate, 2 g/day
Hyperpre-betalipo-proteinemia (very common)	VLDL↑↑↑ β pre β α	Clear, cloudy, or milky	↔↕	↑↑↑	1. Reduction to ideal body weight 2. Carbohydrates restricted to 40% of calories 3. Substitute polyunsaturated fats for saturated fats 4. Restrict alcohol intake 5. Reduce cholesterol intake to 300-400 mg/day	1. Nicotinic acid, 3 g/day 2. Lopid, 600-1200 mg/day
Mixed hyperlipo-proteinemia (rare)	Chylomicrons↑↑ VLDL↑↑↑ chylo β pre β α	Creamy layer over milky plasma	↑↑↑	↑↑	1. Reduction to ideal body weight 2. Reduction of fat to 30% of daily calories 3. Alcohol not recommended 4. Reduce cholesterol intake to 300-400 mg/day	1. Nicotinic acid, 3 g/day 2. Clofibrate, 2 g/day 3. Oxandrolone, 2.5 mg/day 4. Lopid, 600-1200 mg/day

Fig. 33-8   Summary of six types of hyperlipoproteinemias. Abbreviations as in Fig. 33-7.

Hyperchylomicronemia

This lipoprotein disorder is characterized by highly elevated plasma triglyceride concentration, generally greater than 10,000 mg/L, as the result of chylomicronemia. The occasional elevation in cholesterol is secondary to the pronounced elevation in chylomicron levels, since these particles also contain cholesterol. LDL and HDL are often low, whereas VLDL may be slightly elevated. Chylomicron removal is reduced, and subjects have deficiencies in lipase activities, such as postheparin lipolytic activity (PHLA) (specifically, extrahepatic, protamine-inactivated lipoprotein lipase). Primary hyperchylomicronemia usually manifests itself early in childhood. Although this disorder is usually primary and familial, the lipoprotein pattern may be produced by several other disease or metabolic states. Thus secondary forms of this dyslipoproteinemia should be ruled out (see Table 33-2).

Once the obvious secondary causes have been ruled out, the primary disorder can be confirmed by (1) presence of eruptive xanthomas, hepatosplenomegaly, lipemia retinalis, abdominal pain, and pancreatitis early in life, (2) intake of drugs that can cause secondary hypertriglyceridemia, (3) presence of reduced plasma levels of triglyceride lipases, (4) reduction in triglyceride levels and disappearance of chylomicronemia on a fat-free diet, and (5) confirmation by family screening of inheritance as an autosomal recessive trait.

Current lipid-lowering drugs are not effective in lowering serum triglycerides; therefore only a low-fat diet is effective in treating this disorder. Because chylomicrons are produced as a response to the ingestion of fat in the diet, the therapeutic approach is to reduce the amount of dietary fat to 15% of total calories. This intervention technique can result in a decrease in serum triglycerides within 24 hours. The primary goal is to decrease serum triglycerides to less than 5000 mg/L to reduce the patient's risk for acute pancreatitis. The secondary goal is to further reduce triglyceride levels to normalize the HDL-cholesterol levels. The NECP recommendation[10,11] for healthy triglyceride levels is less than 1500 mg/L (Table 33-3).

TABLE 33-3 National Cholesterol Education Program Recommendations for Triglyceride Classification of Risk

Triglyceride (mg/L)*	Risk
Less than 1500	Normal
1510 to 1990	Borderline high
2000 to 4990	High
Greater than 5000	Very high

*To convert mg/L of triglyceride to mmol/L, divide by 886.
From Adult Treatment Panel III: Executive summary of the third report of the National Cholesterol Education Program (NCEP) expert panel on detection, evaluation, and treatment of high blood cholesterol in adults, JAMA 285:2486, 2001.

Hyperbeta-lipoproteinemia

The lipoprotein disorder hyperbeta-lipoproteinemia is characterized by elevated concentration of plasma cholesterol with mostly normal triglyceride levels and clear plasma. Primary hypercholesterolemia can be caused by (1) overproduction of VLDL, (2) increased rate of conversion of VLDL to LDL, (3) LDL enriched with cholesteryl esters, (4) defective LDL structure, and (5) decreased LDL receptor number or activity on each cell. It is estimated that about 50% of the variability in blood cholesterol concentrations in the general population is genetic in basis. The lipoprotein pattern is characterized by an elevation of the LDL with normal VLDL. This lipoprotein disorder is recognized as familial hypercholesterolemia, which exhibits the following features: (1) a deficient number of functional LDL receptors in the fibroblast cultures (the pathognomonic feature), (2) an expression of this lipoprotein disorder in infancy, (3) xanthomatosis in severely affected members, and (4) premature CHD seen by the third and fourth decade.

Before primary hypercholesterolemia can be confirmed, investigators should rule out secondary hyperbetalipoproteinemic disorders, such as hypothyroidism, acute intermittent porphyria syndrome, dysgammaglobulinemia, and obstructive liver disease, as well as factors such as obesity, physical inactivity, and highly saturated fat and cholesterol diets.

Once secondary hyperlipoproteinemia has been ruled out, the primary disorder can be confirmed by (1) family screening, including children; (2) persistent hypercholesterolemia even after 8 weeks on a low-cholesterol (less than 300 mg/day), high–polyunsaturated-fat diet (polyunsaturated fat-to-saturated fat [P/S] ratio of 1:1.2); (3) presence of tendinous xanthomas, xanthelasma, and corneal arcus; and (4) determination of LDL receptor defect or deficiency or other genetically determined molecular defects.

Special treatment is often required for the highly elevated cholesterol levels of familial hypercholesterolemic (FH) individuals (5000 to 15,000 mg/L). In addition to the customary diet and drug approach (see below), most FH patients require plasmapheresis every 3 to 4 weeks for removal of LDL. In extreme cases, liver transplants are required. For non-FH individuals, a *therapeutic lifestyle change (TLC)* is the first treatment step. The TLC diet requires a reduction in saturated fat and cholesterol intake. If high triglycerides, low HDL cholesterol, or a metabolic syndrome are a problem, TLC also stresses weight reduction and physical activity. If the diet cannot sufficiently reduce serum cholesterol, lipid-lowering drugs should be used.

The goal of diet therapy is to reduce serum LDL cholesterol while maintaining a nutritionally adequate diet. The recommended dietary approach can be found in the NECP adult treatment panel (ATP) reports.[8, 9,11] The ATP guidelines recommend two steps of intervention: the step I and step II diets. These diets progressively reduce the intake of total and saturated fat and cholesterol and promote weight loss in patients who are overweight. The step diets reduce other risks for CHD by lowering blood pressure, raising

HDL-cholesterol levels, and reducing the risks for diabetes. LDL- and HDL-cholesterol levels should be monitored after 4 to 6 weeks and then 3 months after beginning step I diet therapy. If the cholesterol goals are not yet achieved, the patient may progress to the step II diet. If the step II intervention still does not achieve the cholesterol goals, drug therapy should be considered. The cholesterol-lowering agents include bile acid sequestrants (cholestyramine or cholestipol), HMG-CoA reductase inhibitors (such as lovastatin [Mevacor], pravastatin [Pravacol], simvastatin [Zocor], fluvastatin [Lescol], atorvastatin (Lipitor), nicotinic acid, and probucol. The effect of lipid-lowering drug therapy should be monitored at 4 to 6 weeks and then again at 3 months.

Combined Hyperlipoproteinemia

Another form of familial hyperlipidemia is combined hyperlipidemia, which is characterized by the following features: (1) no abnormality in the number of functional LDL receptors in the fibroblast culture, (2) absence of the hyperbetalipoproteinemic pattern in children, (3) early expression of hypertriglyceridemia, (4) multiple lipoprotein patterns in affected relatives in successive generations, and (5) hypercholesterolemia in the common hyperbetalipoproteinemic pattern.

Combined hyperlipidemia is the most common of the primary hyperlipoproteinemias. The characteristic feature of this disorder is a scatter of lipoprotein phenotypes within a family. Most commonly, patients have an elevation in both LDL and VLDL; however, within a family, hyperbetalipoproteinemia and hyperpre-beta-lipoproteinemia is also found, affecting different persons. In contrast to familial hyperbeta-lipoproteinemia, patients with familial combined hyperlipoproteinemia generally do not manifest their disease until adulthood. Clinically, these patients have an increased incidence of coronary artery disease (CAD). They also frequently have diabetes, show a tendency for hyperuricemia, and have a low incidence of tendinitis and tuberous xanthomas. These features are suggestive of a closer clinical relation to familial hyperpre-beta-lipoproteinemia than to familial hyperbeta-lipoproteinemia. While the mode of inheritance of combined hyperlipoproteinemia is still in doubt, it is clear that this lipoprotein pattern is a familialy inherited disorder. Remember that patients with hyperbetalipoproteinemia or hyperpre-beta-lipoproteinemia may also be members of a family that has familial combined hyperlipoproteinemia.

Combined hyperlipoproteinemia is further characterized by elevated total cholesterol, LDL cholesterol, triglycerides, and VLDL cholesterol with the absence of floating betalipoprotein. Any secondary hypercholesterolemia and hypertriglyceridemia should be ruled out before confirmation of the primary lipoprotein disorder. Family screening is mandatory for recognition of this lipid abnormality. Accurate diagnosis of the lipoprotein profile also requires an appreciation of the factors that determine triglyceride levels. Studies in free-living populations in the United States have documented increases in triglyceride levels with age and have indicated that as many as one fourth of middle-aged men have triglyceride levels that exceeded previously published cutoff values. Thus, although statistically valid, the critical limits for triglyceride concentrations may not represent physiological limits. Therefore investigators might expect a greater prevalence of combined hyperlipoproteinemia in older age groups.

The possible effects of dietary carbohydrates should not be overlooked when assessing this lipoprotein disorder. It has been shown that fasting hypertriglyceridemia in patients with this metabolic lipoprotein profile could be attributable to an acute increase in dietary carbohydrates. It appears that triglyceride values greater than 4000 mg/L are rare in patients with this lipoprotein pattern. The few reported cases in the medical literature occurred in postmenopausal women.

Lipoprotein electrophoresis is rarely necessary for the diagnosis of this pattern. If the hyperbetalipoprotein profile is present, the elevated cholesterol and the normal triglyceride levels leave little for the lipoprotein electrophoretic pattern to clarify. If the familial combined hyperlipidemic pattern is present, the decisive diagnostic procedure is differentiation of this pattern from either the broad-beta pattern or hyperprebetalipoproteinemic pattern. This task is not easily accomplished with lipoprotein electrophoresis. Also note that the total plasma cholesterol may be normal despite an elevated LDL cholesterol value. This relationship also occurs in familial hypercholesterolemia.

The broad-beta pattern described below is no longer considered unique and has been noted in cases homozygous for familial hypercholesterolemia. The presence of a discrete band attributable to high concentrations of Lp(a), or "sinking" pre-beta-lipoprotein, can cause diagnostic confusion with the familial combined hyperlipidemic profile. When the triglyceride value is normal, the appearance of the broad-beta pattern of electrophoresis is suggestive of the presence of Lp(a). Thus the electrophoretic pattern is insensitive and is not a highly specific tool for differentiating patterns.

Treatment for combined hyperlipoproteinemia should focus on decreasing both the LDL cholesterol and the triglyceride concentrations. The strategy for lowering LDL cholesterol is discussed in the section on hyperbetalipoproteinemia (p. 620). The lowering of triglycerides and VLDL cholesterol is somewhat different. From a dietary standpoint, the focus is on carbohydrates and calories (if the patient is overweight), alcoholic restriction, increased physical activity, and achieving an ideal body weight. Drug therapy is generally indicated in patients with very high triglyceride concentrations (see Table 33-3).[10,11] Both clofibrate and gemfibrozil are effective in lowering triglycerides (thus lowering VLDL or VLDL cholesterol). The drug of choice for combined hyperlipoproteinemia is nicotinic acid, since it is very effective in lowering both cholesterol (LDL cholesterol) and triglycerides (VLDL cholesterol) while increasing HDL cholesterol.

Dysbeta-lipoproteinemia

Dysbeta-lipoproteinemia (also called *broad-beta hyperlipo-proteinemia*) is characterized by an elevation of both plasma cholesterol and triglyceride concentrations and an abnormal LDL (more specifically IDL), which floats in the fraction with a density of 1.006 to 1.019 g/mL. This abnormal LDL often merges with the pre-beta band on electrophoresis to produce a broad-beta band (see Fig. 33-8). For accurate diagnosis of dysbeta-lipoproteinemia, an ultracentrifugal study with measurement of cholesterol and triglyceride in the fractions with a density below 1.006 g/mL is required to document the presence of the floating beta-lipoprotein.

Measurements of the lipid composition of lipoproteins with a density less than 1.006 appear to offer a more reliable means of identifying this dyslipoproteinemia than is afforded by the detection of the presence of floating beta-lipoproteins by electrophoresis alone. The ratio used clinically is that of the cholesterol content of the VLDL divided by the plasma triglyceride concentration. This ratio appears to be most useful for documenting this hyper-lipoproteinemia when the triglyceride level is at least 1500 mg/L, but it may be subject to error when triglyceride exceeds 10,000 mg/L. It has been suggested that if the VLDL cholesterol–to–triglyceride ratio is 0.30 or more, the subject may have dysbeta-lipoproteinemia. However, when the ratio is between 0.25 and 0.29, a diagnosis of possible broad-beta hyperlipoproteinemia should be considered. Confirmation of this disorder is made by finding an apoE isoform pattern of E_2-E_2.

The clinical characteristics of patients with this lipoprotein disorder vary widely as a function of age, sex, degree of adiposity, and presence of associated disorders such as hypothyroidism and alcoholism.

The most characteristic xanthoma in subjects with broad-beta-lipoproteinemia is called *xanthoma striatum palmare* (in the literature, the improper Latin forms *xanthoma striatum palmaris* and *xanthoma striata palmaris* are also used). In their most subtle form these lesions produce an orange or yellowish discoloration of the palmar creases (xanthochromia striata palmaris), a phenomenon most easily detected in patients of fair complexion. When more advanced, these lesions may produce planar elevations and even the virtual obliteration of the palmar and digital creases. Raised lesions can occasionally affect the remaining palmar surfaces and in the severe form produce tuberous, incapacitating xanthomas.

Various forms of CHD have been reported in association with broad-beta hyperlipoproteinemia, which is readily treated by diet and drugs. The form of cardiovascular disease associated with this form of dyslipoproteinemia differs significantly from that associated with familial hyperbeta-lipoproteinemia in that peripheral and even cerebrovascular disease appears to be as common as CHD.

Secondary broad-beta hyperlipoproteinemia has been associated with hypothyroidism, gout, and diabetes mellitus and is found in patients with acute renal failure receiving maintenance hemodialysis.

Hyperpre-beta-lipoproteinemia

The pre-beta form of hyperlipoproteinemia has also been called *endogenous hyperlipemia*, or *carbohydrate-induced hyperlipemia*. The latter term is no longer accepted by most investigators, since carbohydrate induction of hypertrigly-ceridemia is also observed in normolipemic individuals. Endogenous hyperlipemia excludes the rare hyperchylo-micronemia but includes the uncommon mixed endogenous and exogenous hyperlipemia (see below).

By definition, hyperpre-beta-lipoproteinemia is an eleva-tion of VLDL (and triglyceride) levels above an arbitrary cutoff point in the absence of either chylomicrons or the abnormal VLDL of dysbeta-lipoproteinemia. LDL levels are normal, and LDL cholesterol measurement is normal.

A tentative diagnosis of this lipoprotein disorder may be made if the triglyceride concentration is increased, the total cholesterol is normal or moderately elevated, and the standing plasma (at 4° C for 10 to 12 hours) reveals no chylomicrons. The biochemical diagnosis is confirmed if electrophoresis reveals a distinct pre-beta-lipoprotein band and the LDL cholesterol is within normal limits. Keep in mind that the presence of a pre-beta band with normal plasma triglyceride levels occurs with "sinking" pre-beta-lipoprotein, a trigly-ceride-poor, apparently normal lipoprotein variant observed in up to 35% of healthy subjects.

Once the biochemical pattern of hyperpre-beta-lipo-proteinemia has been confirmed (i.e., based on more than one sample under standard conditions), it should be classified according to cause as a primary, either familial or sporadic, or secondary disorder (see Table 33-2).

The diagnosis of the primary disorder depends on the following criteria: (1) a hyperprebetalipoproteinemic electro-phoretic pattern, (2) an increase in VLDL cholesterol, (3) one or more first-degree relatives with this disorder, and (4) no close relative with other primary lipoprotein disorders. Other common features are a normal cholesterol level if the triglyceride level is less than 4000 mg/L, a triglyceride level usually below 15,000 mg/L, and a family history of diabetes.

Since a large proportion of our society imbibes alcohol, a brief consideration of its connection to hyperlipidemia is warranted. Although not regarded as a major cause of hyper-lipidemia, ethanol is known to cause acute but transient hypertriglyceridemia with an elevation in primarily VLDL, causing mainly hyperpre-beta-lipoproteinemia (sometimes mixed hyperlipoproteinemia). In the hypertriglyceridemia produced by ethanol intake, the following features stand out:

1. The hypertriglyceridemia is usually moderate in extent and limited in duration. The level of triglyceridemia rarely exceeds 10,000 mg/L, and the lipemia peaks in 12 to 14 hours and disappears after 25 to 40 hours. This apparently transient effect appears to hold true, especially for normolipemic individuals.
2. This hypertriglyceridemia is, for the most part, the result of increased VLDL and possibly chylomicrons.
3. The fatty liver associated with alcohol intake plays a vital role in the form and extent of the induced

hyperlipoproteinemia, and the resultant changes may be related to the stage of the hepatic damage.

The triglyceride concentration in alcoholic hyperlipidemia is intimately related to the quality and quantity of dietary fatty acid intake. It is well known that simultaneous ingestion of ethanol with fat (as in complex meals or singly as corn oil) produces a prolonged and augmented rise in serum triglyceride concentration.

Although it is obvious that hyperlipemia can be produced by an excessive production and release of lipids (hence lipoproteins) into circulation, by defective removal or clearance of lipids from the blood, or by a combination of these physiological processes, the precise mechanism of ethanol-induced hyperlipemia is still unknown.

The treatment protocol is described in the section on combined hyperlipoproteinemia (p. 621).

Mixed Hyperlipoproteinemia

Another form of hyperchylomicronemia is mixed hyperlipoproteinemia, which is distinguished by the presence of both elevated VLDL and chylomicrons in the plasma of fasting subjects on a regular diet. This disorder can occur as a primary genetic defect; thus it represents a second form of familial hyperchylomicronemia. Triglyceride levels similar to those seen in hyperchylomicronemia may be observed. As in that disorder, the occurrence of abdominal syndromes such as pancreatitis and the physical findings of eruptive xanthomas, lipemia retinalis, and hepatosplenomegaly are related to the level of plasma triglyceride. Although the pathophysiological characteristics of these manifestations probably do not differ from those observed in hyperchylomicronemia, a variety of other differences exist in clinical, genetic, metabolic, and biochemical observations.

In sharp contrast to hyperchylomicronemia, most instances of mixed hyperlipoproteinemia occur in adulthood, although several children with familial hyperlipoproteinemia have been described. Full appearance of the abnormality may not occur until the fifth or sixth decade of life, with females presenting at a later age than males.

Extremely high triglycerides and hyperchylomicronemia are usually not attributable to primary metabolic disorders but are found in the setting of several disorders that can lead to secondary metabolic disorder. These disorders are particularly prone to produce this form of dyslipoproteinemia if they occur in patients with primary hyperprebeta-lipoproteinemias. For example, pancreatitis may be associated with pronounced hyperchylomicronemia, but later when the patient is reevaluated under stable conditions, only mild hypertriglyceridemia may be found. It is also well known that hyperpre-beta-lipoproteinemia can present as this disorder in patients with poorly controlled, insulin-dependent diabetes and in patients with alcoholism.

Although mixed hyperlipoproteinemia is associated with elevated triglycerides (i.e., VLDL and chylomicrons), plasma cholesterol concentrations may be slightly to moderately increased. LDL and HDL cholesterols are usually normal to low. The plasma is usually opaque, and a floating cream layer above the turbid plasma may be observed.

When total triglyceride is over 10,000 mg/L, visual appreciation of a discrete floating "creamy" supernate over turbid plasma becomes difficult. The use of ultracentrifugation (to remove the chylomicrons) or refrigeration test (separation of chylomicrons after standing overnight at $4°$ C) will help differentiate this form of hyperlipoproteinemia. The ultracentrifuge may be used to separate the chylomicrons from the VLDL for individual quantification if needed. A qualitative assessment of the electrophoresis strip is sometimes sufficient to document elevated VLDL and chylomicrons. Since in practice some overlap of VLDL levels may occur between these two lipoprotein patterns, a postheparin lipoprotein lipase measurement should be made as a final characterization. This enzyme should be present in mixed hyperlipoproteinemia. In the absence of a specific assay for the enzyme, a reasonably reliable clue to its presence may be sought by observation of the change in the lipoprotein electrophoresis pattern obtained with a plasma sample drawn 10 minutes after heparin injection (10 U/kg of body weight). The plasma cholesterol-to-triglyceride ratio in this form of dyslipoproteinemia (0.23 ± 0.02) is usually lower than in hyperpre-beta-lipoproteinemia (0.86 ± 0.03) because the chylomicrons incorporate less cholesterol than the VLDL does. Major qualitative difficulties can arise in distinguishing this lipoprotein disorder from hyperpre-beta-lipoproteinemia (endogenous hypertriglyceridemia) because this pattern is often transient, with many subjects losing their chylomicron band with moderate reductions in triglyceride.

Mixed hyperlipoproteinemia is often secondary to a wide variety of diseases, drugs, and dietary habits (see Table 33-2). Since there are many ways of acquiring this form of hyperlipoproteinemia, a careful distinction between primary and secondary causes must be made. A routine history of ethanol intake and estrogen or steroid administration, a urinalysis, and the measurement of a fasting or 2-hour postprandial blood glucose, and liver, thyroid, and renal function tests are all useful in this distinction. Superimposition of poorly controlled diabetes mellitus, excessive alcohol intake, or use of estrogens or estrogen-containing oral contraceptives in an individual with preexisting hyperpre-beta-lipoproteinemia will often produce the mixed pattern. In familial cases, particularly with plasma triglycerides above 15,000 mg/L, lipemia retinalis, hepatosplenomegaly, and eruptive xanthomas may be present.

The biochemical defect in this form of hyperlipoproteinemia is still not clear. The presence of high levels of chylomicrons in the fasting plasma of a subject whose diet contains a usual or low content of fat clearly indicates that clearance mechanisms are inadequate. A primary defect in removal of plasma triglyceride could also explain the elevated VLDL. Establishing that this defect is not simply a variant of hyperchylomicronemia is accomplished by detecting and often quantitating heparin-releasable plasma PHLA from these patients. Thus a different type of problem must lead to this failure in lipoprotein uptake. One possibility is that the synthesis of endogenous triglyceride and the resulting secretion of VLDL from the liver may proceed at an abnormally high rate, sufficient to saturate pathways of removal that are shared by chylomicrons, thereby leading to an elevation of both lipoproteins. Studies using lipoproteins labeled with radioisotopes have indicated that many patients with endogenous hypertriglyceridemia have elevated synthesis of VLDL triglyceride.

Familial hyperchylomicronemia may be divided into hyperchylomicronemia and a mixed form of hyperlipoproteinemia. Both disorders are manifested by significantly elevated triglyceride levels and frequently present with eruptive xanthomas, lipemia retinalis, hepatosplenomegaly, and abdominal pain. Hyperchylomicronemia is caused by a pronounced deficiency of lipoprotein lipase. The triglyceride elevation appears with ingestion of dietary fat and is thus manifested in very young children. The mixed form may be detected in rare instances in childhood, but the usual presentation is in the adult. Mixed hyperlipoproteinemia also differs from hyperchylomicronemia in that lipoprotein lipase is measurable and glucose intolerance and hyperuricemia are commonly associated findings. The only effective treatment for hyperchylomicronemia is a low-fat diet, whereas the mixed form of hyperlipoproteinemia is most effectively treated by diet-induced weight loss and will frequently respond to one of the following drugs: nicotinic acid, norethindrone, oxandrolone, benzafibrate, gemfibrozil, or clofibrate.

Metabolic Syndrome

The ATP III guidelines[9] describe a new disorder called *metabolic syndrome*,[17] which is a constellation of lipid and nonlipid risk factors of metabolic origin. This syndrome is closely linked to a generalized metabolic disorder called *insulin resistance*, in which the normal actions of insulin are impaired (see Chapter 32). Factors characteristic of metabolic syndrome are listed in the following box.

According to a recent survey,[17] metabolic syndrome is highly prevalent in the United States. Among men, whites and Mexican Americans had the highest age-adjusted prevalences of abdominal obesity, hypertriglyceridemia, and low HDL cholesterol concentration. African American men had the highest age-adjusted prevalence of hypertension, and Mexican American men had the highest age-adjusted prevalence of hyperglycemia. Among women, Mexican

Americans and African Americans had the highest age-adjusted prevalence of abdominal obesity. African American women had the highest age-adjusted prevalence of high blood pressure, and Mexican American women had the highest age-adjusted prevalences of hypertriglyceridemia, low HDL cholesterol, and hyperglycemia. The overall, age-adjusted prevalence of metabolic syndrome is 24% in the U.S. population.

The ATP III recognizes metabolic syndrome as a secondary target of risk-reduction therapy after the primary target (LDL cholesterol, see p. 633). The management of metabolic syndrome has a two-fold objective: (1) to reduce the underlying causes (such as obesity and physical inactivity) and (2) to treat associated nonlipid and lipid risk factors. The first-line therapies are weight reduction and increased physical activity, which will effectively reduce the risk factors. Thus, after appropriate control of LDL cholesterol, total cholesterol reduction should focus on weight loss and physical activity.

TRANSFORMATION OF HYPERLIPIDEMIA TO HYPERLIPOPROTEINEMIA
Limitation of Classification of Types of Hyperlipoproteinemia

The limitations and potentials of the lipoprotein-typing system of Frederickson, Levy, and Lees are well recognized.[1,2] However, it should be stressed that plasma lipoprotein patterns are not a substitute for an etiological classification of the hyperlipoproteinemias. The approach of Fredrickson, Lees, and Levy is to be regarded as provisional, pending a more fundamental understanding of the causes of the hyperlipidemias.

Using quantitative measurements of cholesterol and triglyceride alone, we can divide patients into three major groups: those with hypercholesterolemia alone, those with hypertriglyceridemia alone, and those with a combination of the two. Subjects with pure hypercholesterolemia usually have the hyperbetalipoproteinemic pattern and those with pure hypertriglyceridemia without chylomicrons, the hyperprebetalipoproteinemic pattern. Subjects with relatively high cholesterol and triglyceride levels may have dysbetalipoproteinemic or hyperprebetalipoproteinemic patterns or profiles. Although lipoprotein typing is no longer considered necessary or important today, there may be four areas in which the lipoprotein-typing system retains general validity for clinical research purposes:

1. Lipoprotein patterns are useful in sharpening the focus on the diverse metabolic abnormalities that underlie hyperlipidemia.
2. The types of hyperlipoproteinemias so identified are not disease states but are the result of disorders that similarly affect the concentrations of particular lipoproteins.
3. Each lipoprotein type is often associated with certain distinctive clinical features.
4. Each lipoprotein type, irrespective of cause, is generally more successfully handled by a specific diet and therapeutic approach.

FACTORS CHARACTERISTIC OF METABOLIC SYNDROME

Abdominal obesity
Atherogenic dyslipidemia
Elevated triglycerides, small LDL particles, low HDL cholesterol
Raised blood pressure
Insulin resistance (with or without glucose intolerance)
Prothrombotic and proinflammatory states

The lipoprotein-typing system has four major limitations:

1. For distinction of dysbeta-lipoproteinemia, the diagnosis requires substantiation by determination of the ratio of cholesterol in VLDL divided by the VLDL triglyceride, as well as electrophoretic confirmation of beta-migrating VLDL. In addition, in subjects with mixed elevations of cholesterol and triglyceride, quantitation of LDL (LDL cholesterol) is important for accurate distinction.

2. The lipoprotein-typing system has limitations in genetics. No specific type of hyperlipoproteinemia should be considered genotypic; lipid and lipoprotein determinations cannot provide the diagnosis of a specific genetic disorder in a single patient; and increasing evidence suggests strong heterogeneity in lipoprotein patterns in first-degree relatives from families with monogenic familial hyperlipidemia.

3. The lipoprotein-typing system does not cover the evaluation of alpha-lipoprotein. It is now known that a low concentration of HDL cholesterol is an independent risk factor for coronary heart disease, and genetic abnormalities such as hypoalpha-lipoproteinemia, although rare, do exist.

4. Finally, present electrophoretic systems are limited in their ability to resolve other unusual lipoprotein fractions, such as lipoprotein variants, beta-migrating VLDL, and IDL.

From Lipids to Lipoproteins: Laboratory Considerations

In the transformation of hyperlipidemia to hyperlipoproteinemia, lipid analyses and the overnight refrigeration test can be used to determine the lipoprotein profile with a fair degree of accuracy. If the plasma is clear, the triglyceride level is most likely to be either normal or near normal (less than 2000 mg/L). When triglyceride increases to about 3000 mg/L or higher, the plasma is usually hazy to turbid in appearance and is not translucent enough to allow for clear reading of newsprint through the tube. When plasma triglyceride is over 10,000 mg/L, the plasma is usually opaque and milky (lipemic, lactescent). If chylomicrons are present, after an overnight incubation at 4° C a thick homogeneous "cream" layer may be observed floating at the plasma surface. As summarized in Fig. 33-8, a uniformly opaque plasma sample usually denotes a hyperpre-beta-lipoproteinemia. An opaque plasma sample with a cream layer on top is usually consistent with the mixed form of hyperlipoproteinemia. A thick chylomicron cream layer with generally clear plasma infranate is usually consistent with a hyperchylomicronemic profile.

In patients with hypercholesterolemia without hypertriglyceridemia, most often with raised LDL levels, the plasma is clear but may have an orange-yellow tint, since carotene is carried with LDL. After a visual observation that is "simple and free," the diagnosis of the lipid abnormality can be made in as many as 90% of subjects by quantitation of plasma cholesterol and triglyceride alone.

The NECP ATP recommended protocol for the laboratory analyses needed to effectively assess CHD risk and detect common lipoprotein abnormalities includes measurement of total cholesterol, triglycerides, and LDL and HDL cholesterol.[9,13,14] These measurements can be performed by most clinical laboratories (see Methods in CD-ROM). More demanding analytical techniques, such as analytical ultracentrifugation or apolipoprotein and lipoprotein subfraction measurements, may be needed to differentiate atypical lipoprotein abnormalities; these are usually available in specialized research laboratories. LDL cholesterol levels can be measured by use of the preparative ultracentrifuge, but they can be routinely measured directly and are more inexpensively and conveniently estimated by the Friedewald formula:

$$\text{LDL cholesterol} = \text{total cholesterol} - (\text{triglyceride}/5 + \text{HDL cholesterol})$$

This estimation requires measurement of HDL cholesterol by various precipitation techniques and is accurate in patients whose triglycerides are less than 4000 mg/L. Triglyceride concentrations over 4000 mg/L lead to an inconsistency in the VLDL triglyceride calculated value, that is, the VLDL cholesterol-to-triglyceride ratio does not permit division by a fixed number, and the formula cannot be used with great accuracy. In addition, hypertriglyceridemia is a major cause of inaccurate measurements of HDL-cholesterol measured by precipitation methods. The reason is that the triglyceride-rich, Apo B-containing lipoproteins are incompletely precipitated, resulting in falsely elevated HDL cholesterol values.

Secondary Hyperlipoproteinemia

In general, lipoprotein quantification and typing alone will not distinguish the primary from the secondary form of hyperlipoproteinemia (see Table 33-2). Even the diagnosis of a concurrent disorder that is likely to cause secondary hyperlipoproteinemia does not necessarily establish it as the cause of a patient's hyperlipoproteinemia. Reversal of the lipid abnormality accompanying treatment of the suspected causative disorder, however, is compelling evidence of the secondary nature of the hyperlipoproteinemia. Failure of such reversal to occur implies that the hyperlipoproteinemia may be primary and indicates the need for family screening.

Some disorders associated with hyperlipoproteinemia will be obvious from the patient's history and physical examination. Others will require blood or urine tests for diagnosis. If such a screening reveals no abnormalities, it is reasonable to assume that the patient has primary hyperlipoproteinemia. Whether or not the hyperlipoproteinemia is established as familial in origin depends on the results of the family screening.

Other Forms of Dyslipoproteinemias

In the familial lipoprotein disorders discussed in this chapter, one or more of the four lipoprotein fractions (chylomicron, VLDL, beta-migrating VLDL, and LDL) are present in elevated concentrations.

However, there are other lipoprotein abnormalities in addition to the hyperlipoproteinemias reviewed so far. Three genetically determined disorders exist in which one or more of the lipoprotein families are absent from plasma or occur in concentrations that are extremely low.[1] The first of these to be discovered was *abeta-lipoproteinemia*, in which chylomicrons, VLDL, and LDL are missing. The probable inherited defect is one involving synthesis of the major protein moiety of LDL, Apo B. Another disease is *hypobeta-lipoproteinemia* (familial LDL deficiency), in which no lipoproteins are missing but LDL concentrations are far below normal. In the third disorder, *familial hypoalpha-lipoproteinemia*, HDL circulates but contains an abnormal proportion of the two major HDL apolipoproteins. A defect in the synthesis of Apo A-I is the probable locus affected by this rare mutation. With this abnormal high-density lipoprotein, patients with Tangier disease have low plasma HDL concentration, store cholesteryl esters in most parts of the body, and often have neuropathic changes for reasons that are not understood. Their large orange tonsils are an unmistakable feature of the syndrome. All these diseases are usually detected initially because of a common manifestation, hypocholesterolemia.

Finally, although not classified as a dyslipoproteinemia, *hyperalpha-lipoproteinemia* is a condition in which the HDL is elevated in the blood beyond two standard deviations for a given age and sex. This condition is under genetic influence, and these persons appear to have a longer life-span than those with "normal" concentrations of HDL. There are no other clinical symptoms associated with this lipoprotein feature. A more detailed discussion of each of these lipoprotein abnormalities is provided below.

Abeta-lipoproteinemia. The rare disorder abeta-lipoproteinemia has five basic features: undetectable plasma LDL concentration, malabsorption of fat, acanthocytosis, retinitis pigmentosa, and ataxic neuropathic disease. These features, however, are not specific for this lipoprotein condition. Acanthocytosis may occur in other diseases in which lipoproteins are not deficient. In abeta-lipoproteinemia LDL is absent, not merely deficient. The plasma cholesterol concentration does not exceed 800 mg/L and is likely to be no higher than 300 mg/L. This is accompanied by concentrations of triglycerides lower than those seen in any other disease, usually less than 200 mg/L. The total phospholipid concentration is also low, that is, less than 1000 mg/L. Both the phospholipid partition and the fatty acid composition of the plasma lipids are abnormal and are frequently reflected in similar abnormalities in erythrocytes and adipose tissue. The gastrointestinal problems of patients with abeta-lipoproteinemia are stereotypical. Fat malabsorption is present from birth, and the neonatal period is characterized by poor appetite, vomiting, loose voluminous stools, and little weight gain. The neuromuscular manifestations of abeta-lipoproteinemia are devastating. The cause of the neuromuscular abnormalities in abeta-lipoproteinemia is obscure. Attention has focused on the abnormal amount of ceroid pigment (lipofuscin) in the cerebellum and other tissues in this disorder.

Abeta-lipoproteinemia involves a functional disturbance in fat transport. Chylomicrons never enter the plasma, and net transport of endogenous glycerides in VLDL appears to be either absent or sustained at some unchanging minimum level. Heavy feeding of carbohydrate for days, which promotes a brisk rise in the level of plasma glycerides and VLDL in patients with Tangier disease and in nearly all other subjects, fails to do so in patients with abeta-lipoproteinemia. The defect in abeta-lipoproteinemia is not known, although the most likely problem is a failure to synthesize Apo B. The intracellular assembly point of Apo B–containing lipoprotein is another possible site of dysfunction, or the defect may possibly lie in the secretion process. Whichever of these defects may be primary, none of them explains the many secondary manifestations of the disease.

Diagnosis of abeta-lipoproteinemia can be made in a patient with one of the abnormalities listed at the beginning of this section. The possibility of dysglobulinemia producing antibodies to LDL should also be kept in mind. The single most important laboratory test for screening is the plasma cholesterol determination. The finding of a subnormal value, particularly any concentration below 1000 mg/L, should be followed by a triglyceride determination and lipoprotein electrophoresis. The definitive diagnosis depends on immunochemical demonstration of the absence of LDL Apo B in the plasma. In all patients in whom the diagnosis is made, it is also important to check, in all obligate heterozygotes, the concentration of LDL by immunochemical or ultracentrifugal analysis. In familial hypobeta-lipoproteinemia, the heterozygote has lower-than-normal concentrations of LDL and Apo B.

Hypobeta-lipoproteinemia. Apparently unrelated to abeta-lipoproteinemia, hypobeta-lipoproteinemia is a genetic disorder in which plasma LDL concentrations are present at about one tenth of normal concentrations. This lipoprotein abnormality is inherited as an autosomal dominant trait. The plasma total cholesterol concentrations can be as low as those seen in abeta-lipoproteinemia. The percentage of cholesterol esterified is normal. The triglyceride levels may be well within the normal range, but sometimes these are in the lower limits of accurate measurement. The phospholipid concentrations may vary from 100 to 1800 mg/L and are usually in the low-normal borderline region in most patients. Vitamin A and E concentrations are normal or low but, if low, are not decreased to the level seen in abeta-lipoproteinemia. A faint beta-lipoprotein band is visible on electrophoresis. HDL concentrations as measured by precipitation, preparative ultracentrifuge, or analytic ultracentrifuge are normal; VLDL is usually modestly reduced but is present.

LDL is present in serum as measured by immunoprecipitin tests. These measurements have suggested concentrations of LDL that are one eighth to one sixteenth of normal.

Hypoalpha-lipoproteinemia or an alpha-lipoproteinemia. Tangier disease (familial HDL deficiency) is characterized by severe deficiency or absence of normal HDL in plasma and by the accumulation of cholesteryl esters in many tissues throughout the body, including liver, spleen, lymph nodes, thymus, intestinal mucosa, skin, and cornea. A combination of two features is pathognomonic: (1) a low plasma cholesterol concentration in combination with normal or elevated triglyceride levels and (2) hyperplastic orange-yellow tonsils and adenoid tissue. Some persons may exhibit peripheral neuropathy. The small amounts of HDL in Tangier plasma differ qualitatively and quantitatively from normal HDL, particularly with respect to apolipoprotein content (Apo A-I). The disorder appears to be attributable to an autosomal recessive gene affecting HDL synthesis or catabolism. Heterozygotes in families with known homozygotes can usually be identified by low HDL concentrations (50% below normal); they do not develop neuropathy and cholesteryl ester accumulation. Among the lipoprotein-deficiency states (indeed, among all known diseases), the combination of very low cholesterol and elevated triglyceride concentrations gives Tangier disease a unique signature. Some patients may have normal triglyceride levels in the postabsorptive state, however, and may superficially resemble those with LDL deficiency. The plasma total cholesterol level ranges from about 400 to 1250 mg/L, within the range also observed in abeta-lipoproteinemia and hypobeta-lipoproteinemia. Individual variation in the plasma triglyceride levels is considerable and is highly contingent on diet. Substitution of carbohydrate for fat often paradoxically lowers the plasma triglyceride concentration in this disorder. The plasma lipoprotein pattern is distinctive: the alpha-lipoprotein band is absent, irrespective of the support medium used. Immunoelectrophoresis may occasionally generate a faint precipitin line of alpha-globulin mobility against anti-HDL antiserum. Most useful for detecting the small amounts of the A apoproteins is immunoanalysis of plasma with specific antiserums to the A-I and A-II apolipoproteins. The reactivity with anti–Apo A-II is generally stronger than with anti–Apo A-I. Estimation of the cholesterol content of the plasma lipoproteins after sequential preparative ultracentrifugation or after ultracentrifugation and selective heparin-manganese precipitation confirms the paucity of HDL.

In addition to HDL absence or deficiency, the following diseases must be excluded:

1. Familial deficiency of LCAT. In this case, HDL is very low, but the plasma cholesterol level is normal or high, and most of the cholesterol is unesterified.
2. Obstructive liver disease, in which the plasma HDL and Apo A may be reduced to levels as low as those seen in Tangier disease. In this disorder the cholesterol level is not low but high, and most of the cholesterol is not esterified. Appropriate tests of liver function should permit the correct diagnosis.
3. Severe malnutrition or hepatic parenchymal disease in which high-density lipoproteins are decreased. The decrease in cholesterol will also be associated with low triglyceride and LDL levels.
4. Acquired HDL deficiency attributable to dysglobulinemia, including possible development of antibodies to HDL.

5. Other storage diseases associated with foam cells and hepatosplenomegaly. In these conditions HDL levels are higher than those seen in Tangier disease, and typical tonsillar abnormalities are absent.

CLINICAL IMPLICATIONS OF HYPERLIPIDEMIA

Why should there be any concern about hyperlipidemia or hyperlipoproteinemia? Hyperlipidemia is usually a symptomless biochemical state that, if present for a sufficiently long time, may be associated with the development of atherosclerosis and its complications, including myocardial infarctions and vascular diseases. Occasionally hyperlipidemia may be associated with specific overt symptoms or signs directly attributable to the presence of hyperlipidemia. Examples are abdominal pain, pancreatitis, and the cutaneous manifestations of hyperlipidemia, such as xanthomas, corneal arcus, and xanthelasmas.

Coronary Artery Disease

Coronary artery disease (CAD) is almost always the result of atherosclerosis—hardening of the arteries. Coronary atherosclerosis primarily results from the accumulation of fatty deposits in the walls of coronary arteries, which leads to the formation of fibrous tissue in the vessel wall. CAD is the most common type of heart disease and the leading cause of death in the United States and many other countries. In the United States, an estimated 50% of the adult deaths each year are attributable to CAD.[7]

CAD affects middle-aged males; nearly 45% of all heart attacks occur in individuals younger than 65 years of age. Coronary heart disease (CHD) develops in men 60 years of age or younger at approximately twice the rate as that of women, while postmenopausal women have a higher incidence of CHD than premenopausal women of the same age.[18] For both men and women, the incidence of coronary vascular disease (CVD) and the rates of death from atherosclerosis increase with advancing age. About 75% of coronary-related mortalities are the result of atherosclerosis. Each year about 1.25 million Americans are afflicted with myocardial infarction, and about 300,000 bypass operations are performed.[19] The estimated annual cost of CHD to the American public is between $42 billion and $88 billion.[20]

Risk factors associated with coronary artery disease. Although the basic cause of CAD is unknown, scientists have identified several factors associated with a distinct increase in the likelihood that a person will develop a heart attack later in life.[20,21] These risk factors, listed in the box on p. 628 and identified as primary or secondary factors, correlate with the presence of CHD. Some risk factors are unavoidable, such as racial and genetic susceptibility, increased prevalence in males, and increased likelihood of having a heart attack as aging occurs. Many known risk factors are, however, susceptible to behavior modification. Particularly important among these are high blood pressure, cigarette smoking, and elevated serum cholesterol, or more significantly, elevated LDL cholesterol. Approximately 50% of persons who experience heart attacks have one or more of

PRIMARY AND SECONDARY RISK FACTORS ASSOCIATED WITH CORONARY HEART DISEASE (CHD)

Primary

Genetic predisposition for CHD
Family history of premature CHD in first-degree relatives
    (<45 years for males, <55 years for females)
Hypertension
Cigarette smoking
Elevated total cholesterol (LDL cholesterol)
Decreased HDL cholesterol
Elevated triglycerides (VLDL cholesterol, remnant
    lipoproteins)
Increasing age
Male gender

Secondary

Lack of exercise
Obesity
Stress
Diabetes mellitus
Elevated lipoprotein(a)
Elevated homocysteine
Elevated intermediate-density lipoproteins
Renal failure patients receiving hemodialysis
Postmenopausal state
Certain thrombogenic disorders

these three risk factors. According to the Framingham data, there is a clear gradient of CHD incidence rates in relation to serum HDL-cholesterol concentrations. Persons with levels below 350 mg/L have eight times the CHD rate of persons with HDL-cholesterol levels of 650 mg/L or greater.

Important additional risk factors include lipoprotein(a) (Lp[a]), oxidized LDL, small lipoprotein particle size (or dense LDL), fibrinogen, homocysteine, specific apolipoproteins (A-I, B, E isoforms), triglyceride-poor remnant lipoproteins, and stress.[22-28] No degree of risk has yet been assigned to these factors. Other possible factors whose relative importance is still being established include hypertriglyceridemia, level of physical activity, and personality types.

ATHEROSCLEROTIC PLAQUE FORMATION

The healthy blood vessel (artery) architecture consists of an *intima*, lined by endothelium on the inner, luminal side of the vessel, which is bound by the internal elastic lamina to the *media* (Fig. 33-9). The outermost layer is the adventitia, which is bound by the external elastic lamina and exterior to the vessel itself. The intima is the site at which the atherosclerotic lesions form. The endothelium serves as a barrier to blood-borne materials and as a site where at least two mitogens are synthesized and secreted (see p. 630). The tunica media is the muscular wall of the artery that consists of smooth muscle cells held together by a discontinuous basement membrane and by interspersed collagen fibrils and proteoglycan.[21,29,30] The smooth muscle cells that proliferate in the arterial intima to form the advanced lesions of atherosclerosis originate in the media. This smooth muscle cell proliferation represents the *sine qua non* of the lesions of advanced atherosclerosis. The smooth muscle cells, like the endothelium and fibroblasts, contain receptors for LDL and PDGF (see below). One characteristic feature of the smooth muscle cells found in the lesions of atherosclerosis is the accumulation of lipids that results in the formation of highly vacuolated cells, or *foam cells*.

Atherosclerotic plaque formation occurs in three progressive stages: (1) the *fatty streaks*, which gradually develop into raised lesions, called *fatty plaques*; (2) the *fibrous plaque*, which has a proliferation of smooth muscle cells and a collagen-rich fibrous cap that covers a lipid core which is lined by foam cells and surrounds an amorphous extracellular accumulation of cholesteryl esters; and (3) the *complicated lesion*, which can manifest calcification, hemorrhage, ulceration (rupture), and thrombosis (Fig. 33-10). It is the complicated lesion that frequently underlies the acute

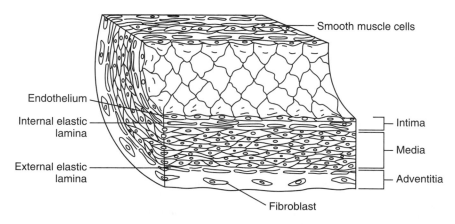

Fig. 33-9   Diagram of a healthy blood vessel (artery) with normal integrity of the intima, media, and adventitia.

clinical event of arterial occlusion that leads to myocardial injury (MI).

The formation and accumulation of foam cells in the intima are the hallmark of the early atherosclerotic lesion. Currently it is believed that most of the foam cells are derived from blood-borne macrophages, though some may come from smooth muscle cells. A pivotal step in the development of foam cells is the accelerated uptake of modified LDL (see below), followed by proliferation of smooth-muscle cells (with and without lipid deposits in their cytoplasm) (Fig. 33-11). The smooth muscle cell proliferation is accompanied by increased synthesis of cellular

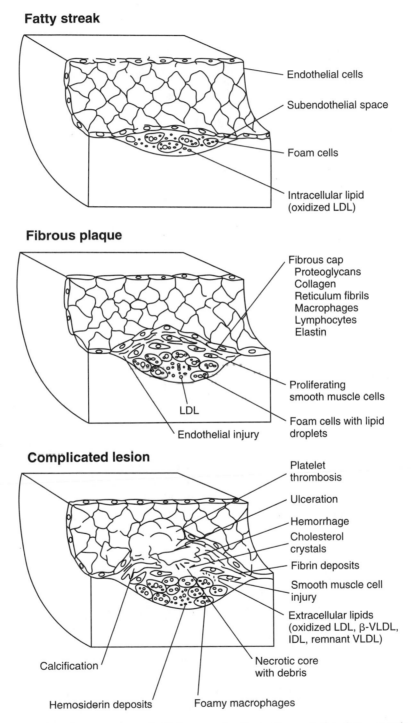

Fatty streak

- Endothelial cells
- Subendothelial space
- Foam cells
- Intracellular lipid (oxidized LDL)

Fibrous plaque

- Fibrous cap
  Proteoglycans
  Collagen
  Reticulum fibrils
  Macrophages
  Lymphocytes
  Elastin
- Proliferating smooth muscle cells
- Foam cells with lipid droplets
- LDL
- Endothelial injury

Complicated lesion

- Platelet thrombosis
- Ulceration
- Hemorrhage
- Cholesterol crystals
- Fibrin deposits
- Smooth muscle cell injury
- Extracellular lipids (oxidized LDL, β-VLDL, IDL, remnant VLDL)
- Necrotic core with debris
- Calcification
- Hemosiderin deposits
- Foamy macrophages

Fig. 33-10 The three stages of atherogenesis: formation of the fatty streak, fibrous plaque, and complicated lesion. Notice the development and accumulation of foam cells in the *fatty streak*, accumulation of smooth muscle cells in the *fibrous plaque*, and formation of calcification, ulceration, thrombosis, and hemorrhage in the advanced or *complicated lesion.*

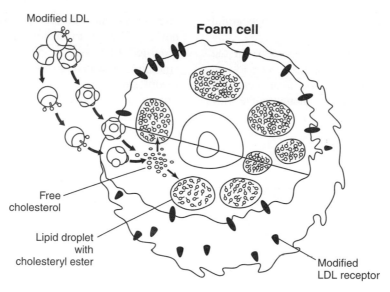

Fig. 33-11   Formation of the foam cell: *macrophage* uptake (ingestion) of *modified LDL* by the modified LDL receptor pathway, which results in the development of large *fat-laden droplets*. This process of foam cell formation is the hallmark of the fatty streak development in atherogenesis.

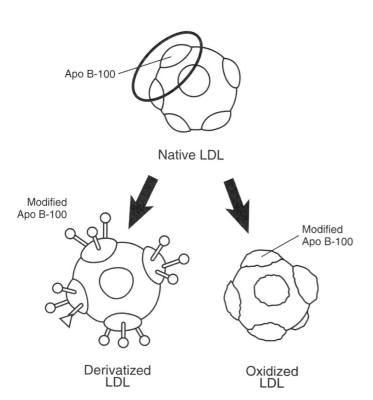

Fig. 33-12   Modification of LDL. Entrapped *native LDL* (in the subendothelial space) can undergo two types of modifications: *derivatization* (malondialdehyde attachment to or glycosylation of Apo B-100) or *oxidation* (degradation of Apo B-100 by superoxides).

elastin, collagen, and proteoglycans, which these cells deposit extracellularly in the developing plaque.

The development of the atherosclerotic lesion is promoted by the secretion of two key blood cells, macrophages and platelets. The macrophages can secrete chemotactic agents (such as interleukin-1, superoxide anion, leukotriene B_4) and growth factors (such as platelet-derived growth factor [PDGF], interleukin-1, fibroblast growth factor, epidermal growth factor, transforming growth factor–β). These two macrophage-derived groups of factors are probably responsible for the promotion of connective tissue proliferation in the blood vessel during the disease process.[21]

The platelets have a smaller role in some atherosclerotic lesions but play a major role in the formation of thrombi. It is usually a mural or occlusive thrombus that leads to an MI. Platelets can also produce the same growth factors as activated macrophages. Thus, at sites of injury in which collagen exposure occurs, numerous vasoactive, stimulatory, and proliferative responses can take place and probably play a role in the initiation of the atherosclerotic lesions.

The initial biochemical step in cell proliferation is the infiltration of lipoproteins (VLDL remnants, LDL, and IDL) into the subendothelial space. Here some lipoproteins are trapped in the intimal ground substance, modified, and ingested by macrophages to form foam cells. The uptake of LDL by the macrophages can be enhanced if the LDL is modified by oxidation or degradation of Apo B by reactive oxygen species (such as free radicals) or via derivitization of the Apo B by glycosylation or through reaction with malonaldehyde[31] (Fig. 33-12).

The fat-laden macrophages, together with varying numbers of lipid-filled smooth muscle cells, develop into the fatty streaks. Most of the lipid in the foam cells is free cholesterol and cholesteryl ester. The fatty streaks are observed early in childhood, and their transformation into the complicated lesions usually takes four to five decades before the appearance of the clinical manifestation of disease, including angina pectoris, MI, or sudden cardiac death.[29] In males, the first MI event usually occurs around 55 years of age, whereas in females there is a 10-year delay, occurring around 65 years of age. This atherosclerotic process can be accelerated by having (1) additional CHD risk factors, (2) endothelial injury, which removes the natural barrier to the entrance of lipoproteins into the arterial wall or causes thrombosis, and (3) a genetic predisposition for primary hypercholesterolemia.

Etiology of Atherosclerotic Lesions

Current thoughts on the pathogenesis of atherosclerotic lesions include the response-to-injury and monoclonal hypotheses. The first theory centers on the premise that an initial injury occurs to the endothelial cell lining of the arterial wall. The endothelial injury, caused by mechanical, chemical, immunological, toxic, or infectious factors, results in an increased uptake of LDL cholesterol. This, in turn, changes the surface characteristics of the endothelial cells and the circulating leukocytes (monocytes and platelets), leading to enhanced adhesion of monocytes to the endothelium.[21] The monocytes are then transformed to macrophages, which now have the ability to take up additional lipids. According to Steinberg et al,[31] oxidized LDL may play a central role in atherogenesis in at least four ways (Fig. 33-13): (1) it acts as a chemoattractant for the blood-borne monocytes to enter the subendothelial space; (2) it causes the transformation of the monocytes to macrophages; (3) it causes the trapping of macrophages in the endothelial spaces by inhibiting their motility; and (4) it is toxic to the endothelial cells. The lipid-laden macrophage forms the foam cells that contribute to the development of the fatty streaks. Also, these activated macrophages can form at least four different growth factors, which may be responsible for the migration of smooth muscle cells and fibroblasts into the intima and for their subsequent proliferation. The platelets, in this hypothesis, are involved in atherogenesis by aggregating and forming mural thrombi at particular anatomical sites where the blood flow properties produce shearing effects and cause some sort of injury to the endothelium. This mechanism causes the platelets to release growth factors (similar to those released by activated macrophages) that may lead to the proliferative smooth muscle atherosclerotic lesions.

Other hemostatic factors have been investigated and have shown to have a reasonable association with ischemic heart disease (IHD).[32] These factors include fibrinogen, factor VII, factor VIII, antithrombin III, plasminogen activator inhibitor 1, Lp(a), and antiphospholipid antibodies. Of these various thrombogenic factors, the most convincing independent risk factor for CVD has been plasma fibrinogen. The Northwick Park Heart Study[32] indicated that the incidence of IHD was more strongly related to fibrinogen levels than to total cholesterol concentrations. The Leigh study[32] also concluded that the association between fibrinogen concentration and IHD was higher than that of total cholesterol, blood pressure, and smoking. Possible mechanisms for the role of fibrinogen as a thrombogenic risk factor include its role as a precursor of fibrin and subsequent thrombosis and its effect on increases in blood viscosity, which affects the blood flow hemodynamic characteristics that can lead to thrombosis.

The second hypothesis associated with the atherogenesis is the monoclonal hypothesis. This premise is based on a single smooth muscle cell that serves as a source of all the cells within the lesion. This benign neoplasm of the arterial wall is derived from a cell that has been transformed by viruses, chemicals, toxins, or some other mutagens.

THE NATIONAL CHOLESTEROL EDUCATION PROGRAM

In the late 1980s, health care workers realized that a unified effort was needed to standardize the approach for the detection and classification of individuals at high risk for CHD and to standardize treatment and monitoring of such individuals. This effort also required a major educational drive to inform both physicians and their patients of CHD risk factors. To fulfill this scientific and educational goal, the federal government and a broad range of professional health care groups worked together to formulate guidelines and recommendations with the intent of reducing CHD in America. This national campaign was called the *National Cholesterol Education Program (NCEP)*.

As a result of this effort, the NIH in 1985[33] and in 1988 (the first NIH Adult Treatment Panel [ATP I[8]of the NCEP]) recommended new medical decision levels for cholesterol and LDL cholesterol. These new guidelines had a significant effect on reducing the CHD morbidity and mortality in the United States, where CHD is still a major disease. To simplify the classification system and to make it more convenient to remember the cutoff levels, the panel eliminated the age and sex stratification once recommended.[33,8] The goals of the NCEP ATP I, II, III programs were to establish criteria that defined the high-risk person for medical intervention and to provide clear guidelines on how to detect, set goals for, treat, and monitor these patients over time. Some of the key features of these landmark reports[8,9,11] on cholesterol are now described.

The ATP I[8] outlined a strategy for primary prevention of CHD in individuals with high levels of LDL cholesterol ($\geq$1600 mg/L) or those with borderline high LDL cholesterol (1300 to 1590 mg/L) and multiple (2+) risk factors. ATP II[11] affirmed the importance of this approach and added a new feature: the intensive management of LDL cholesterol in person with established CHD. For patients with CHD, ATP II[11] set a new, lower LDL cholesterol goal of $\leq$1000 mg/L. ATP III[9] emphasized the need for more intensive LDL-lowering therapy in certain groups of people, in accord with recent clinical trial evidence. The new features of ATP III[9] are as follows:

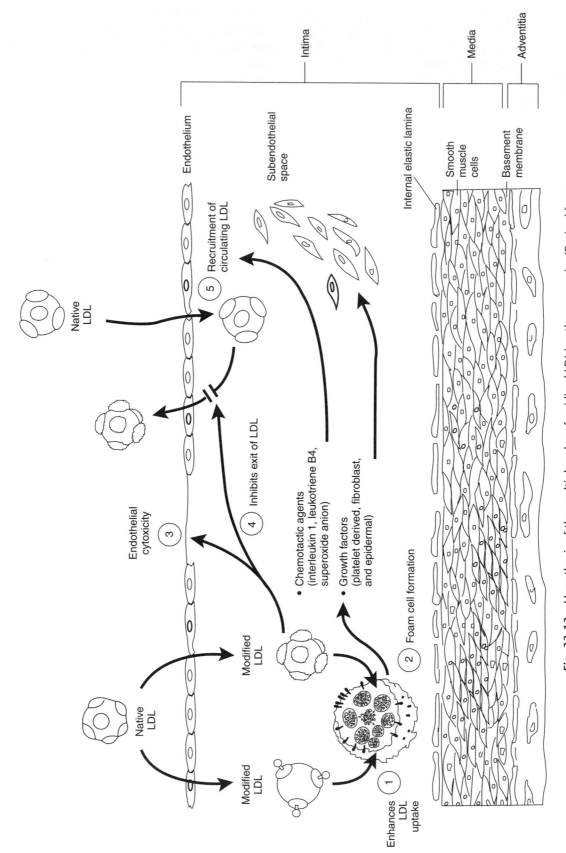

Fig. 33-13 Hypothesis of the multiple roles of *oxidized LDL* in atherogenesis. *(Derived from Steinberg D et al: Beyond cholesterol: modifications of low-density lipoproteins that increase its atherogenicity, N Engl J Med 320:915, 1989.)*

TABLE 33-4 CLASSIFICATIONS OF RISK IN ADULTS BASED ON LOW-DENSITY LIPOPROTEIN CHOLESTEROL

LDL Cholesterol (mg/L)*	Classification of Risk
<1000	Optimal
1000 to 1290	Optimal or above optimal
1300 to 1590	Borderline high
1600 to 1890	High
>1900	Very high

*To convert mg/L of cholesterol to mmol/L, divide by 387 or multiply by 0.002586.
From Adult Treatment Panel III: Executive summary of the third report of the National Cholesterol Education Program (NCEP) expert panel on detection, evaluation, and treatment of high blood cholesterol in adults, JAMA 285:2486, 2001.

- Recommends a complete *lipoprotein profile* (total, LDL, and HDL cholesterol and triglycerides) as the preferred initial test, rather than screening for total cholesterol and HDL cholesterol alone.
- Raises the risk for CHD of individuals with diabetes *without* CHD, most of whom have multiple risk factors, to the risk level of CHD *risk equivalent*, that is, a risk for major coronary events equal to that of established CHD.
- Identifies certain patients with multiple (2+) risk factors as candidates for more intensive treatment.
- Identifies persons with multiple metabolic risk factors (*metabolic syndrome*) as candidates for intensified therapeutic lifestyle changes.
- Identifies LDL cholesterol <1000 mg/L as optimal.
- Raises categorical low HDL cholesterol from <350 mg/L to <400 mg/L.
- Lowers triglyceride classification cutoff point from <2000 mg/L to 1500 mg/L.
- Emphasizes the use of a sliding scale for LDL cholesterol therapeutic goals: zero or one risk factor, <1600 mg/L; two or more risk factors, <1300 mg/L; CHD and CHD risk equivalents, <1000 mg/L.

All adults 20 years of age or older should have a fasting total cholesterol, triglycerides, and lipoprotein profile done every 5 years. For nonfasting individuals, only the values for total cholesterol and HDL cholesterol should be used. If the total cholesterol (≥2000 mg/L) or HDL cholesterol (<400 mg/L) value is abnormal, a follow-up fasting lipoprotein profile is required for the development of therapeutic goals.

The ATP III's more aggressive classification of risk[9] based on total, LDL, HDL cholesterol is defined in Tables 33-4, 33-5, and 33-6. The LDL cholesterol, *not* the total cholesterol, will serve as the primary target of CHD risk assessment and therapy.

Along with lipid and lipoprotein testing, all adults should also be evaluated for the presence or absence of CHD and of

TABLE 33-5 NCEP ATP III RISK CLASSIFICATION FOR HDL CHOLESTEROL LEVELS

Classification of Risk	HDL Cholesterol
Low	<400 mg/L
High	≥600 mg/L

From Adult Treatment Panel III: Executive summary of the third report of the National Cholesterol Education Program (NCEP) expert panel on detection, evaluation, and treatment of high blood cholesterol in adults, JAMA 285:2486, 2001.

TABLE 33-6 RECOMMENDATIONS FROM THE NCEP FOR CHILDREN AND ADOLESCENTS

Total Cholesterol (mg/L)	Classification of Risk	LDL Cholesterol (mg/L)
<1700	Acceptable	<1100
1700 to 1990	Borderline high	1100 to 1290
>2000	High	>1300

NCEP, National Cholesterol Education Program.
From The Expert Panel: Report of the National Cholesterol Education Program Expert Panel on Blood Cholesterol Levels in Children and Adolescents, U.S. Department of Health and Human Services, NIH Publ. No. 91-2732, Bethesda, MD, 1991, U.S. Department of Health and Human Services. Also from Scanu AM: Structural and functional polymorphism of lipoprotein(a): biological and clinical implications, Clin Chem 41:170, 1995.

other major CHD risk factors (Box 33-1, p. 634). The patient is considered to have a *high-risk status* if he or she has any of the following:

1. Definite CHD (i.e., definite prior myocardial infarction or myocardial ischemia)
2. The presence of two or more other CHD risk factors
3. A lipid or lipoprotein abnormality with the presence of one other CHD risk factor

The selection of therapeutic LDL cholesterol intervention strategies requires two additional major therapeutic modalities. The first involves therapeutic lifestyle changes, including a low saturated fat and cholesterol intake diet and/or weight reduction and increased physical activity if the patient has a metabolic syndrome (see p. 624) or life-habit risk factors such as abdominal obesity, atherogenic dyslipidemia (elevated triglyceride, small LDL particles, low HDL cholesterol), elevated blood pressure, insulin resistance (with or without glucose intolerance), and prothrombotic and proinflammatory states. The second major intervention strategy is drug therapy, including statins, bile acid sequestrants, and nicotinic acid.

The ATP III[9] report also emphasizes primary *prevention* of CHD along with LDL-lowering therapy. Therapeutic lifestyle changes are the foundation of clinical primary

BOX 33-1

RISK FACTORS ASSOCIATED WITH THE DEVELOPMENT OF CORONARY HEART DISEASE

Major

Age (years): Male, >45; Female, >55 or premature menopause without estrogen replacement therapy
Family history of premature coronary heart disease
Current cigarette smoking
Hypertension (≥140/90 mm Hg) or on hypertensive medication
Diabetes mellitus
Low HDL cholesterol, <400 mg/L (0.104 mmol/L)

Other

Obesity
Physical inactivity
Atherogenic diet
Elevated Lp(a)
Elevated homocysteine
Elevated triglycerides
Remnant lipoproteins
Metabolic syndrome (high triglycerides, low HDL, abdominal obesity, physical inactivity, insulin resistance, hypertension, high fasting glucose)
Prothrombogenic and proinflammatory factors
Impaired fasting glucose
Subclinical atherosclerotic disease (peripheral arterial disease, abdominal aortic aneurysm, symptomatic carotid artery disease)
Multiple risk factors and 10-year increased risk for CHD

Negative Risk Factors

High HDL cholesterol, >600 mg/L (1.6 mmol/L)

prevention. Nonetheless, some persons at highest risk for CHD, because of high LDL cholesterol concentrations or multiple risk factors, are candidates for LDL-lowering drugs. Secondary prevention with LDL-lowering therapy is also beneficial, and the goal of therapy should be aggressive (i.e., LDL cholesterol <1000 mg/L). Clinical trials have demonstrated that the LDL-lowering therapy reduces total mortality, coronary mortality, major coronary events, coronary artery procedures, and stroke in persons with established CHD. It should be stressed that any person with elevated LDL cholesterol or other form of hyperlipidemia should undergo clinical or laboratory assessment to rule out secondary dyslipidemia before initiation of lipid-lowering therapy.

Additional features of the ATP III report include the following:

- Age (45 years or older for males and 55 years or older in women) is a major CHD risk factor (Box 33-1).
- Delayed use of pharmacological agents for lipid and lipoprotein therapy in most young adult men and premenopausal women with elevated LDL cholesterol levels.
- Enhanced recognition that high-risk postmenopausal women and high-risk older adult patients who are otherwise in good health are candidates for cholesterol-lowering therapy.
- More attention to *HDL cholesterol* as a CHD risk factor, which includes the addition of HDL cholesterol measurements to the initial cholesterol testing. A high HDL cholesterol (greater than 600 mg/L) level has been designated as a negative CHD risk factor, whereas a low HDL cholesterol (less than 400 mg/L) has been designated as a positive CHD risk factor (Table 33-5). In addition, when a physician is selecting a drug for lowering LDL cholesterol, consideration should be given to the effect of the drug on the patient's HDL cholesterol.
- Increased emphasis on *physical activity and weight loss* as components of the dietary therapy of high blood LDL cholesterol.

It should be reiterated that the NCEP ATP strategy is based on the use of *LDL cholesterol* and *HDL cholesterol* as the criteria for the initial classification of the patient's CHD risk, which also depends on other risk factors (Box 33-1) that can influence the final category of risk.

This NIH Expert Panel on Blood Cholesterol Levels in Children and Adolescents[19] recommended the following (see Table 33-6):

- Selective screening of *high-risk children* and *adolescents* who have a *family history of premature cardiovascular disease* or at least one parent with *high blood cholesterol* (>2400 mg/L). Screening was also advocated if the *parents or grandparents*, at 55 years of age or less, underwent diagnostic coronary arteriography and were found to have coronary atherosclerosis. This includes parents or grandparents who have undergone balloon angioplasty or coronary artery bypass surgery or who have suffered a documented MI, angina pectoris, peripheral vascular disease, cerebrovascular disease, or sudden cardiac death.
- *Universal screening* of children and adolescents for high blood cholesterol was *not* advocated.
- The minimum goals of *treatment*—for patients with borderline LDL cholesterol, to lower the level to <1100 mg/L; for patients with high LDL cholesterol, to lower the level to <1300 mg/L. Drug therapy should not be used in children who are less than 10 years of age or in those who have not been prescribed an adequate cholesterol-lowering diet for at least 6 months to 1 year.

The positive and negative CHD risk factors are used as a guide to the type and intensity of cholesterol-lowering therapy that should be used by the physician (Box 33-1). For example, a male patient who is over 45 years or a female patient over 55 years is at higher risk for CHD and should be treated more aggressively. Therefore the goals for lowering serum levels of LDL cholesterol and total cholesterol are more intensive.

It should be stressed that a person with two or more of the positive risk factors listed in Box 33-1 in addition to an elevated LDL cholesterol value would be classified as a high-risk individual for CHD. Keep in mind that a high amount of HDL cholesterol (>600 mg/L) represents a negative risk factor.

Treatment strategies still focus on lowering the high blood level of LDL cholesterol in order to provide primary prevention of CHD.[9] The algorithm of testing and treatment modality for primary prevention in adults *without* evidence of CHD is shown in Figs. 33-14 and 33-15. For example, for a person with a desirable LDL cholesterol (<1000 mg/L), further LDL-lowering therapy is not required. However, emphasis should be placed on controlling other lipid and nonlipid risk factors and on treatment of the metabolic syndrome, if present. If the patient has CHD (or CHD risk equivalents) and an LDL cholesterol level ≥1000 mg/L, three possible approaches are possible:

1. Initiate or intensify *total lifestyle changes (TLC)*—for example, reduction of saturated fat and cholesterol intakes, increased physical activity, weight control—and/or drug therapies specifically to lower LDL cholesterol.
2. Emphasize weight reduction and increased physical activity in persons with the metabolism syndrome.
3. Delay the use or intensification of LDL-lowering

therapies and institute treatment of other lipid risk factors (elevated triglycerides; HDL cholesterol < 400 mg/L) or nonlipid risk factors (see Tables 33-7 and 33-8).

The therapeutic goal is to lower the LDL cholesterol to <1000 mg/L. If the patient has no CHD but has two or more CHD risk factors, intervention should begins if the LDL cholesterol is ≥1300 mg/L. The goal for this patient is to lower the LDL cholesterol to <1300 mg/L. If the patient has no CHD and has fewer than two risk factors, intervention should not begin until the LDL cholesterol is ≥1600 mg/L. The goal for this patient is to lower the LDL cholesterol to <1600 mg/L. For secondary prevention of disease in adults with evidence of CHD or other clinical atherosclerotic disease, lipoprotein analyses are required, and the LDL cholesterol concentration is the key index for classification of CHD risk and therapy. For secondary prevention the optimum LDL cholesterol is <1000 mg/L, a far more aggressive goal than that of the primary prevention group. Persons in this category with LDL cholesterol levels >1000 mg/L should have the appropriate clinical work-up and cholesterol-lowering therapy started.

It cannot be overemphasized that therapy should always start with dietary intervention in order to achieve the LDL cholesterol targets described in Tables 33-4 and 33-6. Weight reduction (if appropriate) and physical activity should be part

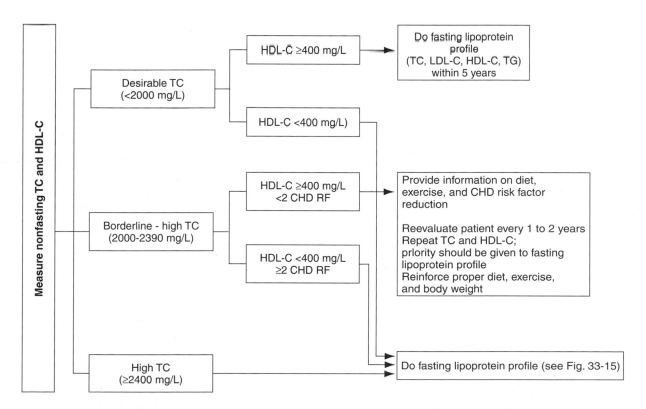

Fig. 33-14 Algorithm of coronary heart disease risk assessment, treatment, and monitoring using the NCEP Adult Treatment Panel III guidelines[52] for primary prevention in adults with and without evidence of CHD. Initial classification of risk is based on nonfasting results of both the *TC* (total cholesterol) and *HDL-C* (high-density lipoprotein cholesterol) concentrations. *RF*, risk factor.

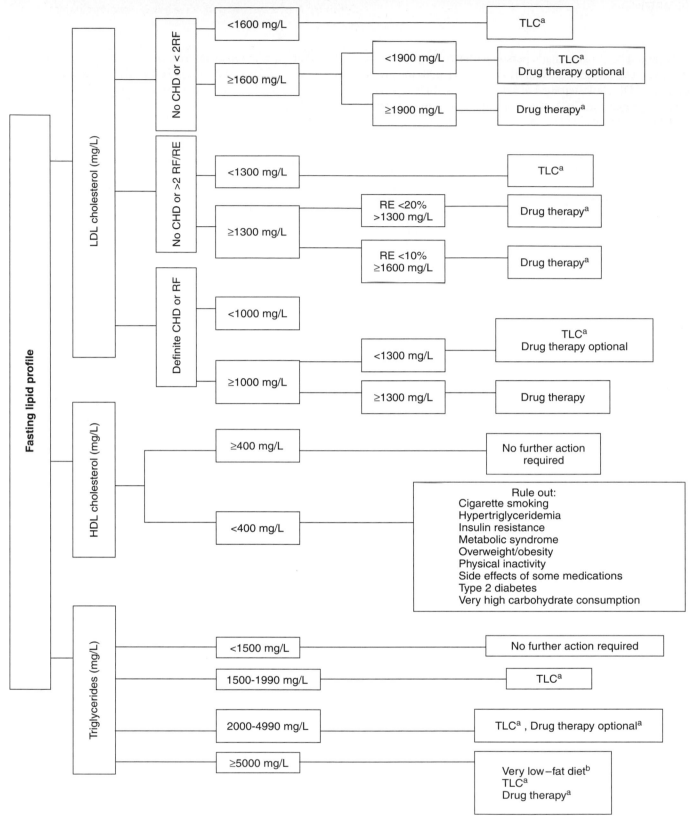

Fig. 33-15 Algorithm of CHD risk assessment, treatment, and monitoring for primary and secondary prevention of CHD in adults with and without evidence of CHD.[14] Classification of risk is based on fasting results on low-density lipoprotein cholesterol (LDL-C), high-density lipoprotein cholesterol (HDL-C), triglycerides (TG) concentrations, and other risk factors. *RF,* Risk factor; *RE,* risk equivalent; *TLC,* therapeutic lifestyle changes. Monitoring LDL cholesterol response to therapy should be evaluated 6, 12, and 16 to 24 weeks after initiation of therapy. If the initial goal is to reduce the risk for acute pancreatitis, rapid reduction of the triglycerides by diet is required; triglyceride monitoring should be done within a few days.

TABLE 33-7   THREE CATEGORIES OF RISK THAT MODIFY LDL CHOLESTEROL GOALS

CHD and Risk Factor Status	LDL Cholesterol Decision Level mg/L (mmol/L)	Treatment Modality
Without CHD and <2 risk factors	>1600 (4.1)	TLC
	>1900 (4.9)	Drug optional
Without CHD and >2 risk factors	>1300 (3.4)	TLC for 3 mo; start drug if LDL is still high
	>1600 (4.1)	Drug
With CHD or CHD risk equivalents	>1000 (2.6)	TLC
	>1300 (3.4)	Drug

TLC, *therapeutic lifestyle changes.*
From Adult Treatment Panel III: Executive summary of the third report of the National Cholesterol Education Program (NCEP) expert panel on detection, evaluation, and treatment of high blood cholesterol in adults, JAMA *285:2486, 2001.*

TABLE 33-8   COMPARISON OF LDL CHOLESTEROL AND NON-HDL CHOLESTEROL GOALS FOR THREE RISK CATEGORIES

Risk Category	LDL-C Goal (mg/L)	Non-HDL C Goal (mg/L)
0 to 1 RF	<1600	<1900
2+ RF and CHD RE ≤20%	<1300	<1600
CHD and CHD RE >20%	<1000	<1900

RF, *risk factor(s);* RE, *risk equivalent (10-year risk for CHD).*
From Adult Treatment Panel III: Executive summary of the third report of the National Cholesterol Education Program (NCEP) expert panel on detection, evaluation, and treatment of high blood cholesterol in adults, JAMA *285:2486, 2001.*

of the intervention process. If the elevated LDL cholesterol persists after an appropriate trial of TLC, drug intervention may be considered. The NCEP report is very specific as to when drug therapy should be used (Table 33-7). More specifically, with fewer than two risk factors, drug intervention should begin only when the LDL cholesterol exceeds 1900 mg/L. If the individual has two or more risk factors or if the 10-year risk is <10%, drug intervention should be initiated if the LDL cholesterol is ≥1600 mg/L; if the 10-year risk is between 10% and 20%, intervention should begin when LDL cholesterol equals or exceeds 1300 mg/L. If the person has CHD or a 10-year risk of greater than 20%, drug intervention should begin when LDL cholesterol is ≥1300 mg/L.

In young adult men (20 to 35 years old) and premenopausal women (20 to 45 years old) who have LDL cholesterol concentrations ≥1300 mg/L, TLC should be instituted. Unlike the ATP II[14] report, which recommended delaying the use of drug therapy, the ATP III[9] guidelines indicate that drugs should be considered when LDL cholesterol is reaches or exceeds 1900 mg/L in young men and women. Young men who smoke and have high LDL cholesterol (1600 to 1890 mg/L) may be candidates for drug intervention. African Americans have the highest overall CHD mortality rate and the highest out-of-hospital coronary death rates of any ethnic group in the United States, particularly at younger ages. However, the present ATP III[9] guidelines do not recommend more aggressive strategies for specific racial and ethnic groups.

Finally, avoid a common mistake when classifying a patient's CHD risk: remember to differentiate secondary from primary dyslipidemias. Some of the more frequently occurring secondary dyslipidemias are listed in Table 33-2. In these cases, it is imperative that the primary condition leading to secondary hyperlipidemia be treated first.

References

1. Fredrickson DS, Lees RS: Familial hyperlipoproteinemia. In Stanbury JB, Wyngaarden JB, Fredrickson DS, editors: *The metabolic basis of inherited disease*, ed 3, New York, 1982, McGraw-Hill.
2. Fredrickson DS, Levy RJ, Lees RS: Fat transport in lipoproteins: an integrated approach to mechanisms and disorders, *N Engl J Med* 276:32, 1967.
3. Gotto AM, Jr., editor: *Plasma lipoproteins*, New York, 1987, Elsevier Science Publishers.
4. Scanu AM, Spector AA, editors: *Biochemistry and biology of plasma lipoproteins*, New York, 1986, Marcel Dekker.
5. Levy RJ et al, editors: *Nutrition, lipids, and coronary heart disease*, New York, 1979, Raven Press.
6. Miller ME, Lewis B, editors: *Lipoproteins, atherosclerosis and coronary heart disease*, New York, 1981, Elsevier Publishing.
7. Naito HK, editor: *Nutrition and heart disease*, New York, 1982, Spectrum Publications, Inc.
8. The Expert Panel: Report of the National Cholesterol Education Program expert panel on detection, evaluation, and treatment of high blood cholesterol in adults, *Arch Intern Med* 148:36, 1988.
9. Adult Treatment Panel III: Executive summary of the third report of the National Cholesterol Education Program (NCEP) expert panel on detection, evaluation, and treatment of high blood cholesterol in adults, *JAMA* 285:2486, 2001.
10. National Heart, Lung, and Blood Institute Consensus Conference on Treatment of Hypertriglyceridemia, *JAMA* 251:1196, 1984.
11. Second Expert Panel: Detection, evaluation, and treatment of high blood cholesterol in adults (Adult Treatment Panel II), *Circulation* 89:1329, 1994.

12. Havel RJ: Familial dysbeta-lipoproteinemia, *Med Clin North Am* 66(2):441, 1982.

13. Lewis LA, Opplt JJ, editors: *Handbook of electrophoresis*, vol 1: *Lipoproteinemia: basic principles and concepts*; vol 2: *Lipoproteins in disease*, Boca Raton, FL, 1980, CRC Press.

14. Lewis LA, editor: *Handbook of electrophoresis*, vol 3: *Lipoprotein methodology and human studies*, Boca Raton, FL, 1983, CRC Press.

15. Scanu AM: Structural and functional polymorphism of lipoprotein(a): biological and clinical implications, *Clin Chem* 41:170, 1995.

16. Rifkind BM, Levy RI, editors: *Hyperlipidemia: diagnosis and therapy*, New York, 1977, Grune & Stratton.

17. Ford ES, Giles WH, Dietz WH: Prevalence of the metabolic syndrome among US adults, *JAMA* 287:356, 2002.

18. Kris-Etherton PM, editor-in-chief: Risk factors for coronary heart disease. In *Cardiovascular disease: nutrition for prevention and treatment*, Chicago, 1990, American Dietetic Association.

19. The Expert Panel: Report of the National Cholesterol Education Program Expert Panel on Blood Cholesterol Levels in Children and Adolescents, U.S. Department of Health and Human Services, NIH Publ. No. 91-2732, Bethesda, MD, 1991, U.S. Department of Health and Human Services.

20. Gotto AM, Jr., Farmer JA: Risk factors for coronary artery disease. In Braunwald E, editor: *Heart disease: a textbook of cardiovascular medicine*, ed 3, Philadelphia, 1988, Saunders.

21. Ross R: The pathogenesis of atherosclerosis. In Braunwald E, editor: *Heart disease: a textbook of cardiovascular medicine*, ed 3, Philadelphia, 1988, Saunders.

22. Naito HK: 18th Annual Symposium, National Academy of Clinical Biochemistry. Atherogenesis: current topics on etiology and risk factors, *Clin Chem* 41:132, 1995.

23. Grundy SM: Role of low-density lipoproteins in atherogenesis and development of coronary heart disease, *Clin Chem* 41:139, 1995.

24. Roheim PS, Asztalos BF: Clinical significance of lipoprotein size and risk for coronary atherosclerosis, *Clin Chem* 41:147, 1995.

25. Malinow MR: Plasma homocyst(e)ine and arterial occlusive diseases: a mini-review, *Clin Chem* 41:173, 1995.

26. Srinivasan SR, Berenson GS: Serum apolipoproteins A-I and B as markers of coronary artery disease risk in early life: the Bogalusa Heart Study, *Clin Chem* 41:159, 1995.

27. Wilson WF: Relation of high-density lipoprotein subfractions and apolipoprotein E isoforms to coronary disease, *Clin Chem* 41:165, 1995.

28. Zilversmit DB: Atherogenic nature of triglycerides, postprandial lipidemia, and triglyceride-rich remnant, *Clin Chem* 41:153, 1995.

29. Strong JP: Natural history and risk factors for early human atherogenesis, *Clin Chem* 41:143, 1995.

30. Wissler RW: Theories and new horizons in the pathogenesis of atherosclerosis and the mechanisms of clinical effects, *Arch Pathol Lab Med* 116:1281, 1992.

31. Steinberg D et al: Beyond cholesterol: modifications of low-density lipoproteins that increase its atherogenicity, *N Engl J Med* 320:915, 1989.

32. Meade TW, Miller GJ, Rosenberg RD: Characteristics associated with the risk of arterial thrombosis and the prethrombotic state. In Fuster V, Verstraete M, editors: *Thrombosis in cardiovascular disorders*, Philadelphia, 1992, Saunders.

33. NIH Consensus Development Conference: Lowering blood cholesterol to prevent heart disease, *JAMA* 253:2080, 1985.

Internet Sites

General

http://www.heartpoint.com/coronartdisease.html
http://www.chestx-ray.com/Coronary/CorCalc.html
http://my.webmd.com/content/dmk/dmk_summary_account_1454
http://familydoctor.org/handouts/239.html
http://www.med.unibs.it/~marchesi/fatoxidationdisorders.html
http://locus.umdnj.edu/nigms/nigms_cgi/cells.flat.cgi?id=2&query=LP&display=diags
www.ohsu.edu/cliniweb/C18/C18.452.494.html
http://www.nlm.nih.gov/medlineplus/ency/article/00396.htm

Biochemistry of Lipids

www.indstate.edu/thcme/mwking/lipids.html
www.indstate.edu/thcme/mwking/cholesterol.html

Lipoproteins

www.lipoproteins.net
www.indstate.edu/thcme/mwking/lipoproteins.html
www.acclakelouise.com/acc99/htm/genest2.htm

Diagnosis and Treatment/Adult Treatment Panel/National Institutes of Health Sites

www.nhlbi.nih.gov/guidelines/cholesterol—National Heart, Lung, and Blood Institute (NHLBI)
www.nhlbi.nih.gov/guidelines/cholesterol/atp3_rpt.htm
http://www.nhlbi.nih.gov/about/ncep/index.htm
www.acsm.org/pdf/certnews/cnwv11n2.pdf—Summary of the National Cholesterol Education Program (NCEP)
www.americanheart.org/presenter.jhtml?identifier=4764—Step I and Step II Diets
www.medal.org/ch13.html—The Medical Algorithms Project, Treatment of Hypercholesterolemia. NCEP Adult Treatment: Panel III (ATP III)

Atherosclerosis

www.americanheart.org
www.nlm.nih.gov/medlineplus/coronarydisease.html

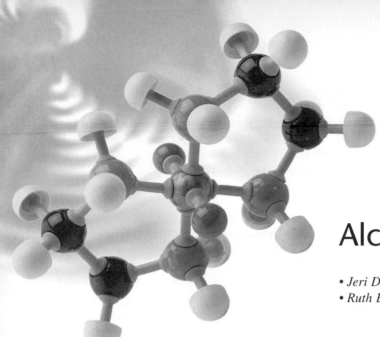

CHAPTER 34

Alcoholism

• *Jeri D. Ropero-Miller*
• *Ruth E. Winecker*

Chapter Outline

Identification of intoxication and alcoholism
   Alcoholic intoxication
   Alcoholism
Biochemical and metabolic alterations
   Ethanol metabolism
   Altered lipid, protein, and carbohydrate biochemistry
Nutritional alterations associated with alcoholism and
   alcoholic liver disease
   Protein-calorie malnutrition
   Vitamin abnormalities
   Mineral abnormalities
Pathology: systemic diseases of the alcoholic
   Mechanisms of organ damage
   Liver
   Pancreas and gastrointestinal tract
   Fetal alcohol syndrome
   Less common systemic involvement
Pathology: trauma and alcohol abuse

Change of analyte in disease
   Enzymes
   Bilirubin
   Proteins
   Lipids
   Carbohydrates
   Mean corpuscular volume (MCV)
Biological markers of alcoholism
   Monoamine oxidase
   Carbohydrate deficient transferrin
   Aldehyde-modified hemoglobin
   Other biological markers
Withdrawal, toxic syndromes, and treatment of
   alcohol dependency
   Withdrawal
   Toxic syndromes
   Treatment

Objectives

• Describe the metabolism of ethanol and the alterations of lipid, protein, and carbohydrate biochemistry that result from excess alcohol consumption.
• List and describe nutritional alterations associated with alcoholism and alcoholic liver disease.
• Describe the systemic diseases associated with alcoholism.
• State expected changes in measurements of the following laboratory analytes in alcoholic liver disease: mean corpuscular volume, serum aspartate aminotransferase, alanine aminotransferase, lactate

dehydrogenase, γ-glutamyltransferase, alkaline phosphatase, 5′-nucleotidase, bilirubin, albumin, globulins, cholesterol, triglycerides, bile acids, and glucose.
• Discuss changes in biological markers caused by chronic alcoholism.
• Describe symptoms of alcohol withdrawal and treatment of alcohol dependency.
• Describe ethanol analysis including specimens and their handling, analytical procedures, and interpretation of results.

Key Terms

addiction Physical and/or psychological dependence on a chemical substance caused by habitual use. Addiction implies risk of harm and the need to stop drug use (see also Chapter 52).

alcoholic beverage A drinkable liquid with an ethanol alcohol content of 0.5% to 95%.

alcoholic cirrhosis Cirrhosis resulting from chronic excess alcohol consumption. The cirrhotic process in the liver is a pathological process in which progressive injury produces fibrotic bands or scar tissue that entraps liver cells and results in loss of normal microscopic lobular architecture (nodular regeneration).

alcoholic hepatitis Acute toxic liver injury associated with excess ethanol consumption. This is characterized by necrosis, polymorphonuclear inflammation, and in many instances Mallory bodies.

alcoholic ketoacidosis The fall in blood pH (acidosis) sometimes seen in alcoholics and associated with a rise in serum ketone bodies (acetone, β-hydroxybutyric acid, and acetoacetic acid).

alcohol withdrawal syndrome The clinical symptoms associated with cessation of alcohol consumption. These may include tremor, hallucinations, autonomic nervous system dysfunction, and seizures.

fatty liver Excessive accumulation of fat in the liver parenchymal cells, primarily neutral lipids, triglycerides, and cholesterol. Fatty liver predictably develops after exposure to a variety of hepatotoxins, of which ethanol (ethyl alcohol) is the most common.

fetal alcohol syndrome A group of fetal abnormalities resulting from maternal alcohol consumption during gestation.

hemochromatosis A disorder of iron metabolism characterized by excess iron deposits in tissues, such as those comprising the liver, pancreas, and heart, leading to organ injury. The organ injury may manifest itself as cirrhosis, diabetes mellitus, or heart failure.

hepatic fibrosis The deposition of collagen and fibrous tissue in the liver before the development of nodular regeneration and cirrhosis.

kwashiorkor A nutritional disease resulting from protein deprivation. Depleted visceral proteins and immunological dysfunction characterize the disease. Total calorie consumption may be deficient, adequate, or even excessive.

Mallory bodies (alcoholic hyalin) An eosinophilic cytoplasmic inclusion that accumulates in the liver cells. It is typically but not always associated with acute alcoholic liver injury (alcoholic hepatitis).

marasmus A nutritional disease resulting from calorie deprivation. It is characterized by weight loss and wasting of muscle mass and fat stores.

tolerance An attenuation of the effects of a drug on the body as a result of prolonged use or large-dose use. Tolerance can result from a metabolic rate increase or a functional change in organ or system sensitivity to a drug. Drug tolerance requires a larger amount of drug to obtain the same effects originally achieved by smaller doses.

Wernicke-Korsakoff syndrome A disease of the central nervous system occurring in alcoholics and attributed to thiamine deficiency. Wernicke's encephalopathy consists of ocular disturbances, ataxia, and impaired mental functions. If untreated, it may become Korsakoff's syndrome, which includes memory impairment, confabulations, and deranged perception of time.

Methods on CD-ROM

Alanine aminotransferase
Albumin
Alcohol
Alkaline phosphatase, total
Aspartate aminotransferase
Bilirubin
Calcium
Drug screen
Folic acid

Gamma-glutamyl transferase
Glucose
Immunoglobulins (IgA, IgG, IgM)
Iron and iron-binding capacity
Lactic acid
Lipids (cholesterol, triglycerides)
Magnesium
Transferrin and carbohydrate-deficient transferring
Vitamin B_{12}

Alcoholism represents one of the most serious worldwide socioeconomic, health, and legal dilemmas. Use of alcohol among Americans is steadily rising. The 1999 National Household Survey conducted by the federal Substance Abuse and Mental Health Services Administration (SAMHSA) estimated that 105 million Americans above the age of 12 (47.3%) used alcohol in the past 30 days. Of this population, 45 million admitted to alcohol consumption of more than five drinks during at least one occasion and another 12.4 million admitted to at least five "heavy drinking" occurrences during the preceding month.[1]

The repercussions of alcoholism are dramatic. An alcoholic individual often experiences problems with psychiatric and physical illnesses, family relationships, finances, employment, and social and legal accountability. The United States spends more than $166 billion a year on alcohol-related illnesses and accidents and loses an estimated $148 billion annually because of related absenteeism and poor job performance.[2,3] Alcohol-related liver disease is the ninth leading cause of death in the United States and the sixth leading cause of death in 35- to 54-year-old men. In fact, an estimated 500,000 Americans suffer from cirrhosis secondary to alcoholism.[4] In addition, the legal system is heavily taxed with enforcement and prosecution of alcohol-related crimes.

Because alcohol is a social beverage that can be consumed by anyone of legal age, it is often erroneously categorized separately from other drugs. Alcohol is, however, a chemical substance capable of producing pharmacological effects consistent with narcotics (heroin and morphine) including central nervous system (CNS) and respiratory depression, and induction of euphoria, **tolerance**, and **addiction**.[5]

The amount of ethanol capable of producing disease depends on a variety of factors, including genetic predisposition, nutritional status, and concomitant viral infection of the liver (viral hepatitis) or other liver disease.[6] For a susceptible person, a disease-contributing dose may be as low as 35 g/day, which is equivalent to the daily consumption of three cocktails made with 100-proof whiskey. However, for most persons the amount of alcohol necessary to produce disease is in excess of 80 g/day for at least 10 to 15 years. An alcoholic beverage is equivalent to 10 g of alcohol, which produces an approximate blood alcohol concentration (BAC) of 25 mg/dL. A standard drink is equivalent to:

Standard drink = 1 oz. (30 mL) 100-proof whiskey (50% w/v)
1.5 oz. (45 mL) 80-proof liquor (40% w/v)
4 oz. (120 mL) unfortified wine (12% w/v)
12 oz. (360 mL) beer (4% w/v)

A disease-associated daily consumption amount represents eight 12-ounce beers, a liter of wine, or a little more than a half pint of 80-proof whiskey.[7] See Chapter 52 for a discussion of the general problem of addiction.

IDENTIFICATION OF INTOXICATION AND ALCOHOLISM
Alcoholic Intoxication

An elevated BAC demonstrates *recent* alcohol ingestion and possible intoxication; however, it cannot be used to diagnose alcoholism. The general signs of ethanol intoxication are listed in the box at left.

The well-established relationship between blood alcohol levels and the physical signs of intoxication is summarized in Table 34-1. The decreased motor function associated with elevated levels of blood alcohol can lead to trauma of the intoxicated person. Individuals experience CNS dysfunction (such as significant impairment of driving skills, including motor, cognitive, and information-processing skills) and signs of intoxication at different BACs. The statutory limit for operation of a motor vehicle is no more than 100 mg/dL (0.1%). However, some states have reduced the legal limit to 80 mg/dL because findings indicate that drivers with BACs of 80 mg/dL or more are eight times as likely to be involved in a vehicular crash than individuals with an undetectable BAC.[5] Moreover, some states have established a "zero tolerance" law for individuals under the legal drinking age, requiring arrest if any alcohol is detected in a minor operating a motor vehicle.

For chronic users of ethanol, the same signs and symptoms listed in the box may not occur until alcohol concentrations are in excess of 100 mg/dL. A current history of alcohol intoxication may lead a physician to suspect chronic alcoholism, but other data must substantiate these suspicions.

Alcoholism

Social identification. An alcoholic is a person who progressively consumes an amount of ethanol (ethyl alcohol, alcohol) capable of producing pathological changes and who exhibits a cumulative pattern of social behaviors associated with drinking including frequent intoxication, physical injury, problems with family and job, and multiple accidents and/or charges of driving under the influence.[8,9] An estimated 75% of Americans drink and 10% of these will experience problems associated with alcoholism at some point. Males are four times more likely to drink than females, but more females drink alone, which may reduce the known incidence rate.[9]

Characteristically, alcoholics may attempt to conceal their excessive drinking, and so the history of consumption may be unreliable. Verification from a spouse is frequently

---

SIGNS OF ETHANOL INTOXICATION

History of alcohol consumption
Odor of alcohol
Nystagmus (rapid, horizontal eye movement)
Visual disturbances
Slurred speech
Poor motor coordination
Loss of inhibition and judgment
Diminished concentration and memory
Diminished pain response
Vomiting/nausea
Depressed level of consciousness

TABLE 34-1	**BLOOD ALCOHOL CONCENTRATIONS AND SYMPTOMS**	
Blood Alcohol Concentration (mg/dL)	*Physical Signs/Symptoms*	*Degree of Intoxication*
<50	Relaxed state	Generally, none
80	Mild euphoria; beginning of sensory-motor impairment; reduced visual acuity	**Legally intoxicated** in some states
100	Euphoria; increased confidence; deficits in attention, judgment, and control; slight sensory-motor impairment	**Legally intoxicated** in all states
100 to 200	Loss of inhibition; reduced visual acuity and visual stability; cognitive impairment; moderate sensory-motor impairment; drowsiness	
200 to 250	Decreased alertness; gross intoxication; numbness; pain threshold altered; increasingly lethargic; effort may be needed to have emotional and motor control	
300 to 350	Vomiting; incontinence; hypothermia; respiratory depression; stupor to coma	
>450	Death may ensue	

necessary to determine an accurate drinking history. The signs and symptoms of current intoxication, such as those listed in the box, and the symptoms of drug withdrawal, may further verify suspicions of chronic alcohol abuse.

Clinical identification. Simple clinical screening tests such as quantity-frequency questions related to alcohol usage patterns, and more formal diagnostic research instruments such as The Alcohol Use Disorders Identification Test (AUDIT), Michigan Alcohol Screening Test (MAST), and the Composite International Diagnostic Interview (CIDI) assist in diagnosing alcohol dependency. The goals of these tests are to assess an individual's consumption behavior and identify alcohol dependency early to initiate therapy, and to promote rehabilitation and relapse prevention.[8,10]

Several laboratory tests have also been proposed for use as diagnostic tools to confirm the excess consumption of ethanol (see pp. 652-653 for details of these tests). Many of these changes in analytes also occur with other disease processes or traumatic states and, therefore, must be interpreted with caution.

BIOCHEMICAL AND METABOLIC ALTERATIONS
Ethanol Metabolism

In humans, ethanol is primarily an exogenous compound consumed in **alcoholic beverages** and readily absorbed from the entire gastrointestinal tract. Ethanol is water- and lipid-soluble; consequently, it readily crosses the blood-brain barrier and the placenta. Alcohol distributes in body tissues and fluids according to water content with an approximate volume of distribution of 0.5 L/kg. Hence, a whole blood ethanol concentration is 1.2 times larger than a plasma ethanol concentration. Food consumption can greatly reduce (by greater than 70%) the efficiency and rate of alcohol absorption. Normally absorption is complete within an hour but food intake can delay absorption 4 to 6 hours.[5]

Metabolism of ethanol is independent of dose and, therefore, is linear (zero-order kinetics) at most concentrations. However, nonlinear (first-order) kinetics has been demonstrated at concentrations lower than 20 mg/dL and at very high BACs.[11] Blood ethanol is cleared by the liver at a constant rate, decreasing at 150 to 200 mg/L per hour in a normal individual and at 300 to 400 mg/L in a chronic alcoholic. This translates to a clearance rate of approximately 3 ounces of ethanol per hour in an average adult; this is an approximate reduction in BAC of 20 mg/dL/hr. Gender affects the biotransformation of alcohol; women demonstrate approximately a 10% lower volume of distribution but a 17% faster metabolic rate.[5,11]

Oxidative processes, located primarily in the liver, degrade most of the absorbed ethanol by the following steps:

$$CH_3CH_2OH \leftrightarrow CH_3CHO \rightarrow CH_3COOH \rightarrow CO_2 + H_2O$$

ethanol acetaldehyde acetic acid carbon dioxide water

At least three hepatic enzyme systems are capable of ethanol oxidation to acetaldehyde: (1) cytosolic alcohol dehydrogenase, (2) microsomal ethanol oxidizing system (MEOS), and (3) peroxidase-catalase located in the peroxisomes. Many other drugs are also metabolized by these metabolic pathways, resulting in the drug interactions that are summarized in Table 34-2. Only 2% to 10% of consumed alcohol is excreted unoxidized through the lungs, urine, or sweat.[6]

Alcohol dehydrogenase (ADH) appears to be the principal pathway for ethanol oxidation.

$$Ethanol \xrightarrow[\text{NAD}^+ \qquad \text{NADH} + H^+]{\text{Alcohol dehydrogenase}} Acetaldehyde$$

The initial step catalyzed by alcohol dehydrogenase appears to be rate limiting for the clearance of ethanol from

TABLE 34-2 DRUG INTERACTIONS OF ALCOHOL

Drug or Drug Class	Pharmacological Effect	Psychological Effect	Mechanism
Amphetamines	Possibly antagonize	None	Unknown
Anticonvulsants (Phenytoin)	Additive at high concentration; antagonistic with chronic consumption	Unknown	Decreases metabolism; increases metabolism
Barbiturates	Synergistic/additive	Additive	Increases absorption; induces MEOS; increases CNS and respiratory depression; cross-tolerance associated
Benzodiazepines	Synergistic/additive	Additive (long-acting); none (short-acting)	Increases absorption; induces MEOS; impairs clearance; increases CNS and respiratory depression
Caffeine	Unknown	Counteracts cognitive and motor impairment of alcohol	Unknown
Cannabinoids	Unknown	Increases psychological effect; additive motor impairment	Unknown
Cocaine	Minor impairment of alcohol; increases toxic effects of cocaine	Increases euphoria; decreases cognitive and motor impairment of alcohol	Produces toxic and active metabolite, cocaethylene
Disulfiram	Increases toxic effects of alcohol	None	Inhibits ADH
Disulfiram-like agents (chloramphenicol, furazolidone, griseofulvin, quinacrine HCl, metronidazole, procarbazine HCl, sulfonylureas [oral antidiabetics], edible mushrooms [*Coprinus atramentarius*], and industrial solvents [oximes, amides, and carbamates])	Increases toxic effects of alcohol	None	Inhibits ADH
Histimine₂-receptor antagonist (ranitidine, cimetidine)	Additive	Increases alcohol effects	Inhibits gastric ADH; inhibits MEOS; increases CNS depression
Naltrexone	Antagonize		
Naloxone	Antagonize		
Opioid analgesics (propoxyphene, heroin)	Additive		Increases CNS and respiratory depression
Phenothiazines	Additive	Unknown	Increases CNS depression
Selective serotonin reuptake inhibitor antidepressants	None or possibly antagonize	None	Unknown
Tricyclic antidepressants	Additive	Additive	Increases absorption; cardiotoxicity; increases CNS depression; hypothermia

Garriott JC, editor: Medicolegal aspects of alcohol, ed 3, Tucson, AZ, 1996, Lawyers & Judges; Ellenhorn MJ et al, editors: Ellenhorn's medical toxicology: diagnosis and treatment of human poisoning, Baltimore, 1997, Williams & Wilkins.

the blood, but is not specific for ethanol. In addition to ethanol, alcohol dehydrogenase oxidizes methanol, retinol (vitamin A), and several other alcohols. This is clinically relevant because alcohol is an administered antidote in the treatment of acute methanol poisoning because it competes with methanol for ADH binding; thus minimizing formation of the toxic methanol metabolite, formaldehyde.[8]

The MEOS, found in the smooth endoplasmic reticulum (SER) of hepatocytes, appears to be a secondary enzyme system for ethanol clearance.

$$\text{Ethanol} \xrightarrow[\text{NADPH} + \text{H}^+]{\overset{\text{Oxygen}}{\underset{\text{NADP}^+ + 2\text{H}_2\text{O}}{\text{MEOS}}}} \text{Acetaldehyde}$$

In the chronic alcoholic, there is an increase in MEOS activity that may result in an increase in metabolism of up to 72%.[11] The induction of MEOS activity is associated with increased activity of various other metabolic components of the SER involved with drug metabolism, such as other enzymes (5'-nucleotidase and γ-glutamyltransferase [GGT]), cytochrome P-450 reductase, and cytochrome P-450. These changes have clinical significance because they render the alcoholic more resistant to the effects of many common sedatives and barbiturates, resulting in the necessity for a larger-than-normal dose when sedation is required. If, however, ethanol and barbiturates are consumed simultaneously, death is possible because competitive enzyme inhibition between the two drugs results in reduced metabolism of barbiturates and abnormally high blood levels of barbiturates.[5] In addition, based on their interactions with alcohol dehydrogenase, some agents can increase BACs (such as pyrazole) whereas others (such as antibiotics) decrease them.[12]

The role of catalase in the biological oxidation of ethanol is minimal.[6] In vitro experiments demonstrate that in the presence of a peroxide (H_2O_2)-generating system, catalase can oxidize ethanol by the following reaction:

$$\text{Ethanol} + \text{H}_2\text{O}_2 \xrightarrow{\text{Catalase}} 2\text{H}_2\text{O} + \text{Acetaldehyde}$$

It appears that the slow rate at which NADPH oxidase or xanthine oxidase generates peroxide prevents catalase from contributing to more than 2% of the in vivo ethanol oxidation.[6]

Altered Lipid, Protein, and Carbohydrate Biochemistry

Lipids. Low or moderate ethanol use (<20 g/day) is associated with an increase in high-density lipoproteins and therefore a decreased risk for coronary artery disease (see Chapter 33).[13,14] However, when ethanol use is excessive (>80 g/day), lipids accumulate in most tissues in which ethanol is metabolized, and such accumulation results in fatty liver, fatty myocardium, fatty renal tubules, and so on.[6] The mechanism appears to be multifactorial, resulting from both increased lipid accumulation and decreased lipid oxidation.[6,15] Although the secretion of serum lipoproteins is low relative to the lipid load accumulating in the liver, the total amount secreted is increased above normal, and alcoholic hyperlipemia may result.[6,16] This syndrome is an acquired type V hyperlipoproteinemia characterized by excessive serum triglycerides, very low density lipoproteins (VLDL), and chylomicrons.[16,17] (See Chapter 33 for more information on acquired and familial hyperlipoproteinemias.)

Protein. Protein turnover can be altered because of excess ethanol intake. As seen with the poor nutritional status of many alcoholics, the rate of protein degradation exceeds the rate of synthesis, resulting in alcoholic myopathy, osteo-pathy, and intestinal atrophy.[18] Approximately 20% of protein synthesis is attributed to the liver and one of the earliest liver changes seen in the alcoholic is the accumulation of protein.[18] This is a consequence of acetaldehyde binding with the tubulin of microtubules, which impairs the secretion of protein from liver cells.[19] This occurs concurrently with fat accumulation and contributes to the development of the enlarged liver (hepatomegaly) that is seen in more than 90% of alcoholics with liver disease.[20]

Carbohydrate. Gluconeogenesis is similarly impaired by ethanol by a variety of mechanisms. Gluconeogenesis is the process whereby glucose is formed from noncarbohydrate sources, that is, glycerol, pyruvate, and several amino acids (see Chapter 32). Because ethanol promotes glycerol-lipid formation and impairs amino acid transport, the availability of glycerol and amino acids for gluconeogenesis is decreased. Glutamic acid dehydrogenase activity is also diminished by elevated NADH levels, decreasing the availability of α-ketoglutarate, which is necessary for the transamination of amino acids before their conversion into glucose. This further impairs gluconeogenesis.

The increase in NADH with a concomitant decrease in NAD$^+$ associated with ADH activity may also produce sequential changes of carbohydrate metabolism with clinical consequences. The increased availability of NADH results in increased lactate production, which decreases its availability for gluconeogenesis and can result in hyperlacticacidemia.[21] The hyperlacticacidemia reduces the capacity of the kidney to excrete uric acid, leading to a secondary hyperuricemia.[22] In susceptible persons this may aggravate or precipitate attacks of gout.[6,23]

NUTRITIONAL ALTERATIONS ASSOCIATED WITH ALCOHOLISM AND ALCOHOLIC LIVER DISEASE
Protein-Calorie Malnutrition

Alcoholic beverages are high in calories. Each gram of ethanol yields 7 kcal, and ethanol may account for up to 10% of the total energy intake of moderate consumers of ethanol and up to 60% for alcoholics. However, alcoholic beverages are low in nutritive value.[5,24,25] In fact, chronic alcoholism has long been associated with both malnutrition and liver disease. Malnutrition in the form of protein-calorie deficiency results from a variety of causes, including: (1) poor dietary intake; (2) malabsorption of consumed nutrients as a result of alcohol-induced gastritis, pancreatitis, or diarrhea; and (3) altered biochemical and physiological processes.

A large percentage of alcoholics suffer from protein-calorie malnutrition (PCM). A diet inadequate in nonprotein calories (such as sugars, starches, and fats) produces **marasmus** (caloric deficit) PCM, whereas a diet inadequate in proteins and essential amino acids results in a **kwashiorkor**-like disease (protein deficit) (see Chapter 37). Intermediate forms of PCM are also common in alcoholics and are termed *marasmic-kwashiorkor*. In a study of 284 alcoholics with **alcoholic hepatitis**, all patients had some degree of protein-calorie malnutrition, and 80% also exhibited marasmic PCM.[26] Measurements of serum prealbumin, transferrin, essential amino acids, glucose, and β-lipoprotein are useful diagnostic and monitoring tools of PCM (see Chapter 37).[9]

Although liver injury can develop in the absence of malnutrition, more severe forms of liver disease are invariably associated with severe malnutrition. Recognition of nutritional deficits appears to be important for the alcoholic with liver disease because correction of these abnormalities by appropriate nutritional therapy may increase survival and accelerate improvement of the liver injury.

Vitamin Abnormalities

Excessive alcohol use commonly leads to vitamin deficiency as a result of poor general nutrition, impaired vitamin metabolism, malabsorption, and hepatic damage.[24,27] Not only is the liver a major storage depot for vitamins but it also converts vitamins into metabolically useful forms (see Chapter 39). Vitamins can be released from necrotic liver cells and lost from the body without adequate replacement. In addition, absorption of fat-soluble vitamins (vitamins A, D, K, and E) by the intestine of alcoholics may be inadequate if pancreatitis or cholestasis, often present in alcoholics, is present (see later discussion).[27] Alcohol consumption can increase the body's need for folic acid, vitamin B_{12}, vitamin E, and vitamin B_6 because of increased nucleic acid synthesis and liver regeneration.[9,27,28] Table 34-3 summarizes alcoholic vitamin deficiencies and gives the incidence of low serum values of vitamins in chronic alcoholics. (See Chapter 39 for a discussion of the biochemistry and physiology of vitamins.)

Vitamin deficiencies in chronic alcoholism are associated with various disease states. Thiamine deficiency can produce brain injuries, including a distinctive neuropsychiatric disorder called **Wernicke-Korsakoff syndrome** in a small number of alcoholics; this syndrome can be genetically predicted.[8,9] Symptoms of this disease include cognitive impairment, ocular abnormalities, ataxia, hypotension, and changes in mental status. A severe deficiency of nicotinic acid leads to pellagra, a condition characterized by cutaneous and mucous membrane abnormalities, CNS aberrations, and gastrointestinal disturbances.[6] Finally, folate and vitamin B_{12} deficiencies contribute to the megaloblastic anemia observed in alcoholics, whereas pure vitamin E deficiency may produce testicular lesions and hypogonadism.[12,24]

Evaluation of an alcoholic's dietary intake of vitamins can help diagnose and treat disease. In the case of vitamin K, biliary obstruction or severe parenchymal liver disease can produce bleeding abnormalities because stores of this vitamin are small. Alcoholics often have prolonged prothrombin time. When these patients are given vitamin K parenterally, some show corrected prothrombin time, indicating vitamin K deficiency. Those who do not improve with vitamin K have liver disease too severe to use the vitamin treatment.[9] Also, the severity of liver disease can be assessed by vitamin evaluation. Because vitamin B_{12} is stored in the liver, the acute liver cell necrosis of alcoholic hepatitis may actually produce a noticeable increase in serum B_{12} levels that parallels the severity of the liver injury.

Mineral Abnormalities (see Chapters 28, 35, 37, and 38)

Mineral abnormalities also occur in chronic alcoholism (Table 34-3). Although not as fully understood, it is assumed that mineral deficiencies arise from similar dietary abnormalities and disease processes. Chronic alcoholics commonly have mineral deficiencies from a single or multiple sources including (1) poor dietary intake (Fe, Zn, Mg^{2+}, Ca^{2+}, P), (2) increased diuresis that is a direct effect of alcohol (Zn, Mg^{2+}), (3) malabsorption (Ca^{2+}), or (4) starvation ketosis and vomiting (Mg^{2+}, P).[12,28,29,30] Many of these nutrients are essential to body function and a deficient state can have alarming consequences. For example, zinc deficiency affects RNA and DNA synthesis, enzymatic processes (ADH), vitamin metabolism (vitamin A), and contributes to hypogonadism.[31,32] Severe depletion of magnesium affects thiamine, indirectly leading to Wernicke-Korsakoff syndrome.[33]

Some minerals are increased in alcoholics. Iron and lead accumulation in the liver may result from the manufacture of ethanol itself. Beer production in iron kettles has led to **hemochromatosis** among the South African Bantu and incidents of lead poisoning have been traced to lead pipes and radiators used to construct homemade stills for the production of "moonshine" whiskey.[5,33] Higher iron and lead content has also been found in wines, possibly resulting from storage containers (i.e., metal-banded wooden barrels) or pest control in vineyards (i.e., lead arsenate compounds).[5,28] Furthermore, a sevenfold iron increase, in the form of erythrocyte ferritin content, has been measured in alcoholics with liver disease. This increase is attributed not only to the iron content of the beverages themselves, but also increased hydrochloric acid secretion of the stomach and inhibition of a coenzyme, pyridoxal kinase, responsible for iron utilization.[28]

PATHOLOGY: SYSTEMIC DISEASES OF THE ALCOHOLIC
Mechanisms of Organ Damage

Ethanol is a direct systemic toxin that produces injury to all tissues, depending on the dose and duration of exposure. The degree of injury varies among organ systems. The liver, the organ that is predominantly responsible for ethanol metabolism, develops the highest incidence and severity of injury.

The product of all three ethanol oxidation pathways described earlier is acetaldehyde. It appears that either ethanol or acetaldehyde induces various organ disorders and biochemical alterations, but not necessarily together. For example, **fetal alcohol syndrome** appears to be an ethanol effect independent of acetaldehyde,[6] whereas **hepatic fibrosis** and collagen formation may be more closely associated with acetaldehyde than with ethanol. Acetaldehyde readily forms adducts with components of cellular membranes. These adducts may directly cause cellular damage or may create new antigenic stimulants.[34]

Liver

Three types of pathological liver conditions develop, forming a continuum of disease from very mild reversible changes to

TABLE 34-3 NUTRITIONAL DEFICIENCY IN THE ALCOHOLIC

Vitamin	Solubility of Vitamin	Effect of Alcohol on Intestinal Absorption	Mechanism of Deficiency	Incidence (%) of Low Serum Values in Chronic Alcoholics	References
A (retinol)	Fat	None	Decreased hepatic conversion of retinol to retinal; deficit in storage and transport; poor dietary intake	12	9, 27, 28
B₁ (thiamine)	Water	Decrease	Poor dietary intake; decreased utilization because of liver disease	30 to 70	9, 27, 28
B₂ (riboflavin)	Water	None	Poor dietary intake	17 to 26	27, 28
Nicotinic acid	Water	Not evaluated		33	29
B₆ (pyridoxine)	Water	None	Abnormal intestinal handling because of enzymatic inhibition	50 to 60	28
Folic acid	Water	None	Poor dietary intake; increased requirements; increased secretion; decreased mucosal uptake and transport of folate	20 to 50	12, 27, 28
B₁₂ (cyanocobalamin)	Water	Decrease	Poor dietary intake; decreased utilization; hepatic release	Rare	27
C (ascorbic acid)	Water	Not evaluated	Poor dietary intake	25	34
D	Fat	None	Malabsorption of lipid secondary to pancreatitis or cholestasis	45	28, 29
K	Fat	None	Poor dietary intake	15	28, 29
E	Fat	None	Hepatic release decreased because of disease; β-lipoprotein deficiency	Unknown	28

Mineral	Effect of Alcohol on Mineral Body Content	Mechanism of Mineral Depletion	Incidence (%) of Low Serum Values in Chronic Alcoholics	References
Iron	Increase	Manufacturing process	Rare	12, 27, 29, 35
	Decrease	Poor dietary intake; malabsorption (species dependent)		
Zinc	Decrease	Poor dietary intake; increased urine loss; destruction of zinc metallo-enzymes	Unknown	30, 35
Lead	Increase	Manufacturing process	Unknown	35
	Decrease	Poor dietary intake		
Magnesium	Decrease	Poor dietary intake; increased urine loss; defects in renal tubular reabsorption; intestinal loss (vomit; diarrhea)	30	12, 29, 30, 33
Calcium	Decrease	Poor dietary intake; malabsorption; increased excretion	10 to 20	27, 29, 40
Phosphorus	Decrease	Poor dietary intake; increased GI loss of phosphate; increased phosphorus entry into cells	30 to 60	27, 29

life-threatening, irreversible disease.[6,35] The interrelationships among these changes are depicted in Fig. 34-1.

Fatty liver. The mildest form of liver damage is characterized by fatty infiltration (alcoholic **fatty liver**) and by some minimum degree of inflammation and necrosis. An overloading of the liver's metabolic functions by alcohol brings about fatty infiltration of the liver, or steatosis. This causes a decrease in fatty acid metabolism and consequently storage of the excess lipids.[6,35] In more severe cases of fatty liver, fibrosis may be present, especially around central venous channels. Clinically this is manifested by liver enlargement (hepatomegaly), tenderness over the liver, and anorexia. Alcoholic fatty liver is usually considered a benign, reversible disease. However, sudden deaths have been observed in a small percentage of alcoholics, presumably from fat emboli.

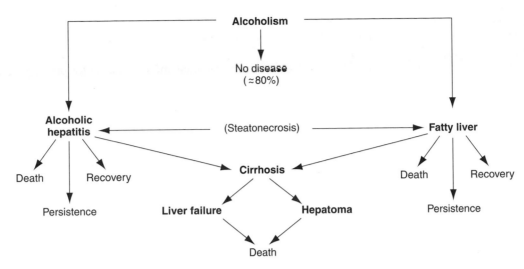

Fig. 34-1 Alcoholic liver disease.

Alcoholic hepatitis. Fatty liver and hepatomegaly also characterize the more severe toxic form of hepatic injury, alcoholic hepatitis. In addition, inflammation and necrosis are more extensive, and fibrosis and iron deposits are prominent features. Alcoholic hepatitis is frequently a crucial stage toward the progression of cirrhotic disease. In the large Veterans Administration Cooperative Study[20] of patients with clinical alcoholic hepatitis, the disease had progressed to cirrhosis in 54.7% of 97 patients in whom histological specimens were available. In a high percentage of patients (76.2%) an irregularly outlined homogeneous meshwork of eosin-staining material could be seen in the cytoplasm of the liver cells **(Mallory bodies** or **alcoholic hyalin).** Although the presence of Mallory bodies is not solely diagnostic for alcoholic hepatitis, because it is seen in Wilson's disease and primary biliary cirrhosis, in an alcoholic with liver disease these histological findings most likely represent alcoholic hepatitis. This damage results from degenerating microfilaments, which then act as immunological irritants and stimulate fibrosis.[34,36] Additionally, substantial iron deposits can be found in the livers of alcoholics.[37] This appears to be unrelated to genetic disorders resulting in iron overload and may be due to increased iron absorption related to folic acid deficiency.[38] This is not a benign finding, however, because there appears to be an inverse correlation between liver iron staining and survival in alcoholic hepatitis and cirrhosis.[39]

The clinical features and complications of alcoholic hepatitis are shown in Table 34-4. None of the symptoms or complications specifically predicts this condition.

Although the histological presentation of hepatitis is the best prognostic indicator of survival, the serum bilirubin level and prothrombin time are the laboratory tests that allow the most reliable prediction of the severity and survival prognosis of liver disease. These tests, however, are not sensitive enough to diagnose minimal disease because in very mild cases results may be normal or near normal. However, as the disease progresses, the usefulness of the tests increases. (See Change of Analyte in Disease section for a comprehensive review of bilirubin and prothrombin time.)

TABLE 34-4 INITIAL CLINICAL FEATURES AND COMPLICATIONS OF ALCOHOLIC HEPATITIS*

Feature or Complication	SEVERITY OF DISEASE		
	Mild	Moderate	Severe
Anorexia[†]	46.2	63.0	65.7
Weight loss[‡]	36.8	27.1	16.2
Fever	18.0	26.2	19.2
Hepatomegaly	85.9	97.1	88.9
Splenomegaly*	24.5	38.6	46.2
Infection	5.2	16.8	8.1
Pancreatitis	13.6	10.3	10.1
Gastrointestinal bleeding	10.4	7.5	14.1
Ascites			
Mild	18.7	19.4	17.2
Moderate	11.0	38.0	45.5
Severe	1.3	20.4	29.3
Combined[†]	31.0	77.8	92.0
Encephalopathy			
Grade 1	17.3	29.6	25.3
Grade 2	4.5	24.1	41.4
Grades 3 and 4	0.7	3.7	0
Combined[‡]	2.5	57.4	66.7
Probability of surviving 1 yr[¶]	0.91 ± 0.027	0.75 ± 0.045	0.46 ± 0.055

From Mendenhall CL et al: Protein-calorie malnutrition associated with alcoholic hepatitis, Am J Med 76:221, 1984.
*The diagnoses of the various complicating features and conditions were not defined in the protocol but were determined by the clinical judgment of the participating investigator. Because n varied among severity groups (mild, 156; moderate, 108; severe, 99), values are expressed as a percentage of total. Data analysis consisted of an overall chi-squared test, which, when significant at the 0.05 level, was followed by Bartholomew's test for order. The hypothesized order was $p_{mild} < p_{moderate} < p_{severe}$ except for weight loss where the presence of ascites reversed the hypothesized order.
[†]$p < 0.005$ (Bartholomew's test).
[‡]The decreasing incidence of weight loss with increasing severity represented an increasing incidence of ascites.
[¶]$p < 0.006$. All pairwise comparisons (mild, moderate, severe) determined by normal distribution test statistics.

Cirrhosis. The end stage of chronic alcoholic liver disease is the development of cirrhosis with extensive liver fibrosis, nodular regeneration, distortion of the liver architecture, and ultimately all the clinical complications of chronic liver disease, liver failure, and death. In some instances cirrhosis may be hard to diagnose clinically, especially when active alcoholic hepatitis with acute necrosis and inflammation are also present. Only a liver biopsy specimen will provide an accurate diagnosis of cirrhosis.[20,35]

Pancreas and Gastrointestinal Tract

The association between alcohol and pancreatitis equals the strong relationship between alcohol and liver disease. In developed countries, alcohol causes 60% to 70% of cases of chronic pancreatitis.[6,40] Although there is a wide range of individual variation, the average duration of alcohol consumption before the initial diagnosis of pancreatitis is made is 18 years in men and 11 years in women. With each approximately 50 g increase in daily alcohol consumption, the risk of developing pancreatitis doubles.[41]

Alcohol stimulates the secretion of at least some acid from the stomach. When acid comes into contact with duodenal mucosa, it stimulates the flow of pancreatic juice.[6,42] The pancreatic juice induced by alcohol early in the disease process has a high concentration of protein, which precipitates and forms protein plugs. These plugs form within the pancreatic ductules and subsequently obstruct the ductules. This obstruction leads to ductular dilation, ductular proliferation, dilation of acinar tissue, and ductal sclerosis.[42] In time, the protein plugs may calcify giving the x-ray picture of chronic calcific pancreatitis. As scarring of the pancreas continues, the protein or enzyme concentration in the pancreatic juice decreases until not enough enzymes are present for food digestion, and malabsorption occurs.[40,42,43] Once pancreatitis has been established, a fairly high percentage of patients who continue to drink have chronic pain.[44] After 80% to 90% of the pancreas has been destroyed, pancreatic insufficiency develops, requiring oral enzyme replacement.[45] In addition to the destruction of enzyme-secreting cells, insulin- and glucagon-producing cells may also be destroyed. When this occurs, the alcoholic develops diabetes mellitus and the need for insulin.

The excess acid secretion combined with the direct toxic effect of ethanol triggers the serious complication of gastrointestinal bleeding seen in many alcoholics. Blood loss occurs in the gastrointestinal tract because of duodenitis, esophagitis, Mallory-Weiss lesions, peptic ulcerations, and esophageal varices. Chronic low-level blood loss is a problem for many alcoholics because it leads to anemia and degeneration of gastrointestinal lesions. These erosions can lead to acute hemorrhagic gastritis, which can result in a fatality unless treatment is promptly initiated.[19]

Fetal Alcohol Syndrome

Alcohol, an established fetal toxin and teratogen, readily crosses the placenta and distributes throughout fetal tissue. Thus, ethanol consumption during pregnancy can result in a wide variety of adverse effects, including spontaneous abortion, premature delivery, low infant birth weight, stillbirth, and poor outcome of the newborn. The last effect includes poor mental and motor development and the fetal alcohol syndrome.

The fetal alcohol syndrome is characterized by a pattern of birth defects such as prenatal and postnatal growth retardation, facial abnormalities, renal and CNS dysfunction, and mental retardation.[46] It has been estimated that the fetal alcohol syndrome is now the leading nongenetic cause of decreased mental acuity in the Western world.[46,47]

Less Common Systemic Involvement

Heart. Excessive consumption of ethanol can lead to alcoholic heart muscle disease (AHMD),[48] which mimics cardiomyopathy in presentation and is often referred to as alcoholic cardiomyopathy.[48] In two large studies of alcoholics totaling 278 cases at autopsy, 11% to 15% had AHMD.[49] Alcoholic cardiomyopathy is typified by cardiomegaly (enlargement of the heart), dilation of the left ventricle, contractile abnormalities, and pathological alterations involving both ventricles culminating in a low output type of cardiac failure.[48] Death often results from gross cardiomegaly and chronic intractable cardiac failure complicated by embolic phenomena.

Central and peripheral nervous system. The most common manifestations of altered brain function in the alcoholic are the symptoms of inebriation, followed in frequency by the withdrawal syndromes of tremor, confusion, hallucinations, delirium tremens, and convulsions. These are usually reversible functional changes. Much less common, but frequently irreversible, are neurological abnormalities resulting from the metabolic disorders associated with protracted steady drinking and, in most instances, nutritional deficiencies.[50] These include Wernicke-Korsakoff syndrome, peripheral neuropathy, amblyopia (loss of vision), cerebellar and cerebral degeneration, central pontine myelinolysis, and progressive dementia with demyelination of the corpus callosum (Marchiafava-Bignami disease). Both clinical and animal studies on mnemonic brain function indicate an ethanol-induced impairment.[51] (Refer to a neurology text for details on each of these syndromes.)

Cancer. Alcoholism is closely associated with a number of malignancies occurring in the liver, pancreas, breast, and upper and lower gastrointestinal tract. Although pure ethanol is not known to be carcinogenic, ethanol promotes or enhances the carcinogenicity of other compounds, possibly by increasing the intracellular concentration of the carcinogen.[52] Primary liver cancer comprises only 2% of all cancers in the United States, but 5% to 10% of alcoholics with **alcoholic cirrhosis** develop hepatic carcinoma.[53] Heavy drinkers have an increased incidence of cancer of the upper digestive tract including the mouth, pharynx, larynx, and esophagus.[19,54,55] A heavy drinker and smoker has a 15 times greater risk of developing oral malignancy than a nondrinker and nonsmoker.[55] Alcohol consumption may also be related to increased incidences of cancer of the pancreas, the breast, and the colon. However, the evidence linking alcohol use and these cancers is less convincing than that of liver and upper gastrointestinal cancers.[52,56,57]

Endocrine effects. The effects of alcohol on the endocrine system vary, depending on whether the alcohol intake is acute or chronic. Acute alcohol use produces an elevated plasma cortisol level, but the response decreases with chronic use of ethanol.[58,59] Occasionally, chronic alcoholics will show clinical features of Cushing's syndrome and high cortisol levels. Abstention causes the cortisol level to return to normal in 2 to 3 weeks.[58]

Some alcoholics have evidence of pituitary insufficiency. Low blood glucose normally produces a rise in cortisol. This response is decreased or absent in 25% of chronic alcoholics because the pituitary gland does not secrete enough adrenocorticotropic hormone to stimulate the adrenal gland.[58] In addition to reduced cortisol levels, low levels of growth hormone and prolactin after low blood glucose stimulation further support pituitary insufficiency.[60] Low testosterone levels present in alcoholics are due to pituitary insufficiency and increased metabolic clearance.[58] Clinically, this results in hypogonadism and feminization in males and menstrual disorders in females with spider veins (radiating lines of capillaries, most often seen on the legs) in both sexes.[58,59]

Hematopoietic effects. The effects of alcohol on the blood and bone marrow are the result of both a direct toxic effect and associated nutritional deficiencies[19] (see Chapters 37 and 39). Not only do alcoholics have low folate levels, but also vitamin B_{12} absorption is inhibited by alcohol. Each of these factors alone or in combination can lead to abnormally large red blood cells and megaloblastic anemia.[12,24]

Iron metabolism is affected by alcohol in several ways. Excess alcohol consumption increases serum and tissue iron, and causes abnormal iron use within the bone marrow. Finally, alcohol excess can cause acute hemolytic anemia. Abstinence can often reverse bone marrow damage and associated iron utilization problems. However, use of disulfiram to achieve abstinence may enhance the persistence of bone marrow damage.[61]

Inhibition of the bone marrow by alcohol can also reduce the number of circulating white blood cells[62] and platelets.[63] Increased susceptibility to infection and bleeding result from alcohol-induced impairment of white blood cell[61] and platelet function. Vitamin K deficiency, seen in alcoholics, causes a prolonged prothrombin time because of the lack of vitamin K–dependent clotting factors normally produced in the liver. When liver disease is severe, inadequate clotting factors are produced even when vitamin K is present.

Immune system. Ethanol affects the immune system in a number of ways. Most patients with alcoholic liver disease have increased circulating B-cell antibodies.[20] Specific antibodies against alcoholic hyalin are present in patients with alcoholic hepatitis, which may explain the frequently observed elevations in serum IgA levels.[52] Primary changes observed in the cell-mediated immune system of alcoholics include a decrease in total numbers of T-cells[64]; impairment of the ability of immune cells to synthesize DNA (lymphocyte transformation); suppression of response to antigens and mitogens; and increase in cytotoxic properties. Clinical manifestations include a low lymphocyte count, anergy to skin tests,[26] altered response to vaccinations,[20,65] and increased susceptibility to infections.

These immunological alterations may be partly responsible for some of the liver cell injury and progression of the disease seen in patients with alcoholic hepatitis and in the increased rate of certain types of cancers in alcoholics.[19,52] Finally, the immune systems of children with fetal alcohol syndrome have been shown to have T- and B-cell deficiencies. This type of immunosuppression could result in the development of leukemias and other tumors and an increase in the susceptibility to bacterial infections.[52]

PATHOLOGY: TRAUMA AND ALCOHOL ABUSE

Every year, hundreds of thousands of people come to the nation's emergency departments and trauma clinics exhibiting mental status changes. These individuals challenge the medical staff and laboratories to determine the immediate cause of their altered mental status, be it trauma, metabolic disorders, infectious agents, or drugs. In 1999, SAMHSA's Drug Abuse Warning Network (DAWN) reported more than 550,000 drug-related hospital emergency department episodes in the United States of which more than 35% involved alcohol. Greater than 33% (3,916 of 11,651) of the drug-related deaths mentioned in DAWN's Annual Medical Examiner's Data showed that alcohol was present in combination with other drugs.[66,67]

An estimated 50% of fatal automobile accidents and 60% of pedestrian deaths caused by automobiles are attributed to alcohol impairment. Vehicular accidents are the most frequent cause of trauma to the alcoholic. Half of all vehicular accidents, accounting for 25,000 deaths and over a half a million injuries a year, are associated with a driver that has a positive blood alcohol.[68] Aviation and boating accidents are 10% and 69% alcohol-related, respectively.[5] Alcohol facilitated crimes are also prevalent in our society, affecting 50% of murder victims, 35% of suicide victims, and an equally high percentage of domestic violence victims.[69] Many of these patients also show evidence of other drugs of abuse. These numbers certainly describe a pathological state that is endemic in American society.

CHANGE OF ANALYTE IN DISEASE (Table 34-5)

Alcoholism takes its toll on the human body, manifesting alcohol-related illnesses and disease. These disease states lead to predictable alterations in enzymes, proteins, lipids, and carbohydrates. Consequently, these analyte alterations can be measured and used to evaluate disease status, treatment effectiveness, and prognosis.

Enzymes

Increases in serum enzyme levels in liver disease may result from leakage of enzymes into the serum because of damaged cell membranes (aspartate aminotransferase, alanine aminotransferase, and lactate dehydrogenase) or from increased

TABLE 34-5 LABORATORY CHANGES AND BIOLOGICAL MARKERS IN CHRONIC ALCOHOLICS

Laboratory Test	Direction of Analyte Change	Incidence of Abnormal Results (%)*†	Sensitivity of Biological Marker (%)‡	Specificity of Biological Marker (%)‡	Advantages of Test	Limitations of Test
Albumin	Decrease	36 to 96				
ALP	Increase	67 to 100			Routine assay Economical	Low sensitivity Nonspecific
ALT (SGPT)	Increase	56 to 73	A: 22 to 50 B: 11 to 40 C: 35 to 47 D: 22 to 50	B: 85 to 98 C: 85 to 86	Routine assay Economical	Low sensitivity Nonspecific
AST (SGOT)	Increase	79 to 98	A: 17 to 85 B: 7 to 56 C: 46 to 50 D: 22 to 50	B: 92 to 97 C: 77 to 82	Routine assay Economical	Low sensitivity Nonspecific
CDT	Increase	Not evaluated	A: 29 to 85 B: 10 to 61 C: 47 to 70 D: 35 to 72	A: 88 to 95 B: 80 to 96 C: 81 to 98 D: 75 to 100	Available commercial assays	Altered by genetic disorders and liver dysfunction Low sensitivity in females May show age differences
Cholylglycine (bile acid)	Increase	85 to 100				
GGT	Increase	Not evaluated	A: 35 to 85 B: 10 to 61 C: 45 to 77 D: 44 to 96	A: 86 to 95 B: 80 to 100 C: 65 to 85 D: 18 to 100	Routine assay Economical	Nonspecific
HAA	Increase	Not evaluated			High sensitivity High specificity Not influenced by age or gender	Investigational only Possible interference with aspirin and/or acetaminophen
IgA	Increase	84 to 98				
IgG	Increase	49 to 83				
IgM	Decrease	17 to 43				
MAO	Decrease	Not evaluated			Possible genetic influence Stable over time	Other drugs influence MAO
MCV	Increase Decrease	73 to 90 2 to 8	A: 22 to 67 B: 12 to 63 C: 27 to 54 D: 33 to 87	A: 93 to 98 B: 77 to 94 C: 85 to 91 D: 63 to 100	Routine assay Economical	Low sensitivity Nonspecific
Total bilirubin	Increase	53 to 100				

ALP, *alkaline phosphatase;* ALT, *alanine aminotransferase;* AST, *aspartate aminotransferase;* CDT, *carbohydrate deficient transferrin;* GGT, *γ-glutamyltransferase;* HAA, *acetaldhyde modified hemoglobin;* IgA, *immunoglobulin A;* IgG, *immunoglobulin G;* IgM, *immunoglobulin M;* MAO, *monoamine oxidase;* MCV, *mean corpuscular volume;* Group A, *heavy drinkers and alcoholics (>40 g/d);* Group B, *primary health care settings and among young populations;* Group C, *medical wards and other hospital settings;* Group D, *patients with liver disease.*
Leevy CM et al: Am J Clin Nutr 17:259-271, 1965.
†*Hazelett SE et al: Evaluation of acetaldehyde-modified hemoglobin and other markers of chronic heavy alcohol use: effects of gender and hemoglobin concentration,* Alcohol Clin Exp Res 22:1813-1819, 1998.
‡*Salaspuro M: Carbohydrate-deficeint transferrin as compared to other markers of alcoholism: a systemic review,* Alcohol 19:261-271, 1999.

enzyme production (alkaline phosphatase and GGT). Interpretation of changes in enzyme concentration must carefully evaluate the patient's therapeutic and drug histories to eliminate contributions from other conditions, drugs, or chemicals.

Aspartate aminotransferase (AST) and alanine aminotransferase (ALT) (see p. 503, Chapter 27). Serum AST and ALT are two enzymes present in the liver and both readily leak from the cells during necrosis and cell injury. Although liver cell necrosis and inflammation characterize alcoholic liver injury, the increase in these enzymes is minimum to moderate, with the rise in AST almost always exceeding that observed in ALT. In alcoholic hepatitis the serum AST is greater than the serum ALT in 90% of the patients.[30] Abnormalities in AST are common and occur early, but the magnitude of the change may not parallel the clinical severity of the liver injury.[70] Although AST is elevated in more than 75% of even the mild cases, the magnitude of the elevation rarely exceeds 10 times the upper limits of normal. ALT values of 200 mU/mL or ALT values that are greater than the AST indicate a chronic, persistent hepatitis or chronic, aggressive hepatitis rather than uncomplicated alcoholic hepatitis. Explanations for this minimum response to injury are inadequate. Because pyridoxal phosphate is required for transamination reactions, deficiency in pyridoxine in some alcoholics may contribute to the apparent low serum levels of these enzymes. AST and ALT concentrations return to normal within weeks of cessation of drinking. Serum AST and ALT are used as biological markers of heavy drinking, many times they are evaluated as a ratio (i.e., AST/ALT) with values greater than two suggesting possible alcoholism. These biliary enzymes are nonspecific because other illnesses such as myocardial infarction, heart failure, muscle injury, and hepatitis demonstrate serum elevation of AST and ALT.[70] These enzymes are easily measured in the laboratory with routine automated chemistry screens.

Alkaline phosphatase (ALP) (see p. 502, Chapter 27). ALP is another enzyme that assists in measuring liver damage. In alcoholic liver disease the increase in ALP activity tends to parallel the changes seen in bilirubin. Increases in ALP can be greater than two to four times the normal range in alcoholics with hepatitis.

γ-glutamyltransferase (GGT)[71,72] (see p. 503, Chapter 27). Increases in serum GGT have been reported in alcoholics with minimum or no liver disease. This has been attributed to microsomal enzyme induction. GGT is one of the first tests to change in individuals regularly consuming six or more drinks on each occasion. GGT correlates best with alcohol ingestion rather than liver damage. Changes in GGT of 30 units or higher may signify risky drinking behavior. Like other liver function tests, GGT concentrations return to normal within weeks of drinking cessation. Consequently, a baseline GGT can readily be measured and serial monitoring showing increases of 20% or more suggest return to heavy drinking.[73] Because all forms of liver disease are associated with increased GGT concentrations, increased GGT determinations alone are nonspecific for detecting alcoholism, and patient history and clinical evaluation are necessary for the diagnosis of alcoholism. Increases in GGT are also associated with other factors such as consumption of other drugs (i.e., phenytoin, benzodiazepines), obesity, and pregnancy.[12]

Bilirubin

Although alcohol does not directly alter bilirubin metabolism, the liver injury produced by alcohol does and, as such, can be used as a marker of reversible cholestasis. Jaundice, the clinical sign of elevated bilirubin, is seen in about 60% of patients with alcoholic hepatitis. Bilirubin elevation, along with a prolonged prothrombin time unresponsive to vitamin K and depressed serum albumin correlate well with the severity of alcoholic hepatitis. The bilirubin and prothrombin time results are used to classify the severity of disease as mild, moderate, or severe. Mild disease is present when the bilirubin is less than 50 mg/L with a normal or only slightly increased prothrombin time. Moderate disease is present when the bilirubin is equal to or greater than 50 mg/L and the prothrombin time is normal to moderately elevated (less than 4 seconds prolonged). Severe disease is present when the bilirubin exceeds 50 mg/L and the prothrombin time is more than 4 seconds prolonged[20] (Fig. 34-1).

Proteins

Prealbumin and albumin. Because serum albumin and prealbumin are synthesized and secreted by the liver, their serum concentrations have been used as tests of liver function. However, serum levels of prealbumin are depressed in PCM and in all forms of liver disease, including those associated with alcoholism. It is not uncommon to find values below 25 g/L in severe kwashiorkor PCM.[9] Prealbumin is considered to be a more sensitive and specific test for PCM than serum albumin. Depressed serum albumin levels in alcoholics may indicate either PCM or liver disease. Of 111 patients with severe alcoholic hepatitis in the Veterans Administration Cooperative Study,[20] 18% had values below 20 g/L, whereas only 1% had values within the normal range. However, many patients with alcoholic liver disease have ascites with expanded extravascular pools. The low serum albumin in these persons may represent a shift of albumin from the intravascular to the expanded extravascular space. In addition, serum albumin forms immunogenic adducts with acetaldehyde, which may be another useful biological marker of chronic alcoholism.[12]

Immunoglobulins. Serum γ-globulin levels change during acute and chronic liver disease in response to antigenic stimulation, reflecting the immune changes associated with alcoholic liver disease. Of the three types of γ-globulins (IgG, IgA, and IgM), IgA is most frequently increased in alcoholic liver disease, being elevated in 90% of cases, with a mean increase of 118%.[20] IgM increases the least and is elevated in 25% of cases. IgG is intermediate at 64% with a mean increase of 25%. Increases in serum γ-globulin levels are nonspecific, therefore, these measurements have little diagnostic value.[9]

Lipids

Triglycerides and cholesterol. Increases in serum triglycerides and cholesterol are frequently observed and are discussed on p. 644.

Carbohydrates

Hyperglycemia. Hepatocellular damage, regardless of its cause, is an important cause of glucose intolerance and may play a major role in the hyperglycemia found in some alcoholics.[6] Acute alcohol ingestion may cause a transient hyperglycemic state based on alcohol's effect on carbohydrate metabolism. Alcohol-induced elevation in cortisol, especially when sufficient to produce pseudo–Cushing's syndrome, is another contributing factor in alcoholic hyperglycemia.[12]

Hypoglycemia. Hypoglycemia occasionally occurs in alcoholics as a result of depletion of liver glycogen stores associated with a state of starvation. Alcohol inhibits hepatic production of glucose and inhibits gluconeogenesis.[12] Hypoglycemia may be profound resulting in coma and death. The patients are stuporous or comatose, smell of alcohol, and are often hypothermic. The diagnosis is made on the clinical findings of hypoglycemia and elevated blood alcohol; lactic acidosis is not uncommon. Other contributing factors include mild adrenocortical insufficiency and a defect in growth hormone secretion.[74] Another form of hypoglycemia occurs when alcohol is consumed with carbohydrates (alcohol-induced reactive hypoglycemia). Alcohol impairs the cell's ability to respond to insulin, and if taken with food can develop into nocturnal hypoglycemia.[73] Finally, alcoholics taking sulfonylurea hypoglycemic agents greatly deplete their blood sugar levels when they coadminister alcohol.[12]

Alcoholic ketoacidotic analytes. Alcoholic ketoacidosis is an uncommon condition occurring in nondiabetic alcoholics that was first described by Dillon, Dyer, and Smelo in 1940.[75] Patients often have abdominal pain, nausea, vomiting, and recent lack of food intake following a binge episode. The patients are acidotic but conscious, with high levels of serum ketones, salt and water depletion, and normal glucose levels. Laboratory findings are consistent with fluid and electrolyte imbalances, acid-base irregularities, and abnormal hematocrit and hemoglobin measurements. Serum insulin concentrations are low with high cortisol levels and mild elevations of growth hormone. Metabolic abnormalities improve with administration of parental hydration and glucose.[21]

Mean Corpuscular Volume (MCV)

MCV is a measure of the size of red blood cells (RBC). As a result of dysfunctional production of RBCs, MCV increases in alcoholics. MCV concentrations greater than 90 m^3 may indicate heavy alcohol consumption. Sensitivity of MCV determinations is higher in women.[12,76]

BIOLOGICAL MARKERS OF ALCOHOLISM

Because it is important to recognize alcoholism before disease occurs, biological markers are used in the laboratory to determine chronic alcohol consumption (Table 34-5). In addition, biological markers may be useful in identifying high-risk individuals at earlier stages and subtyping alcoholics based on genetic and environmental characteristics. More traditional markers of chronic alcoholism include hepatic enzymes (ALT, AST, GGT, ALP) and MCV, discussed earlier. Analytes such as carbohydrate deficient transferrin (CDT), monoamine oxidase (MAO), and acetaldehyde-modified hemoglobin (HAA) have been investigated as potential biological markers of chronic alcoholism. Ideal biological markers should be convenient and easy to measure, persist for an extended period after abstinence, and be a direct result of chronic alcohol consumption and not associated behaviors such as smoking, drug abuse, or nutritional deficiencies.[70] Several biological markers of chronic alcoholism, such as CDT, MCV, and GGT, are often tested in combination for greater sensitivity. In addition, some biological markers are measured serially to monitor relapse in recovering alcoholics. For serial monitoring to be accurate, it is important to obtain a baseline concentration following a documented prolonged abstinence period.[4]

Monoamine Oxidase

Monoamine oxidase is a mitochondrial enzyme present in platelets that oxidizes monoamine neurotransmitters such as norepinephrine, serotonin, and dopamine. Like many other drugs, ethanol has the ability to inhibit MAO activity, with decreases ranging from 20% to 60%. The mechanism by which alcohol indirectly inhibits MAO is unclear, but may be a result of secondary effects of prolonged alcohol consumption on enzymatic cofactors such as iron and riboflavin, or the negative effect of alcohol intake on platelet formation.[77] Inhibition of monoamine oxidase by alcohol is significantly higher in alcoholics when compared to nonalcoholic individuals. Even after 23 days of abstinence, monoamine oxidase activity does not return to normal levels.[70] Differences in MAO activity have been established for subtyped alcoholics; first characterized in the Stockholm Adoption Studies of the early 1980s. Type II alcoholics, who are younger, have a higher degree of heritability, and demonstrate an earlier onset of alcoholism, have a significantly reduced platelet MAO activity in comparison to type I alcoholics and controls.[78]

Carbohydrate Deficient Transferrin

Carbohydrate deficient transferrin (CDT) was initially identified in the serum and cerebral spinal fluid of alcohol abusers in 1978.[79] A CDT test measures asialo-, monosialo-, and disialo-modified isoforms of transferrin. The carbohydrate-deficient moieties are caused by acetaldehyde inhibition of protein glycosylation and increased terminal trisaccharide truncation of serum transferrin molecules.[4,80] These isoforms can be qualitatively separated by isoelectric focusing and quantitated by immunoelectrophoresis, immunofixation, Western blotting, or immunoblotting with laser densitometry.[80] Reported sensitivity for detecting alcohol abuse ranges from 48% to 100% in alcoholics and 22% to 76% in risky drinkers.[81] More than 80% of chronic alcoholics have a CDT level greater than 70 mg/L (20 U/L), however, the elevated CDT concentrations will decline within a few weeks of abstinence.[73] CDT has a high specificity, but false-positives have been demonstrated in individuals who have advanced liver disease, a genetically rare transferrin variant, or a genetic glycoprotein disorder. Moreover, CDT concentrations are affected by age, gender, alcohol consumption pattern (identifies alcoholics more accurately than at-risk drinkers), and liver dysfunction (increased CDT abnormalities with greater liver disease).[76,81] The mechanism by which gender influences CDT concentrations has been associated with hormonal differences. Combined studies demonstrate that moderate alcohol consumption increases estradiol concentrations in postmenopausal women.[12] Furthermore, hormonal changes related to pre- and postmenopausal states, timing of menses, and pregnancy can cause CDT concentrations to fluctuate.[71,72,82] CDT can be as much as 50% less sensitive at detecting alcoholism in women versus men.[80]

Acetaldehyde-Modified Hemoglobin (HAA)

Once acetaldehyde is formed from alcohol metabolism, it can bind to hemoglobin through non-covalent (reversible) and covalent (irreversible) bonds. The irreversible process forms modified hemoglobin known as *acetaldehyde-modified hemoglobin*. HAA concentrations rapidly increase and remain above baseline for up to 2 days following alcohol consumption. Recent studies indicate that HAA concentrations may be positively influenced in populations of specific genotypes. Fifty percent of the Japanese population has a mutant heterozygous gene, low-K_m acetaldehyde dehydrogenase (ALDH2), which causes undesirable effects with alcohol use, such as flushing of the skin and illness. This mutant ALDH2 genotype reduces individuals' capacity to metabolize acetaldehyde and renders them more susceptible to alcoholic liver disease.[83] These findings may support monitoring HAA concentrations in specific genetic populations. HAA can be separated from other hemoglobin forms and detected by high-performance liquid chromatography or an enzyme immunoassay.[81]

Other Biological Markers

Investigators have reported findings for other potential biological markers of chronic alcohol consumption. These markers include catalase, platelet adenylate cyclase, and early detection by alcohol consumption (EDAC) scores. Catalase activity, which may oxidize alcohol to acetaldehyde, has a positive relationship with an individual's ability to consume alcohol, and monitoring catalase activity in an individual may predict alcohol intake.[84] Platelet adenylate cyclase activity is greatly reduced in alcoholics and remains abnormal for periods of 1 to 4 years of abstinence.[70] EDAC tests use routine blood serum panels to calculate a score, which is statistically compared to scores of reference controls. With this information, an individual is categorized as a light or heavy drinker.[85] Presently, these biological markers are investigational and are not routinely measured when evaluating an individual for alcoholism.

WITHDRAWAL, TOXIC SYNDROMES, AND TREATMENT OF ALCOHOL DEPENDENCY
Withdrawal

Most patients only experience minor withdrawal symptoms from alcohol including insomnia, anxiety, and autonomic disturbances (i.e., increased blood pressure, temperature, heart and respiratory rates). Using minimal outpatient treatment, these symptoms generally peak within 48 hours and subside within 5 days.[12] In some instances, medical and psychiatric intervention is necessary because of severe health conditions or toxic syndromes that manifest in some patients.

Toxic Syndromes

There are a number of **alcohol withdrawal syndromes** related to the cessation of ethanol consumption. These include a generalized abstinence syndrome that develops within 6 to 8 hours of abstinence with symptoms that include tremor, agitation, sleep disturbances, nausea, vomiting, weakness, headache, and diaphoresis. Symptoms may continue for 3 to 7 days. This is a minor syndrome and prognosis of the patient is excellent with supportive management of symptoms.[86]

Alcoholic hallucinosis usually develops 24 to 36 hours after cessation of drinking. Symptoms range from delusions to visual and auditory hallucination. Often the patient remains fully oriented and minimal medical intervention is necessary. Benzodiazepines may be administered to alleviate excess anxiety that may occur with the hallucinations.[87] "Rum fits" or grand mal seizures occur with a peak incidence at 24 hours after cessation of ethanol. There is a 3% risk of developing *status epilepticus* but 30% of those experiencing seizures will proceed to delirium tremens.[86]

Delirium tremens is a toxic syndrome with severe symptoms that constitute a medical emergency. Symptoms usually develop within 3 to 5 days after withdrawal of ethanol and usually include confusion, delusions, vivid hallucinations, fever, tachycardia, and seizures. When ethanol withdrawal proceeds to this syndrome the mortality rate is 9% to 15%.[86]

Treatment

Millions of dollars are spent annually to detoxify and rehabilitate chronic alcoholics, who comprise 11% to 16% of the American population. Studies show that patients have a high risk of relapse, with nearly 50% returning to alcohol within 12 months of their detoxification.[88] Because of these statistics, an arsenal of pharmacological, medical, and psychosocial treatments are offered to the public every year.

Pharmacological treatment

Disulfiram (Antabuse). Disulfiram was first introduced for the treatment of alcohol dependence in 1948.[11] Disulfiram acts as a psychological deterrent to prevent alcohol consumption by blocking aldehyde dehydrogenase, leading to an accumulation of toxic acetaldehyde levels when alcohol is consumed. The high concentrations of acetaldehyde produce undesirable effects such as tachycardia, nausea, vomiting, hypotension, headache, anxiety, and flushing, thus making the individual extremely uncomfortable. The "disulfiram effects" may begin within minutes of alcohol ingestion and persist for up to an hour.[12] Disulfiram symptoms may appear with a serum ethanol concentration as low as 10 mg/dL and an individual can lose consciousness at serum ethanol concentrations greater than 120 mg/dL.[11] Disulfiram can be administered orally (200 to 250 mg/day) or as an implant (800 to 1000 mg implant). Implants were first proposed as an answer to compliance issues. Once an alcoholic knows the effects of drinking while taking disulfiram, patient noncompliance of disulfiram treatment may occur. Several controlled clinical trials show that disulfiram therapy modestly reduces drinking frequency but does not improve abstinence rates. Because the duration of action for disulfiram averages 72 hours, patients will fight impulsive inclinations to resume drinking, thereby reducing drinking frequency. The variability of disulfiram implant efficacy suggests that the bioavailability of this drug may be inconsistent.[2] Disulfiram can have life-threatening effects in alcoholics who resume heavy drinking and have medical complications including diabetes, high blood pressure, cirrhosis, or severe heart disease.[12]

Opioid antagonists. Opioid antagonists, such as naltrexone and nalmefene, act at the opioid receptor to inhibit binding of endogenous opioids like β-endorphin and enkephalins. Naltrexone was approved by the Food and Drug Administration (FDA) for the treatment of alcohol dependency in 1994, whereas nalmefene is a newly investigated opioid antagonist because it is less hepatotoxic and is slowly metabolized.[35] Without the binding of endogenous opioids, the individual does not experience desirable CNS effects such as euphoria associated with abused drugs. The naltrexone dose used to treat alcohol dependency is 50 mg/day. Controlled studies of naltrexone therapy report improved abstinence when combined with psychosocial therapy but not with coping skills therapy, lower relapse rates than the placebo-controlled groups (23% to 40% vs. 53% to 80%), and GGT levels in naltrexone-treated patients that were either comparable or lower than placebo-treated patients.[2]

Acamprosate (calcium acetylhomotaurinate). Acamprosate is a synthetic drug with a similar chemical structure to γ-aminobutyric acid (GABA), a neurotransmitter. Administered orally, acamprosate binds selectively to glutamate (GABA$_B$) receptors, which may play a role in CNS effects of alcohol and symptoms of ethanol withdrawal syndromes.[12,88] A recent meta-analysis study conducted by Garbutt et al. indicates that acamprosate reduces drinking frequency but its effect on abstinence was uncertain.[2] Several studies have indicated that the efficacy of acamprosate may be dose dependent, with concomitant use of disulfiram or psychosocial therapy improving relapse rates following detoxification. Tolerance to acamprosate is usually acceptable, with mild to moderate adverse effects including gastrointestinal disturbances, dermatological complications, transient headaches, dizziness, and loss of sex drive. Given at a recommended dose (0.4 to 0.67 g three times daily for up to 1 year), acamprosate does not show signs of abuse potential. Patients have reportedly survived acamprosate overdoses of up to 43 g.[88]

Serotonergic agents. The use of serotonergic agents, including agonists (such as lithium, buspirone) and antagonists (such as ondansetron) has been investigated as possible treatment for alcoholism. Because of the limited effectiveness and possible dangerous side effects, none of these agents are in current use.

Psychosocial therapy. Individual and group counseling sessions are employed in psychosocial therapy to support an alcoholic during rehabilitation, recovery, and pursuit of a new lifestyle. Psychosocial and group therapy aim to assist patients with dealing with their disease; whether it be discussing the patient's difficulties in succeeding with recovery, family and job-related issues, coping skills, self-awareness, and/or understanding the risks of their disease. Many programs include the family and employer in their rehabilitation efforts.[12]

Closed detoxification and inpatient rehabilitation facilities. Inpatient detoxification and rehabilitation facilities offer a place of forced abstinence. The goals of these facilities include diagnosing and treating serious medical and psychiatric disorders, increasing and maintaining motivation for abstinence, and assisting the alcoholic in readjusting to an alcohol-free lifestyle. These facilities are chosen based on the patient's medical and psychiatric needs, history of previous treatment, financial considerations, and social supports. Generally, inpatient treatment begins with supportive care and detoxification. During detoxification, medical treatments may include benzodiazepine therapy to counteract withdrawal symptoms, pharmacological agents to minimize alcohol dependency, and corticosteroids to treat severe acute alcoholic hepatitis if the patient is not immunocompromised.[35] Patients are given thiamine (100 mg three times daily) for several days followed by a thiamine-containing multivitamin for several months. Other care includes physical exam, group therapy sessions, rest, food, and exercise. Inpatient treatments last from 2 to 6 weeks with required outpatient follow-up.[12]

Alcoholics Anonymous and other self-help organizations. Alcoholics Anonymous (AA) and other self-help organizations offer recovering alcoholics a nurturing environment and a model for recovery, a social arena to voice experiences and witness experiences of others, and a mentoring system to closely assist an individual. Some AA groups focus on religion, others discuss the "12 essential steps" to recovery, and others embody a more individualistic approach. Meetings are held daily throughout most major cities at no cost to the attending alcoholic. In addition, AA sponsors other support groups (Alanon and Alateen) that help family members of alcoholics understand this disease.[12]

ACKNOWLEDGEMENTS

With acknowledgments to the previous author, Charles L. Mendenhall.

References

1. SAMHSA's News Release: *1999 National Household Survey,* www.samhsa.gov.
2. Garbutt JC et al: Pharmacological treatment of alcohol dependence: a review of the evidence, *JAMA* 281:1318, 1999.
3. Wiese JG, Shlipak MG, Browner WS: The alcohol hangover, *Ann Intern Med* 132:897, 2000.
4. Lieber CS: Carbohydrate deficient transferrin in alcoholic liver disease: mechanisms and clinical implications, *Alcohol and Alcoholism* 19:249, 1999.
5. Garriott JC, editor: *Medicolegal aspects of alcohol,* ed 3, Tucson, AZ, 1996, Lawyers & Judges.
6. Cotran RS, Kumar V, Collins T, editors: *Robbins pathologic basis of disease,* ed 6, Philadelphia, 1999, Saunders.
7. Rockerbie RA, editor: *Alcohol and drug intoxication,* Victoria, BC, Canada, 1999, Trafford Publishing Service.
8. Ellenhorn MJ et al, editors: *Ellenhorn's medical toxicology: diagnosis and treatment of human poisoning,* Baltimore, 1997, Williams & Wilkins.
9. Beers RE, Berkow R, editors: *The Merck manual of diagnosis and therapy,* ed 17, Whitehouse Station, NJ, 1999, Merck Research Laboratories.
10. Fiellin DA, Reid MC, O'Conner PG: Screening for alcohol problems in primary care, *Arch Intern Med* 160:1977, 2000.
11. Baselt RC, editor: *Disposition of toxic drugs and chemicals in man,* ed 5, Foster City, CA, 2000, CTI.
12. Mendelson JH, Mello NK, editors: *Medical diagnosis and treatment of alcoholism,* New York, 1992, McGraw-Hill.
13. Gaziano JM et al: Moderate alcohol intake, increased levels of high-density lipoprotein and its subfractions, and decreased risk of myocardial infarction, *N Engl J Med* 329:1829, 1993.
14. Kannel WB, Ellison RC: Alcohol and coronary heart disease: the evidence for a protective effect, *Clinica Chimica Acta* 246:59, 1996.
15. Suter PM, Schutz Y, Jequier E: The effect of ethanol on fat storage in healthy subjects, *N Engl J Med* 326:983, 1992.
16. www.merck.com
17. Bennington JL, editor: *Saunders dictionary & encyclopedia of laboratory medicine and technology,* Philadelphia, 1984, Saunders.
18. Preedy VR et al: Protein metabolism in alcoholism: effects on specific tissues and the whole body, *Nutrition* 15:604, 1999.
19. Lieber CS: Hepatic and other medical disorders of alcoholism: from pathogenesis to treatment, *J Stud Alcohol* 59:9, 1998.
20. Mendenhall CL: Alcoholic hepatitis, *Clin Gastroenterol* 10:417, 1981.
21. Fulop M: Alcoholic ketoacidosis, *Endocrin Metab Clin North Am* 22:209, 1993.
22. Olin JS, Devenyi P, Weldon KL: Uric acid in alcoholics, *Q J Study Alcohol* 34:1202, 1973.
23. Newcombe DS: Ethanol metabolism and uric acid, *Metabolism: Clin & Exp* 21:1193, 1972.
24. Tomaiolo PP: Nutritional problems in the alcoholic, *Nutrition* 7:24, 1981.
25. Bunout D: Nutritional and metabolic effects of alcoholism: their relationship with alcoholic liver disease, *Nutrition* 15:583, 1999.
26. Mendenhall CL et al: Protein-calorie malnutrition associated with alcoholic hepatitis, *Am J Med* 76:211, 1984.
27. World MJ, Ryle PR, Thomson AD: Alcoholic malnutrition and the small intestine, *Alcohol and Alcoholism* 20:89, 1985.
28. Watson RR, Watzl B, editors: *Nutrition and alcohol,* Boca Raton, FL, 1992, CRC Press.
29. Elisaf MS, Siamopoulos KC: Mechanisms of hypophosphataemia in alcoholic patients, *Int J Clin Pract* 51:501, 1997.
30. Devgun MS et al: Vitamin and mineral nutrition in chronic alcoholics including patients with Korsakoff's psychosis, *P Br J Nutr* 45:469, 1981.
31. Thomson AD, Majumdar SK: The influence of ethanol on intestinal absorption and utilization of nutrients, *Clin Gastroenterol* 10:263, 1981.
32. Smith JC, Jr, et al: Zinc: a trace element essential in vitamin A metabolism, *Science* 181:954, 1973.
33. Flink EB: Magnesium deficiency in alcoholism, *Alcoholism: Clin Exp Res* 10:590, 1986.
34. Xu D et al: Detection of circulating antibodies to malondialdehyde-acetaldehyde adducts in ethanol fed rats, *Gastroenterology* 115:686, 1998.
35. Walsh K, Alexander G: Alcoholic liver disease, *Postgrad Med J* 76:280, 2000.
36. Fang C et al: Zonated expression of cytokines in rat liver: effect of chronic ethanol and the cytochrome P450 2E1 inhibitor, chlormethiazole, *Hepatology* 27:1304, 1998.
37. Ludwig J et al: Hemosiderosis in cirrhosis: a study of 447 native livers, *Gastroenterology* 112:882, 1997.
38. MacDonald RA, Jones RS, Pechet GS: Folic acid deficiency and hemochromatosis, *Arch Path* 80:153, 1965.
39. Ganne-Carrie N et al: Predictive value of liver iron content for survival in 229 prospectively followed patients with cirrhosis, *J Hepatol* 25(suppl 1):95, 1996.
40. Naruse S, Kitagawa M, Ishiguro H: Molecular understanding of chronic pancreatitis: a perspective on the future, *Molec Med Today* 5:493, 1999.
41. Durbec JP, Sarles H: Multicenter survey of the etiology of pancreatic diseases: relationship between the relative risk of developing chronic pancreatitis and alcohol, protein, and lipid consumption, *Digestion* 18:337, 1978.
42. Niebergall-Roth E, Harder H, Singer MV: A review: acute and chronic effects of ethanol and alcoholic beverages on the pancreatic exocrine secretion in vivo and in vitro, *Alcohol Clin Exp Res* 22:1570, 1998.
43. Sarles H: Chronic calcifying pancreatitis-chronic alcoholic pancreatitis, *Gastroenterology* 66:604, 1974.
44. Ammann RW, Largiader F, Akovbiantz A: Pain relief by surgery in chronic pancreatitis? Relationship between pain relief, pancreatic dysfunction, and alcohol withdrawal, *Scand J Gastroenterol* 14:209, 1979.
45. DiMagno EP, Go VLW, Summerskill WHJ: Relations between pancreatic enzyme outputs and malabsorption in severe pancreatic insufficiency, *N Engl J Med* 288:813, 1973.
46. Stressguth AP, Clarren SK, Jones KL: Natural history of the fetal alcohol syndrome: a 10 year follow-up of eleven patients, *Lancet* 2:85, 1985.
47. Abel EL, Sokol RJ: Incidence of fetal alcohol syndrome and economic impact of FAS-related anomalies, *Drug Alcohol Depend* 19:51, 1987.
48. Preedy VR, Richardson PJ: Ethanol induced cardiovascular disease, *British Med Bull* 50:152, 1994.
49. Schenk EA, Cohen J: The heart in chronic alcoholism: clinical and pathologic findings, *Pathol Microbiol* 35:96, 1970.
50. Gimsing P et al: Vitamin B-12 and folate function in chronic alcoholic men with peripheral neuropathy and encephalopathy, *J Nutr* 119:416, 1989.
51. Tamerin JS et al: Alcohol and memory: amnesia and short-term memory function during experimentally induced intoxication, *Am J Psychiatry* 127:1659, 1971.
52. Mufti SI, Darban HR, Watson RR: Alcohol, cancer and immuno-modulation, *Crit Rev Oncol Hematol* 9:243, 1989.
53. Stuart KE, Anand AJ, Jenkins RL: Hepatocellular carcinoma in the United States: prognostic features, treatment outcome, and survival, *Cancer* 77:2217, 1996.
54. Katz AE: Update on immunology of head and neck cancer, *Med Clin North Am* 77:625, 1993.
55. Kato I, Nomura AMY: Alcohol in the aetiology of upper aerodigestive tract cancer, *Oral Oncol Eur J Cancer* 30B:75, 1994.
56. Fontham ETH, Correa P: Epidemiology of pancreatic cancer, *Surg Clin North Am* 69:551, 1989.
57. Andren-Sandberg A, Dervenis C, Lowenfels B: Etiologic links between chronic pancreatitis and pancreatic cancer, *Scand J Gastroenterol* 32:97, 1997.
58. Noth RH, Walter RM: The effects of alcohol on the endocrine system, *Med Clin North Am* 68:133, 1984.
59. Rivier C: Alcohol stimulates ACTH secretion in the rat: mechanisms of action and interactions with other stimuli, *Alcohol Clin Exp Res* 20:240, 1996.
60. Chalmers RJ et al: Growth hormone, prolactin and corticosteroid responses to insulin hypoglycaemia in alcoholics, *Br Med J* 1:745, 1978.
61. Casagrande G, Michot F: Alcohol induced bone marrow damage: status before and after a 4-week period of abstinence from alcohol with or without disulfiram, *Blut* 59:231, 1989.
62. Liu YK: Leukopenia in alcoholics, *Am J Med* 54:605, 1973.
63. Cowan DH, Hines JD: Thrombocytopenia of severe alcoholism, *Ann Intern Med* 74:37, 1971.

64. Bernstein IM et al: Reduction in circulating T lymphocytes in alcoholic liver disease, *Lancet* 2:488, 1974.

65. Smith WI, Jr, et al: Altered immunity in male patients with alcoholic liver disease: evidence for defective immune regulation, *Alcohol Clin Exp Res* 4:199, 1980.

66. SAMHSA: *DAWN annual emergency department report*, 1999, www.samhsa.gov.

67. SAMHSA: *DAWN annual medical examiner data*, 1999, www.samhsa.gov.

68. Fell JC, Nash CE: The nature of the alcohol problem in US fatal crashes, *Health Educ Q* 16:335, 1989.

69. O'Neal CL, Poklis A: Postmortem production of ethanol and factors that influence interpretation: a critical review, *Am J Forens Med Pathol* 17:8, 1996.

70. Tabakoff B et al: Differences in platelet enzyme activity between alcoholics and nonalcoholics, *N Engl J Med* 318:134, 1988.

71. Sillanaukee P et al: Effect of hormone balance on carbohydrate-deficient transferrin and gamma glutamyltransferase in female social drinkers, *Alcohol Clin Exp Res* 24:1505, 2000.

72. van Pelt J et al: Test characteristics of carbohydrate-deficient transferrin and gamma glutamyltransferase in alcohol-using perimenopausal women, *Alcohol Clin Exp Res* 24:176, 2000.

73. Schuckit MA, editor: *Drug and alcohol abuse: a clinical guide to diagnosis and treatment*, ed 5, New York, 2000, Kluwer Academic/Plenum.

74. Johnston DG, Alberti KGMM: The liver and the endocrine system. In Wright R et al, editors: *Liver and biliary disease*, Philadelphia, 1979, Saunders.

75. Dillon ES, Dyer WW, Smelo LS: Ketone acidosis in nondiabetic adults, *Med Clin North Am* 24:1813, 1940.

76. Mundle G et al: Sex differences of carbohydrate-deficient transferrin, gamma glutamyltransferase, and mean corpuscular volume in alcohol-dependent patients, *Alcohol Clin Exp Res* 24:1400, 2000.

77. Pandey GN et al: Platelet monoamine oxidase in alcoholism, *Biol Psychiatry* 24:15, 1988.

78. von Knorring AL et al: Platelet monoamine oxidase activity in type I and type II alcoholism, *Alcohol Alcohol* 26:409, 1991.

79. Stibler H et al: Abnormal microheterogeneity of transferrin in serum and cerebrospinal fluid in alcoholism, *Acta Med Scand* 204:49, 1978.

80. Salaspuro M: Carbohydrate-deficient transferrin as compared to other markers of alcoholism: a systemic review, *Alcohol* 19:261, 1999.

81. Hazelett SE et al: Evaluation of acetaldehyde-modified hemoglobin and other markers of chronic heavy alcohol use: effects of gender and hemoglobin concentration, *Alcohol Clin Exp Res* 22:1813, 1998.

82. Leusink GL et al: Carbohydrate-deficient transferrin in relation to the menopausal status of women, *Alcohol Clin Exp Res* 24:172, 2000.

83. Takeshita T, Morimoto K: Accumulation of hemoglobin-associated acetaldehyde with habitual alcohol drinking in the atypical ALDH2 genotype, *Alcohol Clin Exp Res* 24:1, 2000.

84. Koechling UM, Amit Z: Relationship between blood catalase activity and drinking history in a human population, a possible biological marker of the affinity to consume alcohol, *Alcohol and Alcoholism* 27:181, 1992.

85. Harasymiw J, Vinson DC, Bean P: The EDAC score in the identification of heavy and at-risk drinkers from routine blood tests, *J Addict Med* 19:43, 2000.

86. Erwin WE, Williams DB, Speir WA: Delirium tremens, *So Med J* 91:425, 1998.

87. Olmedo R, Hoffman RS: Withdrawal syndromes, *Emerg Med Clin North Am* 18:273, 2000.

88. Wilde MI, Wagstaff AJ: Acamprosate: a review of its pharmacology and clinical potential in the management of alcohol dependence after detoxification, *Drugs* 53:1038, 1997.

Internet Sites

www.niaaa.nih.gov—National Institute on Alcohol Abuse and Alcoholism

www.ncadd.org/—National Council on Alcoholism and Drug Dependence (NCADD)

www.aca-usa.org/—American Council on Alcoholism (ACA)

www.medicouncilalcol.demon.co.uk/—The Medical Council on Alcohol

http://alcalc.oupjournals.org

http://www.nlm.nih.gov/medlineplus/alcoholism.html

http://www.nmha.org/infoctr/factsheets/02.cfm

http://www.alcoholismtreatment.org/

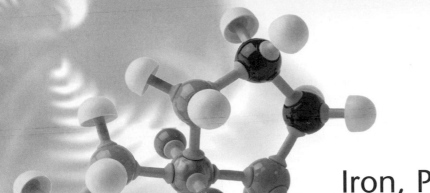

CHAPTER 35

Iron, Porphyrin, and Bilirubin Metabolism

• *William E. Schreiber*

Chapter Outline

Objectives

• List the physiological functions of iron and describe its absorption from the gut and its transport in the body.
• Describe the pathological conditions leading to iron deficiency and overload and describe changes in the

following analytes in iron deficiency anemia, anemia of chronic disease, thalassemia, hemochromatosis, and lead poisoning: ferritin, serum iron, iron-binding capacity, and free erythrocyte protoporphyrin.

- Define porphyria and distinguish between primary and secondary porphyrias.
- List porphyrin analytes that will be elevated in each

of the primary and secondary porphyrias.
- Outline the formation and catabolism of bilirubin.

Key Terms

ampulla of Vater   The junction of the common bile duct and pancreatic duct proximal to their opening into the duodenum.

anemia   A reduction in the quantity of hemoglobin or number of red cells in blood.

bile   The yellow-green fluid secreted by the liver and poured into the duodenum through the bile ducts.

chelate   A chemical compound in which a metallic ion is firmly bound to a chelating molecule.

cholestasis   The stoppage of the flow of bile.

cirrhosis   A liver disease characterized by the loss of the normal microscopic architecture, with fibrosis and nodular regeneration.

erythropoiesis   The production of erythrocytes.

hemolytic anemia   Anemia caused by shortened survival of mature red blood cells.

hypochromic   Referring to erythrocytes that are paler than normal because of a decrease in hemoglobin content.

mean corpuscular hemoglobin (MCH)   The average amount of hemoglobin per red blood cell.

mean corpuscular hemoglobin concentration (MCHC)   The average concentration of hemoglobin per red blood cell.

mean corpuscular volume (MCV)   The average red blood cell volume.

megaloblastic anemia   Anemia characterized by large red blood cell precursors in the bone marrow.

microcytic   Referring to erythrocytes that are smaller than reference interval.

parenchyma   The functional tissue of an organ (excluding the fibrous framework).

pernicious anemia   A **megaloblastic anemia** caused by failure to absorb vitamin B_{12}.

photoisomers   Isomers produced on exposure to light.

photosensitivity   Abnormal reactivity of the skin to sunlight.

porphyrinuria   The presence of excess porphyrin in urine.

reticuloendothelial system   A functional system composed of highly phagocytic cells with both endothelial and reticular attributes, located in blood vessels, lymph nodes, liver, spleen, bone marrow, and other tissues.

sideroblastic anemia   A heterogenous group of anemias in which iron stores of the reticuloendothelial tissues are increased and bone marrow normoblasts contain iron deposits within mitochondria (ringed sideroblasts).

tachycardia   Rapid heart rate.

thalassemia   A heterogeneous group of hereditary hemolytic anemias that have a decreased rate of synthesis of one or more hemoglobin polypeptide chains.

Methods on CD-ROM

Bilirubin
Iron and total iron-binding capacity

Porphobilinogen screening and quantitation
Transferrin and carbohydrate-deficient transferring

Part 1: Iron Metabolism
DISTRIBUTION AND FUNCTION

Iron is one of the most abundant elements on earth, yet only trace amounts are present in living cells. Most of the iron in humans is located within the porphyrin ring of heme, which is incorporated into proteins such as hemoglobin, myoglobin, catalase, peroxidases, and cytochromes. There are also iron-sulfur proteins, such as NADH dehydrogenase and succinate dehydrogenase, in which iron is present in clusters with inorganic sulfur. In all these systems, it is the

ability of iron to interact reversibly with oxygen and to function in electron-transfer reactions that makes it biologically indispensable.

An average adult male has about 4 g of body iron. About 65% to 70% of the total is found in hemoglobin, and about 10% is located in myoglobin and other iron-containing enzymes and proteins. The remaining 20% to 25% consists of a storage pool of iron. By comparison, the average adult woman has only 2 to 3 g of iron in her body. This difference is attributable in part to the much smaller iron reserves in

TABLE 35-1 IRON DISTRIBUTION AND FUNCTION IN A NORMAL ADULT MALE		
Compound	**Function**	**Iron (mg)**
Hemoglobin	O_2 transport, blood	2500
Myoglobin	O_2 storage, muscle	
Enzymes		
Catalase	H_2O_2 decomposition	500
Peroxidases	Oxidation	
Cytochromes	Electron transfer	
Iron-sulfur*	Electron transfer	
Transferrin*	Iron transport	3
Ferritin* and hemosiderin*	Iron storage	600 to 1000

Nonheme iron compounds.

women. Also, women have a lower hemoglobin concentration in blood and a smaller vascular volume than men. Iron distribution is summarized in Table 35-1.

METABOLISM

Daily requirements for iron vary depending on the person's age, sex, and physiological status. Although iron is not excreted in the conventional sense, there is a daily loss of about 1 mg through the normal shedding of skin epithelial cells and cells lining the gastrointestinal and urinary tracts. Small numbers of erythrocytes are lost in urine and feces as well. An iron intake of 1 mg per day is therefore sufficient for men and postmenopausal women. However, since the blood lost in each menstrual cycle drains 20 to 40 mg of iron, women in their reproductive years need 2 mg of iron per day. The diversion of iron to the fetus during pregnancy, blood loss during delivery, and subsequent breast-feeding of the infant consume 900 mg of iron on average. This increases daily iron demands to 3 or 4 mg in pregnant and lactating women.

Absorption

A healthy North American diet contains between 10 and 20 mg of iron per day. Only 5% to 10% of this amount is absorbed, mainly in the duodenum and upper small intestine. Most dietary iron is in the ferric (Fe^{3+}) state, but it must be converted to the ferrous (Fe^{2+}) state before it can enter the intestinal cell. A ferrireductase on the brush border of the enterocyte reduces Fe^{3+} to Fe^{2+}, which is then transported into the cell by a divalent metal transporter (DMT1), as shown in Fig. 35-1. Gastric acid and dietary components that form soluble iron **chelates** (such as ascorbic acid, sugars, and amino acids) keep ingested iron in solution and increase its absorption. Substances that form insoluble complexes with iron—such as phosphates (in eggs, cheese, and milk), oxalates and phytates (in vegetables), and tannates (in tea)—decrease iron absorption. Heme iron, which comes mainly from meat and fish, is processed differently. After it is released from the surrounding polypeptide chain, heme is absorbed intact by the intestinal cell, where the porphyrin

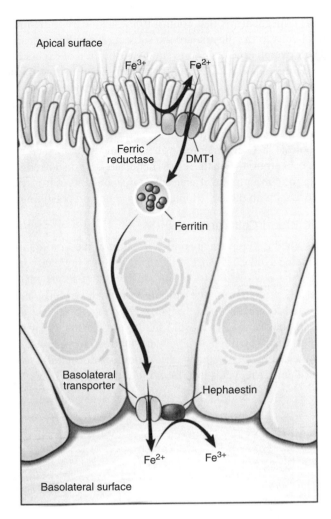

Fig. 35-1 Iron absorption. Dietary iron is reduced from Fe^{3+} to Fe^{2+} at the apical surface of intestinal epithelial cells, then taken into the cells by a divalent metal transporter (DMT1). Within the cell, iron may be stored as ferritin, or it may be transported through the basolateral surface to enter the circulation. The basolateral transporter has not yet been identified. It works in combination with hephaestin, a copper-containing protein that is thought to oxidize Fe^{2+} back to Fe^{3+}. *(From Andrews NC: Disorders of iron metabolism, N Engl J Med 341(26):1986, 1999. Copyright ©1999 Massachusetts Medical Society. All rights reserved.)*

ring is split and iron is liberated. This process is more efficient than the absorption of nonheme iron and is not affected by dietary factors.

Since iron loss is a continuous and largely unregulated process, iron balance is controlled by changes in absorption. The intestinal cells take in considerably more iron than the amount that eventually will enter the circulation. Once inside the intestinal cell, iron is transferred across its basolateral surface into plasma or is incorporated into ferritin for storage. Stored iron can subsequently be mobilized as necessary, but most of this iron is lost when the mucosal cells are shed. New cells take their place, and the cycle of iron buildup starts again.

The mechanisms that control iron transfer from the intestinal cells to the plasma are the subject of ongoing research. Their overall effect is to prevent the absorption of excess iron while maintaining an adequate supply for current needs. The major factors affecting iron absorption are body iron stores and the rate of red blood cell production. When necessary, the efficiency of absorption can increase by threefold or more. Thus iron deficiency, pregnancy, and the accelerated **erythropoiesis** that occurs in some anemias all stimulate increased iron absorption. On the other hand, absorption is reduced after the consumption of unusually large amounts of iron, such as occurs with dietary supplementation or iron poisoning.

Red Blood Cell Turnover

Absorbed iron represents only a fraction of the iron required for heme synthesis. Most of the iron, 20 to 25 mg/day, comes from the destruction of old erythrocytes by tissue macrophages, primarily in the spleen. Within these cells, heme oxygenase breaks open the porphyrin ring to release iron. Macrophages transfer most of the iron to plasma transferrin, which then carries it to the bone marrow for hemoglobin synthesis. In this manner, the **reticuloendothelial system** continuously recycles iron from old red cells into new ones.

Macrophages also maintain a storage pool of iron. When red cell destruction exceeds the rate of production, iron accumulates within macrophages and the storage pool expands. When the balance shifts toward red cell production, macrophages release additional iron from their stores. Infection, inflammation, and malignancy interfere with the release of iron from macrophages and may cause a drop in red cell production despite the presence of adequate iron reserves.

Transport and Cell Uptake

Transferrin, a single-chain glycoprotein with a molecular weight of 79,500 daltons, is the transport protein for iron in blood. Each transferrin molecule has two binding sites for Fe^{3+} that are normally 20% to 50% saturated. The need for a specific carrier protein derives from the toxicity and insolubility of free iron; virtually all plasma iron is protein-bound. Iron transport is a dynamic process, and the half-life of an iron atom in plasma is between 60 and 120 minutes under normal circumstances.

Transferrin delivers iron to cells with specific surface receptors for this protein (Fig. 35-2). After binding to the receptor, the transferrin receptor-transferrin complex is taken

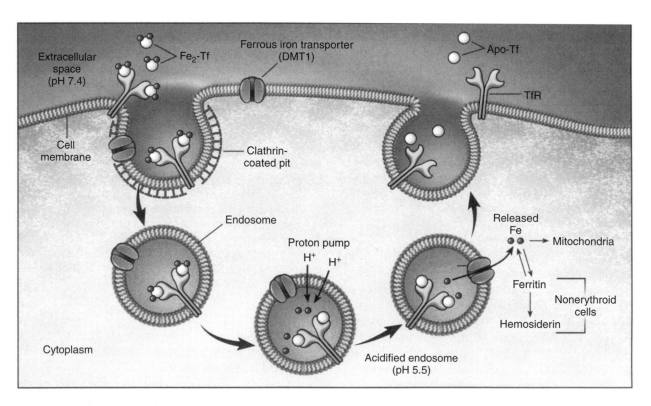

Fig. 35-2 Delivery of iron to cells. Iron-loaded transferrin (Fe_2-Tf) binds to transferrin receptors (TfR) on the cell surface. A portion of the cell membrane is then pinched off to form an endosome, a self-enclosed fragment of the membrane with the Fe_2-Tf-TfR complex inside. Protons (H^+) are pumped into the endosome, releasing iron from transferrin. Iron is transported out of the acidified endosome and into the cytoplasm, where it can enter the mitochondria for heme synthesis or be stored as ferritin. The endosome then fuses with the cell membrane, and iron-free apotransferrin (Apo-Tf) is released into the extracellular space. *(From Andrews NC: Disorders of iron metabolism, N Engl J Med 341(26):1986, 1999. Copyright ©1999 Massachusetts Medical Society. All rights reserved.)*

into the cell by endocytosis and formed into a vesicle. At the acidic pH of the vesicle, iron is released from transferrin. The receptor-transferrin complex is then returned to the cell surface, where both apotransferrin and the receptor become available for additional rounds of iron transport and uptake. Inside the cell, iron is used for heme synthesis within the mitochondria or is stored as ferritin.

Storage

Iron is stored in tissues in either of two forms, ferritin or hemosiderin. Ferritin consists of a multisubunit protein shell, known as *apoferritin*, surrounding a core of up to 4500 iron atoms. The iron in ferritin is deposited within its core as a ferric hydroxyphosphate complex. Ferritin is present in most cells and is a readily mobilized form of storage iron. It serves to package and isolate iron atoms from the intracellular environment, thus preventing any toxic action on cell constituents. Hemosiderin is an insoluble complex derived from ferritin that has lost some of its surface protein and become aggregated. It is present in granules 1 to 2 μm in diameter and is visible by light microscopy after staining tissue sections with Prussian blue dye. Hemosiderin has a higher iron concentration than ferritin, but it releases iron more slowly.

About one third of the body's iron reserves is stored in the liver, one third in the bone marrow, and the remainder in the spleen and other tissues.

PATHOLOGICAL CONDITIONS
Iron Deficiency

When iron intake falls below the amount required for red blood cell production, iron reserves become depleted and, in time, **anemia** develops. Iron deficiency is a common nutritional disorder in humans and is the most frequent cause of anemia. It is estimated that about 3% of adult men, 20% of women in their reproductive years, and 50% of pregnant women are deficient in iron.

The high prevalence of iron deficiency among women is the result of the blood loss that occurs during each menstrual cycle. Bleeding from the gastrointestinal tract is the usual cause of iron deficiency in men. The increased demand for iron in infants and young children, adolescents, and pregnant women may also lead to iron deficiency, especially if these individuals have diets that are low in iron. Impaired absorption of iron after gastrointestinal surgery and in patients with chronic diarrhea or malabsorption also causes depletion of iron reserves.

Iron deficiency develops in stages, the first of which is depletion of storage iron in response to a prolonged negative iron balance. Once iron reserves have been exhausted, biochemical tests of iron metabolism become abnormal. Next, a drop in the hemoglobin concentration of blood is seen, and in time the red blood cells become smaller and paler than normal. In fully developed iron deficiency anemia, a complete blood count reveals a decrease in hemoglobin and in all the red blood cell indices: **mean corpuscular volume (MCV)**, **mean corpuscular hemoglobin (MCH)**, and **mean corpuscular hemoglobin concentration (MCHC)**. Examination of a peripheral blood smear shows erythrocytes that are **hypochromic** and **microcytic** with an abnormal variation in size and shape. No stainable iron is visible in the bone marrow.

Laboratory tests of iron status can distinguish iron deficiency from other causes of hypochromic, microcytic anemia (Table 35-2). The concentration of serum iron decreases, while the total iron-binding capacity (TIBC), which measures the capacity of transferrin for iron, increases. The transferrin saturation, calculated as iron concentration divided by TIBC, is well below its reference interval. A decrease in serum ferritin, which is a reflection of body iron stores, is the single most reliable indicator of iron deficiency. Free erythrocyte protoporphyrin is increased, but this increase is not specific for iron deficiency.

Iron Overload

Hereditary hemochromatosis. Hereditary hemochromatosis is a genetic disorder characterized by a progressive increase in iron stores, leading to organ impairment and damage. Inheritance is autosomal recessive. Among populations of northern European descent, about 10% of people carry the gene and 0.3% are homozygotes. For reasons that are not clearly understood, only a fraction of homozygotes

TABLE 35-2   LABORATORY MEASUREMENTS OF IRON STATUS

	Serum Iron (μg/L)	TIBC (μg/L)	Transferrin Saturation (%)	Serum Ferritin (μg/L)	Free Erythrocyte Protoporphyrin (μg/L)
Reference range	650 to 1750 (men) 500 to 1700 (women)	2500 to 4500	20 to 50 (men) 15 to 50 (women)	20 to 250 (men) 10 to 120 (women)	170 to 770
Iron-deficiency anemia	↓	↑	↓	↓	↑
Anemia of chronic disease	↓	↓	↓	N or ↑	↑
Thalassemia trait	N	N	N	N	N
Sideroblastic anemia	↑	N	↑	↑	N or ↑
Hemochromatosis	↑	↓	↑	↑	N

N, *Normal;* ↓, *decreased;* ↑, *increased.*
TIBC, *Total iron-binding capacity.*

develop the full-blown disease. Men are affected five to ten times more frequently than women because of the protective effect of menstrual blood loss and pregnancy. Symptoms of the disease are not usually apparent before 40 years of age.

The gene responsible for most cases of hemochromatosis encodes a protein known as *HFE* that appears to interact with transferrin and the transferrin receptor to regulate the amount of iron absorbed by cells. Patients with a specific mutation in the HFE gene (C282Y) absorb 4 mg of iron or more per day, even on a usual diet. Iron is deposited directly into parenchymal cells of the liver, pancreas, heart, and other organs. After accumulating for years, the excessive amounts of intracellular iron lead to tissue injury and ultimately organ failure. At this stage, the amount of storage iron may exceed 20 g.

Several organ systems are affected by hemochromatosis. The liver is nearly always enlarged and in time may become cirrhotic, predisposing patients to an unusually high risk for hepatocellular carcinoma. Damage to the islet cells of the pancreas causes diabetes mellitus in about two thirds of patients. Most patients show an increase in skin pigmentation as a result of increased melanin production and iron deposition within the skin. Cardiac damage may be expressed as congestive heart failure or arrhythmias. Testicular atrophy in men is caused by a drop in the production of gonadotropins by the pituitary gland, another site of iron deposition. Arthritis also occurs in up to half of the patients.

In hemochromatosis, the serum iron concentration increases and the TIBC decreases, the opposite of the changes seen in iron deficiency. The transferrin saturation is much higher than the reference interval and is a particularly sensitive index of iron overload. Serum ferritin concentration is increased early in the course of disease, before signs and symptoms become apparent. Measurement of iron content in a liver biopsy specimen has long been considered the definitive test for hemochromatosis. Now that DNA testing for the C282Y mutation is available, most homozygotes can be diagnosed without the need for liver biopsy (see below).

Acquired hemochromatosis. Iron overload can also be an acquired disorder. At first, excess iron is deposited in reticuloendothelial cells of the liver, spleen, and bone marrow. As the iron load increases, its distribution pattern changes, and iron is deposited in the **parenchymal** cells of the liver, pancreas, heart, and other organs. The clinical picture then resembles the hereditary form of hemochromatosis.

Acquired hemochromatosis may be a complication of anemias in which ineffective erythropoiesis occurs, such as β-thalassemia major (see p. 689). Not only is iron absorption increased in this disorder, but patients are treated with multiple blood transfusions, further increasing their iron load. Alcoholics with chronic liver disease may also develop an increase in tissue iron stores, but those with massive iron overload probably have the genetic form of hemochromatosis. Use of medicinal iron supplements does not, by itself, cause hemochromatosis.

CHANGE OF ANALYTE IN DISEASE

The clinical laboratory can measure three iron compartments, accounting for 90% of the total body iron. The largest of these pools is the iron contained in hemoglobin, which is measured as part of a complete blood count. Next largest is the tissue storage compartment, and the serum ferritin concentration is proportional to the size of this pool. Finally, circulating iron is evaluated by measurement of the serum concentrations of iron and its transport protein, transferrin. This combination of hematological and biochemical studies makes it possible to identify disorders of iron metabolism (see Table 35-2).

Hematological Studies

A complete blood count gives the number of erythrocytes per liter, hemoglobin concentration, hematocrit, and red blood cell indices. When the hemoglobin concentration falls below 130 g/L in men, below 120 g/L in women, and below 110 g/L in pregnant women, anemia is present. Iron deficiency causes a hypochromic, microcytic anemia in which cell size (MCV), hemoglobin content (MCH), and the concentration of hemoglobin per cell (MCHC) are all reduced. The peripheral blood smear shows a wide variation in the size, shape, and hemoglobin content of erythrocytes, with a large proportion of cells that are smaller and paler than normal. This clear-cut picture will not be present at the early stages of iron depletion, when both hemoglobin concentration and red cell indices remain normal. Hypochromic, microcytic anemia is characteristic of **thalassemia** trait, **sideroblastic anemia**, and anemia of chronic disease, as well as iron deficiency. Red blood cell parameters thus define the presence or absence of anemia and its morphological character, but other tests are required to identify the cause of anemia. Erythrocyte studies do not contribute to the diagnosis of hemochromatosis.

Serum Iron

The circulating iron pool turns over 10 to 20 times per day, so a typical iron atom spends no longer than 2 hours in plasma. Changes in serum iron concentration of 20% or more may occur suddenly, even in healthy people, because of momentary imbalances in iron inflow and outflow. Diurnal variation occurs, with a fall in iron concentration in the evening; significant day-to-day variations occur as well. All these factors limit the diagnostic usefulness of serum iron measurements. Serum iron values should always be interpreted in combination with TIBC and transferrin saturation.

Total Iron-Binding Capacity (TIBC) and Transferrin Saturation

TIBC measures the maximum amount of iron that serum proteins can bind and is therefore an indirect way of assessing transferrin levels. Transferrin can also be measured directly by immunoassay and converted to TIBC by application of a conversion formula. The serum iron concentration divided by TIBC gives the transferrin saturation.

Causes of abnormal values for TIBC are listed in the box on p. 663. The low serum iron and high TIBC in iron

CHANGES IN TOTAL IRON-BINDING CAPACITY (TIBC)

Decreased by:
   Malignancy
   Inflammation
   Nephrotic syndrome
   Malnutrition
   Megaloblastic and hemolytic anemia
   Hemochromatosis
Increased by:
   Iron deficiency
   Hepatitis
   Pregnancy
   Use of oral contraceptives

deficiency produce a low transferrin saturation; low values may also be seen in pregnancy and chronic disease. High transferrin saturation is characteristic of iron overload and is a sensitive test for hemochromatosis. Thalassemia major, sideroblastic anemia, and acute iron poisoning also cause the transferrin saturation to increase.

Serum Ferritin

A small amount of ferritin circulates in plasma, mostly as iron-free apoferritin. Circulating ferritin is in equilibrium with tissue iron stores and, under most circumstances, accurately reflects the amount of storage iron present. A low serum ferritin concentration is diagnostic of iron deficiency. Ferritin levels drop early in the development of iron deficiency, before serum iron and transferrin saturation become abnormally low. An increase in serum ferritin may be the first indication of iron overload, long before the signs and symptoms of hemochromatosis appear. However, the release of ferritin from damaged tissues in hepatitis, acute inflammatory conditions, and a variety of tumors also dramatically increases the serum ferritin level. In these situations, normal ferritin values can mask the presence of iron deficiency, and examination of' the bone marrow for stainable iron may be required to confirm the diagnosis.

Free Erythrocyte Protoporphyrin

In the course of heme synthesis, small numbers of protoporphyrin molecules bind Zn^{2+} instead of Fe^{2+} to produce zinc protoporphyrin, which then circulates in the mature erythrocyte. A decrease in the iron available to developing red cells increases the formation of zinc protoporphyrin. Measurement of zinc protoporphyrin, usually as free erythrocyte protoporphyrin (FEP), provides an assessment of the iron available for hemoglobin production.

   Both iron deficiency (absolute lack of iron) and chronic disease (impaired use of iron) will increase FEP. Lead interferes with the final step in heme synthesis, and chronic lead poisoning may produce large increases in FEP. Protoporphyria, a hereditary deficiency of ferrochelatase, is

associated with very high FEP values. This assay is most commonly used as a screening test for iron deficiency, but an abnormal result should be followed by more specific tests of iron status.

Molecular Genetics

It is now possible to test for a specific mutation in the HFE gene, C282Y, found in about 80% of patients with hereditary hemochromatosis. Molecular testing can determine whether the patient has two copies (homozygote), one copy (heterozygote), or no copies of this mutation. Homozygotes are at risk for developing iron overload and hemochromatosis; heterozygotes do not accumulate excess iron and are not at risk for the disease. Some patients with clinical and laboratory evidence of hemochromatosis are either heterozygous or negative for the C282Y mutation and are presumed to have a different genetic defect.

Part 2: Heme Synthesis and the Porphyrias

STRUCTURE AND FUNCTION

The porphyrins are a class of molecules that have in common a central, macrocyclic ring structure consisting of four pyrrole units joined by methenyl (=CH—) bridges (Fig. 35-3). The cyclic network of alternating single and double bonds causes porphyrins to absorb visible light; it is this group that imparts a red color to hemoglobin. Porphyrins also fluoresce a reddish-pink color under long-wavelength ultraviolet light, a property that is quite useful when detecting and measuring porphyrins in body fluids. Another unique property is the arrangement of four nitrogen atoms at the center of the ring, enabling porphyrin molecules to chelate metal atoms. In biological systems, iron is the most important metal that complexes with porphyrins.

   Differences in porphyrin structure depend on the type and position of side chains located at the corners of the pyrrole rings. In humans, there are three major porphyrins: uroporphyrin (URO), coproporphyrin (COPRO), and protoporphyrin (PROTO). URO has four propionate and four acetate side chains, whereas COPRO has four propionate and four methyl side chains. These groups may be arranged in four different structural configurations, of which the type III isomer is normally produced. PROTO has two propionate,

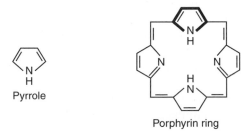

Fig. 35-3 Chemical structures of pyrrole and the porphyrin ring. One of the pyrrole units within the porphyrin ring appears in *boldface*.

two vinyl, and four methyl groups that can be arranged in 15 different configurations. Only the type IX isomer is produced by the body.

Free porphyrins are byproducts of the heme synthetic pathway and have no biological function of their own. Heme, the iron chelate of protoporphyrin, is the prosthetic group for many proteins and enzymes involved in oxygen metabolism and electron-transfer reactions (see Table 35-1). Trace amounts of zinc protoporphyrin also occur naturally, although no physiological role has been assigned to this compound.

METABOLISM

Heme synthesis takes place in all cells but occurs to the greatest extent in the bone marrow (red cell precursors) and liver. There are eight steps in the process, each of which is catalyzed by a different enzyme. It is helpful to consider the pathway in two halves: (1) formation of the ring structure by repeated condensations of precursors (Fig. 35-4) and (2) modification of the side chains and insertion of iron (Fig. 35-5).

Synthetic Pathway

The synthetic pathway begins with the condensation of succinyl CoA and glycine to form delta-aminolevulinic acid (ALA). This reaction, catalyzed by ALA synthase, is the rate-limiting step in heme synthesis. Two ALA molecules then condense to form porphobilinogen (PBG), a pyrrole with propionate and acetate side chains at its corners. Next, four PBG molecules condense in head-to-tail fashion to form a linear tetrapyrrole, hydroxymethylbilane. This unstable intermediate cyclizes spontaneously to form uroporphyrinogen I. In order to produce the physiological type III isomer of uroporphyrinogen, a specific enzyme (uroporphyrinogen III synthase) rearranges the orientation of propionate and acetate side chains on one of the pyrrole units.

At this point the basic ring structure is in place. Modification of the side chains begins with the decarboxylation of the four acetate groups to form coproporphyrinogen III. Two propionate groups are then decarboxylated and dehydrogenated to vinyl groups, producing protoporphyrinogen IX. The bridging carbon atoms are oxidized from methylene ($-CH_2-$) to methenyl ($=CH-$) to yield protoporphyrin IX. In the final step, Fe^{2+} is inserted into the protoporphyrin ring to produce heme.

Three of the intermediates in the heme synthetic pathway are porphyrinogens. They differ from porphyrins in that the bridging carbon atoms are fully reduced and all four nitrogen atoms are protonated. There is no network of alternating single and double bonds, so these compounds are colorless and nonfluorescent. Porphyrinogens that are not used in the regular pathway spontaneously and irreversibly oxidize to the corresponding porphyrins. For this reason, URO, COPRO, and PROTO, and *not* the porphyrinogens, are the major excretion forms.

Regulation

Within the liver, heme synthesis is controlled primarily by changes in the activity of ALA synthase, the first and rate-limiting enzyme. Small amounts of free heme are present within liver cells. An increase in this cellular pool inhibits the activity of ALA synthase, whereas a decrease stimulates the enzyme. Regulation of heme synthesis in red cell precursors appears to involve other enzymes within the pathway, as well as the rate of cellular iron uptake.

The synthetic pathway for heme begins and ends in mitochondria, but four of the intervening steps take place in the cytosol. The intracellular distribution of enzymes is shown in Fig. 35-6. Since erythrocytes lose their mitochondria as they mature, only half of these enzymes can be assayed in circulating red blood cells.

PATHOLOGICAL CONDITIONS

What would happen if the enzymes involved in heme synthesis did not function properly? The answer to that question can be found in the study of the porphyrias, a group of genetically determined disorders of heme synthesis. Deficiencies in seven of the eight enzymes involved in heme synthesis, each leading to a distinct form of porphyria, have been described. Most of the porphyrias are inherited as an autosomal dominant trait. Since the patient has only one gene producing a functional enzyme, about 50% of normal enzyme activity takes place. This partial defect does not cause a deficiency of heme in red blood cells, so patients do not develop anemia. However, porphyrins and their precursors build up behind the deficient enzyme and accumulate in body tissues and fluids. The photosensitizing properties of porphyrins are responsible for the cutaneous signs and symptoms seen in patients with these disorders.

The excretion of excess porphyrins and their precursors is the basis for diagnosing the porphyrias. The route of excretion is a function of solubility. URO, with eight carboxyl groups, is the most water-soluble and is excreted almost entirely in urine. PROTO, with only two carboxyl groups, is excreted exclusively in feces. COPRO, which has four carboxyl groups, is excreted by either route. The porphyrin precursors ALA and PBG are both water-soluble and are eliminated in urine, resulting in **porphyrinuria**.

Traditionally, the porphyrias have been classified as *erythropoietic* or *hepatic*, based on the site of overproduction of the porphyrins and their precursors. A more useful approach is the classification of the porphyrias by signs and symptoms (*neurological* versus *cutaneous*), since this approach allows one to think in terms of clinical presentation.

Neurological Porphyrias

There are three porphyrias characterized by acute attacks of abdominal pain, neurological signs and symptoms, and psychiatric disturbances. The acute attacks, which may last from days to weeks, are accompanied by an increase in the excretion of ALA and PBG in urine. Despite the association of increased levels of porphyrin precursors with the attacks, their biochemical basis remains a mystery. Neither ALA nor PBG has been clearly shown to cause neurotoxicity. ALA is a structural analog of gamma-aminobutyric acid and, at high

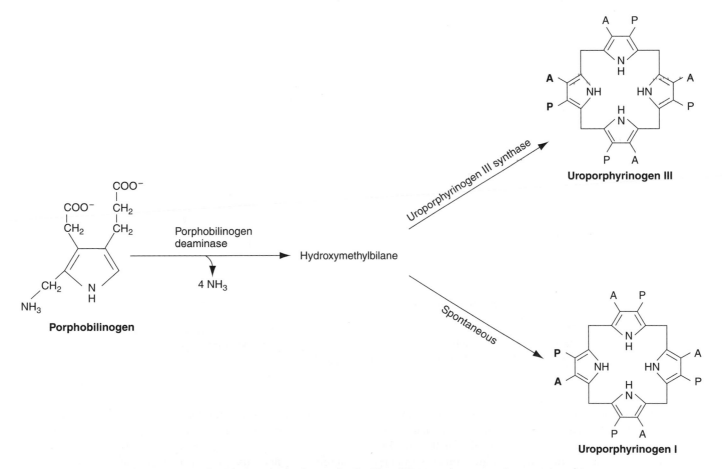

Fig. 35-4 Initial steps in porphyrin synthesis. The difference between the type I and type III isomers of uroporphyrinogen is indicated by the *bolded* side chains. Only the type III isomer is a precursor of heme. *A,* Acetate; *P,* propionate.

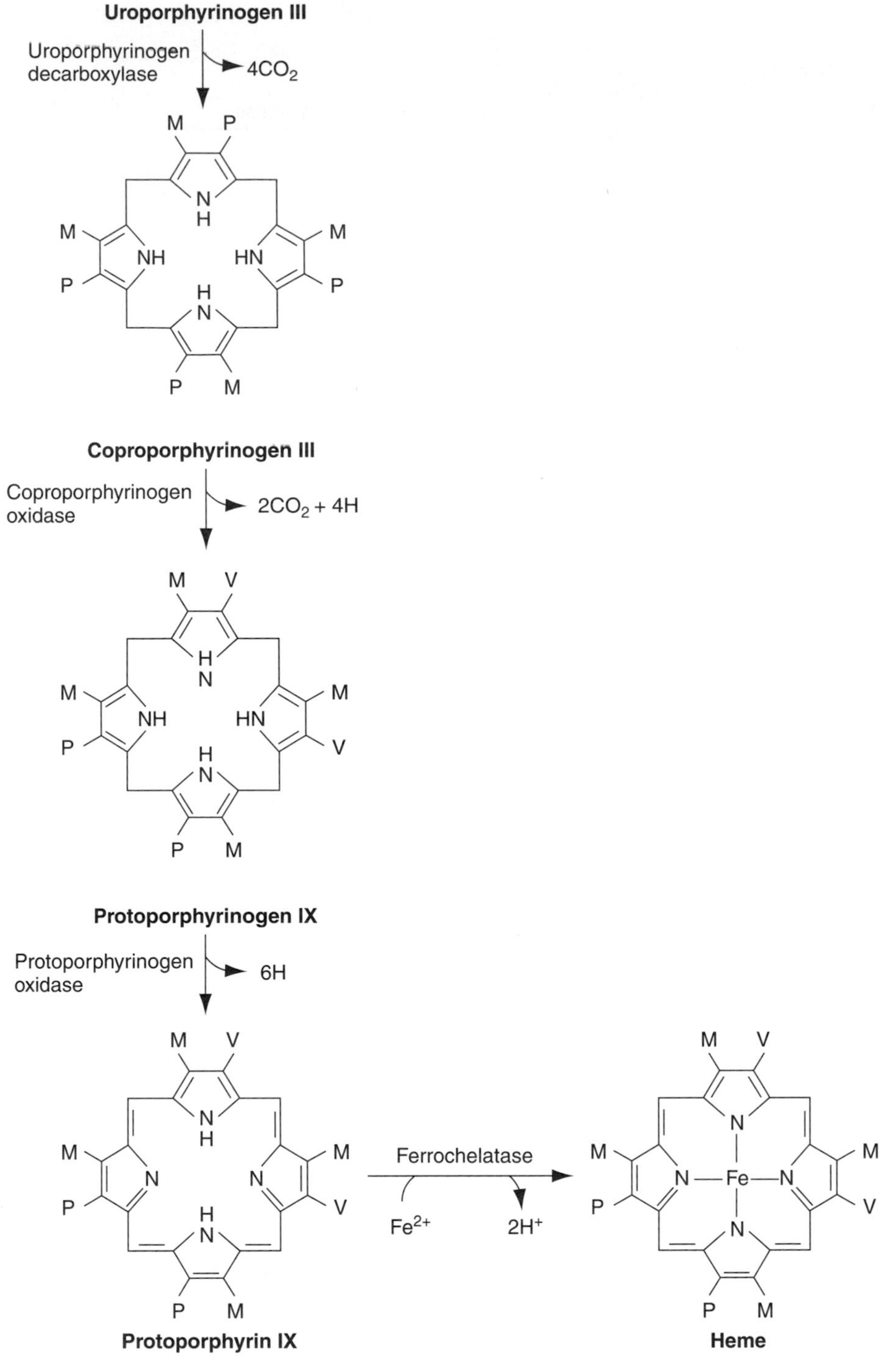

Uroporphyrinogen III

Uroporphyrinogen
decarboxylase → 4CO$_2$

Coproporphyrinogen III

Coproporphyrinogen
oxidase → 2CO$_2$ + 4H

Protoporphyrinogen IX

Protoporphyrinogen
oxidase → 6H

Protoporphyrin IX

Ferrochelatase

Fe^{2+} 2H$^+$

Heme

Fig. 35-5 Latter half of the heme biosynthetic pathway. Note the difference in structure between a porphyrinogen and a porphyrin (compare protoporphyrinogen IX with protoporphyrin IX). *M*, Methyl; *P*, Propionate; *V*, vinyl.

concentrations, could mimic or interfere with the actions of this neurotransmitter. Another theory maintains that heme deficiency within nerve cells is responsible for the attacks. Each enzyme defect is inherited as an autosomal dominant trait.

The signs and symptoms of the neurological porphyrias usually begin during adolescence or early adulthood and

affect women more often than men. Abdominal pain is the most constant finding and is frequently accompanied by constipation, nausea, and vomiting. Abnormalities of the autonomic nervous system include **tachycardia**, hypertension, sweating, and urinary retention. Sensory and motor dysfunction of the peripheral nervous system may be expressed as pain in the extremities, areas of reduced or

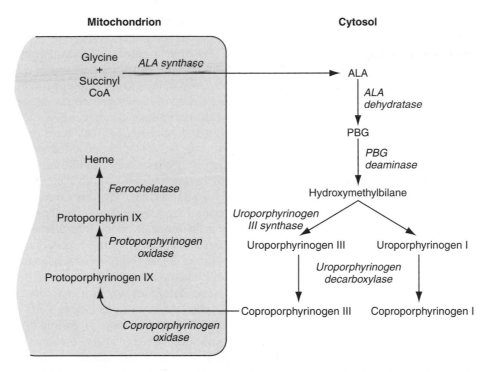

Fig. 35-6 Distribution of the porphyrin pathway between mitochondria and cytosol.

altered sensation, muscle weakness, and paralysis. Visual disturbances, seizures, and coma can also occur, and inappropriate secretion of antidiuretic hormone may contribute to a low serum sodium concentration. Some patients have a history of nervousness, mood disorders, or delusional thinking, suggestive of a primary psychiatric illness.

Acute attacks of neurological porphyria can be precipitated by a variety of drugs. Lists of drugs considered to be safe and unsafe for use in patients with a neurological porphyria have been developed to assist in preventing attacks. Fasting, alcohol consumption, infections, and other factors can also precipitate an attack. Between attacks, the signs and symptoms of porphyria are usually absent. Most

people who carry the gene for one of these porphyrias never have an attack, and their disease remains clinically latent.

The unique features of each of the neurological porphyrias are reviewed below and in Table 35-3,

Acute intermittent porphyria. Acute intermittent porphyria is the most common of the neurological porphyrias, with an estimated prevalence of 1 to 10 per 100,000 population. Patients with this disease have a 50% deficiency of porphobilinogen deaminase, the enzyme that joins four PBG molecules to form uroporphyrinogen. The defect causes ALA and PBG to accumulate, and the partial interruption of the pathway induces the activity of ALA synthase. Consequently, ALA and PBG are excreted in the largest

TABLE 35-3 BIOCHEMICAL AND CLINICAL FEATURES OF THE PORPHYRIAS

	Acute Intermittent Porphyria	Variegate Porphyria	Hereditary Coproporphyria	Porphyria Cutanea Tarda	Protoporphyria	Congenital Erythropoietic Porphyria
Enzyme defect	Porphobilinogen deaminase	Protoporphyrinogen oxidase	Coproporphyrinogen oxidase	Uroporphyrinogen decarboxylase	Ferrochelatase	Uroporphyrinogen III synthase
Inheritance	Autosomal dominant	Autosomal dominant	Autosomal dominant	Autosomal dominant	Autosomal dominant	Autosomal recessive
Abdominal pain, neurological dysfunction	Yes	Yes	Yes	No	No	No
Photosensitivity, cutaneous lesions	No	Yes	Yes	Yes	Yes	Yes
Tissue expression	Liver	Liver	Liver	Liver	Erythroid cells and liver	Erythroid cells

amounts in this porphyria. Since the defect does not involve the porphyrinogen portion of the pathway, porphyrins are not produced in excess, and **photosensitivity** does not occur.

The major laboratory finding in acute intermittent porphyria is an increase in urine ALA and PBG concentrations during acute attacks. However, between attacks these values may revert to normal. When PBG is present at high concentrations in urine, it spontaneously condenses and cyclizes to form uroporphyrinogen (type I isomer), which then oxidizes to URO. Large increases in URO may be present in any of the neurological porphyrias, particularly acute intermittent porphyria. By contrast, fecal porphyrins are normal. Porphobilinogen deaminase can be assayed in erythrocytes and is usually decreased to about 50% of normal, whether the patient is acutely ill or has the unexpressed latent form.

Variegate porphyria. Patients with variegate porphyria may suffer from acute neurological attacks, sensitivity of the skin to sunlight and mechanical trauma, or both. The enzymatic defect is a partial deficiency of protoporphyrinogen oxidase. PROTO and COPRO accumulate in the body, giving rise to photosensitivity and cutaneous lesions. The disease is most common among South African whites and has been traced to a couple who emigrated from Holland in 1688. In an interesting but unproved historical footnote, several authors have speculated that King George III of England suffered from variegate porphyria.

The finding of increased ALA and PBG in urine during acute attacks establishes the presence of a neurological porphyria. Variegate porphyria is distinguished from the other two neurological porphyrias by the increased excretion of PROTO and COPRO in feces.

Hereditary coproporphyria. A partial deficiency of coproporphyrinogen oxidase in this disease causes COPRO to accumulate. In addition to the acute attacks, photosensitivity and skin lesions may occur, though less often than in variegate porphyria. Urinary levels of ALA and PBG are increased during acute attacks. The key diagnostic finding is an increase in the fecal excretion of COPRO.

ALA dehydratase deficiency. Several patients with a nearly complete deficiency of ALA dehydratase have been described. Homozygotes have neurological symptoms but no photosensitivity; heterozygotes are asymptomatic. Significant laboratory findings are increased excretion of ALA and COPRO in the urine.

Cutaneous Porphyrias

The three cutaneous porphyrias have in common an excess of porphyrins in body tissues, including skin. Porphyrin molecules absorb light at about 400 nm, which raises electrons to a higher energy state. As electrons return to their ground state, some of the energy they release may be transferred to molecular oxygen, producing activated oxygen species that can react with membranes and other cellular constituents. The release of proteolytic enzymes from damaged lysosomes may be responsible for cell injury and, ultimately, the photosensitivity and skin lesions seen in these

disorders. Each of the cutaneous porphyrias is briefly discussed below and reviewed in Table 35-3.

Porphyria cutanea tarda. Porphyria cutanea tarda is a skin disorder that does not usually appear until adulthood. The most common type of porphyria, it is caused by a partial deficiency of uroporphyrinogen decarboxylase. Some cases of the disease are clearly familial and inherited as an autosomal dominant trait, but most cases are sporadic and probably represent an acquired deficiency of the hepatic enzyme. Patients may exhibit fragile skin, blister formation, thickening and scarring of sun-exposed skin, and areas of hyperpigmentation. The disease remains dormant until some form of liver dysfunction develops, such as an overload of hepatic iron or alcoholic liver disease. Estrogen therapy may activate the skin lesions. The rare, homozygous form of this disease, called *hepatoerythropoietic porphyria*, produces severe photosensitivity.

The deficiency of uroporphyrinogen decarboxylase in porphyria cutanea tarda causes URO as well as porphyrins with 7, 6, and 5 carboxyl groups to accumulate, and their concentrations in urine are greatly increased. Fecal porphyrins are only mildly elevated, but the presence of isocoproporphyrin, an isomer of COPRO, is distinctive for this porphyria. Red blood cell porphyrins are within the reference interval.

Protoporphyria. Patients with protoporphyria have a partial deficiency of ferrochelatase, the last enzyme in the synthetic pathway for heme. The resulting accumulation of PROTO causes photosensitivity beginning in childhood or adolescence. When exposed to sunlight, patients develop burning, itching, swelling, and redness of the skin. Sun-exposed areas such as the backs of the hands and face are affected, but skin changes are mild and scarring uncommon. A minority of patients develop liver disease or protoporphyrin-containing gallstones, since the liver must excrete the unusually large amounts of PROTO.

In protoporphyria, the concentration of free erythrocyte protoporphyrin is greatly elevated. Fecal PROTO is usually increased as well, although the size of the increase is variable. Urine porphyrins and their precursors are normal.

Congenital erythropoietic porphyria. Congenital erythropoietic porphyria is a rare autosomal recessive disorder caused by deficiency of uroporphyrinogen III synthase. The enzyme defect is not complete, and enough uroporphyrinogen III is synthesized to meet metabolic needs. However, large amounts of the type I isomer series are also produced and are eventually oxidized to form URO I and COPRO I. The disease usually presents in early childhood with extreme photosensitivity. Light-exposed areas of the skin become scarred, and as patients grow older, extensive scarring and mutilation of the fingers, nose, and ears may occur. A unique finding is erythrodontia, the reddish-brown staining of teeth caused by porphyrin deposition. Patients also develop **hemolytic anemia** and enlargement of the spleen. Of all the porphyrias, this one has the worst prognosis.

Patients excrete urine that is pink or red because of the massive amounts of URO and COPRO that are present. Red blood cells contain large amounts of URO and COPRO and fluoresce when examined microscopically under ultraviolet light. Fecal porphyrins are also increased.

Secondary Disorders of Porphyrin Metabolism

Alterations in porphyrin metabolism and excretion can occur in situations other than the porphyrias. Several common examples are described below.

Lead poisoning. Lead poisoning may occur in young children who eat chips of paint containing lead or in adults who are exposed to lead compounds in an industrial setting or those who drink "moonshine" whiskey distilled in lead-containing equipment. The signs and symptoms include abdominal pain and neurological abnormalities that may mimic an acute attack of porphyria. Lead inhibits two enzymes in the porphyrin pathway, ALA dehydratase and ferrochelatase. Consequently, there is an increase in urine ALA (but not PBG) and in the erythrocyte concentration of zinc protoporphyrin; urine COPRO is also increased. Although these findings are typical of lead poisoning, the diagnosis is based on the demonstration of increased concentrations of lead in whole blood.

Iron deficiency. Patients with iron deficiency have an imbalance between protoporphyrin (which is produced in normal amounts) and iron (which is not readily available for heme synthesis). As a result, zinc protoporphyrin accumulates in red blood cells to higher-than-normal levels. Because it is such a widespread condition, iron deficiency is the most common cause of increased red blood cell porphyrins. Physiological states that decrease the availability of iron, such as acute or chronic inflammation, also increase red cell porphyrins. Measurement of zinc protoporphyrin is a useful screening test for iron deficiency, but the diagnosis is confirmed by studies of serum iron, total iron-binding capacity, and ferritin.

Coproporphyrinuria. An increase in urinary COPRO is the most common abnormal laboratory result when urine is screened for porphyrins. Although this finding may indicate a porphyria, it is much more often caused by problems unrelated to heme synthesis, such as liver disease, acute illness, or exposure to toxic compounds. A small (less than twofold) isolated increase in urinary COPRO is usually a nonspecific finding of limited diagnostic value.

CHANGE OF ANALYTE IN DISEASE

The laboratory work-up of a suspected porphyria depends on the clinical presentation. As a rule, screening tests are used to identify increases in PBG and in urine and fecal porphyrins. Positive screening tests should be confirmed by quantitative measurements on a 24-hour urine sample or random feces sample, as well as by the identification of which porphyrins are elevated. Negative screening tests require no further analysis.

The interpretation of results is complicated by several factors. In traditional screening tests, porphyrins are extracted into an acidified organic solvent, and a positive result is indicated by a reddish-pink fluorescence of the extract under long-wavelength ultraviolet light. The screening test for PBG is based on its reaction with *p*-dimethylaminobenzaldehyde to form a reddish-purple compound. Both techniques require subjective judgment as to whether the expected color is present. Moreover, false-positive and false-negative results may be caused by interfering substances in urine and feces. Newer screening tests based on spectrophotometry and spectrofluorometry have eliminated these interferences and provide a numerical value for the amount of PBG or porphyrin that is present in the sample.

Another issue is the variable excretion of porphyrins and their precursors in health and disease. Urine, fecal, and red blood cell porphyrins are typically increased by five- to tenfold in patients with porphyria. The same is true for ALA and PBG in the acute phase of a neurological porphyria. However, some analytes are affected by current disease activity, and the range of values seen in any of the porphyrias can vary greatly. An isolated increase of porphyrins in urine (less than twofold), feces (less than threefold) and red blood cells (less than fivefold) may also occur in people who do not have a porphyria. For these reasons, diagnosis must be based on a combination of clinical presentation, reliable analytical techniques, and careful interpretation of test results.

The key laboratory findings in the porphyrias are summarized in Table 35-4.

Porphobilinogen (PBG)

Urine PBG is elevated in acute intermittent porphyria, variegate porphyria, and hereditary coproporphyria. The screening test for PBG is positive during acute attacks but may be negative between attacks. A positive screening test is confirmed by a quantitative PBG analysis, performed on a 24-hour urine collection.

Delta-Aminolevulinic Acid (ALA)

Urine ALA values parallel the increase in PBG seen in the three neurological porphyrias. ALA excretion is also increased in lead poisoning and hereditary tyrosinemia and is therefore a less specific indicator of porphyria than is PBG. Measurements are performed on a 24-hour urine collection.

Urine Porphyrins

Screening tests for urine porphyrins are usually positive in all of the porphyrias except protoporphyria and the latent phase of acute intermittent porphyria. Positive screening tests are followed by quantitative measurement of total porphyrins in a 24-hour urine sample and identification of the porphyrins that are elevated. A slight-to-moderate increase of urinary COPRO concentration is seen in liver disease, lead poisoning, alcohol ingestion, and acute illness. Larger increases in COPRO or URO are more likely to indicate a porphyria.

Patients with congenital erythropoietic porphyria excrete huge amounts of URO and COPRO. In porphyria cutanea tarda, excretion of URO and a distinctive 7-carboxyl porphyrin, with smaller amounts of 6- and 5-carboxyl porphyrins and COPRO, is diagnostic for this disease. Variegate porphyria and hereditary coproporphyria are characterized by an

TABLE 35-4 LABORATORY DIAGNOSIS OF THE PORPHYRIAS

Porphyria	Urine ALA and PBG* (mg/Day)	Urine Porphyrins (µg/Day)	Fecal Porphyrins (µg/g Dry Weight)	Red Blood Cell Porphyrins (µg/L)
Reference range	ALA: 1.5 to 7.5 PBG: ≤2	URO: ≤50 COPRO: ≤230	COPRO: ≤30 PROTO: ≤60	170 to 770
Acute intermittent porphyria	↑	↑ URO*	N	N
Variegate porphyria	↑	↑ COPRO	↑ PROTO, COPRO	N
Hereditary coproporphyria	↑↑	↑ COPRO	↑ COPRO	N
Porphyria cutanea tarda	N	↑ URO, 7-carboxyl	↑ Isocoproporphyrin	N
Protoporphyria	N	N	↑ PROTO	↑ PROTO
Congenital erythropoietic porphyria	N	↑ URO, COPRO	↑ COPRO	↑ URO, COPRO

N, *Normal;* ↑, *increased.*
May be increased only during acute attack.

excess of COPRO in urine. Patients with acute intermittent porphyria sometimes excrete high levels of URO, produced by the nonenzymatic condensation of PBG molecules in urine. URO may be increased in the other two neurological porphyrias for the same reason.

Fecal Porphyrins

Fecal porphyrins consist of COPRO, PROTO, and several other dicarboxylic porphyrins (meso-, deutero-, and pempto-porphyrin). The amount of porphyrins excreted by this route is a function of diet and the anaerobic flora of the colon. Consequently, increases in fecal porphyrin excretion up to threefold the upper reference limit may be seen in healthy individuals.

Fecal porphyrins are usually increased in all of the porphyrias except acute intermittent porphyria. The most important application of this test is to distinguish variegate porphyria (PROTO and COPRO both elevated) from hereditary coproporphyria (only COPRO elevated). An increase in PROTO is also seen in protoporphyria, whereas patients with congenital erythropoietic porphyria excrete large amounts of COPRO. Fecal porphyrins may be within the reference interval or only slightly increased in porphyria cutanea tarda, but fractionation reveals a range of porphyrins, including URO, 7-carboxyl porphyrin, and isocoproporphyrin, not normally found in feces.

Red Blood Cell Porphyrins

Red blood cell porphyrins other than heme are measured as free erythrocyte protoporphyrin (FEP). Under normal conditions, FEP reflects the concentration of zinc protoporphyrin.

The concentration of red blood cell porphyrins is greatly increased in congenital erythropoietic porphyria (URO and COPRO) and protoporphyria (PROTO) but is normal in other porphyrias. Fractionation of red blood cell porphyrins is not necessary, because these two disorders can be differentiated by urine porphyrin assays and clinical presentation. As previously mentioned, FEP is also increased in iron deficiency and lead poisoning.

Enzyme Assays

Only one enzyme in the synthetic pathway for heme, porphobilinogen deaminase, is routinely measured by clinical laboratories. Its activity is decreased to about 50% of normal in the red blood cells of most individuals with acute intermittent porphyria, whether the disease is latent or in an acute phase. The usefulness of this assay is diminished by two factors. First, there is an overlap of values between patients and healthy individuals at the lower end of the reference interval. Second, a small subset of patients with the disease have normal PBG deaminase activity in erythrocytes, caused by mutations in the gene that do not affect expression of the enzyme in red cells. Despite its shortcomings, PBG deaminase is frequently the only test that can identify asymptomatic individuals who carry the gene for acute intermittent porphyria.

Molecular Genetics

All of the genes that encode enzymes of the heme synthetic pathway have now been identified and their coding sequences determined. This work has led to the discovery of mutations that cause each of the porphyrias. For patients in whom a mutation has been identified, DNA-based testing for the mutation can be offered to all members of the family. Such testing is more definitive than conventional biochemical tests in identifying gene carriers, especially in relatives with no signs or symptoms of porphyria. However, a positive test does not predict whether the course of the disease will be asymptomatic, mild, or severe. Since most of the mutations are limited to only one or several families, and searching for mutations is a labor-intensive process, it is not yet possible to offer molecular testing for the porphyrias on a routine basis. At present, DNA-based testing for these disorders is available only in a limited number of research and specialty laboratories.

Part 3: Bilirubin
FORMATION AND STRUCTURE

Heme is degraded in cells of the reticuloendothelial system (Fig. 35-7). Heme oxygenase, in the presence of molecular oxygen and NADPH, opens the protoporphyrin ring to release iron, carbon monoxide, and a linear tetrapyrrole, biliverdin. Iron is recycled for future heme synthesis, and carbon monoxide is excreted by the lungs. Biliverdin is metabolized one step further; the double bond at the center of the molecule is reduced to form bilirubin.* This yellow-

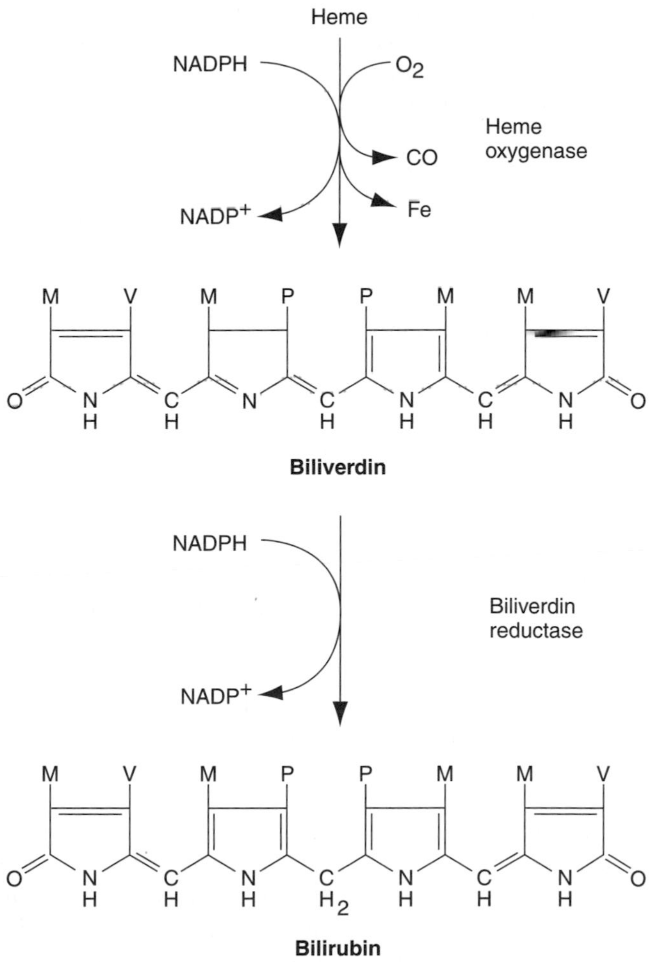

Fig. 35-7 Formation of bilirubin from heme. *M*, Methyl; *P*, propionate; *V*, vinyl.

---

*Bilirubin is more properly referred to as *bilirubin IXα*, since it is derived from the type IX isomer of protoporphyrin and ring cleavage takes place at the α-methene bridge. For convenience, the term IXα is omitted in this section.

orange pigment is the major waste product of heme metabolism.

The structure of bilirubin appears in Fig. 35-7. The molecule consists of two nearly identical halves joined by a methylene ($—CH_2—$) group at its center. There is free rotation about the central carbon atom, which allows the polar groups of bilirubin to form internal hydrogen bonds. The exterior of the molecule is hydrophobic, and this accounts for its very low solubility in aqueous solutions. The double bonds between carbons 4 and 5 in one half of the molecule and carbons 15 and 16 in the other half are normally in the trans or Z-Z conformation. On exposure to light, either of these double bonds can isomerize to a cis conformation, thereby forming E-Z, Z-E, or E-E isomers. A change in geometry interferes with internal hydrogen bonding and makes the molecule more polar. This is the basis for treating jaundiced infants with phototherapy, since **photoisomers** of bilirubin can be excreted directly into **bile** without conjugation.

METABOLISM
Production

The breakdown of heme-containing proteins generates about 250 to 300 mg of bilirubin per day. Approximately 80% to 85% of bilirubin is derived from the hemoglobin in aged erythrocytes. Most of these erythrocytes are destroyed within reticuloendothelial cells in the spleen. A small percentage of erythrocytes are destroyed within the circulatory system as well. The remaining 15% to 20% of bilirubin comes from the destruction of red blood cell precursors in the bone marrow and from the turnover of hemoproteins in other tissues.

Transport

Once bilirubin is released into plasma, it binds very tightly to albumin. Each albumin molecule has one high-affinity binding site for bilirubin and one or two sites of weaker affinity. Transport of bilirubin in the bound state prevents it from crossing cell membranes and entering tissues, where it would exert toxic effects. Certain anionic drugs, such as sulfonamide antibiotics, barbiturates, and salicylates, as well as free fatty acids, compete for the bilirubin-binding sites on albumin. This is not usually a problem in adults, but infants have a lower binding capacity for bilirubin. In the presence of competing substances, bilirubin may be displaced from albumin, cross the blood-brain barrier, and enter brain cells, where it can cause neurological damage.

In addition to the usual reversible binding, bilirubin may also become covalently bound to albumin in patients with impaired hepatic excretion of bilirubin. The covalently bound form, delta-bilirubin, continues to circulate with its albumin carrier until the albumin is removed from the circulation. The mechanism of attachment and physiological purpose of delta-bilirubin, if any, are not known.

Hepatic Uptake, Conjugation, and Excretion

During passage through the microcirculation of the liver, albumin releases bilirubin to hepatocytes (Fig. 35-8). After

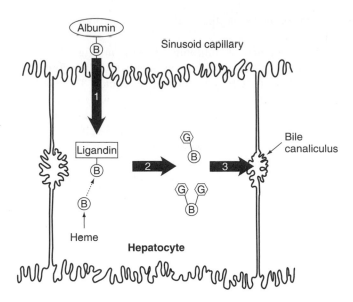

Fig. 35-8 Hepatic metabolism of bilirubin. The indicated steps are (*1*) uptake, (*2*) conjugation, and (*3*) excretion. A small amount of bilirubin is produced by breakdown of heme-containing proteins within hepatocytes. *B,* Bilirubin; *G,* glucuronic acid.

bilirubin diffuses across the cell membrane, it binds to ligandin, a cytosolic protein that binds organic anions. Ligandin does not appear to be involved in the cellular uptake of bilirubin. Its function is probably to prevent the diffusion of bilirubin out of the hepatocyte or into other cellular compartments.

In the endoplasmic reticulum, glucuronic acid residues are added to the propionate side chains of bilirubin. The reaction is catalyzed by bilirubin UDP-glucuronosyltransferase, and UDP-glucuronic acid is the carbohydrate donor. The addition of one or two sugar residues increases the water solubility of bilirubin, so that it can be excreted into the biliary system. About 85% to 90% of bilirubin appears in bile as the diglucuronide, and about 10% to 15% appears as the monoglucuronide. Small amounts of other bilirubin-sugar conjugates (glucosides, xylosides), as well as free bilirubin (water-soluble photoisomers), are also found in bile. Excretion into bile is the rate-limiting step in the hepatic metabolism of bilirubin. It is an energy-dependent process in which bilirubin is transported against a concentration gradient.

Intestinal Transit

After excretion into bile, conjugated bilirubin passes through the hepatic and common bile ducts and into the intestinal lumen. In the distal small intestine and colon, anaerobic bacteria hydrolyze the glucuronic acid residues and reduce bilirubin to a variety of compounds known collectively as *urobilinogens.* Unlike the more polar bilirubin glucuronide, urobilinogens may be reabsorbed by the intestine and enter the portal circulation. More than 90% of reabsorbed urobilinogens are taken up by liver cells and excreted into bile; the remainder are filtered by the kidneys and excreted in urine. Urobilinogens are colorless, but in the presence of air they oxidize spontaneously to the corresponding urobilins. These colored compounds contribute to the normal color of feces and urine.

PATHOLOGICAL CONDITIONS: HYPERBILIRUBINEMIA

Diseases or conditions that interfere with bilirubin metabolism cause a rise in its serum concentration. Jaundice, a yellowish discoloration of the sclera and skin, appears when the serum bilirubin concentration reaches about 25 to 50 mg/L. By itself, hyperbilirubinemia is usually not a threat to health, since adequate mechanisms exist for binding and detoxifying bilirubin. However, hyperbilirubinemia indicates an abnormality in the production or subsequent metabolism of bilirubin.

There are five mechanisms that can lead to hyperbilirubinemia and jaundice:

1. Overproduction
2. Impaired uptake by liver cells
3. Defects in the conjugation reaction
4. Reduced excretion into bile
5. Obstruction to the flow of bile

The first three mechanisms cause an increase in unconjugated serum bilirubin, whereas the latter two mechanisms produce an elevation of both unconjugated and conjugated bilirubin in serum. For a pictorial description of the mechanisms of hyperbilirubinemia, see p. 499.

Overproduction

Increased production of bilirubin is usually the result of accelerated red blood cell breakdown. When the rate of hemolysis exceeds the liver's capacity to clear bilirubin from blood, the patient develops hyperbilirubinemia. Serum bilirubin does not usually exceed 50 mg/L in hemolytic states, and the bilirubin is almost entirely unconjugated. In chronic hemolytic anemias such as sickle cell disease or hereditary spherocytosis, prolonged overproduction of bilirubin may lead to the formation of bilirubin-containing gallstones. Ineffective erythropoiesis, which occurs in thalassemia major, **pernicious anemia**, and other disorders, causes a similar increase in bilirubin production.

Impaired Uptake

The hepatic phase of bilirubin metabolism begins with its uptake by liver cells. Several drugs interfere with this process, possibly by competing with bilirubin for binding to ligandin. Gilbert's syndrome is a hereditary disorder characterized by a small increase in serum unconjugated bilirubin. Some cases appear to involve a defect in hepatic uptake, but more commonly there is a partial deficiency of the conjugating enzyme glucuronosyltransferase. The degree of hyperbilirubinemia in patients with Gilbert's syndrome is variable; it is exacerbated by prolonged fasting. There are no other signs, symptoms, or laboratory abnormalities, and the prognosis is excellent.

Defective Conjugation

Defects in the conjugation reaction may be hereditary, acquired, or developmental. Hereditary deficiency of the conjugating enzyme is known as *Crigler-Najjar syndrome*. In the rare type I disorder, there is a complete absence of glucuronosyltransferase activity. Serum bilirubin levels are exceedingly high from birth, since failure to conjugate bilirubin prevents it from being excreted into bile. Most affected infants die from bilirubin-induced neurological damage before reaching 1 year of age. Patients with type II disease have a partial deficiency of glucuronosyltransferase. The serum concentration of bilirubin is lower than in type I, and neurological complications are unusual. Inheritance is autosomal recessive for the type I disorder and autosomal dominant for type II.

Neonatal jaundice refers to the mild hyperbilirubinemia seen in newborns at 2 to 5 days of life. It is caused in part by immaturity of the glucuronosyltransferase system. Other contributing factors include an increase in red blood cell destruction and possibly a deficiency of ligandin. As the hepatocytes mature, jaundice resolves spontaneously, usually within 7 to 10 days of birth. Glucuronosyltransferase is inhibited by certain drugs, and its activity is decreased in hepatocellular diseases such as hepatitis.

Reduced Excretion

Excretion into bile is the rate-limiting step in bilirubin metabolism; this is also the step most sensitive to injury. Therefore, damage to liver cells is associated with an increase in conjugated bilirubin. Hepatocellular damage also affects uptake and conjugation, which contribute to a rise in unconjugated bilirubin as well. Hepatitis and **cirrhosis** are the most common disorders that produce liver cell injury and jaundice. Some drugs may exert a direct toxic effect on liver cells. Oral contraceptives and other synthetic sex steroids cause a drug-induced **cholestasis** in some people.

The Dubin-Johnson and Rotor syndromes are two hereditary disorders of bilirubin excretion. Both are characterized by increased levels of conjugated bilirubin, whereas other routine liver function tests remain normal. The Dubin-Johnson syndrome is distinguished by the dark pigment that accumulates in hepatocytes. Inheritance of these rare disorders is autosomal-recessive, and the prognosis is excellent.

Obstruction

Mechanical obstruction to the flow of bile is most often produced by gallstones in the common bile duct or by tumors. Cancer of the head of the pancreas compresses the major bile ducts, whereas cancers of the bile duct or **ampulla of Vater** directly occlude the final portion of the biliary tree. Postoperative strictures of the common bile duct narrow this passageway and impair bile flow. Serum bilirubin increases in proportion to the extent of obstruction and is largely conjugated.

CHANGE OF ANALYTE IN DISEASE

An increase in serum bilirubin accompanies a wide variety of pathological states. The majority of diseases or conditions causing jaundice originate in the liver and biliary tree; a smaller percentage are the result of hematological disorders. The clinical laboratory can measure both conjugated and unconjugated fractions of bilirubin. Other first-line laboratory investigations include measurement of aspartate and alanine aminotransferase activities, alkaline phosphatase activity, prothrombin time, and a complete blood count with peripheral smear evaluation. This group of tests can usually identify the pathophysiological basis of jaundice. More specialized tests, such as serological assays for hepatitis or imaging studies of the biliary tree, are then performed to make a specific diagnosis.

Serum Bilirubin

Serum bilirubin consists of unconjugated, conjugated (mono- and diglucuronide) and delta (covalently protein-bound) fractions. The conjugated and delta fractions react in aqueous solution to give the amount of direct bilirubin. Total bilirubin is measured after the addition of an accelerator such as methanol or caffeine that disrupts internal hydrogen bonds and allows the unconjugated fraction to react as well. The unconjugated bilirubin is obtained by subtracting the direct from the total bilirubin. Reference intervals are approximately 3 to 12 mg/L for total bilirubin and 0 to 2 mg/L for direct bilirubin.

Urine Bilirubin

A portion of the conjugated bilirubin in blood is filtered by the kidneys and excreted in urine. Urine bilirubin can easily be tested with commercial dipsticks; it is normally undetectable. The presence of bilirubin in urine indicates an elevation in the conjugated fraction of serum bilirubin.

Urobilinogen

Excretion of urobilinogen in urine is normally 1 to 4 mg/day. Overproduction of bilirubin, as occurs in hemolytic anemia, increases the amount of urobilinogen formed in the intestine and therefore the amount that is reabsorbed and excreted into urine. Hepatocellular disease may also increase urinary urobilinogen by interfering with its uptake and excretion into bile. Processes that reduce the flow of bilirubin into the intestine, such as common bile duct obstruction, limit the formation of urobilinogen and reduce the amount excreted in urine. Urobilinogen can be detected with commercial dipsticks, and an increase provides evidence of a hemolytic cause of jaundice. However, urobilinogen is of little use in the diagnosis of liver disease.

Bibliography

Iron Metabolism

Adams PC et al: Population screening for hemochromatosis: a comparison of unbound iron-binding capacity, transferrin saturation, and C282Y genotyping in 5,211 voluntary blood donors, *Hepatology* 31:1160, 2000.

Andrews NC: Disorders of iron metabolism, *N Engl J Med* 341:1986, 1999.

Brittenham GM: Disorders of iron metabolism: iron deficiency and overload. In Hoffman R et al, editors: *Hematology: basic principles and practice*, ed 3, New York, 2000, Churchill Livingstone.

Conrad ME, editor: Iron overloading disorders and iron regulation, *Semin Hematol* 35:1, 1998.

Fairbanks VF, Beutler E: Iron deficiency. In: Beutler E et al, editors: *Williams hematology*, ed 6, New York, 2001, McGraw-Hill.

Press RD: Hemochromatosis: a "simple" genetic trait, *Hosp Pract* 34:55, 1999.

Roy CN, Enns CA: Iron homeostasis: new tales from the crypt, *Blood* 96:4020, 2000.

Sherwood RA, Pippard MJ, Peters TJ: Iron homeostasis and the assessment of iron status, *Ann Clin Biochem* 35:693, 1998.

Heme Synthesis and the Porphyrias

Bloomer JR: The porphyrias. In Schiff ER, Sorrell MF, Maddrey WC, editors: *Schiff's diseases of the liver*, ed 8, Philadelphia, 1999, Lippincott-Raven.

Elder GH, Hift RJ, Meissner PN: The acute porphyrias, *Lancet* 349:1613, 1997.

Kauppinen R, Mustajoki P: Prognosis of acute porphyria: occurrence of acute attacks, precipitating factors, and associated diseases, *Medicine* 71:1, 1992.

Moore MR et al: *Disorders of porphyrin metabolism*, New York, 1987, Plenum Press.

Schmid R, editor: The porphyrias, *Semin Liver Dis* 18:1, 1998..

Schreiber WE, Jamani A, Armstrong JG: Acute intermittent porphyria in a native North American family: biochemical and molecular analysis, *Am J Clin Pathol* 103:730, 1995.

Thunell S et al: Porphyrins, porphyrin metabolism and porphyrias. I-IV, *Scand J Clin Lab Invest* 60:509, 2000.

Bilirubin

Berg CL, Crawford JM, Gollan JL: Bilirubin metabolism and the pathophysiology of jaundice. In: Schiff ER, Sorrell MF, Maddrey WC, editors: *Schiff's diseases of the liver*, ed 8, Philadelphia, 1999, Lippincott-Raven.

Berk PD, Noyer C, editors: Bilirubin metabolism and the hereditary hyperbilirubinemias, *Semin Liver Dis* 14:321, 1994.

Chowdhury JR, Chowdhury NR: Bilirubin metabolism and its disorders. In: Kaplowitz N, editor: Liver and biliary diseases, ed 2, Baltimore, 1996, Williams & Wilkins.

Dennery PA, Seidman DS, Stevenson DK: Neonatal hyperbilirubinemia, *N Engl J Med* 344:581, 2001.

Sherlock S, Dooley J: *Diseases of the liver and biliary system*, ed 10, Oxford, 1997, Blackwell Science.

Internet Sites

Bilirubin

http://www.mcg.edu/pedson1/ccnotebook/chapter1/neonataljaundice.htm
http://www.mcg.edu/pedson1/ccnotebook/chapter1/breastmilkjaundice.htm
http://www.mcg.edu/pedson1/forhealthprof/neonatology/bilirubin.html
web.indstate.edu/thcme/mwking/heme-porphyrin.html—Indiana University School of Medicine
www.med.monash.edu.au/biochem/thcme/bilirub.html
http://www.umanitoba.ca/faculties/medicine/units/biochem/coursenotes/blanchaer_tutorials/Frank_II/biliOverview.html

Porphyrias

medlib.med.utah.edu/NetBiochem/hi.htm—University of Utah
www.porphyriafoundation.com—American Porphyria Foundation
medic.med.uth.tmc.edu/path/00000884.htm

Heme and Iron Metabolism

http://sickle.bwh.harvard.edu/menu_iron.html—Harvard University, disorders of iron metabolism
http://medlib.med.utah.edu/WebPath/TUTORIAL/IRON/IRON.html—University of Utah, diseases of iron metabolism
www.americanhs.org—American Hemochromatosis Society
www.cdc.gov/genomics/info/perspectives/hemo.htm—Centers for Disease Control and Prevention, hereditary hemochromatosis
http://www.smbs.buffalo.edu/med/hem/iron.html—State University of New York at Buffalo, iron metabolism and deficiency
http://www.med.unibs.it/~marchesi/heme.html
http://www.dentistry.leeds.ac.uk/biochem/thcme/hememetabolism.pdf
www.stargine.com/porphyrins/Mediporph/_mediporphome.html—Medical topics of porphyrias

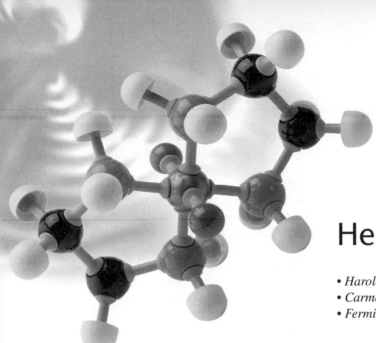

CHAPTER 36

Hemoglobin

- *Harold R. Schumacher*
- *Carmelita Alvares*
- *Fermina M. Mazzella*

Chapter Outline

Objectives

- Describe what is meant by a hemoglobinopathy.
- Describe the Bohr effect.
- Describe the physiological effect of 2,3-biphosphoglycerate.
- List the common hemoglobinopathies and their major biochemical and clinical features.

- Describe the method of sickling in sickle cell anemia.
- Describe the chain structure of fetal hemoglobin and its importance in hemoglobinopathies.

Key Terms

2,3-biphosphoglycerate   A glycolytic intermediate in the red cell that changes the affinity of hemoglobin for oxygen.

anemia   A disorder resulting from low concentrations of hemoglobin in blood.

Bohr effect   The change of oxygen affinity of hemoglobin with pH.

carboxyhemoglobin   Hemoglobin combined with carbon monoxide.

erythropoietin   A renal hormone that stimulates the production of hemoglobin and red blood cells.

fetal hemoglobin   The form of hemoglobin that is present during most of fetal development, also in certain hemoglobinopathies. This form has two α chains and two γ chains.

globins   The polypeptide chains without heme of hemoglobin. It is also used to describe a class of protein molecules.

heme   An iron-containing porphyrin derivative that gives hemoglobin its red color.

heme-heme interaction or **subunit cooperativity**   In general, this describes the effect that the binding of one ligand to a protein has on the binding of other ligands at other sites on that protein. With hemoglobin, the binding of oxygen to one heme group increases the affinity of other heme groups for oxygen, resulting in the sigmoidal curve of oxygen uptake by hemoglobin.

hemichromes   Greenish ferric compounds formed by the oxidation of the heme group and its subsequent covalent binding to the protein.

hemoglobin   A red oxygen-carrying protein found in red blood cells.

hemoglobin A$_1$ A series of hemoglobin derivatives formed by the postsynthetic, nonenzymatic reaction of various sugars with the amino groups of the globin chains of hemoglobin. Hemoglobin A$_{1c}$ (Hb + glucose) is the derivative found in the highest concentration.

hemoglobinopathies   Genetic disorders involving the structure and synthesis of one or more of the globin polypeptide chains.

hemogram   A formula used to differentiate iron deficiency from milder forms of thalassemia.

HPFH (hereditary persistence of fetal hemoglobin) β-Thalassemia, a condition in which the synthesis of the β chains of hemoglobin is diminished.

hypoxia   Low Po_2 in tissues.

methemoglobin   A form of hemoglobin in which the ferrous ion Fe^{2+} of hemoglobin has been oxidized to the ferric state Fe^{3+}.

sickle cell anemia   A chronic, moderate-to-severe hemolytic anemia in persons homozygous for hemoglobin S.

sickle cell disorders   Formation of a morphologic, abnormal sickle cell type caused by the presence of a hemoglobin variant.

sickle cell hemoglobin   A genetically altered globin gene in which valine is substituted for glutamine in the β chain of the hemoglobin, causing reduction in solubility of the hemoglobin molecule.

sulfhemoglobin   A stable compound resulting from the linkage of sulfur to hemoglobin.

thalassemias   A group of disorders in which there is a quantitative defect in the production of globin chains.

α-thalassemia   A group of genetic disorders that result in defective α chain synthesis.

β-thalassemia   A group of genetic disorders that result in defective β chain synthesis.

Methods on CD-ROM

Blood gas analysis (PO$_2$)
Carboxyhemoglobin

Haptoglobin

More than 700 different inherited variants of **hemoglobins** have been described in humans. The majority of these are of no clinical consequence. However, some significantly alter molecular stability or function, resulting in **anemia** or other disease manifestations. Most of the clinical abnormalities are explainable in terms of the structural abnormality. Mutations continue to occur, often resulting in disease states called **hemoglobinopathies**.

All **globin** genes are believed to have arisen from a common globinlike **heme** protein. The earliest duplication of this progenitor gene led to the divergence of myoglobin and the globins that comprise hemoglobin. From this ancestral globin gene diverged the α-globin genes, which include the ζ-gene. The ancient β-globin gene evolved to form hemoglobin gene families. In estimated order of appearance, they are the γ-globin, the ϵ-globin, and the δ-globin genes. Modern globin proteins are the result of an evolutionary process that began more than 700 million years ago (Fig. 36-1).

STRUCTURE AND FUNCTION OF HEMOGLOBIN
Structure

Hemoglobin (Hb) is a red, oxygen-carrying protein found in red blood cells. It is a tetramer of two pairs of different globin chains with a molecular weight of 64,000 D (Fig. 36-2). Each chain carries an iron-containing porphyrin derivative called *heme*, a ferriprotoporphyrin IX in which one iron atom is bound in the center of the porphyrin ring. The polypeptide chains (without heme) are collectively called the *globin* moiety of hemoglobin. Each polypeptide chain is designated by a Greek letter: α (alpha), β (beta), γ (gamma), δ (delta), ε (epsilon), and ζ (zeta). Normal mammalian hemoglobin contains two pairs of chains: two α- and two non-α (β, γ, or δ) chains. The α-chains bind with β-chains to produce normal adult Hb (HbA = $\alpha_2\beta_2$), they bind with the γ-chain to produce fetal Hb (HbF = $\alpha_2\gamma_2$), and they bind with the δ-chain to produce HbA$_2$ (HbA$_2$ = $\alpha_2\delta_2$). The latter accounts for only 2.5% of normal adult Hb. The two early embryonic Hbs, termed Hbs Gower 1 and Gower 2, consist of α-like ζ-chains and β-like ε-chains.

The primary, secondary, tertiary, and quaternary structures of all the hemoglobins have been determined. The β-, γ-, δ-, and ε-chains have similar amino acid sequences, as do the α- and ζ-chains. The α-chain contains 141 amino acid residues, and the β-, δ-, and ε-chains each contain 146.

In all hemoglobin and myoglobin chains, approximately 75% of the amino acids are arranged in an a-helix with three to six amino acids per turn (see Fig. 36-2). The tertiary structure of hemoglobin is depicted in Fig. 36-3. The folding pattern places polar amino acid residues on the outside of the molecule and provides a pocket with a deep hydrophobic niche for the heme ring between the E and F helices in each protein subunit. Many noncovalent bonds are formed between the heme moiety and the surrounding amino acids. An iron atom, in the ferrous (Fe^{2+}) state, in the center of the ferriprotoporphyrin IX ring forms an important bond with the F8, or proximal, histidine via the bound oxygen with the E7, or distal, histidine. This heme iron is critical because oxygenation and deoxygenation occur at this site.

The complete hemoglobin tetramer composed of two α-globin and two non-α-globin chains fits together to form a quaternary structure (Fig. 36-4). The central cavity is filled with water and allows the entrance of small molecules such as **2,3-biphosphoglycerate** (2,3-BPG) and salts. The motion of individual globin chains, including the movement of globin chains relative to one another during oxygenation and deoxygenation, gives hemoglobin its unique ability to serve as a carrier of oxygen. The substitution of a single amino acid can change the secondary, tertiary, and quaternary structures of hemoglobin, causing severe and even fatal pathophysiological changes.

Ontogeny

The hemoglobin composition of a red blood cell (RBC) varies widely depending on when, during gestation or postnatal development, the RBC is produced. The first globin chains formed in embryonic red cells are ε-chains, which

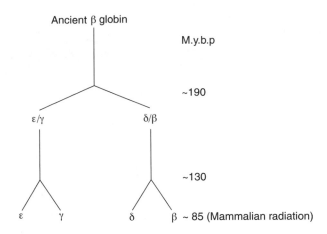

Fig. 36-1 The evolutionary history of the globin gene. *M.y.b.p.*, Million years before present. *(From Steinberg MH, Adams JG III: Hemoglobin A$_2$: origin, evolution and aftermath, Blood 78:2165, 1991.)*

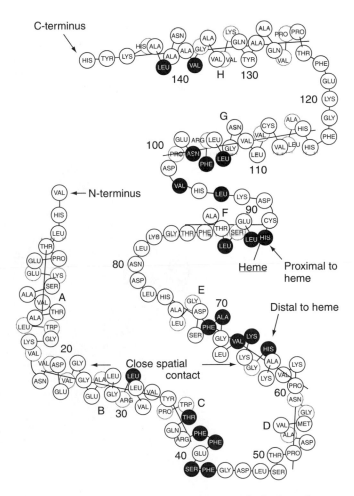

Fig. 36-2 The β-globin chain showing helical and non-helical segments. The helical segments are labeled *A* through *H*, whereas nonhelical segments are designated *NA* for those residues between the N terminus and the A helix, *CD* for residues between the C and D helices, etc. *(From Huisman THJ, Schroeder WA: New aspects of the structure, function and synthesis of hemoglobin, Boca Raton, FL, 1971, CRC Press.)*

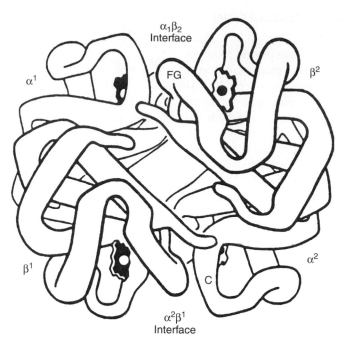

Fig. 36-3 Diagrammatic representation of the tertiary structure of the hemoglobin molecule showing the location of variant hemoglobins that impart physical instability to the molecule. Each chain carries an iron-containing porphyrin derivative called *heme*, a ferriprotoporphyrin IX in which one iron atom is bound in the center of the porphyrin ring. FG corner is shown and represents important area of the molecule that regulates oxygen binding and release. 2,3-Biphosphoglycerate (2,3-BPG) an important oxygen-regulating enzyme is located in central clear area of the molecule. *(From Embury SH et al, editors:* Sickle cell disease: basic principles and clinical practice, *New York, 1994, Raven Press.)*

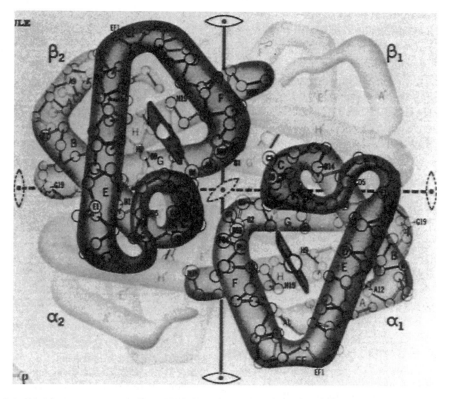

Fig. 36-4 Quaternary structure of hemoglobin. The α_1- and β_2-chains are in foreground, and α_1 β_2 contact is at center. *(From Dickerson RE, Geis I:* The structure and action of proteins, *Menlo Park, CA, 1969, Benjamin/Cummings. Reprinted by permission of Pearson Education, Inc.)*

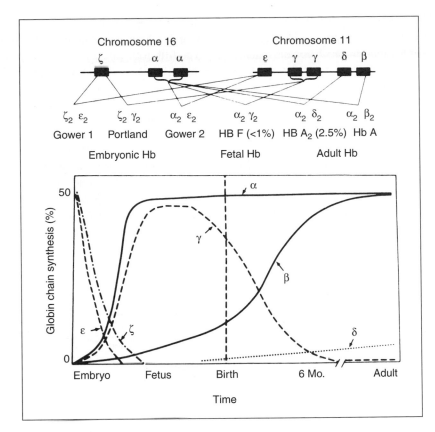

Fig. 36-5   Developmental switching of globin synthesis and the globin chain composition of human hemoglobins. Switching of gene expression within the β-like and α-like gene clusters leads to the synthesis of different hemoglobins in the embryo, fetus, infant, and adult. *Top,* The globin gene–containing chromosomes and their contributions to the hemoglobin molecules of the embryo, fetus, and adult. *Bottom,* Embryonic ε- and ζ-chains rapidly disappear and are replaced by fetal γ- and adult α-chains. γ-Chain synthesis peaks in mid-gestation and reaches its adult level at 6 months of age. There is a progressive rise in β-chain synthesis from the first trimester to its peak at 6 to 12 months of age. The small amounts of δ-chain synthesized peak at about 12 months. *(From Steinberg MH: Hemoglobinopathies and thalassemias. In Stein JH, editor:* Internal medicine, *ed 5, St Louis, 1998, Mosby.)*

resemble β-chains in their primary structure.[1] Almost immediately, the synthesis of ζ-, α-, and γ-chains begins. The sequential activation and inactivation, or switching, among genes within the α- and non-α-globin gene clusters results in the formation of four commonly encountered embryonic hemoglobins. These are Gower 1, $\zeta_2\varepsilon_2$, Gower 2, $\alpha_2\varepsilon_2$, Portland, $\zeta_2\gamma_2$, and fetal hemoglobin, $\alpha_2\gamma_2$. Gower 1 and Gower 2 hemoglobins constitute 42% and 24% of the total hemoglobin, respectively, at 5 weeks of gestation. The rest is **fetal hemoglobin**. Hemoglobin switching during embryonic, fetal, and adult development is shown in Fig. 36-5.

NORMAL HEMOGLOBIN BIOCHEMISTRY
Assembly of Hemoglobin

The α-like globin genes of man are located on the short arm of chromosome 16, between band p 13.2 and the terminus, whereas the β-like genes are located on the terminal portion of the short arm of chromosome 11 (p15).[2] The α and β polypeptide chains of an adult hemoglobin are synthesized in equal amounts, though there may be an excess of α-chains

in the cytoplasm of young red cells. The assembly process starts with the release of α- and β-chains from the ribosomes into the cytoplasm. They immediately incorporate heme (see Chapter 35 for discussion on the synthesis of heme) and form monomer combinations and dimer aggregates followed by the synthesis of tetramers. In the hemoglobinopathies, the concentrations of the two chains, such as βA and βS; βA and βC; and βA and βE, may differ even though their rates of synthesis are the same. There is evidence that the relative rates of assembly in relation to synthesis of hemoglobins A and S may differ because of differences in affinities of βA and βS for α-chains. The α-chains, if in short supply, prefer to combine with normal β-chains rather than with the variant chains,[3] and excess variant chains are then removed by proteolysis.

The synthesis of hemoglobin is normally stimulated by tissue **hypoxia** (low P_{O_2} in tissues). Hypoxia causes the kidneys to produce increased amounts of **erythropoietin** (see p. 484), which in turn stimulates the production of hemoglobin and RBCs.

Functional and Structural Interrelationships

Hemoglobin and oxygen: the oxygen-dissociation

curve. The four subunits of hemoglobin each contain a heme moiety deep in the pocket of the globin chains, leaving one edge of the heme exposed to receive the oxygen. Each of the four heme iron atoms can reversibly bind one oxygen molecule. Because the iron remains in the ferrous form, the reaction is an oxygenation, not an oxidation.

To fulfill its function as a respiratory pigment, hemoglobin must specifically bind oxygen molecules with high affinity, transport them, and unload them at the oxygen tension of tissues. Each gram of hemoglobin binds approximately 1.34 mL of oxygen. The tetrameric structure of hemoglobin is responsible for its unique oxygen-binding capacity and renders it physiologically superior to single hemoglobin sub-

units or to myoglobin. The heme iron has six valence bonds, four of which are occupied by the four pyrrole rings of heme. The fifth iron valency bond attaches heme to globin, leaving the sixth iron valency bond available for a reversible combination with oxygen or other ligands.

The affinity of hemoglobin for oxygen depends on the partial pressure of oxygen (PO_2). A plot of the oxygen content (percentage of hemoglobin saturated with oxygen) against PO_2 in myoglobin subunits results in a hyperbolic oxygen-dissociation curve, but a similar plot using hemoglobin gives a sigmoid curve (Fig. 36-6). The hyperbolic curve indicates appreciable release of oxygen at very low partial pressures only, whereas the sigmoid curve indicates a much earlier release of oxygen even at relatively high oxygen tensions, allowing adequate oxygenation of tissues. The

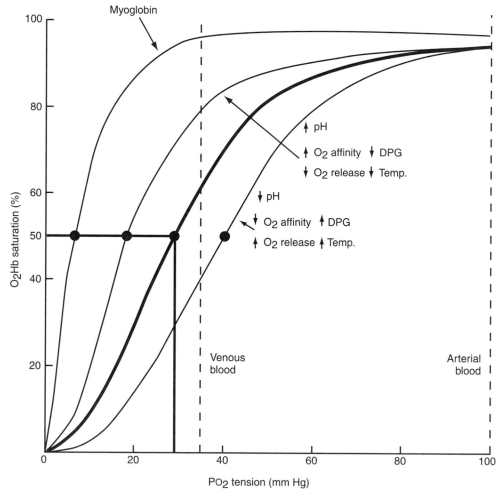

Fig. 36-6 Oxygen-dissociation curves of normal human hemoglobin. *Heavy middle line,* Dissociation curve of normal adult blood (temperature 37° C, pH 7.4, PCO_2 35 mm Hg). *Dots,* P_{50} values, partial pressure of oxygen (27 mm Hg) at which hemoglobin solution is 50% oxyhemoglobin and 50% deoxyhemoglobin. If temperature increases, pH decreases, or carbon dioxide tension (PCO_2) increases, the curve shifts to the right. This shift increases release of oxygen from hemoglobin at given oxygen tension by decreasing its oxygen affinity. If temperature decreases, pH rises, or carbon dioxide tension decreases, oxygen-dissociation curve moves to the left. This shift increases oxygen-binding capacity of hemoglobin at given oxygen tension: thus there is a decrease in oxygen release. *(From Bauer JD: Clinical laboratory methods, ed 9, St Louis, 1982, Mosby.)*

curve has a sigmoid shape because oxygenation of one heme group increases oxygen affinity of the others, a phenomenon called **heme-heme interaction** (or **subunit cooperativity**), which is responsible for the physiologically efficient uptake and release of oxygen. There is a progressive change in oxygen affinity as each heme molecule becomes oxygenated; the affinity for oxygen is low at first but increases as each heme molecule takes up oxygen. In myoglobin, the hyperbolic dissociation curve indicates that each molecule is oxygenated independently. In the lung, at a PO_2 of about 95 mm Hg, arterial blood becomes 97% saturated with oxygen and carries 200 mL of oxygen per 1000 mL of blood. In the capillary bed, venous blood at a PO_2 tension of about 40 mm Hg is still about 75% saturated with oxygen, but is nevertheless able to give up 46 mL of oxygen per 1000 mL of blood. The 75% of hemoglobin returned to the lung in an oxygenated form establishes a large reservoir for improved oxygen delivery to tissues.

The position of the oxygen-dissociation curve is determined by several factors affecting the affinity of hemoglobin for oxygen. The oxygen-dissociation curve is conventionally indexed by the P_{50} value, the PO_2 at which the hemoglobin is 50% saturated with O_2; this normally occurs at a PO_2 of 27 mm Hg. The higher the P_{50}, the lower is the affinity of hemoglobin for oxygen. A decreased P_{50} indicates a shift to the left of the oxygen-dissociation curve, an increased oxygen affinity of hemoglobin, and an impaired oxygen release to tissues. P_{50} is decreased in the presence of (1) a high concentration of HbF, the γ-chain of which binds 2,3-BPG poorly; (2) a modified hemoglobin, such as **methemoglobin** and **carboxyhemoglobin;** (3) certain hemoglobin variants, such as Hb Rainier; and (4) 2,3-BPG-depleted blood found after massive transfusions (see Fig. 36-6). Obviously, 2,3-BPG binding to hemoglobin decreases the affinity of hemoglobin for oxygen (see later discussion). A *shift to the right* indicates a decreased oxygen affinity, which causes the delivery of oxygen to tissues. It is seen in various types of hypoxia, such as that occurring at high altitude, with severe anemia and heart and lung disease.[2]

Oxygen Affinity and Transport

Oxygen affinity and transport depend not only on PO_2 (see earlier discussion) but also on temperature, pH (Bohr effect), and 2,3-BPG concentration.

Bohr effect. The **Bohr effect** expresses the fact that the oxygen affinity of hemoglobin varies with the pH. Protons lower the affinity of hemoglobin for oxygen mass and, conversely, oxygen lowers the affinity of hemoglobin for protons.

$$HB(O_2)_4 + 2H^+ \rightleftharpoons 2HbH^+ + 4O^2 \qquad \textit{Eq. 36-1}$$

At physiological pH in the tissues, about two protons are taken up for every four molecules of oxygen released; whereas in the lungs two protons are liberated again when four molecules of oxygen are bound to hemoglobin. This reciprocal action is known as the Bohr effect and is essential to the mechanism of oxygen transport and the buffering of carbon dioxide (see Chapter 25).

In the physiological pH range, the affinity of hemoglobin for oxygen decreases in the tissues as the acidity increases, and the dissociation curve shifts to the right (see Fig. 36-6). The Bohr effect aids in the transport of oxygen and buffering of carbon dioxide in the acid milieu of the tissues in which carbon dioxide and acid metabolites accumulate and in the more alkaline milieu of the lungs where carbon dioxide is released and oxygen is picked up. Both 2,3-BPG and chloride enhance the Bohr effect.

2,3-Biphosphoglycerate

Other molecules influence the structure and function of hemoglobin. Of the factors that affect oxygen release from hemoglobin (temperature, pH, PO_2, PCO_2, and 2,3-BPG), 2,3-BPG is the most important. It is the most abundant glycolytic intermediate in red blood cells and is present at a concentration equimolar with that of deoxyhemoglobin. In oxyhemoglobin the helices of the β-chains are not open enough to permit firm stereospecific binding of 2,3-BPG within the central cavity of the hemoglobin tetramer to the N-terminal valine, the H21 histidine (position 143), and the EF6 lysine (position 82) of the β-chain. Thus 2,3-BPG binding stabilizes the deoxygenated form at the expense of the oxyhemoglobin form. This, along with other conformational changes in the oxygenated molecule, favors binding 2,3-BPG to the deoxygenated rather than the oxygenated form, reducing the affinity of hemoglobin for oxygen and shifting the oxygen dissociation curve to the right.

$$HBO_2 + DPG \rightleftharpoons Hb \cdot BPG + O_2 \qquad \textit{Eq. 36-2}$$

During anaerobic metabolism, red cells increase production of 2,3-BPG, facilitating oxygen release.

When the pH drops, as in acidosis, the oxygen-dissociation curve moves to the right, but the resulting inhibition of 2,3-BPG corrects the shift by an equal change to the left. An elevated red blood cell pH shifts the dissociation curve to the left, but the rising 2,3-BPG concentration shifts it to the right, returning it to base position (see Fig. 36-6). The common denominator of the 2,3-BPG–Bohr effect is the rate of glycolysis, which is stimulated by alkalosis and suppressed by acidosis because the former stimulates phosphofructokinase activity and the latter suppresses it. 2,3-BPG is formed from 1,3-BPG, an intermediary of the Embden-Meyerhoff pathway (Rappaport-Leubering cycle, see Fig. 32-2).

Other Chemical Derivatives of Hemoglobin

Besides oxyhemoglobin and deoxyhemoglobin (see earlier discussion and Chapter 25), other chemically modified forms of hemoglobin exist.

Hemoglobin A_1. Hemoglobin A_1 is formed by the postsynthetic, nonenzymatic reaction of various sugars with amino groups of the globin chains. HbA_1 actually consists of four principal components, called HbA_{1a1}, HbA_{1a2}, HbA_{1b}, and HbA_{1c}. Hemoglobin A_{1c}, the major sugar derivative, is produced by the reaction of glucose with the terminal amino group (valine) of the β-chain. The glycosylated hemoglobins are useful for the monitoring of diabetes; other hemoglobins are the adducts of glucose-6-phosphate or fructose-1,6-diphosphate and the β-chain. See Chapter 32 for further discussion of glycosylated hemoglobins.

Carboxyhemoglobin. Carbon monoxide (CO) is a ligand that, like oxygen, binds reversibly to the ferrous ion of hemoglobin. However, it forms a toxic compound, carboxyhemoglobin (CO-Hb). It also binds to other heme-containing proteins, such as myoglobin, cytochrome P-450, and cytochrome oxidase.[4] CO combines with hemoglobin more slowly than oxygen, but, because the union is much firmer, the release of CO is 10,000 times slower than the release of oxygen from oxyhemoglobin. Also, the affinity of hemoglobin for CO is 218 times greater than that for oxygen. Because CO and O_2 compete for the same binding sites on heme, the presence of CO reduces the concentration of oxyhemoglobin. At a CO concentration of 0.1% in the inhaled air, more than 50% of the hemoglobin is unavailable for O_2 transport. In the presence of CO, the oxyhemoglobin dissociates more slowly because the iron atoms not bound to CO have a higher affinity for O_2, causing the oxygen-dissociation curve to shift to the left. CO-Hb can be identified in blood by spectroscopic, spectrophotometric, chemical, or gas chromatographic techniques.[5] The presence of CO-Hb in blood does not cause substantial error in pulse oximetry,[6] a determination that has great clinical importance.

Methemoglobin. Methemoglobin (Met-Hb) is a form of hemoglobin (with oxy- or deoxy-forms) in which the ferrous ion (Fe^{2+}) of hemoglobin has been oxidized to the ferric state (Fe^{3+}) to form ferrihemoglobin. Met-Hb cannot bind oxygen reversibly and is unable to act as an effective oxygen transporter. If Met-Hb is present in high enough concentrations (over 30% of total hemoglobin), hypoxia and cyanosis (methemoglobinemia) will result. Normally, a small amount of methemoglobin forms continuously in RBCs; however, this does not normally exceed 1% of the total hemoglobin because the methemoglobin is reduced back to Hb (see p. 690).

After prolonged exposure to the air, the oxyhemoglobin in normal blood is autooxidized and the blood turns brown as methemoglobin is formed. This process is also responsible for the brown color of blood in acid urine.

Hemichromes. **Hemichromes** are greenish ferric compounds with characteristic absorption spectral profiles. During the oxidation of hemoglobin to Met-Hb superoxide anions are formed, and hydrogen peroxide is produced. As a result, more Met-Hb is formed, and oxidative changes occur in the globin protein. These changes, in the heme group and in the protein, alter the stereochemical binding of the heme to the protein, and the heme iron may form ligands with various side chains in the proteins (hemichromes) rather than with the proximal histidine or with oxygen. The heme group can be physically displaced from the protein and precipitate as free ferriheme (or hematin) onto the interior of the RBC membrane. Polypeptide chains also precipitate when they are denatured. These hemoglobin breakdown products form inclusions on the interior of the RBC membrane, called *Heinz bodies*, which are responsible for the lysis of the affected red cells.[7] The steps leading to cell lysis are as follows:

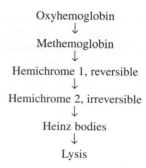

Hematologists use supravital stains to identify Heinz bodies, which are found in a group of anemias known as *Heinz body anemias*.

Sulfhemoglobin. Sulfhemoglobin (S-Hb) is a stable compound resulting from the linkage of sulfur to hemoglobin. The toxic effects of certain drugs on hemoglobin lead not only to the formation of methemoglobin, but also to concomitant S-Hb production.[5]

Sulfhemoglobinemia appears in some persons after exposure to sulfonamides, phenacetin, acetanilid, and trinitrotoluene. It is not clear why Met-Hb is found in the blood of some individuals whereas S-Hb is seen in the blood of others after exposure to these drugs. The structure of S-Hb is unknown, but sulfur is probably linked to heme. The S-Hb complex is stable and irreversible (thus differing from Met-Hb) and does not disappear from the circulation until affected RBCs complete their life cycle. Sulfhemoglobin produces anoxia and cyanosis, which clinically are indistinguishable from the anoxia and cyanosis of Met-Hb. Sulfhemoglobin shows a characteristic absorption of light at 620 nm that does not shift when cyanide is added. Rarely, sulfhemoglobin causes Heinz body formation.

NORMAL HUMAN HEMOGLOBINS (Table 36-1)
Hemoglobin A ($\alpha_2\beta_2$)

Hemoglobin A makes up the major portion (95% to 98%) of the adult hemolysate. Small amounts of HbA are produced in the last 6 weeks of fetal life (see Chapter 40), along with the predominant fetal hemoglobin. During the 6 to 12 months postpartum, the shift to the adult form of hemoglobin is completed (see later discussion).

TABLE 36-1 NORMAL HUMAN HEMOGLOBINS

Designation	Tetrameric Structure	HEMOLYSATE (%) Adult	Newborn
Adult			
HbA	$\alpha_2\beta_2$	95 to 98	20 to 30
HbA$_2$	$\alpha_2\delta_2$	2 to 3	0.2
Fetal			
HbF	$\alpha_2\gamma_2$	<1	80
Embryonic			
Gower 1	$\zeta_2\epsilon_2$	0	0
Gower 2	$\alpha_2\epsilon_2$	0	0
Hb Portland	$\zeta_2\gamma_2$	0	0

Hemoglobin A$_2$ ($\alpha_2\delta_2$)

Hemoglobin A$_2$ is a minor component of hemoglobin that makes its first appearance before the completion of intra-uterine development (0.2% of cord blood hemolysate) and remains at low concentration (2.5%) throughout adult life. Its exact function is unknown but is probably similar to that of HbA.

Fetal Hemoglobin ($\alpha_2\gamma_2$)

Hemoglobin F is the major hemoglobin of fetal life, preceded by the embryonic hemoglobins Gower 1, Gower 2, and Portland. HbF is a mixture of two molecular species in which the γ-chains have either glycine (Gg) or alanine (Ag) at position 136. At birth, the HbF GgAg ratio is about 3:1, whereas in the normal adult the Gg/Ag ratio of the small amount of HbF (less than 1%) is 2:3. In the first months of fetal life, small amounts of HbF are produced along with the Gower hemoglobins, which are replaced by HbF at the end of the second month. From this time to just before birth, the percentage of fetal hemoglobin is about 90%. At birth, the RBCs contain about 70% to 90% HbF, though higher concentrations have been reported. After birth, HbF normally decreases rapidly to about 50% to 70% at the end of the first month, 25% to 60% at the end of the second month, and 10% to 30% at the end of the third month. Between 6 months and 12 months, the HbF concentration falls from 8% to 2%; in the second year it falls to 1.8%; and in the third year it falls to 1%. It finally levels off to the adult level of less than 0.4%, a level not detectable by routine laboratory methods. It is normally slightly increased (up to 3%) during pregnancy.

The functions and molecular characteristics of HbF are as follows:

1. Electrophoretically it is slower than HbA.
2. It resists alkali denaturation, a feature that is the basis of the Singer test for HbF.[7]
3. It is twice as resistant to acid elution as HbA, a characteristic that forms the basis of the Kleihauer elution technique.[8]
4. HbF is oxidized to Met-Hb twice as quickly as HbA, predisposing the newborn to cyanosis.
5. It has a higher oxygen affinity than HbA has, because it binds 2,3-BPG to a lesser degree than adult hemoglobin because of its γ-chain. This characteristic allows oxygen transport across the placental villi, despite their low oxygen concentration (80%).[9]

The molecular properties of HbF allow HbF to function as the primary oxygen carrier for the fetus. The other embryonic hemoglobins have similar properties and are able to combine with oxygen at the low oxygen tension and low pH of interstitial fluid, facilitating fetal growth and development. Embryonic hemoglobins are detectable in red cells by a modification of the Kleihauer method for HbF.

PATHOLOGIC CONDITIONS
Hemoglobinopathies

The inherited disorders of hemoglobin, the hemoglobino-pathies, are genetic disorders involving the structure and synthesis of one or more of the globin polypeptide chains. Hemoglobinopathies may be divided into several over-lapping groups[10]: (1) the structural hemoglobin variants that involve substitution, addition, or deletion of one or more amino acids of the globin chain; (2) the **thalassemias**, a group of disorders in which there is a quantitative defect in globin chain production; (3) combinations of types 1 and 2 that result in complex hemoglobinopathies; and (4) **hereditary persistence of fetal hemoglobin (HPFH)**, an asymptomatic disorder.

Structural Hemoglobin Variants

Nomenclature. Hemoglobins A, F, and S were the first hemoglobins to be discovered and were assigned letters. As additional variants were discovered, they were assigned successive letters of the alphabet beginning with HbC. Subsequently, hemoglobins were discovered so rapidly that the letters of the alphabet were depleted. Therefore, hemo-globins with similar electrophoretic mobility, but with different structures were distinguished by adding (properly as a subscript) the place of discovery of the new hemoglobin, such as HbC$_{Georgetown}$, HbD$_{Punjab}$. Finally, some hemoglobins are called by the names of the families in which they were first discovered, such as Hb$_{Lepore}$. When the exact amino acid substitution of the new variant and the spatial structure of hemoglobin were determined, the expression became more complex. For instance, HbS evolved into the scientific designation: HbS B6 (A3)Glu→Val. This designation reveals that the substitution is located at the sixth position of the amino acid sequence, in the A3 position of the b-chain. It also shows that the glutamine (Glu) has been replaced by a valine (Val). There are over 700 variant hemoglobins identi-fied in humans at present. Some of the more important ones demonstrating clinical disorders are shown in Table 36-2. Excellent tables on nomenclature, molecular structure, clinical manifestations, and electrophoretic mobility of hemoglobin variants are found in reference 11.

Classification

Hemoglobin variants are classified according to (1) mole-cular mechanism, (2) clinical and functional manifestations, and (3) electrophoretic behavior.

Molecular mechanisms responsible for structural hemoglobin variants. Five basic molecular mechanisms are responsible for the structural changes found in most hemoglobin variants: (1) amino acid substitution, (2) deletions and insertions, (3) unequal crossing over (fusion genes), (4) chain elongation, and (5) frame shift variance.[11]

Clinical consequences of structural alterations of hemoglobin molecules. Structural alterations of the hemoglobin molecule are responsible for a wide range of clinical manifestations. Most mutations are asymptomatic because they do not interfere with hemoglobin function. Others produce disease because they affect the stability, shape, or function of the hemoglobin molecule. A person homozygous for an abnormal hemoglobin may have striking clinical manifestations such as **sickle cell anemia**, whereas a

TABLE 36-2 SOME IMPORTANT VARIANT HEMOGLOBINS

Substitution	Name	Property
α-chain variants		
5 (A3) Ala → Asp	J-Toronto	
11 (A9) Lys → Glu	Anantharaj	SE Asia
12 (A10) Ala → Asp	J-Paris	
16 (A14) Lys → Glu	I	Af-Am
23 (B4) Glu → Gln	Memphis	Af-Am with Hb S
30 (B11) Glu → Gln	G-Honolulu	
47 (CE5) Asp → Gly	Umi, Beilinson	Unstable
Asp → His	Hasharon	
57 (E6) Gly → Asp	J-Norfolk	
58 (E7) His → Tyr	M-Boston	Methemoglobinemia
68 (E17) Asn → Lys	G-Philadelphia	Often *cis* to α-thal
78 (EF7) Asn → Lys	Stanleyville-II	With Hb S
85 (F6) Asp → Asn	G-Norfolk	Inc O_2 affinity
Asp → Val	Inkster	With β-thal
87 (F8) His → Tyr	M-Iwate	Methemoglobinemia
92 (FG4) Arg → Leu	Chesapeake	Inc O_2 affinity
112 (G19) His → Asp	Hopkins-II	Unstable
115 (GH3) Ala → Asp	J-Tongariki	*cis* to α-thal
141 (HC3) Arg → Pro	Singapore	
β-Globin variants		
1 (NA1) Val → AcAla	Raleigh	Decr O_2 affinity
7 (A4) Glu → Gly	G-San Jose	Slt unstable
9 (A6) Ser → Cys	Porto Alegre	Inc O_2 affinity, polymerization
16 (A13) Gly → Asp	J-Baltimore	With S, C, β-thal
22 (B4) Glu → Ala	G-Coushata	
Glu → Gln	D-Iran	
26 (B8) Glu → Lys	E	Thal phenotype
42 (CD1) Phe → Ser	Hammersmith	Unstable
61 (E5) Lys → Glu	N-Seattle	With S
63 (E7) His → Arg	Zurich	Unstable
His → Tyr	M-Saskatoon	Methemoglobinemia
67 (E11) Val → Glu	M-Milwaukee-I	Methemoglobinemia
73 (E17) Asp → Asn	Korle-Bu	With S
89 (F5) Ser → Asn	Creteil	Inc O_2 affinity
92 (F8) His → Tyr	M-Hyde Park	Methemoglobinemia
95 (FG2) Lys → Glu	N-Baltimore	
97 (FG4) His → Gln	Malmo	Inc O_2 affinity
98 (FG5) Val → Met	Koln	Unstable
99 (G1) Asp → Asn	Kempsey	Inc O_2 affinity
Asp → His	Yakima	Inc O_2 affinity
Asp → Ala	Radcliffe	Inc O_2 affinity
Asp → Tyr	Ypsilanti	Inc O_2 affinity, asymmetric hybrids
Asp → Gly	Hotel-Dieu	Inc O_2 affinity
Asp → Val	Chemilly	Inc O_2 affinity
102 (G4) Asn → Lys	Richmond	Asymmetric hybrids
112 (G14) Cys → Arg	Indianapolis	Very unstable
121 (GH4) Glu → Gln	D-Los Angeles	With S, Inc O_2 affinity
Glu → Lys	O-Arab	With S, β-thal
136 (H14) Gly → Asp	Hope	Unstable, decr O_2 affinity

TABLE 36-2 SOME IMPORTANT VARIANT HEMOGLOBINS—CONT'D

Substitution	Name	Property
145 (HC2) Tyr → His	Bethesda	Inc O_2 affinity
Tyr → Cys	Ranier	Inc O_2 affinity
Try → Asp	Fort Gordon	Inc O_2 affinity
Tyr → Term	McKees Rocks	Inc O_2 affinity
146 (HC3) His → Asp	Hiroshima	Inc O_2 affinity
His → Pro	York	Inc O_2 affinity
His → Arg	Cochin-Port Royal	
His → Leu	Cowtown	Inc O_2 affinity
Variants having two amino acid substitutions in one chain		
β6 (A3) Glu → Val	C-Harlem	
73 (E17) Asp → Asn		
β6 (A3) Glu → Val	S-Travis	Inc O_2 affinity
142 (H20) Ala → Val		
Variants having extended chains		
α141Term → Gly	Constant Spring	31 amino acids appended to C-terminus
α139-140-1 frame-shift	Wayne	Two terminal amino acids replaced by unique sequence of 10
Fusion genes		
δβ hybrid chain	Lepore	Formed by unequal crossover
Γβ hybrid chain	Kenya	Unequal crossover between Γ and β

From Rucknagel D: Hemoglobinopathies and thalassemias. In Schumacher HK, Rock WA, Stass SA, editors: Handbook of hematologic pathology, *New York, 2000, Marcel Dekker.*

person heterozygous for abnormal hemoglobin (HbA-HbS) is usually asymptomatic. Some hemoglobins (HbC, HbD, HbE) even in the homozygous state produce only mild symptoms, whereas others are responsible for almost specific pathophysiological changes, such as cyanosis and erythrocytosis. Some combinations, such as HbS with HbO$_{Arab}$, are actually more aggressive disease states than either alone. Conversely, other combinations, such as HbS and HbC generate milder symptoms than either Hb alone.

The clinical disorders can be grouped as follows (see Table 36-2):

Hemolytic anemias. Intraerythrocytic crystals of HbS and HbC may form and cause deformity of the RBCs. Such deformities are easily recognized by light microscopy, such as the sickle-shaped cells of sickle cell anemia. Unstable hemoglobins and enzyme abnormalities of the hexose-monophosphate shunt are also responsible for intraerythrocytic Heinz body inclusions. The affected cells are prematurely destroyed in the spleen, resulting in a greatly shortened red cell life span.

HbS adults are functionally asplenic, because of the continuous splenic damage induced by the malformed erythrocytes.

Cyanosis. Amino acid substitution near the heme pocket produces *M-hemoglobins*, which result in methemoglobinemia and cyanosis. Cyanosis may also occur because of hemoglobin mutants that result in increased deoxyhemoglobin, that is, Hb_{Kansas} and $Hb_{Beth\ Israel}$. Both types of hemoglobin show decreased oxygen affinity.

Erythrocytosis. Some amino acid substitutions result in high oxygen affinity and tissue hypoxia. Because of the hypoxia, erythropoietin synthesis is stimulated, resulting in an increased production of RBCs *(erythrocytosis)* and peripheral blood nucleated erythrocytes. Examples are $Hb_{Rainier}$, $Hb_{Chesapeake}$, and $Hb_{Ypsilanti}$.

Hypochromic anemias. Some mutations reduce hemoglobin output. Examples are Hb_{Lepore} and $Hb_{Constant\ Spring}$.

Electrophoretic behavior of hemoglobins. Hemoglobin electrophoresis is the most important laboratory test used to diagnose and classify a hemoglobin abnormality (see p. 692). However, no single hemoglobin test can accurately distinguish an abnormal hemoglobin from a thalassemic disorder.

Sickle Cell Disorders: Sickle Hemoglobin

Sickling disorders are caused by the homozygous form of the sickle cell gene (sickle cell anemia), the heterozygous form of the sickle cell gene (sickle cell trait), and the combination of either with other structural hemoglobin variants or thalassemias.

Sickle hemoglobin (HbS) results when valine is substituted for the normally occurring glutamine residue and intracellular crystals of deoxygenated HbS form, causing the RBC to sickle.

HbS is not the only hemoglobin that causes RBCs to sickle, because RBCs containing $HbC_{Georgetown}$, HbI, and $Hb_{Bart's}$ also sickle. Nevertheless, in America and Africa, HbS is the most common hemoglobin variant, with an incidence of the heterozygous form of approximately 8% in American blacks and 30% in African blacks. HbS can also be found in nonblack inhabitants in the areas bordering Africa. In Africa the high frequency of the sickle cell gene has persisted because heterozygotes for HbS are somewhat protected from malaria because *Plasmodium* organisms fail to grow in HbS-containing RBCs.[12]

Molecular Mechanism of Sickling

The substitution of valine for the normal glutamic acid at position 6 in the β-chain results in a hemoglobin whose deoxy form (deoxy-HbS) polymerizes within the RBCs and forms long fibers readily visible on electron microscopy of red cells from patients homozygous for the $β^S$ mutation. Oxyhemoglobin S does *not* form such fibers.

Several facts about the polymerization are relevant to the pathogenesis of the sickle configuration and to possible therapeutic intervention. The polymerization occurs in two phases. The first of these, the slow-nucleation (or *delay*) phase, reflects the initial association of a few molecules of

TABLE 36-3   VARYING CLINICAL SEVERITY OF THE DIFFERENT SICKLE SYNDROMES

Genotype	% of Hemoglobin S	% of Non-S Hemoglobin	Clinical Severity
SA	30 to 40	60 to 70 (A)	0
SF*	70	30 (F)	0
SS	80 to 90	5 to 15 (F)	++/++++
S-thalassemia	80	20 (A + F)	+/+++
SC	50	50 (C)	+/+++
SO.SD	30 to 40	60 to 70	++/++++

From Bunn HF: Sickle cell anemia and other hemoglobinopathies. In Beck WS, editor: Hematology, Cambridge, Mass 1981, MIT Press.
*Double heterozygous state for hemoglobin S and hereditary persistence of fetal hemoglobin.

deoxy-HbS. This phase varies in duration from milliseconds to a few minutes, depending on several factors including temperature and the presence of hemoglobins other than HbS.

The duration also depends, exponentially, on the concentration of HbS. Thus a prolonged delay time, resulting from a decreased concentration of HbS within the RBC, might permit the deoxygenated cell to traverse the microcirculation without sickling. Factors that favor increasing polymerization of HbS within red cells and thus the severity of the disease have their effect by increasing the relative abundance of deoxy-HbS. Such factors include a decrease in PO_2, increased organic phosphates, increased hydrogen-ion concentrations, and increased temperature.[13] The varying clinical severity of the different sickle syndromes is depicted in Table 36-3.

Pathophysiology of Sickle Cell Disease

HbS is inherited as an autosomal codominant trait. The sickle-shaped cells temporarily or permanently block microcirculation, and the resulting stasis leads to hypoxia and ischemic infarcts of various organs including liver, kidneys, spleen, lungs, heart, bones, and nervous system. Such infarcts lead to increased morbidity and, if located in a vital area, cause death.[14] Based upon studies from numerous laboratories, there is emerging consensus that a key contributor to vasoocclusion may be the increased tendency of sickle red cells to adhere to vascular endothelium.[15,16] Vasoocclusion can occur when the transit time of red cells through the capillaries is longer than the delay time for deoxyhemoglobin-induced hemoglobin polymerization of sickle hemoglobin. Consequently adherence of the sickle red cells to vascular endothelium impedes blood flow and thereby increases capillary transit time. Therefore it has been suggested that increased cell adherence can initiate and propagate vasoocclusion. Factors such as inflammatory mediators that activate endothelial cells and thereby enhance endothelial adversity of sickle red cells thus have potential to trigger vasoocclusive episodes. A partial list of agonists of the endothelium includes TNF-α/β, interferon γ, IL1-β, vascular endothelial growth factor (VEGF), thrombin, histamine, and the effects of hypoxia and reperfusion.

Sickle red cells exhibit increased adherence to endothelial cells in vitro and the extent of in vitro sickle adhesity correlates with vasoocclusive severity.[17] Adhesive ligands identified for sickle red cells include CD36, $\alpha 4\ \beta 1$ integrin, sulfated glycolipid, and the Lutheran blood group antigen. On the endothelial side, cytokine-induced VCAM-1, a ligand for $\alpha_4\beta$, and $\alpha_v\beta_3$ integrin that binds von Willebrand factor and thrombospondin have been shown to mediate sickle cell adherence. Bridging molecules exist that function between the adhesive receptors in the sickle cells and endothelial cells.

In addition to adherence, viscosity plays an important role in both affecting the rate of blood flow (hypoxia) and the production of thrombosis. Studies indicate that the membrane viscosity and deformability in sickle cell disease are markedly altered even when the red cell is fully oxygenated.[18-20] Although internal viscosity of the red cells is of great importance in determining the flow characteristics of the blood, the hematocrit is a major determinant in whole blood viscosity. The effects on the circulation caused by increased viscosity are seen in larger vessels than the effects of adherence and occlusion. Thrombosis can be seen on either the arterial or venous side of the circulation and has been known for many years in the pathophysiology of polycythemia and macroglobulinemia.[21]

Sickled cells have a greatly shortened life span. The ensuing hemolytic anemia is augmented by the inability of the bone marrow to respond adequately to the anemia because of ineffective erythropoiesis. The increased RBC destruction is responsible for hyperbilirubinemia, reticulocytosis, bone marrow erythroid hyperplasia, gallbladder pigment stones, and osteoporosis as a result of the expanding bone marrow.

Sickle cells exhibit oxygen-transport abnormalities.[22] In sickled cells the oxygen-dissociation curve is shifted to the right. The resulting decreased oxygen affinity favors the release of oxygen at higher oxygen tensions but also supports the formation of deoxyhemoglobin and sickling. The shift to the right of the oxygen equilibrium is caused by an elevated 2,3-BPG concentration and by an HbS polymerization-mediated defect.

Sickle Cell Trait (HbAS)

Persons with sickle cell trait are usually asymptomatic and have a normal **hemogram** (RBC profile, including RBC count, mean corpuscular volume [MCV], and mean corpuscular hemoglobin [MCH]) and RBC survival. The demonstration of HbS is usually of no clinical significance, because a normal HbA gene has been inherited along with the HbS gene, but should indicate the need for genetic counseling. There are rare reports of sickling complications in HbAS patients. They include (1) spontaneous hematuria in about 3% of patients and more frequently hyposthenuria because of the impairment of the concentrating power of the kidneys, both signs pointing to sickling within the blood vessels of

the medulla; (2) rupture of the infarcted spleen; (3) sickling crisis at elevated altitudes; and (4) rarely, proliferative retinopathy. Recently, a large study on military personnel with the sickle cell trait undergoing basic training showed a significant increase in sudden death.[23] This was most likely related to dehydration.

Sickle Cell Anemia (HbSS)

Sickle cell anemia is a chronic, moderate to severe, hemolytic anemia in a person homozygous for HbS, having inherited the HbS gene from both parents. The finding of HbSS is useful to differentiate sickle cell anemia from sickle cell-β-thalassemia or HbS hereditary persistence of HbF. The disease is not evident at birth and does not manifest itself until the γ-chains of the newborn are replaced by β^S-chains after 3 to 6 months of life.

The clinical severity of HbSS disease varies from patient to patient. Such variation has been further clarified by the investigation of haplotypes (Fig. 36-7). These genetic variations are of hematological, genetic, and anthropological interest, because they offer new insights in the sickling disorders. Each haplotype has a different combination of 14 cleavage sites for 10 restriction endonucleases in the vicinity of the β-globin locus. Each haplotype, plus genetic modifiers on the X-chromosome, contributes additively to the proportion of HbF, with Senegal and Indian contributing more than Benin, Bantu, and Cameroon. Clinical manifestations may be divided into acute and chronic episodes. Acute problems result from vasoocclusive crises involving several areas, as well as acute hematologic crises (see box below).

Splenic crisis may result from sudden trapping of blood in the spleen. Chronic manifestations of sickle cell disease usually appear after mid-childhood. These include disturbances in growth and development, bone and joint disease, and organ damage involving cardiovascular, pulmonary, hepatobiliary, genitourinary, ocular, and dermatologic systems. Renal failure may occur in many patients with sickle cell anemia, probably as the result of glomerular capillary disease.

Hemoglobin values hover around 70 to 80 g/L accompanied by a greatly elevated reticulocytosis (10%). The hemoglobin electrophoretogram shows absence of HbA (no

---

ACUTE CLINICAL MANIFESTATIONS OF HbSS

Hematological
Accelerated hemolytic anemia
Megaloblastic anemia
Aplastic crisis

Vasoocclusive
Bone and joints
Abdomen, spleen
Lungs
Central nervous system
Back

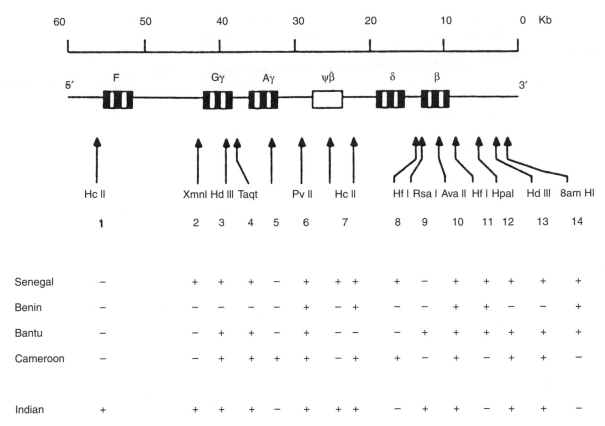

	Hc II		Xmnl	Hd III	Taqt	Pv II	Hc II		Hf I	Rsa I	Ava II	Hf I	Hpal	Hd III	8am HI
	1		**2**	**3**	**4**	**5**	**6**	**7**	**8**	**9**	**10**	**11**	**12**	**13**	**14**
Senegal	–		+	+	+	–	+	+	+	–	+	+	+	+	+
Benin	–		–	–	–	–	+	–	+	–	+	+	–	–	+
Bantu	–		–	+	+	–	+	–	–	–	+	+	+	+	+
Cameroon	–		–	+	+	+	+	–	+	+	–	+	–	+	–
Indian	+		+	+	+	–	+	+	+	–	+	+	–	+	–

Fig. 36-7 Restriction endonuclease polymorphisms in the β-globin cluster. *Top, arrows* point to the cleavage sites for each of the enzymes. *Bottom,* haplotypes defined by the patterns of cleavages typical of the regions where each haplotype is most prevalent. *(From Nagel RL: Origins and dispersions of the sickle gene. In Embury SH et al: Sickle cell disease. Basic principles and clinical practice, New York, 1994, Raven Press.)*

β^A-chains), 80% to 95% HbS, 2% to 4% HbA$_2$, and 2% to 20% HbF. Three outstanding biochemical findings include hyperuricemia in patients with altered tubular function; reduced zinc levels in plasma, red cells, and hair; and high lactate dehydrogenase levels in patients in crisis. Treatment of HbSS is designed to (1) inhibit HbS polymerization, (2) decrease intracellular levels of total Hb, and (3) increase the concentration of HbF. Many drugs have been used to increase HbF, which early on was recognized to interfere with HbS polymerization. The first "hemoglobin switching" agent was a nucleoside analog 5-azacytidine, and was postulated to increase HbF by inducing gene expression. Hydroxyurea is the prototype and promotes HbF production indirectly, perturbing the maturation of erythroid precursors. Butyrates appear to directly modulate globin gene expression by binding to transcriptionally active elements.[24] Hydroxyurea is the cornerstone of treatment for sickle cell disease. Presently, the use of butyrate remains experimental.

Sickle Cell-HbC Disease

Sickle cell-HbC disease has a relatively high incidence (1 in 833 births among blacks in the United States) because HbS and HbC are common hemoglobin variants. The patient inherits one abnormal gene from each parent, and the resulting disease is a mild to moderate hemolytic anemia associated with the same vasoocclusive complications seen in sickle cell disease. However, these complications usually occur with a lower frequency. Because genes in this disease are allelic β-chain mutations, no normal β-chains are formed and HbA is absent.

Peripheral blood smear reveals many target cells, rare sickle cells, and red cells with straight or curved crystals. The hemoglobin values range from 100 to 130 g/L, with only HbC and HbS bands seen on electrophoresis. The reticulocyte count varies from 3% to 10%.

HbC Trait and Disease

HbC trait (HbAC) affects about 3% of American blacks. It is asymptomatic, and the peripheral blood smear is normal except for a few target cells. Electrophoresis patterns show about 30% to 40% HbC, 50% to 60% HbA, 3% to 4% HbA$_2$, and 7% HbF.

Hemoglobin C Disease (HbCC)

The homozygous form is rare, occurring in 1 out of 10,000 American blacks, and is asymptomatic. Upon examination the carrier has features of mild anemia, numerous target cells, and HbC crystals.

Hemoglobin E Trait and Disease

The variant HbE, or B26 Glu → Lys, is the second most common hemoglobin abnormality worldwide. Because of the large influx of refugees from Southeast Asia, an increasing number of patients with HbE are encountered in the United States. HbE trait, though clinically silent, exhibits moderately severe microcytosis and no anemia. The amount of HbE in HbE trait is 30% to 35%. This is lower than expected for a heterozygous condition; for example, 45% HbS is observed in patients with sickle cell trait. This discrepancy is attributable to the thalassemia-like defect of the HbE gene.

Patients with HbE disease exhibit mild microcytic, normochromic anemia with many target cells, conferring a thalassemic phenotype.

Because many Southeast Asians have α- and β-thalassemic gene abnormalities, combinations of HbE with these genes become much more clinically significant. For example, patients with HbE-β⁰ thalassemia have significant anemia and require transfusions; a clinical situation similar to that seen with thalassemia intermedia.[25]

Unstable Hemoglobin Disorder

The unstable hemoglobins are structural variants of HbA, in which the mutant hemoglobin is less stable than normal hemoglobin. Approximately 150 variants of HbA have been shown to be unstable in in vitro tests. However, only 70 have been shown to have significant clinical manifestation, usually hemolysis.[26] The molecular distortion responsible for unstable hemoglobin produces a series of pathophysiological effects that can be evaluated by laboratory methods, though they are not equally expressed by all unstable hemoglobins.

They are (1) hemolytic anemia, (2) increased methemoglobin and sulfhemoglobin production, (3) hemichrome formation, (4) inclusion (Heinz) body formation, (5) altered oxygen dissociation, (6) drug sensitivity, (7) altered electrophoretic mobility (rare), (8) altered response to hemoglobin stability tests, and (9) passage of dark urine. The deeply pigmented urine is caused by mesobilifuscin, a dipyrrole derived from the catabolism of Heinz bodies or free heme.

THALASSEMIAS
Definitions

Thalassemias are inherited hemoglobinopathies resulting from a decreased rate of production of one or more globin chains of hemoglobin.[10,27] They are quantitative hemoglobinopathies that differ from the qualitative hemoglobinopathies by the fact that the structure of the affected globin chain (or chains) is normal, but its synthesis is reduced or absent. The decreased hemoglobin synthesis results in decreased RBC hemoglobin, hypochromia, microcytosis, and a variable degree of hemolysis.

Defective synthesis of one set of globin chains results in excess production of the unaffected pair[10] (imbalanced globin-chain synthesis), which precipitates in the RBCs in the form of inclusion bodies, which cause the hemolysis.

Classification

The older classification of thalassemias as *thalassemia major*, *intermedia*, *minor*, and *minima* describes the clinical severity of the disorder and disregards the genetic makeup. The preferred genetic classification is based on the particular deficient polypeptide chain. In **α-thalassemia**, the synthesis

TABLE 36-4 LABORATORY FINDINGS IN α-THALASSEMIAS

Genotype	Anemia (Hypochromic)	Hb Types		α-Chain Deletions
α-Thalassemia 1 trait	±	Birth:	Hb_Bart's 5% to 10% HbCS 1% to 2%	2
		Adult:	HbA,A₂,F	
α-Thalassemia 1/α-thalassemia 1 (hydrops)	+++	Birth:	Hb_Bart's 80% Traces of HbH and Portland	4
		Adult:	Not compatible with life	
α-Thalassemia 2/trait	±	Birth:	Hb_Bart's 1% to 2% HbCS 1% to 2%	1
		Adult:	HbA,A₂F	
α-Thalassemia 1/α-thalassemia 2 (HbH disease)	± (Inclusions)	Birth:	Hb_Bart's 1% to 15% HbB 4% to 30%	3
		Adult:	HbA,A₂,F HBH 8% to 10%	
α-Thalassemia 1/HbCS (Hb H/CS)	++ (Inclusions)	Birth:	Hb_Bart's HbH, HbCS	2 plus α-chain termination mutation
		Adult:	HbH HbA,A₂,F,CS	
α-Thalassemia 2/HbCS	+	Birth:	Hb_Bart's	1 plus α-chain termination mutation
		Adult:	HbA, CS	
HbCS/HbCS	+	Birth:	Hb_Bart's	α-chain termination mutation
		Adult:	HbA,A₂,F,CS	

of α-chains is diminished, in **β-thalassemia** the synthesis of β-chains is diminished. The major forms of thalassemia are depicted in Table 36-4.

Thalassemias involving γ-, ε-, or ζ-genes may lead to fetal or embryonic death.[27] A thalassemia-like condition that is asymptomatic is HPFH. The inheritance of thalassemia is autosomal and is similar to that of HbS. From the clinical viewpoint, it is recessive because the heterozygous form is asymptomatic. Similar to the HbS(β^S) gene, the thalassemia gene may express itself in homozygous, heterozygous, and doubly heterozygous states.

The clinical range varies from normal to a severe, life-threatening condition and can include growth retardation, hepatomegaly, bone overgrowth, bone pain, and jaundice.

α-Thalassemias

The α-thalassemias are a group of genetic disorders that result in defective α-chain synthesis. The α-thalassemias are more difficult to diagnose because characteristic elevations in HbA_2 or HbF seen in the β-thalassemias are not observed. Diminished α-chain synthesis depresses the production of HbA, HbF, and HbA_2 because they contain α-chains, and it leads to excess β- and γ-chains, which polymerize to the tetrameric forms γ_4 ($Hb_{Bart's}$) and β_4 (HbH). The presence of these hemoglobins is the hallmark of α-thalassemia. Four classical α-thalassemias include α-thalassemia-2 trait (silent carrier) in which one of the four α-globin gene loci fails to function; α-thalassemia-1 trait (mild hypochromic anemia) with two dysfunctional loci; HbH (moderate severe hemolytic anemia) with three loci affected; and $Hb_{Bart's}$ (hydrops fetalis incompatible with life) in which all four loci are affected. α-Thalassemia may also result from the production of $Hb_{Constant\ Spring}$ (HbCS). This hemoglobin is the result of a mutation in the terminal codon of the 3′ portion of DNA that normally stops α-chain production. Therefore, HbCS contains 172 amino acids in the α-chain rather than 141. Production of this elongated α-chain causes an inadequacy of α-chains relative to non-α-chains with a resultant thalassemic condition (Table 36-4).

β-Thalassemias

The β-thalassemias are a group of genetic disorders that result in diminished (β^+ and β^{++} thalassemias) or absent (β^0-thalassemia) β-chain synthesis. They are inherited in a multitude of genetic combinations responsible for a heterogeneous group of clinical syndromes. Like α-thalassemia, β-thalassemia is transmitted as a Mendelian autosomal recessive characteristic. The output of β-chains is reduced or absent because of a defect in transcription of the β-thalassemia genes. Currently point mutations that result in the various β-thalassemias number approximately 90. β-Thalassemia major, also known as *Cooley's anemia*, or *homozygous β-thalassemia*, is a clinically severe disorder caused by the inheritance of two β-thalassemia alleles, one on each copy of chromosome 11. The hypochromic anemia of thalassemia major is so severe that lifetime blood transfusions are usually required.

β-Thalassemias are widely distributed throughout the world but occur most frequently in the Mediterranean population; they also occur in Southeast Asia, the Middle East, India, and Pakistan. In Greeks and in American blacks the β^+-thalassemia is most common, whereas in Italy the β^0 is predominant.

Heterozygous β-thalassemia, whether β^+ or β^0, is an asymptomatic disorder that may or may not be associated with a mild degree of anemia.[27] It is the most commonly found thalassemia in North America.[10,27] Characteristically there is a slight to moderate erythrocytosis of poorly hemoglobinized RBCs. The MCH and the MCV are always strikingly decreased. The mean corpuscular hemoglobin content (MCHC) is variable.

The heterozygous carrier states have also been called *thalassemia minor* and *thalassemia minima*. The designation *thalassemia intermedia* describes clinical manifestations of a form of β-thalassemia more severe than the traits and milder than the homozygous form.

Homozygous β^0-thalassemia leads to complete suppression of β-chain synthesis and to complete absence of HbA. It is the cause of a severe lethal transfusion-dependent hemolytic anemia accompanied by characteristic clinical and hematological findings. Homozygous β^+ thalassemia is a heterogeneous disorder that, on the basis of the amount of HbA synthesized, is best divided into three main types. Type 1, in which 5% to 15% HbA is synthesized, is the Mediterranean and Oriental form characterized by a severe transfusion-dependent anemia. Type 2, of African background, has 20% to 30% HbA and is responsible for a milder disease. Type 3 leads to a mild form of thalassemia intermedia.[27]

Pregnancy may lead to severe anemia in patients with thalassemia trait.[28] The hemoglobin electrophoretogram shows a slightly elevated HbF (1% to 7%) in 50% of cases and a diagnostic elevation of A_2 (3.5% to 7.5%).[22] Distribution of HbF within the RBCs demonstrated by acid elution technique reveals a heterogeneous pattern.

Hereditary Persistence of Fetal Hemoglobin (HPFH)

HPFH consists of a group of rare conditions characterized by continued synthesis of high levels of HbF in adult life. No deleterious effects on patients are observed, and such an absence supports the concept that prevention or reversal of the switch from the fetal hemoglobin to the adult hemoglobin would benefit patients with sickle cell anemia and β-thalassemia. It is considered to be a form of δβ-thalassemia[29] because the persistence of the γ-chain synthesis compensates for the deficient δ- and β-chain production.

Two major types of HPFH exist: (1) pancellular and (2) heterocellular. The pancellular type has very high levels of fetal hemoglobin synthesis and uniform distribution of HbF among all RBCs. It can be further divided by mutation type into deletional and nondeletional forms. HPFH shows ethnic differences in that blacks with heterozygous pancellular deletional disease have HbF ranges between 15% and 35% and contain γ^{Gly} and γ^{Ala} chains in a ratio of 2:3. On the other hand, Greeks with pancellular nondeletional HPFH demonstrate lower HbF levels (10% to 20%) and contain 90% γ^{Ala}.

A few black patients may have homozygous HPFH. All the Hb within the red cells is HbF. These patients demonstrate mild microcytic hypochromic erythrocytes but no anemia.

HPFH-β-thalassemia is similar to the β-thalassemia trait except for a greater proportion and regular distribution of HbF in the RBCs.[30] Some patients with HPFH-δβ-thalassemia may have a more severe clinical condition similar to thalassemia intermedia.

Heterocellular HPFH seems to result from mutations outside the globin gene cluster and results in a variable increase in the number of F cells. HbF levels are usually lower than those in the pancellular forms.

Methemoglobinemia

Methemoglobinemia is classified into acquired and hereditary forms.[5]

Acquired methemoglobinemia. Normal individuals develop methemoglobinemia after exposure to agents that increase methemoglobin production beyond the capacity of the methemoglobin-reducing pathways. Most agents capable of producing methemoglobinemia are aromatic compounds containing amino, hydroxy, or nitro functional groups. Some of the agents responsible for methemoglobinemia include nitrites, nitrates, sulfonamides, aniline dyes (laundry markings), acetanilid, phenacetin, and phenazopyridine HCl (Pyridium). The nitrites and nitrates account for the majority of the occurrences. The blood may be chocolate-brown. Symptoms vary in intensity, depending on the level of methemoglobin.

Hereditary methemoglobinemia. Hereditary methemoglobinemia can be subdivided into two forms: one resulting from mutations leading to NADH methemoglobin reductase deficiency and the other resulting from hemoglobin accumulation because of an amino acid substitution in the globin chain that stabilizes methemoglobin, rendering it poorly susceptible to subsequent reduction. These hemoglobins are termed *M hemoglobins*.

Four metabolic pathways for the reduction of the methemoglobin to hemoglobin are available[31]: (1) the NADH methemoglobin reductase pathway, (2) the reverse (NADPH) methemoglobin reductase pathway, (3) the reduction by ascorbic acid, and (4) the reduction by reduced glutathione. Methemoglobinemia caused by an inherited deficiency of NADH methemoglobin reductase is transmitted as an autosomal recessive trait. M hemoglobins show a recessive inheritance pattern and, unlike many hemoglobinopathies, do not produce hemolytic anemias. The mutation causes the formation of an abnormally stable methemoglobin. This stability is attributable to amino acid substitution in or near the heme pocket resulting in direct heme-globin bonding. Tyrosine is substituted for histidine at or across from the heme-binding site in many of the M hemoglobins. HbM$_{Iwate}$ and M$_{Boston}$ have this substitution in the α-chain, whereas HbS M$_{Hyde\ Park}$ and M$_{Saskatoon}$ have it in the β-chain.

Methemoglobin rarely exceeds 25% to 30% in these individuals. If α-chains are involved, the cyanosis may be present at birth, whereas β-chain substitutions are responsible for cyanosis in later months because of the later appearance of these chains.[32]

Clinically, patients with hereditary methemoglobinemia have erythrocytosis and slate gray cyanosis from birth, which is not associated with cardiopulmonary disease. Methemoglobin concentrations of 10% to 20% of the total hemoglobin produce cyanosis but no other ill effects. Methemoglobin concentrations of 30% may be responsible for headache and dyspnea, and concentrations of 70% and over may be fatal. A low incidence of mental retardation and early death can be observed in cases of methemoglobinemia caused by NADH methemoglobin reductase deficiency, a disease that lends itself to prenatal diagnosis.[32]

CHANGE OF ANALYTE IN DISEASE
Interpretation of Hemoglobin Values

The mean and reference intervals for hemoglobin in healthy adults are 151 (136 to 163) g/L for men and 135 (120 to 150) g/L for women. The values of hemoglobin vary greatly for newborns, infants, children up to puberty, and adults (Table 36-5).

TABLE 36-5   REFERENCE INTERVALS FOR HEMOGLOBIN IN GRAMS PER LITER IN "APPARENTLY HEALTHY" SUBJECTS, WHITE AND BLACK

Subjects	Mean (Reference Interval)
Adult men	151 (136 to 163)
Adult women	135 (120 to 150)
Boys	
Birth	200 (185 to 215)
1 mo	170 (155 to 185)
3 mo	150 (135 to 165)
6 mo	140 (130 to 160)
9 mo	130 (120 to 140)
1 yr	121 (100 to 140)
2 yr	123 (105 to 142)
4 yr	126 (112 to 143)
8 yr	134 (120 to 148)
14 yr	140 (125 to 150)
Girls	
Birth	195 (180 to 210)
1 mo	170 (158 to 189)
3 mo	148 (133 to 164)
6 mo	138 (128 to 148)
9 mo	128 (117 to 139)
1 yr	122 (100 to 140)
2 yr	122 (105 to 142)
4 yr	127 (113 to 142)
8 yr	130 (115 to 145)
14 yr	132 (116 to 148)

From Miale JB: Laboratory medicine: hematology, ed 6, St Louis, 1982, Mosby.

Physiological variations and pathological processes influence hemoglobin concentrations. The physiological variations include age, sex, physical exercise, posture, dehydration, and altitude. The influence exerted by age is readily apparent in Table 36-5. During puberty the male hemoglobin level increases over the female value secondary to the influence of testosterone. Strong exercise raises the hemoglobin level probably through fluid loss, and a transient increase is also experienced after a change from the recumbent to the standing position. Dehydration is responsible for a rise in hemoglobin concentration of such magnitude as to mask a significant anemia. High altitude is responsible for increased hemoglobin levels because of the erythropoietin-stimulating effect of hypoxia.

There are three main causes of anemia: an impaired production, increased destruction, and excessive blood loss. Impaired production occurs with aplastic anemias; increased destruction occurs with the hemolytic anemia; and excessive blood loss usually occurs in iron-deficiency anemia. The reticulocyte count is usually depressed in chronic iron deficiency, reflecting the effect of iron lack on erythropoiesis.

Increased hemoglobin values are encountered in polycythemia vera, erythrocytosis, dehydration, newborn chronic heart and lung disease, high altitude, renal cysts, and numerous erythropoietin-producing tumors, also in cigarette smoking and in chronic lung diseases.

HbF

In normal adults, the concentration of F cells is fairly constant at 0.2% to 0.7%, but there are both genetic and acquired hematological conditions in which the concentration is increased. The genetic disorders include thalassemias (β and $\delta\beta$), hereditary persistence of HbF, sickle cell anemia, and unstable β-chain variants. The acquired conditions include pregnancy at about midterm, recovery from bone marrow depression,[33] leukemias (highest values in Philadelphia chromosome-negative juvenile chronic myelocytic leukemia), thyrotoxicosis, and hepatoma.[9,34,35]

HbA$_{1c}$

HbA$_{1c}$ levels depend on the time-integrated blood levels of glucose (see Chapter 32 for a more detailed discussion). HbA$_{1c}$ levels are decreased in hemolytic anemia because the RBC life span is shortened by lysis[36] and in hemoglobinopathies in which there is decreased HbA (though the percentage of HbA$_{1c}$ in relation to total HbA may be normal).

Carboxyhemoglobin (CO-Hb)

Some carboxyhemoglobin is produced endogenously as 1 mol of CO is generated by the degradation of 1 mol of heme to bilirubin (see Chapter 35). Although this endogenous production of carboxyhemoglobin can present a hazard when exhaled air is concentrated in poorly ventilated, small spaces, the exogenous generation of CO from combustion of organic material in confined spaces causes intoxication. Exogenous CO is derived from the exhaust of automobiles and from industrial pollutants such as coal gas, charcoal burning, and tobacco smoke. In the absence of exogenous CO, the endogenous CO-Hb concentration is 0.2% to 0.8%. Co-Hb levels can be elevated in hemolytic anemias,[37] and in smokers the Co-Hb may vary from 4% to 20%. In smokers who have a greater exposure to CO, the average level may be 10%.[5]

Because of the firm binding of CO to hemoglobin, long exposure to even low CO concentrations can lead to toxic accumulations to which the most oxygen-dependent organs, such as brain and heart, are most susceptible. Mild symptoms such as slight headache and slight dyspnea on exertion can occur at levels of 10% to 15% saturation. At levels of 20% to 30%, the headaches are more severe and are accompanied by impaired vision and judgment. Levels of more than 50% cause increasingly severe symptoms, coma, and convulsions, and levels of 60% and over are usually fatal, though death has occurred at levels as low as 20%. The half-life of elimination of CO is about 4 hours for a person breathing atmospheric air, but in smokers the level may remain high.[38] Chronic exposure to CO may be responsible for a relative polycythemia.[39] Carboxyhemoglobin produces a cherry-red color of the blood and skin. Sometimes the blood may have a violet tinge because of the simultaneous presence of moderate quantities of reduced hemoglobin. Exposure to toxic levels of CO is treated with oxygen, often at elevated pressures (hyperbaric treatment), to displace CO from hemoglobin. Both exposure and therapy are closely followed by blood-gas analysis for CO-Hb.

Oxygen Saturation

Clinically, oxygen saturation is used as an indicator of tissue hypoxia or hyperoxia. Tissue hypoxia is produced by decreased oxygen content of inspired air, as in high altitude, or by decreased alveolar capillary oxygen exchange in the lungs, as in pulmonary fibrosis, emphysema, and chronic heart disease with a left-to-right shunt. Tissue hypoxia is also produced (1) by a defect in the erythrocytic oxygen transport as in severe anemia, (2) when hemoglobin ligands are present that prevent oxygen binding, such as carboxyhemoglobin, sulfhemoglobin, and methemoglobin, (3) in hemoglobinopathies, (4) in inappropriate concentrations of erythrocytic 2,3-BPG, and (5) in intraerythrocytic enzyme deficiencies. Therapeutic hyperoxia must be carefully monitored because of danger of oxygen toxicity. In newborns it can be responsible for retrolental fibroplasia and in adults for hyaline membrane disease of the lungs (adult respiratory distress syndrome).

2,3-Biphosphoglycerate

2,3-BPG and hemoglobin interaction in hypoxia is related to the increased intraerythrocytic levels of deoxyhemoglobin, which binds large amounts of BPG. This binding results in a feedback mechanism that stimulates glycolysis and BPG synthesis. Increased deoxyhemoglobin concentrations raise the pH, which in turn also stimulates the synthesis of BPG. It has been emphasized that there is a reciprocal relationship between hemoglobin and BPG concentrations. Pyruvate kinase deficiency leads to a buildup of BPG, decreased oxygen affinity, and a low hemoglobin concentration. Hexokinase deficiency leads to a decrease in BPG and to a compensatory erythropoietic response with increased hemoglobin values. Many hemoglobin mutations result in an increased oxygen affinity by the abnormal hemoglobin, and some increase this affinity further by impairing BPG binding, such as HbS$_{Shepherds\ Bush}$, HbS$_{Ohio}$, and HbS$_{Little\ Rock}$.

Other Hemoglobins

The HbF concentration can vary from 10% to 90%, and the HbF distribution in the RBCs as determined by the Kleihauer technique can be heterogeneous. Possible abnormal cellular distribution patterns are as follows:

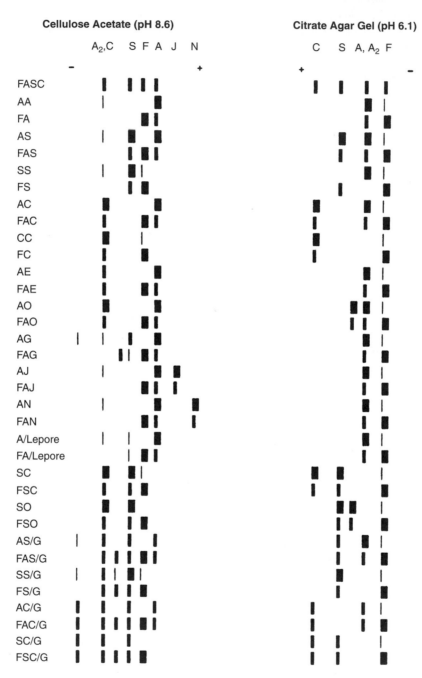

Fig. 36-8 Comparative mobilities in standard electrophoretic methods of hemoglobin of the most common variant hemoglobins. The fetal phenotypes are designated with the letters in descending order of concentration in the blood; for example, FAS=F>A>S. Other hemoglobins migrating with the mobility of Hb S on CAE are Hbs S, D, G-Philadelphia, and Lepore. Those migrating with the mobility of Hb C or A$_2$ are Hbs E, O-Arab, and the G/S hybrid molecule of compound heterozygotes of Hb S and G$_\alpha$ ($\alpha_2{}^G\beta_2{}^S$). The hemoglobin migrating between the positions Hbs S and C is the Hb G derivative of Hb F ($\alpha_2{}^G\Gamma_2$). *(From Embury SH et al: Sickle cell disease. Basic principles and clinical practice, New York, 1994, Raven Press.)*

1. *Separate cell patterns.* RBCs containing HbA or HbF are observed in cases of fetal-maternal hemorrhage if the mother's blood is examined or in cases of maternal-fetal hemorrhage if the infant's blood is examined.
2. *Even distribution.* HbA and HbF are equally distributed in all the red blood cells. This distribution is observed in hereditary persistence of HbF (HPFH).
3. *Uneven distribution.* Red blood cells have varying amounts of HbA and HbF. This pattern is seen in thalassemia, sickle cell disease, Fanconi's anemia, and hereditary spherocytosis.

The HbA_2 concentration may vary from 1.4% to 20%, including low, normal, elevated, and very high values. The concentration of HbA_2 is increased in β-thalassemia, β-chain unstable hemoglobinemias, sickle cell trait, megaloblastic anemias, and hyperthyroidism. Normal or decreased values are seen in α-thalassemias, δβ-thalassemias (Lepore heterozygotes), δ-thalassemia, and HPFH. In Hb_{Lepore} homozygotes, HbA_2 is absent because there is no δ-chain synthesis. HbA_2 is decreased in acquired disorders such as iron deficiency, sideroblastic anemias, and lead poisoning.

In homozygous β-thalassemia, the A_2 value, even if it is low or normal in the patient, will be high in both parents. If the HbA_2 level in the patient is expressed as a percentage of the total hemoglobin, it spans the previously mentioned range from low to high, but if it is expressed in relation to the HbA value only, the ratio is decreased in all cases of β-thalassemia, that is, the A/A_2 ratio is about 10:1 as compared to the normal A/A_2 ratio of about 40:1. If the HbA_2 level is greatly increased, HbF is normal or only slightly elevated and vice versa. In $β^0$-thalassemia, there is a total absence of HbA, and so the patient's hemoglobin consists only of HbF and HbA_2, whereas in $β^+$-thalassemia diminished amounts of HbA are found (5% to 20%). In both these β-thalassemias, free α-chains may be seen close to the application point of the electrophoretogram at alkaline pH. The severe reduction in β-globin chains leads to a β/α ratio of less than 0.25:0.3. Some of the more common hemoglobinopathies evaluated by cellulose acetate, pH 8.6, and citrate agar, pH 6.0 to 6.2, electrophoresis are depicted in Figure 36-8.

Other Related Biochemical Findings

Because of the hemolytic components of the anemia in most hemoglobinopathies, serum unconjugated bilirubin levels are elevated, and haptoglobin is decreased or absent. Serum aspartate aminotransferase, lactate dehydrogenase, and erythropoietin concentrations are also raised. The erythropoietin elevation is responsible for the 20% to 30% increase in erythropoietic marrow and is a result of the anemia and high oxygen affinity of HbF, which further increases the tissue anoxia. The liver involvement (transfusion hemosiderosis) can lead to a bleeding tendency. Gross examination of the urine may show the brown color of dipyrroles caused by excessive hemolysis.

Use of Hemogram Results to Differentiate Iron Deficiency from Thalassemias

Various formulas exist to differentiate iron deficiency from milder forms of thalassemia. One such formula is the discriminant function (DF):

$$DF = MCV - RBC - (5 \times Hb) - 3.4$$

in which MCV is in fL (femtoliters), RBC is in millions/mm^3, and Hb is in g% (g/dL). The 3.4 is an instrument constant and varies with the instrument. A positive DF result is suggestive of iron deficiency, whereas a negative DF result is suggestive of a thalassemia. For example, a patient with MCV of 65 fL, Hb of 13 g/dL, and RBC of 6 million/mm^3: DF = 65 – 6 – (5 × 13) – 3.4 = -9.4. The example indicates a diagnosis of thalassemia minor. A simpler formula is the ratio MCV/RBC. Values of this ratio greater than 13 are associated with iron-deficiency anemia; values less than 13 are associated with thalassemias. In the above example the ratio would be 10.8.

References

1. Bunn HF, Forget BG: *Hemoglobin: molecular, genetic and clinical aspects*, Philadelphia, 1986, Saunders.
2. Hardison R: Hemoglobins from bacteria to man: evolution of different patterns of gene expression, *J Exp Biol* 201:1099, 1998.
3. Shaeffer JR: Evidence for a difference in affinities of human hemoglobin β^A and β^S chains for α chains, *J Biol Chem* 255:2322, 1980.
4. Hawkins M: Carbon monoxide poisoning, *Eur J Anaesthesiol* 16:585, 1999.
5. Nagel RL: Carbon monoxide poisoning, methemoglobinemia and sulfhemoglobinemia. In Schumacher H, Rock W, Stass S, editors: *Handbook of hematologic pathology*, New York, 2000, Marcel Dekker.
6. Bozeman WP, Hampson NB: Pulse oximetry in CO poisoning—additional data, *Chest* 117:295, 2000.
7. Sepulveda W et al: Accuracy of the haemoglobin alkaline denaturation test for detecting maternal blood contamination of fetal blood samples for prenatal karyotyping, *Prenat Diagn* 19:927, 1999.
8. Nelson M et al: A flow-cytometric equivalent of the Kleihauer test, *Vox Sang* 75:234, 1998.
9. Weatherall DJ, Pembrey ME, Pritchard J: Fetal hemoglobin, *Clin Hematol* 3:467, 1974.
10. Clarke GM, Higgins TN: Laboratory investigation of hemoglobinopathies and thalassemias: review and update, *Clin Chem* 46:1284, 2000.
11. Fairbanks VF: Nomenclature and taxonomy of hemoglobin variants. In Fairbanks VF, editor: *Hemoglobinopathies and thalassemias*, New York, 1988, Brian Decker.
12. Destro Bisol G: Genetic resistance to malaria, oxidative stress and hemoglobin oxidation, *Parassitologia* 41:203, 1999.
13. Buihl RW: Physical chemical properties of sickle cell hemoglobin. In Wallach DPH, editor: *The function of red blood cells: erythrocyte pathobiology*, New York, 1981, Alan Liss.
14. Bunn HF: Hemoglobin II, sickle cell anemia and other hemoglobinopathies. In Beck WS, editor: *Hematology*, Cambridge, MA, 1981, MIT Press.
15. Hebbel RP, Mohandas N: Sickle cell adherence. In Embury SH et al, editors: *Sickle cell disease: basic principles and clinical practice*, New York, 1994, Raven.
16. Embury SH et al: Pathogenesis of vasoocclusion. In Embury SH et al, editors: *Sickle cell disease: basic principles and clinical practice*, New York, 1994, Raven.
17. Hebbel RP et al: Erythrocyte adherence to endothelium in sickle cell anemia. A possible determinant of disease severity, *N Engl J Med* 302:992, 1980.
18. Chien S, Usami S, Bertles JF: Abnormal rheology of oxygenated blood in sickle cell anemia, *J Clin Invest* 49:623, 1970.

19. Nash GB, Johnson CS, Meiselman HJ: Mechanical properties of oxygenated red blood cells in sickle cell (HbSS) disease, *Blood* 63:73, 1984.
20. Clark MFR, Mohandas N, Shohet SB: Deformability of oxygenated irreversibly sickled cells, *J Clin Invest* 65:189, 1980.
21. Rosse W: *New views of sickle cell disease. Pathology and treatment*, Washington, DC, 20001, American Society of Hematology.
22. Nagel RL, Bookchin RM: Oxygen transport and the sickle cell. In Wallach DFH, editor: *The function of red blood cells: erythrocyte pathobiology*, New York, 1981, Alan Liss.
23. Kark JA et al: Sickle cell trait as a risk factor for sudden death in basic training, *N Engl J Med* 317:781, 1987.
24. Glauber JG et al: 5′-Flanking sequences mediate butyrate stimulation of embryonic globin gene expression in adult erythroid cells, *Mol Cell Biol* 11:4690, 1991.
25. Fucharoen S, Winichagoon P: Clinical and hematologic aspects of hemoglobin E beta-thalassemia, *Curr Opin Hematol* 7:106, 2000.
26. Rucknagel DL: Hemoglobinopathies and thalassemias. In Schumacher H, Rock W, Stasse S, editors: *Handbook of hematologic pathology*, New York, 2000, Marcel Dekker.
27. Weatherall DJ: Pathophysiology of thalassaemia, *Baillieres Clin Haematol* 11:127, 1998.
28. Najdecki R, Georgiou I, Lolis D: The thalassemia syndromes and pregnancy, molecular basis, clinical aspects, prenatal diagnosis, *Ginekol Pol* 69:664, 1998.
29. Forget BG: Molecular basis of hereditary persistence of fetal hemoglobin, *Ann NY Acad Sci* 850:38, 1998.
30. Weatherall DJ, Clegg JB: Hereditary persistence of fetal haemoglobin, *Br J Haematol* 29:191, 1975.
31. Jaffe ER: Methemoglobinemia, *Clin Hematol* 10:103, 1981.
32. Jaffe ER: Methemoglobinemia, *Clin Hematol* 10:117, 1981.
33. Dover GJ, Boyer SH, Zinkhorn WH: Production of erythrocytes that contain fetal hemoglobin in anemia, *J Clin Invest* 63:173, 1979.
34. Honig GR et al: Juvenile myelomonocytic leukemia (JMML) with the hematologic phenotype of severe beta thalassemia, *Am J Hematol* 58:67, 1998.
35. Rochette J, Craig JE, Thein SL: Fetal hemoglobin levels in adults, *Blood Rev* 8:213, 1994.
36. Bunn HF et al: The biosynthesis of human hemoglobin A_{1c}, *J Clin Invest* 57:1652, 1976.
37. Landau SA, Winchell HS: Endogenous production of ^{14}CO: a method for calculation of RBC life-span in vivo, *Blood* 36:642, 1970.
38. Astrup P: Carbon monoxide inhalation-time for clearance from blood in reversible coma, *JAMA* 230:1064, 1974.
39. Smith JR, Landau SA: Smoker's polycythemia, *N Engl J Med* 298:6, 1978.

Bibliography

Bick RL et al: *Hematology: clinical and laboratory practice*, St Louis, 1993, Mosby.

Brenner MK, Hoffbrand AV: *Recent advances in haematology*, vol 8, New York, 1996, Churchill Livingstone.

Bunn HF, Forget BG: *Hemoglobin: molecular, genetic and clinical aspects*, Philadelphia, 1986, Saunders.

Hoffman R: *Hematology: basic principles and practice*, Edinburgh, 1999, Churchill Livingstone.

Jandl JH: *Blood: textbook of hematology*, Boston, 1996, Little, Brown.

Lee GR et al: *Wintrobe's clinical hematology*, ed 10, Baltimore, 1999, Williams and Wilkins.

Rappaport SI: *Introduction to hematology*, ed 3, Philadelphia, 1997, Lippincott, Raven.

Schumacher HR, Garvin DF, Triplett DA: *Introduction to laboratory hematology and hematopathology*, New York, 1984, Alan Liss.

Schumacher HR, Rock WA, Stass SA: *Handbook of hematologic pathology*, New York, 2000, Marcel Dekker.

Stamatoyannopoulos G et al: *The molecular basis of blood diseases*, ed 3, Philadelphia, 2001, Saunders.

Steinberg M: *Disorders of hemoglobin: genetics, pathophysiology and clinical management*, London, 2001, Cambridge University Press.

Weatherall DJ: *The thalassemia syndrome*, Oxford, 2001, Blackwell Scientific.

Williams W: *Hematology*, ed 6, New York, 2000, McGraw-Hill.

Internet Sites

http://www.hematology.org/—American Society of Hematology

http://www.cooleysanemia.org/—Cooley's Anemia Foundation, for patients with thalassemia

http://www.emory.edu/PEDS/SICKLE/—The sickle cell information center at the Grady System

http://sickle.bwh.harvard.edu/—Joint Center for Sickle Cell and Thalassemic Disorders

http://www.people.virginia.edu/~rjh9u/hemoglob.html

http://web.indstate.edu/thcme/mwking/hemoglobin-myoglobin.html#hemoglobin

http://omlc.ogi.edu/spectra/hemoglobin/index.html

http://cpmcnet.columbia.edu/texts/gcps/gcps0053.html—Congenital disorders: screening for hemoglobinopathies. In U.S. Preventive Services Task Force Guide to Clinical Preventive Services, ed 2, Washington, DC, 1996, U.S. Department of Health and Human Services, Office of Disease Prevention and Health Promotion

http://www.slh.wisc.edu/newborn/guide/disorders6.html—The Wisconsin State Laboratory of Hygiene Health Professionals' guide to newborn screening for hemoglobinopathies

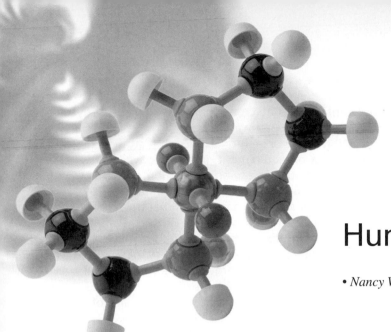

CHAPTER 37

Human Nutrition

• *Nancy W. Alcock*

Objectives

• Discuss the contribution of individual nutrient classes to human metabolism.
• Discuss the importance of nutrition in health and disease.
• Discuss therapeutic nutrition support by enteral and parenteral routes.

• Discuss the role of the laboratory in the support of nutrition programs and in the support of patients with inborn errors of metabolism.
• List the biochemical parameters used to monitor nutritional status.

Key Terms

anabolic Biochemical pathways that synthesize macromolecules such as proteins and nucleic acids.
anthropometric Study of human body measurements, often determining body upper arm circumference, etc.
basal metabolic rate (BMR) The energy expended to maintain the basic physiological functions.
bioavailability Amount (usually expressed as a percentage) of dietary components able to be

absorbed from the gastrointestinal tract, either intact or after degradation.
cachexia Physical wasting caused by starvation and malnutrition.
catabolic Metabolic degradation or breakdown of macromolecules.
diet The food that is ingested orally.
dysphagia Difficulty in swallowing.
enteral feeding Provision of synthetic nutrients to

the gastrointestinal tract through a tube.

essential nutrients   Nutrients required for normal growth and development and for maintaining the adult body in equilibrium, which either cannot be synthesized at all or cannot be synthesized in sufficient amounts. These include vitamins, minerals, trace elements, certain amino acids, and at least two fatty acids.

kilocalorie (kcal)   The amount of energy-producing food equivalent to the energy required to raise the temperature of 1 kg of water from 15° to 16° C.

kilojoule (kJ)   A unit of heat; 1 kJ is equivalent to approximately 0.24 kcal.

kwashiorkor   Malnutrition caused by a diet deficient in protein.

malnutrition   Suboptimal nutrition arising from inadequate or unbalanced intake, bioavailability, or utilization of nutrients.

marasmus   A protein-calorie malnutrition arising from inadequate food intake as the result of partial or complete starvation.

nitrogen balance   The difference between total nitrogen intake and the sum of fecal and urinary nitrogen excretion; an estimate of net synthesis of body proteins.

nutrient   A dietary component used by the body in any metabolic pathway.

nutrition   The branch of science that studies the processes of requirement, intake, bioavailability, absorption, utilization, and excretion of nutrients.

parenteral nutrition   Nutrition administered by a route other than the gastrointestinal tract.

peripheral parenteral nutrition (PPN)   Parenteral nutrition introduced through a peripheral vein.

Recommended Dietary Allowance (RDA)   Suggested daily requirements of some essential nutrients for healthy subjects of various ages as published by the Food and Nutrition Board of the National Research Council.

resting energy expenditure (REE)   Energy expended at resting state, that is, at a **basal metabolic rate (BMR)**.

total parenteral nutrition (TPN)   Parenteral nutrition administered as the sole source of nutrition.

Methods on CD-ROM

Albumin
Iron and iron-binding capacity
Transferrin
Triglycerides

Urea
Vitamin B_{12}
Zinc

The science of **nutrition** is concerned with the qualitative and quantitative aspects of the **diet** and utilization of the dietary components required to sustain health. The major component groups required for human nutrition—carbohydrates, proteins, lipids, minerals, trace elements, vitamins, and fiber—are biochemically well defined. Some **nutrients** can be synthesized by metabolic processes, but others cannot be synthesized and therefore must be specifically provided in the diet. These nutrients are termed *essential* and include the essential amino acids and fatty acids (see below). All the water-soluble vitamins, as well as the fat-soluble vitamins A, E, and K are essential (see Chapter 39). Vitamin D, the fourth fat-soluble vitamin, is required for growing children, but adequate supplies are usually formed from its endogenous precursor, 7-dehydrocholesterol, in the adult human (see Chapter 28). Dietary fat and its absorption are prerequisites for absorption of the fat-soluble vitamins (see Chapter 30).

The variation in requirement of nutrients depends on the age and sex of the individual, on reproductive status, and on the altered nutritional demands associated with disease, injury, and therapeutic interventions. The Food and Nutrition Board of the Commission on Life Sciences, National Research Council, estimates the levels of dietary **essential nutrients** that should be adequate to meet the known nutrient needs of practically all healthy persons. These estimates are reported as **Recommended Dietary Allowances (RDAs)** and are revised from time to time. The latest revision was published in 1989[1] and updated as Dietary Reference Intakes in 1999 and 2001.[2]

Various estimates indicate that at least 40% of hospitalized patients are malnourished (see below). The Joint Commission on Accreditation for Healthcare Organizations (JCAHO) has stressed the importance of a nutrition care plan that addresses detection of **malnutrition**, monitoring the intake of nutrition by the patient, and the route of nutrition delivery. Goals and the means to achieve these goals must be defined for patients at nutritional risk. Although **anthropometric** measurements are first-tier indicators of suboptimal nutrition, nutritional assessment using biochemical parameters can help to alert the physician to deficiencies. Biochemical measurements are of great importance in monitoring the patient's response to nutritional supplementation.

TABLE 37-1 BASIC CLASSES OF NUTRIENTS	
Nutrient	*Chapter Discussed*
Carbohydrate	Diabetes, 32
Lipids	Lipid, 33
Proteins	Liver, 27
Inorganic elements	
Na, K, Cl	Electrolytes and water balance, 24
Ca, Mg, inorganic phosphorus	Bone, 28
Fe^{++} (Fe^{+++})	Iron, porphyrins, bilirubin, 35
Trace minerals	Trace elements, 38
Vitamins	Vitamins, 39
Water	Renal, 26
	Electrolytes and water balance, 24

OBSERVATIONS ASSOCIATED WITH HYPERMETABOLIC STATE

Increased basal metabolic rate (BMR)
Increased nutritional needs
Fever
Increased heart rate and cardiac output
Altered immune system activity
Altered hormone levels, including insulin, glucagon,
    catecholamine, cortisol
Negative nitrogen balance
Synthesis of acute phase proteins

Biochemical and clinical aspects of the essential minerals, electrolytes, trace metals, and vitamins and their function are discussed in detail in relevant chapters (see Table 37-1). References 3 and 4 provide additional details. Discussion here is limited to the previously stated objectives.

NUTRIENT CLASSES
Energy Requirements[5-8]

The World Health Organization defines the energy requirement of an individual as follows: "The level of energy intake that will balance energy expenditure when the individual has a body size and composition, and a level of physical activity, consistent with long-term good health. The energy requirement should also allow the maintenance of economically necessary and socially desirable physical activity. In children and pregnant or lactating women, the energy requirement includes the energy requirements associated with the deposition of tissues or the secretion of milk at rates consistent with good health."[5]

The body is in energy balance when the metabolizable energy intake is equal to the sum of energy expenditure and changes in stored energy. Energy expenditure can be determined by direct calorimetry (heat-generated), indirect calorimetry (from measurement of oxygen consumption and carbon dioxide production), and by isotope-dilution methods using doubly labeled water. An estimate of the expenditure of endogenous energy stores can be quantitated from measurement of the **nitrogen balance**. A positive nitrogen balance is essential for growth of the fetus, placenta, and other associated changes during pregnancy and lactation. Extra energy is required during periods of growth and during physiologically stressful pathological states. Hormones and cytokines, such as tumor necrosis factor, may initiate a heightened metabolic response to injury and infection. The increased metabolism associated with physiological stress is termed the *hypermetabolic state*.[7] Observations associated with hypermetabolic state are listed in the following box.

For individuals with major burns, there is a 180% to 200% increase of the body's normal metabolic rate (MR), for as long as 50 days after the burn. In contrast, peritonitis is associated with an increased MR of 140% or more for 10 to 20 days, while fractures will have a peak in MR at 120% by 7 days. Individuals who are *hypometabolic*, that is starving, will experience a 60% to 70% decrease in MR.

Patients suffering from trauma, burns, and sepsis are often in a hypermetabolic state. The increased metabolic rate, which is proportional to the severity of the condition, results in insulin insensitivity and hyperglycemia. In addition, stored triglycerides are mobilized and oxidized, and if the patient is not fed, stores of fat and protein may be depleted. The loss of adipose tissue (fat) and muscle tissue (protein) results in the wasted appearance of individuals suffering from protein-calorie malnutrition. To meet the increased nutritional needs in these cases, health care providers should give minimal nutritional support at first and then increase this support gradually to maintain body cell mass. Biochemical parameters useful in monitoring such patients are discussed below.

Energy intake at birth is approximately 120 **kilocalories (kcal)**/kg/day (30 kilojoules) for both males and females. During the first 2 years of life there is a gradual drop to 90 to 100 kcal/kg/day. From 2 to 14 years of age energy requirements decrease gradually to approximately 40 kcal/kg/day, with males requiring 5 kcal/kg/day more than females.

Carbohydrates (see Chapter 32)

Carbohydrates are the principal source of energy for the body, contributing 50% to 60% of the total calories.[9] Complex carbohydrates, such as starches and sugars found in fruits and vegetables, are a better source of energy than simple refined sugars and may lower the incidence of hypertension, maturity-onset diabetes, and cardiovascular disease. Excessive carbohydrate intake leads to an increase in body weight, whereas insufficient intake stimulates mobilization of lipid stores with associated ketosis, loss of electrolytes, and dehydration. In a healthy adult, carbohydrate is stored as glycogen, principally in muscle (about 150 g) and in the liver (about 90 g). One gram of carbohydrate provides 4 kcal (1 kj) of energy.

Proteins

Requirements. Dietary proteins are the source of amino acids, the building blocks for synthesis and maintenance of tissue proteins.[10] Some amino acids either cannot be synthesized by the body at all or cannot be synthesized in sufficient amounts to satisfy requirements; it is therefore "essential" that these amino acids be obtained in the diet. The essential amino acids are listed in the box below. The quality of dietary protein is determined from its content of all essential amino acids. For infants, children 10 to 12 years of age, and adults, essential amino acids should make up 43%, 36%, and 10%, respectively, of the total amino acid intake. Good-quality protein is required to replace losses during the acute phase of physiological (hypermetabolic) stress associated with fevers, burns, surgical trauma, fractures, and other pathological states. On the other hand, protein restriction is required to manage acute liver failure and end-stage renal disease.

Nitrogen balance. Nitrogen balance studies are used to assess utilization of dietary amino acids for protein synthesis and the balance between anabolic and catabolic processes. An accurate diet record is used to calculate dietary intake of protein nitrogen. Accurate assessment of nitrogen output requires the measurement of both fecal and urinary nitrogen and a correction for nitrogen losses through sweat, hair, nails, and sloughed cells from the skin. The most accurate quantitative assessment of nitrogen excretion measures total nitrogen excretion. This can be achieved by use of instruments that directly measure total nitrogenous compounds in urine or feces by chemiluminescence after pyrolysis of the sample. Because this technique is not in widespread use, an approximate estimate of nitrogen excretion can be obtained from measurement of urine urea nitrogen (UUN). The UUN must be adjusted by a factor that is intended to account for any other body losses. In an adult, a positive nitrogen balance is associated with general good health. A positive nitrogen balance during periods of growth and development and in pregnancy is necessary. A negative nitrogen balance during periods of starvation, in cachexia, and in many hypermetabolic disease states should alert the physician to consider appropriate nutritional support. The frequency of quantitative measurements is dictated by the patient's response to therapy, but it has been suggested that several assessments per week may be needed during the most catabolic state of an acute illness.[11,12]

Protein deficiency. Conditions of protein deficiency, such as the disease **kwashiorkor**, occur in underdeveloped countries when breast-fed infants are transferred to a high carbohydrate diet. Although kwashiorkor is easily preventable, it can be a fatal disease. The major characteristics of kwashiorkor are listed in the following box.

An overall nutritional deficiency occurs in **marasmus** (wasting away) and appears in children with classic signs of starvation, including the loss of adipose and muscle tissues, which produces a wasted appearance. Overlap may occur between the conditions of kwashiorkor and marasmus, and the two are often indistinct. However, patients with marasmus do not have the severe edema present in kwashiorkor and, by contrast, usually retain their mental alertness.

The Recommended Dietary Allowances for protein for various ages and conditions is shown in Table 37-2. One gram of protein provides 4 kcal of energy.

CHARACTERISTICS OF KWASHIORKOR

Edema ("swollen belly")
Rashes and skin lesions ("flaky paint" dermatosis)
Diarrhea
Thinning and discoloration of the hair
Enlarged, fatty liver
Apathy, lethargy
Retarded physical and cognitive growth
Immunodeficiency

ESSENTIAL AMINO ACIDS

Isoleucine	Phenylalanine	Histidine*
Leucine	Threonine	Arginine*
Lysine	Tryptophan	Taurine†
Methionine	Valine	

*Indicated to be unnecessary for maintenance of nitrogen equilibrium in adults in short-term studies but probably necessary for normal growth of children.
†Required in infants.

TABLE 37-2 RECOMMENDED DIETARY ALLOWANCES FOR PROTEIN FOR VARIOUS AGES

Category	Age (Years) or Condition	WEIGHT (kg)	(lb)	HEIGHT (cm)	(in)	Protein (g)
Infants	0.0 to 0.5	6	13	60	24	13
	0.5 to 1.0	9	20	71	28	14
Children	1 to 3	13	29	90	35	16
	4 to 6	20	44	112	44	24
	7 to 10	28	62	132	52	28
Males	11 to 14	45	99	157	62	45
	15 to 18	66	145	176	69	59
	19 to 24	72	160	177	70	58
	25 to 50	79	174	176	79	63
	51+	77	170	173	68	63
Females	11 to 14	46	101	157	62	46
	15 to 18	55	120	163	64	44
	19 to 24	58	128	164	65	46
	25 to 50	63	138	163	64	50
	51+	65	143	160	63	50
Pregnant						60
Lactating	1st 6 mo					65
	2nd 6 mo					62

From Food and Nutrition Board, National Academy of Sciences, National Research Council: Recommended dietary allowances, revised 1989, Washington, D.C.

Lipids

Lipids are the most energy-dense of the macronutrients, providing 9 kcal/g of fat.[13] Although a typical American diet contains 35% to 45% of calories as fat, the American Heart Association and the Food and Nutrition Board of the National Research Council recommend that fat consumption be reduced to as low as 35% of total calorie intake (see Chapter 33).

In view of the association of saturated fats from animal sources with heart disease, it is recommended that at least 10% of the fat ingested be polyunsaturated. Some fatty acids found in the structural lipids of cells and the mitochondrial membranes cannot be synthesized in sufficient quantity, and their supply is thus essential. The essential fatty acids are linoleic acid, linolenic acid, and arachidonic acid, though there is some question whether linolenic acid is essential. Arachidonic acid accounts for 5% to 10% of the fatty acids in phospholipids of the cell membrane. Approximately 2.7 g/day of the essential fatty acids, linoleic, linolenic, and arachidonic acids, are required for normal health.

Lipids are stored as triglycerides, mainly in adipose tissue. Lipid metabolism and associated diseases are discussed in Chapter 33.

Macrominerals[1,2,14,15]

The Recommended Dietary Allowances for the major inorganic components, the macrominerals, of the diet are shown in Table 37-3. The role of each of the macrominerals is discussed in detail in the relevant chapters, as listed in Table 37-1. Important aspects of the biological roles and symptoms of deficiency or excess of the individual minerals are shown in Table 37-4.[14,15] A discussion of the biological role of trace elements is found in Chapter 38.

Fiber

Fiber, an important component of the diet, comprises plant cell components that cannot be digested by enzymes found in the gut. The more insoluble fibers, such as cellulose and lignin found in wheat bran, are beneficial with regard to colonic function, whereas the more soluble gums and pectins found in fruits and vegetables have been associated with the lowering of blood cholesterol.[16] High-fiber diets are associated with reduced incidence of cancer of the colon, cardiovascular disease, and diabetes mellitus.[16] However, high-fiber diets and their phytate content provide binding sites for the divalent metals calcium, iron, and zinc, making these metals less **bioavailable**. Hence, a requirement for increased intake of these metals should be addressed when high-fiber diets are consumed.

NUTRITION IN HEALTH AND DISEASE[17-18]

The world's general population can be divided into those at risk for malnutrition (likely to become malnourished) and those who are at low risk for becoming malnourished (likely to remain well nourished). Among the former group are those who become at risk for malnutrition because of changing nutritional needs, such as illness or change in socioeconomic status. Included in the latter group are individuals who are obese. These populations are discussed in some detail below.

General Populations

World population.[17,18] Over 800 million people, mostly in the developing world, cannot meet basic needs for energy and protein, while more than two billion people lack essential micronutrients. The malnutrition in these poverty-stricken countries disproportionately affects children; 174

TABLE 37-3   RECOMMENDED DIETARY ALLOWANCES FOR SOME MINERALS AND TRACE ELEMENTS

Category	Age (Years) or Condition	Ca (mg)	P (mg)	Mg (mg)	Fe (mg)	Zn (mg)	I (µg)	Se (µg)
Infants	0.0 to 0.5	400	300	40	6	5	40	10
	0.5 to 1.0	600	500	60	10	5	50	15
Children	1 to 3	800	800	80	10	10	70	20
	4 to 6	800	800	120	10	10	90	20
Males	11 to 14	1200	1200	270	12	15	150	40
	15 to 18	1200	1200	400	12	15	150	50
	19 to 24	1200	1200	350	10	15	150	70
	25 to 50	800	800	350	10	15	150	70
	51+	800	800	350	10	15	150	70
Females	11 to 14	1200	1200	280	15	12	150	45
	15 to 18	1200	1200	300	15	12	150	50
	19 to 24	1200	1200	280	15	12	150	55
	25 to 50	800	800	280	15	12	150	55
	51+	800	800	280	10	12	150	55
Pregnant		1200	1200	300	30	15	175	65
Lactating	1st 6 mo	1200	1200	355	15	19	200	75
	2nd 6 mo	1200	1200	340	15	16	200	75

From Food and Nutrition Board, National Academy of Sciences, National Research Council: Recommended dietary allowances, *revised 1989, Washington, D.C.*

TABLE 37-4   MAJOR ROLE OF MACROMINERALS AND ASSOCIATED ABNORMALITIES

Element	Major Role	Associated Abnormality	Comments
Calcium	Major component with phosphorus of skeletal and dental tissues	Deficiency: rickets in children; osteomalacia in adults; contributes to osteoporosis	Hormonal regulation: parathyroid hormone, vitamin D, calcitonin
Chloride	Important in fluid and electrolyte balance; major extracellular fluid anion; contributes to osmolality	Deficiency may occur as result of vomiting, diarrhea, diuretics, renal disease	
Magnesium	Major pools intracellular, bone; cofactor for many enzymes	Deficiency may occur because of malabsorption, diarrhea, alcoholism	Symptom of deficiency: muscle weakness
Phosphorus	Major component with calcium in skeletal and dental tissue; energy source from ATP Phosphorylated intermediate in metabolic pathways; component of nucleic acids	Deficiency: in children, rickets; in adults, osteomalacia	Parathyroid hormone and vitamin D regulatory mechanisms
Potassium	Major intracellular cation; important in muscle and nerve functions Na^+, K^+-ATPase	Muscle weakness, confusion, paralysis	Hormonal regulation of potassium excretion by aldosterone; urine loss increased by diuretics
Sodium	Major extracellular fluid cation; contributes to osmolality Important in acid-base balance Na^+, K^+-ATPase	Excess may cause hypertension in some individuals	Hormonal regulation of sodium reabsorption by aldosterone

million children under 5 years of age in the developing world are malnourished while 230 million have stunted growth. Associated with the malnutrition and undernutrition are poor physical and mental development, lower resistance to infectious disease, and a high mortality. In developing countries, approximately half of the deaths of children under 5 years of age—about 10 million each year—are associated with malnutrition.

American population. An increased emphasis on wellness has led to suggested improvements in the composition of the American diet to maintain good health and to prolong life. The most recent recommendations of the American Heart Association for a decrease in total fat consumption are described in Chapter 33. The increased consumption of fruits and vegetables, especially citrus fruits, leafy vegetables, tomatoes, and orange-colored vegetables, is recommended because these foods are good sources of vitamins. A reduction in caloric intake has been demonstrated to be beneficial; excessive caloric intake leads to obesity and its accompanying health problems (see below). Populations requiring special consideration of nutritional requirements are shown in Box 37-1. It is important to note that many of these populations include ambulatory individuals who are not acutely ill and may even be completely healthy (such as pregnant women). Many of these populations may become acutely protein-calorie–malnourished as the result of illness or trauma.

Obesity[19,20]

Obesity is generally defined as an excessively high amount of body fat or adipose tissue in relation to lean body mass.[19]

BOX 37-1

CONDITIONS REQUIRING SPECIAL NUTRITION CONSIDERATIONS

Aging
Alcoholism
Cancer
Coronary heart disease
Diabetes
Growth
Hyperlipidemia
Injury, severe (e.g., burns, trauma)
Immunoincompetence
Kwashiorkor disease
Lactation
Low–birth-weight infant
Malabsorption
Marasmus
Obesity
Poverty
Pregnancy
Sepsis

More strictly, obesity is defined by a body mass index (BMI) greater than or equal to 30.0. While protein-calorie malnutrition remains a major problem in developing countries, obesity is a growing problem in affluent societies in all countries. Current prevalence data from a number of countries suggest that obesity is rising and will continue to rise. For example, in most European countries, the obesity prevalence has risen by 10% to 40% in the last 10 years, now ranging from 10% to 20% for men and 10% to 25% for women.

In the United States, the problem of obesity is also growing, with poorer, especially minority populations being at especially high risk. Among U.S. adults between the ages of 20 and 74 years, the prevalence of obesity has nearly doubled from approximately 15% in 1980 to an estimated 20% in 2000.[19-21] The Centers for Disease Control and Prevention (CDC) estimates that 27% of blacks, 21% of Hispanics, and 17% of whites in the United States are obese (see also http://www.cdc.gov/nccdphp/brfss/). The medical consequences of obesity include increased sleep apnea and respiratory problems, non-insulin-dependent (type 2) diabetes, gallbladder disease, cardiovascular problems (hypertension, stroke, and CHD), and endometrial, breast, prostate, and colon cancers. There is a direct relationship between the rise in obesity and the rise of type 2 diabetes (see Chapter 32). Severe obesity in 25- to 35-year-olds is associated with a 12-fold increase in mortality when compared with lean individuals.

Drug-Nutrient Interactions

A comprehensive coverage of the nature of interactions between drugs and nutrients and their consequences is given by Roe.[22] Physicochemical interaction may occur in the gastrointestinal tract and may impair absorption of drug or nutrient, or both. Factors involved may include solubility properties, pH of the milieu, adsorptivity, chelation, gel formation, and ion exchange. Physiological interactions in which gastrointestinal function is altered may alter transit time and hence absorption rate, produce electrolyte imbalance or vasodilation, or have a modifying effect on appetite, resulting in excessive or inadequate food intake. A third category of interaction occurs when pathological changes result from drug toxicity. These interactions may have a pronounced effect on metabolism in general; in particular, they may impair a fetus, the gastrointestinal tract, or other organs such as liver, kidney, brain, blood system. Roe lists 59 specific drugs the absorption of which may be reduced or retarded by food or food supplements, and 24 the absorption of which may be increased by food or by enteral formulas. Although the effects of diet composition on drug metabolism and toxicity have been documented extensively in animal experiments, few studies have been reported in humans. As pointed out by Roe, this is an area in which research is wanting, especially in aging populations where the high prevalence of drug reactions, combined with the frequency of multiple drug prescriptions may involve a diet-related explanation.

Low-protein diets reduce renal plasma flow, creatinine clearance, and renal clearance of drugs such as the anti-uricemic drug allopurinol, which inhibits xanthine oxidase. Basic drugs such as gentamicin are affected by the alkalinizing effect of low-protein diets, presenting a less ionized form of the drug to the kidney and resulting in increased reabsorption. An area requiring further study is the effect of obesity on drug distribution: Should lyophilic drugs be given according to ideal body weight or according to the patient's weight?

Amphetamines are known to decrease appetite. Likewise, digitalis given for long periods at a high level causes nausea and cachexia. Many cancer chemotherapeutic drugs also decrease appetite; in some cases this may be attributable to gastrointestinal ulceration.

The mechanism of action of many drugs appears to be as a vitamin antagonist. Although evidence of this has been provided by in vitro studies and observed in animal experiments for many drugs, confirmation in vivo in humans is often lacking. Table 37-5 lists some drugs that are vitamin antagonists.

The effect of drugs on retention or loss of major minerals in humans is well established and is summarized in Table 37-6.

Institutionalized Populations

Malnutrition in chronic and acute care institutions can be a major problem.[11,12,23-25] The estimated 40% of hospitalized patients who show signs of malnutrition includes individuals who enter the hospital with preexisting chronic conditions (such as individuals with acquired immunodeficiency syndrome [AIDS] or cancer), as well as those who may become acutely ill as the result of their hospital stay (such as trauma patients, surgery and burn patients, and very-low-birth-weight babies).[12,23] Individuals in chronic care facilities (such as nursing homes) may not eat properly and may become chronically malnourished.[24] Cancer patients with cachexia or who have had prior surgery or radiation therapy that interferes with gastrointestinal function will benefit from nutrition support.[26] Progressive weight loss before surgery is an indication for nutrition support before surgery proceeds.

There are both medical (see following box) and economic consequences of protein-energy malnutrition (PEM) in institutionalized patients.[12] The medical complications resulting from PEM are all associated with greatly increased costs to hospitals and nursing homes. These costs result from the increased length of stay (LOS) in intensive care units (ICUs) or regular hospital beds, as well as increased use of medical resources.

MEDICAL CONSEQUENCES OF PROTEIN-CALORIE MALNUTRITION IN INSTITUTIONALIZED INDIVIDUALS

Delayed wound healing
Increased risk for postoperative complications
    Pneumonia
    Wound site infection
Impaired immune function
Increased length of stay in hospitals
Increased death rates

TABLE 37-5 EXAMPLES OF DRUGS THAT ARE VITAMIN ANTAGONISTS*

Drug	Use/Effect	Vitamin Affected
Adriamycin	Cancer chemotherapy; dose-dependent cardiomyopathy, if accumulation >500 mg/m² Histologic pattern resembles that of vitamin E deficiency	Incidence, severity of damage reduced by vitamin E supplementation in animals, not in humans
Alcohol	Impaired utilization of B vitamins	Thiamine administration improves, as in Wernicke-Korsakoff syndrome
Coumarin drugs Warfarin Dicumerol	Anticoagulants	Vitamin K antagonists; high vitamin K intake decreases anticoagulant effects
Hydralazine	Antihypertensive drug	B_6 antagonist; inhibits nicotinamide synthesis
Isoniazid	Antituberculosis drug	B_6 antagonist; inhibits nicotinamide synthesis
Methotrexate	Cancer chemotherapeutic drug	Folate antagonist
Moxalactam	Antibiotic	Decreases vitamin K–dependent clotting factors
Nitrous oxide	Anesthetic; important in cardiac bypass surgery	B_{12} antagonist
Pentamidine	*Pneumocystis carinii* pneumonia therapy	Folate antagonist
Pyrimethamine	Antimalarial agent	Folate antagonist
Sulfasalazine	Antiinflammatory drug	Folate antagonist
Tramterine	Diuretic	Folate antagonist
Trimethroprim	Antibiotic	Folate antagonist

*From Roe DA: Diet, nutrition, and drug interactions. In Shils ME, Olson JA, Shike M, editors: Modern nutrition in health and disease, ed 8, Philadelphia, 1993, Lea & Febinger, with extensive bibliography. It should be noted that demonstration of vitamin antagonism by a drug in vitro in animal models often lacks confirmation in humans.

TABLE 37-6 SOME CLASSES OR INDIVIDUAL DRUGS THAT INFLUENCE MINERAL STATUS

	MINERAL STATUS	
Mineral	Overload	Depletion
Potassium	Succinylcholine increases serum potassium; potassium-sparing diuretics	Laxatives; potassium-losing diuretics; nephrotoxic antibiotics
Sodium	Antacids containing $NaHCO_3$; diazoxide, an antihypertensive, may increase serum sodium	Sodium-losing diuretics
Calcium	Thiazide diuretics–calcium retention; etidronate, a biphosphonate, increases bone mass; pharmacological doses of vitamin D and metabolites–potential hypercalcemia and soft-tissue calcification	Aluminum-containing antacids or parenteral fluids–osteomalacia may occur; corticosteroids; phenobarbital; phenytoin
Magnesium	Magnesium-containing antacids	Nephrotic antibiotics; diuretics; cisplatin
Iron		Aspirin; indomethacin
Zinc		Penicillamine; nephrotic antibiotics

It thus becomes incumbent upon institutions to establish policies that will enable early detection of PEM, early and effective treatment of PEM, and careful monitoring of that treatment.

THERAPEUTIC NUTRITION SUPPORT[27,28]

In all cases of PEM, appropriate nutritional intervention is needed to treat the malnourished patient. The nutritional therapy must be tailored to the needs of the individual patient. The route of nutritional administration depends on the ability of the gut to function effectively; for patients who are unable to receive nutritional care orally, **enteral feeding** or parenteral feeding may be necessary.

Enteral Feeding

Enteral feeding refers to the introduction of nutrients into the gastrointestinal tract through a tube.[27] This method is necessary when patients are unable to consume sufficient food normally. Box 37-2 provides a brief list of conditions in which enteral feeding may be indicated. The availability of a variety of commercial enteral formulas tailored to meet specific circumstances has made this an increasingly practical route for maintaining adequate nutrition. Percutaneous endoscopic gastrostomy and jejunoscopy procedures have simplified the procedures used for guiding placement of the tubes. The placement of the tube is determined by the particular problem; for example, in the presence of recurrent aspiration, the tube must not be placed in the stomach but in the jejunum. Indications for enteral nutrition include burn patients who require increased nutritional support; coma states; partial obstruction of the stomach or small bowel; fistulas of the small bowel or colon; persistent anorexia; and disorders with specific requirements that can be met by the introduction of tailored solutions. A more detailed discussion of enteral feeding is given in reference 27. Whenever possible, enteral feeding is preferred to **total parenteral nutrition (TPN)**, since enteral nutrition enables the patient to maintain a functioning gut, with its contribution to normal metabolic processes. In addition, enteral formulas are simpler to manage and preferable to intravenous administration, or **parenteral nutrition**. However, when enteral feeding is not possible, nutrients must be administered intravenously.

Parenteral Nutrition (PN)[28]

Parenteral nutrition aims to maintain or improve the nutritional status of patients who are unable to obtain the necessary nutrients from normal feeding or from enteral formulae. Parenteral nutrient solutions are intravenously administered either by peripheral vein, that is, by **peripheral parenteral nutrition (PPN)**, or through a central vein in which a central catheter has been maintained (TPN). Isotonic lipid emulsions in 5% or 10% glucose, 5% amino acids, electrolytes, and micronutrients supplying up to 2500 kcal in 3 liters can be administered peripherally.[28] When a critically ill patient is unstable, continued access to a vein is required; hence a central catheter is essential and must be readily available. Total parenteral nutrition allows larger volumes and therefore more nutrients to be administered than can be delivered by the PPN route. Conditions in which patients may benefit from TPN are summarized in Box 37-3. The evidence for a beneficial effect of TPN given preoperatively to malnourished patients is equivocal. However, although

TPN used preoperatively in patients with gastrointestinal tumors improved the postoperative outcome, there has been no evidence that TPN improved treatment tolerance or outcome in patients receiving chemotherapy. Nutritional support by TPN *has* been demonstrated to be advantageous for patients receiving chemotherapy when cachexia is a problem.

Dietary Therapy

Dietary regimes for the treatment of individuals with obesity, hyperlipidemias, or coronary heart disease include a restriction of calories, total fat, saturated fat, and animal protein and an increase in consumption of complex carbohydrates, fiber, and vegetable proteins and in the proportion of polyunsaturated and monounsaturated fats. The intake of cholesterol should be less than 100 mg/1000 kcal.

Nutrition plans for patients with diabetes who are at risk for development of atherosclerosis recommend that carbohydrates supply at least 55% to 60% of calories. Complex carbohydrates should provide at least two thirds of the total. Protein intake should provide 12% to 16% of calories. Fat intake should be reduced to 20% to 25% of calories, no more than 10% of which should be saturated fats. A high-fiber intake that includes as much as 30 to 50 g/day is usually well tolerated and beneficial. Additional detail can be found in Chapter 33.

Dietary intervention is usually required for a number of populations with other medical conditions including obesity, cancer,[26] end-stage renal disease, pregnancy and lactation, and inborn errors of metabolism. Often, dietary therapy will require supplemental pharmaceutical intervention.

NUTRITION AND INBORN ERRORS OF METABOLISM

Inherited metabolic diseases are the result of "inborn errors" in genes that result in alterations in the structure and function of enzymes or protein molecules (see Chapter 47). Elas and

Costa[29] indicate that over 250 genetic disorders have been reported in which there occurs an accumulation, deficiency, or overproduction of the substrates or products involved in normal metabolic pathways. They review approximately 100 of these disorders in which nutritional therapy is an integral component of the treatment of these diseases. Intervention in the first few weeks of life is mandatory for phenylketonuria, galactosemia, isovaleric acidemia, homocystinuria, maple syrup urine disease, argininosuccinic aciduria, and citrullinemia. A description of chemically defined formulas, medications, and dietary guides for many classes of inherited metabolic disorders is also included in reference 29, as well as a comprehensive discussion of the biochemistry, screening procedures, diagnosis, and treatment for many of these diseases.

BIOCHEMICAL PARAMETERS USED TO MONITOR NUTRITIONAL STATUS

Early detection and treatment of PEM in hospitals and chronic care facilities has now become a required standard of care of the Joint Commission on Accreditation of Healthcare Organizations (JCAHO). Institutions are required to have plans to screen for malnutrition within 24 hours after admission of a patient to an institution, to effectively treat the condition, and to monitor the success of that intervention.

General Detection and Monitoring of PEM[11,12]

Assessment of the nutritional status of institutionalized patients and the monitoring of nutritional therapies includes both anthropometric and laboratory measurements. Because anthropometric measurements are a complex task for nonspecialized health care workers, laboratory tests serve increasingly as surrogate markers for PEM.

The properties of an ideal laboratory marker in biological fluids for detecting and monitoring nutritional status are summarized in Box 37-4. Although these properties cannot all be met for every clinical situation, when used in conjunction with considerations of a patient's condition, they enable interpretation of the patient's nutritional status. Routine biochemical screening panels provide data on the patient's status and requirements for carbohydrates and the macrominerals. Although classic cases of micronutrient deficiency (trace minerals and vitamins) are rarely seen in developed

---

BOX 37-4

PROPERTIES OF AN IDEAL NUTRITIONAL MARKER

Is specific for analyte to be measured
Has a high degree of sensitivity
Is indicative of status of a particular analyte
Has very short biological half-life
Responds rapidly to supplementation
Indicates onset and degree of deficiency early

---

countries, they can be found in war-ravaged, poverty-stricken populations. In developed countries, individuals who chronically receive parenteral nutrition may be at high risk for developing a deficiency in micronutrients and may need monitoring of specific nutrients (e.g., zinc, selenium).[11] In most other cases of at-risk populations (see Box 37-1), routine measurement of a micronutrient is rarely needed; monitoring patients for specific signs of a nutrient deficiency (see Chapters 38 and 39) will suffice.

Refeeding Syndrome

In addition to providing information on specific nutrients, these routine biochemical tests can also be useful for assessment of the general response of patients to nutrition therapy. Specifically, by ensuring careful biochemical monitoring, physicians can avoid a negative aspect to nutritional treatment called the *refeeding syndrome*.

The refeeding syndrome describes the negative sequelae that can result when patients who have been chronically starved and severely malnourished receive aggressive nutritional support. This syndrome may begin when the starved individual receives more glucose than can be physiologically processed. Under normal conditions, the maximal rate at which glucose can be metabolized is 2 to 4 mg/kg/min. Under stress, this metabolic rate can increase to 3 to 5 mg/kg/min. If these rates are exceeded, an exaggerated insulin response may occur. In addition to its hypoglycemic effect (see Chapter 32), insulin has strong antidiuretic properties. Thus in an exaggerated insulin response, which can occur if a malnourished patient is treated with excessive glucose, there will be water and salt retention, increasing the vascular space, leading to fluid overload and stress to the heart.

Other biochemical sequelae to the insulin include decreases in serum phosphate, magnesium, and potassium, as the insulin drives these analytes into peripheral cells, primarily muscle cells. In a body that might already be deficient in these nutrients, hypophosphatemia, hypokalemia, and hypomagnesemia may result.

- A deficiency in serum magnesium may reduce the activity of key enzymes in tissue, especially cardiac tissue.
- The hypophosphatemia can lead to decreased cellular levels of ATP and, in red blood cells, of 2,3-diphosphoglycerate (2,3-DPG). The decreased 2,3-DPG alters the shape of red blood cells, decreases the half-life of red blood cells, and alters the binding of oxygen to hemoglobin (see Chapters 25 and 36). This results in a diminished delivery of oxygen to peripheral cells and tissue hypoxia.
- The hypokalemia results in an increased irritability of cardiac tissue and reduced ability of cells to take up glucose.

In a severely protein-malnourished individual, muscles have already been weakened because muscle proteins have been catabolized to amino acids that are consumed in the

TABLE **37-7** LABORATORY TESTS TO MONITOR RESPONSE TO NUTRIENT SUPPLEMENTS

Parameter	Rationale/Comments
Urine urea nitrogen	*Approximates* nitrogen balance in anabolic and catabolic states
Total urine nitrogen	Direct measure of excreted nitrogen
Plasma albumin	Low in malnutrition, affected by redistribution with fluid shifts or retention
Plasma transthyretin* (prealbumin)	Low in malnutrition; half-life of 2 days; reflects hepatic protein synthesis
Plasma transferrin*	Low in malnutrition; half-life of 8 days
Plasma retinol-binding protein*	Low in malnutrition; half-life of 10 hours
Plasma zinc	Low levels (500 µg/L) with skin lesions indicate immunoincompetence
Plasma triglycerides	Essential to monitor hypertriglyceridemia in peripheral parenteral nutrition

*Acute phase reactants, see text.

gluconeogenic pathway to increase the availability of blood glucose for the brain. In this weakened condition, the biochemical stresses listed above act to further reduce the capability of muscles to function, leading to respiratory failure and tissue hypoxia, which in turn leads to congestive heart failure and cardiac arrest. These sequelae of aggressive nutrition therapy can be avoided by careful monitoring of the serum levels of these analytes and a cooperative relationship among the physician, laboratory, and pharmacist.

Nitrogen Balance

Tests that may be used to monitor nitrogen balance and provide some estimates of the liver's protein synthesis capabilities are shown in Table 37-7. Nitrogen balance may be estimated from calculated dietary intake and determination of 24-hour excretion of urine urea. An adjustment factor for estimated fecal and other nitrogen losses, such as creatinine, uric acid, ammonia, and losses to hair, nails, and sweat, is determined from an individual patient's condition. Limitations of this method have been discussed, particularly with the critically ill patient using the factor urine urea $\times 1.25$ grams to estimate total nitrogen have been discussed.[11,30] A more accurate measure of nitrogen excretion can be made by direct analysis of total nitrogen (see above and reference 11).

Protein Synthesis

Interpretation of results of plasma albumin and of specific proteins must take into account the individual patient's condition. Alterations in fluid volume status and fluid shifts into or out of the vascular system produce changes in the concentration of plasma albumin and transferrin. Conditions initiating the acute-phase response, including trauma, infection, malignancy, and myocardial infarction, can affect the levels of specific hepatic proteins. Of the commonly measured specific proteins, ceruloplasmin is a positive acute-phase reactant, and serum levels will be increased because of increased synthesis at the site of injury. At the same time the serum levels of negative-phase reactants are decreased because of enhanced catabolism and decreased synthesis. Hence, a decrease in plasma transthyretin (prealbumin), transferrin, retinol binding protein, and albumin may result, at least in part, in conditions other than malnutrition. Nevertheless, analyses of specific proteins of short biological half-lives are useful in monitoring the response to nutritional supplementation. Half-lives of some of the specific proteins, as well as suggested levels at which supplementation is indicated, are shown in Table 37-8. Response to protein supplementation is reflected most rapidly by an increase in retinal-binding protein, but prealbumin has been found to be more predictive of improved status. Because prealbumin can be readily measured using routine laboratory equipment, its use as a rapid marker to screen for PEM and to monitor treatment has been recommended[11,25] and is being used increasingly for this purpose.

TABLE **37-8** PROTEINS USED IN NUTRITION ASSESSMENT

Protein	Half-Life	Normal Values	Suggested Medical Decision Point
Albumin	21 days	35 to 55 g/L	30 g/L
Transferrin	8 days	2000 to 4000 mg/L	1500 mg/L
Prealbumin	2 days	160 to 350 mg/L	110 mg/L
Retinol-binding protein	10 hours	26 to 76 mg/L	16 mg/L

From Kaplan LA, *general editor:* Laboratory support in assessing and monitoring nutritional status, *National Academy of Clinical Biochemistry's "Standards of Laboratory Practice" series.*

References

1. Subcommittee on the 10th Edition of the RDAs, Food and Nutrition Board, Commission on Life Sciences, National Research Council: *Recommended dietary allowances*, ed 10, Washington, DC, 1989, National Academy Press.
2. Standing Committee on the Scientific Evaluation of Dietary Reference Intakes, Food and Nutrition Board, Institute of Medicine: *Dietary reference intakes for vitamin C, vitamin E, selenium, and carotenoids*, Washington, D.C., 2001, National Academy Press; Standing Committee on the Scientific Evaluation of Dietary Reference Intakes, Food and Nutrition Board, Institute of Medicine: *Dietary reference intakes for vitamin A, vitamin K, arsenic, boron, chromium, copper, iodide, iron, manganese, molybdenum, nickel, silicon, vanadium, and zinc*, Washington, D.C., 2001, National Academy Press; Standing Committee on the Scientific Evaluation of Dietary Reference Intakes, Food and Nutrition Board, Institute of Medicine: *Dietary reference intakes for calcium, phosphorus, magnesium, vitamin D, and fluoride*, Washington, D.C., 1997, National Academy Press.
3. Shils ME et al, editors: *Modern nutrition in health and disease*, ed 9, Philadelphia, 1999, Lea & Febiger.
4. Murray RK et al, editors: *Harper's biochemistry*, ed 23, Norwalk, CT, 1993, Appleton & Lange.
5. World Health Organization: *Energy and protein requirements: report of a joint FAO/WHO/UNU expert consultation technical report*, series 724, Geneva, Switzerland, 1985, WHO.
6. Scrimshaw NS, Waterlow JC, Schürch B, supplement editors: Proceedings of an IDECG workshop held at the London School of Hygiene and Tropical Medicine, UK (31 October-4 November 1994), *Eur J Clin Nut* 50(suppl 1):S1, February 1996 (see also www.unu.edu/unupress/food2/UID01E/UID01E00.htm).
7. Wilmore DW: *Catabolic illness: strategies for enhancing recovery, N Engl J Med* 325:695, 1991.
8. Souba WW, Wilmore DW: Diet and nutrition in the care of the patient with surgery trauma and sepsis. In Shils ME et al, editors: *Modern nutrition in health and disease*, ed 9, Philadelphia, 1999, Lea & Febiger.
9. MacDonald I: Carbohydrates. In Shils ME et al, editors: *Modern nutrition in health and disease*, ed 9, Philadelphia, 1999, Lea & Febiger.
10. Crim MC, Munro HN: Proteins and amino acids. In Shils ME et al, editors: *Modern nutrition in health and disease*, ed 9, Philadelphia, 1999, Lea & Febiger.
11. National Academy of Clinical Biochemistry: Laboratory support in assessing and monitoring nutritional status. In Kaplan LA, general editor: *Standards of laboratory practice series*, Washington, DC, 1994, National Academy of Clinical Biochemistry.
12. Kaplan LA, Bernstein LH: Medical and economic consequences of protein energy malnutrition: CAP check sample, *Clin Chem* 37(4):47, 1997.
13. Linscheer WG, Vergroesen AJ: Lipids. In Shils ME et al, editors: *Modern nutrition in health and disease*, ed 9, Philadelphia, 1999, Lea & Febiger.
14. Nordin BEC, editor: *Calcium in human biology*, London, 1988, Springer-Verlag.
15. Shils ME: Magnesium. In Shils ME et al, editors: *Modern nutrition in health and disease*, ed 9, Philadelphia, 1999, Lea & Febiger.
16. Schneeman BO, Tietyen J: Dietary fiber. In Shils ME et al, editors: *Modern nutrition in health and disease*, ed 9, Philadelphia, 1999, Lea & Febiger.
17. Grantham-McGregor S: A review of studies of the effect of severe malnutrition on mental Development, *J Nut* 125(suppl 8S):2235S, 1995.
18. Philip W et al: The contribution of nutrition to inequalities in health, *Brit Med J* 314:1545, 1997.
19. Stunkard AJ, Wadden TA, editors: *Obesity: theory and therapy*, ed 2, New York, 1993, Raven Press.
20. National Institutes of Health: *Clinical guidelines on the identification, evaluation, and treatment of overweight and obesity in adults*, Bethesda, MD, 1998, Department of Health and Human Services; National Institutes of Health; National Heart, Lung, and Blood Institute.
21. Mokdad AH et al: The continuing epidemics of obesity and diabetes in the United States, *JAMA* 286(10):1195, 2001.
22. Roe DA: Diet, nutrition, and drug interactions. In Shils ME et al, editors: *Modern nutrition in health and disease*, ed 9, Philadelphia, 1999, Lea & Febiger.
23. Coats KG et al: Hospital-associated malnutrition: a re-evaluation 12 years later, *JADA* 93:27, 1993.
24. Breslow RA, Hallfrisch J, Goldberg AP: Malnutrition in tube fed nursing home patients with pressure sores, *J Parent Enteral Nutr* 15:663, 1991.
25. Kaplan LA, Minkowitz, G: Serum prealbumin in institutionalized populations, *Nutrition* 15:51, 1999.
26. Shils ME: Nutrition and diet in cancer management. In Shils ME et al, editors: *Modern nutrition in health and disease*, ed 9, Philadelphia, 1999, Lea & Febiger.
27. Shike M: Enteral feeding. In Shils ME et al, editors: *Modern nutrition in health and disease*, ed 9, Philadelphia, 1999, Lea & Febiger.
28. Shils ME: Parenteral nutrition. In Shils ME et al, editors: *Modern nutrition in health and disease*, ed 9, Philadelphia, 1999, Lea & Febiger.
29. Elsas LJ, Acosta PB: Nutrition support of inherited metabolic disease. In Shils ME et al, editors: *Modern nutrition in health and disease*, ed 9, Philadelphia, 1999, Lea & Febiger.
30. Konstantinides FN et al: Urine urea nitrogen: too insensitive for calculating nitrogen balance in clinical nutrition, *JPEN* 15:189, 1991.

Internet Sites

General

www.nutrition.org.uk—British Nutrition Foundation
www.nutrition.uu.se/studentprojects/group98/micronut/micronut.html
www.who.int/nut/pem.htm—World Health Organization: Nutrition
http://www.fao.org/es/ens/index_en.stm—Click on the "Human Nutrition" button for more information
www.who.int/inf-fs/en/fact119.html—WHO fact sheet on childhood malnutrition
http://www.css.cornell.edu/FoodSystems/nutr%26health.html
http://www.aces.uiuc.edu/~fshn/
http://www.gfhnrc.ars.usda.gov/hnrcnews.htm
http://www.nps.ars.usda.gov/programs/programs.htm?NPNUMBER=107
http://www.nutritionperspectives.com/flash.html—Dade Behring nutrition articles

http://www.ars.usda.gov/—U.S. Department of Agriculture: Agriculture Research Service (Click on Search, type in Nutrition)

Obesity

www.iotf.org/—WHO International Obesity Task Force
www.cdc.gov/nccdphp/dnpa/obesity/—National Center for Chronic Disease Prevention and Health Promotion: Obesity and Overweight
www.nhlbi.nih.gov/guidelines/obesity/ob_home.htm—National Heart, Lung, and Blood Institute Clinical Guidelines on the Identification, Evaluation, and Treatment of Overweight and Obesity in Adults
www.cdc.gov/brfss—National Center for Chronic Disease Prevention and Health Promotion Behavioral Risk Factor Surveillance System

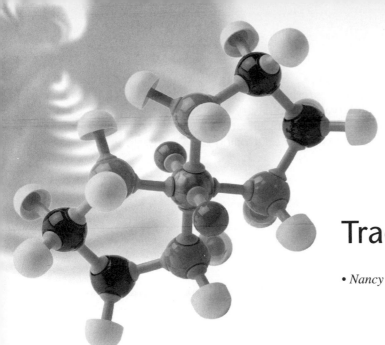

CHAPTER 38

Trace Elements

• *Nancy W. Alcock*

Chapter Outline

Classification
Essential trace elements
   Chromium (Cr)
   Copper (Cu)
   Fluorine (F)
   Iodine (I)
   Manganese (Mn)
   Molybdenum (Mo)
   Selenium (Se)
   Zinc (Zn)

Toxic trace metals
   Aluminum (Al)
   Arsenic (As)
   Cadmium (Cd)
   Lead (Pb)
   Mercury (Hg)
Considerations in assessing trace-element status in humans

Objectives

- Discuss the primary biochemical role of essential trace elements in humans.
- Present the clinical symptoms associated with a deficiency or an excess of essential trace elements.
- Discuss the biological toxicity of trace levels of some metals.
- Discuss considerations in assessing the status of trace metals in humans.

Key Terms

deficiency Status of a nutrient in which an abnormal symptom or biochemical function is reversed by supplementation with the nutrient.

dental caries A condition in which the calcified dentin or enamel, or both, of a tooth is destroyed by the action of microorganisms on carbohydrates.

essential trace element An element that, if removed from the diet, produces a biochemical abnormality that is reversed by supplementation with the element.

metallothionein A 6200-D protein, with approximately 30% of its amino acid residue content composed of cysteine, which firmly binds Cd>Cu>Zn ions. Metallothionein plays an important role in zinc-copper interactions, and its synthesis is readily induced by zinc.

micronutrients Essential food components that are required or present in the body in very small amounts. Includes vitamins and some metals.

RDA Recommended daily allowance of a micronutrient.

toxic trace elements Those elements found in the environment in abnormal amounts that are antagonistic to biochemical processes. When present in tissues in elevated levels, they can be toxic and may eventually be fatal.

trace elements Elements present in the body in very low amounts (micrograms/gram or less). Some are essential; others may be toxic, even at relatively low levels. Most trace elements are metals, exceptions being the halogens iodine and fluorine.

zinc fingers Specific zinc binding (by histidine and cysteine residues) regions that occur at defined intervals of regulatory proteins. These proteins bind to deoxyribonucleic acid (DNA) and regulate gene expression by controlling DNA transcription.

Methods on CD-ROM

Iron and iron-binding capacity
Lead
Zinc

CLASSIFICATION[1]

Trace elements are present in the body in very low amounts, usually less than 1 microgram per gram of tissue. They are part of the **micronutrients** of the body and can be subdivided into four major groupings based on their physiological function.

1. **Essential trace elements** for which a recommended daily allowance (**RDA**) has been established. These elements have been shown to be essential for normal growth, development, and maintenance, and a specific biological role has been identified. The elements in this group that are considered in this chapter are zinc, iodine, and selenium. The RDAs for these elements are listed in Table 38-1. Iron, the most abundant of the essential trace metals, is discussed in Chapter 35. Iron and zinc are transition elements in Mendeleev's original classification of the elements, whereas selenium and iodine are members of the "normal" series in group VI and group VII, respectively.

2. Trace elements for which there is definite evidence of an essential role in human metabolism but for which an RDA has not yet been established. These include the transition metals copper, manganese, chromium, cobalt, and molybdenum and the group VII halogen fluorine. The estimated safe but adequate dietary intakes for these elements are shown in Table 38-2. The only known requirement for cobalt in humans is

TABLE 38-1 RECOMMENDED DIETARY ALLOWANCES ESTABLISHED FOR ZINC, IODINE, AND SELENIUM (THE RDA FOR IRON IS INCLUDED FOR COMPARISON.)

Category	Age (Years) or Condition	WEIGHT kg	WEIGHT lb	HEIGHT cm	HEIGHT in	Iron (mg)	Zinc (mg)	Iodine (µg)	Selenium (µg)
Infants	0.1 to 0.5	6	13	60	24	6	5	40	10
	0.5 to 1.0	9	20	71	28	10	5	50	15
Children	1 to 3	13	29	90	35	10	10	70	20
	4 to 6	20	44	112	44	10	10	90	20 to 30
	7 to 10	28	62	132	52	10	10	120	30
Males	11 to 14	45	99	157	62	12	15	150	40
	15 to 18	66	145	176	69	12	15	150	55
	19 to 24	72	169	177	70	10	15	150	55
	25 to 50	79	174	176	70	10	15	150	55
	51+	77	170	173	68	10	15	150	55
Females	11 to 14	46	101	157	62	15	12	150	40
	15 to 18	55	120	163	64	15	12	150	55
	19 to 24	58	128	164	65	15	12	150	55
	25 to 50	63	138	163	64	15	12	150	55
	51+	65	143	160	63	10	12	150	55
Pregnant						30	15	175	60
Lactating	1st 6 mo					15	19	200	70
	2nd 6 mo					15	16	200	70

From Recommended dietary allowances, ed 10, National Research Council, Washington, D.C., 1989; and Dietary reference intakes vitamin C, vitamin E, selenium, and carotenoids, National Academy Press, Washington, D.C., 2001.

TABLE 38-2   ESTIMATED SAFE AND ADEQUATE DAILY DIETARY INTAKES (UPPER LIMITS OF INTAKE) OF SELECTED TRACE ELEMENTS

Category	Age (Years)	Copper* (mg)	Manganese* (mg)	Fluoride** (mg)	Chromium* (µg)	Molybdenum* (µg)
Infants	0 to 0.5	0.2	0.003	0.7	0.2	15 to 30
	0.5 to 1	0.22	0.6	0.9	5.5	20 to 40
Children and adolescents	1 to 3	0.34[†]	2	1.3	11	25 to 50
	4 to 8	0.44[†]	3	2.2	15	30 to 75
	9 to 13	0.7[†]	6	10	25	50 to 150
	13+	0.9[†]	9 to 11	10	21 to 35	75 to 250
Adults		0.9[†]	11	10	25 to 35	75 to 250

1. Because there is less information on which to base allowances, these figures are not given in the main table of the RDA and are provided here in the form of upper limits of intakes.
2. Since the toxic levels for many trace elements may be only several times the usual intakes, the upper levels for the trace elements given in this table should not be habitually exceeded.
From *Dietary reference intakes for vitamin A, vitamin K, arsenic, boron, chromium, copper, iodide, iron, manganese, molybdenum, nickel, silicon, vanadium, and zinc (2001) and **Dietary reference intakes for calcium, phosphorus, magnesium, vitamin D, and fluoride (1997), Standing committee on the Scientific Evaluation of Dietary Reference Intakes, Food and Nutrition Board, Institute of Medicine, Adapted from the National Academy Press, Washington, D.C.
†Recommended Dietary Allowance (RDA).

as a component of the B_{12} molecule, which is discussed in Chapter 39.

3. Trace elements that are consistently found in tissues or biological fluids in "ultratrace" amounts but that have not yet been shown to be either essential or detrimental at these levels of concentration. These include lithium, nickel, tin, silicon, and vanadium. These are not discussed in this chapter.

4. Trace metals that have no known biological function in humans but that, if present at relatively low levels, cause pathological changes. These **toxic trace elements** include aluminum, beryllium, cadmium, mercury, lead, and arsenic. These are discussed in this chapter. Cadmium, arsenic, and mercury are transition elements, whereas aluminum and lead are members of the normal series in group III and group IV, respectively.

ESSENTIAL TRACE ELEMENTS

The biological role of essential trace elements and some abnormalities arising from a deficiency or excess of the respective elements are shown in Table 38-3. Reference intervals, taken from the literature, for essential trace elements are listed in Table 38-4, and those for toxic metals are given in Table 38-5.

Chromium (Cr)[2-8]

Chromium is a transition element in period 4 of the periodic table of the elements, with an atomic weight of 52.

Biochemistry. Chromium has been demonstrated to be essential for normal carbohydrate, lipid, and nucleic acid metabolism. Trivalent chromium is a potentiator of insulin action.[3] It is postulated that chromium, which is found in cell nuclei, binds to DNA, RNA, and nuclear proteins. It appears to be involved in the maintenance of the structural integrity of the nuclear strands and in the regulation of gene expression.[4] The biologically active form is believed to be

an organic complex containing trivalent chromium, nicotinic acid, and glutathione or its constituent amino acids. However, the exact structure of the complex has not been elucidated as yet. In humans, several signs and symptoms are indicative of chromium deficiency. These include impaired glucose tolerance, elevated circulating insulin, glucosuria, elevated fasting blood glucose, elevated serum triglycerides and cholesterol, encephalopathy, and neuropathy. Brewer's yeast is a good source of the glucose tolerance factor, but only 5% of its total chromium was found to be associated with the insulin-potentiating activity. It is not known exactly how chromium potentiates the action of insulin in vivo. It may bind directly to insulin, or it may act by increasing receptor number or affinity.

Clinical significance.[5] The status of chromium in the body has not been successfully characterized from its concentration in urine or serum. One reason for this is the difficulty associated with its accurate measurement in biological fluids because of contamination. Stainless steel, which contains chromium, is a common source for gross contamination. Anderson[2] suggests that even when chromium analysis is carefully performed, the levels of chromium in serum or urine may not be indicative of the body status. Demonstration of a **deficiency** of chromium has been successful when improvement in glucose or lipid metabolism resulted from the administration of 200 µg of chromium per day to adults over a period of months. Patients receiving long-term total parenteral nutrition (TPN) are at risk for chromium deficiency if their TPN fluids are not supplemented. In the first reported case of chromium deficiency, the patient showed impaired glucose tolerance with normal insulin levels and had elevated fatty acid levels, low respiratory quotient, abnormalities of nitrogen metabolism, and neuropathy. Insulin infusion failed to improve glucose tolerance or respiratory quotient, but these parameters returned to normal after chromium supplementation.

TABLE 38-3 BIOLOGICAL ROLE OF ESSENTIAL TRACE ELEMENTS AND ASSOCIATED ABNORMALITIES

Element	Biological Role	Comments	Deficiency/Abnormality/Toxicity
Chromium	Metabolism of glucose	Potentiates insulin action	Glucose intolerance in deficiency
Cobalt	Component of vitamin B_{12}	No other function known in man	Vitamin B_{12} deficiency; anemia
Copper	Cofactor for oxidase enzymes	90% to 95% plasma copper bound to ceruloplasmin	Inherited diseases: Wilson's, Menkes'
Fluorine	Inhibits dental caries; therapeutically improves quality of hydroxyapatite crystals in bone	Usually supplied as supplement to drinking water	Excessive intake causes fluorosis
Iodine	Component of T_3 and T_4	Concentrated in the thyroid; supplementation by addition to salt common	Iodine deficiency still occurs in various geographic areas
Iron	Component of heme enzymes: hemoglobin, cytochromes	In plasma bound to transferrin; stored as ferritin	Deficiency: hypochromic, microcytic anemia
Manganese	Required for glycoprotein and proteoglycan synthesis	Component of mitochondrial superoxide dismutase	Deficiency not known in man
Molybdenum	Component of sulfite and xanthine oxidases	Essential for production of uric acid	Deficiency reported in TPN patient; inability to metabolize methionine
Selenium	Component of glutathione peroxidase and iodinothyronine-5' deiodinase	Antioxidant properties; selenium and vitamin E act synergistically	Deficiency may occur where soil Se is low and in long-term TPN patients with inadequate supplements
Silicon	Involved in calcification in bone	Role in bone, cartilage, and connective tissue poorly understood	Deficiency: impairment of normal growth in animals; silicosis may occur from industrial exposure
Zinc	Cofactor or component of more than 200 metalloenzymes	Involved in many metabolic processes: protein synthesis; immunological function; growth and development	Deficiency: growth failure, hypogonadism, impaired wound healing; genetic disease: acrodermatitis enteropathica-impaired absorption; toxicity: vomiting, gastrointestinal irritation

TPN, Total parenteral nutrition.

The safe and adequate recommended level of chromium intake is shown in Table 38-2. It is estimated that less than 2% of dietary trivalent chromium is absorbed from the gastrointestinal tract.

Toxicity. Toxicity from trivalent sources of chromium has not been reported in humans. Hexavalent chromium toxicity from industrial exposure through inhalation has been associated with increased incidence of lung cancer.[6] In experimental animals, ingestion as chromate resulted in liver and kidney damage. Chromium in detergents and bleaches may be associated with the occurrence of dermatitis.

Food sources. Chromium is found in brewer's yeast, mushrooms, molasses, nuts, wine, beer, asparagus, prunes, meats, cheeses, and whole grains. It is difficult to assess accurately the chromium content of foods, because preparation for analysis usually involves homogenization in equipment with stainless steel parts and some contamination usually occurs.

Method.[7,8] Graphite furnace flameless atomic absorption spectrometry is the preferred method of analysis. Although a tungsten halogen lamp provides adequate background correction, graphite furnace atomic absorption spectrophoto-metry using Zeeman background correction is the preferred instrumentation.

Reference intervals. Normal, nonsupplemented human adults excrete approximately 0.5 μg of chromium/L of urine and have serum levels <0.5 μg/L.[7,8] Erythrocytes have a concentration of 20 to 36 μg/L.

Copper (Cu)[9-16]

Copper is a transition element in period 4 of the periodic table of the elements, with an atomic weight of 64.

Divalent copper forms complexes with proteins, many of which are enzymes. A group of these constitute copper metalloenzymes with oxidase activity. These include cytochrome oxidase, ferroxidase (ceruloplasmin), superoxidase dismutase, lysine oxidase, dopamine β-hydroxylase, spermine oxidase, tyrosinase, uricase, benzylamine oxidase, diamine oxidase, and tryptophan 3,3-di-oxygenase. In biological systems, copper has the ability to induce the synthesis of **metallothionein** and is intermediate between cadmium and zinc in this activity. Approximately 50% of dietary copper is absorbed, with the process being facilitated by the complexing of copper with amino acids. In

TABLE 38-4 SUGGESTED REFERENCE INTERVALS FOR ESSENTIAL TRACE ELEMENTS

Element	Specimen Type or Source	REFERENCE INTERVAL	
		Concentration	IU
Cr	S	0.12 to 2.1 µg/L	2.3 to 40.3 nmol/L
	RBC	20 to 36 µg/L	384 to 692 nmol/L
	U	0.1 to 2.0 µg/L	1.9 to 38.4 nmol/day
Co	S	0.11 to 0.45 µg/L	1.9 to 7.6 nmol/L
	RBC	16 to 46 µg/L	272 to 781 nmol/kg
	U	1 to 2 µg/L	17 to 34 nmol/L
Vitamin B$_{12}$	S	100 to 700 pg/mL	74 to 516 pmol/L
Cu	S	µg/dL	µmol/L
	Birth to 6 mo	20 to 70	3.14 to 10.99
	6 years	90 to 190	14.13 to 29.83
	12 years	80 to 160	12.56 to 25.12
	Adult (male)	70 to 140	10.99 to 21.98
	Adult (female)	80 to 155	12.56 to 24.34
	Term pregnancy	118 to 302	18.53 to 47.41
	U	3 to 35 µg/day	0.047 to 0.55 µmol/day
F	P	0.01 to 0.2 µg/mL	0.5 to 10.5 µmol/L
	U	0.2 to 1.1 µg/mL	10.5 to 57.9 µmol/L
I	P	0.8 to 6.0 µg/L	102 to 761 µmol/L
T$_4$ free	Newborn	2.6 to 6.3 ng/dL	33.5 to 81.3 pmol/L
	Adult	0.8 to 2.3 ng/dL	10.3 to 31.0 pmol/L
T$_4$ total	S adult	5 to 12 µg/dL	65 to 155 µmmg/L
T$_3$ free (equilibrium dialysis)	S cord blood	15 to 391 pg/DI	0.2 to 6.0 pmol/L
	Children and adults	260 to 380 pg/dL	4.0 to 7.4 pmol/L
	Adult	208 to 674 pg/dL	3.2 to 104 pmol/L
T$_3$ total	Adult	100 to 200 ng/dL	1.54 to 3.08
Mn	S	0.5 to 1.5 µg/L	9 to 27 nmol/L
	B	~11 µg/L	~200 nmol/L
	U	0.2 to 0.5 µg/L	3.6 to 9.0 nmol/L
Mo	S	0.1 to 3.0 µg/L	1.0 to 31.3 nmol/L
Se	S	124.3 to 165 µg/L	1.57 to 2.09 µmol/L
	≥11 years	46 to 143 µg/L	0.58 to 1.81 µmol/L
	Adult	85 to 145 µg/L	1.08 to 1.84 µmol/L
	Toxicity	>400 µg/L	>5.06 µmol/L
	U	7 to 60 µg/L	0.09 to 0.78 µg/L
Zn	S	70 to 120 µg/dL	10.7 to 18.3 µmol/L
	U	300 to 500 µg/day	4.58 to 7.64 µmol

B, Whole blood; IU, standard international units; P, plasma; RBC, red blood cell; S, serum; U, urine.

plasma approximately 95% of copper is bound to ceruloplasmin, an α_2-globulin with ferroxidase activity. Copper is also transported in the plasma loosely bound to albumin. A small fraction of plasma copper is complexed with amino acids.

Although 1.5 to 3 mg/day of dietary copper has been determined to be safe and adequate (Table 38-2), it is estimated that 35% of diets in the United States provide less than 1 mg/day. Excretion of copper occurs mainly in the bile, with urinary excretion normally <40 µg/day.

Clinical significance. A relatively high carbohydrate intake in the American diet accompanied by marginal intake of copper possibly potentiates subclinical copper deficiency.[11] There is evidence that marginal copper deficiency is associated with heart disease, bone and joint osteoarthritis, and osteoporosis. Microcytic, hypochromic anemia, neutropenia, hypothermia, and demineralization have also been associated with copper deficiency. Copper deficiency in humans results in hypercholesterolemia[12] and decreased antioxidant protection. In an X-linked genetic defect seen in 1 in 35,000 to 50,000 infants by 2 to 3 months, Menkes' kinky hair syndrome, absorption of copper from the gastrointestinal tract is impaired. The resulting copper deficiency is manifested by severe cerebellar and cerebral degeneration, subdural hematoma and/or thrombosis of arteries in the brain, osteoporosis, motor delay, and failure to thrive.[13] Many infants with Menkes' syndrome die within the first decade of life, usually by the age of three.

TABLE 38-5 ACCEPTABLE AND TOXIC REFERENCE RANGES FOR TOXIC TRACE METALS

Element	Specimen Type	REFERENCE RANGE Concentration	IU
Al	S	<4 µg/L	148 nmol/L
	U	0.120 mg/day	0.4 to 4 µmol/L
	S toxic	See text	
As	B	2 to 62 µg/L	26 to 826 µmol/L
	U	5 to 50 µg/day	66 to 660 nmol/day
	B acute toxicity; B chronic toxicity	600 to 9300 µg/L	8 to 125 µmol/L
Cd	B	<5 µg/L	<44.6 nmol/L
	U	<3 µg/day	<26 nmol/L
	Toxic	>50 µg/L	>446 nmol/L
Hg	B	<5 µg/L	<24.9 nmol/L
	B (dentists)	5 to 15 µg/L	24.9 to 74.7 nmol/L
	U	<20 µg/day	<99.5 nmol/L
	B toxicity	>50 µg/day	>249 nmol/L
	Hair	<1 µg/g	<4.9 nmol/g
Pb	B (children)	<100 µg/L	<480 nmol/L

B, Whole blood; IU, standard international units; S, serum; U, urine.

Wilson's disease is an inherited autosomal recessive error in copper metabolism that results in excessive accumulation of copper in liver, brain, cornea, and kidneys.[14] Ceruloplasmin levels are low, with elevated levels of nonceruloplasmin-bound copper. Tissue copper deposits may be diminished and then excreted by the intravenous administration of a chelating agent.[14]

Marginal copper deficiency, especially in adults, has so far proved to be difficult to detect biochemically. Milne and Johnson[15] have concluded that diminished cytochrome oxidase activity in leukocytes or diminished superoxide dismutase activity in erythrocytes is likely to be the most reliable index of reduced levels of metabolically active copper.

Plasma copper is not a reliable indicator of copper status. Although long-term copper deprivation, as in treatment by TPN, results in low plasma levels, chronic therapy with corticosteroids and adrenocorticotropic hormone (ACTH) also reduces copper levels. Factors that are associated with elevated serum copper levels include oral contraceptives, pregnancy, and infectious or inflammatory conditions.

Food sources of copper. Most foods contain appreciable amounts of copper. Those rich in copper include shellfish, liver, kidney, egg yolk, and some legumes.

Methods.[16] Flame atomic absorption spectrophotometry for serum or plasma, and graphite furnace flameless atomic absorption spectrophotometry for urine, where concentration is usually less than 40 µg/L, are the preferred methods of analysis.

Reference intervals. Serum or plasma levels vary with age and are higher in adult women than in men (Table 38-4). Most copper is excreted through the bile, and urine levels are usually less than 40 µg/day.

Fluorine (F)[17-21]

Fluorine, atomic weight 19, is the first member of period 2 of the group VII halogens of the periodic table of elements.

Biochemistry. The fluoride anion may substitute for the hydroxyl ion in the hydroxyapatite crystal structure in calcified tissues, bone, and teeth. The production of a "harder" crystal is believed to account for the protective effect of fluoride against **dental caries**.[17] Fluoride has also been used therapeutically, alone or in combination with vitamin D, in the treatment of osteoporosis.

Clinical significance. A direct, inverse association between the incidence of dental caries and the fluoride concentration in drinking water of ≤1 mg/L has long been recognized. Less convincing is a reported beneficial effect of sodium fluoride as a therapy for osteoporosis.[18,19]

Requirement. The daily requirement is 1 to 2 mg/day. Usually a fluoridated water supply with 1 mg/L of fluoride provides the daily requirement.

Food sources. Traces of fluoride are present in most foods. Fluoride can be present in drinking water, either naturally or because of artificial supplementation.

Toxicity. A high intake of fluoride causes *dental fluorosis* characterized by discolored and mottled teeth. Increased bone density and calcification of muscle insertions evident by radiography occur in areas where 10 to 45 mg/L of fluoride is present in water.

Method. An ion-selective electrode[21] method is the preferred method of analysis.

Reference intervals.[21] Reference intervals in plasma are: 0.01 to 0.2 µg/mL; 0.5 to 10.5 µmol/L. Reference intervals in urine are: 0.2 to 1.1 µg/mL; 10.5 to 57.9 µmol/L.

Iodine (I)[22-24]

Iodine, atomic weight 127, is in period 5 of the group VII halogens of the periodic table of elements.

Biochemistry. Although iodine is widely distributed throughout the earth's surface, the sea is the major source of iodine. Iodides, oxidized by sunlight to the volatile elemental iodine, are estimated to provide annually some 400,000 tons of iodine to the atmosphere from seawater. The iodide concentration in seawater, approximately 50 µg/L, is similar to that of human serum.

Iodine is of significance in human biology as a constituent of the thyroid gland's hormones, thyroxine (3,5,3′,5′-tetraiodothyronine, (T_4) and 3,5,3′-triiodothyronine (T_3), which are synthesized by the iodination of tyrosine (see Chapter 44 for details). These hormones are essential for healthy growth, differentiation, and development. Iodine deficiency occurs in areas where soil is depleted of iodide. Uptake by crops is directly proportional to soil content. Iodine-deficiency disease is still a frequent occurrence in various underdeveloped countries.

Clinical significance. Both maternal and fetal thyroid hormones contribute to fetal development. Iodine deficiency during pregnancy may result in spontaneous abortions, stillbirths, an increase in infant or perinatal mortality, congenital abnormalities or neurological cretinism, fetal hypothyroidism, and psychomotor defects. Most areas in the United States screen for neonatal hypothyroidism, which is readily treatable. In the child and adolescent, goiter, mental retardation, and retarded development are prominent signs of hypothyroidism. Myxedematous, or neurological, cretinism is also seen. In adults endemic goiter results from iodine deficiency. Iodine status may be determined by measurement of either serum thyroid hormone levels or urine iodine excretion.[22]

Requirements. Iodine requirements vary with age (Table 38-1).

Food sources. Marine fish and seaweed are rich in iodine.

Toxicity. Prolonged excess of iodine intake (>2 mg/day) results in iodide goiter and myxedema.

Methods. Immunoassay[24] for thyroid hormones and ion-selective electrode methods for iodide are the recommended methods of analysis.

Reference intervals.[23] See Chapter 44 for levels of iodine-containing hormones. Reference intervals for plasma inorganic iodide are 0.8 to 6.0 µg/L. Urine inorganic iodide correlates with plasma level. The lower limit of the reference interval is age dependent: 5 to 10 years, 32.5 µg/g creatinine; adolescents, 50 µg/g creatinine; adults, 75 µg/g creatinine.

Manganese (Mn)[25-29]

Manganese is a transition element in period 4 of the periodic table of the elements with an atomic weight of 55.

Biochemistry. Manganese forms divalent and trivalent salts. It is important for proper metabolism in connective tissue, physical growth and development of reproductive functions, and proper carbohydrate and lipid metabolism. It functions as an enzyme activator, however, and other divalent cations, in particular magnesium, may substitute for manganese. Enzymes that may have high specificity for manganese are glycosyl transferases and mitochondrial pyruvate carboxylase and superoxide dismutase.[25] The total manganese content in adult humans is 12 to 20 mg, of which 25% is in the skeleton. The usual intake ranges from 1.7 to 8.3 mg/day, of which 2% to 15% is absorbed. Absorption occurs in the small intestine and is inhibited by the presence of other divalent cations, including Fe, Ca, and Mg, and by phosphate, fiber, and phytate. Excess manganese is excreted through bile and pancreatic secretions; only a small amount is excreted in the urine.

Clinical significance. Manganese deficiency in humans has not been unambiguously demonstrated. An anecdotal report in association with experimental vitamin K deficiency has not been substantiated.[27] A manganese deficiency has been suspected in hip abnormalities, joint disease, congenital skeletal deformities, and childhood epilepsy. Serum manganese has been reported to be increased in myocardial infarction, in acute hepatitis, and in industrial manganese exposure. Industrial poisoning produces schizophrenia-like psychiatric effects and neurological disorders similar to those of Parkinson's disease. Symptoms arising from a decrease in striatal dopamine present in manganese poisoning can be reversed by administration of L-dopa, the precursor of dopamine.[28]

Requirement. The estimated safe and adequate dietary intake for various ages is shown in Table 38-2.

Food sources. Bran flakes and wheat are rich in manganese. Refined grains and meat contain little manganese.

Toxicity. Manganese toxicity from prolonged industrial exposure results in neurological changes resembling those of Parkinson's disease.[28]

Method. Zeeman graphite furnace atomic absorption spectrophotometry is the preferred analytical procedure. Magnesium nitrate is recommended as matrix modifier.[29]

Reference intervals. Reference intervals in whole blood are approximately 11 µg/L; approximately 200 nmol/L. Intervals in serum are 0.5 to 1.5 µg/L; 9 to 27 nmol/L; and in urine are 0.2 to 0.5 µg/L; 3.6 to 9.0 nmol/L.

Molybdenum (Mo)[30-34]

Molybdenum is a transition element in period 5 of the periodic table of the elements, with an atomic weight of 96.

Biochemistry. Molybdenum is a cofactor of the metalloenzymes xanthine oxidase, sulfite oxidase, and aldehyde oxidase, and thus plays a role in the metabolism of purines to uric acid, the final stages of oxidation of sulfur-containing amino acids, and the oxidation of aldehydes, respectively. Absorption of molybdenum from the gastrointestinal tract may be inhibited by competition from dietary copper if copper intake is high.

Clinical significance. Most of the available evidence on the metabolism of molybdenum results from animal studies. Increased intake of molybdenum inhibits copper utilization; this effect is potentiated by increased sulfate intake. Molybdenum retention is decreased in the presence of excess copper or sulfate.[31] An increase in molybdenum intake is accompanied by increased serum levels of uric acid and the development of gout.

A case of molybdenum deficiency in a patient maintained on TPN was reported.[32] Elevated levels of the amino acid methionine and decreased uric acid excretion and sulfate excretion were corrected by administration of molybdenum, indicating a reduced activity of molybdenum-containing metalloenzymes in the molybdenum-deficient patient.

Requirement. An estimate of the safe and adequate daily intake of molybdenum ranges from 10 µg in infancy to 250 µg in adults.

Food sources. Milk, milk products, organ meats, and dried legumes and cereals contain molybdenum.

Toxicity. A single report from Armenia documented elevated blood levels of molybdenum that were associated with high levels of molybdenum in soil and plants.[33] Symptoms of gout were reported, as well as others that indicated possible involvement of the liver, gastrointestinal tract, and kidney.

Method. Graphite furnace atomic absorption spectrophotometry is the recommended method of analysis for molybdenum.[34]

Reference interval. The reference interval for serum molybdenum is 0.1 to 3.0 μg/L.

Selenium (Se)[35-44]

Selenium is in period 4, group VI, of the periodic table of the elements and has an atomic weight of 79.

Biochemistry.[35] Selenium is a member of the same group of elements as oxygen and sulfur. It is known that in plants selenium is present predominantly as selenomethionine, whereas in animals selenocysteine is the major form. Four selenium atoms are covalently bound to cysteine residues in the enzyme glutathione peroxidase, which has strong antioxidant properties and, in animal models, acts synergistically with vitamin E. Glutathione peroxidase is present in the cytoplasm and mitochondria of tissues. It is also found in erythrocytes, platelets, and plasma. A second enzyme, type 1 iodothyronine deiodinase, has been identified, and it contains one selenium atom per molecule. This selenium-metalloenzyme plays a role in the conversion of T_4 to T_3.[35]

Selenium enters the food chain via plants. Because of the wide variability in the concentration range of selenium in various areas throughout the world, low availability of selenium may occur in some areas, whereas in seleniferous areas excessive selenium is taken up by plants.[37] In human studies, the bioavailability of selenium from wheat, tuna, and mushrooms was 83%, 57%, and 5%, respectively, compared with that of sodium selenite. However, the form in which selenium occurs in foods is still unknown.

Clinical significance. Although no single marker for selenium status has been identified, plasma selenium is an indication of recent ingestion. Erythrocyte and platelet glutathione peroxidase activity correlates well with selenium supplementation in patients maintained on home TPN.[41] Urine selenium varies with intake, and, at very high levels of intake, volatile forms of selenium are exhaled. Nails and hair, which can have a high presence of sulfur- or selenium-containing proteins, have both been assessed for measurement of selenium status. In the United States the use of selenium-containing shampoos precludes the use of hair for such measurement.

Low selenium status has been recognized when intake is below the RDA shown in Table 38-1; chronic ingestion of levels above the RDA produces clinical symptoms. Experimentally selenium has been shown to be protective against mercury, cadmium, and silver toxicity, suggesting a preventive role for the element.

Selenium deficiency has been demonstrated in Keshan (pronounced *kuh-shahn*), a city in Manchuria, China, where soil selenium content is very low.[40] Although Keshan disease, often associated with a cardiomyopathy in children and young females, responded to supplementation by selenium, the selenium deficiency is not considered to be the sole cause of this condition, and the implication of a virus or other agent has been considered. In other areas such as New Zealand, Finland, and Sweden, where low selenium status has been demonstrated, serious detrimental effects of the low soil selenium have not been observed. A second disease associated with low selenium intake in China is Kashin-Bek disease, which causes cartilage degeneration and osteoarthritis in adolescents and preadolescents. Patients maintained on long-term TPN are at risk of developing selenium deficiency if fluids are not supplemented. Numerous such cases have been reported, and several deaths associated with cardiomyopathy have occurred.

Requirement. The RDA for selenium is shown in Table 38-1 and ranges from 10 μg in infants to 75 μg in adults.

Food sources. In decreasing order of magnitude, organ meats and seafood, cereals and grains, dairy products, and fruits and vegetables are sources of dietary selenium.

Toxicity. Selenium toxicity is characterized by dermatitis, loose hair, and diseased nails. Selenium poisoning resulting from excessive intake of supplements results in acute toxicity. Symptoms include a metallic taste, odor of garlic, mucosal irritation, gastroenteritis, paronychia, and reddening of nails, hair, and teeth.[43] There is evidence that chronic ingestion of moderately elevated levels of selenium may be carcinogenic.

Method.[44] Zeeman graphite furnace atomic absorption analysis with nickel nitrate or reduced palladium as matrix modifier is the recommended analysis method.

Reference intervals. Reference intervals in serum[42] vary from region to region depending on the selenium content of the soil of food sources. The mean serum levels (±1 SEM) for adults in the United States are 1.10 (±0.10) μmol/L for men and 1.20 (±0.18) μmol/L for women.

Zinc (Zn)[45-52]

Zinc is a transition element in period 4 of the periodic table of the elements and has an atomic weight of 65.

Biochemistry. Zinc forms stable complexes, called **zinc fingers**, with the histidine and cysteine amino acid residues of proteins, and is a component of more than 200 metalloenzymes. Important among the enzymes are those involved in nucleic acid and protein synthesis, including DNA and RNA polymerases, and reverse transcriptase. Regulatory proteins containing zinc fingers are central to gene expression.

Zinc induces the synthesis of metallothionein, which serves an important regulatory function of zinc and copper metabolism. The protein binds copper more firmly than zinc and forms an unabsorbable complex in the gastrointestinal tract, hence reducing copper absorption. In the liver, induction of metallothionein synthesis is significant in cases of stress and infection when this organ sequesters zinc. Zinc fingers, defined as domains of zinc-binding proteins that also bind to DNA, are involved in the gene expression of metallothionein.

Zinc is an intracellular cation present in all body tissues and fluids and, next to iron, is the second most abundant of the trace metals in humans. Muscle contains 50% to 60% of the 2 g of total body zinc. Bone contains 28% of body zinc stores, and 0.5% is found in blood. Erythrocytes contain 75% to 88% of blood zinc. In the plasma approximately 18% of zinc (normal range 700 to 1200 µg/L) is tightly bound to an α_2-macroglobulin, 80% is loosely bound to albumin, 2% is bound to transferrin, ceruloplasmin, or the amino acids histidine and cysteine, and a small fraction is present as free zinc.

The RDA of 15 mg of zinc for adult males and 12 mg for females is not likely to be provided by many diets consumed in the United States. Red meat is a prime source of bioavailable zinc. Hence, vegetarians are at risk for zinc insufficiency. In addition, the high fiber content of a vegetarian diet binds zinc and hence diminishes its bioavailability. From a usual nonvegetarian diet approximately 20% of zinc is absorbed. Meats, liver, eggs, and seafood enhance absorption, whereas vegetables, whole grain foods, fiber, phytate, calcium, and iron inhibit absorption.

Clinical significance. Because zinc is required for the activity of enzymes that are critical for nucleic acid replication and protein synthesis, it is a necessary component for cell replication. Adequate supplies of zinc are imperative for healthy development of the fetus, and in early pregnancy plasma zinc falls despite increased intake. During pregnancy there is an increase in the plasma zinc fraction bound to α_2-macroglobulin and a decrease in the zinc bound to albumin. Plasma zinc is elevated during lactation.

Zinc deficiency was first described by Prasad et al[47,48] in Iran and Egypt. Male adolescents showed retarded development and hypogonadism. Experimental zinc deficiency in animals is characterized by fetal abnormalities, impaired embryogenesis, impaired brain development, and impaired vision. Acute zinc deficiency in humans, especially in growing children, is apparent from skin lesions especially on body extremities or around orifices, diarrhea, irritability, hair loss, growth retardation, and increased susceptibility to infections. An inherited autosomal recessive abnormality in ability to absorb zinc from the gastrointestinal tract was first described by Moynahan and Barnes.[49] In sickle cell anemia, some cancers, and traumas such as burns, stress, and acute infections, plasma zinc may fall precipitously, probably as the result of its redistribution to other tissues such as liver.

Impaired immunological function is associated with zinc insufficiency. In vitro, stimulation of lymphocytes by phytohemagglutinin and concavalin A is enhanced by zinc. In vivo, a delayed hypersensitive response to skin allergens occurs consistent with the degree of zinc deficiency.

Identification of a reliable marker for assessment of zinc status has yet to be realized. Although abnormal plasma zinc levels are associated with many pathological conditions, plasma zinc concentrations are a poor indicator of the body status of zinc. Plasma levels of zinc may be lowered in response to stress and trauma, but do not reflect intracellular status. Leukocyte zinc has been suggested as a reliable marker, but consistent findings have yet to be reported. Urinary excretion of zinc in response to a zinc challenge has been explored as a marker of zinc nutriture, as has the level of zinc in hair. Further investigation is required before any of these markers can be recommended. The use of stable isotopes of zinc[50] showed that in premenopausal women zinc disappeared more rapidly from the plasma of those women judged to be zinc deficient. In both this and an earlier study, an inverse relationship between serum ferritin and zinc status was suggested. A strong association between zinc and iron nutriture was demonstrated. It is considered that marginal zinc deficiency is common and should be considered a public health problem.[51]

Requirement. The RDA for zinc is shown in Table 38-1. An increase in intake to 30 mg/day is recommended during pregnancy.

Food sources. Seafoods, meat, milk, and eggs are good sources of zinc. Although vegetables contain appreciable amounts of zinc, the presence of high concentrations of fiber and phytate account for zinc's low bioavailability in these food sources.

Toxicity. Epigastric pain, diarrhea, and vomiting have been observed from high zinc intake from food stored in galvanized containers. Supplements of as little as 25 mg of zinc have resulted in diminished absorption of copper, presumably because of competition.

Method.[52] The preferred method for zinc analysis is flame atomic absorption spectrophotometry in serum or plasma, with its erythrocytes, and in urine.

Reference intervals. Reference intervals in serum are 700 to 1200 µg/L; 10.7 to 18.3 µmol/L and in urine are 300 to 500 µg/day; 4.58 to 7.64 µmol/day.

TOXIC TRACE METALS

There are many toxic trace metals. We shall limit our discussion to the ones more commonly monitored.

Aluminum (Al)[53-59]

Aluminum is classified as a period 3 element with an atomic weight of 27.

Basis for toxicity. Aluminum toxicity can result from exposure to industrial sources of aluminum, but most commonly the cause is iatrogenic. Patients who have chronic renal failure are at high risk for aluminum toxicity from two sources. First, these patients use antacids containing aluminum hydroxide to decrease phosphate absorption. Second, aluminum may be present in the dialysate used for chronic dialysis of patients with end-stage renal disease. A second group of potentially vulnerable patients are those receiving TPN. Premature infants who receive TPN are particularly at risk for aluminum toxicity because of their reduced renal clearance. Casein hydrolysates were found to contain high concentrations of aluminum,[53-56] and components such as calcium and phosphate[57] have been shown to contain appreciable aluminum contamination.

In all cases of aluminum toxicity, the brain and the skeleton are the two target organs.[53,54] Although the biochemical basis for the neurotoxic effects of aluminum is uncertain, an association was found between high brain-aluminum concentrations at autopsy and dialysis dementia or dialysis encephalopathy in a large number of patients with renal failure who were undergoing chronic dialysis. By contrast, the finding of elevated brain aluminum in patients with Alzheimer's disease has not been uniformly reported.

Deposition of aluminum along the calcification front in bone has long been recognized. The development of bone pain in dialysis patients can indicate an excessive accumulation of aluminum. Bone morphology in these cases is consistent with osteomalacia (see p. 521, Chapter 28). Another major sign of aluminum toxicity is microcytic anemia.

The use of free amino acids instead of casein hydrolysate considerably reduced the aluminum load from artificially prepared nutrients used for enteral and parenteral nutritional supplements. The finding of varying amounts of aluminum in different batches of the same ingredient, from the same and different manufacturers, accents the need for monitoring the aluminum content of TPN solutions. A working group for standards for aluminum content of parenteral nutrition solutions supports the Food and Drug Administration's proposal for setting a limit of 25 mg of aluminum per liter in large-volume parenteral fluids. It has been recommended that many TPN components, including solutions of minerals, trace metals, and vitamins and heparin, should require a statement of the aluminum content on their label. Other intravenous fluids such as immunoglobulins and albumin also contain variable amounts of aluminum.

Serum levels and indications for treatment. Reference intervals for serum aluminum vary among laboratories because of the ease of contamination. An upper limit of 4 µg/L (0.15 µmol/L) is considered to be within the reference interval. Serum aluminum levels do not necessarily reflect the amount of metal deposited in bone, liver, and brain. Bone pain is a useful clinical indicator of the degree of aluminum toxicity. The effectiveness of chelation therapy with desferrioxamine during dialysis can be monitored by measurement of serum aluminum.

Method. Zeeman graphite furnace atomic absorption spectrophotometry using magnesium nitrate as matrix modifier[53] is the recommended method of analysis.

Arsenic (As)[60-66]

Arsenic is a period 4 element with an atomic weight of 75.

Basis for toxicity. There is evidence that a very small amount of arsenic is essential in humans.[60] Arsenic has been shown to give protection against selenosis.[62] In tissues, arsenic is present in both trivalent and pentavalent states. Organic arsenic compounds containing methyl groups are the most important biochemically. Arsenate may be able to replace phosphate in some biological molecules.

The relative toxicity of oral arsenic trioxide is low: A fatal acute dose is estimated to be 10.2 to 26 nmol (0.76 to 1.95 µg) of arsenic per kilogram of body weight. In animal experiments 10 g/kg of body weight of arsenobetaine produced symptoms that disappeared within an hour.

Arsenic is usually found in all tissues, with skin, hair, and nails showing the highest concentrations,[61] because of arsenic binding to sulfhydryl (—SH) groups of proteins.

Symptoms of acute toxicity in humans from oral intake of arsenic are nausea, vomiting, diarrhea, burning of the mouth and throat, and severe abdominal pain.[62] Chronic exposure to smaller toxic doses causes weakness, prostration, muscle aches, and, in children, loss of hearing at low frequencies. Headaches, drowsiness, and confusion occur both in acute and chronic toxicity. Although the mechanism for the symptoms is not defined, arsenic probably inhibits enzyme activity.

Both the absorption of organic forms of arsenic from the gastrointestinal tract and its excretion in the urine are highly efficient. Urine excretion is an effective mode of monitoring body status.[63] Refined techniques such as high-performance liquid chromatography are required to characterize the form in which arsenic is excreted.

Treatment.[64-66] Treatment of acute poisoning with D-penicillamine, 2,3-dimercapto-1-propanesulfonate, 2,3-dimercaptosuccinic acid, or 2,3-dimercaptopropanol (BAL) has been successful in humans.

Method. The recommended method of analysis is flameless atomic absorption.

Cadmium (Cd)[67-73]

Cadmium is a period 5 element with an atomic weight of 112.4.

Basis for toxicity. The primary organs affected by cadmium toxicity are liver and kidney.[68] Cadmium toxicity may be the result of the formation of cadmium-metallothionein, which prevents the usual binding of zinc and copper to metallothionein, thus preventing the healthy functioning of the target organs.

Clinical significance. Cadmium is present in human infants in very low concentrations, but the metal accumulates rapidly within the first 3 years of life and continues to accumulate up to approximately 50 years of age. The level in blood, which is usually <1 µg/L, is increased about 50% in smokers.[69,70] Urinary excretion is approximately 1 µg/L normally, and higher in smokers.

Only small amounts of cadmium are absorbed from the gut. Absorbed cadmium is stored in the liver and preferentially in the renal cortex. Retention in the liver and kidney is explained by the formation of cadmium-metallothionein in these organs.[71] It is estimated that the biological half-life of cadmium is approximately 30 years. It is postulated that in the kidney low levels of cadmium reduce the number of binding sites in metallothionein for zinc and copper, thus interfering with the usual function of metallothionein in the kidney. Inhalation of cadmium results in renal damage even before impaired lung function is detected, causing a low–molecular-weight proteinuria and a reduced glomerular filtration rate. Osteomalacia (itai-itai disease) in Japanese women has been ascribed to cadmium exposure.[72]

Treatment. Chelation therapy has been found to be efficient immediately after toxic exposure to cadmium but less effective later. Diethylenetriaminepentaacetate probably does not effectively chelate the less accessible intracellular cadmium. However, BAL, if continuously administered, has been shown to increase biliary excretion of cadmium.[73]

Method. The recommended method of analysis is flameless atomic absorption.

Lead (Pb)[74-82]

Lead is considered to be a heavy metal and lies in period 6 of the periodic table of elements. Its atomic weight is 207.

Basis for toxicity. The major source of lead in the environment, apart from industrial waste, is lead-based paint in the interior and exterior of wooden houses. Subsequent removal or decay of the paint leads to soil and water contamination and possible exposure of children to lead contamination. Other potential sources of lead contamination, such as lead pipes that are used for conveying water and lead solder used in food cans, have been largely eliminated.

Several enzymes in the heme synthetic pathway are inhibited, in vitro, by lead (see also p. 669). The cytosolic enzymes δ-aminolevulinic acid synthetase and δ-aminolevulinic acid dehydratase are readily inhibited.[74] However, this effect has not been unequivocally demonstrated in vivo. Anemia is usually present in subjects when the blood-lead level exceeds 400 µg/L (1.92 µmol/L). In both iron deficiency and lead poisoning there is decreased incorporation of ferrous iron into protoporphyrin IX, a step needed for the synthesis of heme, and the replacement of iron by zinc to form zinc protoporphyrin occurs. Erythrocyte protoporphyrin begins to rise at a blood-lead level of 200 µg/L.

Lead absorption by the intestines is increased when a deficiency of iron, calcium, magnesium, zinc, phosphate, or vitamin D is present.[74] The use of dietary supplements of one or more of these nutrients is suggested as preventive or remedial treatment for lead toxicity.

Clinical significance of lead toxicity. Lead toxicity produces neurological, gastrointestinal, renal, immunological, endocrinological, and hematopoietic changes in humans. Children 6 months to 6 years of age are most affected, because they are growing rapidly and lead crosses the blood-brain barrier at an age when brain development is critical. Although the detrimental effects of lead have been recognized for many years, it is now believed that these effects occur at lower blood-lead concentrations than was previously believed. The work of Needleman and others[75,76,79] convincingly demonstrated a lowering of IQ in children with blood lead as low as 100 µg/L. At this level the magnitude of the problem, which affects millions of children, was recognized, and widespread efforts were undertaken to prevent or minimize the possibility of increasing exposure. In 1991 the Centers for Disease Control and Prevention (CDC) published a statement on preventing lead poisoning in young children.[77]

Blood-lead levels.[78,79] Although the level of blood lead considered to be safe is currently <100 µg/L, there is evidence that even lower blood-lead concentrations may be detrimental in growing children. Although no specific action level has been suggested, the CDC has suggested diagnostic evaluation and medical management of children at lead levels of >200 µg/L. Adults are less vulnerable to the neurological damage caused by lead than children are, but a blood-lead level of 300 µg/L or higher in an adult requires evaluation. In New York State, all blood-lead values in children must be reported to the State Department of Health, and values >200 µg/L in children and >400 µg/L in adults are considered critical.

Treatment. The treatment of lead toxicity with chelating agents has included the use of penicillamine, calcium-ethylenediaminetetraacetic acid (Ca-EDTA), and 2,3-dimercaptopropanol. Dimercaptosuccinic acid (Succimer),[80] which may be administered orally, appears to have the fewest side effects. Effectiveness of treatment may be monitored by measurement of urine excretion of lead.[82]

Method.[81-82] Zeeman graphite furnace atomic absorption spectrophotometry is the recommended method of analysis. Matrix modifiers of ammonium dihydrogen phosphate and magnesium nitrate together are effective.

Mercury (Hg)[83-89]

Mercury is a transition element also in period 6 of the periodic table of elements, with an atomic weight of 201.

Biochemistry. Mercury is usually present in all body tissues tested in humans, even in the absence of any identified exposure apart from dental amalgams. In fresh tissue, levels ranged from 0.1 to 0.5 µg/g. The highest levels occur in skin, nails, and hair. The kidneys contain higher mercury concentrations than liver, brain, thyroid, and pituitary do. In populations exposed to industrial mercury, the pituitary and thyroid concentrate mercury to a greater degree than other organs. Elevated tissue levels of mercury are usually associated with an elevation of selenium, with both elements present in a 1:1 molar ratio.

Inorganic mercury is poorly absorbed. However, alkyl derivatives of mercury, especially methyl mercury, formed by the action of microorganisms in sediments in fresh water and seawater, enter the food chain and are approximately 90% absorbed. Mercury vapor is efficiently absorbed by inhalation, and approximately 80% of inhaled mercury is retained.

There is a national effort to reduce the presence of mercury in hospitals and laboratories because these represent a major source of mercury pollution (see p. 30, Chapter 1). In addition, the American Academy of Pediatrics has alerted the public about the exposure of newborns to mercury, which is a common preservative (Thimerosal; contains ~50% mercury by weight) of some vaccines.

The most common food source of mercury is fish, in which the element is present as methyl mercury.[84] In the United States and other countries, limits of 0.1[85] to 0.4[86] mg Hg/kg of fish per day have been established for safe consumption. The red blood cell readily takes up methyl mercury, with a blood cell-to-plasma ratio of approximately 20:1. Populations with a heavy fish consumption may have blood-mercury levels as high as 400 µg/L. Methyl mercury crosses the placenta, and the level in cord blood correlates well with that of the mother,[87] though slightly higher. Inhalation of mercury vapor results in a smaller increase in mercury in red blood cells than is observed from methyl mercury absorption.

Clinical significance. Mercury poisoning affects the central nervous system (CNS). CNS abnormalities associated with mercury poisoning include tremors, incoordination, irritability, moodiness, and depression.[88] Salivation, diarrhea, stomatitis, and impaired vision accompany the neurological abnormalities. The passage of methyl mercury across the placenta is associated with increases in congenital abnormalities, mental retardation, cerebral palsy, and fetal mortality. All these symptoms were present after an incident termed the *Minamata Bay incident*,[84] in which industrial wastes containing mercury were dumped into Minamata Bay. In Minamata disease, increased levels of methyl mercury were found in fetal tissue, most particularly in the brain.

Mercury concentration in hair has been shown to correlate well with blood levels of mercury. The concentration in hair is approximately tenfold higher than the levels seen in blood. Clinical manifestations of mercury intoxication appear at whole blood levels of 200 µg/L, which can result from an exposure of about 0.3 mg of mercury per day as methyl mercury; this is a dosage equivalent to approximately 4 mg of mercury per kilogram of body weight in an adult.

Method.[89] Cold vapor atomic absorption spectrophotometry is the preferred method for analysis of inorganic mercury. Predigestion is required to convert methyl mercury to inorganic mercury.

Critical levels in blood and urine.[86] Critical levels in blood are >20 µg/L; 0.10 µmol/L, in red blood cells >40 µg/L; 0.20 µmol/L, and in urine 150 to 300 µg/L; 0.75 µmol/L.

CONSIDERATIONS IN ASSESSING TRACE-ELEMENT STATUS IN HUMANS

The roles of essential trace elements in biology are summarized in Table 38-3. The status of most of the essential trace elements cannot be assessed from their concentration in whole blood or plasma, the most easily accessible body component, and this remains a problem in patient care. Because it is not possible to assign a threshold for plasma or serum zinc, copper, selenium, chromium, or manganese below which supplementation of the respective element is indicated, other biochemical parameters should be considered concomitantly for assessment of trace-metal nutriture. These include dietary availability, existing conditions that may involve redistribution within the body, genetic disorders, hormonal regulation in the case of iodine, and the functional state of excretory organs. In addition, the presence of clinical signs and symptoms that are usually associated with a deficiency of a trace metal is an important diagnostic finding. Hence, a plasma zinc amount less than 500 µg/L associated with dermatological lesions, especially in a rapidly growing child, is suggestive of severe acute zinc deficiency. Investigation would be necessary to determine if the deficiency resulted from an insufficient dietary intake of zinc or from malabsorption of zinc as occurs in the genetic disorder acrodermatitis enteropathica. In cases of trauma such as burns, a similarly low plasma zinc level indicates redistribution of zinc, and the necessity for zinc supplementation is equivocal. Usually, the main route of excretion of endogenous zinc is the gastrointestinal tract, with contributions from pancreatic secretions and bile. The intestinal absorption of trace metals can be reduced as a result of the competition between zinc, iron, copper, manganese, and other divalent minerals in the diet. Trace-metal absorption may also be decreased in high-fiber diets because of the binding of the metals to phytates.

Although very low levels of plasma copper, such as 300 µg/L, and ceruloplasmin (which binds 60% to 95% of the copper) are indicative of frank copper deficiency, the plasma level is generally not a good indicator of copper status. Hence, functional tests, such as response to antigenic challenge for zinc and measurement of a copper-requiring enzyme such as superoxide dismutase or cytochrome oxidase, are considered to be useful in the assessment of the status of these metals. Serum selenium is an acceptable indicator of recent selenium absorption.

Chromium status is currently best assessed by the patient's ability to metabolize glucose. Excretion of glucose in the urine can be monitored for this purpose. Difficulties with obtaining an accurate (contamination-free) measurement of the very low levels of chromium seen in either serum or urine minimize the value of direct chromium measurements for the assessment of chromium status.

Deficiencies of trace elements in patients maintained on TPN or by enteral feeding are now rare, but consideration must be given to ensure adequate supplementation in these groups of patients, especially when the therapy is over a long term. If periodic estimations of zinc, copper, selenium, or manganese reveal a decrease in the plasma levels of a trace metal when the patient's condition is stable, the possibility of a deficiency should be further explored.

People who consume over-the-counter nutritional supplements may have an intake of trace elements that greatly exceed suggested limits (Tables 38-1 and 38-2). Very often claims of improved health with supplements are not validated by proper studies and these supplements may result in health problems rather than improved health.

An emerging problem is the potential and actual exposure of people to toxic levels of trace metals that rarely were present in the environment. For example, an increasing number of people receive metal implants that contain significant levels of trace metals. The long-range effects of such implants are not known. In addition, *beryllium* is being used with increased frequency in computers, cellular telephones, and dental works. Workers manufacturing these materials are at risk for *berylliosis*, an often-fatal lung disease.

Identification of the biochemical parameters that can be measured to indicate the status of trace elements in the body remains a challenge. Appropriate function tests or tests that measure the activity of an enzyme that has a specific requirement for a particular trace metal that are suitable for routine testing in a clinical chemistry laboratory have yet to be realized.

References

Classification of Trace Elements

1. Subcommittee on the tenth edition of the RDA's Food and Nutrition Board, Commission on Life Sciences, National Research Council: *Recommended dietary allowances*, ed 10, Washington, DC, 1989, National Academy Press .

Essential Trace Elements

Chromium

2. Anderson RA: Chromium. In Wertz W, editor: *Trace elements in human and animal nutrition*, vol 1, ed 5, New York, 1987, Academic Press.
3. Anderson RA et al: Chromium supplementation of human subjects: effect on glucose, insulin, and lipid variables, *Metabolism* 32:894, 1983.
4. Okada S, Tsukada H, Ohba HJ: Enhancement of nucleolar RNA synthesis by chromium (III) in regenerating rat liver, *J Inorg Biochem* 21:113, 1984.
5. Jeejeebhoy KN et al: Chromium depletion: glucose intolerance and neuropathy reversed by chromium supplementation in a patient receiving long-term total parenteral nutrition, *Am J Clin Nutr* 30:531, 1977.
6. Fishbein L: Perspectives of analysis of carcinogenic and mutagenic metals in biological samples, *Int J Environ Anal* 28:21, 1988.
7. Veillon C, Patterson KY, Bryden NA: Determination of chromium in human serum by electrothermal atomic absorption spectrometry, *Anal Chem Acta* 164:67, 1984.
8. Veillon C, Patterson KY, Bryden NA: Chromium in urine as measured by atomic absorption spectrometry, *Clin Chem* 28:2309, 1982.

Copper

9. Genetic and Environmental Determinants of Copper Metabolism, Proceedings of an international conference, Bethesda, Md, March 18-20, 1996, *Am J Clin Nutr* 67:951, 1998.
10. Uauy R, Olivares M, Gonzalez M: Essentiality of copper in humans, *Am J Clin Nutr* 67:952, 1998.
11. Reiser S et al: Indices of copper status in humans consuming a typical American diet containing either fructose or starch, *Am J Clin Nutr* 42:242, 1985.
12. Klevay LM et al: Increased cholesterol in plasma in a young man during experimental copper depletion, *Metabolism* 33:1112, 1984.
13. Danks DM et al: Menkes' kinky hair syndrome: an inherited defect in copper absorption with widespread effects, *Pediatrics* 50:188, 1972.
14. Stremmel W et al: Wilson's disease: clinical presentation, treatment, and survival, *Ann Int Med* 115:720, 1991.
15. Milne DB, Johnson PE: Assessment of copper status: effect of age and gender on reference ranges in healthy adults, *Clin Chem* 39:883, 1993.
16. Alcock NW: Copper. In Pesce AJ, Kaplan LA, editors: *Laboratory medicine: a scientific and management infobase*, v5.0., Cincinnati, 2002, Pesce Kaplan.

Fluorine

17. Krishnamachari KAVR: Fluorine. In Mertz W, editor: *Trace elements in human and animal nutrition*, vol 1, ed 5, New York, 1987, Academic Press.
18. Department of Health and Human Services, Public Health Service: *Review of fluoride benefits and risks*, Report of ad hoc subcommittee on fluoride of the Committee to Coordinate Environmental Health and Related Programs, Washington, DC, 1991, US Government Printing Office.
19. Riggs BL et al: Effect of fluoride/calcium regimen on vertebral fracture occurrence in postmenopausal osteoporosis: comparison with conventional therapy, *N Engl J Med* 306:446, 1982.
20. Riggs BL et al: Effect of fluoride treatment on the fracture rate in postmenopausal women with osteoporosis, *N Engl J Med* 322:802, 1994.
21. Blancke RV, Decker WJ: Analysis of toxic substances: determination of fluoride in plasma and urine by ion specific potentiometry. In Tietz NW, editor: *Textbook of clinical chemistry*, New York, 1986, Saunders.

Iodine

22. Hetzel BS, Maberly GF: Iodine. In Mertz W, editor: *Trace elements in human and animal nutrition*, vol 2, ed 5, New York, 1986, Academic Press.
23. Clugston GA, Hetzel BS: Iodine. In Shils ME, Olsen JA, Shike M, editors: *Modern nutrition in health and disease*, ed 8, Philadelphia, 1993, Lea & Febiger.

24. Larson PR et al: Revised nomenclature for tests of thyroid hormones and thyroid related proteins in serum, *J Clin Endocrinol Metab* 64:1089, 1987.

Manganese

25. Keen CL, Zidenberg-Cherr S: Manganese. In Brown ML, editor: *Newer knowledge in nutrition*, ed 6, Washington, DC, 1990, International Life Sciences Institute, Nutrition Foundation.
26. Hurley LS, Keen CL: Manganese. In Mertz W, editor: *Trace elements in human and animal nutrition*, vol 1, ed 5, New York, 1987, Academic Press.
27. Doisy EA, Jr: Effect of a deficiency in manganese upon plasma levels of clotting proteins in man. In Hoekstra WG et al, editors: *Trace elements in animals*, ed 2, Baltimore, 1974, University Park Press.
28. Cotzias GC et al: Interactions between manganese and brain dopamine, *Med Clin North Am* 60:729, 1976.
29. *Techniques for graphite furnace atomic absorption spectrophotometry*, Norwalk, CT, 1985, Perkin-Elmer Corp.

Molybdenum

30. Nielsen FH: Ultratrace minerals. In Shils ME, Olsen JA, Shike M, editors: *Modern nutrition in health and disease*, ed 8, Philadelphia, 1993, Lea & Febiger.
31. Mills CF, Davis GK: Molybdenum. In Mertz W, editor: *Trace elements in humans and animals*, vol 1, ed 5, New York, 1987, Academic Press.
32. Abumrad NN et al: Amino acid intolerance during prolonged TPN reversed by molybdate therapy, *Am J Clin Nutr* 34:2551, 1981.
33. Koval'skii UV, Iarovaia GA, Shmavonian DM: [Modification of human and animal purine metabolism in conditions of various molybdenum bio-geochemical areas], *Zh Obshch Biol* 22:179, 1961.
34. International Union of Pure and Applied Chemistry (IUPAC): Determination of molybdenum in biological materials, *Pure Appl Chem* 63:1627, 1991.

Selenium

35. Lockitch G: Selenium: clinical significance and analytical concepts, *Crit Rev Clin Lab Sci* 27:483, 1989.
36. Lavender OA, Burke RF: Selenium. In Shils ME, Olsen JA, Shike M, editors: *Modern nutrition in health and disease*, ed 8, Philadelphia, 1993, Lea & Febiger.
37. Robinson MF: Selenium in human nutrition in New Zealand, *Nutr Rev* 47:99, 1989.
38. Ip C: The chemopreventive role of selenium in carcinogenesis, *J Am Coll Toxicol* 5:7, 1986.
39. Ip C, Ganther HE: Activity of methylated forms of selenium in cancer prevention, *Cancer Res* 50:1206, 1990.
40. Ip C et al: Chemical form of selenium, critical metabolites and cancer prevention, *Cancer Res* 51:595, 1991.
41. Lane HW et al: The effect of selenium supplementation on selenium status of patients receiving chronic total parenteral nutrition, *JPEN* 11:117, 1987.
42. Keshan Disease Research Group: Epidemiologic studies on etiologic relationship of selenium and Keshan disease, *Chin Med J* 92:477, 1979.
43. McLaren CS: Clinical manifestations of human vitamin and mineral disorders. In Shils ME, Olsen JA, Shike M, editors: *Modern nutrition in health and disease*, ed 8, Philadelphia, 1993, Lea & Febiger.
44. Jacobson BE, Lockitch G: Direct determination of selenium in serum by graphite furnace atomic absorption spectrometry with deuterium background correction and a reduced palladium modifier: age specific reference ranges, *Clin Chem* 34:709, 1988.

Zinc

45. Hambidge KM, Krebs NF: Zinc. In Mertz W, editor: *Trace elements in humans and animals*, vol 2, ed 5, New York, 1986, Academic Press.
46. Cousins RJ, Hempe JM: Zinc. In Brown ML, editor: *Present knowledge in nutrition*, ed 6, Washington, DC, 1990, International Life Sciences Institute, Nutrition Foundation.
47. Prasad AS et al: Zinc metabolism in patients with the syndrome of iron deficiency anemia, hepatosplenomegaly, dwarfism, and hypogonadism, *J Lab Clin Med* 1:537, 1963.
48. Prasad AS: Discovery and importance of zinc in human nutrition, *Fed Proc* 43:2829, 1984.
49. Moynahan EJ, Barnes PM: Zinc deficiency and a synthetic diet for lactose intolerance, *Lancet* 1:676, 1973.

50. Yokoi K, Alcock NW, Sandstead HH: Iron and zinc nutriture of premenopausal women: associations of diet with serum ferritin and plasma zinc disappearance and of serum ferritin with plasma zinc and plasma zinc disappearance, *J Lab Clin Med* 124:852, 1994.
51. Sandstead HH: Zinc deficiency: a public health problem, *Am J Dis Child* 145:853, 1991.
52. Smith JC, Jr, Butrimovitz GP, Purdy WC: Direct measurement of zinc in plasma by atomic absorption spectroscopy, *Clin Chem* 25:1487, 1979.

Toxic Trace Metals
Aluminum
53. Alfrey AC: Aluminum. In Mertz W, editor: *Trace elements in human and animal nutrition*, vol 2, ed 5, New York, 1986, Academic Press.
54. Ott SM et al: Aluminum is associated with low bone formation in patients receiving chronic parenteral nutrition, *Ann Intern Med* 98:910, 1983.
55. Sedman AB et al: Evidence of aluminum loading in infants receiving intravenous therapy, *N Engl J Med* 312:1337, 1985.
56. Klein GL et al: Aluminum loading during total parenteral nutrition, *Am J Clin Nutr* 35:1425, 1982.
57. Koo WWK et al: Aluminum in parenteral nutrition solutions—sources and possible alternatives, *JPEN* 10:591, 1986.
58. Klein GL et al: Parent drug products containing aluminum as an ingredient or a contaminant: response to FDA notice of intent, *Am J Clin Nutr* 53:399, 1991.
59. Alcock NW, Goeger MP: *Determination of aluminum with Zeeman graphite furnace atomic absorption spectrophotometry.* (In press.)

Arsenic
60. Anke M: Arsenic. In Mertz W, editor: *Trace elements in human and animal nutrition*, vol 2, ed 5, New York, 1986, Academic Press.
61. Smith HS: The distribution of antimony, arsenic, copper, and zinc in human tissue, *J Forensic Sci Soc* 7:97, 1967.
62. Diplock AT, Mehlert A: Arsenic. In Anke M, Schneider HJ, Bruckner C, editors: *Spurenelement—Symposium*, Geneva, Switzerland, 1980, Wiss Publisher, Friedrich-Schiller University, pp 75-81.
63. Tan GKH et al: Excretion of a single oral dose of fish-arsenic in man, *Bull Envir Contam Toxicol* 28:669, 1982.
64. Peterson RG, Rumack BH: D-Penicillamine therapy of acute arsenic poisoning, *J Pediatr* 91:661, 1977.
65. Tadlock CH, Aposhian V: Protection of mice against lethal effects of sodium arsenite by 2,3-dimercapto-1-propane sulfonic acid and dimercaptosuccinic acid, *Biochem Biophys Res Comm* 94:501, 1980.
66. Levine WG, Goodman LS, Gilman A, editors: Heavy metals and heavy metal antagonists. In *Pharmacological basis of therapeutics*, ed 5, New York, 1975, MacMillan.

Cadmium
67. Kostial K: Cadmium. In Mertz W, editor: *Trace elements in human and animal nutrition*, vol 2, ed 5, New York, 1986, Academic Press.
68. Kjellström T: Exposure and accumulation of cadmium in populations from Japan, the United States, and Sweden, *Environ Health Perspect* 28:169, 1979.
69. Smith TJ et al: Cadmium, lead, and copper blood levels in normal children, *Clin Toxicol* 9:75, 1976.

70. Kowal DE et al: Normal levels of cadmium in diet, urine, blood, and tissues of inhabitants of the United States, *J Toxicol Environ Health* 5:995, 1979.
71. Nordberg M: Studies on metallothionein and cadmium, *Environ Res* 15:381, 1978.
72. Tohyama C et al: Urinary metallothionein as a new index of renal dysfunction in "itai-itai" disease patients and other Japanese women environmentally exposed to cadmium, *Arch Toxicol* 50:159, 1982.
73. Klassen CD, Waalkes MP, Cantilena LR: Alteration of tissue disposition of cadmium by chelating agents, *Environ Health Perspect* 54:233, 1984.

Lead
74. Centers for Disease Control and Prevention (CDC): *Preventing lead poisoning in young children—a statement by the CDC*, Atlanta, 1991, Department of Health and Human Services, Public Health Service.
75. Quarterman KA: Lead. In Mertz W, editor: *Trace elements in human and animal nutrition*, vol 2, ed 5, New York, 1986, Academic Press.
76. Burns JM et al: Lifetime low-level exposure to environmental lead and children's emotional and behavioral development at ages 11-13 years, *Am J Epidemiology* 149:740, 1999.
77. Mahaffey KR: Environmental lead toxicity: nutrition as a component of intervention, *Environ Health Perspect* 89:75, 1990.
78. Bellinger DC, Stiles KM, Needleman HL: Low level lead exposure, intelligence, and academic achievement: a long-term follow up study, *Pediatrics* 90:855, 1992.
79. Needleman HL: The current status of low level lead toxicity, *Neurotoxicology* 14:161, 1993.
80. Rogan WJ et al: The effect of chelation therapy with Succimer on neuropsychological development of children exposed to lead, *N Engl J Med* 344:1421, 2001.
81. Parsons PJ, Slavin W: A rapid Zeeman graphite furnace atomic absorption spectrometric method for the determination of lead in blood, *Spectrochim Acta* 48B:925, 1993.
82. Parsons PJ, Slavin W: Electrothermal atomization atomic absorption spectrometry for the determination of lead in urine: results of an interlaboratory study, *Spectrochim Acta* 54B:853, 1999.

Mercury
83. Clarkson TW: Mercury. In Mertz W, editor: *Trace elements in human and animal nutrition*, vol 1, ed 5, New York, 1987, Academic Press.
84. Subaki T, Irukagama K: *Minamata disease: methyl mercury poisoning in Minamata and Niigata, Japan*, Amsterdam, 1977, Elsevier Scientific.
85. Stern AH: Estimation of the interindividual variability in the one-compartment pharmacokinetic model for mercury: implications for the derivation of a reference dose, *Regul Toxicol Pharmacol* 25:277, 1997.
86. US Environmental Protection Agency: *Mercury Study Report to Congress*, EPA-452/R-97-007, Washington, DC, 1997, Environmental Protection Agency.
87. Choi BH: The effects of methyl mercury on the developing brain, *Prog Neurobiol* 32:447, 1989.
88. Swedish Expert Group: Methyl mercury in fish: a toxicological-epidemiologic evaluation of risks report from an expert group, *Nord Hyg Tidsk* 4(suppl.):19, 1971.
89. Magos L, Clarkson TW: Atomic absorption determination total, inorganic and organic mercury in blood, *J Assoc Office Anal Chem* 55:966, 1972.

Internet Sites

General
http://www.nal.usda.gov/—National Agriculture Library Recommended Dietary Allowances (RDA)
http://www.nap.edu/—National Academy Press Division of the National Academy of Sciences
www.toxlab.co.uk—Regional Laboratory for Toxicology: British Health Service
http://hsl.mcmaster.ca/tomflem/nutrition.html—McMaster University nutrition health care information links
http://cchs-dl.slis.ua.edu/—University of Alabama Health Sciences digital library research topics. To find information, type name of element into the search engine
http://www.lhsc.on.ca/lab/metallab/—London Health Sciences Center of Canada trace elements laboratory

http://www.aruplab.com/cgi-bin/htsearch—Type in "Trace Metals"
http://www.seismo.berkeley.edu/geology/labs/epma/trace.htm—Electron Probe Microanalysis Laboratory, Department of Earth and Planetary Science, University of California at Berkeley
www.nin.ca—National Institute of Nutrition of Canada

Chromium
http://www.nap.edu/books/030906354X/html/index.html—National Academy Press Division of the National Academy of Sciences: The Role of Chromium in Animal Nutrition, 1997, online book

Copper
www.nutrition.org—American Society for Nutritional Sciences: To find information, type name of element into the search engine

Wilson's disease

http://www.wilsonsdisease.org/—Wilson's Disease Association International

http://www.niddk.nih.gov/—National Institutes of Diabetes & Digestive & Kidney Diseases: To find information, type *Wilson's disease* into the search engine

http://www.ninds.nih.gov/—National Institute of Neurological Disorders and Stroke: To find information, type *Wilson's disease* into the search engine

Menkes' syndrome

http://www.ncbi.nlm.nih.gov/—National Center for Biotechnology Information: Click on OMIM (Online Mendelian Inheritance in Man) and type *Menkes' syndrome* into the search engine

http://dmoz.org—Open Directory Project, type *Menkes' syndrome* into the search engine for website links

Lead

http://www.cdc.gov/nceh/lead/guide/guide97.htm—Centers for Disease Control and Prevention: Screening Young Children for Lead Poisoning, Guidance for State and Local Officials

http://www.aap.org/—American Academy of Pediatrics: type *lead* into the search engine

http://www.slh.wisc.edu/—Wisconsin State Laboratory of Hygiene, lead proficiency testing program: type *lead* into the search engine

www.wadsworth.org—Wadsworth Center, New York State Department of Health, Certification for Lead Proficiency

Mercury

http://www.aap.org/—American Academy of Pediatrics: type *mercury* into the search engine

http://www.epa.gov/—Environmental Protection Agency: type *mercury* into the search engine

Manganese

http://www.tldp.com/—Townsend letter for doctors and patients

Selenium

www.cc.nih.gov—NIH Clinical Center: type *selenium* into the search engine

www.cce.cornell.edu—Cornell Cooperative Extension: type *selenium* into the search engine

Zinc

http://www.tamu.edu/—Texas A & M University: type *zinc* into the search engine

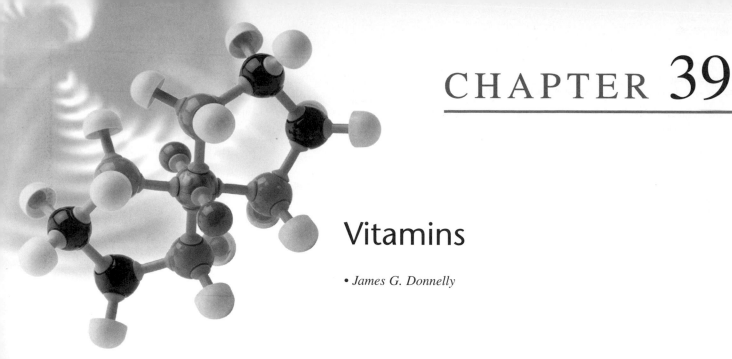

CHAPTER 39

Vitamins

• *James G. Donnelly*

Chapter Outline

General considerations
   Recommended dietary allowances and intakes
Fat-soluble vitamins
   Vitamin A
   Vitamin E
   Vitamin K
   Vitamin D
Water-soluble vitamins
   Ascorbic acid (vitamin C)
   Riboflavin

Pyridoxine
Niacin
Thiamin
Biotin
Pantothenic acid
Vitamin B_{12}
Folic acid
Carnitine
The antioxidant and cancer preventive role of certain vitamins

Objectives

- Define the term vitamin.
- List the fat-soluble vitamins, their functions, and conditions that result from a deficiency.
- List water-soluble vitamins, their functions, and conditions that result from a deficiency.
- Describe the functions of vitamin B_{12} and folic acid and describe disease conditions that are a result of deficiencies of these vitamins.

- Understand the role of absorption, metabolism, and genetics in the development of relative or absolute vitamin deficiencies.
- Understand the role of vitamin deficiencies in the development of disease.

Key Terms

avidin   A glycoprotein in raw egg white with strong affinity for biotin.
carotenoids   Compounds structurally similar to β-carotene (provitamin A) occurring naturally in vegetables and fruits.
dry beriberi   A degenerative neurological disease affecting motor neurons.
flavins   A group of yellow water-soluble pigments

that include riboflavin, flavin adenine dinucleotide (FAD) and flavin mononucleotide (FMN).
pellagra   Niacin deficiency resulting in the 3 "Ds": diarrhea, dementia, and dermatitis.
pyridine nucleotides   A group of nucleotides bearing a pyridine structure and involved in electron transfer reactions: NAD, NADH, NADP, NADPH.

rickets   Skeletal deformities caused by bone softening due to vitamin D deficiency.

scurvy   Severe ascorbic acid deficiency characterized by spongy gums with loosening of teeth, weakened capillary beds, and defective cartilage synthesis.

Wernicke-Korsakoff syndrome   Neurological pathology occurring in alcoholics with severe nutritional deficiencies, particularly thiamin deficiencies.

wet beriberi   Similar to dry beriberi, but also includes left ventricular failure and concomitant edema.

Methods on CD-ROM

Folic acid

Vitamin B_{12}

The vitamins are a diverse group of low–molecular-weight compounds that primarily serve as cofactors to certain enzymes. In addition, certain vitamins have been shown to function as hormones or transcriptional regulators. The antioxidant function ascribed to some vitamins is a controversial one; this may simply be an incidental effect, the result of their labile oxidation status. In general, vitamins can be classed as nutrients that must be obtained from the diet because they are either not synthesized or are synthesized in inadequate quantities to meet metabolic demands. Refer to earlier editions of this text for a more detailed discussion on the historical perspective of the discovery of vitamins.

GENERAL CONSIDERATIONS

In the clinical setting the investigation of vitamin deficiencies is often the primary focus, although there has been a shift to preventing disease by maintaining adequate intake. Both of these efforts require knowledge on the causes of deficiencies beyond inadequacies of diet. Deficiencies can be absolute or can be due to an inability to utilize a vitamin optimally. Absolute vitamin deficiencies are the result of a nutritional deficit, an inability to properly absorb a vitamin, increased metabolism and clearance, or markedly increased utilization. The inability to make use of a vitamin is typically the result of an inherited genotype that results in the synthesis of either a defective enzyme or reduced enzyme quantities. These inherited defects often present with symptoms that can be quite different from an absolute deficiency of the vitamin.

Historically, vitamin deficiencies were defined by overt clinical signs, which often present only after a prolonged and gross insufficiency of the vitamin. However, we are beginning to understand that the clinical appearance of vitamin deficiencies can be a continuum that is dependent on the duration of deficiency, metabolic demand, as well as the cellular concentration and form of the vitamin. It is becoming apparent that different physiological conditions and also certain individual genetic differences in the associated apoenzyme, or possibly at a receptor, can influence an individual's nutritional requirement of a vitamin. This confounds the use of population-based reference intervals that do not account for these genetic differences.

Insufficient nutritional intake resulting in the deficiency of a vitamin often does not occur in isolation. One must also consider the presence of other nutritive deficits, including other vitamins or other essential nutrients (see Chapter 37). Metabolic demand is also an important consideration. Periods with marked growth or repair of tissues such as pregnancy, recovery from surgery, or the presence of a major infection will affect vitamin intake requirements.

Because of the pervasive action of vitamins in metabolic processes, the clinical symptoms of vitamin deficiencies can be nonspecific and vague, often delaying a definitive diagnosis. In many cases clinical and dietary history as well as physical examination can be more informative than biochemical measurements when diagnosing a vitamin deficiency. Vitamin functions and the usual symptoms seen in deficient and toxic states are listed in Table 39-1.

Recommended Dietary Allowances and Intakes

Suspicion of dietary deficiency of a vitamin arises primarily from knowledge of dietary sources and dietary practices likely to provide inadequate intake or absorption. Recommended Dietary Allowances (RDA) were defined by the National Academy of Sciences, Food, and Nutrition Board[1] as the levels of intake of essential nutrients considered to be adequate, on the basis of available scientific knowledge, to meet the nutritional needs of practically all "healthy persons." These levels were defined from information on the daily intake requirements needed to avoid deficiency symptoms and to maintain specific functions. RDA values are generally set high enough to meet the needs of 97.5% of the population. The RDA values were set high because in some cases the actual quantity required for a particular nutrient is not known. RDA values are periodically reviewed and as specific nutritional requirements for various age, sex, and physiological status are identified, the tables are updated. More recently the RDA values have been replaced by dietary reference intakes, or DRIs[2]. DRIs were devised by the Food and Nutrition Board starting in 1996[3] and are based on our current knowledge of a nutritional requirement within specific groups or individuals.[4]

The DRIs contain at least four nutrient-based reference values that are useful for the planning and assessment of

TABLE 39-1   VITAMIN FUNCTIONS AND SYMPTOMS OF DEFICIENCY OR TOXICITY

Vitamin	Function	Clinical Deficiency	Toxicity
Fat-Soluble			
A	Vision, growth, reproduction, mucus secretion, immune responses, cancer prevention (?)	Night blindness, growth retardation, appetite loss, reduced taste, recurrent infections, dermatitis, dry mucous membranes *Late:* bone growth failure, aspermatogenesis, xerophthalmia (dry, thickened, lusterless eyeballs), blindness	*Acute:* raised intracranial pressure and skin desquamation; teratogen *Chronic:* liver damage, skin changes, and exostoses
D	Bone calcification	*Children:* rickets *Adults:* osteomalacia	Anorexia, vomiting, headache, drowsiness, and diarrhea
E	Antioxidant (membrane stability), neurological function, cardiovascular disease prevention	Mild hemolytic anemia, ataxia, loss of tendon reflexes, pigmentary retinopathy	Creatinuria, decreased platelet aggregation, impaired wound healing, anti-inflammatory activity, hepatomegaly, impaired fibrinolysis, potentiation of vitamin K deficiency, coagulopathy
K	Coagulation (gamma-carboxylation of inactive clotting factors—prothrombin, factors II, IX, and X)	Hemorrhage (ranging from easy bruising to massive ecchymoses, mucous membrane hemorrhage, or posttraumatic bleeding)	*Adults:* cardiac and pulmonary signs *Newborns:* hemolytic anemia
Water-Soluble			
B_{12}	Myelin formation, methionine synthesis, folate interconversions, and DNA synthesis	*Early:* cognitive impairment? *Late:* megaloblastic anemias, neurological abnormalities (paresthesias progressing to spastic ataxia)	Infrequent adverse reactions are mostly allergic (possibly related to contaminates or preservatives)
Biotin	Coenzyme for CO_2 carboxylation reactions and for carboxyl group exchange	Dermatitis progressing to mental and neurological changes, nausea, anorexia, peripheral vasoconstriction, or coronary ischemia in some cases	None described
C	Collagen formation, catecholamine synthesis, cholesterol catabolism, antioxidant	*Early:* weakness, lassitude, irritability, vague aches and pains *Late:* scurvy (hemorrhages into skin, alimentary and urinary tracts, other tissues; osteoporotic bones, defective tooth formation, anemia, pyrexia, delayed wound healing)	Increased excretion of oxalate and urate, diarrhea, dyspepsia
Carnitine	Energy metabolism and acyl-group transport	Muscle weakness, fatigue	None known
Folate	One-carbon transfers	Megaloblastic anemia, organic mental changes?	Few reports–mostly allergic reactions
Niacin	Oxidation-reduction (as pyridine nucleotides NAD and NADP)	*Early:* lassitude, anorexia, weakness, digestive disturbances, anxiety, irritability, and depression *Late:* pellagra (dermatitis, mucous membrane inflammation, weight loss, disorientation, delirium, dementia)	Cutaneous flushing, gastric irritation, mild liver dysfunction, jaundice, hyperuricemia, impaired glucose tolerance
Pantothenate	Acyl-group transfer reactions (as part of coenzyme A and acyl carrier protein)	Never spontaneously seen—with chemical agonist: apathy, depression, increased infection, paresthesias (burning sensations), muscle weakness	None described

TABLE 39-1	VITAMIN FUNCTIONS AND SYMPTOMS OF DEFICIENCY OR TOXICITY—CONT'D		
Vitamin	**Function**	**Clinical Deficiency**	**Toxicity**
Pyridoxine	Enzyme systems involving amino acid transaminases, phosphorylases, racemases, decarboxylases, deaminases	*Infants:* irritability, seizures, anemia, vomiting, weakness, ataxia, abdominal pain *Adults:* facial seborrhea	Usually low systemic toxicity Reduced milk production? Sensory neuropathy?
Riboflavin	Oxidative enzymatic reactions	Angular stomatitis (mouth lesions), glossitis (smooth tongue), photophobia, blepharospasm (eyelid spasm), conjunctival congestion and other ocular changes, dermatological changes, neurological alterations (behavior changes, decreased hand grip strength, burning feet in adults, retarded intellectual development and EEG changes in children), and hematological dyscrasia (anemia and reticulocytopenia)	Low toxicity
Thiamine	Decarboxylations, ketol formation	*Infants:* dyspnea and cyanosis, diarrhea, vomiting, wasting, aphonia *Adults:* "dry beriberi" (poor appetite, fatigue, peripheral neuritis) or "wet beriberi" (edema and cardiac failure), Wernicke-Korsakoff syndrome (intelligence disturbance, apathy, ataxia, double vision, nystagmus, drooping eyelids, loss of recent memory)	Anxiety, headache, convulsions, weakness, trembling, neuromuscular collapse

diets. The RDA remains as the first requirement. The second is the *adequate intake (AI)* guideline, which is to be used when an RDA is unobtainable. The AI is based on the recommend intake value for groups of healthy individuals and is derived from experimental or observational sources. The *tolerable upper limit*, or *UL*, is the highest level of a nutrient that can be tolerated in one day without experiencing adverse effects. The fourth value in the DRI is the *estimated average requirement (EAR)*. This is a daily nutrition value that is estimated to suffice for half of a group of healthy individuals. The RDA was replaced as the sole standard for dietary planning because it does not provide nutritional guidelines for nutrients above the acceptable lower limit.[5]

The Food and Nutrition Board also identifies other food constituents that may be needed by humans. However, the validity of the claims that these substances are necessary has not been proven. These food constituents fall into four categories: (1) growth factors that are essential for less differentiated species; (2) substances with either pharmacological activity or no activity whatsoever, covering all compounds with unsubstantiated claims of physiological activity; (3) compounds essential to animals that have not been proven to be essential to humans; and (4) substances that lack scientific proof of nutritional value. This latter category is of interest because many of the "dietary supplements" sold at nutritional outlets fall into this group. A health-conscious population lacking clear direction from scientific bodies[6] is susceptible to the influence of vendors promoting unsubstantiated nutritional value for these compounds. This problem is not limited to Western countries; many non-Western countries have specific food supplements and "medications" touted to maintain or restore health and potency. Unfortunately, many of these supplements are obtained from the unnecessary slaughter of animals, some of which are endangered.

The public's lack of knowledge on the role of vitamins in maintaining health has led to the perception that increased intake of vitamins will provide extra health benefits, such as increased energy, strength, or stamina or the ability to tolerate stress. In most cases such indiscriminate use of vitamin supplements is likely less dangerous than a deficiency of a vitamin, although it is a wasteful and misapplied use of medications.

The tolerable upper intake level (UL)[7] has become a necessary guideline because food fortification and the use of supplements has increased the risk of a person reaching or exceeding the critical level of a vitamin or mineral, which may result in toxic side effects. The tolerable level is derived for the most part through human data, and each vitamin or nutrient is set at a level thought to pose no risk to humans. It is important to consider that most humans have no need to achieve the UL in their diets and that this maximum allowable limit is not intended to be a target value.

Vitamin deficiencies. Vitamin deficiencies are relatively common, and identification of patients at risk for decreased intake, malabsorption, or impaired utilization should be considered for many patient settings. For patients at risk for vitamin deficiencies, the use of supplements on a prophylactic basis is generally accepted.

Vitamin deficiency is more common among individuals living in lower socioeconomic groups, where the condition is usually part of a general malnourished state (see p. 699, Chapter 37), as well as among older adults, alcoholics, and persons with unconventional diets. This last group is represented in all age groups and races and can include patients with psychiatric disorders. Patients with end-stage renal disease (ESRD) also present a special challenge for clinicians because dialysis adversely affects the ability to maintain adequate levels of vitamins.

Biochemical indices of vitamin status can sometimes become abnormal before development of obvious clinical changes, thus allowing some vitamin deficiencies to be detected indirectly. Chemical determination of human vitamin status has been approached in the following ways:

1. Measurement of the active cofactor(s) or precursor(s) in biological fluids or blood cells
2. Measurement of urinary metabolite(s) of the vitamin
3. Measurement of a biochemical function requiring the vitamin (such as enzymatic activity) with and without in vitro addition of the cofactor form
4. Measurement of urinary excretion of vitamin or metabolite(s) after a test load of the vitamin
5. Measurement of urinary metabolites of a substance, the metabolism of which requires the vitamin, after administration of a test load of the substance
6. Measurement of accumulated metabolic byproducts of vitamin deficiencies

Reduced serum concentrations of a vitamin do not always indicate a deficiency that interrupts cellular function, just as values within a reference interval as defined by population studies do not always reflect adequate supply.

Table 39-2 lists representative biochemical data that are usually associated with classical deficiency symptoms. These values are, of course, somewhat affected by the age of the patient and by laboratory methodology. A bibliography of articles regarding methodologies and vitamin functions is provided.[8-15]

Vitamins have historically been classed as either fat- or water-soluble. This classification was adopted, in part, because the absorption of the so-called fat-soluble vitamins depends on the normal fat absorptive processes in the bowel (see Chapter 31 and below). For better or worse, this classification remains to the present date, and we will use it in this chapter. However, to better understand vitamins, greater emphasis

TABLE 39-2 CONCENTRATION OR EXCRETION RATES ASSOCIATED WITH CLASSICAL VITAMIN DEFICIENCY SYMPTOMS*†

Vitamin	Chemical Value
Fat-Soluble	
A	<0.1 mg/L of plasma retinol
	>20% relative dose response (RDR) in plasma
D	See Chapter 28
E	<5.0 mg/L of plasma α-tocopherol
K	Plasma prothrombin time greater than normal
Water-Soluble	
Ascorbic acid (C)	<2.4 mg/L of serum ascorbate
	<3 mg/L of whole blood ascorbate
	<80 mg/L of leukocyte ascorbate
B_{12}	<150 ng/L of serum vitamin B_{12}
	≥24 mg of urinary methylmalonic acid per day
	>0.44 nM serum methylmalonic acid
	>4 mmol/mole of creatinine in urine
	>15 nM serum total homocysteine
Biotin§	<0.7 μg/L of whole blood?
Carnitine	<30 nM plasma total carnitine
	15 μg of urinary biotin per day?
Folate	<140 μg/L of erythrocyte folate
	<3.0 μg/L of serum folate
	≥30 mg of urinary N^5-formiminoglutamic acid (FIGLU) per 8 hours
	>15 nM serum homocysteine
Niacin	≥1 urinary ratio (α-pyridone/N′–methyl-nicotinamide)
Pantothenic acid§	<1.0 mg/L of whole blood pantothenate
	<1.0 mg of urinary pantothenate per day
Pyridoxine (B_6)	≥1.5 AC of erythrocytic AST
	≥1.25 AC of erythrocytic ALT
	<0.8 mg of urinary 4-pyridoxic acid per day
	>25 mg of urinary xanthurenic acid per day
	<30 nM plasma pyridoxal phosphate
Riboflavin (B_2)	>1.4 AC‡ of erythrocytic glutathione reductase
	<0.1 mg of riboflavin per liter of erythrocytes
	<0.12 mg of urinary riboflavin per day
	≥0.08 mg of urinary riboflavin per gram of creatinine
Thiamine	>1.25 AC of erythrocyte transketolase
	<0.1 mg of urinary thiamine per day

*These are general guidelines with reference intervals dependent on age and methodology used.
†Compiled from references 3,4, and 42.
‡AC, Activity coefficient; ratio of activities with and without added cofactor.
§Deficient values for biotin and pantothenate are not well established.

should be placed on their biochemical and physiological properties, both of which are defined by the associated metabolic pathways, rather than by their physicochemical properties, which give little insight into their action.

FAT-SOLUBLE VITAMINS

Because the fat-soluble vitamins (A, E, K, and D) are absorbed as part of the chylomicron complex (see Chapter

33), their absorption depends on the presence of adequate bile and pancreatic secretions, as well as healthy bowel mucosa. Therefore chronic malabsorptive states are often associated with a deficiency of one or more of these vitamins (see Chapters 29 and 30). The malabsorptive states include chronic bowel inflammatory conditions, impaired bile flow, pancreatic insufficiency, and alcoholic liver disease (see Chapter 34). A new acquired form of lipid-soluble vitamin deficiency can occur with the use of gastrointestinal lipase inhibitors, such as Xenical, or the ingestion of non-bioavailable fat substitutes, such as Olestra. Deficiency of this class of vitamins generally develops slowly as stored supplies of vitamins are depleted. Vitamin A can be stored in liver parenchymal cells for a year or longer, and vitamin E can be stored in body fat for several months. Paradoxically, although they are fat-soluble, vitamins K and D appear to be stored only for days or weeks.

Vitamin A

First described in 1909 and found to prevent night blindness in 1925, vitamin A is now known to be made up of three biologically active forms: retinol, retinal, and retinoic acid. These major vitamin A compounds all contain a tri-methyl-cyclohexenyl group and an all-*trans* polyene chain with four double bonds (Fig. 39-1). These compounds are derived directly from dietary sources, primarily as retinyl esters, or from metabolism of dietary **carotenoids** (provitamin A), primarily β-carotene. Major dietary sources of these compounds include animal products (vitamin A) and pigmented fruits and vegetables (carotenoids). Each of these compounds is soluble in organic solvents, with retinoic acid being more polar than the others. Oxidation of retinol or retinal by peripheral cells is irreversible; thus neither retinoic acid nor retinal is metabolically converted to retinol. Vitamin A also has a very important role as a hormone that binds to nuclear hormone receptor proteins. This group of receptors is also associated with the actions of calcitriol and thyroid hormone. The natural ligand for the receptors is the 9-cis-retinoic acid form of vitamin A, which appears to play a role in cellular differentiation, growth, and apoptosis (cell death). The hormonal roles for vitamin A and its derivatives span the entire life of the cell and are of great interest in anticancer therapies.

Metabolism. Enzymes of the small intestinal mucosa convert dietary β-carotene and retinal to the predominant form of vitamin A, retinol (Fig. 39-2). The retinyl esters of dietary animal products are cleaved to retinol by pancreatic and mucosal hydrolases (vitamin A esterases). Once in the mucosal cell, retinol is reesterified, forming retinyl esters (primarily retinyl palmitate) that are transported in lymph chylomicrons to the systemic circulation. After the chylomicrons release their triglycerides, the retinyl esters are transported to the liver where they are stored bound to intracellular retinol binding proteins within the liver.[16] The retinoids are biologically inactive when bound to these proteins; this may serve as a protective mechanism to prevent unwanted or inappropriate retinoid transcriptional activity.

This is supported by the observation that increased exposure to retinoids can lead to dramatic increases in retinoid binding protein.[16] The more polar retinoic acid does not require this lipoprotein transport route but is directly absorbed into the portal circulation. However, this form is not stored in the liver but is excreted through bile as a glucuronide conjugate. The exact role of these water-soluble glucuronide derivatives is unknown; however, they have much reduced toxicity and still have some biological activity. This is of interest for the development of drugs with retinoid activity that have much reduced toxicity.[17,18]

When body demands require mobilization of hepatic vitamin A, the stored retinyl palmitate is hydrolyzed and the free retinol combines with retinol-binding protein (RBP). RBP-retinol is then secreted into the circulation, where it complexes with prealbumin. This large complex then circulates to target tissues that have specific receptor sites for RBP, and retinol is transferred intracellularly to another specific binding protein termed *cytosol-retinol-binding protein (CRBP)*. CRBP-retinol presumably transports the retinol to its functional site within the cell. Retinol metabolism is shown in Fig. 39-2.

Function (see Table 39-1). The only clearly defined physiological role for retinol is its role in vision. Retinol is oxidized in the rods of the eye to retinal, which when complexed with opsin, forms rhodopsin, allowing dim-light vision. In the visual cycle, rhodopsin is reversibly bleached by a photon of light. During this process 11-cis-retinal is converted to all-trans-retinal forcing the dissociation of opsin. Activated rhodopsin stimulates transducin, a G protein, which ultimately decreases the cellular content of cyclic guanosine 3′,5′-monophosphate (cyclic GMP) via the activation of a cyclic-GMP phosphodiesterase. This effect culminates in nervous conduction in the optic nerve to the brain. All-trans-retinal then isomerizes to 11-cis-retinal, which then associates with opsin to reform rhodopsin, completing the visual cycle. When retinal is depleted in the retina, opsin becomes destabilized and is catabolized. This eventually results in the permanent destruction of the rod cells.

In vitamin A deficiency, epithelial cells (cells in the outer skin layers and cells in the lining of the gastrointestinal, respiratory, and urogenital tracts) become dry and keratinized. Thus vitamin A may help to maintain epithelial cells, which provide protection against infectious organisms. Retinoic acid and retinol play a significant role in epithelial differentiation in mucus and keratinizing tissues. Retinoic acid induces mucus production in basal epithelial cells and inhibits keratinization of epithelium, whereas goblet cell formation occurs in the presence of retinoids. The end result is the formation of a healthy, non-stratified non-keratinizing epithelial layer. Because the mucous secretions of the goblet cells are part of the natural immune system, retinoid compounds function to bolster the immune system. Retinoids are also known to stimulate the production of fibronectin and decrease the synthesis of collagenase and keratin in fibroblasts.

The role that retinoids play in cellular differentiation and regulation occurs at the level of nuclear transcription.

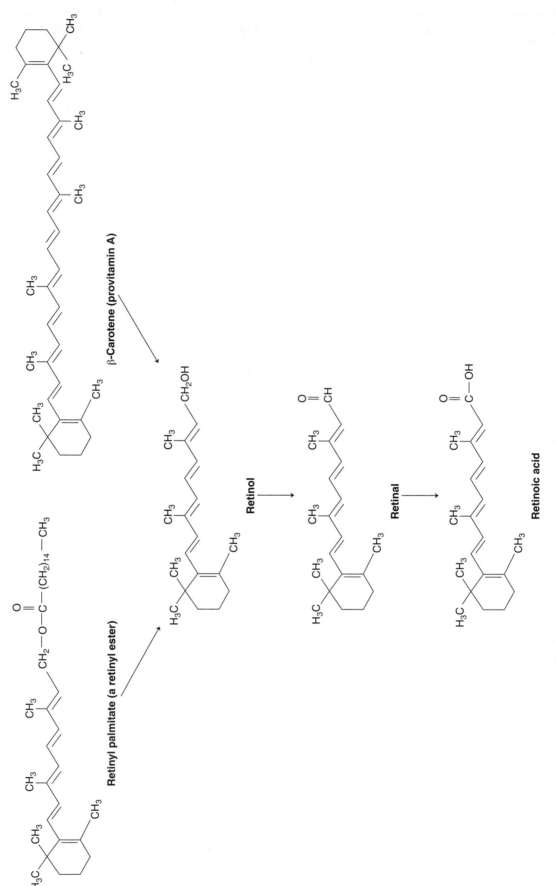

Fig. 39-1 Structures of vitamin A (retinol) with its precursors and metabolites.

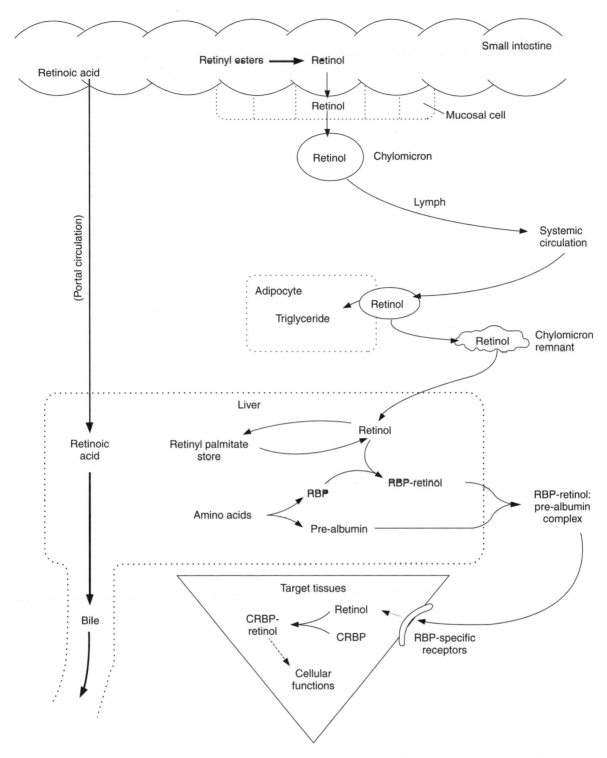

Fig. 39-2 Retinol metabolism. *RBP*, Retinol-binding protein; *CRBP*, cytoplasmic retinol-binding protein.

Two superfamilies of retinoid nuclear receptors have been described. The retinoic acid receptor (RAR) and retinoid X receptor (RXR, since more than one retinoid may naturally bind to the receptor) groups each have alpha, beta, and gamma subtypes. In general, the role of these receptors is to activate the transcriptional machinery of cells, activating specific genes in a concerted manner.

Retinoids most likely affect apoptosis (programmed cell death) by the induction of Bcl-2 mRNA.[19] This is a significant discovery since malignancy often coincides with a loss of apoptotic activity. Many of the classic cancer chemotherapeutic drugs function by triggering apoptosis. Failure of a malignancy to undergo apoptosis is one of the most common reasons for failure of chemotherapeutic treatment. For example, chronic myeloid leukemia (CML) is characterized by clonal expansion and accumulation of a differentiated cell line that lacks the ability to undergo apoptosis at the proper time. All trans retinoic acid has been shown to at least partially restore apoptosis in some patients, which permits the effective use of classic chemotherapeutic agents such as cytosine arabinoside (ARA-C).[20] Another anticancer role for vitamin A may result from its ability to alter cellular differentiation. Premalignant changes in tissues result in the formation of cancerous tissues, only after several specific phenotypic changes have occurred (see pp. 963-964, Chapter 49). Vitamin A has been tested as a chemopreventive agent for head and neck squamous cell carcinoma and Kaposi's sarcoma, among others.[21,22] Results for the modulation of the squamous cell carcinoma cell lines release of angiogenic agents were promising when combined with interferon-alpha. Similarly, patients with Kaposi's sarcoma who were topically treated with 9-cis-retinoic acid showed a slowing of progression of the malignant lesions.

Clinical and chemical deficiency signs. Vitamin A deficiency is a serious nutritional problem in a large part of the world, especially in Africa, Central and South America, Southeast Asia, and the Middle East. Vitamin A deficiency can be fatal, particularly when associated with other nutritional disorders.[23] Clinical signs of vitamin A deficiency can be separated into early and late signs (see Table 39-1). Keratomalacia is an acute sign often seen in children who have a severe deficiency. Keratinization of the respiratory tract with subsequent reduction in mucous secretion can result in respiratory infections, a significant cause for mortality in developing countries. The chemical sign of deficiency is reduction in plasma vitamin A. Generally, retinol values below 0.1 mg/L are associated with clinical symptoms, and values above 0.2 mg/L are not[8,24]; however, values below 0.29 mg/L may be inadequate for post-adolescent persons. Vitamin A itself is not excreted in human urine. Although several metabolites are excreted, they do not seem to reflect the tissue status of vitamin A. One method for assessment of vitamin A status is the relative dose response (RDR) test and a modified version of it (MRDR); these tests measure the increase in plasma retinol after administration of retinyl palmitate (RDR) or dehydroretinol (MRDR). Another functional measure of vitamin A status involves evaluation of the morphology of conjunctival epithelial cells, referred to as conjunctival impression cytology (CIC).[25-27]

Pathophysiology. Because retinol and RBP are secreted from the liver as a 1:1 complex, low plasma concentrations of both are seen in vitamin A deficiency. Adequate concentration of plasma retinol usually indicates dietary and tissue adequacy, but low concentrations do not always indicate dietary deficiency. Factors that reduce hepatic synthesis of RBP or secretion of the RBP-retinol complex also lower plasma concentrations of retinol and RBP, even though dietary intake and the hepatic retinol store are adequate. These states are primarily recognized by the absence of an increase in plasma retinol after oral therapy with vitamin A

and include protein-calorie malnutrition, liver disease, zinc deficiency, and cystic fibrosis.

Pathophysiological conditions that can result in increased retinol and RBP include chronic renal disease and use of oral contraceptives.

Toxicity and therapeutic uses. Retinoids have been used therapeutically to treat a variety of skin disorders including acne (Isotretinoin and tretinoin) and psoriasis (etretinate). Retinoids are known to result in congenital malformations, and women using high-dose retinoid therapy should practice contraception for up to 2 years after discontinuation of the drug. Premature infants are born with lower serum retinol and RBP levels, as well as low hepatic stores of retinol. Newborns are thus treated with vitamin A as a preventive measure.

Vitamin A toxicity, one of the more common hypervitaminosis states, can occur in adults or children. Typically, it is the result of over medication with vitamin supplements but can also result from the use of topical retinoids for acne. Infants are more susceptible to retinoid toxicity than are adults. A well-known, albeit rare, cause of hypervitaminosis A that can be fatal occurs from the ingestion of polar bear liver, which contains up to 1.2% vitamin A by weight. Signs of vitamin A toxicity include dry, itchy skin; dermatitis; fissures of the lips; bone pain; edema; fatigue; renal disorders; intracranial hypertension; and hemorrhage.

Hypervitaminosis A can also result in the development of numerous congenital malformations in the fetus.[28] Indeed, the dose required to cause defects in the fetus can be reached with dietary supplements. Second, as mentioned above, retinoid therapy can result in significant stores of retinoids in fat, which extend the length of time that women of childbearing years should wait before discontinuing contraceptive use.

Vitamin E

A factor in vegetable oils that prevented fetal resorption in deficient rats was isolated in the early 1920s as vitamin E; later it was given the generic name tocopherol and was shown to include several biologically active isomers (Fig. 39-3). The word *tocopherol* is of Greek derivation, meaning an "oil that brings forth in childbirth," but the fertility role of these compounds is still questionable. α-Tocopherol is the predominant isomer in plasma and is the most potent isomer by current biological assays.

Dietary sources of tocopherols include vegetable oils, fresh leafy vegetables, egg yolk, legumes, peanuts, and margarine. Diets suspect for vitamin E deficiency are those low in vegetable oils or fresh green vegetables or those high in unsaturated fats.

Metabolism. The absorption, transport, storage, and metabolism of tocopherols are only partially understood. Absorption is believed to be associated with intestinal fat absorption. Approximately 40% of ingested tocopherol is absorbed. Because of the antioxidant effect of vitamin E, it is thought that physiological requirement for vitamin E increases with increasing polyunsaturated fatty acids in the diet.

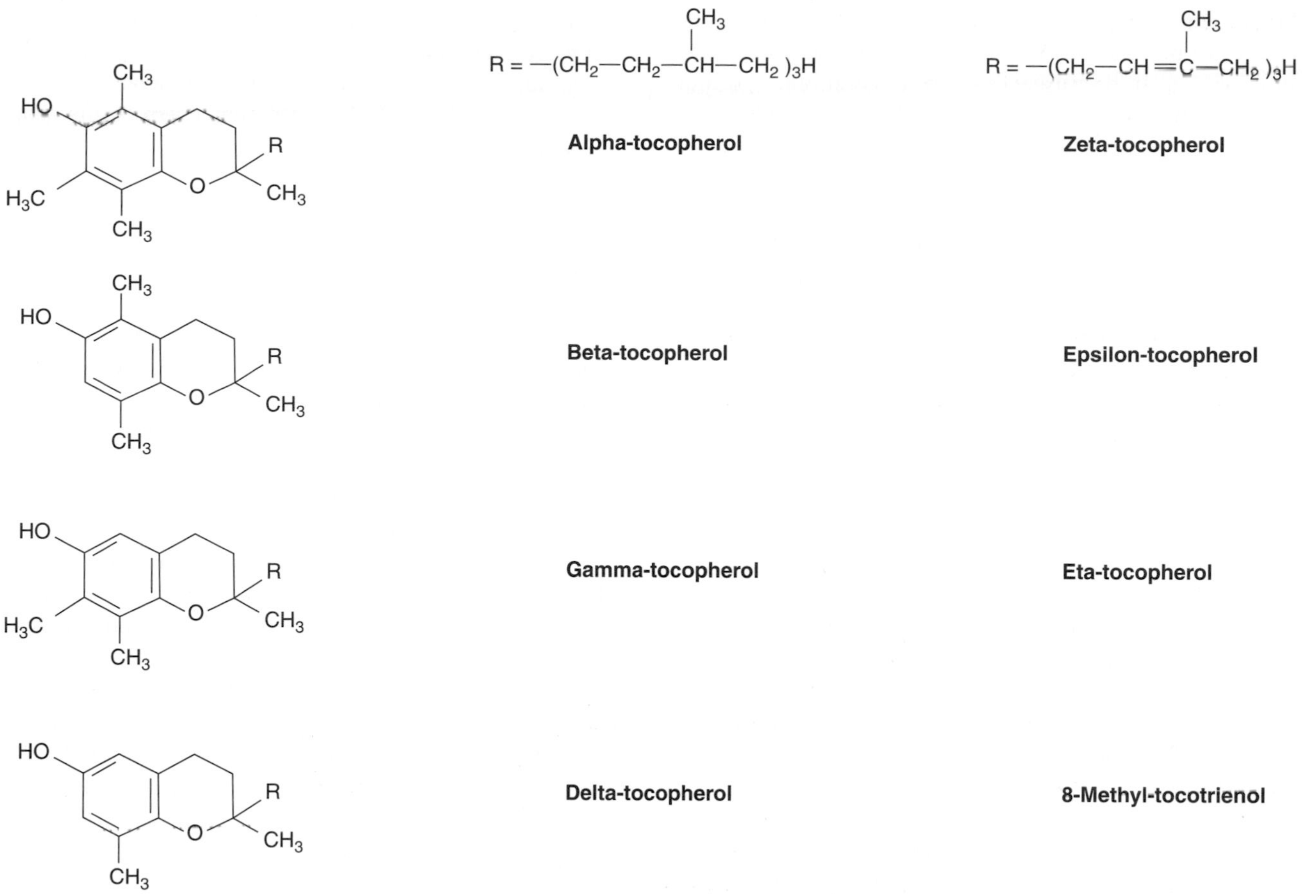

$$R = -(CH_2-CH_2-CH-CH_2)_3H$$
(with CH_3 on the CH)

Alpha-tocopherol

$$R = -(CH_2-CH=C-CH_2)_3H$$
(with CH_3 on the C)

Zeta-tocopherol

Beta-tocopherol

Epsilon-tocopherol

Gamma-tocopherol

Eta-tocopherol

Delta-tocopherol

8-Methyl-tocotrienol

Fig. 39-3 Vitamin E isomers. The structure in the left column is the core ring isomer. The R groups in the second or third columns are the two forms that can be part of the structure. Thus eight forms of the vitamin are described.

Absorbed vitamin E is first associated with circulating chylomicrons and very–low-density lipoproteins (VLDL) and some is transferred to adipose tissue during triglyceride hydrolysis. The remaining vitamin E in chylomicron remnants is transported to the liver. α-Tocopherol is resecreted as a component of liver-derived VLDLs (and perhaps HDLs).[29] Vitamin E is predominantly found in adipose tissue, though increased dietary α-tocopherol acetate is reflected by increased concentrations in all animal tissues, including plasma, erythrocytes, and platelets. A tocopherol-binding protein (TBP) in the hepatic cell cytosol has been described.[29]

Function. Although vitamin E has been shown to function as an antioxidant, protecting unsaturated lipids from peroxidation (cleavage of fatty acids at unsaturated sites by oxygen addition across the double bond and formation of free radicals), it is unclear whether this role is important in the antioxidants of humans[30]; the specific role for this vitamin is uncertain in humans. The role of vitamin E in protecting the erythrocyte membrane from oxidant stress is presently the major documented role of vitamin E in human physiology. There is evidence for preventive roles of vitamin E in retrolental fibroplasia, intraventricular hemorrhage, and mortality of small premature infants.[13] There is now much

evidence that vitamin E plays a neurological role[29] and also may have a preventive role in cardiovascular disease.

Clinical deficiency signs (see Table 39-1). The major symptom of vitamin E deficiency is hemolytic anemia. Although the practice is still controversial, premature newborns are commonly supplemented with vitamin E to stabilize their red blood cells and prevent hemolytic anemia. Patients with conditions resulting in fat malabsorption, especially cystic fibrosis and abetalipoproteinemia, are very suspect for vitamin E deficiency; a relationship has been recognized between vitamin E deficiency and progressive loss of neurological function in infants and children with chronic cholestasis.[31] Vitamin E deficiency can also occur without lipid malabsorption.[29] Animal deficiencies of vitamin E have been studied extensively. The nervous system is particularly sensitive to vitamin E deficiency. Some signs of deficiency include axonal deterioration in the spinal cord with associated gait disturbances and proprioception loss. Reproductive loss also occurs with vitamin E deficiency in animal models. In frank vitamin E loss, animals suffer from a necrotizing myopathy similar to muscular dystrophy. This also occurs in cardiac tissues on a lesser scale. In humans a macrocytic megaloblastic anemia is associated with α-tocopherol deficiency. It is important to understand that this anemia is related to severe protein/caloric deficiency and may not be totally attributable to vitamin E. Premature infants may also be susceptible to a hemolytic anemia resulting from oxidative damage (see above). In addition, a rare genetic disorder that results in a beta-lipoprotein deficiency with concomitant vitamin E deficiency produces acanthocytosis. This disorder also appears to be associated with a malabsorptive state for vitamin E. Steatorrhea also affects α-tocopherol absorption, and subsequently premature erythrocyte destruction occurs.

Chemical deficiency signs. Plasma concentrations of α-tocopherol below 5 mg/L are associated with increased erythrocyte hemolysis in the presence of hydrogen peroxide and are thus designated "deficient."[13,21] There is a strong correlation between plasma α-tocopherol and plasma lipids, indicating that plasma concentrations should be interpreted relative to plasma lipid levels; 0.8 mg of α-tocopherol per gram of total plasma lipids appears to indicate adequate levels of vitamin E in infants. Elevation of plasma total lipids above 15 g/L can apparently shift erythrocyte α-tocopherol to plasma, potentially altering erythrocyte susceptibility despite "adequate" plasma concentrations of α-tocopherol in hyperlipidemic states.[32,33] Breath ethane has been measured as a marker of deficiency.

Pathophysiology. At the present time assessment of vitamin E status is primarily indicated in newborns, in persons with fat-malabsorption states, and in persons receiving synthetic diets. Dietary insufficiency rarely causes vitamin E deficiency.

Decreased serum values have been reported in patients with grand mal seizures[10,34] and in persons exposed to nonsymptomatic doses of organophosphates.[11]

Toxicity. Toxicity may result from chronic voluntary overdoses. Premature infants receiving vitamin E sufficient to sustain serum levels above 30 mg/L have an increased incidence of sepsis and necrotizing enterocolitis. Patients receiving synthetic diets should be monitored to avoid vitamin E toxicity (see Table 39-1).

Vitamin K

Experiments in the mid-1930s led to the discovery of the antihemorrhagic factor later called *vitamin K* (from German *Koagulationsvitamin*). Purification efforts revealed several quinone-containing compounds possessing this antihemorrhagic activity, and the term *vitamin K* is now used as a generic descriptor for menadione and derivatives exhibiting this activity.[35] A large number of these compounds are related to those shown in Fig. 39-4 by number and substituents of polyisoprenoid side chains and degree of saturation.

Major dietary sources of K vitamins are cabbage, cauliflower, spinach, and other leafy vegetables, as well as pork, liver, soybeans, and vegetable oils. Uncomplicated dietary deficiency is considered rare in healthy children and adults, but a study of elderly persons revealed deficiencies in a large percentage that were correctable by oral administration of vitamin K.[36] The two major forms of vitamin K are the phylloquinone (vitamin K_1) and the menaquinones (vitamin K_2). The phylloquinone derivatives of vitamin K are found in plants and constitute the dietary source of vitamin K. Menaquinone forms of vitamin K are produced in grampositive bacteria and represent the bowel-derived source of vitamin K in humans.

Metabolism. In infants vitamin K is absorbed in the colon, where bacterial synthesis is the major source of this

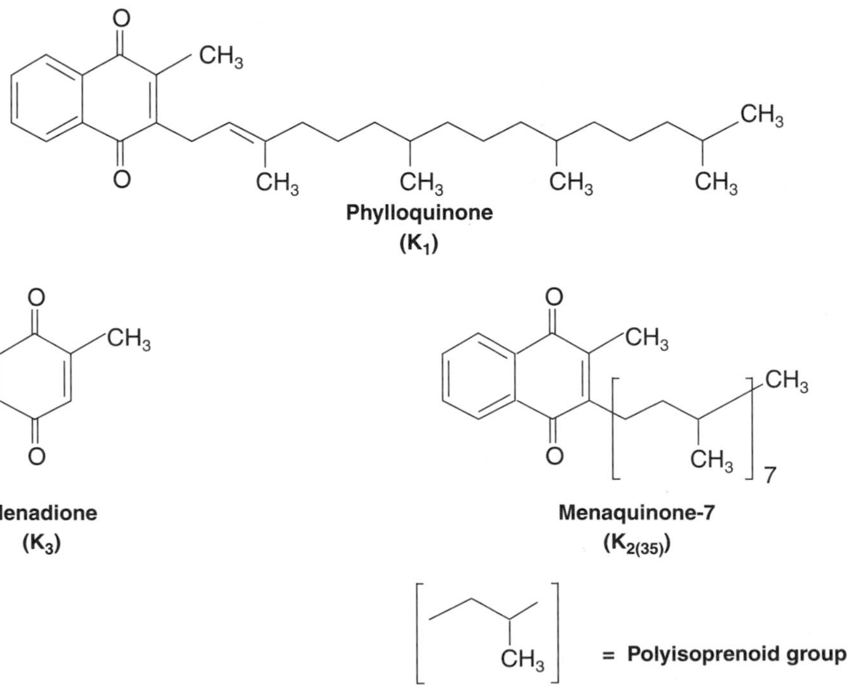

Fig. 39-4   Structures of vitamin K forms.

vitamin. Older children and adults absorb dietary vitamin K in the upper small intestine, where the contribution of intestinal bacteria is insignificant. Absorption of vitamin K in the intestines is chylomicron mediated and is dependent on adequate bile flow. Vitamin K malabsorption states include cystic fibrosis, biliary atresia, cholelithiasis, and obstructive jaundice resulting from hemolytic anemias, as well as other disorders leading to dysfunction of the upper small intestine. Tissue stores of the vitamin diminish through normal metabolism, and the vitamin does not appear to be conserved through recycling. As tissue stores become conjugated with glucuronate, vitamin K is excreted in urine. Depletion of body stores sufficient to manifest deficiency usually requires 3 weeks.

Function. The phytonadione and menaquinone forms of vitamin K are largely inactive. Vitamin K must be reduced to the hydroquinone form to act as a cofactor. First shown to be involved in prothrombin synthesis, vitamin K has also been found to be required for the synthesis of other active clotting factors (factors VII, IX, and X). Vitamin K-dependent γ-carboxylation of glutamic acid residues of inactive precursor proteins occurs in the liver. The conversion of glutamic acid to a γ-carboxyglutamic acid permits the coagulation proteins to bind calcium, which can then serve as an ionic bridge to bind with phospholipids. This is essential to the coagulation pathway. Gamma-carboxylation occurs in the presence of oxygen and carbon dioxide. A microsomal carboxylase enzyme facilitates the conversion of the hydroquinone form to a 2,3-epoxide. The hydroquinone form of vitamin K is regenerated from the 2,3-expoxide via the action of epoxide reductase, which is inhibited by coumarin.

Other proteins that contain gamma-carboxyglutamate include osteocalcin, which is secreted from osteoblasts, and matrix gamma carboxyglutamic acid protein. Serum osteocalcin reflects bone turnover rate. Two other proteins crucial to the anticoagulation regulatory processes, protein S and protein C, also contain carboxygammaglutaminate. These proteins are involved with the deactivation of activated factors V and VIII.

Clinical deficiency signs (see Table 39-1). The primary clinical manifestation of a vitamin K deficiency is an increased tendency to hemorrhage as a result of decreased hemostatic function, primarily from a reduction in active prothrombin as well as other clotting factors. The major signs of hemorrhage are ecchymosis (bleeding under the skin), epistaxis, and intestinal bleeding.

Administration of oral anticoagulants during the first trimester of pregnancy results in fetal bone growth retardation deformities known as *fetal warfarin syndrome*. This congenital syndrome may result from the decrease in the gamma carboxylation of osteocalcin and matrix protein, although this has not yet been proven. The defects are the result of premature calcification of cartilage, which can be associated with breathing problems because of nasal hypoplasia.[37]

Chemical deficiency signs. Direct measurement of vitamin K in blood is not usually performed for adults. Determination of prothrombin time (velocity of clotting after addition of thromboplastin and calcium to citrated plasma) is an excellent index of prothrombin adequacy. This time is prolonged in deficiency of vitamin K and also in liver diseases characterized by decreased synthesis of prothrombin. Deficiency of vitamin K also results in prolongation of the partial thromboplastin time, but the thrombin time is within the reference interval. Immunological measurement of acarboxyprothrombin (protein induced by vitamin K absence; PIVKA-II) is useful in the detection of vitamin K deficiency in neonates and appears to have greater sensitivity than the coagulation tests.[38] Vitamin K status can be directly assessed by HPLC measurement of phylloquinone and menaquinone in plasma or liver tissue.

Pathophysiology. The vitamin K malabsorptive states are described above. The prothrombin reduction seen in patients with alcoholic fatty liver is corrected by administration of vitamin K only if there is associated malnutrition or malabsorption. Vitamin K action is antagonized by coumarin or indanedione anticoagulants. Oral contraceptive use increases the levels of prothrombin and factors VII, IX, and X and apparently reduces the requirement for vitamin K.

Vitamin D

As early as 1822, it was known that **rickets** (muscle hypotonia and skeletal deformities) could be prevented with cod liver oil. A century later, the antirachitic factor of cod liver oil was identified as vitamin D, which was soon shown to have multiple forms. These antirachitic compounds are now collectively termed *vitamin D*. The naturally occurring fish oil vitamin is cholecalciferol (vitamin D_3); it is produced in the skin from ultraviolet activation of 7-dehydrocholesterol. Vitamin D_3 is a prohormone that is converted in the liver to 25-hydroxycholecalciferol (calcidiol), which is further hydroxylated in the kidney to form the hormone 1,25-dihydroxycholecalciferol (calcitriol). Calciferol (vitamin D_2), the primary dietary form (the form used in food fortification), is similarly hydroxylated (see Chapter 28).

Major dietary sources include irradiated foods and commercially prepared milk. Small amounts occur in butter, egg yolk, liver, salmon, sardines, and tuna.

Physiological actions, regulation, and assessment of the hormone forms of vitamin D are discussed in Chapter 28. Concentration of 25-hydroxycholecalciferol in serum reflects overall vitamin D status, since it is an average of dietary and sunlight-induced vitamin D. Concentration of 1,25-dihydroxycholecalciferol in serum is useful in evaluations of disorders of calcium and bone metabolism.[39]

Deficiency results in rickets (in children) or osteomalacia (in adults), both of which are forms of abnormal bone synthesis. Excess dietary intake is common in the United States, creating concern as to the role of hypervitaminosis D in development of arteriosclerosis.[40]

WATER-SOLUBLE VITAMINS

The water-soluble vitamins include the B vitamin group and ascorbic acid. The B vitamin group is large and varied (see following box).

B VITAMIN GROUP

Folic acid
Cobalamin
Thiamine
Pyridoxine
Pantothenic acid
Nicotinic acid
Thiamine
Riboflavin
Choline
Inositol

Although choline and inositol are historically considered part of the B vitamin complex, a detailed description of these two nutrients will not be included in this chapter because their status as vitamins is debatable.

Choline (trimethylethanolamine), a constituent of the phospholipid lecithin, is lipotropic (removes lipid from the liver), functions as a methyl donor in hepatocytes, and is required for acetylcholine synthesis. Inositol is an isomeric form of glucose. Similar to choline, inositol is a constituent of phospholipids in cell membranes. Phosphatidylinositol is also found in lipoproteins in serum. Phosphorylated inositol functions as an intracellular second messenger in response to hormones, neurotransmitters, and autocoids (local and often self-acting hormones).

All water-soluble vitamins are absorbed without the involvement of fat absorption, and excess vitamin is almost immediately excreted in the urine. Thiamine is stored for only a few weeks, and most other B-complex vitamins and ascorbic acid are stored for less than 2 months. Development of deficiency can therefore be quite rapid. Vitamin B_{12}, although a water-soluble vitamin, is stored in the liver for several years. The water-soluble vitamins function as coenzymes, and all except ascorbic acid and biotin must be metabolically converted to active forms.

Ascorbic Acid (Vitamin C)

The symptom cluster known as **scurvy** (swollen gums with loss of teeth, skin lesions, bruising, ecchymosis and weakness in the lower extremities) was clearly described during the time of the Crusades and became commonplace when long sea voyages began. In 1747, a naval surgeon experimenting with diets to cure scurvy identified the efficacy of citrus fruits. This antiscurvy agent, vitamin C, was isolated in 1932 and later given the name *ascorbic acid* (from its antiscorbutic effect). The structures of this water-soluble vitamin and its oxidized form, dehydroascorbate, are shown in Fig. 39-5. By virtue of its ene-diol group, ascorbate is a very strong reducing compound. Although plants and most animals can synthesize this vitamin, humans cannot; thus dietary ingestion is essential.

Major dietary sources include fruits (especially citrus) and vegetables (tomatoes, green peppers, cabbage, leafy greens, and potatoes). Since ascorbate is labile to heat and oxygen, fresh and uncooked foods are highest in ascorbate content.

Metabolism. Ascorbate is absorbed in the small intestine. It is widely distributed in tissues (most concentrated in the adrenal cortex and pituitary) and passes the placenta readily. The normal body store requires several months to deplete before the appearance of symptoms of scurvy. Cerebrospinal fluid (CSF) concentrations are higher than those in plasma. Excess ascorbate and a metabolite, oxalate, are readily eliminated in urine. Generally ascorbate metabolism accounts for about half the urinary oxalate (Fig. 39-5).

Function. Ascorbic acid functions as an electron transfer molecule for enzymes that are involved in selected reductive processes. This is essential for the conversion of proline and lysine in procollagen to hydroxyproline and hydroxylysine, respectively. Thus ascorbic acid is important in formation and stabilization of collagen by hydroxylation of proline and lysine, which are used for cross-linking collagen chains. Ascorbic acid may also be involved in the stimulation of collagen synthesis.[41] This effect may be demonstrated clinically since scurvy is a disease of impaired collagen synthesis. Petechiae formation and subsequent bruising in scurvy is thought to reflect decreased fibrous tissue support for capillary beds, which results in their bursting when stressed. Tyrosine conversion to catecholamines via dopamine β-hydroxylase also requires ascorbic acid. In addition, ascorbic acid is involved in the synthesis of carnitine and steroids.[42] Uptake of the nonheme form of iron in the gut is facilitated by ascorbic acid through the nonenzymatic reduction of ferric iron to the ferrous state. Ascorbic acid is also involved in the generation of peptide hormones such as oxytocin and antidiuretic hormone.[43]

Clinical and chemical deficiency signs. Clinical signs of ascorbic acid deficiency are listed in Table 39-1. Clinical signs of scurvy have been associated with serum ascorbate values below 2.4 mg/L or whole blood ascorbate levels below 3 mg/L. Transient low values, however, do not necessarily reflect a tissue deficiency. Increased ascorbate intake raises serum ascorbate levels to a maximum of about 14 mg/L, at which time renal clearance rises sharply. Leukocyte ascorbate is considered to reflect tissue stores more closely but is technically more difficult to assay. Although plasma vitamin C is predominantly in the ascorbic acid form, leukocyte cell types also contain considerable dehydroascorbic acid. The different vitamin C stores in each leukocyte cell type, the possibility of artifactual interconversion of vitamin C forms, and the numerous assay methodologies have led to widely divergent target values for leukocytes.[44,45] Measurement of urinary ascorbate is not recommended for status assessment because it reflects recent intake and is subject to numerous analytical difficulties. Drugs known to increase the urinary excretion of ascorbate include aspirin, aminopyrine, barbiturates, hydantoins, and paraldehyde. No reliable functional assessment of vitamin C status has yet been described. Assessment approaches and pitfalls have recently been reviewed.[44,45]

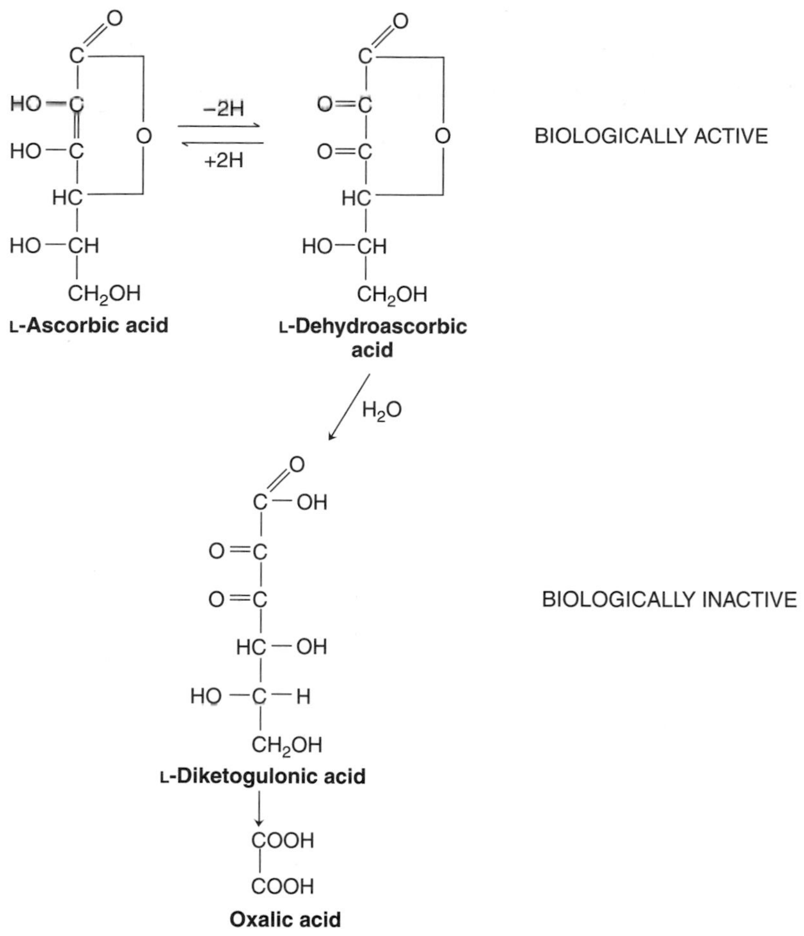

Fig. 39-5   Structures of ascorbic acid and metabolites.

Pathophysiology. Ascorbic acid requirements appear to be increased in chronic illness as well as during pregnancy.

Toxicity and therapeutic uses. The usefulness of ascorbate in preventing colds and cancers has not been scientifically supported (except possibly for gastric and esophageal cancers by prevention of nitrosamine formation)[46] but has led to the practice of megadose intakes of vitamin C. Morbidity and mortality from the common cold is extremely low, and despite the discomfort and lost manpower attributable to frequent colds, the need to use ascorbate as a cure is questioned. Although there is little toxicity associated with this ascorbate, excess intake may interfere with metabolism of vitamin B_{12} and with drug actions (aminosalicylic acid, tricyclic antidepressants, and anticoagulants) and could lead to increased hydroxyl formation, which is itself a contributor to free radicals. A sudden discontinuation of megadose intake can result in rebound scurvy, which is likely the result of the induction of clearance mechanisms of vitamin C.

Riboflavin

This highly pigmented yellow compound consists of flavin, attached to D-ribitol-riboflavin. Its structure and that of its two cofactor-active forms, riboflavin 5'-phosphate (flavin mononucleotide FMN) and flavin adenine dinucleotide

(FAD), are shown in Fig. 39-6. FAD, the most water-soluble of these three **flavins**, exhibits orange fluorescence, whereas the other two fluoresce greenish yellow. Aqueous solutions of flavins are stable to heat and oxidizing agents, but the riboflavin in milk is dramatically reduced on exposure to sunlight.

Foods high in riboflavin include milk, liver, eggs, meat, and some green leafy vegetables. Intestinal organisms synthesize riboflavin, but the distal location of these bacteria may preclude absorption.

Metabolism. Dietary protein complexes of FAD and FMN release these flavins on gastric acidification and proteolysis. After dephosphorylation, they are absorbed in the proximal small intestine and rephosphorylated; they then appear in the circulation weakly bound to albumin and other plasma proteins, including specific riboflavin-binding proteins. The liver and the kidneys quickly take up most flavins, though measurable amounts are found in most tissues. The three flavin forms can be interconverted enzymatically. FAD is the predominant tissue form. Small amounts of flavin are excreted in bile, feces, sweat, and breast milk; urinary flavin excretion is greater. Flavin is excreted in urine mostly in the free riboflavin form; the amount excreted depends on tissue stores and on the amount ingested. The

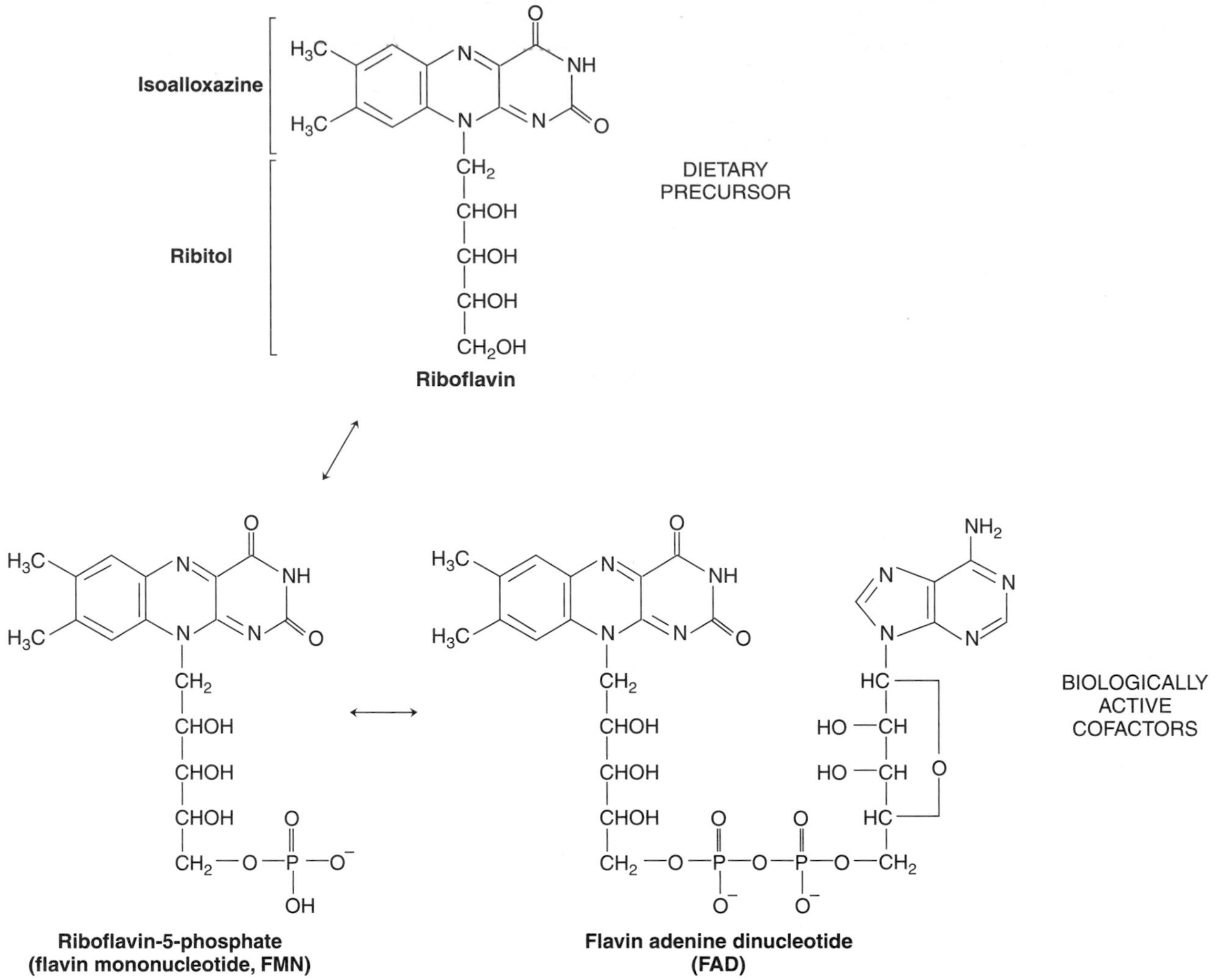

Fig. 39-6 Riboflavin and its active cofactor forms.

body metabolizes only a small amount of the ingested riboflavin. Riboflavin, but not FMN or FAD, is the moiety transferred from plasma into the brain. The flavins in blood are present primarily in the erythrocytes and function in the two FAD enzymes, glutathione reductase and methemoglobin reductase. The fetus obtains free riboflavin derived from maternal erythrocytic FAD through the placenta.

Function. Flavoprotein enzyme systems contain FAD or FMN as prosthetic groups. Most flavoproteins catalyze removal of either a hydride ion or a pair of hydrogen atoms from the substrate. Riboflavin has key roles in respiratory enzymes such as D-amino acid oxidase, pyruvate dehydrogenase, xanthine oxidase, glutathione reductase, and NADH dehydrogenase. In addition, flavins are involved in the metabolism of iron, pyridoxine, and folate; they also play a role in protection against peroxidation, in metabolism of xenobiotics, and in superoxide generation by granulocytes.[47]

Clinical and chemical deficiency signs. Clinical signs of riboflavin deficiency are listed in Table 39-1. Erythrocytic concentrations of riboflavin, FMN, and FAD are more sensitive indices of riboflavin status than flavin measure-

ments in urine or plasma, but these blood indices are altered only late in the progression of deficiency. A functional approach to assessment of riboflavin status involves measurement of the increase in erythrocytic glutathione reductase (EGR) activity after in vitro addition of FAD (EGR index). This EGR index plateaus rapidly and does not continue to increase as deficiency progresses. In subjects deficient in glucose-6-phosphate dehydrogenase (G-6-PD), the EGR index is misleading because the EGR does not lose its coenzyme even in severe riboflavin deficiency.[48]

Pathophysiology. Ariboflavinosis is most commonly encountered when intake is inadequate as a result of poverty. American surveys have indicated inadequate riboflavin nutrition in up to 10% of children, up to 47% of teenagers, and up to 32% of geriatric subjects. Ariboflavinosis can occur as a result of disease states, including prolonged febrile illness, malignancy, hyperthyroidism, cardiac failure, diabetes mellitus, and gastrointestinal diseases. Alcoholics have decreased riboflavin and other nutrients as well. Riboflavin decomposition is accelerated by phototherapy for neonatal jaundice, but the induced deficiency does not appear to limit riboflavin-dependent fatty acid oxidation. Negative nitrogen-balance, seen in all catabolic states (including stress, physical exertion, fasting, prolonged bed rest), results in increased urinary riboflavin excretion. Riboflavin deficiency often occurs concomitantly with deficiencies of other B vitamins. Additionally, riboflavin interacts in metabolic processes involving other vitamins. These interactions can therefore result in a mixed clinical picture and may explain how therapy with one vitamin may improve symptoms of another vitamin deficiency.

Pyridoxine

Vitamin B_6 is known chemically as pyridoxine. Pyridoxal and pyridoxamine were first identified with vitamin activity; then their phosphorylated forms were recognized as active cofactors. The term *vitamin B_6* is reserved for pyridoxine. The structure is shown as pyridoxal phosphate in Fig. 39-7. Pyridoxine occurs mainly in plants, whereas pyridoxal and pyridoxamine are present primarily in animal products. These three pyridine derivatives are metabolically interconverted.

Major dietary sources of vitamin B_6 are meat, poultry, fish, potatoes, and vegetables; dairy products and grains contribute lesser amounts. The predominant food form is pyridoxal phosphate, which is readily lost in food processing.

Metabolism. Pyridoxine does not bind to plasma proteins; pyridoxal and pyridoxal phosphate bind mainly to albumin. Erythrocytes rapidly take up pyridoxine, convert it to pyridoxal phosphate and pyridoxal, and then release pyridoxal into plasma. Metabolism of pyridoxal appears to occur primarily in the liver with formation of 4-pyridoxic acid, which is excreted in urine (Fig. 39-7). Pyridoxal phosphate synthesis depends on a flavin enzyme, which interrelates riboflavin and pyridoxine nutrition. Vitamin B_6 concentration is high in the brain and the CSF; the non-phosphorylated forms enter the CSF, choroid plexus, and brain.

Function. Almost all pyridoxal phosphate-catalyzed reactions involve transformations of amino acids; the major exception is provided by the phosphorylases. Decarboxylation, transamination, and racemization reactions depend on pyridoxine. The pyridoxine cofactor forms act in over 60 different enzyme systems, catalyzing a variety of reaction types, including the clinically relevant transaminases AST and ALT. The best-known functions of the pyridoxine cofactors are their roles in the conversion of tryptophan to 5-hydroxytryptamine (serotonin) and in the separate pathway of tryptophan to nicotinic acid ribonucleotide (the "niacin pathway"), both shown in Fig. 39-8.

Clinical and chemical deficiency signs. Clinical signs of pyridoxine deficiency for infants and adults are listed in Table 39-1. Chemical indices of pyridoxine depletion include reduction in plasma and erythrocyte concentrations of pyridoxine or pyridoxal phosphate. Urinary pyridoxine

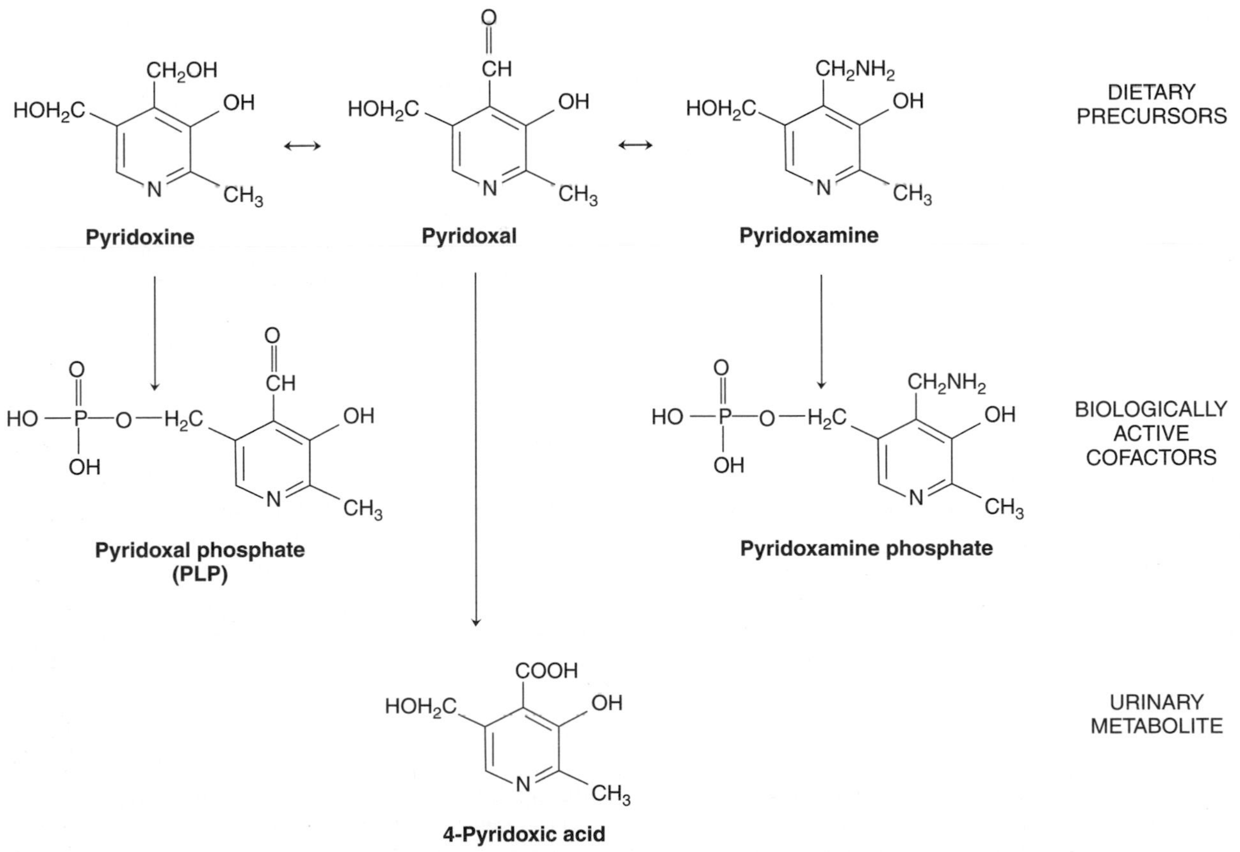

Fig. 39-7 Vitamin B_6 forms and major metabolites.

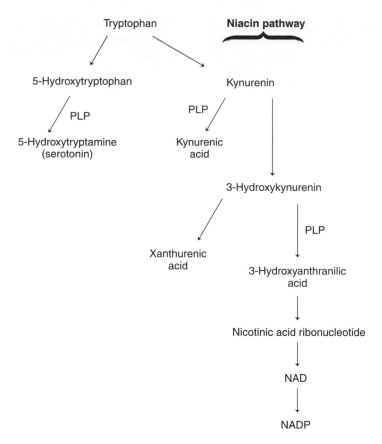

Fig. 39-8 Role of vitamin B_6 in tryptophan metabolism. *NAD*, Nicotinamide adenine dinucleotide; *NADP*, nicotinamide adenine dinucleotide phosphate; *PLP*, pyridoxal phosphate.

(usually representing less than 10% of the pyridoxine intake) and pyridoxic acid, the major urinary metabolite, are also reduced. An oral tryptophan load given to persons suspected of being deficient in pyridoxine results in excretion of several tryptophan metabolites in higher amounts than usual, xanthurenic acid being the one most commonly measured (Fig. 39-8). The involvement of other metabolic and hormonal factors in this pathway necessitates cautious interpretation of the tryptophan challenge test.

The tissue status of pyridoxal phosphate can be assessed by measurement of the increment of erythrocytic aspartate (or alanine) aminotransferase (AST or ALT, respectively) after in vitro addition of the pyridoxal phosphate cofactor. Elevation in the ratio of activity plus or minus pyridoxal phosphate (the EAST index) is suggestive of inadequate tissue stores. Plasmas from normal subjects primarily contain pyridoxal phosphate and 4-pyridoxic acid with lesser amounts of pyridoxal. All the known B_6 vitamins can be measured simultaneously by HPLC. Of the direct measures of B_6 status, plasma pyridoxal phosphate is currently considered most reflective of tissue status. Measurement of plasma pyridoxal phosphate, urinary 4-pyridoxic acid, and an indirect measure (the EAST index or urinary xanthurenic acid) are all recommended to evaluate B_6 status.[49]

Pathophysiology. Conditions that may affect pyridoxine concentrations in the body include celiac disease, ulcerative colitis, lactation, and alcoholism. Certain mental illnesses such as psychoses and schizophrenia have in the past been associated with pyridoxine deficiency; however, to what extent this is simply an associated finding of individuals who have marginal or deficient nutritional intake is uncertain. Pyridoxine requirements increase during pregnancy as a result of fetal demand and hormonal induction of maternal enzymes, which increases maternal requirements. Pyridoxine inadequacy during pregnancy has been linked to suboptimal birth outcomes (infants with low Apgar scores and low birth weight).[50] A novel vitamin B_6 compound (adenosine-N_6-diethylthioether-N_1-pyridoxamine-5α-phosphate) is synthesized by tumor cells; higher concentrations of this B_6 relative in sera from patients with different malignancies indicate that it may be a biomarker of active tumor growth; however, recent literature shows no further development in this area.

Drugs known to antagonize pyridoxine include isonicotinic acid hydrazide (isoniazid, INH), steroids, and penicillamine. Isoniazid combines with pyridoxine to form a hydrazone, which is not available for enzymatic reactions. Thus, because enzymes dependent on pyridoxine as a cofactor can be inactivated, liver function is monitored during isoniazid therapy. The vitamin B_6 compounds are considered to be of low systemic toxicity, although toxicity has been reported with high dosages. Controversy over an antiemetic preparation containing pyridoxine having a teratogenic effect when used to control hyperemesis gravidum is unsubstantiated. However, pyridoxine deficiency in pregnancy *does* confer teratogenic risk.

Niacin

Pellagra (from the Italian, meaning "rough skin") is associated with diarrhea, dementia, and dermatitis (the "three Ds") and has been attributed to poor diet for over two centuries. In 1912, nicotinic acid was extracted from rice polishings and was claimed to have vitamin-like effects, but it was not until 1935 that nicotinic acid (also called *niacin*) was shown to cure black tongue in dogs (a disease similar to pellagra in humans).

Niacin is a simple derivative of pyridine and is extremely stable. The active cofactor forms of NAD and NADP (Fig. 39-9) derived from niacin can also be synthesized in situ from tryptophan (Fig. 39-8), and so sufficient dietary tryptophan can abolish the requirement for niacin. This makes niacin relatively unique with respect to the other vitamins in that we are only partially dependent on diet for a direct source. Sources of niacin include meats and grains, as well as many food products that are supplemented with this vitamin. Corn is especially poor in tryptophan, and part of the niacin in corn is not bioavailable, depending on how the corn is prepared. It has also been noted that high levels of dietary leucine somehow interfere with niacin pathways. The niacin equivalent of tryptophan is approximately 60 mg of tryptophan, equaling 1 mg of niacin. The typical diet has approximately 600 mg of tryptophan, which is not sufficient to meet the nutritional needs for niacin in all adults.

Metabolism. Both niacin and nicotinamide are readily absorbed in the gut. Niacin is transported in blood mainly in erythrocytes. There is little storage of niacin in the body, and urine contains nicotinamide and other metabolites of niacin (Fig. 39-9). Plasma nicotinamide readily enters the CSF, whereas niacin does not. Brain tissue does not express the niacin pathway of tryptophan and so must use plasma nicotinamide from the diet or dephosphorylated forms of the cofactors.

Function. NAD and NADP are involved in a large number of oxidation-reduction reactions catalyzed by dehydrogenases including alcohol, glutamate, glucose-6-phosphate, and glycerol-3-phosphate dehydrogenases. Reduction yields dihydronicotinamide (NADH or NADPH), which has a strong absorption at 340 nm, a feature widely used in assays of **pyridine nucleotide**-dependent enzymes (see Chapter 54).

Clinical and chemical deficiency signs. Clinical signs of niacin deficiency are listed in Table 39-1. Diagnosis of niacin deficiency is usually made with a careful evaluation of the patient's socioeconomic and behavioral status in addition to the clinical picture. Niacin deficiency usually does not occur in isolation, and other nutritional deficits will also be present. The diagnosis of niacin deficiency can usually be confirmed with treatment. Biochemical detection of niacin deficiency is usually not necessary although niacin and several metabolites can be detected in biological fluids. Chemical measures of niacin status primarily involve the two

major urinary metabolites *N'*-methylnicotinamide and *N'*-methyl-2-pyridone-5-carboxylamide. The ratio of 2-pyridone compound to *N'*-methylnicotinamide is reduced in niacin deficiency; reduction in the individual metabolites is also seen.

For some time, pharmacological doses of niacin have been recognized as an efficacious means to reduce mixed dyslipidemias while increasing HDL.[51,52] For example, increased lipoprotein a, or Lp(a) is also treatable with niacin. Large doses of niacin are associated with gastrointestinal discomfort and flushing; however, newer drug combinations and sustained release niacin preparations that can be taken at bedtime will hopefully reduce these side effects and increase compliance.

Thiamine

Thiamine consists of a pyrimidine linked by a methylene group to a substituted thiazole (Fig. 39-10). Thus the name reflects its components of amine and sulfur (*thia-*) groups.

Highly water-soluble, thiamine is easily leached out of foodstuffs being washed or boiled.

Sources of thiamin include yeast, wheat, whole grain and enriched breads and cereals, nuts, peas, potatoes, and most vegetables. In Western society, alcoholics are the most common sufferers of thiamine deficiency, although the elderly[53] and individuals with psychiatric disorders can also be at risk.

Metabolism. Dietary thiamine is absorbed in the intestine by a pH-dependent, carrier-mediated process that is saturated at an oral intake of about 10 mg. About 5% of thiamine appears in the CSF and brain through simple diffusion; the balance is derived through a saturable active transport, most likely through a carrier associated with the choroid plexus. Thiamin is primarily excreted in urine with excretion directly proportional to intake. Thiamine pyrophosphate (TPP) is the predominant moiety in tissues, whereas the major form in plasma is thiamine. Sequestration of thiamine at saturable levels as TPP in tissue is reflected in the differential between erythrocyte and plasma concentrations of this vitamin. Tissues such as liver, heart, and brain have higher concentrations than muscle and other organs.

Function. In its TPP cofactor form, thiamine catalyzes the decarboxylation of α-keto acids (pyruvate and α-ketoglutarate), the oxidative decarboxylation by α-keto acid dehydrogenases, and the formation of ketols. Thiamine pyrophosphate functions in major carbohydrate pathways and also functions in the metabolism of branched-chain amino acids. At one time thiamine triphosphate (TTP) was thought to be an "action" substance released from nerves after electrical stimulation; however, the role of TPP in ion conductance is unsubstantiated.

Clinical deficiency signs. Table 39-1 lists the major clinical signs of thiamine deficiency. The **Wernicke-Korsakoff syndrome** responds to thiamine therapy, and there is evidence for an abnormality of neurotransmitter metabolism, perhaps involving TTP. These patients typically accumulate excessive amounts of pyruvate and lactate in physiological fluids.[54]

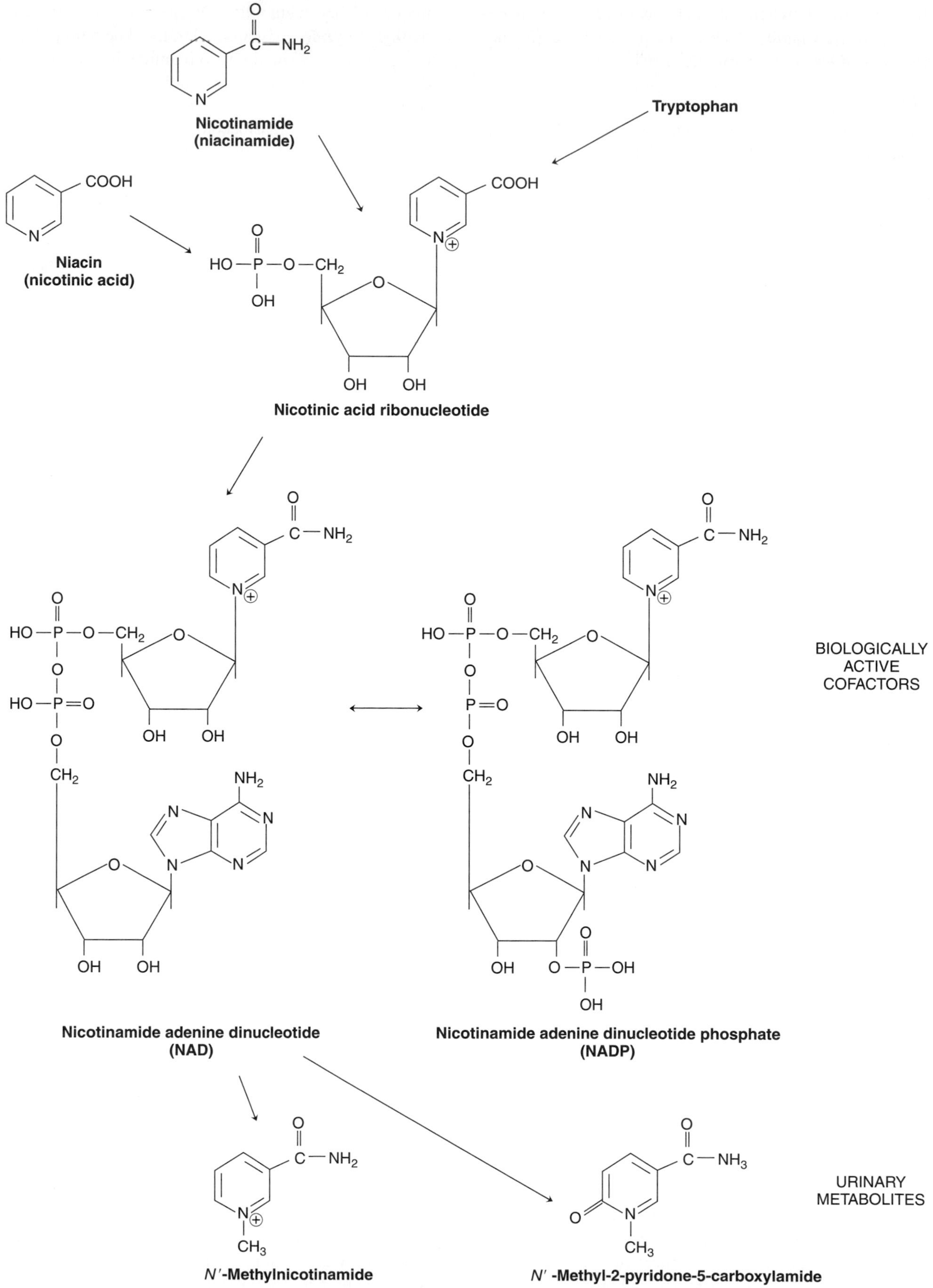

Fig. 39-9 Cofactor forms and metabolites derived from niacin or tryptophan.

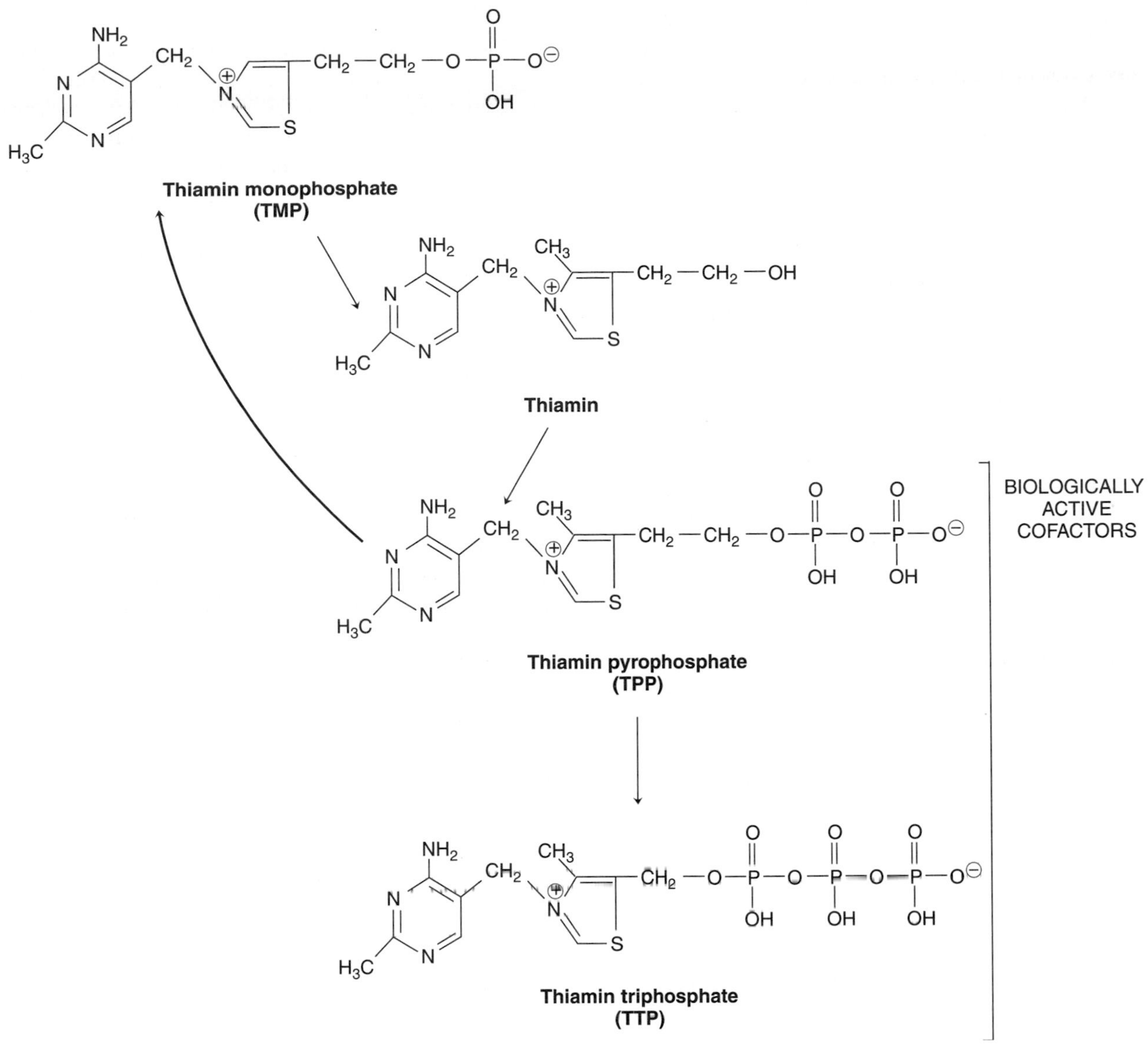

Fig. 39-10 Thiamin and its cofactor forms.

Genetic variations in TPP-dependent enzymes modify the effect of dietary thiamine deficiency. Although most patients with thiamine deficiency do not develop Wernicke-Korsakoff syndrome, mild deficiency leads to impairments in higher integrative functions (including memory). More severe deficiency leads either to **dry beriberi** or **wet beriberi** (see Table 39-1).

Chemical deficiency signs. Chemical indices of thiamine deficiency commonly used are reduction in urinary thiamine, reduction in erythrocyte transketolase (ETK) activity, and stimulation of ETK by in vitro TPP. Prolonged deficiency results in decreased synthesis of the ETK apoenzyme, and so the ETK stimulation test may underestimate the magnitude of deficiency. There is also evidence of reduction of ETK in undernutrition, diabetes, and liver disease without a TPP stimulation effect. As is possible with all proteins, genetic heterogeneity of ETK has been demonstrated in humans. Correlation between ETK stimulation and dietary thiamine or clinical signs is not always seen. There are conflicting reports as to the usefulness of blood thiamine levels; this is possibly related to low concentrations and measurement difficulties. HPLC separates thiamine and its three phosphate esters.

Pathophysiology. The clinical manifestations of thiamine deficiency depend on the degree of depletion. Mild thiamine deficiency is common among elderly persons and alcoholics. Cardiovascular disease associated with thiamine deficiency is relatively common in the elderly or chronic alcoholics. Less commonly, pregnant women are susceptible to a form of cardiac failure that typically presents with high cardiac output that is readily corrected with the administration of thiamine. Paradoxically, thiamine deficiency is thought to be precipitated by furosemide therapy for edema. Thus cardiac failure precipitated or exacerbated by furosemide therapy should be empirically treated with thiamine. Magnesium deficiency, commonly encountered in alcoholics, impairs thiamine activation. This can exacerbate Wernicke's encephalopathy in the already thiamine-depleted alcoholic. Wernicke's encephalopathy is also common in under-nourished AIDS and cancer patients and is characterized by confusion, ataxia, and ophthalmoplegia. This disorder is so common among alcoholics that preventative treatment with intravenous thiamine is often given at hospital admission without clear clinical signs of the disorder.

Korsakoff's psychosis often presents with Wernicke's syndrome. This psychiatric disorder is characterized by memory loss and learning deficits. Confabulation also occurs to compensate for the memory loss. Leigh disease, a necrotizing encephalopathy of childhood, is also associated with decreased brain TTP. Leigh disease is a congenital disorder of oxidative phosphorylation resulting in lesions in numerous areas of the brain, including the stem, optic nerve, and thalamic region. The disease may present early in child-hood with gait problems progressing to severe neurological deterioration. At least three enzyme defects are associated with Leigh disease. Deficiencies of pyruvate dehydrogenase, pyruvate carboxylase, and cytochrome-C oxidase have all been associated with Leigh disease. The common feature is that thiamine dependent oxidative pathways are affected. Treatment can include high-dose thiamine, lipoic acid, and creatine.

Studies have failed to show that oral contraceptive use induces deficiency of thiamine or indeed most vitamins. The time course to thiamine deficiency with a thiamine-deficient diet is relatively short, although predicting the development of deficiency could occur only under controlled experimental conditions. Patients with typical sporadic amyotrophic lateral sclerosis (ALS) reportedly have a very high incidence of decreased CSF thiamine monophosphate with inversion of the thiamine/TMP ratio.[55] The significance of this finding in either the development, progression, or course of ALS has not been established. Some groups susceptible to unrecognized thiamine deficiency are chronically ill children (those receiving nasogastric feeding or intensive chemo-therapy or receiving intensive care for a period of weeks) and individuals suffering from chronic vomiting or behavioral-based eating disorders. Patients who are administered carbo-hydrates or who are treated for hyperglycemia are at risk for thiamine deficiency (as a result of the thiamine consumption that occurs in normal carbohydrate metabolism). Those most at risk are patients who are already nutritionally compromised.

Biotin

The water-soluble coenzyme, biotin (structure shown in Fig. 39-11), was discovered through experimental diets consisting of raw egg whites administered to rats. The cause of biotin deficiency in this diet was **avidin**, a heat-labile component of egg white that binds with biotin with one of the highest noncovalent associations known. The presence of avidin prevents biotin from being absorbed. Numerous foods contain biotin, though no one food is especially rich (up to 2 mg/100 g).

Metabolism. Biotin is absorbed in the proximal half of the small intestine and circulates in blood largely bound to plasma proteins. Forms of excreted biotin in urine include bisnorbiotin, bisnorbiotin methyl ketone, biotin sulfoxide, and biotin sulfone. Little else is known about the catabolic pathways of this cofactor.

Function. Biotin acts as a coenzyme, participating in the metabolic pathways of gluconeogenesis, fatty acid synthesis, and amino acid catabolism. Specifically, biotin functions as a prosthetic group for carboxylation and carboxyl exchange reactions. Important enzymes include acetyl CoA, propionyl CoA, and pyruvate carboxylases, as well as methylmalonyl-oxaloacetic transcarboxylase. Recently, the enzyme biotini-dase has been shown to have biotin transferase activity in addition to its hydrolase activity. Biotin has been observed covalently attached to the nuclear histone proteins. The reason for biotinylation of histones is unclear; however, biotin may play a direct role in the regulation of protein transcription.

Clinical deficiency signs. Pure biotin deficiency is extremely rare. Table 39-1 lists the major signs of biotin deficiency.

Chemical deficiency signs. Dietary deficiency is accompanied by decreased urinary and plasma[56] biotin and increased urinary organic acids, indicating functional defi-ciency of β-methylcrotonyl CoA carboxylase and propionyl CoA carboxylase. Genetic alterations in these carboxylases may result in biotin-dependent states that cause metabolic acidosis and require pharmacological biotin doses; these enzyme deficiencies are confirmed in leukocytes. Genetic deficiency of biotinidase, which can be detected by a blood spot assay, is treated with biotin.[57]

Pathophysiology. With proper modern nutrition, biotin deficiencies are extremely rare. However, biotin deficiency might be suspected in newborns on special diets, patients

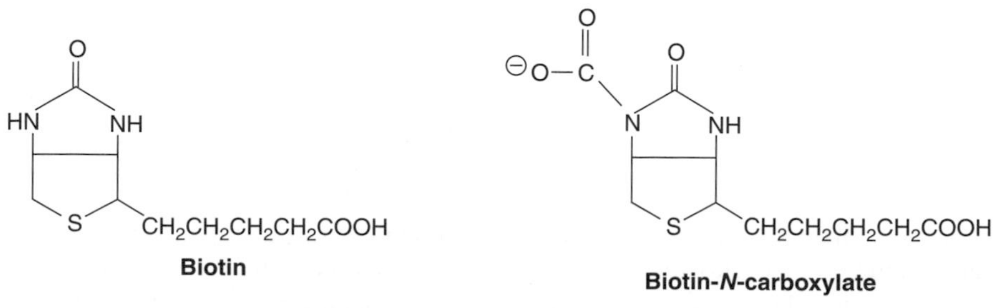

Biotin

Biotin-*N*-carboxylate

Fig. 39-11 Biotin and its active form.

receiving long-term total parenteral nutrition, and occasionally in individuals who practice unusual eating habits, such as the ingestion of raw eggs. Apparent biotin deficiency also occurs with inherited metabolic disorders of biotin metabolism. Biotinidase deficiency or holo-carboxylase synthetase deficiency are autosomal recessive disorders that prevent the completion of biotin dependent pathways.

Pantothenic Acid

Pantothenic acid is the precursor to 4'-phosphopantothenine, a cofactor that is indispensable in fatty acid metabolism. Dietary sources include liver and other organ meats, milk, eggs, peanuts, legumes, mushrooms, salmon, and whole grains. Although many organisms are capable of synthesizing pantothenic acid, there is no evidence that intestinal microorganisms are responsible for part of the human daily requirement of this cofactor.

Metabolism. As shown in Fig. 39-12, pantothenate is metabolically converted to 4'-phosphopantothenine, which becomes covalently bound to either serum acyl carrier protein (ACP) or to coenzyme A. Little is known of pantothenate metabolism. Urinary excretion of pantothenate

decreases with experimental deficiencies. Free pantothenate is the major form in both urine and serum, whereas coenzyme A is the major erythrocytic form. The appearance of various fatty acids in circulation has not proven to be a good indicator of pantothenate deficiency.

Function. Coenzyme A is a highly important acyl-group transfer coenzyme that is involved in a large number of reactions of a great variety of reaction types. Acyl derivatives of coenzyme A are first formed (by thioester linkage), followed by transfer of the acyl group to an acceptor molecule.

Clinical and chemical deficiency signs. No clear-cut case of a pantothenate deficiency has been reported; Table 39-1 lists clinical signs observed in experimentally induced deficiencies. Cellular levels of coenzyme A remain unchanged in pantothenate deficiency, indicating a pantothenate conserving process that minimizes the effects of reduced nutritional intake.

Pathophysiology. Low urinary excretion and reduced blood levels of pantothenate have been reported in patients with chronic malnutrition and alcoholism. The clinical significance of pure pantothenate deficiency is unclear. No toxicity from increased intake is known.

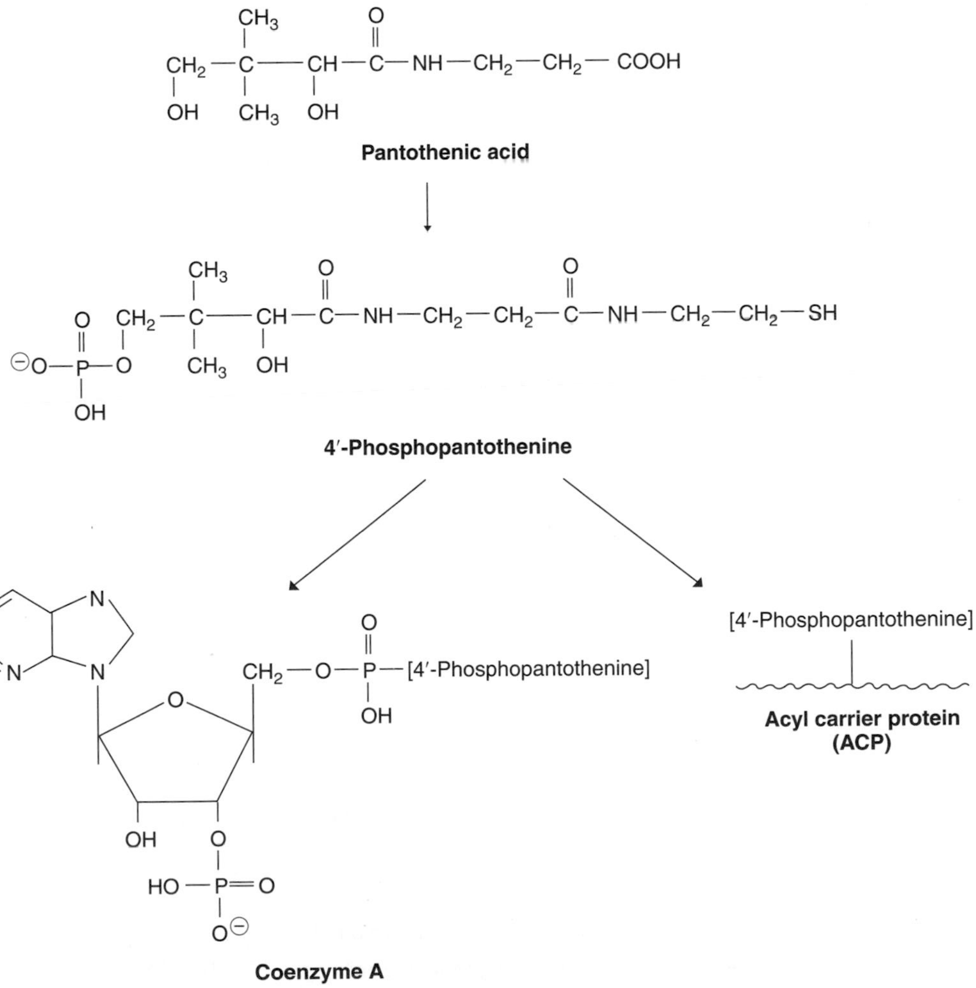

Fig. 39-12 Pantothenic acid and its active cofactors.

Vitamin B$_{12}$

Vitamin B$_{12}$, an isolate from liver extracts, was shown to reverse some forms of pernicious anemia. Another compound isolated from leafy vegetables was shown to reverse other types of pernicious anemia. Purification of this substance led to its identification as pteroylglutamic acid, more commonly known as *folic acid*. Thus similar clinical symptoms were found to result from deficiencies of two totally different structures (Figs. 39-13 and 39-14), neither of which could replace the other. The clinical similarities and the metabolic interactions of vitamin B$_{12}$ and folic acid usually dictate their simultaneous assessment.[58] This is of particular importance when administering one or the other vitamin since methyl-trapping, that is, sequestration of folate, can occur when cobalamin (vitamin B$_{12}$) is administered. Conversely, symptoms of cobalamin deficiency can be masked by folate administration.

Vitamin B$_{12}$ bears a corrin ring (containing pyrroles similar to porphyrin) linked to a central cobalt atom. Different corrinoid compounds, or cobalamins, are distinguished by the substituent linked to the cobalt, with methylcobalamin and 5′-deoxyadenosylcobalamin being the two known coenzyme forms.

Dietary sources of vitamin B$_{12}$ are primarily of animal origin (meat, eggs, milk). Total vegetarian diets are therefore likely settings for deficiency. Animals can derive some of their vitamin B$_{12}$ from intestinal microbial synthesis. The average daily diet contains 3 to 30 mg of vitamin B$_{12}$, of which 1 to 5 mg is absorbed. The frequency of dietary deficiency increases with age, occurring in a substantial proportion of older adults,[59] particularly when cobalamin status is assessed by the measurement of intracellular release of the metabolites of cobalamin metabolism, methylmalonic acid, homocysteine, and cystathionine. Direct measurement of cobalamin, B$_6$, and folate demonstrated deficiency of one or all B vitamins in 30% of adults aged 65 to 75 years and 55% in adults older than 75 years.[60] All the more striking was the occurrence of B vitamin deficiency in these two aged populations when cobalamin metabolites were used as an indicator of deficiency. Deficiency of cobalamin and the

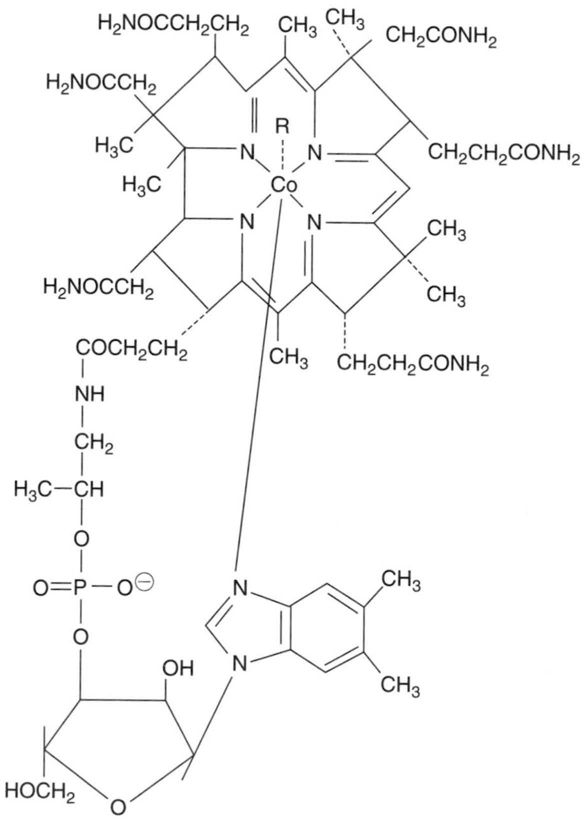

	R		
(Me-B$_{12}$)	CH$_3$	**Methylcobalamin**	ACTIVE COFACTOR FORMS
(Ado-B$_{12}$)	5′-Deoxy-adenosine	**Deoxyadenosyl-cobalamin**	
(OH-B$_{12}$)	OH	**Hydroxocobalamin**	DIETARY FORMS AND THERAPY
(CN-B$_{12}$)	CN	**Cyanocobalamin**	

Fig. 39-13   Vitamin B$_{12}$ forms.

other B vitamins was 55% and 90% in each of the respective groups. This observation demonstrates two important concepts in monitoring vitamin status; first, measurement of accumulated metabolites can be a sensitive indicator of intracellular deficiency and second, there is a reciprocal relationship of age to poor nutritive intake and absorption. Poor nutritional intake appears to be a larger determining factor for folate deficiency[61] when compared with cobalamin deficiency in the elderly. Care must be taken when interpreting studies from diverse geographical locations as diet, socioeconomic status and general health of the elderly population can vary widely between regions.

Metabolism. Most vitamin B_{12} absorption is through a complex with intrinsic factor (IF), a protein secreted by gastric parietal cells (Fig. 39-15). Gastric parietal cell release of hydrogen ion is also essential for the liberation of cobalamin from exogenous binding proteins. The IF- B_{12} complex binds with specific ileal receptors. IF-antibodies, which prevent binding of vitamin B_{12} to IF, are considered blocking antibodies, while binding antibodies can combine with either free IF or the IF- B_{12} complex, thus preventing attachment of the complex to ileal receptors. Parietal cell antibodies have also been identified as a cause of pernicious anemia.

Released from the IF complex within the mucosal cell, vitamin B_{12} circulates in plasma bound to specific transport proteins and is deposited in liver, bone marrow, and other tissues. There is a significant enterohepatic circulation of vitamin B_{12}. As a result of this biliary reabsorption, several years may be required for a strict vegetarian to become clinically deficient. Deficiency becomes evident significantly sooner in a person who has normal B_{12} stores but lacks IF.

Cobalamin is transported by a family of binder proteins called the *transcobalamins*. Transcobalamin II (TC II) appears to be the major serum protein transporting vitamin

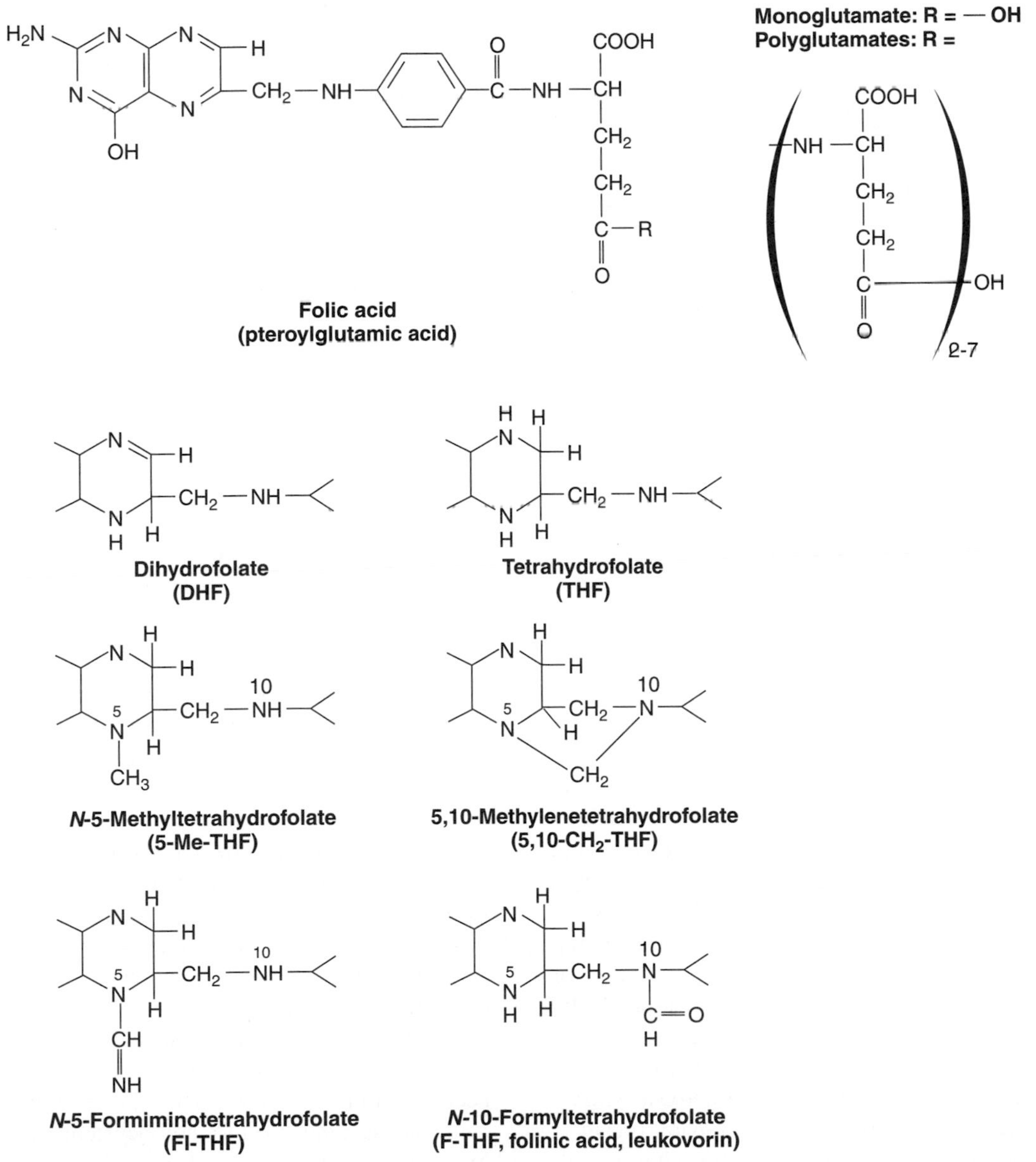

Fig. 39-14 Structures of folic acid forms.

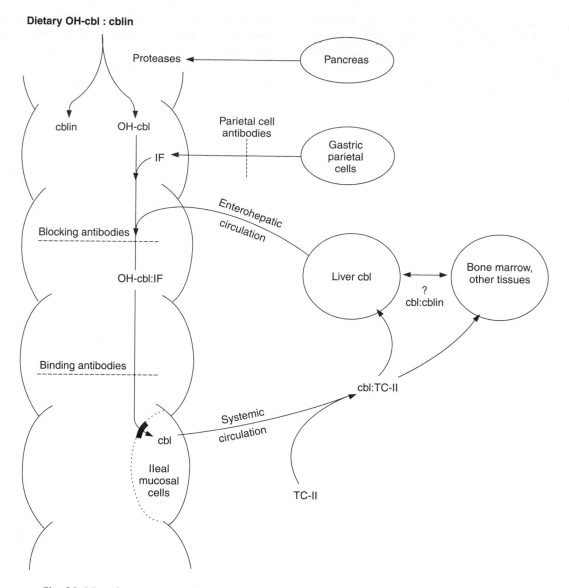

Fig. 39-15 Absorption of dietary vitamin B_{12} and its transport to storage sites. *cblin*, Cobalophilin; *cbl*, cobalamin; *IF*, intrinsic factor; *OH-cbl*, hydroxycobalamin; *TC II*, transcobalamin II.

B_{12} to tissues. TCI (previously named *cobalophilin, R,* or *rapidly migrating protein,* or *binding protein*) is found in high concentrations in secondary granules of granulocytes. It is also produced in glandular endothelial cells,[62] particularly in the digestive system, bronchial glands, renal proximal tubules, prostate, uterus, Fallopian tubes, sweat glands, and mammary glands. The role of this protein is not understood; however, it is thought to be involved in local immunological defense.[62] One speculation is that granulocytic degranulation of TCI blocks bacterial use of the local concentration of cobalamin, thereby preventing bacterial replication. Little is known about the role of TCIII. Plasma contains all types of transport proteins and the three forms of vitamin B_{12} (hydroxycobalamin, methylcobalamin, and deoxyadenosyl-cobalamin); however, TCII is the predominant transport protein. Absorption and transport of this vitamin are illustrated in Fig. 39-15.

Functions. There are two distinct known roles for cobalamin. The deoxyadenosylcobalamin form (AdoCbl) is a cofactor for the enzyme methylmalonyl CoA mutase, which is responsible for the conversion of methylmalonyl CoA to succinyl CoA. An absolute deficiency of cobalamin or congenital lack of the enzyme results in accumulation of the intermediate methylmalonyl CoA and subsequent hydrolysis to methylmalonic acid. The second important reaction involves methylcobalamin, which functions as a methyl-donor for methionine synthase. A deficiency of methylcobalamin (MeCbl) will result in the accumulation of homocysteine, the precursor to methionine. A lack of functional methionine synthase or methionine synthase reductase will also cause an accumulation of homocysteine. Folate deficiency will also cause an accumulation of homocysteine since methyltetra-hydrofolate is responsible for the de novo methylation of cobalamin to sustain the reaction.

Methionine, obtained from remethylated homocysteine, is necessary for the generation of adenosylmethionine, which bears a high-energy methyl group. This methyl group participates in over one hundred intracellular reactions. Notably, intact DNA synthesis requires adequate methylation activity to ensure the incorporation of thymidine and not uridine. The insertion of uridine in the DNA double strand increases the need for DNA repair, placing the organism at increased risk for flawed DNA replication. Dietary deficiency of the precursor of these two coenzyme forms results in deficiencies of both active cobalamins. Genetic deficiencies of enzymes in either pathway are known. In the few case reports of inherited deficiency of TC II, symptoms of pancytopenia and failure to thrive develop within a few months of birth. Several large studies have shown a racial difference in serum vitamin B_{12} levels, with blacks maintaining higher B_{12} levels than whites.[63]

Clinical and chemical deficiency signs. Table 39-1 lists signs of vitamin B_{12} deficiency. Diagnostic tests for vitamin B_{12} deficiency include measurement of serum B_{12} by microbiological or radioligand assay methods, measurement of urinary or serum methylmalonic acid or total homocysteine, and the Schilling test (see p. 557).

Early serum B_{12} competitive-binding methods used B_{12} binders with variable purity and binding specificity, yielding unreliable results; there are numerous reports of cobalamin deficiency in patients with normal serum cobalamin concentrations. Analysis of serum methylmalonic acid concentration, by gas chromatography-mass spectrometry, appears to be a more sensitive and specific indicator of cobalamin deficiency than direct measures of serum cobalamin. However the cost of this assay prohibits its use as first-line test in the assessment of cobalamin deficiency. Urinary methylmalonic acid excretion has been recommended as a sensitive screening test for undetected cobalamin deficiency among the elderly and the newborn. Uremic patients show elevated serum methylmalonic acid apparently unrelated to cobalamin status. This may be a function of the form and location of cobalamin or it may reflect decreased methylmalonyl CoA mutase activity. Hyperhomocysteinemia is seen in deficiency of B_{12}, folate, or vitamin B_6. It is likely not an early indicator of B_6 status and does not appear to be superior to serum methylmalonic acid as an index of B_{12} deficiency.

An invasive and largely unused test for cobalamin deficiency is the deoxyuridine suppression test, which is based on the observation that preincubation of normal bone marrow with an appropriate concentration of deoxyuridine severely suppresses the subsequent incorporation of tritiated thymidine into DNA. This suppression is subnormal with bone marrow from patients deficient in either vitamin B_{12} or folate and is correctable in vitro by addition of the appropriate deficient vitamin.

Pathophysiology. Inadequate secretion of intrinsic factor may accompany lesions of the gastric mucosa, gastric atrophy, gastrectomy, iron deficiency, and some endocrine disorders. The IF-B_{12} complex may be inadequately formed in pancreatic insufficiency because there is insufficient pancreatic protease activity to split the dietary vitamin B_{12} from cobalophilin in the duodenum. The IF-B_{12} complex may be inadequately absorbed in ileal malfunction (sprue, enteritis, ileal resection, neoplasias, and granulomas). The term *pernicious anemia* is now most commonly applied to vitamin B_{12} deficiency resulting from lack of IF. Antibodies to IF and to parietal cells are common in pernicious anemia patients, in their healthy relatives, and in patients with other autoimmune disorders. Blocking antibodies can result in normal or high serum B_{12} levels in patients with pernicious anemia. Hyperhomocysteinemia is an independent risk factor for premature vascular disease and is associated with suboptimal status of B_6, B_{12}, or folate.

In addition to deficiencies of cobalamin, congenital defects of the enzymes directly and indirectly involved with cobalamin transport and metabolism can present in childhood with a wide range of clinical signs, including megaloblastic anemia, developmental delay, and failure to thrive. Eight genetic disorders are characterized by somatic cell (fibroblast) hybridization (complementation) studies. These are the cbl complementation inherited disorders named *cblA-H*. Each of the disorders can be determined by the biochemical picture in the child and by the correction (complementation) of the disorder in cultured fibroblasts fused to other characterized cell lines. For example, a cbla will be corrected by fusion to all other cbl cell lines with the exception of cblA. A description of the cbl, complementation disorders is beyond the scope of this chapter and interested readers should read Fenton and Rosenberg's chapter in reference.[64]

Folic Acid

Structural relatives of pteroylglutamic acid (folic acid) are the metabolically active compounds usually referred to as folates (see Fig. 39-14). Up to eight glutamate residues may be found in these naturally occurring compounds. The glutamate residue number may function as a "handle" for the channeling of folate from enzyme to enzyme. Channeling is the movement of cofactor or substrate from enzyme to enzyme within a biochemical complex without equilibration to the external environment. This serves to conserve a rare cofactor or substrate and to prevent degradation if it is unstable. Also, it is thought that the various enzymes that use folate as a cofactor preferentially have affinity to a specific number of glutamate residues attached to the folate molecule. Therefore if cells control the number of glutamate residues added to the folate cofactor, efficient and coordinated use of the species can be facilitated.[65]

Food folates are primarily found in green and leafy vegetables, fruits, and organ meats. Excessive heating of foods and use of large quantities of water when boiling vegetables results in folate destruction. Because the intake of folate is insufficient in the diets of many individuals living in Western cultures, particularly pregnant women, many countries are now supplementing cereal and grain foods, as well as flours, with folate.

Metabolism. The naturally occurring folate polyglutamates are hydrolyzed to monoglutamate forms before absorption (which occurs primarily in the proximal jejunum) by the intestinal mucosal cells. After this, folate enters the liver through the portal circulation. Enterohepatic recirculation is required for distribution of folate to the general circulation. While the liver converts some folate monoglutamates to polyglutamates for its own use, folate that is excreted to bile as N^5-methyltetrahydrofolate (MeTHF) is the primary source of folate available to tissues. The enzyme responsible for the synthesis of methyltetrahydrofolate is methylenetetrahydrofolate reductase (MTHFR). This methylated form of folate is reabsorbed from the gut but is not taken up by the liver and therefore becomes the major circulating form of folate. Serum folate (MeTHF), in the monoglutamate form, readily enters the choroid plexus and the CSF. Folic acid, on the other hand, is readily transported from CSF to plasma. A folate-binding protein has been identified in the choroid plexus, probably accounting for the high CSF/plasma ratio. The CSF form is mainly MeTHF; brain folates are predominantly polyglutamate forms of dihydrofolate (DHF). Folate catabolism involves cleavage of the pterin ring, followed by acetylation to form the excreted product, *p*-acetamidobenzoylglutamic acid.

Function. Folate (MeTHF) is a cofactor for enzymatic reactions involving one-carbon transfers. After cellular uptake, the MeTHF is converted to THF while transferring a carbon to homocysteine to yield methionine. As mentioned previously, this reaction requires vitamin B_{12}. In the absence of vitamin B_{12}, the folate is essentially trapped in the MeTHF form, making it unavailable for other reactions, including the synthesis of thymine for DNA (Fig. 39-16).

Clinical and chemical deficiency signs. The major clinical symptom of frank and prolonged folate deficiency is megaloblastic anemia. Other indices of deficiency are, in order of occurrence, moderate hyperhomocysteinemia, low serum folate (see Table 39-2), hypersegmentation of neutrophils, high urinary formiminoglutamic acid (FIGLU; a histidine metabolite accumulating in absence of folate), low erythrocyte folate, macro-ovalocytosis, megaloblastic marrow, and finally anemia. The deoxyuridine suppression test, discussed with vitamin B_{12}, is also an index of folate status. The urinary FIGLU test requires ingestion of an oral load of histidine, followed by a timed urine collection, and can be abnormally high in deficiencies of either folate or vitamin B_{12}. Because most folate storage occurs after the vitamin B_{12}-dependent step, erythrocyte folate can also be reduced in deficiency of either B_{12} or folate. As indicated in the discussion of vitamin B_{12}, homocysteine elevation in serum or urine occurs in folate deficiency. Total homocysteine is generally measured, which is the sum of all homocysteine species, both free and protein-bound forms. Homocysteine measurements should be interpreted in conjunction with the determination of folate and cobalamin status.

Pathophysiology. Folate requirement increases during pregnancy and lactation. The increase is the result of elevated

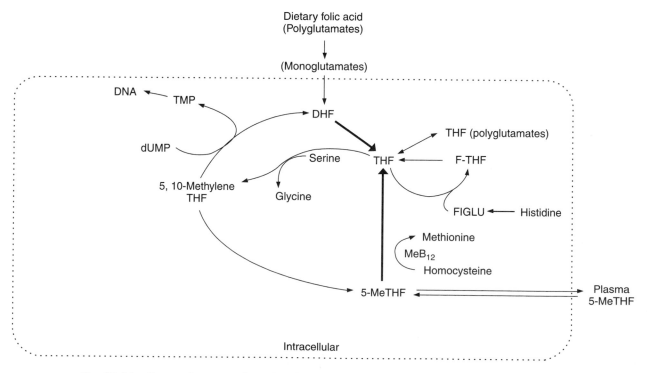

Fig. 39-16 One-carbon transfer using folic acid forms as cofactors. *DHF,* Dihydrofolate; *DNA,* deoxyribonucleic acid; *dUMP,* deoxyuridine monophosphate; *FIGLU,* formimino-L-glutaric acid; *F-THF,* folinic acid; *MeB$_{12}$,* methylcobalamin; *5-MeTH,* N^5-methyltetrahydrofolate; *THF,* tetrahydrofolate; *TMP,* thymidine monophosphate.

demand in the rapidly growing tissues of the placenta and fetus and the newborn. The increase during lactation partially results from the presence in milk of high-affinity folate binders, which likely serve to concentrate folate in milk for the infant. Other conditions that may result in an increased need for folate include hemolytic anemias, iron deficiency, prematurity, and malignant neoplasia—particularly neoplasias in which bone marrow infiltration is present. End-stage renal disease patients receiving dialysis treatment rapidly lose folate and pyridoxine. Folate deficiency as a result of malabsorption can occur in sprue, celiac disease, and inflammatory bowel diseases. Intestinal transport of folate is pH-sensitive at the micro-environmental level. Conditions that can interfere with intestinal transport include not only inflammatory bowel disease but also some of the drugs used to treat it, notably sulfasalazine.

Genetic alterations in most of the folate-interconverting enzymes have been reported. The best-described genetic defect is in the gene for MTHFR and consists of a C677T transition, resulting in a thermolabile phenotype in the expressed enzyme. Approximately 12% of Caucasians are homozygous for this defect. A second defect is found at allele 1298 on this gene, A1298C. This mutation has nearly the same allele frequency of the C677T mutation in Caucasians, and some cases of combined dual 677/1298 mutations have been reported,[66,67] which may result in spontaneous abortion or neural tube defects.[67,68] Both mutations result in reduced MTHFR activity, which in turn decreases the quantity of folate delivered to bile and subsequently to systemic circulation. Coupled with the marginal intake of folate in diets, these polymorphisms likely play a significant role in the development of hyperhomocysteinemia.[69,70] Maintaining a plasma folate concentration above 15 nmol/L (6.6 ng/mL) would have a significant effect on reducing the occurrence of hyperhomocysteinemia in adults.[69,70] This is the first instance of a reference interval that takes into account the genetic influence on nutrient handling. Several rare cases of folate transport defects have been described, involving children who are unable to transfer folates from the lumen of the gut to blood and, in some cases, into CSF. Failure to thrive and mental retardation are common in these children. Remarkably, neural tube defects have not been described in these cases. This suggests that maternal-placental-fetal transfer of folate does not depend on the transport systems found in the postgestational state. Folate deficiency of dietary origin commonly occurs in the elderly.[71]

Phenytoin (Dilantin) therapy accelerates folate metabolism. Alcohol interferes with folate's enterohepatic circulation, whereas the chemotherapeutic agent methotrexate inhibits the enzyme dihydrofolate reductase.

The therapeutic form of folate is 5-formyl-THF (also known as *leucovorin, citrovorum factor,* or *folinic acid*). This form of folate can bypass MeTHF and enter the cycles of folate's one-carbon transfer reactions (see Fig. 39-16). This feature is useful in the "leucovorin rescue" of pediatric cancer patients given high-dose methotrexate therapy with toxic levels of methotrexate. The use of folate supplements prior to conception and early pregnancy is now recommended to reduce the occurrence of neural tube defects.[72] As noted at the start of this section, government-mandated grain and cereal supplementation should also help to reduce the risk of development of neural tube defects.

Carnitine

Carnitine, including L-carnitine and its fatty acid esters (acylcarnitines) (Fig. 39-17), is described as a "conditionally essential" nutrient.

Major dietary sources are meat, poultry, fish, and dairy products. Foods of plant origin generally contain very little carnitine (exceptions being peanut butter, asparagus, and avocados). Average diets provide more than half the human requirement; strict vegetarian diets provide only 10% of the total available carnitine. Most of the dietary carnitine is absorbed.

Metabolism. De novo synthesis involves *N*-tri-methyl-lysine residues of proteins; the biosynthetic rate is determined by the available supply of these *N*-tri-methyllysine residues. Synthesis occurs in liver, brain, and kidney, with storage primarily in muscle. Carnitine is not degraded but is excreted mainly in the urine both as free and esterified forms.

Function. L-carnitine facilitates entry of long-chain fatty acids into mitochondria for oxidation and energy production.[73] As shown in Fig. 39-18, coenzyme A esters of the long-chain fatty acids (acyl-S-CoA) are transesterified to L-carnitine by means of catalysis by an enzyme of the mitochondrial outer membrane, CPT I (carnitine palmitoyltransferase I). Once inside the inner membrane, the long-chain fatty acid is once again transesterified (by CPT II), yielding the CoA ester, which can enter the beta-oxidation pathway for energy production.[74] The carnitine "transporter" can then leave the mitochondria to be reused, or it can serve its other known role and carry out short- and medium-chain fatty acids that accumulate in normal or abnormal metabolism.

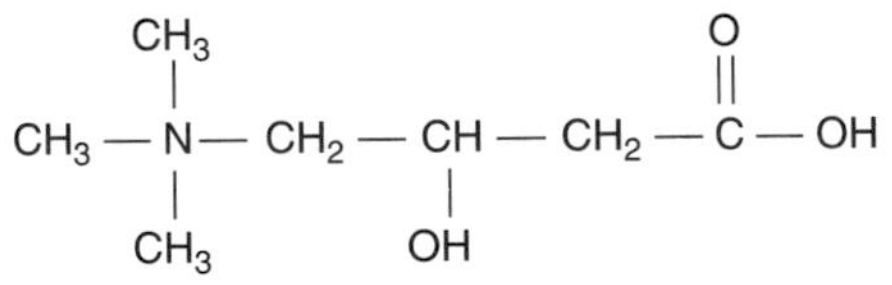

L-Carnitine

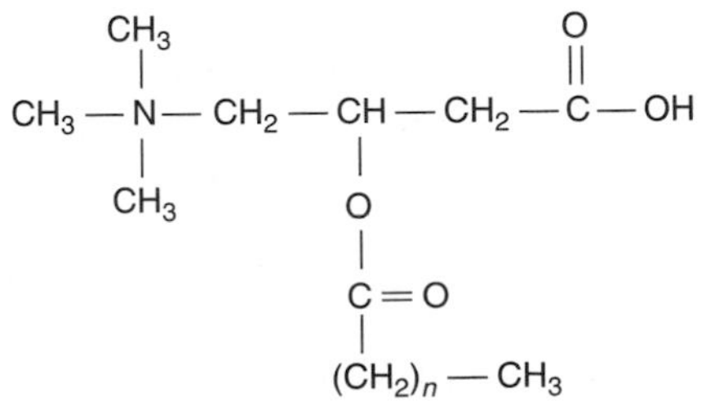

Acylcarnitine

Fig. 39-17 L-Carnitine and fatty acid esters.

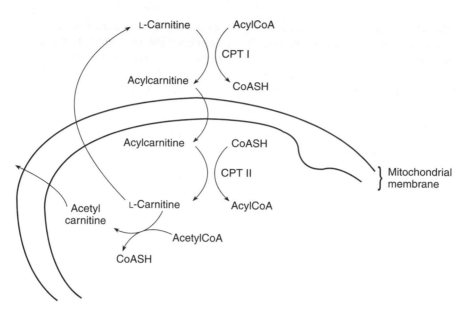

Fig. 39-18 Carnitine transport of acyl groups.

The carnitine esters may be excreted in urine or distributed in tissues; some may be used for specific purposes.

Chemical deficiency signs. The major signs of carnitine deficiency are muscle weakness and fatigue. Chemical indices of deficiency include decreased total or free carnitine in serum, urine or tissues. Total carnitine is measured after hydrolysis of ester forms to free carnitine; acylcarnitines represent the difference between these two measures. Short- and long-chain esters can be distinguished by differing solubility. Characterization of individual esters is helpful in recognizing disorders of fatty acid metabolism; techniques include gas chromatography-mass spectrometry and fast atom bombardment mass spectrometry. Abnormally high ratios of acylcarnitines to free carnitine are seen in disorders of fatty acid oxidation and also in ketosis (excess acetylcarnitine).

Pathophysiology. Human deficiency can be either hereditary (systemic carnitine deficiency, myopathic carnitine deficiency) or acquired. Acquired deficiency can be caused by inadequate intake, increased requirement (pregnancy and breast feeding), or increased urinary loss (valproic acid therapy). Infants, patients following a course of long-term parenteral nutrition, and perhaps children are groups most vulnerable to deficiency as judged by decreased circulating levels and altered indicators of energy metabolism. Patients receiving hemodialysis may lose carnitine in the dialysis fluid. Excessive loss is also seen in Fanconi syndrome. These secondary deficiencies may result in muscular dysfunction. Primary deficiencies show muscle weakness and fatigue and may also have cardiac and hepatic involvement. Carnitine therapies are being evaluated for these circumstances and also in patients with disorders of ammonia metabolism. The three-carbon ester propionyl-L-carnitine has been shown to protect the ischemic heart from reperfusion injury. Function of patients with Alzheimer's disease has been reportedly improved by treatment with acetyl-L-carnitine. Mechanisms for these processes are not yet clear.[74]

Primary carnitine deficiency is very rare. In this inherited disorder lipid metabolism is affected, and both cardiac and skeletal muscles have fat deposits. Muscle weakness, cardiomyopathy, and hepatic disturbances can occur with this disorder.

THE ANTIOXIDANT AND CANCER PREVENTIVE ROLE OF CERTAIN VITAMINS[75-80]

Free radicals are highly reactant molecules generated during ordinary metabolism and from certain drugs or xenobiotics (foreign chemicals). Exposure to ultraviolet radiation, cigarette smoke, and other environmental pollutants increases the body's burden of free radicals. These short-lived free radicals can damage membranes, enzymes, and DNA. An array of antioxidant defenses exists in cells and tissues to prevent formation or limit the effects of free radicals. Free radicals have been implicated as a possible cause of cancer and cardiovascular disease. Vitamins C and E and β-carotene protect against cancer of the lung and other epithelial tissues through a variety of mechanisms. Human intervention trials testing the efficacy of these compounds as anticancer agents are ongoing. Recent evidence indicates that low-density lipoprotein (LDL) apoprotein may be modified by a free radical-driven lipid peroxidation process. The resultant modified ApoB protein has altered receptor affinity leading to macrophage scavenging and initiation of the atherosclerotic lesion. This peroxidation may be prevented by the endogenous vitamin E carried in LDL lipid. Consumption of antioxidants is associated with delayed development of various forms of cataracts. Clinical trials indicate improved immune responses in the elderly upon supplementation with vitamins C, E, and A or β-carotene. Vitamin A supplementation decreases the morbidity and mortality associated with measles infection in children. In addition to specific antioxidant compound assessments, measures of overall oxidant status include breath pentane, electron spin resonance, and measures of base damage to DNA.

Studies have not conclusively demonstrated a cancer protective role for vitamins when taken as a supplement. Indeed, the role of vitamin supplements in the prevention of cancer is most likely limited to individuals with marginal nutritional intake. On a more mechanistic basis, folate deficiency and changes to the MTHFR gene (polymorphisms) are associated with cancer. The role of the MTHFR enzyme is to balance the needs of folate-methylating pools with the need to synthesize thymidine. Thymidine requires methyl-enetetrahydrofolate while the methylation pathways require 5,10-methyltetrhydrofolate. When thymidine is depleted due to either folate deficiency or enhanced methylating status because of the presence of wild type MTHFR (MTHFR 677CC), there is increased uridylate incorporation into DNA forcing DNA excision and repair. Moreover, decreased methylation of DNA affects DNA transcription through the masking of transcriptional sites. Each effect opposes the other; however, there is no indication that one or the other is more mutagenic than the other, although excision and repair of DNA is known to influence carcinogenesis.

References

1. Food and Nutrition Board: *Recommended dietary allowances*, ed 10, Washington, DC, 1989, National Academy of Science.
2. Dietary reference intakes, *Nutr Rev* 55:319, 1997.
3. Committee on Scientific Evaluation of Dietary Reference Intakes, Food and Nutrition Board, Institute of Medicine: Origin and framework of the development of dietary reference intakes, *Nutr Rev* 55(9):332-334, 1997.
4. *Dietary reference intakes for thiamin, riboflavin, niacin, vitamin B_6, folate, vitamin B_{12}, panthenoic acid, biotin and choline*, Report of the Standing Committee on the Scientific Evaluation of Dietary Reference Intakes and its Panel on Folate, Other B Vitamins, and Choline and Subcommittee on Upper Reference Levels of Nutrients Food and Nutrition Board Institute of Medicine, 2000.
5. Brussaard JH et al: Approach of the U.S. Food and Nutrition Board to daily nutrient requirements: a useful basis for the European discussion on risk assessment of nutrients? Report on a workshop organized by the European Academy of Nutritional Sciences (EANS) and TNO Food and Nutrition Research Institute, 11 December 1998, Brussels, *Eur J Clin Nutr* 53(10):786, 1999.
6. Position of the American Dietetic Association: Food fortification and dietary supplements, *J Am Diet Assoc* 101:115, 2001.
7. Walter P: Towards ensuring the safety of vitamins and minerals, *Toxicol Lett* 120:83, 2001.
8. Pesce AJ, Kaplan LA: *Methods in clinical chemistry*, St Louis, 1987, Mosby.
9. Labbe RF, editor: Clinics in laboratory medicine, vol 1, *Laboratory assessment of nutritional status*, Philadelphia, 1981, Saunders.
10. Briggs MH, editor: *Vitamins in human biology and medicine*, Boca Raton, FL, 1981, CRC Press.
11. Calabrese EJ: Nutrition and environmental health, vol 1, *The vitamins*, New York, 1980, Wiley & Sons.
12. Brewster MA, Naito HK, editors: *Nutritional elements and clinical biochemistry*, New York, 1980, Plenum Publishing.
13. Pereira GR, Zucker A: Nutritional deficiencies in the neonate, *Clin Perinatol* 13:175, 1986.
14. Rosenthal MJ, Goodwin JS: Cognitive effects of nutritional deficiency, *Adv Nutr Res* 7:71, 1985.
15. Snodgrass GR: Vitamin neurotoxicity, *Molec Neurobiol* 6:41, 1992.

Vitamin A
16. Jessen KA, Satre MA: Mouse retinol binding protein gene: cloning, expression, and regulation by retinoic acid, *Mol Cell Biochem* 211:85, 2000.
17. Formelli F, Barua AB, Olson JA: Bioactivities of N-(4-hydroxyphenyl) retinamide and retinoyl beta-glucuronide, *FASEB J* 10:1014, 1996.
18. Goswami BC et al: Topical retinoyl beta-glucuronide is an effective treatment of mild to moderate acne vulgaris in Asian-Indian patients, *Skin Pharmacol Appl Skin Physiol* 12:167, 1999.
19. Agarwal N, Mehta K: Possible involvement of Bcl-2 pathway in retinoid X receptor alpha-induced apoptosis of HL-60 cells, *Biochem Biophys Res Commun* 230:251, 1997.
20. Stagno F et al: In vitro apoptotic response of freshly isolated chronic myeloid leukemia cells to all-trans retinoic acid and cytosine arabinoside, *Acta Haematol* 104:57, 2000.

21. Lingen MW, Polverini PJ, Bouck NP: Retinoic acid and interferon alpha act synergistically as antiangiogenic and antitumor agents against human head and neck squamous cell carcinoma, *Cancer Res* 58:5551, 1998.
22. Walmsley S et al: Treatment of AIDS-related cutaneous Kaposi's sarcoma with topical alitretinoin (9-cis-retinoic acid) gel. Panretin gel North American Study Group, *J Acquir Immun Defic Syndr* 22:235, 1999.
23. Rao VG, Sugunan AP, Sehgal SC: Nutritional deficiency disorders and high mortality among children of the Great Andamanese tribe, *Natl Med J India* 11:65, 1998.
24. Garry PJ: Vitamin A. In Labbe RF, editor: Clinics in laboratory medicine, vol 1, *Laboratory assessment of nutritional status*, Philadelphia, 1981, Saunders.
25. Shamberger RJ: Vitamin A alterations in disease. In Brewster MA, Naito HK, editors: *Nutritional elements and clinical biochemistry*, New York, 1980, Plenum Publishing.
26. Sklan D: Vitamin A in human nutrition, *Prog Food Nutr Sci* 11:39, 1987.
27. Underwood BA: Methods for assessment of vitamin A status, *J Nutr* 120(suppl 11):1459, 1990.
28. Dolk HM et al: Dietary vitamin A and teratogenic risk, *Eur J Obstet Gynecol Reprod Biol* 83:31, 1999.

Vitamin E
29. Sokol RJ: Vitamin E and neurological deficits, *Adv Pediatr* 37:119, 1990.
30. Bland J: Lipid antioxidant nutrition. In Brewster MA, Naito HK, editors: *Nutritional elements and clinical biochemistry*, New York, 1980, Plenum Publishing.
31. Sokol RJ et al: Frequency and clinical progression of the vitamin E deficiency neurologic disorder in children with prolonged neonatal cholestasis, *Am J Dis Child* 139:1211, 1985.
32. Farrell PM, Bieri JG: Megavitamin E supplementation in man, *Am J Clin Nutr* 28:1381, 1975.
33. Bieri JG, Evarts RP, Thorp S: Factors affecting the exchange of tocopherol between red cells and plasma, *Am J Clin Nutr* 30:686, 1977.
34. Ogumekan AO: Vitamin E deficiency and seizures in animals and man, *Can J Neurol Sci* 6:43, 1979.

Vitamin K
35. Suttie JW: Role of vitamin K in the synthesis of clotting factors. In Draper HH, editor: *Advances in nutritional research*, vol 1, New York, 1977, Plenum Publishing.
36. Hazell K, Baloch KH: Vitamin K deficiency in the elderly, *Gerontol Clin* 12:10, 1970.
37. Howe AM, Webster WS: The warfarin embryopathy: a rat model showing maxillonasal hypoplasia and other skeletal disturbances, *Teratology* 46:379, 1992.
38. Motohara K, Endo F, Matsuda I: Screening for late neonatal vitamin K deficiency by acarboxyprothrombin in dried blood spots, *Arch Dis Child* 62:370, 1987.

Vitamin D
39. Holick MF: The use and interpretation of assays for vitamin D and its metabolites, *J Nutr* 120(suppl 11):1464, 1990.

40. Taylor CB, Peng S: Vitamin D—its excessive use in the U.S.A. In Brewster MA, Naito HK, editors: *Nutritional elements and clinical biochemistry*, New York, 1980, Plenum Publishing.

Ascorbic Acid

41. Davidson JM et al: Ascorbate differentially regulates elastin and collagen biosynthesis in vascular smooth muscle cells and skin fibroblasts by pretranslational mechanisms, *J Biol Chem* 272:345, 1997.
42. Englard S, Seifter S: The biochemical functions of ascorbic acid, *Annu Rev Nutr* 6:265, 1986.
43. Lew RA, Smith AI: Identification and characterization of an amidating enzyme in ovine heart, *Clin Exp Pharmacol Physiol* 20:231, 1993.
44. Jacob RA: Assessment of human vitamin C status, *J Nutr* 120(suppl 11):1480, 1990.
45. Washko PW et al: Ascorbic acid and dehydroascorbic acid analyses in biological samples, *Anal Biochem* 204:1, 1992.
46. Mirvish SS: Effects of vitamins C and E on N-nitroso compound formation, carcinogenesis and cancer, *Cancer* 58:1842, 1986.

Riboflavin

47. Komindr S, Michaels GE: Clinical significance of riboflavin deficiency. In Brewster MA, Naito HK, editors: *Nutritional elements and clinical biochemistry*, New York, 1980, Plenum Publishing.
48. Bates CJ: Human riboflavin requirements and metabolic consequences of deficiency in men and animals, *World Rev Nutr Diet* 50:215, 1987.

Pyridoxine

49. Leklem JE: Vitamin B_6: a status report, *J Nutr* 120(suppl 11):1503, 1990.
50. Shuster K, Bailey LB, Madan CS: Vitamin B_6 status of low-income adolescent and adult pregnant women and the condition of their infants at birth, *Am J Clin Nutr* 34:1731, 1981.

Niacin

51. Wahlqvist ML: Effects on plasma cholesterol of nicotinic acid and its analogues. In Briggs MH, editor: *Vitamins in human biology and medicine*, Boca Raton, FL, 1981, CRC Press.
52. Glueck CJ: Nonpharmacologic and pharmacologic alteration of high-density lipoprotein cholesterol: therapeutic approaches to prevention of atherosclerosis, *Am Heart J* 110:1107, 1985.

Thiamine

53. Flint DM, Prinsley DM: Vitamin status of the elderly. In Briggs MH, editor: *Vitamins in human biology and medicine*, Boca Raton, FL, 1981, CRC Press.
54. Blass JP: Thiamin and the Wernicke-Korsakoff syndrome. In Briggs MH, editor: *Vitamins in human biology and medicine*, Boca Raton, FL, 1981, CRC Press.
55. Poloni M et al: Inversion of T/TMP ratio in ALS: a specific finding? *Ital J Neurol Sci* 7:333, 1986.

Biotin

56. Roth KS et al: Serum and urinary biotin levels during treatment of holocarboxylase synthetase deficiency, *Clin Chem Acta* 109:337, 1981.
57. Wolf B et al: Biotinidase deficiency: initial clinical features and rapid diagnosis, *Ann Neurol* 18:614, 1985.

Vitamin B_{12} and Folic Acid

58. Steinkamp RC: Vitamin B_{12} and folic acid: clinical and pathophysiological considerations. In Brewster MA, Naito HK, editors: *Nutritional elements and clinical biochemistry*, New York, 1980, Plenum Publishing.

59. Elsborg L, Lung V, Bastrup-Madsen P: Serum vitamin B_{12} levels in the aged, *Acta Med Scand* 200:309, 1976.
60. Herrmann W et al: Role of homocysteine, cystathionine and methylmalonic acid measurement for diagnosis of vitamin deficiency in high-aged subjects, *Eur J Clin Invest* 30:1083, 2000.
61. Howard JM et al: Dietary intake of cobalamin in elderly people who have abnormal serum cobalamin, methylmalonic acid and homocysteine levels, *Eur J Clin Nutr* 52:582, 1998.
62. Kudo H et al: Distribution of vitamin B_{12} R binder in normal human tissues: an immunohistochemical study, *J Histochem Cytochem* 35:855, 1987.
63. Saxena S, Carmel R: Racial differences in vitamin B_{12} levels in the United States, *Am J Clin Pathol* 88:85, 1987.
64. Fenton WA, Rosenberg LE: Inherited disorders of cobalamin transport and metabolism. In Scriver CR et al, editors: *The metabolic and molecular bases of inherited disease*, vol II, ed 7, New York, 1995, McGraw-Hill.
65. Donnelly JG: Folic acid, *Crit Rev Clin Lab Sci* 38(3):183, 2001.
66. Isotalo PA, Donnelly JG: Prevalence of methylenetetrahydrofolate reductase (MTHFR) mutations in venous thrombosis patients: evidence for natural selection of MTHFR allelic patterns, *Mol Diagn*, 5(1):59, 2000.
67. Isotalo PA, Wells GA, Donnelly JG: Neonatal and fetal methylenetetrahydrofolate reductase genetic polymorphisms: an examination of C677T and A1298C mutations, *Am J Human Gen* 67:986, 2000.
68. Weisberg I et al: A second genetic polymorphism in methylenetetrahydrofolate reductase (MTHFR) associated with decreased enzyme activity, *Mol Genet Metab* 64(3):169, 1998.
69. Donnelly JG, Isotalo PA: Occurrence of hyperhomocysteinemia in cardiovascular, hematology and nephrology patients: contribution of folate deficiency, *Ann Clin Biochem* 37:304, 2000.
70. Donnelly JG, Isotalo PA: Non-fasting reference intervals for the Abbott IMx™ Homocysteine and AxSYM™ plasma folate assays, *Ann Clin Biochem* 37:390, 2000.
71. Infante-Rivard C et al: Folate deficiency among institutionalized elderly: public health impact, *J Am Geriatr Soc* 34:211, 1986.
72. Bailey LB: Folate status assessment, *J Nutr* 120(suppl 11):1508, 1990.

Carnitine

73. Rebouche CJ: Carnitine function and requirements during the life cycle, *FASEB J* 6:3379, 1992.
74. Tanphaichitr V, Leelahagul P: Carnitine metabolism and human carnitine deficiency, *Nutrition* 9:246, 1993.

Vitamins as Antioxidants

75. Roe CR et al: Carnitine homeostasis in the organic acidurias, *Prog Clin Biol Res* 321:383, 1990.
76. Bendich A: Physiological role of antioxidants in the immune system, *J Dairy Sci* 76:2789, 1993.
77. Cheeseman KH, Slater TF: An introduction to free radical biochemistry, *Br Med Bull* 49:481, 1993.
78. Perera FP et al: Molecular epidemiology of lung cancer and the modulation of markers of chronic carcinogen exposure by chemopreventive agents, *J Cell Biochem* 17F(suppl):119, 1993.
79. Manson JE et al: Antioxidants and cardiovascular disease: a review, *J Am Coll Nutr* 12:426, 1993.
80. Taylor A: Cataract: relationship between nutrition and oxidation, *J Am Coll Nutr* 12:138, 1993.

Internet Sites

www.asns.org/—American Society for Nutritional Sciences
www.faseb.org/ascn—American Society for Clinical Nutrition
www.asns.org/sinr/index.htm—Society for International Nutrition Research
http://vm.cfsan.fda.gov/list.html—United States Food and Drug Administration Center for Food Safety and Applied Nutrition
www.nalusda.gov/fnic/—Food and Nutrition Information Center of the National Agriculture Library
http://books.nap.edu/books/—Dietary reference intakes report. This site takes you to the Crawler List of all NAP searchable open books: go to 0309065542

www.nalusda.gov/fnic/etext/—This site takes you to the National Agriculture Library Food and Nutrition Information Center e-text list. Go to 000105 on the index of /fnic/etext document list. Select *Dietary Reference Intakes for Thiamin, Riboflavin, Niacin, Vitamin B_6, Folate, Vitamin B_{12}, Pantothenic Acid, Biotin, and Choline*
http://web.indstate.edu/thcme/mwking/vitamins.html—Indiana State University Terre Haute Center for Medical Education: Introduction to Vitamins

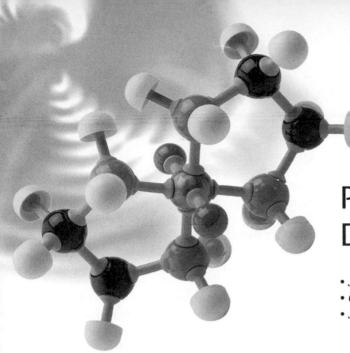

CHAPTER 40

Pregnancy and Fetal Development

• *John F. Chapman, Jr.*
• *Catherine A. Hammett-Stabler*
• *Jane E. Phillips*

Chapter Outline

Objectives

- Describe amniotic fluid including its formation, functions, and normal constituents.
- Describe the usual healthy and pathological maternal biochemical changes that occur during pregnancy.
- Describe fetal biochemical changes that occur during prenatal development.
- Describe pathological conditions associated with pregnancy or the perinatal period and list expected levels of significant laboratory analytes.

Key Terms

anencephaly   A defective development of the brain wherein the cerebral and cerebellar hemispheres are absent.

blastocyst   An early stage in embryonic development characterized by a fluid-filled cavity within the cell mass covered by the trophoblast.

ectopic pregnancy   Pregnancy occurring outside the uterine cavity, most commonly in the fallopian tubes.

hematopoietic   Related to the process of formation and development of the various types of blood cells.

keratinization   The process in skin development and differentiation whereby keratin, a proteinaceous substance, is produced.

lamellar bodies   The physical form of pulmonary surfactant extruded from type II pneumocytes.

meningomyelocele   A protrusion of the membranes and spinal cord resulting from a defect in the vertebral column.

oligohydramnios   The presence of less amniotic fluid than is usual for a given gestational age.

polyhydramnios   The accumulation of an excessive amount of amniotic fluid.

spina bifida   A developmental abnormality characterized by defective closure of the spinal cord.

transudation The passage of a substance through a membrane as a result of a difference in hydrostatic pressure.

trophoblast   The cell layer covering the blastocyst, which erodes the inner lining of the uterus during the process of implantation. Trophoblastic cells do not become part of the embryo itself but contribute to the formation of the placenta.

Methods on CD-ROM

α-Fetoprotein
Bilirubin
Creatinine
Glucose

β-Human chorionic gonadotropin (β-hCG)
Magnesium
Uric acid
Urine protein, total

ANATOMICAL AND PHYSIOLOGICAL INTERACTION OF MOTHER AND FETUS
Fertilization and Implantation of the Ovum

Chapter 45 reviews the biochemical changes required for the successful development and release of an ovum. After ovulation, the ovum is expelled into the peritoneal cavity where it is moved into either of the two fallopian tubes by the action of the ciliated epithelial cells of the fimbriated tentacles. Fertilization normally occurs either before the ovum enters the tube or shortly thereafter. Approximately 3 days are required for transport of the fertilized ovum through the tube and into the cavity of the uterus. An additional 2 to 5 days are required for implantation of the ovum in the endometrium of the uterus. Thus, implantation of the developing ovum, the **blastocyst**, typically occurs 5 to 8 days after fertilization. Implantation results from the proteolytic digestion of the endometrium by the **trophoblasts** covering the surface of the blastocyst (Fig. 40-1). Once implantation is complete, both trophoblastic and endometrial cells proliferate rapidly in a coordinated fashion, forming the placenta and its membranes. The placenta serves both to separate the foreign body, the *fetus*, from the maternal host, and to provide an interface between the fetal and maternal circulatory systems. Through this interface, nutrients from maternal blood are delivered to the fetus, and fetal wastes are delivered to the mother for eventual disposal.[1]

As the demands for nourishment and oxygen by the rapidly growing embryo increase, the trophoblast increases its surface area by forming villi. The surface area of these villi is enormous, and from the villi the fetal circulation of the placenta is established. The innermost membrane, the amnion, immediately surrounds the embryo and is filled with fluid. This fluid, referred to as the *liquor amnii*, or *amniotic fluid*, bathes the fetus, thereby preventing desiccation, and buffers the fetus against physical shocks. The blood in the placenta is derived from the fetal circulation.

Fetal Growth and Nutrition

Fetal growth is dependent on the availability of essential nutrients, which are delivered to the fetus from the maternal/uterine circulation via the placenta. Placental transfer of nutrients is not passive, but rather is a dynamic process controlled by hormonal signals from both maternal and fetal somatotrophic axes. Growth hormone (GH) and insulin-like growth factor (IGF-1) produced from maternal and fetal sources are pivotal regulators in this process. Placental size

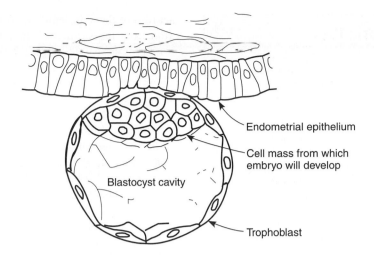

Fig. 40-1   Attachment of blastocyst to endometrial wall.

and architecture, developmental and pathologic processes, and interaction of maternal and fetal somatotrophic mechanisms act in concert to regulate placental-fetal nutrient exchange.[2,3]

Unlike the *infant* whose diet is a complex mixture of carbohydrates, fats, and proteins, the *fetus* has a diet consisting largely of glucose and sufficient quantities of amino acids to satisfy the nitrogen requirements of protein synthesis. Also included are small amounts of essential fatty acids, ketones, vitamins, and minerals. Although glucose provides most of the energy needed for the formation of tissues, amino acids can serve as an alternative source of oxidizable fuel. Ketones may also serve as alternative fetal energy sources and as precursors for proteins and lipids during periods of maternal fasting.

The amount of glucose available to the fetus depends on the concentration of glucose in maternal blood, which is regulated by the action of numerous hormones, including insulin and the placental hormone, human chorionic somatomammotropin (also called *human placental lactogen,* or hPL).

Glucose passes readily from the maternal to the fetal circulation by means of "facilitated diffusion," crossing the placenta at a faster rate than would be expected on physiological grounds alone. A rise in the glucose concentration in maternal blood is followed rapidly by a comparable increase in its concentration in fetal blood. The two levels do not become equal, however, and a concentration gradient from mother to fetus is always present. In addition, the placenta consumes a significant proportion of glucose to meet its own energy requirements.

Because glucose levels in the fetus mirror those in the mother, there is usually little need for the fetus to regulate its own blood glucose concentrations. Mechanisms for doing so do develop during the fetal period, but, except in infants of hyperglycemic diabetic mothers, these mechanisms are largely dormant until birth, when the supply of glucose through the placenta ends abruptly. Nevertheless, two important processes are active from an early stage. The first

is the storage of glucose as glycogen or fat to provide for the metabolic needs of the newborn until feeding begins. The second is the control of the rate at which glucose is used by the growing tissues, and this is attributable primarily to the action of insulin secreted by the fetal pancreas beginning at 8 to 9 weeks of gestational age.

Role of Placenta in Gas Exchange

To meet its metabolic needs the fetus is completely dependent on a continuous delivery of oxygen across the placenta. Transplacental exchanges, including those of gases, depend on both perfusion and permeability. Placental perfusion is a composite of uterine and umbilical blood flows, whereas permeability is a characteristic of the placental membrane. Under healthy conditions with well-oxygenated maternal blood, oxygen transport across the placenta is primarily regulated by blood flow. However, maternal placental or fetal blood flows and O_2 capacities may be altered by as much as 50% without significant effect on fetal uptake of oxygen. To meet the increasing demands of the growing fetus, uterine blood flow and placental membrane permeability increase during gestation. In the presence of maternal hypoxia, oxygen transport across the placenta becomes limited primarily by the permeability of the placental membrane.[4]

Carbon dioxide rapidly diffuses across the placenta in either direction. This allows the fetus to maintain a normal P_{CO_2} and the mother to eliminate carbon dioxide. The placenta has limited permeability to bicarbonate ions. The placenta therefore allows the fetus to dispose of carbon dioxide while protecting it from maternal metabolic acidosis.

Formation of Amniotic Fluid

The volume of blood in the amniotic sac, which surrounds the developing embryo, increases throughout pregnancy until it reaches a maximum volume at about 36 weeks of gestation (Table 40-1). Many maternal and fetal abnormalities can produce **oligohydramnios** or **polyhydramnios** states. Amniotic fluid volume and composition at any point in time is the result of a dynamic balance between production and

TABLE 40-1   AMNIOTIC FLUID VOLUME IN NORMAL PREGNANCY

Gestational Age (Weeks)	Volume of Fluid (mL)
12	5 to 200
14	50 to 200
16	150 to 300
18	200 to 400
20	225 to 775
22	300 to 500
24	500 to 675
26	500 to 700
28	500 to 875
30	400 to 1300
32	400 to 1375
34	500 to 1350
36	525 to 1500
38	300 to 1525
40	325 to 1450
42	600

removal. Amniotic fluid originates from multiple sources, including the placenta, fetal kidneys, skin, membranes, lungs, and intestine. The relative contribution of each source depends on the stage of fetal development. In the first half of pregnancy, amniotic fluid forms as a transudate from the skin surface of the fetus. The composition of amniotic fluid is similar to that of extracellular fluid, and the amniotic fluid should be considered as an extension of the fetal extracellular fluid space. Later in pregnancy, fetal kidneys and lungs assume the major role in the formation of amniotic fluid, and its volume now depends on a balance between fetal urination and volume of amniotic fluid that is swallowed.[1]

Fluid moving from the trachea and pharynx into the esophagus can enter the amniotic cavity. This provides an explanation for the appearance of pulmonary surfactant in amniotic fluid. Respiratory movements by the fetus readily mix fluid with surfactant because the movements produce a tidal volume exchange (in and out) of about 600 to 800 mL/day[2] through the fetal lungs throughout the third trimester.

Amniotic fluid disappearance is in part affected by fetal swallowing. It is estimated that between 200 and 450 mL of amniotic fluid per day flows out from the amniotic cavity by this route, accounting for about half of the daily urine production of the fetus. Because the amniotic cavity gains a fluid volume of no more than 10 mL/day in the third trimester (the total solute concentration always remains in the normal range), a sizable quantity of urine must be reabsorbed by other pathways.[3,5]

BIOCHEMISTRY OF AMNIOTIC FLUID[6]
Water, Electrolytes, and Nitrogenous Products

Because of the shift in the source of amniotic fluid that occurs about midway through pregnancy, constituents of amniotic fluid also change during gestation. Before **keratin-**

ization of the skin, amniotic fluid can result as a **transudation** from the surface of the fetus. After keratinization and with progressive development of the renal system, fetal urine makes a more prominent contribution to the amniotic fluid compartment. The biochemical composition of amniotic fluid therefore reflects the routes of formation of the fluid and is related to the developmental stage of the fetus.

Amniotic fluid is isotonic during early pregnancy but by term becomes moderately hypotonic (mean total solute concentration, 255 mOsm/kg of water) compared with fetal and maternal plasma. This changing concentration of amniotic fluid reflects the maturation of fetal renal function. The osmotic and oncotic pressures in fetal and maternal tissues cause the transfer of water from mother to fetus to amniotic fluid and then back to the mother. It has been calculated that the net transfer of water from mother to fetus reaches 20 to 25 mL/day in late pregnancy.[6]

Amniotic fluid concentrations of nitrogenous products of metabolism, creatinine, urea, and uric acid increase toward the end of the term (see later discussion) but are many times lower than concentrations found in maternal urine. The composition difference between amniotic fluid and maternal urine is readily measurable and can be used to determine whether a sample obtained from vaginal leakage or an errant amniocentesis is amniotic fluid.

Proteins

Proteins derived from many sources have been identified in amniotic fluid. Under healthy conditions, amniotic fluid proteins of fetal origin come from the skin, the urinary and gastrointestinal tracts (urine and meconium, respectively), and the respiratory tract. Proteins from the respiratory tract are part of the proteolipid product secreted by type II epithelial cells of the fetal lung. These products function as components of the lung surfactant system[7] (see later discussion).

At least four surfactant protein (SP) species have been described: SP-A, B, C, and D. These differ in molecular weight and charge and possibly function. Proteins of maternal origin can enter amniotic fluid by transudation across the amnion. Under abnormal circumstances, unusual avenues for protein exchange can occur, such as central neural tube development defects, which increase the α-fetoprotein levels in amniotic fluid (see later discussion).

More than 50 enzymes have been identified in amniotic fluid,[4,5] but the origin of many of these enzymes and their significance in the fluid are not understood. The enzymes fall into two categories: those having an activity greatest early in pregnancy (12 to 20 weeks) and those active at the later stage of pregnancy (35 to 40 weeks). Acetylcholinesterase, an enzyme of fetal origin, is used in the diagnosis of neural tube defects.

Hormones

Examples of the hormones that have been identified in amniotic fluid are listed in the box on p. 757. This list includes hormones (such as the catecholamines) derived from

HORMONES IDENTIFIED IN AMNIOTIC FLUID

Protein and Polypeptide
Adrenocorticotropic hormone
Angiotensin
Endorphin
Follicle-stimulating hormone
Growth hormone
Human chorionic gonadotropin
Human placental lactogen
Insulin
Luteinizing hormone
Oxytocin
Prolactin
Relaxin
Renin
Somatomedin
Somatostatin
Thyrotropin
Thyroxine

Steroids
Estradiol
Estriol
Estrone

Prostaglandins
E_2
$F_{2\alpha}$

steroids, peptides, and amino acids. Although many of these hormones are products of urinary or biliary excretion from the fetus, a few have clinical usefulness and are discussed later. A more extensive list is available.[4,5]

MATERNAL BIOCHEMICAL CHANGES DURING PREGNANCY

Human Chorionic Gonadotropin

The urine and serum of pregnant women contain high concentrations of human chorionic gonadotropin (hCG), produced by the trophoblast, and provide the basis of tests for the diagnosis of pregnancy. Specific and sensitive analytical methods for the β-chain subunit of hCG permit the detection of pregnancy as early as 8 days after ovulation (1 day after implantation). Human chorionic gonadotropin concentrations climb early in pregnancy, reaching a maximum by 8 to 10 weeks of gestation (Fig. 40-2).

Human chorionic gonadotropin is one of a family of closely related glycoprotein hormones that regulate reproductive and metabolic functions. This family includes follicle-stimulating hormone (FSH), luteinizing hormone (LH), and thyroid-stimulating hormone (TSH). These hormones are composed of two polypeptide subunits referred to as α- and β-chains, and each contains carbohydrate; thus the term *glycoprotein* is used. The α-chains of hCG, LH, FSH, and TSH are similar in their amino acid sequences, a finding that accounts for the immunological similarity of these protein hormones.[8]

The β-chains of the glycoprotein hormones each have a unique amino acid sequence, which gives these hormones their biological specificity. Human chorionic gonadotropin has amino acid sequences in both the α- and β-chains that are virtually identical to those in LH, differing to a significant degree only in carbohydrate content, with hCG containing about 30% carbohydrate by weight and LH approximately half that amount. This similarity allows hCG to be used instead of LH for such purposes as ovulation induction. The carbohydrate-content difference perceptibly influences the metabolic patterns of these hormones; thus the biological half-life of hCG is about 6 hours, whereas the biological half-life of plasma LH is 12 to 45 minutes. These differences in metabolic clearance correlate well with our understanding of the functions of these hormones, with LH regulating the complicated process of ovulation and subsequent formation of the corpus luteum and hCG providing continued stimulation of the corpus luteum to ensure uninterrupted progesterone production until the placenta can provide sufficient progesterone to maintain the pregnancy (see Chapter 45 for details).

Estrogens

A substantial increase in estrogen excretion accompanies pregnancy. The predominant estrogen produced is estriol, not the usual ovarian estrogens estradiol or estrone (Fig. 40-3).

Estrogen formation proceeds in an obligatory sequence of reactions that converts cholesterol to progestin, then to androgens, and then to estrogens (see Chapter 45). In the ovary, this sequence occurs solely within that organ. In pregnancy, for this sequence to lead to estriol formation, a complementary relationship is needed between the placenta, the fetal adrenal cortex, and the fetal liver. This unique interrelationship is referred to as the *fetoplacental unit*[9] (Fig. 40-4). The rationale behind this interdependence is that certain enzymes develop uniquely in the fetus but not in the placenta, whereas other enzymes develop in the placenta but not in the fetus. For the pregnancy to proceed as intended, the biosynthetic activities of fetal enzymes must complement those of the mother. An imbalance in this system may produce metabolic abnormalities that could cause natural abortion of the fetus.[9,10]

The fetal adrenal gland synthesizes dehydroepiandrosterone (DHEA), which is converted to 16α-hydroxy-DHEA by the fetal liver. The 16α-hydroxy-DHEA is converted to estriol by placental aromatizing enzymes. In addition, the placenta possesses a very active sulfatase. Sulfation/desulfation of estriol appears to be integrally involved in the transfer of steroids from the placenta, because, in conditions in which the placental sulfatase is absent, low maternal estriol levels are characteristically observed.[11]

Estriol, from precursors produced in the fetus, constitutes over 90% of the known maternal estrogens of pregnancy. It is metabolized to both sulfate and glucuronide conjugated forms by maternal liver. These conjugates are the primary excretory forms of estriol. Concentrations in maternal serum increase with advancing gestation and reach nearly 40 ng/mL

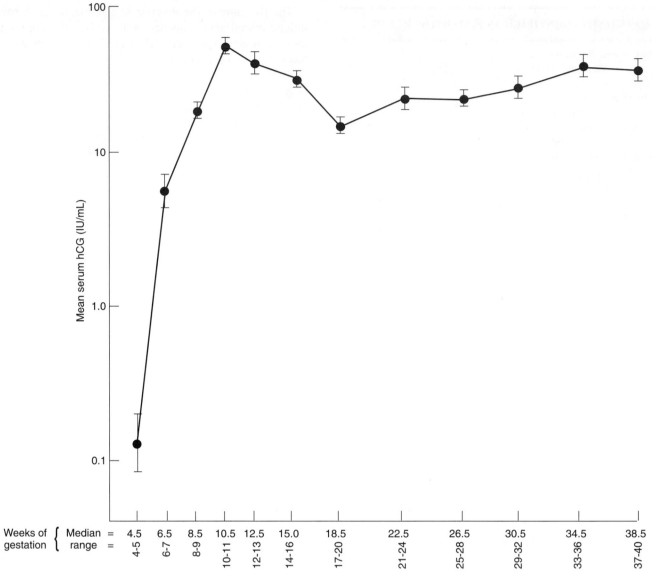

Weeks of gestation { Median = / range = }

Median =	4.5	6.5	8.5	10.5	12.5	15.0	18.5	22.5	26.5	30.5	34.5	38.5
range =	4-5	6-7	8-9	10-11	12-13	14-16	17-20	21-24	25-28	29-32	33-36	37-40

Fig. 40-2 Serum chorionic gonadotropin (hCG) concentrations during pregnancy. *(From Goldstein DP et al: Am J Obstet Gynecol 102:110, 1968.)*

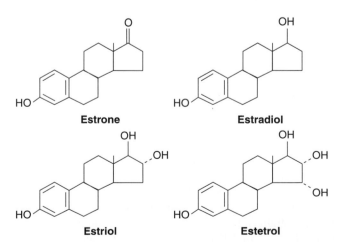

Fig. 40-3 Structures of estrogens. *Dashed lines,* α-stereo-configurations; *solid lines,* β-stereoconfigurations of hydroxyl groups.

at the end of the term. In Fig. 40-5, the patterns of a normal increase in plasma estriol and the patterns seen with a diabetic patient, with fetal death, and with growth retardation are shown. Estriol is also found in amniotic fluid.[12]

The functional role for estriol in pregnancy has prompted much speculation. In many biological test systems, estriol is a weak estrogen, demonstrating only a hundredth of the potency of estradiol and one tenth of the potency of estrone per unit weight. However, estriol can be demonstrated to be equipotent to estradiol in its ability to promote uteroplacental blood flow. For this reason, its role in pregnancy may be to ensure optimum blood flow in the gravid uterus.

It has been suggested that levels of the estrogen *estetrol* (Fig. 40-3) offer more information than estriol levels about the status of the fetus in utero.[13] However, clinical evaluations of fetal well-being have not shown a clear advantage of estetrol over estriol.[14,15,16]

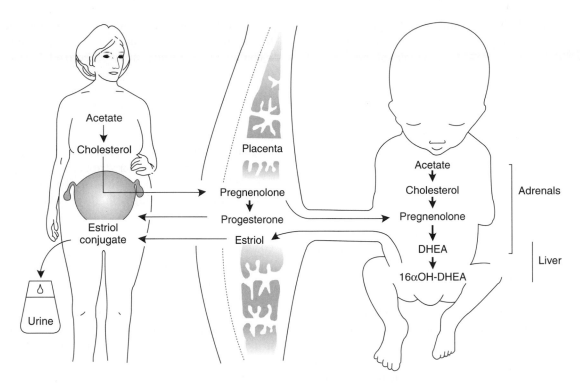

Fig. 40-4 Schema of fetoplacental unit. *DHEA,* Dehydroepiandrosterone; *16α-OH-DHEA,* 16α-hydroxydehydroepiandrosterone.

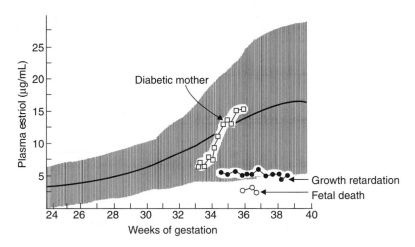

Fig. 40-5 Mean *(solid line)* and estimated fifth and ninety-fifth percentiles *(shaded area)* for plasma unconjugated estriol during normal pregnancy. Estriol patterns from three actual pregnancy conditions are shown.

Thyroid

Although maternal thyroid disease can occur in pregnancy (see Chapter 44), the changes in the maternal serum levels of thyroid hormones are a normal response to meet the immediate needs of the mother and the developing fetus.[17] The increase in maternal thyroid hormone requirements is such that women who are hypothyroid need 25% to 50% more thyroxine (T_4) to maintain normal thyrotropin (TSH) concentrations. In areas of iodine sufficiency, the maternal thyroid increases 10% to 20% in volume during pregnancy.[18,19] The increased requirements are related both to

the needs of the developing fetus and to the physiological changes observed with the mother. The fetal thyroid follicles become apparent about 8 to 10 weeks after conception, but animal and human studies suggest that thyroid hormones have important roles before this time.[20,21] For example, rat brain tissue contains triiodothyronine (T_3) and T_4 before either is produced by the fetal thyroid. In addition, it appears that when these hormones are absent or insufficient during this time, mental and neurological abnormalities result.[22] So for the first few weeks of gestation T_3 and T_4 and iodide are provided either by placental transfer or by placental deiodination. In addition, physiological changes associated with pregnancy, such as an increase in the maternal glomerular filtration rate, lead to an increased clearance of the thyroid hormones, iodide, and the smaller binding protein, albumin.

Although many of the initiating mechanisms are unknown, hCG and estriol play roles in maintaining the levels of maternal thyroid hormone production needed to ensure a healthy fetus. hCG has some TSH-like activity (about 1/4000 the thyrotropic activity of pituitary TSH) and the large amounts of hCG produced by the placenta stimulate the maternal thyroid gland, leading to an increase in T_4 and T_3 production. At the same time, the increased estriol stimulates the maternal liver to synthesize more thyroid-binding globulin (TBG) and to increase the number of carbohydrate residues of the protein (sialylation) to reduce its renal clearance. By the end of the first trimester, maternal serum TBG levels almost double and remain elevated throughout pregnancy. The net result of these events is that although the amount of *total* T_4 and T_3 increases in maternal serum, the *free* hormone concentrations usually remain within the reference intervals and the pregnant woman is euthyroid. In the second and third trimesters the maternal pituitary increases the release of TSH in response to the decreasing hCG levels.

Serum Lipids

Hyperlipidemia develops during a healthy pregnancy and may be the result of alterations in hormone levels. Pregnant women have greatly increased total serum lipid concentrations that increase progressively throughout pregnancy, with highest levels in the second and third trimesters.[23]

Interestingly, these levels stabilize to prepregnancy levels after pregnancy, thus lending further support for the role of pregnancy-related hormones in regulating serum lipid levels. All components of the serum lipids are increased, but the triacylglyceride fraction shows the largest proportionate rise. High-density lipoprotein/low-density lipoprotein (HDL/LDL) ratios decrease with increasing duration of pregnancy, and HDL levels remain decreased 1 year after pregnancy. Oral contraceptives may have some effect on HDL levels, but more thorough studies are needed.

Serum Proteins and Liver Function

The total concentration of serum proteins decreases by about 1 g/L during pregnancy. Most of the decrease occurs during the first trimester. The decrease is mainly in serum albumin. Levels of α_1-, α_2-, and β-globulins rise slowly and progressively during pregnancy. γ-Globulin probably decreases slightly. The maternal antibody (IgG) component, which is the major immunoglobulin transferred to the fetus, falls progressively. Throughout pregnancy fibrinogen increases progressively, and values at term are 30% to 50% above nonpregnant levels. Clotting factors VII, VIII, IX, and X are also increased, whereas prothrombin and factors V and XII are reduced. Alterations that occur in the levels of clotting factors and plasminogen are probably brought about by estrogen action on the liver.

Under the influence of increased estrogens, the maternal liver increases the synthesis of transcortin (corticoid-binding globulin). This results in total cortisol levels increasing during pregnancy, almost doubling by late pregnancy. However, the levels of free, active cortisol are normal.

Several liver function tests change as a consequence of healthy pregnancy. For example, nonspecific alkaline phosphatase activity in serum nearly doubles during a pregnancy with a healthy mother and fetus and can reach levels that would be considered abnormal in the nonpregnant woman. Much of this increase is attributable to isoenzymes of this enzyme originating from the placenta.[24]

Glucosuria

Glucosuria is common in healthy, pregnant women. Glucose excretion rises very early in pregnancy, reaching a peak between 8 and 11 weeks of gestation. The degree of glucosuria varies thereafter. The cardinal feature of the glucosuria of pregnancy is a conspicuous variability both from day to day and during the course of a day. The cause of glucosuria in pregnancy appears to be the reduced efficiency of the kidneys to reabsorb glucose.[25]

From these comments it can be seen that pregnancy is potentially diabetogenic. Diabetes mellitus may be aggravated by pregnancy, and clinical diabetes may appear in some women only during pregnancy. The renal processing of glucose during pregnancy is of particular interest because of the frequent appearance of clinical glycosuria and the necessity to differentiate this "renal glycosuria" from that of pregnancy-aggravated diabetes mellitus, or *gestational diabetes*.

Because of the many variables associated with an altered renal physiology in pregnancy, blood glucose levels should be used to monitor pregnant diabetic women because urine testing can yield misleading values. Screening for gestational diabetes by a glucose challenge test has become routine for newly pregnant women. It is important to maintain blood glucose within the reference interval to prevent perinatal morbidity associated with gestational hyperglycemia. See later discussion and Chapter 32 for additional information on gestational diabetes.

FETAL BIOCHEMICAL CHANGES DURING PRENATAL DEVELOPMENT
Liver Function

Fetal liver contains a large number of hematopoietic cells that disappear after birth. In very early fetal life, the liver is the major blood-forming organ, but by 22 to 24 weeks of gestation the bone marrow has assumed the major responsibility for the formation of blood. Because of widely varying amounts of the different cell types in the newborn liver, enzyme-activity patterns are considerably different from the adult.

The fetal yolk sac and later the fetal liver produce α-fetoprotein (AFP), which is released into the fetal circulation. It passes from the bloodstream by way of the urine to amniotic fluid. It is usually removed from amniotic fluid by fetal

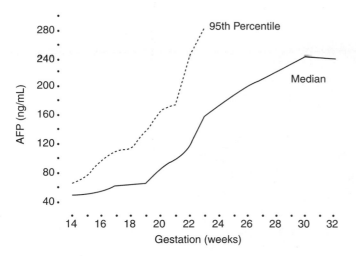

Fig. 40-6 Median and ninety-fifth percentile of α-fetoprotein, *AFP*, in maternal serum. *(From Crandall BF: In Kirkpatrick AM, Nakamura RM, editors:* Alpha-fetoprotein: laboratory procedures and clinical applications, *New York, 1981, Masson.)*

swallowing. α-Fetoprotein appears in maternal serum throughout gestation (Fig. 40-6), where it can be easily measured to screen for neural tube defects.

The fetus's need for increased quantities of amino acids for protein synthesis is satisfied by placental transport. This is an active process against a concentration gradient that depends on placental blood flow and, to a lesser degree, on the concentration of amino acids in the maternal plasma.

Because maturation of the fetal liver is not complete by the time of birth, some jaundice regularly occurs in virtually every newborn during the first week of life. This is known as *physiological jaundice*. The yellow pigmentation, or jaundice, is caused by bilirubin that comes from the normal destruction of red blood cells. However, because the immature fetal liver has not developed its full capability to clear bilirubin from the blood, jaundice occurs (see pp. 498 and 673 for details).

Renal Function

The primary function of the mammalian kidney is to maintain water and electrolyte homeostasis. This is accomplished by selective excretion or retention of water and solutes as conditions dictate. In the fetus, body water and electrolyte balance are maintained largely by the placenta. For this reason fetuses without functional kidneys often show no water or electrolyte abnormalities. Thus the full development of mature renal function occurs when it is needed–after birth.

Organic nitrogenous compounds such as urea, uric acid, and creatinine (Fig. 40-7) gradually increase in amniotic fluid as the renal system of the fetus matures. In early pregnancy these compounds are present in amniotic fluid in concentrations similar to concentrations in maternal and fetal blood. Concentrations increase gradually to become significantly higher than levels in maternal or fetal blood. A sharp rise in creatinine at about the thirty-seventh week of gestation elevates the amniotic fluid concentrations of urea and creatinine to levels two to three times higher than those of the reference interval of serum in healthy persons.[26]

Lung Development

At birth there is an abrupt physiological transition that requires the newborn infant to assume vital functions that were previously handled by the maternal circulation. The lung is shifted from a fluid-filled organ to a gas-exchange system in a few brief minutes. This functional transition is

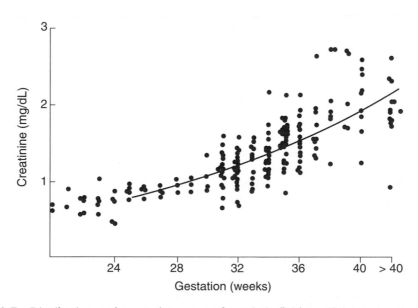

Fig. 40-7 Distribution and regression curve of amniotic fluid creatinine concentration in milligrams per deciliter. *(From Lind T: In Fairweather DVI, Eskes TKAB, editors:* Amniotic fluid: research and clinical application, *ed 2, Amsterdam, 1978, Excerpta Medica.)*

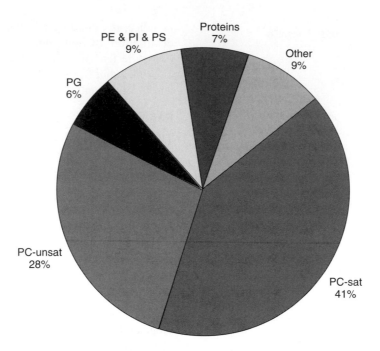

Fig. 40-8   Composition (by weight percent) of human surfactant. *PC-sat,* Saturated phosphatidylcholine; *PC-unsat,* unsaturated phosphatidylcholine; *PE,* phosphatidyl-ethanolamine; *PG,* phosphatidylglycerol; *PI,* phosphatidylinositol; *PS,* phosphatidylserine. Proteins include 3.8% SP-A (SP-B and SP-C detected but not quantified). *(From Hallman M: Rev Perinatal Med 6:197, 1989.)*

possible only if sufficient maturation of the fetal lung has occurred during development. The fetal lung maturation process appears to consist of two distinct components: (1) the morphological development of fetal lungs and (2) the synthesis, storage, and release of pulmonary surfactant. In the latter process, the control mechanisms for synthesis and storage of pulmonary surfactant appear to be distinct from those responsible for surfactant release.[27] Thus, functional lungs should have developed alveoli with adequate surface area and vascularization for gas exchange, and sufficient surfactant must be available to sustain the ventilatory movements needed for pulmonary function. These processes are highly organized and are coordinated by the timing of anatomical and biochemical events.

Surfactant facilitates pulmonary function in at least two ways: it maintains alveolar stability by preventing collapse of the terminal respiratory tree, and it reduces the pressure that is needed to distend the lungs in the initial phase of inspiration. Infants who develop the respiratory distress syndrome (RDS) have a higher surface tension at the alveolar air-liquid interface as a result of a pulmonary surfactant deficiency.

Human surfactant is composed principally of phospholipid that contains highly saturated fatty acid moieties.[28] The major constituents and their relative concentrations are shown in Figs. 40-8 and 40-9. In addition to the highly unusual saturated lecithins, other important constituents of the surface-active system include phosphatidylglycerol and the SPs mentioned previously. These proteins may serve a key role in enabling surfactant function by enhancing the rapidity

with which surfactant can spread to form a monolayer along the air-water interface of the alveolus. Although functional differences between the individual SPs are incompletely described, recent evidence indicates that surfactant protein B (SP-B) may be the most important of the proteins in pulmonary surfactant.[29] This is believed to be the result of the unique interaction of this protein with phospholipid moieties in surfactant. This interaction adds stability to the surfactant monolayer, thus increasing the ability of this layer to resist surface tension and prevent alveolar collapse. Detailed accounts of the function and biochemical composition of pulmonary surfactant have been published.[30,31,32]

Surfactant is formed in the large alveolar epithelial cells known as type II pneumocytes, which comprise about 10% of the cells of the lung. Although the biosynthetic pathways for the individual phospholipids are well described, much remains to be learned about the factors responsible for their regulation. Synthesis and storage begin between 24 and 28 weeks of gestational age. Beginning at about 32 weeks, this material is released from the type II pneumocytes in the form of specialized unique structures called **lamellar bodies** (LB). This term describes the concentrically wound, or "onion-like," structure of these particles when viewed with the electron microscope. Once in the alveolar air space, LBs unravel to form tubular myelin. Tubular myelin then remains in the alveolar space where it eventually spreads into a surfactant monolayer at the air-liquid interface with the alveoli. During normal respiration up to 50% of the surface-active material is reabsorbed and subsequently re-released

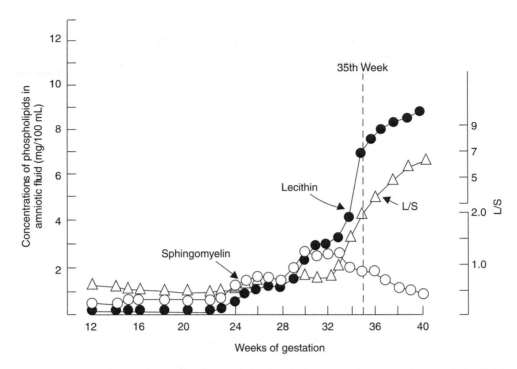

Fig. 40-9   Lecithin, sphingomyelin, and lecithin/sphingomyelin ratios in amniotic fluid during normal pregnancy. *(Modified from Gluck L, Kulovich MV:* Am J Obstet Gynecol *115:539, 1973.)*

by the type II pneumocytes. The complex synthesis and degradation of pulmonary surfactant is shown in Figure 40-10.

Hemoglobln

Embryos have a hemoglobin that is unique to the embryonic stage of development. This is replaced during fetal life by fetal hemoglobin (HbF) and finally by adult hemoglobin (HbA).[33] The pattern of hemoglobins formed during development is presented in Fig. 40-11. Fetal hemoglobin has been found to constitute 34% of the total in an embryo just less than 7 weeks of age.[34]

By approximately 10 weeks of gestation, the embryonic hemoglobins decrease to 10% of the total hemoglobin present. Before the end of the first trimester (less than 12 weeks) the HbF has increased to approximately 90% of the total, with the remaining percentage constituted by HbA. From this point, the percentage of HbF remains constant until about the thirty-sixth week of gestation, when there is a decline. The decline is primarily caused by an increase in HbA synthesis rather than by a decrease in HbF. Sharp increases in HbA are seen in reticulocytes and erythrocytes by birth. The developmental changes in **hematopoietic** sites, the red cell morphology, and the hemoglobin types are shown in Fig. 40-12.

The physiological differences in the hemoglobins are summarized by Kleihauer[33] and include differences in affinities for oxygen; resistance to acid, base, and heat denaturation; and electrophoretic and chromatographic properties. The higher affinity that fetal hemoglobin has for oxygen is

reflected in the fetal oxyhemoglobin saturation curve, which lies to the left of the maternal oxyhemoglobin curves under standard conditions. In fact, when oxygen is diffusing from maternal blood with a P_{CO_2} of about 34 mm Hg to fetal blood at a P_{CO_2} of about 30 mm Hg, the oxygen is actually moving against a concentration gradient.

Bilirubin

Erythrocyte destruction precedes the formation of bilirubin. Biliverdin is the principal and initial degradation product of hemoglobin and an important intermediate pigment in the formation of bilirubin (see Chapters 27 and 35 for details). These relationships are presented in simplified terms:

$$\text{Hemoglobin} \longrightarrow \text{Biliverdin} \xrightarrow{\text{Biliverdin reductase}} \text{Bilirubin}$$
$$\searrow \text{Globin}$$

Plasma concentrations of bilirubin are usually low in the fetal circulation except in unusual circumstances, as in severe *erythroblastosis fetalis* (see p. 768). Even in circumstances in which the rapid breakdown of erythrocytes leads to accelerated bilirubin production, as in severe maternal-fetal blood group incompatibility, cord blood bilirubin rarely exceeds 50 mg/L. This fact attests to the rapid, efficient transfer of this pigment across the placenta and the equally efficient disposal of fetal bilirubin by the mother.

After birth, the newborn loses the placental mechanism for bilirubin removal. As a result, there is a modest accumulation of unconjugated bilirubin in the plasma. The jaundice resulting from this change in physiological circumstance is

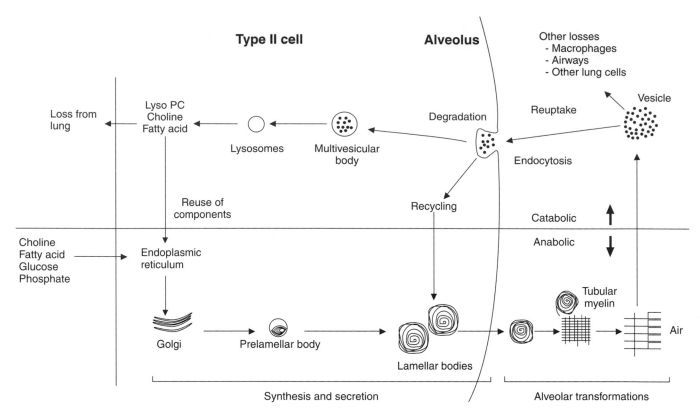

Fig. 40-10   Illustration of surfactant metabolism. The anabolic synthetic and secretory pathways link with the alveolar transformation of lamellar bodies to tubular myelin that forms the functional surfactant monolayer. During the newborn period, the majority of surfactant is taken up by type II pneumocytes and recycled. *(From Jobe AH, Ikegami M: Surfactant metabolism,* Clin Perinatol *20:687, 1993. With permission.)*

related to the limited uptake, conjugation, and excretion of bilirubin by the immature liver. The degree of neonatal jaundice occurring at birth depends on the maturity and health of the fetal liver at birth. A discussion of the transport and liver metabolism of bilirubin can be found in Chapter 35.

PATHOLOGICAL CONDITIONS ASSOCIATED WITH PREGNANCY AND PERINATAL PERIOD
Placental Disorders

Adequate exchange across the placenta between the maternal and fetal circulations is essential for normal fetal growth and metabolism. Less than optimum quantities of nutrients result in small-for-gestational-age fetuses, whereas excessive quantities of nutrients, as with maternal diabetes, result in large-for-gestational-age infants.

Few pathological conditions involving the placenta exist in which the monitoring of chemicals by the laboratory is useful. One such example is the hydatidiform mole. Molar tissue is a developmental anomaly of the placenta that has the potential for malignant growth. It is the most common lesion antecedent to choriocarcinoma. Because the mole is trophoblastic tissue, hCG is produced, resulting in a positive pregnancy test result. If serum or urinary hCG levels exceed values typical of specific times in pregnancy, a mole may be

suspected. However, because of the variations in gonadotropin values possible for normal pregnancy, no single value can be established as the borderline between normal and abnormal. Because highly sensitive and specific methods are available for monitoring serum hCG, this hormone is useful in monitoring the response of hydatidiform moles to therapy. Recent studies indicate that structural variants of hCG, with distinct oligosaccharide glycosylation patterns, occur in a variety of pregnancy-related disorders, including choriocarcinoma and hydatidiform mole.[35,36]

Ectopic Pregnancy

Usually fertilization occurs in the fallopian tubes, where the fertilized egg migrates down the tube and enters and implants in the uterus. Occasionally implantation takes place outside the uterus. In 99% of such cases, implantation occurs in the fallopian tube itself. Any implantation outside the uterus is called an **ectopic pregnancy**, and an implantation that occurs in the tube is called a *tubal pregnancy*. An ectopic pregnancy can be caused by endocrine imbalances, residual effects stemming from tubal infections, especially recurring salpingitis, or retrograde movement of the embryo from the uterus to the fallopian tube.[37] The incidence of ectopic pregnancy has risen from 4.5 cases per 1000 pregnancies in

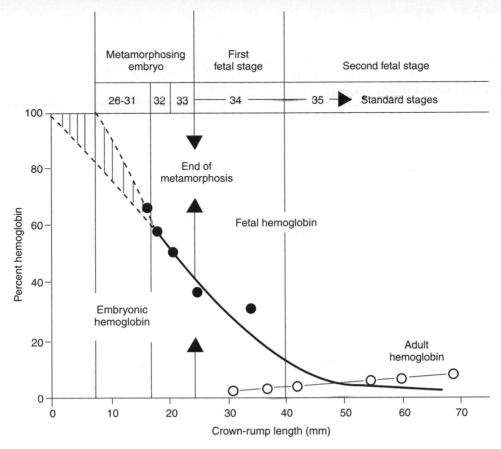

Fig. 40-11 Relationship between hemoglobin types and developmental stages in early human life. *Dashed lines and hatched area*, expected development. *(From Kleihauer E: In Stave U, editor:* Perinatal physiology, *New York, 1978, Plenum.)*

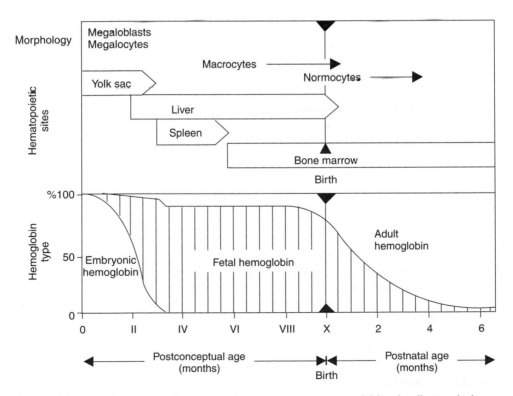

Fig. 40-12 Developmental changes in hematopoietic sites, red blood cell morphology, and hemoglobin types. *(From Kleihauer E: In Stave U, editor:* Perinatal physiology, *New York, 1978, Plenum.)*

1970 to 19.7 per 1000 pregnancies in the 1990s. Risk factors include a previous occurrence of pelvic inflammatory disease (infections with *Chlamydia trachomatis* and *Neisseria gonorrhoeae* are most common), tubal surgery, or ectopic pregnancy, and infertility treatment.

Clinical symptoms include lower abdominal pain and vaginal bleeding, although the former is highly variable in intensity and perceived location. Amenorrhea is not a characteristic feature. Before rupture of the fallopian tube occurs, tubal pregnancies usually give a positive pregnancy test. However, because compromised placentas (i.e., those in the process of abruption, degeneration, or penetration of the tubal wall) cannot produce chorionic gonadotropin in usual quantities, the tests may turn negative and become misleading. Early diagnosis is important to reduce morbidity, mortality, and to preserve fertility (see later discussion).

Premature Delivery

Preterm labor, defined as labor occurring before 37 weeks of gestation, is a prevalent and expensive complication of pregnancy in the United States. It affects approximately 8% to 10% of births and is the leading cause of perinatal morbidity and mortality. For unknown reasons, the incidence is becoming more common in the population, even while advances in the care of preterm babies are improving. These facts contribute to a cost of over $3 billion per year to manage premature birth and preterm babies.[38] Babies born before the thirty-seventh week are at risk for morbid complications, including pulmonary immaturity with resultant RDS and intraventricular hemorrhage. In addition, premature rupture of membranes (PROM) can increase the risk of fetal infection.

Symptoms of preterm labor include vaginal bleeding and spotting, increased vaginal discharge, abdominal cramping, and back pain. Because these are relatively nonspecific clinical findings, it is difficult to diagnose with absolute certainty. Patients are usually hospitalized for observation and many times, the symptoms subside. If preterm labor advances, tocolytic agents (such as magnesium sulfate), which can slow or halt uterine contractions, can be used over the course of several days to delay labor. This allows time in which the physician can administer corticosteroids in an attempt to induce fetal lung maturity. In some cases the patient is not in labor, but the membranes have ruptured and this can cause preterm delivery. Causes of premature labor and PROM are listed in the box and can be grouped as maternal, fetal, and infectious. Although these risk factors can guide the physician in deciding which patients to monitor closely, using them to assess risk of premature labor has proven to be of limited value. Currently, two tests are used in the clinic that have a proven high positive predictive value for preterm labor, the first being ultrasonography to measure cervical length. Pregnant women with a cervical dimension of 1.5 cm or less display an increased risk of premature birth.[39,40]

The second test is for fetal fibronectin (fFN), a large, extracellular glycoprotein that is produced by the chorion

---

RISK FACTORS ASSOCIATED WITH PRETERM BIRTH

Maternal
History of preterm birth (most significant risk factor)
Maternal age, less than 18 and greater than 40 years
Maternal weight, less than 100 lb
Non-white race
Maternal behaviors, including smoking and cocaine, amphetamine, or alcohol use
Multiple gestation
No prenatal care
Cervical incompetence
Exposure to DES (diethylstilbestrol)
Placenta previa
Retained intrauterine device

Fetal
Chromosomal abnormalities
Intrauterine fetal death
Intrauterine growth retardation

Infectious
Acute pyelonephritis
Bacterial vaginosis
Gonorrhea
Group B streptococcus
Chorioamnionitis
Chlamydia

---

and found in fetal membranes, decidua, and amniotic fluid, but not in blood or urine. The detection of fFN in vaginal fluids can indicate the loss of membrane integrity. This protein is further discussed under Change of Analyte in Disease.

Toxemia

Toxemia of pregnancy is characterized by hypertension (blood pressure over 140/90 mm Hg), edema, proteinuria, consumptive coagulopathy, sodium retention, hyperreflexia *(preeclampsia)*, and possibly convulsions *(eclampsia)* beginning after 20 weeks of gestation.[41] This syndrome affects approximately 0.35 to 0.42 million pregnancies in the United States each year, making this one of the most common medical conditions associated with pregnancy.

Preeclampsia tends to occur mostly (85%) in nulliparous women (those having first pregnancies), though women with hypertension predating a pregnancy have a 25% risk of developing preeclampsia. It is believed that the precipitating cause of pregnancy hypertension is a compromised utero-placental blood flow. Management includes bed rest, dietary restriction of salt, and the carefully controlled use of magnesium sulfate to prevent eclamptic convulsions.[42] Although the exact etiology of toxemia is unknown at present,[41,42] the only satisfactory "cure" is delivery, and for this reason information about the pulmonary status of the fetus is of considerable importance. The frequent association of toxemia with maternal diabetes and with vascular disease provides a basis for the correlation of this condition with small-for-gestational-age fetuses. Routine tests for serum uric acid, creatinine, and urine protein are the most common laboratory means of monitoring the toxemic pregnancy. Important adjunct tests are magnesium levels to monitor magnesium sulfate therapy and the test of fetal lung maturity.

Maternal Diabetes (also see Chapter 32)

There is an increased association of intrauterine deaths, congenital malformations, and perinatal mortality and morbidity in fetuses of diabetic women. For this reason, the pregnant diabetic woman is monitored closely throughout the course of her pregnancy. Monitoring is especially critical in the month immediately after conception, because maintaining a euglycemic state in diabetic women at the time of conception greatly reduces fetal morbidity and mortality (see p. 595). The fetal pancreas does not ameliorate maternal diabetes, because insulin does not cross the placenta.[43] Exogenous insulin therapy and diet are therefore necessary for management of the diabetic mother's insulin-deficient state.

As placental size increases, increasing amounts of human placental lactogen (HPL) and other factors that modify or oppose the action of insulin are produced. HPL may be the cause of the increased insulin requirements of pregnancy.[44,45]

Opposing the effect of HPL, maternal pancreatic-cell hyperplasia frequently occurs with pregnancy, increasing the production of maternal insulin. Thus, normal insulin-glucose homeostasis is maintained when there is an increased glucose demand by the fetus.

When insufficient insulin is available to maintain normal glucose homeostasis, maternal hyperglycemia results. This in turn increases the blood glucose of the fetus, which although it produces a fetal hyperinsulinemia, results is unusually large babies (macrosomia). These infants are at increased risk for becoming diabetics in later life. At delivery, when the fetus is deprived of the maternal glucose source, the excess insulin in the newborn rapidly decreases the blood glucose levels so that the newborn becomes hypoglycemic. Life-threatening hypoglycemic crises are frequently encountered in untreated infants of diabetic mothers. When this happens, glucose must be administered to the newborn until a proper glucose-insulin balance can be achieved.

In pregnancies complicated by diabetes, a significant increase in the incidence of the RDS has been noted, though this is by no means a universal finding.

Intrahepatic Cholestasis of Pregnancy

Intrahepatic cholestasis of pregnancy (ICP) is the most frequent liver disorder of pregnancy, with an incidence of between 1:1000 to 1:10,000 pregnancies. Mild to severe itching beginning in the third trimester is the major clinical complaint of the mother. The itching is caused by the increase in serum bile acids, which is the key diagnostic finding of the disease. ICP is associated with increased risk of premature birth and stillbirth (perinatal mortality can be as high as 1%). If ICP is diagnosed, it is best treated by early delivery of the fetus. Diagnosis can be made by seeing an increase in hepatic enzymes associated with complaints of itching, and most importantly, by an increase in serum bile acids.

Fetal Lung Immaturity

The last of the organ systems to mature sufficiently to support extrauterine life is the lungs. Fetal lung immaturity, or the RDS, occurs most often when insufficient lung surfactant is present.[46] Infants with RDS require increased respiratory effort. The tremendous effort needed to inflate uncooperative lungs often results in the grunting, nasal flaring, and substernal retractions that are characteristic physical signs in these infants. The greater expenditure of energy that is required to breathe can result in the death of weak, premature newborns.

Therapy for newborns with RDS is basically supportive, although techniques and outcomes continue to improve, as exemplified by current mortality rates from RDS of about 50% compared with 80% mortality in the 1960s.[47] Clinical management is aimed at effective management of pulmonary exchange of oxygen and carbon dioxide, acidosis, and circulatory insufficiency.

The effect of administration of pulmonary surfactant from exogenous sources (human, mammalian, and artificially synthesized) has been investigated in infants with RDS. Several recent studies have established clear benefits from surfactant replacement therapy in reducing the severity of pulmonary damage and mortality from RDS.[48,49]

Glucocorticoids stimulate the process of pulmonary maturation, and it is well established that prenatal administration of maternal dexamethasone or betamethasone can promote lung development and reduce the risk and/or severity of RDS between 30 and 33 weeks gestational age.[50,51] Interestingly, only about 15% of eligible pregnancies actually receive hormonal therapy.[52] Intrauterine infection, diabetes, and severe preeclampsia represent contraindications to antenatal steroid administration. The potential risks of glucocorticoid administration and the short window of therapeutic response (24 hours to 7 days) are probably largely responsible for its limited use.

Although the therapies discussed demonstrated significant reductions in RDS morbidity and mortality, no ideal preventative therapy has yet been developed for infants with RDS. Thus obstetrical management efforts continue to be directed toward prevention of the syndrome in premature infants through delivery management based, in part, on antenatal assessment of lung maturation. Because the status of fetal surfactant synthesis and release correlates so well with the probability of lung maturity at delivery, amniotic fluid tests that assess the quantity or quality of pulmonary surfactant present before delivery are used widely for obstetrical management. These tests are discussed in detail in the next section.

Fetal Hemolytic Disorders (Rh Problems)

Hepatic excretory capacity does not become fully mature until nearly 4 weeks postpartum in full-term human infants. The hepatic processing of bilirubin therefore falls short of the maximum before that time. When uptake and conjugation of bilirubin are forced to operate at rates exceeding the capacity of the liver to excrete the quantity formed, as in infants with severe hemolytic disease, unconjugated bilirubin accumulates in liver and serum.

Hemolytic disease of the newborn. This condition can be caused by antigen incompatibilities between the fetus and mother, most often involving the antigens of the Rh, ABO, or other minor blood groups of the red blood cells (RBCs). Fetal RBC antigen incompatibility, arising from an Rh-negative mother and an Rh-positive father, is the most common cause of fetal hemolytic disease, the rapid destruction of fetal RBCs. If the fetus is also Rh-positive, fetal cells entering the maternal circulation may elicit a maternal antibody response to the Rh blood factor. The IgGs cross the placenta into the fetus where they destroy fetal red blood cells. This condition can vary from subclinical, to mild anemia, to the life-threatening condition of erythroblastosis fetalis.[53] The risk for more severe disease increases with subsequent pregnancies.

The healthy fetus generates approximately 35 mg of bilirubin from the catabolism of 1 g of hemoglobin. The high maternal-to-fetal plasma protein gradient facilitates rapid transplacental extraction of unconjugated fetal bilirubin and at the same time suppresses glucuronide conjugation by the fetal liver. The transferred bilirubin is so efficiently conjugated and excreted by the mother that it is uncommon for the neonate to have an elevated cord blood bilirubin level. However, in severe erythroblastosis, particularly if coupled with placental deterioration, unconjugated bilirubin levels can run as high as 80 mg/L. Fetuses receiving intrauterine transfusions are often born with high levels of conjugated bilirubin, probably arising from stimulation of fetal glucuronide formation coupled with decreased placental permeability to the bilirubin glucuronide.

Also unique to the newborn and related to developmental immaturity is the tissue toxicity of unconjugated bilirubin, especially to the brain. In the adult, serum bilirubin elevations are viewed as an important clinical or laboratory sign of disease or altered physiological state. In the newborn, hyperbilirubinemia has a dual significance as a clinical sign and also as a toxin.

Conjugated bilirubin is highly water soluble and is therefore readily excreted in fluids. Unconjugated or indirect bilirubin, on the other hand, is insoluble in aqueous solution but highly soluble in lipids. Under healthy circumstances, unconjugated bilirubin is bound to plasma albumin, and this binding prevents the entrance of free or unbound indirect bilirubin into the lipid-rich central nervous system. When the albumin-binding capacity is exceeded, unbound, unconjugated bilirubin readily passes into the central nervous system cells. Unconjugated bilirubin is toxic to the central nervous system and causes necrosis, a pathological process referred to as *kernicterus*. Surviving infants may have mental retardation, hearing deficits, or cerebral palsy. Many affected infants, particularly those of low birth weight, may have no neonatal symptoms but later in childhood can develop hearing deficits, perceptual handicaps, and hyperkinesis.

Usually there is no detectable bilirubin in amniotic fluid when fetus and mother are healthy.[54] However, a newborn who demonstrates significant elevations of unconjugated bilirubin in serum, as in erythroblastosis fetalis, frequently also passes bilirubin into the amniotic fluid as a fetus. The route by which bilirubin is transferred into amniotic fluid from the fetus is unclear. Measuring the concentration of amniotic bilirubin (the A_{450} test, see later discussion) is used to assess the risk for fetal complications resulting from erythroblastosis fetalis.

Newborns with severe Rh hemolytic disease are clearly at risk for life-threatening anemia or hyperbilirubinemia. Following delivery and stabilization, cord blood hematologic and biochemical tests should be performed. These generally include: direct and total bilirubin, direct Coombs, blood type, hemoglobin, reticulocyte count, and nucleated RBCs. The results of these tests are used to determine the need for continued close monitoring versus immediate exchange transfusion.

Spina Bifida and Anencephaly

Spina bifida and **anencephaly** are relatively common (approximately 5 per 10,000 live births) neural tube defects (NTD) that constitute a large portion of the serious congenital malformations in humans. In spina bifida there is a midline defect of the spine that results in a protrusion of the meninges or spinal cord or other neural elements, that is, a **meningomyelocele**. In anencephaly the brain is a disorganized mass of neural tissues, and the forebrain, overlying meninges, cranial vault, and skin are all absent. Most anencephalic infants are stillborn, and those born alive survive for only several hours. Failures to close the ventral wall of the developing fetus also occur.

It is possible to identify women who are at increased risk for carrying fetuses with NTD by measurement of maternal serum α-fetoprotein levels.[55] Population *screening* for NTD by measurement of maternal serum α-fetoprotein levels has become widely accepted in the United States. Prenatal *diagnosis* of NTDs by measurement of α-fetoprotein and fetal-specific acetylcholinesterase levels in amniotic fluid has become routine in recent years. Approximately 80% of open spina bifida cases and 95% of anencephaly cases are detectable by measurement of maternal serum α-fetoprotein during 16 to 18 weeks of gestation. In addition, anencephaly specifically affects estriol formation. The absence of fetal pituitary function and fetal adrenal hypoactivity and reduced ACTH levels result in very low rates of production of DHEA from the fetal adrenal glands. Because this androgen is a precursor to estriol, levels of estriol are characteristically low.

Down Syndrome

Down syndrome (DS), or trisomy 21, is the most common genetic cause of mental retardation, with an approximate occurrence of 1:700 births. In 1984 Merkatz et al[56] reported an association of low maternal serum α-fetoprotein with trisomy 21. Elevated maternal serum hCG and decreased unconjugated E_3 levels have also been associated with an increased risk for Down syndrome.[57,58] Most recently, inhibin A, a hormone that is produced by the granulosa cells of the ovaries in non-pregnant women and by the developing placenta (see p. 855), have been found to be significantly elevated in DS pregnancies.[59] DS is usually not an inherited condition and does not run in families so it is difficult to predict which pregnancies will be affected.

CHANGE OF ANALYTE IN DISEASE

Over the past two decades significant advances elucidating the course of growth and development of the fetus have been made. Part of this newfound knowledge has been possible through the development and application of improved analytical techniques and the improved safety of amniocentesis through ultrasound visualization. Application of much of this knowledge has dramatically altered the course of management of problem or "high-risk" pregnancies. Fig. 40-13 indicates the multifaceted array of its applications.

Three clinical problem areas have been the primary beneficiaries of amniocentesis: (1) the management of Rh-antigen incompatibility of mother and fetus, (2) the identification of the earliest possible time in pregnancy that delivery can be performed with minimal risk of lung immaturity, and (3) the identification of developmental or genetic disorders. Genetic disorders are discussed in Chapter 47.

Human Chorionic Gonadotropin

Human chorionic gonadotropin (hCG) is used to identify and follow both trophoblastic disease and the course of normal pregnancy. In a healthy pregnancy, urinary levels of hCG rise to a range of 20,000 to 100,000 U/day and then decrease to a range of 4000 to 11,000 U/day later in the pregnancy. Pregnancy can be detected by analysis of urinary hCG about a week after a missed menses. By using assays of serum hCG, particularly with sensitive and specific methods for the hCG β-chains, pregnancy can be detected as early as a few days after conception. In cases of hydatidiform mole, urinary hCG titers rise to over 300,000 U/day. After molar evacuation, these values drop within 1 month, and in about 90% of cases hCG is not detectable by urinary assay after 3 months. In cases in which trophoblastic tissue remains, such as retained choriocarcinoma, values remain elevated, and serial assays of urine or serum hCG are of great value in determining the results of treatment, usually chemotherapy.

On a molecular basis, hCG shows about 1/4000 the thyrotropic activity of pituitary TSH. If hCG levels are very high, thyroid-stimulating activity is possible. For this reason, the levels of hCG attained in molar pregnancies are believed to be the reason hyperthyroidism is often associated with molar pregnancies. If hCG values exceed 100,000 U/day in urine or 300 U/mL in serum, the presence of hyperthyroidism and hydatidiform mole should be suspected.

Levels of hCG are often low for gestational age with ectopic pregnancies. Positive pregnancy tests have been obtained in only 50% of ectopic pregnancies. A negative test

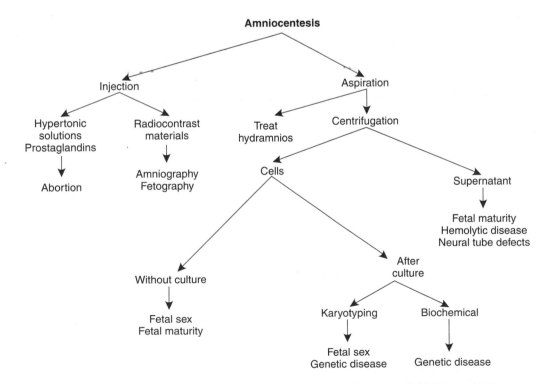

Fig. 40-13 Clinical applications of amniocentesis. *(From Pritchard JA, MacDonald PC: In Pritchard JA, MacDonald PC, editors:* Williams obstetrics, *ed 16, New York, 1990, Appleton-Century-Crofts.)*

result therefore does *not* exclude ectopic pregnancy. Newer, more sensitive immunoassays may improve the diagnosis of ectopic pregnancies. Serial, quantitative hCG levels that show an increase of less than 60% in 48 hours are strongly suggestive of an ectopic pregnancy.[37] Low levels of maternal serum hCG have also been associated with fetal trisomy 18, a lethal condition in which 75% of affected fetuses are spontaneously lost in the third trimester.[60] Unlike in trisomy 18, maternal serum hCG levels have been shown to be increased in trisomy 21 (Down syndrome).[61] In addition, women with a diagnosis of threatened abortion who have low hCG levels for the estimated time of gestation have been shown to have complete abortions.

hCG and Progesterone in Ectopic Pregnancy

The diagnosis is most effectively made using serial β-hCG measurements collected 48 hours apart in combination with transvaginal utlrasonography.[62-64] Although the mean plasma hCG concentration is lower for an ectopic pregnancy than for a viable intrauterine pregnancy, there is no definitive concentration that distinguishes between the two. If the pregnancy is proceeding normally, the β-hCG concentrations are expected to increase by 66% or greater during the first 5 weeks of gestation. It should be noted that this rate may not be found in about 15% of normal pregnancies. For about 85% of ectopic pregnancies, the rate of increase of hCG is significantly less. A prospective study by Sheppard et al[65] reported a 36% sensitivity and 63% to 71% specificity. After week 5 the rate of hCG increase slows and so the test becomes less useful after this time. It should be noted that this test cannot distinguish the failing intrauterine pregnancy from an ectopic pregnancy.

Other biochemical tests have been evaluated: creatine kinase, fetal fibronectin, and progesterone levels have received considerable attention. Of these, progesterone continues to have some interest because low serum concentrations are found in many ectopic pregnancies. Again there is no single progesterone concentration that can be recommended as a cutoff. Although about half of ectopic pregnancies had levels below 20 ng/mL, at least 2% had levels above 25 ng/mL.[66] If progesterone level is to have value, the cutoff must be established by individual laboratory and must be available as a stat test.

Estriol

Low serum or urinary estriol levels, or, more importantly, declining estriol levels, carry an unfavorable prognostic significance[67] (see Fig. 40-5, showing serial estriol values during various pregnancies). As a rough guideline, a decline of 30% to 50% from the mean of 3 previous days indicates probable impending danger to the fetus. Because of the pronounced diurnal variation in estrogen formation, maintaining a consistent time of day for sampling (particularly when measuring estrogen levels in urine) is important.

Serum or urinary estriol levels that are greater than the 95th percentile should be suggestive of the possibility of twins. Estriol values are good predictors of impending fetal death in hypertensive disease, renal disease, and diabetes. Conditions associated with chronically low serum estriol levels include toxemia, anencephaly, placental sulfatase deficiency, Down syndrome, and trisomy 18. In these cases, serum unconjugated estriol is usually preferred over urine or total serum estriol because it is unconjugated estriol produced by the fetus that has the best clinical correlation. Estriols are not helpful in monitoring erythroblastosis fetalis.

Fetal Fibronectin

Fetal fibronectin (fFN) is believed to play a role in adhesion of the developing embryo to the interior surface of the uterus. It is found in vaginal secretions during the early weeks of pregnancy as the gestational sac implants into the uterine wall. Past 24 weeks gestation, it does not appear again in cervicovaginal secretions unless there is a disturbance of choriodecidual junction or a rupture of the placental membranes.[68]

The fFN test is used to monitor women at risk of preterm labor.[69] To measure fFN, clinicians swab the posterior fornix of the vagina, store the swab in a buffer solution, and the swab is analyzed for the presence of the protein. Samples must be tested within 3 days of collection.

When fFN is not detected (≤ 50 ng/mL) labor is unlikely within the next 7 to 14 days. Negative predictive values have been reported to be as high as 99%.[70] Other factors contributing to labor are not measured using fFN, leading to false-negative results. Conversely, a high level of fFN can be caused by something other than impending labor. It has been shown that increases in fFN can correlate with chorioamnionitis and the presentation of sepsis in the infant at birth.[70] The predictive value of the test is short term, lasting between 1 and 2 weeks so repeat testing of women at high risk for preterm labor is judicious. The high negative predictive value of the fFN test can save money because physicians can choose not to intervene and to send the patient home. This also saves on the expense of tocolytic ($MgSO_4$) and steroid therapy and decreases the risks to the baby.

Tests of Fetal Lung Maturation

Antenatal laboratory tests for fetal lung maturity (FLM) are used by the obstetrician to predict the likelihood of RDS subsequent to preterm delivery. Typically these tests include biochemical or biophysical evaluations of amniotic fluid for the presence of surfactant components derived from maturing fetal lungs. These tests have been designed either to quantify specific surfactant-associated phospholipids (biochemical approach) or to measure the surface-active effects of these pulmonary surfactant components in the amniotic fluid sample (biophysical approach). Other methods that do not seem to fit neatly into either group have been developed. Over the years an enormous number of FLM methods have been developed, though most of these have never gained widespread acceptance for routine use. Some of the more popular, or promising, FLM methods are described next.

Biochemical assays

The lecithin-to-sphingomyelin ratio (LSR) test.

Gluck and Kulovich[71] were the first to correlate the relative concentrations of lecithin and sphingomyelin in amniotic fluid to the functional status of the fetal lung, and the lecithin/sphingomyelin ratio (LSR) they described was the first laboratory test for fetal lung maturity to be widely accepted. Rather than quantifying lecithin and sphingomyelin directly, the test is used to determine the ratio of these compounds after thin-layer chromatography (TLC). This semiquantitative approach was designed to provide faster analysis times than quantitative TLC, to be relatively independent of usual and sometimes significant variations in the volume of amniotic fluid during pregnancy, and to diminish the effects of variations in the extraction recovery of lipids. Using TLC methods of the type originally proposed by Gluck, LSR values of 2 or greater have been found to correlate with fetal lung maturity. Before 34 weeks of gestation, lecithin and sphingomyelin are present in amniotic fluid in approximately equal amounts, but at about 34 weeks the concentration of lecithin begins to rise rapidly compared to sphingomyelin. When the concentration of lecithin in amniotic fluid becomes at least twice that of the sphingomyelin, the likelihood of respiratory distress after delivery is minimal.

Because early reports suggested that a greater risk of RDS is associated with the diabetic pregnancy, values of 2.5 or greater have often been used for these pregnancies. The validity of this approach has been questioned by some, however, because no consistent gestation age–matched differences in LSR results have been observed between diabetic and nondiabetic pregnancies in many recent studies.[27]

The clinical predictability of the LSR, like most FLM tests, varies widely. Reported sensitivities and specificities for this test range between 80% and 85%.[72] This variability is likely to result from poor analytical standardization, differences in study populations, inherent lack of consistency in the diagnosis of RDS, and the use of different reference values.

Gluck and Kulovich[71] and others have reported that in certain pathological pregnancy conditions pulmonary maturation appears to be accelerated, whereas in others it is delayed. Diseases in which FLM may be delayed include diabetes mellitus and hemolytic disease in the fetus. Maternal hypertension and premature rupture of the membranes with delayed delivery have been reported to hasten maturation through increased surfactant production by the fetal lung. However, the exact nature and extent of the effects of these and other maternal and fetal complications on the results obtained for the LSR and most other FLM tests remain largely speculative.

Pathophysiological factors that alter the overall rate of lung maturation might be expected to affect these processes individually and to differing extents. This proposed effect has been termed the *uncoupling phenomenon* by some[27] and refers to the apparent uncoupling of phospholipid synthesis from clinical outcome. An emerging concept is that FLM tests measure surfactant, *but* lung maturation requires (1) surfactant production *and* release and (2) morphological development of lung tissue (differentiation, such as production of lung connective tissue and vascularization). Processes (1) and (2) are usually synchronized; however, some disease states may cause morphological development to occur faster or slower than surfactant development. In these cases FLM tests, which measure only one component of this process (surfactant release), may not correctly reflect fetal pulmonary status. As an example, β-methasone administration at 30 to 32 weeks of gestational age promotes lung maturation as evidenced by decreased incidence of RDS. However, standard FLM tests do not typically reflect any change from pretreatment levels because the β-methasone effect is believed to be mostly on morphological development and secondarily on increased surfactant synthesis. This concept is important because it makes the point that lung maturation is a very complicated process with many interrelated factors and is not just surfactant related. In situations in which alterations in morphological factors were predominant in the lung-maturation process, the relationship between FLM test results and the status of fetal lung development could be altered such that the surfactant-based tests lose their usual significance. If this should indeed be the case, the use of altered FLM reference values, as has been the practice for diabetes and other maternal or fetal diseases, would seem to be without foundation unless the nature and extent of specific surfactant-related alterations can be determined.

Contamination of samples with blood tends to produce falsely elevated values for very immature samples and falsely lowered values for very mature samples. Meconium, vaginal secretion, and maternal urine contamination can also produce false results. Also RDS can develop in an asphyxiated neonate, despite a mature LSR.

The LSR was the first laboratory procedure designed to assess fetal lung maturity directly, and largely because of this historical fact, it has come to be considered by many as the "standard" test for fetal lung maturity. Over the years, however, numerous modifications of the original procedure have been proposed in an effort to overcome many perceived practical and analytical deficiencies. Unfortunately, this activity has led to the development of many unique TLC methods for determining the ratio of lecithin to sphingomyelin in amniotic fluid, each of which may produce substantially different LSR values. Up to now, there is no standard method for the LSR, and many problems persist, including poor interlaboratory and intralaboratory reproducibility and excessive analysis time. In addition, there are still many questions about specific components of the general procedure such as phospholipid extraction, TLC solvent systems, TLC plates, and detecting systems (see later discussion).

Because the LSR method is believed to be less successful in predicting fetal lung maturity in diabetic pregnancies, tests for other surface-active lipids or surfactant proteins have been developed for use either with the LSR or solely as independent tests. These efforts to improve on the clinical reliability of the LSR have led to the development of the *lung profile*,[73,74] which consists of the two-dimensional TLC determination and combined interpretation of the LSR, phosphatidylglycerol (PG), phosphatidylinositol, and the percentage of acetone-precipitable lecithin. Unfortunately, the marginal improvements in clinical reliability associated with this method may be offset by extremely long analysis times and the requirement for high levels of technical expertise.

Phosphatidylglycerol. Because phosphatidylglycerol (PG) does contribute to the functional properties of surfactant, tests for this phospholipid came to be popular as an adjunct to the LSR. Functional lung maturity is clearly associated with measurable quantities of PG[75]; however, the absence of PG does not necessarily mean that RDS is inevitable. Collective experience with the PG test indicates that, whereas the predictive value of the presence of PG is nearly 100% for lung maturity, the predictive value of the absence of PG in predicting RDS may be so low as to be virtually uninformative. Because PG appears to be but a very small constituent of blood, the measurement of PG is especially valuable at times when fetal lung status must be predicted from blood- or meconium-contaminated amniotic fluid samples. The measurement of PG is also considered important when evaluating the maturity of fetuses of diabetic mothers, because the LSR and other FLM tests may be less reliable in these cases. When amniotic fluid obtained from leakage into the vagina is the most readily accessible sample, PG is the only phospholipid that should be measured. If a proper vaginal pool sample is obtained, false-positive results are rare, though there have been rare reports of local PG production by vaginal flora. Creatinine or urea values should be obtained on vaginal pool samples suspected of being heavily contaminated with maternal urine to help determine the nature of the sample. PG has been measured by one- or two-dimensional TLC procedures, though both are time-consuming and some TLC methods may be subject to comigration of other phospholipids or interfering substances with the PG spot.[76]

A slide agglutination assay for PG (AmnioStat-FLM, Irvine Scientific, Irvine, California) employs antiserum specific for PG, can be applied to vaginally collected samples, and is rapid. This test is relatively simple to perform, and has good specificity but poor sensitivity.

Biophysical assays. The methods in this group were originally so classified because they were designed to measure some specific biophysical property of pulmonary surfactant in the amniotic fluid sample. As mentioned recently by Dubin,[77] however, this classification has, over time, come to include a group of fundamentally dissimilar assays that have in common the primary property of not fitting into the biochemical category. They are generally easier, faster, and cheaper to perform than traditional TLC techniques.

Foam-stability assays. The shake test and foam stability index (FSI) test are based on the observation that ethanol acts as a competitive antifoaming surfactant that overcomes the foam-stability effects of most nonpulmonary surfactants in amniotic fluid. Pulmonary phospholipid surfactants, however, are capable of producing a surface tension lower than 29 dynes/cm, thus allowing stable foam formation in ethanolic solutions after vigorous shaking. This is the basis for the shake test[78] for assessing fetal lung maturity. The end point of this test is the formation of a continuous ring of bubbles at the meniscus of a tube that was shaken vigorously and that contained equal volumes of 95% (v/v) ethanol and amniotic fluid. This value was roughly equivalent to over 30 mg of dipalmitoyl phosphatidylcholine per liter, and was found to be highly predictive of FLM. In 1978, Sher et al[79] reported a modification of the original *shake test*, named the *foam stability index* (FSI), that allowed the semiquantitative measurement of varying amounts of surfactant, primarily dipalmitoyl phosphatidylcholine, in concentrations ranging from 15 to 30 mg/L. The reported clinical performance of this test is generally quite good. Drawbacks of this test include the subjective nature of the foam reading and the test's susceptibility to a wide variety of foam-producing contaminants. Because of this, particular care must be taken to ensure that sample containers and glassware for the test are clean and that the reagents and amniotic fluid samples are not contaminated with blood, meconium, excessive numbers of leukocytes, or vaginal secretions.

Fluorescence polarization assays. The TDx Fetal Lung Maturity Assay (TDx-FLM) test is a fluorescence polarization assay designed for use on the Abbott TDx Analyzer (Abbott Laboratories Diagnostics Division, Irving, TX 75015). This test employs a unique fluorescent probe (PC16)[80] that, when added to amniotic fluid, partitions between endogenous albumin (high fluorescence polarization) and phospholipid surfactant (low fluorescence polarization). The overall polarization measured by the analyzer reflects the ratio of surfactant to albumin in the sample, and this value is highly correlated with lung maturity. Recent clinical evaluation demonstrated sensitivity and specificity for TDx-FLM test equal to or exceeding that of the LSR.[81] Either version of this test is precise, requires minimal sample preparation and sample volume and can be performed in less than 30 minutes. The TDx-FLM version employs standardized reagents and calibrators.

Lamellar bodies. Because the lamellar bodies (LBs) are the structural form of pulmonary surfactant extruded by the type II pneumocytes, the concentration of lamellar bodies in amniotic fluid has been evaluated for use in FLM assessment. Early approaches were generally based on ultracentrifugation to separate the LB fraction of the sample followed by quantitation of the phospholipid content of this fraction.[82] Although the clinical performance of this approach was generally quite good, the hardware requirements and procedural complexity exceeded the capabilities of most clinical laboratories.

More recently, Dubin[83] has reported on the measurement of LBs by refractive index matched anomalous diffraction (RIMAD) and resistive-pulse counting[84] techniques. The RIMAD technique consists in the measurement of the difference in the optical density of amniotic fluid diluted 1:2 in glycerol (reference cuvette) and in saline (test cuvette). Light scattering caused by the lamellar bodies occurs in the test cuvette but not in the glycerol blank because the refractive index of glycerol very closely matches that of the lamellar bodies. Because the light absorbance of common chromogens, such as methene pigments, is independent of the refractive index, any interference should be the same in both the reference and the test cuvettes and should thus be corrected for in a dual-beam spectrophotometer. The net effect is an increase in measured absorbance at 650 nm resulting from the light scattering alone. Using the absorbance (A) difference criterion of A = 0.056, this test has been shown to correlate well with the lamellar body number density (LBND) and fetal lung maturation.[83] Quantitation of LBND by resistive-pulse counting techniques using the platelet channel of commercial cell counters also represents a promising new approach to FLM testing. Lamellar body number density values of 40,000/μL and 26,000/μL, in uncentrifuged and centrifuged specimens respectively, demonstrate strong predictive concordance with other accepted measures of FLM.[84] This method possesses the advantages of little or no sample preparation, relative freedom from common interfering substances, and rapid, semiautomated performance. Because of their procedural simplicity and rapid turnaround times, both of the LB procedures described here appear to be useful tests in the initial screening for FLM.

FLM testing/interpretive strategies. Biochemical or biophysical procedures for FLM can provide important clinical information. However, the low prevalence of RDS causes a high proportion of false-positive predictions of immaturity throughout gestation for all FLM tests. Given this reality, testing strategies for the purpose of enhancing the predictive value of test results that are positive for respiratory *immaturity* have been developed.[81,85,86] Such strategies rely heavily on the availability of rapid methods for FLM that can be performed in a sequential, or cascade, fashion without substantially lengthening the total turnaround time for results. Typically the easiest and fastest tests are performed first, followed by additional tests until the first mature result is obtained or all tests in the cascade indicate immaturity. Occasionally there is a clinical need to be relatively certain that RDS will not occur after delivery that could be delayed if necessary. In these cases, the requirement for multiple mature test results that indicate fetal maturity, higher reference values, or results from markers that are positive only after fetal maturity is well established, such as PG, are sometimes employed to enhance the predictive value of test results.

Traditionally, the clinical interpretation of FLM test results has been based on the use of referent values, or cutoffs, for lung maturity determined from clinical studies. This practice, although well established for FLM testing, is known to possess certain limitations. Because no FLM test yet devised can discriminate the probability of RDS versus lung maturity with perfection, any given referent value represents an unavoidable compromise between sensitivity and specificity.

In some cases, multiple referent values have been used in an attempt to overcome these shortcomings. This practice may result in improved predictability at the high and low extremes of test results, but typically generates a substantial "indeterminate" middle range that is clinically uninformative. An alternate interpretive approach has recently been reported by a working group of the National Academy of Clinical Biochemistry (personal communication). In this study of 312 subjects from six US hospitals, the investigators employed multiple regression techniques to derive joint odds ratios and probabilities for RDS risk based on Abbott TDx-FLM II S/A values and gestational age at sampling. In this approach, no specific referent values for maturity are assumed or used for test interpretation. Instead, the calculated joint odds ratios and probabilities for RDS are reported for various TDx-FLM II result/gestational age combinations. Using this approach, the investigators were also able to generate odds ratios and probabilities for the likelihood of mild versus moderate or severe RDS.

Testing for Hemolytic Disease (Isoimmunization)

Amniotic fluid bilirubin (ΔA_{450}). The findings of a maternal anti-Rh (D) antibody titer (indirect Coombs' test) of 1 to 8 or more, or a history of hemolytic disease with previous infants, warrants an investigation into the likelihood of hemolytic disease in the fetus. The investigation entails repeated amniocentesis and measurements of bilirubin pigment in the amniotic fluid. The absorbance of bilirubin, when measured using a continuously recording spectrophotometer, is demonstrable as a broad increase in absorbance around 450 nm (Fig. 40-14). The magnitude of the increase in absorbance above the baseline value (ΔA_{450}) usually, but not always, correlates well for any gestational age with the intensity of the hemolytic disease.

Liley[87] developed a graph that reasonably allows the prediction of the severity of hemolytic disease and the recommendation of clinical management (Fig. 40-15). The higher the ΔA_{450}, the more severe is the hemolytic disease relative to the gestational age of the pregnancy. In general, a

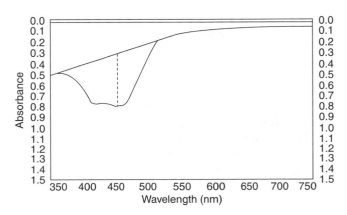

Fig. 40-14 Spectrum of bilirubin. *Dashed line,* Absorbance at 450 nm. *(From Queenan JT: Clin Obstet Gynecol 14:505, 1971.)*

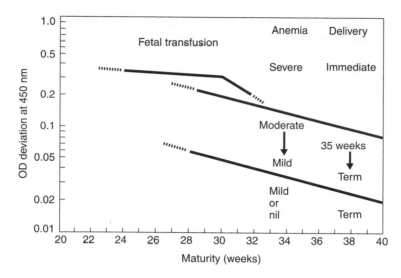

Fig. 40-15   Relationship of absorbance at 450 nm, gestational age of amniotic fluid associated with fetal anemia, and suggested clinical management. *OD,* Optical density (absorbance). *(From Liley AW:* Am J Obstet Gynecol *86:485, 1963.)*

decreasing amniotic fluid bilirubin trend is a good prognostic indicator that a fetus will survive, whereas a horizontal or rising bilirubin level indicates that there is severe erythroblastosis fetalis. The main source of error is the fetus with polyhydramnios, because it can cause a false-low bilirubin determination. In addition, maternal hyperbilirubinemia or sickle cell disease may result in elevations of bilirubin in amniotic fluid in the absence of fetal hemolytic disease.

Cord Blood/Venous Bilirubin

Transient neonatal hyperbilirubinemia (unconjugated) is observed in approximately 60% of term and approximately 80% of preterm infants. As described previously, this is usually the result of excess neonatal production combined with an immature hepatic bilirubin conjugation system. Generally, bilirubin values that do not exceed 120 mg/L during the first week of life in an otherwise healthy infant are considered nonpathological. The box lists bilirubin levels for which pathological causes should be sought.[88] Infants with significant bilirubin elevations may be treated with phototherapy or exchange transfusion. Specific recommendations for treatment are somewhat controversial and typically vary for premature versus mature infants, breast-feeding status (which promotes an increase in bilirubin levels), birth weight, and possibly race. Although somewhat controversial, detailed treatment guidelines for management of hyperbilirubinemia in healthy term infants have been published.[89]

In newborn term infants with a positive-reacting Coombs' test, a cord total bilirubin value greater than 50 mg/L in the first 24 hours after birth suggests the need for an immediate exchange transfusion. This procedure effectively removes antibody-coated RBCs that would eventually contribute to an even higher bilirubin load. For mildly affected full-term infants, exchange transfusion may be indicated if the rate of bilirubin rise suggests that a concentration of greater than 200 mg/L will be achieved

Glucose Screening and Monitoring (see also pp. 760 and 767)

Two issues exist with respect to pregnancy and diabetes. The first deals with the identification of gestational diabetes.[90] Not only are a significant number of pregnancies affected by gestational diabetes, but many of these women may go on to develop diabetes while not pregnant. At risk are women who develop glycosuria, have a positive family history of diabetes, have a history of large-for-gestational-age infants, have had a stillbirth, a parity of five or more, and are obese, or over age 35. Because of the adverse effects of diabetes on the fetus, the American College of Obstetrics and Gynecology recommends that all women undergo diabetes screening by 24 to 28 weeks gestation. The American Diabetes Association also recommends screening unless the woman is considered low-risk (maternal age < 25 years, ethnicity other than African American, Hispanic, or Native American).[90] See p. 596, Chapter 32, for details of the recommended screening procedure.

The second issue deals with careful monitoring and control of the pregnant diabetic. A number of studies using humans and animal models have shown that high maternal glucose, high fetal glucose and insulin, or a combination of these, delays both the biochemical and morphological

---

BILIRUBIN VALUES TYPICALLY ASSOCIATED WITH PATHOLOGICAL CAUSES

Serum bilirubin >50 mg/L during first 24 hours of life
Serum bilirubin levels rising more than 50 mg/L/day
Term infants with serum bilirubin (unconjugated) values >120 to 130 mg/L
Preterm infants with serum bilirubin (unconjugated) values >150 mg/L

development of the fetal lung. The exact mechanisms involved remain to be determined, but in vitro studies suggest the high glucose concentrations block the movement of lipids from fibroblasts to type II cells.[91] When diabetic mothers are in good or strict metabolic control, there is little difference in the lung development of their fetuses compared to nondiabetic mothers. It is interesting to note that the fetuses of mothers who are poorly controlled but who have more than five episodes of hypoglycemia per week are often found to have accelerated lung maturation, quite possibly because of the stress on the fetus.[92]

The pregnant diabetic is at risk for other complications as well, including hypertension, infection, acidosis, and nephropathy, and should be monitored carefully to detect these conditions early.[93] Frequent self-monitoring of blood glucose using a reliable point-of-care device is encouraged. Not only is elevated glucose a concern, but as indicated above, recognition of episodes of hypoglycemia may be useful in identifying fetal stress. Blood glucose goals in the pregnant diabetic woman include a fasting capillary glucose concentration of 550 to 650 mg/L or a venous plasma concentration of 630 to 750 mg/L, and a 1-hour postprandial blood glucose level less than 1200 mg/L or a venous plasma concentration of less than 1400 mg/L. Although some recommend monitoring hemoglobin A_{1c} (HbA_{1c}) at frequent intervals, it is important to realize that the levels of glycated hemoglobin reflect both changes in glucose tolerance and changes in red cell mass and survival time during pregnancy. This results in an initial decrease in HbA_{1c} followed by a rise during the third trimester.[94] Thus it should be remembered that the HbA_{1c} level may be lower than when the patient is not pregnant. Miller found an increased risk of congenital anomalies (ventricular septal defects, anencephaly, etc.) when the HbA_{1c} was greater than 8.5%.[95]

Because diabetic nephropathy in association with hypertension presents a risk of fetal death, urinary microalbumin and creatinine clearance should be monitored. A creatinine clearance below 50 mL/min has been associated with fetal demise. Because there is an increased risk of hypothyroidism with these patients, early screening is recommended (see p. 841).

Renal Function Tests (see also pp. 489-490)

During a healthy pregnancy, renal blood flow and the glomerular filtration rate are significantly increased above nonpregnant levels. With the development of pregnancy-induced hypertension, renal perfusion and glomerular filtration are reduced. Most often, therefore, the creatinine or urea concentration in plasma is not appreciably elevated. The plasma uric acid concentration is much more commonly elevated, especially in women with more severe renal disease. The elevation is a result primarily of decreased renal clearance of uric acid by the kidney, a decrease that exceeds the reduction in glomerular filtration rate and creatinine clearance.

α-Fetoprotein

α-Fetoprotein (AFP) is a glycoprotein with molecular weight of approximately 68,000 D and physicochemical properties similar to albumin. Several AFP isoforms have been identified, yet their clinical relevance has not been elucidated. It has been speculated that individual isoforms may be associated with phases of development, neoplastic disease, congenital disease, and a variety of biochemical processes. Unlike other analytes, elevations or decreases in AFP levels do not directly confirm a pathological process. However, this analyte is unique as an identifier of patients at risk for having fetuses with a variety of birth defects, as well as malignant disease in men and nonpregnant women.

Elevated maternal serum AFP levels are associated with an increased risk for NTDs, whereas decreased levels are associated with an increased risk for Down syndrome. However, because maternal AFP levels are dependent on numerous factors, including gestational age, maternal weight and age, race, insulin-dependent diabetes, multiple pregnancies, and drug ingestion, the results are not diagnostic. Thus maternal serum AFP levels are most useful in identifying (*screening*) those pregnant women who require additional testing (such as ultrasonography and amniocentesis) to exclude the possibility of an affected fetus.

Maternal serum α-fetoprotein results are routinely reported as a multiple of the normal median (MoM) for the relative gestational week once the value has been normalized for the factors mentioned above. Spina bifida, anencephaly, gastroschisis, and omphalocele are among the differential diagnoses at 15 to 20 weeks of gestation when both the maternal serum and amniotic fluid AFP levels are above 2.0 MoM and the amniotic fluid acetylcholinesterase levels are increased. When there is increased risk because of maternal age and the maternal serum AFP levels are below 0.4 MoM, Down syndrome is suspected.

Screening for Down Syndrome in the First and Second Trimesters

The principal factor in assessing the risk of having a child with DS is maternal age, which increases the risk of cell division anomalies. Although only 1 case occurs in 1250 pregnancies at maternal age 19, the risk increases to 1 in 100 births by the age of 40.[96] But because far more pregnancies occur in the third and fourth decade of life, the majority of Down babies are born to younger mothers. Screening tests are not diagnostic for DS, but will identify which patients should undergo more definitive tests. The diagnostic tests for the presence of trisomy 21 are amniocentesis or chorionic villus sampling, which isolate fetal cells for karyotypic analysis (see p. 915, Chapter 47). Currently all pregnant women over the age of 35 are advised to undergo one of these two procedures, which are expensive and also carry a slight risk of miscarriage. Younger mothers can be screened using serum screening tests.

Until recently, the screening test used most commonly to rule out DS was the triple screen performed early in the second trimester (15 to 20 weeks of gestation), in which levels of AFP, hCG, and unconjugated estriol (uE_3) in maternal serum are measured. AFP is synthesized in the fetal liver, hCG is manufactured by the placenta, and uE_3 is the major sex hormone produced during pregnancy (see earlier discussion). In the case of DS, AFP and uE_3 levels are low and hCG is elevated. The triple screen can detect DS with an accuracy of 60% and a false-positive rate of 5%. New tests have been suggested for increasing the sensitivity of DS screening. These include the measuring of serum inhibin A, pregnancy-associated protein-A, degraded hCG molecules, and the ultrasound measurement of fetal nuchal translucency (measuring the area between fetal skin and tissues at the back of the neck).[97] In all DS screening programs, analyte MoM values are adjusted for the gestational age, the mother's weight, race, and the number of fetuses,[97] and a likelihood ratio for the presence of DS is calculated. These data are combined with maternal age to determine which patients should undergo further testing.

Magnesium

Women with toxemia of pregnancy or premature labor are often treated with high levels of magnesium sulfate ($MgSO_4$). These women, usually under hospital care, must be closely monitored for excessive hypermagnesemia (>80 mg/L).

Bile Acids

Liver function tests are not routinely measured during a normal pregnancy. However, if a pregnant women shows signs suggestive of intrahepatic cholestasis of pregnancy (ICP), the measurement of serum bile acids is needed for the diagnosis of this disorder. Measurement of total bile acid is sufficient for this purpose.

ACKNOWLEDGMENTS

The editors wish to acknowledge Paul T. Russell, the author of the previous versions of the methods Amniotic Fluid Bilirubin and Fetal Lung Maturity Assessment: Amniotic Fluid Analysis, Lecithin-to-Sphingomyelin Ratio, Phosphatidyl Glycerol.

References

1. Heikinheimo O, Gibbons WE: The molecular mechanisms of oocyte maturation and early embryonic development are unveiling new insights into reproductive medicine, *Mol Human Reprod* 4:745, 1998.
2. Bauer MK et al: Fetal growth and placental function, *Mol Cell Endocrinol* 140:115, 1998.
3. Hay WW: Placental transport of nutrients to the fetus, *Hormone Res* 42:215, 1994.
4. Carter AM: Factors affecting gas transfer across the placenta and the oxygen supply to the fetus, *J Develop Physiol* 12:305, 1989.
5. Gilbert WM, Brace RA: Amniotic fluid volume and normal flows to and from the amniotic cavity, *Semin Perinatol* 17:150, 1993.
6. Sandler M, editor: *Amniotic fluid and its clinical significance*, New York, 1981, Marcel Dekker.
7. Weaver TE: Pulmonary surfactant-associated proteins, *Gen Pharmacol* 18:1, 1987.
8. Pierce JG, Parsons TF: Glycoprotein hormones: structure and function, *Annu Rev Biochem* 50:465, 1980.
9. Vinson GP: *The adrenal cortex*, Englewood Cliffs, NJ, 1992, Prentice Hall.
10. Foye WO, Lemke TL, Williams DA: *Principles of medicinal chemistry*, ed 4, Baltimore, 1995, Williams & Wilkins.
11. France JT, Seddon RJ, Liggins GC: A study of a pregnancy with low estrogen production due to placental sulfatase deficiency, *J Clin Endocrinol Metab* 36:1, 1973.
12. Schindler AE, Siiteri PK: Isolation and quantitation of steroids from normal human amniotic fluids, *J Clin Endocrinol Metab* 28:1189, 1968.
13. Kundu N et al: Sequential determination of serum human placental lactogen, estriol, and esterol for assessment of fetal morbidity, *Obstet Gynecol* 52:513, 1978.
14. Notation AD, Tagatz GE: Unconjugated estriol and 15a-hydroxyestriol in complicated pregnancies, *Am J Obstet Gynecol* 128:747, 1977.
15. Burton PJ, Waddell BJ: Dual function of 11β-hydroxysteroid dehydrogenase in placenta: modulating placental glucocorticoid passage and local steroid action, *Biol Reprod* 60:234, 1999.
16. Miller WL: Steroid hormone biosynthesis and actions in the materno-feto-placental unit, *Clin Perinatol* 25:799, 1998.
17. Burrow GN, Fisher DA, Larsen PR: Mechanisms of disease: maternal and fetal thyroid function, *N Engl J Med* 331:1072, 1994.
18. Glinoer D et al: Regulation of maternal thyroid during pregnancy, *J Clin Endocrinol Metab* 71:276, 1990.
19. Lowe TW, Cunningham FG: Pregnancy and thyroid disease, *Clin Obstet Gynecol* 34:72, 1991.
20. Glinoer D, Delange F: The potential repercussions of maternal, fetal, and neonatal hypothyroxinemia on the progeny, *Thyroid* 10:871, 2000.
21. Klein RZ, Mitchell ML: Maternal hypothyroidism and child development. A review, *Horm Res* 52:55, 1999.
22. Koibuchi N, Chin WW: Thyroid hormone action and brain development, *Trends Endocrinol Metab* 11:123, 2000.
23. van Stiphout WAHJ, Hofman A, de Bruijn AM: Serum lipids in young women before, during, and after pregnancy, *Am J Epidemiol* 126:922, 1987.
24. Studd JW, Wood S: Serum and urinary proteins in pregnancy. In Wynn RM, editor: *Obstetrics and gynecology annual*, New York, 1976, Appleton-Century-Crofts.
25. Davison JM: The urinary system. In Hytten F, Chamberlain G, editors: *Clinical physiology in obstetrics*, Oxford, UK, 1980, Blackwell Scientific.
26. van Geuns HJ, van Kessel H: Creatinine in amniotic fluid and fetal renal function. In Fairweather DVI, Eskes TKAB, editors: *Amniotic fluid: research and clinical application*, ed 2, Amsterdam, 1978, Excerpta Medica.
27. Spillman T, Cotton DB: Current perspectives in the assessment of fetal pulmonary surfactant status with amniotic fluid, *CRC Rev Clin Lab Sci* 27:341, 1989.
28. Hallman M: Recycling surfactant: a review of human amniotic fluid as a source of surfactant for treatment of respiratory distress syndrome, *Rev Perinatal Med* 6:197, 1989.
29. Cochrane CG, Revak SD: Pulmonary surfactant protein B (SP-B): structure-function relationships, *Science* 254:566, 1991.
30. Martin RJ, Fanaroff AA, Skalina MEL: The respiratory system. In Fanaroff AA, Martin RJ, editors: *Behrman's neonatal/perinatal medicine*, St Louis, 1987, Mosby.
31. Reynolds MS, Wallander KA: Use of surfactant in the prevention and treatment of neonatal respiratory distress syndrome, *Clin Pharmacol* 8:559, 1989.
32. Gibson AT: Surfactant and the neonatal lung, *Br J Hosp Med* 58:381, 1997.
33. Kleihauer E: The hemoglobins. In Stave U, editor: *Perinatal physiology*, New York, 1978, Plenum.
34. Hecht F, Jones RT, Koler RD: Newborn infants with Hb Portland 1, an indicator of α-chain deficiency, *Ann Hum Genet* 31:215, 1967.
35. Lustbader JW, Lobel Land Wu H: Structural and molecular studies of human chorionic gonadotropin and its receptor, *Recent Prog Hormone Res* 53:395, 1998.
36. Kobata A, Takeuchi M: Structure, pathology and function of the N-linked sugar chains of human chorionic gonadotropin, *Biochim Biophys Rev* 1445:315, 1999.
37. Lehner R et al: Ectopic pregnancy, *Arch Gynecol Obstet* 263:87, 2000.
38. Weismiller DG: Preterm labor, *Am Fam Phys* 59:593, 1999.

39. Iams JD et al: The length of the cervix and the risk of spontaneous premature delivery, *N Engl J Med* 334:567, 1996.

40. Hartmann K et al: Cervical dimensions and risk of preterm birth: a prospective cohort study, *Obstet Gynecol* 93:504, 1999.

41. Roberts JM, Redman CRG: Pre-eclampsia: more than pregnancy-induced hypertension, *Lancet* 341:1447, 1993.

42. Redman CRG, Roberts JM: Management of pre-eclamsia, *Lancet* 341:1451, 1993.

43. Posner BI: Insulin metabolizing enzyme activities in human placental tissue, *Diabetes* 22:552, 1973.

44. Klopper A: Placental metabolism. In Hytten F, Chamberlain G, editors: *Clinical physiology in obstetrics*, Oxford, UK, 1991, Blackwell Scientific.

45. Carl J, Christensen M, Mathiesen O: Human placental lactogen (HPL) model for the normal pregnancy, *Placenta* 12:289, 1991.

46. Cotran RS, Kumar VK, Collins T, editors: *Robbins pathologic basis of disease*, Philadelphia, 1999, Saunders.

47. Rudolph A, editor: *Rudolph's pediatrics*, Englewood Cliffs, NJ, 1996, Appleton & Lange.

48. Dekowski SA, Holtzman RB: Surfactant replacement therapy: an update on applications, *Pediatr Clin North Am* 45:549, 1998.

49. Hudak ML et al: A multicenter randomized masked comparison trial of synthetic surfactant versus calf lung surfactant extract in the prevention of neonatal respiratory distress syndrome, *Pediatrics* 100:39, 1997.

50. Moya FR, Gross I: Combined hormonal therapy for the prevention of respiratory distress syndrome and its consequences, *Semin Perinatol* 17:267, 1993.

51. Robertson B: Corticosteroids and surfactant for prevention of neonatal RDS, *Ann Med* 25:285, 1993.

52. Taeusch HW, Ballard RA: *Avery's diseases of the newborn*, Baltimore, 1998, Williams & Wilkins.

53. Doyle JJ et al: Hematology. In Avery GB, Fletcher MA, MacDonald MG, editors: *Neonatology: physiology and management of the newborn*, Philadelphia, 1999, Lippincott Williams & Wilkins.

54. Liley AW: The administration of blood transfusions to the foetus *in utero*, *Triangle* 7:184, 1966.

55. Sundaram SG et al: Alpha-fetoprotein and screening markers of congenital disease, *Reprod Med* 12:481, 1992.

56. Merkatz IR et al: An association between low maternal serum alpha-fetoprotein and fetal chromosome abnormalities, *Am J Obstet Gynecol* 148:886, 1984.

57. Cheng EY et al: A prospective evaluation of a second trimester screening test for fetal Down syndrome using maternal serum alpha-fetoprotein, hCG, and unconjugated estriol, *Obstet Gynecol* 81:72, 1993.

58. Haddow JE et al: Prenatal screening for Down's syndrome with use of maternal serum markers, *N Engl J Med* 327:588, 1992.

59. Haddow JE et al: Second trimester screening for Down's syndrome using maternal serum dimeric inhibin A, *J Med Screen* 5:115, 1998.

60. Palomaki GE et al: Prospective intervention trial of a screening protocol to identify fetal trisomy 18 using maternal serum alpha-fetoprotein, unconjugated oestriol, and human chorionic gonadotropin, *Prenatal Diagn* 12:925, 1992.

61. Mancini G et al: hCG, AFP, and uE$_3$ patterns in the 14-20th weeks of Down syndrome pregnancies, *Prenatal Diagn* 12:619, 1992.

62. Tenore JL: Ectopic pregnancy, *Am Fam Physician* 61:1080, 2000.

63. ACOP practice bulletin. Medical management of tubal pregnancy, no 3, *Int J Gynaecol Obstet* 65:97, 1999.

64. Gracia CR, Barnhart KT: Diagnosing ectopic pregnancy: decision analysis comparing six strategies, *Obstet Gynecol* 97:464, 2001.

65. Shepperd RW et al: Serial beta hCG measurements in the early detection of ectopic pregnancy, *Obstet Gynecol* 75:417, 1999.

66. Buckley RG et al: Serum progesterone testing to predict ectopic pregnancy in symptomatic first-trimester patients, *Ann Emerg Med* 36:95, 1999.

67. Little B, Billar RB: Endocrine disorders. In Romney SL et al, editors: *Gynecology and obstetrics: the health care of women*, New York, 1980, McGraw-Hill.

68. Andersen HF: Use of fetal fibronectin in women at risk for preterm delivery, *Clin Obstet Gynecol* 43:746, 2000.

69. Goldenberg RL et al: The preterm prediction study: fetal fibronectin, bacterial vaginosis, and peripartum infection. NICHD Maternal Fetal Medicine Units Network, *Obstet Gynecol* 87:656, 1996.

70. Stetzer BP, Mercer BM: Antibiotics and preterm labor, *Clin Obstet Gynecol* 43:809, 2000.

71. Gluck L, Kulovich MV: Lecithin/sphingomyelin ratios in amniotic fluid in normal and abnormal pregnancies, *Am J Obstet Gynecol* 115:539, 1973.

72. Dubin SB: Assessment of fetal lung maturity by laboratory methods, *Clin Lab Med* 12:603, 1992.

73. Kulovich MV, Hallman MB, Gluck L: The lung profile I: normal pregnancy, *Am J Obstet Gynecol* 135:57, 1979.

74. Kulovich MV, Gluck L: The lung profile II: complicated pregnancy, *Am J Obstet Gynecol* 135:64, 1979.

75. Bent AE et al: Assessment of fetal lung maturity: relationship of gestational age and pregnancy complications to phosphatidylglycerol levels, *Am J Obstet Gynecol* 139:664, 1981.

76. Spillman T et al: Removal of a component interfering with phosphatidylglycerol estimation in the "Helena" system for amniotic fluid phospholipids, *Clin Chem* 30:737, 1984.

77. Dubin SB: The laboratory assessment of fetal lung maturity, *Am J Clin Pathol* 97:836, 1992.

78. Clements JS et al: Assessment of the risk of respiratory distress syndrome by a rapid test for surfactant in amniotic fluid, *N Eng J Med* 286:1077, 1972.

79. Sher G et al: Assessing fetal lung maturation by the foam stability index assay, *Obstet Gynecol* 52:673, 1978.

80. Russell JC: A calibrated fluorescence polarization assay for assessment of fetal lung maturity, *Clin Chem* 33:1177, 1987.

81. Herbert WNP, Chapman JF, Schnoor MM: Role of the TDx FLM assay in fetal lung maturity, *Am J Obstet Gynecol* 168:808, 1993.

82. Duck-Chong CG: Lamellar body phospholipid content of amniotic fluid: a possible index of fetal lung maturity, *Am J Obstet Gynecol* 136:191, 1979.

83. Dubin S: Determination of lamellar body size, number density and concentration by differential light scattering from amniotic fluid: physical significance of A$_{650}$, *Clin Chem* 34:938, 1988.

84. Dubin S: Characterization of amniotic fluid lamellar bodies by resistive-pulse counting: relationship to measures of fetal lung maturity, *Clin Chem* 35:612, 1989.

85. Garite TJ, Freeman RK, Nageotte MP: Fetal maturity cascade: a rapid and cost effective method for fetal maturity testing, *Obstet Gynecol* 67:619, 1986.

86. Herbert WNP, Chapman JF: Clinical and economic considerations associated with testing for fetal lung maturity, *Am J Obstet Gynecol* 155:820, 1986.

87. Liley AW: Amniocentesis and amniography in hemolytic disease. In Greenhill JP, editor: *Yearbook of obstetrics and gynecology, 1964-1965 series*, St Louis, 1964, Mosby.

88. Kaplan LA, Tange SM, editors: *Guidelines for the evaluation and management of the newborn infant*, Washington, DC, 1998, National Academy of Clinical Biochemistry.

89. American Academy of Pediatrics, Provisional Committee for Quality Improvement and Subcommittee on Hyperbilirubinemia: Practice parameter: management of hyperbilirubinemia in the healthy term newborn, *Pediatrics* 94:558, 1994.

90. Expert Committee on the Diagnosis and Classification of Diabetes Mellitus: Report of the Expert Committee on the Diagnosis and Classification of Diabetes Mellitus, *Diabetes Care* 20:1183, 1997.

91. Gewolb IH, Torday HS: High glucose inhibits maturation of the fetal lung in vitro. Morphometric analysis of lamellar bodies and fibroblast lipid inclusions, *Lab Investigation* 73:59, 1995.

92. Zapata A, Grande C, Hernandez-Garcia JM: Influence of metabolic control of pregnant diabetics on fetal lung maturity, *Scand J Clin Lab Invest* 54:431, 1994.

93. Javanovic L: Medical emergencies in the patient with diabetes during pregnancy, *Endocrinol Metab Clin North Am* 29:771, 2000.

94. Worth R: Glycosylated hemoglobin in normal pregnancy: a longitudinal study with two independent methods, *Diabetologia* 28:76, 1985.

95. Miller E: Elevated maternal hemoglobin A$_{1c}$ in early pregnancy and major congenital anomalies in infants of diabetic mothers, *N Eng J Med* 304:1331, 1981.

96. King D: New methods facilitating Down's syndrome screening, ADVANCE for Medical Laboratory Professionals, www.advanceforal.com.

97. McDowell G et al: Enhanced second trimester maternal serum screening for Down syndrome: addition of dimeric inhibin A, ADVANCE for Medical Laboratory Professionals, www.advanceforal.com.

Internet Sites

http://www.babycenter.com/pregnancy/fetaldevelopment/
http://www.pregnancy.about.com/cs/pregnancy/
http://www.dartmouth.edu/~obgyn/mfm/PatientEd/—Dartmouth-Hitchcock Medical Center, Division of Maternal Fetal Medicine, Patient Education
http://www.fpnotebook.com/—Family Practice Notebook
http://www.atlanta-mfm.com/clindisc/vol4no5.html—Atlanta Fetal-Medicine PC Clinical Discussion, volume 4, number 5, May 21, 1996

http://www.w-cpc.org/index.htm—Westside Pregnancy Resource Center
http://www.ibd.nrc.ca/english/s_clinical_fetal.htm—Institute for Biodiagnostics, National Research Council of Canada
http://www.docboard.org/me/rules/allch078.htm—Maine Board of Licensure in Medicine: Medical Board Rules 2. Procedure: Assessment of fetal maturity prior to repeat cesarean delivery or elective induction of labor
http://www.acog.org/—The American College of Obstetricians and Gynecologists. Type *diabetes* into the website's search engine

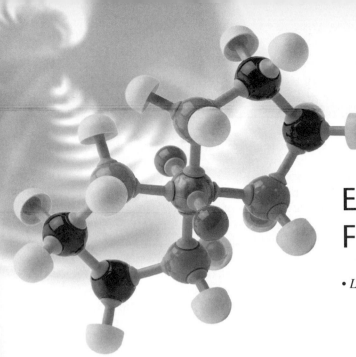

CHAPTER 41

Extravascular Biological Fluids

• *Lewis Glasser*

Chapter Outline

Serous fluids
Formation
Change of analyte in disease

Synovial fluid (synovia)
Normal synovial fluid
Change of analyte in disease

Objectives

- Define serous fluid and describe the formation of serous fluids.
- Differentiate transudate and exudate based on cause, mode of formation, and protein and enzyme levels.
- List analytes of serous fluids that may be markers of disease conditions.

- Define synovial fluid and describe a normal synovial fluid.
- Describe changes in synovial fluid in pathological conditions.

Key Terms

arthritis   Inflammation of a joint.

ascites   Pathological accumulation of serous fluid in the peritoneal cavity.

chyle   Fatty lymph fluid originating from the intestinal lymphatics. Chyle is milky white in appearance.

colloid osmotic pressure of plasma   The difference in osmotic pressure between plasma and interstitial fluid that drives water into the bloodstream from the interstitial spaces.

effusion   Pathological accumulation of fluid in a body cavity.

empyema   The presence of pus in a body cavity, usually the pleural cavity.

epicardium   The visceral layer of pericardium.

exudate   A fluid with a high concentration of protein that accumulates in a body cavity when capillary permeability is increased.

gout   An inflammatory arthritis of the joint secondary to crystallization of monosodium urate in the joint.

hemothorax   Blood in the pleural cavity secondary to rupture of the blood vessels.

hyaluronic acid   A high–molecular-weight polymer made up of repeating units of the disaccharide *N*-acetylglucosamine and glucuronic acid.

hydrostatic pressure   The lateral pressure of water within a vessel that tends to drive fluid out of the capillaries into the interstitial space.

joint   An articulation between bones.

neuroarthropathy   Disease of a joint secondary to a disease of the nervous system.

osmotic pressure   The force with which a solvent passes through a semipermeable membrane.

osteoarthritis   A degenerative form of arthritis that is primarily a disease of the bones with joint involvement.

osteochondromatosis   A joint disease characterized by the development of cartilaginous nodules in the synovial tissues.

paracentesis   Aspiration of fluid from a body space.

parapneumonic effusion   An accumulation of fluid in the pleural space secondary to pneumonia.

parietal membrane   The wall of a cavity.

pericardium   The sac enclosing the heart.

peritoneum   The serous membrane lining the abdominal cavity and the organs of the abdominal cavity.

permeable   Allowing the passage of fluid through a membrane.

pigmented villonodular synovitis   A disease of the joints of unknown cause characterized by fingerlike proliferative growths of the synovial tissue with hemosiderin deposition within the synovial tissue.

pleura   The serous membrane lining the inner surface of the thorax, the diaphragm, and the outer surface of the lungs.

pseudogout   An inflammatory arthritis of the joint secondary to crystals of calcium pyrophosphate.

psoriatic arthritis   A chronic destructive joint disease that occurs in some patients with the skin disease psoriasis.

Reiter's syndrome   A syndrome of unknown cause characterized by inflammation of the joints, urethra, and conjunctivae.

rheumatoid arthritis   A chronic progressive inflammatory disease of unknown cause involving multiple joints.

serous fluid   Fluid having the characteristics of serum.

synovial fluid   Joint fluid.

systemic lupus erythematosus (SLE)   A multisystem disease that is caused by an autoimmune reaction and involves mostly the skin, kidneys, joints, and serosal membranes.

thoracentesis   Removal of fluid from the pleural cavity.

transudate   Fluid with a low concentration of protein that has accumulated in a body cavity.

visceral membrane   The outer wall of an organ.

Methods on CD-ROM

Albumin
Alkaline phosphatase
Amylase
Creatinine
Glucose

Lactate dehydrogenase and lactate dehydrogenase enzymes
Osmolality
Total serum protein
Triglycerides
Urea

SEROUS FLUIDS

In this chapter the term **serous fluids** is restricted to pleural, pericardial, or peritoneal fluid. The word *serous* is derived from *serum* and accurately expresses the derivation of the body fluids from plasma. Body fluids are designated by a variety of medical terms. Pleural fluid (thoracic or chest fluid) is obtained by surgical puncture of the chest wall (**thoracentesis**). **Empyema** refers to pus in the pleural cavity. Peritoneal fluid is frequently designated by the non-anatomical term *ascitic fluid*. *Ascites* is derived from the Greek word *askos* (meaning "wineskin, belly") and describes the bloated abdomen of the patient afflicted with a massive accumulation of peritoneal fluid. **Paracentesis** is aspiration of fluid from a cavity, and *abdominal paracentesis fluid* is synonymous with *peritoneal fluid*. Whole blood in the body cavities is designated with the prefix *hemo-*, as in **hemothorax**. A *chylous effusion* refers to the accumulation of lymph (**chyle**) in the body cavity.

Formation

Normal formation. Each body cavity is lined by a thin serosal membrane. The lining of the body wall is the **parietal membrane**, and the outer lining of the organs is the **visceral membrane**. The two membranes, which together form the serosal membrane, are continuous, and the space between them is the body cavity (Fig. 41-1). The serosal membrane is composed of a thin layer of connective tissue containing numerous capillaries and lymphatics and a superficial layer of flattened mesothelial cells.

Serous fluid is an ultrafiltrate of plasma derived from the rich capillary network in the serosal membrane. Its formation is similar to the production of extravascular interstitial fluid anywhere in the body. Three factors are important: hydrostatic pressure, colloid osmotic pressure, and capillary **permeability**. **Hydrostatic pressure** drives fluid out of the capillaries and into the body cavities. Impermeable protein molecules in the plasma exert a force that counteracts the hydrostatic pressure and causes capillaries to absorb fluid. This force is called the **colloid osmotic pressure (COP)** and is proportional to the molar concentration of protein. Lymphatics also play an important role in the absorption of water, protein, and particulate matter from the extravascular space. In the thoracic (chest) cavity, fluid is formed at the parietal **pleura** because the high hydrostatic pressure of the

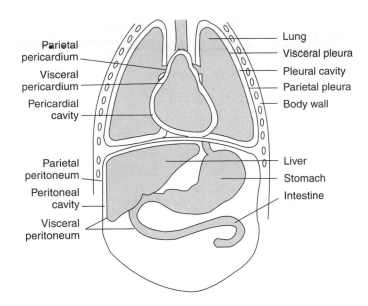

Fig. 41-1 Relationships of serous membranes, body cavities, and viscera. The heart is enclosed in the pericardial sac. The outer layer of pericardium is called *parietal pericardium.* Lining the exterior surface of the heart is visceral pericardium, which is also called *epicardium.* Parietal peritoneum lines the wall of the abdominal cavity. Visceral peritoneum invests stomach, liver, and intestines. The peritoneal cavity is the space between the two layers of peritoneum.

systemic circulation exceeds the colloid osmotic pressure, and fluid is reabsorbed at the visceral pleura, where capillary colloid osmotic pressure exceeds the low hydrostatic pressure of the pulmonary circulation (Fig. 41-2). Normally there is less than 15 mL of fluid in each pleural cavity, 10 to 50 mL in the pericardial sac, and less than 50 mL in the peritoneal cavity.[1]

Abnormal formation. Effusions will form when the normal physiological mechanisms responsible for the formation or absorption of serosal fluid are impaired. Thus, fluid will accumulate if capillary permeability increases,

hydrostatic pressure increases, colloid osmotic pressure decreases, or lymphatic drainage is obstructed. Hydrostatic pressure is increased in congestive heart failure, a frequent cause of effusions. Hypoproteinemia decreases the colloid osmotic pressure. A decreased plasma protein can be secondary to decreased synthesis or increased loss of protein. Albumin, synthesized in the liver, is the most important protein in the maintenance of colloid osmotic pressure. Diseases of the liver may impair albumin synthesis; the liver disease most frequently associated with hypoproteinemia and effusions is cirrhosis. Hypoalbuminemia is also caused

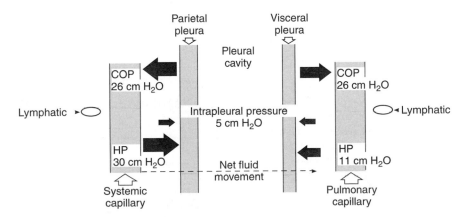

Fig. 41-2 Pleural fluid is formed at the parietal pleura because net forces for flow of fluid out of the systemic capillaries exceed net colloid osmotic pressures. Fluid moves toward the visceral pleura where net colloid osmotic pressure exceeds outward forces because of low hydrostatic pressure in pulmonary capillaries. Lymphatics play a role in absorption of water, protein, and particulate matter. *COP,* Colloid osmotic pressure; *HP,* hydrostatic pressure.

by an increased loss of serum protein, which occurs in the nephrotic syndrome. Capillary permeability increases if the pleural surfaces are inflamed. Increased capillary permeability also results in loss of protein from the vascular space, so the physical forces that lead to excess fluid formation are accentuated. Conditions causing an increase in capillary permeability include inflammatory diseases, infection, and metastatic tumors. If the lymphatics are obstructed, a protein-rich fluid will accumulate. Neoplasms of the lymph nodes frequently produce pleural effusions. The causes of effusions and the underlying pathogeneses are listed in Table 41-1.

Change of Analyte in Disease

Transudates and exudates. Serous effusions are designated as **transudates** or **exudates**, depending on the protein content of the fluid. The distinction is important because transudates are not caused by inflammations but by disturbances of hydrostatic or colloid osmotic pressure, whereas exudates are caused by increased capillary permeability secondary to diseases that directly involve inflammation of the surfaces of body cavities. Distinguishing between transudates and exudates involves the use of arbitrary medical decision levels that have been empirically determined. The higher the protein content, the more likely it is that the fluid is caused by a process that alters the capillary permeability and involves the surfaces of the body cavity. Measuring the specific gravity will indirectly measure the protein concentration. Pleural fluids are classified as exudates if the specific gravity is greater than 1.015 g/mL or the total protein is 30 g/L or greater. Measurement of total protein is preferable to measurement of specific gravity. The distinction between exudates and transudates in pleural fluids is even more precise if the fluid protein is compared with the serum total protein. A ratio is calculated by dividing the concentration of the protein in the fluid by the concentration of the protein in the serum; a ratio of 0.5 or greater is indicative of an exudate.[2] The distinction is further improved if a large protein molecule such as lactate dehydrogenase (LD) is used as a marker of capillary permeability. Pleural fluid-to-serum LD ratios of 0.6 or greater are diagnostic of exudates.[2] The differences between transudates and exudates in pleural effusions are summarized in Table 41-2. Different cutoff values are used for peritoneal fluid. Protein levels greater than 25 g/L classify the fluid as an exudate.[1] Use of the difference between the serum and peritoneal fluid albumin concentrations provides significantly better discrimination between transudative and exudative ascites than use of the total protein levels; differences less than 11 g/L correlate with malignant effusions.[3,4]

Glucose. Pleural fluid glucose concentrations are similar to plasma glucose levels in normal fluids and transudates. Glucose is decreased in exudates, such as those seen with bacterial infection, tuberculosis, neoplasia, and rheumatoid disease.[5,6] A pleural fluid glucose concentration less than 600 mg/L or a difference between the plasma and fluid glucose concentrations of more than 300 mg/L is clinically

---

TABLE 41-1 CAUSES OF EFFUSIONS

Cause	Finding	Pathogenesis
Transudates		
Congestive heart failure	↑ HP	Systemic and pulmonary venous hypertension
Hepatic cirrhosis	↑ HP	Portal and inferior vena cava hypertension
	↓ COP	Hypoalbuminemia
Nephrotic syndrome	↓ COP	Hypoalbuminemia
Exudates		
Pancreatitis	↑ CP	Inflammation secondary to chemical injury
Bile peritonitis	↑ CP	Inflammation secondary to chemical injury
Rheumatoid disease	↑ CP	Inflammation of serosa
Systemic lupus erythematosus	↑ CP	Inflammation of serosa
Infections (bacterial, tuberculosis, fungal, viral)	↑ CP	Inflammation secondary to microorganisms
Infarction (myocardial, pulmonary)	↑ CP	Inflammation secondary to extension of process to serosal surface
Neoplasms	↑ CP	Increased permeability of capillaries supplying tumor implants; pleuritis secondary to obstructive pneumonitis
	↓ LyD	Lymphatic obstruction secondary to lymph node infiltration
Chyle		
Trauma Surgery Neoplasms Idiopathic	↓ LyD	Disruption of lymphatic ducts

COP, *Colloid osmotic pressure;* CP, *capillary permeability;* HP, *hydrostatic pressure;* LyD, *lymphatic drainage.*

TABLE 41-2 DIAGNOSTIC CRITERIA OF TRANSUDATES AND EXUDATES IN PLEURAL FLUID

Test	Transudate	Exudate
Appearance	Clear	Cloudy
Fibrinogen	No clot	Clots
Specific gravity	<1.015	≥1.015
Total protein	<30 g/L	≥30 g/L
Total protein (fluid/serum)	<0.5	≥0.5
Lactate dehydrogenase (fluid/serum)	<0.6	≥0.6
Glucose	~ Serum	Often <600 mg/L

significant. Only low glucose levels are diagnostically useful, and the various diseases associated with low glucose levels are also associated with normal values. Any etiological diagnosis on the basis of a low glucose level alone is unreliable. Two mechanisms are operative in producing low values. One is increased glucose use, and the second is a relative block in the transport of glucose from the blood to the fluid. The latter occurs in rheumatoid effusions.[7] Interpretation of low glucose concentrations in peritoneal and pericardial fluid is similar to that in pleural fluid.

pH. Measurement of pleural fluid pH is clinically useful in the management of patients with **parapneumonic effusions**. Patients with pneumonia develop effusions because the infectious process extends to the visceral pleura, causing exudation of fluid into the pleural space. Complications of parapneumonic effusions include loculation and pus in the pleural cavity. Fluids are divided into potentially benign and complicated effusions on the basis of the pH. Fluids with a pH greater than 7.30 resolve spontaneously, whereas a pH less than 7.20 indicates a need for tube drainage.[8] A cautionary note: the specimen must be collected anaerobically in a heparinized syringe, stored on ice, and measured at 37° C. There is a significant relationship between pleural fluid pH and glucose concentration.[9]

Lipid. Chyle is a milky-white emulsion of fatty lymph fluid originating from the intestinal lymphatics. The accumulation of chyle in the pleural space is rare. Even less frequent is chyle accumulation in the peritoneal or pericardial cavities. Chylous fluid accumulates because of the disruption of the thoracic duct. Chylomicrons found on lipoprotein analysis are the best evidence for a chylous effusion. Triglyceride values above 1100 mg/L are highly suggestive of chylous effusion.[10] Cholesterol values do not distinguish between chylous and nonchylous effusions.

Analytes as markers for organs. Chemical substances can serve as markers for the specific organ involved in the pathogenesis of the effusion. The rationale for these tests is easily understood when one considers the anatomical location of the viscera and normal biochemistry (Fig. 41-3). Analytes that have been used as markers include amylase, pH, alkaline phosphatase, urea nitrogen, and creatinine. Pleural effusions accompany most cases of esophageal rupture. The perforation allows secretions from both the oral cavity and stomach to contaminate the effusion fluid. Pleural fluid amylase levels can be elevated, and the levels are higher than the serum amylase. Electrophoretic studies indicate that the amylase is from the saliva.[11] Another indicator of esophageal perforation is the pH of the pleural fluid. Normal gastric juice has a pH below 3.5. Leakage of gastric contents through the esophageal tear will acidify the pleural fluid.[12,13] A pH below 6.0 is clinically significant. The measurement may be performed at the bedside by use of pH reagent paper.

Amylase is a well-accepted marker of pancreatic disease. In acute pancreatitis, amylase-rich fluid seeps into the peripancreatic tissue and causes a chemical peritonitis, with the formation of small amounts of peritoneal fluid in most cases. One study reports fluid amylase levels of 27,800 ± 7560 U/L

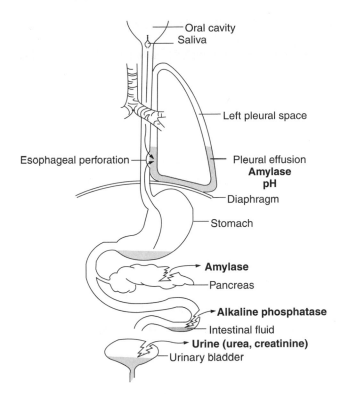

Fig. 41-3 Chemical determinations of body fluids as markers for specific organ involvement.

(15,030 ± 4086 Somogyi units/dL).[14] The fluid levels are higher and persist longer than the corresponding blood amylase levels.[15] Pancreatic ascites is the chronic accumulation of massive amounts of fluid in association with pancreatitis. It is not certain whether the fluid represents leakage of pancreatic secretions from ruptured ducts or exudation of fluid from the serosal surfaces secondary to chemical irritation.[16] In pancreatic ascites, peritoneal fluid amylase concentrations range from 680 to 129,500 U/L (370 to 70,000 Somogyi units/dL).[17] Pleural effusions are present in 15% of cases of pancreatitis. Increased amylase levels are caused by transdiaphragmatic lymphatic drainage or seepage of the enzyme across the diaphragm.[17] In a rare case pleural fluid is present because of a direct communication between the pleural and peritoneal cavities.[18]

Alkaline phosphatase has been shown to be a marker enzyme for pathological processes of the small intestine. The source of the enzyme can be leakage of alkaline phosphatase-rich fluid from the intestinal contents or extravasation from the wall of the intestine.[19] The enzyme is elevated in peritoneal serous effusions in association with intestinal perforation and infarctions of the small bowel and in peritoneal blood in patients with physically induced injuries of the small intestine.[20] The values are higher than corresponding peripheral blood levels.

Both urea nitrogen and creatinine are helpful in the differential diagnosis of a ruptured urinary bladder after abdominal trauma. Extravasated urine will have high levels of both urea nitrogen and creatinine. The former is freely diffusible and will also elevate the blood urea nitrogen; however, the **peritoneum** is relatively impermeable to creatinine, and blood levels of creatinine will not increase. In uncomplicated serous effusions, the fluid urea nitrogen and creatinine are low. If the physician inadvertently aspirates urine from the bladder, both urea nitrogen and creatinine will be high, but their concentrations in the blood will be within the reference interval.

SYNOVIAL FLUID (SYNOVIA)

Joints are articulations between bones. Freely movable joints are composed of hyaline articular cartilage and a fibrous capsule lined on its inner surface by a membrane (Fig. 41-4). **Synovial fluid** fills the joint cavity and acts as a lubricant, keeping to a minimum the friction between bones during movement or weight bearing. The fluid also provides the sole nutrition for cartilage. Synovial fluid enters the cartilage by diffusion and by a spongelike effect when the cartilage is compressed and relaxed. The term *synovia*, coined by Paracelsus, is derived from the Greek *syn* ("with"), along with *oon* (from the Latin *ovum*, meaning "egg") and *-ia* (probably "condition"), suggesting the fluid's resemblance to raw egg white.

Synovial fluid is a dialysate of plasma mixed with **hyaluronic acid**. Ultrafiltration in the rich vascular network in the synovial tissue produces this fluid, whereas hyaluronic acid, a mucoprotein, is secreted into the dialysate by synovial cells.

Normal Synovial Fluid

The fluid volume in the normal joint depends on the size of the structure. The knee joint usually contains 0.1 to 3.5 mL of fluid.[21] Normal synovial fluid is rarely obtained; if it is obtained, the fluid is clear or pale yellow with a specific gravity close to that of plasma. The viscosity is high relative to that of water because of the protein-polysaccharide complex, hyaluronic acid, which constitutes 99% of the mucoproteins present in the fluid. Hyaluronic acid, a long-chain, high–molecular-weight polymer made up of repeating units of acetylglucosamine and glucuronic acid, is destroyed in inflammatory states by hyaluronidase, an enzyme contained in the neutrophils. When this occurs, the fluid viscosity decreases significantly, giving the clinician a bedside test for the presence of inflammatory fluid.

Synovial protein concentrations are related to the molecular weight of each protein because of the dialytic effect in the synovia. Thus, albumin is present in relatively higher concentrations than are the higher–molecular-weight globulins. Fibrinogen is not present because of its high molecular weight, so normal synovia does not coagulate. Glucose and uric acid diffuse freely into the synovia and in the fasting state are as concentrated in synovia as in plasma.

The characteristics of normal synovia are summarized in Table 41-3.[22-25]

Change of Analyte in Disease

Physical and chemical changes that occur in the synovia during disease reflect basic pathological processes occurring in the joint. A pathological classification of synovial fluids and the diseases associated with each category are summarized in Table 41-4. The laboratory tests discussed in this section include viscosity, fibrinogen, total protein, complement, glucose, and uric acid.

Clinically there is no need for a sophisticated measurement of viscosity. Instead, it may be measured at the time of

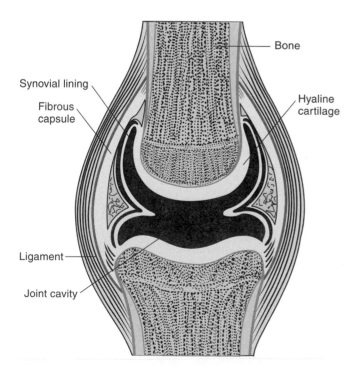

Fig. 41-4 Diagram of normal synovial joint. *(From Beck EW: Mosby's atlas of functional human anatomy, St Louis, 1982, Mosby. Courtesy Ernest Beck.)*

Labels: Bone; Synovial lining; Fibrous capsule; Hyaline cartilage; Ligament; Joint cavity

TABLE 41-3 PHYSICAL AND CHEMICAL CHARACTERISTICS OF NORMAL SYNOVIA

	Mean	Range
Volume (mL)*	1.1	0.13 to 3.5
Relative viscosity at 38° C	235	5.7 to 1160
Hyaluronic acid (g/L)	3600	1700 to 4050
Total protein (g/L)	17.2	10.7 to 21.3
Immunoglobulins (mg/L)		
IgG	4530	330 to 8500
IgA	740	270 to 1770
IgM	370	0 to 840
Fibrinogen (mg/L)	0	0
Complement (CH_{50} U/mL)	20†	16 to 25
Glucose (mg/L)	‡	650 to 1200
Uric acid (mg/L)	‡	25 to 72

* Knee.
†Values are approximately 10% of plasma values.
‡Fasting values are similar to plasma values.

TABLE 41-4 PATHOLOGICAL CLASSIFICATION OF SYNOVIAL FLUIDS

Test	Noninflammatory	Inflammatory	Septic	Hemorrhagic
Volume (mL)	>3.5	>3.5	>3.5	>3.5
Color	Yellow	Yellow-white	Yellow-green	Red-brown
Viscosity	High	Low	Low	Low
Leukocytes (cells/μL)	200 to 2000	2000 to 100,000	10,000 to >100,000	>500
Neutrophils (%)	<25	>50	>75	>25
Glucose (mg/L)	~ Serum	>250 mg/L lower than serum	>250 mg/L lower than serum	~ Serum
Culture	Negative	Negative	Positive	Negative
Diseases	Osteoarthritis	Gout	Bacterial infection	Hemophilia
	Osteochondritis dissecans	Pseudogout	Fungal infection	Trauma
	Osteochondromatosis	Psoriatic arthritis	Tuberculous infection	Pigmented villonodular synovitis
	Traumatic arthritis	Reiter's syndrome		
	Neuroarthropathy	Rheumatoid arthritis		
		Systemic lupus erythematosus		

aspiration by placing a finger at the tip of the syringe and stringing out the fluid. Noninflammatory fluids will "string out" longer than 4 cm. An alternative method is to drip fluid off the needle and syringe and observe it. Generally, if the fluid strings, it is a noninflammatory fluid; if it drips similar to water, the fluid is the result of inflammation. The depolymerization of the hyaluronic acid by neutrophil hyaluronidase decreases the viscosity in inflammatory disease.

The mucin clot test (Ropes's test) is seldom advocated but is frequently described in the literature. This test reflects the degree of hyaluronate polymerization and is performed by dropping fluid into a dilute acid solution and determining the quality of the clot. Although the test is often mentioned without critical comment in discussions of synovia, the quality of the information obtained by use of this test is inferior to that obtained by use of other procedures, and therefore the test should be considered obsolete.

Normal synovia contains no fibrinogen, but because inflammatory synovitis permits the passage of high–molecular-weight proteins into the fluid, fibrinogen can be present and spontaneous clotting can occur. Thus anticoagulants are necessary when specimens are collected for microscopic and bacteriological examination.

In synovia, unlike in serous fluids, total protein concentration is not used to distinguish noninflammatory from inflammatory fluids because the leukocyte count is used to make that distinction. Thus, total protein is not included in the routine examination of synovial fluids; however, its measurement can be helpful in interpreting complement levels.[26] Complement proteins are usually present at lower concentrations in synovial fluid than in serum. In systemic inflammatory conditions, complement behaves as an acute-phase reactant, and there is hypercomplementemia. In some conditions, such as Reiter's disease, the joint fluid complement concentration has been reported to be even higher than that of the serum.

In systemic immune complex diseases such as **systemic lupus erythematosus (SLE)**, complement is consumed widely and can be low in both the serum and synovial fluid.

In other diseases, such as **rheumatoid arthritis** and viral synovitis, complement is consumed locally in the synovia whereas serum levels are usually normal or high.

Measurement of C_3 and C_4 by precipitation methods is preferable to measuring CH_{50}, which will be falsely low if the fluid sits out at room temperature. A decreased C_4 level is suggestive of a classical pathway activation by immune complexes and is more sensitive than C_3 or CH_{50}. C_3 and CH_{50} are low in both classical and alternative pathway activation of complement and are suggestive of more profound systemic activity. The proper approach to interpreting complement levels in synovia is controversial. For practical purposes compare synovia and serum complement levels and consider synovia complement low if it is less than 30% of serum levels. However, in SLE and other severe immune complex diseases both levels may be low. In such a situation one can compare the synovia and serum complement levels with total protein in each fluid.

Interpretation of synovial glucose levels requires knowledge of the patient's simultaneous serum glucose. This is best done in the fasting state, but such preparation is not always clinically feasible. In the ideal situation after an 8-hour fast, the difference between serum and synovia is less than 100 mg/L; levels 250 mg/L or more below the serum level are suggestive of inflammation, and differences greater than 400 mg/L are suggestive of sepsis. In the nonfasting state, synovial glucose levels less than half of serum levels should definitely arouse suspicion of a septic process. Rarely, such findings are noted in rheumatoid arthritis effusions. Lactic acid and succinic acid have been advocated for use in the diagnosis of septic arthritis; however, these tests have not gained general acceptance.[27]

Serum uric acid levels are important in the diagnosis of **gout**. The synovial fluid uric acid concentration is similar to that of serum, and measurement of uric acid in synovial fluid is of no diagnostic value[28]; however, formation of monosodium urate crystals and their identification by polarized light microscopy in synovia is central to the diagnosis of gouty arthritis.

References

1. Krieg AF, Kjeldsberg CR: Cerebrospinal fluid and other body fluids. In Henry JB, editor: *Clinical diagnosis and management by laboratory methods*, Philadelphia, 1991, Saunders.
2. Light RW et al: Pleural effusions: the diagnostic separation of transudates and exudates, *Ann Intern Med* 77:507, 1972.
3. Pare P, Talbot J, Hoefs JC: Serum-ascites albumin concentration gradient: a physiologic approach to the differential diagnosis of ascites, *Gastroenterology* 85:240, 1983.
4. Rector WG, Jr, Reynolds TB: Superiority of the serum-ascites albumin difference over the ascites total protein concentration in the separation of "transudative" and "exudative" ascites, *Am J Med* 77:83, 1984.
5. Light RW, Ball WC, Jr: Glucose and amylase in pleural effusions, *JAMA* 225:257, 1973.
6. Carr DT, Mayne JG: Pleurisy with effusion in rheumatoid arthritis, with reference to the low concentration of glucose in pleural fluid, *Am Rev Respir Dis* 85:345, 1962.
7. Dodson WH, Hollingsworth JW: Pleural effusion in rheumatoid arthritis: impaired transport of glucose, *N Engl J Med* 275:1337, 1966.
8. Sokolowski JW, Jr, et al: Guidelines for thoracentesis and needle biopsy of the pleura, *Am Rev Resp Dis* 140:257, 1989.
9. Sahn SA, Good JT: Pleural fluid pH in malignant effusions, *Ann Intern Med* 108:345, 1988.
10. Staats BA et al: The lipoprotein profile of chylous and nonchylous pleural effusions, *Mayo Clin Proc* 55:700, 1980.
11. Sherr HP et al: Origin of pleural fluid amylase in esophageal rupture, *Ann Intern Med* 76:985, 1972.
12. Dye RA, Lafaret EG: Esophageal rupture: diagnosis by pleural fluid pH, *Chest* 66:454, 1974.
13. Abbott OA, Mansor KA, Logan WD: Atraumatic so-called spontaneous rupture of the esophagus, *J Thorac Cardiovasc Surg* 59:67, 1970.
14. Geokas MC et al: Studies on the ascites and pleural effusion in acute pancreatitis, *Gastroenterology* 58:950, 1970.
15. Keith LM, Zollinger RM, McCleery RS: Peritoneal fluid amylase determinations as an aid in diagnosis of acute pancreatitis, *Arch Surg* 61:930, 1950.
16. Donowitz M, Kerstein MD, Spiro HM: Pancreatic ascites, *Medicine* 53:183, 1974.
17. Salt WB, Schenker S: Amylase—its clinical significance: a review of the literature, *Medicine* 55:269, 1976.
18. Goldman M, Goldman G, Fleischner FG: Pleural fluid amylase in acute pancreatitis, *N Engl J Med* 266:715, 1962.
19. Lee YN: Alkaline phosphatase in intestinal perforation, *JAMA* 208:361, 1969.
20. Delany HM, Moss CM, Carnevale N: The use of enzyme analysis of peritoneal blood in the clinical assessment of abdominal organ injury, *Surg Gynecol Obstet* 42:161, 1976.
21. Ropes MW, Rossmeisl EC, Bauer W: The origin and nature of normal human synovial fluid, *J Clin Invest* 19:795, 1940.
22. Shmerling RH et al: Synovial fluid tests: what should be ordered? *JAMA* 264:1009, 1990.
23. Shmerling RH: Synovial fluid analysis: a critical reappraisal, *Rheum Dis Clin North Am* 20:503, 1994.
24. Pekin TJ, Zvaifler NJ: Hemolytic complement in synovial fluid, *J Clin Invest* 43:1372, 1964.
25. Pruzanski W et al: Serum and synovial fluid proteins in rheumatoid arthritis and degenerative joint diseases, *Am J Med Sci* 265:483, 1973.
26. McCarty DJ: Synovial fluid. In McCarty DJ, Koopman WJ, editors: *Arthritis and allied conditions, a textbook of rheumatology*, ed 14, Philadelphia, 2001, Lea & Febiger.
27. Borenstein DG, Gibbs CA, Jacobs RP: Gas-liquid chromatographic analysis of synovial fluid: succinic acid and lactic acid as markers of septic arthritis, *Arthritis Rheum* 25:947, 1982.
28. Baker DG: Chemistry, serology, and immunology. In Gatter RA, Schumacher HR: *A practical handbook of joint fluid analysis*, ed 2, Philadelphia, 1991, Lea & Febiger.

Internet Sites

www.arthritis.org—Arthritis Foundation

www.niams.nih.gov/—National Institute of Arthritis and Musculoskeletal and Skin Diseases

www.arthritis-research.com—Arthritis Research

www.vh.org/Providers/TeachingFiles/PulmonaryCoreCurric/PleuralEffusion/PleuralEffusion.html—Virtual Hospital: Adult Pulmonary Core Curriculum: Pleural Effusions and Chemical Pleurodesis

www.aafp.org/afp/20000415/2391.html—American Academy of Family Physicians: Knee Effusions: A Systematic Approach to Diagnosis

http://medicine.creighton.edu/forpatients/pleuraleff/pleuraleff.html—Creighton University School of Medicine: Pleural Effusions

www.postgradmed.com/issues/1999/05_01_99/rubins.htm—Postgraduate Medicine: Evaluating Pleural Effusions

www.uwcme.org/courses/rheumatology/rheumlab/synovial.html—University of Washington School of Medicine: Synovial Fluid Analysis

www.nlm.nih.gov/medlineplus/ency/article/003629.htm—National Library of Medicine: Synovial Fluid Analysis

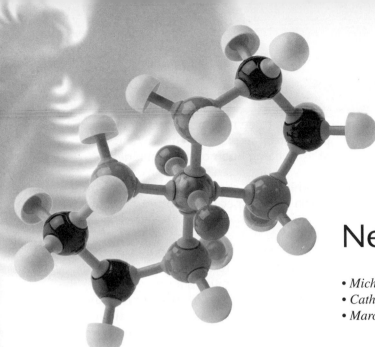

CHAPTER 42

Nervous System

- *Michael D. Privitera*
- *Cathy Cao*
- *Marcia Kaplan*

Chapter Outline

Objectives

- Define the blood-brain barrier and its physiological function.
- Describe the function and composition of cerebrospinal fluid (CSF) and list the major changes to CSF that are seen in disease states.
- List the major neurotransmitters and define their function.
- List the major causes of coma or altered mental status.

Key Terms

affective disorder   A disorder of mood regulation manifested clinically by episodes or sustained periods of depression or mania or both.

antiepileptic drugs   Medications given therapeutically to prevent seizures of various types. Many of these drugs are used widely for various nervous system disorders like pain, headache, or bipolar disorder.

antipsychotic drugs   Drugs that are used for the reversal or attenuation of psychotic symptoms (hallucinations, delusions, and disorders of cognition).

anxiety disorders   Chronic disorder characterized by inappropriate, pervasive, continuous, or paroxysmal feelings of worries or fear.

bipolar affective disorder   Affective disorder in which episodes of depression and mania are episodically present in the same patient.

blood-brain barrier   The barrier between the brain and the blood that allows the brain to maintain a cerebrospinal fluid composition different from that of blood.

cerebrospinal fluid (CSF)   Clear, colorless fluid contained within the four ventricles of the brain, the subarachnoid space, and the spinal cord.

coma   A state of unconsciousness from which patients cannot be aroused, even by the strongest stimuli.

depression   A mood disturbance often described as being sad, blue, hopeless, low, "down in the dumps," or irritable, accompanied by pervasive loss of interest or pleasure in almost all usual activities or pastimes.

epilepsy   A disorder characterized by a tendency to have seizures.

IgG index   The ratio (CSF IgG × Serum albumin)/ (Serum IgG × CSF albumin) used as an indicator of the source of elevated cerebrospinal fluid protein.

mania   A periodic disturbance of mood in which the mood is elevated, expansive, or irritable, accompanied by hyperactivity, pressure of speech, flight of ideas, inflated self-esteem, and decreased need for sleep.

meninges   The three membranes covering the brain and spinal cord: the dura, arachnoid, and pia.

meningitis   Inflammation of the meninges, often caused by viral or bacterial infections.

neurotransmitter   A chemical substance released by one neuron onto a specific receptor on an adjacent cell that alters the physiological functioning of the cell.

receptor   A protein complex embedded in the cell membrane that binds to a particular neurotransmitter and initiates a series of events that alter the membrane's physiological functioning.

reuptake   A process by which neurons conserve their own neurotransmitter by recovering it from the synaptic cleft for storage and subsequent rerelease.

schizophrenia   A chronic psychotic illness with delusions, hallucinations, and disorders of cognition that has lasted more than 6 months and from which full recovery is not expected.

seizure   A sudden and transient disturbance of mental function or body movements that results from an excessive electrical discharge of a group of brain cells.

stroke   Sudden onset of symptoms caused by acute ischemia in the brain resulting from hemorrhage, embolism, or thrombosis, and evidenced by loss of neurological functions.

subarachnoid space   The space between the arachnoid and pia membranes.

synapse   The structural junction of two neurons where chemical messages are carried from the presynaptic neuron to the postsynaptic receptor by neurotransmitters.

unipolar affective disease   Affective disorder in which episodes of depression alone occur without episodes of mania.

ventricles   Four cavities within the brain filled with cerebrospinal fluid and lined by the pia and the choroid plexus.

xanthochromia   A yellow coloring of the cerebrospinal fluid caused by the presence of breakdown products of hemoglobin.

Methods on CD-ROM

Barbiturates
CSF proteins
Drug screen
Glucose
Lithium

Serum protein electrophoresis
T_3 uptake
Thyroxine
Tricyclic antidepressants
TSH

BASIC NEUROANATOMY

The central nervous system (CNS) consists of the brain and spinal cord. The brain includes the two cerebral hemispheres, which are roughly mirror images of one another; the brainstem, a narrow structure through which all the pathways entering and leaving the two hemispheres must pass and that contains the centers that control breathing, heart rate, eye movements, and many other critical functions; and the cerebellum, a rounded structure about the size of a baseball that helps control movement and balance (Fig. 42-1). The lower brainstem flows into the spinal cord. The spinal cord is the point of exit for nerves on their way out to the muscles they control and the point of entry for sensory fibers returning from the body's sensory organs. All the nerves outside the CNS are collectively called the *peripheral nervous system*.

The two cerebral hemispheres are built around a connecting system of hollow spaces called the *ventricular system*. The **ventricles** are filled with **cerebrospinal fluid (CSF)** (Fig. 42-2).

The brain and spinal cord are both covered by a double membrane called the **meninges** (Fig. 42-3). Its inner membrane, the *arachnoid*, lies next to the outermost covering of the brain and spinal cord, the *dura*. The dura is a tough, nonelastic membrane that essentially wraps the brain and spinal cord in a nondistensible sac. The brain, blood, and CSF are thus sealed within a space the volume of which is fixed. The space between the pia and the arachnoid is called the **subarachnoid space** and communicates directly with the ventricular system.

PHYSIOLOGY AND BIOCHEMISTRY
Formation of Cerebrospinal Fluid

The ventricular system and the subarachnoid space are filled with CSF. The total volume of CSF in adults is about 150 mL. CSF is constantly produced and reabsorbed at a rate of approximately 500 mL/day (0.35 mL/min). This means the total amount of CSF is replaced every 6 to 8 hours.

CSF is produced in the ventricles by a specialized sponge-like structure called the *choroid plexus*. Beginning in the lateral ventricles, where it is formed, CSF circulates into the third ventricle and then into the fourth ventricle. It leaves the fourth ventricle by three small openings, or foramina, to circulate through the intracranial and spinal subarachnoid spaces. Circulation may be blocked in any of the ventricles or at the foramina between them, leading to an *obstructive hydrocephalus* (accumulation of fluid in the brain).

New CSF is constantly produced and is absorbed at the arachnoid villi and granulations to keep volume constant. These arachnoid villi and granulations are scattered along the entire inner table of the skull and down the spinal canal to the points at which the spinal nerves exit the dura. Thus CSF reabsorption can occur along the entire neuraxis. If absorption is impaired (as after meningeal inflammation, bacterial meningitis, or subarachnoid hemorrhage), CNS pressure and CSF volume both rise; this is called a *communicating hydrocephalus*.

Factors that determine the rate at which CSF is formed and absorbed are complex and not completely understood. Any increase in the size of one component (i.e., brain, CSF, or blood) leads to a sharp increase in pressure within the system unless there is a corresponding decrease in the volume of one of the other two components. With increased CSF pressure

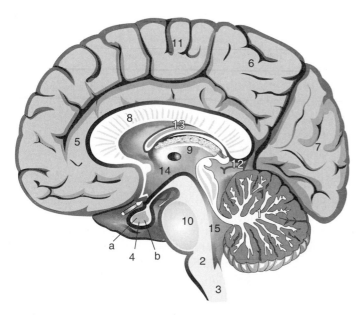

Fig. 42-1 Scheme of functional or motor-control areas of brain (right hemisphere, medial view). *1*, Cerebellum; *2*, medulla oblongata; *3*, spinal cord; *4*, pituitary gland: *a*, anterior lobe, *b*, posterior lobe; *5*, frontal lobe; *6*, parietal lobe; *7*, occipital lobe; *8*, corpus callosum; *9*, thalamus; *10*, pons; *11*, cerebrum; *12*, pineal body; *13*, fornix; *14*, third ventricle; *15*, fourth ventricle. (*From Beck EW: Mosby's atlas of functional human anatomy, St Louis, 1982, Mosby. Courtesy Ernest Beck.*)

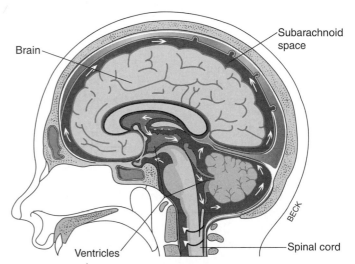

Fig. 42-2 Scheme of brain showing relationships of ventricles and subarachnoid space with rest of brain. (*From Beck EW: Mosby's atlas of functional human anatomy, St Louis, 1982, Mosby. Courtesy Ernest Beck.*)

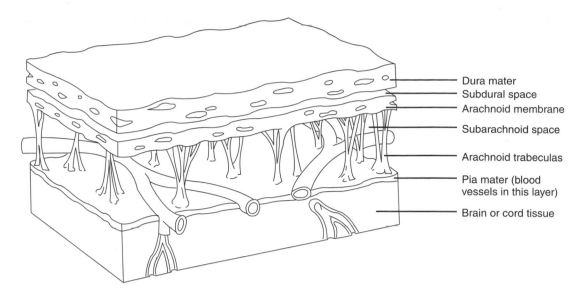

Fig. 42-3   Scheme of meninges. Arrangement may be compared with an underground parking garage. Dura and arachnoid form roof with pia membrane as floor. CSF flows in subarachnoid space. *(From Prezbindowski KS:* Guide to learning anatomy and physiology, *St Louis, 1982, Mosby.)*

the brain may suffer from direct effects of the abnormally high pressure or from having its blood flow decreased.

Blood-Brain Barrier

The term **blood-brain barrier** refers to a physiological barrier separating the brain and CSF from substances borne in the blood. The blood-brain barrier allows brain and CSF composition to be maintained at levels quite different from those of blood with respect to proteins, ions, and other molecular elements. The blood-brain barrier is extremely important in clinical practice. It determines the access of antibiotics to the brain and meninges and contributes to the exquisite control exercised over the brain's chemical milieu despite simultaneous changes occurring in the peripheral blood.

The extracellular fluid (ECF) compartment of the brain is in relatively free communication with the CSF, whereas a barrier exists between capillary blood and the ECF compartment–CSF combination.

Factors that significantly influence the access of substances to brain and CSF include molecular weight, protein binding, and lipid solubility. With molecular weight, entry is inversely related to size, hence the 1:200 CSF-to-plasma ratio of albumin (molecular weight, 69,000 D). Drugs that are highly protein bound enter the CSF much less readily than unbound smaller molecular weight substances. For example, phenytoin is 90% protein bound and 10% free in blood. Only 10% of the total measured blood phenytoin level is easily able to enter the CNS, and only that 10% is "active." Calcium, magnesium, and metabolites such as bilirubin are also highly protein bound and thus relatively restricted from CSF. Highly lipid-soluble substances such as carbon monoxide, neuroactive drugs, and alcohol readily enter

the CNS. Substances that are highly ionized at physiological pH are relatively excluded. Highly polar substances, such as some amino acids, enter slowly and require an active-transport mechanism.

The blood-brain barrier is readily permeable to water but not to electrolytes. The major cations, sodium and potassium, require hours to reach equilibrium with CSF after changes in peripheral blood. Changes in blood osmolality are followed by parallel CSF changes after a lag time of a few hours.

In the case of drugs, their pK_a, or *ionic dissociation constant*, is important in determining how readily they cross the blood-brain barrier. pK_a refers to the pH at which 50% of a compound is ionized. A nonionized drug is relatively lipid soluble and so more freely enters the CNS. The polar-ionized fraction is relatively excluded.

Finally, the characteristics of the blood-brain barrier can be dramatically altered by disease states. Penicillin, an acidic substance, is normally excluded from the CNS after parenteral injection, and yet it is an effective agent for treating **meningitis**. The reason is that meningeal inflammation alters (damages) the blood-brain barrier, allowing greater access of drugs, such as penicillin, that normally would not reach infected tissue.

Some specific factors that alter permeability of the blood-brain barrier are as follows:

1. Inflammation can increase the ease of entry into the nervous system of macromolecules such as albumin and penicillin.
2. Neovascularity, in association, for example, with tumor, trauma, or ischemia, alters the blood-brain barrier. This may be caused by defects in the new vessels or by their immaturity.

3. Toxins can change blood-brain barrier characteristics, and some agents used in radiographic studies increase the permeability of the barrier by direct toxic effects. When they are injected in hyperosmolar concentrations, the effect is greater.
4. Finally, the blood-brain barrier of the immature nervous system is more permeable to a variety of substances. For infants younger than 6 months of age, CSF protein concentration is normally as high as 1000 mg/L.

Functions of Cerebrospinal Fluid

Why should the brain be suspended in and bathed by this distinctive fluid? First, CSF provides mechanical support to the brain. Second, CSF probably functions to help remove metabolic products from the brain, a function that is poorly understood but probably important in both healthy and diseased states. Third, there is some evidence that CSF transports biologically active compounds that may function as chemical messengers. Finally, it plays an important role in maintaining the chemical environment of the brain. Although its communication with the plasma compartment is tightly regulated, CSF seems to be in relatively free communication with the brain's extracellular fluid compartment, which aids brain cells themselves. The following section examines the composition of CSF more closely.

Composition of Cerebrospinal Fluid

The ionic and molecular composition of CSF differs from that of plasma for some components and is the same for others (see box). Changes in serum sodium are followed by corresponding changes in CSF sodium so that after a lag time of about 1 hour sodium values are nearly the same. However, CSF potassium is lower than plasma potassium, and furthermore potassium is maintained within a very narrow concentration range in CSF despite wide fluctuations in plasma values. Active transport in and out of the CSF space appears to be largely responsible for maintaining these differences. Chloride and magnesium are somewhat higher in CSF than in plasma, and bicarbonate is somewhat lower.

CSF glucose normally ranges from 450 to 800 mg/L (2.5 to 4.44 mmol/L), that is, between 60% and 80% of the blood glucose concentration after equilibration. Blood and CSF glucose equilibrate only after a lag period of about 4 hours, and so CSF glucose at any given time reflects blood glucose levels during the past 4 hours. When a lumbar spinal puncture (LP) is performed and CSF glucose is to be determined, a simultaneous sample of peripheral blood must also be drawn. CSF glucose is altered by certain disease processes, as is discussed later. Equilibrated CSF glucose is definitely abnormal when it is less than 40% of the simultaneous blood glucose value; values less than 400 to 450 mg/L are almost always abnormal.

The expected percentage of CSF glucose to blood glucose (60% to 80%) falls as blood glucose rises. That is, a CSF-to-blood ratio of 0.5 is expected when blood glucose values reach 5000 mg/L and a ratio of 0.4 if blood glucose level reaches 7000 mg/L.

Proteins found in the CSF ordinarily originate from serum and reach the CSF space by pinocytosis across the capillary endothelium. The normal ratio of serum to CSF protein is 200:1 (with serum equal to 70 g/L and CSF equal to 350 mg/L).

CHARACTERISTICS OF NORMAL SPINAL FLUID

Total volume: 150 mL
Color: Colorless, like water
Transparency: Clear, like water
Osmolarity at 37° C: 281 mOsm/L
Specific gravity: 1.006 to 1.008
Acid-base balance:

pH	7.31
Pco_2	47.9 mm Hg
HCO_3^-	22.9 mEq/L

Sodium: 138 to 150 mEq/L
Potassium: 2.7 to 3.9 mEq/L
Chloride: 116 to 127 mEq/L
Calcium: 2.0 to 2.5 mEq/L (40 to 50 mg/L)
Magnesium: 2.0 to 2.5 mEq/L (24.4 to 30.5 mg/L)
Lactic acid: 1.1 to 2.8 mmol/L
Lactate dehydrogenase: Absolute activity depends on method; approximately 10% of serum value
Glucose: 450 to 800 mg/L
Proteins: 200 to 400 mg/L
   At different levels of spinal tap:

Lumbar	200 to 400 mg/L
Cisternal	150 to 250 mg/L
Ventricular	150 to 100 mg/L

Normal values in children:

Up to 6 days of age	700 mg/L
Up to 4 years of age	244 mg/L

Electrophoretic separation of spinal fluid proteins (% of total protein concentration):

Prealbumin	2% to 7%
Albumin	56% to 76%
α_1-globulin	2% to 7%
α_2-globulin	3.5% to 12%
β- and γ-globulin	8% to 18%
γ-globulin	7% to 12%
IgG	10 to 40 mg/L
IgA	0 to 0.2 mg/L
IgM	0 to 0.6 mg/L
κ/λ ratio	1

Erythrocyte count:

Newborn	0 to 675/mm^3
Adult	0 to 10/mm^3

Leukocyte count:

<1 year of age	0 to 30/mm^3
1 to 4 years of age	0 to 20/mm^3
5 years of age to puberty	0 to 10/mm^3
Adult	0 to 5/mm^3

Brain Metabolism

The brain's metabolic rate is one of the highest of any of the body's organs, whether the body is awake or asleep. But unlike most other organs, which store and reserve some supplies of energy to sustain themselves, the brain has almost no energy reserve. It depends entirely on an uninterrupted supply of glucose and oxygen delivered by peripheral blood. The brain uses glucose almost exclusively to supply its energy needs (see Chapter 32). To get an idea of just how hungry the brain is and how dependent it is on a constant, swift flow of blood, consider that under resting conditions total cerebral blood flow equals 15% to 20% of cardiac output (or about 500 mL per 100 g of brain per minute). Although *total* cerebral blood flow remains remarkably constant, discrete areas within the brain show striking variability; gray matter receives three to four times the blood flow compared to white matter. Moreover, *regional* blood flow is known to vary during performance of certain tasks, with regional flow increasing in the appropriate areas during tasks such as hand movement, speaking, or mental problem solving. Blood flow is also altered in response to disease states, as in **stroke**.

Neurotransmitter Systems

Neurons (nerve cells) within the CNS process information arriving from multiple internal and external sources. To maintain physiological and psychobiological homeostasis, CNS neurons communicate both with one another and eventually with effectors outside the CNS by means of **neurotransmitters** released by each neuron on to specific **receptors**. Neurons are characterized by the anatomical distribution, by the path of projection to their areas of innervation, and by the nature of the neurochemical hormone or transmitter that they synthesize and release (Fig. 42-4).

The function of the neurotransmitter is to propagate an electrical impulse from one neuron to another. The electrical impulse travels down a neuron causing the release of a neurotransmitter from presynaptic vesicles in which the neurotransmitter is synthesized and stored. Subsequently several thousand molecules of neurotransmitter are released into the synaptic cleft, the space between the presynaptic and postsynaptic neurons. There they bind to transmitter-specific receptors of the postsynaptic neurons and produce either an excitatory or inhibitory impulse. Enzymes in the synaptic cleft break down neurotransmitters. Both the metabolites and the parent compounds bind to receptors on the presynaptic membrane, where they are again taken back into the presynaptic neuron (**reuptake**) for formation of new neurotransmitter.

Norepinephrine. Norepinephrine is formed in presynaptic noradrenergic neurons from the substrate tyrosine by means of the intermediary products of dopa and dopamine (Fig. 42-5). Norepinephrine produces an excitatory response at postsynaptic receptors. It is either broken down in the cleft to 3-methoxy-4-hydroxyphenylglycol (MHPG) or taken up into the presynaptic neuron where it is metabolized by a cytoplasmic enzyme called *monoamine oxidase*, and the breakdown product is resynthesized to norepinephrine. By this mechanism most of the norepinephrine released into the synaptic cleft is recovered by the noradrenergic neuron. MHPG also crosses the blood-brain barrier, enters the circulatory system, and is excreted into urine; approximately 50% of urinary MHPG is derived from the CNS.

Dopamine. Dopamine is formed by the same metabolic pathway as shown in Fig. 42-5 in dopaminagenic neurons that lack the enzymes for further metabolism of dopamine into norepinephrine. These neurons project from the brainstem to the limbic system and frontal cortex. Dopamine appears to be mainly inhibitory in action. There now appear to be five to seven different types of dopamine receptors; these subtypes may have significance in pharmacological treatment of mental disorders. Dopamine is metabolized to homovanillic acid and is excreted into urine.

Acetylcholine. Acetylcholine, the first demonstrated neurotransmitter, is formed in presynaptic cholinergic neurons from acetyl CoA, a ubiquitous metabolite, and choline,

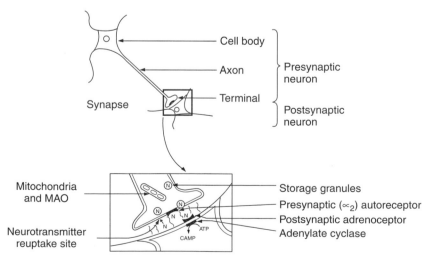

Fig. 42-4 Norepinephrine neuron, synapse, and postsynaptic connections.

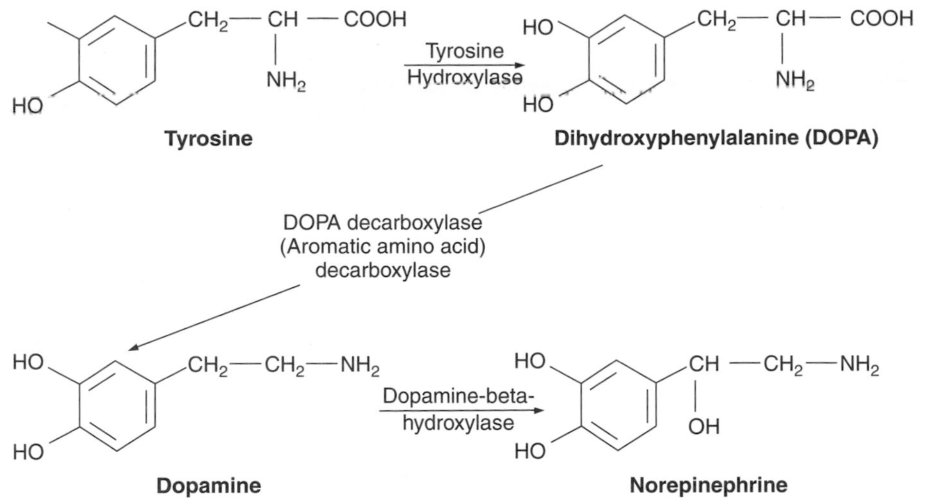

Fig. 42-5 Enzymatic pathway for synthesis of dopamine and norepinephrine. *(From Kaplan H, Sadock B: Clinical psychiatry, Baltimore, 1988, Williams & Wilkins.)*

which is derived from lipid metabolism. The essential enzyme for this reaction is choline acetyltransferase.

Once released from presynaptic vesicles into the synaptic cleft, acetylcholine binds to postsynaptic receptors and acts as an excitatory neurotransmitter. It is broken down by the enzyme acetylcholinesterase in the synaptic cleft. Ten percent of all **synapses** in the central and peripheral nervous system use acetylcholine. The synapses are located in all the neuromuscular junctions, the major portion of the autonomic nervous system, and in brain areas such as motor pathways, the hippocampus, which is part of the limbic system, and the basal ganglia.

Serotonin (5-hydroxytryptamine, 5-HT). Serotonin is formed in presynaptic serotoninergic neurons from the amino acid tryptophan, by means of hydroxytryptophan. Most serotoninergic neurons originate in the raphe nuclei in the pons from where projections run diffusely throughout the brain and spinal cord. The raphe nuclei are part of the reticular formation, which regulates general arousal. Serotonin binds to the postsynaptic hydroxytryptamine receptor, where it produces an excitatory response. Both serotonin and its metabolite 5-hydroxyindoleacetic acid (5-HIAA) are taken up into the presynaptic neuron.

GABA (γ-aminobutyric acid). GABA is formed from the amino acid glutamic acid by decarboxylation. GABA is used as a neurotransmitter by 30% to 40% of all synapses in the brain and is diffusely located throughout the brain, brainstem, and spinal cord. It acts as an inhibitory neurotransmitter. The postsynaptic GABA receptor complexes also bind drugs like phenobarbital, valproate and benzodiazepines. Tiagabine, one of the new **antiepileptic drugs**, is believed to enhance the activity of the GABA system by binding to recognition sites associated with the GABA uptake carrier. This results in reduced GABA reuptake thereby increasing the GABA concentration available to the receptor.

Other neurotransmitters. A variety of other substances make up the majority of neurotransmitters in the CNS, but their clinical significance is poorly understood at the present time. Such substances are glutamate, an amino acid that has excitatory function in synapses in the brain; glycine, another amino acid that has inhibitory function in the spinal cord; endogenous opioids, such as endorphin and enkephalin; and substance P, which is found in neuronal pathways transmitting pain. Most recently, two gases, nitrous oxide and carbon monoxide, have been shown to act as neurotransmitters.

PATHOLOGICAL CONDITIONS: NEUROLOGICAL

Loss of neural function with resulting disease states is caused by abnormalities of the neurotransmitter biochemical pathways. For example, in the early stages of Alzheimer's disease there is a large decrease in choline acetyltransferase activity along with degeneration of neurons using acetylcholine. Loss of acetylcholine activity in the hippocampus may explain the hallmark symptom of early memory loss in Alzheimer's disease, because the hippocampus is involved in acquisition of memory. In Huntington's disease there is degeneration of cholinergic neurons in the basal ganglia, contributing to the movement disorder and dementia seen in Huntington's disease. Dysfunction of GABA-ergic systems is postulated in idiopathic generalized **epilepsy**, Huntington's disease, and **anxiety disorders**. Clinical disease states attributable to dopaminergic neuron dysfunction vary according to the anatomical location of the dysfunctional neurons. Dopaminergic neuron dysfunction in pathways from the brainstem to the frontal cortex and limbic system may contribute to clinical symptoms of **schizophrenia**, whereas dysfunction of dopaminergic neurons that project from the brainstem to the corpus striatum is important in movement disorders such as Parkinson's disease.

Damage to *discrete* (focal) areas of the brain or spinal cord produces predictable circumscribed signs and symptoms, such as paralysis of an arm, leg, or side of the body, loss of ability to speak or comprehend spoken language, incoordination, and visual or sensory loss. *Diffuse* impairment of cerebral tissue, on the other hand, leads to a different characteristic clinical picture. Failure of various intellectual functions such as attention, concentration, judgment, memory, problem-solving ability, and insight are early findings with mild diffuse disease. Other symptoms include changes in alertness beginning with clouding of consciousness and proceeding to drowsiness, stupor, and **coma**. Excessive synchronized nerve transmission can cause sudden transient abnormalities of mental function or body movement, called **seizures**. Seizures can accompany both diffuse and focal brain damage.

Various disease states tend to produce either focal or diffuse brain damage, and so the pattern of deficits described above is often helpful to the clinician in working backward toward a specific diagnosis. Some examples of conditions that cause focal damage are stroke caused by arterial occlusion or hemorrhage; trauma; cerebral abscess; and tumors. Many of these conditions also cause changes in the CSF by damaging the blood-brain barrier (elevating CSF protein) and stimulating inflammatory changes (with leukocytosis), tissue necrosis (elevating CSF protein and cell count), or shedding of tumor cells (observed in cytological specimens).

Examples of conditions associated with diffuse cerebral dysfunction (encephalopathic states) are anoxia, generalized ischemia, hypoglycemia, sepsis, thyroid abnormalities, disseminated intravascular coagulation, and the entire group of toxic and metabolic derangements. The diagnosis of these states often rests on laboratory findings.

Some of the clinical and pathological changes commonly found in many conditions are briefly discussed.

Coma

Coma is a state of unconsciousness from which the patient cannot be aroused. A coma is but one aspect of altered states of consciousness that can be present in patients. *Confusion* is the least altered state, in which there is disorientation with respect to time, associated drowsiness, and altered attention span. *Stupor* is a state in which the patient is unresponsive but can be aroused back to a near-normal state with appropriate stimuli.

A patient with an altered mental state, as seen in an emergency department, must first be given any life support, such as ventilation, necessary to maintain vital functions. The next step is to determine the underlying cause of the altered mental status. Readily treatable causes can be corrected by procedures, such as administration of dextrose to relieve coma caused by severe hypoglycemia. Table 42-1 lists the most important causes of coma and altered mental states, which include metabolic, structural, or infectious causes. Many of these causes are described in detail later.

Intracranial Bleeding

Bleeding from a vessel on the surface of the brain, such as an arterial aneurysm, pours blood between the brain's surface and the pia and arachnoid layers and is called a *subarachnoid hemorrhage*. Blood thus mingles with CSF, and red blood cells appear on examination of the CSF. Furthermore, because blood is an extremely irritating substance when it escapes from its usual vascular channels, it may provoke an inflammatory response in the meninges, called a *chemical meningitis*, and leukocytes will be shed into the CSF by the irritated meninges. Because meninges are pain sensitive, a subarachnoid hemorrhage typically causes acute, severe headache.

Infectious Diseases

Both the type of invading bacterial or viral organism and the intracranial structures they invade help determine CSF changes seen in the infectious process. The CSF parameters that reflect CNS invasion by an infectious agent are white blood cell (WBC) count and differential, glucose, and to a lesser extent protein concentration.

Meningitis is an inflammation of the meninges leading to several clinical patterns. Bacterial, or *purulent*, meningitis is

TABLE 42-1 SOME CAUSES OF COMA AND ALTERED MENTAL STATES

Type	Cause	Laboratory Findings
Metabolic	Alcoholism	Increased blood ethanol, metabolic acidosis, and ketosis
	Hyperosmolar coma	Blood glucose $\geq$5000 mg/L, no ketosis, dehydration
	Diabetic ketoacidosis	Increased blood glucose, ketosis, acidosis, dehydration
	Metabolic acidosis of other origin	Decreased pH, increased lactic acid
	Hypoglycemia	Decreased blood glucose (<500 mg/L)
	Hypercalcemia or hypocalcemia	Changes in calcium levels; hypomagnesemia can be found with hypocalcemia
	Drugs	Presence of any of many drugs on serum or urine toxicology screen, often at very high levels
Systemic metabolic diseases	Hepatic coma	Increase in blood ammonia, increased liver function tests
	Uremic coma	Increased serum urea, creatinine with metabolic acidosis
	Ischemia; cardiac, pulmonary	Lactic acidosis
	Hypothyroidism, hyperthyroidism	Abnormal thyroid function tests
Encephalopathy	Intracranial hemorrhage	Blood in CSF
Trauma		None, or blood in CSF if traumatic hemorrhage is present
Infectious	Bacterial, viral	Decreased CSF glucose, increased protein
Psychiatric		None

associated with a CSF polymorphonuclear (PMN) leukocytosis, with cell counts ranging from a very few to many thousands of PMNs. The CSF glucose levels may be depressed to strikingly low values, and CSF protein concentrations may be elevated. Later in the course of illness lymphocytes can become prominent or dominant, especially if the infection has been partially treated with antibiotics. Partial treatment of bacterial meningitis that fails to eradicate the infection can produce confusing findings and may make diagnosis difficult.

Viral meningitis causes a predominantly or exclusively lymphocytic leukocytosis. Red blood cells may be seen with herpes simplex encephalitis. CSF glucose levels usually remain within the healthy reference interval but may be decreased in mumps, herpes simplex, or herpes zoster encephalitis. Protein is usually within the healthy reference interval or slightly elevated in these diseases.

Fungi also invade the CNS and may cause no change in CSF other than a lymphocytosis and increased protein concentration. Glucose levels usually remain within the healthy reference interval.

Viral encephalitis is a viral infection of the brain parenchyma. Viral encephalitis is characterized by acute fever, headache, altered mentation, and evidence of parenchymal involvement: seizures, focal cerebral symptoms or signs, stupor or coma, and a signs of increased intracranial pressure. In the United States, the common pathogens are herpes simplex virus-1 (HSV-1), arbovirus, enterovirus, measles, and mumps. HSV-1 encephalitis is the most common viral encephalitis; it manifests with fever, headache, focal or generalized seizures, behavioral changes, amnestic syndrome, and aphasia. CSF is under normal or elevated pressure, with lymphocytic pleocytosis, the cell count of 10 to 1000 WBC/µl; red blood cells (RBCs) and **xanthochromia** also may be present. Protein is elevated, and glucose is normal or decreased. Cultures and serology are important diagnostic tools for identifying specific viral agents. Herpes viral (human cytomegalovirus [CMV], HSV, varicella zoster virus [VZV], Epstein-Barr virus [EBV]), enteroviral, Jacob-Creutzfeldt (JC) viral, and measles viral nucleic acid can be detected by polymerase chain reaction (PCR) from CSF specimens.

The presence of bacteria should be determined by Gram stain and culture of CSF. Viruses can be sought with appropriate serological tests or culture, and fungi can be found with culture or immunological procedures and with appropriate staining. For example, carefully performed India ink staining may reveal *Cryptococcus* species.

The CSF findings in syphilis depend on the stage of illness, disease activity, and whether previous treatment was given in adequate amounts. Pleocytosis is lymphatic or mononuclear in character, with white cell counts in the range of 100 to 1000/µL. CSF protein levels may be elevated. CSF Venereal Disease Research Laboratory (VDRL) and serum fluorescent treponemal antibody (FTA) tests are usually positive, and oligoclonal bands may be present.

Organisms can invade the brain substance, in which case the term *encephalitis* is used. CSF findings are comparable to findings in meningitis or may be quite minimal.

Abscess formation in the brain may produce no CSF changes even though a potentially deadly infection is present.

Finally, any of the above conditions can and frequently do lead to increased CSF pressure. This is especially true of meningitis, which obstructs the usual flow of CSF, causing an obstructive hydrocephalus. Meningitis can also impair CSF absorption, causing a communicating hydrocephalus.

A variety of organisms that do not usually cause serious infections in healthy individuals may produce life-threatening infections in patients whose immune system is compromised. Patients at risk for these "opportunistic" infections include those with acquired immunodeficiency syndrome (AIDS), cancer, or those taking immunosuppressant drugs for other reasons (e.g., to treat an immune-mediated disease like myasthenia gravis).

AIDS is caused by the human immunodeficiency virus (HIV). Direct HIV invasion of the nervous system may produce neurological manifestations but AIDS also predisposes affected individuals to opportunistic infections and unusual malignant tumors that can involve the nervous system. Opportunistic infections, AIDS-related neoplasms, or HIV can affect the brain, spinal cord, or peripheral nerves; usually multiple sites are affected by multiple causes. With direct HIV infection of the CNS, oligoclonal bands and elevated protein concentrations are usually present in the CSF. The most common CNS tumors are lymphoma and metastatic Kaposi's sarcoma. Common infections are toxoplasmosis, progressive multifocal leukoencephalopathy, fungal and mycobacterial granulomas, and HSV encephalitis.

Lyme disease, first identified in 1975 by a cluster of cases in Old Lyme, Connecticut, is caused by a spirochete *(Borrelia burgdorferi)* and is spread through tick bites. Clinical symptoms include arthritis, meningitis, radiculitis, neuropathy, and in late stages, concentration, memory, and sleep disorders. The diagnosis is made by organism-specific IgG or IgM in the serum, but CSF typically shows elevated WBCs and protein levels, and the presence of oligoclonal bands.

Prion diseases are a group of transmissible neurological degenerative diseases that have characteristic pathological changes that led to the early designation of spongiform encephalopathy. They result from the accumulation of an abnormal amyloid form of a host-encoded proteins-resistant protein (PrP, or *prion*), specified by a gene on chromosome 20. The most common prion disease in human is Creutzfeldt-Jacob disease (CJD). The clinical features are progressive dementia, behavior changes, and abnormal movements. The average time of survival is approximately 7 months. Routine examination of CSF is usually normal. An important new immunoassay that detects a class of 14-3-3 proteinase released into the CSF from damaged neurons, has been proved extremely useful in the diagnosis.

Inflammatory Diseases

Multiple sclerosis and sarcoidosis are inflammatory CNS diseases of unknown cause. *Multiple sclerosis (MS)* is a disorder of unknown cause usually affecting young adults.

MS produces numerous areas of demyelination in the CNS and is characterized by a waxing and waning but usually progressive course. The diagnosis of MS is best made by magnetic resonance imaging (MRI) by which approximately 90% of patients show white matter lesions. Examination of CSF, however, can clarify the diagnosis in many cases. Five major CSF abnormalities are seen in MS: (1) an elevation of up to 40 cells/mm^3 of WBCs, (2) an elevation of protein up to 1000 mg/L, (3) elevation in IgG, (4) presence of oligoclonal bands, and (5) elevation in myelin basic protein. However, none of these CSF abnormalities are specific for multiple sclerosis.

Sarcoidosis is a generalized disease of unknown cause that may affect the nervous system. Serum angiotensin-converting enzyme (ACE) is usually elevated and CSF shows elevations in protein concentration, cells, and occasionally decreased glucose levels.

Further information regarding infectious disorders of the nervous system can be found in general textbooks of neurology or infectious disease (see the bibliography).

Ischemia

Although immensely dependent on glucose for its energy source, the brain's own glucose reserves are small. With oxygen available and the brain's metabolic needs supplied by respiration using only glucose stored in the brain itself, those stores supply the brain's needs for only 2 to 3 minutes. If *both* glucose and oxygen are cut off (as in ischemia) glycolysis becomes the dominant source of energy, and glucose stores in the brain can support its energy metabolism for only about 14 seconds. When energy metabolism ceases, the integrity of cellular membranes fails, potassium begins leaking from the cells, osmotic balance is lost, fluid rushes into the damaged cells, and within seconds cells begin to die.

The term *ischemia* can be defined as inadequate blood flow to a tissue. In the brain, ischemia can be present for many reasons. For example, if the heart stops, total cerebral blood flow ceases; if the blood pressure drops low enough, the flow of blood becomes inadequate; and if a single large vessel such as the carotid artery becomes narrowed, too little blood passes through. If an embolus or an atherosclerotic plaque occludes a cerebral blood vessel, the tissue that it irrigates becomes ischemic. Other blood vessels usually try to supply the area and make up the difference, but if the area of brain supplied by an occluded vessel cannot be supplied with blood from surrounding vessels, the cells in that area die. This is called a cerebral *infarction*, or a *stroke*.

Stroke

When a stroke occurs, the functions served by the infarcted region are damaged. For example, if the area controlling strength and movement in one extremity or one side of the body is infarcted, that extremity or side becomes weak or paralyzed. If the area subserving speech is damaged, the patient may lose the ability to talk or to comprehend what is heard. The dying or dead area of brain may release protein into the CSF. Because blood vessels in the area are also damaged by ischemia, some bleeding may occur. Only a few cells may appear in the CSF, if only a little blood has escaped from the area, or the CSF may become frankly bloody if an actual hemorrhage occurs in the damaged area. Finally, as the brain begins to clear away the damaged tissue, some WBCs may appear in the CSF. In summary, then, after a stroke that has not involved significant hemorrhage, the CSF can be either normal or more likely contain an elevated protein level, a few RBCs, and possibly some WBCs.

Diffuse Cerebral Ischemia and Hypoxia

If total cerebral circulation stops, as in cardiac arrest, consciousness is lost within 6 to 8 seconds. On the other hand, if oxygen supply becomes inadequate but circulation continues, the clinical result is usually a feeling of light-headedness followed by mental confusion in mild cases, proceeding to loss of consciousness, seizures, and coma with moderate to severe hypoxia. Precipitating events include pulmonary edema, carbon monoxide poisoning, pulmonary embolism, strangulation, respiratory failure during mechanical ventilation, and exposure to ambient air at high altitudes. Failure to restore cerebral circulation and oxygenation within 4 to 5 minutes after their total cessation may result in cell death and irreversible damage.

Neuromuscular Diseases (see also Chapter 31)

The term *neuromuscular disease* refers to disorders that affect peripheral nerves, neuromuscular junctions, or muscle cells, typically causing weakness, sensory loss, or loss of autonomic function. A detailed discussion of these disorders is beyond the scope of this chapter, but laboratory aids in their diagnosis will be discussed.

Peripheral nerve disorders are either hereditary or acquired. The diagnosis of hereditary *neuropathies* usually requires nerve biopsy for histological evaluation of the nerve; however, neuropathy resulting from porphyria is frequently associated with elevated levels of δ-aminolevulinic acid and porphobilinogen in urine. Guillain-Barré syndrome (acute idiopathic demyelinating polyneuropathy) and its chronic form cause weakness and loss of reflexes, and have a characteristic CSF finding of elevated protein levels without elevated cell counts. Other causes of neuropathy in which laboratory diagnosis is essential include diabetes (see Chapter 32), hypothyroidism (see later discussion), vasculitis, uremia (see Chapter 26), hepatic dysfunction (see Chapter 27), or heavy metal (arsenic, lead, mercury, and thallium) poisoning. Infectious causes of neuropathy include AIDS, Lyme disease, herpes zoster, diphtheria, and leprosy. Amyloidosis causing neuropathy can be secondary to a plasma cell dyscrasia or because of hereditary amyloidosis.

Myasthenia gravis is a disorder of the neuromuscular junction in which antibodies are directed against the acetylcholine receptor. Patients have fluctuating weakness typically affecting the face, limbs, and eye movements. Approximately 85% of patients with active myasthenia show elevated acetylcholine receptor antibody titers.

Muscular disorders can be hereditary or acquired. Hereditary forms are genetic myopathies, usually caused by a disturbance of a structural protein. Duchenne's muscular dystrophy and Becker's muscular dystrophy are caused by absence or deficiency of dystrophin that causes progressive destruction of muscle. The serum concentration of creatine kinase (CK) is markedly elevated in these illnesses; levels greater than 10,000 U/L are common. The dystrophin gene is located on the X chromosome. The diagnosis is confirmed by obtaining DNA studies revealing depletion in the dystrophin gene or muscular biopsy proving absence or reduced dystrophin.

Several familial muscular illnesses, including hyperkalemic and hypokalemic periodic paralysis and myotonia congenital are now recognized to be caused by abnormalities in ion channels (particularly sodium and chloride). This group of diseases is characterized by attacks of generalized weakness, dystonia, and elevated or decreased serum potassium concentrations. Myoglobinuria occurs when necrosis of the muscle is acute and myoglobin from muscle escapes into the blood and then into the urine.

Mitochondrial disorders are inherited diseases affecting the CNS and muscles caused by disturbances in mitochondrial function that produce neurological damage and abnormalities in the muscle. They are clinically characterized by muscle weakness, exercise intolerance, seizures, myoclonus, and stroke. Blood lactate levels are elevated. Muscle biopsy shows "ragged-red fibers" and abnormalities in the mitochondria under the electron microscope.

Polymyositis and dermatomyositis are termed *inflammatory myopathies*, and are believed to be abnormalities of the autoimmune system. Dermatomyositis is an illness in which weakness is associated with a characteristic skin rash. It is the most common form of myositis in childhood. Serum CK concentrations are usually elevated at the range of several hundreds to a thousand IU/mL. Blood tests also provide evidence of an altered immune state with development of unusual antibodies, including Jo-1 antibody and anti Mi-2 antibody. The muscle biopsy reveals perifascicular atrophy that may be diagnostic. Polymyositis occurs at any age, produces widespread weakness, often more proximally than distally. CK levels may be markedly elevated; anti-Jo-1 antibodies are found in one fifth of patients. The muscle biopsy shows muscle fibrosis associated with inflammatory reactions.

Neoplastic and Paraneoplastic Syndromes

Neoplasms affecting the CNS can be present in neural tissue (brain, cranial nerves, spinal cord, or peripheral nerves) or related structures (skull, meninges, blood vessels, pituitary or pineal glands). Carcinomatous meningitis refers to invasion of the CSF and meninges by neoplastic cells. If the neoplasm arises directly from these structures, it is termed *primary;* it is termed *metastatic* if it has spread from a neoplasm elsewhere in the body. The symptoms that develop with various types of nervous system tumors are related to the nature of the tumor, its size, and its location.

Approximately one third of patients with cerebral tumors develop seizures.

Paraneoplastic syndromes are neurological disorders associated with cancer, but not caused by a direct effect of the tumor mass or its metastases. The presence of the antibodies in many patients suggests that immune mechanisms participate in these disorders. The antibodies found in neoplastic syndromes are different from each other but have some common characteristics. Most are polyclonal immunoglobulin G (IgG) that fix complement. They react predominantly or exclusively with both target neurological tissue and the underlying tumor. Antibodies often identify a subset of patients with a specific clinical syndrome and a specific tumor. The anti-Yo antibody is found in patients with paraneoplastic cerebellar degeneration and gynecological tumors; the anti-Hu antibody is found in patients with limbic encephalitis, sensory neuropathy, and small cell lung cancer. Anti-Ri antibody is found in patients with opsoclonus-myoclonus syndrome, breast, and gynecological cancer. Anti-voltage-gated calcium channel antibody is found in Lambert-Eaton myasthenic syndrome and small cell lung cancer.

Modern imaging techniques such as MRI and computerized tomography (CT) can identify nervous system neoplasms with extraordinary accuracy. Laboratory diagnosis, however, can still be useful for certain neoplasms. The diagnosis of carcinomatous meningitis is made by examination of the CSF for neoplastic cells. Elevated CSF β-glucuronidase and carcinoembryonic antigen (CEA) are also found in some cases.

Epilepsy

A seizure is a sudden and transient disturbance of mental function or body movements that results from an excessive electrical discharge by a group of brain cells. There are two main types of seizures: *focal onset* and *generalized onset*. Focal onset seizures begin in a discrete region of the brain and then have varying degrees and patterns of spread. Generalized onset seizures begin throughout the brain at once. The clinical manifestations of the seizure depend on the areas of the brain involved. For example, a focal onset seizure involving the motor cortex may manifest as twitching of one hand, whereas a seizure involving the temporal lobe may show alteration in consciousness with staring and memory loss (known as a *complex partial seizure*). Staring spells of generalized onset are known as *absence* or *petit mal seizures*. Either focal onset or generalized onset seizures may spread to involve the entire brain and cause a *generalized tonic clonic seizure* with generalized motor activity, sometimes called a *convulsion* or *grand mal seizure*.

Focal onset seizures are usually caused by some localized abnormality of the brain that can sometimes be identified by using brain-imaging procedures such as CT or MRI. Frequent causes of focal onset seizures include: stroke, brain tumors, birth injuries, or severe head injury. Generalized seizures can be idiopathic (no obvious cause) or symptomatic resulting from a generalized insult to the brain such as drug overdose, renal failure, encephalitis, or illicit drugs. The type and duration of treatment are determined by the seizure type and presumed cause. Each person who has seizures needs a careful evaluation by a physician searching for an underlying cause that can be corrected.

Persons with seizures are usually prescribed antiepileptic drugs (AEDs) for months or even for the rest of their lives in an attempt to stop or at least reduce the frequency of seizures. Once treated most persons with seizures obtain excellent control and can live normal lives, and often the medication can be stopped after some period of time. However, about 30% to 40% of persons with seizures will obtain inadequate seizure control or have unacceptable side effects from AEDs.

Intoxication With Drugs and Poisons

Many drugs and poisons affect the nervous system directly, producing confusion, drowsiness, stupor, coma, seizures, or psychotic states. Drugs may also cause respiratory depression, alter the systemic metabolic balance, or otherwise indirectly damage the nervous system. In many cases, the differential diagnosis of these states requires laboratory confirmation of the presence of an offending drug or toxin. When specific drugs are known or suspected to be available to the patient, the search is simplified.

Physical findings may raise suspicion of a certain class of drugs; for example, small pupils are suggestive of the presence of opiates, and widely dilated pupils are suggestive of drugs with atropine-like effects such as tricyclic antidepressants or amphetamines with adrenergic actions. Unfortunately, many cases of intoxication involve multiple substances, whether "street" drugs or medications. For these cases or because the circumstances surrounding an ingestion are unclear, a *toxic screen* for common substances is necessary.

Metabolic Diseases

A variety of metabolic disorders can affect the nervous system and usually present with episodic confusion, stupor, or coma. Metabolic diseases affecting mental status include respiratory acidosis, hypoglycemia, ketoacidosis, nonketotic hyperosmolar coma, hepatic failure, renal failure, renal dialysis, and electrolyte disturbances. *Anoxic encephalopathy* occurs when there is a lack of oxygen delivery to the brain, caused by failure of respiration, circulation, or both. Mild degrees of hypoxia may produce only transient confusion, whereas severe degrees may cause coma sometimes with permanent brain injury. *Hypercapnia* (elevated pressure of CO_2 in the blood) can produce alterations in level of consciousness. *Hypoglycemia* is an infrequent cause of CNS symptoms unless it is severe (plasma glucose below 250 to 300 mg/L [1.4 to 1.7 mmol/L]) as may occur with insulin overdose, acute severe alcohol intoxication, or various conditions in children and neonates. Hyperglycemia uncommonly causes stupor or coma except when severe ketoacidosis or hyperosmolar nonketotic hyperglycemia occurs (see Chapter 32). Hepatic failure can cause impaired consciousness by elevating serum ammonia. Altered consciousness in patients with renal insufficiency can be attributable to uremia or to a *disequilibrium syndrome* associated with dialysis. Altered consciousness sometimes accompanied by seizures may result from a variety of electrolyte disturbances including (but not limited to) metabolic acidosis, hypernatremia and hyponatremia, hypokalemia, and hypocalcemia.

Endocrine Diseases

Adrenal disease. Inadequate release of cortisol affects the brain in ways that are complex and not well understood. In chronic untreated hypoadrenalism, apathy, **depression**, fatigue, and even mild delirium are common. Stupor and coma usually occur only when there is an abrupt severe worsening of chronic illness, the so-called *addisonian crisis*. Other metabolic derangements secondary to the hypoadrenalism such as hyponatremia, hyperkalemia, hypoglycemia, and hypotension may occur and produce additional CNS dysfunction.

Excess glucocorticoid products and the administration of steroid medications are associated in some patients with disturbances of mood (depression, elevation, or hypomania), mild confusion, delusion, hallucinations, impaired insight, and grossly inappropriate behavior.

Hypothyroidism. In the fetus and during infancy hypothyroidism can cause irreversible brain damage and profound mental retardation (cretinism) unless the condition is corrected without delay. Chronic hypothyroidism is associated with depression or lability of mood, listlessness, confusion, and sometimes delusions and hallucinations (see Chapter 44). Peripheral neuropathy and unsteady gait related to impaired cerebellar functions also occur together with abnormal deep tendon reflexes. For obscure reasons, elevated CSF protein is a common finding in hypothyroidism. Severe hypothyroidism (myxedema coma) may cause decreased body temperature, slowed respiration, and hypometabolism, usually occurring in a setting of chronic hypothyroidism on which some acute event is superimposed, such as infection, surgery, trauma, or congestive heart failure. Because myxedema coma is rapidly fatal, correct diagnosis and prompt treatment are essential.

Signs of thyroid hypermetabolism (thyrotoxicosis) distinguish the state of thyroid excess that is associated with disturbances in thinking and emotion. Because the clinical appearance of thyroid disease can mimic psychiatric disease or CNS dysfunction, thyroid function tests are frequently ordered from psychiatric and emergency areas of the hospital.

PATHOLOGICAL CONDITIONS: PSYCHIATRIC
Schizophrenia

Description. Approximately 1% of the population is affected with the mixed group of chronic psychotic disorders termed *schizophrenia* that usually start in young adulthood and persist throughout life. Schizophrenia disease patterns include active phases in which illogical thinking, delusions (fixed false beliefs), auditory hallucinations (often with threatening content), and bizarre behavior may be prominent.

Because of the chronic nature and the frequent gradual decline in the schizophrenic patient's ability to function appropriately and independently, the cost of care to society is tremendous. In the current classification of psychiatric disorders (DSM–IV) several subtypes, including disorganized, paranoid, undifferentiated, catatonic, and residual type are described.

Pathophysiology. The cause of this disorder remains unknown, and theories include developmental abnormalities and aberrant neurotransmitter function. Unlike some forms of psychiatric illness that seem to result from childhood experience and stressful life circumstances, schizophrenia runs in families and has a genetic and biological basis.[1,2] Increased production of neurotransmitters in the mesolimbic dopaminergic pathway appears to be correlated with hallucinations and delusions (referred to *as positive symptoms*), whereas decreased production in the mesocortical dopaminergic pathway is postulated to be associated with the withdrawn, asocial behavior (referred to as *negative symptoms*) and gradual decline in function in chronic schizophrenic patients.[3] Supporting this concept is the observation that at postmortem examination the neurons of substantial numbers of chronic schizophrenic patients have an increased number of dopamine-related postsynaptic receptors.

Treatment. Antipsychotic medication ameliorates and stabilizes schizophrenic disorder; however, these medications do not cure the disease and typically must be taken for life. The mechanism by which these medications act on schizophrenic symptoms is poorly understood but they all share the blockade and antagonism of dopamine receptors to a variable extent. The antipsychotic drugs (also known as neuroleptics) available for the past 50 years are now known as *conventional antipsychotics*. The conventional agents probably are effective because of blockade of dopamine receptors but also cause adrenergic and cholinergic blockade that leads to sedation, orthostatic hypotension, dry mouth, urinary retention, and constipation.

The conventional agents primarily block dopamine D-1 receptors, which cause unwanted muscular side effects (called *extrapyramidal side effects* or EPS) and probably cause tardive dyskinesia (TD), a chronic movement disorder that begins after some period of use of the antipsychotics. EPS include muscle stiffness and rigidity, often in the jaw. Patients taking these medications may appear to have Parkinson's symptoms such as difficulty initiating movements and a masklike face. Patients experiencing EPS are given anticholinergic agents such as trihexphenidyl (Artane) or benztropine (Cogentin) to relieve the muscle stiffness.

TD often involves dystonic movements of the mouth and tongue. Another dangerous side effect is the neuroleptic malignant syndrome, which if untreated can be lethal; it is characterized by mental status changes, fever, muscle rigidity, elevated WBC count, and elevated creatine phosphokinase (CPK) levels. Some of the typical antipsychotics (haloperidol and fluphenazine) are available in injectable depot forms that are effective for up to 4 weeks after a single injection.

Newer antipsychotic or neuroleptic agents are known as *atypical antipsychotics*, because they are designed to block dopamine D-2, D-3, and D-4 receptors. These include olanzapine, risperidone, quetiapine and ziprasidone. By avoiding D-1 blockade, these atypical agents rarely cause EPS and seem much less likely to cause TD. The atypical antipsychotics affect serotonin receptors, which confer effectiveness in treating depressive and anxiety symptoms. They also block histamine receptors, which may cause weight gain and sedation.

Affective Disorders

Description. The **affective disorders** are diseases of mood regulation. Clinical symptoms may be depression, **mania** (abnormally elevated mood), or **bipolar affective disorder** (mood alternating between depression and mania). Depression may be seen in either unipolar (termed *unipolar affective disorder*) or bipolar disorder and is accompanied by changes in neurovegetative functions such as sleep, appetite, motivation, psychomotor regulation, and energy, as well as distinct cognitive effects with loss of concentration and capacity to make decisions. Major depression causes loss of enjoyment of usual activities, feelings of worthlessness, and severe hopelessness that may lead to suicidal thoughts or actions. Major depression or bipolar depression may be accompanied by psychotic symptoms such as hallucinations and delusions, often of a persecutory nature. *Dysthymic disorder* is a milder form of depression that is chronic, lasting at least 2 years, and *cyclothymia* refers to a milder form of bipolar mood swings that are not as severe as those seen in bipolar affective disorder.

Major depression and bipolar affective disorder tend to run in families and have a genetic and biological basis,[4,5] whereas dysthymia and cyclothymia may result from stressful life events and maladaptive behavior. There is evidence from epidemiological studies of identical twins compared with fraternal twins that there is a substantial genetic background for many psychiatric illnesses.

Pathophysiology. The monoamine theory of depression has been popular for many years, and states that depression results from deficits in norepinephrine, serotonin, dopamine or all three. The first available treatment for depression was the tricyclic antidepressants, compounds that increase transmission of both serotonin and norepinephrine in the CNS. Norepinephrine affects mood, cognition, sexual function, sleep, and attention via projections from the locus ceruleus (an area of norepinephrine neurons in the brainstem) to the frontal cortex. Depressed patients have been shown to have abnormally low levels of CSF norepinephrine and urinary MHPG, half of which has its origin from CNS norepinephrine metabolism. Patients with decreased urinary MHPG excretion often respond to antidepressants that selectively inhibit the reuptake of norepinephrine into the presynaptic neuron. As a consequence of this reuptake inhibition, more norepinephrine is available in the synaptic cleft to act on the postsynaptic receptor, correcting the central norepinephrine deficiency. Reboxetine, a pure norepinephrine reuptake inhibitor, is being tested for use in the United States, but has been shown to be effective as an antidepressant in Europe.

Evidence for the role of serotonin in depression comes from numerous reports of diminished quantities of its metabolite, 5-HIAA, in the cerebrospinal fluid of depressed patients; furthermore 5-hydroxytryptophan (5-HT), a precursor of serotonin, is an effective antidepressant only in depressed patients with decreased cerebrospinal fluid 5-HIAA. Low levels of 5-HIAA have also been found in primates with higher levels of aggression and in nonsuicidal patients with high levels of aggression,[6,7] linking depression with aggression and impulsivity.

Many investigators are searching for a neuroanatomical and biochemical basis for the affective disorders, probably a complex chain of events that may or may not involve neurotransmitter deficits. There may be problems in the molecular events taking place after the neurotransmitter stimulates its receptor, with one possible defect occurring in the maintenance of brain-derived neurotrophic factor (BDNF). Patients with major depression have been found to have reduced volume of the left hippocampus compared with normal.[8] The loss of BDNF may lead to loss of brain cells in critical brain areas, leading to depression.[9] Depression may also be related to disruption of the pituitary-hypothalamic axis, possibly because of excessive hypothalamic secretion of corticotrophin-releasing factor (CRF) and excessive adrenal gland production of cortisol, with loss of the normal feedback mechanism. This may be related to observations that depressed patients are less likely to show normal suppression of cortisol production when given dexamethasone.[10] A recent study showed a positive correlation between nonsuppression of cortisol after dexamethasone and completed suicide[11] (see later discussion about DST). CRF antagonists are being investigated as new treatments for depression.

Treatment. The tricyclic antidepressants and monoamine oxidase inhibitors were once the only medications available for the treatment of depression. Though very effective, these medications caused significant unwanted side effects such as dizziness, constipation, dry mouth, increased sweating, and tachycardia. The tricyclics can be dangerous in patients with coronary artery disease because they can cause arrhythmias, and are fatal in overdose. Since the introduction of fluoxetine (Prozac) in 1988, which was equally effective but without the side effects of the tricyclics, the first-line treatment of depression is now the selective serotonin reuptake inhibitors (SSRIs), which include fluoxetine, sertraline, paroxetine, fluvoxamine, and citalopram. These medications work by blocking reuptake of serotonin on the presynaptic side of the synapse, leading to more serotonin available in the synaptic cleft. The subsequent generation of antidepressants includes the serotonin and norepinephrine reuptake inhibitors or SNRIs, agents that affect reuptake of both monoamines. These include venlafaxine, nefazodone, and mirtazapine. Bupropion is the only agent currently used that seems to affect dopamine transmission as well as that of norepinephrine (Table 42-2).

The tricyclics include amitriptyline, nortriptyline, imipramine, desipramine, protriptyline, and clomipramine. These agents variably bind to both presynaptic and postsynaptic noradrenergic and serotoninergic receptors in the synaptic cleft. The mechanism of action of these medications appears to be a competitive blockade of these receptors, which become unavailable for norepinephrine and serotonin to bind to, resulting in increased availability of neurotransmitter. Antidepressant drugs that are relatively selective in inhibition of neuronal reuptake of norepinephrine include desipramine, protriptyline, and the tetracyclic maprotiline. Pharmacological agents such as amitriptyline, trazodone, and clomipramine, which are effective in the treatment of depression, have been shown to inhibit selectively the neuronal reuptake of 5-HT from the synapse.

The monoamine oxidase inhibitors work by irreversibly inhibiting cytoplasmic monoamine oxidase A and B in the presynaptic neuron and thus inhibiting the breakdown of norepinephrine, serotonin, and dopamine. This inhibition takes place within 5 to 10 days after starting medication and makes more neurotransmitter available for neuronal transmission (see later discussion).

For many years the first-line treatment for bipolar affective disorder was lithium, which has nonspecific membrane-stabilizing properties. It remains the first-line treatment for bipolar disorder that includes episodes of euphoric mania, called *bipolar type I*. Psychiatrists increasingly recognize the existence of other forms of bipolar illness including bipolar type II, which is characterized by episodes of severe depression alternating with mild or hypomania or spells of irritability and anger. Valproate (Depakote), an antiepileptic medication with mood-stabilizing properties, is now the first-line treatment for this form of bipolar disorder and for bipolar disorder primarily manifest as depression. Olanzapine (Zyprexa), an atypical antipsychotic, is now FDA-approved for treatment of bipolar disorder. Carbamazepine

TABLE 42-2   SITES OF ACTION OF SOME ANTIDEPRESSANTS

	REUPTAKE BLOCKADE		RECEPTOR BLOCKADE		
	NE	*5-HT*	*Muscarinic ACh*	*H1*	*H2*
Imipramine	+	+	++	±	±
Desipramine	+++	±	±	-	-
Trimipramine	±	±	++	++	?
Amitriptyline	±	++	+++	++	++
Nortriptyline	++	±	+	±	±
Protriptyline	+++	±	+	+++	-
Amoxapine	++	±	+	±	?
Doxepin	+	±	++	+++	+
Maprotiline	+++	-	+	±	?

From Kaplan H, Sadock B: Clinical psychiatry, Baltimore, 1988, Williams & Wilkins. ACh, Acetylcholine; H, histamine; 5-HT, 5-hydroxytryptophan; NE, norepinephrine.

(Tegretol and others) is another antiepileptic drug effective in mania, and several recently introduced antiepileptic medications including gabapentin (Neurontin), lamotrigine (Lamictal), and topiramate (Topamax), are useful as adjunctive treatments.

Anxiety Disorders

Anxiety disorders are defined as pervasive chronic or paroxysmal feelings of apprehension that are often accompanied by physical signs such as dizziness, sweating, shortness of breath, increased heart rate, tingling or numbness of the mouth or extremities, and agitation or restlessness.

The spectrum of anxiety disorders includes *generalized anxiety disorder*, which is chronic rather than experienced as spells. Generalized anxiety disorder frequently disrupts the individual's capacity to fall asleep because of excessive worrying and tension. *Panic disorder* is defined as circumscribed anxiety attacks that may occur at any time including on awakening from sleep. Patients with panic disorder often have such fear of another attack occurring that they may have difficulty leaving their homes, or agoraphobia. *Obsessive-compulsive disorder* is characterized by obsessions, pervasive, ruminative worries, often quite implausible (such as fearing that the environment is somehow contaminated by blood) and compulsions, or repetitive acts meant to undo the obsessive fear (such as repeatedly washing the hands to overcome the imagined contamination). Both the obsessions and compulsions are beyond the person's ability to control, but are responsive to behavioral desensitization treatment. Phobias are irrational fears of specific places, objects, or activities, such as heights, elevators, snakes, insects, or driving on highways. Some phobias involve social activities such as speaking, eating, writing, or using the bathroom in public.

The pathophysiological characteristics of anxiety disorders are poorly understood at the present time, and a variety of biological, genetic, and behavioral theories exist. Research into neurotransmitter systems is focused on the noradrenergic, serotonergic and GABA-ergic systems. Drugs such as benzodiazepines increase the affinity of GABA for the receptor complex.

Treatment. As with depression, the first-line pharmacological treatment for the anxiety disorders is now the SSRIs, because they are effective and safe. The serotonergic medications are uniquely effective for obsessive-compulsive disorder, which does not respond to noradrenergic antidepressants like the tricyclics, with the exception of clomipramine, which has prominent serotonergic activity.

Generalized anxiety disorder and panic disorder also respond to drugs that affect the noradrenergic system and down-regulate its activity. Such drugs are β-adrenergic receptor blockers, tricyclic antidepressants, monoamine oxidase inhibitors, and benzodiazepines, in addition to the SSRIs. Benzodiazepines bind to specific receptor sites throughout the brain and spinal cord. These binding sites are coupled to a GABA-benzodiazepine receptor complex that mediates the anxiolytic, sedative, and antiepileptic action of these agents. Because of the potential for tolerance and addiction, the benzodiazepines should not be considered first-line treatment for the anxiety disorders.

FUNCTION TEST
Dexamethasone Suppression Test

Cortisol, the major corticosteroid hormone, is secreted by the adrenal glands in a circadian rhythm, with a peak occurring in the early morning hours. Production of this hormone is regulated by the release of pituitary ACTH, which in turn is under the control of CRH (corticotrophin-releasing hormone) that is produced by the hypothalamus (see pp. 822 and 823 for details). Under physiological conditions cortisol production is suppressed by the presence of even small amounts of exogenous corticosteroids such as dexamethasone.

The dexamethasone suppression test was originally used for the evaluation of the hypothalamic-pituitary axis in Cushing's syndrome (see p. 886). It was subsequently shown that a subgroup of depressed patients who mainly displayed features of unipolar depression or depression with psychosis had an abnormal response to the dexamethasone suppression test; that is, unsuppressed cortisol levels after dexamethasone administration. It has further been shown that the normalization of the dexamethasone suppression test after treatment of depression correlates with the degree of clinical response. On the other hand, depression in the absence of dexamethasone suppression normalization carries with it the risk of early relapse, should antidepressant medication be discontinued.

Description of test. In the dexamethasone suppression test 1 mg of dexamethasone (a synthetic corticosteroid) is administered orally around bedtime and plasma cortisol levels are measured at 4 and 11 PM the following day (see p. 892). Plasma cortisol levels of over 50 μg/L are abnormal and are suggestive that depression will respond to antidepressant medications. The best predictive value of this test appears to be in the setting of patients who suffer from unipolar depression with psychotic or melancholic features. The test is not used routinely but may be helpful in selected cases.

CHANGE OF ANALYTE IN DISEASE: NONDRUG ANALYTES (Table 42-3)
Appearance of Cerebrospinal Fluid

CSF is normally crystal clear and free from all pigmentation, that is, "clear and colorless." It should be examined in a glass tube in comparison to a tube of water while both are held in white light against a pure white background. It is best to look down the long axis of the tube. At least 1 mL of fluid should be observed.

An RBC count of 500/mm^3 gives a pink or yellow tinge to the fluid. WBC counts of 200/mm^3 will give a slightly cloudy appearance. Xanthochromia (a yellow tinge) will appear when blood has been mixed with CSF. This yellowing does not occur immediately but requires from 2 to 4 hours. A *traumatic* lumbar puncture occurs when the lumbar puncture needle pierces small blood vessels near the spinal cord coverings and blood enters the CSF collection tubes. Because blood in the CSF may represent subarachnoid

TABLE 42-3	CHANGE OF ANALYTE IN CNS DISEASE

Disease	Glucose	Total Protein	IgG	IgG Index	Xanthochromia	Lactic Acid
Stroke (cerebral) infarction)	N	↑	N	↓	N, ↑	N, ↑
Hemorrhage	N	N, ↑↑	N	N	↑↑	N
Epilepsy	N	N	N	N	N	N
CNS tumor	N, ↓	↑	N, ↑	↓	N, ↑	N, ↑
Infection						
Fungal, bacterial	↓	↑	↑	↑	N	↑
Viral	N	N	↑	↑	N	N
Coma	↑↑ hyperosmolar ↓ hypoglycemia	↑ (trauma)	N	N	N, ↑ (trauma) N	N
Meningitis, viral	N	N, ↑	N, ↑	↑	N	N

N, *Little or no change;* ↑, *increase;* ↑↑, *large increase;* ↓, *decrease.*

bleeding or may be simply the result of a traumatic lumbar puncture (a common occurrence), the CSF sample should be centrifuged immediately. If this is done promptly, bleeding that is caused by a traumatic lumbar puncture should produce no xanthochromia. Xanthochromia indicates that the bleeding may have occurred at least 2 to 4 hours before observation of the sample. As many as 10% of patients with subarachnoid hemorrhage actually have clear CSF at 12 hours, but beyond that time 100% will show xanthochromia if the sample is examined carefully. A more sensitive technique, such as second derivative spectrophotometry, can increase the ability to detect low levels of xanthochromia.

Protein concentrations greater than 1500 mg/L will also give a slightly xanthochromic appearance to CSF. Hemoglobin from hemolyzed RBCs will appear in CSF after about 10 hours. When a patient is jaundiced (i.e., when serum bilirubin is elevated, as it may be in liver failure), bilirubin may enter the CSF. However, this requires serum bilirubin levels of at least 100 to 150 mg/L before CSF xanthochromia is found.

Proteins of Cerebrospinal Fluid

In disease states the local production or modification of proteins within the CNS may lead to diagnostically useful changes in CSF protein patterns. In general, diseases that interrupt the integrity of the capillary endothelial barrier lead to an increase in total CSF protein. Examples are brain tumor, purulent (bacterial) meningitis, cerebral infarction, and trauma.

Immunoelectrophoresis allows further fractionation of CSF protein constituents. The major *immunoglobulins* in CSF are IgG, IgA, and IgM (with only trace amounts of IgD and IgE). Of all these, IgG is quantitatively the most important. It is often useful to know whether an elevated IgG value is caused by local production of that immunoglobulin within the CNS (as may be the case in some demyelinating diseases such as multiple sclerosis) or by the leakage of IgG

across a damaged blood-brain barrier (as in some infections). Because the normal serum IgG is 15% to 18% of total serum protein and normal CSF IgG is 5% to 12%, the ratio of IgG to total protein is sometimes used to estimate the source of IgG elevation. That is, if the ratio in a sample more nearly approximates the ratio ordinarily found in serum, the IgG is suspected to have been somehow transferred into the CSF from serum. But this is a crude and not especially reliable estimate. A more widely used measure currently is the IgG-albumin index. The formula for determining it is as follows:

$$\text{IgG index} = \frac{\text{IgG (CSF)} \times \text{Albumin (serum)}}{\text{IgG (serum)} \times \text{albumin (CSF)}}$$

The upper reference interval for this index must be determined for each laboratory, but generally it ranges between 0.25 and 0.85. The **IgG index** is elevated in diseases in which there is increased CNS IgG production and an intact blood-brain barrier (as in multiple sclerosis). The IgG index is decreased when the blood-brain barrier is compromised, allowing serum proteins to cross into the CSF (as in strokes, tumors, and some forms of meningitis).

Myelin basic protein (MBP) concentration increase in serum is a potential indicator of demyelination. Myelin is a complex substance that surrounds many CNS axons like the insulation on a wire cable and is necessary for normal conduction of nerve impulses down the axon.

Demyelinating diseases are a group of disorders in which the primary insult is some form of damage to the myelin coating of CNS axons. MBP is a constituent of normal myelin, and has been found to be elevated in a variety of conditions involving myelin damage. Initially it was believed that MBP was specific for multiple sclerosis, but it is now known to be elevated in many CNS disorders.

γ-Globulin Synthesis

Elevations of CSF γ-globulin may be caused by changes in serum proteins, such as the small–molecular-weight Bence

Jones proteins seen in multiple myeloma, which cross the blood-brain barrier and appear in the γ-fraction of CSF proteins. However, there is evidence that local CNS immunoglobulin production occurs in many diseases. Examples include multiple sclerosis, subacute sclerosing panencephalitis (a rare devastating process of myelin damage that occurs in children and young adults in association with greatly elevated CSF measles titers), many chronic and acute infections (neurosyphilis, tuberculous meningitis, abscess, viral meningoencephalitis, and sarcoidosis), and some brain tumors. As a practical point, in those settings in which CSF total protein rises as a result of increased permeability of the blood-brain barrier, the addition of serum protein (which normally contains 15% to 18% γ-globulin) raises the CSF γ-fraction. It thus becomes difficult to estimate the upper reference interval for γ-globulin as a percentage of total protein when total protein is significantly elevated. In any case, when CSF γ-globulin is elevated, a clinician may order a simultaneous serum protein electrophoresis to help determine the source of the increased CSF γ-fraction.

Oligoclonal Bands

The γ-fraction of CSF is composed of a variety of immunoglobulins. Agarose gel electrophoresis performed on concentrated CSF can demonstrate elevation of a population of proteins within the γ-range. When these proteins all share the same electrophoretic mobility they are called *oligoclonal bands*. The population of γ-proteins that separates as oligoclonal bands is believed to derive from a few clones of immunocompetent cells. The appearance of oligoclonal bands has been reported in 79% to 90% of patients with multiple sclerosis and in a variety of CNS inflammatory conditions. Interestingly, this change in the composition of the γ-fraction may occur without any increase in the total γ-globulin concentration.

A final practical point should be made about protein determinations in CSF. When there is blood in the CSF from a traumatic lumbar puncture or bleeding within the nervous system, it is expected that the blood will elevate the CSF protein value. The CSF protein level can still be determined by correcting for the amount of blood present. Simply allow 10 mg/L of protein for every 1000 RBCs/mm^3. For example, if the red cell count is 10,000 in the CSF sample and its total protein is 1000 mg/L, the corrected total protein equals 900 mg/L. The cell count should be performed as rapidly as possible after lumbar puncture, preferably in the first half hour and certainly not later than 2 hours, because hemolysis will occur after that time.

Glucose in Cerebrospinal Fluid

Determination of CSF glucose helps distinguish bacterial from viral meningitis; the glucose value is often quite *low* (less than 40% to 45% of simultaneously analyzed serum glucose) in bacterial meningitis and tuberculous meningitis and is generally normal in viral disease. Carcinomatous meningitis (widespread infiltration of the meninges by tumor cells) also drives CSF glucose values below the normal range.

Thyroid Function Tests

Diseases of the thyroid gland can result in changes of mood that are difficult to distinguish from psychiatric illnesses. Therefore, as part of the diagnostic evaluation of patients newly admitted to psychiatric wards, thyroid tests are ordered to rule out thyroid imbalance as a cause (see p. 838 for recommended thyroid testing).

Toxicology Screen

One of the causes of abnormal behavior is the presence of drugs or toxins in the affected patient. A urine drug screen is frequently ordered by emergency unit physicians to establish drugs as a cause of acute psychoses. These are usually focused to search for a limited number of abused stimulant drugs, such as amphetamines, cocaine, and phencyclidine. Less frequent causes of abnormal behavior or neurological symptoms are the result of heavy metal poisoning. In these cases, analyses of blood lead and urine mercury may be requested.

3-Methoxy-4-hydroxyphenylglycol (MHPG) and 5-Hydroxyindoleacetic acid (5-HIAA)

In years past, investigators attempted to subtype depression based on levels of neurotransmitters that could be measured in the CSF, blood, and urine. This concept followed from the monoamine theory of depression and was intended to help in choosing among medications available at the time, basically the tricyclics and monoamine oxidase inhibitors. Since then, newer generations of effective antidepressants with more benign side effect profiles, managed care pressures to treat patients with as few hospital days as possible, and lack of improved clinical outcomes resulting from such testing have meant that CSF analysis of 5-HIAA and 24-hour urine collections for MHPG are strictly research procedures.

CHANGE OF ANALYTE IN DISEASE: THERAPEUTIC DRUG MONITORING

Therapeutic drug monitoring (TDM) is essential in optimally managing many neurological and psychiatric disorders. The clinician can more readily assess efficacy, toxicity, drug interactions, or the effect of generic substitution when the plasma concentration of the drug is known (see Chapter 56). More advanced tests, such as unbound plasma concentration or measurement of active metabolites, can further refine patient management.

Antiepileptic Drugs

Among neurologists, measurement of plasma concentrations of antiepileptic drugs (AEDs) is probably the most widely used laboratory test. Table 42-4 presents pharmacokinetic data on the most commonly used AEDs. The *therapeutic range* is an important concept but should be used only as a general guide in patient management. The goal of treatment is control of seizures without toxic side effects, and many patients achieve this goal with plasma concentrations of AEDs either below or above the "therapeutic range." Furthermore, several recent studies show that most patients taking a single AED can tolerate plasma concentrations above the therapeutic range and obtain improved seizure control.[12] AEDs are now widely used for nervous system disorders other than epilepsy like pain, headache, and bipolar disorder. It is unknown whether AED "therapeutic range" for these disorders is the same as for epilepsy treatment. Thus, AED plasma concentrations can be quite useful to the clinician; however, decisions about patient management should always combine information about the patient's clinical state with plasma-concentration data.

Plasma concentrations of AEDs should always be interpreted with knowledge of whether the patient has taken the drug over a long enough period to have reached a steady-state concentration, especially with AEDs that have a longer half-life (Table 42-4). This is even more important in the case of phenytoin, which shows saturable metabolism and can have a half-life that ranges from a few days to several weeks, depending on the plasma concentration. AEDs with a shorter half-life (valproate or carbamazepine) may show substantial variation between peak and trough concentrations. Carbamazepine plasma concentrations may fall after the first 2 to 3 weeks of use because of the drug's induction of liver enzymes that speed its metabolism. Plasma concentrations of AEDs that cause toxicity are generally close to concentrations that are needed for seizure control; thus, frequent plasma AED determinations may be necessary when generic AED substitutions are used.

Measurement of non–protein bound (free) AED plasma concentrations are useful when patients receive phenytoin or valproate in combination with other drugs, in patients with renal or hepatic failure, or in patients with hypoalbuminemia. In these instances the free plasma drug concentration may increase and produce toxic symptoms while the total plasma concentration remains unchanged. Active metabolites of primidone, carbamazepine (especially carbamazepine 10,11-epoxide), and possibly valproate can produce toxicity, and measurement of these metabolites may improve patient management in selected cases. The new AED, oxcarbazepine, is rapidly metabolized to a mono-hydroxy derivative bypassing production of carbamazepine 10, 11-epoxide, and thus avoiding some of the toxicity associated with use of carbamazepine.

Antipsychotic Medication

Antipsychotics, also known as *neuroleptics*, are a heterogeneous group of medications used to treat psychosis associated with schizophrenia, depression, dementia, and nonspecific agitation. They may also be useful in a variety of movement disorders such as Huntington's disease, tic disorders, and Tourette's syndrome.

Neuroleptics include the drug class phenothiazines, all of which share the three-ring phenothiazine structure but differ in the side-chain varieties (Table 42-5).

Clozapine (a dibenzodiazepine), quetiapine (a dibenzothiazine), olanzapine (a thienobenzodiazepine), risperidone (a benzisoxazole), and ziprasidone (a benzothiazolylpiperazine) are all atypical compounds in use in the United States. None of these medications require therapeutic blood levels for effective dosing, but patients receiving clozapine are

TABLE 42-4 COMMONLY USED ANTIEPILEPTIC DRUGS

Antiepileptic Drug	Trade Name	"Recommended" Therapeutic Range (μg/mL)*	Approximate Time to Steady State (Days)	Protein Binding	Other
Phenytoin	Dilantin	10 to 20	3 to 21[†]	High	
Carbamazepine	Tegretol Carbatrol	4 to 12 (10 to 11 epoxide)	3 to 5	Medium	Active metabolite
Primidone	Mysoline	5 to 12	1 to 2	Low	Metabolized to PEMA and phenobarbital
Phenobarbital		10 to 40	15 to 25	Low	
Valproate	Depakene	50 to 100	2 to 5	High	Saturable protein binding
Divalproex	Depakote	50 to 120			
Ethosuximide	Zarontin	40 to 100	7 to 13	Low	Associated with aplastic anemia and hepatic failure
Felbamate	Felbatol	NE	4 to 5	Low	
Gabapentin	Neurontin	NE	1 to 2	None	Not liver metabolized
Topiramate	Topamax	NE	4 to 5	Low	
Tiagabine	Gabitril	NE	1 to 2	High	
Lamotrigine	Lamictal	NE	4 to 5	Low	Concentrations increased twofold when used with valproate
Levetiracetam	Keppra	NE	1 to 2	None	Not liver metabolized
Oxcarbazepine	Trileptal	NE	2 to 3	Low	Rapidly metabolized to active compound
Zonisamide	Zonegran	NE	10 to 15	Low	

NE, Not established.
*See text under Antiepileptic Drugs.
[†]Exhibits saturable metabolism, so time to steady state increases as plasma concentration increases.

followed with bimonthly WBC counts because of the risk of aplastic anemia associated with this compound.

Another major group of neuroleptics are the butyrophenones such as droperidol, haloperidol, and pimozide, which have structures dissimilar to those of the phenothiazines. At present haloperidol is the most widely prescribed conventional neuroleptic in the United States. Atypical antipsychotics, with their lower risk of EPS and TD, may soon replace the conventional antipsychotics for most patients.

There is no correlation between blood concentrations of neuroleptic drugs and clinical response.

It has been suggested that a plasma level of 5 to 20 ng/mL is the optimal therapeutic window for haloperidol treatment of psychotic symptoms and schizophrenia. Haloperidol levels above 20 ng/mL are linked to subjective and objective medication side effects such as dysphoria, hypotension, and parkinsonian effects (extrapyramidal), which may interfere with a therapeutic response. In clinical practice, blood concentrations of neuroleptics are rarely obtained.

Antidepressant Medications

The selective serotonin reuptake inhibitors include fluoxetine, sertraline, paroxetine, fluvoxamine, and citalopram. The norepinephrine-serotonin reuptake inhibitors include venlafaxine, mirtazine, and nefazodone. The only dopaminergic antidepressant is bupropion.

Typical doses and side effects of these medications are listed in Table 42-5. Therapeutic drug monitoring is not typically useful with these medications. The possibility exists for interactions based on cytochrome P-450 enzyme subtypes used to metabolize each drug. For instance, the competition for SSRI metabolism by CYP 3A4 means that if tricyclics are used concurrently, blood concentrations of the tricyclic will rise by as much as 50%. Blood monitoring is not necessary as a rule but clinicians must be alert to reported side effects and must use caution in giving tricyclics to any patient with compromised myocardium.

Tricyclic antidepressants. Apart from reuptake blockade of serotonin and norepinephrine, the tricyclic antidepressant medications block α-adrenergic, muscarinic, and histaminic receptors to a variable degree resulting in the medication side effects such as orthostatic hypotension, dry mouth, constipation, and sedation (Table 42-5). Tricyclic antidepressants are absorbed from the gastrointestinal tract to a variable and incomplete degree. Protein binding appears to be 75%, and the medications are highly lipid soluble. In the liver, tertiary amines (amitriptyline and imipramine) are desmethylated to secondary amines (nortriptyline and desipramine) that are active metabolites. Half-life lies between 10 hours and 70 hours and can be even longer as with nortriptyline and protriptyline. Steady-state plasma levels are achieved within 5 to 7 days, and once-a-day dosage is possible.

TABLE 42-5   ANTIDEPRESSANT MEDICATIONS

Medication	Typical Dose Range (mg)	Dosing	Common Side Effects
Fluoxetine	5 to 80	Once daily, usually AM	Insomnia, agitation in patients with anxiety, emotional blunting
Paroxetine	5 to 80	Once daily, usually at night	Sedation, possible weight gain
Sertraline	12.5 to 250	Once daily	+/- Agitation in anxious patients
Fluvoxamine	25 to 300	Once daily, usually at night	Insomnia or sedation
Citalopram	10 to 80	Once daily	Sedation
Venlafaxine extended release	37.5 to 375	Once daily, usually AM	Sweating, insomnia, early nausea
Bupropion sustained release	100 to 450	Twice daily, second dose before 6 pm	Agitation, insomnia, no antianxiety effect
Nefazodone	50 to 600	Twice daily, though may be given once at night only	Agitation (mCPP metabolite may be anxiogenic) or sedation
Mirtazapine	15 to 90	Once daily at night	Sedation, weight gain
Tricyclics (imipramine, clomipramine, desipramine, amitriptyline, nortriptyline)	10 to 150 for nortriptyline, 10 to 300 for all others	Once daily, usually at night	Dry mouth, increased heart rate, orthostatic hypotension, dizziness, constipation, increased sweating, blurred vision, weight gain
Monoamine oxidase inhibitors	30 to 60 for Parnate 60 to 90 for Nardil	Three times daily	Dry mouth, blurred vision, constipation, weight gain, orthostatic hypotension; hypertensive crisis if combined with tyramine-containing foods or serotonergic/stimulant medications
Trazodone	25 to 600	Once daily, at night	Sedation; often used as hypnotic in subtherapeutic doses

The dosage range for most tricyclic antidepressants usually lies between 50 and 300 mg/day, depending on age, body weight, and liver and renal function. The notable exceptions are nortriptyline and protriptyline, both of which have dosage requirements between 50 and 150 mg/day. The linkage between plasma levels of tricyclics and their clinical response appears clearest in patients with major depression. For most tricyclic antidepressants, the relationship between response and plasma level appears sigmoidal (Fig. 42-6). Yet, for nortriptyline and to a lesser extent protriptyline, the relationship is curvilinear, and when plasma levels are above the therapeutic range the clinical response falls dramatically and side effects are more prominent.

Monoamine oxidase inhibitors. There are two classes of monoamine oxidase inhibitors (MAOIs): the *hydrazine class*, which includes isocarboxazid and phenelzine, and the *nonhydrazine class*, which includes tranylcypromine. The clinical effects of these and other antidepressant medications take 2 to 3 weeks to develop for reasons that are not understood. MAOIs are completely absorbed in the gastrointestinal tract. Metabolism occurs in the liver by acetylation. The half-life is extremely variable because up to 50% of Caucasians and more than 50% of people of Asian descent are slow acetylators. Dosage range is from 30 to 60 mg/day for isocarboxazid and tranylcypromine and 45 to 90 mg/day for phenelzine.

The side effects and dietary restrictions required for patients receiving the MAOIs has limited use of this class of drug. Tyramine, which is usually broken down in the gastrointestinal tract by monoamine oxidase A, must be eliminated from the diet, otherwise rapid and dangerous elevation of blood pressure can occur. Tyramine is found in large quantities in cured foods such as beer, wine, cheese, and sausage. Another factor limiting use of MAOIs is the potential for dangerous interactions with other antidepressants. MAOIs cannot be used concurrently with the SSRIs, nefazodone, venlafaxine, mirtazapine, or bupropion. If these drugs are being used, they must be tapered off before starting an MAOI. This is not a serious problem for drugs with shorter half-lives, but the long half-life of fluoxetine means that the patient must be off fluoxetine for at least 4 weeks before beginning an MAOI. Tricyclics can be combined with the MAOIs, typically with the tricyclic started first and the MAOI added. There is no relationship between MAOI plasma level and response rate.

Anxiolytics

As mentioned above, the SSRI and SNRI medications, as well as the tricyclics and MAOIs, all are effective anxiolytics, and the newer agents are now used as first-line treatment for the anxiety disorders. Only the serotonergic medications are helpful in obsessive-compulsive disorder. The benzodiazepines and buspirone are sometimes used as sole treatment for the anxiety disorders, but more commonly as adjunctive treatment for anxiety, affective, and psychotic disorders. Benzodiazepines are also used to aid in alcohol withdrawal.

All benzodiazepines share the same three-ring structure, but differ mainly in substitutions on the heptagonal ring. There are three established subgroups: (1) the 2-ketobenzodiazepines including chlordiazepoxide, diazepam, and prazepam, which are oxidized in the liver to desmethyldiazepam (active metabolite) with a half-life of 60 hours, (2) the 3-hydroxybenzodiazepines (oxazepam, lorazepam, and temazepam), metabolized in the liver with a half-life of 9 to 15 hours, and (3) the triazolobenzodiazepines (alprazolam and triazolam), metabolized in the liver with a 3- to 8-hour half-life. Oxazepam is the safest benzodiazepine to use in

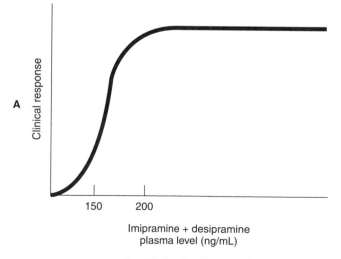

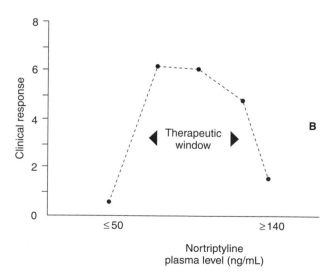

Fig. 42-6 **A,** Sigmoidal relationships between clinical response and imipramine plus desipramine plasma levels. **B,** Curvilinear relationship between clinical response and nortriptyline plasma levels. *(From Schatzberg AF, Cole JO, DeBattista C: Manual of clinical psychopharmacology, ed 3, Washington, DC, 1997, American Psychiatric Press [www.appi.org].)*

patients with liver disease, because it is excreted by the kidney after glucuronidation.

The most common side effects include sedation at low doses, ataxia at higher doses, and respiratory suppression at toxic doses. Generally, it is believed that these drugs have a wide safety margin and overdose only rarely leads to lethal outcome. An important recent development is the availability of a benzodiazepine antagonist, flumazenil, which can be used acutely in benzodiazepine overdose.

Maximum doses for the individual benzodiazepines differ widely, from 6 mg/day for alprazolam to 200 mg/day for chlordiazepoxide. Unlike other psychiatric medications discussed in this section, benzodiazepines have potentially strong addictive properties causing psychological and physical drug dependence and possible withdrawal upon cessation of the drug. Therapeutic plasma concentrations of benzodiazepines have not been established, except for clonazepam, which is also used as an antiepileptic.

Apart from the benzodiazepines, buspirone is the other commonly used class of anxiolytics. It is a nonbenzodiazepine, nonsedating anxiolytic. This drug probably does not act directly through the GABA receptor complex. It is believed that dopaminergic pathways might mediate its anxiolytic effects. The daily dosage ranges from 5 to 40 mg. Side effects upon use include nausea and headaches. Plasma levels are not in use at the present time.

Mood Stabilizers

This group of drugs includes lithium carbonate, carbamazepine, valproate, olanzapine, lamotrigine, gabapentin, and topiramate. Their therapeutic use in psychiatry is for treatment of bipolar disorder, schizoaffective disorder, intermittent explosive disorder, posttraumatic stress disorder, and unstable behavior related to personality disorders.

Physiologically, *lithium* ions are indistinguishable from sodium and replace sodium along cell membranes. The exact mode of lithium action is unknown. Because lithium replaces sodium throughout the whole body, its side effects may involve most organ systems. Neurological effects such as tremor, ataxia, confusion, sedation at higher and toxic levels, and encephalopathy in conjunction with haloperidol administration have been described. Long-term lithium treatment can result in hyperthyroidism from a nontoxic goiter. Renal effects such as polyuria with secondary polydipsia, renal diabetes insipidus, and interstitial nephritis are also occasionally seen.

Dosage range is 600 to 2100 mg/day in two or three divided doses. Plasma levels should be measured approximately 12 hours after the previous dose to obtain a trough value. Plasma levels from 0.8 to 1.5 mEq/L have been shown to produce a therapeutic response in the treatment of acute mania. Slightly lower lithium levels have been recommended for maintenance treatment of bipolar disorders and treatment of other conditions. The maintenance plasma level of lithium used is often limited by subjective side effects and by development of thyroid or renal impairment. Lithium is frequently used in conjunction with other mood stabilizers in patients with severe forms of bipolar disorder.

Carbamazepine, valproate, lamotrigine, gabapentin, and topiramate are used as antiepileptics but recently have found increasing use in psychiatry for disorders such as rapid cycling bipolar disorder, depressed bipolar disorder, and intermittent explosive disorder. Although these medications may be used in addition to lithium, and can be used in combination with one another, only valproate and carbamazepine are recommended for use as first-line medication.

The dosage and plasma level ranges, particularly for valproate and carbamazepine, are similar to their use as antiepileptics. (For dose ranges and side effects see Table 42-4.)

References

1. Kendler KS et al: Outcome and family study of the subtypes of schizophrenia in the west of Ireland, *Am J Psychiatry* 151:849, 1994.
2. Kety SS et al: Mental illness in the biological and adoptive relatives of schizophrenic adoptees: replication of the Copenhagen study in the rest of Denmark, *Arch Gen Psychiatry* 51:442, 1994.
3. Davis K et al: Dopamine in schizophrenia, *Am J Psychiatry* 148:1474, 1991.
4. Kendler KS, Thornton LM, Gardner CO: Genetic risk, number of previous depressive episodes, and stressful life events in predicting onset of major depression, *Am J Psychiatry* 158:582, 2001.
5. Blackwood DHR, Visscher PM, Muir WJ: Genetic studies of bipolar affective disorder in large families, *Br J Psychiatry* 178(suppl 41):s134, 2001.
6. Higley JD et al: Excessive mortality in young free-ranging male non-human primates with low cerebrospinal fluid 5-hydroxyindoleacetic acid concentrations, *Arch Gen Psychiatry* 53:537, 1996.
7. Stanley B et al: Association of aggressive behavior with altered serotonergic function in patients who are not suicidal, *Am J Psychiatry* 157:609, 2000.
8. Bremner JD et al: Hippocampal volume reduction in major depression, *Am J Psychiatry* 157:115, 2000.
9. Stahl SM: Essential psychopharmacology, ed 2, Cambridge, UK, 2000, Cambridge University Press.
10. Zobel AW et al: Cortisol response in the combined dexamethasone/CRH test as predictor of relapse in patients with remitted depression: a prospective study, *J Psychiatric Res* 35:83, 2001.
11. Coryell W, Schlesser M: The dexamethasone suppression test and suicide prediction, *Am J Psychiatry* 158:748, 2001.
12. Lesser RP et al: High-dose monotherapy in treatment of intractable seizures, *Neurology* 34:707, 1984.

Bibliography

Beckman H, Goodman FK: Antidepressant response to tricyclics and urinary MHPG in unipolar patients, *Arch Gen Psychiatry* 32:17, 1975.
Binder SR et al: Standardization of multi-wavelength UV detector for liquid chromatography–based toxicological analysis, *J Chromatogr* 550:449, 1991.
Fishman RA: *Cerebrospinal fluid in diseases of the nervous system*, Philadelphia, 1980, Saunders.
Garvey M et al: Response of depression to very high plasma levels of imipramine plus desipramine, *Biol Psychiatry* 30:57, 1991.
Kaplan H, Sadock B: *Clinical psychiatry*, Baltimore, 1988, Williams & Wilkins.

Pesce AJ, Kaplan LA: *Laboratory medicine: a scientific and managerial infobase*, V5.O, Cincinnati, 2003, Pesce Kaplan Publishers.

Peter JG: *Use and interpretation of tests in neuroimmunology*, Santa Monica, CA, 1991, Specialty Laboratories.

Plum F, Posner JB: *The diagnosis of stupor and coma*, ed 3, Philadelphia, 1980, FA Davis.

Rowland LP, editor: *Merritt's textbook of neurology*, ed 8, Philadelphia, 1989, Lea & Febiger.

Schildkraut JJ et al: Biochemical discrimination of subgroups of depressive disorders based on differences in catecholamine metabolism. In Usdin E, Hanin I, editors: *Biological markers in psychiatry and neurology*, New York, 1982, Pergamon Press.

van Putten T et al: Haloperidol plasma levels and clinical response, *Am J Psychiatry* 149:500, 1992.

Wu AHB et al: Evaluation of the triage system for emergency drugs-of-abuse testing in urine, *J Anal Toxicol* 17:241, 1993.

Internet Sites

http://www.ninds.nih.gov/—National Institute of Neurological Disorders and Stroke

http://www.nimh.nih.gov/—National Institute of Mental Health

http://www.nimh.nih.gov/publicat/depressionmenu.cfm—NIMH publications on depression

http://www.mic.ki.se/Diseases/c10.html—Karolinska Institute Library, Stockholm, Sweden

http://www.vh.org/Providers/Teaching Files/CNSInfDisR2/IDCNSHomePg.html—University of Iowa Virtual Hospital: Infectious Diseases of the Central Nervous System

http://www.nda.ox.ac.uk/wfsa/html/u05/u05_010.htm—World Federation of Societies of Anaesthesiologists: The Autonomic Nervous System

http://www.kumc.edu/instruction/medicine/anatomy/histoweb/nervous/nervous.htm—University of Kansas Medical Center, Department of Anatomy and Cell Biology: Nervous System

http://weavernt.med.utah.edu/kw/neuro.html—Knowledge Weavers, Spencer S. Eccles Health Sciences Library at the University of Utah: Neuroanatomy

http://www.merck.com/pubs/mmanual/section14/sec14.htm—The Merck Manual, Section 14: Neurological Disorders

http://www.drada.org/—Depression and Related Affective Disorders Association

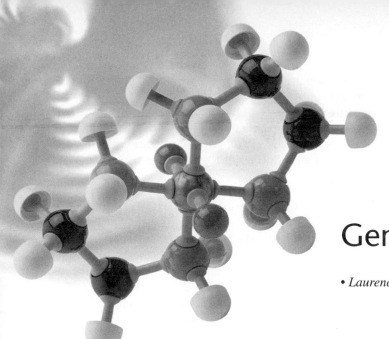

CHAPTER 43

General Endocrinology

• *Laurence M. Demers*

Chapter Outline

Objectives

- Describe the mechanism of action of steroid and peptide hormones.
- Describe the regulatory control of hormone biosynthesis and release.
- List the hypothalamic factors and the pituitary hormones they control.

- Describe the pathological conditions of pituitary deficiency and excess.
- List the major hormones that provide an assessment of pituitary function.

Key Terms

acromegaly A pathological state in adults that is associated with hypersecretion of growth hormone.

adenohypophysis The anterior lobe of the pituitary gland, which secretes trophic hormones.

amenorrhea The absence of a menstrual cycle and menstrual period.

autocrine factor A cellular factor that interacts with receptors that are found on the same cell that released the factor.

bioavailable hormone A hormone in the circulation, whether free or weakly bound to plasma proteins, that is available for tissue receptor binding and cell uptake.

cytokines Peptides synthesized and released by white blood cells and tissue macrophages that stimulate or suppress the functional activity of lymphocytes, monocytes, neutrophils, fibroblast cells, and endothelial cells.

endocrine gland   A specialized gland that releases hormones into the circulation, affecting a tissue or organ at a distal site.

feedback loop   A loop integrating two endocrine glands by means of a positive or negative hormone signal.

galactorrhea   An uncontrolled secretion of fluid from the breast.

G-protein   A regulatory protein found in the membrane of all mammalian cells that acts to transmit an extracellular hormone signal to inner membrane factors as part of a cell-membrane transduction signaling system.

hormone   A chemical substance released by an endocrine gland into the circulation.

hormone transport   The mechanism by which hormones are carried in the bloodstream, bound to protein carriers.

intracrine factor   A cytosolic factor made by a cell that travels to the nucleus and binds to a specific receptor on DNA to regulate gene activity.

juxtacrine factor   A membrane-bound growth factor that interacts with the membrane receptor of a neighboring cell by direct cell-to-cell contact.

neurohypophysis   The posterior part of the pituitary gland that is an extension of the central nervous system.

paracrine factor   A factor that is released by one cell in a tissue and binds to receptors of a different cell in that same tissue.

peptide hormones   Hormones that are made from amino acids by specialized endocrine glands and are released into the circulation to interact with membrane-bound receptors of other tissues and organs.

pituitary adenoma   A tumor of the pituitary that produces excess amounts of a particular pituitary hormone.

pituitary portal circulation   The vascular channel connecting the hypothalamus with the anterior pituitary.

pulsatile release   The release of hypothalamic and pituitary hormones in short bursts, or pulses, during the course of a 24-hour day. The amplitude and frequency of the pulse is unique to each hormone.

receptors   Specific cytosolic and membrane proteins that bind a hormone or growth factor with high specificity and affinity.

releasing factors   Peptides synthesized by the hypothalamus and released into the portal circulation to affect pituitary hormone synthesis and secretion.

steroids   Hormones that are made by endocrine glands from cholesterol and that have as a basic structure the cyclopentanophenanthrene nucleus.

Methods on CD-ROM

Follicle-stimulating hormone (FSH)
Luteinizing hormone (LH)

Thyroid-stimulating hormone (TSH)

FUNDAMENTALS OF ENDOCRINOLOGY

The endocrine system comprises part of the extracellular communication system within the body that links the brain to organs and functions that control body metabolism, growth and development, and reproduction. The other two major components of this communication system, the central nervous system and the immune system, are also linked to the endocrine system as part of the brain's overall control of bodily function. The endocrine system itself functions through an elaborate network of chemical messengers called **hormones** that are produced by highly specialized endocrine organs. The location of the **endocrine glands** is shown in Fig. 43-1. The hormones enter the circulation to effect their action at a site usually distant from their site of production. Hormones interact with specific **receptors** within or on the target cell, conferring the selectivity of hormone action. The traditional definition of endocrinology, that is, the study of hormone action distal to the site of hormone production, has become obscured in recent years because we now recognize the important local, or autocrine, effects of hormone metabolism and action within a given endocrine gland or tissue. In addition, many growth factors produced locally by specific cells elicit a network of cellular communication akin to the hormone receptor interactive event. Many of the biological effects of hormones are produced at the target site through local metabolism of hormone precursor substances. The local biosynthesis of estrogen from steroid precursor substrates such as androstenedione and the formation of triiodothyronine from T_4 are examples of local hormone synthesis at the target cell.

Control of the endocrine system is affected primarily by its linkage to the central nervous system through the hypothalamus and pituitary glands. This aspect of the endocrine system is referred to as the neuroendocrine system and involves an intimate relationship between neurosecretory chemicals formed in the brain and hormonal factors produced by

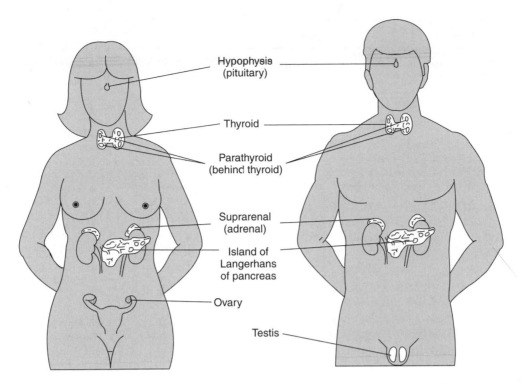

Fig. 43-1 Location of endocrine glands. *(From Toporek M: Basic chemistry of life, St Louis, 1980, Mosby.)*

the endocrine organs located within the brain. It is now evident that the immune system also acts at nerve centers of the brain to facilitate the orchestration of hormone signals, both positive and negative, by the elaboration of a network of **cytokine** factors produced both by endocrine tissues and immunocompetent cells residing in the brain.

The Chemical Nature of Hormones

Hormones are divided into basically two broad classes, peptides and **steroids**. Most hormones are amino acid and peptide in nature, ranging from complex carbohydrate-polypeptide molecules, such as human chorionic gonadotropin, to single amino acid moieties such as the catecholamines. Steroids are all derived from cholesterol and are subdivided into two types, those containing an intact cyclopentanophenanthrene nucleus, such as adrenal and gonadal steroids, and those such as vitamin D that have an alteration in the B ring of the basic phenanthrene nucleus. It is the chemical makeup of the hormone that is integral to its ability to interact with a specific tissue-based receptor to bring about hormone action. For example, the simple lack of a methyl group between the A and B rings of a steroid molecule, along with a saturated A ring, determines the difference between a female steroid hormone such as estradiol and the male hormone testosterone. It is this subtle chemical difference and the presence of highly specific protein receptors in tissues that allow the hormone to recognize a particular tissue or organ and invoke its biological effect. A list of the major peptide and steroid hormones and their primary sites of action is shown in Table 43-1.

Mechanisms of Hormone Action

All hormones act on their respective target glands and tissues through highly specific binding proteins, called *receptors*, located either on the surface of the cell membrane or within the cytosol of the target cell. The binding of a hormone to its specific receptor serves as an initial signal to a cell. An amplification of the signal then ensues, involving many intermediate messenger signals. These signals ultimately impact on the nucleus of the target cell to elicit an alteration in gene expression, resulting in the synthesis of a specific mRNA message and new protein synthesis. Figs. 43-2 and 43-3 provide examples of hormone binding and the mechanism of hormone action as they are currently understood.

Steroid hormones. All steroid hormones interact with their target cells by binding to specific protein receptors located in both the cytoplasmic and nuclear fractions of the cells (Fig. 43-2). Each steroid-responsive tissue contains a finite concentration of receptor protein with an affinity constant that is greater than that of other steroid binders such as the transport proteins. Transport proteins, which are found in the circulation, carry steroids from the organ of synthesis to the target organ or tissue. The higher affinity of the receptor protein enables the tissue to sequestrate a specific steroid from the hormone's specific carrier protein as the tissue is perfused with blood containing the circulating steroid.

Steroids enter the cell primarily through diffusion, bind to the receptor molecule, and produce a conformational change in the receptor structure. This conformational change in the receptor activates the receptor complex, forming a trans-

TABLE 43-1 STEROID AND PEPTIDE HORMONES

Hormone	Source	Target Organ	Circulating Level	Biological Effect
Steroid Hormones				
Androgens				
Testosterone (dihydrotestosterone)	Testis	Accessory sex glands	3.0 to 10.0 ng/mL	Male, secondary sex characteristics, protein anabolism
DHEAS (dehydroepiandrosterone sulfate)	Adrenal	Liver, fat tissue	1500 to 4000 ng/mL	Androgen substrate
Estrogens				
Estradiol	Ovary	Accessory sex glands, liver, brain	50 to 300 pg/mL	Female, secondary sex characteristics
Estrone	Ovary, fat tissue	Accessory sex glands	50 to 200 pg/mL	Estradiol substrate
Progesterone	Ovary	Uterus, breast, brain	5 to 20 ng/mL	Pregnancy hormone
Adrenal steroids				
Cortisol	Adrenal	Liver, muscle, brain, fat tissue	50 to 250 µg/L	Gluconeogenesis, immune system control
Aldosterone	Adrenal	Kidney	50 to 300 ng/L	Salt homeostasis
Peptide Hormones				
Anterior pituitary				
TSH (thyroid-stimulating hormone)	Anterior pituitary	Thyroid gland	0.4 to 4.0 µU/mL	Biosynthesis of thyroid hormones
ACTH (adrenocorticotropic hormone)	Anterior pituitary	Adrenal	25 to 80 pg/mL	Biosynthesis of adrenocortical hormones
FSH (follicle-stimulating hormone)	Anterior pituitary	Ovary/testis	5 to 20 mIU/mL	Follicular development, ovary and sperm formation, testis
LH (luteinizing hormone)	Anterior pituitary	Ovary/testis	5 to 25 mIU/mL	Corpus luteum, ovary Leydig cell, testis
Prolactin	Anterior pituitary	Mammary gland, uterus, ovary, testis	5 to 20 ng/mL	Mammary gland development, ovary and testis steroid production
GH (growth hormone)	Anterior pituitary	All tissues	2 to 5 ng/mL	Tissue growth, fat and carbohydrate metabolism
Posterior pituitary				
AVP (arginine vasopressin)	Posterior pituitary	Kidney	2 to 8 pg/mL	Water homeostatis
Oxytocin	Posterior pituitary	Breast, uterus	1 to 5 pg/mL	Milk secretion, uterine contractility
Calcitropic hormones				
PTH (parathyroid hormone)	Parathyroid	Bone, kidney, intestine	10 to 55 pg/mL	Calcium homeostasis
Calcitonin	Thyroid	Bone	0 to 50 pg/mL	Calcium regulation
Pancreatic hormones				
Insulin	Pancreas	Most tissues	6 to 25 µU/mL	Carbohydrate metabolism
Glucagon	Pancreas	Liver	50 to 100 pg/mL	Glycogenolysis
Gastrointestinal hormones				
Gastrin	Stomach	Stomach	30 to 150 pg/mL	Acid secretion
Secretin	Small intestine	Stomach, pancreas	0 to 50 pg/mL	Stomach and pancreatic fluid secretion
Thyroid hormones				
T_4 (thyroxine)	Thyroid	All tissues	40 to 120 µg/L	Basal metabolism
T_3 (triiodothyronine)	Thyroid	All tissues	800 to 2200 ng/L	Basal metabolism

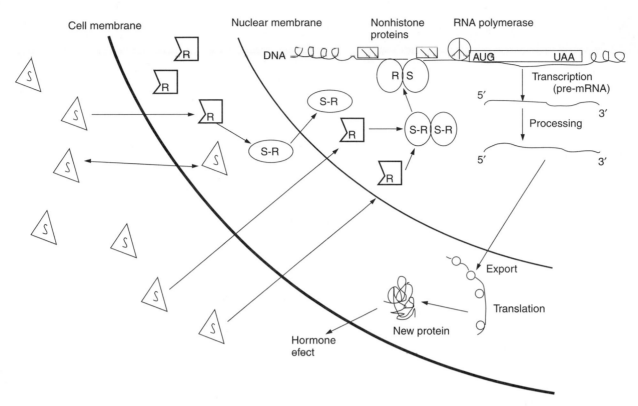

Fig. 43-2 Current proposed mechanism of action of steroid hormones (estrogens, androgens, progesterone, glucocorticoids, aldosterone). Steroids, *S*, diffuse across the plasma membrane and bind to a cytosolic protein receptor, *R*. Steroid binding activates the receptor complex, which then translocates to the nucleus of the cell, where it interacts with chromatin at a specific binding site on DNA called the *steroid-response element*. This binding activates the transcription of specific genes involved in steroid hormone action. Transcription of messenger RNA then takes place with the eventual synthesis of specific proteins by the cells that are linked to steroid hormone action.

formed receptor-steroid activated complex. This complex has a high affinity for nuclear binding sites on chromatin and binds to both regulatory and nonregulatory DNA sequences in the 5′ end of the responsive gene element. Binding of the transformed receptor-steroid complex to the regulatory elements of the gene results in gene activation and subsequently the synthesis of specific proteins. The net result is altered cell metabolism, which can lead to cell growth and differentiation and the secretion of specific cell products. All steroid hormones interact with their receptor complexes in a similar fashion. Thus the interaction is much the same for a cortisol-activated event as it is for estrogen acting to promote uterine cell growth.

Although we speak of cytosol receptors for steroids, it is important to understand that thyroid hormone also exerts its biological effect through a cytosol-receptor complex with translocation of the complex to the nucleus in a fashion quite similar to that of the steroid hormones. Under certain circumstances, the measurement of tissue steroid receptor levels is used for determining the course of treatment for certain malignancies. In the case of breast cancer, estrogen and progesterone tissue receptor levels are important prognostically, and they facilitate categorization of the

subtype of breast cancer. Normal breast tissue contains very small amounts of estrogen and progesterone-receptor proteins. Certain forms of breast cancer demonstrate an increase in the level of breast tissue steroid-receptor protein. These breast cancers are termed *hormone-dependent*. They require a particular modality of antihormonal therapy for the patient. Hormone ablative therapy (reduction of hormone levels) thus becomes an alternative means of chemotherapy for the patient. This therapy is based on the use of drugs that either inhibit the binding of estrogen to its receptor or inhibit the biosynthesis of estrogenic hormones. Thus the measurement of breast tissue steroid-receptor protein content has proved to be an important clinical tool in categorizing the subtype of hormone-dependent breast cancer and helping to select appropriate antihormonal therapy for these patients.

Peptide hormones. **Peptide hormones** interact with cellular receptors located on the surface of the cell membrane, in contrast to the intracellular cytoplasmic receptors that bind steroid and thyroid hormones. The receptor protein for peptide hormones comprises three areas, or domains—an extracellular hormone-binding domain, a transmembrane spanning domain, and the intracellular kinase domain. The receptor mechanism located in the cell membrane appears to

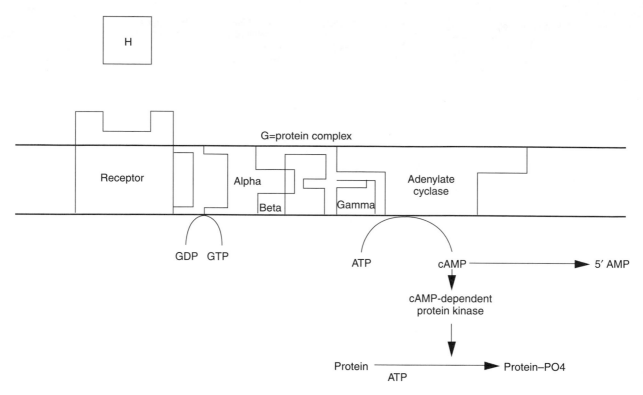

Fig. 43-3 Current proposed mechanism of action of peptide hormones. Peptide hormones bind to a specific receptor on the external domain of the plasma membrane. Hormone binding causes activation of a G-protein complex in the cell membrane that is coupled to and activates the enzyme adenylate cyclase. When the catalytic component of adenylate cyclase is activated, ATP is converted into cyclic AMP, which in turn activates cAMP-dependent protein kinase, resulting in protein phosphorylation and expression of the peptide hormone effect.

be much more complex than the cytosolic-based receptor mechanism. The signaling mechanism involved with peptide hormone-receptor interaction includes postreceptor cascade events that involve multiple effector systems such as the cyclic nucleotides, arachidonic acid metabolites, **G-proteins**, and inositol phospholipids. These signaling systems act as secondary messengers that transmit the signal of the initial receptor-hormone interaction to other areas of the cell. In many cases, when the hormone binds to the extracellular domain of the membrane-bound receptor, a membrane-bound intermediate signal is activated that translates the signal to an intracellular event. This membrane-bound signal transducer is often a guanine nucleotide-binding regulatory protein (G-protein). The G-protein is coupled to the adenylate cyclase and phospholipase enzyme systems that activate subsequent intracellular protein kinases to transmit the biological response. Some receptor systems contain the effector component as part of the intrinsic structure of the receptor. Most of the growth factors, such as insulin, insulin-like growth factor, and epidermal growth factor, interact with a surface receptor that has inherent protein tyrosine kinase enzyme activity within the intracellular domain of the receptor. An example of the G-protein-membrane receptor complex and the activation sequence by a peptide hormone is shown in Fig. 43-3.

Regulatory Control of Hormone Synthesis and Release

Feedback control mechanism. A unique feature of the endocrine system is its ability to regulate itself by providing negative or positive feedback stimuli to each gland that produces a secretory hormone. All hormone production comes under some form of feedback control. A "feedback" control system requires two production units, in which the product of one unit directly affects the production of the other unit. The products of the two units comprise the two halves of a continuous **feedback loop**. The product of one unit usually causes the second unit to increase the production of its product. The second unit's product "feeds back" to the original unit to control the output of that unit. Most often, the feedback is negative; that is, the product of the second gland causes a decrease in the hormone release from the first gland. This negative-feedback loop, in turn, results in a diminished stimulation of the second gland. Under normal physiological conditions, the overall effect of the two parts of the feedback loops in the endocrine system is to maintain relatively constant levels of circulating hormones.

Hormone feedback to the hypothalamus-pituitary axis from endocrine glands is the most well-known feedback loop; however, other feedback loops exist in endocrinology—for example, calcium feedback to the parathyroid glands to

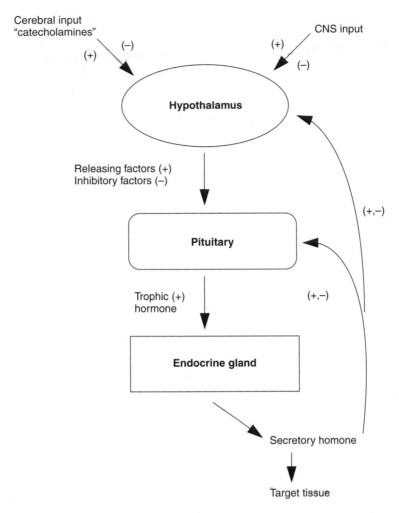

Cerebral input
"catecholamines"

CNS input

(+) (−)

(+) (−)

Hypothalamus

Releasing factors (+)
Inhibitory factors (−)

Pituitary

(+,−)

Trophic (+)
hormone

(+,−)

Endocrine gland

Secretory homone

Target tissue

Fig. 43-4　Regulatory feedback loops of the hypothalamic-pituitary–target organ axis. The hypothalamus receives neural and sensory input to produce pituitary hormone-releasing and inhibitory peptides and factors. The pituitary responds by releasing trophic hormones that act on specific endocrine glands or tissues to promote primary gland hormone synthesis and release. The secretory hormone from the endocrine organ negatively feeds back to the higher centers of control to maintain a homeostatic balance of hormone in the circulation.

reduce PTH secretion and glucose feedback control of pancreatic insulin secretion. When studying endocrine feedback control, however, the paradigm is usually the hypothalamic-pituitary-endocrine gland axis (Fig. 43-4). Hormone output from the target endocrine gland, such as the thyroid gland, adrenal gland, or the gonads, is controlled primarily by negative feedback to the hypothalamus and the pituitary, which maintain central nervous system (CNS) control over the circulating level of each gland's hormone. When circulating hormone levels decline, the hypothalamus rapidly senses the decline in hormone output and increases its production of hypothalamus-based **releasing factors** that enter the portal circulation in the brain to stimulate pituitary hormone synthesis and secretion and reestablish normal hormone output. This stimulus is termed a *positive-feedback loop*. Conversely, when the hormone output from the endocrine gland becomes excessive, the high levels of circulating

hormone feedback negatively to the hypothalamic-pituitary axis, reducing the synthesis of the hypothalamic releasing factors and hence pituitary hormone secretion. The reduced pituitary secretion in turn reduces the original stimulation of the target glands to maintain hormone levels.

Negative-feedback control predominates in endocrinology, though positive feedback is also important. An example of positive feedback is the ovarian estrogen-pituitary positive-feedback event, occurring at the midpoint of the monthly menstrual cycle, in which estradiol stimulates the ovulatory surge of pituitary gonadotropin release. Each target organ controls its own biosynthetic rate and increases the synthesis of hormone when needed through attenuation of the negative-feedback loop that decreases hypothalamic-pituitary secretions. Examples of the feedback and stimulus loops that tie the hypothalamic pituitary axis to the primary endocrine organ or tissue are shown in Figs. 43-5 through 43-9.

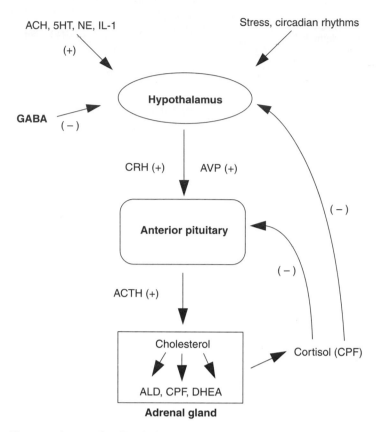

Fig. 43-5 The regulatory feedback loop of the hypothalamic-pituitary-adrenal axis. Several neurotransmitters, including acetylcholinesterase (*ACH*), 5-hydroxytryptamine (*5-HT*), norepinephrine (*NE*), and the cytokine interleukin-1 (*IL-1*), have a positive effect on the release of corticotropin-releasing factor (*CRH*) from the hypothalamus. Gamma-aminobutyric acid (*GABA*) has a negative influence. Stress and circadian rhythm also influence the release of *CRH* from the hypothalamus. Both CRH and arginine vasopressin (*AVP*) stimulate the pituitary to release adrenocorticotropin (*ACTH*), which in turn stimulates the adrenal gland to synthesize and release three major classes of hormones (aldosterone, *ALD*; cortisol, *CPF*; and dehydroepiandrosterone, *DHEA*). Cortisol is the only adrenal steroid to feed back negatively to the hypothalamic-pituitary axis to control its own biosynthetic rate.

The hypothalamic and pituitary hormones are secreted in cyclic patterns that vary in duration. Studies in recent years have focused on the pulsatile and circadian release of the pituitary hormones. It is now evident that virtually all hypothalamic and pituitary hormones are synthesized and released in a minute-to-minute pulsatile fashion. For example, in both men and women, pituitary release of FSH and LH occurs every 30 to 40 minutes as a consequence of the **pulsatile release** of gonadotropin-releasing hormone (GnRH) from the hypothalamus.

Overlaying this shorter, pulsatile cycle, pituitary hormone secretion also exhibits a cyclic change in secretion rates that occurs over a 24-hour period, termed a *circadian rhythm*. The frequency and magnitude of the pulsatile release are different for the individual pituitary hormones. For example, in the case of pituitary ACTH secretion, there is a character-istic circadian rhythm during the course of the 24-hour day, with a much higher output in the early morning hours and a nadir around midnight. Growth hormone output exhibits increased amplitude and frequency during periods of REM sleep, a period from about midnight to 4 a.m. In women, there is the added factor of menstrual cyclicity of the pituitary reproductive hormones LH and FSH, which occurs over the course of a 30-day menstrual cycle (see Chapter 45). Pulsatility and variable hormone secretory behavior are important considerations in interpreting the circulating levels of hormones within the context of the normal biological rhythms.

Control of hormone availability. Hormones are potent, biologically active compounds. The physiological activity of hormones is controlled by changing their rates of synthesis and release. In addition, however, two other mechanisms act by limiting the hormones' availability after they have been released into the circulation. These mechanisms are rapid catabolism (breakdown) and sequestration.

Catabolism-peptide hormones. Except for the thyroid hormones, peptide and amino acid-derived hormones are water-soluble and are found free in plasma. However,

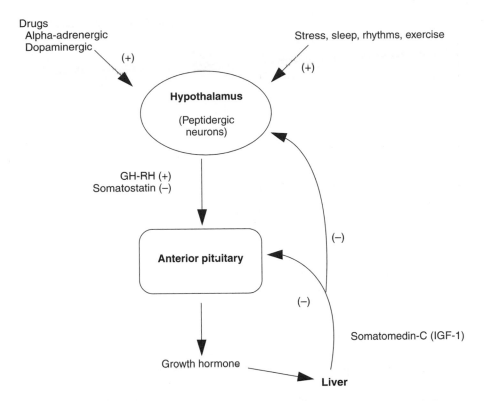

Fig. 43-6 The regulatory feedback loop of the hypothalamic-pituitary–growth hormone axis. Growth hormone release from the pituitary is driven primarily by growth hormone–releasing hormone (*GH-RH*) from the hypothalamus. GH-RH release from the hypothalamus is positively influenced by alpha-adrenergic and dopaminergic drugs and by stress, sleep patterns, and exercise. Growth hormone acts on the liver to produce somatomedin-C, or insulin-like growth factor (*IGF-1*). This factor in turn negatively feeds back to the hypothalamic-pituitary axis to maintain homeostatic control over growth hormone secretion.

rapid catabolism of these hormones to inactive compounds by tissue and plasma enzymes reduces the availability of the original intact hormone and gives it a relatively short half-life. For example, PTH is released from parathyroid glands as an 84-amino acid, intact peptide. Within a few minutes, it is acted upon by proteolytic enzymes in the circulation to reduce this hormone to inactive fragments. Thus control of plasma circulatory levels of active hormone becomes a balance between new hormone synthesis and release from tissues and the metabolic inactivation of existing hormone.

Sequestration-free and bound transport of steroid and thyroid hormones. Immediate control of the activity of steroid and thyroid hormones in plasma is exercised by sequestration of most of the steroid and thyroid hormones into a protein-bound, inactive form. Since steroid hormones are themselves water-insoluble, plasma proteins also serve as the transport medium for these hormones. The transport/binding proteins, which are synthesized in the liver, are listed in Table 43-2. Generally three circulating pools of hormones exist, listed here in order of increasing bioavailability: those bound to specific proteins with high affinity for the hormone; those bound to proteins with low affinity for the hormone; and those totally free in the plasma. An

TABLE 43-2 HORMONE TRANSPORT PROTEINS

Protein	Hormone
CBG (cortisol-binding globulin)	Cortisol
SHBG (sex hormone–binding globulin)	Estradiol, testosterone
TBG (thyroid-binding globulin)	T_3, T_4
TBPA (thyroxine-binding prealbumin)	T_4
VDBG (vitamin D–binding globulin)	Vitamin D
ALB (albumin)	All hormones

example of the binding of testosterone to its respective carrier proteins is shown in Fig. 43-10.

In the case of thyroid hormone, three different proteins, each with different binding affinities, participate in the transport of T_4 and T_3 in the circulation: thyroxine-binding globulin, thyroxine-binding prealbumin, and albumin (see Chapter 44). Speculation exists that hormones bound to proteins with high affinity represent a circulating storage form of the hormone that is not immediately bioavailable to the target organ. When hormone is transferred from the free

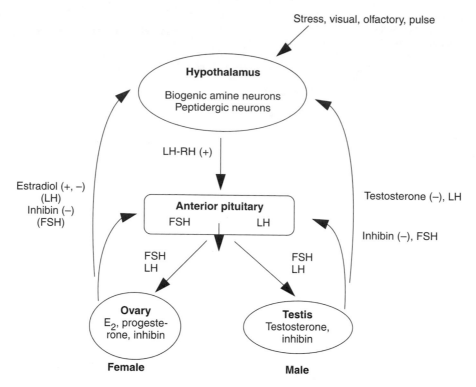

Fig. 43-7 The regulatory feedback loop of the hypothalamic-pituitary-gonadal axis. Biogenic amine and peptidergic neurons in the hypothalamus respond to neural and sensory input from the brain to elicit the release of gonadotropin hormone (*LH-RH*). This input can be visual and olfactory in origin and occurs in a pulsatile fashion. Stress can override these inputs in a negative fashion. LH-RH in turn acts on the pituitary to synthesize and release the gonadotropins *FSH* and *LH*. In the female, FSH causes ovarian follicular development and the production of estradiol, whereas LH causes corpus luteum development and the secretion of progesterone. Estradiol feeds back both negatively and positively to the hypothalamic-pituitary axis to control the menstrual cycle and LH secretion. FSH-release feedback control is orchestrated by an ovarian peptide called *inhibin*. In the male, FSH causes testicular spermatogenesis, whereas LH stimulates testosterone production by the testes. Testosterone negatively feeds back to the hypothalamic-pituitary axis to control LH release, whereas a testicular peptide, inhibin, feeds back to control FSH release.

or weakly bound form to its tissue receptor, the hormone equilibrium shifts from the storage form to the more weakly bound form to maintain appropriate availability of free hormone within the circulation (see below).

Free and Protein-Bound Hormone Transport

Several proteins serve as carriers of hormones in plasma and also serve as a form of hormone storage within the circulation (see above). Albumin and prealbumin serve as general transport proteins for the steroid hormones and thyroid hormones. Binding of thyroid hormones and steroid hormones to albumin and prealbumin is weak, however, with an affinity constant that is much lower than that of the tissue receptor. Thus the hormones bound to albumin and prealbumin are a weakly bound form of free hormones and are considered to be readily bioavailable to tissues—a phenomenon in contrast to the previous belief that only hormones absolutely free of carrier proteins could gain access to tissue receptors. This new concept has led to the description of free

hormone as inclusive of free and weakly bound hormone.

In addition to general, low-affinity, transport proteins such as albumin, there exist specific transport proteins. These specific transport proteins have a high affinity for the hormones they carry, which closely parallels the binding and specificity characteristics of intracellular receptors; thus they significantly influence the metabolic clearance rate for hormones. Several important considerations underscore the role of all the transport proteins that carry hormones in the circulation. The high-affinity binding proteins act as reservoirs for the storage and transport of hormones in the circulation. Once free or weakly bound hormone enters the tissue, rapid circulatory adjustments are made in the free hormone level through an exchange and reequilibration between specific transport protein-bound hormone and weakly bound transport protein-bound hormone. The overall decline in circulatory hormone is then eventually compensated for through activation of positive feedback to higher centers of control, like the hypothalamic-pituitary axis. This keeps a

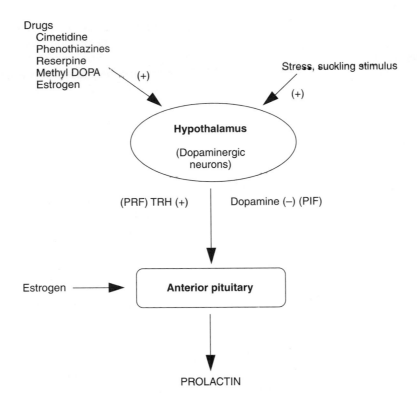

Fig. 43-8   The regulatory feedback loop for prolactin secretion. Prolactin release from the pituitary is under tonic inhibitory control from hypothalamus-derived dopamine, or prolactin inhibitory factor (*PIF*). Thyrotropin-releasing hormone (*TRH*) in turn is stimulatory to prolactin release. Prolactin release is affected by many factors that influence dopamine release. Drugs, estrogen, and stress are overriding factors that can produce an augmentation in prolactin release from the pituitary. Estrogen can directly sensitize the pituitary to release prolactin.

sufficient amount of life-sustaining hormones such as thyroxine and cortisol available continuously with a significant circulating reservoir available as soon as it is needed.

Many laboratories now measure **bioavailable** (i.e., free and albumin- or prealbumin-bound) **hormone**, in contrast to previous measurements, which included only the free concentration of hormone. An example of the utility of measuring both the free and weakly bound hormone can be seen in the measurement of free and weakly bound testosterone (see Fig. 43-10). Testosterone is carried in the circulation bound tightly to its specific carrier protein, sex hormone-binding globulin (SHBG), and bound weakly to albumin. Only a small (<10%) fraction of the testosterone in the circulation is actually free. When blood perfuses an organ containing testosterone receptors, both the free and albumin-bound fractions of testosterone are available for immediate binding to an available receptor. Hence the term *bioavailable testosterone* is used to describe the free and albumin-bound fraction of total hormone in the circulation.

Some steroid hormones, like dehydroepiandrosterone (DHEA), a major androgenic steroid produced by the adrenal gland, lack a specific transport protein. To compensate for the lack of a specific carrier protein for this steroid, DHEA is sulfated at the 3-hydroxyl position of the basic steroid molecule. This step increases the solubility of this steroid for general transport in the circulation. Thus DHEA circulates primarily as a sulfated derivative (i.e., DHEA-S) in the blood.

Local Hormone and Growth Factor Action

The classical understanding of endocrinology and hormones states that a hormone is produced by a specialized gland in one part of the body and travels through the bloodstream to a distant site to elicit a biological effect. The recent discovery of a family of peptide growth factors, however, has challenged the current perception of classical endocrinology. Like hormones, these growth factors can be extracellular regulators of cell growth and function. The major difference is that growth factors' actions are local and rely on cell-to-cell communication within the tissue and cellular environment.

Terms such as *autocrine* and *paracrine effect* have been coined to describe the local synthesis and release of growth factors that interact with receptors on neighboring cells within the same tissue (paracrine effect) or with receptors from the same cell that release the growth factor (autocrine effect) (Fig. 43-11).

The gastrointestinal tract is a prime example of local regulatory interactions between hormones, growth factors,

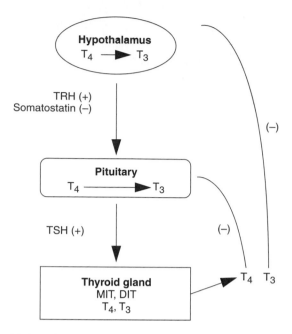

Fig. 43-9 The regulatory feedback loop of the hypothalamic-pituitary-thyroid axis. The hypothalamus secretes thyrotropin-releasing factor (*TRH*) to stimulate the synthesis and release of *TSH* from the pituitary. TSH in turn stimulates the thyroid gland to grow, vascularize, and produce the thyroid hormones tetraiodothyronine (*T_4*) and triiodothyronine (*T_3*). T_3 is primarily formed from T_4 outside the thyroid gland. T_4 (through hypothalamic and pituitary conversion to T_3) and T_3 (directly) feed back to the hypothalamic-pituitary axis to maintain a homeostatic balance of circulating thyroid hormone.

and neurotransmitters that influence cell function through cell-to-cell communication (see Chapter 30). An analogy to this system of communication is the cytokine network of communication that exists between the lymphoid cells of the immune system and the cells of a particular tissue, such as the tissue macrophage and an epithelial cell.

Two additional terms have been used to describe growth factor communication within the local cellular environment. **Intracrine factor** refers to an intracellular cytosolic factor that travels to the nucleus in the same cell to bind to a specific receptor within the DNA-binding region of chromatin. The term **juxtacrine factor** refers to direct cell-to-cell communication elicited by growth factors that are still anchored to each cell's membrane. When the cells come into contact with each other, this membrane-bound growth factor directly influences its neighboring cell. As the family of growth factors continues to expand, a reclassification of the nomenclature will be needed to assign hormones, growth factors, and neural peptides to their proper location and function.

THE HYPOTHALAMIC-PITUITARY AXIS
Hypothalamus

The hypothalamus exerts control over pituitary function by both direct neurostimulation and neurosecretion events of the hypothalamus. The anatomic positioning of the hypothalamus at the base of the brain with both neural and anatomic connection to the pituitary through the pituitary stalk and the portal circulation ensures the close interdependence of these two important organs. The pituitary is anatomically confi-

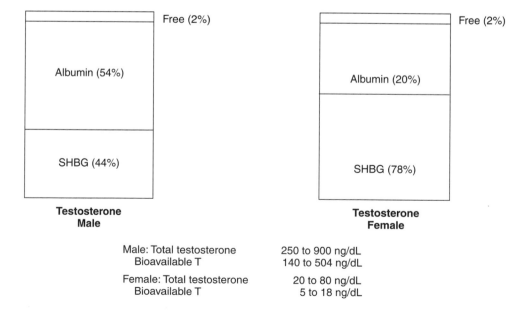

Male: Total testosterone	250 to 900 ng/dL
Bioavailable T	140 to 504 ng/dL
Female: Total testosterone	20 to 80 ng/dL
Bioavailable T	5 to 18 ng/dL

Fig. 43-10 Free and weakly bound testosterone. Testosterone circulates bound to two proteins: a specific binding protein, sex hormone–binding globulin (*SHBG*), and albumin. Only a small fraction of testosterone circulates in a free state. Total testosterone levels are a combination of SHBG-bound, albumin-bound, and free testosterone. The bioavailable form of circulating testosterone, the form that "sees" the tissue receptor, is composed of the free fraction and that bound to albumin. Thus bioavailable testosterone is the biologically active form of the hormone found in the circulation.

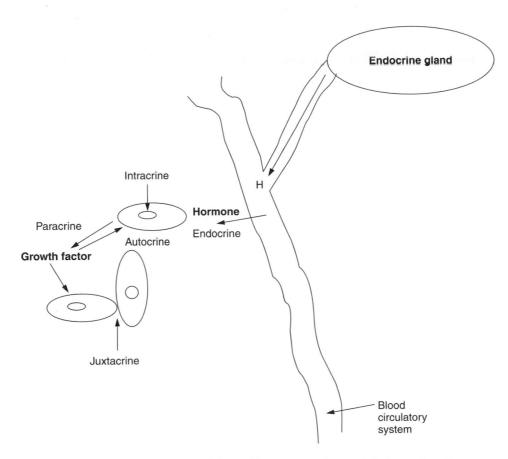

Fig. 43-11   Local and systemic modalities of hormone and growth factor action. Hormones, *H*, are the chemical messengers released into the circulation by endocrine glands to effect a response.

gured with a posterior and an anterior lobe (Fig. 43-12). The hypothalamus directly innervates the posterior lobe (**neuro-hypophysis**), and hypothalamic stimulation causes the posterior pituitary to release stored peptide hormones such as arginine vasopressin (AVP) and oxytocin. These two hormones are synthesized by the neurosecretory cells of the hypothalamus and are stored in the neurohypophysis. In contrast, the anterior lobe (**adenohypophysis**) responds to hypothalamus-derived neuropeptides, which, when released directly into the **portal circulation**, cause the release of the corresponding pituitary hormones (see Table 43-1).

In addition to the classical hypothalamic releasing factors, there exists a hypothalamic peptide, somatostatin, which exerts a negative influence on TSH, GH, and several other hormone secretions, including gastrointestinal and pancreatic hormones. Somatostatin is a peptide synthesized not only by the hypothalamus but also within the lumen of the gastrointestinal tract and the pancreas. Different isoforms are synthesized in the brain and gastrointestinal tract. This neurohormone exerts a profound inhibitory effect on both the synthesis of GH and TSH and the secretion of these hormones from the pituitary. Somatostatin inhibits virtually all endocrine secretions (including gastrin, insulin, glucagon, and secretin) of the gastrointestinal tract, pancreas, and gallbladder. Its primary role is to attenuate hypersecretion of

these hormones in pathological states; for example, endocrine-secreting tumors such as insulinomas and carcinomas. Somatostatin analogs have been used as effective therapeutic agents to treat endocrine-secreting pituitary tumors such as **acromegaly** and pancreatic tumors such as insulinomas.

Neurohypophysis

The neurosecretions of vasopressin and oxytocin have specialized roles in mammalian physiology that involve water-conserving (antidiuretic) and nonvascular smooth muscle contracting properties, respectively. Arginine vaso-pressin (AVP) is the major homeostatic factor that maintains normal water concentration in the blood, keeping plasma volume and blood osmolality tightly controlled. Control of blood volume plays an important role in the maintenance of normal blood pressure (see p. 900). The release of AVP occurs immediately in response to increases in plasma osmolality, and AVP acts in the kidney to increase water reabsorption by the distal kidney tubules and the collecting ducts. AVP also participates in volume regulation. A sudden reduction in blood volume of greater than 10%, as occurs with a massive hemorrhage, can evoke a rapid release of AVP. Volume receptors for AVP are located in the heart and carotid sinus. Under normal conditions, AVP is released in response to changes in plasma osmolality. Severe volume

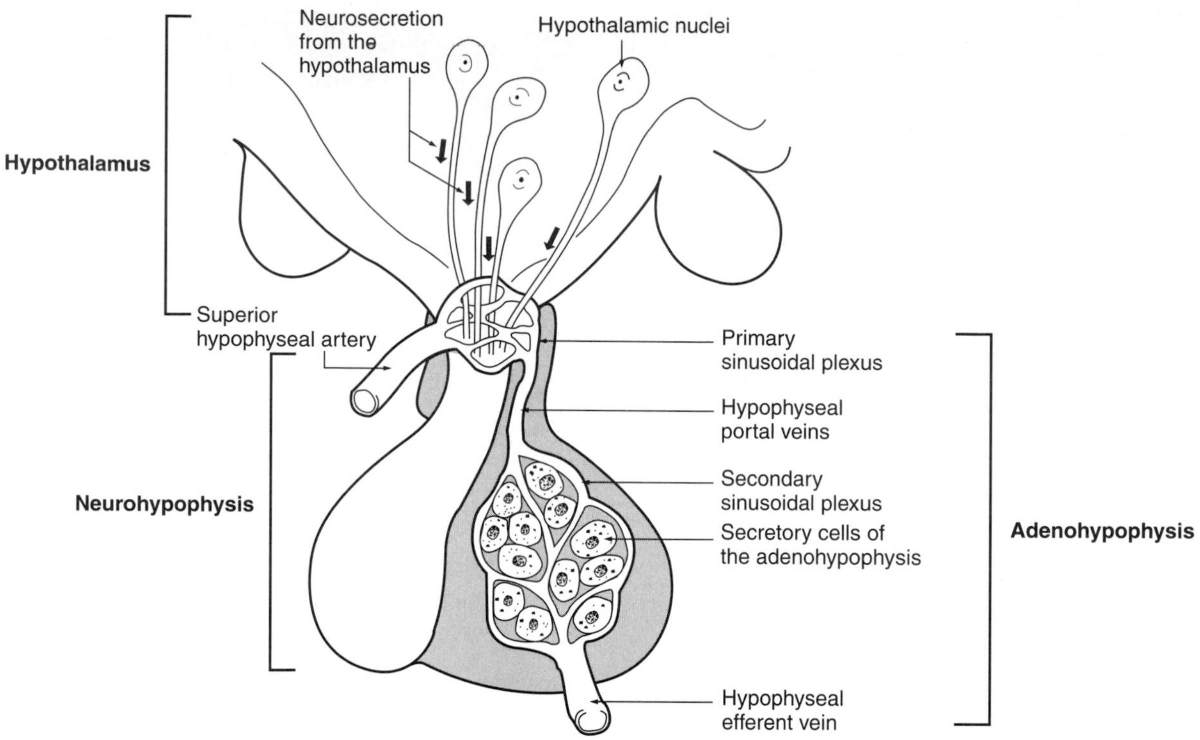

Fig. 43-12   Sinusoidal portal system of pituitary gland.

depletion, however, can override the influence of osmolality on AVP release.

Oxytocin appears to have a role in mammalian physiology that transcends reproductive behavior. Release of oxytocin is generally brought about through a neurogenic reflex transmitted primarily from nerve endings in the nipple of the breast. The stimulus is transmitted through the spinal cord, midbrain, and ultimately to the hypothalamus. Suckling of the breast induces the release of oxytocin, which causes contraction of epithelial cells that encircle mammary acini. This produces expulsion of milk from the milk ducts of the breast, termed *milk letdown*, which is a key event in breast-feeding. Oxytocin also plays a role in the induction of labor in pregnancy by stimulating the nonvascular smooth muscle of the uterus to contract. Although the exact signal precipitating the onset of human labor has not yet been identified, oxytocin receptors in the uterus translate the oxytocin signal to produce rhythmic myometrial contractile changes and the physical events of labor. The secretion of oxytocin from the posterior pituitary occurs independent of AVP secretion; thus it is believed that both fall under independent control mechanisms.

Adenohypophysis

The anterior lobe of the pituitary is responsible for the secretion of trophic hormones that govern virtually the entire endocrine system. As noted previously, pituitary cell differentiation, proliferation, and hormone synthesis are controlled by neurosecretory factors of hypothalamic origin. All the releasing factors are peptides except dopamine (Table 43-3), a neurotransmitter that is also synthesized and released from the hypothalamus and plays an important regulatory role over pituitary hormone secretion. Dopamine is believed to be the major regulator of prolactin secretion, exerting a continuous and sustained inhibition on its release from the pituitary. In addition to its effect on prolactin, dopamine also inhibits the secretion of TSH, FSH, LH, and GH.

Although each hypothalamic releasing factor has a targeted hormone, some integration of hormone release does occur. For example, TRH causes synthesis and release of not only TSH but prolactin as well. Similarly, LH-RH stimulates the release of both FSH and LH. Only CRH and GH-RH act through a single pituitary hormone release mechanism. All releasing factors interact with the pituitary through the same receptor mechanism used by other peptide hormones. Although they are generally restricted to the portal circulation, several releasing factors have been measured in blood and urine. Direct target organ effects have been described for LH-RH in the ovary and testis. The exact physiological meaning of this interaction is still unclear.

PATHOLOGICAL CONDITIONS

Diseases and disorders of the hypothalamic-pituitary axis can strike at any age and can produce a myriad of symptoms that are often subtle in presentation. Many early forms of endocrine disease are detected only with provocative testing. Bacterial infections, tumors, and head trauma are the most usual causes of alterations in central hormone regulation in the young. In older adults, vascular disease, inflammatory diseases, and nutritional deficiencies are additional causes of neuroendocrine disorders (Box 43-1). Associated with these diseases are deficits in the autoregulatory feedback loop from

TABLE 43-3 HUMAN HYPOTHALAMIC NEUROSECRETORY FACTORS

Vasopressin	cys-tyr-phe-gln-asn-cys-pro-arg-gly-NH$_2$ (1084.38 daltons)
Oxytocin	cys-tyr-ile-gln-asn-cys-pro-leu-gly-NH$_2$ (1007.35 daltons)
CRH	ser-glu-glu-pro-pro-ile-ser-leu-asp-leu-thr-peh-his-leu-leu-arg-glu-val-leu-glu-met-ala-arg-ala-glu-gln-leu-ala-gln-gln-ala-his-ser-asn-arg-lys-leu-met-glu-ile-ile-NH$_2$ (4758.14 daltons)
GH-RH	try-ala-asp-ala-ile-phe-thr-asn-ser-tyr-arg-lys-val-leu-gly-gln-leu-ser-ala-arg-lys-leu-leu-gln-asp-ile-met-ser-arg-gln-gln-gly-glu-ser-asn-gln-glu-arg-gly-ala-arg-ala-arg-leu-NH$_2$ (5040.40 daltons)
LH-RH	pglu-his-trp-ser-tyr-gly-leu-arg-pro-gly-NH$_2$ (1182.39 daltons)
TRH	pglu-his-pro-NH2 (362.42 daltons)
Somatostatin	ala-gly-cys-lys-asn-phe-phe-trp-lys-thr-phe-thr-ser-cys (1638.12 daltons)
Dopamine	3,4-dihydroxyphenylmethylamine

CRH, *Corticotropin-releasing factor*; GH-RH, *growth hormone–releasing hormone*; LH-RH, *luteinizing hormone–releasing hormone*; p-, *pyrido-*; TRH, *thyrotropin-releasing hormone*.

BOX 43-1

DISORDERS OF THE HYPOTHALAMIC-PITUITARY AXIS

Hypopituitarism	*Hyperpituitarism*
Congenital	Hypothalamic
Gene deletions	Irradiation
Aplasia, hypoplasia	Infection
Disconnection of pituitary	Tumor
stalk	Primary pituitary
Septo-optic dysplasia	Hyperplasia or
Hypoxia	adenoma
Acquired	Hypersomatotropism
Infections	Acromegaly
Trauma	Starvation
Radiation	Infection
Neoplasms	Adrenocorticotropin
Drugs	Pituitary adenoma
Surgery	Addison's disease
Functional defects	Thyrotropin
Isolated hormone deficiency	Primary hypothyroidism
Severe illness	Hypergonadotropism
Multiple hormone defects	Primary organ failure
Secondary hypothyroidism	Hyperprolactinemia
Secondary hypoadrenalism	Pituitary stalk section
Hyposomatotropism	Pregnancy
Hypogonadotropic	Pituitary adenoma
hypogonadism	Hypothyroidism

the target organs. The loss of circadian rhythm, for example, of ACTH secretion with bacterial infection brings about subsequent compromise in pituitary-adrenal function. This effect can be subtle but nevertheless important, since cortisol production is a key factor in the control of immune cell function. Because we cannot easily determine the local hormone environment of the portal circulation, we rely on the measurement of pituitary hormones in the systemic circulation to provide a clinical picture of events at the hypothalamic level in health and disease.

Abnormalities of hormone secretion are usually defined in terms of the serum levels of the hormone, that is, high or low levels, and the endocrine gland directly demonstrating the abnormality. In addition, the disease is defined by whether the hormone abnormality is the result of the endocrine gland producing the hormone (primary disease), a disease of the pituitary gland controlling the primary gland (secondary disease), a disease of the hypothalamus controlling the pituitary (tertiary disease), or an inability of the hormone's target tissue to respond to the hormone (end-organ, or quaternary, disease). For example, increased levels of thyroxine resulting from a pituitary gland producing excessive TSH defines secondary hyperthyroidism.

Pituitary Hormone Deficiency

Deficiencies in a specific pituitary cell type can result in primary pituitary failure. A list of primary causes of hypopituitarism can be found in Box 43-1.

Secondary pituitary failure can occur as a result of a deficiency or excess in one or more hypothalamic releasing factors brought on by infection, brain tumors, head trauma, brain surgery or a congenital defect. Hypothalamic tumors, such as a craniopharyngioma, or inflammatory episodes in the brain, such as meningitis, can result in inappropriate synthesis of certain hypothalamic releasing factors, leading to a decrease in pituitary hormone synthesis and release. Hypothalamic hypothyroidism, for example, is a deficiency syndrome of TRH secretion that is initially diagnosed by observing a suppressed circulating level of TSH of unknown etiology. Provocative testing in the form of an intravenous TRH stimulation test can help determine whether the suppressed TSH level is due to hypothalamic disease or is a result of pituitary dysfunction. An isolated deficiency in LH-RH is the most common form of hypothalamic releasing hormone deficiency and is caused by a congenital defect in the development of LH-RH–containing neurons in embryonic life. A deficiency in growth hormone-releasing hormone (GH-RH) is yet another example of a hypothalamic disorder that results in idiopathic dwarfism. This disorder is typically diagnosed by observing inappropriate blood levels of circulating growth hormone before and after provocative testing. Deficiencies in the availability of TRH, LH-RH, GH-RH, and CRH have all been described in patients and are usually categorized as tertiary endocrine disease.

Pituitary Hormone Excess

Primary hyperpituitarism. Pituitary hypersecretion is most commonly caused by the presence of a **pituitary adenoma** or benign tumor of pituitary origin. Prolactin-secreting pituitary adenoma is by far the most common form of pituitary disease. Prolactin, the secretion of which is usually under continuous negative control by the neurosecretory factor dopamine, is produced and secreted uncontrollably in large amounts by pituitary prolactinomas. Prolactin-secreting tumors are diagnosed more readily in women, since disruption of the normal menstrual cycle and **amenorrhea** usually herald a potential problem early in the manifestation of the disease. Women with prolactinomas can also manifest **galactorrhea**, that is, an abnormal secretion of fluid from the nipple of the breast. Males who develop a prolactinoma, in contrast, are less fortunate and usually do not present at a microadenoma stage as females do. Growth of the prolactin-secreting pituitary tumor usually continues in the male without overt symptoms, and the tumor eventually reaches the size of a macroadenoma before symptoms appear. Headache, impotence, and visual-field disturbances as a consequence of tumor extension that compresses the optic nerve are the classical symptoms that result from a pituitary macroadenoma. The diagnosis of a prolactinoma is usually confirmed by the appearance of blood levels of prolactin in excess of 200 ng/mL.

Growth hormone– and ACTH–producing pituitary tumors are also relatively common pituitary disorders, though of lower prevalence than prolactin-secreting tumors. Growth hormone excess is characterized by the development of acromegalic features, including soft tissue and cartilaginous growth, that result in the characteristic facial features of gigantism. This growth hormone-excess disease entity is called *acromegaly*. The major effect of growth hormone is to induce the synthesis of an insulin-like growth factor (IGF-1) by the liver. In patients with acromegaly, IGF-1 levels are raised to a greater extent than those of growth hormone itself. The recent availability of commercial immunoassays for IGF-1 has allowed for the routine measurement of this circulating growth factor for the diagnosis and management of patients with acromegaly.

Pituitary adenomas hypersecreting ACTH are also common and lead to the condition known as Cushing's disease (see Chapter 46). This syndrome is associated with bilateral adrenal hyperplasia and clinical manifestations of cortisol overproduction as a consequence of excessive ACTH. TSH-producing pituitary adenomas leading to thyroid gland hyperstimulation have also been described but are much less common than the previously mentioned pituitary adenomas.

Secondary hyperpituitarism. Pituitary hypersecretion can be induced by numerous factors including neurogenic tumors of the hypothalamus. Overproduction of releasing factors will hyperstimulate the pituitary, leading to an excessive pituitary hormone release that overrides the usual negative-feedback mechanisms. LH-RH hypersecretion associated with precocious puberty, GH-RH-secreting ganglio-cytomas causing acromegaly, and CRH-secreting tumors producing Cushing's disease are examples of releasing factor hypersecretion and secondary causes of hyperpituitarism. Hypothalamus-based disorders are relatively rare, however, compared with the hypersecretion that occurs with primary pituitary disease.

Inappropriate release (hypersecretion) of AVP can bring about excessive water retention and a dangerous expansion of plasma volume. Brain injury resulting from physical trauma, infection, or tumors in the brain can bring about excessive AVP release, leading to the clinical condition known as *SIADH* (syndrome of inappropriate secretion of antidiuretic hormone). The ectopic production of AVP by certain tumors can also lead to inappropriate water retention. The thirst mechanism in the brain is also linked to AVP secretion from the neurohypophysis. Both drinking behavior and AVP release are believed to be activated by similar hyperosmotic stimuli resulting in repletion of plasma water in states of dehydration. SIADH is associated with dilutional hyponatremia and the production of urine that is hypertonic relative to plasma, despite normal renal and adrenal function. Clinically, SIADH is associated with symptoms of muscle weakness, malaise, and poor mental status, ultimately progressing to convulsions.

TESTS OF HYPOTHALAMIC AND PITUITARY FUNCTION

Evaluation of pituitary disease is very often difficult because of subtle disease presentation. The diagnosis usually requires some form of provocative testing of gland function either by suppressing or stimulating the pituitary gland through exogenous hormone treatment, or provocation of symptoms with stress or exercise. These challenge tests are then followed by measurement of specific pituitary hormones. For each suspected type of pituitary adenoma a specific testing protocol is usually employed to confirm the clinical suspicion. Many factors, however, must be considered when one is interpreting these functional tests. The pulsatile nature of pituitary hormone secretion, the time of day the test is performed, whether stress or infection might be present, and the concentration of circulating hormone are all factors that affect the interpretation of pituitary function tests. In addition, clinical laboratories have access to a wide variety of immunoassays with differing specificities and sensitivities that affect interpretability of provocative hormone testing.

ACTH Excess

Dexamethasone suppression tests (see p. 891). The existence of a tumor secreting ACTH is usually suspected when an abnormal elevation in urine or blood cortisol levels is observed. In these patients, cortisol determinations are made after a low-dose dexamethasone suppression test. A lack of cortisol suppression is suggestive of a pituitary tumor. One then gives a higher dose of dexamethasone that will elicit a modest but still incomplete suppression of cortisol output in the patient with a functional pituitary adenoma. Cortisol output in patients with ACTH from an ectopic (nonpituitary) source will not be suppressed by either low- or high-dose dexamethasone.

GH Deficiency

Insulin challenge test. The most commonly performed challenge test for a growth hormone problem is the insulin challenge test used to determine the presence of a GH deficiency in young children. Most pediatric endocrinologists use a combination of insulin-induced hypoglycemia, which produces a form of stress through carbohydrate sensing, and the drug levodopa (L-dopa), which acts in the CNS to induce pituitary release of GH. Insulin is usually administered first, and blood is collected for the assessment of GH at 30-minute intervals for 90 minutes. This is followed by the administration of L-dopa over the subsequent 120 minutes with the additional collection of blood for GH measurement every 30 minutes. Because of the influence of stress, baseline levels can be slightly raised because of the venipuncture and can sometimes cause misinterpretation of the results. The recent availability of the releasing factor GH-RH for clinical use has allowed for a better clinical work-up of patients with a subtle manifestation of pituitary growth hormone deficiency. Administration of GH-RH and the measurement of GH are useful in discerning growth deficiencies that are of hypothalamic origin.

Secondary Hypogonadism

LH-RH challenge. LH-RH is usually given intravenously to stimulate pituitary secretion of FSH and LH; low FSH and LH levels after this challenge are suggestive of hypopituitary function. LH-RH analogs are available for use in provocative testing and in the treatment of a variety of reproductive disorders and malignancies, such as endometriosis and prostate cancer.

CHANGE OF ANALYTE IN DISEASE
Prolactin

The pulsatile secretion of prolactin has little effect on its measurement or interpretation for the diagnosis of a prolactinoma because of the high levels of prolactin that are usually achieved in this disease. Prolactin hypersecretion is usually established simply by the observation of an elevated basal level. A prolactin level above 200 ng/mL is virtually diagnostic of a prolactinoma. Mild elevations of prolactin (25 to 50 ng/mL), however, can easily be achieved in response to the stress of venipuncture or simply after physical examination and examination of the breasts. Repeated measurements of mild elevations of prolactin will confirm the presence of a prolactinoma. Levels up to 150 ng/mL, which are elevated approximately tenfold, can be achieved in normal individuals who are receiving certain medications. The phenothiazines and antiulcer medications, such as Tagamet, can produce a significant increase in prolactin secretion, and so a careful drug history is important when assessing a patient with raised levels of prolactin. A CAT scan of the pituitary of a patient with raised prolactin levels is usually required to confirm the presence of a pituitary tumor.

ACTH

Patients with an ACTH-producing pituitary adenoma are usually diagnosed through an elevation in basal blood cortisol levels; ACTH measurements are not routinely needed in these cases. ACTH measurements are more commonly used for patients requiring _localization_ of the tumor within the pituitary before surgical removal of the pituitary adenoma. In these cases, blood samples are collected from the petrosal sinus. Occasionally patients with a suspected ectopic source of ACTH, from an ACTH-producing tumor, are candidates for blood ACTH measurements. The highest values for ACTH are usually found in patients producing this peptide from a tumor source. The dexamethasone suppression test is used for this diagnosis (see above). Sustained high levels of ACTH can be helpful in establishing the presence of a nonpituitary source for ACTH. Tumors of the lung, particularly oat cell carcinoma, are commonly associated with nonpituitary sources of ACTH. Blood levels of ACTH in a patient with a pituitary adenoma rarely exceed 1000 pg/mL; however, with an ectopic source the levels are frequently in excess of this concentration. Pancreatic tumors are also commonly associated with ectopic ACTH release.

ACTH measurements are not routinely used. The short half-life of ACTH, stringent collection requirements because of the lability of this peptide (antiproteases are required in the collection vial), and the need for immediate sample storage at $-20°$ C are factors that impede the routine use and the interpretation of an ACTH result.

Growth Hormone

Growth hormone is secreted in healthy individuals in a pulsatile fashion, with the greatest amounts produced during rapid-eye-movement sleep. During the day, blood levels of GH can range from undetectable to 5 ng/mL. However, GH levels can be greatly influenced by stress and also by the recent ingestion of food, with carbohydrates suppressing and proteins stimulating GH secretion. Thus a single determination of GH is not particularly useful in establishing either inadequate or excessive release of GH from the pituitary. When a GH deficiency is suspected, provocative testing is usually required to confirm this suspicion (see above).

One method to evaluate the possibility of pituitary hypersecretion of growth hormone in a patient suspected of having acromegaly is to measure the concentration of somatomedin C, or IGF-1. The concentration of this liver factor, which mediates the effects of growth hormone, is raised in the circulation in patients with acromegaly, and its measurement can be useful to confirm the diagnosis in borderline cases. IGF-1 measurements are also helpful in monitoring therapy of patients treated for acromegaly.

TSH

The availability of ultrasensitive TSH assays has greatly enhanced the usefulness of TSH measurements for the diagnoses of both hypofunction and hyperfunction of the pituitary-thyroid axis. Before the advent of these highly sensitive tests, TRH stimulation tests were important provocative tests that helped distinguish hypothalamic from pituitary disease as the cause of the thyroid dysfunction. This is particularly important when hyperthyroidism and euthyroidism are being distinguished. The newer highly sensitive TSH assays can reasonably be expected to distinguish between depressed and normal TSH secretion, thus obviating, in most patients, the need to carry out TRH provocative testing. Basal TSH level becomes the important parameter to determine when the adequacy of pituitary TSH release is being assessed. A basal serum TSH level of less than 0.05 μ/mL, for example, indicates with virtual certainty that primary hyperthyroidism exists for whatever clinical reason. TRH testing has been quietly abandoned for the most part and has been reserved for establishing the differential diagnosis of suspected hypothalamus-based thyroid disease in patients who have a complex disease presentation (see p. 842). Patients who have a TSH level in excess of 10 μ/mL are strongly suspected of having hypothyroidism, and when the TSH level exceeds 25 μ/mL, the diagnosis is usually established as primary hypothyroidism.

FSH/LH

Of all the pituitary hormones influenced by pulsatile release, the gonadotropins are the most affected. In males, this pulsatility doesn't interfere with the clinical utility of gonadotropin measurements, since the assessment of primary gonadal disease is the usual reason for determining gonadotropin levels in the male. Testosterone measurements provide the initial biochemical indication for the diagnostic work-up of the hypogonadal male. Measurement of the gonadotropins with LH-RH provocative testing can be useful in the diagnosis of males with hypogonadotropic hypogonadism, or secondary hypogonadism (see above).

In women, the situation is more complex because the menstrual cycle, menopausal status, and the pulsatility and frequency of hypothalamic LH-RH secretion all affect the interpretation of serum FSH and LH levels. A single gonadotropin measurement is of little practical use in the female unless one simply wants to determine the probability of menopause. In this case, use of FSH is a better test to confirm menopause than LH. In dealing with the more intricate cases of infertility, amenorrhea, and the many disorders that influence the hypothalamic-pituitary-ovarian axis, multiple blood measurements of the gonadotropins are necessary to pinpoint the disorder (see p. 859). An alternative to this is the use of timed urine gonadotropin measurements, which can effectively integrate the pulsatile secretion of gonadotropins and concentrate the gonadotropins for use in the different clinical diagnoses. Pediatric endocrinologists routinely use urinary gonadotropin measurements to diagnose delayed puberty, precocious puberty, and functional disorders of the pituitary-ovarian and pituitary-testicular axis in young girls and boys.

In general, dynamic testing of pituitary function takes on the uniqueness of the specific disorder. With the current clinical availability of the four hypothalamic releasing factors, GH-RH, CRH, LH-RH, and TRH, direct pituitary responses can now be monitored by the measurement of the corresponding pituitary peptide. This allows the clinician to distinguish between hypothalamic and pituitary disease and determine adequacy of the hypothalamic-pituitary-endocrine axis.

Bibliography

Besser GM: *Clinical endocrinology*, ed 2, St Louis, 1994, Mosby.
Besser GM, Thorner MO: *Clinical endocrinology* (including CD-ROM), ed 3, St Louis, 2002, Mosby.
DeGroot LJ, Jameson JL: *Endocrinology*, ed 4, Philadelphia, 2001, Saunders.
Hall R: *Color atlas of endocrinology*, ed 2, St Louis, 1990, Mosby.
Wilson JD, Foster DW: *Williams' textbook of endocrinology*, ed 9, Philadelphia, 1998, Saunders.
Yen SSC et al: *Reproductive endocrinology*, ed 4, Philadelphia, 1999, Saunders

Internet Sites

www.endo-society.org—The Endocrine Society Home Page
www.mic.ki.se/Diseases/c19.html—Karolinska Institute (a list of sites providing information on a wide variety of endocrine disorders)
www.aace.com/—American Association of Clinical Endocrinologists
www.niddk.nih.gov/health/endo/endo.htm—National Institute of Diabetes & Digestive & Kidney Diseases

www.euro-endo.org—European Federation of Endocrine Societies
http://www.slis.ua.edu/dls/cchs/main/clinical/endocrinology/general.htm
http://www.hormoneproblems.com/Gen_Endo.htm
http://www.mednets.com/sendocri.htm
http://www.vetmed.ucdavis.edu/PHR/Therio/General%20Male%20Endocrinology.pdf

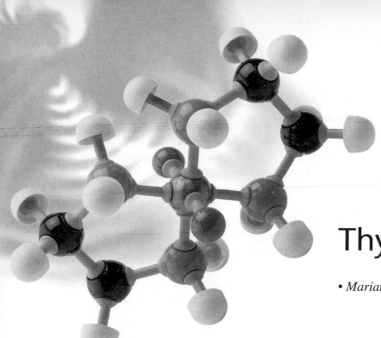

CHAPTER 44

Thyroid

• *Mariano Fernandez-Ulloa*

Objectives

• Describe the synthesis, transport, function, and regulation of thyroid hormones.
• Describe pathological conditions resulting in hyperthyroidism or hypothyroidism.
• State the importance of the analysis of the free hormone levels of T_4 and T_3 and the meaning of the free thyroxine measured.

• Describe the thyroid function tests and which analytes are used.
• State the diagnostic value of the following laboratory tests in assessing thyroid conditions: T_4, T_3, FT_4, T_3RU, FTI, and TSH.

Key Terms

androgen Natural or synthetic substance (usually a hormone) that produces masculinizing effects.

antimicrosomal antibody An antibody against thyroid peroxidase, the principal antigen in thyroid microsomes.

C-cells Calcitonin-secreting cells of the thyroid.

calorigenesis Production of heat and energy.

cretinism Hypothyroid condition caused by congenital lack of thyroid hormone secretion and characterized by impaired physical and mental development.

DIT Diiodotyrosine.

exocytosis The opposite of endocytosis; the release from cells of particles too large to diffuse through the plasma membrane.

factitial Produced by artificial means; unintentionally produced.

follicular cells Thyroid hormone–producing cells arranged in units of spherical vesicles.

goiter Enlargement of the thyroid gland.

Graves' disease Immune disorder caused by the binding of antibodies to thyroid-stimulating hormone (TSH) receptors, resulting in an unregulated increase in thyroid hormone production and release.

Hashimoto's thyroiditis Inflammatory process of the thyroid caused by a derangement of the immune system, which may or may not lead to abnormal thyroid function.

hyperthyroidism Metabolic and clinical state caused by an increase in circulating active thyroid hormone.

hypothyroidism Metabolic and clinical state caused by decreased levels of circulating active thyroid hormone or increased tissue resistance; primary—decreased thyroid function caused by disease of the thyroid gland; secondary—decreased thyroid function caused by disease of the pituitary gland; tertiary—decreased thyroid function caused by disease of the hypothalamus.

iatrogenic Any adverse condition resulting from the actions of a physician.

interstitium Pertaining to the intercellular spaces of a tissue.

iodine trapping The ability of the thyroid gland to sequester iodine against a concentration gradient.

medullary carcinoma (thyroid) Cancer of the C-cells.

MIT Monoiodotyrosine.

monodeiodination Loss or removal of a single iodine atom.

multinodular goiter Enlarged thyroid containing numerous superficial and deep indurations.

organification Incorporation of ionic form of iodine into the molecular structure of tyrosine.

parafollicular C-cells Calcitonin-secreting cells located between follicles.

prohormone A compound requiring chemical transformation to become an active hormone.

radioiodine thyroid uptake Measurement of thyroid functions based upon percentage of ^{123}I or ^{131}I accumulation after a known dose is administered orally.

resin-uptake test Measurement of the number of available binding sites of plasma thyroid hormone–transporting proteins.

rT$_3$ Reverse T$_3$, triiodothyronine with iodine in positions 3, 3′, and 5′.

solitary nodule Localized enlargement of a portion of the thyroid gland.

struma ovarii Rare teratoid tumor of the ovary composed almost entirely of thyroid tissue.

T$_3$ Thyroid hormone with iodine atoms in positions 3, 5, and 3′ (triiodothyronine).

T$_4$ Thyroxine, a thyroid hormone with iodine atoms in positions 3, 5, 3′, and 5′ (tetraiodothyronine).

thyroglobulin A glycoprotein of molecular weight 660,000 D produced by the follicular cells and containing the precursors of T$_3$ and T$_4$.

thyroid colloid The material found within the follicles of the thyroid and containing thyroglobulin and thyroid hormone.

thyroid hormone–binding ratio (THBR) Current terminology for the T$_3$ or T$_4$ resin-uptake tests.

thyroiditis A general term for inflammation of the thyroid gland.

thyrotoxicosis Condition caused by excess thyroid hormone secretion; often used as synonym for hyperthyroidism.

thyrotropin A synonym for thyroid-stimulating hormone (TSH).

thyroxine-binding globulin (TBG) A glycoprotein of α-mobility that transports thyroid hormone in the blood.

transthyretin Thyroxine-binding prealbumin, a protein that transports thyroid hormone in the blood.

TRH (thyrotropin-releasing hormone) A hypothalamic tripeptide that promotes release of TSH.

trophic action Stimulation of cell reproduction and enlargement.

trophoblastic tumor Tumor originating from extraembryonal cells of ectodermic nature located in the blastocyst.

TSH (thyroid-stimulating hormone, thyrotropin) A glycoprotein composed of α- and β- subunits that is released from the pituitary. TSH promotes thyroid hormone production and release.

TSI Thyroid-stimulating immunoglobulin.

Wolff-Chaikoff effect   Decreased formation and release of thyroid hormone in the presence of excess iodine.

Methods on CD-ROM

Thyroid-stimulating hormone (TSH)
Thyroxine (T_4)

T_3 uptake

In the last few years there has been a large increase in knowledge about thyroid function, the impact of thyroid dysfunction on health, and the use of laboratory tests to assess thyroid function. Much of this information has been summarized in a number of excellent practice guidelines published by professional societies.[1-4] More importantly, these guidelines are available on Internet sites, where updated versions can be easily reviewed. The reader is strongly urged to visit these Internet sites, which are listed after the references and in the CD-ROM, to obtain additional information.

ANATOMY

The thyroid is usually formed of two lobes, one on either side of the neck. The thyroid gland consists of two types of cells, follicular and parafollicular (Fig. 44-1). **Follicular cells** are arranged spherically in a single layer with an apical end

facing the center of the follicle and a basal end facing the **interstitium**. Follicular cells produce thyroid hormone, which is then stored in the central portion of the spherical follicle in a material called **thyroid colloid**. The interstitium contains the blood supply and parafollicular cells. Parafollicular cells secrete the hormone calcitonin. For this reason they are called **parafollicular C-cells** or simply **C-cells**.

THYROID PHYSIOLOGY

The thyroid gland has as its main function the production and secretion of metabolically active hormones that are essential for the regulation of various metabolic processes. Thyroid hormones are produced within the cells of the follicles from the amino acid tyrosine and the halogen element iodine. The two most important thyroid hormones are thyroxine (T_4), which contains four iodine atoms, and triiodothyronine (T_3), which contains three iodine atoms (Fig. 44-2).

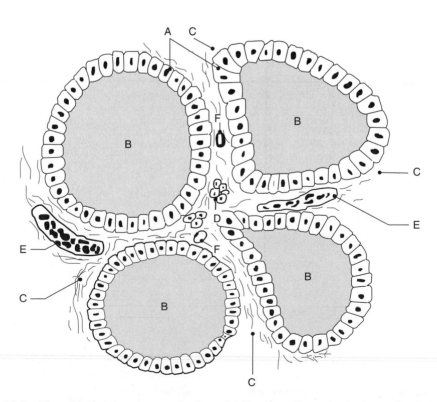

Fig. 44-1   Thyroid gland structure consists of follicular cells, *A;* enclosing colloid, *B;* and parafollicular C-cells, *D,* in the interstitium, *C. E,* Venule; *F,* capillary.

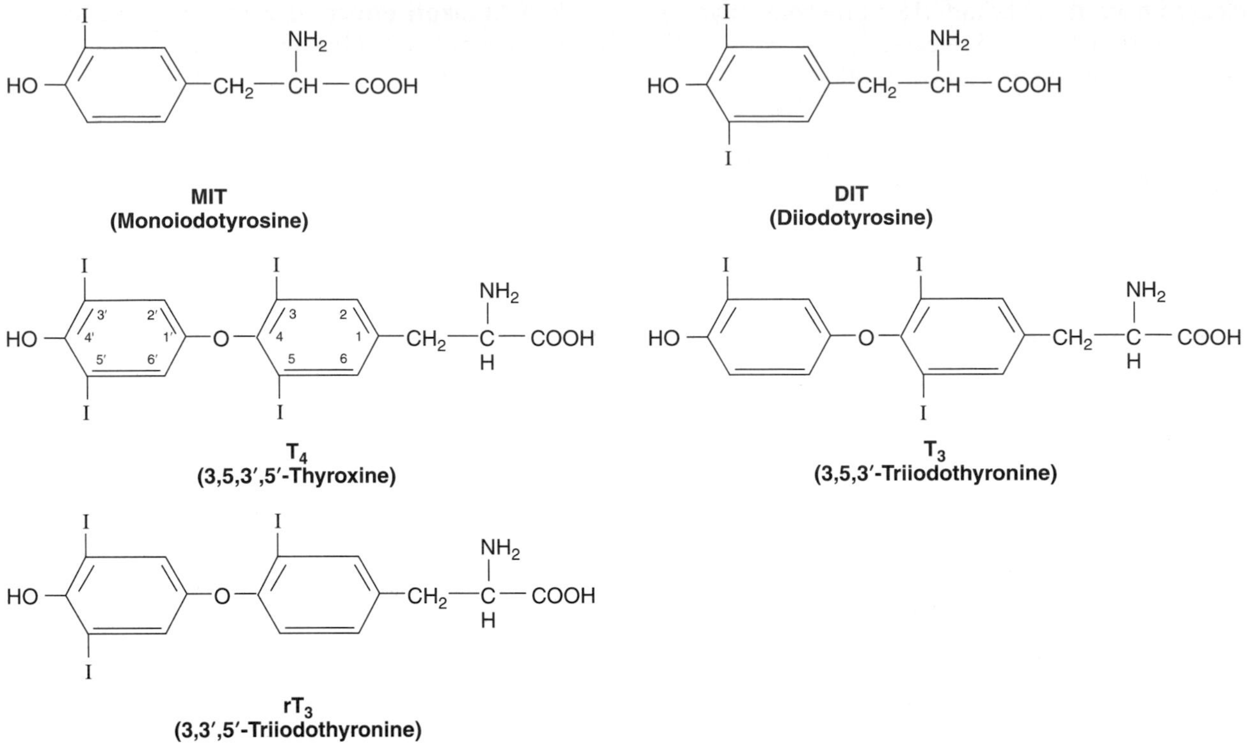

Fig. 44-2 Chemical structure of thyroid hormones and iodinated precursors and metabolites.

Thyroid hormones are released from the colloid and secreted into circulation in response to stimulation of the thyroid gland by the pituitary hormone called **thyroid-stimulating hormone (TSH, thyrotropin)**.

Metabolism of Iodine and Thyroid Hormone Synthesis

Iodine is a natural component of many foods, and in the United States it is provided in adequate amounts by a well-balanced diet. Extra amounts of iodine are currently provided by the ingestion of iodine-enriched foods and numerous "vitamin pills." The daily intake of iodine varies widely in different parts of the world. In the United States daily iodine intake ranges from 250 to 700 μg or more. In countries such as Japan, intake may reach several milligrams per day, whereas in some areas of Africa, South America, Asia, and Europe daily intake may be as low as 50 μg.

Under physiological conditions, iodine, which is reduced to iodide (I^-) in the gastrointestinal tract, is absorbed in the small bowel and then enters either the excretory or metabolic pathways (Fig. 44-3). Between 60% and 80% of the ingested iodine is excreted by the kidneys. Small amounts are excreted through the intestinal route. Fecal excretion is derived mostly from hormones degraded by the liver and excreted into the bowel by the biliary tract. The remainder of the iodine is distributed into the extracellular and thyroid compartments. The intrathyroid iodine compartment contains about 90% of the total body iodine and can amount to as much as 6000 to 12,000 μg. The extracellular compart-

ment contains most other iodine, except for a small but important amount that is found in cells. The metabolism of iodine is closely related to the process of thyroid hormonogenesis, which necessitates two separate metabolic processes that run simultaneously within the follicular cells. One of these processes leads to the formation of the protein **thyroglobulin**. The second is geared towards the production of the thyroid hormone itself and is closely related to the intracellular metabolism of iodine.

Classically, intrathyroidal iodine metabolism and thyroid hormone formation have been divided into the following stages: (1) **iodine trapping** or uptake of iodine by the follicular cells, (2) **organification** (iodination), (3) coupling, (4) storage, and (5) secretion (Fig. 44-4). During trapping, thyroid cells concentrate iodine from the blood against high chemical and electrical gradients, which requires an active energy-dependent mechanism at the level of the cell membrane.[5]

This trapping mechanism for iodine has been exploited for many years in clinical tests to assess thyroid function. Radioactive iodine is given orally to patients, and its degree of concentration in the thyroid is subsequently measured. Various physiological and pharmacological factors influence trapping. The most important factor is TSH, which stimulates trapping of iodine. Iodine excess inhibits the transport of iodine; iodine deficiency stimulates it.

Organification is the process by which iodine is incorporated into thyroid hormone.[6] Normally the thyroid organifies about 75 μg of iodide per day. The iodine used comes from

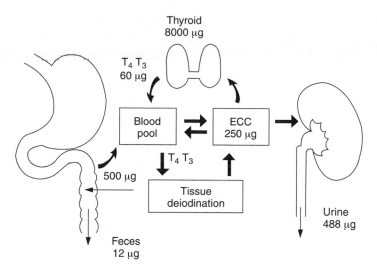

Fig. 44-3 Iodine metabolic pathway in a 24-hour period. *ECC,* Extracellular compartment.

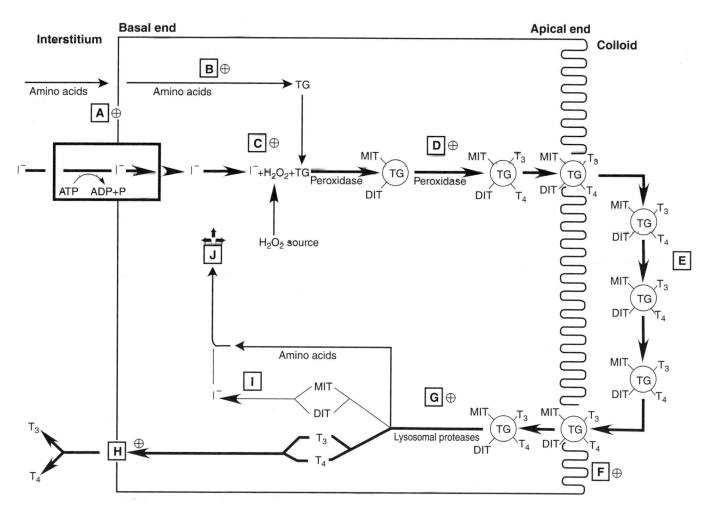

Fig. 44-4 Thyroid cell. Schema depicting stages of thyroid hormonogenesis and intrathyroidal iodine metabolism. *A,* Iodine transport; *B,* thyroglobulin (*TG*) synthesis; *C,* iodide organification; *D,* intrathyroglobulin oxidative coupling; *E,* storage; *F,* endocytosis; *G,* hydrolysis; *H,* hormone secretion; *I,* intrathyroidal deiodination; *J,* recycling. Steps influenced by the thyroid-stimulating hormone (*TSH*) are indicated by the symbol ⊕.

both trapping and from the intrathyroid deiodination of stored thyroid hormone precursors. For iodide to be incorporated into the tyrosine amino acid, it is first oxidized in the presence of a peroxidase enzyme into a reactive form that combines with the protein thyroglobulin.[6]

Thyroglobulin, a glycoprotein with a molecular weight of about 660,000 D, is synthesized intracellularly, carried within secretory vesicles towards the apical portion of the follicular cells, and discharged into the lumen by a process of **exocytosis**. The intracellular thyroglobulin serves as a preformed matrix containing 140 tyrosine residues to which reactive iodine is attached to form monoiodotyrosine (**MIT**) and diiodotyrosine (**DIT**); some iodination also occurs in the colloidal thyroglobulin. After their formation, enzymatic coupling of MIT and DIT takes place to form intrathyroglobulin triiodothyronine (T_3), and thyroxine (T_4). Coupling appears to occur between two iodotyrosine residues located in separate thyroglobulin chains or within folds of the same protein strands. Iodinated thyroglobulin serves as a storage pool of thyroid hormone. Thyroglobulin from these stores is degraded, forming the thyroid hormones, which are finally released into the circulation.

When TSH stimulates the thyroid, a series of cellular and biochemical changes takes place in the gland, all directed toward the synthesis and release of thyroid hormone.[7] Droplets of thyroglobulin-containing colloid are engulfed by the follicular cells of the thyroid gland and then digested by lysosomal proteases, releasing MIT, DIT, T_3, and T_4. Intracellular MIT and DIT are immediately deiodinated, and their iodine is reused in subsequent thyroid hormone synthesis. The T_3 and T_4 are resistant to intrathyroid deiodination and are immediately secreted. The daily secretion of thyroid hormone includes about 80 to 100 μg of T_4 and about 7 μg of T_3.[8] Small amounts of reverse T_3 (**rT_3**) are also secreted by the thyroid.

A low dietary intake of iodine causes a depletion of intrathyroidal deposits of iodine, resulting in an initial decrease of thyroid hormone secretion that in turn leads to an increase of TSH secretion (see later discussion). TSH causes thyroid gland growth (hyperplasia and hypertrophy), which compensates for the iodine deficiency and, at least temporarily, restores the normal levels of circulation hormone. A persistent low ingestion of iodine causes **goiter** associated with **hypothyroidism** (see p. 842).

Transport of Thyroid Hormones

After they are released into the bloodstream, the thyroid hormones are transported in two forms, protein bound and free. The free hormone, which is most readily available for cellular uptake and is thus the physiologically active fraction, represents only a small fraction (less than 0.1%) of the total plasma thyroid hormone content. The bound hormone is metabolically inactive and serves as a large, stable reservoir of hormone, and thus a constant supply of hormone is available to tissues.

Thyroid hormones are bound to three plasma proteins.[9] The most important of these is the **thyroxine-binding globulin**

(**TBG**), which is a 55,000-D glycoprotein synthesized in the liver. The second most important is thyroxine-binding prealbumin (TBPA), also called **transthyretin**, which has a molecular weight of 50,000 D. The third transporting protein is albumin. The role of each of these binding proteins in the transport of T_3 and T_4 is related to their relative affinities for each of the thyroid hormones and on their relative concentrations in plasma. Almost all the circulating T_4 (99.98%) is bound to these plasma proteins. Under physiological circumstances, TBG transports 60% to 75% of total T_4. TBPA and albumin transport 15% to 30% and 10% of T_4, respectively. As is true for T_4, most (99.7%) plasma T_3 circulates in the bound form. The affinity of TBG for T_3 is lower than its affinity for T_4, and binding of T_3 to TBPA is negligible. T_3 is mostly bound to TBG and to a lesser extent to albumin.

T_4 has different affinities for each of its binding proteins, which must be compared to its affinity to the intracellular T_4 receptor (see later discussion). T_4's affinity for TBG is greater than its affinity for the T_4 receptor. T_4's affinity for albumin, however, is weaker than its affinity for the T_4 receptor. Thus there are three pools of protein-bound T_4 in decreasing order of amount of T_4 bound: high-affinity, low-availability (TBG); medium-affinity, medium-availability (TBPA); and low-affinity, high-availability (albumin). This allows a rapid shifting of T_4 among all pools as described in the following equation and ensures a constant availability of T_4 to target cells:

$$\overbrace{\text{TBG-}T_4 \rightleftharpoons \text{TBPA-}T_4 \rightleftharpoons \text{Albumin-}T_4}^{\textbf{Protein bound }T_4} \rightleftharpoons \text{Free }T_4 \rightleftharpoons$$
$$\text{Intracellular receptor-}T_4$$

Abnormalities of the binding proteins may result in abnormal total (bound) hormone concentrations in the blood even when normal amounts of free hormone are present. Because both T_4 and T_3 are bound to TBG, changes of TBG levels affect total serum T_4 and T_3 levels. Changes in TBG concentrations in blood have an indirect effect on the negative-feedback mechanisms of thyroid hormone regulation (Table 44-1). An increase in levels of TBG binding results in an immediate increase in the amount of thyroid hormone that is protein bound, with a subsequent decrease in circulating free hormone. The decrease in free thyroid hormone immediately triggers the secretion of TSH, which results in increased thyroid hormone production and release. All of these changes are transient, and a new equilibrium with preservation of the normal thyroid status is quickly reached. Decreases of TBG serum levels cause the opposite biological changes.

Metabolism of Thyroid Hormones

Circulating T_3 and T_4 are either incorporated into the intracellular pool, where they undergo partial transformations and exert their metabolic effects, or are degraded and eliminated by excretory organs.

Although all circulating T_4 originates in the thyroid gland, the more metabolically important T_3 originates from both direct thyroid secretion (about 20%) and peripheral conversion of T_4 to T_3 by **monodeiodination** (about 80%).[7] The total daily production of T_3 from all sources ranges from 22 to 47 μg. T_3 has been established as the main active hormone at the cellular level. The role of T_4 as a hormone with direct biological activity has been questioned, and some workers consider T_4 to be a **prohormone**. However, T_4 is believed to have some direct biological activity, albeit much less than T_3.

The thyroid hormones are metabolized through deiodinative and nondeiodinative mechanisms. The following are some of the most important metabolic steps (Fig. 44-5):

1. Both T_4 and T_3 exert their biological effects by binding to specific intracellular receptors and are subsequently degraded through successive deiodinations.
2. Deiodination accounts for 80% to 85% of the metabolism of T_4 and T_3.[10]

TABLE 44-1 PHYSIOLOGICAL RELATIONSHIP BETWEEN THYROXINE-BINDING GLOBULIN (TBG) AND SERUM THYROID HORMONE CONCENTRATIONS

Biological Modulators	Initial Biochemical Changes	Intermediate Biological Response	Final Equilibrium Conditions
Increased TBG Pregnancy Oral contraceptives	Increased TBG levels, decreased saturation Augmented binding of hormone (T_4, T_3) Decreased free T_4, T_3	Decreased negative-feedback mechanism Increased serum TSH Increased T_4 and T_3 production	Increased TBG Elevated serum T_4 and T_3 levels Normal TBG saturation Normal free T_4 and T_3
Decreased TBG Androgens Malnutrition Liver disease	Decreased TBG, increased saturation Diminished binding of hormone (T_4, T_3) Increased free T_4 and T_3	Increased negative-feedback mechanism Decreased serum TSH Decreased T_4 and T_3 production	Decreased TBG Decreased T_4 and T_3 Normal TBG saturation Normal free T_4 and T_3 serum

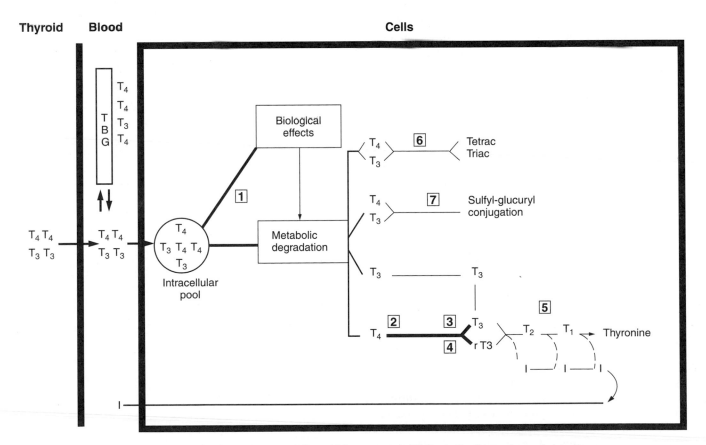

Fig. 44-5 Metabolic pathways of thyroid hormone. *1*, Biological effects through binding to intracellular receptors; *2*, main deiodinative pathway for T_4; *3*, conversion of T_4 into T_3; *4*, conversion of T_4 into rT_3; *5*, serial deiodinations of T_3 and rT_3; *6*, deamination and decarboxylation pathway; *7*, conjugative pathway.

3. About 35% to 50% of the T_4 undergoing deiodination is converted to T_3.[10,11]

4. About 50% to 65% of the deiodinated T_4 is converted into rT_3.[11]

5. Most of the T_4, T_3, and rT_3 are metabolized through a chain of successive deiodinations, resulting in the formation of iodinated intermediary metabolites and ultimately thyronine.

6. Both T_4 and T_3 undergo oxidative deamination and decarboxylation of the alanine side chains to form the acetic acid analogs tetrac and triac.[8]

7. Small amounts of free T_4 are eliminated in the bile and urine.

8. Small amounts of T_3, rT_3, and indirectly T_4 are metabolized by being conjugated with glucuronic acid and sulfate and excreted in the bile.

Conversion of T_4 to active T_3 by monodeiodination of the outer ring is one of the most important metabolic pathways of T_4. In T_3, iodine atoms are located at positions 3 and 5 of the inner (nonphenolic) ring and at position 3' of the outer (phenolic) ring (Fig. 44-2). Two types of 5'-deiodinases have been identified. Type 1, 5'-deiodinase maintains the plasma T_3 concentration and is found in the liver and kidney. Its activity increases in hyperthyroidism and decreases in hypothyroidism. There is a reduced amount of type 1, 5'-deiodinase activity in severe illness, fasting states, and significant hepatic disease. Reduced activity is also seen in the fetus and secondary to certain medications, including propylthiouracil (PTU), propranolol, and excess glucocorticoids. Type 2, 5'-deiodinase maintains the local T_3 concentrations in the tissue in which it is present. It predominates in the brain, pituitary, placenta, and brown fat and is under noradrenergic control. Its activity increases in hypothyroidism, maintaining the constant intracellular T_3 levels, and decreases in **hyperthyroidism** as a compensatory mechanism. Decreased amounts of both types of 5'-deiodinases may be caused by the administration of iodinated radiographic contrast material or by the administration of amiodarone, an antiarrhythmic drug that causes inhibition of T_4 monodeiodination.

If the inner ring of T_4 undergoes monodeiodination, the product is *reverse T_3* (rT_3), which is metabolically inactive. In rT_3, the iodine atoms are found in position 3 of the inner ring and positions 3' and 5' of the outer ring. Almost all rT_3 derives from inner ring monodeiodination of T_4.

Mechanisms of Action

Mechanisms of action of the thyroid hormones at the cellular level have been the focus of intensive research. Initially the thyroid hormone appears both to bind to cell membrane receptors and to cross the cell membrane by direct diffusion. Once inside the cell, the thyroid hormone binds to a cytosol receptor and then nuclear receptor sites (thyroid receptors [TRs], α and β). Although TRα and TRβ receptors are widely expressed in most tissues, the degree of expression varies considerably. The greater hormonal potency of T_3 appears to be related to its higher binding affinity to its receptors compared to that of T_4. The T_3 nuclear receptors are the gene products of the *c-erb*, a protooncogene. Mutations of these sites are believed to be the cause for familial thyroid hormone resistance.

TRs have two separate binding domains. The DNA domain binds to specific sequences of the effector genes, causing either stimulation or inhibition of gene transcription. Once the T_3-nuclear receptor complex binds to sites on DNA, messenger ribonucleic acid (mRNA) is formed and directs the synthesis of proteins and enzymes responsible for metabolic functions.[12] Other postulated mechanisms of action at the cellular level are (1) mitochondrial activation, (2) stimulation of Na^+,K^+-adenosine triphosphatase (ATPase) activity,[13] (3) stimulation of cell membrane functions, probably through a specific receptor, and (4) interaction with the adrenergic system.

Control and Regulation of Thyroid Function

Hypothalamic-pituitary-thyroid axis (HPTA). The HPTA is a group of physiologically interrelated neuroendocrine and endocrine organs that regulate and control the secretion of thyroid hormone (Fig. 44-6). The ultimate effector in this axis is the thyroid gland, which produces,

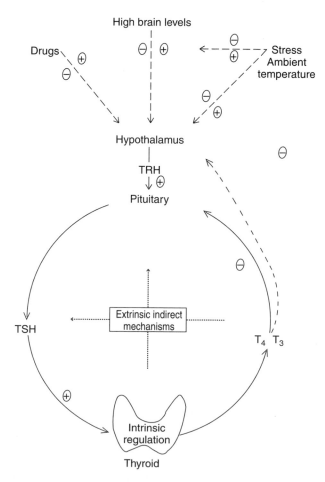

Fig. 44-6 Hypothalamic-pituitary-thyroid axis (HPTA). Stimulatory, ⊕, or inhibitory, effect of agent.

stores, and secretes the hormones thyroxine and triiodothyronine. The hypothalamus, located in the brain, acts as a crucial regulating organ (see also Chapter 43).

Thyrotropin-releasing hormone (TRH) is a tripeptide produced in the paraventricular nucleus of the hypothalamus and secreted into the venous system, which then drains into the pituitary. The TRH attaches to receptor sites in the pituitary, where it causes increased production and secretion of thyroid-stimulating hormone (TSH). TSH is a glycopeptide structurally composed of two subunits, α and β. The β subunit confers on TSH the specific physiological properties that differentiate it from other pituitary glycopeptides. TSH is released from the pituitary into the bloodstream. At the thyroid, TSH attaches to specific cell membrane receptors thereby activating adenylate cyclase and increasing intracellular levels of cyclic AMP (cAMP). The increased levels of cAMP have two main actions. The first, trophic, action is the stimulation of cell reproduction and hypertrophy. The second effect is the stimulation of production and secretion of thyroid hormone by the thyroid cell.

In healthy persons an increase in blood TRH levels affects the blood levels of TSH and thyroid hormone (Fig. 44-7). After the intravenous administration of synthetic TRH, blood levels of TSH begin to increase within 10 minutes, reach a maximum at 15 to 45 minutes, and return to normal base levels in 1 to 4 hours.[14] Elevations of TSH after the administration of TRH result in increases in serum T_4 and T_3. The initial increases in T_3 are higher (75% increase over basal levels) than those in T_4 (15% to 50% over basal levels). The T_3 and T_4 levels subsequently drop slowly. The **TSH** (and occasionally T_3 and T_4) responses to intravenous administrations of synthetic TRH are occasionally used for diagnostic purposes (see p. 842).

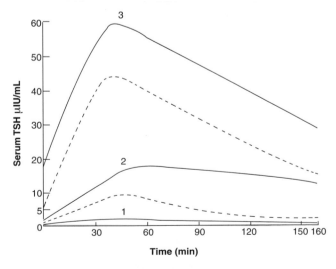

Fig. 44-7 Changes in serum TSH levels in response to TRH (given at 0 minutes). The upper and lower ranges of normal responses are shown by the *dashed lines.* Serum TSH changes after TRH challenge in pituitary, *1;* hypothalamic, *2;* and primary hypothyroid, *3,* disease are also shown.

Negative-feedback system on pituitary secretion of TSH. The most important regulation of TSH production is the thyroid hormone status. Increased levels of thyroid hormones in blood inhibit TSH secretion by the pituitary (negative feedback). The mechanism of this inhibitory effect appears to involve circulating free T_3 and T_4. The pituitary and hypothalamus glands are also able to convert T_4 directly to T_3. This locally generated T_3 then acts with circulating T_3 on the pituitary gland cells to inhibit the secretion of TSH in response to TRH and on the hypothalamus to reduce TRH output. Conversely, decreased levels of thyroid hormone result in increased secretion of TRH and TSH.

An important fact about the normal negative feedback system is that there is an inverse, log-linear relationship between the serum levels of TSH and free T_4. That is, a small, linear change in the free T_4 concentration results in a logarithmic change in the opposite direction of the concentration of TSH as the negative feedback system attempts to maintain normal levels of free T_4. Thus the very small changes of free T_4 concentration (within the reference interval) that might be associated with mild cases of thyroid dysfunction, with no apparent clinical symptoms (*subclinical* hypothyroidism or hyperthyroidism, see later discussion), could be paired with an abnormal serum TSH concentration. Because an abnormal TSH is usually the first indication of thyroid dysfunction, many guidelines recommend a TSH-based approach for screening ambulatory patients for thyroid disease (see later discussion).

Other factors affecting thyroid function. Thyroid function is finely regulated by both extrinsic and intrinsic mechanisms. The extrinsic direct mechanism is the HPTA. The extrinsic indirect mechanisms, which include neurogenic, metabolic, and pharmacological mechanisms, exert inhibitory and stimulatory effects centrally at all levels of the HPTA and peripherally on the metabolism of the thyroid hormones (see later discussion). The intrinsic mechanisms are those that act within the thyroid cells, ensuring that adequate amounts of intrathyroid hormone are produced. These mechanisms are closely dependent on the availability and effects of iodine.

Rapid and large increases of iodine cause an inhibition of the formation and release of thyroid hormone. This inhibition is known as the **Wolff-Chaikoff effect**.[15] If the thyroid continues to be exposed to increased concentrations of iodine, the inhibitory effects of excess iodine on hormone formation and release decrease and eventually cease.[15]

Other effects of excess iodide include blunting of responses to TSH-receptor activation, decreased production of hydrogen peroxide resulting in a decrease of coupling reactions, and inhibition of colloid reabsorption. These responses decrease the production and release of thyroid hormone. Iodine also decreases the vascularity of the thyroid gland. Occasionally, excess of iodide can cause hyperthyroidism; a condition called the *Jodbasedow effect.*

Effects of drugs and other compounds on thyroid function. Various drugs and substances may interfere with thyroid function. Their pharmacological effects may take place at one or several levels (Table 44-2). For example, the drug amiodarone causes elevations of free and total T_4, decreased T_3, and increased rT_3.[16] Various other drugs affect TBG levels and hormone binding and thus total T_3 and T_4 determinations (see box, p. 837).

An important possible interferent of TSH assays is *h*eterophilic *a*nti-*m*ouse *a*ntibodies (HAMAs). Depending on the nature of the assay, HAMAs can cause artifactually increased or decreased TSH measurements. Abnormal TSH values that have no clinical correlation should be verified by another method.

Interrelationships Between Thyroid Gland and Other Functions

Various physiological factors indirectly influence thyroid function and the effects of thyroid hormones. The effects of sex hormones and sex type on thyroid function are variable. Thyroid disease is known to predominate in females. Estrogens cause an increase in TBG and therefore total serum T_3 and T_4 content, whereas **androgen** hormones have the opposite effect. On the other hand, states of decreased (hypothyroidism) and increased (hyperthyroidism) thyroid function are asso-

ciated with alterations of the reproductive system, abnormalities of the menstrual cycle, delayed or precocious puberty, infertility, and growth retardation.

The newborn has lower levels of total T_3 and higher levels of total T_4 and rT_3 than adults have.[17] Immediately after birth there is an increase of TSH, with corresponding elevations of total T_3 and total T_4 that reach their zenith the second day after birth and then gradually decrease toward normal adult levels by the end of the first year of life. There is also a slow progressive decrease of T_3 levels in adults during the aging process.

Striking changes in thyroid function occur during pregnancy (see also Chapter 40). The normal placenta produces significant amounts of nonthyroid hormones (especially estrogens), which stimulate the synthesis of TBG, increasing serum TBG levels. In addition, human chorionic gonadotropin (hCG) has very weak TSH-like activity as the result of similarities of structure for both hormones.[18] However, the very high levels of hCG that occur in pregnancy produce a significant TSH effect. Both total T_4 and, to a lesser extent, total T_3 levels in serum increase during pregnancy because of these increases in TBG concentration[19] and may be as much

TABLE 44-2 EFFECTS OF VARIOUS DRUGS ON THYROID FUNCTION

Mechanism of Action	Drug	Effects
Hypothalamic stimulation	Amphetamine	Increased T_4, T_3, and free T_4
Inhibition of TSH secretion	Dopamine	Decreased TSH
	Levodopa	Blunted TSH response to TRH
	Glucocorticoids	
	Bromocriptine	
Enhanced TSH secretion	Metoclopramide	Increased TSH response to TRH
Blocking of iodine trapping	Perchlorate	Block production of T_4 and T_3
	Thiocyanates	
	Nitroprusside	
Inhibition of organification	Propylthiouracil	Decreased T_4 and T_3 production
	Methimazole	
	Sulfonylureas	
	6-Mercaptopurine	
Inhibition of release of T_4 and T_3	Lithium	Mild transient decrease of T_4, T_3
		Induction of goiter
Decreased conversion of T_4 and T_3		
Decreased type I 5'-deiodinase	Propylthiouracil	Decreased T_3
	Propanolol	
	Glucocorticoid excess	
Decreased type I and II 5'-deiodinase	Amiodarone	Decreased T_3
	Telepaque (iopanoic acid)	
	Oragrafin (ipodic acid sodium calcium salt)	
Increased degradation	Phenobarbital	Slight decrease of T_4 and T_3 and increase in TSH
Modulation of excess of β-adrenergic receptors	β-Adrenergic blockers	Blunted adrenergic-related effects of T_3 and T_4
Decreased hormone protein-binding to TBG	Salicylates	Decreased T_3 and T_4
	Phenytoin	Increased T_3RU
	Fenclofenac	
	Furosemide	

From Kaplan MM: *Med Clin North Am* 69:863-880, 1985; Oppenheimer JH, Schwartz HL, Surks MI: *J Clin Invest* 51:2493-2497, 1972; Singer I, Rotenberg D: *N Engl J Med* 289:254-260, 1973; Cavalieri RR et al: *Metabolism* 29:1161-1165, 1979.

CAUSES OF ABNORMALITIES IN THYROXINE-BINDING GLOBULIN (TBG)

Quantitative

Increased TBG serum levels
Pregnancy
Estrogen therapy
Clofibrate treatment
Oral contraceptives
Perphenazine
Abuse of heroin or
   methadone
Acute hepatitis
Hypothyroidism
Neonatal period
Acute intermittent porphyria
Genetic TBG excess

Decreased TBG serum levels
Androgens
Anabolic agents
Cirrhosis
Acute illness
Surgical stress
Severe chronic illness
Severe hypoproteinemia
Protein malnutrition
Nephrotic syndrome
Hyperthyroidism
Corticosteroid therapy
L-Asparaginase therapy
Active acromegaly

Klinefelter's syndrome
Cushing's syndrome
Down syndrome
Type III hyperlipidemia
Chronic metabolic acidosis
Genetic deficiency
   (usually X-linked)

Qualitative
Genetic
Genetically determined
   increase in binding
   affinity
Genetically determined
   decrease in binding
   affinity
Drugs competing with T_4 and T_3 for TBG-binding sites
Phenytoin
   (diphenylhydantoin,
   Dilantin)
Dicumarol
Heparin (causes release of
   fatty acids, which affect
   hormone binding to TBG)
Atromid S
Aspirin
Phenylbutazone

as one and one half times higher by 16 weeks gestation than in the nonpregnant state, although TSH levels are generally lower in the first trimester of pregnancy. Levels of free hormone remain normal in early pregnancy, but decrease by 20% to 40% below nonpregnancy values by the second and third trimesters.

In fasting states, changes in levels of thyroid hormone in serum occur within 24 to 48 hours. Initially serum T_3 decreases rapidly; if fasting is maintained; the decrease slows, becoming more gradual. The decrease in T_3 levels is caused by decreased peripheral conversion of T_4 to T_3. Concomitantly there is an increase in rT_3 levels. Chronic decreased caloric intake also results in a decline in thyroxine-binding prealbumin (TBPA), probably caused by decreased hepatic production.

General Metabolic and Physiological Effects of Thyroid Hormone

Increases and decreases in hormone production result in states of hyperfunction (hyperthyroidism) and hypofunction (hypothyroidism), respectively. The clinical presentation of hyperthyroidism or hypothyroidism reflects the basic effects of thyroid hormone on various organs and metabolic systems.

Table 44-3 depicts some general effects that thyroid hormone has on various metabolic functions and systems. The effects of thyroid hormone can be classified according to their clinical expression into (1) general metabolic effects, (2) growth and maturation effects, and (3) organ-specific effects. Generally speaking, both intermediary metabolic pathways and specific metabolic pathways are stimulated by the thyroid hormone, resulting in increased oxygen consumption and **calorigenesis**. Thyroid hormone has important actions as a promoter of cell differentiation, growth, and maturation. Deficiency of thyroid hormone in early life results in severe impairment of physical growth, maturation, and brain development. The third class of thyroid hormonal effects represents many direct effects exerted on specific organs and systems, such as the brain and heart. Finally, increased thyroid function is associated with an elevated catecholamine (hyperadrenergic) state important in the genesis of some symptoms of hyperthyroidism.

Decreased thyroid hormone results in deposition of mucoproteins and mucopolysaccharides in various tissues such as the skin, muscles, and heart. This phenomenon partly explains the thick skin, muscle weakness, enlarged heart, and symptoms of heart failure seen in hypothyroidism.

The developing fetus requires thyroid hormone for normal brain development.[20] The fetus is dependent upon the mother for thyroid hormone until midgestation, when it begins to produce the hormones. Insufficient first trimester levels of maternal thyroid hormone have been demonstrated to increase the risk for mental[21] and psychomotor deficits in the newborn.[22] Because early intervention may prevent the long-term effects of maternal hypothyroidism,[23] screening of pregnant women has been advocated (see later discussion).[24]

Thyroid Function in Nonthyroid Disease (NTD)

Certain conditions do not directly alter the output of hormone by the thyroid but rather interfere with the normal transport and metabolism of thyroid hormones. These conditions, including those abnormalities in thyroxine-binding globulin (see box), produce changes in standard blood tests of thyroid function but are generally *not* accompanied by true thyroid dysfunction. The disorders are of clinical importance because they may mimic true thyroid disease or confound the diagnosis of concomitant thyroid dysfunction.

Many acutely ill, hospitalized individuals have abnormal measures of thyroid function, either TSH or free hormones, in the absence of overt thyroid dysfunction. This entity of nonthyroid disease (NTD, or *sick euthyroid*) may result from improper control over the release of TRH from the hypothalamus.[25] NTD can be very confusing to physicians who need to determine if the underlying cause of an acute illness might be thyroid disease. In these cases, discussions with the laboratory can be very important (see later discussion, p. 846).

Malnutrition, renal, and hepatic dysfunctions are the three most important nonthyroid factors leading to abnormalities of thyroid function tests. States of malnutrition are often seen in chronic and debilitating diseases. The most conspicuous physiological abnormality found in malnourished patients is the impaired peripheral conversion of T_4 to T_3.[26] As a result, serum total and free T_3 concentrations decrease significantly while the serum total T_4 concentration stays relatively stable. The levels of rT_3 may double.

TABLE 44-3 BASIC PHYSIOLOGICAL EFFECTS OF THYROID HORMONE AND THEIR RELATIONSHIP WITH SYNDROMES OF THYROID DYSFUNCTION

System	Thyroid Hormone Effects	USUAL SYMPTOMS	
		Hyperthyroidism	Hypothyroidism
Metabolic	Increased calorigenesis and O_2 consumption	Heat intolerance	Cold intolerance
	Increased heat dissipation	Flushed skin	Dry and pale skin
	Increased protein catabolism	Increased perspiration	Coarse skin
	Increased glucose absorption and production (gluconeogenesis)	Increased appetite and food ingestion	Lethargy
	Increased glucose use	Muscle wasting and proximal weakness	Generalized weakness
		Weight loss	Weight gain
		Onycholysis (nail disease)	Voice coarsening, slow speech
		Lid lag	Myxedema
		Proptosis (exophthalmos)	
Cardiovascular	Increased adrenergic activity and sensitivity	Palpitations	Slow heart rate (bradycardia)
	Increased heart rate	Fast heart rate (tachycardia)	Low blood pressure
	Increased myocardial contractility (inotropy)	Bouncy, hyperdynamic arterial pulses	Heart failure
	Increased cardiac output	Shortness of breath	Heart enlargement
	Increased blood volume	Atrial fibrillation	
	Decreased peripheral vascular resistance	Widened pulse pressure ($\uparrow$ systolic BP, $\downarrow$ diastolic BP)	
Central nervous	Increased adrenergic activity and sensitivity	Restlessness, hypermotility	Apathy
		Nervousness	Mental sluggishness
		Emotional lability	Depressed reflexes
		Fatigue	Mental retardation
		Exaggerated reflexes	
		Tremor	
Gastrointestinal (GI)	Increased motility	Hyperdefecation	Constipation

BP, *Blood pressure.*

The liver plays an important role in the metabolism of thyroid hormones by its production of thyroxine-binding proteins, conversion of T_4 to T_3 or rT_3, and removal of thyroid hormones. Alterations in these functions can occur in liver disease, resulting in abnormal test results in the absence of thyroid disease.

The kidneys have two main functions in relation to the thyroid: the first concerns iodine metabolism, because the kidneys represent a major pathway of iodine elimination; the second is the prevention of excessive losses of thyroxine-binding globulins in the urine. Kidney disease can result in either decreased iodine clearance and excretion, with the secondary increases in blood and interstitial pools of iodine seen in renal failure, or the augmented loss of thyroxine-binding proteins seen in the nephrotic syndrome. Finally, although it plays a less important role than that of the liver, the kidney has the metabolic function of converting T_4 to T_3. In acutely and severely ill patients, the serum T_3 may be undetectable, the serum T_4 greatly reduced, and the serum TSH normal or mildly increased. As the patient recovers, there is an approximate increase in TSH until free T_4 and free T_3 return to normal.

PATHOLOGICAL CONDITIONS
Screening

Most thyroid testing occurs in screening situations. Either a physician needs to exclude thyroid disease as the possible cause for a patient's symptoms, or the physician has raised concerns about the possibility of thyroid disease because of certain symptoms (such as cardiac disease) or older age, which is associated with increased prevalence of thyroid disease.[1-4] Most current guidelines[1-4] recommend that screening for thyroid disease be performed using a second- or third-generation TSH assay (see later discussion and CD-ROM). An abnormal TSH result should be followed up by measurement of free T_4.

When screening for disease, results are often obtained in which the more sensitive test, TSH, is outside of the reference interval but the free T_4 or free T_3 results are within the reference interval. When the patients in these cases are without clinical symptoms of thyroid disease, the situations may be termed *subclinical* hypothyroidism or hyperthyroidism. Although overt thyroid disease may not be seen until more extremely abnormal TSH levels are achieved, the value of detecting subclinical thyroid disease is becoming increasingly apparent, and is discussed more fully later under hyperthyroidism.

Monitoring

Once a diagnosis of hypothyroidism or hyperthyroidism has been made (see later discussion), patients must be monitored to determine the success of therapy. The patient's thyroid status is usually unstable following the initiation of therapy and the most sensitive indicator of thyroid function, TSH, usually does not reliably indicate the new thyroid status very well. So during the initial 3 months of therapy, serum free T_4 levels should be used to track thyroid status.

Hyperthyroidism

Causes. Hyperthyroidism refers to the clinical syndrome caused by an excess of circulating active thyroid hormone. Hyperthyroidism is caused by numerous pathological conditions that have as a common denominator an increase in circulating thyroid hormone (see box below).

Graves' disease, which occurs in 0.4% of the US population, is caused by an immunological disorder in which serum autoantibodies bind to TSH receptors in the thyroid cell and stimulate the production and release of thyroid hormone. These antibodies comprise a heterogeneous group of serum immunoglobulins that belong to the IgG fraction and are generically termed *thyroid-stimulating immunoglobulins* **(TSI)**[27] because of their ability to stimulate function in thyroid cells. The long-acting thyroid stimulator (LATS)

CAUSES OF HYPERTHYROIDISM

Primary Hyperthyroidism
Primary thyroid abnormalities
   Toxic multinodular goiter (Plummer's disease)
   Thyroid adenoma
   Thyroid carcinoma
   Struma ovarii (ovarian teratoma with thyroid elements)

Secondary Hyperthyroidism
Endogenous: increased serum levels of TSH (thyroid-stimulating substances), resulting in thyroid hyperactivity:
   Graves' disease
   Neonatal hyperthyroidism
   Pituitary tumors (TSH-secreting)
   Trophoblastic tumors
      Hydatidiform mole
      Choriocarcinoma
      Embryonal carcinoma of testes
Exogenous:
   Iatrogenic
   Factitious hyperthyroidism (Jodbasedow effect)

Thyroiditis
Subacute thyroiditis (early phase)
Lymphocytic (Hashimoto's) thyroiditis
Radiation
Postpartum thyroiditis (early phase)

---

antibody was the first TSI described and is present in about 60% of patients with Graves' disease.

Graves' disease is characterized clinically by the presence of diffuse goiter (enlarged thyroid gland), symptoms and signs of hyperthyroidism (Table 44-3), ophthalmopathy, and, occasionally, pretibial (swelling of the shins) edema. Graves' ophthalmopathy is characterized by a myxedematous (swelling observable by pressing on the tissue) infiltration of the tissues and muscles of the orbit, resulting in protrusion of the eyes and ocular muscle dysfunction. The ophthalmopathy may exist without accompanying thyroid hyperfunction. TSI can cross the placenta and can cause transient neonatal hyperthyroidism. This condition occurs in about 1% to 2% of pregnancies in women with a background of Graves' disease.

Toxic **multinodular goiter** is a frequent cause of hyperthyroidism and usually appears in patients with preexisting nodular goiters. Nodular goiters are discrete portions of the thyroid gland that are no longer under normal feedback control and secrete excess amounts of thyroid hormone. This condition occurs more frequently in elderly patients and is not accompanied by ophthalmopathy or pretibial edema.

Thyroid adenomas are benign tumors that do not respond to the normal control mechanism and can occasionally produce excess thyroid hormone. Patients with adenomas have thyroid nodules that concentrate radioactive iodine avidly (hot nodules). It should be emphasized that most adenomas do not cause thyroid hyperfunction. Thyroid cancer is a rare cause of hyperthyroidism.

Thyroiditis is a general term used to describe an inflammation of the thyroid gland. All forms of thyroiditis can potentially cause hyperthyroidism because large quantities of hormone can be released from the inflamed and disrupted follicles. *Subacute thyroiditis* and its variant, *painless thyroiditis*, are considered to be caused by a viral infection of the gland and have two phases. The early phase is characterized by active inflammation of the thyroid, which results in enlargement and tenderness of the gland and clinical and laboratory findings of thyroid hyperfunction caused by release of hormones.[28,29] During the late phase, recuperation takes place and function usually returns to normal. Some patients may evolve through an intermediary state of hypothyroidism. *Chronic lymphocytic thyroiditis* **(Hashimoto's thyroiditis)** is occasionally associated with an overactive thyroid state but more often results in hypothyroidism.

Postpartum thyroiditis occurs in 3.9% to 8.2% of women after delivery.[30,31] Similar to subacute thyroiditis, there may be three phases beginning with a painless **thyrotoxicosis** with greatly diminished radioactive iodine uptake. This typically occurs 1 to 3 months postpartum and lasts for 1 to 2 months.[30] The thyroid gland often becomes enlarged. The patient may then develop hypothyroidism before recovery. Fatigue and depression are common symptoms. Postpartum thyroiditis is believed to be attributable to an autoimmune process and thyroid autoantibodies may be present.[32]

A sudden release of hormone may be seen after irradiation of the thyroid gland (*radiation thyroiditis*). Thyroid hyperfunction caused by this radiation thyroiditis as suggested by elevations of serum T_3 and T_4 is usually mild and self-limited.

Exogenous hyperthyroidism is caused by the administration of excessive thyroid hormone by the physician (**iatrogenic**) or as a result of surreptitious intake of thyroid hormone by patients (**factitial**).

Tumors originating from the trophoblast, or outer cellular layer of the forming embryo, can secrete large amounts of hCG. This hormone has been found to have a weak thyroid-stimulating action. As a result, **trophoblastic tumors** may cause an increased secretion of thyroid hormones. Secondary hyperthyroidism caused by pituitary tumors that secrete high levels of TSH is a rare occurrence.

Some iodine-deficient patients develop hyperthyroidism after replacement of iodine either through diet or after the administration of radiographic iodine contrast material. This condition, known as the Jodbasedow phenomenon, is postulated to occur in patients with occult Graves' disease or multinodular goiter.

Laboratory findings. Graves' disease is the classic example of hyperthyroidism. Its laboratory abnormalities (Table 44-4) include (1) elevation of thyroid hormones in serum, (2) decreased serum levels of TSH, and (3) blunted responses to TRH (see p. 842). In addition, patients with Graves' disease may have elevated serum levels of thyroglobulin and thyroid-stimulating immunoglobulin. In general there is a disproportionately higher rate of production of T_3 in Graves' disease. Patients at risk for postpartum thyroiditis will have antithyroperoxidase antibodies present in the first trimester of pregnancy.

As many as 5% of people with thyroid disease have been described with symptoms of hyperthyroidism and normal total T_4 and free T_4 concentrations, normal or mildly elevated

thyroidal radioactive iodine uptake, and elevated T_3 levels in blood. This syndrome, termed *T_3 thyrotoxicosis*, may be present in patients with Graves' disease. It has also been observed in 5% of patients with toxic nodular goiter, in patients with previous iodine deficiency after iodine ingestion, and in patients with recurrent hyperthyroidism after treatment with radioactive iodine, thyroid-blocking agents, or surgery. T_3 thyrotoxicosis appears to be caused by increased intracellular conversion of T_4 to T_3.

A less frequently found entity (a prevalence of approximately 5%), *T_4 toxicosis*, refers to a condition in which the T_3 is normal or only mildly elevated and T_4 is quite elevated. This condition is seen most often in patients with an alteration in conversion of T_4 to T_3 as a result of chronic debilitating diseases or in patients acutely exposed to large amounts of iodine (such as x-ray contrast media).

Neonatal hyperthyroidism refers to a state of increased thyroid function seen in newborn infants of mothers whose serum may contain TSI. This condition is postulated to be caused by transplacental transfer of maternal TSI.[33] Its course is benign with spontaneous remission.

There is increasing evidence that s*ubclinical hyperthyroidism* is associated with harmful effects, including cardiovascular disease, neurological disease,[34,35] and generally long-term increased mortality.[36] Cardiovascular disease and increased mortality were often found at TSH values between 0.1 and 0.4 µU/mL, levels not usually associated with overt hyperthyroidism. Physicians screening for possible thyroid disease or monitoring patients undergoing treatment may need to respond to these borderline low TSH values, especially those in elderly patients, to ensure that there are no long-term effects of subclinical hyperthyroidism.

Treatment. The treatment of hyperthyroidism can be aimed at eliminating excess functioning thyroid tissue

---

TABLE 44-4   HYPERTHYROIDISM: LABORATORY FINDINGS IN VARIOUS CLINICAL CONDITIONS

Clinical Entity	T_4	T_3	FT_4	T_3RU	FT_4I	TSH	TRH Stimulation	TSI	Thyroid [123]I Uptake
Graves' disease	↑	↑	↑	↑	↑	↓, U	Blunted	↑	
Euthyroid Graves' disease	N	N	N	N	N	N	Blunted, N	+	N
Toxic multinodular goiter	↑	↑	↑	↑	↑	↓, U	Blunted	−	↑, N
Toxic adenoma	↑	↑	↑	↑	↑	↓, U	Blunted	−	↑, N
T_3 toxicosis	N	↑	N	N, ↑	N	↓, U	Blunted	+, −	N, ↑
Hyperthyroidism in pregnancy	↑	↑	↑	N, ↓	↑	↓, U	Blunted	+, −	*
Neonatal hyperthyroidism	↑	↑	↑	↑	↑	↓, N	Blunted	+	*
Subacute thyroiditis	↑, N	↑, N	↑, N	↑, N	↑, N	N, ↓, U	Blunted, N	−	↓, N
Exogenous hyperthyroidism with T_4	↑	↑	↑	↑	↑	↓, U	Blunted	−	↓
Trophoblastic tumors	↑	↑	↑	↑	↑	↑, N, ↓	Blunted	−	↓, N, ↑
Pituitary TSH-secreting tumors	↑	↑	↑	↑	↑	↑	N, ↑	−	↑
Pseudohyperthyroidism	↑	↑, N	↑, N	↑, N	↑, N	↑, N	N	−	N or ↑

FT$_4$, Free thyroxine; FT$_4$I, free thyroxine index; N, normal; TRH, thyrotropin-releasing hormone; T$_3$RU, triiodothyronine resin-uptake test; TSH, thyroid-stimulating hormone; TSI, thyroid-stimulating immunoglobulins; U, undetectable.
↑, Elevated; ↓, decreased; +, present; −, absent; *, test contraindicated or not recommended.

(surgery or radioiodine); inhibiting the production of thyroid hormone using thyroid-blocking drugs such as propylthiouracil (PTU), methimazole, saturated solution of potassium iodide (SSKI), or Lugol's solution; inhibiting thyroid hormone release from the thyroid (SSKI, Lugol's solution); or suppressing the symptoms of hyperthyroidism (β-adrenergic receptor blockers). All these methods are currently used, and the choice depends on the cause of the hyperthyroidism, special clinical situations, and the physician's personal preferences.

Hypothyroidism

Causes. A clinical state of hypothyroidism develops whenever insufficient amounts of thyroid hormone are available to tissues. By and large the most common group of entities causing hypothyroidism are those that involve the thyroid gland itself (see box below).

Hashimoto's thyroiditis is probably the single most common cause of hypothyroidism. It is believed to result from a derangement of cellular and humoral components of the immune system.[37] The most important characteristic of Hashimoto's thyroiditis is the presence of a defect in organification, accompanied by lymphocytic infiltration of the gland with concomitant loss of thyroid tissue. These elements of the disease are reflected clinically by the presence of an enlarged thyroid gland, thyroid hypofunction, and the presence in serum of antithyroid antibodies. The **antimicrosomal** (antiperoxidase) **antibody** is found in 90% to 95% of patients with Hashimoto's thyroiditis.

Causes of Hypothyroidism

Primary Thyroid Dysfunction
Parenchymal damage
  Thyroiditis
    Chronic lymphocytic (Hashimoto's) thyroiditis
    Subacute thyroiditis
  Therapeutic ablation
    After ^{131}I therapy
    After surgery
  Thyroid dysgenesis
    Aplasia
    Dysplasia
  Thyroid infiltration
    Tumors
    Iodine deficiency (endemic goiter)
    Iodine excess (>6 mg/day)
    Thyroid-blocking drugs (lithium, sulfonamides, etc.)
  Congenital and acquired defects of hormone synthesis and
    thyroglobulin metabolism defects
  Abnormal hormonogenesis

Pituitary Hypothyroidism (TSH Deficiency)

Hypothalamic Hypothyroidism (TRH Deficiency)

Reduced Peripheral Response to Thyroid Hormone

Hypothyroidism can result from various other conditions. It often follows surgical thyroidectomy or therapy with radioiodine for treatment of Graves' disease. Developmental abnormalities and tumors and other infiltrative disorders that displace and destroy thyroid tissue can occasionally cause hypothyroidism. Congenital defects in hormonogenesis and the effect of drugs can also result in hypothyroidism. Pituitary and hypothalamic disease are rare conditions that occasionally lead to hypothyroidism caused by inadequate TRH or TSH secretion.

As mentioned earlier, there is now evidence that maternal hypothyroidism can result in harmful effects to the developing fetus. Although screening pregnant women for subclinical or overt hypothyroidism has been advocated,[24] there are both clinical[24] and laboratory problems with screening. The National Academy of Clinical Biochemistry has recommended that laboratories develop gestation week–specific reference intervals for TSH and thyroid hormones.[2]

Laboratory findings. Regardless of the cause, the laboratory findings in hypothyroidism are characterized by decreased total serum T_4, T_3, FT_4, FT_4I, and T_3RU. The degree of abnormality of these tests varies widely, depending on the cause of hypothyroidism and stage of the disease.

Some distinctive laboratory findings can be found in Table 44-5. For example, hypothyroidism caused by intrinsic thyroid disease (primary hypothyroidism) is characterized by elevated TSH levels and exaggerated TSH response to TRH stimulation. Low or borderline normal levels of TSH and TRH test responses characterize hypothyroidism caused by pituitary (secondary) and hypothalamic (tertiary) disease, as noted earlier. Hypothyroidism in the neonatal period can lead to severe retardation of the growth and maturation of the central nervous system (**cretinism**). Routine screening of neonates for hypothyroidism is an important tool for the early diagnosis of hypothyroidism.[38] TSH-blocking antibody, which has been found in the serum of patients with atrophic thyroiditis, may be transmitted across the placenta and cause temporary hypothyroidism in the newborn. Disappearance of

---

TABLE 44-5 Laboratory Findings in Hypothyroidism

Type	T_4	T_3	T_3RU	FT_4I	TSH	TRH Stimulation*	Ab
Primary	↓	↓, N	↓, N	↓	↑	↑	†
Secondary	↓	↓	↓	↓	↓, N	↓	—
Tertiary	↓	↓	↓	↓	↓, N	N	—
Peripheral unresponsiveness	↑	↑	N	↑ or N	↑ or N	N or ↑	

*Assessed by response of serum TSH to TRH administration.
†10% of normal population has acute antiperoxidase antibody, with females more than males.
Ab, Antibodies to thyroid microsomal peroxidase; N, Normal; ↑, elevated; ↓, decreased. See Table 44-4 for abbreviations.

the antibody is associated with remission of the hypothyroid state.

Treatment. The treatment of hypothyroidism consists in thyroid hormone replacement given orally, which reverses the abnormal laboratory findings and clinical symptoms and signs, provided that there are no abnormalities in the transport and peripheral use of thyroid hormones. The most common agent used is levothyroxine (T_4), which is converted peripherally to T_3. The average replacement dose in most adults is 1.6 μg/kg body weight.

Goiter

Goiter is a generic reference to an enlargement of the thyroid gland. It may be associated with a hyperthyroid, hypothyroid, or euthyroid state. Diffuse goiter is characterized by uniform enlargement of the thyroid gland. In multinodular goiter the thyroid gland is enlarged in a nonuniform fashion, resulting in nodules located both superficially and deep within the gland.

Solitary Nodule

A **solitary nodule** refers to the presence of a solitary localized enlargement of a portion of the thyroid gland. Although most of these nodules represent benign conditions, such as cysts, localized hemorrhages, focal thyroiditis, and adenomas, they may also represent malignant tumors of the thyroid. External radiation therapy used in the past for acne and enlarged tonsils and other conditions of the head, neck, and chest has been associated with an increased risk for the development of both thyroid cancer and benign thyroid neoplasms.[39]

Thyroid Cancer

The most common primary malignant thyroid tumors originate from the epithelial cells of the follicles. Patients with thyroid cancer usually do not display significant abnormalities of thyroid function. These tumors often release thyroglobulin into the circulation, where it may be followed as a tumor marker. Rarely, a patient may have an antithyroglobulin antibody, which invalidates the use of the thyroglobulin assay. Because other thyroid diseases can also result in increased levels of thyroglobulin, this parameter is most useful for following the activity of thyroid cancer once a specific diagnosis has been made and treatment has been instituted. However, the clinician must be confident antibodies to thyroglobulin have not confounded the thyroglobulin measurements.

A different type of thyroid cancer originates from the parafollicular C-cells of the thyroid and is termed **medullary carcinoma**. These tumors secrete calcitonin, a hormone that lowers blood calcium, which is a useful tumor marker for diagnosing and following the clinical course of these patients.

Peripheral Resistance to Thyroid Hormone

Cases of abnormally high T_4 and T_3 hormone levels have been described in patients with otherwise normal baseline TSH concentrations and a normal or increased response to TRH stimulation. Clinical features of this disease vary. They range from euthyroid to an expression of thyroid deficiency.

TESTS OF THYROID FUNCTION

The iodine-concentrating property of the thyroid is used to estimate thyroid function and to obtain functional anatomical images of the gland. For these studies tracer amounts of a radioiodine (iodine-123 or iodine-131) are administered to the patient. γ-Rays emitted by the radioiodine concentrated in the thyroid are detected by specially designed imaging and counting devices and transformed into **radioiodine thyroid uptake** percentages and images of the gland. ^{123}I is the preferred radioisotope because it produces better images and delivers lower radiation doses to the patient's thyroid. Serum samples for hormone radioassays that are obtained after the administration of radioactive materials to the patient must be checked for residual radioactivity before the assay is started or spurious results may be obtained.

Thyroid Iodine Uptake

The thyroid iodine-uptake test measures the percentage of an administered dose of radioiodine that is concentrated in the thyroid by the trapping and organification mechanisms. This measurement may be obtained at various intervals after radioiodine administration. Imaging and counting of the radioiodine are usually performed 4 to 24 hours after the radioisotope dose. For ^{123}I the dose is approximately 200 μCi. Theoretically the amount of radioiodine in the thyroid at a given time reflects thyroid hormone synthesis and secretion and therefore reflects the functional status of the thyroid. Graves' disease is characterized by an elevated radioactive-iodine uptake. Low thyroid uptakes are found not only in hypothyroidism but also in certain conditions actually associated with thyroid hyperfunction, including (1) thyrotoxicosis factitia caused by exogenous thyroid hormone, (2) subacute thyroiditis, (3) iodine-induced hyperthyroidism, (4) chronic lymphocytic thyroiditis, and (5) ectopic thyroid tissue.

TRH Stimulation Test

The TRH stimulation test takes advantage of the interrelationship between the TRH and TSH secretions. Normally, after the intravenous administration of TRH, there is an increase of TSH levels in blood, which in turn elicits an elevation of T_3 and T_4 serum levels.[15,40] Various factors influence the TSH response to TRH stimulation. Abnormal responses to TRH stimulation are of two types. The first type is characterized by lower-than-normal responses of serum TSH to TRH stimulation. In these cases the TSH response to TRH is said to be blunted. A blunted response is usually associated with pituitary dysfunction. The second type of abnormal response manifests as higher-than-normal increments of serum TSH after TRH stimulation and is associated with primary hypothyroidism. Responses of TSH to TRH in various clinical conditions are depicted in Fig. 44-7. Falsely low TSH responses may be associated with depression, with excessive use of glucocorticoids, and serious illnesses.

The main clinical applications of the TRH stimulation test are (1) diagnosis of subclinical and early biochemical hyperthyroidism, (2) evaluation of patients with ophthalmopathy without overt hyperthyroidism, and (3) diagnosis of hypothalamic and pituitary hypothyroidism. A significant increment in TSH eliminates the diagnosis of hyperthyroidism except in the extremely rare patient with the TSH-induced form of this disease.

TSH Stimulation Test

Administration of exogenous TSH will stimulate all phases of thyroid function, which will be reflected by increases in the uptake of radioiodine by the thyroid and increases in blood levels of thyroid hormone. The TSH stimulation test is performed by monitoring the thyroidal radioiodine uptake before (baseline value) and after the administration of bovine TSH for three consecutive days. Normally there is an increase of serum T_4 and radioiodine uptake to more than $1\frac{1}{2}$ times the baseline value in response to TSH administration. The chief use of this test has been to differentiate primary hypothyroidism (decrease of serum T_4 and decrease in radioiodine uptake) from secondary or tertiary hypothyroidism. The TSH stimulation test has been replaced largely by TSH determinations in serum and by the TRH stimulation test.

Triiodothyronine (T_3) or Cytomel Suppression Test

This test is performed by a determination of 24-hour thyroid radioiodine uptake before (baseline value) and then after the oral administration of T_3 for 7 to 10 days.[41] Images of the thyroid gland and thyroid radioisotope uptake determinations are obtained simultaneously. The purpose of this test is to establish the presence of thyroid tissue that has become autonomous and unresponsive to TSH changes. Normally the administration of thyroid hormone (T_3 or T_4) suppresses the secretion of TSH by the pituitary gland. The subsequent absence of TSH results in diminished thyroid concentration of radioiodine. A thyroid gland that is overactive is often autonomous, and so suppression of TSH production by administration of exogenous thyroid hormone is not followed by corresponding declines of thyroid radioiodine uptake. Normally a drop in thyroid uptake (suppression) to 30% to 50% of the baseline value occurs after T_3 administration. Failure to repress the thyroid uptake indicates an autonomous gland.

Perchlorate-Discharge Test

The perchlorate-discharge test detects defects of iodine organification present in conditions such as Hashimoto's thyroiditis and congenital goiters. It is also used to determine the degree of organification defect caused by certain thyroid-blocking drugs used for treatment of hyperthyroidism to assess their therapeutic effects.

CHANGE OF ANALYTE IN DISEASE

Thyroid function can be assessed by determination of various analytes in blood. Tables 44-4 to 44-6 summarize the changes of some analytes in various disease states.

Serum T_4 (see Methods on CD-ROM)

Elevations in total serum T_4 can occur as a result of increased hormone synthesis, increased hormone release from the thyroid cells, or increased binding capacity of plasma proteins, especially TBG. Increased hormone secretion is most frequently seen in states of hyperthyroidism. Causes of hyperthyroidism are listed in the box on p. 839.

Increased T_4 release from the thyroid gland because of cellular damage occurs in subacute thyroiditis, Hashimoto's thyroiditis, and after radiation. Increased levels of serum TBG from various causes (see box, p. 837) produce elevations of total serum T_4. These conditions are not accompanied by hyperthyroidism.

Serum T_3

In general, elevations of serum T_3 are proportionally greater than the increases of T_4 found in most states of hyperthyroidism. Thus routine measurements of total serum T_3 are not necessary. In approximately 5% of cases, elevations of T_3 occur while serum T_4 levels remain normal. This condition is termed T_3 *thyrotoxicosis*. Total T_3 measurements are needed to monitor the treatment of thyroid disease in these cases.

Free Hormone Levels: Estimates or Direct Measurements

Thyroid hormones in the blood are distributed into two compartments: protein-bound and unbound, or free, compartments (Fig. 44-8). Variations in total thyroid hormone in blood can result from changes in the concentration of binding protein. Hypothyroidism and hyperthyroidism occur only if a

TABLE 44-6	THYROID-FUNCTION TESTS IN NONTHYROID DISEASES (NTD)								
	T_4	T_3RU	FT_4I	Free T_4	Free T_3	T_3	rT_3	TSH	TBG
General NTD*	N, ↓	↑, N	↓, N	N, ↑	↓, N	↓, N	↑, N	N	↓, N
Acute hepatitis	N, ↑	↓	N, ↓	N, ↑	N, ↓	↓, N	↑	N	↑
Chronic active hepatitis	N, ↑	↓	N, ↓	N, ↑	N	N	↑	N	↑
Alcoholic cirrhosis	N, ↓	N, ↑	N, ↑	N, ↑	↓	↓	↑	N	↓, N
Renal failure	N, ↓	N	N, ↓	N, ↓	↓	↓	N	N	N
Acute psychiatric illness	N, ↑	—	N, ↑	N, ↑	N	N	—	N	—

Normal thyroid function in patients with very complex problems; findings in individual patients may vary widely.
N, *Normal;* ↑, *augmented;* ↓, *diminished.*
*Includes all patients with NTD.

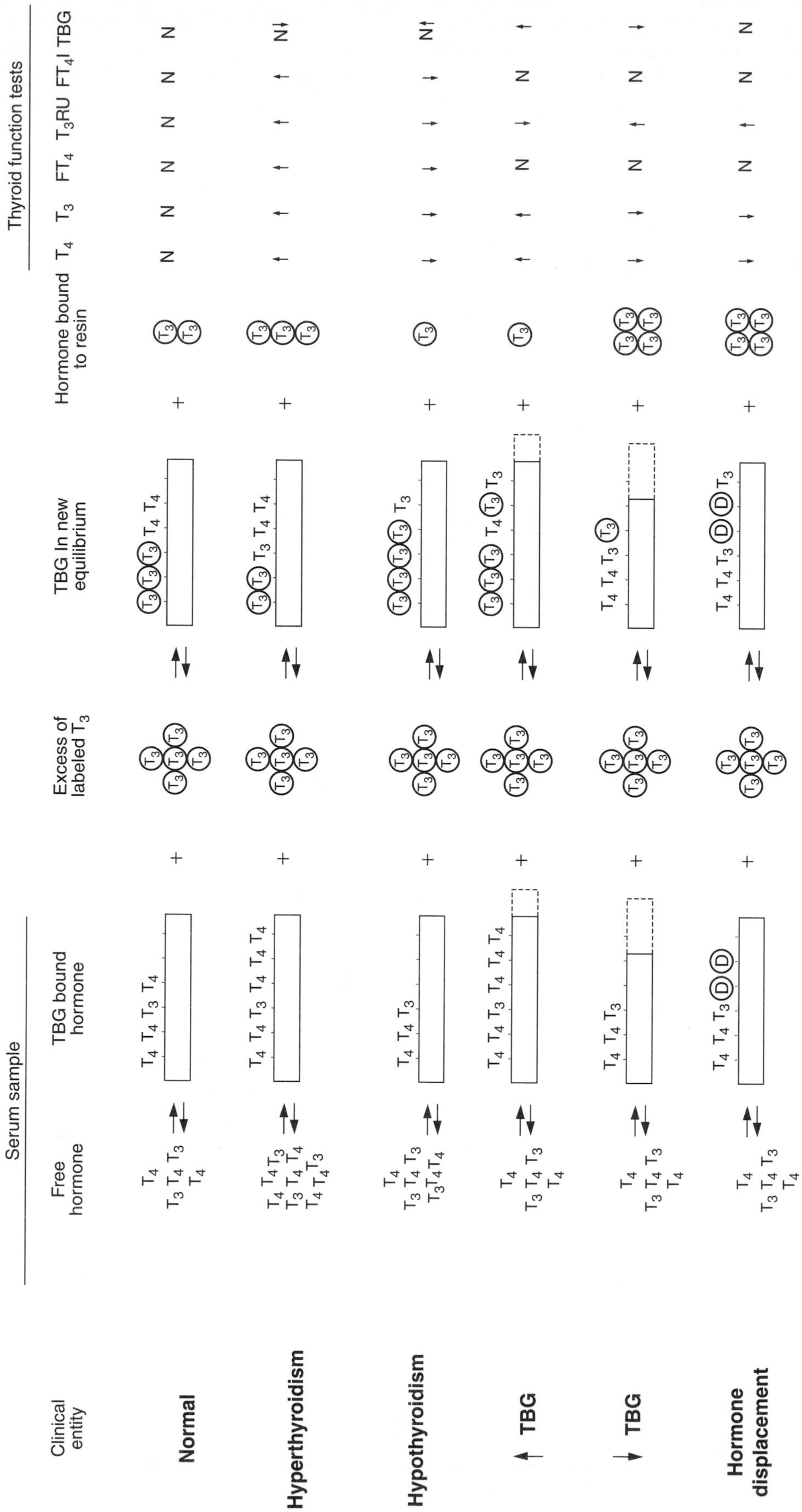

Fig. 44-8　Interrelationships between serum *TBG* (thyroxine-binding globulin), the *T₃RU*, and other thyroid function tests. *D*, Drugs occupying binding sites on TBG; *FT₄I*, free thyroxine hormone index.

net persistent decrease or increase of free unbound thyroid hormone exists in the blood. Because of the limited utility of total thyroid hormone measurements, in 1990 the American Thyroid Association recommended that free thyroid hormones be either measured directly or estimated indirectly.[42] Blood level determinations of total T_4 and T_3 are clinically meaningful only if the functional levels of thyroid hormone–binding protein in blood are known. This is achieved by use of the **resin-uptake test**, which does not measure a specific analyte per se but measures the functional state (ability to bind hormone) of the hormone-binding proteins (such as TBG).

Resin-Uptake Test (T_3RU or T_4RU)

The resin-uptake test is an estimate of the number of available binding sites on the plasma thyroid hormone–transporting proteins, especially TBG, which is the most important transporter of thyroid hormones. Samples of patient serum are mixed with labeled thyroid hormone (T_3 or T_4). The amount of labeled hormone that remains unbound in the mixture is inversely proportional to the number of available binding sites (Fig. 44-8). This unbound hormone is separated from the mixture when a relatively low-affinity binder, such as a resin, is added to the system (Fig. 44-8). The resin is then separated from the serum, and the amount of labeled hormone bound to the resin (resin uptake) is determined. In the classic uptake procedure, the amount of resin uptake is directly proportional to the degree of saturation of T_4-binding sites on carrier proteins (see later discussion).

In cases of increased TBG in plasma, although free thyroid hormone levels are normal, the total T_4 is increased, because the total number of binding sites in TBG is increased. Labeled T_4 or T_3 will find an increased pool of TBG (available binding sites), and less labeled hormone will remain free to bind to resin. Therefore the resin uptake is low. The opposite changes occur in states of decreased TBG. Conditions that cause abnormalities of the binding sites (TBG) are listed in Table 44-2 and the box on p. 837. Certain drugs (salicylates, phenytoin, furosemide, and fenclofenac) compete with thyroid hormone for the TBG-binding sites. This phenomenon is reflected by normal free T_4, low total T_4, and high resin-uptake values.

In hyperthyroidism, free thyroid hormone in plasma increases. This results in complete or almost complete saturation of binding sites in TBG, which in turn results in fewer molecules of labeled hormone bound to TBG and increased amounts of free labeled hormone. This results in an increased resin uptake.

Recently, there has been an attempt to change the nomenclature from T_3 (T_4) resin-uptake test to **thyroid hormone–binding ratio (THBR)** to avoid confusion with direct measurements of serum T_3 (T_4).[43]

Free Thyroxine Hormone Index (FT$_4$I)

It is the free hormone that induces metabolic and biological effects in target cells. The free T_4 index (FT$_4$I) indirectly estimates the level of free T_4 in blood and adjusts for most interferences caused by binding-protein abnormalities.[44] The FT$_4$I is determined from total T_4 and resin-uptake values obtained on the sample. The FT$_4$I is calculated as follows:

$$FT_4I = \frac{\text{Total serum T4} \times \% \text{ T uptake of patient serum}}{\% \text{ T uptake of pooled reference serum}}$$

As expected, most alterations of binding proteins produce reciprocal changes in resin uptake and total serum T_4 or T_3, resulting in normal values of the FT$_4$I, whereas true alterations of free thyroid hormone content cause concordant, unidirectional changes of the FT$_4$I. The FT$_4$I is elevated in hyperthyroidism (Table 44-4) and is decreased in states of hypothyroidism (Table 44-5).

The calculation of the free T_3 index is similar to that used for the FT$_4$I, except that total serum T_3 is used.[45] It has similar applications and significance as the FT$_4$I. The FT$_3$I may be helpful to exclude T_3 toxicosis in some patients taking oral contraceptives in whom isolated serum T_3 increases are found without corresponding elevations of T_4. In general, the FT$_3$I offers no advantages to the FT$_4$I and is used less frequently in clinical practice.

Free T_4 (FT$_4$) and Free T_3 (FT$_3$)

Serum FT$_4$ correlates very well with secretion and metabolism rates of T_4. FT$_4$ and FT$_3$ levels tend to parallel changes in total T_4 and total T_3 concentrations. Measurement of the free hormone levels is useful in routine clinical practice and in instances in which other test results are borderline or conflicting. Elevations and decreases of free T_4 and free T_3 theoretically are true reflections of hyperthyroidism and hypothyroidism. However, the results are dependent on the analytical method used to measure "free" hormone and clinically have been less useful than originally hoped.

Thyroxine-Binding Globulin (TBG)

Many diseases produce alterations of TBG (see box, p. 837) and other thyroid hormone–transporting proteins in plasma. Changes in concentrations of such proteins affect the total plasma concentrations of T_4 and T_3 (Fig. 44-8). Because most of the T_4 and T_3 is bound to TBG, changes in this protein level are clinically important. Quantitative abnormalities are those characterized by absolute increases or decreases of TBG levels in plasma. Consequently, the total amount of thyroid hormone transported in plasma will increase (increased TBG) or decrease (decreased TBG).

Qualitative abnormalities of TBG refer to those stemming from alterations of the hormone-binding affinity rather than from absolute changes of TBG amounts in plasma. The binding affinity of the TBG may be increased or decreased in intrinsic TBG defects. Various compounds and drugs may strongly bind to TBG and result in displacement of thyroid hormone from binding sites. The result is decreased total serum T_4 and T_3 (Fig. 44-8) and increased free T_4 and free T_3.

Serum Thyroid-Stimulating Hormone (TSH)

A principal use of thyroid-stimulating hormone (TSH) determinations in serum is the diagnosis of hyperthyroidism and hypothyroidism. Patients with untreated hypothyroidism stemming from intrinsic thyroid defects (primary hypothyroidism), regardless of the cause, have elevated serum levels of TSH. Patients with hypothyroidism caused by pituitary lesions (secondary) or hypothalamic (tertiary) lesions have normal or low TSH levels. Differentiation between secondary and tertiary hypothyroidism is accomplished by use of the TRH stimulation test.

Most patients with hyperthyroidism have low or undetectable TSH levels in serum, reflecting the inhibitory effects of high levels of circulating thyroid hormone on the hypothalamic-pituitary axis.

Analytical improvements have dramatically enhanced the clinical utility of TSH determinations. Automated immunometric assays (IMAs) for TSH measurement have generally replaced the less sensitive radioimmunoassay (RIA) method. Clinicians often refer to the updated techniques as either second-generation (functional sensitivity approximately 0.1 μIU/mL) or third-generation (functional sensitivity approximately 0.01 μIU/mL) assays. Because of the increased sensitivity of second- and third-generation TSH assays, the very low TSH levels encountered in patients with hyperthyroidism can be easily discriminated from those levels found in euthyroid states.[46] The diagnosis of hypothyroidism can also be made earlier and with more certainty by finding an elevated TSH by an IMA method. The specificity of TSH-IMA is also greater than TSH-RIA because the former employs antibodies to the β-subunit of TSH, resulting in less cross-reactivity with LH, FSH, and hCG, which have α-subunits that are similar to those of TSH. With the availability of the third-generation TSH assays, TSH levels can now be used as accurate indicators of thyroid suppression in patients with thyroid carcinoma or thyroid nodules treated with thyroid hormone.[47]

Immunoglobulins

It has been suggested that immunological abnormalities play an important role in thyroid pathological conditions.[28] Antibodies against components of thyroid cells are found in many patients with thyroid disease. High levels of antibodies against thyroglobulin or thyroid peroxidase are found frequently in patients with Hashimoto's thyroiditis. High titers of thyroid-stimulating immunoglobulins may be found in Graves' disease.

TSH-receptor antibodies may differ in their actions. They may (1) displace TSH without activating the receptor, (2) activate the receptor and mimic TSH, (3) block the action of TSH and cause atrophy of the gland, or (4) stimulate growth of the thyroid gland without increasing secretion of thyroid hormone. The presence of antithyroglobulin antibody interferes with the measurement of serum thyroglobulin. TSH-blocking antibody may be transmitted across the placenta in patients with atrophic thyroiditis and cause temporary hypothyroidism in the newborn.

Laboratory Findings in Nonthyroid Disease (NTD)

The abnormal changes in thyroid test results that may be seen in patients with NTD are listed in Table 44-6. These changes can mimic thyroid disease or modify and confound laboratory findings in patients with thyroid disease. Chronic and acute diseases that alter laboratory tests of thyroid function are more frequent than thyroid disease. These conditions include patients with general chronic debilitating diseases and patients with specific conditions, namely, alcoholic cirrhosis, hepatitis, renal failure, and acute psychiatric illness.

As a group, euthyroid patients with NTD have either normal or low total T_4, normal or low FT_4I, normal or low total T_3 and free T_3, normal or high rT_3, normal or high T_3RU, and low or slightly high TSH levels in serum.[42,48-50] The free T_4 index (FT_4I), which is often a reliable indicator of thyroid function, is usually normal but may also be low in patients with NTD.

Low total T_4, low FT_4I, and low or subnormal T_3 levels indicate the possible presence of hypothyroidism in patients with NTD. The presence of high serum levels of rT_3 is useful in excluding hypothyroidism in this circumstance.[37]

Liver disease is characterized by abnormalities of protein synthesis, including the thyroid-binding proteins, and by alterations of T_4 metabolism. Alcoholic liver cirrhosis is accompanied by decreased binding capacity of thyroid hormones, resulting in high T_3RU[51] (Table 44-6). Total T_4 is usually normal or low,[50] and free T_4 is slightly elevated. There is depressed deiodination and conversion of T_4 to T_3 with decreased serum levels of T_3 and occasionally free T_3.

Acute hepatitis is characterized by an increase of the serum TBG[52] (Table 44-6), which results in increased levels of total T_4 and decreased T_3RU. Chronic active hepatitis also produces some changes in blood hormone levels. These include (1) increased T_4, (2) low free T_4 index, (3) decreased free T_4, (4) normal serum TSH, and (5) abnormally increased TSH response to TRH.[53]

In patients with renal failure the most common findings are decreased total and free T_3 in the serum,[54] caused by diminished peripheral conversion of T_4 to T_3. Serum thyroxine-binding protein, T_3RU, and total T_4 usually are normal. However, the total T_4 and free T_4 may be slightly low.[55] Diminished total T_4 can result from renal failure with severe catabolic states, probably caused by decreased thyroxine-binding proteins in serum. Concentration of TSH in serum is normal.

There is a selective increase in T_4 in patients with an acute psychiatric illness. The reason for the increase is not known, but it is postulated that there is an acute redistribution of T_4 out of the liver, which contains one third of the total body pool of T_4 outside of the thyroid. T_4 levels typically normalize in 1 to 2 weeks after the acute psychiatric event.[56]

Association of NTD with hyperthyroidism is found occasionally. In these situations there is a disproportionate increase of T_4 in serum with only modestly elevated or normal T_3 levels. This is caused by a decreased peripheral conversion of T_4 to T_3 concomitant with the increased T_4 production.

The guidelines produced by the National Academy of Clinical Biochemistry[2] recommend that whenever possible, laboratory determinations of thyroid function in hospitalized patients should be delayed until the illness has been resolved and the patient is no longer receiving medications that could possibly interfere in the measurements. However, if it is critical to exclude thyroid disease as the underlying cause of the illness, measurements of thyroid hormone must be made in conjunction with a measurement of TSH by a third-generation assay. However, an abnormal free T_4 result should be confirmed by a total T_4 measurement.

Laboratory Findings after Therapeutic Interventions for Thyroid Disease

The two most frequently found clinical situations that require closely monitored treatment are hyperthyroidism and hypothyroidism.

Graves' disease, when successfully treated surgically, results in normalization of T_4, T_3, T_3RU, FT_4I, and TSH. In patients treated with antithyroid drugs, such as propylthiouracil (PTU), improvement of thyroid function tests may be occasionally seen as soon as 2 weeks after initiation of treatment. Because of the blocking effect of PTU on conversion of T_4 to T_3, a disproportionately rapid decrease in T_3 may be seen in some cases.

Therapy with ^{131}I is now used more frequently to treat hyperthyroidism. After this treatment, laboratory tests show a decrease of T_4, T_3, T_3RU, and FT_4I in approximately 6 to 10 weeks. Residual radioactivity in the serum must be considered when radioassay methods are used within 90 days of therapy.

Patients treated for thyrotoxicosis by any of the methods may follow one of three courses. Ideally normal thyroid function ensues and is reflected by normal laboratory values. Occasionally patients remain hyperthyroid, and abnormal laboratory tests persist. More often patients become hypothyroid with low T_4, T_3RU, and FT_4I values. The earliest indication of the ensuing hypothyroidism is a depressed T_4 followed by an elevation of TSH levels as the hypothalamic-pituitary axis recovers. The TSH may remain elevated with normal T_4 levels, a condition known as *biochemical hypothyroidism*. Patients with treated Graves' disease may develop a hyperthyroid status with normal or subnormal T_4 values but elevated T_3 levels.

The treatment for hypothyroidism is thyroid hormone replacement. During the monitoring of thyroid hormone replacement, it is important to keep in mind the effect that changes in TBG levels produce on thyroid hormone levels. Laboratory tests should therefore include those that indirectly or directly assess TBG levels, such as the T_3RU, FT_4I, and TBG determinations. With the development of the sensitive TSH-IMAs, it is most practical to diagnose hypothyroidism by detection of an elevated serum TSH. After thyroid hormone replacement therapy for hypothyroidism, it is necessary to wait at least 6 weeks before reevaluating the TSH response to therapy. When preparations containing T_4 and T_3 are used, normalization of both T_3 and T_4 values is expected. When preparations containing only T_3, such as liothyronine (Cytomel), are used, T_3 values become normal or slightly elevated, but the T_4 values may remain mildly depressed. Normalization of T_4 and T_3 values is accompanied by a corresponding decline in TSH levels. When monitoring patients on T_4 replacement, it is important to take into consideration the fluctuation of serum levels caused by the oral administration of the preparation. Increases of T_4 from baseline levels can be observed 2 to 10 hours after ingestion of T_4-containing medications.[57] More accurate interpretation of serum T_4 levels is accomplished by measurement of serum T_4 levels after this peak absorption period, that is, at least 10 hours after dosage.

References

1. Ladenson PW et al: American Thyroid Association guidelines for detection of thyroid dysfunction, *Arch Intern Med* 160:1573, 2000.
2. Demers LM, Spencer CA: Laboratory medicine practice guidelines: laboratory support for the diagnosis and management of thyroid disease, National Academy of Clinical Biochemistry, www.nacb.org.
3. Cobin RH et al: AACE/AAES medical/surgical guidelines for clinical practice: management of thyroid carcinoma, *Endocrine Pract* 71:1203, 2001.
4. Vanderpump MPJ et al: Consensus statement for good practice and audit measures in the management of hypothyroidism and hyperthyroidism, *Br Med J* 313:539, 1996.
5. Wolff J: Transport of iodide and other anions in the thyroid gland, *Physiol Rev* 44:45, 1964.
6. DeGroot LJ, Niepomniszcze H: Biosynthesis of thyroid hormone: basic and clinical aspects, *Metabolism* 26:665, 1977.
7. Dumont JE: The action of thyrotropin on thyroid metabolism, *Vitam Horm* 29:287, 1971.
8. Chopra IJ et al: Pathways of metabolism of thyroid hormones, *Recent Prog Horm Res* 34:521, 1978.
9. Woeber KA, Ingbar SH: The interactions of the thyroid hormones with binding protein. In Greer MA, Solomon DH, editors: *Thyroid, American handbook of physiology*, vol 3, Washington, DC, 1973, American Physiological Society.
10. Chopra IJ: An assessment of daily production and significance of thyroidal 3,3′,5′-triiodothyronine (reverse T_3) in man, *J Clin Invest* 58:32, 1976.
11. Schimmel M, Utiger RD: Thyroidal and peripheral production of thyroid hormones, *Ann Intern Med* 87:760, 1977.
12. Oppenheimer JH, Samuels HH, editors: *Molecular basis of thyroid hormone action*, New York, 1983, Academic Press.
13. Edelman IS, Ismail-Beigi F: Thyroid thermogenesis and active sodium transport, *Recent Prog Horm Res* 30:235, 1974.
14. Erfurth EM et al: Normal reference interval for thyrotropin response to thyroliberin: dependence on age, sex, free thyroxine index and basal concentrations of thyrotropin, *Clin Chem* 30:196, 1984.
15. Wolff J: Iodide goiter and pharmacologic effects of excess iodide, *Am J Med* 47:101, 1969.
16. Mason JW: Amiodarone, *N Engl J Med* 316:455, 1987.
17. Abuid J, Stinson DA, Larsen PR: Serum triiodothyronine and thyroxine in the neonate and the acute increases in these hormones following delivery, *J Clin Invest* 52:1195, 1973.
18. Talbot JA et al: The nature of human chorionic gonadotropin glycoforms in gestation thyrotoxicosis, *Clin Endocrinol* 55:33, 2001.
19. Selenkow HA, Birnbaum MD, Hollander CS: Thyroid function and dysfunction during pregnancy, *Clin Obstet Gynecol* 16:66, 1973.
20. Boyages SC: The neuromuscular system and brain in hypothyroidism. In Braverman LE, Utiger RD, editors: *Werner & Ingbar's the thyroid: a fundamental and clinical text*, ed 8, Philadelphia, 2000, Lippincott Williams & Wilkins.
21. Haddow JE et al: Maternal thyroid deficiency during pregnancy and subsequent neuropsychological development of the child, *N Engl J Med* 341:549, 1999.

22. Pop VJ et al: Low maternal free thyroxine concentrations during pregnancy are associated with impaired psychomotor development in infancy, *Clin Endocrinol* 50:147, 1999.

23. Radetti G et al: Psychomotor and audiological assessment of infants born to mothers with subclinical thyroid dysfunction in early pregnancy, *Minerva Pediatr* 52:691, 2000.

24. Editorial: Should all women be screened for hypothyroidism? *Lancet* 354:1224, 1999.

25. Van den Berhe G: Novel insights into the neuroendocrinology of acute illness, *Eur J Endocrinol* 143:1, 2000.

26. Portnay GI et al: The effect of starvation on the concentration and binding of thyroxine and triiodothyronine in serum and on the response to TRH, *J Clin Endocrinol Metab* 39:191, 1974.

27. McKenzie JM, Zakarija M, Sato A: Humoral immunity in Graves' disease, *Clin Endocrinol Metab* 7:31, 1978.

28. Christiansen NJB et al: Serum thyroxine in the early phase of subacute thyroiditis, *Acta Endocrinol* 64:359, 1970.

29. Dorfman SG et al: Painless thyroiditis and transient hyperthyroidism without goiter, *Ann Intern Med* 86:24, 1977.

30. Roti E, Emerson CH: Clinical review 29: postpartum thyroiditis, *J Clin Endocrinol Metab* 74:3, 1992.

31. Gerstein HC: How common is postpartum thyroiditis? *Arch Intern Med* 150:1397, 1990.

32. LiVolsi VA: Postpartum thyroiditis: the pathology slowly unravels, *Am J Clin Pathol* 100:193, 1993 (editorial).

33. McKenzie JM, Zakarija M: Pathogenesis of neonatal Graves' disease, *J Endocrinol Invest* 2:183, 1978.

34. Sawin CT et al: Low serum thyrotropin concentrations as a risk factor for atrial fibrillations in older persons, *N Engl J Med* 331:1249, 1994.

35. Kalmijn S et al: Subclinical hyperthyroidism and the risk of dementia. The Rotterdam Study, *Clin Endocrinol* 53:733, 2000.

36. Parle JV et al: Prediction of all-cause and cardiovascular mortality in elderly people from one low serum thyrotropin result: a 10-year cohort study, *Lancet* 258:861, 2001.

37. Brown J et al: Autoimmune thyroid disease—Graves' and Hashimoto's, *Ann Intern Med* 88:379, 1978.

38. Dussault JH et al: Preliminary report on a mass screening program for neonatal hypothyroidism, *J Pediatr* 86:670, 1975.

39. Maxon HR III et al: Clinically important radiation-associated thyroid disease: a controlled study, *JAMA* 44:1802, 1980.

40. Snyder PJ, Utiger RD: Response to thyrotropin-releasing hormone (TRH) in normal man, *J Clin Endocrinol Metab* 34:380, 1972.

41. Werner SC, Spooner M: A new and simple test for hyperthyroidism employing l-triiodothyronine and the 24 hour ^{131}I uptake method, *Bull NY Acad Med* 31:139, 1955.

42. Surks MI, Chopra IJ, Mariash CN: American Thyroid Association guidelines for the use of laboratory tests in thyroid disorders, *JAMA* 263:1529, 1990.

43. Larsen PR et al: Committee on Nomenclature, American Thyroid Association: revised nomenclature for tests of thyroid hormones and thyroid-related proteins in serum, *J Clin Endocrinol Metab* 64:1089, 1986 (letter to the editor).

44. Stein RB, Price L: Evaluation of adjusted total thyroxine (free thyroxine index) as a measure of thyroid function, *J Clin Endocrinol Metab* 34:225, 1972.

45. Sawin CT, Chopra D, Albano J: The free triiodothyronine (T_3) index, *Ann Intern Med* 88:474, 1978.

46. Toft AD: Use of sensitive immunoradiometric assay for thyrotropin in clinical practice, *Mayo Clin Proc* 63:1035, 1988.

47. Schlumberger M et al: Post-operative surveillance of differentiated thyroid carcinoma: contributions of the ultra-sensitive TSH assay, *Presse Méd* 16:1791, 1987.

48. Wartofsky L: The low T_3 or "sick euthyroid syndrome": update 1994, *Endocrinol Rev* 3:248, 1994.

49. Kapstein EM: Thyroid hormone metabolism and thyroid diseases in chronic renal failure, *Endocrinol Rev* 17:45, 1996.

50. Stockigt JR: Guidelines for the diagnosis and monitoring of thyroid disease: nonthyroidal illness, *Clin Chem* 42:188, 1996.

51. Inada M, Sterling K: Thyroxine turnover and transport in Laënnec's cirrhosis of the liver, *J Clin Invest* 46:1275, 1967.

52. Tabei A, Shimoda S: Increased TBG-T_4–binding capacity in acute hepatitis, *Folia Endocrinol* 49:1025, 1973.

53. Schussler GC, Schaffner F, Korn F: Increased serum thyroid hormone binding and decreased free hormone in chronic active liver disease, *N Engl J Med* 299:510, 1978.

54. Spector DA et al: Thyroid function and metabolic state in chronic renal failure, *Ann Intern Med* 85:724, 1976.

55. Lim VS et al: Thyroid dysfunction in chronic renal failure, *J Clin Invest* 60:522, 1977.

56. Cavalieri RR: The effects of nonthyroid disease and drugs on thyroid function tests, *Med Clin North Am* 75:27, 1991.

57. Maxon H et al: Variation in serum thyroxine concentrations with time after oral replacement dose, *Clin Nucl Med* 12:369, 1987.

Internet Sites

www.thyroid.org—American Thyroid Association
www.endo-society.org—The Endocrine Society
www.thyroid.about.com—About Network
www.thyroid.ca—Thyroid Foundation of Canada
www.thyroidmanager.org—Thyroid Disease Manager
http://the-thyroid-society.org/—The Thyroid Society
www.4women.gov/faq/thyroid_disease.htm—National Women's Health Information Center

http://www.focusonthyroid.com/Script/Main/hp.asp
http://www.tsh.org
http://www.aace.com/clin/guidelines/—American Association of Clinical Endocrinologists
www.nacb.org—National Academy of Clinical Biochemistry: Draft Guidelines of Laboratory Support for Diagnosis and Monitoring of Thyroid Disease

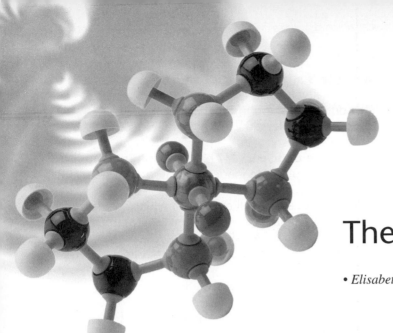

CHAPTER 45

The Gonads*

• *Elisabeth Nye*

Chapter Outline

Objectives

- Describe the normal development of the male and female gonads.
- Describe the hypothalamic-pituitary-gonadal axis and its regulation.
- Outline the pathways of biosynthesis, transport, and metabolism of sex hormones.

- Describe the hormonal changes that regulate the menstrual cycle and discuss the investigation of absent/abnormal menstruation.
- Describe the etiology and investigation of male hypogonadism.
- Discuss evaluation of the infertile couple.

Key Terms

androgens   Sex steroid hormones responsible for the development of the male secondary sex characteristics.

anovulation   Failure of the ovary to produce ova.

corpus luteum   Transient endocrine organ, arising from the granulosa and theca cells of the ovarian follicle, that secretes progesterone during the luteal phase of the menstrual cycle.

cryptorchidism   Failure of the testes to descend into the scrotum.

dihydrotestosterone   Metabolite of testosterone with potent androgenic activity.

diploid   Cell containing the full complement of 46 chromosomes.

dysfunctional uterine bleeding (DUB) Unpredictable menstrual bleeding in association with anovulatory cycles.

---

*With acknowledgment to the previous author, Karen Nickel.

dysmenorrhea   Cramping and pain associated with menstruation.

endometrium   Tissue forming the inner lining of the uterus.

epididymis   Elongated, cordlike structure of the testis that contains ducts capable of storing spermatozoa.

estrogens   Sex steroid hormones responsible for the development of the female secondary sex characteristics. Estradiol is the most bioactive.

fallopian tube   Long, slender tubes that extend from the uterus towards the ovaries.

fecundability   The probability of achieving pregnancy within one menstrual cycle (20%-25% per cycle).

gonadotropins   Glycoprotein hormones (FSH and LH) that are secreted by anterior pituitary cells (gonadotropes) and stimulate the gonads.

gonadotropin-releasing hormone (GnRH) Decapeptide hormone that is secreted by hypothalamic neurons and stimulates gonadotropin secretion by the pituitary.

gynecomastia   Glandular enlargement of the mammary glands in males.

haploid   Cell containing 23 chromosomes, the haploid number.

hirsutism   Excess terminal (thick, pigmented) body hair occurring in a male distribution in women.

hypogonadism   Abnormally low activity of the gonads.

infertility   Involuntary failure to conceive after 1 or more years of unprotected intercourse.

inhibin   Glycoprotein hormones secreted by the testes and the ovary whose principal role is probably to exert negative feedback on pituitary FSH secretion.

in vitro fertilization (IVF)   Assisted reproductive technique in which oocytes are extracted, fertilized in the laboratory, and embryos are transferred transcervically into the uterus.

Kallmann syndrome   Inherited defect in hypothalamic gonadotropin releasing hormone (GnRH) secretion causing hypogonadotropic hypogonadism.

Klinefelter's syndrome   Sex chromosome abnormality in males (XXY) producing primary hypogonadism and infertility.

Leydig cells   Interstitial cells of the testes that produce testosterone.

luteal phase deficiency   Abnormal corpus luteum function resulting in inadequate progesterone production.

meiosis   Process of cell division in which specialized cells called *gametes* are produced (spermatozoa in males and ova in females), which contain half the diploid number of chromosomes, that is, the haploid number.

menarche   Onset of menstruation.

menopause   Cessation of menstruation.

mosaicism   Tissue of unlike genetic constitution is mingled.

polycystic ovary syndrome (PCOS)   Condition characterized by hyperandrogenism, menstrual irregularities, and anovulation.

premature ovarian failure   Amenorrhea, infertility, estrogen deficiency, and elevated gonadotropins in a woman less than 40 years old.

premenstrual syndrome (PMS)   Behavioral changes associated with the menstrual cycle.

pseudohermaphroditism   Conditions in which the individual has sex chromosomes and gonads characteristic of one sex but some phenotypic features (such as external genitalia) of the other sex.

sex hormone–binding globulin   A protein produced by the liver that binds testosterone and estradiol in blood.

spermatozoa   Male reproductive cell produced in the testes.

testicular feminization syndrome   Failure of virilization in a genetic and gonadal male because of an X-linked defect in the androgen receptor.

testosterone   Principle male sex hormone.

Turner syndrome   Chromosomal abnormality (45,X) in girls associated with gonadal dysgenesis.

virilization   Development of male phenotypic features in a female.

Methods on CD-ROM

Alpha-fetoprotein
Dehydroepiandrosterone and its sulfate
FSH

LH
Prolactin

NORMAL OVARY AND OVARIAN FUNCTION
Early Development of the Ovary

Fetal ovary. Formation of the gonads occurs early in fetal development; primordial germ cells can be identified in the 4.5 day old human blastocyst. Sexual differentiation (dimorphism) becomes apparent by 42 days gestation. In male embryos, the developing gonad switches to the male pattern and seminiferous cords can be identified in the fetal testes. In the absence of a Y chromosome, ovarian development will occur. The fetal ovary is composed of three principal cell types: (1) coelomic epithelial cells, which differentiate into granulosa cells; (2) mesenchymal cells, which give rise to the ovarian stroma; and (3) primordial germ cells. The primordial germ cells (oogonia) proliferate in the fetal ovary by successive mitotic divisions, reaching the maximal number of 6 to 7 million oogonia by the 20th week of gestation. Thereafter, the number of germ cells decreases (a process known as *atresia*), so that only about 1 million are present at birth, about 400,000 are present at **menarche**, and only a few remain by **menopause**.

After mitotic division, the oogonia are converted to primary oocytes, which begin a unique form of cell division called **meiosis**. Meiosis involves two cell divisions (meiosis I and II), in which only the first is preceded by duplication of the chromosomes. Gonadal germ cells contain the full complement of 46 chromosomes, the **diploid** number. After the process of meiosis, however, specialized cells called *gametes* are produced, which contain only half the diploid number of chromosomes (the **haploid** number). Reproduction involves the fusion of male and female gametes to form a zygote, which will once again contain the diploid number of chromosomes. In the female fetus, meiosis I is initiated by the primary oocytes during the second trimester of gestation, but the process is arrested in the diplotene (resting) phase when each cell contains a duplicated set of chromosomes. Meiosis I does not resume until after menarche, at which time it will proceed in an individual ovum just before ovulation. In the fetal ovary, the primary oocytes become surrounded by a layer of primitive granulosa cells, and together these make up the primordial follicle.

The primordial genital ducts, the wolffian ducts (male) and müllerian ducts (female), temporarily coexist in all embryos during the ambisexual period of development (up to 8 weeks). The critical factors in determining which of the duct structures stabilize or regress are two secretions from the testes: antimüllerian hormone and **testosterone**. In the absence of these factors, the wolffian duct system regresses and müllerian duct development takes place. The **fallopian tubes**, the uterus, and the upper third of the vagina develop from the müllerian ducts.

Childhood and premenarchal ovary. After birth, the ovaries increase in size and weight, from about 250 mg to 4000 mg by menarche. The hormonal regulation of both male and female reproductive function is dependent on a complex system involving the hypothalamus, the pituitary and the gonads. As will be discussed later in more detail, the hypothalamus secretes a decapeptide hormone, **gonadotropin-releasing hormone (GnRH)**, which stimulates the anterior pituitary to secrete the glycoprotein hormones, luteinizing hormone (LH) and follicle-stimulating hormone (FSH) (the **gonadotropins**). Plasma gonadotropin levels vary markedly during different stages of life in females. During the second trimester of pregnancy, fetal gonadotropin concentrations rise progressively to very high levels. As the fetal hypothalamic-pituitary axis matures, becoming progressively more sensitive to the suppressive effects of high levels of estrogen and progesterone secreted by the placenta, the plasma gonadotropin concentrations decrease to virtually undetectable levels by birth. Following delivery, with removal of the placenta, plasma gonadotropin levels once again increase markedly because of the abrupt decrease in estrogen and progesterone levels. Elevated gonadotropin levels persist for the first few months, decreasing to low levels again by 1 to 3 years. During the childhood years, the hypothalamic-pituitary axis remains highly sensitive to the negative feedback effects of gonadal steroids so that gonadotropin levels remain low despite the low levels of circulating gonadal steroids.

Puberty is characterized by three major events: (1) adrenarche, the onset of adrenal **androgen** secretion; (2) decreased sensitivity of the hypothalamic-pituitary axis to negative feedback by gonadal steroids, leading to increased activity of the GnRH-secreting hypothalamic neurons and increased pituitary gonadotropin secretion; and (3) gonadarche, increased ovarian estrogen secretion and the onset of ovulatory cycles. The increase in secretion of adrenal androgens occurs before maturation of gonadotropin secretion. Plasma levels of androstenedione, dehydroepiandrosterone (DHEA), and dehydroepiandrosterone sulfate (DHEAS) begin to increase in children age 6 to 8 years. Pulsatile secretion of GnRH is critical in the initiation of puberty. In girls, FSH levels increase earlier than LH. As a consequence of the increased FSH concentrations, plasma estradiol levels (more than 90% derived from the ovary) increase progressively throughout puberty. Estradiol accelerates linear growth and stimulates development of female secondary sex characteristics (breast growth, maturation of the urogenital tract, and development of the female body habitus). Adrenal androgens regulate axillary and pubic hair development. The culmination of puberty is the advent of cyclic, regular (and hence ovulatory) menses; however, the age of menarche is influenced by many factors including general health, nutrition, body weight, and genetic factors.

Ovary of the Reproductive Years

Structural organization of the mature ovary. Mature human ovaries are paired, oval-shaped organs with a combined weight during the reproductive years of 10 to 20 g (average 14 g). The ovaries are attached to the posterior surface of the broad ligament by a fold of peritoneum called the *mesovarium* and lie in proximity to the posterior and lateral pelvic wall. Blood vessels, nerves, and lymphatics reach the ovaries via the mesovarium, entering each organ via the hilum (depression).

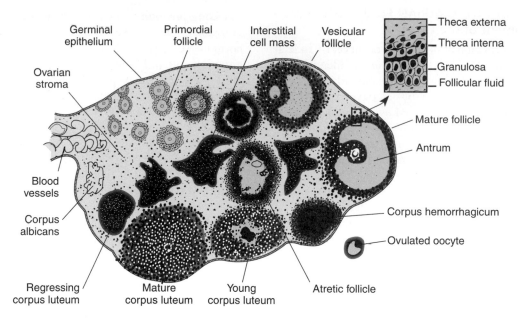

Fig. 45-1 Diagram of ovary, showing sequential development of a follicle and formation of corpus luteum. Section of wall of a mature follicle is enlarged at upper right. *(From Gorbman A, Bern HA: A textbook of comparative endocrinology, New York, 1962, Wiley & Sons.)*

Histologically, the ovary consists of three distinct regions: an outer cortex containing the germinal epithelium and the follicles; a central medulla consisting of stroma; and a hilar area around the mesovarium attachment. Ovarian follicles can be divided into two functional types: nongrowing (or primordial) and growing. The majority of follicles remain nongrowing throughout the reproductive period. Following recruitment of a growing follicle, significant changes in growth, structure, and function occur. The follicle undergoes five histologically distinct stages of development: primary, secondary, tertiary, mature (or graafian), and atretic (death of the graafian follicle because of abortion of the ovum). When mature, an ovarian follicle consists of three layers of cells: the theca externa, the theca interna, and the granulosa cells (Fig. 45-1). The oocyte is contained within, surrounded by an accumulation of granulosa cells and a cavity containing antral fluid. As the follicle matures, the oocyte also grows, accumulating nutritional stores and completing the process of meiosis I. The mature graafian follicle is then ready to release the ovum by the process of ovulation. The average time period for development of a primary follicle to the point of ovulation is 10 to 14 days. Recruited primordial follicles either develop into a dominant, mature graafian follicle destined to ovulate, or they degenerate and die via the process of atresia.

After rupture of the follicle and release of the ovum, clotting leads to the formation of the corpus hemorrhagicum. The granulosa and theca cells of the follicle then proliferate to form the **corpus luteum**. The corpus luteum is a transient endocrine organ that predominantly secretes progesterone for about 14 days. The purpose of the corpus luteum is to prepare an estrogen-primed **endometrium** for acceptance of a newly fertilized ovum and the establishment of early pregnancy. In the absence of a pregnancy, the luteum begins to degenerate about 4 days before the next menses, and it is eventually transformed into a fibrous scar, the corpus albicans.

The hypothalamic-pituitary-ovarian axis: an overview. Cyclic ovarian function depends on appropriately timed secretion of the anterior pituitary gonadotropins, FSH and LH, in response to hypothalamic GnRH. Coordination of the menstrual cycle also depends on the positive and negative feedback relationships between the ovarian hormones, estrogen and progesterone, and GnRH, FSH and LH secretion (Fig. 45-2). The release of pituitary FSH and LH requires the constant pulsatile secretion of GnRH from the hypothalamus. The gonadotropins are glycoproteins composed of two polypeptide chains, designated alpha and beta. The alpha chain is common to both, whereas the beta subunit is unique, thus ensuring specific biological activity for each hormone.

The release of FSH and LH is affected both positively and negatively by estrogen and progesterone. Whether estrogen or progesterone stimulate or inhibit gonadotropin secretion depends on the concentration of the hormone and the duration of exposure of the pituitary. Estrogen exerts its inhibitory effect on both the hypothalamus and pituitary. Some inhibition of FSH and LH release occurs at low levels of estrogen, but it is more complete at high concentrations. Progesterone in high concentrations inhibits gonadotropin secretion by suppression of hypothalamic GnRH release. In addition to these negative feedback effects, female gonadal steroids also have a positive effect on pituitary gonadotropin secretion. The positive feedback is triggered by a sharply rising plasma level of estrogen and is critical in promoting the LH surge required to initiate ovulation. The two essential attributes

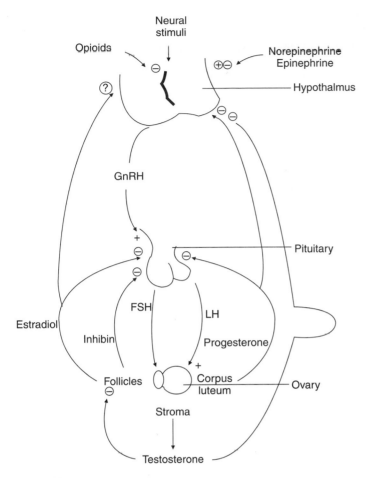

Fig. 45-2 Diagram of hypothalamic-pituitary-ovarian axis. *FSH,* Follicle-stimulating hormone; *GnRH,* gonadotropin-releasing hormone; *LH,* luteinizing hormone; +, positive effect; –, negative effect. *(Modified from Greenspan FS: Basic and clinical endocrinology, East Norwalk, CT, 1991, Appleton & Lange.)*

are (1) estradiol concentrations of more than 700 pmol/L (200 pg/mL) and (2) maintenance of elevated estradiol levels for at least 48 hours. Progesterone at low concentrations can also stimulate LH release but only after the pituitary has been exposed to prolonged high levels of estrogen.

Hypothalamic-pituitary regulation of ovarian function is also influenced by neural stimuli from the central nervous system. The hypothalamus receives both neural and hormonal signals, which can affect GnRH secretion and the menstrual cycle. This type of input can disrupt the pattern of GnRH secretion and lead to **anovulation** and amenorrhea. These manifestations may be observed in situations of chronic stress or profound weight loss.

Ovarian steroid hormones. The ovarian steroid hormones belong to a large family of steroid compounds, whose composition is based on a four ring structure containing three cyclohexane rings and one cyclopentane ring (Fig. 45-3). Steroid hormones have diverse biological effects that depend on the nature of numerous chemical modifications of the basic steroid structure, such as unsaturation of carbon-carbon bonds within the rings or the attachment of

hydroxyl or ketone groups to specific carbon atoms. Ovarian hormones are classified on the basis of their structure and principal biological function and consist of three major types: **estrogens**, progestagens, and androgens.

Estrogens. The naturally occurring estrogens are C_{18}-steroids. They are characterized by an attached hydroxyl group (estradiol) or ketone group (estrone). The principal and most potent estrogen secreted by the ovary is estradiol-17α. In contrast, relatively small amounts of estrone are actually secreted by the ovary; most originates from extraglandular conversion of androstenedione (and to a lesser extent estradiol) in peripheral tissues, mainly adipose tissue. Increased extraglandular estrone formation can occur in simple obesity or in conditions such as polycystic ovary syndrome in which increased androstenedione secretion occurs. Estrogen formed by this route can then interfere with normal feedback mechanisms and cause disturbances in the menstrual cycle. Estrogens promote the development of the female secondary sex characteristics, uterine growth, thickening of the vaginal mucosa, thinning of the cervical mucus and development of the ductal system of the breast.

Progestagens. The progestagens are C_{21}-steroids and include pregnenolone, progesterone, and 17-hydroxyprogesterone (17-OHP). Pregnenolone is the precursor of all the ovarian steroid hormones (see Fig. 45-3). Progesterone is the primary secretory product of the corpus luteum and is required for the induction of secretory activity in an estrogen-primed uterus, implantation of a fertilized ovum and maintenance of early pregnancy. The corpus luteum also secretes 17-OHP; however, this steroid has little or no biological activity.

Androgens. The ovarian thecal cells, and to a lesser extent the stromal cells, produce a variety of C_{19}-steroids in small amounts, including dehydroepiandrosterone (DHEA), androstenedione, testosterone, and **dihydrotestosterone**. Only testosterone and dihydrotestosterone are true androgens capable of interacting with the androgen receptor. The major C_{19}-steroid produced is androstenedione, some of which is released into plasma, the remainder being converted into testosterone or estrogen within the ovary. Circulating androstenedione can also be converted to testosterone or estrogen in extraglandular tissues.

Biosynthesis of ovarian steroid hormones. All steroid hormones are derived from cholesterol (see Fig. 45-3). Cholesterol may be synthesized de novo within the ovary or derived from preformed sources (i.e., circulating plasma lipoproteins or stored lipid in adipose tissue). The primary source is the uptake of plasma low-density lipoprotein (LDL) cholesterol. Little hormone is stored in the ovary, so secretory activity is closely related to synthetic activity and substrate availability. All the main steroid-producing cells of the ovary (i.e., the granulosa, theca, and corpus luteum cells) contain the full complement of enzymes required for the synthesis of any of the ovarian steroid hormones. However, the predominant steroid produced differs among the cell types. The granulosa cells mainly produce estrogen, the thecal and stromal cells secrete androgens, and the corpus

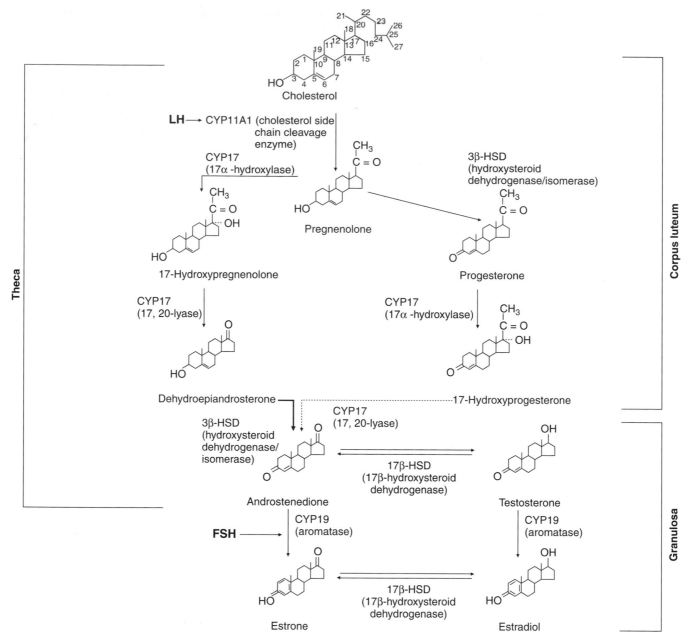

Fig. 45-3 Principal pathways of steroid hormone biosynthesis in the human ovary. Although each cell type of the ovary contains the complete enzyme complement required for the formation of estradiol from cholesterol, the amounts of the various enzymes and consequently the predominant hormones formed differ among the cell types. The major enzyme complements for the corpus luteum, theca, and granulosa cells are shown in *brackets*; these cells produce predominantly progesterone and 17-hydroxyprogesterone (corpus luteum), androgen (theca), and estrogen (granulosa). The major sites of actions of LH and FSH in mediating this pathway are shown by the *horizontal arrows*. The *dotted line* emphasizes that the metabolism of 17-hydroxyprogesterone is limited in the human ovary. *(From Wilson JD et al:* Williams' textbook of endocrinology, *ed 9, Philadelphia, 1999, Saunders.)*

luteum produces progesterone and 17-OHP. Several factors determine which steroid is secreted by each cell type, including gonadotropin levels and the relative numbers of cell gonadotropin receptors, the local expression of steroidogenic enzymes, and the availability of LDL cholesterol. Both FSH and LH are required for estrogen synthesis. The

rate-limiting step in ovarian steroidogenesis is the initial conversion of cholesterol to pregnenolone. This process is regulated by LH, which stimulates thecal cell uptake of LDL cholesterol and the subsequent synthesis of pregnenolone. FSH controls the conversion of androgens to estrogens. In response to LH, the thecal cells produce androstenedione and small amounts of testosterone. These steroids diffuse into the granulosa cells, in which (in response to FSH) they are aromatized to produce estrone and estradiol-17α.

Transport of steroid hormones. After secretion, the gonadal steroids circulate either in a free (unbound) state or weakly or strongly bound to plasma proteins. Steroid transport molecules include specific globulins and albumin. **Sex hormone-binding globulin** (SHBG) is a β-globulin synthesized by the liver, which exhibits high-affinity, low-capacity binding. Albumin has a low affinity but a high capacity. Approximately 60% of plasma estradiol is bound to albumin, 38% is bound to SHBG, and 2% to 3% is free. Progesterone binds strongly to cortisol-binding globulin (CBG) and weakly to albumin. The general consensus is that the biological activity of steroid hormones is proportional to the concentration of free hormone in plasma, *not* the concentration of protein-bound hormone. However, the globulin-binding proteins may have specific functional properties related to tissue delivery in addition to steroid transport. The metabolic clearance rate of gonadal steroids is inversely related to the binding affinity for SHBG; therefore alterations in the concentration of SHBG can affect gonadal steroid metabolism and target tissue activity. The level of SHBG may be altered by a variety of clinical conditions. SHBG concentrations are increased by estrogens (pregnancy, oral contraceptive pills, hormone replacement therapy) and hyperthyroidism; they are decreased by androgens, hypothyroidism, and obesity.

Mechanisms of action of steroid hormones. Steroid hormones have a low molecular weight and diffuse readily across cell membranes down a concentration gradient because of their high lipid solubility. Most steroid receptors are localized within the cell nucleus. After nuclear binding, conformational changes occur within the hormone-receptor complex, exposing high-affinity DNA-binding sites that can then interact with chromosomal DNA to alter rates of gene transcription. This process is followed by mRNA synthesis, transport of the mRNA to the ribosomes in the cytoplasm and synthesis of the appropriate proteins that direct cell function. Low levels of steroid hormones produce specific biological effects because of the high affinity, specificity, and concentration of steroid receptors within cells. Specificity is partially determined by the relative numbers of receptors within a cell; for example, in estrogen target tissues such as the uterus, estrogen action is greater and more prolonged because each target cell contains large numbers of estrogen receptors.

Metabolism of ovarian hormones. Plasma estradiol is rapidly converted in the liver to estrone. Some of this estrone reenters the circulation; however, the majority is further metabolized to estriol or 2-hydroxyestrone, conjugated, and then excreted by the kidney. Progesterone is rapidly cleared, having a half life of about 5 minutes. It is converted in the liver to pregnanediol, conjugated to glucuronic acid, and excreted via the kidneys.

Nonsteroidal hormones. Steroidogenesis and the development of the dominant follicle in each menstrual cycle

in the ovary are modulated by many local nonsteroidal factors, such as cytokines, growth factors, and neuropeptides. More recently, the inhibin-related family of multifunctional glycoproteins has been identified. These hormones act locally to influence the development of the ovarian follicle, but they are also present in the circulation and play an important role in the regulation of gonadotropin secretion.[7,16]

Two forms of **inhibin** have been identified: namely, inhibin A ($\alpha_A\beta_A$) and inhibin B ($\alpha_B\beta_B$). These glycoproteins are dimers of two subunits linked by disulfide bonds. One subunit, termed the α *subunit*, is common to both forms of inhibin, whereas β subunits are specific for each hormone. In the male, the principal circulating form of inhibin is inhibin B. In the female, serum levels of both inhibin A and B fluctuate during the menstrual cycle. Inhibin A levels are low in the early follicular phase and rise in the late follicular phase to reach maximal concentrations during the luteal phase. The changes in inhibin B levels parallel those of FSH, in that they rise rapidly at the onset of the follicular phase, peak just after the midcycle FSH rise and then progressively fall during the remainder of the luteal phase. These cyclical changes in inhibin concentrations suggest that circulating inhibin B is produced by the granulosa cells during follicular development, whereas inhibin A is secreted mainly by corpus luteum cells. The major local effect of ovarian inhibin is to increase theca cell androgen production. Granulosa cells secrete inhibin into follicular fluid, enabling it to diffuse into thecal cells and positively modulate LH-induced androgen synthesis. Circulating inhibins (A and B) contribute to the ovarian-pituitary negative feedback relationships by decreasing FSH secretion.

The activins are disulfide-linked dimers of the β subunits of inhibin.[7] Three forms have been identified: namely activin A ($\beta_A A\beta_A A$), activin B ($\beta_B B\beta_B B$), and activin AB ($\beta_A A\beta_B B$). All the activins have the capacity to stimulate FSH secretion from the pituitary gland; however, their precise roles have yet to be determined. The activins appear to act primarily at a local level. Plasma activin A concentrations do not change significantly during the menstrual cycle, suggesting that circulating activin is not important in the regulation of pituitary FSH secretion. In the ovary, however, locally produced activin A may augment the effects of FSH as it has been shown to enhance the proliferation of cultured granulosa cells and induce the expression of FSH receptors. Gonadotropes produce activin B in the pituitary, where it may act directly to increase FSH secretion.

The Menstrual Cycle

The development of regular, ovulatory menstrual cycles depends on the complex interactions between the hypothalamus, pituitary, ovaries, and genital tract. The menstrual cycle is usually divided into two phases: the follicular, or proliferative, phase and the luteal, or secretory, phase (Fig. 45-4). The length of the menstrual cycle is defined as the period dating from the onset of one instance of menstrual bleeding (day 1) until the onset of the next. The average normal cycle length is 28 days. The greatest variability in

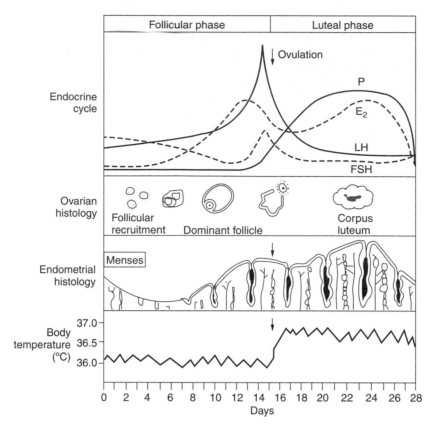

Fig. 45-4 The hormonal, ovarian, endometrial, and basal body temperature changes and relationships throughout the normal menstrual cycle. *E_2,* estradiol; *FSH,* follicle-stimulating hormone; *LH,* luteinizing hormone; *P,* progesterone. *(From Braunwald E et al: Harrison's principles of internal medicine, ed 15, New York, 2001, McGraw-Hill.)*

cycle length occurs following menarche and preceding menopause, as a result of inadequate follicular development resulting in anovulatory cycles. The variation in the length of the menstrual cycle between individual women is due to variability in the length of the follicular phase, from 10 to 16 days. In contrast, the duration of the luteal phase (approximately 14 days) is remarkably constant.

Follicular phase. The initiation of follicular growth begins during the last few days of the luteal phase of the preceding menstrual cycle. During this period, the corpus luteum is degenerating, and plasma progesterone and estrogen levels are declining. With the reduction in negative feedback, FSH concentrations increase, stimulating the growth of new follicles and estrogen secretion. During menstruation, levels of estrogen, progesterone, and LH are relatively constant and low, whereas FSH concentrations are rising. Several follicles are recruited during days 1 through 4 of the menstrual cycle in response to FSH. Selection of the dominant follicle occurs between cycle days 5 and 7. This follicle then continues to grow, releasing unknown factors that suppress the maturation of the other recruited follicles. During the early follicular phase, FSH levels continue to rise. However, estrogen concentrations increase in parallel with follicular growth, thereby exerting a negative feedback effect on hypothalamic and pituitary hormone secretion and resulting in a fall in FSH levels by the midfollicular phase. In contrast, LH levels are low in the first part of the follicular phase, but they begin to rise in the midfollicular phase as a result of the positive feedback effects of the rising estrogen concentrations.

Ovulation. Just before ovulation, estrogen secretion by the preovulatory follicle increases dramatically, initiating the LH surge. LH enhances follicular progesterone secretion, which stimulates the midcycle increase in FSH release. The onset of the LH surge occurs 34 to 36 hours before release of the ovum from the follicle. The peak LH level occurs about 10 to 12 hours before ovulation. Ovulation usually occurs at around day 14 in a 28-day cycle. Immediately before the LH peak, estrogen levels fall precipitously, slowly rising again after ovulation. The precise mechanism of follicular rupture is unknown. Just before ovulation, the follicle becomes extensively vascularized and proteolytic enzymes such as collagenase and plasmin digest collagen in the follicular wall, leading to thinning and distention. Prostaglandin concentrations reach a peak in follicular fluid just before ovulation and are thought to play a role in the rupture of the follicle.

Luteal phase. After ovulation, the ruptured follicle undergoes changes in structure and function to become the corpus luteum. The corpus luteum is the site of steroid secretion by the ovary during the luteal phase, producing predominantly progesterone and some estrogen. Progesterone produced by the corpus luteum begins to increase

3 days after ovulation, and the rising progesterone levels rapidly inhibit LH secretion. Progesterone concentrations reach a maximum about 8 to 9 days after the LH peak. Estrogen levels also increase during the luteal phase and, together with progesterone, cause the progressive decline in LH and FSH concentrations. In the last few days of the luteal phase, as the corpus luteum begins to regress, the levels of estrogen and progesterone decrease. The loss of negative feedback results in rising FSH levels once more and the recruitment of a new batch of follicles for the next cycle.

The effect of ovarian hormones on the uterus/ endometrium. The fluctuations in estrogen and progesterone levels during the menstrual cycle produce characteristic changes in the endometrium (the tissue lining the uterus) (Fig. 45-4). In the initial phase, these changes relate to preparation of the endometrium to receive and implant a fertilized ovum. During the follicular phase of the menstrual cycle, the rising levels of estradiol stimulate the reconstruction of the endometrium following the preceding menstrual period. This phase of endometrial growth is termed the *proliferative phase*, during which endometrial thickness increases from about 0.5 mm to approximately 3.5 to 5.0 mm. Following ovulation, the endometrium responds to the combined effects of estradiol and progesterone. The overall endometrial thickness remains constant, but individual components continue to grow, so there is a progressive increase in the tortuosity of the endometrial glands and intensified coiling of the spiral blood vessels. This phase corresponds with the luteal phase of the menstrual cycle but is called the *secretory phase* because of the significant increase that occurs in endometrial gland secretion. The endometrial glands secrete many substances, including numerous peptide growth factors, cytokines, and prostaglandins, the functions of which have yet to be fully elucidated. Implantation of a fertilized ovum (now a blastocyst) occurs about six days after ovulation and by this stage the endometrium is of sufficient depth, vascularity, and nutritional richness to support the early development of the placenta (i.e., invasion of the trophoblastic cells to create the trophoblast-maternal blood interface). The peak endometrial gland secretory activity coincides with the time of blastocyst implantation.

In the event of successful implantation, human chorionic gonadotrophin (hCG) is produced by the trophoblastic cells, and the corpus luteum will thereby be maintained. If this does not happen, the corpus luteum begins to regress about 9 days after ovulation and estrogen and progesterone levels decrease. The withdrawal of these hormones initiates several events within the endometrium. Arteriolar vasomotor changes result in rhythmic vasoconstriction and vasodilation in the spiral vessels. Each successive vasoconstrictive spasm is more severe, ultimately leading to tissue necrosis and interstitial hemorrhages due to capillary breakdown. As ischemia and tissue weakness progresses, bleeding into the endometrial cavity occurs and menstruation begins.

Premenstrual syndrome. Many women experience a variety of cyclic premenstrual symptoms that occur after ovulation and disappear after menstruation. The most frequently encountered symptoms include abdominal bloating, anxiety, breast tenderness, crying spells, depression, fatigue, irritability, headache, thirst, and appetite changes, all occurring during the last 7 to 10 days of the menstrual cycle. In some women, the combination of symptoms known as the **premenstrual syndrome (PMS)** is more severe for unknown reasons. Although the cause is unknown, prevention of ovulation by the use of oral contraceptives is often helpful. Other treatments that may relieve some symptoms include drug therapy with bromocriptine (a dopamine agonist), prostaglandin synthetase inhibitors (nonsteroidal antiinflammatory agents), mild diuretics, or antidepressants if symptoms are severe.

Dysmenorrhea. Dysmenorrhea, or painful menstruation, is very common, affecting at least 50% of women at some time during their reproductive life. Primary dysmenorrhea is associated with ovulatory cycles and is caused by uterine smooth muscle contractions induced by prostaglandins, especially prostaglandin $F_{2\alpha}$, formed in the secretory endometrium. Patients with primary dysmenorrhea often have additional symptoms, which can include headache, nausea and vomiting, diarrhea, and emotional disorders. This form of dysmenorrhea can often be treated by prevention of ovulation by oral contraceptives or by the use of prostaglandin synthetase inhibitors. Secondary dysmenorrhea is associated with a variety of conditions such as endometriosis, pelvic inflammatory disease, congenital defects in uterine development, and the presence of intrauterine devices. Secondary dysmenorrhea sometimes requires surgical therapy; however, about 80% of women with either form of dysmenorrhea experience some relief with the use of prostaglandin synthetase inhibitors. A further benefit of these agents is a reduction in the amount of blood lost with menstrual flow.

Menopause

Menopause is the permanent cessation of menstruation resulting from the loss of ovarian follicular function. Clinically, menopause is recognized as having occurred after 12 consecutive months of amenorrhea, so the time of the final menses is determined retrospectively. Perimenopause, or the climacteric, includes the period immediately prior to menopause, when the endocrinological, biological, and clinical features of approaching menopause commence, and the first year after menopause. The mean age at which menopause occurs is about 51 years.[10] There is no correlation between the age of menarche and the age of menopause. Socioeconomic circumstances, race, parity, and weight have no effect on the timing of menopause, but women who smoke may experience an earlier menopause.

The major underlying pathophysiology of menopause is the loss of ovarian follicles.[3] Ovarian primordial follicle numbers decrease steadily with increasing age up to about the age of 38, but their number then declines much more rapidly during the last decade of reproductive life. At the time of menopause itself, few if any follicles can be found in the ovaries. The ovary of the postmenopausal woman is reduced in size, weighs less than 2.5 g, and is wrinkled in appearance. Microscopically, the cortical area is reduced because of follicular loss, the stroma becomes hyperplastic, and interstitial and hilar cells are more prominent.

The normal menstrual cycle is characterized by the changing levels in plasma gonadotropins, the ovarian steroids, and the inhibins, as described above. No endocrine event clearly differentiates the time just before and just after the final menses. FSH levels begin to rise a year or two before the final menses, often coinciding with the onset of cycle irregularity, but estradiol levels are well maintained until just a few months before the cessation of menses. It is only after a woman has experienced more than 3 months of amenorrhea that the rise in FSH is accompanied by a substantial fall in estradiol levels. Indeed, during perimenopause, FSH concentrations may be raised to the postmenopausal range during some cycles but return to premenopausal levels during subsequent cycles. Thus, in menstruating women, laboratory measurement of FSH cannot reliably determine menopausal status.[10] LH levels remain largely unchanged during the perimenopausal period.

A major hormonal event of the menopausal transition is a decline in inhibin B levels during the first half of the cycle. This decrease in inhibin B produces a reduction in negative feedback on the pituitary, thereby allowing a rise in FSH sufficient to stimulate follicular development and maintain dominant follicle function and estradiol production for as long as possible. The observed fall in inhibin B levels in older women may reflect a decrease in the size of the recruited cohort of follicles at the onset of each cycle or a decrease in the ability of granulosa cells to secrete inhibin B. As cycles become irregular, menstrual bleeding may occur at the end of an inadequate luteal phase or after an estradiol peak without subsequent ovulation or corpus luteum formation. However, ovulation and the formation of a functional corpus luteum can occur, and the perimenopausal woman is not safe from unexpected pregnancy until elevated levels of both FSH and LH can be demonstrated. In the postmenopausal state, there is a 10- to 15-fold increase in circulating FSH levels, a 4- to 5-fold increase in LH, and more than a 90% decrease in circulating estradiol. Inhibin levels are undetectable postmenopausally. FSH levels are higher than LH because LH is cleared from the blood much more rapidly (their respective half lives are about 30 minutes for LH and 4 hours for FSH). Gonadotropin levels reach a maximum some 1 to 3 years after the final menses. Elevated levels of both FSH and LH in association with prolonged amenorrhea constitute conclusive evidence of ovarian failure.

The classical symptoms of menopause such as hot flushes, vaginal dryness, and urinary frequency are thought to result from falling or low estradiol levels. Hot flushes are a sensation of warmth, commonly accompanied by skin flushing and perspiration. They can be occasional or frequent, last from seconds to an hour and be associated with mild warmth or profound sweating. Hot flushes diminish spontaneously as time from menopause increases, but often the primary indication for treatment is to relieve distressing symptoms. In some women, hot flushes are a major problem, disrupting work, sleep, or daily activities. Other clinical consequences of the postmenopausal state include significantly increased risks of developing coronary heart disease and osteoporosis. Postmenopausal women are estimated to have a two-fold higher risk of developing coronary heart disease than premenopausal women, after adjustment for age. The adverse change in age-adjusted plasma lipid and lipoprotein profiles that occurs after menopause is a significant factor in this association. A causal relationship between menopause and osteoporosis is evident from the higher rates of osteoporotic fractures observed in postmenopausal women and the loss of bone mineral density that has been documented after menopause. Longitudinal cohort studies suggest that the maximal changes in bone mineral density occur during late perimenopause and early postmenopause, corresponding to the time of maximal decrease in circulating estradiol levels.[3]

Hormone replacement therapy (HRT) can therefore be directed at symptom relief or at prevention or treatment of the above diseases associated with the postmenopausal state. Doses, routes of administration, and duration of treatment can vary according to the indication for therapy. A progestagen must be used in combination with estrogen in a woman with an intact uterus, in order to prevent endometrial hyperplasia and the associated risk of endometrial malignancy. Systemic estrogens can be given orally, transdermally, vaginally, by intramuscular injection, and via slow-release pellets implanted subcutaneously. Non-oral administration of estrogen can be useful because it avoids first-pass liver metabolism. Transdermal patches are most commonly used; estrogen injections are suboptimal since they produce wide fluctuations in concentration. In oral hormone replacement regimens, estrogen, and progesterone may be given cyclically (with progestagen given for 10 to 12 days of each cycle) or as continuous combined preparations. Continuous unopposed estrogen may be used in women who have had a hysterectomy. Estrogen replacement therapy is the most effective treatment for hot flushes, and there is a dose-dependent relation between estrogen dose and suppression of such symptoms. Systemic or locally applied topical estrogen preparations can be used to treat vaginal dryness and may improve urinary symptoms.

Cohort studies suggested that estrogen replacement (with or without a progestagen) reduces the relative risk of coronary heart disease in unselected postmenopausal women. This effect has not been substantiated in more rigorous studies; however, as a recent large randomized placebo-controlled trial showed that 4 to 5 years of continuous combined estrogen and progesterone in postmenopausal women with preexisting coronary artery disease did not reduce the incidence of coronary events.[10] There is stronger evidence that HRT protects against osteoporosis; a large number of cohort studies have shown that HRT increases bone mineral density and reduces fracture rates in postmenopausal women. Estrogens may exert positive effects on the central nervous system, possibly reducing the incidence and severity of Alzheimer's type dementia and maintaining normal cognitive function in postmenopausal women. Estrogen therapy is not without drawbacks, however. Side-effects such as nausea and breast tenderness can be problematic, particularly in older women, and many women dislike the concept of ongoing regular or irregular menstrual bleeding. Several meta-analyses have shown that estrogen treatment, especially long-term (greater than 10 years), is associated with a small increase in the relative risk of developing breast cancer.[6] It is also associated with an increased risk of deep venous thrombosis and gallbladder disease. Selective estrogen receptor modulators (SERMS), such as raloxifene, are an attractive alternative to conventional estrogen therapy that may offer the benefits without the risks. Some of these compounds act as estrogen antagonists in human reproductive tissues but are partial agonists on the skeletal system and on serum lipoproteins. Raloxifene treatment has been shown to significantly reduce the relative risk of vertebral fracture in women with established osteoporosis, to have favorable effects on plasma lipids, to have minimal effects on uterine tissue, and to perhaps reduce the risk of breast cancer in postmenopausal women.[6]

PATHOLOGICAL STATES
Amenorrhea

As described above, normal menstrual function depends on the complex hormonal interactions between the hypothalamus, pituitary, and ovaries. An intact outflow tract and the existence and development of the endometrium are also required for normal menstrual flow. Abnormalities in any of these hormonal or anatomical systems may cause amenorrhea (absence of bleeding). The clinical problem of amenorrhea may be defined by the following criteria:

1. No period by age 14 in the absence of growth or development of secondary sex characteristics (primary amenorrhea)
2. No period by age 16, regardless of the presence of normal growth and development with the appearance of secondary sex characteristics (primary amenorrhea)
3. In a woman who has been menstruating, the absence of periods for a length of time equivalent to a total of at least three of the previous cycle intervals or 6 months of amenorrhea (secondary amenorrhea)

The assessment of a patient with amenorrhea requires a careful history and examination. Pregnancy must always be ruled out. In the following sections, the various disorders that may cause amenorrhea and how the clinical laboratory contributes to the diagnostic process will be described. The causes of amenorrhea are shown in Box 45-1 and a proposed clinical workup summarized in Fig. 45-5.

Disorders of the outflow tract or uterus. Congenital abnormalities of the organs that develop from the müllerian duct system must always be considered in the evaluation of primary amenorrhea. Many different müllerian anomalies can occur, including imperforate hymen, obliteration of the vaginal orifice, absence of the uterine cavity or endometrial lining, or absence of the uterus itself or the cervix. Some

---

> ### BOX 45-1
> #### CAUSES OF AMENORRHEA
>
> **Disorders of the Outflow Tract or Uterus**
> Müllerian duct anomalies/complete müllerian agenesis
> Complete/partial androgen insensitivity (testicular feminization syndrome)
> Endometrial destruction (Asherman syndrome)
>
> **Disorders of the Ovary (Primary Hypogonadism)**
> Gonadal dysgenesis (Turner syndrome, mosaics 45,X/46,XX, 47,XXX)
> Resistant ovary syndrome
> Premature ovarian failure (idiopathic, autoimmune, postirradiation, or chemotherapy)
>
> **Disorders of the Anterior Pituitary (Secondary Hypogonadism)**
> Prolactin-secreting pituitary tumor
> Other pituitary tumors
> Granulomatous infiltration (sarcoidosis, histiocytosis)
> Lymphocytic hypophysitis
> Pituitary apoplexy (Sheehan syndrome)
>
> **Central Nervous System Disorders**
> Kallmann syndrome
> Hypothalamic infiltrative disease (sarcoidosis, histiocytosis, hemochromatosis)
> Hypothalamic tumors (craniopharyngioma)
> Cranial irradiation

of these anomalies are apparent on physical examination; others can be identified via pelvic ultrasound. Patients with complete müllerian agenesis have an absent vagina and varying uterine abnormalities, ranging from virtual absence of the uterus with the presence of rudimentary uterine tissue only, to a morphologically normal uterus. Ovarian function is normal in these patients; hence growth and development are also normal. Complete androgen insensitivity (testicular feminization syndrome) produces congenital absence of the uterus and a blind-ending vaginal canal. The patient with testicular feminization has a female phenotype (appearance), including some breast development at puberty, but is a genetic and gonadal male with failure of **virilization**. Resistance to the action of fetal testicular testosterone means that the male wolffian duct system cannot develop, but antimüllerian hormone produced by the fetal testes acts normally and hence the female müllerian duct system develops abnormally. The chromosomal karyotype is XY, and testicular tissue is present, sometimes intra-abdominally but frequently within an inguinal hernia as antimüllerian hormone mediates testicular descent. The incidence of malignant neoplasia in these gonads is high, and they must be surgically removed. This disorder is genetically transmitted by means of a maternal X-linked recessive gene, which encodes the intracellular androgen receptor. These patients have normal to

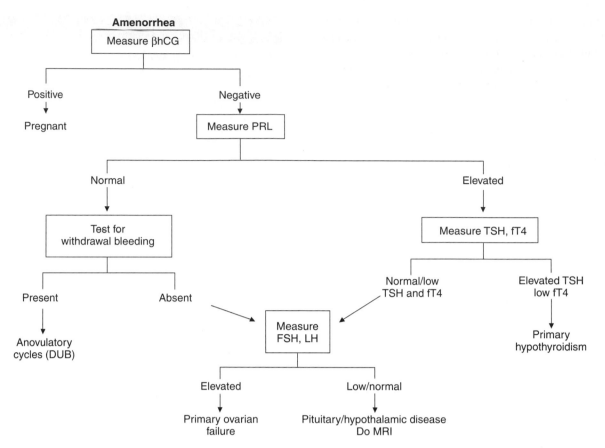

Fig. 45-5 Clinical approach to the investigation of amenorrhea. *βhCG*, human chorionic gonadotropin; *DUB*, dysfunctional uterine bleeding; *FSH*, follicle-stimulating hormone; *fT4*, free thyroxine; *LH*, luteinizing hormone; *MRI*, magnetic resonance imaging; *PRL*, prolactin; *TSH*, thyroid-stimulating hormone.

slightly high male plasma testosterone levels and high LH levels. Incomplete androgen insensitivity occurs more rarely. These individuals also have a female phenotype, but show some evidence of androgen effect, such as clitoral enlargement.

Secondary amenorrhea can occur after destruction of the endometrium (Asherman syndrome). This condition is usually the result of an overly aggressive curettage resulting in intrauterine scarring and adhesions. Rarely, it may occur after an infection related to an intrauterine device (IUD) or a severe generalized pelvic infection.

Disorders of the ovary (primary hypogonadism). Patients with abnormal gonadal development (gonadal dysgenesis) can present with primary or secondary amenorrhea. Several different chromosomal karyotypes are associated with gonadal dysgenesis, including 45,X (**Turner syndrome**), mosaics (e.g., 45,X/46,XX), deletions of the short or long arms of X, 47,XXX, and not uncommonly, the normal female karyotype of 46,XX. These individuals have high plasma gonadotropin levels as a result of the lack of ovarian estrogen secretion and negative feedback on the pituitary. All patients presenting with primary or secondary amenorrhea in conjunction with high gonadotropin levels should have a karyotype determination. Although women with chromosomal defects are more likely to present with primary amenorrhea,

individuals with **mosaicism** may have some functional gonadal tissue giving rise to various degrees of sexual development and transient menstrual cyclicity. Identifying the presence of a mosaic form with a Y chromosome present is critical. Gonadal tissue in these patients must be surgically removed, because the presence of any testicular component within the gonad carries with it a significant risk of malignant tumor formation. A normal female phenotype does not exclude the presence of a Y chromosome; about 30% of mosaic patients with a Y will not develop signs of virilization.

Turner syndrome (an abnormality in or absence of one of the X chromosomes), is relatively common (about 1 in 7000 live female births) and has several well-defined clinical characteristics. The presence of short stature, a webbed neck, shield chest, and increased carrying angle at the elbow in association with hypergonadotropic hypoestrogenic amenorrhea virtually confirms the diagnosis. A karyotype must still be performed, however, since 20% to 30% of patients presenting with the classical clinical features of Turner's syndrome are mosaics. In comparison with gonadal dysgenesis, the resistant ovary syndrome is a rare clinical entity. Such patients present with primary amenorrhea in conjunction with high gonadotropin levels and a normal karyotype, but ovarian development occurs and a full-thickness biopsy of the ovary can demonstrate the presence of follicles.

Premature ovarian failure is typically defined as amenorrhea, **infertility**, estrogen deficiency, and elevated gonadotropins in a woman less than 40 years of age. It affects 1% of women by the age of 40 and 0.1% by age 30 years.[15a] Normal menopause is irreversible, whereas premature ovarian failure is associated with intermittent ovarian function in about 50% of cases. Affected women may intermittently produce estrogen and ovulate despite the presence of high gonadotropin levels. Premature ovarian failure can present as primary or secondary amenorrhea. Patients with secondary amenorrhea may experience symptoms of estrogen deficiency, such as hot flushes. The underlying etiology of premature ovarian failure is unknown in most cases; presumably the ovarian follicles undergo a process of accelerated atresia. It may be associated with autoimmune endocrine disorders such as primary adrenal failure (Addison's disease), type 1 diabetes mellitus, and hypothyroidism, or it may follow follicle destruction by infections (such as mumps virus) or physical insults such as irradiation or chemotherapy. Young women with premature ovarian failure, which may occur before peak adult bone mass is achieved, are estrogen-deficient for a much longer period than women who undergo a natural menopause. The associated risks of osteoporosis and cardiovascular disease are therefore significantly increased, and appropriate hormone replacement therapy in these patients is critically important. Long-term surveillance is necessary, and hormone replacement should be continued at least until the average age of natural menopause. There is a 5% to 10% chance of spontaneous pregnancy in young women, and fertility is not adversely affected by concurrent hormone replacement therapy. The efficacy of hormone ovulation induction regimens in women who fail to conceive naturally is variable in patients with premature ovarian failure, depending on whether there is potentially functioning ovarian tissue.

Disorders of the anterior pituitary (secondary hypogonadism). Several disorders of the pituitary can result in estrogen deficiency and amenorrhea. In this instance, plasma gonadotropin levels will be low (or within the reference range, which is also evidence of gonadotrope dysfunction in view of the coexisting estrogen deficiency), and estrogen concentrations will be low. This situation is termed *hypogonadotropic hypogonadism*. Pituitary tumors may directly decrease gonadotropin secretion by the destruction of pituitary gonadotropin-producing cells or secrete prolactin, which is thought to disturb GnRH neuron function. Granulomatous (sarcoidosis, histiocytosis) and autoimmune (lymphocytic hypophysitis) disorders can cause gonadotrope destruction. Pituitary apoplexy (spontaneous infarction or necrosis) can occur in the setting of a preexisting pituitary tumor or following severe postpartum hemorrhage and shock (Sheehan syndrome). Pituitary tumors comprise approximately 10% of all intracranial tumors, and prolactin-secreting tumors are the most common. Pituitary cells of all types can be transformed into adenomatous lesions, and pituitary tumors may secrete one or more hormones or be nonfunctioning. Pituitary tumors usually grow slowly, and when they enlarge, they typically extend superiorly and may impinge on the optic chiasm. Patients may therefore present with the effects of excess hormone secretion, with symptoms of **hypogonadism** or with mass effects such as visual field defects.

Women with hyperprolactinemia commonly have amenorrhea and/or galactorrhea; therefore all patients presenting with such symptoms should have a serum prolactin measurement. Not all women with hyperprolactinemia have a prolactinoma, however, because pituitary stalk transection (associated with head injury), hypothalamic granulomatous diseases, hypothyroidism, renal failure, and stress may all be associated with elevations in serum prolactin. Prolactin secretion is normally regulated via inhibitory hypothalamic dopaminergic pathways. Many drugs have some inhibitory action on the dopamine receptor or deplete central dopamine levels, for example phenothiazines, metoclopramide, opiates, and the monoamine oxidase inhibitors. All these drugs have the potential to produce mild to moderate increases in serum prolactin. The assessment of any patient with hyperprolactinemia therefore requires that a thorough drug history be taken. All patients with elevated prolactin levels in association with amenorrhea and/or galactorrhea require radiological imaging of the pituitary. Magnetic resonance imaging (MRI) is the method of choice if available, since it is more sensitive than computer tomography (CT) in the detection of small pituitary tumors. As with other pituitary tumors, prolactinomas can be categorized as microadenomas (<10 mm in diameter) or macroprolactinomas (>10 mm). The serum prolactin level roughly correlates with the size of the tumor; a small elevation in prolactin in association with a large pituitary tumor probably reflects stalk compression rather than tumor prolactin secretion. First-line therapy for these tumors is pharmacological. Biochemically and in terms of tumor shrinkage, prolactinomas have a high response rate to treatment with the dopamine agonists, bromocriptine, or the longer-acting cabergoline.

Central nervous system disorders. If a pituitary lesion has been excluded, hypothalamic disorders resulting in failure of the normal pulsatile GnRH secretion must be considered, since these may also produce the clinical syndrome of hypogonadotropic hypogonadism. Deficient GnRH secretion may occur in isolation, as part of a congenital or inherited disorder, or it may result from a variety of structural and functional hypothalamic lesions.[14] In the developing fetus, the GnRH and olfactory neurons originate outside the central nervous system and must migrate up the nasal septum, through the cribriform plate to the forebrain and ultimately to the arcuate nucleus of the hypothalamus. A defect in the formation and migration of GnRH neurons is called *isolated hypothalamic hypogonadism* or *congenital isolated GnRH deficiency*. When this condition is associated with anosmia (the inability to smell) and agenesis of the olfactory bulbs, it is called **Kallmann syndrome**. This genetically heterogenous disorder is most commonly inherited as an autosomal-dominant trait but may be autosomal-recessive or X-linked. It is four times more common in males and can be associated with other anomalies such as cleft lip and palate, sensorineural deafness, and renal agenesis. The clinical features of GnRH deficiency typically become apparent at puberty, a time when there is normally a marked increase in GnRH secretion. Affected women present with primary amenorrhea and failure to develop secondary sex characteristics. There are other rare syndromes with a genetic basis in which hypogonadotropic hypogonadism is associated with several other characteristic clinical features, such as the Prader-Willi, Laurence-Moon, and Bardet-Biedl syndromes. These disorders are usually evident in early childhood.

Structural lesions of the hypothalamus can also interfere with the normal pattern of GnRH synthesis, secretion or stimulation of pituitary gonadotropes. In children, the most common tumor resulting in hypogonadotropic hypogonadism is a craniopharyngioma. In adult patients, gliomas, meningiomas, and germinomas may cause hypothalamic dysfunction. Rarer causes include involvement of the hypothalamus by infiltrative disorders such as hemochromatosis, sarcoidosis, and histiocytosis. Previous cranial irradiation for the treatment of central nervous system tumors or leukemia may result in a gradual deterioration in hypothalamic-pituitary function. Functional forms of hypogonadotropic hypogonadism also exist, in which the disturbance in GnRH secretion is of a transient rather than permanent nature. In susceptible women, amenorrhea may be precipitated by stress, significant weight loss and undertaking regular strenuous exercise. In these circumstances, treatment is ideally directed at the underlying cause, but cyclic hormone replacement therapy or the oral contraceptive pill can be used to protect against osteoporosis. GnRH suppression due to exogenous anabolic steroids is also reversible, although recovery can take some weeks after steroid withdrawal.

Evaluation of amenorrhea. A thorough history and examination is mandatory in the assessment of a patient with amenorrhea. Any history of psychological stress or severe weight loss, abnormal growth or development, galactorrhea, visual problems, a previous curette and a family history of genetic disorders is highly relevant. Abnormalities of the vagina, the absence of secondary sex characteristics, clinical features suggestive of Turner syndrome, evidence of androgenization, and body weight can be assessed during the physical examination. Further investigation depends to some extent on the history and examination findings; for example, in a young woman with primary amenorrhea and abnormal development, the initial investigations should include a karotype and pelvic ultrasound. The presence of normal secondary sex characteristics implies that estrogen production was adequate in the past. The progestin withdrawal test provides a functional assessment of current estrogen status in women with normal outflow tract. A course of a progestagen with no estrogenic activity, such as oral medroxyprogesterone acetate 10 mg daily for 5 days, is administered. The presence of vaginal bleeding within 7 days after the end of progesterone treatment indicates that the patient is producing sufficient estrogen to stimulate endometrial growth.

Pregnancy should be ruled out in all patients with amenorrhea by measuring a plasma βhCG level (human chorionic gonadotropin), a glycoprotein produced by the developing placenta. Clinical laboratory tests also help considerably in differentiating between primary ovarian pathology and the pituitary/hypothalamic causes of amenorrhea. In women with primary ovarian failure or gonadal dysgenesis, the plasma gonadotropin levels are elevated. Decreased or normal levels of FSH and LH in conjunction with low estrogen levels indicate a defect in pituitary or hypothalamic function. All patients with hypogonadotropic hypogonadism or a history of galactorrhea should have a serum prolactin measurement. In patients with unexplained hypogonadotropic hypogonadism and/or an elevated prolactin level, an MRI (or CT, if MRI is unavailable) of the pituitary should be performed. Patients with severe hypothyroidism may occasionally present with amenorrhea and/or galactorrhea; therefore all such patients should also have serum thyroxine and thyroid-stimulating hormone (TSH) measurements. A GnRH stimulation test has been described, in which a bolus of 100 µg GnRH is administered intravenously and plasma LH and FSH levels are measured at 30 and 60 minutes; however, the clinical usefulness of such testing in adult patients is not established. Clomiphene citrate normally stimulates hypothalamic GnRH release, resulting in increased pituitary secretion of FSH and LH. Oral clomiphene may be given to women on days 2 to 6 of her menstrual cycle and a doubling of plasma LH levels over the next 10 days indicates normal hypothalamic function. In practice, these dynamic stimulation tests are rarely used in the evaluation of patients with hypogonadotropic hypogonadism.

Dysfunctional Uterine Bleeding

Between menarche and menopause, almost every woman experiences one or more episodes of abnormal uterine bleeding, defined as any bleeding pattern that differs in frequency, duration, or amount from the pattern observed during a normal menstrual cycle. Abnormal bleeding may occur during ovulatory cycles. The cycles occur regularly, but the duration or amount of bleeding differs from normal. Excessive or prolonged bleeding may be due to pathological abnormalities of the uterus, such as leiomyomas or endometrial polyps, or to a coagulation disorder. Regular ovulatory cycles characterized by spotting or light bleeding may be due to intrauterine adhesions or cervical scarring. Intermenstrual bleeding or spotting is often caused by endometrial or cervical lesions.

Uterine bleeding during anovulatory cycles is unpredictable with respect to amount, onset and duration, and is known as **dysfunctional uterine bleeding (DUB)**. DUB is usually painless because of the absence of ovulation. This disorder reflects a disruption in the normal maturation and development of the endometrium. In the absence of ovulation, there is inadequate corpus luteum progesterone support of the estrogen-primed endometrium, and therefore bleeding occurs at unpredictable and irregular intervals. The continued exposure of the endometrium to estrogen, unopposed by progesterone, causes a hyperplastic endometrium, and women with untreated DUB are at increased risk for endometrial cancer. DUB occurs in normal women at the extremes of reproductive life (i.e., postmenarche), as anovulatory cycles precede the development of regular ovulatory cycles, and perimenopausally, as follicle depletion leads to anovulatory cycles. In women of reproductive age, the most common cause of chronic anovulation in the presence of adequate estrogen levels is polycystic ovary syndrome.

Polycystic ovary syndrome. **Polycystic ovary syndrome (PCOS)** is a complex disorder that is typically characterized by infertility, **hirsutism**, obesity, and various menstrual disturbances, such as amenorrhea, oligomenorrhea, or DUB. Classic PCOS, as originally described by Stein and Leventhal, is associated with enlarged, sclerotic ovaries with thickened capsules, containing multiple atretic follicles (creating the so-called polycystic appearance) and rare or absent corpora albicans, reflecting the lack of ovulation. The presence of this ovarian morphology alone, however, is insufficient to make the diagnosis of PCOS, because it has been described in 20% to 25% of normal women with regular ovulatory cycles and no evidence of hyperandrogenism. The key features of PCOS are therefore the presence of menstrual irregularity in association with hyperandrogenism, which may be evident clinically (as hirsutism, acne, or male pattern balding) or biochemically (as elevated serum androgen levels). Hirsutism is defined as excess terminal (thick, pigmented) body hair in a male distribution.[2] It is commonly observed on the upper lip, the chin, around the nipples, and along the linea alba of the lower abdomen. Severe hyperandrogenism may cause increased muscle mass, a deepening voice, and clitoromegaly; however, these signs of virilization are more commonly associated with androgen-secreting ovarian or adrenal tumors. Not all women with PCOS are overweight, but at least 50% are obese and some of these women will resume more regular menstrual cycles after relatively small amounts of weight loss. PCOS is also associated with hyperinsulinemia due to a relative insulin resistance, which exists independently of body weight but is exacerbated by obesity. About 20% of obese women with PCOS develop impaired glucose tolerance or overt non–insulin-dependent diabetes mellitus by the age of 40.

In normal women, androgens are produced by the adrenal gland and the ovary, as well as from peripheral conversion of less potent androgens to more potent androgens by enzymes such as 5-α-reductase located in the skin and fat tissue. The principal source of androgen in PCOS is the ovary. Women with PCOS may have elevated plasma levels of androstenedione, testosterone and/or dehydroepiandrosterone (DHEA), but there is considerable individual variation and the androgen levels may be completely normal. Dehydroepiandrosterone sulfate (DHEAS) is derived mostly from the adrenal gland, and therefore it acts as a marker of adrenal, *not* ovarian, androgen hypersecretion. Testosterone is the most potent circulating androgen, although its activity is determined by the amount of binding to sex hormone-binding globulin (SHBG) because only the free hormone fraction is biologically active. Androgens and insulin suppress SHBG production by the liver, so women with PCOS tend to have low SHBG levels. This can mask the degree of testosterone excess when total testosterone levels are measured. Free testosterone assays are neither widely available nor particularly reliable; therefore the free androgen index (ratio of total testosterone to SHBG) may be used to estimate free testosterone activity. In women with PCOS, total testosterone levels may be normal but the free androgen index may be elevated. Women with PCOS generally have estradiol levels within the normal range for the early follicular phase but elevated estrone levels. These estrogens are partly derived from the numerous small follicles in the polycystic ovary and partly from the peripheral aromatization of androgens to estrogens in fat cells. Some women with PCOS have abnormal gonadotropin levels, suggesting a disturbance in the normal pituitary-ovarian relationship. The characteristic pattern is of relatively high LH levels in conjunction with normal or low FSH levels, resulting in an elevated LH to FSH ratio. About 15% to 20% of women with PCOS also have mildly elevated plasma prolactin levels.

Other disorders associated with androgen excess. The most frequent symptom of hyperandrogenism is hirsutism, a relatively common presenting complaint in women. Over 95% of hirsute women will have the more benign conditions of idiopathic hirsutism, which is often familial and is associated with a normal menstrual cycle, or PCOS. However, these conditions should be diagnosed after the exclusion of more serious and potentially life-threatening causes of hirsutism. The causes of hirsutism, the majority associated with hyperandrogenism and menstrual irregularity, are shown in Box 45-2. The less common causes of hirsutism can generally be distinguished from idiopathic hirsutism and PCOS by specific clinical features and biochemical tests. A history of abrupt onset, short duration (less than 1 year), or progressively worsening hirsutism, particularly if associated with signs of virilization, strongly suggests an androgen-secreting ovarian or adrenal tumor. Such patients usually have very high plasma testosterone levels. High levels of DHEAS indicate an adrenal tumor, although a low DHEAS level does not rule out a tumor with 100% sensitivity, as there are some reports of adrenal carcinomas

---

BOX 45-2

CAUSES OF HIRSUTISM

Idiopathic (including familial)
Drug-induced (anabolic steroids, minoxidil, phenytoin)
Ovarian
    Polycystic ovary syndrome
    Androgen-secreting ovarian tumors
Adrenal
    Late-onset (nonclassical) 21-hydroxylase deficiency
    Congenital adrenal hyperplasia
    Androgen-secreting adrenal tumors
Cushing syndrome

that lack sulfating activity. In addition, DHEAS secretion decreases after about 30 years of age, so serum levels must be interpreted according to age-specific normal ranges. Transvaginal ultrasound is an effective means of identifying ovarian tumors, but abdominal computer tomography or magnetic resonance imaging is required to search for an adrenal mass. The late-onset (nonclassical) form of adrenal 21-hydroxylase deficiency, producing congenital adrenal hyperplasia (CAH), should be considered in women with an early onset of hirsutism, hyperkalemia or a family history of CAH. This diagnosis may be ruled out by measuring 17-hydroxyprogesterone (17-OHP), a precursor of cortisol that is converted to 11-deoxycortisol by the 21-hydroxylase enzyme. Plasma levels of 17-OHP increase during the luteal phase, so sampling for a basal 17-OHP level should be performed during the follicular phase in menstruating women. In patients with borderline basal 17-OHP levels, the diagnosis may be confirmed by demonstrating an exaggerated 17-OHP response to adrenal stimulation with exogenous synthetic ACTH. Testing for Cushing's syndrome should be considered in hirsute women with symptoms and signs suggestive of cortisol excess, such as progressive weight gain with a predominantly central distribution, purple striae, easy bruising, muscle weakness, mood changes, and hypertension. Screening tests include measuring 24-hour urinary excretion of free cortisol and performing an overnight dexamethasone suppression test (see Chapter 46).

Ovarian Hyperfunction

Ovarian neoplasms are organized according to a complex histological classification. Almost any tumor of the ovary may produce an endocrine effect, either through functional activity of the tumor cells themselves or via an effect on reactive non-neoplastic stromal cells. The majority of clinically functioning tumors are of the sex cord stromal type or germ-cell tumors. Sex cord stromal tumors are thought to be derived from the specialized ovarian stroma; this group includes the granulosa, theca, Sertoli-Leydig, and lipoid cell tumors. The granulosa tumor is the most common malignant functioning tumor of the ovary. Granulosa tumors are almost always estrinizing, although rarely these tumors produce testosterone and are virilizing. The symptoms differ with the age of the patient: prepubertal girls present with precocious puberty, women in their reproductive years experience disturbances in menstruation, and postmenopausal women present with irregular vaginal bleeding secondary to endometrial hyperplasia. Functioning thecomas are also almost always estrinizing, whereas Sertoli-Leydig and lipoid cell tumors are more often virilizing. In all instances, primary ovarian hyperfunction results in suppression of LH and FSH secretion as a result of increased negative feedback effects on the pituitary.

NORMAL TESTES AND TESTICULAR FUNCTION
Early Development

The early development of the gonads up to about 42 days gestation is identical in male and female embryos. By this time, in male embryos, the fetal testes become apparent histologically with the development of seminiferous cords in the genital ridge. As in the ovary, there are three principal cell types involved in the formation of the testes: (1) coelomic epithelial cells, which differentiate into the Sertoli cells; (2) mesenchymal cells, which give rise to the interstitial (Leydig) cells; and (3) the primordial germ cells. A portion of the Y chromosome is essential for normal male gonadal development. The testes-determining factor has been mapped to a segment on the short arm of the Y chromosome, and the gene isolated from this locus has been called the *sex-determining region Y (SRY)*. Male wolffian duct development is dependent on testicular production of testosterone and antimüllerian hormone. Histological development of the testis is essentially complete by the end of the third month of gestation. Descent of the testes from the abdomen to the scrotum occurs later; this process is not complete until the seventh month of gestation. Testicular descent depends in part on hormonal factors, such as antimüllerian hormone and androgen, but also on the normal development of abdominal musculature and intra-abdominal pressure. Each testis contains approximately 3×10^5 primordial germ cells, which remain quiescent until puberty, when they divide by mitosis to form spermatogonia. Unlike ovarian germ cells, testicular germ cells do not begin the process of meiosis until puberty. As previously described, the process of meiosis involves two cell divisions; in the male this ultimately yields cells called *spermatids*, which contain the haploid (23) chromosome number.

Fetal pituitary LH and placental hCG are both important in the regulation of testosterone secretion from the fetal testes, although the precise control of testosterone production is not completely understood. In the male embryo, the secretion of testosterone by the testes and the level of plasma testosterone begin to rise at the end of the second month of gestation, reaching a maximal level shortly thereafter that is maintained until late in gestation but decreases before birth. At birth, the plasma testosterone level is only slightly higher in males than in females. Shortly after birth, the plasma testosterone level rises in the male infant, remaining elevated for about 3 months but falling to low levels by 1 year. The plasma level then remains low (although higher in males than females) until puberty, when it again increases in boys, reaching adult male levels by about age 17. As in girls, the hypothalamic-pituitary axis in prepubertal boys is highly sensitive to the negative feedback effects of gonadal steroids, in this instance testosterone, and plasma gonadotropin levels remain low until puberty. However, although basal secretion is low in prepubertal children, the pituitary gonadotropins are secreted in a pulsatile manner, the pulses occurring at 2- to 3-hour intervals. Sleep-associated surges in LH secretion, and to a lesser extent surges in FSH secretion, in response to bursts of GnRH release from the hypothalamus herald the onset of puberty. Later in puberty, pulsatile gonadotropin secretion occurs throughout the day and night, and plasma gonadotropin levels become more sustained, as do the resulting increases in plasma testosterone and dihydrotestosterone concentrations. In boys, the anatomic and functional changes of puberty are primarily the result of testicular androgens. Androgens stimulate the development of male secondary sex characteristics and the male body physical appearance, accelerating linear growth and initiate spermatogenesis in the testes.

The Mature Testes

Structural organization. The adult testes are spheroid organs located within the scrotum. The extra-abdominal location of the testes serves to maintain the testicular temperature about 2° Celsius below the core body temperature. The process of spermatogenesis is exquisitely sensitive to alterations in temperature, and temporary increases in systemic or local temperature are frequently followed by brief decreases in sperm production.

The macroscopic structure of the testes is shown in Fig. 45-6. The testes contain two functional units: (1) a network of tubules for the production and transport of sperm to the excretory-ejaculatory ducts and (2) a system of interstitial cells (**Leydig cells**) that constitute the major endocrine component of the testes, since they are responsible for the production of testicular androgens (predominantly testosterone).

Within each testis there are about 250 pyramidal lobules that contain coiled seminiferous tubules separated by fibrous septa; this component accounts for 80% to 90% of the testicular mass. The seminiferous tubules are lined with Sertoli cells and germ cells (spermatogonia). The Sertoli cells are large cells, with a basal portion that lies adjacent to the outer basement membrane of the spermatogenic tubule and an inner extensive branching cytoplasm. The process of spermatogenesis takes place within a network of Sertoli cell cytoplasm, and the differentiating spermatocytes and spermatids are encompassed by the Sertoli cells (see Fig. 45-6). Thus these cells are thought to provide the necessary environmental conditions for germ cell maturation. Spermatogenesis commences after puberty, when the tubules and interstitial cells become mature. Each germ cell (spermatogonium) undergoing differentiation gives rise to 16 primary spermatocytes, each of which enters meiosis to give rise to four spermatids. Cell division stops after the formation of the spermatids, but a complex series of developmental changes must still occur in order to transform these conventional cells into the highly specialized **spermatozoa** capable of flagellar-derived motility. The pituitary gonadotropins play vital roles in the process of spermatogenesis. FSH acts directly on the Sertoli cells in the spermatogenic tubule, whereas LH influences spermatogenesis indirectly by increasing testosterone synthesis in the adjacent Leydig cells. FSH is essential for the initiation of spermatogenesis, but full maturation of spermatozoa also requires adequate local production of testosterone.

The process of spermatogenesis takes approximately 70 days from the beginning of the differentiation of the spermatocyte to the completion of a motile sperm. The seminiferous tubules empty into a highly convoluted network of ducts called the *rete testis*. Spermatozoa are then transported into a

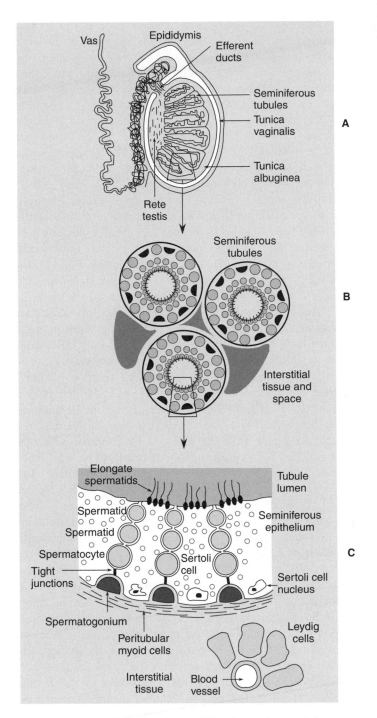

Fig. 45-6 **A,** Human testis, epididymis, and vas deferens showing efferent ducts leading from the rete testis to the caput epididymis and the cauda epididymis continuing to become the vas deferens. **B,** Cross-section through a seminiferous tubule showing central lumen, seminiferous epithelium, and interstitial space containing Leydig cells. **C,** Anatomical relationships in the seminiferous epithelium between germ cells (spermatogonia, spermatocytes, and spermatids), Sertoli cells, peritubular myoid cells, and Leydig cells. *(From Weatherall DJ et al: Oxford textbook of medicine, ed 3, Oxford, UK, 1996, Oxford University Press.)*

single duct, the **epididymis**. During their 12- to 21-day passage through the epididymis, the spermatozoa undergo the further maturation required for effective fertilization. The epididymis also serves as a reservoir for sperm, which then enter the vas deferens and are propelled into the ejaculatory duct. In addition to the spermatozoa and secretory products of the testes, the ejaculatory ducts receive fluid from the seminal vesicles. These glands are the source of seminal fructose, which serves as the energy source for spermatozoa, as well as phosphorylcholine, ascorbic acid, and prostaglandins. About 60% of the seminal fluid volume derives from the seminal vesicles. The ejaculatory ducts terminate in the prostatic urethra. There, the remaining 20% of the seminal fluid is added by the prostate gland. Constituents of prostatic fluid include spermine, citric acid, fibrinolysin, prostate specific antigen, and acid phosphatase. Fluid is also added to the seminal plasma by the Cowper glands and the urethral glands during its transit through the penile urethra.

The hypothalamic-pituitary-testicular axis: an overview. As in the female, the control of gonadal function in the male begins with the pulsatile release of GnRH from the hypothalamus. GnRH is then transported via the hypothalamic-pituitary-portal system to the anterior pituitary, where it stimulates the release of LH and FSH. The relative amounts of LH and FSH that are released from the pituitary depend on the frequency of GnRH pulses and the negative feedback signals from the testes. At a suboptimal pulse rate of GnRH, FSH is preferentially released, whereas a higher pulse frequency of GnRH results in more prominent LH secretion. The major regulator of testosterone production is LH, which specifically binds to high-affinity plasma membrane receptors on the Leydig cells, stimulating testosterone synthesis and secretion. Because of the pulsatile pattern of LH release from the pituitary and its relatively short half-life (30 minutes), plasma LH concentrations normally vary widely in normal men, and a single plasma sample may not provide an accurate estimate of mean LH levels. Plasma FSH levels are more constant because FSH responses to GnRH are more delayed and of a lesser magnitude, and it has a significantly longer circulating half-life (4 hours) in comparison with LH. FSH released into the systemic circulation binds specifically to the Sertoli cells, where it has several effects, including increased synthesis of androgen-binding protein and the aromatase enzyme complex, which converts testosterone to estradiol, and increased production of inhibin. During puberty, FSH also stimulates Sertoli cell mitosis and promotes their maturation.

The secretion of LH is controlled by the negative feedback action of gonadal steroids on the hypothalamus and pituitary. It has been shown in normal males that both testosterone and estradiol may contribute to this inhibition. This may reflect the conversion of testosterone to estrogen within the brain and pituitary, but small amounts of estradiol are normally secreted directly by the testes and the inhibitory effects of testosterone and estradiol may be independent. Both gonadal peptide and steroid hormones are involved in the negative feedback inhibition of FSH secretion. Testosterone can inhibit the secretion of both LH and FSH, but the glycoprotein hormone inhibin primarily inhibits the secretion of FSH. Unlike women, who have fluctuating levels of both inhibin A and B during the menstrual cycle, the major circulating form of inhibin in men is inhibin B. Inhibin B is produced by the Sertoli cells, where it may have some local actions within the testes, but its principal role is to feedback on the pituitary to inhibit FSH secretion.[7] In the testes, both FSH and testosterone are necessary for normal inhibin production. The activins (dimers of the β subunit of inhibin) may regulate pituitary FSH secretion and may have local actions within the testes. Activin α_A and β_B subunits have been localized to the Sertoli cells, and animal studies suggest that activin A may modulate germ cell and Sertoli cell proliferation in the developing testes.[7]

Testosterone synthesis and secretion. The testis is the primary site of androgen production in the male, and the major circulating androgen is testosterone. As stated earlier, all steroid hormones are derived from cholesterol (see Fig. 45-3). In the testes (as in the ovary), cholesterol may be synthesized *de novo* or derived from the systemic circulation by receptor-mediated uptake of low density lipoprotein (LDL). The rate-limiting step in testosterone synthesis is the conversion of cholesterol to pregnenolone. LH regulates the rate of this enzymatic reaction and thus controls the overall rate of testosterone synthesis. The daily production rate of testosterone in normal adult men is approximately 6 mg, but only about 25 μg of testosterone is stored in the testes, indicating that the testes are continuously synthesizing and releasing testosterone into the circulation. There is a diurnal rhythm in circulating testosterone levels in adult men, with the highest levels in the early morning, followed by a progressive fall throughout the day, reaching the lowest levels at night during the first few hours of sleep. Peak and nadir values may differ by about 30%, and ideally testosterone concentrations should be measured in the morning. Although testosterone is the major hormone produced, small amounts of dihydrotestosterone, androstenedione, 17-hydroxyprogesterone, progesterone, estradiol, and pregnenolone are also secreted by the testes. Testicular estradiol secretion contributes about 20% to 30% of the total circulating estradiol, the remainder being derived from peripheral, extraglandular aromatization of androgenic substrates, such as androstenedione. The functions of plasma pregnenolone, progesterone, and 17-hydroxyprogesterone in the male are not known.

Testosterone transport. Of the circulating testosterone in normal men, less than 4% is free (not protein-bound), 1% to 2% is bound to cortisol-binding globulin, approximately 50% is loosely bound to albumin, and the remainder (about 45%) is bound with high affinity to sex hormone-binding globulin (SHBG). SHBG levels are increased by estrogens and decreased by androgens; therefore the normal level of SHBG is about 30% to 50% lower in men compared with women, and SHBG levels may be elevated in testosterone-deficient men. In many clinical situations, measurement of the total testosterone concentration (usually by immuno-assay) is satisfactory. However, when circulating SHBG levels are altered, this can be reflected by an increase or decrease in the measured total testosterone level. For example, obesity is associated with decreased SHBG levels, and a low total testosterone level in an obese man may be misinterpreted as evidence of androgen deficiency.

The degree of testosterone affinity to its binding proteins produces three serum pools: free testosterone (non–protein-bound), bioavailable testosterone (free, plus that bound loosely to albumin), and testosterone bound tightly to SHBG. Because the non–SHBG-bound portion of circulating testosterone is thought to represent the biologically active fraction, methods for estimating the non–SHBG-bound or free testosterone level are available.

Extraglandular metabolism of androgens. Testosterone mediates androgenic effects but also serves as a circulating precursor for the formation of two types of active metabolites. Testosterone can undergo irreversible reduction to generate 5α-reduced steroids, most significantly dihydro-testosterone (DHT), a key intracellular mediator of androgen action. The concentration of circulating DHT in adult men is approximately 10% that of testosterone; about 25% of this is directly secreted by the testes, and the remainder arises from the conversion of testosterone in tissues such as the liver, kidney, muscle, prostate, and skin. There are two isoenzymes that convert testosterone to DHT, 5α-reductase types 1 and 2. The type 1 isoenzyme is found in the liver and skin; the type 2 enzyme predominates in the male urogenital tract, in which 5α-reduction is a prerequisite for normal androgen-mediated function. Only a small fraction of the DHT generated in target tissues appears in plasma; it is mainly metabolized by 3α reduction to 5α-androstane 3β-17β-diol, which then enters plasma and is further metabolized by glucuronide conjugation and other pathways.

Most of the estrogens in the circulation in normal adult men are derived from the aromatization of testosterone to 17β-estradiol and androstenedione to estrone. Estrogen formation requires sequential hydroxylation, oxidation, and removal of the carbon at position 19 and aromatization of the A ring of the steroid. Prior 5α-reduction of the steroid A ring prevents completion of aromatization, so DHT or other 5α-reduced steroids are not aromatized. The aromatase enzyme complex is active in many tissues, including muscle, liver, and kidney, but the most significant is probably adipose tissue. The overall rate of aromatization increases with age and adiposity. In addition to these pathways, testosterone is also metabolized to inactive excretory metabolites, including 17-ketosteroids and a series of polar compounds, including diols, triols, and conjugates.

The androgen receptor. Cytoplasmic androgen receptors (ARs) are widely expressed in genital and nongenital tissues and mediate the cellular effects of testosterone and DHT. The AR binds DHT with a higher affinity than testosterone. Like other members of the steroid hormone receptor superfamily, the AR contains a steroid-binding domain, a DNA-binding domain, and a transcription-regulating domain. Following androgen binding, the receptor dimerizes and proceeds to the nucleus to bind to DNA-target sequences and initiate or decrease transcription of androgen-responsive genes. The AR is encoded by a gene located on the X chromosome; therefore females can be carriers of mutant AR genes, which when transmitted to male offspring, produce androgen insensitivity syndromes.

Numerous AR mutations, in both the steroid-binding and DNA-binding domains, have been described that cause complete or partial androgen insensitivity. The AR gene contains a segment of CAG repeats in exon 1 that codes for glutamine. Men with spinal and bulbar muscular atrophy (Kennedy disease) have an expansion of this segment to 40-60 triplet repeats as compared with an average of 21 in normal men. Such men develop **gynecomastia**, clinical signs of androgen deficiency and small testes, in association with increased LH and testosterone levels indicative of androgen insensitivity. The mutations are thought to impair activation of androgen-responsive genes.

PATHOLOGICAL STATES
Hypogonadism

Male hypogonadism may be defined as a failure of the testes to produce testosterone, spermatozoa, or both. As in women, hypogonadism may be caused by primary gonadal failure or an abnormality within the hypothalamic-pituitary axis (Box 45-3, and see Fig. 45-7 for clinical workup). The clinical presentation of hypogonadism in males is directly related to the time of development of androgen deficiency. Androgen deficiency during the second to third months of fetal development can cause sexual ambiguity and male **pseudohermaphroditism**. In prepubertal hypogonadism, absence of testosterone production by the testes is associated with persistent infantile genitalia, a barely palpable prostate, poor secondary sexual development and lack of secondary sex characteristics, delayed bone age, and eunuchoidal skeletal proportions (crown-to-pubis/pubis-to-floor ratio is decreased, arm span is considerably greater than height). These body proportions result from a failure of epiphyseal fusion and continued growth of long bones. Prepubertal hypogonadism is usually not apparent until the time of puberty, when the normal pubertal changes, including genital and secondary sexual development, fail to occur. Postpubertal hypogonadism results in more subtle clinical manifestations. For example, there may be diminished beard growth and thinning of body hair, a decrease in strength and muscle mass, loss of libido, and softened testes of decreased volume. Older males may be unaware of any of these changes.

Disorders of the testes—primary hypogonadism. Primary hypogonadism due to testicular dysfunction is characterized by low serum testosterone concentrations in conjunction with high gonadotropin levels, reflecting the absence of negative feedback on the hypothalamic-pituitary axis. Abnormal testicular function may result from a genetic disorder, from defects in testosterone synthesis or metabolism, from abnormalities in the androgen receptor, or from direct gonadal damage.

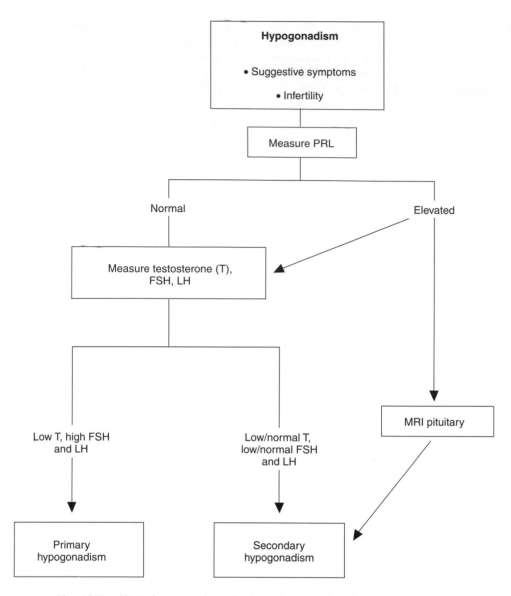

Fig. 45-7 Clinical approach to the investigation of male hypogonadism.

The most common genetic disorder causing primary hypogonadism in men is **Klinefelter's syndrome**, which is associated with the chromosomal pattern of 47,XXY and occurs in about 1 in 400 men. The phenotypic manifestations of Klinefelter's syndrome are characteristic for the classic form of the disorder, in which all cell lines carry the XXY karyotype. Many men with this syndrome have a mosaic form, in which some cell lines are XXY and others are XY, so the clinical presentation is variable. This disorder rarely presents before puberty because the only early physical finding is the presence of very small testes (less than 1.5 mL after age 6). After puberty, the other characteristic features appear, including gynecomastia, abnormalities in skeletal proportions with exaggerated growth of the lower extremities (decreased crown-to-pubis/pubis-to-floor ratio but no abnormality in arm span/height ratio), reduced androgen-dependent hair growth, central adiposity, poor muscle mass with reduced strength, and infertility. In patients with Klinefelter's syndrome, testosterone concentrations range from abnormal low to the normal range, but postpubertal gonadotropin levels are always elevated, even when the testosterone is normal. Other genetic disorders associated with primary hypogonadism include XX males (majority due to translocation of the SRY gene to the X chromosome), XY/XO gonadal dysgenesis, Ullrich-Noonan syndrome, and myotonic dystrophy.

There are several different enzymes involved in testosterone synthesis that may be defective, resulting in testosterone deficiency with or without cortisol deficiency. The enzymes potentially affected include 20,22-desmolase, 3β-hydroxydehydrogenase, 17α-hydroxylase, 17,20-desmolase, and 17-ketosteroid reductase. The majority of these enzyme defects are associated with ambiguous genitalia at birth in association with a normal male XY karyotype. The 5α-reductase deficiency syndrome is an autosomal recessive disorder that also occurs in males with a normal XY sex

BOX 45-3

CAUSES OF MALE HYPOGONADISM

Primary Hypogonadism
Genetic disorders
   Klinefelter's syndrome
   XX males
   XY/XO gonadal dysgenesis
   Ullrich-Noonan syndrome
   Myotonic dystrophy
Enzymatic defects involving testosterone synthesis
   5α-reductase deficiency
Androgen receptor defects
   Androgen resistance (testicular feminization syndrome)
   Kennedy syndrome
Testicular damage
   Cryptorchidism
   Infection
   Testicular trauma or torsion
   Irradiation
   Chemotherapy

Secondary Hypogonadism
Hypothalamic disorders
   Kallmann syndrome
   Cranial irradiation
   Systemic illness
Pituitary disorders
   Prolactin-secreting pituitary tumor
   Other pituitary tumor
Hemochromatosis
Lymphocytic hypophysitis
Histiocytosis

chromosome pattern. It arises from an absence or low activity of the 5α-reductase enzyme, producing a defect in the conversion of testosterone to DHT. The testes function normally with respect to androgen and antimüllerian hormone production, so the müllerian structure regresses and the normal wolffian system forms, but at birth, these individuals appear to be girls with moderately ambiguous genitalia. At puberty, however, testosterone production by the testes is normal, producing an overall dramatic masculinization with development of a male body habitus and hair distribution and penile enlargement. However, those tissues that respond primarily to DHT, such as the scrotum, prostate, and testes, remain prepubertal.

Abnormalities in the androgen receptor have been previously discussed. Complete lack of function results in the testicular feminization syndrome, in which an XY individual has the female phenotype. Variants of this syndrome occur, depending on the degree of receptor defect. *Kennedy syndrome*, in which primary hypogonadism is associated with a specific muscular dystrophy, is caused by a polynucleotide repeat expansion in the AR gene. The AR sequence is normal, but an expanded polyglutamine region suppresses receptor activity.

Primary hypogonadism manifesting after puberty is frequently the result of testicular damage. Men who are infected with mumps virus during or after puberty have about a 50% chance of developing orchitis, and as many as 60% of these will be infertile because of extensive seminiferous tubule damage. **Cryptorchidism** (undescended testes) usually results in failure of testicular function on the affected side and frequently of the nonaffected side also, producing primary hypogonadism. Similarly, unilateral testicular trauma or torsion may also cause complete testicular failure, although the mechanism by which the physically undamaged testis is affected is not clear. Therapeutic irradiation and chemotherapy may also damage the testes. Spermatogonia are exquisitely sensitive to radiation, with damage being evident after only 15 rad.[17] With doses greater than 100 rad, extreme oligospermia or azoospermia develops. The likelihood of germ cell recovery is dose-dependent, and permanent failure may occur after high-dose therapy even if the testes are shielded. The main chemotherapeutic drugs that cause infertility are the alkylating agents, such as cyclophosphamide, but other drugs can also cause germ cell depletion, including chlorambucil, cisplatin, doxorubicin, and vinblastine. The toxic effects of chemotherapeutic drugs can be additive, and some combination regimens have particularly profound effects on spermatogenesis.

Secondary hypogonadism—hypogonadotropic hypogonadism. Secondary hypogonadism is characterized by low testosterone concentrations in association with gonadotropin levels that are subnormal or within the reference range, indicating failure of the pituitary to respond normally to a lack of negative feedback. Hypogonadotropic hypogonadism may be caused by congenital or acquired defects. As in primary hypogonadism, the clinical presentation of the acquired disorders will depend on whether the individual has gone through puberty and whether other anterior or posterior pituitary hormone deficiencies are present.

The classic example of congenital hypogonadotropic hypogonadism is Kallmann syndrome, in which there is a defect in hypothalamic GnRH secretion. This syndrome is characterized by isolated gonadotropin deficiency and anosmia or hyposmia. Other associated anomalies, such as cleft lip and palate, sensorineural deafness, and cardiac abnormalities, have also been described. *Kallmann syndrome* is most commonly inherited in an autosomal dominant manner, but autosomal-recessive and X-linked modes of inheritance have been reported. The incidence of this syndrome is about 1 in 10,000 male births. These men typically present with failure to go through puberty in association with eunuchoid skeletal proportions. Testicular development remains at prepubertal levels, although unlike Klinefelter's syndrome, the testes are of normal prepubertal size. Basal gonadotropin levels are low normal or undetectable, testosterone levels are low, and serum prolactin levels are normal. If gonadotropin deficiency is the only abnormality and the other clinical features such as anosmia are absent, Kallmann syndrome can be very difficult to distinguish from delayed puberty. Congenital gonadotropin deficiency is also associated with a number of rare genetic syndromes, such as Prader-Willi, Laurence-Moon, and Bardet-Biedl syndromes, which are usually evident in early childhood.

Gonadotropin deficiency may result from numerous acquired disorders that cause pituitary dysfunction (see Box 45-3). Pituitary tumors, granulomatous diseases affecting the pituitary, autoimmune lymphocytic hypophysitis, and hemochromatosis can directly inhibit gonadotropin secretion by damaging the gonadotropin secreting cells. Prolactin secreting pituitary tumors can cause hypogonadism without anatomic destruction of gonadotropes; the elevated prolactin is thought to interfere with GnRH neuron function. In men, 80% of prolactinomas are macroadenomas, whereas in women over 80% are microadenomas. This difference may result from earlier detection in women, in whom hyperprolactinemia is associated with menstrual cycle disturbances and galactorrhea. In contrast, the symptoms of hypogonadism in adult men are often nonspecific. All men with an elevated prolactin level should undergo an MRI of the pituitary. Secondary hypogonadism also occurs in association with any severe systemic illness, in severe uremia, and after therapeutic cranial irradiation.

Testicular Hyperfunction

Testicular tumors account for only about 1% of cancer deaths in American men, but they are the second most common malignancy (after leukemia) in men aged 20 to 35 years. An increased incidence of testicular tumors occurs in men with cryptorchidism, **testicular feminization syndrome** (androgen resistance), and Klinefelter's syndrome. Tumors of the testis may originate from several cell types in the seminiferous tubules or the interstitial tissue, but most testicular neoplasms are germ-cell tumors. Germ-cell tumors are classified histologically as seminomas or nonseminomas, although approximately 30% of germ-cell tumors contain mixed elements. They usually present as a painless scrotal mass. Biochemical markers in serum are often useful in the diagnosis of germ-cell tumors and in the detection of residual or recurrent disease following treatment. Overall, about 25% to 30% of germ-cell tumors produce human chorionic gonadotropin (hCG), α-fetoprotein (AFP), or both, although the presence of large amounts of hCG or AFP in the serum generally indicates a nonseminomatous tumor. Only a relatively small percentage of seminomas are secretory, whereas about 60% of nonseminomatous germ-cell tumors produce significant amounts of hCG, AFP, or both. Non–germ-cell tumors are rare. Only 3% of testicular tumors originate from the Leydig cells; 90% of these are benign, and they usually produce steroid hormones (testosterone or estrogen). The production of excessive amounts of androgenic hormones in adult males produces few symptoms, but an estrogen-secreting tumor may cause gynecomastia. In prepubertal boys, excessive testosterone production causes precocious puberty. Primary hypergonadism is characterized by abnormally high testosterone (or estrogen) concentrations in association with suppressed gonadotropin levels.

Secondary hypergonadism may also occur in the setting of altered hypothalamic-pituitary function, resulting in increased LH/FSH secretion. Premature activation of the hypothalamic-pituitary-gonadal axis produces gonadotropin-dependent precocious puberty in children. In boys, the initial symptom/sign is testicular enlargement; this is followed by further secondary sex development and accelerated linear growth. The most common cause of this disorder is a hypothalamic hamartoma. These non-neoplastic congenital malformations contain ectopic GnRH neurons, which are not subject to the normal CNS regulation that inhibits activity prior to puberty, and therefore they may function as autonomous GnRH-pulse generators and initiate puberty. Many other CNS abnormalities, including space-occupying lesions in the region of the third ventricle and high-dose cranial irradiation administered for childhood tumors, can also result in gonadotropin-dependent precocious puberty, probably via disruption of inhibitory input to the hypothalamus.

Erectile Dysfunction

Erectile dysfunction (ED) is defined as difficulty obtaining or maintaining a penile erection sufficient to permit vaginal penetration and satisfactory conclusion of sexual intercourse. Epidemiological data suggest a high prevalence of ED; in the Massachusetts Male Aging Study, 9.6% of men between ages 40 and 70 years suffered from complete erectile dysfunction, and a further 25% admitted to moderate dysfunction.[15] Recognition that ED frequently stems from an organic cause and the availability of better therapies have revolutionized the approach to this disorder. The normal erectile process depends on a complex array of autonomic and somatic nerves that innervate the penis, together with an adequate arterial blood supply. Psychogenic and interrelationship factors are also important components in normal sexual function. ED can be associated with many systemic diseases, such as diabetes mellitus, aortoilial atherosclerosis, hypertension, previous treatment for benign prostate hypertrophy or prostate cancer, and many neurological disorders. Numerous drugs that act on the central or autonomic nervous system have been associated with ED, including anticholinergic, antidepressant, antipsychotic, and antihypertensive drugs. Differentiating between psychogenic and organic (neurogenic or vascular) causes of ED can be difficult, particularly as the former may frequently arise from the latter. The assessment of a man with ED naturally requires a thorough history and examination. A complete blood count and routine serum chemistries will detect many of the systemic diseases associated with ED. Androgen deficiency and hyperprolactinemia must also be excluded by measuring serum testosterone (preferably a morning sample), LH, FSH, and prolactin levels.

The treatment of erectile dysfunction depends to some extent on whether there is an underlying endocrine cause. For example, testosterone replacement therapy should be considered in androgen deficient men, while those with hyperprolactinemia may require dopamine agonist therapy and/or pituitary surgery. Other therapies for ED are more generic, in that they may be used to treat ED regardless of the underlying cause. These include intracavernosal prostaglandin injection, vacuum constrictor devices, penile prostheses, and the oral drug sildenafil. Sildenafil (Viagra) is a selective inhibitor of cGMP-specific phosphodiesterase type 5 (PDE5), which enhances nitric oxide-mediated vasodilation in the corpus cavernosum by inhibiting cGMP breakdown, thus facilitating smooth muscle relaxation. Nitric oxide release from the noradrenergic noncholinergic nerves that innervate the cavernosal smooth muscle is triggered by sexual stimuli. Therefore, sildenafil potentiates erections induced by physiological mechanisms, and unlike intra-cavernosal prostaglandins, it cannot independently invoke an erection.[15] Sildenafil is an effective therapy; clinical trials have shown that about 70% of men with erectile dysfunction of all etiologies will experience significant improvement. The drug is also generally well tolerated. However, there are potential side effects relating to the presence of the PDE5 enzyme in tissues other than cavernosal smooth muscle. The most common side effects of headache and facial flushing result from a blockade of PDE5 in vascular smooth muscle. Dyspepsia may occur, as PDE5 is present in the gastro-esophageal junction cells. A transient alteration in color vision is an uncommon side effect of sildenafil, which results from limited inhibition of PDE6. This enzyme subtype is found in the retina and is involved in the conversion of photon energy to a neuronal signal. Sildenafil is probably safe in patients with mild to moderate cardiovascular disease, but it is specifically contraindicated in patients taking nitrate drugs, because the two agents have a synergistic action that can produce a precipitous drop in blood pressure.

EVALUATION OF THE INFERTILE COUPLE

Infertility is the involuntary inability to conceive, whereas sterility is the permanent inability to reproduce. Primary infertility exists if no pregnancy has occurred after attempts at conception for 12 months. Secondary infertility implies that a previous pregnancy has occurred, regardless of the outcome of that pregnancy. Fecundability is the probability of achieving pregnancy within one menstrual cycle, about 20% to 25% per cycle. Approximately 10% to 15% of American couples experience infertility. Many couples, however, presenting for assistance with fertility would ultimately conceive without any medical intervention. Overall, about 15% of couples fail to achieve pregnancy in 1 year, but only 6% fail by the end of 2 years. Thus it is reasonable to commence a basic evaluation and consider low-cost therapies after 1 year, but reserve the use of expensive, specialized techniques until 2 or more years of infertility have occurred.

According to The National Center for Health Statistics, approximately 8.4% of women in the United States between the ages of 14 and 44 years are infertile. About 45% experience primary infertility, and 25% experience secondary infertility at some point during their reproductive lives. The age of the couple has a definite impact on fertility. The incidence of infertility increases with increasing age of the female partner and to a lesser extent the male partner. The peak biological fertility in women is in the late teens and early 20s. Male fertility also declines after the age of 25

years, but the decline is less marked. Thus, delaying child-birth until later in life significantly reduces the probability of conception. The frequency of sexual intercourse also affects the conception rate.

In general, 40% of the time infertility is attributable to female factors, 40% is due to male factors, 10% results from combined male and female factors, and 10% remains unexplained. A thorough history and physical examination of both partners is always essential in the evaluation of the infertile couple.

Female Infertility

There are many potential causes of infertility in women (Box 45-4). Several of these, such as congenital abnormalities of the vagina or uterus, gonadal dysgenesis, and premature ovarian failure, have already been discussed in preceding sections. The most common causes of infertility in women, however, are tubal pathology and disturbances in ovulation. Normal function of the fallopian tubes is critical to reproduction because the sperm and ovum must unite for fertilization to take place. Any history of pelvic inflammatory disease, endometriosis, septic abortion, ruptured appendix, tubal surgery, or ectopic pregnancy suggests there may be tubal damage. Tubal disease may be evaluated radiologically (hysterosalpingogram) or by laparoscopy.

Disorders of ovulation, ranging from anovulation to luteal phase deficiency, account for about 15% of all infertility problems. The investigation and differential diagnosis of amenorrhea and dysfunctional uterine bleeding has been previously discussed. Assessment of ovulation may be done by measurement of daily basal body temperature (BBT). The LH surge (and hence ovulation) typically occurs within 2 to 3 days of the BBT nadir, although this relationship may not always be reliable. Luteal phase deficiency (also termed *short luteal phase*) results from insufficient progesterone production from the corpus luteum to support the normal endometrial maturation changes required for implantation of the embryo. Endometrial biopsy is a traditional method of evaluating luteal function, but this procedure has some drawbacks in that it is relatively invasive, the biopsy must be appropriately timed within the cycle, and abnormal findings

---

BOX 45-4

CAUSES OF FEMALE INFERTILITY

Structural problems
    Tubal pathology
    Uterine abnormalities
Disorders of ovulation
    Anovulation—polycystic ovary syndrome
    Luteal phase deficiency
    Hypogonadism—primary or secondary
Functional problems
    Suboptimal cervical mucus
    Autoimmunity—antisperm antibodies

should be confirmed by successive biopsies in two consecutive cycles to make the diagnosis conclusive. Serum progesterone measurements are a more convenient method of assessing luteal function. A midluteal phase progesterone level of greater than 6.5 ng/mL (21 nmol/L), or preferably greater than 10 ng/mL (30 nmol/L), suggests ovulation and normal luteal function. However, progesterone is secreted in a pulsatile fashion, and a single value may not reflect luteal function adequately. Therefore, midluteal phase progesterone measurements may need to be repeated over several cycles.

Uterine abnormalities are rarely a factor in infertility. Intramural and submucosal tumors (myomas) may distort the uterine cavity or obstruct the tubal lumen or endocervical canal. Infertility and pregnancy loss are thought to result from faulty implantation and compromised placental vascular supply. Uterine scarring (Asherman syndrome) may produce infertility via similar mechanisms. Suboptimal changes in the quality of cervical mucus at midcycle have also been implicated in infertility. Cervical mucus is normally thick and opaque, except at midcycle when it should become thin, watery, and acellular to facilitate sperm penetration. In the postcoital test, sperm motility is assessed in a sample of cervical mucus.

Male Infertility

The medical history of the male partner should focus on identifying factors that are known to impair erectile or testicular function (Box 45-5). Many chronic systemic illnesses are associated with decreased testicular function and reduced sperm production.[12] Symptoms that suggest primary or secondary hypogonadism must be specifically sought. Key aspects of the physical examination include the degree of virilization, any evidence of gynecomastia, and testicular size and consistency.

Any of the causes of primary or secondary hypogonadism previously discussed may present as infertility (see Box 45-3.). Bilateral or unilateral cryptorchidism is commonly associated with infertility (about 70%) even if orchiopexy has been performed.[17] Testicular varicoceles are relatively common, with an incidence of around 10%. About 50% of

men with varicoceles will have reduced semen quality, some show biochemical evidence of testicular dysfunction, and many have impaired fertility. Ejaculatory dysfunction may cause infertility. Retrograde ejaculation can occur if there is dysfunction of the sympathetic nerves that mediate closure of the bladder neck sphincter during ejaculation. A postejaculation urine specimen will demonstrate abundant sperm. Diabetic neuropathy, prostatic resection, and extensive pelvic surgery are most commonly associated with retrograde ejaculation.

Sperm transport can also be impaired if there are abnormalities of the duct system, such as those associated with mutations in the gene responsible for cystic fibrosis (CF). The cystic fibrosis transmembrane conductance regulator gene, located on the short arm of chromosome 7, encodes for a membrane protein that functions as an ion channel and also influences the formation of the ejaculatory duct, seminal vesicle, vas deferens, and the distal two-thirds of the epididymis. Over 400 different mutations in this gene have been described, and these are associated with a spectrum of clinical manifestations[13] (see Chapter 47). Congenital bilateral absence of the vas deferens is common in men who have CF, but it can also occur in isolation without the other features of CF. Congenital unilateral absence of the vas deferens may be an incomplete form of the bilateral disorder. In polycystic kidney disease, dilated cysts of the seminal vesicles may cause obstruction to semen transport. In addition to mumps virus, which causes a primary orchitis, other infective agents can also produce infertility. A variety of organisms, such as *Neisseria gonorrhea*, *Chlamydia trachomatis*, *Mycobacterium tuberculosis*, *Ureaplasma urealyticum*, and coliform bacteria, can cause chronic epididymitis or prostatitis, which may reduce sperm count or motility directly or result in post-infection ductal damage.

Autoimmunity has been postulated as a cause of infertility. Antibodies to the basement membrane of the seminiferous tubule and, more commonly, to sperm themselves have been described. Whether such antibodies play a directly causative role in infertility is still unclear, because the presence of antisperm antibodies does not correlate with specific abnormalities in the semen analysis. Furthermore, not all men who are antibody-positive are infertile, and a decrease in antibody titer is not always associated with improved fertility. As previously discussed, treatment with chemotherapeutic drugs or radiation may result in infertility.

Not all cases of male infertility can be explained by the above conditions, and up to 40% of cases have been classified as idiopathic infertility. However, sequencing of the human genome has led to a new understanding of the genes that regulate spermatogenesis and many instances of so-called idiopathic infertility may be caused by previously unidentified, subtle genetic defects. Several genes located on the long arm of the Y chromosome have been described that are involved in spermatogenesis. In men with major defects in spermatogenesis and apparently normal chromosome analysis, microdeletions involving genes on the long arm of the Y chromosome have been demonstrated.[13] The presence

---

BOX 45-5

CAUSES OF MALE INFERTILITY

Structural problems
    Congenital absence of the vas deferens
    Infective epididymitis causing ductal damage
    Cryptorchidism
Hypogonadism
    Primary—testicular damage of any cause
    Secondary—pituitary/hypothalamic disease
Genetic—Y chromosome microdeletions
Functional problems
    Retrograde ejaculation
    Autoimmunity—antisperm antibodies

of microdeletions in the Y chromosome has clinical implications if the technique of intra-cytoplasmic sperm injection (ICSI) is to be used, because the genetic defect will be transmitted to any male offspring. Testing for Y chromosome microdeletions is undertaken in IVF/ICSI units, but the currently available screening methods using specific gene probes will not identify all men with microdeletions.

Semen analysis is a critical part of the evaluation of an infertile man. Semen quality is assessed according to sperm count, motility, morphology, and semen volume. Each of these parameters is scored as having good, poor, or equivocal probability of fertility to provide an overall analysis, since no single semen characteristic (except azoospermia) has an absolute correlation with infertility. A total sperm count of less than 20 million/mL, motility less than 40%, normal oval morphology less than 40%, or semen volume less than 1.0 mL are all associated with impaired fertility. At least three samples collected over a 2 to 4 month period should be analyzed, because semen characteristics can vary considerably in normal men, making interpretation of a single sample difficult. Functional assays, such as the sperm penetration assay, which uses hamster ova to assess the fertilizing capacity of sperm, are laborious and only occasionally used.

Testicular function is also assessed by measuring serum testosterone, LH, and FSH levels. Four different patterns may be observed in infertile men: (1) normal values for all three hormones; (2) elevated serum gonadotropins and a low testosterone level suggesting severe primary testicular failure; (3) an elevated FSH, normal LH, and low/normal testosterone, implying a milder form of primary hypogonadism; and (4) low/normal serum gonadotropins and low testosterone levels indicating secondary hypogonadism. Prolactin levels should be measured in any patient with biochemical evidence of secondary hypogonadism. A biochemical profile consistent with primary hypogonadism in conjunction with any clinical features suggestive of Klinefelter's syndrome should prompt a karyotype assessment. Differentiating between primary and secondary gonadal failure is important as spermatogenesis can sometimes be restored in the secondary syndromes by treatment with gonadotropin or GnRH. A testicular biopsy can provide direct information about the degree of spermatogenesis in the region sampled. This procedure is not commonly indicated but may be useful in demonstrating obstructive azoospermia and enabling sperm retrieval for ICSI.

Infertility Treatment

Ovulation induction. Clomiphene citrate is the first-line treatment in women with absent or infrequent ovulation and dysfunctional uterine bleeding (oligomenorrhea). Documentation of anovulation via basal body temperature readings is not essential prior to treatment, but thyroid dysfunction and an elevated serum prolactin level (or pregnancy if there has been no recent menstrual flow) must be excluded; if these are present, a specific treatment for an underlying disorder may be indicated. In women with amenorrhea, particularly those who fail to have withdrawal bleeding following the administration of progesterone, an estrogen deficiency secondary to hypogonadism (either primary or secondary) must be suspected and serum estradiol, LH, and FSH levels must be measured. Estrogen deficient women rarely ovulate in response to clomiphene, and usually other treatment modalities are pursued at the outset. Ideally, a semen analysis should also be performed before any ovulation induction therapy to exclude azoospermia.

Clomiphene is an orally active, nonsteroidal agent that has a similar structure to estrogenic compounds but has only a weak biological estrogenic effect. Its structural similarity is sufficient for it to be bound to estrogen receptors, where it remains bound for much longer periods than endogenous estrogens (weeks versus hours) and acts to inhibit the process of receptor replacement, thereby reducing the concentration of estrogen receptors. Centrally, this results in a lowering of estrogen-related negative feedback on the hypothalamic-pituitary axis, which responds by increasing GnRH, LH, and FSH secretion. Thus, clomiphene does not directly stimulate ovulation but acts to enhance the normal gonadotropin-dependent events that bring it about. Clomiphene treatment is therefore commenced on day 5 of a menstrual cycle, following either spontaneous or induced bleeding, and continues through days 5 to 9, amplifying the normal rise in gonadotropins at a time when the dominant follicle is being selected. If given earlier, multiple follicles may undergo maturation, increasing the risk of multiple pregnancies. Clomiphene may be purposely administered early in IVF programs in order to produce more than one oocyte per cycle for collection.

In the initial cycle the dose used is 50 mg/day, but if no ovulation occurs, the dose may be increased to 100 mg or even higher in subsequent cycles if the woman continues to be anovulatory. The ovulatory surge can occur from 5 to 10 days after the last day of clomiphene administration. The couple is advised to have intercourse every second day for 1 week, beginning 5 days after the last day of medication. About 50% of patients achieve pregnancy with the 50-mg dose and another 20% with the 100-mg dose.

Human menopausal gonadotropin (hMG), used in conjunction with hCG, can stimulate ovulation in anovulatory patients who have potentially functioning ovarian tissue. This treatment is usually used only after failure with maximal doses of clomiphene, because it is expensive, requires careful monitoring, and is associated with the potentially dangerous ovarian hyperstimulation syndrome. Typically, follicular stimulation is achieved by 7 to 14 days of continuous hMG, given as a single daily intramuscular injection. Usually the higher dose hMG preparation (containing 150 IU of FSH and LH) is used initially, unless the patient has PCOS, in which case the lower hMG dose is used (75 IU of each gonadotropin), since these patients are more responsive.

Serial estrogen measurements are used to determine the optimal time for administering the ovulatory dose of hCG. The timing of the sample for estrogen measurement in relation to the preceding injection of hMG must also be taken into account. If the hMG was administered between 5 PM and 8 PM the previous night and the sample collected early the following morning, then an estradiol level of 1000 to 1500 pg/mL (3700 to 5500 pmol/L) is optimal. Higher levels indicate a significant risk of ovarian hyperstimulation. Transvaginal ultrasound may also be performed to assess follicular growth and development. Administration of a single intramuscular injection of 10,000 IU of hCG (which is structurally and biologically similar to LH) stimulates ovulation. The couple is instructed to have intercourse on the day of hCG injection and daily for the next 2 days. On occasion, GnRH may be given (0.5 mg subcutaneously for 2 weeks) prior to a cycle of hMG in order to suppress endogenous pituitary gonadotropin secretion if disturbed hypothalamo-pituitary-ovarian function is thought to be interfering with successful ovulation induction. In this instance, the aim is to produce a hypogonadal state with estradiol levels less than 25 pg/mL (90 pmol/L) before giving hMG.

Pulsatile GnRH administration is the most physiological means of ovulation induction and is particularly effective in women with hypothalamic amenorrhea; for example, women with Kallmann syndrome. The advantages of GnRH treatment are that the normal feedback mechanisms controlling endogenous gonadotropin secretion are maintained, thus minimizing the amount of biochemical monitoring required and undoubtedly contributing to the low incidence of ovarian hyperstimulation and multiple births observed with this therapy. The major drawback is that it must be given in repeated subcutaneous or intravenous injections via a programmable portable pump for a period of about 3 weeks.

Assisted reproduction. *Assisted reproductive technology (ART)* refers to all techniques that involve direct retrieval of oocytes from the ovary. A complete evaluation of both partners is mandatory before embarking on any ART therapy. The first developed, and still the most common procedure, is **in vitro fertilization (IVF)**, but many other techniques are currently available; some are listed below. These procedures can overcome many of the barriers to fertility, but only at the expense of invasive, costly, and time-consuming protocols. In virtually all cases, ovulation induction protocols as described above are used to increase the number of oocytes available for collection in a cycle.

IVF—In vitro fertilization: extraction of oocytes, fertilization in the laboratory, transcervical transfer of embryos into the uterus

GIFT—Gamete intrafallopian tube transfer: the placement of oocytes and sperm into the fallopian tube

ZIFT—Zygote intrafallopian transfer: the placement of fertilized oocytes into the fallopian tube

ICSI—Intracytoplasmic sperm injection (of a single spermatozoa)

References

1. Agrawal R, Holmes J, Jacobs HS: Follicle-stimulating hormone or human menopausal gonadotropin for ovarian stimulation in in vitro fertilization cycles: a mate-analysis, *Fertil Steril* 73(2):338, 2000.
2. Azziz R, Carmina E, Sawaya ME: Idiopathic hirsutism, *Endocr Rev* 21(4):347, 2000.
3. Burger H: The endocrinology of the menopause, *J Steroid Biochem Mol Biol* 69:31, 1999.
4. Carr BR: Disorders of the ovaries and female reproductive tract. In Wilson JD et al, editors: *Williams' textbook of endocrinology*, Philadelphia, 1998, Saunders.
5. Clark RV: Male infertility. In Becker KL, editor: *Principles and practice of endocrinology and metabolism*, Philadelphia, 2001, Lippincott Williams & Wilkins.
6. Cosman F, Lindsay R: Selective estrogen receptor modulators: clinical spectrum, *Endocr Rev* 20(3):418, 1999.
7. De Kretser DM et al: The roles of inhibin and related peptides in gonadal function, *Mol Cell Endocrinol* 161:43, 2000.
8. De Kretser DM: Morphology and physiology of the testis. In Becker KL, editor: *Principles and practice of endocrinology and metabolism*, Philadelphia, 2001, Lippincott Williams & Wilkins.
9. Filicori M, Cognigni GE: Roles and novel regimens of luteinizing hormone and follicle-stimulating hormone in ovulation induction, *J Clin Endocrinol Metab* 86(4):1437, 2001.
10. Greendale GA, Lee NP, Arriola ER: The menopause, *Lancet* 353:571, 1999.
11. Griffin JE, Wilson JD: Disorders of the testes and the male reproductive tract. In Wilson JD et al, editors: *Williams' textbook of endocrinology*, Philadelphia, 1998, Saunders.
12. Handelsman DJ: Testicular dysfunction in systemic disease, *Endocrinol Metab Clin North Am* 23(4):839, 1994.
13. Hargreaves TB: Genetic basis of male infertility, *Brit Med Bull* 56(3):650, 2000.
14. Hayes FJH, Seminara SB, Crowley WF: Hypogonadotropic hypogonadism, *Endo Metab Clin North Am* 27(4):739, 1998.
15. Holmes S: Treatment of erectile dysfunction, *Brit Med Bull* 56(3):798, 2000.
15a. Kalantaridou SN, Davis SR, Nelson LM: Premature ovarian failure, *Endocrinol Metab Clin North Am* 27(4):989, 1998.
16. Pezzani I et al: Influence of non-gonadotrophic hormones on gonadal function, *Mol Cell Endocrinol* 161:37, 2000.
17. Plymate S: Hypogonadism, *Endocrinol Metab Clin North Am* 23(4):749, 1994.
18. Ory SJ, Barrionuevo MJ: The differential diagnosis of female infertility. In Becker KL, editor: *Principles and practice of endocrinology and metabolism*, Philadelphia, 2001, Lippincott Williams & Wilkins.
19. Speroff L, Glass RH, Kase NG: Female infertility. In Speroff L, Glass RH, Kase NG: *Clinical gynecologic endocrinology and fertility: test, self-assessment and study guide on CD-ROM (for Windows & MacIntosh)*, Baltimore, 2001, Williams & Wilkins.
20. Speroff L, Glass RH, Kase NG: The uterus. In Speroff L, Glass RH, Kase NG: *Clinical gynecologic endocrinology and fertility: test, self-assessment and study guide on CD-ROM (for Windows & MacIntosh)*, Baltimore, 2001, Williams & Wilkins.
21. Speroff L, Glass RH, Kase NG: Induction of ovulation. In Speroff L, Glass RH, Kase NG: *Clinical gynecologic endocrinology and fertility: test, self-assessment and study guide on CD-ROM (for Windows & MacIntosh)*, Baltimore, 2001, Williams & Wilkins.
22. Speroff L, Glass RH, Kase NG: Amenorrhea. In Speroff L, Glass RH, Kase NG: *Clinical gynecologic endocrinology and fertility: test, self-assessment and study guide on CD-ROM (for Windows & MacIntosh)*, Baltimore, 2001, Williams & Wilkins.
23. Winters SJ: Evaluation of testicular function. In Becker KL, editor: *Principles and practice of endocrinology and metabolism*, Philadelphia, 2001, Lippincott Williams & Wilkins.

Internet Sites

Amenorrhea

http://www.advancedfertility.com/amenor.htm—Advanced Fertility Center of Chicago

Polycystic Ovary Disease

www.pcosupport.org/—Polycystic Ovarian Syndrome Association
http://www.wdxcyber.com/dxinf001.htm—Women's Diagnostic Cyber

Infertility/Fertility

http://www.inciid.org/—The InterNational Council on Infertility Information Dissemination, Inc.

http://www.womens-health.com/health_center/infertility/—Women's Health Interactive
http://www.fertilityuk.org/—This site is an online version of the book Fertility

Premenstrual Syndrome

http://www.pms.org.uk/—National Association for Premenstrual Syndrome

Klinefelter's Syndrome

http://www.akac70.care4free.net/home.html—Klinefelter's Syndrome Association UK
http://www.e-testicles.com/—Altruis Biomedical Network

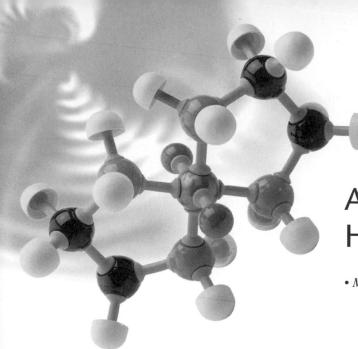

CHAPTER 46

Adrenal Hormones and Hypertension

• *Morris R. Pudek*

Chapter Outline

Objectives

- List the principal glucocorticoids, mineralocorticoids, adrenal androgens, and medullary hormones and state their physiological effects.
- Describe the synthesis, transport, catabolism, and regulation of glucocorticoids, mineralocorticoids, adrenal androgens, and medullary hormones.
- Describe each of the following pathological conditions, including diagnostic laboratory results: Cushing's syndrome, hyperaldosteronism, congenital adrenal hyperplasia, Addison's disease, and pheochromocytoma.

- Describe each of the following adrenal function tests and the interpretation of results: clonidine suppression test, overnight and 2-day dexamethasone suppression tests, ACTH stimulation test, CRH stimulation test, bilateral petrosal sinus sampling, captopril suppression test, and metyrapone test.
- Describe some of the factors regulating blood pressure and list the major causes and complications of hypertension.
- Describe the minimum laboratory evaluation for the

initial work-up of a patient with hypertension and the indications for testing for secondary hypertension.

- List some of the most important metabolic complications associated with antihypertensive therapy.

Key Terms

Addison's disease   Primary adrenal insufficiency, most commonly the result of an autoimmune adrenalitis.

adrenal cortex   The outer portion of the adrenal gland, which produces various steroid hormones.

adrenal medulla   The inner portion of both adrenal glands, which produces catecholamines.

adrenocorticosteroids   Refers to all steroids secreted by the adrenal cortex.

adrenocorticotropic hormone (ACTH)   A polypeptide hormone secreted by the anterior pituitary gland, which primarily stimulates the synthesis and release of glucocorticoids from the adrenal cortex.

adrenocorticotropic hormone (ACTH) stimulation test   An initial screening test used in the assessment of adrenal insufficiency. Also called *short ACTH* or *rapid ACTH* stimulation test.

adrenoleukodystrophy   An inherited X-linked disorder in the metabolism of very long chain fatty acids that can lead to severe neurological problems and primary adrenal insufficiency.

captopril suppression test   A test that is useful in the investigation of Conn's syndrome. Captopril is an angiotensin-converting enzyme inhibitor and blocks the formation of angiotensin II, which normally results in a fall in aldosterone.

catecholamines   Epinephrine and norepinephrine, which are produced in the adrenal medulla and are responsible for maintenance of blood pressure.

chromaffin cells   Cells found in the adrenal medulla and other sites throughout the body that produce catecholamines.

clonidine suppression test   A function test used in the diagnosis of pheochromocytoma.

congenital adrenal hyperplasia   Also known as **adrenogenital syndrome**. A group of hereditary diseases that result from enzyme deficiencies in the steroid hormone production pathways.

Conn's syndrome   Another name used to denote primary hyperaldosteronism.

corticosteroid-binding globulin   Also known as **transcortin**. A protein that binds and transports the majority of cortisol in the circulation.

corticotropin-releasing hormone (CRH)   A hypothalamic polypeptide that stimulates ACTH secretion.

Cushing's disease   A form of Cushing's syndrome specifically attributable to an ACTH-secreting pituitary adenoma.

Cushing's syndrome   A range of specific symptoms resulting from the elevation of blood glucocorticoid levels from primary or secondary causes.

dexamethasone suppression test   A function test that is used in the diagnosis and differentiation of various causes of Cushing's syndrome.

glucocorticoids   A group of steroid hormones secreted by the adrenal cortex that have multiple physiological effects including regulation of carbohydrate metabolism. Cortisol is the major glucocorticoid in humans.

hyperaldosteronism   Increased secretion of aldosterone from the adrenal cortex either because of elevated blood renin levels or autonomous adrenocortical secretion (Conn's syndrome).

hypoadrenalism   Adrenal insufficiency resulting in decreased output of steroid hormones from the adrenal cortex.

metyrapone stimulation test   An adrenal function test that can be used in the assessment of both hyperadrenal and hypoadrenal function. Metyrapone blocks 11-hydroxylase activity, and the response is usually determined by measurement of 11-deoxycortisol in serum.

mineralocorticoids   Steroid hormones secreted by the adrenal cortex that stimulate the resorption of sodium and the excretion of potassium in the distal tubules of the kidneys. Aldosterone is the major mineralocorticoid in humans.

pheochromocytoma   A tumor of the chromaffin cells, usually located in the adrenal medulla, that results in hypersecretion of epinephrine and norepinephrine.

primary hypertension, also called **essential hypertension**   It is an elevated systemic arterial pressure for which no cause can be found; it is often the only significant clinical finding.

renin-angiotensin system   This system is responsible for the regulation of aldosterone secretion from the adrenal cortex.

secondary hypertension   Elevated blood pressure associated with several primary diseases, such as renal, endocrine, and vascular diseases.

zona fasciculata   The middle portion of the adrenal cortex in which glucocorticoids and various sex hormones are produced.

zona glomerulosa   The outer portion of the adrenal cortex in which the mineralocorticoids are produced.

zona reticularis   The innermost portion of the adrenal cortex, next to the adrenal medulla, that acts in concert with the zona fasciculata.

Methods on CD-ROM

Catecholamines (plasma)
Catecholamines (urine)
Cortisol
Dehydroepiandrosterone and its sulfate

Homovanillic acid
Metanephrines
Vanillylmandelic acid

Part 1: The Adrenal Hormones

ANATOMY

The adrenal glands are situated at the upper pole of each kidney (Fig. 46-1). In the adult the adrenal cortex, which constitutes 90% of the gland volume, is made up of three distinct layers. The outer layer is called the **zona glomerulosa**. The wide middle layer and the inner layer are called the **zona fasciculata** and the **zona reticularis**, respectively. These three layers secrete steroid hormones that may have **mineralocorticoid**, **glucocorticoid**, or androgen functions. The gland is highly vascular with a complex venous circulation that is believed to play a role in regulating steroid hormone synthesis.

The **adrenal medulla** consists of sheets of irregular cells with small nuclei called **chromaffin cells**. These cells synthesize and secrete the **catecholamines**.

PHYSIOLOGY OF ADRENAL HORMONES

All adrenal steroids secreted by the **adrenal cortex (adrenocorticosteroids)** have the same basic cyclopentanoperhydrophenanthrene nucleus consisting of three six-carbon hexane rings and one five-carbon ring. The numbering of the carbon atoms is indicated in Fig. 46-2. The steroid molecules with 21 carbon atoms and a hydroxyl group at the carbon-17 position are termed *17-hydroxysteroids*. The steroid structures with 19 carbon atoms with a ketone group at C-17 are termed *ketosteroids*.

There are three major functional groups of steroids secreted by the adrenal cortex. These are the mineralocorticoids secreted by the zona glomerulosa and the glucocorticoids and androgens secreted by the zona reticularis and zona fasciculata. Relatively minor differences in the chemical structure result in major differences in the physiological function of these steroid molecules.

The adrenal medulla secretes the catecholamines. These molecules are not related in structure to the adrenal steroids and have very different physiological functions.

Glucocorticoids

The glucocorticoids (primarily cortisol in humans) are synthesized and secreted by the zona fasciculata and the zona reticularis. These steroid molecules are involved in the regulation of carbohydrate, protein, and lipid metabolism. Cortisol at high concentrations also demonstrates mineralocorticoid activity. Some of the more important physiological effects of the glucocorticoids are summarized in the box. These hormones are essential for life, especially when the human body is subjected to a stress such as surgery, major illness, or severe trauma. Cortisol concentrations increase greatly during these stresses, with the output of cortisol from the adrenal glands increasing from 10 to 30 mg/day in the nonstressed state to as high as 300 mg/day. Stress induces the release of numerous mediator substances such as catecholamines and kinins that can affect cardiovascular function, and, if unchecked, can lead to cardiovascular collapse. The

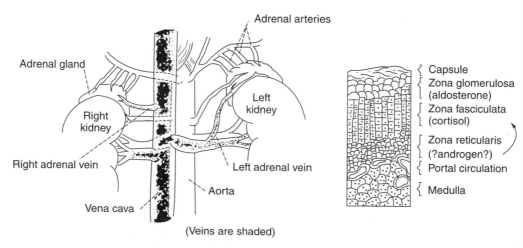

Fig. 46-1   Adrenal gland anatomy and histology. *(From Ryan W:* Endocrine disorders, *St Louis, 1980, Mosby.)*

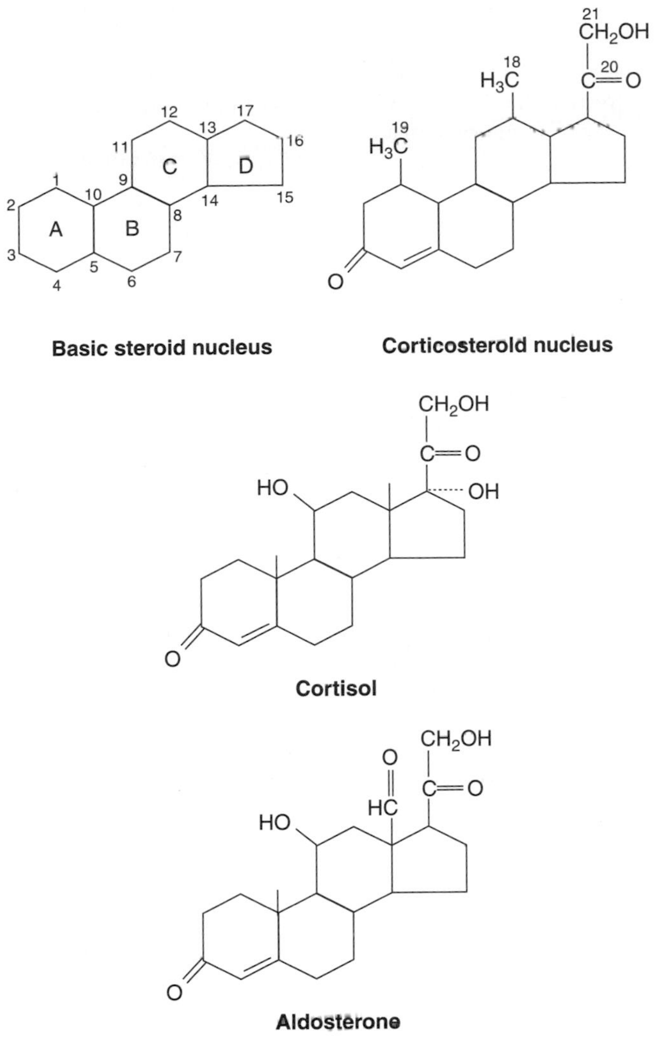

Fig. 46-2 Structures of adrenocortical hormones.

glucocorticoids block mediator production and action and prevent them from becoming life threatening.

Intermediary metabolism. The overall metabolic action of glucocorticoids is catabolic, promoting protein and lipid breakdown and inhibiting protein synthesis in muscle, connective tissue, adipose tissue, and lymphoid cells. Wound healing is inhibited, and osteoporosis is promoted. Glucocorticoids, however, have an anabolic effect on liver metabolism. The effects of cortisol are antagonistic to those of insulin, increasing the concentration of glucose by stimulating gluconeogenesis. The amino acids and glycerol released by the catabolic action of cortisol on protein and fat are used as gluconeogenic substrates. Cortisol increases the synthesis and activity of numerous enzymes in the liver that are involved in amino acid and glucose metabolism. Cortisol decreases glucose utilization by muscle and promotes lipolysis in adipose tissue. Paradoxically central fat stores are increased in states of cortisol excess. The net effect is increased production and conservation of glucose for use by essential tissues, such as the brain and red blood cells, at the expense of "less essential" tissues during times of stress or starvation.

Blood pressure. Cortisol also contributes to the maintenance of normal blood pressure through several mechanisms. Cortisol increases urine flow by stimulating GFR and decreasing water resorption. At high concentrations, however, cortisol can act like a mineralocorticoid, promoting sodium and water retention and causing hypokalemia. Cortisol interacts avidly with the mineralocorticoid receptor. In fact, free serum cortisol levels are 150-fold higher than free serum aldosterone levels; therefore the mineralocorticoid receptor is saturated by cortisol in most tissues except the kidney. Renal cells rapidly convert cortisol to cortisone, allowing aldosterone to be the predominant regulator of renal sodium resorption and potassium excretion. Also, in high concentrations cortisol may have additional contributions to maintaining blood pressure homeostasis. These include increasing angiotensinogen (renin substrate) synthesis by the liver; increasing the vascular reactivity to vasoconstrictors; maintaining the activity of the enzyme responsible for converting norepinephrine to epinephrine in the adrenal medulla, which can affect cardiac output; decreasing the activity of the vasodilatory kinin and prostaglandin systems; and promoting movement of sodium from the cellular compartment to the vascular compartment resulting in extracellular fluid volume expansion.

Immune function. The hematological effects of cortisol are multiple, stimulating erythropoiesis and causing leukocytosis through decreasing the movement of polymorphonucleocytes out of the vascular compartment, resulting in neutrophilia, lymphocytopenia, monocytopenia, and eosinopenia. Glucocorticoids also suppress the inflammatory and immune response by stabilizing lysosomes, interfering with leukocyte migration, and inhibiting phagocytosis. Some of the glucocorticoid action is mediated through its effects on the production and actions of mediators such as the interleukins and interferons.

Miscellaneous functions. Cortisol has a number of miscellaneous physiological effects, many of which are seen at high serum concentrations. These are listed in the box on p. 880.

The molecular basis for steroid hormone actions is described in Chapter 43.

Mineralocorticoids

Aldosterone is the primary product of the zona glomerulosa with approximately 200 mg produced per day, roughly 1/100th the amount of cortisol synthesized daily. The major physiological functions of aldosterone are (1) regulation of extracellular fluid volume and (2) regulation of potassium metabolism. Its actions are mediated through a high-affinity mineralocorticoid receptor found in a variety of tissues. Its most important action is in the cells of the renal distal convoluted tubule where it promotes sodium resorption in exchange for excretion of potassium. Sodium diffuses passively through the sodium channels within the cell membrane to the apical membranes of the epithelial cells. Aldosterone action increases the number of open sodium channels via methylation of the channels' proteins. Aldoste-

---

PHYSIOLOGICAL FUNCTIONS OF CORTISOL

Effects on Intermediary Metabolism
Increases gluconeogenesis
Increases glycogen synthesis
Increases lipolysis
Increases blood glucose levels
Decreases glucose utilization

Effects on Protein Metabolism
Increases protein catabolism
Decreases protein synthesis

Effects on Blood Pressure
Increases urine flow by increasing glomerular filtration rate (GFR)
At high concentrations acts like aldosterone
Increases synthesis of angiotensinogen
Increases reactivity to vasoconstrictors
Enhances conversion of norepinephrine to epinephrine in adrenal medulla
Modulates effects of kinins and prostaglandins
Promotes movement of sodium out of cells
High concentrations inhibit antidiuretic hormone (ADH) release

Effects on Immunological and Inflammatory Responses
Decreases antibody formation
Decreases circulating lymphocytes, eosinophils, and monocytes
Decreases production and inhibits actions of interleukins and interferons
Stabilizes lysosomes
Inhibits leukocyte migration
Inhibits phagocytosis

Miscellaneous
Bone: Inhibits bone formation, increases reabsorption, enhances PTH action, and decreases GI calcium absorption
Growth: Decreases growth by inhibiting release of growth hormone and somatomedin C (IGF-1)
Gonads: Inhibits response of pituitary to GnRH, decreasing release of gonadotropins and gonadal steroids
Central nervous system: Chronic high cortisol levels associated with irritability, depression, psychosis, loss of memory and concentration, and decreased libido. Chronic low levels associated with apathy, depression, and decreased appetite.
Thyroid: Increased cortisol inhibits TSH

---

rone also increases potassium conductance through specific channels and increases the synthesis of sodium-potassium ATPase in the basolateral membranes that generate the electrochemical gradient to drive diffusion. Water passively follows the transported sodium through the membranes (see Chapter 24).

Cortisol and other corticosteroids such as corticosterone and deoxycorticosterone have some mineralocorticoid activity that can become clinically significant when serum levels of these compounds are elevated. This can occur with the high cortisol levels seen in **Cushing's syndrome**. In fact cortisol has equivalent affinity for the mineralocorticoid receptor; however, the kidney cells express high concentrations of 11-β-hydroxysteroid dehydrogenase, which rapidly converts cortisol to cortisone inactivating its mineralocorticoid activity. Aldosterone in turn has weak glucocorticoid activity, but its concentration is too low to have any physiological effect.

Adrenal Androgens

The predominant androgens secreted by the adrenal cortex are dehydroepiandrosterone sulfate (DHEA-S), dehydroepiandrosterone (DHEA), and androstenedione. Small amounts of testosterone (T) and dihydrotestosterone (DHT) are also secreted. The average daily production rate of DHEA-S is approximately 30 mg in young men and 20 mg in young women. The half-life of DHEA-S is between 8 and 11 hours, whereas it is only 30 to 60 minutes for the unconjugated androgens. Adrenal androgen production reaches a peak between 20 and 30 years of age and then gradually falls with age to about 20% of peak levels after 70 years. This is in contrast to cortisol production, which does not change with age. DHEA-S is also the principal steroid of the fetal adrenal, but the serum levels of DHEA-S fall rapidly after birth and then slowly rise in mid-childhood as the zona reticularis matures (adrenarche). At their peak, at age 20 to 30 years, circulating levels of DHEA-S are 20 times higher than those of cortisol because of increased secretion rates and decreased metabolic clearance. DHEA and DHEA-S levels decrease during illness, depression, and other stresses.

The biological effects of the adrenal androgens are either direct or indirect. These steroids can be converted by peripheral tissues to the primary sex hormones; testosterone, DHT, and estradiol. Adrenal androgens are the major source of testosterone in females. Some direct effects of DHEA have been determined. DHEA can inhibit the enzyme glucose-6-phosphate dehydrogenase, an important factor controlling the synthesis of NADPH, which is required for many important biological reactions including lipogenesis. DHEA may also be involved with many other broad-based physiological effects, including immune regulation, through possible direct effects on production of cytokines and by acting as a neurosteroid to modulate γ-aminobutyric acid and N-methyl aspartate receptors in the hippocampus area of the brain.

DHEA-S may have an important antiglucocorticoid role and DHEA-S deficiency may result in relative glucocorticoid excess, with impaired memory and negative mood effects. There is now evidence that DHEA-S can improve psychological well being, lean body mass, and may have beneficial effects on bone turnover. The evidence is insufficient to support the general use of DHEA-S in the elderly as an antiaging hormone but there is support for its use in women with **Addison's disease** who have traditionally only been treated with glucocorticoid and mineralocorticoid replacement therapy. Women with primary or secondary adrenal insufficiency have very low DHEA and DHEA-S levels and experience loss of axillary and pubic hair and osteoporosis. Patients not treated with replacement DHEA retain normal longevity, but have lower strength and stamina. Studies have shown psychological and sexual function benefits when DHEA was given, resulting in normalization of DHEA-S, androstenedione, and low-normal testosterone levels. Also improved were serum levels of IGF-1; serum low-density lipoprotein (LDL) cholesterol levels decreased. Negative effects include acne and hirsutism in a small percentage of women.

Catecholamines

The naturally occurring catecholamines are norepinephrine (NE, noradrenaline), epinephrine (E, adrenaline), and dopamine. The main secretory products of the adrenal medulla are epinephrine and norepinephrine. Production of catecholamines is not restricted to the adrenal medulla, however, and synthesis of these hormones also occurs in the neurons of the sympathetic and central nervous systems (CNS) and in scattered groups of chromaffin cells found in other regions of the abdomen and neck. Norepinephrine is the principal product synthesized in the CNS, and epinephrine is the principal catecholamine produced by the adrenal glands.

Physiological actions of the catecholamines are diverse. Norepinephrine functions primarily as a neurotransmitter. Both norepinephrine and epinephrine influence the vascular system, whereas epinephrine affects metabolic processes such as carbohydrate metabolism. The biological actions of the catecholamines are initiated through their interaction with two different types of specific cell membrane receptors, the α-adrenergic and β-adrenergic receptors. These receptors have different affinities for norepinephrine and epinephrine and cause opposing physiological effects. Norepinephrine primarily interacts with α-adrenergic receptors, whereas epinephrine interacts with both α- and β-receptors.

Stimulation of α-adrenergic receptors results in vasoconstriction, decreased insulin secretion, sweating, piloerection (hair standing on end), and stimulation of glycogenolysis in the liver and skeletal muscle leading to an increase in blood glucose concentration. Stimulation of β-receptors, however, leads to vasodilation; stimulation of insulin release; increased cardiac contraction rate; relaxation of smooth muscle in the intestinal tract; bronchodilation by relaxation of smooth muscles in bronchi; stimulation of renin release, which enhances sodium resorption from the kidney; and enhanced lipolysis.

BIOSYNTHESIS
Adrenocorticosteroids

All adrenal steroid synthesis begins with cholesterol. Cholesterol in the adrenal tissue may be synthesized in situ from acetate or may come from cholesterol made in the liver and transported to the adrenal glands by LDL.

The biosynthetic pathway leading to the three major groups of adrenal steroids is outlined in Fig. 46-3. Several of the reactions in steroidogenesis involve cytochrome P-450 enzymes, which are heme-containing enzymes that transfer electrons from NADPH to perform hydroxylation reactions using molecular oxygen. The rate-limiting step in the synthesis of all steroids is the conversion of cholesterol to pregnenolone. The enzyme responsible for this side chain cleavage step (cholesterol desmolase) is a product of the gene CYP11A1. This step is stimulated by adrenocorticotropic hormone (ACTH) in the zona fasciculata and zona reticularis and by angiotensin II and III in the zona glomerulosa. The pathway leading to progesterone is common to both aldosterone and cortisol synthesis. The conversion of pregnenolone to progesterone is catalyzed by 3-β-hydroxysteroid dehydrogenase. In the zona reticularis and zona fasciculata, progesterone is hydroxylated at the 17, 21, and 11 positions to form cortisol. The enzymes responsible are gene products of CYP17, CYP21A2, and CYP11B2, respectively. Under normal circumstances, 10 to 30 mg of cortisol is synthesized per day.

Aldosterone is biosynthesized in the zona glomerulosa from cholesterol by the action of four enzymes; cholesterol desmolase (CYP11A1), 3-β-hydroxysteroid dehydrogenase, 21 hydroxylase (CYP21A2), and aldosterone synthetase (CYP11B2). Cortisol requires a 17 hydroxylation (CYP17), which is only expressed in the zona fasciculata, whereas aldosterone synthetase is only expressed in the zona glomerulosa.

The androgens are derived from the major pathway of steroid biosynthesis after cleavage of the side chain attached to carbon 17 in ring D. See Chapter 45 for a description of the synthesis of androgens. The adrenal gland production of androgens is significant, indirectly generating 60% of the circulating testosterone in females, mainly through peripheral tissue conversion of testosterone precursors.

Catecholamines

The biochemical pathway leading to the synthesis of the catecholamines is outlined in Fig. 46-4. The rate-limiting step is the hydroxylation of the amino acid tyrosine leading to the formation of dihydroxyphenylalanine (dopa). This step is inhibited by both epinephrine and norepinephrine. Tyrosine comes from the diet or from hydroxylation of phenylalanine. Dopa is decarboxylated to form dopamine, which is a major end product in the CNS where it functions as a neurotransmitter. Dopamine is stored in granules that are present in both neurons and the adrenal medulla. Within the granules, dopamine β-hydroxylase converts dopamine to norepinephrine. Finally, the norepinephrine is released from the storage granules, and phenylethanolamine N-methyltransferase (PNMT) methylates the norepinephrine to form epinephrine. PNMT, which is found only in the adrenal medulla, is induced by glucocorticoids (cortisol). High concentrations of cortisol within the adrenal are required for the induction of PNMT in the adrenal medulla. Exogenous steroids suppress endogenous cortisol and reduce the high concentration of cortisol around the medulla, reducing the

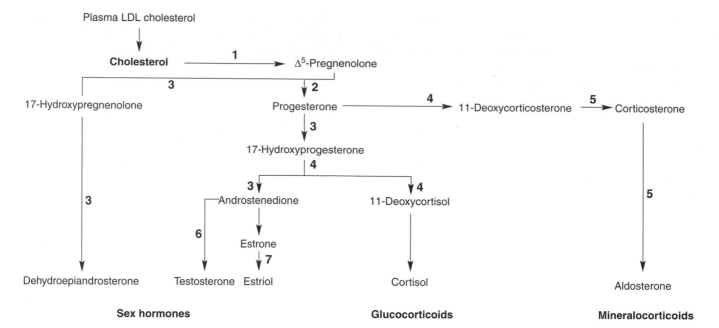

Fig. 46-3 Principal pathways of adrenal steroidogenesis. The letters represent the different enzymes responsible for catalysis of each of the biochemical transformations. Notice that the same enzyme may be responsible for more than one type of reaction. *1,* Mitochondrial cytochrome P-450scc catalyzes the side chain cleavage of cholesterol. *2,* 3-β-hydroxysteroid dehydrogenase bound to the endoplasmic reticulum also catalyzes Δ^5-Δ^4 isomerase activity. *3,* P-450c17 is responsible for both 17-hydroxylase activity and 17,20-lyase activity, which cleaves off the remaining side chain at C-17 position. *4,* P-450c21 catalyzes 21-hydroxylation of progesterone and 17-hydroxyprogesterone. *5,* Mitochondrial P-450c11 catalyzes three different reactions: 11-hydroxylation, 18-hydroxylation, and 18-methyloxidase. *6,* 17-Ketosteroid reductase is found mainly in the testes and ovaries. *7,* P-450aro mediates the aromatization of ring A and is located mainly in the ovaries.

production of epinephrine. Adrenocortical insufficiency of whatever cause is associated with reduced epinephrine secretions from the adrenal. The hormones of the adrenal medulla are stored complexed with proteins (chromogranin A, dopamine-β-hydroxylase) and adenosine-5'-triphosphate (ATP) in chromaffin granules. Nerve stimulation results in release of the stored catecholamines from these vesicles by the process of exocytosis.

TRANSPORT AND CATABOLISM
Adrenocorticosteroids

In plasma, aldosterone and cortisol are bound to plasma proteins to different degrees. Aldosterone exists approximately 40% in the free state, whereas approximately 4% of cortisol is free in solution. Albumin and **corticosteroid-binding globulin** (CBG, **transcortin**, cortisol-binding globulin) account for most of the binding of these two steroids. CBG is a high-affinity, low-capacity steroid binder, binding 90% of the cortisol under normal circumstances, whereas albumin is a low-affinity, high-capacity binding protein. The proportion of cortisol in the free state greatly increases as the concentration of cortisol exceeds the binding capacity of CBG (approximately 550 nmol/L). The binding

affinity of CBG for cortisol is reduced in areas of inflammation. This increases the concentration of free cortisol, therefore increasing its effectiveness at that site. CBG levels are increased in hyperestrogenic states such as those found in pregnant women and in women taking estrogen-containing birth control pills. The free cortisol levels remain normal under these circumstances because of a compensatory increase in total cortisol. Aldosterone is much less affected by these hormonally induced changes.

Steroid catabolism is quite complex, and only a brief discussion of it is necessary for the understanding of the pathogenesis and laboratory investigation of adrenal disorders. The liver and the kidneys catabolize most steroids. Examples of the types of reactions that are carried out include further hydroxylation of the steroid nucleus, conjugation with glucuronic acid, and reduction of the double bond in ring A. These transformations increase the water solubility of the steroids, allowing for their excretion into the urine. Normally only a small portion of aldosterone and cortisol (less than 1%) is excreted unmetabolized into the urine.

The amount of cortisol directly secreted into the urine is related to the proportion of cortisol that circulates in the free form. CBG is saturated at high physiological concentrations

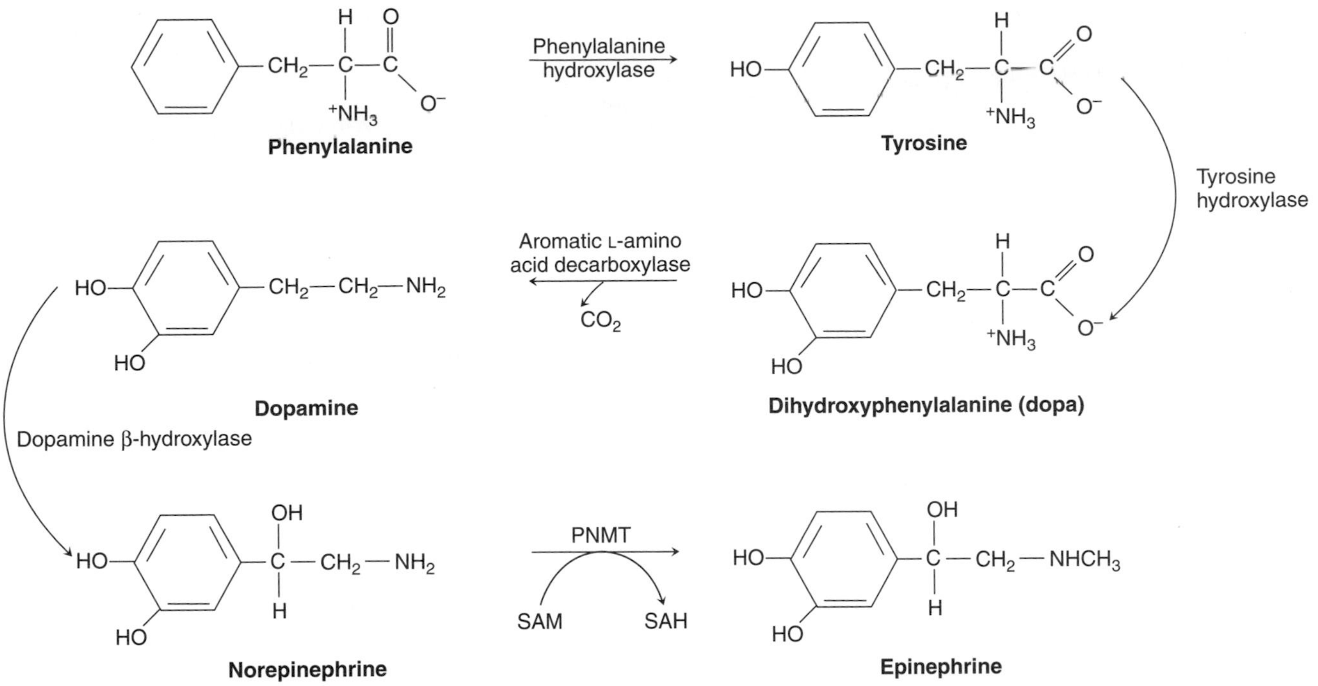

Fig. 46-4 Synthesis of medullary hormones. *PNMT,* Phenylethanolamine N-methyltransferase; *SAH,* S-adenosyl homocysteine; *SAM,* S-adenosylmethionine. *(From Orten JM, Neuhaus OW:* Human biochemistry, *St Louis, 1982, Mosby.)*

of cortisol. Therefore any increase in cortisol above this level results in a pronounced increase in the amount of cortisol excreted into the urine, making urinary free cortisol a valuable test in the investigation of Cushing's syndrome, as is discussed later.

Catecholamines

The catecholamines are stable within the storage granules of the adrenal medullary cells. However, when they are released they are rapidly degraded by two enzymes: catechol-O-methyltransferase (COMT) and monoamine oxidase (MAO) (Fig. 46-5). Only a small fraction of catecholamine output (2%) is excreted unmetabolized as free catecholamines into the urine. COMT is present in many tissues, especially liver and kidney, and in erythrocytes. This enzyme methylates the C-3 hydroxyl group of norepinephrine and epinephrine, resulting in normetanephrine and metanephrine, respectively. Approximately 20% of catecholamines are excreted into the urine as metanephrines. Most catecholamines, however, are further converted to vanillylmandelic acid (VMA) by the combined action of COMT and MAO; the latter is a

ubiquitous enzyme that deaminates these amines. The measurement of free catecholamines, metanephrines, and VMA in the urine may be useful in the diagnosis of adrenal medullary disease. A large proportion of catecholamine metabolites appear in the urine as sulfate conjugates.

CONTROL AND REGULATION
Glucocorticoids

Cortisol released from the adrenal cortex is regulated by the hypothalamic-pituitary-adrenal axis (Fig. 46-6 and Chapter 43). The hypothalamus synthesizes a 41–amino acid polypeptide, **corticotropin-releasing hormone (CRH)**, which is carried by the circulation to the anterior pituitary gland. There it causes the release of adrenocorticotropic hormone (ACTH), a 39–amino acid polypeptide. The first 18 amino acids are essential for biological activity. The ACTH molecule interacts with membrane receptors of the cells of the adrenal cortex and through its second messenger, cyclic AMP, stimulates the rate-limiting step in steroidogenesis (the conversion of cholesterol to pregnenolone) leading to cortisol secretion. The free circulating cortisol acts in a negative-

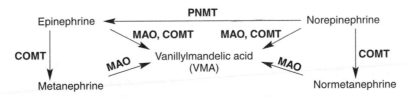

Fig. 46-5 Metabolism of medullary hormones (see text for description of abbreviations).

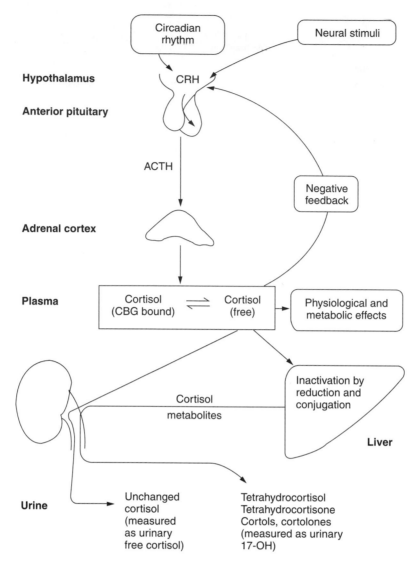

Fig. 46-6 Control and metabolism of glucocorticoids. *(From Toft A:* Diagnosis and management of endocrine diseases, *St Louis, 1981, Blackwell Scientific.)*

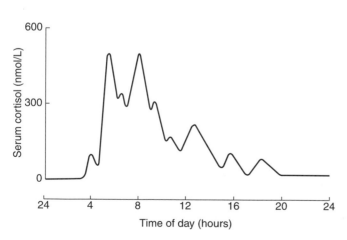

Fig. 46-7 Variation of serum cortisol concentration during 24-hour period in normal individual.

feedback manner to control the release of ACTH from the pituitary gland. Overriding this system of negative-feedback control are the higher centers of the brain, which establish the normal diurnal variation of cortisol (Fig. 46-7). Serum cortisol levels are normally highest in the morning on waking and lowest in the late evening. This pattern is mainly affected by the sleep-wake cycle of the individual. If the sleep-wake cycle is altered, several days are required for the pattern to change. The circadian pattern of ACTH release is controlled by means of CRH secretion from the hypothalamus. Short-term release of cortisol is episodic, following the pattern of ACTH pulses by about 2 to 3 minutes. Stress is another factor that can override the negative feedback of cortisol on ACTH release. Stress stimulates release of neurogenic amines, which in turn stimulates the release of CRH. The inflammatory cytokines, tumor necrosis factor α, interleukin-1, and interleukin-6 also stimulate the release of ACTH. ACTH levels can increase up to tenfold in times of stress,

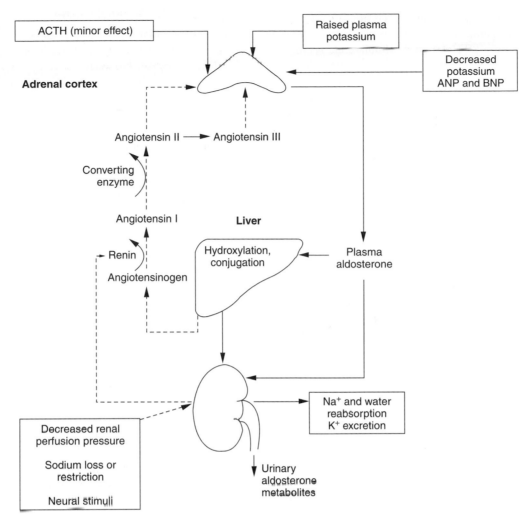

Fig. 46-8   Control and metabolism of aldosterone. *(Modified from Toft A:* Diagnosis and management of endocrine diseases, *St Louis, 1981, Blackwell Scientific.)*

resulting in high levels of cortisol. Hypoglycemia, which is a form of chemical stress, can also increase CRH release, ultimately leading to an increase in cortisol. This effect is mediated by glucose receptors in the hypothalamus.

Mineralocorticoids

In normal individuals three main factors control the secretion of aldosterone from the zona glomerulosa: (1) the **renin-angiotensin system**, (2) potassium, and (3) ACTH. Under normal circumstances, the renin-angiotensin system predominates. Recently described natriuretic peptides, atrial natriuretic peptide (ANP) and B-type natriuretic peptide (BNP), from the heart may exhibit part of their physiological function through inhibition of aldosterone release (see Chapters 24 and 31). Fig. 46-8 outlines the normal regulation of aldosterone secretion. A more detailed description is found in Chapter 24.

Renin is a proteolytic enzyme stored by specialized cells in the wall of the afferent arteriole of the glomerulus. These cells are associated with the *macula densa*, which is part of the juxtaglomerular apparatus. There are two forms of renin

in the circulation, active renin and its precursor, prorenin. Active renin can only be released from the juxtaglomerular apparatus. Prorenin concentration in the circulation is 10 times higher on average than active renin. There are also extrarenal sources of prorenin. A drop in blood pressure or serum sodium concentration results in the release of renin. Renin cleaves a peptide bond in circulating angiotensinogen, a protein secreted by the liver, releasing a decapeptide called *angiotensin I*. Angiotensin I in turn is cleaved by angiotensin-converting enzyme (ACE), forming an octapeptide called *angiotensin II*. Angiotensin II is a potent vasoconstrictor that increases blood pressure directly. This peptide also stimulates aldosterone release through its interaction with a membrane-bound receptor of the G-protein type on the surface of cells in the zona glomerulosa. Aldosterone, acting through the mineralocorticoid receptor within kidney tubular cells, facilitates sodium retention and potassium loss. Finally, angiotensin II is converted to a heptapeptide, *angiotensin III*, by a carboxypeptidase. Angiotensin III still retains the capacity to stimulate aldosterone release but has little pressor activity.

Potassium stimulates aldosterone secretion directly at the adrenal level. Hyperkalemia stimulates and hypokalemia inhibits renin release. ACTH can also stimulate aldosterone secretion directly; however, this is only an acute phenomenon that is short lived. There is normally a circadian rhythm in plasma aldosterone concentration with highest values occurring in the morning. In addition, there are alterations in aldosterone levels with postural changes. Plasma levels range from 50 to 150 ng/L (140 to 420 pmol/L) in healthy individuals when recumbent and from 150 to 300 ng/L (420 to 840 pmol/L) when upright. Approximately 150 to 200 µg of aldosterone is secreted per day under normal circumstances. Dopamine, serotonin, γ-melanocyte-stimulating hormone (γ-MSH), β-endorphin, and an unidentified pituitary aldosterone-stimulating factor also participate in aldosterone regulation.

Several drugs can have physiological effects on the renin-aldosterone system. Nonsteroidal antiinflammatory agents and β-blockers can decrease both aldosterone and renin levels. Potassium-sparing diuretics and ACE inhibitors can result in increased renin with decreased aldosterone. Thiazide diuretics and laxatives can increase the concentration of both.

Adrenal Androgens

Androgen secretion is partially regulated by ACTH but not by gonadotropins. ACTH stimulation is variable, and dexamethasone (a synthetic corticosteroid) administration decreases adrenal androgen production to a dissimilar degree when compared to cortisol. In other instances, as at adrenarche or puberty, or with aging or severe illness, cortisol and androgen production diverge, and such divergence indicates that other factors are playing a role in the regulation of adrenal androgen secretion. These factors may include the arrangement of the blood supply to the adrenal cortex, intrinsic properties of the adrenocortical cells, and other unknown factors exogenous to the adrenal, such as factors from the pituitary.

Catecholamines

The synthesis of epinephrine and norepinephrine is regulated by the intracellular concentrations of these hormones by negative-feedback inhibition, as stated previously. The catecholamines are released from the adrenal medulla in response to hypotension, hypoxia, exposure to cold, muscular exertion, pain, and emotional disturbances.

PATHOLOGICAL CONDITIONS

In this section the causes and clinical features associated with the disorders of the adrenal cortex and the adrenal medulla are discussed. In general, the gland may hyperfunction and produce excess quantities of bioactive molecules, or the gland may hypofunction and secrete too little of certain important molecules that may be essential for the normal maintenance of life. The pathological cause of these disorders may be neoplastic, hyperplastic, vascular, inflammatory, autoimmune, infectious, hereditary, or idiopathic.

Disorders of the Adrenal Cortex

Hyperadrenalism. There are three basic conditions associated with hyperadrenalism, each of which may have more than one cause. These are Cushing's syndrome, resulting from excess cortisol production; primary **hyperaldosteronism**, or **Conn's syndrome**; and congenital adrenal hyperplasia caused by an enzymatic block in the steroid synthetic pathway.

Cushing's syndrome. *Cushing's syndrome* is the term used to describe any condition resulting from an increased concentration of circulating glucocorticoid, usually cortisol. The most common cause of excess cortisol is iatrogenic, resulting from high doses of cortisol or other glucocorticoids used in the management of a wide variety of clinical problems. The most common noniatrogenic causes are, in order, pituitary tumors (60%), ectopic ACTH (20%), and adrenal adenoma and adrenal carcinoma (combined 20%). The estimated prevalence of Cushing's syndrome is approximately 1:10,000 women and 1:30,000 men. The most common cause of Cushing's syndrome in children is adrenal tumors.

Cushing's syndrome may be divided into two broad categories: ACTH dependent and ACTH independent. ACTH-dependent Cushing's syndrome is caused by excess ACTH and results in bilateral adrenal hyperplasia. This is most commonly caused by autonomous ACTH secretion by a benign pituitary adenoma, also called **Cushing's disease**. This condition is much more common in women than in men (female/male ratio 7:1 or 8:1). Ectopic sources of ACTH include carcinoma of the lung (oat cell or small cell) (50%), thymic cancer (10%), pancreatic cancer (10%), neural crest tumors (5%), bronchial carcinoid (2%), medullary carcinoma of the thyroid (5%), and miscellaneous tumors (18%). It is now known that many nonendocrine tissues of the body can synthesize small amounts of proopiomelanocortin (POMC), the precursor to ACTH. Very few tissues can actually metabolize POMC and release bioactive ACTH. Most lung tumors produce POMC, but only 3% of these have the right proteolytic enzymes to release active ACTH, thus causing Cushing's syndrome.

In ACTH-independent Cushing's syndrome, serum ACTH levels are low because of the negative inhibition that results from the increased cortisol production of adrenal adenomas and carcinomas. Adrenal carcinoma has a particularly bad prognosis, with most patients dying within 3 years despite surgical intervention. Adrenal neoplasms are usually unilateral. In adults, about half of these are malignant, whereas in children neoplasms of the adrenal are more often malignant.

Rare causes of Cushing's syndrome include ectopic CRH secretion, macronodular adrenal hyperplasia (elevated ACTH and elevated cortisol), primary pigmented nodular hyperplasia (a familial autoimmune disorder analogous to Graves' disease), and gastric inhibitory polypeptide (GIP)–dependent cortisol hypersecretion (food-dependent Cushing's syndrome). In this last rare disorder there is ectopic expression of GIP receptors by the adrenal cells, with normal increases in serum GIP (see Chapter 30) stimulating cortisol secretion.

Cushing's syndrome in advanced stages may be easy to recognize (see the box). In early stages of the disease, however, patients can have a wide variety of clinical symptoms that may be confused with other common problems such as essential hypertension, glucose intolerance, depression, and obesity. The laboratory plays a major role in sorting out the diagnosis. Central obesity is a characteristic redistribution of adipose tissue with increased deposition around the face (moon facies), in the supraclavicular region, in the interscapular region (buffalo hump), and in the mesenteric bed (truncal obesity). The reason for this is not known. Less common findings include neuropsychiatric dysfunction, pigmentation, acne, and hypokalemic alkalosis. Polyuria may be seen because cortisol in high concentrations may suppress antidiuretic hormone (ADH) release. The neuropsychiatric problems include depression, manic behavior, psychoses, and attempts at suicide.

The catabolic effect of glucocorticoids on protein metabolism can account for the bruising, striae (stretch marks), osteoporosis, and muscle weakness. Hypertension and hypokalemia can be explained by the mineralocorticoid actions of excess cortisol. Hirsutism, acne, and menstrual dysfunction, a result of excess androgen production, may most dramatically be seen in some cases of adrenal carcinoma. Hyper-

pigmentation sometimes occurs in association with ectopic ACTH when the high levels of ACTH, which has some melanocyte-stimulating hormone (MSH) activity, causes generalized hyperproduction of melanin. Some patients may also suffer from impotence, decreased libido, and infertility.

There are some key clinical clues that might suggest an ectopic source for the ACTH. Some patients may not have some of the physical findings of Cushing's syndrome because of the rapid onset of symptoms, which can be seen with oat cell carcinoma. Symptoms are more common with the slow growing tumors such as bronchial, thymic, or pancreatic carcinoids. Because of the very high ACTH and cortisol levels seen in some of these patients they may be hyperpigmented, have more profound hypokalemia, and demonstrate glucose intolerance, weakness, and edema. Other signs associated with the malignant disease such as anorexia and weight loss may also be obvious. Opportunistic infections may be a key feature of ectopic ACTH because of the immunosuppressive effects of large concentrations of cortisol. Pneumocystic pneumonia is a possible complication.

In summary, frequent findings include truncal obesity (buffalo hump, supraclavicular fat pads), facial fullness (moon face), glucose intolerance, gonadal dysfunction, hirsutism, acne, hypertension, proximal muscle weakness, skin atrophy (easy bruising, stretch marks) and psychiatric problems. Less common findings at diagnosis include osteoporosis, edema, polyuria and polydipsia, and fungal infections. Some patients have only isolated findings and diagnosis can be missed for a long time. Other laboratory abnormalities associated with Cushing's include neutrophilia, leukocytosis, increased cholesterol, and hypercoagulability. Any child with recent weight gain and stunted linear growth should be investigated for Cushing's syndrome.

Recently there has been increased recognition of subclinical Cushing's syndrome associated with adrenal incidentalomas. The prevalence of incidentally discovered adrenal masses is approximately 1% of the population. It is estimated that 75% of these are nonfunctional, whereas 10% may hypersecrete cortisol bringing the prevalence of subclinical Cushing's syndrome to as high as 1/1000 of the population. By definition these individuals should be asymptomatic, however, there is a high prevalence of central obesity, hypertension, and diabetes. Often these problems resolve when the tumor is removed despite no clear biochemical evidence of functionality of the tumor.

Hyperaldosteronism

Primary autonomous hypersecretion of aldosterone by the zona glomerulosa is mainly caused by two disorders: (1) an adrenal adenoma producing aldosterone (APA), or Conn's syndrome (approximately 70% of cases), and (2) idiopathic hyperaldosteronism (IHA) caused by bilateral hyperplasia (approximately 30% of cases). Primary adrenal hyperplasia, which is indistinguishable biochemically from APA, may account for 1% to 2% of patients with this problem. Carcinomas secreting aldosterone are even more rare (<1%). A rare form of primary hyperaldosteronism, glucocorticoid-

---

MAJOR CAUSES AND CLINICAL FEATURES OF CUSHING'S SYNDROME

Causes
ACTH independent
  Adrenal adenoma
  Adrenal carcinoma
ACTH dependent
  Pituitary adenoma secreting ACTH (Cushing's disease)
  Ectopic ACTH
  Ectopic corticotropin-releasing hormone
Nodular hyperplasia
  Macronodular hyperplasia
  Primary pigmented nodular hyperplasia
  Gastric inhibitory polypeptide–dependent Cushing's
    syndrome
Iatrogenic
  Glucocorticoid therapy
  ACTH therapy

Clinical Features
Central obesity
Hypertension
Glucose intolerance
Plethoric facies
Purple striae
Menstrual dysfunction
Muscle weakness
Hirsutism
Bruising
Osteoporosis
Psychiatric problems

remediable aldosteronism (GRA), also called *dexamethasone suppressible hyperaldosteronism*, but now officially renamed *familial hyperaldosteronism type 1* (FH-1), has clinical features of Conn's syndrome but results from an ectopic expression of aldosterone synthase (AS), the gene product of CYP11B2. A chimeric gene is formed at meiosis between two homologous genes on chromosome 8, CYP11B1 and CYP11B2. Aldosterone synthase, normally only expressed in the zona glomerulosa is now partially expressed in the zona reticularis and as a result is now under ACTH control rather than angiotensin II control. Another genetic cause of hypertension includes apparent mineralocorticoid excess (AME). In this case an enzyme in the kidney, 11 β-hydroxy-steroid dehydrogenase type 2, fails to inactivate cortisol. Cortisol is now free to interact with the mineralocorticoid receptor, causing hypertension and hypokalemia. Both of the above hereditary causes of hypertension are treatable with dexamethasone.

The major clinical feature of hyperaldosteronism is hypertension. The estimated prevalence of this disorder in the hypertensive population varies from 0.05% to as high as 2.0%. More recent estimates suggest that this condition may in fact be a common cause of hypertension, accounting for as much as 5% to 15% of the hypertensive population. This high prevalence may be a function of the selected population examined and the revised testing protocols used to identify these patients. The hypertension associated with primary hyperaldosteronism can be explained by the actions of aldosterone that result in retention of sodium and water and decreased plasma potassium levels (see Chapter 24). The most consistent laboratory finding in patients with primary aldosteronism is hypokalemia. Spontaneous hypokalemia is found in 80% to 90% of patients. Administration of sodium chloride for several days will provoke hypokalemia in the remainder. The prevalence of primary hyperaldosteronism in patients with hypertension and spontaneous hypokalemia is more than 50%. The degree of hypokalemia is affected partly by the sodium intake. Many patients with hypokalemia do not experience symptoms (see box below). Abnormal glucose tolerance can be observed in more than half the patients. Hypokalemia impairs insulin release from the β-cells of the pancreas. The hallmark of primary hyperaldosteronism is inappropriately elevated aldosterone in the presence of suppressed plasma renin activity.

Hyperaldosteronism may also result from secondary causes. In these situations the adrenal gland is not autonomously secreting aldosterone but is responding to enhanced production and release of renin from the kidney, which may be triggered by sodium loss, decreased renal perfusion, renal artery stenosis, or vascular volume depletion. Rarely the hypersecretion of renin may be inappropriate, as in *Bartter's syndrome*, a kidney defect in chloride resorption, or in patients with renin-secreting tumors. In contrast to primary aldosteronism in which renin is decreased, plasma renin is elevated in secondary aldosteronism.

Congenital Adrenal Hyperplasia

Congenital adrenal hyperplasia (CAH), or **adrenogenital syndrome**, describes a group of inborn errors of metabolism that are caused by deficiencies of enzymes in the biosynthetic pathways leading to cortisol and aldosterone production. There are at least six distinct inheritable defects in this pathway, the most common of which is a 21-hydroxylase deficiency, which accounts for 95% of all cases of CAH. These enzyme defects lead to diminished production of cortisol, which results in increased levels of ACTH. This, in turn, stimulates adrenal hyperplasia and steroid production as the body attempts to overcome the enzyme deficiency. The block is usually partial, and the patient may be capable of maintaining normal levels of cortisol and aldosterone under normal circumstances at the expense of the accumulation of steroid precursors that are diverted down other metabolic pathways. Commonly there is hypersecretion of various androgens including DHEA and androstenedione, which after peripheral conversion to testosterone, may lead to precocious puberty in males and varying degrees of masculinization and sexual dysfunction in females.

Symptoms in CAH are related to both the decrease in the final product of metabolism and the accumulation of its precursors. In the case of 21-hydroxylase deficiency, there is an accumulation of 17-hydroxyprogesterone and other precursors. These compounds may exhibit antimineralocorticoid activity by binding to the mineralocorticoid receptor, which can exacerbate the salt-wasting tendency. Plasma renin levels increase in response, triggering greater demand for aldosterone synthesis, which also requires 21-hydroxylase activity. Severely affected individuals come to medical attention within 1 to 4 weeks of birth. Their nonspecific symptoms, such as poor appetite, vomiting, lethargy, and failure to thrive, may be mistaken for formula intolerance, colic, sepsis, pyloric stenosis, etc. On physical examination the child may appear gray or mottled with an unobtainable blood pressure value. If the deficiency is partial, the salt-losing tendency is compensated; as little as 2% of normal enzyme activity is sufficient to prevent salt wasting. If the loss of enzyme activity is more complete, more severe salt wasting will occur and an addisonian crisis (see p. 890) is

---

MAJOR CAUSES AND CLINICAL FEATURES OF PRIMARY HYPERALDOSTERONISM (CONN'S SYNDROME)

Causes
Adrenal aldosterone-producing adenoma, APA (70% of cases)
Idiopathic hyperaldosteronism, IHA (30% of cases)

Clinical Features
Hypertension
Symptoms resulting from hypokalemia
   Muscle weakness
   Polyuria and polydipsia
   ECG changes
   Glucose intolerance

more likely. The non–salt wasting variant of this condition, seen in two thirds of patients with this disorder, is primarily characterized by the problems associated with increased androgens. The less severe deficiencies may not become clinically apparent until after puberty. Without treatment the excess androgen results in precocious development in both males and females with rapid growth, pubic hair, and acne at an early age. There is also premature epiphyseal closure. Additional problems for females include clitoromegaly, deepening voice, increased muscle mass, failure of breast development, primary amenorrhea, and facial hair.

The 21-hydroxylase deficiency is inherited through an autosomal recessive trait with an estimated heterozygote frequency of approximately 1 in 50 of the population. The approximate frequency of homozygous 21-hydroxylase deficiency causing CAH is 1 in 10,000 births (male/female ratio 1:1). Mild, nonclassic 21-hydroxylase deficiency is much more common, with a prevalence of 1 in 1000 in the general population. The prevalence is much higher in some populations; for example, among Ashkenazi Jews it may be as high as 1 in 30. Because of the high incidence of non-classic CAH, some have questioned whether it is a true disease or simply a common genetic variant (polymorphism). Heterozygous carrier estimates for nonclassic CAH may be as high as 10% of the population.

A deficiency of 11-hydroxylase (gene product of CYP 11B1) is the second most common cause of CAH, affecting 1 in 100,000 newborns. However, the prevalence is much higher in Jewish immigrants from Morocco (1 in 5000). Again, depending on the severity of the deficiency, cortisol production may or may not be adequate. A unique feature of this enzyme deficiency is the accumulation of 11-deoxy-corticosterone, a precursor in the aldosterone pathway. This steroid and its metabolites promote sodium resorption and therefore can cause hypertension. Approximately two thirds of patients with this deficiency have an elevated blood pressure in the first few years of life along with other complications of hypertension. The majority also have hypo-kalemia, muscle wasting, and cramping. Excess androgen production is also a problem leading to masculinization, abnormal genitalia in females, rapid somatic growth, premature closure of epiphyses, short adult stature, acne, premature adrenarche, amenorrhea, and precocious puberty. Nonclassic forms of 11-hydroxylase deficiency also occur but are much less common than nonclassic 21-hydroxylase deficiency.

Treatment for both of these forms of CAH is simply glucocorticoid replacement therapy. Female patients in addition require surgical correction for ambiguous genitalia. Male patients tend to respond well to therapy, whereas female patients, despite adequate therapy, have a high incidence of sexual identity disorders, infertility, hirsutism, and virilization.

High cortisol concentrations within the adrenal gland are required to induce the enzyme responsible for conversion of norepinephrine to epinephrine within the adrenal. Therefore an additional feature associated with CAH is the reduced output of epinephrine from the adrenal because of the lower concentrations of cortisol within the adrenal gland. Exogenous glucocorticoid therapy may also exacerbate this deficiency because endogenous production by the adrenal will be suppressed.

Hypoadrenalism. Adrenal hypofunction or insufficiency can be caused by (1) primary adrenal disease, involving the entire adrenal cortex; (2) secondary adrenal insufficiency caused by decreased levels of CRH or ACTH, as a result of pituitary or hypothalamic disease; or (3) long-term suppression of the hypothalamic-pituitary-adrenal axis by gluco-corticoids, which leads to adrenal atrophy. Secondary adrenal insufficiency resulting from decreased ACTH or CRH is discussed further in Chapter 43.

Addison's disease. Primary adrenal hypofunction or insufficiency, also known as *Addison's disease*, is relatively rare (estimated prevalence 1 in 50,000). A major cause of Addison's disease today, accounting for 70% of all cases, is autoimmune adrenalitis with circulating adrenal antibodies. This disorder may be associated with other autoimmune disorders such as Hashimoto's thyroiditis, hypoparathyroidism, diabetes mellitus, pernicious anemia, vitiligo, and primary ovarian failure. Polyglandular autoimmune disease type II (Schmidt's syndrome) is a form of Addison's that occurs most commonly in females age 20 to 40. A rarer form, type I occurs in children and is associated with chronic mucocutaneous candidiasis and hypoparathyroidism. In both forms an adrenal autoantibody is directed frequently against the enzyme 21-hydroxylase. Other causes of primary adrenal failure are listed in the box. Tuberculosis was the leading cause of adrenal failure in the first half of this century.

Symptoms of Addison's disease begin to appear after about 90% of the adrenal cortex has been destroyed (see box below). The disease usually develops slowly with progressive loss of cortisol and increasing ACTH levels, resulting in hyperpigmentation of the patient because of the melanocyte-

---

MAJOR CAUSES AND CLINICAL FEATURES OF PRIMARY ADRENAL INSUFFICIENCY

Causes	*Clinical Features*
Autoimmune adrenalitis	Muscle weakness
Granulomatous disease	Fatigue
Tuberculosis	Weight loss
Histoplasmosis	Orthostatic hypotension
Sarcoidosis	Pigmentation
Neoplastic infiltration	Anorexia
Hemochromatosis	Addisonian crisis
Amyloidosis	Fever
Bilateral adrenalectomy	Dehydration
Infarction	Nausea
Infectious disease	Hypotension
Drugs (metyrapone,	Shock
ketoconazole, mitotane)	Abdominal pain
Adrenoleukodystrophy	
Congenital adrenal hyperplasia	

stimulating hormone properties of ACTH. Because of coincident aldosterone deficiency, there is sodium loss and potassium retention. Hypoglycemia may be present because of cortisol deficiency. These symptoms may be vague and nonspecific. However, some patients may be seen with an acute life-threatening disease that is termed an *addisonian crisis* after stress caused by illness, surgery, or trauma. An addisonian crisis is a result of an acute deficiency of both mineralocorticoids and glucocorticoids. An addisonian crisis, the signs of which are listed in the box, can rapidly evolve into circulatory shock. Hyperkalemia and hyponatremia are common laboratory findings along with hemoconcentration and elevated urea levels resulting from fluid loss. The hyperkalemia may be severe enough to induce cardiac arrhythmias and cardiac arrest.

Congenital adrenal hyperplasia, discussed in the previous section, can result in primary adrenal insufficiency. Certain drugs, such as metyrapone used in the treatment of Cushing's syndrome, *o,p'*-DDD (mitotane) used in the treatment of adrenal cancer, and other therapeutic agents such as ketoconazole and etomidate, which interfere with steroid synthetic pathways, all have the potential to cause primary adrenal insufficiency.

The X-linked form of **adrenoleukodystrophy** (ALD) should also be considered in the differential diagnosis of primary adrenal insufficiency in the male patient. It occurs more frequently than recognized, with up to 40% of males with Addison's disease having this problem. The defect is caused by a deficiency of a peroxisomal enzyme (lignoceroyl CoA ligase), which results in decreased oxidation and therefore accumulation of very long chain fatty acids (VLCFAs). Pathological changes are found in the adrenal cortex, testes, CNS white matter, and the peripheral nervous system. The cells of the adrenal gland in the zona fasciculata and zona reticularis tissues become swollen with lamellar inclusions consisting of cholesterol esters of VLCFAs and eventually atrophy and die. Patients with ALD may present with adrenal insufficiency alone, both neurological and adrenal problems, or neurological problems alone. The neurological problems include emotional lability, failure at school, and hyperactivity that progresses to visual impairment, diffuse cerebral demyelination, seizures, mental deterioration, and death.

The primary adrenal insufficiency in ALD is mainly the result of diminished cortisol reserve. Primary gonadal insufficiency is a problem in 20% of patients with decreased testosterone and increased gonadotropins. Bone marrow transplantation may arrest progression of the disease in those with mild neurological disorder at the time of treatment.

Patients with secondary adrenal insufficiency do not usually experience symptoms related to hypoaldosteronism because aldosterone synthesis and secretion depend on the renin-angiotensin system rather than on ACTH. Hyperpigmentation is also not a feature of this disorder. However, patients with secondary adrenal insufficiency may show other signs of hypothalamic or pituitary disease including concomitant hypogonadism and hypothyroidism. Symptoms common to both primary and secondary disease of the adrenal cortex include weakness, hypoglycemia, weight loss, and gastrointestinal discomfort.

Patients prescribed glucocorticoid therapy for 3 weeks or less generally only experience transient hypothalamic-pituitary-adrenal axis suppression. In cases of long-term treatment, dosages need to be tapered gradually.

Disorder of the Adrenal Medulla: Pheochromocytoma

Pheochromocytoma, a relatively rare, usually benign tumor arising from chromaffin cells, results in hypersecretion of the catecholamines epinephrine and norepinephrine. It is estimated that at least 0.1% of patients with persistent diastolic hypertension may have this tumor. Although it is a rare cause of hypertension, it is important to diagnose because it is surgically curable, and, even more significantly, it can cause death from acute hypertensive attacks. Despite its rarity (prevalence in patients with adrenal incidentalomas ranges from 2% to 13%), all patients with an adrenal mass need to be screened for this condition. This tumor can occur as an isolated problem at any age; for example, 10% of pheochromocytomas are reported in children. Overall incidence is estimated at 1 to 2 per 100,000. The autopsy incidence is considerably higher at 0.3%. Pheochromocytomas are most commonly discovered in the third to fifth decades of life.

Approximately 90% of pheochromocytomas occur in the adrenal glands, with the remainder occurring in extraadrenal chromaffin cells, anywhere from the base of the brain to the lower abdomen. Approximately 10% of pheochromocytomas are bilateral or multiple, and approximately 10% are malignant. Pheochromocytomas also occur as an inheritable disorder. In this case they may be associated with multiple endocrine neoplasia (MEN) type 2A syndrome, which manifests as pheochromocytoma, hyperparathyroidism, and medullary carcinoma of the thyroid, or MEN type 2B, which manifests as multiple mucosal neuromas, medullary carcinoma of the thyroid, and pheochromocytoma. Approximately 50% of patients with MEN 2A or B will develop a pheochromocytoma. There is also a significant association with neurofibromatosis (von Recklinghausen's disease), with up to 5% of patients developing a pheochromocytoma, and with von Hippel-Lindau disease with 20% of patients possibly affected. MEN 2A and 2B result from mutations in the RET protooncogene.

Pheochromocytomas may release their hormones in a sustained or episodic fashion. Clinically the most significant finding is persistent or paroxysmal hypertension; other common findings are summarized in the box on p. 891. Many of the symptoms may be persistent or episodic, although some patients are totally asymptomatic. Episodes can be as infrequent as once every few weeks or as frequent as 20 to 30 times daily, with attacks persisting for less than a minute or for as long as a week. The symptom pattern depends on the specific catecholamine secreted by the tumor. Rarely, hypotension may be the clinical problem. This is the case if the tumor primarily secretes epinephrine, dopa, or dopamine. Some patients may first come to the physician with cardiac

MAJOR CAUSES AND CLINICAL FEATURES OF PHEOCHROMOCYTOMA

Causes

Benign adrenal chromaffin cell tumor (80%)

Malignant adrenal chromaffin cell tumor (10%)

Extraadrenal chromaffin cell tumor (10%)

Clinical Features

Episodic or sustained hypertension

Headache

Sweating

Palpitations with or without tachycardia

Nervousness

Weight loss

Nausea

Weakness or fatigue

Less common:

Flushing

Dyspnea

Dizziness

---

hypertrophy or cardiac failure. It must be emphasized that the clinical symptoms are often subtle. A high degree of clinical alertness is required from the physician. The symptoms are not specific for pheochromocytoma. A common cause of death in patients with unsuspected pheochromocytoma is hypertensive or hypotensive crisis precipitated by surgery. Paroxysmal attacks may be precipitated by palpation of the tumor, postural changes, emotional trauma, and even rarely micturition (in the case of a rare bladder tumor).

CHANGE OF ANALYTE IN DISEASE (Table 46-1)
Hyperadrenalism

Cushing's syndrome. In the laboratory investigation of Cushing's syndrome, the first step is to establish that the patient actually has autonomous cortisol production, or Cushing's syndrome. Once this is established, the next step is to differentiate the cause of the Cushing's syndrome.

One of the simplest and most important tests to perform initially is the overnight **dexamethasone suppression test**. Dexamethasone is a synthetic glucocorticoid that is 30 times as potent as cortisol, and it does not cross-react in standard immunoassays for cortisol. The patient is given a tablet containing 1 mg of dexamethasone and instructed to take it at 11 PM and come to the laboratory for plasma cortisol determination at 8:00 the following morning. A morning cortisol level less than 140 nmol/L (50 µg/L) usually excludes any cause of hypercortisolism. This is a normal response. Levels greater than 280 nmol/L (100 µg/L) indicate hypercortisolism. This test has a reported sensitivity of 95% to 98% for Cushing's syndrome. The specificity is not as good, and false-positive results can be seen in patients with some forms of mental depression, stress-induced hypercortisolism, pseudo–Cushing's syndrome resulting from chronic alcoholism, and increased levels of cortisol-binding globulin associated with pregnancy or the use of birth control pills. False-positive results are also seen in patients receiving drugs such as phenytoin or rifampin that increase the rate of clearance of dexamethasone. However, the dexamethasone suppression test remains an ideal screening test for Cushing's syndrome, because false-negative results are a more serious problem than false-positive results in screening procedures. To minimize false-negative results, some centers lower the expected cortisol suppression to below 85 nmol/L (30 µg/L).

Another useful initial investigative test is the estimation of a 24-hour urine free cortisol level. This is in essence a direct measure of the amount of cortisol that is not bound to plasma

---

TABLE 46-1   CHANGE OF ANALYTE WITH DISEASE

Disease	24-hour Urinary Free Cortisol	17-OHCS	Plasma ACTH	Urinary Aldosterone	Plasma Aldosterone	Plasma Cortisol	Plasma Renin Activity	Urine or Plasma Catecholamines	Urine Vanillylmandelic Acid and Metanephrine
Hypercortical Disease									
Primary Cushing's syndrome	↑	↑	↓			±			
Cushing's disease (secondary)	↑	↑	±			±			
Ectopic ACTH	↑	↑	↑			±			
Primary hyperaldosteronism				↑	↑		↓		
Secondary hyperaldosteronism				↑	↑		↑		
Hypocortical Disease									
Primary	±	↓	↑			↓			
Secondary	±	↓	↓			↓			
Pheochromocytoma								↑	↑

↑, Elevated; ±, variable response; ↓, diminished.
ACTH, Adrenocorticotropic hormone; 17-OHCS, 17-hydroxycorticosteroid.

protein and is thus excreted unmetabolized in the urine over a 24-hour period. This test also has good sensitivity (95%) for Cushing's syndrome. However, some claim the sensitivity is closer to 90%. This is largely a function of the method used for urine free cortisol determination and the decision levels. A 24-hour urine cortisol determination is required along with a urine creatinine determination to ensure the adequacy of collection. It is also suggested by some that up to three separate 24-hour collections be carried out because of the variability of cortisol output. The measurement of other steroid metabolites in urine that reflect glucocorticoid output, such as 17-hydroxycorticosteroids and 17-ketogenic steroids, is not considered reliable. Immunoassays for urine free cortisol are not specific enough for accurate estimation. Metabolites of cortisol and their conjugated products cross-react with the antibodies employed and therefore consistently overestimate the true urine free cortisol concentration. Even if an extraction step is included to remove the more water-soluble conjugates, results may be twice as high as the true value. The most accurate way to determine urine free cortisol is by high-performance liquid chromatography (HPLC) analysis.

A traditional test that is no longer part of the standard work-up for Cushing's syndrome is the morning and afternoon serum cortisol determination. Plasma cortisol values usually display diurnal variation, with the highest levels occurring in the morning and the lowest levels in the early evening. Evening values are usually less than 50% of the early morning concentrations. Classically, samples are drawn at 8 AM (reference interval 140 to 660 nmol/L, 50 to 239 µg/L) and 4 PM (reference interval 50 to 330 nmol/L, 18 to 119 µg/L). Many patients with Cushing's syndrome will not show this diurnal variation and will have elevated concentrations at both times. However, the release of cortisol is episodic, and there is considerable overlap between healthy individuals and patients with Cushing's syndrome. To differentiate patients with Cushing's syndrome from healthy patients it is best to take the sample at the time when cortisol is usually at its lowest concentration in the circulation. This time happens to be at midnight, and because it is not always practical to draw blood at this time, the more practical time of 4 PM is often chosen. Midnight plasma cortisol levels greater than 420 nmol/L (152 µg/L) are highly suggestive of hypercortisolism. Levels >50 nmol/L are 100% sensitive for Cushing's. Loss of diurnal variation can also occur with stress, anorexia, obesity, and emotional disturbances, or it may be secondary to sedatives, stimulants, or psychotropic or antiepileptic drugs.

Another variation of the overnight dexamethasone suppression test is the low-dose dexamethasone suppression test, which can also be used to confirm that the patient has Cushing's syndrome. This test is more time consuming and is not included in some of the recent protocols for this disorder. Some now suggest that the high-dose dexamethasone suppression test, which is discussed below, should be done first. In the classic low-dose dexamethasone suppression test the patient is given a total dose of 2 mg of dexametha-

sone per day for 2 days in 0.5-mg doses every 6 hours. This dose is equivalent to about four times the usual adrenal output. During the second day a 24-hour urine specimen is collected for urine free cortisol. Plasma cortisol measurements may also be performed. Patients with Cushing's syndrome generally will not show significant suppression of cortisol output with this dose of dexamethasone. Normal patients should show greater than 50% suppression of the urine cortisol output present before the test. Urine cortisol excretion usually falls to less than 50 nmol/day (18 µg/day) and morning serum cortisol to less than 140 nmol/L (50 µg/L). For higher sensitivity a normal result could be set at <50 nmol/L for serum cortisol. Generally obesity can be excluded as the cause of the increased cortisol with this test but false-positive results may still be seen with psychiatric illness, alcoholism, stress, glucocorticoid resistance, decreased absorbance of dexamethasone, drugs that stimulate liver metabolism (phenytoin, phenobarbital), and in people who don't follow instructions for performing the test. False-negative results are associated with chronic renal failure and hypothyroidism.

Once Cushing's syndrome has been confirmed the cause of the disease needs to be determined. There are several possible approaches that can be used to determine the cause of Cushing's syndrome. A high-dose dexamethasone suppression test can be performed. This can be done as an overnight procedure using 8 mg of dexamethasone, or it can be carried out over 2 days, giving a total of 8 mg of dexamethasone per day divided into four doses of 2 mg every 6 hours. The response can be assessed by measurements of plasma cortisol or 24-hour urine free cortisol. Patients who have pituitary tumors secreting excess ACTH (Cushing's disease) will show greater than 50% suppression of the glucocorticoid output after the high-dose dexamethasone suppression test because pituitary tumors remain responsive to negative feedback, though requiring higher levels of corticosteroid than normal. Patients with adrenal tumors or ectopic sources of ACTH will fail to show suppression of glucocorticoids. Anomalous responses, however, do occur. Higher doses of dexamethasone, up to 32 mg, have been used in some studies to confirm lack of suppression.

Plasma ACTH levels, which can be measured by radioimmunoassay, are essential in determining the specific cause of Cushing's syndrome. ACTH is a labile polypeptide hormone, and special precautions are required in its handling. Plasma samples should be collected on ice, and the plasma should be separated in a refrigerated centrifuge and stored frozen. ACTH is now measured by two-site immunometric assays that have better precision, specificity, and sensitivity than a traditional competitive radioimmunoassay. However, the new assays do not measure fragments of ACTH and do not react well with "big" ACTH, a precursor to ACTH that is produced by some tumors. Less specific radioimmunoassays may be better in these situations. ACTH levels in the upper half of the reference interval (<11.4 pmol/L) and up to twice the upper limit of normal are consistent with a pituitary cause of Cushing's syndrome. Nondetectable levels of ACTH (less than 2 pmol/L) are suggestive of an adrenal tumor. Very high levels of ACTH (greater than 50 pmol/L) are suggestive of an ectopic source, such as a malignant tumor. There is overlap in the plasma concentrations of ACTH associated with ectopic and pituitary causes of Cushing's syndrome.

The **metyrapone stimulation test** has also been used to delineate the cause of Cushing's syndrome. Metyrapone acts by inhibiting the enzyme 11-hydroxylase and therefore blocking the synthesis of cortisol. In healthy patients, the cortisol level drops, and ACTH levels will increase because of loss of negative-feedback inhibition from cortisol. The response to metyrapone can be determined by measurement of either serum or plasma 11-deoxycortisol or urine 17-hydroxycorticosteroids. The following protocol is recommended: First measure the baseline serum cortisol and 11-deoxycortisol values in serum at 8 AM. Give the patient 750 mg of metyrapone every 4 hours for 24 hours, and then repeat the measurement of serum cortisol and 11-deoxycortisol. In Cushing's syndrome caused by a pituitary tumor the ACTH response remains intact, and 11-deoxycortisol levels increase to levels greater than 200 nmol/L. Levels of 11-deoxycortisol that are less than this are consistent with an adrenal tumor or ectopic ACTH. Some investigators have suggested that this test may be better than the high-dose dexamethasone suppression test in determining the cause of Cushing's syndrome; however, most laboratories do not perform this protocol because of the lack of ready availability of an 11-deoxycortisol assay.

If ACTH is suppressed in a patient with Cushing's syndrome, a CT scan is usually successful in identifying the adrenal lesion. Adrenal adenomas are usually obvious because the adjacent normal adrenal tissue and the contralateral adrenal have become atrophic. With adrenal carcinoma the gland is usually very large, with dimensions that exceed 6 cm. Other features that help distinguish between adrenal adenoma and carcinoma include increased androgen production associated with adrenal carcinoma; benign tumors may respond to ACTH and malignant tumors are usually pleomorphic and invasive.

The most difficult causes of Cushing's to differentiate are ectopic ACTH production and a pituitary adenoma. This differentiation was not necessary until the 1970s because bilateral adrenalectomy was standard treatment for both. Starting in the late 1970s transsphenoidal surgery became the treatment of choice for pituitary adenoma. It subsequently became clear that not all patients with an apparent pituitary adenoma had this problem. Patients with bronchial carcinoids most often had biochemical parameters, including ACTH and high-dose dexamethasone suppression test results, which were similar to those patients with Cushing's disease. These slow-growing tumors were not radiologically apparent for years in some cases. Pituitary imaging techniques may give high rates of false-positive (10% pituitary incidentalomas) and false-negative results (up to 40% of patients with pituitary adenoma not visible on MRI even with gadolinium enhancement). False-negative results are usually a problem with small pituitary tumors. The false-positive

results occur because of the high incidence of nonfunctional pituitary tumors. CT scan of the abdomen generally reveals bilateral adrenal enlargement in ACTH-dependent Cushing's, nodular hyperplasia in 10%, and normal adrenal size is seen in up to 30% of cases. Nuclear medicine scintigraphic imaging studies with indium-labeled pentetreotide can be used to visualize ectopic sources of ACTH that express somatostatin receptors. Labeled cholesterol may be useful with some malignant adrenal tumors and PET scans may help identify adrenal tumors and ectopic ACTH sources.

There was some hope that the corticotropin-releasing hormone (CRH) stimulation test would be more helpful. In principle, ACTH-secreting pituitary tumors usually retain CRH receptors whereas ectopic sources of ACTH should theoretically not express CRH receptors, and after the administration of 100 µg of CRH, pituitary tumors should respond with a brisk increase in ACTH release. Patients with other causes of Cushing's syndrome should theoretically show no response. Unfortunately, as with the previously discussed tests, false-positive and false-negative results do occur. The overall diagnostic accuracy of the CRH stimulation test is approximately 90%, which is only marginally better than that of the high-dose dexamethasone suppression test.

The test that is now considered definitive in the differentiation of pituitary causes of Cushing's syndrome from other causes is bilateral inferior petrosal sinus sampling after CRH administration. In this test a radiologist inserts catheters into both inferior petrosal sinuses, which drain from the anterior pituitary. Venous samples are drawn before and 2, 5, and 10 minutes after 100 µg of CRH has been administered intravenously. The ACTH gradient between the inferior petrosal sinus and peripheral venous sites after CRH stimulation is greater than 2 or 3 if the patient has a pituitary tumor. The average gradient seen in patients with a pituitary tumor secreting ACTH is about 50. A gradient of less than 2 indicates a nonpituitary source of ACTH. Because samples are taken simultaneously from the right and left sinuses, it is possible to localize the tumor to the right or left side of the anterior pituitary in about 80% of cases. This is useful information for subsequent surgical procedures. If there is no identifiable lesion, the surgeon may remove only the left or right side of the pituitary, thereby lessening the risk of panhypopituitarism.

The petrosal sinus sampling procedure is demanding and requires a skilled radiologist and complications may arise. Therefore not everyone agrees that this test should be performed routinely in all patients who are suspected of having pituitary tumors. Data from the National Institutes of Health (NIH) indicate that a 50% suppression of cortisol output by high-dose dexamethasone may be inadequate to confirm that the patient has a pituitary tumor. They recommend that for the confirmation of the diagnosis of a pituitary tumor the urine free cortisol be decreased by 90% from baseline value. In NIH experience, no patient with ectopic ACTH experienced cortisol suppression to this degree. The more invasive petrosal sampling protocol described earlier may then be reserved for those patients who show only partial suppression of urine cortisol excretion.

Pituitary Cushing's syndrome is much more common in women than in men, with a female-to-male ratio of 7 or 8 to 1, whereas with ectopic ACTH the ratio is approximately equal. Forty percent of men with Cushing's syndrome may have an ectopic source of ACTH. As mentioned earlier, the presence of bronchial carcinoids can cause confusion in the diagnostic protocol. Petrosal vein sampling for ACTH helps to resolve this confusion. Localizing bronchial carcinoids remains a problem because they are small and slow growing. These tumors are benign but have malignant potential and must eventually be found. Localization of ectopic sources of ACTH can be one of the most difficult tasks in endocrinology despite the availability of many imaging tools.

Miscellaneous tests for the investigation of Cushing's syndrome. Measurement of salivary cortisol has been proposed for the investigation of Cushing's syndrome; the

sample is collected at 11 PM, which is the usual nadir of cortisol secretion. Salivary cortisol shows a strong correlation with free plasma cortisol. Other new tests have been developed to aid in the distinction of mild Cushing's from pseudo–Cushing's syndrome. A 48-hour low-dose dexamethasone suppression test is followed by an immediate CRH stimulation test. In this test cortisol should remain suppressed in normals and pseudo–Cushing's syndrome but not in those with Cushing's syndrome.

Another test to help distinguish ectopic ACTH from a pituitary source is the combined desmopressin plus CRH stimulation test. A dramatic rise should be seen in the case of a pituitary tumor but not with an ectopic tumor. The problem is at this time there are insufficient data to confirm the validity of this approach.

In summary, if a patient is suspected of having Cushing's syndrome, begin with an overnight dexamethasone suppression test. Confirm a positive result with a 24-hour urine free

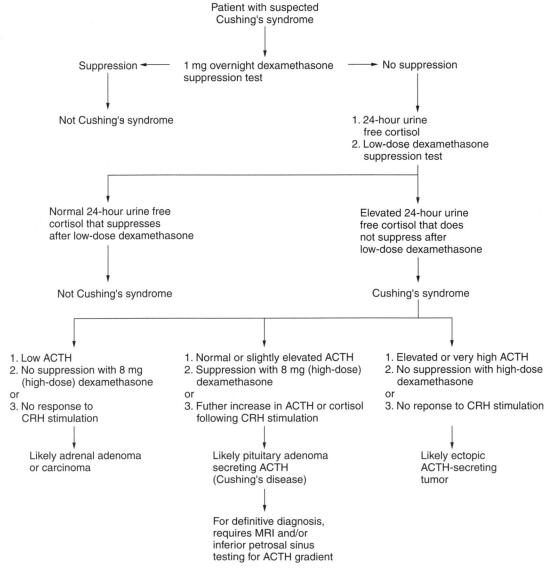

Fig. 46-9 Laboratory protocol for the investigation of Cushing's syndrome. See text for details.

cortisol with or without a subsequent low-dose dexamethasone suppression test. To determine the cause of Cushing's syndrome, ACTH measurements and the urine and serum cortisol responses to high-dose dexamethasone are useful. In centers in which CRH testing is available, measurement of the ACTH response to CRH administration can be used in determining the cause of the excess cortisol. Finally, if the results of the investigation are not definitive, bilateral petrosal sinus sampling for ACTH after CRH administration should provide a definitive diagnosis. See Fig. 46-9 for an outline of the diagnostic protocol. The most common classic approach has been outlined in this figure but there are almost as many variations as there are endocrinologists.

Primary hyperaldosteronism. Conn's syndrome, or primary hyperaldosteronism, is a rare cause of hypertension (although some recent reports suggest that it might not be so rare). The classic investigation process leading to a diagnosis for this disorder is costly and time consuming, and therefore patients with hypertension should be investigated for this disorder only when indicated. A scheme for the investigation of primary hyperaldosteronism is outlined in Fig. 46-10. The laboratory should play a major part in advising on the collection and handling of the specimens required for these expensive investigations to ensure a successful outcome. The simplest method for screening for this disorder is the measurement of serum and urine potassium when the patient is not receiving diuretics. Primary aldosteronism should be suspected in all patients with spontaneous hypokalemia. It should also be suspected in those who become hypokalemic on a high-salt diet or in those who develop hypokalemia very quickly when taking diuretics. If the potassium is low, the next step in the investigation is to determine 24-hour urine potassium and sodium values. Values of serum potassium of less than 3.5 mmol/L along with a urine potassium excretion rate of greater than 30 mmol/24 hours are not usually seen with essential hypertension but are commonly seen with primary hyperaldosteronism. The 24-hour urine sodium should be ≥100 mmol/L for the urine potassium result to be valid; a low sodium intake may decrease potassium excretion and yield a false-negative result. This screen is not entirely reliable because a serum potassium level within the reference interval may be seen in some patients with primary hyperaldosteronism. The test may have to be repeated on two or three occasions.

The confirmation of the diagnosis of primary aldosteronism is dependent on the demonstration in serum of both a suppressed renin concentration and an increased aldosterone. Diuretics and spironolactone should be discontinued for at least 4 weeks before assessment of the patient.

Aldosterone is generally measured under conditions that will ordinarily suppress its secretion. This can most simply be carried out by prescribing for the patient a regimen that entails a moderately large sodium intake for 1 week (>100 mmol/day). Plasma aldosterone is then measured in the morning with the patient in a supine position. A second specimen, drawn 4 hours after the patient assumes an upright position, is used for measurement of plasma aldosterone and renin activity. The diagnosis of primary aldosteronism is confirmed if the supine plasma aldosterone is >150 ng/L (420 pmol/L) and the upright renin activity is <1 ng/mL/

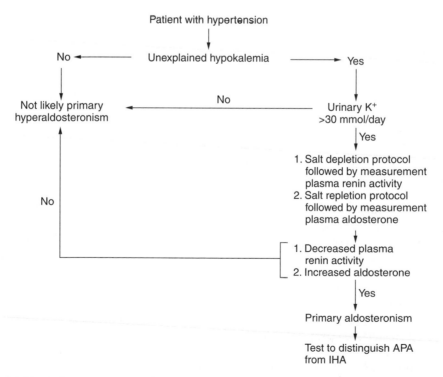

Fig. 46-10   Laboratory protocol for the investigation of a patient with suspected primary hyperaldosteronism (Conn's syndrome). Alternative approaches may be used (see text).

hour. A simultaneous measurement of aldosterone in a 24-hour urine collection should be >65 mg/day in a patient with Conn's syndrome.

Another approach is to measure supine plasma aldosterone before and after infusion of 2 L of normal saline over a 4-hour time span. Normal patients and patients with essential hypertension will have plasma aldosterone suppressed to <50 ng/L (140 pmol/L). This test is not advised in patients with evidence of heart failure. Because the patient must be carefully monitored, this is an expensive test to perform.

Plasma renin activity may also be measured after challenge with a low-salt diet (<20 mmol/day) for 3 days, or after a 1-day low-salt diet followed by ingestion of 40 mg of furosemide taken three times during the day. A plasma sample is taken the following day after 4 hours in the upright position. This procedure causes salt and water depletion. Normal patients and patients with essential hypertension will respond with an increase in renin activity, whereas patients with primary hyperaldosteronism will not respond, and renin activity will remain low.

Low plasma renin activity may also be seen with congenital adrenal hyperplasia caused by 11-hydroxylase deficiency, excessive licorice ingestion, and low-renin essential hypertension.

If the results are ambiguous, the **captopril suppression test** may be useful. Captopril is a drug used to treat some patients with hypertension. Its primary mechanism of action is inhibition of angiotensin-converting enzyme, which converts angiotensin I to angiotensin II. Patients without Conn's syndrome will respond with a drop in plasma aldosterone, but patients with Conn's syndrome will not suppress the aldosterone levels. Aldosterone is usually measured 2 to 3 hours after a 25 mg oral dose of captopril. The expected response is that plasma aldosterone should decrease to <100 ng/L (<280 pmol/L).

Once the diagnosis of primary aldosteronism has been established, the cause of the disorder must be determined so that the proper course of treatment can be chosen. Surgical adrenalectomy is indicated for aldosterone-producing adenoma (APA), whereas medical therapy is required for idiopathic hyperaldosteronism (IHA). Several tests can be used to accomplish this task. The availability and accuracy of these tests vary, and a direct approach employing radiological imaging is limited because lesions associated with primary aldosteronism may be small (<2 cm). Also, non-functioning adrenal masses are quite common and may give false-positive results. The overall accuracy of imaging is only 75%. Slightly better results are seen when biochemical responses to posture change are used. In patients with APA, aldosterone levels may drop after assumption of an upright posture, whereas in patients with IHA, aldosterone usually rises. This indicates that plasma renin activity (PRA) may still be involved in aldosterone regulation in patients with IHA despite the low PRA levels. Another biochemical difference that can be measured involves 18-hydroxycorticosterone. The level of this substance is higher in patients with APA than in patients with IHA. This test has limited availability.

Adrenal imaging with radioactively labeled iodocholesterol can accurately locate the tumor in 90% of patients with APA. The ^{131}I-labeled cholesterol should be administered after dexamethasone treatment to reduce uptake by healthy adrenal tissue.

The best procedure for localizing the lesion is bilateral adrenal venous sampling. The ratio of the ipsilateral to contralateral concentration of serum aldosterone is usually greater than 10:1. The success of this procedure is dependent on the ability of the radiologist to place the catheter accurately. The results can be improved by simultaneous determination of ACTH-stimulated cortisol from both adrenal veins, which should be symmetrical. Although this test is considered the standard, it is usually reserved for those cases in which the simpler tests are inconclusive.

After adrenalectomy for APA, 70% of patients are normotensive 1 year later. Drugs such as amiloride and spironolactone have been used to treat IHA. Surprisingly, some patients respond to angiotensin-converting enzyme inhibitors. Such a response again indicates that angiotensin II may be playing a role in IHA.

The previous, classic approach to screening, confirmation, and localization of the tumor in Conn's syndrome often begins with the detection of hypokalemia, although it is estimated that 7% to 38% of patients do not have hypokalemia. Because of this some investigators have suggested that all hypertensive patients unresponsive to medical treatment be screened by determining their random serum/plasma aldosterone to plasma renin activity ratio (ARR). An abnormal ratio (using reference intervals established with the methods used in the laboratory) result should be confirmed with an acute saline suppression test as described earlier. It is also recommended that to diagnosis Conn's syndrome, in addition to an elevated ARR, the plasma aldosterone level must also be increased above the normal reference interval. This extra precaution is needed because an increased ARR may be seen when the plasma renin activity is low and there is a low normal aldosterone concentration. Elevated ARR may also be seen in patients with chronic renal disease and hyperkalemia, which stimulates aldosterone secretion directly. The ARR should only be used as a screening procedure.

An advantage of the ARR is that there are no posture restrictions when drawing the sample; generally the patient only needs to be seated for the blood draw. The test may be performed while the patient is taking antihypertensive medications except for spironolactone. However, ACE inhibitors may falsely increase the PRA in some patients with primary hyperaldosteronism. A suppressed PRA in the presence of an ACE inhibitor, however, is a strong indicator of primary aldosteronism.

A problem in the localization and confirmation of Conn's syndrome is the presence of adrenal incidentalomas, which can lead to a false diagnosis of adrenal adenoma when the actual diagnosis is bilateral hyperplasia. Another concern is that in the presence of hypokalemia the aldosterone may be suppressed, giving a false impression of an appropriate level

increases or normal levels of norepinephrine and dopamine. This last pattern is seen only in association with adrenal tumors. Some malignant pheochromocytomas may secrete large amounts of dopamine primarily. This is the result of a deficiency of dopamine-β-hydroxylase in malignant cells. The reference intervals for urine norepinephrine, epinephrine, and dopamine are up to 470, 160, and 3300 nmol/day, respectively. An increase in urine norepinephrine is one of the more specific findings associated with pheochromocytoma when a value greater than 900 nmol/day (approximately twice the upper reference level) is used as the decision level. At this concentration, specificity of the assay is greatly improved without loss of sensitivity. Urine norepinephrine measurements are especially useful when the patient has episodic hypertension of short duration. A random urine sample collected shortly after the attack may indicate abnormal catecholamine excretion, whereas the metabolite concentrations may be normal. The results for all these urine metabolites must be normalized for urine creatinine.

There has been considerable interest in plasma catecholamine measurements, especially in combination with the clonidine suppression test. The analysis of plasma catecholamines is very difficult because the concentrations are very low and the compounds very labile. Many conditions can cause elevations of plasma catecholamines into the range seen in patients with pheochromocytoma, including volume depletion, anxiety, exercise, anorexia, smoking, renal failure, obesity, and several drugs such as L-dopa and methyldopa. Sensitivity of plasma catecholamine measurements for the diagnosis of pheochromocytoma may be as high as 95%, but the specificity is suboptimal. Using higher, more specific decision levels results in a drop in sensitivity. With plasma catecholamines, despite precautions to minimize stress during the evaluation period, a significant portion of patients with essential hypertension may have plasma norepinephrine concentrations in the equivocal range that could be the result of increased activity of the sympathetic nervous system (SNS). Before collection of blood for plasma catecholamine determination, the patient should be resting in a supine position with an indwelling catheter for one half hour to avoid stress related to the collection procedure.

The measurement of catecholamines in a 24-hour urine sample has several advantages. Urine collections induce minimal stress in the patient, and integration of production of catecholamines over 24 hours minimizes fluctuations in SNS activity. In addition, the considerably higher concentrations of analyte in a urine sample make the procedure less technically demanding.

The clonidine suppression test may be of some use in difficult diagnoses. Plasma catecholamines are measured before and 3 hours after the administration of 0.3 mg of clonidine. Patients with pheochromocytoma show no suppression, whereas patients with essential hypertension suppress their catecholamine levels into the reference interval. Best results are obtained with methods that are specific for free catecholamines. If conjugated catecholamines, which have longer half-lives, are included, false-positive results may occur. A recent modification of this protocol involves measurement of urine catecholamines in a timed urine specimen after administration of clonidine. Clonidine may cause severe hypotension and patients must be observed closely during a clonidine challenge test. Glucagon and histamine have both been used in combination with measurement of the plasma catecholamine response in patients with episodic attacks of pheochromocytoma to precipitate an attack and facilitate the diagnosis. This is a potentially dangerous protocol and is very rarely employed.

There have been recent claims that the single best test for investigation and confirmation of pheochromocytoma is plasma free normetanephrine and metanephrine by HPLC. A recent study screening for familial forms of pheochromocytoma showed that the tests discussed earlier only had a sensitivity of 50% to 75%, whereas fractionated free plasma metanephrines had a sensitivity of 97%. The rationale for this is that there is a high concentration of COMT within the chromaffin cells, therefore 90% of metanephrine and more than 25% of normetanephrine in the circulation comes from the adrenal glands. In contrast, only 7% of plasma norepinephrine comes from the adrenals, the rest from the SNS. Because of its small contribution to the total pool, a several fold increase in norepinephrine output is required to be diagnostically significant. The problem with urine metanephrines is that most are sulfate conjugated via sulfotransferase from metabolism within the gut before excretion. The theoretical advantage for the determination of fractionated plasma metanephrines is the reduced interference from increased SNS activity.

No single test or 24-hour urine sample may be sufficiently sensitive to define the diagnosis of pheochromocytoma. If clinical suspicion is high, it is appropriate to analyze more than one urine sample and to measure free catecholamines and the metabolites. Tumors larger than 50 g secrete a preponderance of metabolites because of intratumor metabolism. Tumors smaller than 50 g secrete a larger proportion of free catecholamines directly into the circulation. In our laboratory we have seen patients with very large adrenal tumors whose free catecholamine output was well within normal limits but whose catecholamine metabolite values (metanephrine and VMA) were strikingly abnormal. Appropriate patients should be screened with 24-hour urinary fractionated free catecholamines and fractionated urine metanephrines, analyzed by HPLC combined with electrochemical detection. In the future the determination of fractionated plasma metanephrines by HPLC may become the most important test in the investigation of pheochromocytoma for the reasons already indicated. For some patients, these tests may have to be performed on more than one occasion. In patients with episodic hypertension, an analysis of a random urine sample for fractionated free catecholamines may be useful. In very difficult cases, a clonidine suppression test combined with plasma catecholamine measurements may be useful.

To localize the tumor before surgery, CT scans, venous sampling for catecholamines, radioisotope imaging with metaiodo[^{131}I]benzylguanidine, and MRI, are all useful techniques.

It is important to diagnose pheochromocytomas early because of the potential for a life-threatening hypertensive crisis, which may be triggered by a surgical procedure, major trauma, or certain drugs used in the treatment of depression or hypertension. The indications for testing for pheochromocytoma include the list of signs and symptoms described in the previous section. An adrenal mass, which may be an incidental finding on an abdominal CT scan, must be considered a potential pheochromocytoma, and this diagnosis must be ruled out before any surgical procedure is performed. Pheochromocytoma should also be considered in any patient with a history of hypertension after general anesthesia or trauma. Finally, monitoring for pheochromocytoma should be initiated in patients with medullary carcinoma of the thyroid or a family history of MEN type 2A or type 2B, von Hippel-Lindau syndrome, or neurofibromatosis.

Part 2: Hypertension
DEFINITION AND CRITERIA

Chronic hypertension is a common health problem in industrialized countries, with approximately 25% of the adult population affected. In the United States, African Americans are 1.5 to 2 times more likely to have hypertension than the general population. The higher the individual's blood pressure the greater the risk is for developing heart disease, stroke, renal failure, and peripheral vascular disease. The risk for development of these complications extends down to blood pressure values below the population mean. Therefore, any definition of hypertension is purely arbitrary. Other factors such as cigarette smoking and hyperlipidemia increase the risk for hypertension-associated complications.

The World Health Organization (WHO) and the Joint National Committee on Detection, Evaluation, and Treatment of High Blood Pressure (JNC VI) guidelines have defined the criteria for hypertension. These have been subdivided into several categories. Healthy categories include optimal (<120/80), normal (<130/85), and high normal (130 to 139/85 to 89). Stages of increasing hypertension include Stage I (mild, 140 to 159/90 to 99), Stage II (moderate, 160 to 179/100 to 109), and Stage III (severe, >180/110). The stages are defined by the higher of the systolic or diastolic pressure (Table 46-2). It is important not to make the diagnosis of hypertension on the basis of a single measurement, because the stress of visiting a physician may be sufficient to elevate blood pressure in some persons.

It is important to recognize hypertension, because it is treatable, and treatment reduces the incidence of complications. Laboratory testing can be used to monitor the course of some of the complications of hypertension and also, importantly, to screen patients for potentially curable secondary hypertension. This may save the hypertensive patient from life-long expensive medical therapy; the extent of medical therapy may itself be associated with complications.

TABLE 46-2 CLASSIFICATION OF HYPERTENSION (JNC VI)*

Category	Systolic (mm Hg)	Diastolic (mm Hg)
Optimal	<120	<80
Normal	<130	<85
High normal	130 to 139	85 to 89
Stage I (mild)	140 to 159	90 to 99
Stage II (moderate)	160 to 179	100 to 109
Stage III (severe)	≥180	≥110

*Joint National Committee on Detection, Evaluation, and Treatment of high blood pressure. The stage is defined by the higher of the systolic or diastolic pressure.

FACTORS REGULATING NORMAL BLOOD PRESSURE

To better understand the pathophysiology of hypertension, it is necessary briefly to review factors responsible for normal blood pressure regulation. Cardiac output and peripheral vascular resistance are the primary determinants of systemic blood pressure. Cardiac output is determined by plasma volume, cardiac stroke volume (the volume of blood expelled from the heart with each contraction), heart rate, and myocardial contractility. Peripheral vascular resistance is a function of the balance of humoral vasoconstriction (to increase blood pressure) and vasodilation (to decrease blood pressure), adrenergic activity, and arteriole smooth muscle tone. Ordinarily blood pressure is adjusted to maintain sufficient organ perfusion without producing organ or vascular damage. Several systems play a role in modulating cardiac output and peripheral vascular resistance. These are the arterial baroreceptor reflex, the body fluid or plasma volume regulatory system, and vascular autoregulation.

Baroreceptors in the aortic arch and carotid arteries sense the perfusion pressure and wall tension, through the afferent autonomic nervous system. These then signal the brainstem to modulate efferent adrenergic and vagal nerve activity, which in turn regulates myocardial contractility, heart rate, and peripheral vascular resistance. The release of antidiuretic hormone from the hypothalamus is regulated by plasma osmolality and blood pressure. This hormone enhances water resorption by the kidney. The renin-angiotensin system stimulates aldosterone release when blood pressure or sodium concentration drops and leads to sodium and water conservation. Angiotensin II generated by this cascade is also a potent vasoconstrictor. This system has been described in greater detail earlier in this chapter.

The arterioles have the intrinsic capability to alter muscular tone in response to local perfusion pressures. With this vascular autoregulatory system, when cardiac output rises, the arterioles constrict to protect capillaries and tissues from hyperperfusion. Endothelin, a vasoconstrictor, plays a central role in blood pressure homeostasis. Nitrous oxide (see later discussion) and prostacyclin are locally produced vasodilators. The balance of these factors affects blood pressure.

TABLE 46-3	FACTORS THAT REGULATE BLOOD PRESSURE	
Factor	**Site of Synthesis**	**Mechanism and Sites of Action**
Arterial Baroreflex Activators		
Epinephrine	Adrenal medulla	Vasodilation of arterioles of skeletal muscle; vasoconstriction of arterioles of skin, mucous membranes, and viscera; increases in rate and force of cardiac contraction
Norepinephrine	Terminals of sympathetic nervous system	General vasoconstriction
Body Fluid Volume Regulators		
Antidiuretic hormone (ADH)	Neurohypophysis	Enhanced water reabsorption; increased plasma volume
Aldosterone	Adrenal cortex	Renal tubular sodium reabsorption; increased plasma volume
Renin	Juxtaglomerular cells of kidney	Converts angiotensinogen to angiotensin I
Angiotensin-converting enzyme	Lung	Converts angiotensin I to angiotensin II (potent vasoconstrictor, stimulates aldosterone production)
Vascular Autoregulation	Tissue/organ specific	Local mechanisms to maintain constant tissue perfusion

All these systems work together when there is a change in blood pressure. Table 46-3 summarizes some of the factors that play a role in regulating blood pressure. Through our understanding of the physiology of blood pressure control, newer specific therapeutic agents have evolved for treating hypertension.

PATHOLOGICAL CONDITIONS

In the majority of patients the cause of the hypertension is unknown. Definable or secondary causes such as renal vascular disease, chronic renal failure, and endocrine abnormalities are uncommon and account for 5% to 10% of cases at most. Unknown genetic and environmental factors may play a role in the approximately 95% of patients with **essential**, or **primary**, **hypertension**. There is evidence that salt intake, alcohol intake, and obesity have important influences.

It is beyond the scope of this chapter to delve into the many theories behind the mechanisms leading to primary hypertension. It can be most simply stated that the final common pathway is increased peripheral arteriolar vasoconstriction. The initiating factor is not known.

Primary Hypertension

The two broad categories in hypertension are *primary*, or *essential*, hypertension and **secondary hypertension**. The cause of primary hypertension is unknown, and it is improbable that there is a single cause to explain the diversity of hemodynamic pathophysiological derangements in this condition. Hereditary and environmental factors (salt intake, stress, obesity, and alcohol) clearly play a role. Central obesity, insulin resistance, and hyperinsulinism are all linked to high blood pressure. Alcohol consumption of more than 10 mL per day increases both diastolic and systolic blood pressure in a linear relationship with the amount consumed. There are genetic subtypes of individuals who are especially sensitive to dietary factors such as sodium and calcium intake, with increased calcium intake associated with decreased risk of hypertension.

The SNS and the renin-angiotensin system have often been implicated as the source of the problem. A high resting pulse rate is sometimes an early predictor of subsequent hypertension. Up to 40% of all hypertensive individuals have higher than normal catecholamine output as is reflected by increased plasma norepinephrine concentrations. Plasma renin activity is usually normal in hypertensives, but it may be suppressed in some (approximately 25%) and elevated in others (approximately 15%). The malignant (accelerating) phase of hypertension is nearly always accompanied by increased renin.

Initially there may be a single derangement, but hypertension appears to beget hypertension, and other mechanisms become involved as the hypertension continues over time. This may explain why secondary hypertension is not always cured when the primary defect has been corrected.

Many other factors have been implicated. Whether these are causative or simply epiphenomenal is not known. There are reported defects in sodium transport across cell walls either attributable to Na^+, K^+-ATPase dysfunction or because of increased sodium permeability. It is also speculated that hypertension may result from a deficiency of vasodilators rather than an excess of vasoconstrictors. Nitric oxide, produced by nitric oxide synthetase (NOS), is a potent vasodilator. There are three forms of NOS, endogenous NOS, neuronal NOS, and inducible NOS. It is now known that inducible NOS can be stimulated by cytokines, contributing to hypotension seen in septic shock. Exercise and statins can increase endogenous NOS. In chronic renal failure inhibitors of NOS are known to accumulate. There is increasing evidence that a number of mechanisms can lead to interruption of the NOS pathway leading to hypertension. At this point there is no single unifying hypothesis.

Secondary Hypertension

Although secondary causes of hypertension account for only 5% to 10% of all cases, they are important to recognize because of the possibility of a more specific medical therapy or surgical cure. Table 46-4 summarizes the major causes of hypertension.

Renal disease. A leading cause of secondary hypertension is renal disease. Glomerulonephritis, pyelonephritis, polycystic renal disease, renin-secreting tumors, and chronic renal failure are all associated with hypertension.

Renovascular hypertension. Stenosis, or occlusion of one or both main renal arteries or branches, can cause hypertension by stimulating release of renin from the juxtaglomerular cells of the affected kidney. Greater than 60% occlusion is required to have a significant hemodynamic effect. In patients who are older than 50 years of age, atherosclerosis is the most important cause of renal artery stenosis, while in younger patients fibromuscular dysplasia is the leading cause. Overall, fibromuscular dysplasia accounts for less than 10% of renal artery stenosis and mainly affects women in the 15 to 50 age bracket. It is a progressive disease and can lead to renal atrophy in more than 20% of cases. Renovascular hypertension, or renal artery stenosis, is the most frequent cause of curable secondary hypertension, but it is discovered in only about 2% of hypertensive patients. Renovascular hypertension should be suspected when hypertension develops rapidly in those less than 30 or more than 55 years of age, or when there is sudden worsening of previously stable hypertension. The most important physical finding is a systolic-diastolic bruit in the epigastrium, but this sign is present in only 50% of patients.

Drug-induced hypertension. Many drugs may cause hypertension. Oral contraceptives may cause a mild degree of hypertension through an increase in the liver production of angiotensinogen (renin substrate). Oral contraceptives may also cause, directly, some degree of sodium retention. Licorice (glycyrrhizic acid and glycyrrhetinic acid) and carbenoxolone, inhibitors of 11-β-hydroxysteroid dehydrogenase, prevent the inactivation of cortisol to cortisone in the renal tubular cells, resulting in increasing levels of cortisol-induced mineralocorticoid activity. Nasal decongestants can cause hypertension through vasoconstriction. Administered glucocorticoids given in excess will also increase mineralocorticoid activity. Cyclosporin, tricyclic antidepressants, and illicit drugs such as cocaine and amphetamines are some other examples of drug-induced causes of hypertension.

Coarctation of the aorta. Coarctation of the aorta is usually first identified in childhood. In this condition there is an arterial defect with a fibrous aortic stricture reducing blood flow to the lower body and extremities. The result is restricted blood flow to the kidneys and, as a consequence, activation of the renin-angiotensin system. These patients will then have upper extremity hypertension relative to the lower extremities. A soft bruit, louder in the back, is often heard over the coarctation site. Femoral pulses are diminished and delayed when compared to the brachial pulses.

Endocrine causes of hypertension. Several adrenal disorders are associated with hypertension. These include Cushing's syndrome, pheochromocytoma, and Conn's syndrome. The adrenogenital syndrome, resulting from 11-hydroxylase deficiency (a hereditary cause of hypertension), Liddle syndrome, and apparent mineralocorticoid excess (AME type 1 and AME type 2) are other causes of hypertension that can occur with hypokalemia. The causes, clinical features, and laboratory investigation of these problems are summarized in the first section of this chapter. Other endocrine disorders that may be associated with hypertension are acromegaly, primary hyperparathyroidism (50% are hypertensive), hypothyroidism (rarely hypertensive), renin secreting tumors, and thyrotoxicosis (high systolic blood pressure).

COMPLICATIONS OF HYPERTENSION

Blood pressure may gradually rise over many years, and the patient may remain asymptomatic for a long time. Hypertension is usually discovered during a routine physical examination. Unfortunately it is too often discovered after vital organ injury has already occurred, such as ischemic injury to the brain after a stroke or cardiac injury after a myocardial infarct. Headache and light-headedness, symptoms sometimes associated with hypertension, are seen in less than 25% of patients, and the physical examination is usually unremarkable. Years of uncontrolled hypertension may produce damage to several vital organs, in particular the eyes, the brain, the heart, the kidneys, and the aorta.

In the eyes, retinal hemorrhages, exudates, and papilledema may occur. Hypertension is a very important risk factor for stroke. Peripheral resistance in hypertension is high, a condition that increases afterload on the left ventricle, causing left ventricular hypertrophy. Hypertension also accelerates atherogenesis. Long-standing hypertension induces both vascular and glomerular damage in kidneys, causing nephrosclerosis. The renal blood vessels show fibrous atherosclerotic thickening and narrowing of the lumen. The kidneys'

TABLE 46-4 PRINCIPAL CAUSES OF HYPERTENSION

Cause	Relative Incidence (%)
I Primary hypertension	90 to 95
II Renal disease	4 to 5
III Renovascular hypertension	2 to 5
IV Drug- or exogenous agent–induced hypertension	<2
Oral contraceptives	
Sympathetic amines (decongestants)	
Licorice	
High-dose corticosteroids	
V Endocrine	<2
Conn's syndrome	
Cushing's syndrome	
Pheochromocytoma	
Primary hyperparathyroidism	
Hypothyroidism	
Hyperthyroidism	
Acromegaly	
Congenital adrenal hyperplasia (17-hydroxylase and 11-hydroxylase deficiencies)	
VI Coarctation of the aorta	<1

ability to regulate blood flow becomes impaired. Glomerulosclerosis also is initiated with resulting increase in proteinuria (see Chapter 24). This will eventually lead to the loss of the GFR and end-stage renal disease. Large-vessel atherosclerosis, including that of the aorta, is accelerated by hypertension. Aortic aneurysm and intramural dissection may occur. Aneurysms evolve slowly and may be asymptomatic, whereas a dissection is always a painful episode often accompanied by shock.

CHANGE OF ANALYTE WITH DISEASE

Once hypertension has been identified in a patient through multiple determinations of blood pressure, a simple minimum evaluation should be initiated. See the box below for a summary. This evaluation serves three main purposes: (1) to exclude treatable causes of secondary hypertension, (2) to detect evidence of organ damage, and (3) to identify other risk factors that may accelerate cardiovascular disease. This evaluation mainly involves inexpensive, high-volume laboratory tests. The choice of these tests is justified below.

Urinalysis. Routine urinalysis can detect proteinuria, hematuria, and glycosuria. Proteinuria and hematuria may be attributable to hypertensive nephrosclerosis or to intrinsic renal disease, which may in fact be the cause of the hypertension. A renal biopsy is required to distinguish the cause if an abnormality is observed. The presence of proteinuria in a hypertensive patient may be suggestive of a bad prognosis. There has been some interest in diagnosing this problem earlier using sensitive assays for albumin (microalbuminuria) analogous to diabetic nephropathy. There is accumulating evidence that an increased albumin excretion rate is predictive of future cardiovascular disease in hypertensives as well as renal problems. It may be possible to reverse the process, for example, by the use of angiotensin-converting enzyme inhibitors or angiotensin II receptor blockers. The presence of glycosuria, which is suggestive of diabetes mellitus, will affect the choice of antihypertensive therapy. For example, thiazide diuretics are contraindicated in diabetes because they can exacerbate glucose intolerance. It is also possible that the glucose intolerance may be secondary to other endocrine causes of hypertension such as pheochromocytoma, Cushing's syndrome, or acromegaly.

Sodium. An elevated sodium value is not a sensitive or specific test, but it may be elevated in some patients with primary hyperaldosteronism. Another consideration is that serum sodium may be decreased in hypertensive patients receiving thiazide or loop diuretics. This test is therefore also important for monitoring patients undergoing diuretic therapy.

Potassium. The finding of a low potassium value is a very important clue in a hypertensive patient not receiving medication, suggestive of the possibility of either primary (Conn's syndrome) or secondary (i.e., renal artery stenosis) hyperaldosteronism. Also, serum potassium levels may be raised in patients with acute or chronic renal failure and lowered in patients receiving diuretics. See Table 46-5 for causes and renin/aldosterone findings in patients with hypertension and hypokalemia.

Creatinine. Creatinine is a specific screen for renal impairment that may be caused by hypertension or be the cause of hypertension. Creatinine should be assessed on presentation and annually in all hypertensives.

Calcium. The serum calcium level is elevated in primary hyperparathyroidism, which is one of the causes of hypertension. About 50% of patients with this problem will be hypertensive. It is of interest that despite this connection the blood pressure most often does not normalize after surgical cure. Another consideration is that thiazide diuretics can rarely cause hypercalcemia and thus should be excluded before pursuing the diagnosis of primary hyperparathyroidism.

Uric acid. Uric acid value is elevated in about 40% of patients with essential hypertension. The connection is unclear but is more common in patients with renal failure. Uric acid levels may also be elevated by thiazide diuretics, in some cases leading to gout.

Glucose. An elevated fasting plasma glucose value greater than 1400 mg/L (7.0 mmol/L) on two or more occa-

---

> **MINIMUM EVALUATION OF THE HYPERTENSIVE INDIVIDUAL**
>
> Complete history and physical examination
> Serum creatinine, sodium, potassium, glucose, uric acid, cholesterol, and triglyceride concentrations
> Hemoglobin
> Urinalysis
> Electrocardiogram

> **TABLE 46-5 CAUSES OF HYPERTENSION AND HYPERKALEMIA CHARACTERIZED BY PLASMA RENIN ACTIVITY (PRA) AND ALDOSTERONE LEVELS (ALDO)**
>
> | *Finding* | *Conclusion* |
> |---|---|
> | Increased PRA, increased ALDO | Secondary hyperaldosteronism from: Renovascular hypertension Diuretic use Renin-secreting tumor Malignant hypertension Coarctation of the aorta |
> | Decreased PRA, increased ALDO | Primary hyperaldosteronism |
> | Decreased PRA, decreased ALDO | Congenital adrenal hyperplasia Exogenous mineralocorticoid DOC-producing tumor Cushing's syndrome 11-β-OSHD deficiency Liddle syndrome Licorice ingestion |
>
> *DOC, deoxycorticosterone; 11-β-OSHD, 11-β-hydroxysteroid dehydrogenase.*

sions is sufficient to diagnose diabetes mellitus. About 50% of diabetics have hypertension, and up to 10% of hypertensive patients are diabetic. Calcium-channel blockers and angiotensin-converting enzyme inhibitors are the preferred antihypertensive drugs in diabetics. Thiazide diuretics and β-blockers should be avoided.

Cholesterol. The presence of hyperlipidemia is an important risk factor for atherosclerosis along with hypertension. The presence of hyperlipidemia is a contraindication for the use of some antihypertensive medications, such as β-blockers and thiazide diuretics, which may exacerbate the lipid problem. Patients with risk factors for cardiovascular disease need to be treated very aggressively (see Chapter 33).

Electrocardiogram. An electrocardiogram should be obtained in all cases to assess cardiac status as a baseline parameter and to determine if left ventricular hypertrophy is present.

Chest x-ray film. A chest x-ray film may identify aortic dilation or elongation and rib notching, which may occur in coarctation of the aorta.

γ-Glutamyltranspeptidase. This is an optional test that serves as a screen for alcohol abuse. Alcohol consumption may elevate blood pressure acutely and chemically. One ounce of alcohol per day, equivalent to about two drinks, will raise the systolic blood pressure by an average of 2 to 6 mm Hg.

SECONDARY STUDIES

Clues from the history, physical examination, and basic laboratory studies may indicate a possible secondary cause for the hypertension. Some of these clues include:

1. Abrupt onset of severe hypertension, or onset before 25 years of age or after 50 may be suggestive of pheochromocytoma or renovascular disease.
2. A history of palpitations, anxiety attacks, sweating, hyperglycemia, and weight loss may be suggestive of pheochromocytoma.
3. An abdominal bruit may be suggestive of renovascular disease.
4. Bilateral upper abdominal mass on physical examination may imply polycystic kidney disease.
5. Abnormal renal function test results may be suggestive of renal insufficiency.
6. Hypokalemia, or easily provoked hypokalemia, in an untreated hypertensive should be a trigger to look for primary hyperaldosteronism (Conn's syndrome) or other cause of hypertension and hypokalemia.

The investigation of adrenal disorders with associated hypertension is discussed earlier in this chapter. Other endocrine causes of hypertension are suspected on clinical grounds, and laboratory investigations for these disorders are reviewed in other chapters. The focus at this point will be on the investigation of renovascular hypertension.

Renovascular hypertension. In renovascular hypertension, or renal artery stenosis (RAS), there is decreased perfusion of the affected kidney, which leads to activation of the renin-angiotensin system. However, when hypertension

is sustained, the plasma renin activity may drop because of decreased responsivity to prolonged stimulation, thus explaining the limitations of the measurement of renin activity for the diagnosis of this condition. Peripheral vein renin measurement has low predictive accuracy for RAS; results may be influenced by medications and other conditions. RAS is not easily distinguishable from essential hypertension. Clues include decreased potassium, abdominal bruit, duration of hypertension, and age of onset. These are suggestive but have low predictive value. Many patients with RAS have coexisting essential hypertension, which persists despite successful revascularization.

The standard screening test for renal vascular hypertension has been the rapid-sequence intravenous pyelogram (IVP). Abnormalities of contrast excretion and kidney shape and size may be suggestive of this disorder. The definitive test for surgically correctable renal artery stenosis until recently has been the combination of a renal angiogram and renal-vein renin determinations. The angiogram can identify the stenotic lesion, whereas the bilateral renal vein catheterization and subsequent measurement of renin activity confirm the functional significance of the observed lesion. The narrow renal artery supplies less blood to the affected kidney, and renin secretion will be higher on this side. A renal-vein renin ratio of greater than 1.5:1 is associated with cure or amelioration of hypertension after angioplasty or surgical intervention in a high proportion of cases. Before performance of this test the patient must not be receiving β-blockers, which may suppress renin, and should be on a low-salt diet for 4 days.

Another screening procedure is the captopril renogram, which provides an indirect measure of the GFR and its dependence on angiotensin II. In this test renal uptake of radiolabeled diethylenetriaminepentaacetic acid (DTPA) or o-iodohippurate sodium (Hippuran) is measured before and after ACE inhibition with captopril. An abnormal result indicates that the stenosis is functionally significant and will respond to revascularization. This test has replaced renal-vein renin assessment in some centers. Pharmacological screening with an ACE inhibitor is another sensitive but not highly specific means of assessing patients suspected of having renovascular hypertension. Administration of the ACE inhibitor (i.e., captopril) normally leads to an increase in plasma renin activity and a drop in blood pressure. This response is exaggerated in patients with renovascular hypertension. False-positive results can be a problem.

Angioplasty is the initial treatment of choice for renal artery stenosis. It works best in younger patients with fibromuscular dysplasia. If angioplasty is unsuccessful or if restenosis occurs, the angioplasty procedure may be repeated. If this fails, surgical revascularization should be attempted.

DRUG THERAPY

Although medical therapy is beyond the scope of this chapter, it is of value to summarize briefly the major classes of drugs used in the initial treatment of hypertension, primarily focusing on the metabolic complications that may result from their use. Some patients receive several of these drugs. In recent years there has been a gradual shift from dependence on diuretics and β-blockers to use of ACE inhibitors and calcium-channel blockers to control blood pressure because of the lower incidence of side effects. Effectiveness of drug therapy is best assessed by routine monitoring of blood pressure and patient history.

Diuretics. The group of approximately 50 different drugs called *diuretics* promotes the formation and excretion of urine to reduce extracellular fluid volume. In large doses they can cause hypovolemia, electrolyte imbalance, and prerenal failure. Diuretics can also be associated with sexual dysfunction in males. Metabolic side effects include hypokalemia, hypomagnesemia, hyperuricemia, hyperglycemia, and hyperlipidemia. Despite these disadvantages, diuretics are effective and inexpensive, and most side effects are minimal if the patient is properly managed.

β-Adrenergic receptor blockers. Drugs that block β-adrenergic receptors decrease the rate and force of cardiac contractions, among other effects. If the patient has diabetes mellitus, chronic occlusive peripheral arterial disease, or chronic obstructive pulmonary disease, cardioselective β-blockers should be used. These do not completely eliminate complications in the above patients, however. Like diuretics, β-blockers can cause sexual dysfunction and some metabolic disturbances such as impaired glucose tolerance or decreased high-density lipoprotein cholesterol and increases in serum total cholesterol and triglycerides. β-Blockers also have the potential of blunting the patient awareness of hypoglycemia, which can be a disadvantage in diabetics. Most of these effects are primarily elicited at higher dosages.

Angiotensin-converting enzyme (ACE) inhibitors. ACE inhibitors block the conversion of angiotensin I to angiotensin II, which is a stimulator of aldosterone release and a potent vasoconstrictor. This group of drugs has a low reported incidence of side effects. ACE inhibitors neither cause sexual dysfunction in males nor adversely affect lipids, glucose, or uric acid, although they tend to increase potassium. ACE inhibitors reduce proteinuria in patients with diabetic nephropathy and may retard glomerulosclerosis by selectively dilating the efferent arteriole, reducing glomerular capillary pressure without compromising blood flow. ACE inhibitors can cause acute renal failure in patients with severe renal artery stenosis and, in very large doses, can cause nephrotic syndrome, nephritis, and leukopenia.

Angiotensin II receptor blockers. The recent literature has suggested that this group of drugs is very effective in controlling blood pressure in diabetics, slowing the progression of, and even reversing, microalbuminuria; analogous to ACE inhibitors, but with fewer side effects. They have fewer nonrenal side effects than any other antihypertensive drug class. Hyperkalemia is less frequent than with ACE inhibitors, but still may occur, especially in patients with declining renal function or in combination with potassium sparing diuretics or β-blockers.

Calcium antagonists. Calcium antagonists are potent peripheral vasodilators and reduce blood pressure by decreasing peripheral resistance. Verapamil has a direct effect on the myocardium. Calcium antagonists do not have adverse metabolic side effects but are as expensive as ACE inhibitors. Potential side effects include constipation, edema, orthostasis, negative inotropic effects, and tachycardia. Short-acting calcium-channel blockers can adversely affect cardiovascular outcomes. The long-acting formulations are more effective antihypertensive agents.

Bibliography

General

Loriaux DL: The adrenal glands. In Becker KL, editor: *Principles and practice of endocrinology and metabolism*, ed 3, Philadelphia, 2001, Lippincott Williams & Wilkins.

Orth DN, Kovacs WJ: The adrenal cortex. In *Williams textbook of endocrinology*, ed 9, Philadelphia, 1998, Saunders.

Williams GH, Dluhy RG: Disorders of the adrenal cortex. In Braunwald E et al, editors: *Harrison's principles of internal medicine*, ed 15, New York, 2001, McGraw-Hill.

Winter WE: Laboratory approaches to diseases of the adrenal cortex and adrenal medulla. In *Handbook of diagnostic endocrinology*, 1999, AACC Press.

Mineralcorticoids

Cartledge S, Lawson N: Aldosterone and renin measurements, *Ann Clin Biochem* 37:262, 2000.

Ganguly A: Primary aldosteronism, *N Engl J Med* 339:1828, 1998.

Ghose RP, Hall PM, Bravo EL: Medical management of aldosterone producing adenomas, *Ann Intern Med* 131:105, 1999.

Kaplan NM: Cautions over the current epidemic of primary aldosteronism, *Lancet* 357:953, 2001.

Steigerwalt SP: Unravelling the causes of hypertension and hypokalemia, *Hosp Pract* 30:67, 1995.

Stewart PM: Mineralocorticoid hypertension, *Lancet* 353:1341, 1999.

White PC: Disorders of aldosterone biosynthesis and action, *N Engl J Med* 331:250, 1994.

Glucocorticoids

Abdu TAM et al: Comparison of low dose short synacthen test (1 μg), conventional dose short synacthen test (250 μg) and insulin tolerance test for the assessment of the hypothalamic-pituitary-adrenal axis in patients with pituitary disease, *J Clin Endocrinol Metab* 84:838, 1999.

Arlt W et al: DHEA replacement in women with adrenal insufficiency, *N Engl J Med* 341:1013, 1999.

Aron DC, Findling JW, Tyrrell JB: Glucocorticoids and adrenal androgens. In Greenspan FS, Gardner DG, editors: *Basic and clinical endocrinology*, ed 6, New York, 2001, Lange Medical Books/McGraw-Hill.

Boscaro M et al: Cushing's syndrome, *Lancet* 357:783, 2001.

Davies JS et al: Diagnostic dilemmas in Cushing's syndrome, *Ann Clin Biochem* 37:85, 2000.

Findling JW, Raff H: Diagnosis and differential diagnosis of Cushing's syndrome, *Endocrinol Metab Clin North Am* 30:729, 2001.

Henzen C et al: Suppression and recovery of adrenal response after short term high dose glucocorticoid treatment, *Lancet* 355:542, 2000.

Krasner AS: Glucocorticoid-induced adrenal insufficiency, *JAMA* 202:671, 1999.

Newell-Price J, Grossman A: Diagnosis and management of Cushing's syndrome, *Lancet* 353:2087, 1999.

Oelkers W: Adrenal insufficiency, *N Engl J Med* 335:1206, 1996.

Perry LA, Grossman AB: The role of the laboratory in the diagnosis of Cushing's syndrome, *Ann Clin Biochem* 34:345, 1997.

Reincke M: Subclinical Cushing's syndrome, *Endocrinol Metab Clin North Am* 29:43, 2000.

Streeten DHP: What test for hypothalamic-pituitary adrenocortical insufficiency? *Lancet* 354:179, 1999.

Turpeinen U et al: Determination of urinary free cortisol by HPLC, *Clin Chem* 43:1386, 1997.

Walsh JP, Dayan CM: Role of biochemical assessment in management of corticosteroid withdrawal, *Ann Clin Biochem* 37:279, 2000.

Werbel SS, Ober KP: Acute adrenal insufficiency, *Endocrinol Metab Clin North Am* 22:303, 1993.

Adrenal Androgens

Achermann JC, Silverman BL: DHEA replacement for patients with adrenal insufficiency, *Lancet* 357:1381, 2001.

Arlt W et al: DHEA replacement in women with adrenal insufficiency, *N Engl J Med* 341:1013, 1999.

Kroboth PD et al: DHEA and DHEAS: a review, *J Clin Pharmacol* 39:327, 1999.

Oelkers W: DHEA for adrenal insufficiency, *N Engl J Med* 341:1073, 1999.

Adrenal Incidentalomas

Bailey RH, Aron DC: The diagnostic dilemma of incidentalomas, *Endocrinol Metab Clin North Am* 29:91, 2000.

Barzon L et al: Risk factors and long term follow-up of adrenal incidentalomas, *J Clin Endocrinol Metab* 84:520, 1999.

Kievit J, Haak HR: Diagnosis and treatment of adrenal incidentaloma, *Endocrinol Metab Clin North Am* 29:69, 2000.

Linos DA: Management approaches to adrenal incidentalomas, *Endocrinal Metab Clin North Am* 29:141, 2000.

Mantero F, Arnaldi G: Management approaches to adrenal incidentalomas, *Endocrinol Metab Clin North Am* 29:107, 2000.

Ross NS, Aron DC: Hormonal evaluation of the patient with an incidentally discovered adrenal Mass, *N Engl J Med* 323:1401, 1990.

Congenital Adrenal Hyperplasia

Speiser PW: Congenital adrenal hyperplasia owing to 21-hydroxylase deficiency, *Endocrinol Metab Clin North Am* 30:31, 2001.

Therrell BL: Newborn screening for congenital adrenal hyperplasia, *Endocrinol Metab Clin North Am* 30:15, 2001.

White PC: Steroid ll-β-hydroxylase deficiency and related disorders, *Endocrinol Metab Clin North Am* 30:61, 2001.

Catecholamines and Pheochromocytoma

Eisenhofer G: Free or total metanephrines for diagnosis of pheochromocytoma: what is the difference? *Clin Chem* 47:988, 2001.

Eisenhofer G et al: Plasma normetanephrine and metanephrine for detecting pheochromocytoma in von Hippel-Lindau disease and multiple endocrine neoplasia type 2, *N Engl J Med* 340:1872, 1999.

Gerlo EA, Sevens C: Urinary and plasma catecholamines and urinary catecholamine metabolites in pheochromocytoma: diagnostic value in 19 cases, *Clin Chem* 40:250, 1994.

Goldfien A: Adrenal medulla. In Greenspan FS, Gardner DG, editors: *Basic and clinical endocrinology*, ed 6, New York, 2001, Lange Medical Books/McGraw-Hill.

Landsberg L, Young JB: Pheochromocytoma. In Braumwald E et al, editors: *Harrison's principles of internal medicine*, ed 15, New York, 2001, McGraw-Hill.

Pacak K et al: Recent advances in genetics, diagnosis, localization and treatment of pheochromocytoma, *Ann Intern Med* 134:315, 2001.

Scully RE et al: Case records of the Massachusetts General Hospital, *N Engl J Med* 344:1314, 2001.

Young WF: Pheochromocytoma and primary aldosteronism: diagnostic approaches, *Endocrinol Metab Clin North Am* 26:801, 1997.

Hypertension

Boudewijn G et al: Diagnostic tests for renal artery stenosis in patients suspected of having renovascular hypertension: a meta-analysis, *Ann Intern Med* 135:401, 2001.

Don BR, Schambelan M: Endocrine hypertension. In Greenspan FS, Gardner DG, editors: *Basic and clinical endocrinology*, ed 6, New York, 2001, Lange Medical Books/McGraw-Hill.

Feldman RD, Campbell N, Larochelle P: 1999 Canadian recommendations for the management of hypertension, *CMAJ* 161(12 suppl):S1, 1999.

Harvey JM, Beevers DG: Biochemical investigation of hypertension, *Ann Clin Biochem* 27:287, 1990.

Hollenberg NK, editor: *Hypertension: mechanisms and therapy*, vol 2, *Atlas of heart disease*, Philadelphia, 1995, Current Medicine.

Massie BM: Systemic hypertension. In Tierney LM, McPhee SJ, Papadakis MA, editors: *Current medical diagnosis and treatment*, ed 41, New York, 2002, Lange Medical Books/McGraw-Hill.

Safian RD, Textor SC: Renal artery stenosis, *N Engl J Med* 344:431, 2001.

Sixth Report of the Joint National Committee on Detection, Evaluation and Treatment of High Blood Pressure (JNC-VI), *Arch Intern Med* 157:2413, 1997.

Sobel BJ, Bakris GL: *Hypertension: a clinician's guide to diagnosis and treatment*, ed 2, Philadelphia, 1999, Hanley & Belfus.

Stewart PM: Dexamethasone-suppressible hypertension, *Lancet* 356:697, 2000.

Thomas GD, Zhang W, Victor RG: Nitric oxide deficiency as a cause of clinical hypertension, *JAMA* 285:2055, 2001.

Warnock DG, Bubien JK: Liddle syndrome: clinical and cellular abnormalities, *Hosp Pract* 15:95, 1994.

Internet Sites

http://www.medhelp.org/nadf/—National Addison's Disease Foundation

http://arbl.cvmbs.colostate.edu/hbooks/pathphys/endocrine/adrenal/index.html—Colorado State Hypertextbook: The Adrenal Gland: Introduction and Index

http://web.indstate.edu/thcme/mwking/hormone-table.html—Indiana University: Medical Biochemistry

http://www.pslgroup.com/dg/6a3da.htm—Doctor's Guide Publishing Limited: article on hypertension

http://www.wfubmc.edu/hypertension/—Wake Forest Baptist Medical Center: Hypertension and Vascular Disease

http://cgap.ucdavis.edu—Canine Genetic Analysis: A Research Focus on the Statistics & Molecular Genetics of Diseases in Dogs, Department of Animal Science, University of California-Davis

http://www.cancer.gov/cancer_information/—National Cancer Institute Information

http://www.nlm.nih.gov/medlineplus/adrenalglanddisorders.html—Medline Plus: Adrenal Gland Disorders

http://www.ash-us.org/—American Society of Hypertension

http://www.who.int/en/—World Health Organization

http://www.medhelp.org/—Med Help International: Virtual Medical Center for Patients

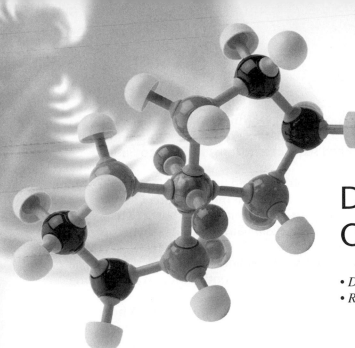

CHAPTER 47

Diseases of Genetic Origin*

• *Donald L. Rucknagel*
• *Richard Wenstrup*

Chapter Outline

Genetic basis of inheritance
Chemical basis
Single gene patterns of inheritance
Human genome project: implications for human health
Uses of the DNA sequence of the human genome
Connexins
Pathological disorders associated with abnormal chromosomes
Aneuploidy
Structural abnormalities of chromosomes
Sex chromosome abnormalities
Cytogenetic methods
Chromosomal markers of disease

Pathological disorders associated with biochemical changes
Lysosomal storage diseases
Disorders of intermediary metabolism
Genetic screening
Role of mass screening
Detection of heterozygote carriers
Prenatal diagnosis
Alpha-fetoprotein testing
Maternal serum alpha-fetoprotein screening
Amniotic fluid determination of alpha-fetoprotein
Methods of analysis

Objectives

- Briefly describe the chromosome abnormality associated with the following pathological disorders: Down syndrome, Turner's syndrome, Klinefelter's syndrome, chronic myelogenous leukemia, Fanconi anemia, and fragile X syndrome.
- Briefly describe the metabolic disorder in each of the following and state the primary abnormal clinical chemistry results:
  Gaucher's disease
  Niemann-Pick disease
  Tay-Sachs disease
  Hurler's syndrome
  Phenylketonuria

  Maple-syrup urine disease
  Galactosemia
  Fanconi syndrome
  von Gierke's disease
  Vitamin D–resistant rickets
  Wilson's disease
  Familial hypercholesterolemia
  Lesch-Nyhan syndrome
  Leber's optic atrophy and myopathies caused by mitochondrial mutations
  Zellweger's cerebrohepatorenal syndrome
- Describe the role of genetic screening in the diagnosis of genetic disease.

---

*The authors would like to acknowledge the previous contribution of Thaddeus E. Kelly.

Key Terms

allele   One of various forms of a gene that may appear at a specific locus.

amniocentesis   A transabdominal aspiration of the uterus by syringe to obtain amniotic fluid.

aneuploidy   A chromosomal abnormality caused by the addition or absence of an entire chromosome.

autosomal   Pertaining to any of the 22 chromosomes except the X and Y chromosomes.

Barr body   The condensation of nuclear (genetic) material of the inactivated X chromosome.

chromosome   Nuclear structure containing a linear array of genes. Humans have 23 pairs of chromosomes.

dominant trait   A trait that is expressed or determined by the heterozygous presence of an allele at the locus on the chromosome.

Down syndrome   A condition characterized by mental retardation and physical abnormalities caused by trisomy of chromosome 21.

dysmorphogenesis   Physical defects caused by intrinsically altered embryonic development.

exon   The portion of a gene that codes for the amino acid sequence of a protein.

fluorescence in situ hybridization (FISH) technique   Hybridization of short sequences of fluorescent-labeled, single-stranded DNA probes, complementary to the desired test DNA sequences. The probes bind to the complementary DNA in intact chromosomes, allowing visualization within those chromosomes of the location of the test sequences of DNA (http://helios.bto.ed.ac.uk/bto/glossary/s.htm#s).

frameshift mutations   Insertions or deletions of multiples of one or two base pairs, resulting in the formation of nonsense or chain-terminating codons that produce complex insertions or deletions in the amino acid sequence of the gene product.

galactosemia   A toxicity syndrome associated with intolerance to dietary galactose and characterized by deficiency of the enzyme galactose-1-phosphate uridyl transferase.

gene   The smallest biological unit of heredity, located on specific sites of specific chromosomes. For example, a *structural* gene is a non-regulatory gene that contains the encoding for one specific protein.

gene clones   Colonies of bacteria derived from a single progenitor bacterium containing plasmids into which a human gene or DNA fragment has been spliced.

Guthrie test   A microbiological assay for serum phenylalanine; used to screen for phenylketonuria.

haplotype   The alleles of linked genes contributed by either of the biological parents.

heteronuclear RNA (hnRNA)   The initial RNA transcription product of a gene containing both coding sequences (exons) and noncoding sequences (introns).

heteroplasmic   Pertaining to presence of both abnormal and normal mitochondria in cells.

heterozygous   Pertaining to a state in which a pair of alleles are dissimilar at both positions of the same locus.

homozygous   Pertaining to a state in which a pair of alleles are the same at both positions of the same locus.

intron (intervening base sequence)   A noncoding sequence of DNA composed of a few or several thousands of base pairs interposed within or between the coding sequences (see **exon**) in structural genes.

karyotype   The chromosomal makeup of a nucleated cell.

Lesch-Nyhan syndrome   A rare X-linked error of purine metabolism characterized by mental retardation and self-mutilation. There is a deficiency of the enzyme hypoxanthine-guanine phosphoribosyl transferase.

locus   The particular location on a given chromosome occupied by a structural gene.

lyonization   A process of random inactivation of an X chromosome to compensate for the double-gene dosage of two X chromosomes in females.

lysosomal storage diseases   Recessively inherited disorders, each of which is the result of a deficiency of a specific acid hydrolase.

monosomy   Absence of one chromosome from an otherwise diploid cell. Only known disorder is absence of X chromosome in Turner's syndrome.

nondisjunction   The failure of one of a pair of chromosomes to go to each daughter cell during division; instead both go to one daughter cell.

phenylketonuria (PKU)   An autosomal, recessively inherited disorder resulting from a defect in conversion of phenylalanine to tyrosine because of a phenylalanine hydroxylase deficiency.

polymerase chain reaction   An analytic method whereby repeated replication of a restricted sequence of DNA or RNA is mediated in vitro by DNA polymerase or reverse transcriptase, resulting in a many-fold amplification of the region of interest. See Chapter 48 for additional information.

polymorphism   The occurrence in a population (or among populations) of several phenotypic forms, such as eye color, associated with alleles of one gene or homologues of one chromosome.

preimplantation genetic diagnosis   Genetic analysis of a single cell by removal from cultured blastocysts after in vitro fertilization.

recessive trait   The expression of a trait requiring that both alleles at a locus contain the same genetic variant.

restriction endonuclease   Enzymes that cleave DNA wherever specific sequences of four to nine base pairs occur.

single nucleotide polymorphisms (SNPs)   The most common genetic variations, occurring once every 100 to 300 bases. Used to identify disease genes by examining associations between a disease and specific SNP differences for a given population. (From the NIH website http://www.ornl.gov/hgmis/publicat/primer2001/dictionary.html).

Tay-Sachs disease   Infantile form of a recessive hereditary disorder caused by a defect in lipid metabolism in which sphingolipids accumulate in the brain, resulting in progressive mental and physical degeneration. The disease occurs primarily in children of Ashkenazic Jewish ancestry.

trait   An observable feature of an organism that is visually apparent or apparent from laboratory-derived information.

translocation   The movement of a portion of one chromosome into the structure of another.

trisomy   Presence of one additional chromosome of a specific pair in an otherwise diploid cell (2n + 1 chromosomes). See **Down syndrome**.

Turner's syndrome   A condition consisting of absent ovarian function, short stature, and physical anomalies; most commonly caused by a 45,X **karyotype**.

X-linked   Pertaining to a trait carried on the X chromosome.

Y body   The large fluorescent body observed on the Y chromosome when stained with a fluorescent dye.

Methods on CD-ROM

Alpha$_1$-antitrypsin
Alpha-fetoprotein

Ceruloplasmin
Cholinesterase

GENETIC BASIS OF INHERITANCE

In the 1860s, after a series of simple experiments, Gregor Mendel proposed two laws regarding the transmission of traits across generations. In the first law, Mendel stated that the segregation of factors determining a **trait** followed predictable patterns and that one could anticipate the proportion of offspring expressing various forms of a given trait. The second law, the law of independent assortment, stated that the inheritance of one trait had no effect on the inheritance of a second trait. Approximately 40 years later, aided by the capability of observing cellular division under the microscope, it was recognized that the behavior of **chromosomes** during cellular division was consistent with the predictions made by Mendel regarding the segregation of traits. We now recognize that the factors described by Mendel are genes and that these are carried by chromosomes, the segregation of which can be observed in cellular division.

A large number of inherited diseases have been shown to be caused by the structural abnormality of a protein that is the product of a defective **gene**. The genes responsible for most of the major inherited diseases have now been cloned and their DNA sequenced, some without the protein involved being identified first. The following is not a comprehensive review but, rather, uses specific examples to illustrate the current state of our knowledge of inherited diseases.

Chemical Basis

Genes are composed of DNA and, occasionally (in viruses), RNA. DNA and RNA are composed of nucleotide sequences. See Part IV of Chapter 53 for a more complete chemical description of DNA and RNA. A triplet code of nucleic acid base pairs encodes for a single amino acid; a sequence of triple base pairs determines the sequence of amino acids in a polypeptide chain. A gene might be defined as the amount of DNA equivalent to a polypeptide chain. Eukaryotic genes are more complex than those of bacterial or viral genes, however, and contain blocks of nucleotides, composed of several hundred to many thousands of base pairs inserted into the coding sequence. These inserted sequences, called *intervening sequences*, or **introns (intervening base sequences)**, are transcribed along with the coding sequences (**exons**) to form **heteronuclear RNA (hnRNA)** in the nucleus of the cell. To convert hnRNA to messenger RNA, the hnRNA must be processed, whereby a cap is applied to the 5′ end, the intron (noncoding sequences) transcripts are deleted from the hnRNA, and a polyadenylate tail is attached to the 3′ end. The resulting RNA, messenger RNA, serves as a template for polypeptide chain synthesis (see Part I, Chapter 53). Genes of higher organisms occupy specific locations on chromosomes and code for polypeptides that have specific physiological functions. Each polypeptide may function as a single

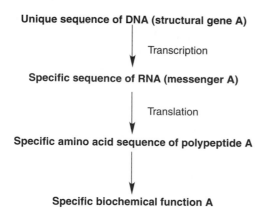

Fig. 47-1 Sequence of events from a structural gene leading to a specific, normal biochemical function.

protein or combine with other polypeptides to form a hetero-polymeric functional unit. However, the basic premise remains that one structural gene encodes a unique polypeptide with a specific function (Fig. 47-1). A change in the DNA sequence of an **exon** of a structural gene, a mutation, will result in a structurally altered polypeptide.

Most mutational changes are single base-pair substitutions that produce single amino acid substitutions in the resultant protein or polypeptide chain. Depending on its location in the molecule an amino acid substitution may profoundly affect function or may be silent. Other mutational changes that have been documented are insertions or deletions of blocks of DNA, **frameshift mutations** caused by insertions or deletions of multiples of one or two base pairs, formation of nonsense chain-terminating codons that interfere with heteronuclear RNA processing to produce complex insertions or deletions in the amino acid sequence of the gene product. Finally, some mutational changes interfere with the regulatory DNA sequences on either side of a gene to alter the rate

TABLE 47-1 DISEASES CAUSED BY VARIOUS GENETIC MUTATIONS

Protein Type	Consequences of Mutation	Example
Enzyme	Loss of enzyme activity	Phenylketonuria
Hemoglobin	Altered protein aggregation	Sickle cell disease
Structural protein (cartilage collagen)	Defective bone matrix	Osteogenesis imperfecta
Receptor	Altered metabolic regulation	Familial hyper-cholesterolemia
Membrane protein	Altered membrane transport	Cystinuria
Coagulation protein	Defective coagulation	Hemophilia
Carrier protein	Inability to transport compound	Hemochromatosis

at which ordinarily normal gene sequences are transcribed. The prototype for such changes is the β-thalassemia mutation of the hemoglobin β-chain loci. The kind of disease that results from such a mutation depends on the function of the polypeptide. Examples are illustrated in Table 47-1. The specific methods employed to detect mutations are discussed below and more fully in Chapter 48.

The genetic material of human cells is diploid in that each gene is represented twice, one of each pair occupying a specific location, or locus, on each of a pair of similar, or homologous, chromosomes. The chromosomes segregate during meiosis, reducing the chromosome number from a diploid to haploid number. Humans have a chromosomal or modal number of 46 in somatic cells and 23 in gametes. Virtually every structural gene locus has a series of variations, or **alleles**, that may occur. In most instances these alleles were created by mutations consisting of a single nucleotide change in the structure of the gene and thus a single amino acid substitution in the gene product. Many of these gene products are equally functional but may be recognized by different electrophoretic or immunological properties of the gene product. On the long arm of chromosome 1 is the locus for the Duffy blood group. At that locus, various alternative forms of the gene, or alleles, may occur, giving rise to different Duffy blood types. The two most common alleles at the Duffy blood group locus are designated *a* and *b* (i.e., Fy^a and Fy^b respectively). The gene products for the *a* and *b* alleles of the Duffy blood group are recognized by standard blood-typing techniques. When the alleles at a given locus are the same, the person is said to be **homozygous** at that locus. Thus a person with the *a* allele at both positions on the pair of 1 chromosomes for the Duffy blood group is homozygous *a*. When the pair of alleles are dissimilar, such as the Duffy allele *a* and *b*, the person is a **heterozygote**.

A series of allelic mutations may impart a range of functional consequences on the polypeptide gene product. For example, many different mutations occur in the structural gene for the β chain of hemoglobin. This series of alleles results in functional changes in β-hemoglobin chains that range from insignificant (no disease) to lack of the gene product and severe disease, β-thalassemia.

Single Gene Patterns of Inheritance

The chromosomes in the pairs numbered 1 to 22, ranging in size from the largest to the smallest, are called *autosomes*, and the chromosomes in the remaining pair are called the *sex chromosomes* (X and Y). When a trait is determined by the presence of one variant allele at the locus on an autosome, that trait is inherited as an **autosomal dominant trait**. A person exhibiting that trait can be either homozygous (two variant alleles) or **heterozygous** (one variant allele) for that trait. When the expression of the trait requires that both genes consist of the same variant allele, the trait is said to be an autosomal **recessive trait**. The terms *dominant* and *recessive* refer to the trait in question, not to the genes determining that trait. Whether a trait is classified as dominant or recessive can depend on the definition of what constitutes presence of the disease. For example, if the investigator studies families with the sickle cell gene only by detecting morphological sickling, the disease would be classed as dominantly inherited because only one gene would be sufficient to cause the trait. If, on the other hand, only measurement of the total hemoglobin concentration is used, the disease is classed as an autosomal recessive disorder because heterozygotes and homozygotes for the normal allele would be indistinguishable. When electrophoresis is used, all three genotypes are definable, and the trait is classified as codominantly inherited. One parent may transmit an autosomal dominant disorder to his or her offspring since a dominant disorder is determined by the presence of a single allele, but an autosomal recessively inherited disorder requires inheritance from both parents. It can be seen from Fig. 47-2 that a person may inherit the carrier state for sickle cell disease by inheriting the disease gene from a single parent, but sickle cell disease occurs only when the disease gene is inherited from both parents. In general, the disorders that are characterized by altered biochemical metabolism and are diagnosable through biochemical means are conditions that are recessively inherited.

The two sex chromosomes of the human male consist of an X chromosome and a Y chromosome. The human female has two X chromosomes. The enzyme glucose-6-phosphate dehydrogenase (G-6-PD) is coded for by a gene on the X chromosome. Because a female has two X chromosomes and a male has one X chromosome, it might be expected that a female would make twice as much G-6-PD as a male does. On the average, however, females and males make equal amounts of G-6-PD. A gene dosage compensation occurs by a mechanism called **lyonization**, or random inactivation of the X chromosome. During early embryonic development of the 46,XX female, one of the two X chromosomes is randomly inactivated; it no longer produces gene products. Because this is a random process, each female is a mosaic, or mixture, of cells in which one or the other, but not both, of the X chromosomes is functioning (Fig. 47-3). The presence of a Y chromosome is associated with maleness, and its absence is associated with femaleness. The Y chromosome carries a factor called the *testis determining factor (TDF)*, which induces the embryonic gonad to develop into a testis; in its absence the gonad develops as an ovary. There are no other genes residing on the Y chromosome that have been shown to code for proteins. The X chromosome carries many structural genes and codes for proteins similar to those coded for by autosomes.

The difference in the sex chromosome constitution of males and females is the basis for the particular pattern of inheritance that is known as **X-linked**. If there is a mutation on the single X chromosome of a male, that male will always transmit that mutant gene to all of his daughters and to none of his sons. A heterozygous female may give either of her X chromosomes, one of which has the normal gene and one of which has the mutant gene, to a son or daughter. If the mutation on the X chromosome results in a disease when present in the heterozygous state of the female, the trait is known as an *X-linked dominant disorder* and will be observed in both males and females. Because the single X of the male carries a mutation, the disease is usually more severe in the male than in the female who has a mutant gene and a normal gene. If the mutation is not expressed as a recognizable trait in the heterozygous state of the female, the disorder is referred to as *X-linked recessively inherited*. Males will manifest the disorder, and females will carry but not manifest the gene for the disorder. Females are carriers

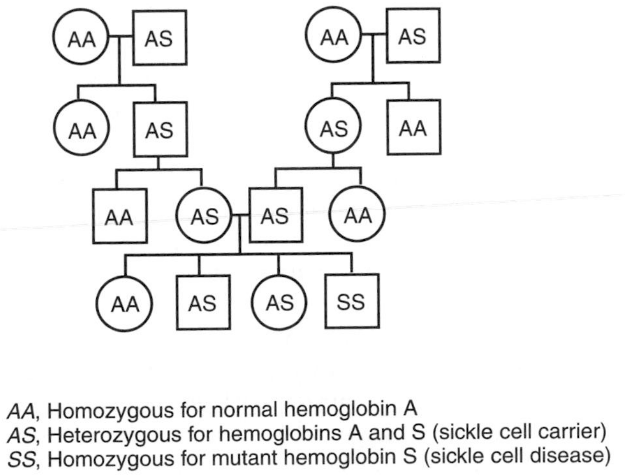

AA, Homozygous for normal hemoglobin A
AS, Heterozygous for hemoglobins A and S (sickle cell carrier)
SS, Homozygous for mutant hemoglobin S (sickle cell disease)

Fig. 47-2 Pedigree that demonstrates segregation of single-gene mutations. Heterozygous state (carrier for sickle-cell disease in this example) is inherited from a single parent, whereas homozygous state (a person affected with sickle cell disease in this example) requires inheritance of a mutant gene from each parent.

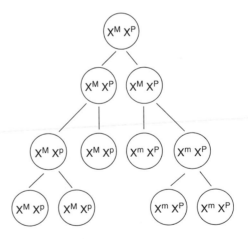

X^M, Active maternally derived X chromosome
X^P, Active paternally derived X chromosome
X^m, Inactive maternally derived X chromosome
X^P, Inactive paternally derived X chromosome

Fig. 47-3 Random inactivation of the X chromosome in the 46,XX female. Once an X chromosome is inactivated, that particular X is inactivated in all subsequent progeny of that cell.

for hemophilia and Duchenne muscular dystrophy, but the disease occurs among males who have a single copy of the mutant gene. Tests can identify the carrier female for most X-linked recessive diseases. In general these tests demonstrate a partial expression in females of the defect seen in affected males.

Numerous traits, such as height and intelligence, and isolated birth defects, such as cleft lip and congenital heart disease, are determined by the joint action of many genes and the environment. This mode of inheritance is called *multifactorial causation*. Such traits are familial and have a major genetic input but do not segregate in families in a manner similar to that seen for autosomal dominant and recessive traits. An expressed trait is the consequence of numerous genes received from each parent and a variable environmental influence that determines the expression of the trait. In addition to isolated birth defects seen in infants, multifactorial causation is responsible for many common diseases of adults. Examples include insulin-independent diabetes mellitus, osteoarthritis, gout, and certain forms of hypertension and coronary artery disease.

A system of describing the chromosomal location of the gene abnormality has been devised using the traditional karyotyping nomenclature and the Human Genome Project information. The chromosome location is expressed as the chromosome number, followed by an indication of whether the gene is on the larger (q) or smaller (p) arm of the chromosome, followed by the karyotyping band number.

Human Genome Project: Implications for Human Health

In 1990, an international effort was initiated to map, sequence, and characterize the entire human genome. The National Human Genome Research Institute (NHGRI) and the Department of Energy (DOE) funded the US arm of the project, the roles of which are as follows: (1) to decipher the complete sequence of the human genome; (2) to develop efficient sequencing technology; (3) to identify the variations in human DNA that underlie disease susceptibility, particularly **single nucleotide polymorphisms (SNPs)**; (4) to interpret the function of the DNA sequence on a genomic scale; (5) to analyze the genome of key model organisms, such as *Drosophila*, yeast, the roundworm, and mouse; (6) to examine the ethical, legal, and social implications of genome research (ELSI); (7) to develop bioinformatics tools and computational strategies for the collection, storage, and analysis of human genome project data; and (8) to train scientists for research in genomic science.

The ultimate goal of the project was to map and characterize all known human genes. That result has already led to far-less-than-expected estimates of the total number of human genes (approximately 30,000). The second major goal is to develop a map of single nucleotide polymorphisms (or SNPs) that can be used to identify heritable susceptibility to common disease, as well as susceptibility to pathological reactions to a host of environmental and pharmacological agents. In the future, these SNPs may also allow pharma-

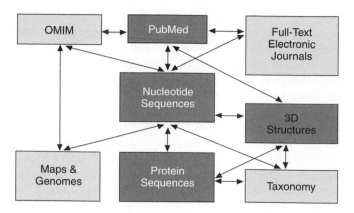

Fig. 47-4   Screen capture of the Human Genome Website and the relationships of the various databases available.

INFORMATION AVAILABLE ON THE OMIM WEBSITE FOR GENETIC DEFECTS

OMIM number
Common name—Example: GAUCHER DISEASE, TYPE 1
Gene map locus, for example 1q21
Explanation of the OMIM number
Clinical features
Links to references
Links to PubMed (see CD-ROM)
Links to gene map

---

ceutical researchers to predict drug efficacy in individuals. A long-term goal is to develop mapped panels of the 30,000 SNPs, spread evenly throughout the genome, that can be assayed after immobilization as arrays on silicone chips. These SNP arrays would then be used with high throughput technology to detect disease or disease susceptibility in individuals.

The large body of information about inherited disorders and the clinical results of these disorders can be related to the proteins affected and thus to the base nucleotide changes. All of this information has been integrated into a large set of interacting databases by the National Center for Biotechnology Information (NCBI), which can be accessed from the NCBI website (http://www.ncbi.nlm.nih.gov/genome/guide/human/). The interaction of these databases is depicted in Fig. 47-4.

One of the databases, Online Mendelian Inheritance in Man (OMIM), catalogs all known genetic defects and/or alleles (www.ncbi.nlm.nih.gov/entrez/query.fcgi?db=OMIM).

The tables in this chapter represent only a small portion of the information available for classifying these genetic diseases. A brief description of the available data is given in the box above.

Fig. 47-5 is a screen capture of a search for lipidoses on the OMIM website, from which you can search for specific diseases or a class of diseases. In this example, lipidoses are described.

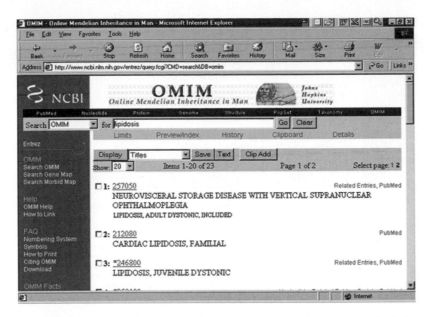

Fig. 47-5 Screen capture of the NCBI website shows the result of a search for information on the lipidoses.

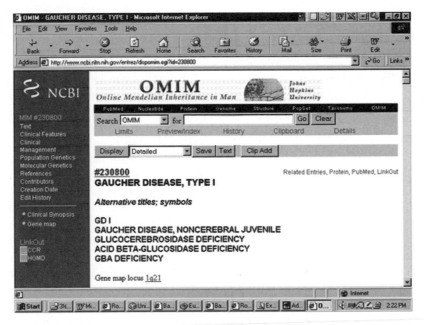

Fig. 47-6 Screen capture of detailed information obtained by clicking on the OMIM number from the search. Each OMIM entry is given a unique six-digit number whose first digit indicates the mode of inheritance of the gene involved. A detailed description of the numbering system is available at the OMIM website.

Fig. 47-6 is a screen capture of detailed information obtained by clicking on the OMIM number from the search. Each OMIM entry is given a unique 6-digit number whose first digit indicates the mode of inheritance of the gene involved. A detailed description of the numbering system is available at the OMIM website.

Fig. 47-7 is a screen capture of detailed genome map of the region where Gaucher's disease is located.

Development of these technologies will fundamentally change the interface between genomic science and clinical medicine. Where once genetics was primarily the province of those studying relatively rare mendelian disorders, new genome-based applications are likely to emerge that will make analysis of human genomic information highly relevant for the practice of general medicine. It is not unreasonable to expect that within the near future, a physician may assay a patient's genome for thousands of **polymorphisms** and use that information to predict the likelihood of complex common diseases, such as arthrosclerosis, arteriosclerotic heart disease, stroke, cancers, and arthritis. That same information

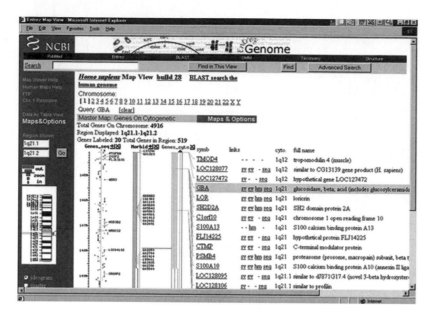

Fig. 47-7 Screen capture of detailed genome map of region where Gaucher's disease is located.

would help the clinician and patient predict the appropriate medication.

Attendant to the tremendous advantages that clinical use of genomic science may bring is the specter of misuse of private genetic information. The establishment of standards for privacy and ethical use of genetic information will be an important social goal in the near future.

USES OF THE DNA SEQUENCE OF THE HUMAN GENOME

Under the aegis of the Genome Project, an ordered set of oligonucleotide sequences, one mapping approximately every 10 million base pairs, was established; 350 such sequences span the entire genome. Starting with families with inherited diseases and using standard linkage studies, investigators can locate the gene in question between two such markers. The sequence of the gene in question can then be compared with the reference sequence to establish whether a gene variation is present. The identity of the candidate protein can also be established by comparing it with the sequence of identified genes in the computerized GenBank database.

Connexins

A more detailed example of how knowledge of gene sequences will be used in genetics in the 21st century is provided by the role of connexins in both nonsyndromic and syndromic hereditary deafness. Connexins are a family of proteins contributing to gap junctions, clusters of proteins in cell outer membranes that create channels for various small molecules to rapidly pass from cell to cell. The gap junctions involved in deafness are believed to be involved in transporting potassium between auditory hair cells and support cells of the cochlea. Two subsets have been identified, alpha and beta (Kumar and Giluda, 1996).

One or more connexin (Cx) molecules may aggregate to form a connexin hexamer, which comprises a connexon, or channel in a cell. Connexons of one cell connect or dock with connexons of a juxtaposed cell to form a gap junction. Gap junctions occur in most cell types throughout the body. Initially these junctions were thought to allow molecules below molecular weights of 1000 to diffuse passively. However, there may be some specificity as to what molecules are transferred from one cell to another.

The connexin molecules are numbered according to their molecular weights in kilodaltons; the genetic loci are designated GJB (for gap junction beta) 1 to 6. Four of the six connexin loci have been found to be associated with deafness in addition to approximately 20 non-connexin other loci that contribute to nonsyndromic deafness. GJB2 at chromosome 13q12 encodes the protein Cx26 with a molecular weight of 26 kilodaltons. As of the year 2000, over 50 mutant alleles at this locus were identified that are transmitted with both dominant and recessive modes of inheritance. These include missense, chain termination, frame shift, and splice site mutations. A deletion of one G nucleotide in a sequence of 6Gs between nucleotides 30 and 35 accounts for 80% of autosomal recessively inherited deafness in Mediterraneans; approximately 3.5% of these populations are heterozygotes. Among Ashkenazi Jews and Sephardic Jews from North Africa, Iran, and Iraq, the frequency of heterozygotes varies from 0.7% to 3.5%. Four percent of Ashkenazi Jews are heterozygous for another deletion of a T at nucleotide 167. Among Japanese persons, 1% to 2% have a deletion of a C at nucleotide 235. GJB6, also on 13q12 close to GJB2, encodes Cx30; alleles at this locus are transmitted as autosomal dominant traits.

GJB3 on chromosome 1p33-p35 encodes Cx31, having both autosomal dominant and recessive alleles. Some mutations of this gene are associated with erythrokeratodermia. Cx32 encoded by GPB1 is X-linked. Charcot-Marie-Tooth, a neurological disease that includes deafness, is a recessively inherited allele at that locus. Alleles at these loci can be identified by either amplifying critical regions with the **polymerase chain reaction** or by sequencing the entire gene.

It is hoped that knowledge of the mutational abnormality will result in development of therapeutic agents to restore hearing or to correct the genetic defect (gene therapy). However, judging from the length of time that has elapsed since the knowledge of the abnormality in sickle cell anemia, the road to effective gene therapy for most genetic diseases is apt to be long and arduous.

PATHOLOGICAL DISORDERS ASSOCIATED WITH ABNORMAL CHROMOSOMES
Aneuploidy

Disorders that occur as the result of a chromosome abnormality involve a change in the gene dosage for a large number of genes rather than a change in the gene structure. This produces a change in the blueprint for the structural development of the embryo. Such an abnormality can come about in two ways. First, there is the presence or absence of an entire chromosome, an **aneuploidy**. This is exemplified by the presence of an extra 21 chromosome in trisomy 21, which causes **Down syndrome**, and by the presence of a single X chromosome resulting in **monosomy**, which occurs in **Turner's syndrome**. **Trisomy** means the presence of three copies of a chromosome rather than the normal two, and monosomy means the presence of a single copy. Second, there are structural alterations in chromosomes that result in the loss or addition of part but not all of a chromosome. A variety of structural abnormalities of chromosomes can lead to such a deviation from the normal amount of chromosomal material.

Chromosomal abnormalities involving the autosomes, whether they involve a partial or a complete loss or addition of a chromosome, always result in altered morphogenesis expressed as major and minor birth defects and altered mental development in the form of mental retardation. The altered physical development in a chromosomally abnormal embryo is called **dysmorphogenesis**; the individual physical abnormalities are called *dysmorphic features*. In Down syndrome these features include small ears, unusual creases on the palms, upward slant of the eyes, small head size, congenital heart disease, and short stature.

Down syndrome is an easily recognized combination of major and minor physical abnormalities associated with mental retardation. It occurs as the specific result of the presence of a triple dose of chromosome 21 material. This occurs most commonly as trisomy 21, the presence of three separate 21 chromosomes as the result of meiotic **nondisjunction**. Meiosis is the special form of cell division that occurs in germ cells that produce ova or sperm. This division reduces the chromosome number from 46 to 23, with one member of each pair of chromosomes being represented. Nondisjunction is the failure of one of a pair of chromosomes to go to each daughter cell during division; instead both go to one daughter cell (Fig. 47-8). The frequency of nondisjunction increases with maternal age. For that reason, prenatal diagnosis through **amniocentesis** with cytogenetic study is recommended for women 35 years of age or older. This form of Down syndrome does not occur with an increased familial incidence.

Structural Abnormalities of Chromosomes

A familial form of Down syndrome occurs with a structural abnormality known as a *Robertsonian translocation*. This **translocation** is formed by the fusion of the centromeres, most commonly of chromosomes 14 and 21. A carrier of a 14/21 translocation will have a total chromosomal number of 45. However, the translocation chromosome contains the normal amount of chromosomal material of two separate chromosomes and the carrier is phenotypically normal. Meiosis in a translocation carrier can result in a variety of different gametes. Among the offspring of carriers of a 14/21 translocation, one may observe normal infants with 46 normal chromosomes, phenotypically normal infants with 45 chromosomes and a translocation similar to the parent, and infants with 46 chromosomes of which there are two normal

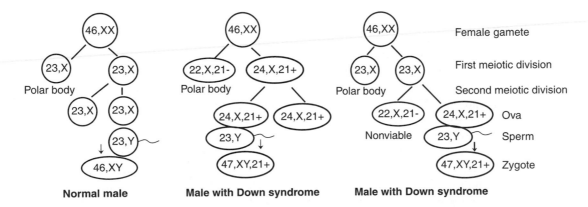

Fig. 47-8 Meiotic nondysjunction. *Left,* Normal meiosis of an ovum fertilized by a normal sperm yielding a normal zygote. *Center,* Error in first cell division of meiosis results in an aneuploid ovum that when fertilized yields a 47,XY,21+ male with Down syndrome. *Right,* Error has occurred in second cell division of meiosis with same result.

Gametes			Zygotes	Phenotype
	14,21			
	t14/21		45,XX,t14/21	Carrier
Ovum	14, 21			
Sperm	14, 21		46,XX	Normal
Ovum	t14/21			
Sperm	14, 21		45,XX,t14/21	Normal (carrier)
Ovum	t14/21, 21			
Sperm	14, 21		46,XX,t14/21	Down syndrome

Fig. 47-9 Translocation 14/21. Carrier has 45 chromosomes with one normal 14, one 21, and genetic content of a 14 and 21 contained in translocation. A person with Down syndrome as a result of such a translocation has two separate 21s and a third 21 as part of translocation. Such a person has a total of 46 chromosomes but genetic content of three number 21s, that is, trisomy 21.

21 chromosomes and the material of a third 21 present in the translocation (Fig. 47-9). Such children have typical Down syndrome. The translocation may occur in multiple members of a family, each of whom is a carrier at increased risk for having a child with Down syndrome. The familial and sporadic forms of Down syndrome can be differentiated by chromosomal studies. For that reason, it is advisable that each person with Down syndrome undergo chromosomal analysis to determine whether there is an increased risk that other family members will have children with Down syndrome.

Sex Chromosome Abnormalities (see also Chapter 45)

Alterations in the number of sex chromosomes are common, and several types of aneuploidy can occur. These conditions were originally recognized through the use of buccal smear for **Barr body** analysis. Each X chromosome in excess of 1 in the cell nucleus is inactivated and is seen microscopically as a Barr body. Named for its discoverer, a Barr body is the nuclear condensation of the inactivated X chromosome and appears as a clump inside and adjacent to the nuclear membrane (Fig. 47-10). The cells of a normal male contain only one X chromosome; thus no Barr body is present. Cells of a normal female contain two X chromosomes and demonstrate a single Barr body.

Abnormalities of sex chromosomes in females occur most commonly as a 45,X and a 47,XXX karyotype. The former is the most common chromosomal finding in Turner's syndrome. This disorder has three major features: short stature, minor dysmorphic abnormalities and congenital malformations, and sexual infantilism. The sexual infantilism occurs as a result of fibrosis of the infantile ovary, and so at the time of puberty there are neither follicles nor hormone-producing cells present. In its classic form this syndrome is diagnosed by buccal smear, which will show the absence of Barr bodies. However, a variety of X-chromosome abnorma-

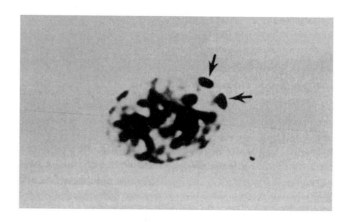

Fig. 47-10 Barr body. This cell has two Barr bodies seen as nuclear condensations just inside nuclear membrane at 3-o'clock position (*arrow*). Two Barr bodies would be seen in a male with 48,XXXY and a female with 47,XXX.

lities may result in Turner's syndrome; for that reason, a full lymphocyte karyotype should always be done regardless of the findings on buccal smear. The 47,XXX karyotype is not associated with significant clinical abnormalities.

The most common abnormalities of sex chromosomes in males include the 47,XXY and 47,XYY karyotypes. Klinefelter's syndrome (47,XXY) has three major clinical findings: minor to no dysmorphic abnormalities, normal to mild retardation in cognitive function, and failure of testicular development with secondary sexual infantilism and a eunuchoid body habitus. Because of the lack of testosterone production at the age of puberty, such males may respond to ovarian estrogens with breast enlargement or gynecomastia. Surgical correction of gynecomastia and testosterone replacement therapy will correct most of the problems associated with this disorder. There is considerable controversy regarding the type and frequency of clinical manifestations associated with the 47,XYY karyotype. Males with the

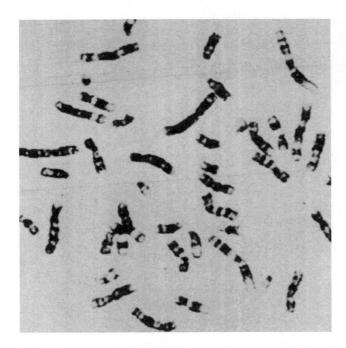

Fig. 47-11 Metaphase spread. Chromosomes as seen through microscope in a spread stained by G-banding technique.

TABLE 47-2 BUCCAL SMEAR FINDINGS IN SEX CHROMOSOME ABNORMALITIES

Karyotype	Sex	Barr Body	Y Body
46,XX	F	+	0
46,XY	M	0	+
45,X	F	0	0
47,XXX	F	++	0
48,XXXX	F	+++	0
49,XXXXX	F	++++	0
47,XXY	M	+	+
47,XYY	M	0	++
48,XXYY	M	+	++
49,XXXXY	M	+++	+

47,XYY karyotype are physically and sexually normal, but some studies have suggested that an increased proportion of men with this karyotype exhibit sociopathic behavior.

Cytogenetic Methods

The most common method of chromosome analysis involves the culture of peripheral lymphocytes. These are mature cells circulating in the peripheral blood that are not actively undergoing cell division. Such cells can be stimulated to divide by the addition of a **mitogen** to the culture medium. The most commonly used mitogen in human cytogenetics is phytohemagglutinin (PHA). Lymphocytes in the presence of PHA are commonly cultured for 72 hours. Toward the end of the culture period, colchicine is added to the culture. This agent acts as a microtubular poison and thereby disrupts the mitotic spindle during cell division. Thus cells can be arrested in metaphase, the only time during cell division when chromosomes can be easily visualized and studied (Fig. 47-11). At the end of the culture period the cells can be harvested, spread on a slide, and stained with a number of fluorogens or chromogens. When special fixative techniques are used, the chromosomes take on a banded appearance. These bands are specific for each chromosome and allow detailed analysis of the structure of each chromosome.

The normal Y chromosome contains a large fluorescent segment in the long arm. If a buccal smear from a 46,XY male is stained with a fluorescent dye, a bright fluorescent spot called the *F body*, or **Y body**, will be revealed. The use of Giemsa staining for Barr bodies and fluorescent staining for Y bodies allows determination of the sex-chromosome constitution from a buccal smear. The recognition of Barr bodies and Y bodies is sufficiently subjective that an accurate determination requires an experienced technician, using control cells from a normal male and female. The expected findings of Barr body and Y body determination on a buccal smear for normal and abnormal sex chromosomal constitutions are shown in Table 47-2. Recently, techniques have been developed for hybridizing RNA or DNA (see Chapter 48) labeled with chromogenic enzymes or fluorochromes to chromosome preparations that have been fixed during metaphase. Labeling the molecular probes with different colored fluorochromes allows complex karyotypic abnormalities, including single-copy genes, to be defined. Genes hybridized with probes for the constituent genes labeled with fluorochromes of complementary colors will appear as a third color. The use of **fluorescent in situ hybridization**, or **FISH technique**, has added another dimension to karyotypic analysis.

Fluorescent in situ hybridization is the hybridization of short sequences of single-stranded DNA probes, complementary to the desired test DNA sequences within the intact chromosomes. The probes bind to the complementary DNA, and the labeled fluorescent tags allow visualization of the location of the test sequences of DNA (Fig. 47-12). One advantage of the FISH technique is that it can be performed on nondividing cells. Because each chromosome can be painted a different color, this technique is used to determine whether an individual has the correct number of chromosomes.

Whole chromosome probes are collections of smaller probes, each of which hybridizes to a different sequence along the length of the same chromosome. Using these libraries of probes, it is possible to paint an entire chromosome and generate a spectral karyotype. This full color image of the chromosomes makes it possible to distinguish between the chromosomes based on their colors, rather than based on their dark and light banding patterns, as with traditional karyotyping.

Microarray analysis is another technology used for the study of the human genome (see www.ncbi.nlm.nih.gov/About/primer/microarrays.html). Microarray analysis works by exploiting the ability of a given mRNA molecule to bind specifically to, or hybridize to, the DNA template from which it originated. The hybridization can be observed or

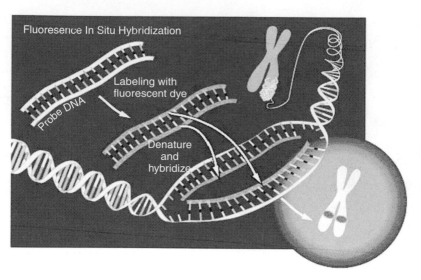

Fig. 47-12   Schematic representation of the FISH technique. *(From the NIH website.)*

quantified by labeling the hybridizing RNA or cDNA with a fluorescent probe. The DNA fragments on the target surface are arranged in a precise manner or array so that every position in the array represents a known sequence. The reaction is quantified by a recording of the fluorescence intensity at each position. The intensity is related to the amount of each gene's expression. With this technology it is possible to map the gene expression of healthy and diseased cells.

Chromosomal Markers of Disease

The analysis of the chromosomes in dividing cells may reveal abnormalities of three types: first, a change in the amount of chromosomal material present as in aneuploidy or partial duplication or deletion; second, no alteration in the amount of chromosomal material but chromosomal changes that are diagnostic of specific disease states; third, nonspecific changes in chromosomal structure or number that reflect the consequences of environmental influences such as drugs or radiation or the abnormal chromosomal behavior seen in malignant cells.

Improvements in culture techniques and staining of chromosomes have revealed that malignant cells often demonstrate a consistent and specific chromosomal abnormality that is of major diagnostic assistance. Such an abnormality is best exemplified by the Philadelphia chromosome (Ph[1]) found in the majority of persons with chronic myelogenous leukemia (CML). The Philadelphia chromosome represents a deletion in chromosome 22, which renders it a small acrocentric chromosome (Fig. 47-13). The deleted material is most often translocated to chromosome 9. Thus there is no loss or gain of chromosomal material, but there is a structural rearrangement. The Philadelphia chromosome is confined to the malignant cells of the bone marrow, and analysis for the Philadelphia chromosome is done on bone marrow aspirate. The breakpoints of these chromosomes have been cloned into bacteria using recombinant DNA technology. The translocation creates a fusion gene, the 5′ portion of which is

derived from the c-*Abelson* oncogene that is usually present in the long arm of chromosome 9; the 3′ end is derived from a gene in the break-cluster region on chromosome 22. The resulting fusion protein is a truncated protein kinase. The clinical expression of the associated malignancy is correlated with the precise location of the translocation. The translocations accompanying many malignancies include oncogenes, immunoglobulins, and various cell receptors.

A second type of chromosomal marker used diagnostically is that of chromosomal breakage. This is most dramatically illustrated in Fanconi anemia. Persons with this form of autosomal, recessively inherited, aplastic anemia demonstrate a pronounced increase in the frequency of spontaneous chromosomal breaks and gaps in cultured peripheral lymphocytes. Aplastic anemia occurs as a result of failure of the bone marrow to produce blood cells. Studies of cultured somatic cells from persons with Fanconi anemia imply four different genetic mechanisms that are believed to affect DNA repair proteins. Thus the various dysmorphic features are believed to be the result of multiple somatic mutations resulting from defective repair of DNA.

The autosomal recessively inherited disorder Bloom's syndrome is also characterized by a sharp increase in the frequency of sister chromatid exchanges in cultured lymphocytes. Bloom's syndrome is typically characterized by intrauterine growth retardation and short stature thereafter. Such patients have increased skin sensitivity to ultraviolet rays and a significant risk for malignancies, including leukemia during late childhood and early adult years.

A fourth type of specific chromosomal marker is the fragile X chromosome recognized in one X-linked form of mental retardation. The characteristic findings in this disorder include postpubertal enlargement of the testes; large, simply formed ears; a jovial personality; and moderate to severe mental retardation. Approximately 10% of female carriers for this form of X-linked mental retardation show a mild form of mental retardation. The culture of lymphocytes

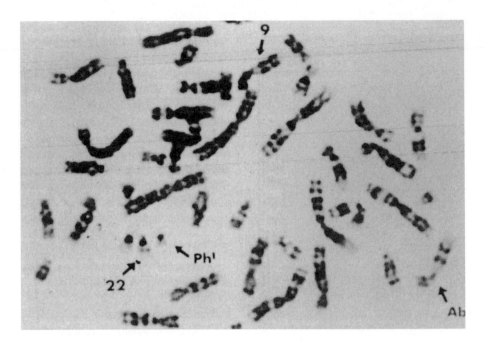

Fig. 47-13 Philadelphia chromosome. A metaphase spread with banded chromosomes shows small number 22, or Ph[1] chromosome, and normal 22 + normal chromosome 9 and chromosome 9(Ab) involved in 9/22 translocation producing Ph[1] chromosome.

with the standard growth media used for cytogenetic studies will not demonstrate the fragile X chromosome. However, the use of media that are deficient in folic acid will show a fragile X chromosome in a significant percentage of cells from an affected male. The designation *fragile X* is used because the X chromosome in these males appears to have a break at the end of the long arm.

The mode of inheritance of the fragile X syndrome has several unusual features. Carrier females have only mild mental retardation, never severe mental impairment. In affected males, the defect appears to be progressively more severe in subsequent generations of the same family, and the age of onset is progressively earlier. The fragile X site has now been cloned, and the basic defect has been shown to be a defect of amplification of DNA. In the normal population, a highly polymorphic sequence of 5 to 54 CGG triplet repeats is found between the 5′ end of the chromosome and the fragile X gene (called the *FMR-1 gene*). Carriers in affected families have an abnormally increased number of triplets. The threshold for clinical expression of the gene defect is approximately 80 triplets. The offspring of individuals with more than 50 repeats are at increased risk for larger amplifications. Severely affected individuals may have up to 4000 tandem copies of the CGG triplets, with severity being proportional to the number of repeats. The number of triplets transmitted by males to their daughters is stable. A many-fold amplification can occur during a single meiosis in a female carrier. Although the FMR-1 protein is expressed in brain and testicle, its function is still not known.

Similar defects in amplification are found in spinal and bulbar muscular atrophy, or Kennedy disease, in which the 11 to 31 CAG repeats normally present in the first exon of the gene for the androgen receptor are represented by a polyglutamine stretch in the protein. In myotonic dystrophy 5 to 30 copies of a GCT repeat are normally present in the untranslated region between the 3′ end of the chromosome and the termination codon of a gene designated the myotonin protein kinase (MT-PK) gene on chromosome 19. Huntington's disease is also caused by perturbed amplification of sequences found between the 5′ end of the chromosome and the Huntington gene on chromosome 7. Additional information on the effect of amplification of repeat sequences can be found in Chapter 48.

PATHOLOGICAL DISORDERS ASSOCIATED WITH BIOCHEMICAL CHANGES
Lysosomal Storage Diseases

Lysosomal storage diseases are recessively inherited disorders, each of which is the result of a deficiency of a specific acid hydrolase. These acid hydrolases are located within membrane-bound cytoplasmic organelles called *lysosomes*. If there is a complete or nearly complete deficiency of a specific hydrolase, the macromolecular compound that it normally degrades will accumulate within tissue. The primary organs affected will depend on the tissue distribution of the macromolecular compound. These organs include (1) the reticuloendothelial system, (2) the central nervous system (CNS), and (3) the skeleton and connective tissues and other somatic tissues. In a given disorder the clinical manifestations may be apparent in only one or in any combination of these three organ systems. The box on p. 920 lists a classification scheme for lysosomal storage diseases.

Varying degrees of deficiency or altered activity of a hydrolase may result in several different clinical syndromes

CLASSIFICATION OF LYSOSOMAL STORAGE DISEASE

Mucopolysaccharidoses
Mucolipidoses (ML)
    ML I (now called sialidosis)
    ML II or I-cell disease
    ML III or pseudo-Hurler polydystrophy
    ML IV
Gangliosidoses
    G_{M1} gangliosidosis or generalized gangliosidosis
    G_{M2} gangliosidosis
        Tay-Sachs disease
        Sandhoff disease
Leukodystrophies
    Metachromatic leukodystrophy
    Krabbe's disease
    Adrenoleukodystrophy
Glycoproteinosis
    Mannosidosis
    Fucosidosis
    Sialidosis
    Aspartylglucosaminuria
Others
    Ceramidosis
    Cholesterol ester storage disease
    Pompe's disease or glycogen storage disease II

occurring as a result of the same enzyme deficiency. This is demonstrated by deficiency of the hydrolase α-L-iduronidase. Deficiency of this enzyme results in the accumulation of the glycosaminoglycans, dermatan sulfate and heparan sulfate. In its most severe form with the greatest degree of enzyme deficiency, Hurler's syndrome occurs with severe skeletal, somatic, and central nervous system manifestations and death by 5 to 8 years of age. In its mildest form, deficiency of this enzyme results in Scheie syndrome, with normal height, life expectancy, and intelligence but with skeletal, ocular, and cardiac abnormalities. An intermediate form, known as *Hurler-Scheie syndrome*, is intermediate in its clinical manifestations.

Reticuloendothelial system involvement. The two disorders in which involvement of the liver and spleen is most prominent and may represent the major manifestation are Gaucher's and Niemann-Pick diseases. Gaucher's disease occurs as a result of the deficiency of the acid hydrolase β-glucosidase.

$$Ceramide\text{-}\beta\text{-}glucose \xrightarrow{\beta\text{-Glucosidase} + H_2O} Ceramide + Glucose$$

Deficiency of this enzyme results in the lysosomal accumulation of the phospholipid glucosylceramide. This disorder occurs in several forms. The most severe form is known as *neuronopathic Gaucher's disease* (type 2) in which, although liver and spleen enlargement occur, massive accumulation of phospholipids within the central nervous system predominates, and affected infants die within the first year of life. The other extreme is illustrated by the adult form

of Gaucher's disease (type 1) recognized by hepatosplenomegaly, in which good general health and normal life expectancy occur. Before the use of enzyme assays for specific diagnoses, Gaucher's disease was most often recognized by the demonstration of Gaucher cells (large macrophages) in a bone marrow aspirate. Because the gene for ceramide glucosidase has been cloned, diagnosis with an accuracy heretofore impossible is allowed. Gaucher's disease is prevalent in Ashkenazi Jews. A mutation at nucleotide 1226 accounts for 73% of the mutant alleles (gene frequency, 0.035) in this population. Additional alleles account for a total-population heterozygote frequency of 8.9% and a disease incidence at birth of 1:450. The enzyme, ceramide glucosidase, is now available commercially, though at great cost. Use of this enzyme as a therapeutic agent can allow mobilization of the accumulated ganglioside from bone and liver. However, reversal of the neurological disease is still not possible.

The second disorder in this group, Niemann-Pick disease, also occurs in several forms ranging from a severe infantile to a mild adult disease. This disorder occurs as a result of a deficiency of sphingomyelinase.

$$Sphingomyelin \xrightarrow{Sphingomyelinase + H_2O} Ceramide + Phosphorylcholine$$

Niemann-Pick disease is also associated with enlargement of the liver and spleen. The disease can be diagnosed by the demonstration of storage cells on bone marrow aspirate that represent macrophages with lysosomes engorged with sphingomyelin. The acid sphingomyelinase gene has been cloned and mapped to chromosome 11p15; numerous mutations have been defined at the molecular level. See the OMIM website to search for detailed information on **gene clones** and these diseases.

CNS predominance. The lysosomal storage diseases that affect primarily the CNS clinically involve gray matter or white matter initially. When the initial accumulation is within white matter, the disorder is known as a *leukodystrophy*, and motor abnormalities are seen early in the course of the disease. The most commonly recognized leukodystrophy is metachromatic leukodystrophy, in which neural tissue demonstrates a particular metachromatic staining property resulting from the lysosomal accumulation of sulfated galactosylceramide. The deficient enzyme is called *arylsulfatase A*, or *cerebroside sulfate sulfatase*. Several screening tests are available for this disorder and include the examination of urine for metachromatic granules.

$$Ceramide\text{-}\beta\text{-}galactose\text{-}3\ sulfate \xrightarrow{Sulfate\ acrylsulfatase\ A + H_2O} Ceramide\text{-}\beta\text{-}galactose + Sulfate$$

In normal urine, adequate amounts of this enzyme are present for a simple colorimetric assay of arylsulfatase activity. The presence of an adequate amount of enzyme activity will exclude this diagnosis, but lack of enzyme activity is not diagnostic and indicates that more specific assay systems should be used. The specific diagnosis of metachromatic leukodystrophy requires the demonstration of arylsulfatase A deficiency in homogenized peripheral leukocytes or cultured skin fibroblasts. Arylsulfatase occurs in two lysosomal forms known as A and B. The use of cellulose acetate electrophoresis is a second diagnostic method. In metachromatic leukodystrophy, a normal arylsulfatase B band will be observed, and no A band will be recognized.

The best-known lysosomal storage disease resulting in macromolecular compound accumulation initially within gray matter is **Tay-Sachs disease**. This disorder occurs as a result of the accumulation of G_{M2} ganglioside (Fig. 47-14) within the CNS. In the classical form it results in early regression of CNS function, and so by 1 year of age children with this disease have delayed cognitive development, impaired hearing and sight, and a characteristic cherry-red spot found on funduscopic examination. The accumulation of G_{M2} ganglioside within the CNS occurs as a result of deficiency of the acid hydrolase N-acetyl-β-D-galactosaminidase. Many variant juvenile and adult-onset forms have been defined, often appearing as the late onset of cerebellar ataxia or convulsions. The activity of N-acetyl-β-D-galactosaminidase is assayed with an artificial substrate, either a glucosamine or a galactosamine. Therefore the enzyme activity so measured is based on hexosaminidase. Hexosaminidase occurs as a heat-labile form, hexosaminidase A, a heteropolymer of α and β subunits, and a heat-stabile form, hexosaminidase B, a homopolymer of β subunits. Tay-Sachs disease is usually characterized by the specific deficiency of hexosaminidase A. Sandhoff's disease is associated with numerous mutations of the β gene. Measurement of enzyme activity with and without heat inactivation gives levels of hexosaminidase B and total hexosaminidase, respectively. The difference between the two determinations is thus the calculated level of hexosaminidase A, or the heat-labile form. A so-called associated activation protein has been found to be a small protein that forms a complex with G_{M2} ganglioside, making it accessible to the hexosaminidase. Mutations of the gene coding for this protein may impair the functional activity of both the A and B enzymes and also affect the disease.

Because Tay-Sachs disease occurs most commonly among Ashkenazi Jews, this target population can be screened for carrier detection. Determination of the percentage of hexosaminidase A present as a function of total hexosaminidase activity represents the most accurate screening method for detecting carriers of Tay-Sachs disease. In the establishment of a screening assay system for Tay-Sachs disease carriers, it is necessary that each laboratory determine its reference values and values for Tay-Sachs disease carriers. Confirmation of the carrier state requires study of hexosaminidase A activity in peripheral leukocytes and additional family studies if necessary to resolve questionable results. The use of such carrier tests among Ashkenazi Jews and subsequent use of prenatal diagnosis have significantly reduced the incidence of Tay-Sachs disease in the United States.

Application of recombinant DNA technology to the study of Tay-Sachs disease has greatly expanded understanding of the clinical heterogeneity of the disease that has been evident. The structural genes for the α and β subunits of hexosamidase and the activator proteins are on chromosomes 15, 5, and 5, respectively. Of the 3% of Ashkenazi Jews who are heterozygotes for this disease, approximately 73% have an insertion of four nucleotide base pairs in exon 11 to create a frameshift mutation; 15% have a G-to-C substitution in the first nucleotide of intron 12 to create a splicing abnormality; 4% have a glycine 269 substitution by serine at the 3′ end of exon 7, which is responsible for adult-onset disease, and 8% have either false-positive results or have a heterogeneous group of other mutations. The presence of multiple mutations, all of eastern European Ashkenazic origin, argues for some selective advantage for heterozygote formation rather than a "founder effect" (passing on original mutations) as the explanation for the high frequency. Eighty percent of non-Jewish heterozygotes have other mutations.

Connective tissue and skeletal predominance. Lysosomal storage diseases in which involvement of connective tissue, especially the skeletal system, predominates are referred to as *Hurler-like disorders*. With skeletal system involvement, there may also be CNS or reticuloendothelial involvement. Table 47-3 lists a classification of lysosomal disorders that are seen with this phenotype.

Hurler's syndrome represents the prototype of diseases involving glycosaminoglycan metabolism and resulting in

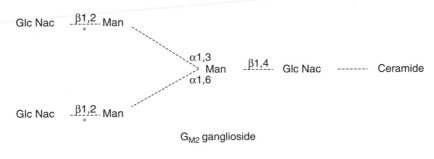

*Cleaved by hexosaminidase A (N-acetyl-β-1,2-galactosaminidase)

Fig. 47-14 Tay-Sachs disease. G_{M2} ganglioside accumulates in the gray matter of brain because of deficiency of N-acetyl-β-1,2-galactosaminidase (hexosaminidase A). *Glc Nac*, N-Acetylglucosamine; *Man*, mannose.

a connective tissue disorder. This form of α-L-iduronidase deficiency is characterized by multisystem involvement that is usually apparent by 6 months of age (Fig. 47-15). It follows a rapidly progressive course thereafter, with all organ systems involved and mental deterioration predominating late in the disorder; death ultimately occurs between 5 and 8 years of age. These diseases were classified initially on the basis of the urinary pattern of mucopolysaccharide or glycosaminoglycan excretion. In Hurler's syndrome massive amounts of dermatan sulfate and heparan sulfate are excreted in the urine. Mucopolysacchariduria is detected by a variety of screening tests, including a urine spot test called the *toluidine blue test*.

Recognition of the clinical phenotype and the presence of a positive urine screening test are followed by the study of mucopolysaccharide metabolism in cultured fibroblasts and the assay of specific hydrolases that can cause the mucopolysaccharidoses. Inorganic sulfate added to tissue culture media is exclusively incorporated into cultured fibroblasts as sulfated glycosaminoglycans. The use of radioactive sulfate allows the recognition of accumulation of these sulfated compounds within cultured fibroblasts and therefore provides direct evidence for tissue accumulation of glycosaminoglycans. A specific diagnosis can be pursued by the assay of the individual hydrolases that, when deficient, result in a mucopolysaccharidosis. The pattern of mucopolysacchariduria

and the specific acid hydrolase deficient in the mucopolysaccharidoses are shown in Table 47-4.

Another disorder that results in a Hurler-like clinical picture is *mucolipidosis II*, or I cell disease. Children with this disease are clinically similar to those with Hurler's syndrome but are diagnosed at an earlier age and follow a more rapid downhill course, with death by 3 to 5 years of age. There is no mucopolysacchariduria. When cultured skin fibroblasts from affected children were first analyzed under phase microscopy, a sharp increase in cytoplasmic inclusions was noted, hence the name *I cell*, or *inclusion cell*, *disease*. Lysosomal hydrolases are glycoproteins. Each lysosomal enzyme has a unique structural gene that codes for the protein component of the glycoprotein. There is, however, commonality in the posttranslational modification of these proteins to form the oligosaccharide component of the glycoproteins. It has been recognized that mannose-6-phosphate sugars in the oligosaccharide chain of the glycoprotein structure of acid hydrolases are required for their appropriate intracellular localization. This is accomplished through several posttranslational enzymatic steps in the modification of the oligosaccharide chain. Deficiency of a transferase involved in such posttranslational modifications represents the primary molecular defect in I cell disease. Cultured skin

---

TABLE 47-3   HURLER-LIKE DISORDERS

Disorders	Screening Test
Mucopolysaccharidoses	Urinary screening for mucopoly-sacchariduria
Mucolipidoses	
ML II and ML III	Serum levels of acid hydrolases
	Urinary bound sialic acid
Glycoproteinosis	Urinary oligosaccharide TLC
	Urinary bound sialic acid

IA—Glc Nac—GA—Glc Nac—IA—Glc Nac
  *   *

Dermatan sulfate

IA—Gal Nac—GA—Gal Nac—IA—Gal Nac
  *   *

Heparan sulfate

*Site of hydrolysis by α-L-iduronidase in oligosaccharide chain of dermatan and heparan sulfate

Fig. 47-15 Hurler's syndrome. Deficiency of lysosomal hydrolase α-L-iduronidase results in widespread accumulation of both heparan and dermatan sulfate. *GA*, Glucosamine; *Gal Nac*, N-acetylgalactose; *Glc Nac*, N-acetylglucosamine; *IA*, iduronic acid.

TABLE 47-4   MUCOPOLYSACCHARIDOSES

Eponym	Number	Mucopolysacchariduria	Enzyme Deficiency
Hurler	HPS I-H	DS, HS	α-L-Iduronidase
Scheie	MPS I-S	DS, HS	α-L-Iduronidase
Hurler-Scheie	MPS I-H/S	DS, HS	α-L-Iduronidase
Hunger	MPS II	DS, HS	Iduronide sulfate sulfatase
Sanfilippo	MSP III-A	HS	Heparan-N-sulfate sulfatase
Sanfilippo	MPS III-B	HS	α-Glucosaminidase
Sanfilippo	MPS III-C	HS	Acetyl-CoA:α-glucosaminide N-acetyltransferase
Morquino A	MPS IV-A	KS	Galactosaminyl-6-sulfate sulfatase
Morquino B	MPS IV-B	KS	α-Galactosidase
Maroteaux-Lamy	MPS VI	DS	Galactosaminyl-4-sulfate sulfatase (arylsulfatase B)
Sly	MPS VII	DS or HS or DS, HS	β-Glucuronidase

DS, *Dermatan sulfate*; HS, *heparan sulfate*; KS, *keratan sulfate*.

fibroblasts from affected children show deficient levels of numerous acid hydrolases in cultured cells. The ultimate defect resides in the abnormal intracellular localization of these hydrolases. The urine of patients with I cell disease shows increased levels of lysosomal hydrolases and an increase in the amount of sialic acid oligosaccharides. The measurement of covalently bound sialic acid in urine is a relatively simple procedure and represents an excellent screening test for a large number of lysosomal storage diseases.

Disorders of Intermediary Metabolism

Disorders of intermediary metabolism occur as a result of three basic mechanisms: an enzyme deficiency with defective substrate conversion, a membrane transport defect resulting in failure of absorption or excessive excretion of a compound, and defects in receptors involved in mediating metabolism. The biochemical basis for the resulting disease occurs as a result of (1) accumulation of a substrate to levels that become toxic, (2) deficiency through lack of production or excessive loss of a needed compound, and (3) conversion of an accumulated compound to an altered metabolite that itself is a toxic material (Fig. 47-16). In general, defects in intermediary metabolism result in alterations of compounds with a molecular weight lower than those seen in lysosomal storage diseases. As a result, they are more likely to result in more acute manifestations and are less likely to be associated with the striking physical features that dominate in the lysosomal storage disorders. Defects in intermediary metabolism result in a disruption of normal metabolic process and often produce an elevated urinary excretion of a normal metabolite or the urinary excretion of an abnormal metabolite. Therefore urine screening tests are the principal means of recognizing the presence of such a disorder, prompting more specific diagnostic assays.

   Aminoacidopathies. Table 47-5 is a list of the more common amino acid disorders and their clinical chemical characterizations. **Phenylketonuria (PKU)** is the best known and best understood of the amino acid disorders. This autosomal recessively inherited disorder occurs as a defect in phenylalanine conversion to tyrosine because of a deficiency of the enzyme phenylalanine hydroxylase (PAH).

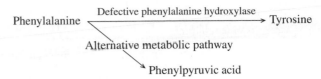

The deficiency of phenylalanine hydroxylase results in a shunting of phenylalanine metabolism to several ketoacids, the principal one being phenylpyruvic acid. This disease occurs in approximately 1 in 15,000 live births. The enzymatic activity is restricted to the liver, and therefore diagnosis is accomplished through demonstration of alterations in phenylalanine metabolism.

   Ferric chloride screening of the urine in the newborn had been used both for diagnosis and dietary management from early infancy; for the former it has been supplanted by the **Guthrie test**, in which a bacterial inhibition assay is used to detect an elevated level of phenylalanine. In newborn screening a Guthrie test is considered positive when the phenylalanine level exceeds 60 mg/L. Approximately 1 in 10 to 1 in 20 infants with a positive Guthrie screening test will in fact have phenylketonuria. Many state newborn screening programs now employ gas chromatography combined with tandem mass spectroscopy that allows automation for more accurate, efficient and rapid analysis with fewer false positive results. The values denoting normal and pathological findings are a function of the instrumentation and methodology employed and whether the sample is procured at 24 or 48 hours after birth. The specific diagnosis of phenylketonuria after a positive screening test requires the demonstration of plasma levels of phenylalanine greater than 200 mg/L on two consecutive days while normal feedings are given. After institution of dietary restriction in phenylalanine intake, urine screening tests will revert to normal. Subsequent monitoring of children on dietary management requires quantitative plasma determinations of phenylalanine levels.

   The gene for phenylalanine hydroxylase (PAH) has been mapped to chromosome 12q22-q24.1. Approximately 50 **haplotypes** have been defined on the basis of seven restriction fragment length polymorphisms. The most prevalent base variation among whites is a G-to-A substitution in intron 12; this mutation is on haplotype 3, and the combination is

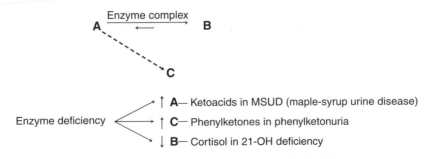

Fig. 47-16 Enzyme deficiency. Deficiency of enzyme in metabolic pathway may produce clinical symptoms because of accumulation of substrate, *A*; lack of production of product, *B*; or shunting of substrate to alternative pathway with production of a toxic compound, *C*.

TABLE 47-5   INBORN ERRORS OF INTERMEDIARY METABOLISM OF AMINO ACIDS

Condition	Defective Enzyme	Biochemical Features	Clinical Features	Treatment
Alkaptonuria*	Homogentisate oxygenase	Urinary excretion of homogenetisic acid	Urine darkens; ochronosis; arthritis in later life	Not known
Phenylketonuria†	Phenylalanine 4-hydroxylase	Phenylalanine accumulates in blood, CSF, etc.; urinary excretion of phenylpyruvic acid and related compounds	Severe mental deficiency, epilepsy, abnormal EEG, eczema, behavioral disorders	Diet low in phenylalanine beginning at early age
Albinism‡	o-Diphenol oxidase (tyrosinase)	Lack of melanin in skin, hair, and eyes	Photophobia, nystagmus, carcinomas of the skin	None known
Goitrous cretinism (several types)	(1) Tyrosine iodinase (2) Coupling enzyme (3) Deiodinase	Lack of thyroid hormone	Cretinism, goiter	Thyroxine or triiodothyronine
Maple-syrup urine disease (leucinosis)	Enzyme responsible for oxidative decarboxylation of α-ketoisocaproic, α-keto-β-methyl-n-valeric and α-ketoisovaleric acids	Leucine, isoleucine, and valine accumulate in blood, CSF, etc.; urinary excretion of the 3 keto acids and related compounds	Cerebral degeneration; usually early death, milder form with partial enzyme deficiency, symptomless except during infections, etc.	Diet low in leucine, isoleucine, and valine
Cystinosis	Cystine reductase (?)	Cystine is deposited in reticuloendothelial system; aminoaciduria, glucosuria, proteinuria, phosphaturia, dilute urine	Dwarfism, photophobia, renal acidosis, hypokalemia, vitamin-resistant rickets; death before puberty; a benign (nonrenal?) variant occurs in adults	Palliative: potassium salts, alkalis, vitamin D; diet low in cystine and methionine (efficacy doubtful)
Homocystinuria	L-Serine dehydratase	Urinary excretion of homocystine	Mental retardation, retinal defects, dislocated lenses, malar flush, thromboses	Diet low in methionine, high in cystine; pyridoxine
Hyperglycinemia (several types)	(Uncertain, depends on type)	Glycine accumulates in blood, etc.; urinary excretion of glycine and, in one type, methylmalonic acid	Neonatal lethargy and ketosis, neutropenia, hypo-γ-globulinemia; mental retardation	Diet low in protein
Oxalosis	Excessive conversion of glycine to oxalic acid	Calcium oxalate accumulates in kidneys, heart, bone marrow, and cartilages	Nephrocalcinosis leading to progressive renal failure	None known
Histidinemia	Histidine ammonialyase	Urinary excretion of β-imidazolylpyruvic acid and related compounds	Speech defects; mental retardation in some	Diet low in histidine
Familial tyrosinemia	Fumarylacetoacetase	Tyrosine levels in blood and urine raised; urinary excretion of phenolic acids related to tyrosine; generalized aminoaciduria; glucosuria; fructosuria	Rapidly enlarging liver; jaundice; hypoprothrombinemia; death common in infancy; survivors may have vitamin D-resistant rickets and acidosis	Diet low in tyrosine and phenylalanine (efficacy doubtful)
Hyperprolinemia				
Type I	Pyrroline-5-carboxylate reductase	Hyperprolinemia; urinary excretion of proline, glycine, and hydroxyproline	Mental retardation convulsions, renal disease, deafness	None known
Type II	Pyrroline-5-carboxylate dehydrogenase			
Hydroxyprolinemia	3-Hydroxypyrroline-5-carboxylate reductase (?)	High levels of hydroxyproline in blood and urine	Mental retardation (?)	None known
Citrullinemia	Argininosuccinate synthetase	High blood and urinary levels of citrulline; blood ammonia increased; urea excretion normal	Mental retardation, epilepsy, vomiting, ammonia intoxication	Diet low in protein

From Geigy scientific tables, ed 7, Summit, NJ, 1970, Ciba-Geigy Corp.
*Incidence 1 in 100,000.
†Incidence varies from 1 in 3200 to 1 in 10^7 according to locality.
‡Incidence 1 in 13,000.

TABLE 47-5 INBORN ERRORS OF INTERMEDIARY METABOLISM OF AMINO ACIDS—CONT'D

Condition	Defective Enzyme	Biochemical Features	Clinical Features	Treatment
Argininosuccinic-aciduria	Argininosuccinate lyase	Urinary excretion of argininosuccinic acid; high blood and CSF ammonia levels; urea excretion normal	Mental retardation, convulsions, hair abnormalities, ammonia intoxication	Diet low in protein
Hyperammonemia Type I Type II	Ornithine carbamolytransferase Carbamolyl-phosphate synthase	Blood ammonia about 10 mg/L; urea excretion normal	Mental retardation, ammonia intoxication	Diet low in protein(?)

widely distributed throughout Europe. The PAH mutations seen in African Americans are distributed among five haplotypes, one common and one rare in whites, the other three unique to African Americans. Some mutations are found on more than one haplotype, reflecting either a new mutation or a chromosomal cross-over.

Maple-syrup urine disease was so named because of the obvious odor of urine in affected infants. This disease occurs in roughly one in 250,000 live-born infants. Many disorders of amino acid metabolism are characterized by unusual odors, usually the result of the excessive urinary excretion of an organic acid. The three branched-chain amino acids, leucine, isoleucine, and valine, undergo transamination, transketolation, and decarboxylation through a common pathway (Fig. 47-17). Maple-syrup urine disease occurs as a result of a deficiency in the multicomponent enzyme branched-chain ketoacid decarboxylase. This enzyme activity resides in two proteins, E1 (composed of subunits E1α and E1β) and E2. The gene for E1a has been cloned and assigned to chromosome 19; E2 is located on chromosome 1. Mutants of all three loci have been defined.

Deficiency of ketoacid decarboxylase results in the elevated urinary excretion of the ketoacid analogs of these three branched-chain amino acids and gives positive ferric chloride and dinitrophenol hydrazine screening tests. The plasma is characterized by elevations in the levels of leucine, isoleucine, and valine. This disorder is screened for in the newborn using a bacterial-inhibition assay system, similar to the Guthrie test, which detects elevated levels of plasma leucine in the newborn. After the diagnosis, special diets that restrict the intake of isoleucine, leucine, and valine combined with careful monitoring can provide adequate control of this disease. Affected children who are not detected by newborn screening within the first month of life generally become acutely ill with hypoglycemia and ketoacidosis. Without early recognition and treatment, death most commonly occurs; in those infants whose complex diet is instituted late, significant mental retardation results.

Homocystinuria is generally recognized in late childhood because of physical abnormalities, with or without mental retardation. Homocystine is an intermediate amino acid in the metabolism of methionine to cystine. The most common form of homocystinuria occurs because of a deficiency of the enzyme cystathionine synthetase, resulting in elevated plasma and urinary levels of homocystine. The elevation in plasma levels of homocystine results in conversion of most of this substance to methionine. Thus one can screen for homocystinuria in newborn blood by analyzing plasma levels of methionine. This condition results in clinical manifestations through two mechanisms: (1) the elevated levels of homocystine have been shown to be toxic to vascular endothelium and account for the thromboembolic phenomenon

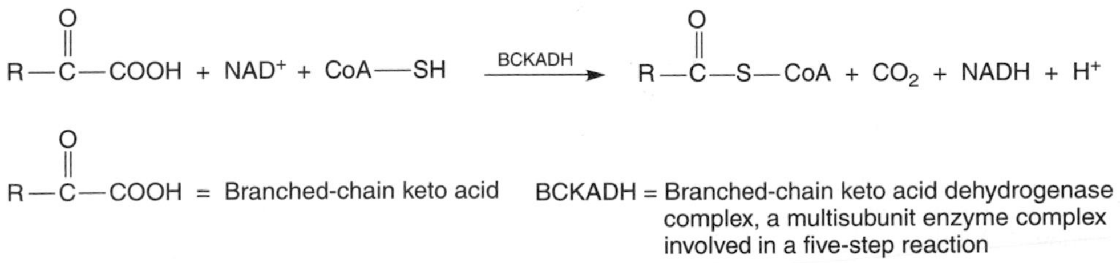

$$R-\underset{\underset{O}{\|}}{C}-COOH + NAD^+ + CoA-SH \xrightarrow{BCKADH} R-\underset{\underset{O}{\|}}{C}-S-CoA + CO_2 + NADH + H^+$$

$$R-\underset{\underset{O}{\|}}{C}-COOH = \text{Branched-chain keto acid}$$

BCKADH = Branched-chain keto acid dehydrogenase complex, a multisubunit enzyme complex involved in a five-step reaction

Fig. 47-17 Maple-syrup urine disease. Branched-chain keto acid decarboxylase enzyme complex when deficient results in elevation of branched-chain amino acids valine, isoleucine, and leucine, as well as their keto acid analogs.

(plugging of brain or lung blood vessels by blood clots) of this disease, and (2) the failure of production of cystine results in a deficiency of this essential amino acid in connective tissue, specifically collagen, metabolism. The enzymatic activity of cystathionine synthetase requires as its cofactor the B vitamin pyridoxine. Different mutations in the gene locus for cystathionine synthetase result in two distinct forms of homocystinuria. In approximately half the patients with cystathionine synthetase deficiency, a sufficient enhancement of residual enzyme activity can be achieved by the addition of therapeutic doses of pyridoxine to the diet essentially to cure the disease.

Cyanide-nitroprusside is used as a urine-screening test for this disease. Nitroprusside combines with sulfhydryl-containing amino acids to produce a red color. The cyanide reduces disulfide bonds and gives a positive screening result. Homocystinuria and cystinuria give a positive cyanide-nitroprusside reaction, whereas silver nitroprusside, which does not reduce the disulfide bond of homocystine, gives a positive result only when cystinuria is present.

Organic acidurias.
The metabolism of amino acids involves several intermediate steps. During each step organic acids are produced. A defect in the subsequent metabolism of these compounds results in disorders characterized by a severe metabolic acidosis. Among this group of disorders, the ketotic hyperglycinemia syndrome is composed of several defects in propionic acid and methylmalonic acid metabolism. Odd-numbered fatty acids and the amino acids leucine, isoleucine, valine, threonine, and methionine lead to the production of propionyl CoA, which is converted to methylmalonyl CoA. Methylmalonyl CoA is converted into succinyl CoA, which can then enter the tricarboxylic acid cycle (Fig. 47-18). Within the first few weeks of life, infants with these disorders usually manifest severe ketoacidosis, which may be accompanied by hypoglycemia. The urine yields a strongly positive dinitrophenol hydrazine reaction, and amino acid analysis reveals striking elevations in glycine in the urine. If methylmalonic acid is not found in the urine, a presumptive diagnosis of propionicaciduria can be made. A definitive diagnosis of this disorder can be further pursued through the demonstration of the presence of methylcitrate in the urine, the gas-liquid chromatographic analysis of organic acids in the urine, or the assay of propionyl CoA carboxylase in cultured cells. The conversion of propionyl CoA to methylmalonyl CoA uses biotin as a cofactor, which may in

therapeutic doses enhance residual enzyme activity. The conversion of methylmalonyl CoA to succinyl CoA involves the metabolism of B_{12}, which in therapeutic doses can also result in significant biochemical improvement. In those instances in which vitamin therapy does not result in a significant therapeutic response, a low-protein diet is used.

The use of gas chromatography-tandem mass spectroscopy for routine newborn screening enables detection of many more abnormalities of organic acid metabolism.

Defects in carbohydrate metabolism.
Galactosemia is a toxicity syndrome associated with an intolerance to dietary galactose. This recessively inherited disorder occurs as a result of a deficiency of the enzyme galactose-1-phosphate uridyltransferase.

$$\text{Galactose-1-phosphate} + \text{UDP-glucose} \xrightarrow{\text{Gal-1-P uridyltransferase}} \text{UDP-galactose} + \text{Glucose-1-phosphate}$$

Lactose, composed of galactose and glucose, is the major disaccharide in mammalian milk. Hydrolysis of lactose by the intestine results in the release of the monosaccharides glucose and galactose. The main pathway of galactose metabolism in humans involves the conversion of galactose to glucose by epimerization of the hydroxyl group at the carbon-4 position. The reaction catalyzed by galactose-1-phosphate uridyltransferase involves galactose-1-phosphate with UDP-glucose, yielding UDP-galactose and glucose-1-phosphate. The UDP-galactose can by further conversion yield UDP and glucose-1-phosphate. Humans are thus capable of metabolizing large amounts of galactose. However, with deficiency of the transferase enzyme, galactose is reduced to galactitol and oxidized to galactonate. It is the presence of these two intermediate products of galactose metabolism that has direct toxic effects and results in the clinical manifestations of galactosemia. The classic clinical presentation of galactosemia is one of failure to thrive in early infancy complicated by vomiting and diarrhea. In addition, these infants show deranged hepatic function with jaundice and hepatomegaly. Severe hemolysis can also occur, and cataracts may be noted shortly after birth. Without dietary therapy, retarded mental development can be apparent in the newborn after only a few months of age. Many states have instituted newborn screening for galactosemia using the disk of blood collected for the Guthrie test to assay for galactose-1-phosphate uridyltransferase. Metabolic screening tests of the urine from acutely ill infants should include a test

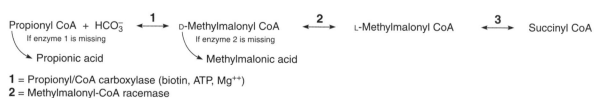

1 = Propionyl/CoA carboxylase (biotin, ATP, Mg^{++})
2 = Methylmalonyl-CoA racemase
3 = Methylmalonyl-CoA mutase

Fig. 47-18 Propionic aciduria and methylmalonic aciduria. This sequence of metabolism of organic acids can be interrupted at several points, each of which results in a specific organic aciduria.

for reducing substances in the urine. Urine dipsticks impregnated with glucose oxidase are specific for glucose. Such a urine screening would be negative in most infants with galactosemia. An infant with the aforementioned clinical manifestations who has a negative dipstick urine test result for glucose but a positive copper sulfate test result (such as Clinitest) for reducing substances in the urine has strong presumptive evidence for galactosemia. Dietary control of the disease in the first few years of life can result in normal growth and development.

A second defect in galactose metabolism occurs as a result of deficiency of the enzyme galactokinase:

$$\text{Galactose} + \text{ATP} \xrightarrow{\text{Galactokinase}} \text{Galactose-1-phosphate} + \text{ADP}$$

This disorder is recognized most commonly after a screening of urine metabolites of patients with cataracts. Deficiency of galactokinase results in the accumulation of galactitol as an end product in galactose metabolism. This compound accumulates within the lenses and is responsible for the cataracts. There are no hepatic or other systemic manifestations of this defect. One can assay the enzyme in red blood cells, and the excretion of galactose and galactitol in urine will give a positive reducing substance reaction. Early recognition of this disorder and the elimination of galactose from the diet will prevent the development of cataracts.

Lactic acidosis is a commonly observed complication of many diseases that result in increased anaerobic metabolism. Primary abnormalities in carbohydrate metabolism leading to lactic acidosis are rare. Anaerobic metabolism and defective carbohydrate metabolism may give rise to elevations in both pyruvic and lactic acid. However, because pyruvate is shunted rapidly to lactate and most clinical laboratories perform lactate assays but not pyruvate assays, lactic acidosis rather than pyruvic acidosis is more commonly recognized and referred to. A primary abnormality in pyruvate metabolism or in muscle mitochondrial metabolism of glucose will result in an increased pyruvate and lactate level after a glucose load. Patients with lactic acidosis in whom no abnormality in tissue blood perfusion or oxygenation is apparent may require additional tests to rule out a primary abnormality in carbohydrate or pyruvate metabolism.

Glycogen-storage diseases. The glycogen-storage diseases combine two different types of metabolic defects. First, because of the alterations in glycogen metabolism, inadequate glucose stores are available for metabolic needs, and symptoms of acute hypoglycemia occur. Second, the accumulation of glycogen results in the long-term, chronic effects of a storage disease. Table 47-6 lists a classification scheme of the glycogen-storage diseases.

The classic form of glycogen-storage disease is von Gierke's disease, which occurs as a result of a deficiency of glucose-6-phosphatase. All metabolic sources of blood glucose are channeled through the intrahepatic formation of glucose-6-phosphate (see Chapter 32). Glucose in this form cannot be transported outside the liver cell. Thus the formation of glucose from amino acids through gluconeogenesis or the conversion of other carbohydrates into glucose uses the intermediate of glucose-6-phosphate. With a deficiency of glucose-6-phosphatase, the only carbohydrate available to maintain blood glucose is the glucose metabolite glucose-1-

---

TABLE 47-6 INBORN ERRORS OF GLYCOGEN DEPOSITION OR UTILIZATION

Condition	Cori Type	Biochemical Features	Clinical Features
Glucose-6-phosphatase deficiency (von Gierke's disease)	1	Normal glycogen accumulates in liver and kidney	Hepatomegaly, hypoglycemia; stunted growth with retarded bone age, etc.
Idiopathic generalized glycogenosis (Pompe's disease)	2	Normal glycogen accumulates in all organs	Cardiac failure, muscle hypotonia, neurological disorders, death in infancy
Dextrin-1,6-glucosidase (debrancher) deficiency (limit dextrinosis; Forbes' disease)	3	Abnormal glycogen with short branches deposited in liver and sometimes skeletal and cardiac muscle	Hepatomegaly, hypoglycemia; less severe than von Gierke's disease
α-Glucan-branching glycosyltransferase (brancher) deficiency (amylopectinosis; Andersen's disease)	4	Abnormal carbohydrate with long inner and outer branches deposited in liver, spleen, and lymph nodes	Hepatic cirrhosis; death within 2 years of birth
Glycogen phosphorylase (glycogen phosphorylase of the muscle) deficiency (McArdle syndrome)	5	Moderate accumulation of normal glycogen in skeletal muscles; lactate and pyruvate levels in blood fall during exercise	Generalized muscular fatigability and pain
Glycogen phosphorylase (hepatic glycogen phosphorylase) deficiency (Hers' disease)	6	Normal glycogen accumulates in liver; phosphorylase content of liver and leukocytes reduced	Hepatomegaly; relatively benign
Deficiency of UDP glucose glycogen glycosyltransferase (glycogen synthetase)	7	Liver glycogen almost completely absent	Severe fasting hypoglycemia

From Geigy scientific tables, ed 7, Summit, NJ, 1970, Ciba-Geigy Corp. From Field RA. In Stanbury JB et al, editors: The metabolic basis of inherited disease, ed 2, New York, 1966, McGraw-Hill, p 141; Hers HG: Adv Metab Disord 1:1, 1964; Control of glycogen metabolism, Ciba Foundation symposium, London, 1964, Churchill.

phosphate. A simplified scheme of glycogen metabolism and the consequences of glucose-6-phosphatase deficiency are shown in Fig. 47-19. Infants with type I glycogen-storage disease, glucose-6-phosphatase deficiency, usually have recurring episodes of hypoglycemia within the first few days of life that are often accompanied by ketoacidosis and lactic acidosis. If there is no elevation in blood glucose after administration of glucagon, a defect in glycogen metabolism must be assumed. Specific diagnosis of type I glycogen-storage disease requires a liver biopsy for the demonstration of glucose-6-phosphatase deficiency. Children with type I glycogen-storage disease are unable to maintain an adequate blood glucose for more than 2 to 2½ hours after a normal feeding. The management of infants with this disorder cannot be satisfactorily accomplished through the use of frequent oral feedings. For that reason, nasogastric tubes and feeding gastrostomies have been used to improve the management of this disease during the first few years of life.

Pompe's disease, or type II glycogen-storage disease, is a condition that is entirely different from the remainder of the glycogen-storage diseases. This disorder is the result of a defect in lysosomal degradation of glycogen. The deficient enzyme is α-glucosidase, an acid hydrolase similar to the deficient enzyme of other lysosomal storage diseases. Deficiency of this enzyme results in widespread systematic lysosomal storage of glycogen and is seen in infancy with hepatomegaly, cardiomegaly, and central hypotonia. The disease follows a rapidly downhill course, with death by 1 to 2 years of age. This alteration of glycogen metabolism does not affect normal glucose homeostasis. Diagnosis of this form of glycogen-storage disease is indicated by lysosomal accumulation of glycogen demonstrated on muscle or liver biopsy. The enzyme α-glucosidase can be assayed in peripheral lymphocytes or in cultured skin fibroblasts to make a specific diagnosis. Because this enzyme is present in cultured cells, prenatal diagnosis exists for this form of glycogen-storage disease.

Transport defects. There are many conditions that lead to altered metabolic states as a result of a defect in membrane transport of metabolites rather than as a result of an enzyme deficiency in a metabolic pathway. After glomerular filtration of plasma, the selective reabsorption of metabolites through the renal tubules occurs so that urine ultimately contains only waste products and nonwaste products are conserved. Single gene-determined components of the plasma membrane of the renal tubule are responsible for the selective reabsorption of individual compounds. One selective renal tubular reabsorption mechanism exists for the four amino acids cystine, lysine, ornithine, and arginine. Homozygotes for a mutation involving this reabsorptive system have a pronounced renal loss of these four amino acids. The condition is known as *cystinuria* because it is the renal loss of cystine that contributes to the clinical disorder. Cystine is less soluble in acidic urine than in alkaline urine. With an increased renal loss of cystine, this amino acid precipitates out to form stones in renal papillae and the collecting system. Cystinuria is seen in early childhood as a form of chronic renal insufficiency, usually first manifesting as growth retardation. Metabolic screening of urine because of failure to thrive or short stature will detect cystinuria through a positive cyanide-nitroprusside reaction.

Several conditions exist in which there is defective renal transport of amino acids; these are shown in Table 47-7.

Vitamin D–resistant rickets, or hypophosphatemic rickets, represents a defect in renal tubular reabsorption of phosphate. This condition is inherited as an X-linked dominant disorder. As a result, its effect is quite variable in hetero-

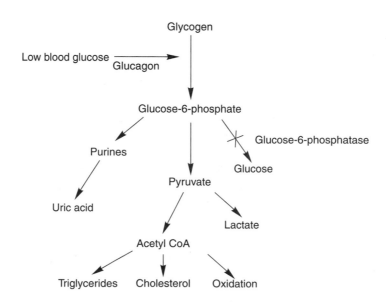

Fig. 47-19 Glycogen-stored disease type 1 (von Gierke's disease). Use of glycogen to form free glucose requires hepatic action of glucose-6-phosphatase to transport glucose extracellularly.

TABLE 47-7   ERRORS IN RENAL AMINO ACID TRANSPORT

Disorder	Urine Analysis	Findings
Cystinuria	Urine cyanide-nitroprusside	Renal failure resulting from cystine stones
Hyperdibasic aminoaciduria	Elevated urinary lysine, ornithine, arginine	Autosomal dominant asymptomatic
Fanconi's syndrome	Elevated urinary amino acids, bicarbonate, phosphate, glucose, potassium, uric acid	Growth failure in primary form, occurs secondarily in Wilson's disease and galactosemia
Glucoglycinuria	Glucosuria, glycinuria	Autosomal dominant asymptomatic
Hartnup disease	Elevated neutral and ring amino acids	Asymptomatic with good nutrition, especially nicotinic acid
Familial renal iminoglycinuria	Elevated urine proline, hydroxyproline, glycine	Autosomal recessive asymptomatic
Lowe (oculocerebrorenal) syndrome	Renal aminoaciduria, proteinuria, aciduria, phosphaturia	X-linked recessive cataracts, mental retardation, and hypotonia

zygous females who may show no clinical manifestations or who may exhibit moderate short stature and evidence of rickets. In affected males there is hypophosphatemia and hyperphosphaturia with short stature and bowing of the legs accompanying the roentgenographic evidence of rickets. Definitive diagnosis is made by demonstration of a greatly elevated 24-hour urine phosphate excretion. This disorder is called *vitamin D–resistant rickets* because massive doses of vitamin D will not correct the altered plasma and urine levels of calcium and phosphate. With regular intake of the maximum gastrointestinal tolerance of phosphate, males with this condition can have significant improvement of rickets and enhancement of their adult height. Phosphate is rapidly cleared from plasma when taken orally, and replacement therapy must include ingestion of phosphate every 4 hours. This disease is the first to be found that is the result of a mutation of a hormone receptor; in this case, the vitamin D_3 intracellular receptor.

Disorders of mineral metabolism. The most common and best-known disorder involving mineral metabolism is *Wilson's disease*, or *hepatolenticular degeneration*, in which copper is accumulated in pathological quantities. This autosomal, recessively inherited disorder involving copper metabolism is often observed symptomatically as cirrhosis in adolescents or as a psychiatric disorder in older teenagers or young adults. The gene responsible for Wilson's disease has been identified as ATP7B on chromosome 13. The Wilson's disease locus is at the junction of bands q14.3 and q21.1. This gene codes for a P type copper-transporting ATPase with characteristics of the P type copper-transporting ATPase responsible for Menkes' disease. Derangements in tissue and urinary levels of copper are diagnostic for the disease. Clinically this disorder is characterized by a triad of findings: a peculiar neurological syndrome, cirrhosis of the liver, and Kayser-Fleischer rings of the cornea. The neurological abnormalities take two forms. The first is lenticular degeneration (loss of cerebellar function), which is also known as the *dystonic* form (abnormal movement and tone of muscles) of the disease. The second neurological form is pseudosclerosis, which involves flapping tremors of the wrist and shoulders associated with rigidity and spasticity. The hepatic involvement of this disease is first manifest as an enlarged liver with associated splenomegaly. Thereafter the course is similar to that of chronic hepatitis. Ultimately the disease progresses to the full-blown picture of cirrhosis. The Kayser-Fleischer ring is still considered as the single most definitive clinical diagnostic finding of this disease. It is a ring of a golden-brown or greenish discoloration that appears at the margin of the cornea near the limbus.

Several laboratory approaches to the diagnosis of Wilson's disease are possible. Most but not all patients with this disorder will have a depressed plasma level of ceruloplasmin. Ceruloplasmin is a metalloglycoprotein containing copper. It acts as an oxidase in the enzymatic oxidation of iron from the ferrous to the ferric state. Early in the course of the disease the 24-hour urine level of copper may be within the normal reference interval or slightly increased, but the copper level is uniformly strikingly elevated in advanced stages of the disorder. Once clinical suspicion of this disorder is established, one diagnostic approach is the 24-hour urine measurement of copper followed by a second 24-hour urine measurement of copper during administration of penicillamine. With increased tissue levels of copper the chelating agent penicillamine will result in a striking increase in copper excretion. In some reports, the most definitive and in some cases the only assured way of making a diagnosis is by liver biopsy and tissue analysis of copper content. However, with the improved understanding, it is expected the definitive diagnosis will be by molecular genetic analysis. Wilson's disease can be essentially controlled by the long-term administration of penicillamine. Patients who have serious side reactions to penicillamine can be treated with zinc sulfate, which blocks metallothionine receptors in the gut, preventing reabsorption of copper excreted in the bile.

A second disorder of copper metabolism is known as *Menkes' syndrome*, or *kinky-hair disease*. This disorder is an X-linked recessive neurological disease that is seen in early infancy characterized by failure to thrive, lethargy, hypothermia, and myoclonic seizure activity. Affected male infants have pallid skin and a characteristic facial appearance. The hair may appear normal at birth, but thereafter a characteristic pattern develops. The hair lacks luster and is somewhat depigmented; it also has a steely feel. Children with Menkes' syndrome have low serum levels of copper and ceruloplasmin. However, attempts at treatment through copper administration have been unsuccessful. The responsible gene change has been located at Xq12-q13. The gene codes for an ATPase copper-transport protein ATP7B.

Disorders of urea cycle and hyperammonemias. The principal end product of nitrogen metabolism in humans is urea. Protein metabolism results in the production of ammonia, which enters the urea cycle (Fig. 47-20) in the synthesis of carbamyl phosphate and leaves through the urea produced in the conversion of arginine to ornithine. Within this cycle there have been recognized five distinct enzymatic deficiencies, each of which results in hyperammonemia. Disruption of the urea cycle does not produce acidosis, ketosis, or hypoglycemia but manifests itself clinically as the direct toxic effect of ammonia on the CNS. The clinical diagnosis should be suspected in infants with CNS depression after protein intake, a condition that should prompt an analysis of a blood ammonia level. The degree of hyperammonemia is massive and in itself does not indicate a particular disorder but rather an interruption in the urea cycle. Quantitative determination of plasma and urine amino acids may show elevations in amino acids suggestive of defects in earlier steps in the urea cycle or demonstrate the specific compound elevated in the latter steps of the urea cycle. Carbamyl phosphate synthetase and ornithine transcarbamylase deficiencies require liver biopsy for specific diagnosis using an enzymatic analysis. Citrullinemia, argininosuccinicaciduria, and argininemia are diagnosed by demonstration of an elevation of these substrates through chromatographic analysis of urine or plasma. The enzyme defect in these latter three conditions is demonstrated in cultured skin fibroblasts.

Receptor defects. Receptors are discrete gene products that function as membrane-bound or cytoplasmic agents required for the transport of specific compounds across membranes or as the intracellular regulators of metabolic activity. Knowledge about receptor function has been greatly enhanced through the study of single gene disorders that result in specific receptor defects. Such genetic disorders are illustrated by the conditions familial hypercholesterolemia and testosterone-resistant syndromes (testicular feminization syndrome).

Familial hypercholesterolemia (see Chapter 33) is a dominantly inherited disorder that is the most common single gene cause of coronary artery disease and myocardial infarction in young adults. In humans, low-density lipoprotein (LDL) is the carrier for most of the cholesterol in plasma. After cholesterol is synthesized within the liver, it is transported within LDL particles to cells, where it is internalized through the binding of the LDL molecules to a specific cell surface receptor. After binding of LDL molecules to the cell surface receptors, an endocytotic vesicle is formed, which fuses with lysosomes. Within the lysosome the LDL molecules are degraded to free amino acids, eventually unesterified free cholesterol. As adequate amounts of cholesterol are internalized, there is suppression of 3-hydroxy-3-methylglutaryl coenzyme A reductase (HMG-CoA reductase), which causes a reduction in cellular cholesterol synthesis. Conversely, an intracellular requirement for cholesterol stimulates HMG-CoA reductase activity. The familial hypercholesterolemia disorder results from a mutation affecting the LDL receptor. With a reduced number of cell surface receptors for LDL cholesterol and thus reduced uptake of cholesterol, there is inadequate suppression of HMG-CoA reductase activity. This results in stimulation of further cholesterol synthesis. The net result is familial, or type IIa, hypercholesterolemia. There are rare persons who are homozygous for a defect in the LDL receptor. During early childhood such persons have greatly elevated levels of plasma cholesterol and severe coronary artery disease, usually leading to death at adolescence. Study of cultured skin fibroblasts from homozygously affected persons

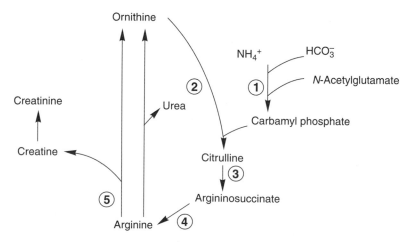

Fig. 47-20 Urea cycle defects. Five primary hyperammonemias include type *1*, or carbamyl phosphate synthetase deficiency; type *2*, or ornithine transcarbamyltransferase deficiency; type *3*, or citrullinemia caused by argininosuccinate synthetase deficiency; type *4*, or argininosuccinicaciduria caused by argininosuccinase deficiency; type *5*, or hyperargininemia caused by arginase deficiency.

allowed elucidation of the defect in LDL receptors and the concomitant effect on the regulation of HMG-CoA reductase activity. As a result of this work, it was possible to show that the more common heterozygous form of autosomal dominant hypercholesterolemia represented a partial defect in LDL receptors and regulation of HMG-CoA reductase activity.

The term *testicular feminization syndrome* is an older designation for a disorder involving an abnormality in testosterone metabolism. Affected individuals are phenotypic females who develop female secondary sexual characteristics at puberty but fail to undergo menarche. A laparotomy in such a person will show absence of a uterus and the presence of intra-abdominal testes. Chromosome analysis reveals a normal male 46,XY karyotype. These chromosomal males embryologically develop the external genitalia of a female because of a cellular resistance to the action of testosterone. There is normal testosterone generation by the testes, but there is an unresponsiveness of target tissues to testosterone. The action of testosterone (androgens) on target cells is mediated by specific cytoplasmic receptors. Dihydrotestosterone combines with a cytosol-binding protein (the receptor) to form a hormone-protein complex that is transported into the cell nucleus, where it exerts its action on chromatin. A defect in the receptor results in an inability of target cells to respond to the testosterone.

Disorders of purine metabolism. The best known disorder involving a defect in purine metabolism is the **Lesch-Nyhan syndrome**. Affected males are seen with manifestations of self-mutilation, mental retardation, and cerebellar dysfunction. Their urine contains excessive amounts of uric acid crystals. The hyperuricemia characteristic of this X-linked recessively inherited disorder is the result of a deficiency of hypoxanthine-guanine phosphoribosyltransferase (HGPRT). This enzyme is involved in the metabolism of the purine nucleotides guanylic acid (GMP) and inosinic acid (IMP). These two purines regulate the activity of several enzymes involved in purine metabolism, including HGPRT. The deficiency of this enzyme results in an accelerated rate of purine biosynthesis, and because of the lack of HGPRT activity, increased amounts of hypoxanthine and xanthine are synthesized, which are readily converted in the liver by xanthine oxidase to massive amounts of uric acid. Allopurinol inhibits xanthine oxidase to lower the serum and urinary levels of uric acid in these patients, but this does not alter the CNS abnormalities that are part of the disorder.

When cells deficient in HGPRT are cultured, they are resistant to the effects of purine analogs such as 8-azaguanine and 6-mercaptopurine, which inhibit the growth of normal cells. Because of lyonization, the female carrier for this X-linked condition has cells with HGPRT and cells without HGPRT, fibroblasts will grow in both normal media and media with one of these purine analogs. Cells from a noncarrier female will grow in the normal media but not in media with the analog. This selective medium system has proved to be a powerful tool in the detection of carriers for the Lesch-Nyhan syndrome. As prenatal diagnosis is available, study of females in a family in which this condition

has occurred is important for genetic counseling. The gene for HGPRT seems to be susceptible to a large number of mutations, ones that may be seen on a single individual or within a family ("private" mutations). This makes the diagnosis of this disorder by molecular means more difficult.

Mitochondrial disorders. Each cell contains hundreds of mitochondria, which are subcellular organelles responsible for a large number of metabolic functions, including most oxidative processes. Many of the proteins and enzymes contained within the mitochondria are coded by the mitochondrial genome, a double-stranded circle of DNA, 16.6 kilobases (kb) in length. Since mitochondria also have their own protein synthesis machinery and a genetic code slightly different from the one used by the nuclear genes, it is appropriate that the translation apparatus (including 22 transfer RNAs and two ribosomal RNAs) also be encoded in the mitochondrial DNA. Thirteen subunits of the respiratory chain, which is responsible for producing ATP, are encoded in the mitochondrial DNA, including the proteins composing the NADH-coenzyme Q reductase (complex I), the cytochrome-*b* subunit of coenzyme Q–cytochrome-*c* (complex III), three subunits of cytochrome-*c* oxidase, and two subunits of ATPase (complex IV). The remaining subunits of these complexes are encoded by nuclear genes. Numerous diseases recognized to be consistent with a sex-limited, or maternal, mode of inheritance have been found to be caused by mutations in genes encoded by the mitochondrial DNA.

A classic example of a maternally inherited mitochondrial disorder is *Leber's optic atrophy*. Because mitochondria are inherited only from the mother, females transmit the disease to sons and daughters; more males are affected than females, but males never transmit the disease to their offspring. One seventh of the mothers of affected males are themselves affected. In 1988, Wallace et al demonstrated that this disease was caused by an error in the mitochondrial gene encoding the NADH-dehydrogenase subunit 4.

Other point mutations underlie mitochondrial myopathies (muscle disorders). These are characterized by syndromes given the acronyms MELAS (myopathy, encephalopathy, lactic acidosis, and stroke-like episodes) and MERRF (myoclonus epilepsy and ragged red fiber). In these cases mutations occur in genes coding for tRNAs. Mutational changes may also consist of large deletions or duplications of the same genes, such as in *Kearns-Sayre syndrome* (progressive ophthalmoplegia, ptosis, proximal myopathy, pigmentary retinopathy, ataxia, and heart block), in which a deletion of 4.9 kb of DNA removes several tRNA genes from mitochondria, primarily in muscles, or in *Pearson syndrome* (sideroblastic anemia, exocrine pancreatic dysfunction, lactic acidosis), in which large insertions or deletions are found in mitochondria in all tissues. The mutant phenotype is found in both normal and abnormal mitochondria in **heteroplasmic** individuals. The clinical manifestations are influenced by the proportion of mutant mitochondria in relevant tissues in heteroplasmic individuals. The proportion can vary from cell type to cell type and with age of the individual in ways that are not yet clear. Although disease severity appears correlated with proportion of affected mitochondria in specific tissues, sufficient exceptions have been observed to indicate that much remains to be learned about the biology of mitochondria.

Peroxisomal disorders. Peroxisomes are subcellular organelles that contain oxidizing enzymes called *peroxidases*. The *Zellweger cerebral hepatorenal syndrome* (CHR; craniofacial dysmorphology, abnormalities of the hands and feet, polycystic kidneys, and intrahepatic dysgenesis) is the prototypic peroxisomal abnormality. Elevated pipecolic acid, abnormalities in very-long-chain fatty acid metabolism (impaired beta-oxidation), and absence of peroxisomes all indicate that the fundamental defect may be a structural abnormality of this organelle. Indeed, a gene for a peroxisomal assembly factor–1 (PAF1) has been cloned and found to contain a point mutation in a Japanese family with a child with CHR syndrome. *Neonatal adrenoleukodystrophy* and *infantile Refsum's disease* may be additional examples of this class of defect. Inasmuch as peroxisomes contain over 40 enzymes and up to eight complementation groups have been identified in the CHR syndrome, additional genes may also be implicated in defective peroxisome biogenesis.

GENETIC SCREENING
Role of Mass Screening

Screening tests play a major role in the diagnosis and population study of genetic disease (Table 47-8). A screening test is not designed as a primary diagnostic tool. Rather, its purpose is to identify a subpopulation of persons in whom definitive diagnostic testing would be cost-beneficial. In general, the more specific a particular screening test, the greater its cost, thus reducing its utility for screening large populations. A definitive diagnostic test for a given entity is one that has a sensitivity and specificity of close to 100%. The *sensitivity* of a test is a measure of how frequently the test will detect a disorder under question. The *specificity* of a test is a measure of how well the test will be negative in the absence of a disorder (see Chapter 20 for details). The sensitivity and specificity that are required of a screening test depend on the population to be studied and the purpose for which the screening test is undertaken. This is best illustrated when one considers the purposes for screening tests: (1) screening tests for the early detection of disease in the pre-symptomatic state when effective therapy exists (phenylketonuria or penicillin prophylaxis for sickle cell anemia), (2) carrier detection for inherited disease, especially in the context of prenatal diagnosis (Tay-Sachs disease), and (3) epidemiological studies of the frequency of a given disorder within the population (47,XXY or 47,XYY karyotype). If a disease can be effectively treated when detected early and if the consequences of nondetection are unacceptable, it is desirable to have a test with maximum sensitivity in order to detect all possibly affected persons. Those persons identified through a positive screening test can undergo additional testing with more specific assays that will establish a specific diagnosis. For a disease in which successful treatment is not readily available for the clinical manifestations, less-sensitive screening tests may be used. Lowering the sensitivity can improve the specificity of the test. The few persons with the disease who are missed by the screening test will not be unduly compromised. Most states now employ isoelectric focusing as their primary screen for abnormal hemoglobins, especially HbS. Quantitation of the percentage of HbS by HPLC of abnormal samples allows more definitive differentiation of sickle cell trait from sickle cell–β^+-thalassemia

---

TABLE 47-8   GENETIC SCREENING TESTS

Nature of Screening Test	Condition(s) Screened For	Definitive Diagnostic Test
Buccal smear for Barr bodies	Numerical abnormalities of the X chromosome	Peripheral blood lymphocyte karyotype
Serum assay for percent hexosaminidase A	Carriers for Tay-Sachs disease	Hexosaminidase A in peripheral leukocytes
Semiquantitative blood phenylalanine levels	Phenylketonuria among newborn infants	Quantitative plasma level of phenylalanine by tandem GC/MS
Maternal serum alpha-fetoprotein determination	In utero detection of neural tube defects and Down syndrome	Amniocentesis for chromosomes, alpha-fetoprotein, and acetylcholinesterase
Hemoglobin IEF or HPLC	Carriers for thalassemia	Hemoglobin electrophoresis or chromatography
Stool for trypsin activity	Cystic fibrosis among newborns	Sweat test at 1 month of age
Serum CK levels in males with delayed walking	Duchenne muscular dystrophy	Restriction analysis
Galactose-1-UDP transferase	Galactosemia	DNA
Hemoglobin IEF or HPLC for black infants	Sickle cell disease	Hemoglobin electrophoresis, IEF, HPLC, or DNA analysis
Serum methionine	Homocystinuria	Quantitative plasma amino acids
Bleeding and clotting times in preoperative evaluation	Hemophilia A	Plasma factor VIII levels

IEF, isoelectric focusing; HPLC, high-performance liquid chromatography.

inasmuch as the cost of locating children for repeated testing may dictate a more definitive initial analysis. Sickle cell trait is sufficiently common, however, that detection of all heterozygotes is feasible and useful for genetic counseling purposes. Detecting all heterozygotes among adults for β-thalassemia would be very expensive.

Detection of Heterozygote Carriers

During the past 20 years considerable information about the specific molecular abnormalities underlying many genetically determined disorders has been amassed. In recessively inherited disorders, knowledge of the molecular defect can be used for the detection of carriers through demonstration of a partial expression of the molecular defect in heterozygous individuals. The accuracy of these carrier detection tests generally is directly proportional to the accuracy of the assay system that measures the specific molecular defect of the disorder under question. Some assay systems used for the detection of carriers of recessively inherited disorders are listed in Table 47-9. Biochemical abnormalities have been seen in cystic fibrosis (CF), most notably an elevation in the chloride content of sweat. The gene for CF is genetically linked to that for the enzyme paraoxonase and has been cloned by positional cloning and mapped to chromosome 7. This gene, known as the *cystic fibrosis transmembrane conductance regulator (CFTR)*, is large, encoding a protein of 1480 amino acid residues (see below and Chapter 48). Its structure indicates that it is a membrane chloride-transport regulator, defects of which allow water and chloride to leak from the cells involved, resulting in the viscous secretions associated with the disease. The most severe mutation, dF508, is characterized by deletion of a phenylalanine codon at that amino acid position 508 of the gene. This allele accounts for 70% of the mutations at this locus, and homozygotes for this allele constitute approximately 57% of persons with CF. The majority of the remainder of CF patients are compound heterozygotes with mutations that can involve a large number of additional alleles.

TABLE 47-9   CARRIER DETECTION FOR GENETIC DISEASES

Disease	Carrier Test	Findings
Sickle cell disease	Hemoglobin electrophoresis	S and A hemoglobin bands
Tay-Sachs disease	Serum hexosaminidase (Hex) A and total assay	% Hex A <45%
Hurler syndrome	α-L-Iduronidase assay	Level <50% control
Duchenne muscular dystrophy	Serum CK assay	Elevated levels
Hemophilia A	Factor VIII assay DNA genotyping	Low level Genotype of carriers in family

CK, *Creatine kinase.*

This creates a substantial public health dilemma. Population mass screening using allele-specific oligonucleotide hybridization that will detect a high proportion of heterozygotes will be very expensive. Use of a smaller number of oligonucleotides will decrease sensitivity.

Prenatal Diagnosis

Once the prevalence of a disease is shown to be high enough to justify the investment involved in establishing a method to detect that disease, the diagnostic method must meet several criteria before it can be used successfully in prenatal diagnosis. First, there must be a means of identifying couples at sufficient risk for a particular condition to warrant incurring the risks and costs of amniocentesis and other diagnostic procedures. Parents may be determined to be at risk for producing an offspring with genetic disease because they have at least one child with a genetic birth defect that has a significant recurrence risk; because they are determined, by previous carrier detection, (guided perhaps by knowledge of their racial or ethnic origin) to be carriers for an autosomal, recessively inherited disorder; or because of the age of the mother.

Second, the disorder under question should by its nature warrant prenatal diagnosis. At present this is generally true, since almost all conditions for which a prenatal diagnosis is available are severe disorders for which there is no effective therapy for affected infants.

Third, the accuracy of the diagnostic method used should be well established because there is little margin for error with these studies. For diagnoses of many genetic disorders and biochemical disorders using cultured amniotic fluid cells, the laboratory receives a 20 to 30 mL sample of amniotic fluid for a one-time opportunity of establishing a culture and performing a limited number of assays. The results of these assays will be used to determine whether the pregnancy will be continued. In such circumstances, it is essential to have supreme confidence in the diagnostic systems used.

The recombinant DNA techniques that have proved so useful in the study of gene structure and function have provided the means for accurate prenatal diagnosis of several conditions. The best-known example is the test for the prenatal diagnosis of sickle cell disease. With this disease it has been possible to combine the use of **restriction endonucleases** that recognize the specific nucleotide change of the mutant sickle cell gene with probes that bind to that portion of the hemoglobin gene that codes for the beta-globin chain. Use of the polymerase chain reaction is more sensitive and faster and does not require use of radioisotopes. The allele specific oligonucleotide (ASO) hybridization allows detection of base-pair abnormalities that are not detectable by use of restriction endonuclease analysis. The reverse ASO employs multiple DNA fragments (oligonucleotides) for various thalassemic base substitutions that are bound to a single membrane and then hybridized by labeled genomic DNA. The reverse ASO technique allows testing for multiple mutations simultaneously. In all these techniques, neither the culturing of amniotic fluid cells nor special studies on the parents are required, provided that the parents are known carriers for sickle cell disease. It is possible to imagine a time when probes and restriction endonucleases will exist for the diagnosis of all genetic disorders. See Chapter 48 for a more detailed description of these techniques.

The box below lists the various diagnostic modalities used in prenatal diagnoses and provides an example of each. A very large number of diseases are now diagnosable using DNA obtained by amniocentesis, by chorionic villus biopsy, or through **preimplantation genetic diagnosis** (Kanavakis, Traeger-Synodinos, 2002). The more commonly diagnosed diseases are Charcot-Marie-Tooth disease 1A, congenital adrenal hyperplasia, cystic fibrosis, Duchenne/Becker muscular dystrophy, familial adenomatosus polyposis coli, fragile X syndrome, hemochromatosis, hemophilia, Huntington's disease, Lesch-Nyhan syndrome, Marfan's syndrome, myotonic dystrophy, neurofibromatosis, sickle cell anemia, spinal muscular atrophy (type I), Tay-Sachs disease, thalassemias, and Wiscott-Aldrich disease.

METHODS OF PRENATAL DIAGNOSIS

Cultured amniotic fluid cells
  Cytogenic
    Chromosome analysis (trisomy 21)
  Biochemical
    Hexosaminidase assays for Tay-Sachs disease
  Morphological analysis
    Electron microscopy for mucolipidosis IV
  Substrate analysis
    Radioactive copper in Menkes' syndrome
Uncultured amniotic fluid cells
  Restriction endonuclease analysis
    Beta-hemoglobin gene study in sickle cell disease
  Genetic polymorphisms for linkage diagnosis
    HLA determination and 21-hydroxylase deficiency
Amniotic fluid analysis
  Quantification of marker components
    Alpha-fetoprotein for open neural tube defects
  Analysis of abnormal metabolites
    Methylmalonate in methylmalonicaciduria
  Genetic polymorphisms for linkage diagnosis
    Secretory status and myotonic dystrophy
Imaging techniques
  Ultrasonography
    Autosomal recessive polycystic kidneys
  Roentgenography
    Skeletal dysplasia—achondrogenesis
  Fetoscopy
    Polydactyly in Ellis–van Creveld syndrome
Fetal sampling
  Fetal blood sampling
    Factor VIII antigen assay in hemophilia A
  Skin biopsy
    Histological appearance in epidermolysis bullosa
      dystrophica

ALPHA-FETOPROTEIN TESTING
Maternal Serum Alpha-Fetoprotein Screening
(see Chapter 40)

Alpha-fetoprotein (AFP) is a plasma protein made by the fetal liver. The plasma of a nonpregnant woman contains virtually no detectable AFP. During pregnancy, the maternal serum AFP level is related to the level of AFP in the amniotic fluid. Any fetal condition that results in increased passage of fetal plasma into amniotic fluid will increase the maternal serum level of AFP. Such conditions include open neural tube defects, such as anencephaly or meningomyelocele; abdominal wall defects, such as gastroschisis or omphalocele; and renal loss of plasma proteins from congenital nephrotic syndrome. These disorders can be screened for by the measurement of the AFP concentration in maternal serum. However, elevated levels of maternal serum AFP are also indicative of pregnancy complications in the absence of a fetal malformation; such complications include fetomaternal transfusion, increased risk of premature delivery, increased risk for fetal death, and the presence of twins.

From empirical experience it has been found that expression of the level of AFP in multiples of the median (MoM) leads to a better correlation with infant risk than does the use of standard deviations of the mean. Many screening programs use 2.5 MoM as the upper limit of the reference interval for maternal serum; this is roughly equivalent to 5 SD above the mean. The amount of AFP produced by the fetus is relatively consistent from pregnancy to pregnancy, but the level of maternal serum AFP will vary with the maternal blood volume. It is necessary to adjust for this by correcting for maternal weight. Other factors that affect the maternal serum level are diabetes and race. The level of maternal serum AFP varies with gestational age, increasing gradually during the time appropriate for screening, 15 to 22 weeks of pregnancy. The maternal serum level in MoM is based on the median determination for each gestational week of pregnancy, and interpretation requires accurate dating of the pregnancy.

Retrospective analysis of maternal serum screening for elevated AFP levels showed a correlation between low levels of AFP and the presence of a fetus with Down syndrome. This correlation was subsequently confirmed in a series of prospective studies so that, currently, low levels of maternal serum AFP are considered an indication for amniocentesis and determination of the fetal karyotype. An independent correlation also exists between maternal age and the risk for a fetus with Down syndrome; a maternal age of 35 years or older is the most common indication for prenatal diagnostic testing by amniocentesis or chorionic villus sampling. Levels of maternal serum AFP can be expressed as a risk for Down syndrome for specific maternal ages. Thus, if a woman's age and her low level of AFP combine to generate a risk equivalent to that of a 35-year-old woman, she is offered prenatal diagnosis.

Amniotic Fluid Determination of Alpha-Fetoprotein

Maternal serum AFP determination is a screening test considered applicable to all pregnancies. In the case of an

TABLE 47-10 INBORN ERRORS OF PURINE AND PYRIMIDINE METABOLISM

Condition	Defective Enzyme or System	Biochemical Features	Clinical Features	Incidence and Genetics
Gout (hyperuricemia)	Excessive synthesis of uric acid from precursors	Concentration of uric acid is increased in serum and often in urine	Acute arthritic attacks, chronic arthritis with urate deposition in tissues; urinary urate calculi causing kidney damage; asymptomatic in 80% of cases	Hyperuricemia in 1% to 2%, clinical gout in 2 to 4/1000; probably autosomal-dominant with variable and sex modified expression
Xanthinuria	Deficiency of xanthine oxidase and defective renal tubular reabsorption of xanthine	Xanthine is excreted in large amounts	Xanthine calculi in urinary tract	Rare recessive
Oroticaciduria	Absence of orotidine-5′-phosphate pyrophosphorylase or decarboxylase, or of both	Orotic acid accumulates and is excreted in urine	Severe megaloblastic anemia, orotic acid crystalluria	Very rare; recessive
β-Aminoisobutyricaciduria	Deficiency of a catabolic enzyme	High urinary excretion of β-aminoisobutyric acid	Harmless	0% to 46%, depending on ethnic group; recessive

From Geigy scientific tables, ed 7, Summit, NJ, 1970, Ciba-Geigy Corp.

TABLE 47-11 LIPIDOSES

Condition	Lipid Accumulating	Site	Clinical Features	Age at Which Symptoms Appear	Genetics
Gaucher's disease Type I—Juvenile Type II—Infantile Type III—Cerebral	Glucocerebro-side	Spleen, liver, bone marrow, leukocytes; brain in (II) and (III); lung in (III)	I. Hematologic abnormalities, hyperplenism, bone lesions, skin pigmentation, pingueculae II. Hepatosplenomegaly, cerebral degeneration III. Similar to type I, neurologic abnormalities	I. 1 to 60 years II. First or second half year of life III. 6 to 20 years	Autosomal recessive; frequency of type I, II, and III is 0.04 in Ashkenazi Jews
Tay-Sachs disease (infantile amaurotic familial idiocy)	Ganglioside G_{M2} (G_0), amino glycolipid	White and gray matter of the brain	Cherry-red spot, retina of eye; progressive cerebral degeneration; death at age 2 to 3 years	Usually 4 to 6 months, sometimes earlier	Autosomal recessive; TSD carrier frequency 0.0324 in Ashkenazi Jews
Neimann-Pick disease type C	Intracellular accumulation of cholesterol	Viscera and CNS	Neurologic abnormalities, ataxia, grand mal seizures	2 to 3 years	Autosomal recessive
Metachromatic leukodystrophy; many allelic variants	Glactosphingo-sulfatides	Brain, kidney, urine, gallbladder	Cerebral and cerebellar degeneration; spasticity; dementia; death after 1 to 6 years	1 to 2 years, death before 5 years	Autosomal recessive
Fabry's disease	Galactosylgaleto-sylceramide	Skin, kidney, cerebrovascular	Acroporethesia; kidney dysfunction; cerebro-vascular GI, heart	Usually adult	Autosomal recessive

Modified from Geigy scientific tables, ed 7, Summit, NJ, 1970, Ciba-Geigy Corp.; data from OMIM database (http://www.ncbi.nlm.nih.gov/omim/).

abnormal result, further testing in the form of ultrasonography and amniocentesis is offered. Normally, AFP determinations are done any time amniotic fluid samples are taken as with amniocentesis for advanced maternal age. A close correlation exists between the level of amniotic fluid AFP and the aforementioned fetal conditions; additionally, these structural defects can often be visualized by ultrasonography. If AFP is elevated in maternal serum and, upon amniocentesis, in amniotic fluid but no fetal defect is discovered by ultrasonography, electrophoresis of amniotic fluid acetylcholinesterase will reveal a specific band if an open neural tube defect is present. Amniotic fluid levels of AFP also vary with gestational age; levels are expressed as MoM with the median established for each gestational week of pregnancy between 16 and 26 weeks.

Methods of Analysis

Each disease caused by an inborn genetic error results in a unique defect in a protein or enzyme function, or both. The consequence of this defect is a singular pattern of analyte change in biological fluids. Tables 47-4 to 47-11 list the pathognomonic analyte changes for many of these genetic defects; the major clinical findings for each disease are also given.

Bibliography

Caskey CT et al: Triplet repeat mutations in human disease, *Science* 256:784, 1992.

de Grouchy J, Turleau C: *Clinical atlas of human chromosomes*, ed 2, New York, 1984, Wiley & Sons.

Kelly TE: *Clinical genetics and genetic counseling*, ed 2, St Louis, 1986, Mosby.

King RA, Rotter JI, Motulski AG: *The genetic basis of common diseases*, ed 2, New York, 2002, Oxford University Press.

McKusick VA: *Mendelian inheritance in man*, ed 11, Baltimore, 1998, Johns Hopkins University Press (www.ncbi.nlm.nih.gov/entrez/query.fcgi?db=OMIM).

Neufeld EF: Natural history and inherited disorders of a lysosomal enzyme, beta hexosaminidase, *J Biol Chem* 264:10927, 1989.

Poulton J: Mitochondrial DNA and genetic disease, *Dev Med Child Neurol* 35:833, 1993.

Sack GH: *Medical genetics*, New York, 1999, McGraw-Hill.

Scriver CR et al: *Metabolic and molecular basis of inherited disease*, vol 1-4, ed 8, New York, 2001, McGraw-Hill.

Scriver CR, Rosenberg LB: *Amino acid metabolism and its disorders*, Philadelphia, 1973, Saunders.

Shimozawa N et al: A human gene responsible for Zellweger syndrome that affects peroxisome assembly, *Science* 255:1132, 1992.

Simpson JL: *Disorders of sexual differentiation*, New York, 1976, Academic Press.

The human genome, *Science* 291(5507):1145, 2001.

Thomas GH, Howell RR: *Selected screening tests for genetic metabolic diseases*, St Louis, 1973, Mosby.

Connexins

Kanavakis E, Traeger-Synodinos J: Preimplantation genetic diagnosis in clinical practice, *J Med Genet* 39:6, 2002.

Kumar NM, Gilula NB: The gap junction communication channel, *Cell* 84:381, 1996.

Rabionet R, Gasparini P, Estivill X: Molecular genetics of hearing impairment due to mutations in gap junction genes encoding beta connexins, *Hum Mut* 16:190, 2000.

Tekin M, Arnos KS, Pandya A: Advances in hereditary deafness, *Lancet* 358:1082, 2001.

Mitochondrial Disorders

Johns DR: Mitochondrial DNA in disease, *N Engl J Med* 333:638, 1995.

Internet Sites

http://www.accessexcellence.org/AB/IWT/Gene_Therapy_Overview.html

http://www.bioscience.org/atlases/disease/genedis/glossary.htm

http://www.ornl.gov/hgmis/publicat/primer2001/index.html—Genomics and Its Impact on Medicine and Society: A 2001 Primer Accessed 2/8/2002 Human Genome Project, US Department of Energy

http://www.genome.gov/glossary.cfm—Glossary of Genetic Terms, National Human Genome Institute, National Institutes of Health (US)

http://www.ncbi.nlm.nih.gov—National Center for Biotechnology Information home page, part of the National Library of Medicine

http://www.ncbi.nlm.nih.gov/Genomes/—National Center for Biotechnology Information, Genome Biology page, part of the National Library of Medicine

http://www.ncbi.nlm.nih.gov/disease—National Center for Biotechnology Information, Genes and Disease page, part of the National Library of Medicine

http://www.ncbi.nlm.nih.gov/entrez/query.fcgi?db=OMIM

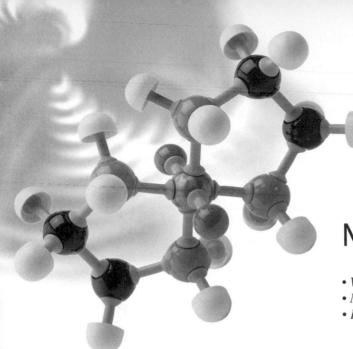

CHAPTER 48

Molecular Diagnostics

- *W. Edward Highsmith, Jr.*
- *Niel T. Constantine*
- *Kenneth J. Friedman*

Chapter Outline

Objectives

- Review the structure of DNA, and describe how its properties of complementary base pairing and digestion by specific nucleases can be used to identify specific sequences of DNA.
- List the major clinical uses of techniques to identify specific DNA sequences.

- Describe the Southern blot technique.
- Describe the polymerase chain reaction.
- Compare and contrast specific and scanning mutation detection methods.

Key Terms

base pairing The process by which purine and pyrimidine bases bind through hydrogen bonds. The bases pair in a specific complementary fashion: adenine with thymine (or uracil) and guanine with cytosine.

base sequence The exact order of purine bases (guanine and adenine) and pyrimidine bases (cytosine and thymine or uracil) found in nucleic acids. The order defines the primary amino acid sequence of the gene products, which are proteins.

complementary DNA (cDNA) DNA that contains an exact sequence of bases that will pair to a strand

of DNA or RNA through base pairing. cDNA can be used as a probe for detecting specific sequences.

denaturation The process by which double-stranded nucleic acid separates to form single strands. Heat, salts, or chemicals can accomplish denaturation. Also termed *melting*.

double-stranded DNA Two complementary strands of DNA that are bound together through base pairing.

gene The smallest biological unit of heredity, located at specific sites on specific chromosomes. A structural gene contains the encoding for one specific protein.

hybridization   The process by which complementary single strands of nucleic acid form double-stranded complexes of nucleic acid through base pairing.

melting temperature   The temperature at which one half of a population of identical DNA species exists in double-stranded form and one half exists in the single-stranded (denatured) form. The melting temperature is dependent on the ionic strength of the solution.

polymerase chain reaction   A process by which complementary DNA strands are enzymatically synthesized and repeatedly copied ("amplified").

polymerases   A class of enzymes that synthesize DNA from an existing template. Polymerases require a primer to begin synthesis, ribonucleotide or deoxyribonucleotide triphosphates as reactants, and magnesium as a cofactor.

probe   A sequence of complementary DNA or RNA that is labeled with a radioisotope, enzyme, or other marker. Probes are used to detect specific sequences of nucleic acid by hybridization.

restriction endonucleases   Class of nucleases (usually bacterial) that act within a strand of DNA at specific base sequences to cleave the DNA.

restriction site   The base sequence that a particular restriction endonuclease recognizes and cleaves.

single-stranded DNA   A length of DNA that is not paired to its complementary strand.

Southern transfer   A process by which electrophoretically separated, denatured DNA is transferred from the electrophoretic gel (usually agarose) onto a nitrocellulose filter or membrane for subsequent hybridization analysis.

stringency   The conditions under which a hybridization experiment is conducted. High stringency conditions (low ionic strength, temperature at about DNA melting temperature) allow the hybridization of only perfectly base-paired strands. Low stringency conditions (high ionic strength, temperature less than DNA melting temperature) allows hybridization of homologous, but not perfectly base-paired, strands.

viral load   The number of circulating viral particles, generally expressed as genome copies/mL or IU/mL.

The smallest unit of inheritance, the **gene**, codes for specific protein chains, each with a specific function in cell physiology. Chemically, genes are composed of both ribonucleic acid (RNA) and deoxyribonucleic acid (DNA, see later discussion; also, see Part IV of Chapter 53 for a general discussion); in this chapter we will focus on DNA. The **base sequences** are grouped into informational units of three bases, called *codons*. Each triplet sequence comprising a codon either codes for a specific amino acid or serves a regulatory function, such as stopping or starting protein chain synthesis. Structurally, the base sequence that composes a gene is linked to other genes, to regulatory sequences, and to (apparently) functionless DNA sequences. DNA is associated with a large number of proteins that serve regulatory functions and also to package the genetic material into larger units called *chromosomes*.

As the number of genes identified and implicated in a variety of human diseases grows (see Chapter 47), the clinical laboratory faces new challenges. Disease or abnormal states can occur when genes are damaged, and this damage usually results from chemical changes to the genes, called *mutations* (see later discussion). The laboratory now utilizes the techniques and technology of molecular biology to identify and characterize specific gene mutations associated both with single-gene disorders, such as cystic fibrosis or Duchenne's muscular dystrophy; and polygenic disorders, such as cancer and atherosclerosis. Additionally, molecular techniques receive wide use for the detection of infectious agents, including organisms that are difficult to culture or are present in low numbers.

DNA STRUCTURE

Fig. 48-1 shows the unique arrangement of sugar, phosphate, and the purine and pyrimidine bases that form the double-helical structure known as DNA. Particular sequences of this structure form the *gene*, which codes for a specific protein (see Chapter 53, Part I).

Human DNA consists of two strands of base sequences that are bound to each other by hydrogen bonding between the bases of each single strand of DNA (Fig. 48-1). The bases bind to each other in a specific, or *complementary*, fashion. Adenine binds only to thymine, whereas guanine binds only to cytosine. Thus one chain of **double-stranded DNA** has a base sequence that is complementary to the other strand. A single strand of DNA will bind to another single DNA strand if the strands contain a high proportion of complementary sequences. For example, if a mixture consists of single strands of DNA-A and its complementary strand and an excess of other noncomplementary DNA strands, strand A will *only* form double-stranded complexes with its complementary strand and none other. In the laboratory the process of allowing complementary single strands of DNA to form double-stranded DNA is called **hybridization**. Hybridization can also be performed between single strands of DNA and complementary strands of ribonucleic acid (RNA). For analysis of a specific DNA base sequence, a known copy of that base sequence is prepared. This copy of **complementary DNA (cDNA)**, known as a DNA **probe**, is labeled in some fashion to allow monitoring of the hybridization reaction. The basis of the techniques described later in the chapter hinge on the hybridization properties of a specific sequence

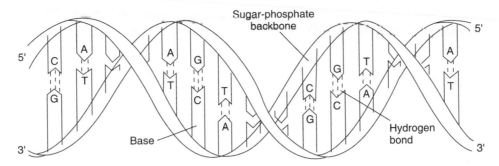

Fig. 48-1   Structure of DNA. DNA molecule is a double helix that consists of two sugar-phosphate backbones with four bases: cytosine (C), guanine (G), adenine (A), and thymine (T) attached. *C* and *G* residues and *A* and *T* residues on opposite strands pair through hydrogen bonding. *(Reprinted with permission from LeGrys V, Leinbach SS, Silverman L: CRC Crit Rev Clin Lab Sci 25:255, 1987. Copyright CRC Press, Inc, Boca Raton, FL.)*

of bases that make up a single strand of the double-stranded helix of DNA.

Mutations and Gene Expression

A genetic mutation is a stable change in the DNA structure that usually is caused by a change in the base sequence that comprises a codon. The base change usually results in a change in the code and the information residing in that code. A mutation occurring in the portion of DNA that codes for a protein usually results in a change in the amino acid structure of that protein. This change can result in no change in the function of the protein, a total loss of function, or a partial loss of function. It is the partial or total loss of function that usually results in a pathological state. The effect of a loss of function can be direct, such as the conformation dysfunction of hemoglobin that results in the disease sickle cell anemia (see Chapter 36), or indirect, such as the loss of function of regulators of gene expression that can result in cancers (see Chapter 49).

Mutations can occur by a wide variety of mechanisms. For the purposes of the discussion of cancer and inherited disease, mutations can be divided into germline and somatic events. A germline mutation is one that is present in all cells of the body and is passed from generation to generation by meiosis (creation of germ cells—sperm and egg) and sexual reproduction. Somatic cell mutations are those mutations that arise in tissue cells, generally as a result of some environmental insult or DNA replication error; they are not passed on to subsequent generations. For additional information on genetic inheritance, see Chapter 47.

Abnormal expression of genes can also result from inheritable changes to the chemical structure of genes that are not a result of a change of a base in a codon triplet. Methylation of the nucleotide bases is a postsynthetic modification to DNA that affects the expression of genes. Abnormal patterns of DNA methylation can cause abnormal gene expression (transcription) and disease states. Repeat base sequences that have no apparent informational content regarding protein structure exist throughout the DNA. The expansion of the number of repeats in a gene has been associated with specific

diseases, and this change in the gene structure is inheritable (see p. 962).

TECHNIQUES OF DNA ANALYSIS

Several core technologies are central to the modern practice of molecular biology. The first takes advantage of the ability of complementary strands of DNA to find each other in solutions containing a complex mixture of DNA and bind together to form the familiar DNA double helix. This specific binding is termed *hybridization*, and forms the basis for almost all types of DNA detection methods. The second set of techniques that are crucial for manipulation and detection of specific nucleotide sequences involve a large number of enzymes that are commercially available. One set of these enzymes is the **restriction endonucleases**, which *in vivo* are involved in DNA metabolism and repair, or in bacterial host defense, and provide the molecular tools with which nucleic acids can be manipulated with extraordinary specificity. Other sets of enzymes that are broadly used are the **polymerases**, both DNA and RNA polymerases and reverse transcriptase. These enzymes are used *in vivo* to replicate DNA, to make RNA copies of DNA sequence, and, by retroviruses, to make DNA copies of RNA genomes. The third set of core techniques in modern molecular biology is the detection methods. These methods are required to possess extreme specificity, not for the chemical structure of DNA, which is identical for all genes, but for the sequence of the bases, which determines the information that a particular piece of DNA is carrying. Further, because specific gene sequences form only a tiny fraction of the whole human genome and because DNA is typically available only in microgram amounts, these methods must possess extreme sensitivity. The first of these methods to be described and widely adopted is the **Southern transfer**. The second is the **polymerase chain reaction** (PCR).

Restriction Digestion and Gel Electrophoresis

A specific property of DNA (and RNA) is its susceptibility to enzymes called *nucleases*. Nucleases hydrolyze the phospho-diester bonds that connect bases within a nucleic acid strand, resulting in cleavage of the strand. Certain nucleases have very high substrate specificity and will cleave a DNA strand only at specific base sequences, often as small as four to eight bases in length. Because these nucleases are employed by bacteria to restrict entry of foreign DNA into their cells, they are called *restriction endonucleases*. The sequences that the enzymes recognize and cleave are referred to as **restriction sites**. These enzymes require Mg^{2+} ion for activity. More than 400 enzymes recognizing different restriction sites have been identified. Most of these are commercially available.

Restriction endonucleases are critical reagents in laboratories investigating DNA base sequences because they cleave the double-stranded nucleic acid only at specific points. After these endonucleases degrade DNA into a series of many smaller fragments, specific sequences can be more readily identified by the hybridization technique. To aid in the identification of a specific base sequence, the fragments can be first separated into molecules of differing molecular size. This is accomplished by either agarose or polyacrylamide (or their derivatives) gel electrophoresis (see Chapter 8).

The most common method for the visualization of DNA after electrophoretic size separation is by staining with the intercalating agent ethidium bromide, or the binding agent SYBR Green (Molecular Probes, Eugene, OR.). These compounds, when in solution, are free to lose energy acquired via incident radiation by increased rotation and collision with solvent molecules. However, when a molecule of ethidium bromide or SYBR Green is bound to the DNA double helix, these motions are lost, and the molecule rids itself of excess energy by fluorescence. The fragments of DNA generated by restriction enzyme digestion are equimolar with respect to each other, giving an easy method for determining the completeness of a given restriction digestion reaction. The hybridization of the separated fragments is then achieved by the Southern transfer technique.

Southern Transfer

Currently, Southern analysis is used in the clinical laboratory to detect large structural changes in DNA sequences that are not amenable to analysis by PCR. An example is the mixed lineage leukemia (MLL) gene at chromosome 11q23. Because this gene has been associated with translocation to more than 40 different chromosomes and genes, it is difficult to design PCR strategies that will detect all MLL rearrangements. Other uses for Southern analysis include examples of genetic disease in which abnormal alleles cannot be efficiently amplified or detected by PCR because of the large gene size or high G and C content of the gene. One such example is the fragile X syndrome.

For many gene targets of clinical interest PCR has supplanted Southern analysis because it is much less costly, labor intensive, and has a much quicker turnaround time. However, in some cases the diagnostic sensitivity of PCR test strategies is not as high as for Southern transfer–based methods. Examples include detection of immunoglobulin gene rearrangements in leukemia and lymphoma and the detection of gene deletions in the dystrophin gene in Duchenne muscular dystrophy. In both cases, PCR will detect most (greater than 95%), but not all, pathological events. Thus Southern transfer analysis still retains a place in the clinical laboratory.

Blood samples for analysis are collected with acid-citrate-dextrose (ACD) or ethylenediaminetetraacetic acid (EDTA) anticoagulant and white cells are then isolated from each sample. DNA is extracted from the white cells and incubated with a restriction endonuclease to cleave the DNA into smaller fragments. The digested DNA sample is applied to an agarose gel and electrophoresed to separate the fragments according to size. The fragments are then treated with alkali to separate the double-stranded DNA into single strands; this process is termed **denaturation**. The separated, denatured fragments are then transferred from the gel onto another support medium, such as a nitrocellulose or nylon membrane (the *Southern blot* procedure). The fragment or fragments containing the DNA sequence of interest are identified by incubating the membrane with a labeled DNA probe that contains sequences complimentary to the sequence of interest. The label can be a radioisotope, an enzyme, or a fluorescent dye. The complementary sequence of the probe permits it to hybridize to the sample DNA containing the linked probe sequences. In the case of radiolabeled cDNA, the membrane is then incubated with x-ray film to expose areas (bands) on the film where the probe has bound to the sample DNA, resulting in an autoradiogram (Fig. 48-2).

The procedure described requires 7 to 10 days from DNA extraction from whole blood to development of the autoradiogram. Usually DNA is extracted on the first day, digested with restriction endonucleases on day 2, electrophoresed overnight on day 3, and hybridized on days 4 and 5. The membrane is then placed in an x-ray cassette with x-ray film for 1 to 4 days and then developed. Alternative, nonisotopic detection methods that use colorimetric or luminescent detection are gaining in popularity because they reduce the time required for band visualization and technologist exposure to ionizing radiation. These methods employ a second incubation step using an enzyme-coupled antibody to a hapten that has been incorporated into the probe DNA instead of phosphorus-32. The action of the enzyme then generates the colored or chemiluminescent material from a colorless or inactive substrate. Several nonisotopic detection systems for use with Southern transfer are commercially available; examples are the GENIUS kit from Boeringer-Mannheim (colorimetric) and the ECL system from Amersham (chemiluminescent).

Polymerase Chain Reaction (PCR)

Although the Southern procedure combines reasonablesensitivity with excellent specificity, it is technically demanding, requires the use of hazardous, high-energy β-emitters, such as ^{32}P, and has a long turnaround time. Several of the objections to the Southern procedure can be addressed by use of the polymerase chain reaction (PCR). PCR is a technique for the rapid, *in vitro* amplification of specific DNA sequences. The introduction of PCR into clinical laboratories has revolutionized the practice of clinical molecular diagnostics.

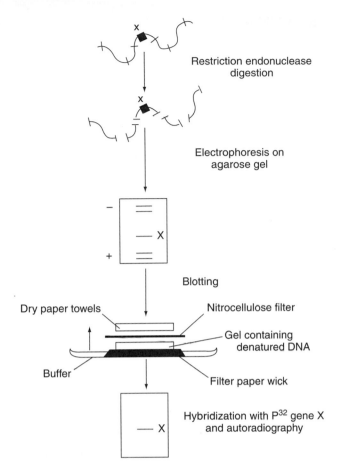

Restriction endonuclease
digestion

Electrophoresis on
agarose gel

Blotting

Dry paper towels   Nitrocellulose filter

Gel containing
denatured DNA

Buffer

Filter paper wick

Hybridization with P³² gene X
and autoradiography

Fig. 48-2 Identification by Southern blot hybridization of DNA fragment containing gene X. DNA was digested with restriction endonuclease, and resulting fragments were fractionated according to size by electrophoresis in agarose gel. DNA fragments in gel were denatured and blotted to nitrocellulose filter as a result of flow of buffer through gel and nitrocellulose filter to dry paper towels. Subsequent hybridization of DNA on filter to ³²P-labeled gene X probe and autoradiography revealed single DNA fragment containing gene X. *(Reprinted with permission from LeGrys V, Leinbach SS, Silverman L: CRC Crit Rev Clin Lab Sci 25:255, 1987. Copyright CRC Press, Inc., Boca Raton, FL.)*

Knowledge of the base sequence of the region of DNA flanking the gene of interest is required for PCR. Two synthetic oligodeoxynucleotides (primers), typically 20 to 30 bases in length, are prepared (or purchased) such that one of the primers is complementary to an area on one strand of the target DNA 5′ to the sequences to be amplified, and the other primer is complementary to the opposite strand of the target DNA, again 5′ to the region to be amplified. A schematic is shown in Fig. 48-3.

To perform the amplification, the sample DNA is placed in a tube along with a large molar excess of the two primers, all four deoxynucleotide triphosphates (dNTPs), buffer, magnesium ion, and a thermostable DNA polymerase. The most commonly used polymerase is isolated from the thermophilic organism, *Thermus aquaticus*. This enzyme,

termed *Taq polymerase*, has its optimal activity at 72° C, but can survive for short periods at temperatures up to 95° C without being irreversibly denatured. The reaction is first heated to 95° C to melt the test DNA from a double-stranded to a single-stranded form. The temperature is then decreased, typically to 50° to 60° C, to allow annealing, or hybridization, of the primers to their complementary sites on the **single-stranded DNA**. It should be noted that the vast molar excess of the primers, and their small size, ensures that the hybridization is between the sample DNA and the primers, and not between the two stands of the test DNA. The temperature is then increased to 72° C, the temperature optimum for Taq polymerase. The polymerase extends the primers in the 5′ to 3′ direction of each strand by incorporating the dNTPs into the growing complementary DNA strands. It is crucial that the polymerase extend far enough along each strand to create a new binding site for the opposite primer. After holding the temperature at 72° C for a period of time sufficient to synthesize a new DNA strand from one primer to the binding site of the other (typically 15 to 60 seconds), the process of temperature cycling is repeated. After heating to denature the newly formed DNA, the temperature is again decreased to allow annealing of the primers, this time to the newly synthesized binding sites as well as those on the original template DNA. The temperature is again increased to 72° C to extend the four bound primers (see Fig. 48-3). As the temperature changes are repeated, the DNA between the two primers is synthesized. The amount of DNA produced is exponential with respect to cycle number. After 30 cycles of annealing, extension, and denaturation, 2^{30} (or approximately 10^9) copies of the DNA will have been generated.

In a typical experiment starting with 100 to 1000 ng of human DNA, 30 cycles of amplification will produce enough DNA to be visualized on an ethidium bromide–stained gel. Because each cycle takes 2 to 5 minutes, amplification of a specific sequence can easily be accomplished in several hours. After amplification, the DNA can be analyzed by one of several techniques, depending on the specific problem.

PCR-Based Techniques and Applications

The application of PCR can be grouped into two broad categories: mutation detection techniques, which are used to investigate the actual base sequence at a particular locus; and quantitative methods in which PCR-based techniques are used to quantify specific nucleic acid sequences. Mutation detection strategies can be further grouped into specific or scanning technique.

Specific mutation detection techniques. Specific mutation detection entails straightforward, and largely routine, procedures by which DNA samples may be analyzed for previously identified mutations using an assay designed for maximum specificity. This approach targets known mutations in potentially large cohorts of patients or small panels of specific mutations in disorders characterized by one or a few common alleles. Results from these types of analyses may confirm or establish clinical diagnoses. Furthermore, in families at risk for a particular genetic disease, specific or

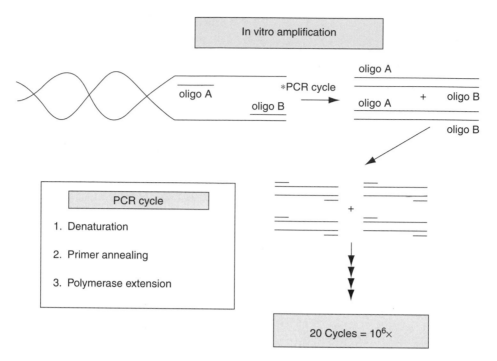

Fig. 48-3 Schematic representation of the first cycle of a PCR reaction. *(Reprinted with permission from Highsmith WE, Jr, Silverman LM: Bull Lab Med 104:1, 1989.)*

targeted mutation detection allows for rapid screening of an entire family for the mutation identified in the patient, thereby permitting accurate carrier determinations that aid reproductive decisions. Rapid testing of large numbers of patients permits an assessment of the mutation's frequency among disease-causing alleles, thereby determining which mutations are most prevalent in different patient populations and guiding the creation of effective clinical mutation testing panels.

The specific mutation detection methods can themselves be divided into those that use gel electrophoresis or hybridization-based methods. Both types of approaches are robust and, in experienced hands, yield reproducible results. Both types of systems are in widespread use in clinical and research laboratories. One criterion for choice between these general platforms is the cost incurred per sample analyzed. In our experience, when the number of samples to be analyzed at one time (samples per batch) is low, electrophoretic methods are often the most cost effective to develop, validate, and implement. However, when the number of samples per batch is larger (more than 8 to 12 samples), then the hybridization-based techniques, many of which can be adapted to 96-well microplate formats, are often more cost effective.

Restriction endonuclease digestion. Mutations represent a change in the local DNA sequence, and may involve single nucleotide substitutions, small deletions or insertions, or more complex rearrangements. Beyond their potential for clinical consequences, gene mutations may also, by virtue of their changes in nucleotide sequence, create novel restriction endonuclease recognition sites or destroy preexisting ones. For example, a DNA fragment harboring a mutation might

not be cleaved with a particular restriction enzyme that usually cleaves normal, wild-type DNA. Conversely, a different mutation might create a novel restriction site not present in the wild-type DNA. In either case, mutated DNA produces a distinct restriction digestion pattern relative to that seen with nonmutated DNA when the digestion products of PCR-amplified DNA are compared after electrophoresis on either agarose or polyacrylamide gels. An example of this commonplace approach applied to mutation detection in cystic fibrosis is shown in Fig. 48-4.

The use of restriction enzymes to distinguish between alleles is one of the most common techniques used in clinical molecular laboratories. This method has advantages over approaches associated with radioisotope usage and their collateral costs and concerns. The large variety of restriction endonucleases that are commercially available represents a substantial resource to molecular laboratories, and the wide variety of recognition sequences associated with these enzymes affords the investigator with many choices for designing straightforward mutation detection strategies.

Despite this large supply of different restriction endonucleases, less than half of known DNA sequence variants independently alter restriction digestion patterns for a commercially available enzyme. Additionally, some enzymes are either unreliable or prohibitively expensive for use in routine, repetitive analyses. Other confounding factors are restriction enzymes with overly common recognition sites.

PCR-mediated, site-directed mutagenesis (PSM). When confounding factors impede the design of facile restriction-based assays, laboratories may employ a modification of

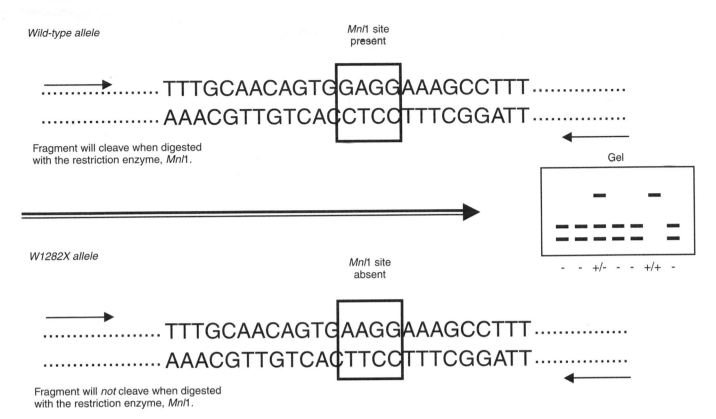

Fig. 48-4 Restriction endonuclease–mediated detection of the CF mutation, W1282X. The restriction recognition site, CCTC/GAGG for the endonuclease MnI1 is present in the normal CFTR gene exon 20. The W1282X mutation ablates this site. *Arrows*, PCR primer. Gel at right shows W1282X-negative (–), W1282X heterozygote (+/–), and W1282X homozygote (+/+) patterns.

this approach. PSM is a technique by which a novel allele-specific restriction digestion pattern can be purposefully generated in association with virtually any mutation. This strategy is known by a variety of names other than PSM, including restriction site–generating PCR (RG-PCR) or amplification-created restriction site (ACRS). These techniques, identical in approach, involve the design of one PCR primer that abuts the mutation locus and includes typically one or two nucleotides mismatched relative to the template DNA. If properly designed, the mutagenic primer will retain sufficient complementarity to anneal specifically to its target DNA and support efficient amplification. All PCR products generated will include not only the mutation locus under study, but will also incorporate the base change inherent to the mutagenic primer. The combination of the mutation and the novel base change of this primer engineers the creation of a novel restriction pattern where none was previously present. This methodology has been applied to a wide variety of clinically important mutations. An example of the application of PSM to the detection of the α-1-antitrypsin Z allele is shown schematically in Fig. 48-5.

Amplification refractory mutation system (ARMS). In this method, also known as *allele-specific PCR*, primers are designed that amplify only one of the alleles present at the locus of interest. This is accomplished with primers that are substantially mismatched relative to one allele, but have sufficient complementarity to anneal to, and amplify, the other allele. Typically ARMS is designed to amplify one allele, whereas a separate reaction is specific for the other allele at that locus. Although this assay avoids the need for a restriction enzyme, it is predicated on high allele-specificity of amplification and requires two PCR reactions per patient sample, one each for the normal and mutant alleles. An example of this technique for detection of the common connexin26 hereditary hearing loss allele, 35delG, is shown in Fig. 48-6.

Allele-specific oligonucleotide hybridization (ASO, or dot blot). In this technique, DNA is amplified by PCR and spotted onto two nylon membranes. Each membrane is then hybridized with one of two synthetic, radiolabeled oligonucleotides that span the region of DNA containing a specific mutation. One oligonucleotide has the sequence complementary to the wild type, or normal DNA sequence, whereas the other is perfectly complementary to the mutant allele. Under appropriate conditions of temperature and salt concentration (**stringency**), hybridization occurs only when the probe and the target DNA are perfectly base-paired. Thus the normal oligonucleotide binds only the normal amplified target, but the mutant oligonucleotide hybridizes only with the mutant allele. Detection is usually by autoradiography. Variants of

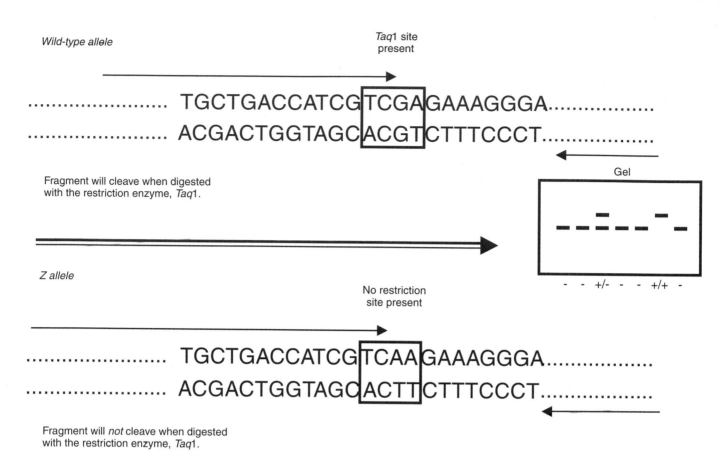

Fig. 48-5 PSM-mediated detection of the α-1-antitrypsin Z mutation. A novel restriction site (TCGA/AGCT) for the endonuclease Taq1 is present in the normal sequence amplified with a PSM primer that mutagenizes a single base. The Z mutation in concert with the mutagenized nucleotide destroys the novel Taq1 restriction site. *Arrows,* PCR primers. Gel at right shows Z-negative (–), Z heterozygote (+/–), and Z homozygote (+/+) patterns.

this procedure include nonisotopic detection and hybridization in microtiter trays instead of on a membrane.

Reverse dot-blot. The reverse dot-blot is a variant on the ASO technique in which the allele-specific oligonucleotides (normal and mutant) are bound to a nylon membrane or immobilized in the wells of a microtiter tray. Amplification of the sample DNA is performed as usual but with one of the PCR primers labeled at the 5′ end with a biotin molecule. The amplified DNA is hybridized with the ASOs bound to the surface of a microtiter tray well under the appropriately stringent conditions for allele-specific hybridization. After the hybridization and washing steps, avidin conjugated to alkaline phosphatase is bound to the biotin. Detection of the hybrids is by monitoring the action of the enzyme on a substrate to produce a colored, insoluble product. This system is the basis for the Roche Amplicor series of products.

Real-time PCR. Instruments with both thermal cycling and fluorescence quantification capabilities have introduced automation to PCR analysis. These instruments allow for the quantification of a fluorescent signal from each PCR reaction vessel during the PCR reaction. This strategy entails the use of a short DNA probe with a 'reporter' dye attached to one end and a quenching agent linked to the other end. This probe is designed to perfectly match one allele at a particular locus but be mismatched relative to other alleles. As the polymerase advances during the extension phase of the PCR reaction, the 5′ to 3′ exonuclease activity of the polymerase digests any probe in its path, releasing the reporter dye from the quencher and generating a fluorescent signal (Fig. 48-7). If the probe is mismatched relative to the template, its affinity for the template will be greatly reduced under appropriately stringent conditions, and probe not bound to the template will neither be digested nor generate a signal. A similar probe may be designed to detect the other alleles, and these assays may be pooled as long as each probe carries a different, separately detectable, reporter dye. This chemistry is compatible with real-time PCR instrumentation from several vendors, including those manufactured by Perkin-Elmer, Roche, BioRad, and Cephiad. Thus the hybridization probe step, which before the development of real-time PCR instruments and chemistries required separate manipulations, can now be accomplished at the same time as the PCR reaction. This platform has been useful for both nucleic acid quantification and specific mutation detection. The 5′ exonuclease

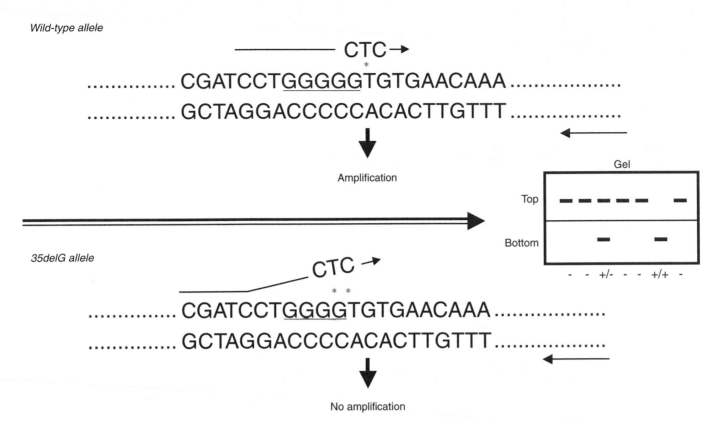

Fig. 48-6 ARMS-based assay for the connexin26 hereditary deafness allele, 35delG. *Top*, A forward primer supports amplification of the wild-type allele, despite a single base mismatch (*) at the penultimate base. *Bottom*, This same primer is mismatched at two 3′ bases (**) relative to the 35delG mutant template (with a missing G/C base pair) and will not support amplification (*top half of gel*). A similar assay that amplifies only the mutant allele may also be designed (*bottom half of gel*). 35delG-negative (–), 35delG heterozygote (+/–), and 35delG homozygote (+/+) patterns are shown.

assay (TaqMan) allelic discrimination protocol enables high-throughput genotyping using real-time PCR.

Another specific mutation detection chemistry that uses the real-time PCR platform is fluorescence resonance energy transfer (FRET) probe analysis. Similar to TaqMan chemistry, this technology uses fluorescence resonance energy transfer between two fluorophores. In FRET probe analysis, two oligonucleotide probes, each labeled with a different fluorescent dye, are designed such that when each probe is hybridized to its complementary sequence, the two fluorescent dye molecules are in close physical proximity. The probes are designed such that one probe, termed the *sensor probe*, overlays the site of the mutation and either forms a perfect DNA duplex or a heteroduplex. The other probe, termed the *anchor probe*, is designed to hybridize to a nonpolymorphic site and is designed to have a **melting temperature** several degrees higher than the perfectly matched sensor probe. The two fluorescent dyes are chosen such that the emission spectrum of one dye overlaps the excitation spectrum of the second dye. When the first dye is irradiated at its absorbance maximum, it transfers its energy via a nonradiative mechanism, FRET, to the second dye. This

dye, now elevated to an excited state, returns to the ground state by emission of a photon at its characteristic emission wavelength. At low stringency, both the sensor and anchor probes hybridize efficiently, and illumination energy is efficiently transferred from the first to the second dye. However, as the temperature is slowly increased, the mismatched sensor probe melts before the perfectly matched probe (Fig. 48-8). Thus mutations are identified by differences in their melting curve profile compared to the wild-type allele. These differences can be seen in a plot of fluorescence intensity versus temperature; however, the data are easier to interpret when displayed as the first derivative. Although FRET probe analysis is compatible with most of the real-time PCR instruments currently available, it was developed for use with the Light Cycler (Roche). Using this instrument, which features very rapid cycle times, a batch of up to 32 samples can be analyzed for the presence of specific mutations in as little as 30 minutes.

Flow cytometry. A novel strategy currently available is the Luminex-100/Lab Map System (Luminex Corp, Austin, TX). Luminex-100 is a microsphere-based flow cytometry assay that allows high throughput sample processing for

Probe matches template

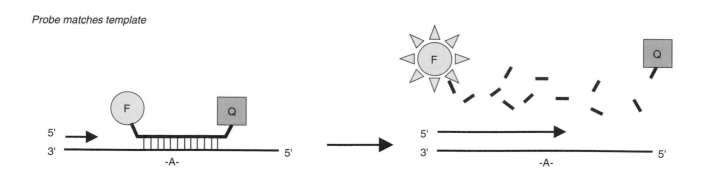

Probe mismatched to template

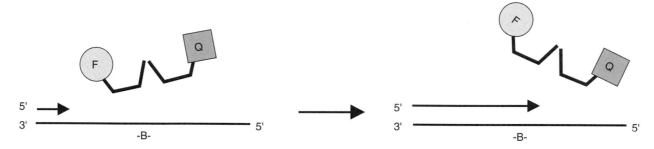

Fig. 48-7   TaqMan mutation detection. The TaqMan probe hybridizes to the wild-type allele and is degraded by the 5′ to 3′ exonuclease activity of Taq polymerase. The starburst figure depicts fluorescence of the fluorophore (*F*) after release from the effect of the quencher (*Q*). The probe does not bind to the mutant allele, the probe is not degraded, and fluorescence is not observed.

simultaneous detection of multiple sequence variants. Polystyrene microspheres are internally dyed with two spectrally distinct fluorochromes. An array is created consisting of 100 different microsphere sets, each set distinguishable by its internal dye ratios. Therefore each set of microspheres can carry a different DNA probe, that is, for one allele at particular genetic locus, and be mixed with many other spectrally distinct microspheres in a multiplex reaction.

Oligonucleotide probes are bound to the surface of microspheres and hybridized with biotin-tagged complementary PCR fragments derived from multiplex reactions amplifying several loci simultaneously. The spheres are then incubated with a fluorochrome that binds the biotin tag. Microspheres are interrogated individually in a rapidly flowing fluid stream as they pass by two separate lasers. High-speed digital signal processing classifies each microsphere based on its spectral address and quantifies the fluorescence-labeled PCR fragment on the surface (Fig. 48-9). Thousands of microspheres are interrogated per second, resulting in an analysis system capable of analyzing and reporting up to 100 different reactions in a single reaction tube in a few seconds. Approximately 1 hour is required for this system to analyze 96 samples arranged in a microtitre plate for multiple alleles.

Mutation scanning techniques. Mutation scanning methods interrogate DNA fragments for all sequence variants present. By definition these strategies are not predicated on specificity for specific alleles but rather are designed for highly sensitive detection for all possible variants. In principle, all sequence variants present will be detected without regard to advance knowledge of their pathogenic consequences. Once evidence for a sequence variant is found, the sample must be sequenced to determine its molecular nature. Only when combined with appropriate genetic data and *in vitro* functional studies, can investigators distinguish disease-causing mutations from polymorphisms without clinical consequence. In the research laboratory, mutation screening is a critical and obligatory final step toward identifying genes that underlie genetic disease. In the clinical laboratory, these methods are applied toward the detection of mutations in diseases marked by significant allelic heterogeneity.

Single-stranded conformational polymorphism analysis (SSCP). The SSCP process involves PCR amplification of the fragment of interest, denaturation of the double-stranded PCR product with heat, and electrophoresis on a non-denaturing polyacrylamide gel. During electrophoresis the single-stranded DNA folds into a three-dimensional

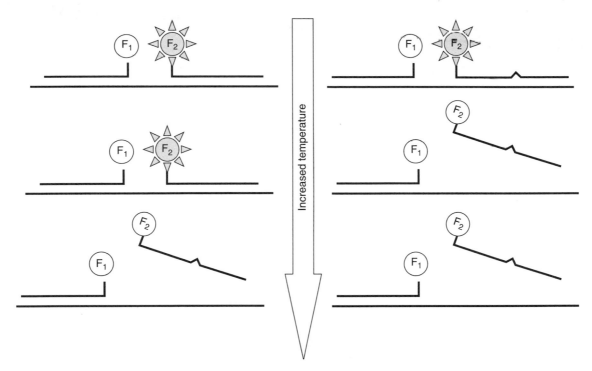

Fig. 48-8　FRET probe specific mutation detection. *Left panel,* Both probes form perfectly base-paired double-stranded DNA. *Right panel,* One probe has a mismatch and melts earlier when the temperature is increased. The starburst figure depicts fluorescence of the second fluorophore (F_2) when it is in close physical proximity to the first fluorophore (F_1) and can be excited by FRET.

structure that is defined by its primary sequence. If a mutation is present, the three-dimensional shape that the single-stranded DNA folds into will be different. The electrophoretic mobility is a function of the shape of the migrating molecule. Thus, if the sequence of a sample PCR product is different from that of a reference fragment, even by a single nucleotide, it is likely that one of the strands, if not both, will adopt different three-dimensional conformations and exhibit unique electrophoretic mobilities. The presence of a mutation or polymorphism within the PCR product will be apparent through band shifts in either one or both single-stranded fragments, compared with DNA fragments without sequence variants (Fig. 48-10). Multiple bands of altered mobility may arise from a single mutation due to the presence of multiple conformers that are equally stable under the specific electrophoretic conditions.

Heteroduplex analysis. Many mutation screening strategies are predicated on heteroduplex formation. Two single-stranded fragments of DNA such as recently synthesized PCR products will form fully matched, stable homoduplex structures at appropriate chemical and temperature conditions if they have 100% sequence complementarity. DNA fragments with high, but incomplete, sequence complementarity will also form duplex structures, but these fragments may have subtly altered conformational properties and become substrates for specific chemical and enzymatic reactions. When amplifying a DNA fragment from an individual heterozygous for a nucleotide substitution, the final PCR product

will include both homoduplex structures for each allele and heteroduplexes derived from the imperfect annealing of dissimilar fragments. Whenever heterozygosity is established, direct sequence analysis or other methods are used to identify the underlying mutation or polymorphism. When heteroduplexes are detected in large genes, DNA sequencing efforts may be targeted more effectively.

The conformational changes associated with heteroduplex structures often lead to fragments with altered electrophoretic mobility. Under the appropriate conditions these heteroduplex fragments are separable from homoduplex forms, thereby establishing heterozygosity for a sequence variant in that sample. A method that exploits the differential migration of homoduplexes from heteroduplexes uses mutation detection enhancement (MDE) gels (BioWhittaker Molecular Applications, Rockland, ME). This proprietary gel matrix is formulated to enhance the electrophoretic separation between homoduplex and heteroduplex fragments in a straightforward manner. After PCR, DNA products are renatured slowly to enhance heteroduplex formation and are subsequently electrophoresed on MDE gels. The gel is then stained for DNA to resolve the fragments (Fig. 48-11). Differential migration of the heteroduplex and homoduplex fragments is directly related to the subtle structural differences between them.

Heteroduplex analysis by MDE gel electrophoresis is a simple, low-cost technique for mutation screening predicated on detecting mutations in the heterozygous state, and some

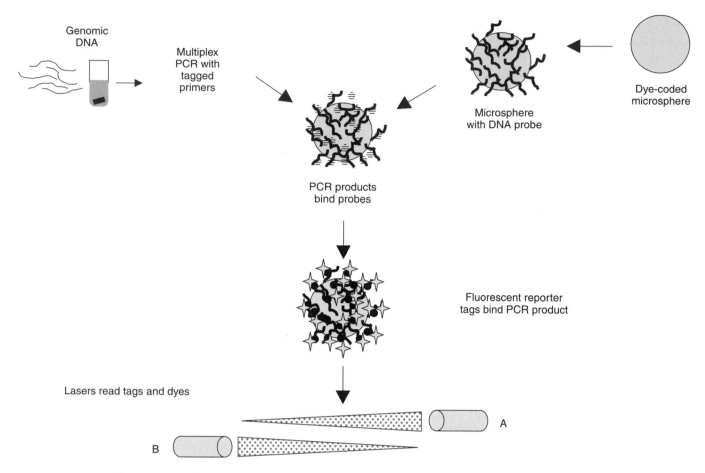

Fig. 48-9 High throughput flow cytometry platform for multiplex genotyping. The Luminex-100 protocol associates particular probes with uniquely dye-coded microspheres. After multiplex PCR using biotin-tagged primers, products are mixed with multiple populations of microspheres, each with their own probe. PCR products bind only to microspheres bearing the cognate probe. Fluorescent reporter tags bind the biotin. Flow cytometry through laser readers identifies microspheres by their dye code and quantifies the amount of fluorescent-tagged PCR products present on each.

SSCP strategies use MDE gels claiming higher analytical sensitivity. Importantly, no heteroduplex-based strategies have utility for detecting mutations present in the homozygous state. To overcome this limitation, DNA of a known genotype can be mixed with the patient sample before amplification; or, a PCR product of known genotype can be mixed with the patient's PCR product to ensure the generation of heteroduplexes if the patient is homozygous for a mutation.

Chemical and enzymatic cleavage. Heteroduplex DNA may be cleaved in a sequence-specific manner using either chemical or enzymatic agents. Chemical cleavage of DNA mismatches (CCM) involves agents that modify specific bases when present in the single-stranded form. In imperfectly annealed, double-stranded heteroduplex fragments, the nucleotide mismatch manifests as a very localized single-stranded region with bases vulnerable to chemical modification. Hydroxylamine modifies unpaired cytosines, whereas osmium tetroxide modifies unpaired thymines. Thus every possible single-base mismatch, as well as small insertions and deletions,

will be subject to chemical alteration. Piperidine is then added to cleave the mismatched products, which are then electrophoresed to resolve the digested fragments.

An enzymatic protocol to effect mismatch-directed cleavage using T4 endonuclease VII avoids the chemical toxicity of the CCM reagents. *In vivo*, T4 endonuclease VII resolves the Holiday structures produced during replication of bacteriophage T4. These structures are similar to heteroduplexes, and heteroduplexes caused by single-base mismatches are substrates for the enzyme. Enzyme mismatch cleavage (EMC) uses this enzyme to recognize and cleave mismatched fragments, allowing the digestion products to be separated by electrophoresis, thereby permitting mutations to be identified (Fig. 48-12). As with CCM, some positional information is also generated.

Denaturing gradient gel electrophoresis (DGGE). The differential conformational properties of heteroduplex fragments may be exploited by other methodologies. As a result of their mismatched bases, heteroduplexes denature into

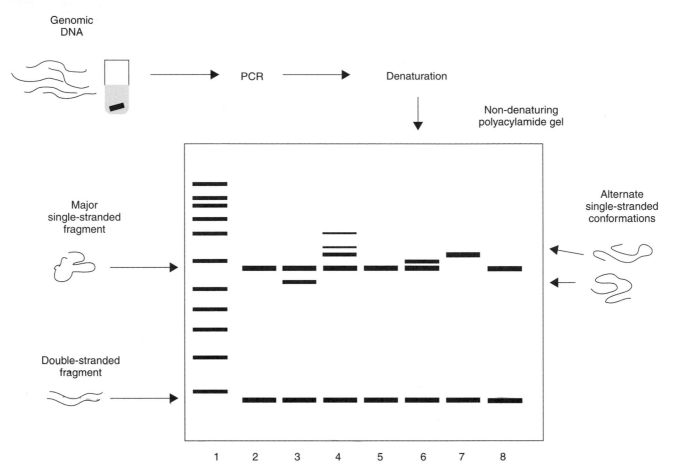

Fig. 48-10 Single-stranded conformational polymorphism analysis (SSCP or SSCA). PCR product is denatured, placed on ice, and electrophoresed on non-denaturating poly-acrylamide gels. *Lane 1*, Size marker. *Lanes 2, 5*, and *8*, No bands of altered mobility are seen in samples with the wild-type sequence. *Lanes 3, 4, 6*, and *7*, Bands of altered mobility establish the presence of sequence variants. Different variants may yield different electrophoretic patterns. Multiple bands reflect distinct fragment conformations.

single strands more readily than the cognate homoduplexes. DGGE uses a chemical gradient within the electrophoretic gel to take advantage of this difference. The chemicals involved, typically urea or formamide, serve to denature the PCR fragments from double- to single-stranded fragments. PCR of heterozygous samples using specially designed primers to optimize denaturation behavior and electrophoresis yields heteroduplex fragments with altered denaturation properties. Once denaturation of a fragment begins, its electrophoretic mobility through the gel slows dramatically. The appearance of these slowly migrating bands on DGGE gels is indicative of heterozygosity for a DNA sequence variant in the underlying sample. The melting process is sensitive not only to the nature of the mismatch and the underlying mutation, but also to the sequence of the fragment as a whole. A similar approach using a temperature rather than chemical gradient (TGGE) has also been described.

Denaturing high-performance liquid chromatography (DHPLC). Automated mutation detection technologies have made significant strides in recent years, and automation of heteroduplex detection is no exception. DHPLC is a column-based platform for detecting heteroduplexes in a high-throughput manner with minimal operator involvement. This approach is well suited to evaluating large numbers of samples (~150/day) for variants in a given DNA fragment. Unlike DGGE, no special primers are required. For DHPLC, PCR products are eluted from a column with buffer containing an ion-pairing reagent such as triethylammonium acetate (TEAA) that masks the DNA fragments' charge and binds them to the hydrophobic column packing. In this manner, size and conformation, not charge, influence elution from the column. The DNA fragments pass through the column with an increasing gradient of acetonitrile. Heteroduplexes that are partially melted elute from the column sooner than homoduplexes under appropriate denaturing conditions based on a temperature derived from readily available DNA melting software. Homoduplexes elute as single peaks. The presence of mutations or polymorphisms will elicit the formation of one or more heteroduplex conformations, which typically elute earlier than the homoduplexes (Fig. 48-13).

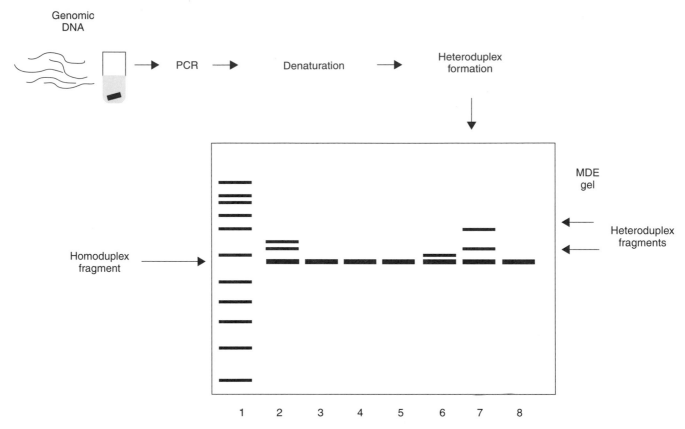

Fig. 48-11   Heteroduplex analysis on MDE gels detects heterozygosity for DNA sequence variants. A genomic DNA is amplified and heteroduplex formation is subsequently enhanced by slow renaturation. Samples are then electrophoresed on MDE gels and stained. *Lane 1*, Size marker. *Lanes 3, 4, 5,* and *8*, No heteroduplexes seen. *Lanes 2, 6,* and *7*, Distinct heteroduplex patterns belie the presence of heterozygosity for discrete sequence variants. Lanes 2 and 7 each have two heteroduplexes, one being sense-normal annealed to antisense mutant, the other being antisense-normal annealed to sense-mutant. These two different heteroduplexes do not resolve in Lane 6.

Although the profile associated with a given mutation or polymorphism is typically reproducible between samples and repeat runs, direct sequencing is recommended to confirm the identity of the sequence variant.

Protein truncation test. As the human genome sequence has been elucidated, much interest now lies in the area of proteomics, or how gene products (proteins) interact. Cell-free expression systems can be used as a bridge between genomics and proteomics by converting nucleic acid sequence into protein sequence. An application of these *in vitro* expression systems for the detection of mutations is referred to as the *protein truncation test* (PrTT). This assay is useful for the detection of those mutations that alter the reading frame of the expressed protein, so-called truncating mutations, which lead to a shortened protein product. This method is particularly useful in interrogating large genes that are frequently altered by nonsense and frameshift mutations (the result of small insertions or deletions), in addition to large deletions. Examples of the underlying disorders include familial adenomatous polyposis, Duchenne and Becker's muscular dystrophy, neurofibromatosis type 1, and hereditary

breast and ovarian cancer defined by the tumor suppressor genes BRCA1 and BRCA2 (see below).

The method involves reverse transcription PCR (RT-PCR) in which total RNA is used to produce cDNA. PCR amplification, using a forward primer that includes appropriate signals for transcription and translation (Fig. 48-14) results in a functional protein-coding segment. Coupling the product with an *in vitro* translation/transcription system that includes RNA polymerase, radiolabeled amino acids, ribosomes, transfer RNAs, and tRNA synthases completes protein synthesis. Transcription and translation of the PCR product results in a labeled protein product. The product can be sized by SDS-polyacrylamide gel electrophoresis. A novel, lower molecular–weight band indicates the presence of a truncated polypeptide, representing a truncating mutation in that sample. The position of the band indicates the relative size of the product, from which the position of the mutation in the coding sequence can be extrapolated. Confirmation of the mutation is achieved by sequencing.

Missense mutations do not usually result in size alterations of proteins; therefore, other procedures must be used for mis-

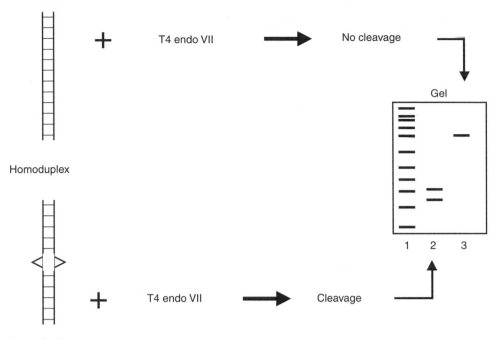

Fig. 48-12 T4 endonuclease VII–mediated cleavage (EMC). Homoduplex PCR fragments have no localized single-stranded domains and will not be cleaved by Endo VII. They will generate a single uncut band after electrophoresis (*Lane 2*). Heteroduplex PCR fragments will be cleaved by Endo VII, giving cleaved fragments (*Lane 3*). *Lane 1*, Size marker.

sense detection, so to achieve maximum analytical sensitivity PrTT analysis is often combined with other scanning techniques. Using this approach, the sensitivity for BRCA1 and BRCA2 mutation detection can approach 90%.

CANCER (see also Chapter 49)

Cancer is defined as an autonomous proliferation of cells with metastatic potential. It is the metastatic and invasive potential that differentiates cancer, or a malignant neoplasm, from benign neoplasms, such as adenomas. Although the disease state of cancer and its ultimate lethality was known to the ancients (cancer derives its name from the crablike tracts of dilated blood vessels seen on the trunk in advanced disease), only recently have significant inroads been made toward understanding the mechanisms of carcinogenesis (the development of cancer) at a fundamental level. Within the last decade, using the tools of the new science of molecular biology, a picture of the exquisite interplay of genes and gene products that serve to regulate cell growth and proliferation has begun to emerge. When one or more of these gene products fails to fulfill its intercellular task, uncontrolled growth can result. The mechanism that brings about failure (inactivity or inappropriate activity) of these protein growth regulators is the occurrence of a mutation, or a change in the DNA coding for that particular protein. Mutations occur by a wide variety of mechanisms. A broad classification system that is useful in discussions of cancer and inherited disease divides mutations into germline and somatic events. A germline mutation is one that is present in all cells of the body and is passed from generation to generation by meiosis (creation of germ cells, sperm and egg) and sexual reproduction. Somatic cell mutations arise *de novo* in tissue cells, generally as a result of some environmental insult or DNA replication error. Although certain rarer types of cancer are associated with germline transmission of mutant genes, the vast majority of cancers are caused by somatic mutations. Among the thousands of genes in the human genome, mutation of only a few of them is necessary or sufficient to cause the deregulation of cell growth. According to our present understanding, there exist two broad classes of genes with these properties— the oncogenes and the tumor suppressor genes.

Oncogenes (see also Chapter 49)

The oncogenes were the first class of genes shown to be involved in the transition from normal, well-regulated cells, to the wildly proliferating, uncontrolled cell mass that characterizes cancer. An oncogene is defined as a gene that, when activated inappropriately, results in uncontrolled growth of a cell population. Because only one copy of the gene needs to be mutated for the genotype to affect the phenotype (malignant versus normal), oncogenes are said to act in a dominant fashion. Although the first oncogenes discovered were of viral origin, it is now clear that the majority of oncogenes are the result of mutations of the normal cell's regulatory genes. These normal genes are referred to as *protooncogenes*. The biochemical activities of protoonco-

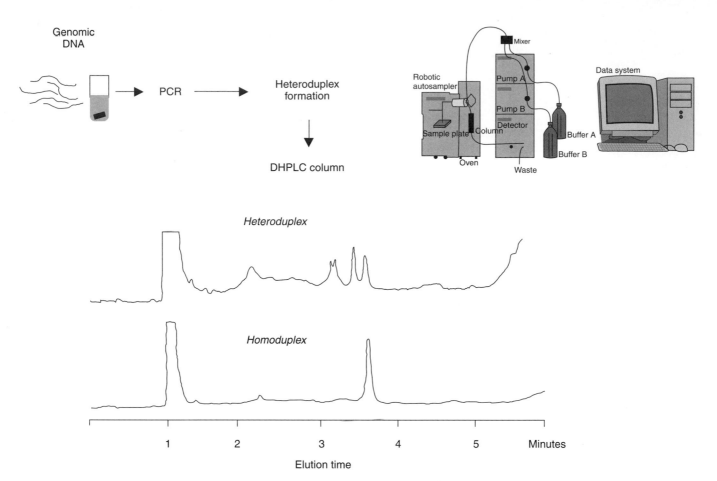

Fig. 48-13 Denaturing high-performance liquid chromatography (DHPLC). Heteroduplex PCR products generate distinctive electrophoretic profiles under appropriate melting conditions. The rapid detection of heteroduplexes helps target sequencing efforts more efficiently. *(Figure adapted with permission of Eric Gerber, Varian Analytical Instruments.)*

genes generally fall into one of three categories: (1) protein kinases and phosphorylases, (2) GTP binding proteins (G-proteins) and signal transduction proteins, and (3) transcription factors. When activated inappropriately, protein kinases and phosphorylases initiate phosphorylation cascades, with the result often being cell division. Examples include the erbB oncogene, which is a mutant form of the epidermal growth factor receptor and the raf1 gene, a serine kinase, which is thought to link signals generated at the cell membrane to nuclear proteins, which regulate cell division.

The G-proteins are part of signal transduction pathways. These pathways connect events at the cell surface, such as the binding of a hormone to its receptor. The G-proteins are activated by the binding of GTP and inactivated by the hydrolysis of GTP to GDP. The activated G-proteins interact with second messenger systems, such as adenyl cyclase and cyclic AMP to stimulate RNA transcription. A well-known example of a G-protein oncogene is the *ras* family of oncogenes. Although normal G-proteins possess a GTPase activity that serves to terminate the signal transduction, the G-protein products of these mutant genes are incapable of hydrolyzing GTP, and thus are inappropriately maintained in an active state.

Several protooncogenes code for transcription factors, and thus directly modulate gene expression. The *myc* family of oncogenes is perhaps the most well studied system. *Myc* is overexpressed in a number of different types of tumors and serves to deregulate the production of cellular growth factors.

There are several mechanisms that result in activated protooncogenes. The common mechanisms are (1) overproduction of the protooncogene caused by loss of the ability to regulate that gene, (2) increased number of copies of the protooncogene, caused by amplification of that gene, and (3) activation of a protooncogene by chromosomal translocation in which the promotor region for a constitutively produced gene is brought into position to regulate a protooncogene. Although several of these mechanisms have been studied, and some are common in particular types of cancer, the most common alteration of function or stability of a protooncogene is via a small mutation in the DNA coding for that gene.

The presence of activated forms of several oncogenes has been associated with poor prognosis, for example, amplification of *N-myc* in neuroblastoma or the activation of *ras* genes in a variety of tumors. A compelling question is, what is the utility of detecting mutant oncogenes in particular tumors and the relationship between genotype and pheno-

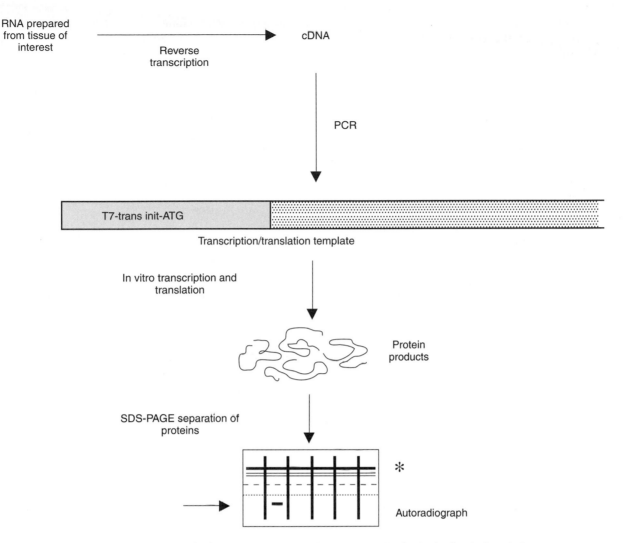

RNA prepared from tissue of interest → Reverse transcription → cDNA

PCR

T7-trans init-ATG

Transcription/translation template

In vitro transcription and translation

Protein products

SDS-PAGE separation of proteins

Autoradiograph

Fig. 48-14 Diagram of the protein truncation test. RNA is typically isolated from peripheral blood lymphocytes from whole blood collected in the presence of ACD or EDTA anticoagulants. (The quality of RNA isolated from tissue depends on rapid freezing of tissue to −70° C or below.) Coupled *in vitro* transcription/translation kits, using a rabbit reticulocyte extract, are commercially available. A labeled amino acid, usually ^{35}S-lysine, is added to the *in vitro* assay to label the synthesized proteins for autoradiography. The *asterisk* identifies the full-length, non-truncated protein. The *arrow* adjacent to the autoradiograph indicates the presence of a band of lower than expected molecular weight, representing a truncated protein.

type? The ability to answer this question will require methods appropriate for very large-scale clinical trials.

Tumor Suppressor Genes

The existence of a class of genes that could act as suppressors of tumor growth was postulated before they were actually shown to exist. After observing familial cases of bilateral retinoblastoma (RB) and comparing those cases with sporadic (nonfamilial) cases of unilateral RB, Knudson proposed that two "hits," or mutational events, were needed for the initiation of tumor growth. In the cases of familial RB, a germline mutation in one tumor suppressor allele was postulated. In this case, there was a much higher probability of tumor initiation, because the individual is born with

one "hit." Therefore, somatic mutations that "hit" or render nonfunctional the remaining normal allele would be tumorigenic. In contrast, in a normal individual (one not born with a mutant RB gene) that same somatic event would not lead to the initiation of a tumor because one functional allele would still be present. Tumor initiation would take place in a normal individual only if two somatic events occurred at the same locus. Because tumor initiation is not observed with a single abnormal allele, it is said that tumor suppressor genes act as recessive alleles.

Since the cloning of the RB gene and the proof of the two-hit hypothesis, a large number of recessively acting tumor suppressor genes have been identified. A partial list includes the Wilm's tumor gene (WT), p53, the neurofibromatosis type

1 and 2 genes (NF1 and NF2), the adenomatous polyposis coli gene (APC), and the deleted in colon cancer gene (DCC). As a rule, they have been identified by searching for genes in chromosomal locations that are commonly deleted in cancer.

Because tumor suppressor genes cause uncontrollable cell growth only by mutations that destroy the function of the gene, it seems reasonable that mutations that give rise to premature "stop" codons (those that instruct translation of the RNA messages) appearing in the reading frame of the gene would be over-represented. This has been observed and influences methodological choices in the clinical analysis for the inactivation of these genes in clinical samples.

Familial Cancer Syndromes

Extensive epidemiological evidence demonstrates that a number of cancers have a higher incidence in relatives of patients than in the general population. Many but not all of these cancers follow straightforward Mendelian inheritance patterns (generally autosomal dominant with reduced penetrance or, rarely, autosomal recessive) (see Chapter 47). These genes are thought to involve germline defects in single genes. On the other hand, familial cancers in which mendelian inheritance patterns cannot be demonstrated (i.e., relatives with risk levels that are elevated relative to the general population, but far less than the risk predicted for single-gene disorders) are most likely the result of multiple factors. It is difficult to separate the increased risk in these families into genetic and environmental factors; undoubtedly, both are important.

Together there are more than 50 recognized mendelian disorders in which the risk of cancer is very high, sometimes approaching 100%. A particularly striking aspect of the inherited cancer syndromes is that multiple primary tumors often occur, whereas more than one tumor in a sporadic case is rare. The genes responsible for some of the cancer syndromes have been identified, including those responsible for adenomatous polyposis coli (colon cancer), familial breast cancer (BRCA1 and 2), neurofibromatosis type 1 (neurofibromas) and type 2 (acoustic neuroma), and Li-Fraumeni syndrome (cancer of multiple tissues). The majority of these genes belong to the class of tumor suppressor genes. However, germline mutations of oncogenes, such as mutations in the RET oncogene in hereditary medullary thyroid carcinoma, have also been described. Although, as previously discussed, tumor suppressor genes act at the cellular level in a recessive manner (the phenotypes of cells with one or with two normal copies of a tumor suppressor gene are indistinguishable, i.e., the cell is normal), the inheritance pattern is dominant with reduced penetrance. Reduced penetrance refers to the fact that not all patients who receive a mutated gene at birth go on to develop cancer. The resolution of this apparent paradox is the realization that the inherited trait results in the increased probability of developing a cancer because of the individual having inherited one "hit."

Although the numbers of individuals affected by a specific Mendelian familial cancer is small, in aggregate the numbers are significant, totaling approximately 5% of total cancers. The ability to detect germline tumor suppressor gene mutations is of extreme importance to families who are shown to have high rates of a cancer of this type. For these families, it is crucial to identify the causative mutation in the relevant gene and then trace that mutation through the family. Individuals who are found not to carry the mutation are relieved of their concerns. Individuals who are found to carry the mutation before the onset of symptoms benefit from increased surveillance, the objective being to identify tumors while they are small and can be treated effectively.

Sporadic Cancers

The great majority (95%) of cancers appear to arise without the inheritance of a mutant tumor suppressor gene. Rather, they arise *de novo* as a result of mutations in somatic (non-germline) cells. Observations in some cancers support a linear view of carcinogenesis (i.e., first a mutation occurs in gene A, followed by a mutation in gene B, followed by a mutation in gene C, etc.). Examples of cancers that seem to follow a linear progression include colon cancer and follicular lymphoma. Observations in other types of cancer, breast and lung cancer for example, suggest a stochastic, or web-of-causation model. In this theory, the order of gene mutation is not important; mutation of any protooncogene or tumor suppressor gene can serve as a first hit. It is not necessary for the first mutational event to be followed by a mutation of a specific gene; rather, the mutation of some number of genes (a number unknown at the present time) is necessary for the development of a malignant phenotype. Further, the identity of those genes is not fixed; there are a large number of genes that can, in theory, act in concert when mutated to allow the cell to grow in an uncontrollable fashion.

Because tumors vary widely in their characteristics (aggressiveness, response to a given therapeutic intervention, etc.), it is not unreasonable to search for correlations between the genotype of the tumor (the set of genes that are mutated and the types of mutations that they harbor) and the phenotype (the observed behavior of the tumor). Although the ability to make genotype/phenotype correlations is in its infancy, the identification of cancer-associated mutations and their correlation with clinical phenotype will yield important insights into the functional characteristics of both oncogene and tumor suppressor proteins. Ultimately these structure/function relationships will contribute to understanding the role these gene products play in cell growth and development and assist in the development of therapeutic strategies for modifying or bypassing abnormal function. A striking example is the drug STI571 that was designed by molecular modeling to inhibit the tyrosine kinase activity of the bcr/abl fusion protein in chronic myelogenous leukemia. The anti-leukemia effects of this compound have been demonstrated in clinical trials, and it is currently marketed under the name Gleevec by Novartis Pharmaceuticals.

Among the first genes for which genotype/phenotype correlations have emerged is p53. This protein has multiple roles in the normal cell. It is associated with both the transcriptional activation of cellular growth factors and the down-regulation of growth-suppressor genes. Further, p53 has been recently shown to mediate the apoptotic (programmed cell death) pathway that is activated in response to severe cellular damage. Protein p53 was originally classified as an oncogene. The majority of the mutations discovered for p53 met the standard criteria for an oncogene; that is, its effect was manifest in a dominant fashion. It was also shown that p53 functions as an oncogene in some tumors, depending on the nature of the mutation; it functions as a mutated tumor suppressor gene in others. More than 1700 mutations have been described in the p53 gene, the majority (approximately 80%) being missense mutations.

The identity of specific p53 mutations may have implications for therapy. In the case of a long lived p53, the apoptotic pathway is still viable; therefore, therapeutic maneuvers aimed at causing enough cellular damage for the cells to undergo programmed death (i.e., radiation therapy) are effective. Conversely, in the complete absence of p53, the apoptotic pathway cannot be engaged, resulting in a radiation resistant phenotype. Recently it has been shown that p53 plays a central role in the process of developing a blood supply (angiogenesis) for large metastatic tumors. Knowledge of p53 mutations will likely be critical in the proper application of emerging therapies in these cases, such as angiostatin, which blocks angiogenesis and can cause tumors to shrink by limiting their blood supply. The use of p53 mutation profiling in cancer is, however, still a research technique. Tests for p53 mutations still must be shown to provide independent clinical information in controlled clinical trials before they become routine procedures in the clinical laboratory.

Translocations in Leukemia and Lymphoma

One set of assay targets that have been validated and are analyzed as part of routine patient care are a variety of recurrent chromosomal translocations in leukemia and lymphoma. Detection of specific translocations is often required for the diagnosis of a specific leukemia or lymphoma. For example, many hematopathologists require cytogenetic or molecular evidence of the t(9:22) translocation to make a diagnosis of chronic myelogenous leukemia. The presence of other translocations may not have the same high sensitivity, but can help make the diagnosis when identified. For example, the presence of the t(14:18) translocation, present in approximately 80% of follicular lymphomas, will identify most, but not all cases of this malignancy.

The recurrent translocations seen in leukemia and lymphoma act via several mechanisms, which are becoming better defined. One mechanism is the activation of tyrosine kinases by translocation. The prototype example of this mechanism is the constitutive activation of the tyrosine kinase activity of the ABL oncogene (chromosome 9) when it is translocated to the BCR gene on chromosome 22. The t(9:22) translocation joins the 5′ end of the BCR gene to the 3′ end of the ABL gene, resulting in a BCR-ABL fusion protein that retains tyrosine kinase activity, but is divorced from the regulatory sequences in the amino terminal domain of the ABL gene. This kinase activity affects the survival and growth of hematopoietic cells through activation of multiple signal transduction pathways, including the RAS, JUN kinase, and STAT pathways.

A common mechanism in leukemia and lymphoma is the dysregulation of a transcription factor by the translocation of its gene to a chromosomal position in which the transcription factor is placed under the control of a strong promotor. An example of this type of mechanism is the constitutive expression of the *myc* oncogene, a transcription factor on chromosome 8, when it is translocated to control of the IgH promotor on chromosome 14 in the t(8:14) translocation; an event characteristic of Burkitt's lymphoma and B-cell leukemia. Other examples of activation of transcription factors by translocation to immunoglobulin promotor loci include activation of BCL6 by translocation to the IgH locus on chromosome 14 in the t(3:14) translocation in diffuse B-cell lymphoma and activation of *myc* by translocation to the Igκ locus of chromosome 2, in the t(2:8) translocation. Genes other than transcription factors can be dysregulated by translocation. Examples include activation of cyclin D1 by translocation to chromosome 14 and constitutive expression of the antiapoptotic gene BCL2 by translocation to the IgH locus.

In addition to their diagnostic utility, the presence of unique molecular identifiers for a malignant clone can be used to monitor the efficiency of therapy. This use, termed *detection of minimal residual disease*, has gained popularity in recent years. An example of this application is the serial quantification over time of the BCR-ABL fusion mRNA by quantitative RT-PCR in chronic myelogenous leukemia. Decreasing levels during chemotherapy indicates tumor killing, whereas rising levels after a chemotherapy-induced remission indicates resurgence of the disease. The advent of quantitative PCR and RT-PCR using real-time analysis will likely make these assays part of the standard of care. One issue to be addressed, however, is the level of analytical sensitivity required for monitoring of anticancer therapy. The analytical sensitivity of very sensitive PCR platforms may be too sensitive, with many patients who display clinical remission still being PCR positive for the molecular marker. Further studies to define the appropriate cut-off values will be very helpful.

INFECTIOUS DISEASE

Nowhere has the revolution in DNA diagnostics had more profound effects than in the detection of infectious agents. Currently, the clinical use of molecular methods has had its major impact on the detection of organisms that are difficult or impossible to culture, especially viruses, but also including organisms such as *Mycobacterium* species and fungi. Molecular diagnostics can provide superior information because of better sensitivity and specificity. In addition, molecular diagnostics can provide a diagnosis in 24 hours as compared to days or even weeks by traditional testing.

Detection of infectious agents by molecular methods presents different problems than the analysis of endogenous

DNA sequences. The target sequences do not have homology to human sequences, so detection methods relying on hybridization by probes or amplification of the target DNA provide good results. However, although the samples for analysis are more varied than the serum or plasma samples typically submitted to the clinical chemistry laboratory, the opportunity for sampling error is large, and sample preparation protocols are key. Contamination can be a particular problem when detecting organisms that survive in the environment. More than 50% of house dust, for example, is composed of desquamated human skin. Assays for nonculturable dermatophytes such as human papillomaviruses (HPV) are highly susceptible to contamination from such sources.

Two of the most successful applications of molecular techniques have been the quantification of human immunodeficiency virus (HIV) viral load and the analysis of HIV drug resistance.

Human Immunodeficiency Virus Viral Load and Drug Resistance Testing

HIV viral load. The quantitative assessment of the number of viral particles in patient's blood, or **viral load**, is now accepted as a standard practice in the management of patients infected with HIV. Measurement of the viral load is a predictor of the progression time to AIDS and death. Thus, clinicians use the viral load as a tool to monitor response to therapy, with the goal of obtaining and maintaining as low a viral load as possible. In addition to being a tool for monitoring response to therapy, there is a dose-response relationship with viral load and the risk of transmission of HIV to sexual partners and in perinatal transmission.

HIV RNA is detectable in plasma about 2 weeks after infection, making it the earliest marker for HIV infection. During early infection, RNA levels generally peak at about 1 million copies/mL, decrease by 2 to 3 logs with some fluctuation, and subsequently reach a "set point" by 6 months. HIV-infected individuals generally have set points of 1000 to 10,000 copies/mL of plasma, and once established, the set points remain fairly constant for months to years. Patients whose HIV RNA viral load levels exceed 100,000 copies/mL within 6 months of seroconversion are tenfold more likely to progress to AIDS within 5 years than those with less than 100,000 copies/mL. Current medical consensus suggests that physicians maintain their patients' plasma RNA levels at less than 10,000 copies/mL, and optimally, below the analytical limits of detection. Antiviral treatment should be initiated or changed if the patient has a viral load level greater than 10,000 copies/mL. Guidelines for the use of antiretroviral agents are posted on the US Department of Health and Human Services HIV/AIDS Treatment Information Service website at www.hivatis.org.

Currently, there are three viral load assay systems marketed to clinical laboratories in the United States. The Roche Amplicor Monitor is a PCR-based test; the Organon Teknika NucliSens HIV-1 QT uses nucleic acid sequence based–amplification (NASBA) for viral quantification; and the Bayer Versant HIV RNA uses a signal amplification,

branched chain DNA (bDNA) strategy. Each of these three viral load tests has similar detection limits, and they are all expensive—about $80 per test, excluding labor. Although the three assays show good correlation with each other, they all show substantial inherent variation in intraassay, interassay, interlaboratory, and intermethod testing with coefficients of variations ranging from 10% to 40%, depending on the viral load. Further, because the numerical results of any one test are not necessarily the same as the other tests, it is recommended that laboratories performing viral load testing consistently use the same type of assay to monitor patients' viral load over time. A fourth test, the Procleix HIV-1/HCV assay, developed and manufactured by Gen-Probe, Inc. and marketed by Chiron, Inc., is based on transcript mediated amplification (TMA).

The HIV reverse transcriptase enzyme is an RNA-dependent DNA polymerase that creates phosphodiester bonds between nucleoside bases to synthesize DNA based on an RNA template. Current anti-HIV therapy is based on inhibitors of nucleoside reverse transcriptase (NRTIs). Acquisition of viral mutations leading to the growth of viral strains that have a resistance to antiretroviral drugs can occur in fully compliant patients, but is accentuated by missing doses of drug. Several factors may promote the development of resistance. Most importantly, the population of HIV virus that infects an individual consists of numerous subspecies of genetic variants that evolve from the population of virus that was initially transmitted to the individual. The vast array of subspecies of HIV within one individual provides HIV with a survival advantage by increasing the possibility that one of its mutated variants will be resistant to a specific drug or a combination of agents. Selective pressure from antiretroviral therapy and immunological responses of the host promotes the replication and propagation of certain variants regardless of their original proportion in the HIV population. Under a specific selective pressure, those strain(s) possessing mutations that provide a survival advantage proliferate and emerge as the predominant quasispecies.

The detection of specific mutations can indicate presence of a strain of HIV resistant to the current drug therapy. The evaluation of the genetic composition of HIV has progressed from an epidemiological tool for research into a clinically useful laboratory test that health care professionals may use to select and tailor the appropriate antiretroviral agents to manage HIV disease progression.

HIV drug resistance: phenotype testing. Phenotypic resistance assays evaluate the amount of drug necessary to inhibit HIV replication in cultured T lymphocytes and therefore directly measure, under controlled laboratory conditions, the level of resistance of the HIV population derived from an individual patient to each of the anti-HIV drugs currently available. As a direct and quantitative measure of resistance, phenotyping is considered the reference method for the determination of resistance of HIV to drugs.

To provide phenotype data, these assays insert PCR-amplified reverse transcriptase and protease genes from the clinical isolate of the infected individual into a laboratory-derived molecular clone containing standardized HIV envelope and accessory genes. The recombinant virus is then grown in viral culture in the presence of varying concentrations of the drug being evaluated, enabling an assessment of the phenotypic characteristics expressed by the inserted genes. In addition, a wild-type virus is grown alongside the recombinant test clone as a control. Resistance is measured in terms of the IC_{50}, the concentration of drug that inhibits replication of the virus by 50%. A fourfold or higher shift between the IC_{50} of the clone and the wild-type virus indicates drug resistance. These assays may be preferred in the management of individuals with multiple drug treatments because they measure susceptibility directly, and results are easier to interpret because these assays measure how an individual strain of HIV will replicate in the presence of a particular drug or treatment regimen. The interpretation of drug susceptibilities is analogous to the antibiotic sensitivity testing of bacteria. Phenotypic analysis assesses the total effect of any mutations and mutational interactions that confer resistance to the currently available antiretroviral agents by the subspecies of HIV within an individual.

The disadvantages of phenotypic assays include their insensitivity for detecting minor species and the restricted availability of such assays. In addition, these tests are typically more expensive (usually $800 to $1000 per test) and have a lengthy turnaround time (2 to 3 weeks). The assay procedures are labor-intensive, lengthy, cumbersome, and technically demanding. Lastly, clinically significant cutoff values may be ill-defined because thresholds to define susceptibility are arbitrary, nonstandardized, and do not vary based on achievable drug concentrations; however, newer decision points are currently being evaluated. No commercial kits are available for HIV phenotype analysis and few, if any, laboratories have developed this highly specialized test in-house. There are two reference laboratories that offer HIV phenotyping tests: ViroLogic, Inc. (San Francisco, Calif.) markets their test under the trade-name PhenoSense; and Virco (Mechelan, Belgium) markets their test in the United States and Europe under the name Antivirogram.

Virco offers an interpretive service, the *Virtual* Phenotype, that is based on a correlative database of more than 100,000 HIV phenotypes and genotypes. Initially the RT and protease gene sequences of the virus are established with a DNA sequencing–based genotyping assay (see later discussion). The sequence is analyzed by computer software that identifies mutations that confer resistance to any of the drugs, and then scans the database for similar genotypes from previous samples that may match the patterns of mutations. Once any matches are identified, the phenotypes of these samples are retrieved from the database, and for each drug, an interpretive evaluation is then provided. Although the database was developed using the Virco genotyping system, the *Virtual* Phenotype is also available via secure Internet to laboratories who use other genotyping products, including procedures developed in-house by individual laboratories. When combined with high-quality DNA sequence data, sound clinical judgment, and the patient's antiretroviral drug history,

the *Virtual* Phenotype may help physicians use genotype information optimally and more effectively.

HIV drug resistance: genotype testing. Genotypic antiretroviral resistance testing (GART) by DNA sequence analysis of the reverse transcriptase and protease genes and the identification of specific mutations is the most common method of evaluating HIV drug resistance. Those mutations that alter the efficacy of drug binding to its active site are referred to as primary mutations. As a result of primary mutations, higher concentrations of drug are generally required to inhibit the activity of the enzyme. Although viruses with primary drug resistance mutations can replicate in the presence of the drug, in many cases the fitness of the virus is compromised by these mutations. Secondary mutations are defined as those mutations that supplement the action of the primary mutations by increasing viral fitness. In the absence of primary mutations, secondary mutations generally lack any effect on the level of resistance demonstrated by the virus.

GART results are usually difficult to interpret. There are several methods of assisting a practitioner with interpreting genotypic information. One approach is the virtual phenotype approach (see earlier discussion of *Virtual* Phenotype, Virco, Inc.), which uses an extensive database of genotype-phenotype correlations. In a rules-based approach, the information provided by genotyping is presented as a categorical resistant or sensitive prediction based on a rules algorithm. The Resistance Collaborative Group (RCG) is a panel of experts that formed in 1999 in the United States to review and advise the FDA regarding the role of resistance testing in the development of new drugs. This group developed the rule-based interpretation, also known as the data analysis plan (DAP analysis), of genetic information, which relies on currently defined mutations or sets of mutations (stored in a computer database) that confer resistance. A preliminary version of online rules-based interpretation software is currently available at Stanford University's website http://hivdb.stanford.edu.

There are several analytical platforms currently in use for GART testing. The first uses Sanger sequencing on automated DNA sequence analyzers. Several vendors have developed total HIV genotyping systems, which include PCR amplification reagents, DNA sequencing reagents and hardware; and software that provides a rules-based interpretation of the sequence and generates a user-friendly, easily interpreted report. These systems are available from Visible Genetics (TruGene HIV-1 Genotyping Assay, Visible Genetics, Inc., Toronto, Ontario) and Applied Biosystems (ViroSeq HIV-1 Genotyping System, Applied Biosystems, Foster City, Calif.). An alternative approach is the line probe assay, available from Innogenetics (INNO-LiPA HIV-1 RT, Innogenetics, Inc., Atlanta, Ga.). This system uses a large set of oligonucleotide probes complementary to known sequence variants associated with drug resistance immobilized on a nylon membrane in a reverse dot-blot format. The advantage of this system is that it has higher sensitivity to minor species, has a much shorter turnaround time, and requires significantly less technical expertise than does DNA sequencing. A disadvantage is that, as new mutations are identified, new strips that incorporate the new probes must be devised, validated, and manufactured.

GENETIC DISORDERS

Abnormal variants of normal DNA sequences are associated with diseases of genetic origin (see Chapter 47). Molecular techniques can be used to make prenatal diagnoses of these diseases, giving prospective parents the opportunity to seek genetic counseling. Online Mendelian Inheritance in Man (OMIM) is an Internet accessible, comprehensive catalogue of human genes and genetic disorders maintained by the National Library of Medicine (www.ncbi.nlm.nih.gov).

In general, genetic disorders can be grouped into the following categories: chromosomal abnormalities, multifactorial disorders, and single gene disorders. The discussion in this chapter centers on single gene disorders.

Single gene disorders are inherited in one of the following patterns: autosomal dominant, autosomal recessive, or X-linked. The terms *autosomal* and *X-linked* refer to the chromosomal location of the disease-causing gene, or mutant gene. Generally, in X-linked disorders, males with the mutant gene express the disorder, whereas females with the same gene are carriers and are usually disease free. Examples of X-linked disorders include Duchenne muscular dystrophy and hemophilia. *Dominant* disorders are expressed whether an individual is heterozygous or homozygous; *recessive* disorders are expressed only when an individual is homozygous for a mutant gene. Examples of the former are the autosomal dominant disorders achondroplasia and Huntington disease; examples of the latter are the autosomal recessive disorders cystic fibrosis, sickle cell anemia, and phenylketonuria. Individuals who are heterozygous for these recessive disorders are carriers.

The number of disease-associated genes that have been identified in the past several years is impressive; theoretically, direct tests could be developed for all of these disorders. Although tests are available for many of them, *allelic heterogeneity* prevents the use of a few simple tests for diagnosis or carrier detection in all patients or families. Allelic heterogeneity refers to the observation that, although single disorders are typically caused by mutations in single genes, the range of disease-associated mutations in that gene is very large. An exception to this rule is sickle cell anemia. Every case of sickle cell anemia is caused by the same mutation, an A to T mutation in codon 6 of the β-globin gene. More typical are the mutational spectra of cystic fibrosis (CF) and Duchenne muscular dystrophy (DMD). There is one mutation (a three base-pair deletion termed ΔF508) in the cystic fibrosis transmembrane conductance regulator (CFTR) gene that accounts for approximately 70% of disease alleles in populations derived from Northern Europe. However, more than 1000 different mutations have been described on CF genes that do not contain the most common mutation. A database of CFTR mutations is maintained at the Department of Genetics, Hospital for Sick Children, Toronto, Canada (www.genet.sickkids.on.ca). In the case of DMD, large deletions in the dystrophin gene account for approximately 60% of cases of DMD. Although many of these deletions are clustered in two hot spots, they are heterogeneous, with few affected boys sharing the same deletion. The nondeletion cases are heterogeneous as well, with only a single report of two apparently unrelated boys sharing the same point mutation. Thus, even after a disease gene has been identified, it still may not be possible to provide a direct test that provides complete information in any given family. A list of available genetic tests and laboratories that offer them is maintained at www.genetests.org/. A very large database of human gene mutations, including links to over 100 gene-specific databases is maintained at the Institute of Medical Genetics, Cardiff, Wales (http://archive.uwcm.ac.uk/uwcm/mg/hgmd0.html).

Bibliography

General

Coleman WB, Tsongalis GJ, editors: *Molecular diagnostics for the clinical laboratorian*, Totowa, NJ, 1996, Humana Press.

Dracopoli NC et al, editors: *Current protocols in human genetics*, New York, 1994, Wiley & Sons.

Farkas DH, editor: *Molecular biology and pathology: a guidebook for quality control*, New York, 1993, Academic Press.

Farkas DH: *DNA simplified II: the illustrated hitchhiker's guide to DNA*, Washington, DC, 1999, AACC Press.

Killeen A, editor: *Molecular pathology protocols*, Totowa, NJ, 2000, Humana Press.

Silverman LM, Heim R, editors: *Molecular pathology*, Durham, NC, 1994, Carolina Academic Press.

Cancer Genetics

Cho Y et al: Crystal structure of a p53 tumor suppressor-DNA complex: understanding tumorigenic mutations, *Science* 265:346, 1994.

Coleman WB, Tsongalis GJ, editors: *The molecular basis of human cancer*, Totowa, NJ, 2001, Humana Press.

Hodgson SV, Maher ER: *A practical guide to human cancer genetics*, New York, 1993, Cambridge University Press.

Knudson AG: Chasing the cancer demon, *Annu Rev Genet* 34:1, 2000.

Levine AJ: The tumor suppressor genes, *Annu Rev Biochem* 62:623, 1993.

Srivastava S, Henson DE, Gazdar A, editors: *Molecular pathology of early cancer*, Washington, DC, 1999, IOS Press.

Vogelstein B, Kinzler KW, editors: *The genetic basis of human cancer*, New York, 1998, McGraw-Hill.

Infectious Disease and HIV

Hirsch MS et al: Antiretroviral drug resistance testing in adult HIV-1 infection: recommendations of an International AIDS Society-USA panel, *JAMA* 283:2417, 2000.

International perspectives of antiretroviral resistance, special issue, *J Acquir Immune Defic Syndr* (suppl 1), 2001.

MacArthur RD: Drug resistance: an updated, user-friendly guide to genotype interpretation, *AIDS Reader* 10:652, 2000.

Naber SP: Molecular pathology: diagnosis of infectious disease, *N Engl J Med* 331:1212, 1994.

Rersing DH et al, editors: *Diagnostic molecular microbiology: principles and applications*, Washington, DC, 1993, American Society for Microbiology.

Saag MS et al: HIV viral load markers in clinical practice, *Nat Med* 2:625, 1996.

Vlahov D et al: Prognostic indicators for AIDS and infectious disease death in HIV-infected injection drug users, *JAMA* 279:35, 1998.

Genetics

The human genome, special issue, *Nature* 409:745, 2001.
The human genome, special issue, *Science* 291:1145, 2001.
Kerem B-S et al: Identification of the cystic fibrosis gene: genetic analysis, *Science* 245:1073, 1989.

Pena SDJ et al, editors: *DNA fingerprinting: the state of the science*, Boston, 1993, Birkhäuser Verlag.
Prior TW: Perspectives and molecular diagnosis of Duchenne and Becker muscular dystrophies, *Clin Lab Med* 15:927, 1995.
Strachan T, Read AP: *Human molecular genetics*, ed 2, New York, 1999, Wiley.
Zielenski J, Tsui LC: Cystic fibrosis: genotypic and phenotypic variations, *Annu Rev Genet* 29:777, 1995.

Internet Sites

www.genetests.org
www.hivatis.org—US Department of Health and Human Services HIV/AIDS Treatment Information Service
http://hivdb.stanford.edu—Stanford University
www.ncbi.nlm.nih.gov—National Library of Medicine

www.genet.sickkids.on.ca—Department of Genetics, Hospital for Sick Children, Toronto, Canada
http://archive.uwcm.ac.uk/uwcm/mg/hgmd0.html—Institute of Medical Genetics, Cardiff, Wales

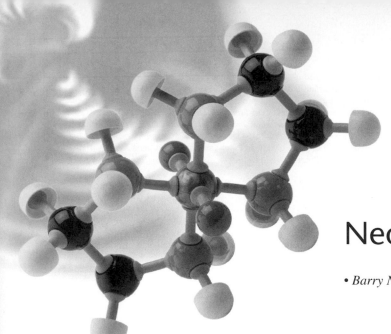

CHAPTER 49

Neoplasia

• Barry N. Elkins

Chapter Outline

Objectives

- Briefly describe the biological factors that can result in cancer.
- List the roles of laboratory tests in the assessment of cancers.

- Define and describe an ideal tumor marker.
- List commonly used chemical and cellular markers and state their clinical significance in relation to cancers.

Key Terms

carcinoembryonic antigen (CEA)   A glycoprotein produced by or associated with cancer cells that is also expressed by fetal cells. Small levels are detected in healthy individuals. Detection is by immunochemical analysis.

carcinogen   An agent, usually a chemical, that transforms a cell from a normal to a cancerous state.

cocarcinogen   An agent that by itself does not transform a normal cell into a cancerous state but in concert with another agent can effect the transformation.

confirmation   Use of a subsequent test with very high specificity to verify the observation of a less specific test (e.g., a biopsy to verify a mass as a tumor).

dedifferentiation The process by which cells go from the more specific to the more general in nature. Usually such cells lose their morphological architecture and ability to synthesize specific cell components (e.g., estrogen receptors).

dissemination The phase of cancer in which the cells spread to various parts of the body distant from the site of origin.

estrogen receptor The specific tissue membrane receptor in breast tissue that binds estrogens. Its presence in breast cancer signifies a differentiated tumor.

heterogeneity Variation in gene expression among cancer cells. Differences between cells exist, and not all cells within a tumor are positive for the same antigen or respond to the same drug.

induction phase The period during which a normal cell becomes transformed into a cancerous cell.

in situ Confined to the site of origin. Used to describe cancer cells that are localized at their place of origin.

invasion The process by which malignant cells move into deeper tissue and through the basement membrane, thereby gaining access to blood vessels and lymphatic channels.

metastases Cancer cells that have spread to other organs and formed colonies that are growing and often invading the organ.

monitoring Measurement of a biochemical marker of cancer after a confirmed diagnosis; used to evaluate the presence or growth of the cancer (e.g., the use of carcinoembryonic antigen to monitor colorectal cancer).

neoplasia Literally, "new growth"; the unrestricted growth of cells resulting in cancer.

oncogene A gene whose protein product can cause the development of a cancer when the protein is present (or absent) in abnormal amounts.

Pap (Papanicolaou) smear A common screening test for cancer, in which cells from the cervix are examined for cytological abnormalities consistent with cancer.

staging A process of diagnosis in which the pathologist determines the position of cancer in the progressive cycle of phases: induction, in situ, invasion, and dissemination.

transformation In oncology, the process by which a normal cell becomes malignant, that is, cancerous.

tumor marker A term that mistakenly implies that certain molecules can be used to diagnose or monitor the presence or growth of a cancer. Usually such markers are not specific for cancer.

Methods on CD-ROM

Alpha-fetoprotein
CEA

Prostatic acid phosphatase and prostate-specific antigen

CANCER INCIDENCE IN THE UNITED STATES

Increasing longevity, presence of **carcinogens** in the environment, and other factors have changed the incidence of cancer in the United States. Table 49-1 presents percentages of cancer cases and deaths by organ site and gender, as tabulated in the year 2001 in the United States. The sites associated most strongly with cancer deaths in males of all ages are, in descending order, lung, blood and lymphoid tissues, prostate, colorectal area, urinary tract, and pancreas. In females of all ages the most common cancer sites are breast, lung, colorectal area, blood and lymphoid tissues, ovary, pancreas, and uterus. Carcinogens in tobacco are believed to be responsible for the alterations in cellular genetic material (deoxyribonucleic acid, or DNA) that lead to lung cancer, whereas ingested carcinogens cause similar DNA lesions that lead to colorectal cancer. The distribution of deaths by organ site is affected by geographical factors as well. For example, in Japan, unlike in the United States, esophageal and stomach cancers are the most common types of malignancy. In Western countries cancer is the second greatest cause of death. Approximately one in five persons in the United States will die of cancer.

CANCER: NATURE OF THE DISEASE

The clonal theory of carcinogenesis states that cancers derive from an original cell that has undergone **transformation**. This transformed cell, or clone, is a normal cell whose genetic material has been altered such that the cell and its progeny lose those regulatory functions that govern cell replication and cell death. By an evolutionary, multistep process, cells derived from the initially modified cell begin to multiply, uncontrolled by the usual local inhibitory systems, often invading other parts of the body. This last phase, called **metastases**, is usually the cause of death by cancer.

Several points of evidence have led scientists to believe that more than one gene must be altered before a malignant cell is formed. First, the relationship between cancer and age is an experiential one; that is, as an individual ages, the likelihood of cancer increases. Time is needed to allow the accumulation of genetic damage, which can lead to the transformed state (see below). Second, cancer cells can be shown to have multiple genetic lesions. Third, cancer is more likely to occur in cells that proliferate. Thus cancer of the heart is very rare, but cancers of the white blood cell are very common. Because white blood cells proliferate, there is far

TABLE 49-1   ESTIMATED NEW CANCER CASES AND DEATHS IN 2001 IN THE UNITED STATES BY SITE AND SEX*

| | SEX | | | |
| | MALE (%) | | FEMALE (%) | |
Site	Cases	Deaths	Cases	Deaths
Breast	NA	NA	31	15
Colon and rectum	10	10	11	11
Blood and lymphoid tissue (leukemias and lymphomas)	8	9	7	8
Respiratory system	16	33	13	26
Oral cavity	3	2	2	1
Ovary	NA	NA	4	5
Pancreas	2	5	2	6
Prostate	31	11	NA	NA
Skin	5	2	4	1
Urinary tract	9	6	4	3
Uterus	NA	NA	8	4
Stomach	2	3	1	2
Liver and gallbladder	2	4	1	3
Other	11	16	11	15

Data supplied by the American Cancer Society website: www.cancer.org.

TABLE 49-2   CLASSES OF ONCOGENES AND THEIR DERIVED PROTEIN PRODUCTS

Class of Factor	Factor	Gene Product
Growth factors	*sis*	PDGF B, chain growth factor
Protein tyrosine kinase	*sic*	Membrane associated, receptor protein tyrosine kinase
Receptors lacking protein kinase activity	*mas*	Angiotensin receptor
Membrane-associated G-proteins	H-*ras*	Membrane-associated GTP-binding/GTPase
Cytoplasmic protein kinase	*rat/mil*	Cytoplasmic protein kinases
Cytoplasmic regulators	*crk*	SH-23 protein
Nuclear transcription cofactors	*myc*	Sequence-specific, DNA-binding protein

greater potential for the expression of genetic lesions and for the process of cell division to become unregulated.

Etiology

Sager[1] has described the cause of cancer as a multistage genetic process. The stages include:

- Initial DNA damage
- Chromosome breakdown and rearrangement; gene replication
- Selection of successfully growing mutant cells

The initial changes in cellular DNA can be caused by a variety of carcinogens, including radiation, chemicals, viruses, and unknown agents. This leads to faulty growth control and loss of chromosome stability. The chromosome breakage and rearrangement occur in several continuous phases after the initiation of cell division. This is later manifested in terms of aberrant chromosomal transpositions, which lead to genomic rearrangements (see Chapter 47).

The changes in the DNA and chromosomes result in a new pattern of gene expression, creating a new phenotype, in which previously quiescent genes are now expressed, previously expressed genes are now quiescent, or there is overexpression of certain key genes. It is now believed that the earliest changes in gene expression that can lead to a transformed cell occur in genes that normally regulate cell growth and cell death.[2] These newly expressed or suppressed regulatory genes are known as **oncogenes**.[3] A list of the cell-derived oncogene products by class is presented in Table 49-2. Assays that detect oncogenes in human cancer tissues

are rapidly becoming available (see Chapter 47). These assays may be potentially useful for the prediction of the development of oncogene-associated cancers in high-risk groups.[4]

A cell that has been transformed has only the *potential* for developing into a cancer. The expression of the cancer phenotype requires cell division, which can be induced by additional genetic damage or can result from a natural induction of cell division. This can be seen in the inverse relationship between the development of breast cancer and the age at which a woman first carries a pregnancy to near term. This relationship is likely the result of the one-time induction of breast epithelial cell hyperplasia that occurs in a first pregnancy. The later in life that the first pregnancy occurs, the greater the likelihood of the accumulation of a cancer phenotype in breast epithelium.

As cancer cells multiply, there may be additional phenotypic changes in the now unstable genetic material. As a result, a process of natural selection allows the most "successful" cancer cell to proliferate the most and to dominate the cancer mass. As the environment surrounding the cancer changes, such as occurs as a result of therapy, the selection process continues.

Diversity of Cancer Cells

Variation of gene expression. There is a broad range of possible combinations of gene expression in the human cell. It varies from normal cells to the most atypical cancer cells. As a result of the genetic changes described above, cancer cells develop new combinations of gene expression and therefore new phenotypes. The phenotypic variation occurs not only from cancer cells to normal cells, or from cancer type to cancer type, but also within particular cancer types and even within a single tumor. For example, in patients with cancer of the breast there is a **heterogeneity** of genes expressed by various cells; that is, not all cells express the same genes. An example is the heterogeneous expression in breast tumors of the gene for the **estrogen receptor** (see below).

Variable gene expression and its manifestations. Variable gene expression leads to biological and biochemical diversity of cancer cells; consequently various tumor-specific markers are not necessarily elaborated by all cancer cells of the same type or even by a single cancer over time. This fact is clinically very important in an investigator's determination of which analyte to follow in **monitoring** patients with known malignancy. The cellular diversity within a single tumor also means that a cancer's clinical manifestation, such as a tumor's response to therapy, may change with time.

Clinical Manifestations

The clinical manifestations of cancer vary widely, depending on the type of tumor, the tissue affected, and the stage of tumor development. For example, cancer of the gastrointestinal tract is manifested by obstruction, hemoptysis, and bloody stools. Cancer of the lung is manifested by hypoxia, chest pain, and often various neurological symptoms. The clinical manifestations are related to the physiological function of the organ with the primary cancer and the effect of the cancer on other organs as well. For example, cancer of an endocrine gland can result in production of excess hormone with many systemic hormonal effects. New symptoms are seen with the spread (metastasis) of the cancer cells to other organs. Cancer spreads through the lymphatic system and the bloodstream, resulting in liver, bone, and pulmonary metastases.

Time as a Factor: Cancer as a Long-Term Process

Cancer is a long-term process and progresses through four obligatory phases: an induction phase, an **in situ** phase, an invasion phase, and a **dissemination** phase. During the *induction phase*, which can last up to 30 years or more, the cells are exposed to one or more carcinogens. These environmental carcinogens may include radiation or various toxins. It has been estimated that approximately three-fourths of all human cancers may be caused by these environmental factors.

It is now believed that a period of many years after exposure may be necessary before a carcinogen is able to have its effect on the host. The histological changes begin with severe dysplasia, eventually leading to cancer. Obviously, not everyone who is exposed to the same carcinogen will develop cancer. Additional factors that play a role in deciding who may get cancer include individual (genetic) or tissue susceptibility, the presence of other carcinogens or **cocarcinogens**, the site at which the carcinogen may act, the duration of exposure (see above), and of course, the nature, amount, and concentration of the carcinogen under question. Often the time between the induction phase and the clinically apparent cancer can be as long as 20 years.

After induction there is the *in situ phase*. This phase represents that time during which the transformed cell actually develops into a cancer, but the cancer remains localized in the original site and does not invade other tissues.

Clonal selection (see above) for those cancer cells that grow most successfully occurs during this phase.

The third phase is called the *invasion phase*. During this phase the malignant cells multiply and invade into the deeper tissues through the basement membrane, thereby gaining access to blood vessels and lymphatic channels.

The fourth stage is the *dissemination phase*. During this phase, which lasts 1 to 5 years, the invading cancer spreads to various parts of the body distant from the site of origin, often through the blood and lymphatic systems. One factor limiting tumor growth during this phase is the formation of a new blood supply. This process, termed *angiogenesis*, is regulated by the presence of vascular endothelial growth factor (VEGF).[5,6] (See references 5 and 6 for detailed discussions of this topic.)

Early detection of cancer, before metastatic spread, is critical to improve success in treating the disease. In fact, it would be ideal to detect cancer during the induction phase; unfortunately, however, this is impossible because prior to the in situ phase, an investigator cannot be certain whether cancer will actually develop in the individual. The next best approach, then, is to detect the cancer during the in situ phase. This has been done with great success in patients with cancer of the cervix, in which the **Pap (Papanicolaou) smear** technique has been of great benefit. When in situ cancer of the cervix is detected, the prognosis is excellent. Most cancers are detected during the invasion phase. If dissemination has not yet occurred, the prognosis is reasonable. Detection of local spreading with or without involvement of the lymph nodes often leads to a cure. However, if dissemination has already occurred, the prognosis is very poor.

Invasion by Cancer Cells of Surrounding Tissue

Several factors play a role in determining the cancer's ability to invade the surrounding tissue. Such factors include increased motility of the cells, increased pressure within the tumor caused by active multiplication of the cells, elaboration by the cancer of lytic substances, lack of intercellular bridges found between all normal cells, decreased cohesiveness between cells, and eventual spread of the tumor cells to the regional lymph nodes. However, when the metastases are still microscopic (micrometastases), the clinician's ability to detect them is very poor. It has been estimated that approximately half the patients who appear to be clinically free of metastases do in fact have unrecognized distant micrometastases at the time of initial diagnosis and treatment.

Change in Cell Division

Cancer is often manifested by a change in cellular division rate. Although most cancers are associated with an increased rate of cell division, there are examples, such as nephroma, in which this is not always the case.

Dedifferentiation of Cells

A common phenomenon of cancer is **dedifferentiation**, in which cells go from a more specific cell type to a more general cell type by the process of clonal selection. Thus it is not uncommon for cancer cells to synthesize various compounds that are normally present only in the embryonic or fetal stage. On the other hand, as cells dedifferentiate, they may lose certain specific cellular properties such as receptor activity or enzyme activity. These phenotypic changes can be used as prognostic indicators.

Chromosomal Changes in Cancer

Chromosomal changes in cancer have been extensively studied in patients with leukemia, and various types of leukemia are often confirmed on the basis of these chromosomal changes.

The colorectal cancer model of tumorigenesis.
A stepwise model of colorectal tumorigenesis involving gene mutations and chromosome changes was developed in 1990 and has since been validated. Subsequent work has discovered additional genetic events and specific molecular pathways affected by these mutations. This model, reviewed by Chung[7] and summarized here, may serve as a general description for the development of cancer cells. In this model the following sequential steps must occur for the development of colorectal cancer.

1. Mutations in the adenomatous polyposis coli (APC) tumor-suppressor gene occur early in the development of polyps.
2. Oncogenic K-*ras* mutations arise during the adenomatous stage
3. Mutations of TP53 and deletions on chromosome 18q coincide with transition to malignancy.

The APC/beta-catenin pathway.
The APC gene encodes a protein which, when mutated, results in either familial adenomatous polyposis (FAP) or Gardner's syndrome; it also plays a critical role in sporadic colon cancer. The APC tumor-suppressor gene is mutated in more than 70% of all colorectal cancers. The mutated APC protein causes a disruption of the APC/beta-catenin complex and increased cytoplasmic levels of free beta–catenin, which translocate to the nucleus, where it activates several oncogenes.

The DNA mismatch repair pathway.
Mutations in five different genes have been identified with the Hereditary Nonpolyposis Colorectal Cancer (HNPCC) Syndrome. Each of the genes encodes a protein involved in DNA mismatch repair, the enzymatic proofreading process which corrects base pair mismatches arising during DNA replication. These gene defects presumably cause tumor development as a result of widespread mutations that are unable to be repaired.

Summary.
About 85% of colorectal tumors show chromosome instability but stability of microsatellite DNA. In the development of these tumors, a normal cell is converted to an early, noncancerous adenoma by mutation in the APC/beta-catenin pathway. Subsequent overexpression of specific mutated genes (COX2 and K-*ras*) and additional mutations in the p53 gene and chromosome 18q deletions promote the development of carcinoma. The other 15% of tumors are characterized by microsatellite DNA instability. In these tumors, a normal cell is again converted to an early adenoma by mutation in the APC/beta-catenin pathway. Ultimately, these mutations result in the development of carcinoma.

Factors identified in promotion of metastasis.
The process of metastasis requires a number of biological and chemical alterations to the cancer cells.[8-11] This includes reduced expression of cellular adhesion molecules (cadherins) and increased degradation of the extracellular matrix components by metalloproteases and serine proteases, which allow the cells to detach from one another and move from the primary tumor mass. Finally, interactions among tumor cells and cells of the surrounding environment, mediated by cytokines and growth factors lead to the establishment of metastases.

OVERVIEW OF ROLES OF LABORATORY TESTS

Laboratory tests can serve four major functions in the field of **neoplasia:** detection or screening, **confirmation**, classification (**staging**), and monitoring.

Detection (Screening)

Table 49-3 lists several screening tests for early detection of cancer.[12] The quality of a screening test is usually expressed by its clinical sensitivity and specificity (see p. 372). The observations from the screening tests are divided into negative and positive results. Each person examined is classified as either a diseased or a nondiseased person.

A rigid classification of test results into positive and negative results may sometimes be too simplistic. Outcomes of screening tests can usually be ordered from very negative to very positive. The latter approach allows for a more sophisticated test interpretation in actual screening programs. For example, patients whose results are not negative but also are not alarming enough to justify immediate diagnostic

TABLE 49-3 SCREENING TEST FOR EARLY DETECTION OF CANCER

Site	Test
Bladder	Cytological analysis of urine
Breast	Mammography, physical examination, self-examination
Cervix	Papanicolaou smear, pelvic examination
Colon and rectum	Testing stool for occult blood, sigmoidoscopy
Hodgkin's disease	Physical examination and roentgenography
Lung	X-ray, cytological analysis of sputum
Oral cavity	Visual examination
Prostate	Prostate-specific antigen, digital palpation by rectum
Skin	Visual inspection
Stomach	Photofluorography, saline wash, and cytological examination of gastric contents, examination of stool for occult blood

From Habbema JDF, van Oortmarssen GJ, van der Maas, PJ. In Statland BE, Winkel P, editors: Laboratory measurements in malignant disease, *vol 2 Philadelphia, 1982, Saunders, Vashi AR, Oesterling JE: Mayo Clin Proc 72:337, 1997.*

action can be scheduled for earlier repeat screenings.[13] Another example is a stepwise screening policy in which only individuals with positive results at the first screening test are subject to further diagnostic testing.[14]

Sometimes the use of more than one screening test may seem advantageous. However, assessment of the sensitivity and specificity of a combination of screening tests based on data available for the individual tests is complicated by the fact that usually the tests are not independent in a statistical sense. In general, it is more effective to combine two tests that are complementary (i.e., directed at different anatomical or biochemical features of the tumor) than to combine tests directed at the same types of features. Examples of complementary tests include sputum cytological examination and chest x-ray examination for lung cancer screening.[15] On the other hand, palpation and mammography in breast cancer screening are examples of two related tests. They both detect tumors largely on the basis of size. One study[16] showed that when mammography was performed, the physical examination proved to be almost completely redundant.

Confirmation

Additional tests are used to confirm the suspicion of cancer based on clinical symptoms or signs. Tests that tend to confirm the presence of a cancer include, for example, bone marrow examination for leukemia, urinary catecholamines for pheochromocytoma, and alpha-fetoprotein for testicular cancer. The confirmatory results must be above a certain decision level.[17] For a laboratory test result to be confirmatory, it should possess 100% diagnostic specificity, that is, contain no false-positive results. For example, all cases in which the catecholamine level is above a certain value should be associated with pheochromocytoma.

Classification and Staging

Classification of tumors is used to describe the degree of tumor differentiation. Tumors are classified as *well differentiated*, *moderately well differentiated*, and *poorly differentiated*. Poorly differentiated tumors are more aggressive and have a poorer prognosis. Surgical pathologists have developed various staging approaches based on the size and extent of invasion of surrounding tissues by the tumor, the number of cancer cell-positive lymph nodes, and the presence or absence of metastases. This has been called the *TNM* (tumor, nodes, metastases) system.[18] The purpose of such staging is to give reasonable estimates of prognosis (i.e., recurrence of cancer), appropriate response to therapy, or the likely course of the disease. In addition to staging based on gross or microscopic pathological data, it would be of great value to have biochemical tests that could classify cancers appropriately. It has been suggested that an elevated serum prostatic acid phosphatase level can indicate the presence of metastatic prostate cancer.

Monitoring

The most important function of laboratory tests in cancer is that of monitoring the course of the disease or its response to

therapy. Winkel et al[19] have developed various strategies to monitor patients known to have breast cancer, addressing the problem of predicting on the basis of sequential values whether a patient would have recurrence of this disease. Other approaches were advanced in the mid-1980s to monitor patients on the basis of **carcinoembryonic antigen (CEA)** in colon cancer,[20] prostate-specific antigen (PSA) for prostate cancer,[21] and others. An increased CEA or PSA value may indicate a need to modify treatment. It is assumed that the CEA- or PSA-producing tumor has reached clinical proportions when the serum values for PSA or CEA reach a certain threshold.

All four major functions—screening, confirming, classifying, and monitoring—are possible roles for laboratory tests for neoplasia.

DEFINITION OF THE IDEAL TUMOR MARKER

Coombes and Neville[22] have suggested that the *ideal* **tumor marker** should fulfill the following criteria:

1. Be easy and inexpensive to measure in readily available body fluids
2. Be specific to the tumor studied and commonly associated with it
3. Have a stoichiometric relationship between plasma level of the marker and tumor mass
4. Have an abnormal plasma level, urine level, or both, in the presence of micrometastases, that is, at a stage at which no clinical or presently available diagnostic methods reveal their presence
5. Have plasma levels, urine levels, or both, that are stable and not subject to wild fluctuations
6. If present in the plasma of healthy individuals, exist at a much lower concentration than that found in association with all stages of cancer

Obviously, much additional research must be done before such ideal tumor markers can be found. However, it is important to recognize that the evaluation of an ideal tumor marker should relate to the clinical setting. To this end, it has been suggested that all tumor markers should also comply with the following major criteria[23]:

1. They should prognosticate a higher or lower risk for eventual development of recurrence.
2. They should change as the current status of the tumor changes over time.
3. They should precede and predict recurrences before they are clinically detectable.

In addition, if a tumor marker is to be used to detect very early stages of cancer, a treatment for that cancer must be available. It might be unethical to detect cancers for which no effective treatment is available (see below).

All tumor markers should be analyzed both according to the criteria that Coombes and Neville have presented and according to the considerations just mentioned. For a tumor marker to be of some value, it must give information beyond that readily seen on the basis of physical examination or history, and it must give this information with a reasonably long lead time to allow appropriate therapy to be given in a timely manner. Lead time is the time elapsed between the point when a test result is positive and the time when the disease is clinically evident or advanced.

ETHICS OF TESTING

Even when a tumor marker can be used to detect the presence of disease, it may not always be beneficial to use it. Prostate cancer, for example, is present in about 40% of males 50 to 70 years of age, but only about 4% of these men will die from this disease itself. The reason is that prostate cancer is usually slow-growing and in most cases it is more likely that a patient will die from some other cause, rather than from the prostate cancer. The standard treatments for early prostate cancer (brachytherapy, external radiation, and surgical intervention, all with or without chemotherapy) can result in unwanted side effects, including impotence, incontinence, and the need for colostomy. In addition, a significant number of patients can die from the treatments themselves.

Thus the ethical question arises: should any tumor marker whose use does not decrease the morbidity and mortality associated with a type of cancer be used for routine clinical care? Should PSA be used to detect prostate cancer when the therapy may result in unnecessary morbidity and its effect on the longevity of patients is unproved? See below for a more detailed discussion of PSA screening.

CHANGE OF ANALYTE IN DISEASE
Classes of Biochemicals Used as Tumor Markers
(Table 49-4)

This section is a review of several biochemical tests that have been used either as primary tumor markers or as secondary tests to note invasion or dissemination of cancer. The types of analytes are listed in the box at right and are discussed in

terms of their clinical usefulness and applications. The goal of this chapter is to provide a discussion of assays that are commonly in use or have potential value. The Food and Drug Administration (FDA) regulates which tumor markers can be used. The current FDA-approved list of protein tumor markers includes CEA, AFP, PSA, PAP, CA-125, CA-15-3 and CA-27-29; the only tumor marker currently approved for screening of the general population is PSA. As large clinical trials are completed, other such markers will be approved. Reviews that cover some of these assays in greater depth are recommended for further reading (see, for example, references 23, 24 and 25).

Oncofetal Antigens

Many of the oncofetal antigens are measured in the laboratory by use of solid-phase immunometric assays, employing second antibodies labeled with enzymes, fluorescent, or chemiluminescent compounds. These proteins are *not* recommended for cancer screening.

The tumor markers discussed previously are antigenic proteins with several distinct antigenic sites. Immunoassay characteristics for these markers are based on antibody affinity and antibody specificity, and the specificity of the assay depends on the recognition of one or more of the antigenic determinants. Obviously, antibodies from different reagent vendors will react differently with the antigen. Since these antigens are glycoproteins and the carbohydrate portion of the molecule may differ from patient to patient, antibodies from different vendors may also react differently

---

TABLE 49-4   CLASSES OF BIOCHEMICALS USED AS TUMOR MARKERS

Class of Biochemical	Examples	Use
Increased production of endogenous biochemicals	Hormones, enzymes, polyamines, and so on	Confirmation, diagnosis, monitoring
Synthesis of biochemicals of previously quiescent genes	Oncofetal proteins, cell surface antigens, enzymes	Monitoring, prognosis
Receptors	Estriol receptor (breast cancer), androgen receptor (prostate cancer)	Prognosis, treatment
Modification of usual cell or organ function	Gamma-glutamyl transferase (GGT) or 5'-nucleotidase	Diagnosis

---

EXAMPLES OF TUMOR MARKERS

Oncofetal Proteins
Carcinoembryonic antigen (CEA)
Alpha-fetoprotein (AFP)
Human chorionic gonadotropin (hCG)
SCC (squamous cell carcinoma) antigen

Mucin Glycoproteins (Carbohydrate Antigen)
CA-125
CA-19-9
CA-15-3 and CA-27-29

Enzymes
Prostate-specific antigen (PSA)

Hormones and Hormone Receptors
ACTH and all other endocrine hormones
Breast estrogen and progesterone receptors

Cell Surface Proteins (Other Than Receptors)
Beta$_2$-microglobulin

Cellular Markers
Oncogenes, such as N-ras
Suppressor genes, such as p53
BRCA1 and BRCA2
c-erB-2 (HER-2)/neu

from one patient to the next. Therefore, when patients are being monitored, the assay used should be from the same manufacturer during the monitoring period. Otherwise, analytically significant changes may occur during serial monitoring as a result of a change in the source of the tumor marker reagent. If it is necessary to change the vendor source, individual patient parallel studies should be performed in which at least two specimens are analyzed by both methods so that the physician can compare individual patient results.

Carcinoembryonic antigen. CEA is a glycoprotein present in colonic adenocarcinoma and fetal gut; it was first described by Gold and Freedman.[26] The detection of CEA in various tissues or serum is complicated by the presence in these tissues of CEA cross-reacting antigens.

In general, CEA plasma levels increase with increasing age and smoking. This has prevented the use of CEA levels for the purpose of general screening.[27] The results of screening programs confined to subpopulations with higher-than-average risk of developing cancer have been equally discouraging.[28] Thus, neither the sensitivity nor the specificity of CEA justifies its use for the definitive diagnosis of cancer.[29]

In specific situations, however, CEA has proved to be of diagnostic value. CEA is useful, for example, for the detection of primary colorectal cancer[30] when used in combination with a barium enema and with radioiodide imaging for the detection of carcinoma metastatic to the liver. According to the consensus statement of the National Cancer Institute,[29] only values five to ten times the upper normal reference limit in patients with symptoms should be considered strongly suggestive of the presence of cancer. In some cancers, including colorectal and breast cancer, the plasma level of CEA and the frequency of elevated values are positively correlated with the severity of the disease as assessed by clinical staging. Currently, CEA is approved only for monitoring of colorectal cancer.

Postoperative monitoring of plasma CEA levels for the detection of recurrence or metastases has proved valuable in colorectal cancer.[31] Evidence suggests that patients with initial low CEA values who develop hepatic metastases as seen by a rising CEA can be cured by surgery (32). However, there is little evidence available to indicate that monitoring all patients diagnosed with colorectal cancer leads to improved patient outcome or quality of life.[32]

CEA is not approved for breast cancer because postoperative CEA levels are less frequently elevated in patients with breast cancer who eventually develop overt metastatic disease than in corresponding patients who undergo surgery for colorectal cancer. In only 10% to 15% of patients with breast cancer does the plasma CEA level rise to values above 10 mg/L.[33]

Alpha-fetoprotein and human chorionic gonadotropin. Alpha-fetoprotein (AFP) is an oncofetal glycoprotein. In early embryonic life it is a predominant component of the serum proteins. It is first synthesized by the yolk sac and later by the fetal liver. Later in life it is mainly produced in the liver. AFP was first recognized as a tumor marker by Abele in 1963.[34]

Serum AFP values should be less than $10\,\mu g/L$ in healthy subjects. In benign hepatic disorders, moderate elevations $(40\,\mu g/L)$ may be seen. Values above $400\,\mu g/L$ are almost always associated with hepatocellular carcinoma, germ cell carcinoma (such as testicular carcinoma), chronic aggressive hepatitis, or subacute hepatic necrosis. Currently, AFP is approved only for use with testicular carcinoma and hepatocellular carcinoma.

Human chorionic gonadotropin (hCG) is a glycoprotein hormone[35] that can be secreted in large amounts by the trophoblastic tissue of tumors of the placenta and the testes. Specific and sensitive assays have revealed that many other cancers can also secrete hCG. However, available data[36] clearly show that hCG determinations are of no value in screening for cancer.

The main clinical use of AFP and hCG is related to the diagnosis, therapy, and follow-up study of germ cell tumors.[37] Table 49-5 presents the World Health Organization (WHO) classification of germ cell tumors and associated markers in tissue and serum. In general, AFP and hCG provide the most information about tumor status when they are persistently elevated. The absence of a marker does not preclude the presence of germ cell tumors.

TABLE 49-5 WHO CLASSIFICATION OF GERM CELL TUMORS AND ASSOCIATED TUMOR MARKERS

| | IMMUNOHISTOCHEMISTRY | | SEROLOGY | | |
WHO Classification	AFP	hCG	AFP	hCG	Comments
Seminoma (S)	−	±	No	± Yes	hCG in giant cells
Embryonal carcinoma (EC)	+	+	± Yes	± Yes	hCG in giant cells AFP controversial, may occur in undiagnosed yolk sac elements
Yolk sac tumor (YST)	+	−	± Yes	No	
Choriocarcinoma (CC)	−	+	No		
Teratoma (TT)	−	−	No?	No?	

From Norgaard-Pedersen B, Hangaard J. In Statland BE, Winkel P, editors: Laboratory measurements in malignant disease, *Philadelphia, 1982, Saunders.*
AFP, alpha-fetoprotein; hCG, human chorionic gonadotropin.

Carbohydrate antigen–19-9. Carbohydrate antigen–19-9 (CA-19-9) occurs in tissue as a monosialoganglioside and in serum as mucin, a high–molecular-weight, carbohydrate-rich glycoprotein. Results of clinical studies indicate that the CA-19-9 level in serum or plasma of patients with an intra-abdominal carcinoma frequently is increased. It is correlated most strikingly with cancer of the pancreas, for which early studies have shown a sensitivity of 90% and a specificity of 85%. CA-19-9 also may be increased with other adeno-carcinomas such as lung, gastric, biliary, and colonic.

Carbohydrate antigen–125. Serum carbohydrate antigen–125 (CA-125), a glycoprotein antigen, is elevated in the serum of patients with ovarian cancer. Increased concentrations of CA-125 were found in many patients with epithelial ovarian cancer and in ovarian teratoma. Changes in CA-125 concentrations in serum during chemotherapy mirrored the progress of the disease as assessed by clinical and radiological evidence. It should be noted that CA-125 provides no real assistance for diagnosis; however, it does have value as a marker for monitoring responsiveness to chemotherapy.

Carbohydrate antigen–15-3 and 27-29. Serum carbo-hydrate antigen–15-3 (CA-15-3), a glycoprotein antigen, is elevated in the serum of patients with breast cancer. Changes in CA-15-3 concentrations in serum after surgery or during chemotherapy mirrored the progress of the disease as assessed by clinical and radiological evidence. Just as with the CA-125 antigen, CA-15-3 provides no actual diagnostic assistance, but it does have possible value as a marker for monitoring responsiveness to chemotherapy. It should also be noted that a third of breast cancer patients with metastatic disease have CA-15-3 levels within the reference range. The CA-27-29 antigen is detected by an antibody specific for the protein core of the same antigen detected by the antibody to CA-15-3.[38] Recent comparisons between CA-27-29 and CA-15-3 suggest that CA-27-29 discriminates primary breast cancer patients from healthy subjects more accurately than does CA-15-3.

Enzymes

Schwartz[39] reviewed the use of enzyme tests in the management of patients with cancer. As with many putative tumor markers discussed in this chapter, the use of enzyme markers is fraught with difficulties. Not all patients with a particular cancer type have elevations in an enzyme (poor sensitivity); furthermore, many noncancerous diseases are associated with elevations of many of these enzymes. Thus the most frequent uses of these enzymes are as objective markers to give semiquantitative estimates of response to therapy or as prognostic indicators. However, enzyme markers have generally been replaced by the oncofetal markers and are rarely used today. An exception to this is PSA, which is an extracellular protease.

Prostate-specific antigen (PSA) exists in serum in several molecular forms, including a free or noncomplexed form, and complexes of PSA with serine protease inhibitors alpha$_1$-antichymotrypsin (ACT) and alpha$_2$-macroglobulin (which

is not detectable with current assays).[40] Total PSA is a combination of all immunodetectable forms in serum, primarily free PSA and PSA-ACT. The complexed form is the predominant form found in serum. Stenman et al in 1991 demonstrated that complexed PSA is higher in patients with prostate cancer than in patients with BPH.[41] Christensson et al[42] has shown that the percent free PSA is lower in patients with cancer and is a more accurate means of discriminating between benign and malignant prostate disease.

In 1997 Vashi and Oesterling[40] showed that percent free PSA improved the clinical sensitivity of the total PSA measurement in the range of 2.5 to 4.0 ng/mL total PSA and that the specificity of the total PSA test was improved in the range of 4.1 to 10 ng/mL. They recommended that a prostate biopsy was needed when the total PSA was in the 4.1 to 10.0 ng/mL range only when the free PSA was less than 24%. They further recommended a cutoff of less than 19% as a biopsy indicator if the total PSA was in the 3.0 to 4.0 ng/mL range. Other calculations, including PSA density (coupled with transrectal ultrasound measurement of prostate volume) and PSA velocity (rate of increase for multiple measurements), as well as age-specific reference ranges, have been suggested as possible approaches to improve PSA specificity.

PSA is also used to monitor response to therapy in treated patients. Serum PSA should fall to undetectable limits within 1 to 3 months in patients with prostate cancer restricted to the prostate gland who have undergone prostatectomy. In patients treated with internal or external radiation, PSA may take several years to reach a baseline level, which may not approach undetectable limits. A continuous rise in PSA level after treatment indicates local recurrence or distance meta-stasis; since the cancer is generally so slow-growing, the rise may not occur for several years. A recent review of clinical trials[43] suggests that the Gleason score (the histopathological grade by which prostate adenocarcinoma is classified) is a better indicator of disease recurrence than is pretreatment PSA.[43]

Both the American Cancer Society and the American Urologic Association recommend that PSA be used in combination with a digital rectal examination to screen for prostate cancer. These groups recommend screening for all men between the ages of 50 and 75 who have a life expec-tancy of 10 years or more and for other men at high risk. This high-risk group includes all African-American men, as well as all men over the age of 40 who have had two relatives diagnosed with prostate cancer. However, the American College of Preventive Medicine recommends that PSA not be used as a screen for the diagnosis of prostate cancer, but rather that men in the groups described by the American Cancer Society be given relevant information about PSA so that they can make their own decisions about screening.

The utility of any screening for prostate cancer is thus controversial, since the proper treatment for this disease, when it is detected early, has not been determined. Although some clinicians believe that "watchful waiting" is sufficient for some prostate cancers, others call for immediate, curative intervention, especially for small, early prostate cancers in men with a life expectancy of more than 10 years. Since prostate cancer is generally slow-growing, and since the PSA test itself has been widely available for only about 10 years, ongoing clinical trials have not been of sufficient duration (10 to 20 years) to provide conclusive data that screening actually improves patient outcome. This ethical question will be resolved through ongoing clinical trials.[44]

Collagen-Breakdown Products

In patients with bone metastases of an osteolytic nature, there is an increase in urinary excretion of both hydroxyproline and hydroxylysine. In fact, hydroxyproline excretion in urine is often the first sign of bony metastases in certain malignancies.

Cellular Markers

Several markers associated with the plasma membrane, cytoplasm, or nuclei of the lymphoid cell have been identified. Various techniques, which tend to be immunological in nature, have been used to detect cellular markers; these techniques include cell rosetting, immunofluorescence, and immunoenzymatic testing. The rosetting technique is based on a reaction between an indicator cell (usually an erythrocyte) and the lymphoid cell to form rosettes in cases in which the lymphoid cell carries a particular membrane marker. By such techniques, the cells may be mixed directly or the indicator cell may first be coded with antibody or complement to demonstrate receptors for the Fc part of immunoglobulin or complement components. The use of flow cytometry in combination with immunofluorescence has proved to be a powerful technique for detecting cell markers.

It appears that the various antigens demonstrated by these techniques are not tumor-specific antigens but rather are tumor-associated differentiation antigens, which represent the expression of oncofetal antigens that are not normally expressed by differentiated cells.

Lymphocytic leukemias and non-Hodgkin lymphomas have been subdivided into clinical subgroups on the basis of biochemical cell markers. The most striking evidence of the value of typing lymphocytes with a panel of markers comes from studies of acute lymphocytic leukemia (ALL). Table 49-6 gives the five prognostically distinct groups of ALL and the relevant markers for each. The groups are ordered according to prognosis. Cells of the B cell type are characterized by the presence of surface membrane immunoglobulin (SmIg), as are normal mature B cells. The cells of the T cell type are characterized by the presence of sheep erythrocyte receptors and human thymocyte antigen, as are mature T cells. The cells of the pre-B cell type are characterized by a cytoplasmic IgM heavy chain but no SmIg, which corresponds to the characteristics of an early stage during the B cell differentiation.

The terminal deoxynucleotidyltransferase and the common ALL antigen are of value not only for classification of ALL (Table 49-6), but also in distinguishing between acute lymphoblastic and myeloblastic leukemia. ALL may be

TABLE 49-6 PHENOTYPIC HETEROGENEITY OF ALL

ALL	E	HTA	SmIg	Cyμ	CALLA	HLA-DR	TdT
Common ALL	–	–	–	–	+	+	+
Pre-B ALL	–	–	–	+	+	+	+
Null-ALL	–	–	–	–	–	+	+
T-ALL	+	+	–	–	–	–	+
B-ALL	–	–	+	–	–	+	–

From Plesner T, Wilken M, Avenstrøm S. In Statland BE, Winkel P, editors: Laboratory measurements in malignant disease, Philadelphia, 1982, Saunders. ALL, Acute lymphocytic leukemia; B-ALL, B cell type of acute lymphoblastic leukemia; CALLA, common ALL antigen; Cyμ, cytoplasmic IgM heavy chain; E, sheep erythrocyte receptor; HLA-DR, human Ia-like antigen; HTA, human thymocyte antigen or antigens; SmIg, surface membrane immunoglobin; T-ALL, T cell type of acute lymphoblastic leukemia; TdT, terminal deoxynucleotidyltransferase.

classified into B cell leukemia (95%), which is characterized by low-density monoclonal surface membrane immunoglobulins (usually IgM or IgM and IgD with one light chain) and the more rare, but also more aggressive, T-ALL (5%). The cells of the last type form E rosettes and have T antigens but lack SmIg.

Steroid Receptor Analysis

Both estrogen and progesterone receptor assays are useful in the assessment of the prognosis of patients with breast cancer.[45] These procedures evaluate the relative concentration of receptors for estrogen and progesterones in breast tumor excised during surgery. Individuals who are positive both for estrogen and progesterone receptors tend to have a longer survival time and thus a better prognosis than individuals who are deficient in these receptors. The estrogen receptor appears to be the most important of the two factors. The presence or absence of steroid receptors can help determine the type of therapy. For those women devoid of receptors, a more aggressive therapy may be used, whereas women with the estrogen receptors can be treated with anti-estrogen therapy with great success.

Hemostasis-Related Factors

Plasma fibrinogen levels are generally elevated in patients with cancer. However, in patients with disseminated intravascular coagulation (DIC), hypofibrinogenemia has also been noted. As expected, DIC is also associated with decreased values for antithrombin III (AT III). Consequently, in patients with DIC associated with cancer, AT III values will be decreased.

Increased fibrinolytic or fibrinogenolytic activity has been reported in patients with cancer. Consequently the fibrinogen-degradation products (FDP) are often elevated in the plasma or urine in patients with cancer. It is noteworthy that plasminogen activators are often elevated in patients with cancer.

Other Markers

Several other markers are currently being used on an investigational basis for cancers of various organ sites. For colorectal cancer, they include cyclin D1, Bcl-2, cytokeratin-19, pyruvate kinase type tumor M2, and CA-72-4.[46-48] Potential new markers for bladder cancer include nuclear matrix protein 22 (NMP22) and bladder tumor antigen (BTA).[49] New breast cancer markers include tissue polypeptide–specific (TPS) antigen[50] and histological demonstration of c-erB-2 (HER-2)/neu gene amplification.[51]

Genetic Screening for Breast Cancer

A number of epidemiological studies have documented that a positive family history of breast cancer is a positive predictor of increased risk for this disease. See reference 52 for a detailed complete review of this subject. At least eight genes have been identified that may contribute to an inherited susceptibility to breast and ovarian cancer, the most important of which are BRCA1 and BRCA2. Approximately 5% of breast and ovarian cancers can be attributed to families with mutations in the BRCA1 gene; this gene has been linked to the 17q21 locus and is thought to be a tumor suppressor gene. It may also be associated with increased risk for ovarian, colon, and prostate cancers. Although numerous mutations in this gene are associated with breast cancer, one specific mutation has a very high frequency among Ashkenazi Jewish women, and may account for 16% of breast cancers and 39% of ovarian cancers diagnosed in this population before the age of 50.

Approximately 3% of breast and ovarian cancers have been attributed to families with mutations in the BRCA2 gene; this gene has been linked to the 13q12-13 locus and is also associated with increased risk for pancreatic cancer and male breast cancer. As with BRCA1, one specific mutation of the BRCA2 gene accounts for a significant number of breast and ovarian cancers in Ashkenazi women, and another specific mutation accounts for a significant number of breast and ovarian cancers in Icelandic women.

DNA testing to identify individuals and families who carry these mutations is available. Although this testing is not recommended for asymptomatic individuals in the general population, it may be used, with appropriate genetic counseling, for members of high-risk families with well-defined syndromes.

CONCLUSIONS

The scope of the tumor marker problem is too large to be covered in one chapter in a textbook of clinical chemistry. More important than merely enumerating all the assays available is emphasizing that the challenge for any candidate tumor marker is that it be clinically useful in the management of patients with the disease or suspected of having the disease and that its use contributes to the improvement of the patient's disease. Although clinical trials are under way to test old and new tumor markers, there is still no clear evidence (with a few exceptions) that the use of any of these markers improves patient quality of life or patient outcome. Indeed, considering the significant morbidity associated with treatment of prostate cancer, it has been suggested that the use of tumor markers to screen the general population for prostate cancer is not warranted. There may, on the other hand, be psychological benefits to cancer patients monitored with tumor markers. The patient whose tumor marker value goes to baseline levels and then does not increase can realistically expect a cure or a lengthy remission. The patient whose tumor marker value is initially high and does not go to baseline levels or begins to rise after dropping to baseline, may be better able to cope with the expected outcome. It is hoped that with completion of ongoing clinical trials, current markers will be shown to benefit cancer patients and additional markers that prove to be of clinical use will be made available.

References

1. Sager R: Explorations on the origin of cancer, *Focus* 2/3:1, 1983.
2. Aaronson SA: Growth factors and cancer, *Science* 254:1146, 1991.
3. Cantley LC et al: Oncogenes and signal transduction, *Cell* 64:281, 1991.
4. Niman HL: Detection of oncogene-related proteins with site-directed monoclonal antibody probes, *J Clin Lab Anal* 1:28, 1987.
5. Liekens S, DeClercq E, Neyts J: Angiogenesis: regulators and clinical applications, *Biochem Pharmacol* 61:253, 2001.
6. Breier G: Functions of the VEGF/VEGF receptor system in the vascular system, *Semin Thromb Hemost* 26:553, 2000.
7. Chung DA: The genetic basis of colorectal cancer: insights into critical pathways of tumorigenesis, *Gastroenterology* 119: 854, 2000.
8. Liotta LA, Kohn EC, Invasions and metastasis. In Holland, JF et al: editors: *Cancer medicine*, Baltimore, 1997, Williams & Wilkins.
9. Liu W et al: Endothelial cell survival and apoptosis in the tumor vasculature, *Apoptosis* 5:323, 2000.
10. Pasche B: Role of transforming growth factor beta in cancer, *J Cell Physiol* 186:153, 2001.
11. Kurschat P, Mauch C: Mechanisms of metastasis, *Clin Exp Dermatol* 25:482, 2000.
12. Habbema JDF, van Oortmarssen GJ: Performance characteristics of screening tests. In Statland BE, Winkel P, editors: *Laboratory measurements in malignant disease*, vol 2, Philadelphia, 1982, Saunders.
13. EVAC: *Rapport eerste screeningsronde*, Leidschendam, 1980, Ministerie van Volksgezondheid en Milieuhygiene.
14. Tabar L, Gad A: Screening for breast cancer: the Swedish trial, *Radiology* 138:219, 1981.
15. Woolner LB et al: Mayo Lung Project: evaluation of lung cancer screening through December 1979, *Mayo Clin Proc* 56:544, 1981.
16. Shapiro S: Evidence on screening for breast cancer from a randomized trial, *Cancer* 39:2772, 1977.
17. Statland BE: *Clinical decision levels for lab tests*, Oradell, NJ, 1983, Medical Economics Co.
18. Rubin P: *Clinical oncology for medical students and physicians*, ed 5, New York, 1978, American Cancer Society.
19. Winkel P et al: Predicting recurrence in patients with breast cancer from cumulative laboratory results: a new technique for the application of time series analysis, *Clin Chem* 28:2057, 1982.
20. Ravry M et al: Usefulness of serial serum carcinoembryonic antigen (CEA) determinations during anticancer therapy or long-term follow-up of gastrointestinal carcinoma, *Cancer* 34:1230, 1974.
21. Chan DW: PSA as a marker for prostatic cancer, *Clin Chem* 33:1916, 1987.
22. Coombes RC, Neville AM: Significance of tumor-index substances in management. In Stoll BA, editor: *Secondary spread in breast cancer*, Chicago, 1978, William Heinemann Medical Books.

23. Rej R et al: Clinical laboratory testing in cancer patient diagnosis and management, *Clin Chem* 39:2359, 1993.

24. Sell S, editor: *Serological cancer markers*, Totowa, NJ, 1992, Humana Press.

25. Bidart J-M et al: Kinetics of serum tumor marker concentrations and usefulness in clinical monitoring, *Clin Chem* 45:1695, 1999.

26. Gold P, Freedman SO: Demonstration of tumor-specific antigens in human colonic carcinomata by immunological tolerance and absorption techniques, *J Exp Med* 121:439, 1965.

27. *CEA as a cancer marker*, vol 3, no 7, Bethesda, MD, 1981, National Institutes of Health, Consensus Development Conference Summary.

28. Holyoke ED, Chu TM, Murphy GP: CEA as a monitor of gastro-intestinal malignancy, *Cancer* 35:830, 1975.

29. Costanza ME et al: Proceedings: carcinoembryonic antigen: report of a screening study, *Cancer* 33:583, 1974.

30. McCartney WH, Hoffer PB: The value of carcinoembryonic antigen (CEA) as an adjunct to the radiological colon examination in the diagnosis of malignancy, *Radiology* 110:325, 1974.

31. Wanebo HJ et al: Preoperative carcinoembryonic antigen level as a prognostic indicator in colorectal cancer, *N Engl J Med* 299:448, 1978.

32. Duffy MJ: Carcinoembryonic antigen as a marker for colorectal cancer: is it clinically useful? *Clin Chem* 47: 624, 2001.

33. Statland BE, Winkel P: Usefulness of clinical chemistry measurements in classifying patients with breast cancer, *CRC Crit Rev Clin Lab Sci* 26:255, 1982.

34. Sell S, Becker FF: Alpha-fetoprotein, *J Natl Cancer Inst* 60:19, 1978.

35. Vaitukaitis JL: Secretion of human chorionic gonadotropin by tumors. In *Carcino-embryonic proteins*, vol 1, New York, 1979, Elsevier/North Holland, pp 447-455.

36. Braunstein GD: Human chorionic gonadotropin in nontrophoblastic tumors and tissues. In Talwar GP, editor: *Recent advances in reproduction and regulation of fertility*, Amsterdam, 1979, Elsevier/North Holland Biomedical Press.

37. Anderson CK, Jones WG, Ward A: *Germ cell tumors*, London, 1981, Taylor and Francis.

38. Gion M et al: Comparison of the diagnostic accuracy of CA27.29 and CA15.3 in primary breast cancer, *Clin Chem* 45:630, 1999.

39. Schwartz MK: Enzyme tests in cancer. In Statland BE, Winkel P, editors: *Laboratory measurements in malignant disease*, Philadelphia, 1982, Saunders.

40. Vashi AR, Oesterling JE: Percent free prostate-specific antigen: entering a new era in the detection of prostate cancer, *Mayo Clin Proc* 72:337, 1997.

41. Stenman U-H et al: A complex between prostate-specific antigen and alpha$_1$-antichymotrypsin is the major form of prostate-specific antigen in serum of patients with prostate cancer: assay of the complex improves clinical sensitivity for cancer, *Cancer Res* 51:222, 1991.

42. Christensson A et al: Serum prostate-specific antigen complexed to alpha$_1$-antichymotrypsin as an indicator of prostate cancer, *J Urol* 150:100, 1993.

43. Stamey TA: Preoperative serum prostate-specific antigen (PSA) below 10 µg/L predicts neither the presence of prostate cancer nor the rate of postoperative PSA failure, *Clin Chem* 47:631, 2001.

44. Carter HB et al: Longitudinal evaluation of prostate-specific antigen levels in men with and without prostate disease, *JAMA* 267:2215, 1992.

45. Pertschuk LP et al: Immunohistologic localization of estrogen receptors in breast cancer with monoclonal antibodies, *Cancer* 55:1513, 1985.

46. Bhatavdekar PM et al: Molecular markers are predictors of recurrence and survival in patients with Dukes B and Dukes C colorectal adenocarcinoma, *Dis Colon Rectum* 44:523, 2001.

47. Holubec L, Jr, et al: The significance of CEA, CA 19-9 and CA 72-4 in the detection of colorectal carcinoma recurrence, *Anticancer Res* 20:5237, 2000.

48. Hardt PD et al: Tumor M2-pyruvate kinase: a promising tumor marker in the diagnosis of gastro-intestinal cancer: *Anticancer Res* 20:4965, 2000.

49. Oge O et al: Comparison of BTA stat and NMP22 tests in the detection of bladder cancer, *Scand J Urol Nephrol* 34:349, 2000.

50. Einarsson R, Lindman H, Bergh J: Use of TPS and CA 15-3 assays for monitoring chemotherapy in metastatic breast cancer patients, *Anticancer Res* 20:5089, 2000.

51. Mark HF et al: HER-2/neu gene amplification in stages I-IV breast cancer detected by fluorescent in situ hybridization, *Genet Med* 1:98, 1999.

52. Greene MH: Genetics of Breast Cancer, *Mayo Clin Proc* 72:54, 1997.

Internet Sites

http://www.cancer.org/—American Cancer Society

http://www.cancer.gov/—National Cancer Institute

http://www.cancer.gov/cancer_information/—CancerNet (current, comprehensive cancer information)

http://www.cancer.gov/clinical_trials/—Cancer Trials

http://cis.nci.nih.gov/—Cancer Information Service

http://medlib.med.utah.edu/WebPath/NEOHTML/NEOPLIDX.html—The Internet Pathology Laboratory for Medical Education, Florida State University College of Medicine

http://edcenter.med.cornell.edu/CUMC_PathNotes/Neoplasia/Neoplasia.html—Cornell University Medical College

http://www.tmc.tulane.edu/classware/pathology/medical_pathology/New_for_98/Neoplasia_new/5t_Answered/Neoplasia_Cases.html#Case1

http://medlib.med.utah.edu/WebPath/EXAM/MULTGEN/NEOFRM.html

http://www.merck.com/pubs/mmanual_home/sec13/149.htm

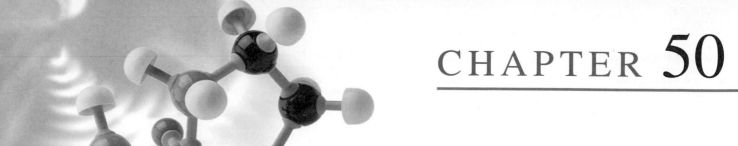

CHAPTER 50

Laboratory Evaluation of the Transplant Recipient and Donor

• Rita R. Alloway

Chapter Outline

Objectives

- Outline the laboratory testing performed before transplantation in potential living related and cadaver kidney donors, liver donors, heart donors, and pancreas donors and in potential transplant recipients.
- Define the different types of rejection seen in transplant patients with regard to timing, organ involvement, and diagnosis.

- List the most important components of the laboratory evaluation of the following transplant types: kidney, pancreas, liver, heart.
- List the immunosuppressive agents that are assessed by therapeutic drug monitoring.
- Define the pretransplant immunological assays used to predict the compatibility of a donor with a potential recipient.

Key Terms

allograft   Refers to organs or cells from another person, which may or may not have the same histocompatibility antigens as the recipient.

antibody   A class of serum proteins induced after contact with antigen. An antibody binds specifically to the antigen that induced its formation. Most antibodies are present in the γ-globulin fraction of serum.

antigen   Any molecule that can be recognized by the immune system. In general, immunoglobulins recognize and bind to intact antigens.

azathioprine and **6-mercaptopurine**   Purine analogs that act on small lymphocytes and dividing cells, thereby blocking development of organ-rejecting T-cells.

B-cells   Lymphocytes that develop in the fetal liver and subsequently in the bone marrow. They respond to antigenic stimuli by dividing and differentiating into plasma cells under the control of cytokines released by T-cells.

CD markers   System of nomenclature used for leukocyte surface molecules as identified by monoclonal antibodies. More than 80 individual molecules are recognized by this series, and some of them are found on cells other than leukocytes.

corticosteroids   Agents that have numerous immunosuppressive and antiinflammatory effects. They interfere with antigen presentation, inhibit the primary antibody response, and reduce the number of circulating T-cells.

cyclophosphamide   A drug that prevents DNA replication by covalently adding to the DNA through an alkylation reaction. It acts primarily on lymphocytes and strongly inhibits antibody responses.

cyclosporine   Cyclosporine binds to an immunophilin, cyclophilin, and this complex binds to the calcium-dependent calcineurin, which results in the inhibition of transcription of cytokines inhibiting early stage T-cell activation.

cytokines   Substances released by leukocytes and other cells that control the development of the immune response. Often termed the *hormones of the immune system*, they modulate the differentiation and division of hematopoietic stem cells and activation of lymphocytes and phagocytes.

cytotoxicity   A general term for the ways in which lymphocytes, mononuclear phagocytes, and granulocytes can kill target cells.

histocompatibility complex   The complex of glycoproteins on the surface of cells that is used by the immune system to define self and nonself.

human leukocyte antigen (HLA)   The major histocompatibility complex. It is divided into seven main groups: A, B, C, Class III, DR, DQ, and DP.

immunosuppression   Measures used to reduce immune responses after transplantation to prevent graft rejection. Most are not specific for the transplant antigens.

interleukin-2 (IL-2)   A cytokine that is an essential T-cell growth factor required for division of antigen-activated T-cells.

interleukin-2 receptor antibodies   Basiliximab (a chimeric mouse-human IL-2 receptor antibody) and Daclizumab (a humanized-mouse IL-2 receptor antibody) bind to the CD25 α-chain subunit of the IL-2 receptor on activated T-cells. This renders T-cells unable to bind with IL-2 and thus unable to proliferate in response to this cytokine.

major histocompatibility complex (MHC)   A large group of genes including those encoding the class I and II MHC molecules that are involved in presentation of antigen to T-cells.

mycophenolate mofetil (MMF)   An ester prodrug of mycophenolic acid (MPA), which upon absorption is rapidly hydrolyzed to the active form, MPA. MPA reversibly binds and inhibits inosine monophosphate dehydrogenase (IMPDH), an enzyme essential for *de novo* purine synthesis, thus inhibiting DNA and RNA synthesis and subsequent synthesis of T-cells and B-cells.

OKT3   A murine monoclonal antibody directed against the CD3 receptor on human T-cells. It is used to prevent and treat acute rejection after transplantation.

polyclonal antilymphocyte agents   Immuno-suppressive antibodies made by injecting human lymphoid material (spleen, thymus, lymph node) into an animal (horse, goat, sheep, rabbit) that makes an antibody response against the human tissue. The animal immune globulin is purified and used to prevent or treat rejection in human transplant patients.

rejection   A reaction induced by recipient T-cells that recognize allogeneic MHC molecules. The T-cells can activate graft-infiltrating mononuclear cells, damaging the graft.

sirolimus (Rapamycin, Rapamune)   Sirolimus binds to a specific immunophilin FKBP similar to tacrolimus, but does not exert its immunosuppressive effects by calcineurin inhibition. Sirolimus binds to the enzyme, target of rapamycin (mTOR), and inhibits translation of several cytokines essential for T-cell regulation and proliferation.

T-cells   Lymphocytes that develop in the thymus and whose role is to recognize antigens originating from within cells of the host as self and foreign antigen as nonself.

tacrolimus (FK506)   Tacrolimus binds to an immunophilin FKBP and this complex binds to the calcium-dependent calcineurin, which results in the inhibition of transcription of cytokines inhibiting early stage T-cell activation.

tissue typing   The technique used to determine the major histocompatibility specificities carried on an individual's cells.

tolerance   The acquisition of nonresponsiveness to a molecule that is normally recognized by the immune system.

Solid-organ transplantation has become the therapy of choice for end-stage diseases of the kidney, liver, and heart. Advances in surgical techniques and diagnostic capabilities, progress in immunology and histocompatibility analysis, development of more specific and potent immunosuppressive agents, improvements in donor management and organ preservation, and new antimicrobial agents have all contributed to the success of transplanting solid organs. Reflecting these improvements, the total number of each type of transplants continues to rise in the United States (Table 50-1).

The term *graft* is used to describe a transplanted organ. *Allografts* refer to tissue that is taken from one individual and used for a second individual. An allograft from a relative is termed a *living related donor graft* (LRD). Allografts from individuals who have been declared legally dead ("brain dead") are termed *cadaver allografts*. Transplants are high-risk medical procedures.

The major factor limiting transplantation is the shortage of organs. By the end of 1999, the waiting list for solid-organ transplants in the United States exceeded 72,000. This represented a continued rise in the demand for transplants, despite the plateau of cadaveric donors. In cases of heart and liver disease, failure to receive a timely transplant results in death. The overall percentage of registrants who died while waiting for a transplant increased in 1999 to 6.4%. The highest death rates were for lung and heart-lung recipients at 11.6% and 15%, respectively.

As transplantation technique has progressed, the role of the clinical laboratory has become more clearly defined. This chapter is a description of the utility of monitoring both transplant donors and recipients of solid organs.

PRETRANSPLANT EVALUATION

No transplant is performed without a thorough clinical investigation of both the donor and the recipient. Each organ has specific criteria that must be reviewed before the transplant is performed.

Live Donor (Kidney)

Allograft survival rates are greater when the graft is obtained from a live donor (LD) rather than from a cadaver donor. A second important advantage of LD transplants is the elective nature of the procedure, sparing the recipient the long waiting period on dialysis that frequently occurs when waiting for a suitable cadaveric transplantation. A third reason for the continued use of living donors is the shortage of cadaver donors. The option of living donation has become more appealing with the accessibility of laparoscopic donation. Kidney donors undergoing the laparoscopic procedure have shorter hospitalizations, less postoperative pain, and quicker return to work when compared to their open nephrectomy donor counterparts. Because most living donors are genetically related to the recipient, this may impart an immunological advantage and improve long-term graft survival. Regardless of the donor being related or nonrelated, living donor allografts are associated with an improved long-term graft survival.

The potential donor and recipient must be tested to demonstrate ABO blood type compatibility. Another immunocompatibility test, termed a *cytotoxic* **T-cell** *crossmatch*, must be performed between the donor and the recipient. This ensures that the recipient has no preformed **antibodies** against the donor. All potential donors must be emotionally stable and must fully understand the process of donating a kidney. Potential donors are meticulously evaluated to ensure that they are in excellent general health and that there are no contraindications to the removal of one kidney (Box 50-1). One goal of this evaluation is the detection of unsuspected disease in the donor, such as diabetes, hypertension, anemia, renal calculi, or malignancy. Another goal is to detect infections that may be transmitted to the recipient. The goal of the remainder of the studies is to assess whether the renal function and structure of the potential renal allograft are completely normal. The age of the potential living related donor is obviously important. Minors are not eligible for kidney donation, but older donors, up to 70 years of age, may be used if in excellent health. Kidney donors who have been monitored for up to 20 years after donation exhibit a slight reduction in glomerular filtration rate and a mild increase in urine protein excretion without an increase in hypertension.

Cadaver Donor

Cadaver donors are previously healthy individuals who suffer irreversible brain death. Once they are declared legally dead, to sustain cardiovascular function they are maintained on a ventilator and clinically managed with appropriate fluids and medications until the organs are removed. An extensive review of each donor's medical history and physical status is necessary, as well as rigorous laboratory testing to ensure optimal organ function. The laboratory studies obtained upon admission are important and establish baseline values of the individual organ systems. The United Network for Organ Sharing (UNOS) has established mandatory laboratory tests (Box 50-2), though additional tests may occasionally be requested. For example, if the donor's heart or lungs are being considered for transplantation, an echocardiogram, ECG, chest x-ray film, and measurement of troponin levels may be ordered at the time of the evaluation.

TABLE 50-1 TRANSPLANTS PERFORMED IN THE UNITED STATES IN 1999	
Type of Transplant	*Number Performed*
Kidney	12,400
Live recipient donor	4474
Cadaver	7926
Liver	4586
Heart	2162
Pancreas	1861
Lung	873
Heart-lung	48
Total	21,516 (all organ transplants)

BOX 50-1

MEDICAL EVALUATION OF THE POTENTIAL LIVE KIDNEY DONOR

Complete history and physical examination
Laboratory studies*
  Complete blood count
  Serum urea and creatinine, sodium, potassium, chloride, bicarbonate
  Fasting blood glucose (glucose tolerance if family history of diabetes)
  Serum calcium, phosphorus, uric acid
  Liver function tests including bilirubin, alkaline phosphatase, transaminases
  Fasting lipids including cholesterol, triglycerides, high-density lipoproteins, low-density lipoproteins
  Prothrombin time, partial thromboplastin time
  Antibodies to cytomegalovirus (CMV), Epstein-Barr virus (EBV), human immunodeficiency virus (HIV), *Treponema pallidum*
  Hepatitis B antigen and antibody, hepatitis C antibody
  Urine analysis and microscopy
  Urine culture
  24-hour urine for creatinine, protein, calcium, uric acid
Electrocardiogram
X-ray studies
  Chest x-ray film
  Intravenous pyelography
  Renal arteriogram

There are no absolute acceptable ranges for these laboratory tests. The aim is to ensure that the potential donor is in excellent general health with no contraindication to the removal of one kidney and no potential infections or malignancies to transmit to the recipient.

BOX 50-2

UNITED NETWORK FOR ORGAN SHARING: MANDATORY LABORATORY TESTING OF THE POTENTIAL CADAVER DONOR

Complete blood count
Electrolytes
Blood gases
ABO typing
Hepatitis screen
Syphilis screen (VDRL or RPR)
Screen for antibodies to: HIV, HTLV-1, cytomegalovirus
Blood and urine cultures if hospitalized more than 72 hours
Renal specific*
  Serum creatinine and urea
  Urinalysis
Liver specific*
  Liver enzymes: transaminases and alkaline phosphatase
  Total and direct bilirubin
  Prothrombin time and partial thromboplastin time
Heart specific*
  12-lead electrocardiogram
  Consultation with cardiologist
  Chest x-ray film
Pancreas specific*
  Serum amylase
  Serum lipase
  Glucose

There are no absolute acceptable ranges for these lab tests. The aim is to ensure that organs function after transplant and no infections or malignancies are passed from donor to recipient.

Kidney. Most cadaver kidney donors are between 2 and 70 years of age. However, kidneys from newborns and donors older than 70 years of age have been successfully transplanted. A thorough past and present medical history of the donor is necessary. The laboratory studies should include those listed in Box 50-2, with specific attention placed on the results of serum creatinine and urea levels and on urinalysis. Only patients with laboratory values that are within the reference intervals, or patients with laboratory values or clinical findings that are returning to normal after management, are usually accepted as cadaveric kidney donors.

Liver. Donor livers from individuals up to 70 years of age can safely be used. Older donors who are healthy enough to remain hemodynamically stable after brain death can become acceptable donors. Social history and the cause of death are often valuable pieces of information for potential liver donors. Laboratory testing includes those tests listed in Box 50-2 with particular attention to bilirubin, AST, ALT, and alkaline phosphatase. Moderate elevations in liver function studies are acceptable, especially if the trend is toward the reference range.

Pancreas. In general, donors who are acceptable for renal or liver transplants are also acceptable as pancreas donors. The primary contraindications for the acceptance of a donor for pancreas transplantation are a history of diabetes and acute or chronic pancreatitis. Hyperglycemia is frequently seen after severe head trauma or as a result of the administration of glucose-containing solutions. These factors are not a contraindication if the patient has no history of diabetes. In questionable cases, glycosylated hemoglobin levels may demonstrate that long-term pancreas function has been normal. An elevated serum amylase is not necessarily indicative of pancreatic trauma. Direct visualization of the pancreas is the best way to assess pancreatic injury in trauma cases. Evidence of pancreatic trauma precludes retrieval. The age of the potential donor is generally not a factor for pancreatic transplants, though age criteria are slightly more restrictive than for kidney transplants.

Heart. The donor's cardiac assessment combines the history, physical examination, and diagnostic tests. Contraindicating problems include prominent blunt chest trauma, prolonged hypotension, cardiac arrest, and premorbid cardiac symptoms. If blunt trauma or cardiac arrest occurred, the measurement of serum troponin levels, in addition to a chest x-ray film and ECG, may help in judging the severity of myocardial damage. Generally individuals older than 50 years of age are not considered as cardiac donors.

Recipient

A detailed medical and psychological evaluation of all potential transplant recipients is essential. Patients must be sufficiently healthy and motivated to undergo the surgical procedure, to withstand the potential problems of immunosuppressive agents, and to comply with a complex and demanding medical regimen.

Renal. The pretransplantation evaluation example of the recipient of a kidney is listed in Box 50-3. The purpose of this evaluation is to detect any problem that may reduce the chance of success of the procedure and to take corrective measures when necessary. Not all patients with end-stage renal disease are candidates for transplantation. Patients of advanced age or with prominent systemic illness are generally not acceptable candidates. The American Society of Transplant Physicians has published a list of absolute contraindications to renal transplantation. They include active infection, advanced cardiovascular disease, advanced pulmonary disease, severe chronic liver disease, malignancy, acute vasculitis or glomerulonephritis, uncorrectable lower urinary tract disease, primary oxalosis, age greater than 70 years, morbid obesity, severe psychosocial problems, drug or alcohol abuse, and positive current T-cell crossmatch. A more complete review (see Abbas et al in the Bibliography) of the evaluation of renal transplant candidates and clinical practice guidelines was recently published that more specifically addresses the issues related to these absolute contraindications.

Other recipients. Similar laboratory evaluations are used to assess potential liver, heart, pancreas, and lung transplant recipients. The primary goal is to ensure that the patient is healthy enough to survive the surgery and posttransplantation complications associated with life-long **immunosuppression**. Obviously, advanced cardiac disease is not a contraindication to heart transplantation but is a contraindication to liver transplantation. Active infection, malignancy, severe psychosocial problems, and any active drug or alcohol abuse are contraindications to all transplants.

CLINICAL AND PATHOLOGICAL DIAGNOSIS OF TRANSPLANT REJECTION

Allograft **rejection** is the destruction of a transplanted organ resulting from an immune attack mounted by the recipient's body. The rejected organ loses function. The process of monitoring the health of a transplanted organ includes a large component of laboratory testing.

The diagnosis of transplant rejection is often an exclusionary process by which the clinician rules out other posttransplantation complications. For example, kidney rejection must be differentiated from the nephrotoxic effects of the drugs **cyclosporine** or **tacrolimus**, which are used to suppress the recipient's immune response. Liver allograft rejection must be differentiated from drug-induced hepatic injury, surgical complications, and hepatitis. Although biochemical and immunological testing and clinical symptoms may be strongly suggestive of organ rejection, a definitive diagnosis is made through histological examination of the transplanted organ. This is an invasive procedure that requires a biopsy in which a core of tissue is removed from the allograft for microscopic examination.

Allograft rejection can be caused by T-cells of the immune system, the antibodies produced by **B-cells**, or both. The differentiation between these processes is based on clinical presentation, timing of the event, and histological examination. *Hyperacute rejection*, defined as organ rejection beginning within minutes of transplantation, occurs because antibodies against the donor tissue are already present in the recipient. Clinical manifestations are noted immediately after the blood supply of the graft is restored. *Acute cellular rejection* is a T-cell–mediated process and is the most common form of rejection. It can occur at any time after transplantation but is most common in the first 6 months after transplantation. *Chronic rejection* is a slow, progressive loss of organ function that generally follows episodes of acute cellular rejection. The course of chronic rejection is generally months to years.

Kidney

Hyperacute rejection of the kidney is a rare occurrence with current crossmatching techniques. Clots form in the renal arteries, followed by necrosis of the renal cortex. Acute cellular rejection ranges from mild to severe forms, depending on the degree of renal damage (Box 50-4). Chronic rejection results in a progressive, irreversible deterioration of renal function that now is commonly referred to as *chronic allograft nephropathy* recognizing the other nonimmunological factors affecting long-term graft loss, such as hypertension, diabetes, drug toxicity, etc.

BOX 50-3

PRETRANSPLANTATION EVALUATION OF THE RENAL RECIPIENT

Complete history and physical examination
Dental evaluation
Gynecological evaluation
Laboratory studies*
    Serum creatinine, urea, AST, ALT, bilirubin, and alkaline phosphatase
    Hepatitis B antigen and antibody, hepatitis C antibody
    Antibodies to CMV, HIV, and EBV
    Urine culture
X-ray studies
    Chest x-ray film
    Upper gastrointestinal series
    Barium enema (age >40 years)
    Gallbladder ultrasound scan
    Voiding cystourethrogram
    Mammography (female >40 years)

There are no absolute acceptable ranges for these laboratory tests. The aim is to ensure that the potential recipient is sufficiently motivated to undergo the surgical procedure and to withstand the potential problems of immunosuppressive agents.

BOX 50-4

BANFF CRITERIA (1997) OF ACUTE RENAL ALLOGRAFT REJECTION*

Banff criteria diagnostic categories for renal allograft biopsies
1. Normal
2. Antibody-mediated rejection. Rejection demonstrated to be due, at least in part, to anti-donor antibody.
   A. Immediate (hyperacute)
   B. Delayed (accelerated acute)
3. Borderline changes: "suspicious" for acute rejection. This category is used when no intimal arteritis is present, but there are foci of mild tubulitis (1 to 4 mononuclear cells/tubular cross-section).
4. Acute/active rejection

Type (Grade)	Histopathological Findings
IA	Cases with significant interstitial infiltration (>25% of parenchyma affected) and foci of moderate tubulitis (>4 mononuclear cells/tubular cross-section or group of 10 tubular cells)
IB	Cases with significant interstitial infiltration (>25% of parenchyma affected) and foci of severe tubulitis (>10 mononuclear cells/tubular cross-section or group of 10 tubular cells)
IIA	Cases with mild to moderate intimal arteritis (v1)
IIB	Cases with severe intimal arteritis comprising >25% of the luminal area (v2)
III	Cases with "transmural" arteritis and/or arterial fibrinoid change and necrosis of medial smooth muscle cells (v3 with accompanying lymphocytic inflammation)

5. Chronic/sclerosing allograft nephropathy (Glomerular and vascular lesions help define type of chronic nephropathy; chronic/recurrent rejection can be diagnosed if typical vascular lesions are seen)

Type (Grade)	Histopathological Findings
I (mild)	Mild interstitial fibrosis and tubular atrophy without (a) or with (b) specific changes suggesting chronic rejection
II (moderate)	Moderate interstitial fibrosis and tubular atrophy (a) or (b)
III (severe)	Severe interstitial fibrosis and tubular atrophy and tubular loss (a) or (b)

6. Other, specify (changes not considered to be due to rejection, i.e., posttransplant lymphoproliferative disorder, nonspecific changes, acute tubular necrosis, etc.)
7. Insufficient specimen

International standardization of criteria for the histological diagnosis of renal allograft rejection developed by a group of renal pathologists, nephrologists, and transplant surgeons meeting in Banff, Canada, 1997.
*Histological grading may or may not correlate with biochemical indices such as serum creatinine.

TABLE 50-2 GRADING OF ACUTE CELLULAR LIVER ALLOGRAFT REJECTION*

Grade	Description
Consistent with rejection	Lymphocytic or mixed portal infiltrate with minimal bile duct damage (<50%) and no endothelialitis
Mild rejection	Mild portal infiltrates with endothelial and biliary epithelial hypertrophy and damage
Moderate rejection	Lymphocytic or mixed portal infiltrate with significant bile duct damage (>50%), with or without endothelialitis
Severe rejection	Lymphocytic or mixed portal infiltrates, arteritis, paucity of bile ducts, central hepatocellular ballooning with confluent dropout of hepatocytes

*Histological grading may or may not correlate with biochemical indices such as AST, ALT, and bilirubin.

Liver

Hyperacute rejection of liver allografts rarely occurs in ABO-compatible donors. However, the paucity of donors has made ABO-incompatible liver transplantation more common, thus increasing the risk for this type of rejection. Acute cellular rejection of liver allografts is characterized by portal inflammation with a predominant lymphocytic infiltrate. The severity of rejection (Table 50-2) determines the therapy implemented. Hepatic chronic rejection, or *vanishing bile duct syndrome*, is characterized by progressive cholestasis and deteriorating liver function. Bile duct injury is the result of a vascular arteriopathy that diminishes the blood supply to the biliary tree.

BOX 50-5

MARYLAND PANCREAS BIOPSY GRADING SCHEME*

1. Grade 0—Normal
2. Grade I—Inflammation of undetermined significance
   Sparse, purely septal mononuclear inflammatory infiltrates
   No venous endothelialitis or acinar involvement identified
3. Grade II—Minimal rejection
   Purely septal inflammation with venous endothelialitis (attachment of lymphocytes to the endothelium with associated endothelial damage and lifting of the endothelium from the basement membrane)
   In the absence of venous endothelialitis a constellation of at least three of the following four histological features:
   (a) Septal inflammatory infiltrates composed of a mixed population of small and large ("activated") lymphocytes
   (b) Eosinophils
   (c) Acinar inflammation in rare (up to two) foci[†]
   (d) Ductal inflammation (permeation of inflammatory cells through the ductal basement membrane)
4. Grade III—Mild rejection
   Septal inflammatory infiltrates composed of a mixed population of small and large ("activated") lymphocytes with associated acinar inflammation in multiple (three or more) foci[†]
   Eosinophils, venous endothelialitis, ductal inflammation, and evidence of acinar single cell injury may be seen depending on sampling
   The latter is manifested as cellular drop-out (apoptosis-pyknotic cell death), or necrosis (oncotic cell death)
5. Grade IV—Moderate rejection
   Arterial endothelialitis and/or necrotizing arteritis (vasculitis). Features described in Grade III are usually present
6. Grade V—Severe rejection
   Extensive acinar lymphoid or mixed inflammatory infiltrates with multicellular focal or confluent acinar cell necrosis
   Depending on sampling, vascular and ductal lesions may be demonstrated

*http://tpis.upmc.edu/tpis/pancreas/CrejOver.html
[†]Inflammatory focus is defined as a collection of at least 10 mononuclear cells.

TABLE 50-3 INTERNATIONAL SOCIETY OF HEART TRANSPLANTATION STANDARD CARDIAC BIOPSY GRADING*

Grade	Description
0	No rejection
1A	Focal perivascular or interstitial infiltrate without myocyte damage
1B	Diffuse but sparse perivascular and/or interstitial infiltrate without myocyte damage
2	One focus only with aggressive infiltration and/or focal myocyte damage
3A	Multifocal infiltrates and/or myocyte damage
3B	Diffuse inflammatory process with myocyte damage
4	Diffuse aggressive polymorphous infiltrate ± edema ± hemorrhage ± vasculitis with necrosis

*Histological grading does not correlate with biochemical indices such as creatine phosphokinase and lactate dehydrogenase.

Heart

Hyperacute rejection in cardiac allografts is extremely rare but has been noted in both ABO- compatible and ABO-incompatible transplants. Because of the rapidity of this process, patient and graft survival is generally poor. Acute cellular rejection is detected by serial endomyocardial biopsies. The grade of the severity of acute cellular rejection is based on the criteria established by the International Society of Heart and Lung Transplantation (Table 50-3). Chronic rejection generally manifests itself as accelerated arteriosclerosis.

Pancreas

Routine biopsy of the pancreas to diagnose rejection is less frequently performed because of the morbidity associated with this procedure and the anatomical proximity of the pancreas. However, the use of tissue biopsy to diagnose rejection in the pancreas is extremely important because of the lack of biochemical markers for pancreas rejection. Typically, by the time an abnormality in serum glucose has been observed, extensive organ damage has already occurred, and reversibility of the rejection episode is decreased. Therefore, aggressive pancreas biopsy and treatment procedures have been associated in improved pancreas graft survival rates. The University of Maryland has published a Pancreas Biopsy Grading Scheme (Box 50-5) that allows for more uniform evaluation of these biopsies.

In the case in which a kidney is transplanted in conjunction with the pancreas, a biopsy of the kidney may be taken as a surrogate marker for rejection in the pancreas.

LABORATORY MONITORING OF THE TRANSPLANT RECIPIENT

The clinical development of acute rejection of a transplanted organ generally results in progressive allograft destruction with accompanying organ dysfunction. Histopathological examination of transplanted tissue remains the standard for the determination of rejection after it has become clinically apparent. However, the continued success of organ transplantation is largely the result of the use of laboratory tests to detect early signs of rejection and to monitor treatment. These tests measure biochemical markers that reflect organ allograft damage and organ function.

Kidney

The laboratory evaluation of posttransplantation renal function employs the same tests routinely used to monitor glomerular and tubular function. Rejection remains an important cause of renal dysfunction after kidney transplant, but cyclosporine or tacrolimus nephrotoxicity, recurrent disease, infection, and vascular complications can cause renal dysfunction in these patients. Routine analysis of serum creatinine and urea remains the most practical clinical measure of renal function. Elevations in serum creatinine are often the initial presentation of posttransplantation renal complications. Both the degree of creatinine elevation and the rate of rise are important in the diagnosis. The rate of increase in serum creatinine, in combination with other clinical and histopathological findings (Table 50-4), can be used to differentiate acute rejection from cyclosporine/tacrolimus nephrotoxicity. Other serum chemistry results may have some utility in this differential diagnosis.

Cyclosporine/tacrolimus (calcineurin inhibitor) induced tubular dysfunction can cause elevations in serum potassium, bicarbonate, and uric acid while causing a decrease in serum magnesium. Abnormalities (increases and decreases) in the urinary excretion of sodium and potassium are consistent with cyclosporine nephrotoxicity. Functional tests such as renal manometry, ultrasonography, magnetic resonance imaging, and radionuclide scans may further delineate the cause of renal allograft dysfunction.

Pancreas

Because the pancreas is usually transplanted in combination with the kidney, biochemical markers of renal function are often used as early indicators of the status of the pancreatic transplant. Increases in serum amylase and glucose occur very late in the process of pancreas rejection and remain largely unreliable as indicators of early allograft rejection. If pancreas transplants are performed so that the pancreatic enzymes drain into the bladder, falling urinary amylase levels have been shown to correlate with early pancreatic transplant dysfunction. The frequency of this testing is a prominent factor in its sensitivity for detecting allograft rejection. Most centers initially monitor urinary amylase levels daily or at least three times per week. Other pancreatic enzymes such as trypsinogen may also be of value. Pancreatic fluid cytological findings may also be of diagnostic value; an increase in lymphocytes and blast cells is indicative of rejection, whereas a predominance of neutrophils is more characteristic of infection. Functional tests that evaluate insulin response to a glucose load may also be useful in the assessment of pancreatic reserve.

TABLE 50-4 COMPARISON OF ACUTE REJECTION VERSUS CYCLOSPORINE (CYA) NEPHROTOXICITY

Parameter	Acute Rejection	CYA Nephrotoxicity
Clinical		
Onset	<60 days	Variable
Fever >37.5° C	+	-
Weight gain >0.5 kg	+	±
Oliguria	++	±
Biochemical		
Creatinine	Rapid rise (>3 mg/L/day)	Gradual rise (1 to 2 mg/L/day)
BUN:creatinine	<20:1	>20:1
Potassium (serum)	Increased	Increased ++
Bicarbonate (serum)	Decreased +	Decreased ++
Uric acid (serum)	No change	Increased +
Magnesium (serum)	No change	Decreased +
Sodium (urine)	Decreased ±	Decreased ++
Cyclosporine* trough level	Low, <150 ng/mL	High, >400 ng/mL
Lymphocytes (urine)	++	-
Pathological		
Biopsy	Endovasculitis	Arteriolopathy
	Tubulitis	Tubular vacuolation and mitochondria
	Interstitial edema	Minimal edema
	Glomerulitis	Interstitial fibrosis
	Diffuse infiltrates	Focal infiltrates
Diagnostic Tests		
Ultrasonography	Increased graft cross-sectional area	Normal graft cross-sectional area
Magnetic resonance imaging	Swelling	Normal
Radionuclide	Decreased perfusion	Decreased tubular function
	Patchy arterial flow	Normal or decreased perfusion

A + indicates a positive response, and a - indicates no response.
*TDx whole blood, monoclonal assay.

Liver

Biochemical markers are routinely used in monitoring liver allograft function. The various tests used to evaluate liver function can be divided into two categories: (1) *static tests*, which allow the assessment of liver function indirectly by measuring substances produced by the liver, and (2) *dynamic tests*, which directly measure the metabolic and clearance capacities of the liver.

Static tests. In general, the serum levels of bilirubin, alkaline phosphatase, aspartate aminotransferase (AST), and alanine aminotransferase (ALT) are routinely used liver function tests. These tests are evaluated daily during the first few weeks of the posttransplantation period. Testing frequency decreases as stable graft function is demonstrated and increases when liver dysfunction occurs. Other tests of serum analytes, such as lactate dehydrogenase (LD), 5'-nucleotidase (5-NT), and γ-glutamyltransferase (GGT) are considered secondary tests and may not be part of standard post–liver transplantation monitoring. Small incremental increases in standard liver tests do not necessarily indicate liver allograft rejection. However, serial increases of >25% over several days are considered a reliable indicator of liver allograft dysfunction.

The results of the liver function tests, such as bilirubin, alkaline phosphatase, AST, and ALT, do not always indicate transplant rejection, because elevation in test results are also associated with other clinical conditions (Table 50-5). For example, although serum bilirubin and alkaline phosphatase are progressively elevated with development of acute cellular rejection, both are also elevated during cholestasis secondary to biliary obstruction, drug toxicity, injury resulting from the process of preserving an organ before transplantation, and infection. Early elevations in serum aminotransferases may occur with rejection but elevations become progressively higher (>2 times the upper limit of normal) in severe cases. Acute elevations in AST and ALT are also reflective of ischemic hepatocellular injury, necrosis, and hepatitis. Serum markers of hepatic synthetic function (serum proteins, serum ammonia, and coagulation factors) generally become abnormal as the result of long-standing progressive liver disease or severe fulminant hepatic failure. In general, static tests are sensitive early indicators of liver allograft dysfunction but are not specific for rejection.

Dynamic tests. Dynamic tests of liver function have been developed in an attempt to measure the functional status of the liver. Dynamic tests assess the liver's ability to clear or metabolize various substrates. Several of these tests have been extensively evaluated as part of the clinical assessment of liver transplant donors and recipients (Table 50-6).

The state of hepatocellular oxygenation is reflected by the ratio of serum acetoacetate (AcAc) to β-hydroxybutyrate (HB), known as the ketone body ratio (KBR). As the oxygenation state of the liver decreases and the NAD/NADH ratio decreases, more HB is formed from AcAc. Clinically, a KBR of <0.7 is associated with diminished hepatocellular function in both liver allograft donors and recipients.

The hepatic clearance of exogenous substances has also been evaluated for assessing liver status. Indocyanine green (ICG) is removed from blood by the liver and is excreted unchanged into the bile. Its removal from blood is primarily reflective of hepatic blood flow. Another measure of hepatocellular metabolism is galactose-elimination capacity (GEC), which is the saturation of the enzyme responsible for galactose elimination from blood. Lidocaine metabolism and the formation of its primary oxidative metabolite monoethylglycinexylidide (MEGX) reflect both hepatic cytochrome P-450 activity and hepatic blood flow. MEGX formation has been clinically correlated with varying degrees of liver function in both donors and recipients. Other exogenous agents that have been evaluated as potential dynamic markers of liver function include antipyrine, caffeine, lorazepam, and debrisoquine. A limitation of these dynamic tests is that they appear to be a sensitive indicator of liver injury but not of liver regeneration after transplantation. The role of dynamic monitoring of the posttransplantation liver recipient requires further clinical evaluation.

Surgical innovations have made possible the more complex procedure of living liver donation. After an extensive

TABLE 50-5 RELATIVE CHANGES IN LABORATORY VALUES AFTER LIVER TRANSPLANTATION

Clinical Condition	Bilirubin	Alkaline Phosphatase	AST	ALT
Rejection				
Mild	++	++	+	+
Moderate	++	++	++	++
Severe	+++	+++	+++	+++
Other Conditions				
Cholestasis	++	++	±	±
Ischemic necrosis	++	++	+++	+++
Hepatitis	+	+	++	++

ALT, *Alanine aminotransferase;* AST, *aspartate aminotransferase.*

TABLE 50-6 DYNAMIC LIVER FUNCTION TESTS

Test	Functional Assessment	Utility
Lidocaine metabolism	Cytochrome P-450 activity, liver blood flow, monoethylglycinexylidide formation	Assessment of potential donor and recipient before transplantation and assessment of recipient after transplantation
Indocyanine green clearance	Liver blood flow	Assessment of potential recipient before transplantation
Galactose elimination	Hepatocellular function by means of enzymatic saturation capacity	Assessment of potential donor before transplantation
Acetoacetate/β-hydroxybutyrate ratio (ketone body ratio)	Reduction/oxidation function, hepatocellular respiration	Assessment of potential donor before transplantation and recipient after transplantation

work-up of both the donor and recipient, the donor undergoes a hepatectomy that removes specific segments of the liver determined to be safest for the donor, and most optimal for the recipient. Unlike other organs, the liver will regenerate in both the donor and recipient and compensate for the reduced size liver in both patients. Living donor liver transplantation in children has proven to be remarkably safe and effective for both donors and recipients and has helped make death on the waiting list for these children a rare event. Since its introduction in 1990, many of the technical and ethical issues have been addressed, and the procedure has become routine. Adult-to-adult living liver donation is currently being approached cautiously until critical issues such as long-term safety to the donor, ethical issues of donation, and a clear need are resolved.

Heart

The use of biochemical markers for the evaluation of cardiac allograft complications is limited by the mechanism of rejection of this organ. In noncardiac allografts, injury to epithelial cells is the cause of the observed biochemical alterations. Unlike the kidney, liver, or pancreas, the heart lacks epithelial cells as a primary target for rejection. Thus in cardiac allograft recipients, changes in levels of analytes used to measure cardiac function, such as creatine kinase, myoglobin, LD, and AST, have no clinical correlation with rejection. Electrocardiography, echocardiography, and radionuclide scanning are only of value in determining functional status late in rejection and are not reliable indicators of early allograft rejection. Because of the lack of sensitive and specific markers of rejection, routine serial endomyocardial biopsies are the standard for posttransplantation cardiac allograft monitoring.

PHARMACOLOGICAL MONITORING

The continued improvement of immunosuppressive therapies for transplant recipients depends on appropriate pharmacological monitoring of these therapies and optimal adjustment of the multiple immunosuppressive drug regimens. The available choices for immunosuppressive therapy have expanded and now include not only irradiation, steroids, and antimetabolites **azathioprine** and **cyclophosphamide**, but also **mycophenolate mofetil**, cyclosporine, tacrolimus, **sirolimus**, and the polyclonal and monoclonal antilymphocyte agents, such as **OKT3**, basiliximab, and daclizumab (Box 50-6). The availability of new immunosuppressive agents has geometrically increased the number of potential immunosuppressive regimen combinations. To the prescriber's advantage, the advent of newer, more potent immunosuppressive agents allows the prescriber to individualize immunosuppressive regimens not only based upon allograft function and survival, but also on the development of drug toxicities and side effects.

Immunosuppressive protocols vary extensively with organ type, patient status, and the treatment philosophies of the physician and transplant center. Posttransplantation immunosuppressive therapy can involve single, double, triple, or even

---

BOX 50-6

COMMON IMMUNOSUPPRESSIVE PROTOCOLS

Monotherapy
Cyclosporine
Tacrolimus
Sirolimus

Double Therapy
Cyclosporine/tacrolimus and prednisone
Sirolimus and prednisone
Prednisone and azathioprine/mycophenolate mofetil
Sirolimus and azathioprine/mycophenolate mofetil
Cyclosporine/tacrolimus and azathioprine/mycophenolate mofetil
Cyclosporine/tacrolimus and sirolimus

Triple Therapy
Prednisone and azathioprine/mycophenolate mofetil and cyclosporine/tacrolimus
Prednisone and azathioprine/mycophenolate mofetil and sirolimus
Prednisone and sirolimus and cyclosporine/tacrolimus
Azathioprine/mycophenolate mofetil and cyclosporine/tacrolimus and sirolimus

Quadruple Therapy
Antibody therapy (OKT3/ATG/basiliximab/daclizumab) and prednisone and azathioprine/mycophenolate mofetil and cyclosporine/tacrolimus
Antibody therapy (OKT3/ATG/basiliximab/daclizumab) and prednisone and azathioprine/mycophenolate mofetil and sirolimus
Antibody therapy (OKT3/ATG/basiliximab/daclizumab) and prednisone and sirolimus and cyclosporine/tacrolimus
Antibody therapy (OKT3/ATG/basiliximab/daclizumab) and azathioprine/mycophenolate mofetil and cyclosporine/tacrolimus and sirolimus

---

quadruple drug therapy (Box 50-6 lists examples of potential drug combinations).

Corticosteroids (see also Chapter 46)

Corticosteroids were among the earliest compounds found to have immunosuppressive activity. The binding of the glucocorticoids to their receptors blocks the synthesis or release of lymphokines and **cytokines**. This results in an inhibition of T-cell response to stimulation, a redistribution of lymphocytes from the vascular to the lymphatic system, and a decrease in the number of circulating T-cells and B-cells. The cellular immune response is blunted, but almost no immunosuppressive effect is seen in the humoral response (antibody production).

Total steroid dosing is generally quite high (100 to 500 mg/day) in the immediate posttransplantation period but is reduced to 10 to 20 mg daily within 2 weeks after transplantation. Often additional doses of intravenous or oral corticosteroids are used to treat acute rejection episodes. Because the liver and kidney are the major organs that metabolize glucocorticoids, dysfunction of these organs may require modification of the dosage.

The acute adverse effects associated with corticosteroids include hypertension, glucose intolerance, hyperlipidemia caused by altered lipid metabolism, negative calcium balance and bone disease, growth retardation in children, weight gain, psychological changes, reduced wound healing, and cataracts. These acute adverse effects may be new symptoms or seen as an aggravation of preexisting conditions. The acute effects are most often dose related and diminish as the patient progresses to lower doses. Adverse effects associated with long-term glucocorticoid therapy lead to cushingoid appearance, osteoporosis or avascular bone necrosis, and cardiovascular disease secondary to hypertension and hyperlipidemia.

The hepatic metabolism of corticosteroids can be affected by multiple drug interactions. Inducers of cytochrome enzymes can increase the oxidative capacity of the liver and cause decreased levels of steroids for a given dose, whereas inhibitors of cytochrome enzymes tend to spare the circulating steroids from degradation and elimination. No specific monitoring of corticosteroids is routinely performed. Dosing is typically driven by protocols, to minimize side effects, and by the immune response of the patient.

Because of the toxicities of corticosteroids and the development of more potent immunosuppressive agents, a resurgence of interest in protocols designed to avoid or withdraw corticosteroids has occurred. The benefits of eliminating steroids and their toxicities must be weighed against the risk of precipitating acute or chronic rejection. With current immunosuppressive agents, this risk of rejection appears to be minimal, but the benefits of toxicity elimination are more difficult to quantitate. Currently extensive, long-term investigations are ongoing to address these issues.

Azathioprine, Cyclophosphamide, Mycophenolate Mofetil

Azathioprine is a prodrug for **6-mercaptopurine**, which is a potent inhibitor of cellular proliferation. It inhibits purine metabolism and thus interferes in nucleic acid replication. Azathioprine diminishes the clonal expansion of lymphocytes, resulting in suppression of bone marrow function and the cellular immune response, but is not specific to lymphocytes. Azathioprine is administered orally once a day. Standard dosages are in the range of 1 to 2 mg/kg/day. Dosages may need to be reduced if myelosuppression occurs. If significant leukopenia (reduced white blood cell levels) occurs, azathioprine therapy may be temporarily or permanently discontinued. Azathioprine therapy is monitored primarily by following the white blood cell (WBC) count. Generally, full doses of azathioprine are maintained while the WBC count remains above 5000/mm^3. Dosages are reduced by half if the WBC count decreases into the 3000 to 5000/mm^3 range and discontinued when the WBC count falls below 3000 WBC/mm^3, at least until the leukopenia is resolved. Acute administration of granulocyte colony–stimulating factor (G-CSF) may be used to alleviate the myelosuppression.

Cyclophosphamide is a nitrogen mustard precursor, which is activated in the liver. It acts as an alkylating agent and disrupts cell division, having the greatest effect on rapidly dividing cells such as lymphocytes. It is more toxic and less well tolerated than azathioprine. Its use as an immunosuppressant is generally limited to cases of azathioprine intolerance, usually resulting from hepatotoxicity.

Mycophenolate mofetil (Cellcept, MMF) is a prodrug of mycophenolate (MPA) that reversibly bonds and inhibits inosine monophosphate dehydrogenase (IMPDH). IMPDH is an enzyme essential for the conversion of amino acids to nucleotides. This inhibition of *de novo* purine nucleotide synthesis inhibits DNA and RNA synthesis and subsequent synthesis of T-cells and B-cells. MMF may be an improvement on the antimetabolite azathioprine because of its cell type specificity for lymphocytes. Standard dosages are in the range of 2 to 3 g/day. Dosages may need to be reduced if myelosuppression occurs. If significant leukopenia (reduced WBC levels) occurs, MMF therapy may be temporarily or permanently discontinued. MMF therapy is monitored primarily by following the WBC count. Generally, full doses of MMF are maintained while the WBC count remains above 5000/mm^3. Dosages are reduced by half if the WBC count decreases into the 3000 to 5000/mm^3 range and discontinued when the WBC count falls below 3000 WBC/mm^3, at least until the leukopenia is resolved. An alternative means of monitoring therapy is by measuring MPA levels. Therapeutic drug monitoring of MPA is not routinely used because of the difficult sampling schema (5 samples over 2 hours), lack of correlation with toxicity and efficacy, and lack of routine availability of MPA assay.

Cyclosporine

Cyclosporine transformed the practice of transplantation from an experimental procedure to the treatment of choice for end-organ failure. It is an 11-residue cyclic peptide that is chemically neutral and mostly hydrophobic. Cyclosporine is formulated for oral administration in an olive oil solution or gel capsule and for intravenous (IV) administration as a surfactant dispersion. Recently the gel capsule microemulsion formulation has become available generically and is known as cyclosporine, modified. The avidity of cyclosporine for hydrophobic surfaces has caused concern. Dosage can be dangerously reduced because of the drug's adsorption to plastic drinkware, nasogastric feeding tubes, and IV lines. Cyclosporine is believed to cause immunosuppression by inhibiting the synthesis and release of **interleukin-2** (IL-2) and other lymphokines. Cyclosporine accomplishes this by inhibiting early calcium-dependent events in signal transduction during T-cell activation.

Pharmacokinetics. Absorption of cyclosporine after oral dosing is quite variable. Approximately one third of the dose is absorbed, but its bioavailability can range from 5% to 90%. Dietary fat and excretion of bile fluids aid the absorption in the gut. Patients with diarrhea, nausea, vomiting, or reduced bile secretion may have a significantly reduced bioavailability of orally administered cyclosporine. Peak blood levels occur 2 to 6 hours after oral dosing.

Cyclosporine is widely distributed in tissues. Because of its hydrophobic nature it is tightly bound and can be detected in tissue as long as 2 weeks after discontinuation of therapy. Approximately 10% of cyclosporine in the blood is carried in leukocytes, whereas 40% to 60% is carried in the red blood cells; the balance is carried in the plasma bound to lipoproteins.

Binding to erythrocytes is nonlinear, temperature dependent, and may change with hematocrit. This variability in distribution within blood fractions necessitates that whole blood anticoagulated with EDTA be the specimen customarily used for clinical analysis.

Cyclosporine undergoes extensive hepatic metabolism. Many changes occur at the extended side chains, but little or no modification occurs on the cyclic core configuration. The microsomal oxidases, especially the cytochrome P-450IIIA4 isoenzyme, are responsible for metabolism. These oxidases are present in intestinal mucosa and play a significant role in gut metabolism of cyclosporine. Most metabolites identified have undergone oxidation or N-demethylation.

Elimination of cyclosporine is primarily through hepatobiliary excretion with elimination in the feces. Urinary concentrations of cyclosporine and metabolites account for less than 10% of the administered dose.

Adverse effects. Serious adverse effects related to cyclosporine treatment are dose-related nephrotoxicity, hypertension, neurotoxicity, gingival hyperplasia, hirsutism, hyperlipidemia, and glucose intolerance. Many of these side effects are similar to side effects of corticosteroid treatment, adding to their severity. There are general risks of over-immunosuppression as well, with an increased risk of chronic viral infections, which, although mostly innocuous in the general population, can be a threat to the transplant patient. Both acute and chronic nephrotoxicity can occur. In the early posttransplantation time when the cyclosporine dosage and levels are highest, the probability of occurrence of acute cyclosporine-induced nephrotoxicity is greatest. This toxicity manifests as a reduction in renal blood flow, glomerular filtration rate, and urine output. It may be difficult to distinguish this nephrotoxicity from acute rejection in renal transplants (Table 50-4). Decreasing the cyclosporine dose can usually reverse these short-term effects. Long-term administration of cyclosporine and the associated renal vasoconstriction can lead to a nephropathy characterized by interstitial fibrosis. Secondary to the chronic nephropathy are hypertension and hyperuricemia. Decreasing the cyclosporine dose or switching to noncalcineurin inhibitors as alternative therapies are the most commonly used strategies for dealing with these chronic side effects.

Drug interactions. The pharmacokinetic and pharmacodynamic properties of cyclosporine may be affected by many drugs commonly used to treat transplant recipients (Box 50-7). Drug interactions with cyclosporine may occur as a result of an alteration of the pharmacokinetic parameters, an alteration of the physiological or pharmacological effect, or a combination of these effects. The most common mechanisms for these drug interactions are induction or inhibition of the cytochrome P-450 system, which results

in a reduction or an increase in blood cyclosporine levels, respectively. Close monitoring of the patient is suggested when the administration of drugs known to interact with cyclosporine is initiated or stopped. This monitoring includes the assessment of organ function and known adverse effects of cyclosporine, and the measurement of cyclosporine blood concentrations.

Monitoring. Since its introduction, monitoring of cyclosporine has been used by most transplant centers to optimize immunosuppression while minimizing toxicity. Evolving technology for monitoring cyclosporine and changes in immunosuppressive protocols have made it difficult to establish appropriate therapeutic ranges (Table 50-7). Therapeutic ranges are often specific to each institution with different ranges developed for each organ type, for various times after transplantation, for various immunosuppressant combinations, and for patient individualized therapy during episodes of toxicity or rejection. It remains very difficult to interpret an individual immunosuppressant concentration without a full understanding of the patient and specifics surrounding the dose and level. Box 50-8 offers an example of the variable ranges based upon these factors. Similar ranges exist for other immunosuppressive agents that undergo therapeutic drug monitoring, for the same reasons. Clinical response does not correlate with dose because of the variability in cyclosporine pharmacokinetics and pharmacodynamics. Frequent monitoring of cyclosporine levels is particularly valuable when following the progress of individual patients. The assay techniques vary from institution to institution, but assays specific for the parent drug are recommended. Whole blood is the matrix of choice and trough level monitoring is the standard of practice. Frequent inpatient monitoring early after transplantation is performed in many centers with daily monitoring preferred. The frequency of monitoring decreases after discharge and generally occurs whenever the patient is evaluated in the outpatient clinic. Early after transplantation this may occur as often as three times per week, but much

---

BOX 50-7

CYCLOSPORINE, TACROLIMUS, SIROLIMUS DRUG INTERACTIONS (NOT AN INCLUSIVE LIST)

Decreased Levels	*Increased Levels*	*Nephrotoxic Synergy*
Carbamazepine	Diltiazem	Acyclovir
Isoniazid	Erythromycin	Aminoglycosides
Phenobarbital	Fluconazole	Amphotericin B
Phenytoin	Itraconazole	Cotrimoxazole
Rifampicin	Ketoconazole	Furosemide
Nafcillin	Metoclopramide	Ganciclovir
	Methylprednisolone	H_2-antagonists
	Nicardipine	Melphalan
	Verapamil	Nonsteroidal antiinflammatory agents
		Vancomycin

TABLE 50-7 CYCLOSPORINE ASSAY METHODS COMMERCIALLY AVAILABLE

Assay	Sensitivity	Manufacturer
mFPIA	25 ng/mL	Abbott Laboratories Inc. (TCx)
EMIT	40 ng/mL	Dade Behring, Inc. (Emit)
mRIA	10 ng/mL	DiaSorin Inc. (CYCLO-Trac)

BOX 50-8

CYCLOSPORINE WHOLE BLOOD TDx MONOCLONAL ASSAY THERAPEUTIC RANGES AT THE UNIVERSITY OF CINCINNATI

Kidney and Kidney-Pancreas Transplants
<6 months (250 to 375 ng/mL)
>6 months (100 to 250 ng/mL)

Liver Transplants
<1 month (350 to 450 ng/mL)
2 to 6 months (250 to 350 ng/mL)
>6 months (170 to 240 ng/mL)

Cardiac Transplants
<6 weeks (300 to 420 ng/mL)
6 to 12 weeks (180 to 300 ng/mL)
>12 weeks (120 to 180 ng/mL)

later it may only occur three or four times per year. The amount of monitoring generally increases when physiological changes occur in the transplant recipient (rejection, infection, drug toxicity, and so forth).

Because of the interpatient and intrapatient variability of cyclosporine pharmacokinetic parameters and resulting drug exposure, it is well accepted that the area under the curve (AUC) monitoring more accurately reflects the exposure of a patient to the drug. However, drawbacks of any type of AUC monitoring are increased time and costs, which are formidable barriers to routine clinical practice. Several recent studies have been carried out that suggest 2-hour peak cyclosporine concentrations or C-2 concentrations more accurately correlate with cyclosporine AUC than cyclosporine troughs or C-0. Therapeutic C-2 concentrations are assay specific, but typically range between 1000 to 2000 ng/mL for most automated immunoassay methods. Routine conversion in transplant clinics from cyclosporine trough to C-2 monitoring has also been met with resistance because of logistical concerns, and the need to separate the true science of this approach from the marketing aspects by the reagent manufacturer. Logistical concerns center around the narrow window for accurate sampling times (i.e., within 15 minutes of 2 hours after drug dosage) and the assay used within the institution to measure cyclosporine. When using the C-2

approach to cyclosporine monitoring, the cyclosporine assay must accurately measure much higher cyclosporine concentrations. In addition, levels previously considered to be alert values now may be the actual target C-2 level.

Oral doses of 4 to 8 mg/kg/day are typically required to achieve these target levels, whereas IV doses are typically one third of the oral doses. Dosing based upon body weight is only used to initiate therapy, and subsequent dose changes are made in response to therapeutic drug monitoring mechanisms.

Tacrolimus

Tacrolimus (FK506), a novel macrolide immunosuppressant, is a powerful and selective anti–T cell agent that has a similar mode of action to cyclosporine. Tacrolimus binds to an immunophilin FKBP and this complex binds to the calcium-dependent calcineurin, which results in the inhibition of transcription of genes coding for cytokines, inhibiting early stage T-cell activation. Tacrolimus is approximately 100 times more potent than cyclosporine and has proven to be more effective than cyclosporine in preventing and treating rejection in various organ transplant types.

The pharmacokinetics of tacrolimus exhibit many of the same features that cyclosporine exhibits. The drug is poorly, erratically, and incompletely absorbed in the gut, though its absorption appears to be less dependent on the availability of bile than is that of cyclosporine. In plasma, the drug binds primarily to α_1-acid glycoprotein, whereas in whole blood it is mainly found in erythrocytes. Tacrolimus is metabolized by the microsomal cytochrome P-450 system of the liver and the small intestine. After hepatic metabolism, the biliary route eliminates more than 95% of the drug. Drug interactions between tacrolimus and drugs inhibiting/inducing the cytochrome P-450 pathway are very similar to those occurring with cyclosporine. In addition, those drugs causing nephrotoxicity typically are synergistic with tacrolimus; such drugs include aminoglycosides, nonsteroidal antiinflammatory agents, etc.

Nephrotoxicity, neurotoxicity, and hyperglycemia are significant side effects associated with tacrolimus therapy. Nausea, vomiting, and diarrhea are common side effects that also occur that are different from those of cyclosporine. In earlier clinical trials, new-onset diabetes developed more commonly with tacrolimus than with cyclosporine. However, in more recent trials lower target tacrolimus concentrations and lower total steroid doses have eliminated this difference. Common neurological side effects associated with tacrolimus include tremor, paresthesia, insomnia, headache, photophobia, and seizures. When compared to cyclosporine, tacrolimus results in less hypertension, hyperlipidemia, and cosmetic side effects than cyclosporine-treated patients.

Variability in blood concentrations because of erratic pharmacokinetics and drug interactions together with the dose-dependent immunosuppressive effects and toxicities justify careful monitoring of this drug. The correlation between tacrolimus concentrations and efficacy or toxicity is still unclear. However, unlike cyclosporine, tacrolimus trough concentrations accurately reflect tacrolimus AUC

TABLE 50-8 TACROLIMUS ASSAY METHODS COMMERCIALLY AVAILABLE		
Assay	Sensitivity	Manufacturer
ELISA	0.18 ng/mL	DiaSorin Inc. (Pro-Trac II)
EMIT	1.5 ng/mL	Dade Behring, Inc. (Emit)
MEIA	1.5 ng/mL	Abbott Laboratories Inc. (IMx Tacrolimus II)

concentrations. Many transplant centers are targeting whole blood trough levels from 5 to 20 ng/mL. Several methods for tacrolimus assays are commercially available (Table 50-8). However, when used in conjunction with more potent immunosuppressive agents, tacrolimus concentrations of <5 ng/mL may be targeted. In such cases, assays with sensitive and specific lower limits of quantitation to 0.5 ng/mL are necessary.

Oral doses of 0.05 to 0.2 mg/kg/day are typically required to achieve these target levels. IV doses are typically one third of the oral doses and are rarely used because of the increase in nephrotoxicity. Dosing based upon body weight is commonly used to initiate therapy, whereas dose changes are made in response to therapeutic drug monitoring mechanisms.

Sirolimus (Rapamune, Rapamycin)

Sirolimus was first discovered as an antimicrobial agent, and later identified to have potent immunosuppressant activities. Sirolimus binds to a specific immunophilin FKBP similar to tacrolimus, but does not exert its immunosuppressive effects by calcineurin inhibition. Sirolimus binds to the enzyme, target of rapamycin (mTOR), and inhibits translation of the messenger RNA for several cytokines essential for T-cell regulation and proliferation.

Sirolimus exhibits much of the same pharmacokinetic interpatient and intrapatient variability as cyclosporine and tacrolimus. The oral absorption of sirolimus is approximately 14%, with the peak concentration occurring approximately 2 hours post dose. Sirolimus is metabolized by the CYP3A4 enzyme system, and its drug-interaction potential is similar to that of cyclosporine and tacrolimus. Of note, upon coadministration of sirolimus with tacrolimus and cyclosporine, sirolimus concentrations are increased. The half-life of sirolimus is more than 50 hours, which allows for once daily dosing, but necessitates a loading dose to more quickly achieve steady state concentrations. Like cyclosporine and tacrolimus, a high-fat meal increases the AUC, whereas hepatic impairment prolongs the half-life.

Leukopenia, thrombocytopenia, and hyperlipidemia are the most common side effects reported with sirolimus. Effective strategies to manage these toxicities include dosage reduction and the addition of HMG-coreductase inhibitors to aid in the treatment of hyperlipidemia.

The dose of sirolimus ranges from 2 to 15 mg/day. A loading dose of 6 to 15 mg followed by daily doses of 2 to 6 mg/day result in target sirolimus trough concentrations of 10 to 20 ng/mL. Because of the long half-life of this agent, daily sirolimus level monitoring is not necessary. Weekly levels may be necessary in the early post transplant period, followed by monthly levels. At present there is no automated assay available, the current target levels are achieved by HPLC/MS/MS analysis.

Polyclonal Antilymphocyte Preparations

Polyclonal antilymphocyte agents were first used in clinical transplantation in 1967. An antihuman immunoglobulin is prepared from the serum of horses, rabbits, or goats immunized with human lymph nodes, thymus, or spleen. The effect of these agents is dependent on timing and dose. A transient but significant immunosuppression is gained by removal of lymphocytes from circulation. This therapy is used most often to reduce the activity of the highly stimulated immune system during the first few days after transplantation and during serious rejection episodes.

Antilymphocyte agents are generally administered intravenously. Monitoring lymphocyte counts, total T-cell counts, or T-cell subsets such as CD2+ or CD3+ cells can assess the progress and effectiveness of antilymphocyte therapy. Lower T-cell counts are a general indication of immunosuppression through lymphocyte elimination. Efficacy of treatment with polyclonal antilymphocyte preparations may be compromised by the patient's development of antibodies to the animal source of the antisera.

Currently commercially available antilymphocyte agents include ATGAM, a horse antithymocyte globulin, and thymoglobulin, a rabbit antithymocyte globulin. Thymoglobulin is a more potent and effective agent in preventing and reversing ongoing acute rejection.

OKT3

Monoclonal antilymphocyte antibodies have better specificity than polyclonal preparations. Instead of targeting all lymphocytes or thymocytes, a specific subset of cells can be chosen for suppression. The mouse monoclonal antibody, OKT3, is used widely to prevent and treat acute rejection. OKT3 is usually administered intravenously (5 mg/day) for 7 to 14 days. Its most noted adverse effect has been termed the *cytokine release syndrome*. Symptoms include fever, pulmonary edema, dyspnea, and progressive hypotension. A further consideration in the use of OKT3 is that the patient may develop antibodies to the mouse protein (human antimouse antibody, HAMA). This response may occur as early as 3 to 10 days after the patient's first exposure to OKT3, but it generally does not appear until after cessation of therapy. The elicited antibodies may be isotypic, in which case there is no therapeutic interference; or they may be idiotypic, in which case they neutralize the OKT3 activity.

OKT3 therapy can be monitored by several means. Measurement of lymphocyte subsets, specifically CD3+ cells, is the primary monitor of OKT3 efficacy. CD3+ counts below a range of 10 to 50/mm^3 are considered indicative of effective immunosuppression. The serum concentration of OKT3 can be measured by various immunoassays and by flow cytometry. A trough OKT3 serum level of 500 to 1200 ng/mL is usually considered to be therapeutic. The presence of a high-titer HAMA response leads to reduced efficacy and is a contraindication to possible OKT3 retreatment. The HAMA titer is assessed by enzyme-linked immunosorbent assay (ELISA) technology during and after treatment.

In an effort to circumvent the cytokine release syndrome associated with animal derived antithymocyte preparations, humanized or chimeric antibodies have been developed. Many antibody agents are in development; however, at present, two have become commercially available. These antibodies are antibodies directed against the interleukin-2 (IL-2) receptor. Basiliximab (a chimeric mouse-human **IL-2 receptor antibody**) and daclizumab (a humanized-mouse IL-2 receptor antibody) bind to the CD25 α-chain subunit of the IL-2 receptor on activated T-cells. This renders T-cells unable to bind with IL-2 and thus unable to proliferate in response to this cytokine. These antibodies have proven to be effective in preventing, but not treating acute rejection episodes and are most commonly used in the early posttransplant period to prevent acute rejections. To date, there have been no significant adverse events associated with the administration of these agents. Dosage for basiliximab is typically 20 mg on postoperative day 0 and 4, whereas daclizumab is dosed 1 mg/kg pretransplant, and every other week for five total doses. The subsequent mean IL-2 receptor suppression is 36 days for basiliximab and 120 days for daclizumab. Monitoring is typically not performed with these agents.

IMMUNOLOGICAL MONITORING
Human Leukocyte Antigen Testing

The host immune system discriminates self from nonself by recognizing the **human leukocyte antigens (HLA)** on the major **histocompatibility complex**. HLA matching, or histocompatibility testing, is used to help predict the compatibility of donor tissue with a potential recipient. The HLAs, which mediate transplant rejection, are divided into two molecular groups: class I HLA molecules and class II HLA molecules. Class I HLA is composed of two antigenic loci, HLA-A, and HLA-B, which are found on the surface of most cells. Similarly, class II HLA has three primary antigenic loci: HLA-DR, HLA-DQ, and HLA-DP, but these **antigens** are found primarily on B-lymphocytes and macrophages. Each antigenic locus has two antigenic haplotypes, which are identified for typing.

In general, a complement-dependent lymphocyte **cytotoxicity** test is used for **tissue typing**. The unknown tissue, a lymphocyte, is exposed to a broad panel of standardized antisera of known HLA specificity. If the antisera bind to the cell, complement is fixed, and the lymphocyte is killed, and such a response indicates that the HLA of the cell is similar to that of the known antisera. Class I HLA are typed as a mixed lymphocyte preparation, whereas class II antigens generally require a B-lymphocyte–enriched preparation for adequate typing. The process of HLA typing generally takes several hours, which may be a rate-limiting step in using this test in the clinical setting.

The clinical implications and utility of HLA typing vary depending on the organ transplanted. In general, HLA typing is used clinically only for the matching of renal allograft donors and recipients. Six antigen matches of a cadaveric donor and a recipient are linked automatically through United Network of Organ Sharing (UNOS). All other matches are based on a combination of HLA match, crossmatch negativity, panel reactive antibody status (see later discussion), medical urgency, geographical location, and length of time on the recipient waiting list.

Early data indicated that short-term and long-term kidney allograft survival was strongly influenced by HLA-A, HLA-B, and HLA-DR matching. Although the introduction of cyclosporine has reduced the effect of HLA matching on short-term graft survival, long-term survival still appears to be HLA dependent. It has been estimated that the half-life for HLA-matched kidney transplants from cadaveric donors is twice that for unmatched donors (17.3 years versus 7.8 years; see Cecka et al in the bibliography). The use of HLA matching has been demonstrated to improve graft survival in patients with heart transplants. However, the shortage of organs, combined with a minimal preservation time, have made HLA typing impractical in this population. There appears to be a limited benefit to HLA matching in liver allograft recipients, though some evidence indicates a possible detrimental effect on graft survival with no HLA matching. Limited data exist regarding the effects of HLA matching on pancreas and lung allograft survival.

Panel Reactive Antibody Testing

Panel reactive antibody (PRA) testing is performed as frequently as once per month for assessment of anti-HLA antibodies in transplant candidates. The appearance of these antibodies is generally the result of blood transfusions, pregnancy, and previous transplants. PRA testing uses a serological assay of complement-mediated lymphocytotoxicity. Recipient serum is reacted with a reference panel of cells representing known HLA specificities. The result is expressed as a percentage, with 100% representing sensitization against the entire panel of HLA antibodies. Priority is given to kidney transplant recipients with a negative T-cell crossmatch who are highly sensitized over those patients with lower sensitization. PRA test results are not usually used in heart and liver transplants for assessment of donor and recipient compatibility.

Lymphocyte Crossmatch

The lymphocyte crossmatch is used to detect donor-specific cytotoxic antibodies in the recipient. Purified donor lymphocytes are reacted against the sera of recipients. Both a T-cell and a B-cell crossmatch are performed. A positive crossmatch can allow prediction of the likelihood of hyperacute rejection. Renal transplants are not performed when there is a positive crossmatch. The urgency of heart transplants requires that surgery be performed before crossmatch results are usually available. If a positive crossmatch is found in a patient with a heart transplant, increased immunosuppression including plasmapheresis is usually instituted. Crossmatches have little predictive value in liver transplant recipients.

Mixed Lymphocyte Cultures

Although serological testing of HLA differences provides an initial indication of donor-recipient compatibility, a more specific test has been developed to assess the degree of antigenic incompatibility. This procedure, known as the *mixed lymphocyte culture (MLC) test*, allows evaluation of the degree of histocompatibility of the primary activating antigen, the class II HLAs. MLC testing is based on the principle that two cells of different HLA composition will activate and proliferate upon exposure whereas HLA identical cells will remain unstimulated. The greater the degree of antigenic disparity, the greater amount of cellular activity and therefore potential for graft rejection. In general, the two cell types in question are incubated for 5 or 6 days, allowing them to interact and activate each other. The degree of cellular DNA synthesis, as determined by radiolabeling, is equivalent to the relative amount of T-lymphocyte activation. Because of the length of time required to perform the test, the primary clinical use of MLC testing is in the evaluation of potential living related donors.

POSTTRANSPLANT MONITORING

Transplantation has experienced enormous progress as witnessed by extremely low current rejection rates, and current patient and graft survival. Although several factors have resulted in this advance, the major contribution has been the introduction of more effective immunosuppressive regimens. Additionally, refinements in the diagnosis and treatment of posttransplant complications, such as infections,

malignancy, recurrent disease, and comorbid conditions have played an important role. As mortality rates decline, the reasons for death have changed. Currently death from cardiovascular disease is the most common cause of posttransplant mortality. This presents new challenges in the clinical care of the transplant patient. During this posttransplant period monitoring of not only the transplanted allograft remains important, but adherence to monitoring strategies developed to improve the overall quality and length of life are important. This includes various monitors for hypertension, diabetes, hyperlipidemia, infectious complications, and osteoporosis, just to name a few. Posttransplant management will continue to become a more important factor in achieving and improving the long-term success of transplantation.

CONCLUSION

The role of the clinical laboratory in the transplantation process has become well defined. Successful transplantation depends on a multidisciplinary approach including surgery, medicine, nursing, radiology, pathology, pharmacy, nutrition, and psychiatry. The monitoring of transplant donors and recipients crosses and joins these many areas. Although the demands and responsibilities that transplantation puts on clinical laboratories may be great, the rewards seen in patient successes are far greater. Future advances in transplant science include new procedures (small bowel transplant, pancreatic islet transplants), new immunosuppressive agents (leflunomide metabolites, FTY720, ISATX, mycophenolate sodium, SDZ-RAD, etc.), and new solutions to previously unsolvable problems (xenotransplantation and **tolerance** induction). As the field of transplant science grows, the responsibilities of the laboratory will change to meet each new development.

Bibliography

2000 *Annual Report*, US Scientific Registry of Transplant Recipients and the Organ Procurement and Transplantation Network.

Abbas AK, Lichtman AH, Pober JS, editors: *Cellular and molecular immunology*, Philadelphia, 1994, Saunders.

Drachenberg CB et al: Evaluation of pancreas transplant needle biopsy, *Transplantation* 63:1579, 1997.

First MR, editor: Post transplant management in the 21st century: new challenges in clinical care, *Graft* 2(suppl 2), 1999.

Flye MW, editor: *Principles of organ transplantation*, Philadelphia, 1989, Saunders.

Ghobrial RM, Amersi F, Busuttil RW: Surgical advances in liver transplantation: living related and split donors, *Clin Liver Dis* 4:553, 2000.

Kahan BD, Ponticelli C: *Principles and practice of renal transplantation*, Malden, MA, 2000, Martin Dunitz.

Kahan BD et al: Therapeutic drug monitoring of immunosuppressant drugs, (in press).

Kasiske B et al: *The evaluation of renal transplant candidates: clinical practice guidelines*, AJT 2(suppl 1):5, 2001.

Klintmalm G: A review of FK506: a new immunosuppressive agent for the prevention and rescue of graft rejection, *Transplant Rev* 8:53, 1994.

Phillips MG, editor: *Organ procurement, preservation and distribution in transplantation*, Richmond, VA, 1993, William Byrd Press.

Racusen LC et al: The Banff 97 working classification of renal allograft pathology, *Kidney Int* 5:713, 1999.

Rossi SJ et al: Prevention and management of the adverse effects associated with immunosuppressive therapy, *Drug Safety* 9:104, 1993.

Terasaki PI, Cecka JM, editors: *Clinical transplants 1999*, Los Angeles, 1994, UCLA Tissue Typing Laboratory.

Yatscoff RW: Laboratory support for transplantation, *Clin Chem* 40:2166, 1994.

Zand MS, editor: Care of the well transplant patient, *Graft* 4, 2001.

Internet Sites

http://www.a-s-t.org/—American Society of Transplantation

http://www.ashi-hla.org/aboutfiles/aboutframe.html—American Society for Histocompatibility and Immunogenetics (ASHI)

http://www.transweb.org/

http://www.kidneytransplant.org/—University of Southern California, Department of Surgery, Kidney Transplant Program

http://www.kidneytransplant.org/patientguide/pretransplantevaluation.html

http://worldnet.medbiq.org/clinicalresources/hearttransplant.jsp

http://www.nlm.nih.gov/—National Library of Medicine's Medline encyclopedia

http://tpis.upmc.edu/tpis/pancreas/—University of Maryland's Pancreas Biopsy Grading Scheme http://www.kidneyatlas.org/book5/adk5-11.ccc.QXD.pdf—Examples of immunosuppressive protocols and mechanisms

http://cnserver0.nkf.med.ualberta.ca/cn/Schrier/Volume5/ch9/ADK5-09_7-9.pdf

www.unos.org—United Network of Organ Sharing

http://www.wadsworth.org/labcert/blood_tissue/—New York State Department of Health, Wadsworth Center, Division of Laboratory Certification, Blood and Tissue Resources

http://www-med.stanford.edu/shs/txp/livertxp/livingdonation.html—Stanford University Living Liver Donor Program

http://www.hopkinsmedicine.org/cardiology/heart/—Johns Hopkins Cardiomyopathy and Heart Transplant Service

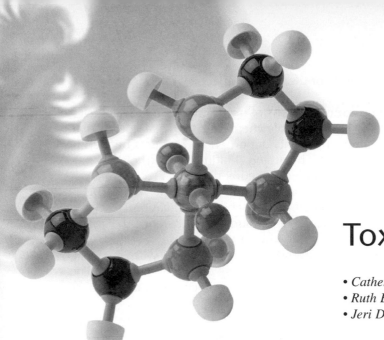

CHAPTER 51

Toxicology

- *Catherine A. Hammett-Stabler*
- *Ruth E. Winecker*
- *Jeri D. Ropero-Miller*

Chapter Outline

Objectives

- Define toxicology, poison, toxicity, and $LD5_0$.
- Describe the factors that influence toxicity.
- Describe how pharmacokinetics change in overdose.

- List and describe frequently encountered poisons.
- Describe the laboratory's role in the toxicological evaluation of a patient.

Key Terms

abused drugs Potentially addictive compounds such as alcohol, cocaine, and marijuana that are taken to stimulate or induce pleasure.

acute toxicity The rapid onset (in seconds, minutes, hours) of a harmful effect following exposure to a toxic agent.

analgesics A class of drugs that reduce pain.

antidepressants A class of drugs that alleviate depression.

antidote Any agent that counteracts the effects of a poison.

benzodiazepines A group of antianxiety/sedative drugs.

biotransformation The biochemical modifications of chemicals as they pass through the body.

chiral drugs Drugs (stereochemical isomers) with four different chemical groups attached to a carbon atom, resulting in nonsuperimposable structures.

(The term *chiral* is based on the Greek word for hand.)

chronic toxicity   The appearance of harmful effects weeks, months, or years following an exposure or repeated exposures to a toxic material.

club drugs   Drugs made popular by their use in the club scene; examples include MDMA, gamma hydroxybutyrate.

cutoff concentration   The administratively chosen concentration used to determine whether a drug test result is positive or negative. Results equal to or greater than the cutoff concentration are reported as positive. Results less than this concentration are reported as negative.

cytochrome P450 isoenzymes   A superfamily of enzymes responsible for much of drug and toxin biotransformation, usually by oxidation.

dose   The amount of a substance given to a patient or received internally into the body.

drug confirmation   The process of verifying the identity of a drug or a drug metabolite by the use of a second test method with greater sensitivity and specificity (see drug screen and screening).

drug interaction   The ability of one drug to change the effect of another drug by altering its metabolic fate or by enhancing or opposing its activity at the site of action.

drug screen   A test that qualitatively identifies the presence of one or more drugs or classes of drugs.

enantiomers   Stereochemical isomers of a compound that are precise mirror images of each other. These isomers demonstrate the ability to rotate polarized light in opposite, but equal, directions. Those that rotate polarized light to the right (clockwise) are designated as *d* or (+) and those left (counterclockwise) are designated as l or (−).

forensic toxicology   A branch of the discipline of toxicology concerned with the medical and legal aspects of the harmful effects of chemicals or poisons.

hypnotics   A class of drugs often used as sedatives.

inhalants   Volatile chemicals, such as toluene, that are components of household products but can be abused by breathing (huffing/sniffing) of their fumes, leading to neural damage.

LD$_{50}$ The amount of a substance that will cause death in half the test animal population.

lethal dose   The amount of a substance that will cause death following exposure.

opiates or **opioids**   A class of drugs with chemical structures similar to those of heroin and morphine. Synthetic opioids include meperidine, oxycodone, and others.

screening test   A rapid test used to separate samples into those considered presumptively positive for specified drugs and those considered negative.

synergistic effects   The situation in which the total effect of two drugs is much greater than the sum of the effect of each drug alone.

therapeutic dose   The amount of a substance that will produce a desired pharmacological effect.

toxicant or **poison**   A substance that, when taken in sufficient quantity, will cause sickness or death.

toxicogenetics   The study of the genetic control of processes involved in the detoxification of poisonous substances (similar to pharmacogenetics).

toxicokinetics   The quantitative study of a toxicant's disposition in the body of an affected person over time (similar to pharmacokinetics).

toxicology   The study of the adverse effects of chemicals or physical agents on living organisms.

window of detection   The period of time over which a toxin or its metabolites can be detected in a given sample. The term is commonly used to designate the length of time over which a drug of abuse (or the primary metabolite) is detected in urine.

Methods on CD-ROM

Acetaminophen
Drug screen

Lead
Salicylates

DEFINITIONS

Literally meaning the "study of poisons," the term **toxicology** is derived from the word *toxic*, which traces its origins to the Latin *toxicus*, meaning "poisonous," and the Greek *toxikón*, referring to the **poisons** into which arrows were dipped. From these origins, it can be correctly deduced that early toxicologists focused on identifying, understanding, and using different poisons. Since that time, the field has expanded into a broad and diverse science, integrating many disciplines, including chemistry, biology, physiology, pathology, pharmacology, and genetics. So today, the meaning of *toxicology* has evolved into *the study of the adverse effects of chemical or physical agents on living organisms*. These chemical and physical agents originate from many sources and can be synthetic or natural.

From this it is not surprising that within toxicology we find specialized branches, including those of clinical, forensic, environmental, and occupational toxicology. While each can be defined, there are areas of overlap, and more than occasionally, a situation begins in one area before moving to another. Furthermore, because anything can become a poison, other disciplines may cross into toxicology. For example, *clinical toxicology* focuses on the pathological processes that are caused by the exposure to a chemical and includes the medical evaluation and treatment of the patient. The substances encountered range from illicit street drugs to therapeutic drugs to household products to plants and animal-derived substances. When a patient receiving a drug for therapeutic purposes receives too much drug and exhibits symptoms of toxicity, a process that may have started as therapeutic drug monitoring (discussed in Chapter 56) becomes clinical toxicology. The legal aspects of a poisoning are considered in the area of **forensic toxicology**. This area has expanded from investigations of causes of death (medical examiner or postmortem investigations) and criminal investigations to include probation- and parole-related testing, workplace drug testing, and performance (athletic) testing. Extending our previous example, if the patient was given excessive drug by an individual *intending harm*, then a legal investigation may ensue and the case may enter the forensic arena. Since state and federal laws have been enacted to deter drug use in the workplace, many clinical laboratories have expanded their services to include some forensic toxicology. Workplace drug testing overlaps into *occupational toxicology*, the discipline concerned with the effects of chemicals encountered in the home and workplace. Safety and accident prevention are major concerns of occupational toxicology, and studies have found the use of some drugs to contribute to workplace accidents. Many physicians involved in occupational medicine review, interpret, and investigate results produced by workplace drug testing laboratories. *Environmental toxicologists* are concerned with the harmful effects of chemicals contaminating the atmosphere, soil, water, or food chain. These toxins range from pesticides to industrial waste to bacteria to radioactivity. Many times environmental exposures take place over long periods of time until the individual, or a family member, notices a symptom and seeks medical care.

THE POTENTIAL FOR TOXICITY
The Dose Makes the Poison

The observation made by Paracelsus (c. 1493-1541) is true even today: "All substances are poisons; there is none which is not a poison. It is the **dose** that makes a thing *not* a poison." What becomes clear as one studies toxicology is that *everything* is potentially toxic, but that the *potential* of toxicity depends on the *dose* and the *conditions* under which a person is exposed to the substance. For example, sarin, a nerve gas, is a very potent poison, and yet there is a level below which exposure to this chemical will not cause death. This is the reason why some of the biological and chemical terrorist attacks have resulted in few deaths or gone essentially unnoticed by the general public. At or shortly after release, the toxin was diluted to levels below which few adverse reactions were noticed.[1] On the other hand, a substance as

apparently safe as pure water will, when ingested in sufficient quantity, cause an incapacitating electrolyte imbalance and possibly death.[2] This may be the contributing factor to some of the symptoms observed for users of current **club drugs**. These individuals are encouraged to drink extreme amounts of water, and it has not been unusual to find serum sodium concentrations below 120 mmol/L![3,4] Both of these examples lie on extreme ends of the spectrum of poisonings, so let's consider a third example, iron. Iron is necessary for life; it is the key component of hemoglobin involved in oxygen transport and a cofactor in numerous enzymatic reactions. But iron has a dark side—it is one of the most common poisons to young children.[5] When taken as an overdose, iron is corrosive and causes hemorrhage, ulceration, and gastritis. Additionally, it inhibits key enzymes involved in coagulation, decreases oxidative phosphorylation, and generates the formation of free radicals. In other words, it is quite possible to have too much iron.

Toxicologists find it useful to be able to compare chemicals in terms of *toxicity*. Toxicity is a relative term, and comparisons can be done in several ways. When a population is exposed to increasing doses of a chemical, observed responses can be plotted as shown in Fig. 51-1 (dose response curve). The responses recorded must be defined. For one chemical, hepatotoxicity may be the concern, whereas for another chemical, cardiac arrhythmia may be of concern. There will be a dose, albeit possibly very small, below which no effect or response is observed. This is known as the *threshold dose*. This concept is important because it implies that there is a no-observed-effect level (NOEL), or a safe level of exposure for all toxins.[6-9] What is also seen in these experiments is that not all individuals within the population are affected identically. Usually only a portion of the population is affected at a given dose, but as increasing amounts of the agent are given, the dose becomes great enough so that

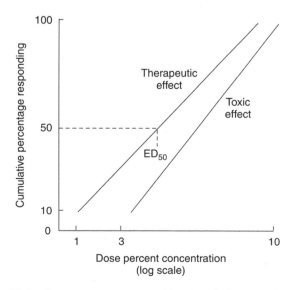

Fig. 51-1 Dose response curve. Results of therapeutic and toxic effects on a population. ED_{50}, Effective dose for 50% of population.

the entire population is affected. This is analogous to the dose response curves observed with therapeutic drugs. The reasons for such individual variability in response include age, gender, ethnicity, health status, and genetic factors. All of these factors contribute to the distribution of the effect of an agent on a population.

Since the most serious harmful effect is death, a drug's **lethal dose** is of particular significance, and the *median lethal dose*, or **LD$_{50}$**, is often considered a useful measure for comparison. Table 51-1 shows the LD$_{50}$ for a selected number of drugs and chemicals. This parameter, initially determined in animal models, represents the dose that causes death to 50% of the population studied. The data determined in these studies are then extrapolated to estimate the equivalent dose for humans. In some cases, the human LD$_{50}$ has been verified from literature reports of exposures.

There are limitations to toxicity studies; some animal test species will be more sensitive to a toxin than are humans, whereas others will be less sensitive. Most chemicals produce more than one effect or response, and not all responses will be observed equally between exposed populations. Finally, and perhaps most important, these experiments are designed to determine acute, not chronic, effects. Chronic toxicities are often not the same as acute responses to an exposure. Still, grouping compounds by the LD$_{50}$ or another response is a useful means to compare the relative amounts or doses required to cause a harmful effect.

Physical Properties of the Toxin

In the simplest of terms, before a chemical can exert a toxic effect, it must gain entry into the body. Thus the physical state of the compound (gas, liquid, or solid) influences the potential of its toxicity. Most inhaled gases and inhalants are quickly absorbed via the lungs. In contrast, liquids are not easily inhaled unless in a vaporous state or aerosol form. Liquids can, however, be absorbed through the skin. Usually, solids must be ingested and dissolved before they produce an effect. A few compounds (such as mercury) exist in a liquid form but have a significant gaseous phase under normal atmospheric conditions. With these, an adequate amount of the compound may be present in the gaseous phase to induce toxicity by inhalation of the vapor.

Unless injected intravenously, all compounds must cross membrane barriers to reach the systemic circulation and eventually travel to the site of action. Three basic mechanisms are involved in this movement: passive diffusion, active transport, and facilitated diffusion. *Passive diffusion* is the primary means by which most drugs and toxins cross membranes. This mechanism does not require the expenditure of energy or the participation of carrier proteins but instead depends on the concentration of the compound on each side of the membrane and the ability of the molecule to move across the membrane. How readily a molecule moves across the membrane depends on its molecular size, pKa (ionization), and lipid solubility. Compounds in the ionized form and those that have greater solubility in water do not move very readily across lipid membranes. If a toxin becomes ionized, it may very well be trapped at that site. *Active transport* requires a carrier molecule and the use of energy, because it is often moving the toxin across a membrane against a concentration gradient. This is one way in which compounds of lesser lipid-solubility are transported. Although *facilitated transport* also involves the use of a carrier protein, the protein is typically embedded within the membrane lipid bilayer. Unlike active transport, this process does not require the expenditure of energy; it is, however, rather competitive since protein-binding sites are limited. Occasionally, toxins are transported via pinocytosis or phagocytosis, two additional mechanisms that play relatively minor roles in membrane transport.

Stereochemistry and Chiral Pharmacology

A number of chemicals exist as stereoisomers. This means they are identical in terms of atomic makeup but differ in the three-dimensional arrangement of the atoms (Fig. 51-2) around a chiral center. Pairs of stereoisomers that are mirror images of each other are known as **enantiomers**. These **chiral drugs** are chemically identical compounds having the same physiochemical properties (melting point, solubility, etc.), but when placed in solution, they rotate polarized light in opposite, but equal, directions. The compounds are designated as *d* or (+) if the light is rotated right, and *l* or (–) if the light is rotated left.

When mixtures of chiral drugs are introduced into biological systems, the differing three dimensional structures will not be recognized equally by receptors, proteins, and enzymes. As a result, they will differ in terms of pharmacological action and toxicity (Table 51-2). If the isomers have more

TABLE 51-1 Approximate LD$_{50}$ of Selected Chemicals

LD$_{50}$ (mg/kg)	Chemical	Species (Route)
190,000	Water injection)	Mouse (intraperitoneal
29,700	Sucrose	Rat (oral)
14,200	Saccharin	Rat (oral)
11,900	Ascorbic acid	Rat (oral)
7000	Niacin	Rat (oral)
5000	Cimetidine	Rat (oral)
4700	Ethylene glycol	Rat (oral)
3000	Sodium chloride	Rat (oral)
1489	Cyclosporine	Rat (oral)
290	Malathion	Rat (oral)
192	Caffeine	Rat (oral)
51	Nicotine	Rat (oral)
24	Sarin	Human (percutaneous)
20	Arsenic trioxide	Rat (oral)
6.4	Sodium cyanide	Rat (oral)
1.4	Arsenic trioxide	Human (oral)
0.65	Aldicarb	Rat (oral)
0.42	Sarin	Mouse (percutaneous)
0.14	VX (nerve agent)	Human (percutaneous)

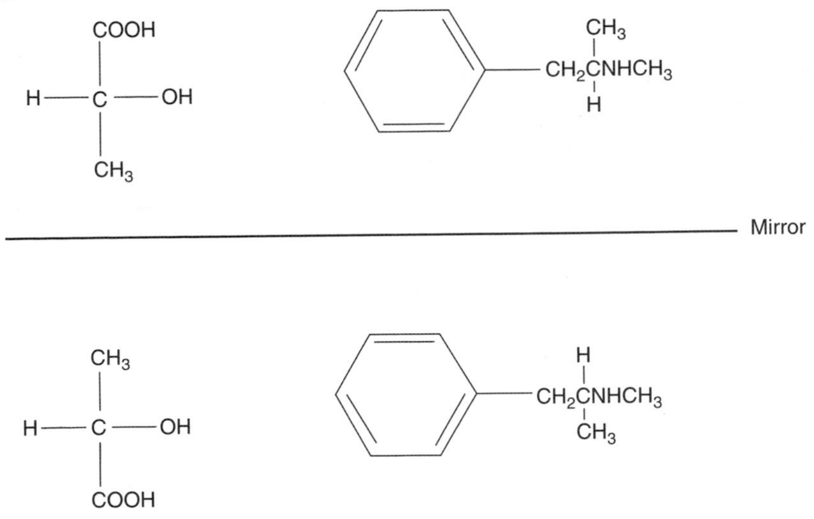

Fig. 51-2 Stereochemistry: Enantiomers. The enantiomeric pairs for lactic acid and methamphetamine are shown. When solutions of these are placed in plane polarized light, the *d* or (+) forms rotate the light to the right whereas the l or (–) forms rotate the light to the left.

TABLE 51-2 COMPARISON OF PHARMACOLOGICAL AND TOXICOLOGICAL DIFFERENCES BETWEEN ENANTIOMERIC PAIRS

Compound	Properties of l-Form	Properties of d-Form
Carnitine		Produces symptoms of myasthenia gravis
Dopa	Anti-Parkinson's activity	Induces granulocytopenia
Ephedrine	Decongestant, bronchodilator, pressor activity, naturally occurring as ephedra in plants (ma huang)	Decongestant, bronchodilator (pseudoephedrine)
Fenfluramine	Does not suppress appetite	Appetite suppression (dexfenfluramine)
Methamphetamine	Decongestant	CNS stimulation
Norepinephrine	Increases blood pressure	Less pressor activity
3-Methoxy-*N*-methylmorphinan	Narcotic activity (levomethorphan)	Cough suppression (dextromethorphan)
3-Hydroxy-*N*-methylmorphinan	Narcotic activity (levorphanol)	Minimal narcotic activity (dextromethorphan)
Sotalol	Beta-blocker	Class III antiarrhythmic

than one asymmetric or chiral center and thus are not mirror images of each other, the pairs are known as *diastereoisomers*.

To illustrate the importance of stereochemistry in toxicology, consider that *l*-methamphetamine is used as a nasal decongestant, whereas its enantiomer, *d*-methamphetamine is an illegal drug with considerable abuse potential. Both compounds have the same chemical structure but clearly possess very different pharmacological activities. Numerous prescribed drugs (Table 51-2) are found as mixtures (racemic) of both enantiomers. In some cases, both compounds possess desired activities, and therefore mixtures may be desirable or advantageous. However, as we have seen with methamphetamine, this is often not the case. Stereospecific chromatographic and electrophoretic techniques are capable of distinguishing enantiomers in biological samples.[10] In contrast, diastereoisomers are usually easily separated from each other.

Duration and Frequency of Exposure

A close relationship exists between dose and time. For many toxins, the length of time over which exposure occurs and the frequency of exposure determine the onset and severity of symptoms observed. This relationship gives rise to two different types of toxicity that must be distinguished from each other: **acute toxicity** and **chronic toxicity**. *Acute toxicity* refers to the ability of a chemical to cause harm as a result of a one-time exposure. For example, acute toxicity occurs when a child ingests some medication or household product. The exposure is sudden, often involves large doses, and may become a medical emergency. *Chronic toxicity* represents the situation in which the exposure occurs repeatedly over a period of time. The dose is usually lower than that necessary to cause an acute response. Chronic exposure is of most concern for those chemicals that are metabolized slowly (i.e., they have a long elimination half-life [$t_{1/2}$]) or deposited in tissues such as bone or fat. In these circumstances, there is a slow accumulation of the substance over time and the effects may be apparent only after many years of exposure. Chronic toxicity cannot be predicted from the responses observed following acute toxicity and may, in fact, affect different organ systems. An acute exposure to a high dose of arsenic by accidental ingestion will produce symptoms of gastric distress, respiratory failure, and possibly death within hours to days. On the other hand, a silversmith may be exposed to low doses of arsenic over many years before having neurological symptoms.[11] The severity of symptoms will vary depending on the agent and on the individual's ability to metabolize and excrete the agent. Occasionally, patients experience a delayed hypersensitivity reaction. In these cases, the patient experiences a severe anaphylactic reaction when exposed to a substance, often at a dose normally considered nontoxic. Typically, the patient has been previously exposed to that substance, or something very similar, and presensitized.

Routes of Administration

The route of exposure to a toxin determines how much of it enters the body and which organs are exposed to the largest dose. Absorption is partially governed by the physical and chemical characteristics of the compound, but the organ exposed plays a key role as well. The skin (dermal), the lungs (inhalation), and the gastrointestinal tract (oral) are the three primary routes of exposure, but it is important to remember that chemicals may enter through other routes such as the eyes, mucous membranes, rectum, or by injection. Although the skin is the most readily accessible organ, for many toxins it provides an efficient barrier of protection, thereby preventing or minimizing exposure. As a result, when the skin is the route of exposure, the potential for toxicity may be the lowest. The route of exposure may also determine the rate of metabolism and excretion of a toxin. For example, some toxins ingested orally are transported via the hepatic portal vein directly to the liver, the primary organ of metabolism, where they undergo extensive metabolism before reaching the circulation (the first-pass effect discussed in Chapter 56 [TDM]). The relationship between the route of exposure and the potential for toxicity can be seen in Table 51-3.

Not only does the route of exposure influence absorption and distribution of the toxin, which affect the rate at which symptoms begin, but the route also influences the intensity and duration of symptoms observed. Consider the routes used to administer cocaine, a drug used medically for its anesthetic effects and illegally for its euphoric effects. The intensity and duration of these effects are related not only to the dose administered but also to the route of administration. When used as an anesthetic, cocaine is administered topically. The dose is low, but this route of administration does not allow enough drug to be absorbed to cause the euphoric effect desired by those using the drug illegally. To achieve euphoria, the user must ingest the cocaine by routes that allow rapid absorption or sufficient dose to reach the central nervous system. When the drug is ingested by either insufflation (snorting) or smoking, the rapid absorption and distribution produces an intense, but brief, high. If the drug is administered by intravenous injection (a rarely used route for this drug), the onset, intensity, and duration of effect would be similar. If absorption is slowed, as happens when cocaine is ingested orally, the duration of the effect is longer but the intensity lower.[12]

Toxicokinetics and Toxicogenetics

Normally occurring physiological differences among individuals contribute to the potential of toxicity. As discussed in Chapter 56, drugs ingested for therapeutic purposes are highly biotransformed by the body. These series of events, collectively known as *pharmacokinetics*, include liberation, absorption, distribution, metabolism, and excretion. Pharmacokinetic processes change throughout life in response to normal changes in physiology and disease. Since these pharmacokinetic parameters govern how much of a dose reaches the target tissues, it makes sense that such changes will also affect toxicity. In general, newborns and older adults are most susceptible to toxicity because both groups metabolize and clear toxins at a slower rate compared with children and younger adults.[13-17] Typically the newborn's liver function will not reach maturity for several months, after which metabolism and the ability to detoxify may actually exceed that of most healthy adults. The metabolic rate of older patients may be one-half to one-third as rapid as that of younger adults. Additionally, the normal diurnal patterns of tubular secretion and glomerular filtration seen in younger adults all but disappears around age 65 to 75.[16, 17]

Body composition in terms of fat-to-muscle ratio varies between males and females and between age groups as well. Thus, the volume of distribution of a toxin may be larger within one group compared with another. Recognizing these differences is important when assessing toxicity following an exposure. Children and smaller adults will likely experience toxicity from smaller doses compared with larger men. Even if a dose is adjusted for size, metabolism or clearance may be slower in newborns or older adults because of differences in organ function.

The toxic actions of chemicals may create some distinct differences for **toxicokinetics**. In the case of an overdose

TABLE 51-3 RELATIONSHIP BETWEEN THE ROUTE OF EXPOSURE AND LD$_{50}$ (MG/KG)

	CHEMICAL		
Route of Exposure	Ethanol	Caffeine	Diphenhydramine
Oral	7060	224	114
Subcutaneous	6000	275	99
Intramuscular	—	200	60
Intravenous	1440	58	20
Dermal	20,000	—	60

with a therapeutic drug, it is not unusual for one or more of the known pharmacokinetic processes to be altered. For example, when many therapeutic drugs are taken with other drugs or as an overdose, the known pharmacokinetic parameters (e.g., half-life, clearance) change. Some toxins delay gastric emptying while others induce diuresis. In many cases of overdose, selective uptake processes involving binding proteins become saturated. When these protective mechanisms are exceeded, the amount of free drug increases and becomes available to act at the various target tissues. (Remember, free drug is active!)

Most discussions of toxicokinetics focus on metabolism. We often think of metabolism as the body's detoxification mechanism, and in most cases, this is true. However, there are a number of drugs or chemicals that are not particularly toxic but whose *metabolites* are toxic. Hence preventing the formation of the toxic metabolites becomes an important part of patient treatment. Often in an overdose, the enzymes involved in metabolism become saturated. In some cases, secondary metabolic pathways are available when this occurs. An overdose of acetaminophen is a good example: when the dose saturates the primary metabolic pathway, the secondary pathway begins to dominate. Unfortunately, this pathway is responsible for the production of a highly toxic metabolite (see Analytes section).

Finally, toxicokinetics also change throughout life in response to health. Changes in organ function due to disease or changes in nutritional status or even hormonal status will also affect how an individual responds to a toxin.

Just as pharmacogenetics (see Chapter 56) is proving a useful tool in therapeutic drug monitoring (TDM), **toxicogenetics** can be used to explain some differences observed among individuals exposed to the same toxin at the same dose under the same conditions.[18-31] Many (but *not all*) metabolic processes take place in the hepatic microsomes via **cytochrome P450 isoenzymes** (CYP450). The cytochrome P450 gene family has evolved over billions of years to accommodate the metabolism of environmental chemicals, food toxins, and drugs. The resulting superfamily of enzymes catalyzes a wide variety of oxidative and reductive reactions and actively transforms a chemically diverse group of substrates. In humans, twelve CYP450 families have been identified and a number of distinct CYP450 isoenzymes may exist within a single cell. The CYP1, 2, and 3 families encode the enzymes involved in most drug **biotransformations**, while the gene products of the remaining CYP450 families are involved in the metabolism of endogenous compounds such as steroids and fatty acids. Table 51-4 describes some of the commonly encountered toxins in the clinical laboratory and the CYP family responsible for their metabolism. In many cases, more than one CYP450 is involved in the metabolism of a substance.[22-29] As can be seen, the table is far from complete—the metabolism rates of many substances by a particular CYP450 isoenzyme have been determined in

---

TABLE 51-4 COMMON DRUGS AND TOXINS METABOLIZED VIA THE CYTOCHROME P450 ISOENZYMES

Cytochrome P450 Enzyme	Drug/Toxin Substrate Metabolized	Inhibitors	Inducers
CYP1A2	Amitriptyline, caffeine, clozapine, haloperidol, imipramine, MDMA, naproxen, phenacetin, phencyclidine, propranolol, theophylline, warfarin	Amiodarone, cimetidine, ciprofloxacin	Tobacco
CYP1B1	Tobacco carcinogens (lung)		
CYP2A6	Nicotine, nitrosamines, aflatoxin		
CYP2C9	Amitriptyline, celecoxib, ibuprofen, naproxen, phenytoin, tolbutamide, warfarin	Amiodarone, fluconazole, fluvastatin, isoniazid, phenylbutazone	Rifampin, secobarbital
CYP2C19	Amitriptyline, diazepam, haloperidol, imipramine, nicotine, omeprazole, phenytoin	Cimetidine, felbamate, indomethacin, ketoconazole	Prednisone
CYP2D6	Amitriptyline, amphetamine, codeine, desipramine, dextromethorphan, haloperidol, heroin, imipramine, methadone, methamphetamine, MDMA, *p*-methoxyamphetamine, nortriptyline, oxycodone, propranolol	Celecoxib, chlorpheniramine, cimetidine, clomiprimine, cocaine, methadone, pentazocine	Amitriptyline, desipramine, imipramine, nortriptyline
CYP2E1	Acetaminophen, caffeine, ethanol, felbamate, fluoxetine, halogenated anesthetics (halothane, isoflurane), halogenated hydrocarbons, isoniazid, methanol, nitrosoamines, propanol, pyrazole, theophylline	Disulfiram, fluoxetine	Ethanol, isoniazid
CYP3A	Carbamazepine, cocaine, cyclosporine, MDMA, phencyclidine, tacrolimus	Midazolam, erythromycin, methadone	Phenobarbital, dexamethasone

Cytochrome P450 Drug Interaction Table (http://medicine.iupui.edu/flockhart); Tanaka E, Terada M, Misawa S: Cytochrome P450 2E1: its clinical and toxicological role, J Clin Pharm Ther 25:165, 2000.

animal models but have not been included here unless also shown to metabolize the drug in humans. Similar tables can be found in a number of reference texts and on the World Wide Web.[29] These resources are a useful toxicological tool, because by identifying an inhibitor, one can often explain a more severe toxic reaction observed in a given patient.[30-31]

Genetic polymorphisms are responsible for many of the differences observed among individuals concerning toxin metabolism. Table 51-5 identifies some of the enzymes for which genetic differences have been identified in humans and some of the agents that may trigger an abnormal response in an affected individual.[30-32] Occasionally gross structural changes are found, such as gene deletion or duplication, but most genetic changes are found to involve single nucleotide polymorphisms (SNPs, see Chapter 47). The location of

the SNP will partially determine its impact on metabolism. Those that occur within the open reading frame of a gene may result in premature termination of transcription, amino acid substitutions, or inappropriate mRNA splicing. Polymorphisms of this type usually lead to decreased or absent catalytic activity of the protein product, although amino acid substitutions can lead to increased activity of the enzymes. SNPs within the regulatory domain of genes can result in altered transcriptional activity of the gene and may include both over- and underexpression of the native gene product. Those occurring within less critical regions may have no effect at all.

The attempt to use known pharmacokinetic or toxicokinetic data is often complicated by the fact that the exact chemical, dose, or time of exposure may be unknown and

TABLE 51-5   EXAMPLES OF IDENTIFIED GENETIC ABNORMALITIES*

Enzyme Affected	Drug/Toxin	Observed Abnormal Response	Frequency
[1]Acetylaldehyde dehydrogenase	Ethanol	Flushing, heart palpitations, vomiting, nausea	1:2 (Japanese)
[1]Acetylcholinesterase	Succinylcholine	Prolonged muscle relaxation, apnea	1:3000
[1]Alcohol dehydrogenase	Ethanol	Flushing, heart palpitations, vomiting, nausea	1 to 5:25 (Caucasian) 1:2 (Japanese)
[1,2]Dihydropyrimidine dehydrogenase	Fluorouracil (5-FU)	Neurotoxicity, myelotoxicity	1 to 3:100 (Caucasian)
[2]CYP2C9	Warfarin	Hemorrhaging	7 to 14:50 (Hh) 1 to 5:500 (HH)
	Phenytoin	Nystagmus, ataxia, drowsiness, nausea, arrhythmias	
	Glipizide, tolbutamide	Hypoglycemia	
	Losartsan	Reduced antihypertensive effects	
[2]CYP2C19	Omeprazole	Enhanced cure rates when taken with clarithromycin	3 to 6:100 (Caucasian)
	Diazepam	Prolonged sedation	8 to 23:100 (Asian)
[2]CYP2D6	Antiarrhythmics	GI disturbances, diplopia, blurred vision	1 to 2:10 (PM)
	Antidepressants	Toxicity in PM, inefficacy in URM	1 to 10:100 (URM)
	Antipsychotics	Tardive dyskinesia	
	Opioids	Respiratory depression, constipation, dependence	
	β-adrenoceptor antagonists	Increased β-blockade (heart failure, broncospasm)	
	Debrisoquine	Orthostatic hypotension	
	Sparteine	Nausea, diplopia, blurred vision	
[2]Glucose-6-phosphate dehydrogenase	Aspirin, chloroquine, quinidine	Hemolytic anemia	
[2]Plasma pseudocholinesterase	Succinylcholine	Prolonged apnea	3:200
[2]N-Acetyltransferase	Sulfonamides	Hypersensitivity	4 to 7:10 (Caucasian)
	Amonafide	Myelotoxicity in URM	1 to 2:10 (Asian)
	Procainamide, hydralazine, isoniazid	Drug-induced systemic lupus erythematosus	
[1]Thioprine methyltransferase	6-mercaptopurine, thioguanineazathioprine	Myelotoxicity	3:100
[3]UDP-glucuronosyltransferase (UGT1A1)	Tolbutamide, rifycin, acetaminophen	Hyperbilirubinemia	23:100 (African) <3:100 (Japanese and Asian)
[2,3]UDP-glucuronosyltransferase (UGT1A1)	Irinotecan, ethinyl estradiol Lorazepam	Diarrhea, myelosuppression Jaundice	1:10

*PM, poor metabolizer; URM, fast/ultrarapid metabolizer; GI, gastrointestinal; Hh, heterozygote; HH, homozygote.
[1]Tanaka E: Update: genetic polymorphism of drug metabolizing enzymes in humans, J Clin Pharm Therapeut 24:323, 1999.
[2]Meyer UA: Phamacogenetics and adverse drug reactions, Lancet 356:1667–1671, 2000.
[3]Burchell B et al: Drug-mediated toxicity caused by genetic deficiency of UDP-glucuronosyltransferases, Toxicol Letters 112:333, 2000.

few poisons are "pure." Household products, cosmetics, pharmaceutical preparations, and street drugs all contain impurities or contaminants. In some cases the "primary" compound of exposure is not toxic, but the chemicals added as solvents, preservatives, or buffers are toxic.[33] Finally, reported exposures typically involve more than one agent.

Interactions

When a patient is exposed to two chemicals, their actions may not be independent; that is, one chemical may affect the action, metabolism, or clearance of the other. When drugs are involved, this phenomenon is called **drug interaction**. The effects of interactions between chemicals (toxic or therapeutic) may not be obvious, and much information about these phenomena has been gathered from anecdotal case reports. Some of these interactions can be explained by studying the enzymes involved in the metabolism of the compounds. It is not unusual for a drug to inhibit the activity of an enzyme involved in the metabolism of another drug or to induce the synthesis of another enzyme. In other cases, two drugs or chemicals may compete for metabolism by the same enzyme, for protein binding, or for excretion. One typically will be more efficiently metabolized, more tightly bound to the protein, or excreted. This means the other remains unchanged for a longer period, or is displaced from its normal carrier protein, or is excreted poorly. Many types of interactions have been noted, and it is not possible to provide a comprehensive list here. Stockley[34] has listed the types of interactions, though he notes that "interactions which occur when drugs are given concurrently are often the result of not a single mechanism, but of two or more mechanisms acting in concert . . . ." Table 51-6 provides this listing with an example of each type of interaction. Drug or chemical interactions may also be more intense in patients who have chronic or acute pathological processes such as congestive heart failure, diabetes, or cirrhosis.[35-38]

Important drug interactions are observed between ethanol and other agents that affect the central nervous system. Ethanol is frequently involved in drug interactions because of its wide usage and its wide range of depressant effects on the central nervous system (see Chapter 34, Alcoholism). For example, the concomitant use of the barbiturates and alcohol can have deleterious effects. The lethal dose of barbiturates is almost 50% lower when combined with alcohol. This same effect occurs with concomitant use of alcohol and agents such as chloral hydrate, paraldehyde, glutethimide, meprobamate, and other tranquilizers.[39] Drug interactions of this type are referred to as **synergistic effects**. This is a toxic situation in which the total effect of two drugs used concomitantly is much greater than the sum of the two drugs' effects when used alone.

Sites and Mechanisms of Toxicity

There are many ways in which toxic agents can cause harmful effects. These can be classified according to the organ(s) affected by the toxin (Fig. 51-3) or by the mechanism of action exerted on the target organ. Both of these will determine whether the toxic effect observed is subtle or dramatic. For some therapeutic drugs, the mechanisms through which the drugs exert their beneficial pharmacological effects at a **therapeutic dose** are intensified at toxic doses. For instance, the pharmacological action of **opiates**, depression of the central nervous system, occurs when the compounds bind to specific receptors. The degree of CNS depression depends on the dose. For other therapeutic drugs the symptoms of toxicity are unrelated to and very different from the desired beneficial effects.

The site most involved in detoxification, the liver, is also the site most vulnerable to chemical induced toxic injury. This is in part related to the vast blood supply of this organ. At any one time approximately 10% to 15% of the total body blood supply will be found in the liver, so it is very difficult

---

TABLE 51-6 EXAMPLES OF CLASSES OF DRUG INTERACTIONS

Action	*Example*
Drugs with similar effects	Multiple nephrotoxic drugs such as gentamicin and cephalosporin yield increased nephrotoxicity.
Drugs with opposing effects	Hypnotics and caffeine result in antagonism to the hypnotic effect.
Absorption interactions	Tetracycline and iron (Fe^{++}) supplement result in decreased oral uptake of drug.
Drug displaced interactions	Theoretical displacement of bound drug from albumin yields increased free-level drug.
Drug Metabolism Interactions	
Enzyme induction	Barbiturates stimulate microsomal oxidation of drugs such as dicumarol, resulting in lower plasma levels.
Enzyme inhibition	Cimetidine blocks the CYP450 oxidation pathway, slowing theophylline metabolism and resulting in a longer-half-life and higher plasma levels.
Altered Excretion Interactions	
Changes in urine pH	Acid urine enhances basic drug excretion. The reverse is true for acidic drugs.
Competition for active tubular secretion	Probenecid decreases the active secretion of drugs such as penicillin, thus increasing serum levels.
Interactions at adrenergic neurons	Tricyclic antidepressants prevent the uptake of guanethidine into neurons, thus blocking its antihypertensive effect.

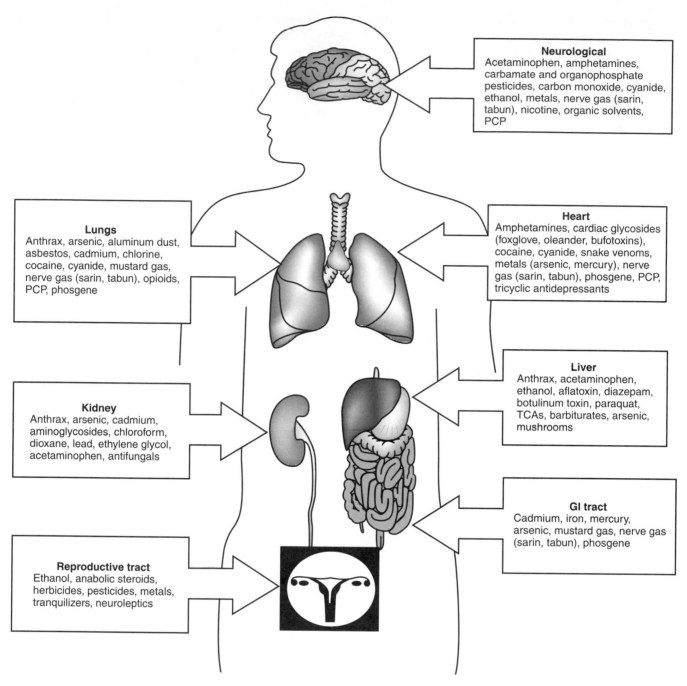

Neurological
Acetaminophen, amphetamines, carbamate and organophosphate pesticides, carbon monoxide, cyanide, ethanol, metals, nerve gas (sarin, tabun), nicotine, organic solvents, PCP

Lungs
Anthrax, arsenic, aluminum dust, asbestos, cadmium, chlorine, cocaine, cyanide, mustard gas, nerve gas (sarin, tabun), opioids, PCP, phosgene

Heart
Amphetamines, cardiac glycosides (foxglove, oleander, bufotoxins), cocaine, cyanide, snake venoms, metals (arsenic, mercury), nerve gas (sarin, tabun), phosgene, PCP, tricyclic antidepressants

Kidney
Anthrax, arsenic, cadmium, aminoglycosides, chloroform, dioxane, lead, ethylene glycol, acetaminophen, antifungals

Liver
Anthrax, acetaminophen, ethanol, aflatoxin, diazepam, botulinum toxin, paraquat, TCAs, barbiturates, arsenic, mushrooms

GI tract
Cadmium, iron, mercury, arsenic, mustard gas, nerve gas (sarin, tabun), phosgene

Reproductive tract
Ethanol, anabolic steroids, herbicides, pesticides, metals, tranquilizers, neuroleptics

Fig. 51-3 Site of toxicity for various agents.

for the organ to avoid exposure to a circulating toxin. Hepatic injury takes many forms from cellular degeneration and necrosis to cirrhosis or cholestasis to vascular injury. Also because of the unique morphology of the organ, the location(s) of the toxic injury may range from particularly focused areas to sites scattered throughout the organ to the most serious situation, in which the entire organ shows damage. Not all hepatocellular toxicity leads to cell death. In fact, cells may exhibit a variety of morphological changes, from swelling to condensed mitochondria in the nucleus, and survive. Fortunately the organ is very resilient to toxic insults. If the injury is not extensive, the organ can regenerate and thus essentially "heal itself"!

Another set of organs frequently susceptible to injury are the kidneys. Not unexpectedly, the primary contributing factor relates to the fact that these two organs receive about 25% of the cardiac output. Another contributing factor lies in the kidneys' ability to concentrate substances as water and sodium are reabsorbed from the glomerular filtrate. Finally, the concentrated substances are transported to the tubular cells, where they accumulate. Overall the kidneys aren't as actively involved in drug/toxin metabolism as is the liver, but there are areas of these organs where numerous metabolizing enzymes are present. For example, a significant amount of CYP450 activity is found in the proximal tubule, one of the sites particularly susceptible to injury.[40]

Pulmonary damage can occur as **toxicants** are inhaled or as the chemical is circulated through the lung. The types of pulmonary injury includes irritation, fibrosis, and destruction of gas-exchanging surfaces (emphysema). As with other organs, some metabolism does take place in the lungs, particularly in the Clara cells of the terminal bronchioles.[41]

Neurotoxicity can be a slow, insidious process or a dramatic one. At the molecular level a chemical may interfere with protein synthesis so that the production of neurotransmitters are enhanced or reduced. Alternatively, a chemical might alter the flow of sodium, potassium, or chloride across ion channels in membranes, thus disrupting transmission of nerve impulses. In other cases, intermediates in signal transduction pathways such as protein kinases and nitric oxide may also be adversely affected. With chronic exposure, it may be difficult to determine whether the symptoms are related to toxicity or a neurodegenerative disease such as Parkinson's or Alzheimer's.[42-46]

Reproductive toxicity involves all stages of reproduction from the development of ovum or sperm to parturition and lactation. Because of the complicated physiological interactions on which the reproductive system depends, many targets for toxicity exist. Unfortunately, exposure to reproductive toxins often occurs through the workplace; this is an area of focus for environmental and occupational toxicologists.[47-49] For example, workers exposed to the fungicide dibromochloropropane were found to have higher rates of sterility, the cause of which was determined to be related to damage to the Sertoli cells of the male reproductive tract.[50] Cadmium is usually associated with nephrotoxicity, but chronic, low level exposure to the metal through occupational settings or from smoking is associated with decreased sperm and ova formation.[51] In some cases, select chemicals or their metabolites are thought to mimic hormones.[52]

The type of organ damage observed relates to the molecular actions of the toxin. Toxins behaving as corrosives or caustics can cause outright cellular injury and destruction, whereas others are subtle. In numerous cases, the chemical substitutes itself as a substrate for an enzyme that is needed for basic cellular function as is the case with organophosphate pesticides. The irreversible binding of these chemicals to cholinesterases prevents the enzyme from hydrolyzing acetylcholine released from nerve endings. Acetylcholine accumulates in nerve cells and overstimulates specific receptors throughout the central and peripheral nervous system. Cyanide exerts its toxic effect by interrupting electron transport in the mitochondrial cytochrome chain. When cyanide binds to the heme group of the final cytochrome in the pathway, the heme molecule is unable to bind oxygen. Electron transfer to molecular oxygen is blocked and cell death occurs. Arsenates and some herbicides act by blocking oxidative phosphorylation. These uncoupling agents allow electron transport to take place but prevent phosphorylation of ADP to ATP. This action increases oxygen consumption, causing heat production and extreme hyperthermia.

When the action of a toxin involves its reaction with the genetic material within the cell, the DNA or RNA for example, the chemical is classified as a genetic toxin. Depending on the mechanism involved and the outcome, the chemical may be further classified as a carcinogen, mutagen, or teratogen. Chemical *carcinogens* are those toxins found to promote cancer within a living organism, whereas *mutagens* and *teratogens* induce genetic changes that become inheritable. The relationship between the occurrence of specific types of cancer and occupational exposure to a chemical was first made in the mid-1700s. Shortly after Hill reported an increased incidence of nasal cancer among snuff users, Sir Percival Pott correlated an increased incidence in scrotal cancer among chimney sweeps.[53] Today we know that in both cases polycyclic aromatic hydrocarbon products, such as benzo(a)pyrene, are the responsible carcinogens. A full discussion of the mechanisms through which chemicals produce genetic changes is beyond the scope of this chapter.

In summary, it is not unusual to find several mechanisms involved in the overall toxicity of a single compound; as a result several organ systems may be adversely affected (see Fig. 51-3). For some toxins the type of injury is distinctive, that is, the microscopic examination of the affected tissue obtained by biopsy will often assist in the identification of, or exclusion of, a toxin.[54]

THE TOXICOLOGY LABORATORY

Most clinical laboratories perform some toxicology testing. The extent of the service varies considerably, depending on a combination of the available personnel and equipment and the medical services supported. A few patients present to the emergency department with a reliable history of exposure, but in many cases, the symptoms of the patient could be the result of disease or trauma instead of a toxin. Though firm identification or exclusion of a toxin is often the desire of the clinician, since everything is potentially toxic, this is neither practical nor possible in every case. Fortunately (for the laboratory), most poisonings involve readily available drugs or chemicals, and most poisonings will be managed symptomatically. Identification is most useful when an **antidote** is available, a specific treatment is indicated, or symptoms are delayed. And so identification represents a small and limited role for most laboratories. Identification of an agent, if present, may provide reassuring information to the clinician, but other laboratory tests may be even more important to the overall management of the patient.[55-57]

Choice of Samples and Methods

The choice of sample depends on a combination of factors. When collecting a sample, the clinician must understand the limitations of the matrix chosen with respect to the purpose of testing, the methods to be used for testing, and the interpretation of the data.

Serum (or blood) is the sample of choice for those analytes where there is a good relationship between the dose found in the body and toxicity. Examples of these include acetaminophen, salicylate, ethanol, carbon monoxide, and certain therapeutic drugs. For an antidote to be administered in the proper amount, it is usually necessary to know how much toxin is circulating in the blood. A list of toxins and antidotes is seen in Table 51-7. Again, for these situations, serum is the sample of choice. Although serum should theoretically be the best sample for the assessment of a patient intoxicated with any drug, some limitations apply with those drugs exhibiting an effect on the central nervous system and those for which the dose-response relationship changes with addiction or tolerance.

Urine is most useful when screening for past exposure. Unless significant renal toxicity is evident, urine is a readily available, easily collected (noninvasive) specimen. For this reason, it is a commonly used sample in the workplace, in rehabilitation clinics, and in athletic testing. It should be remembered that few drugs are found in their original form in urine samples. What is measured is a metabolic end-product, and its presence reflects an exposure that took place in the past. Only in few situations (e.g., the screening for heavy metal exposure) does the presence of a toxin relate to clinical symptoms. Thus it becomes important for the toxicologist to know the length of time (**window of detection**) compounds or metabolites will be detectable in the urine. Not finding a compound in the urine may mean the person was not exposed, or it could mean the exposure was so recent that metabolism to the detected product has yet to occur or that the exposure was so far in the past that elimination is complete.

Other less frequently used samples of importance include saliva, breath, meconium, hair, and nails. Saliva has been of interest because the sample is easily collected and, for a number of drugs, reflects the concentration of drug in the blood. Drugs that are measured in saliva include ethanol, cocaine, amphetamines, barbiturates, **benzodiazepines**, nicotine, phencyclidine, and cannabinoids.[58] Law enforcement personnel have used breath as a sample for the detection of ethanol for many years. Recently, point-of-care devices used for this testing have become popular in emergency and clinical settings. Aspects of ethanol testing using these applications are discussed in Chapter 34, under Alcohol.

Meconium, the complex intestinal contents of the fetus, accumulates from approximately week 12 of gestation until birth. Drugs and drug metabolites are incorporated into meconium when the fetus swallows amniotic fluid containing drugs that have crossed the placenta.[59, 60] Meconium is usually passed by the neonate within 5 days following birth. It is precisely because an infant's first bowel movement usually does not occur until after birth that many researchers feel meconium serves as a final depository for drugs to which the fetus was exposed. Consequently, meconium may offer improved sensitivity for detection of prenatal drug exposure.[60, 61] Finally, unlike urine, meconium has an advantage as a laboratory specimen for newborns because of its relative ease of collection.

Keratinized matrices, such as hair and nails, are yet other specimen types that can be used to detect toxins. Principally, clinical applications of hair and nail analyses include detection of heavy metals, antifungal drugs, and drugs of abuse. Hair and nails offer complementary advantages to more traditional matrices, such as a longer window of detection (weeks to years), less invasive collection procedures, ease of storage (no preservatives or cooling environment required), and stability of analytes within the matrix. However, interpretations of hair and nail results must be performed cautiously because of limited research, lack of meaningful reference ranges, potential for environmental contamination, and other uncertainties that surround these less used matrices.

Toxicology testing uses all available techniques. What method is optimal for a given laboratory depends on, again, the purpose of the testing and the analyte. "Spot tests" using colorimetric or spectrometric methods are described for a few drugs and though rapid, inexpensive, and easy to perform, they are the least sensitive and they are nonspecific. Some of the chemicals required for analysis are considered hazardous and interpretation of the result may be subjective. Techniques such as thin layer chromatography (TLC), gas chromatography (GC), and high-pressure liquid chromatography (HPLC) are useful when testing single samples for multiple chemicals. These methods offer an additional advantage in being adaptable for multiple matrixes (urine, blood, serum, etc.). However, when considering one of these techniques for use in a laboratory, the laboratory director must take into account the level of technical skill available and the response time required. Some chromatographic methods require extensive sample preparation and analysis time and therefore may not be suitable for laboratories with few samples, minimal staff, or rapid response needs.

In contrast, immunoassays techniques are useful when rapid turnaround times are required for a **screening test** or large numbers of samples are to be tested. A range of formats is available, from point-of-care devices to fully automated, high-throughput platforms. For many clinical laboratories, the latter methods offer the ability to perform toxicology testing because they are easy to use, they provide acceptable turn-around times, and the systems are used for other laboratory testing. Along with these advantages have come

TABLE 51-7	EXAMPLES OF POISONS AND ANTIDOTES
Poison	**Antidote**
Acetaminophen	N-acetylcysteine (NAC, Mucomyst)
β-Blockers	Glucagon
Digoxin	Digibind
Ethylene glycol/methanol	4-Methylpyrazole (fomepizole), ethanol
Heavy metals (arsenic, mercury, lead)	Dimercaprol (BAL), EDTA, D-penicillamine, succimer
Iron, aluminum	Deferoxamine
Nitrites, analins, local anesthetics	Methylene blue
Opiates	Naloxone (Narcan)
Organophosphates	Atropine, 2-PAM
Super-warfarins	Phytonadione (vitamin K_1)

limitations that affect the use of these methods within the medical setting, particularly when they are used to test for drugs of abuse in urine (DAU).[57]

In the case of immunoassays, confusion can arise if the specificity of the given test is not fully understood and its subsequent limitations in the medical setting are not appreciated. For some immunoassays, specificity is less than that needed for clinical applications, but for others, the opposite is true. It is imperative that this information is available to the staff of the toxicology laboratory and that staff members understand the limitations of the assays they use for testing.

Mass spectrometry coupled to GC or HPLC is considered the gold standard for identification. As will be discussed, these methods provide the positive identification so important to forensic testing. Finally, remember that *everything is toxic* and that not all toxins can be measured using immunoassay or chromatographic techniques. For example, atomic absorption and inductively coupled plasma-emission spectroscopy are used for metal analysis.

Suicide Versus Accidental Exposures

A useful resource to the toxicologist is the annual report of the American Association of Poison Control Centers (AAPCC).[62] This report lists all toxic exposures reported by participating emergency departments around the country. For the last few years, the number of such exposures have exceeded 4.5 million and resulted in over a million emergency department visits. Of the poison exposures involving children (defined as under age 17 years), most are accidental (Fig. 51-4), in contrast to those involving adults. Again, it is important to remember that most poisonings involve agents

that are readily available. What is "available" depends on the location and the age of the victim, although **analgesics** top the list for both children and adults. The medications and household products involved in pediatric cases are often those that are found in most households and are accessible to the unattended child. It is noteworthy that as more women have begun receiving hormone replacement therapy, hormones and hormone antagonists have made their debut on the pediatric list. On the other hand, as shown in Fig. 51-4, most poisonings involving adults are intentional, many of these being the result of attempted suicides.

Although the number of exposures reported to the AAPCC is impressive, it is important to remember that not all emergency departments participate and so not all exposures are reported through this program. This is further emphasized by the fact that the AAPCC has consistently recorded less than 1000 fatalities annually. In contrast, by reviewing additional death statistics (Table 51-8) one can see that poisons contribute to the cause of death in about 11% of suicides (all ages). This table again emphasizes that readily available drugs or chemicals are used in these attempts, with **antidepressants** or over-the-counter medications demonstrating the highest frequency. About 5% of suicides involve another poison, carbon monoxide. And again, this exposure involves a readily available source—the automobile.[63]

Drugs in the Emergency Setting

The most frequent use of toxicology screens involves the patient who is exhibiting changes in his or her mental status. When a comatose, confused, or bizarrely acting patient is seen in an emergency department, a drug overdose is one

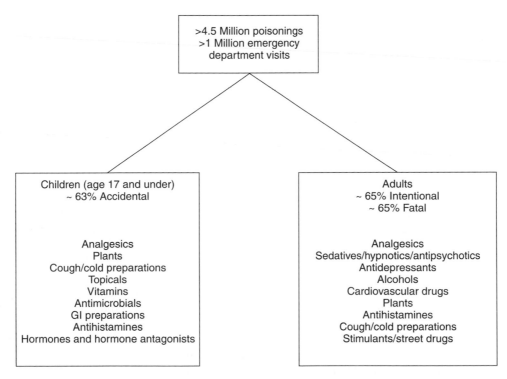

Fig. 51-4   Comparison of poisonings in adults and children. *(From www.AAPCC.org)*

TABLE 51-8 SUMMARY OF POISONING-RELATED DEATHS

Toxin	NCHS Accidental Deaths (%)[1]	NCHS Suicidal Deaths (%)[1]	AAPCC Accidental Deaths (%)[2]	AAPCC Suicidal Deaths (%)[2]	DAWN Accidental Deaths (%)[3]	DAWN Suicidal Deaths (%)[3]
Agricultural preparations (pesticides/ herbicides, rodenticides)	8 (0.1)	28 (0.5)	8 (1.9)	11 (1.3)		
Alcohols (ethanol, methanol, isopropyl)	300 (2.8)		48 (11.3)	66 (8.0)		
Amphetamines			15 (3.5)	9 (1.1)	754 (11.8)	184 (9.9)
Analgesics (opioids, acetaminophen, salicylates, etc.)	3141 (29.1)	508 (9.0)	142 (33.4)	229 (27.7)	5364 (84.0)	1004 (53.8)
Antiinfectives (antibiotics, etc.)	43 (0.4)		3 (0.7)	2 (0.2)		
Cocaine			44 (10.4)	14 (1.7)	3187 (49.9)	455 (24.4)
Gases (pipeline, carbon monoxide, inhalants/aerosols, etc.)	546 (5.0)	2291 (40.6)	38 (8.9)	18 (2.2)	42 (0.7)	12 (0.6)
Hallucinogens (LSD, PCP)	3				71 (1.1)	16 (0.8)
Heavy metals	35 (0.3)	2	1 (0.2)	1 (0.1)		
Household products (cleaning agents, disinfectants, paint, varnish, antifreeze, etc.)	10 (0.1)		9 (2.1)	32 (3.9)		
Psychotropic agents (antidepressants, psychostimulants, etc.)	331 (3.1)		7 (1.6)	152 (18.4)	742 (11.6)	607 (32.5)
Sedatives/hypnotics (barbiturates, benzodiazepines, etc.)	131 (1.2)	823 (14.6)	24 (5.6)	99 (12.0)	1137 (17.8)	819 (43.9)
Total Deaths	10801	5637	425	827	6383	1867

1. National Center for Health Statistics (NCHS), http://www.cdc.gov/nchs/datawh/statab/unpubd/mortabs/gmwki.htm. 1998. General mortality worktable I (GMWKI) provides the total number of deaths for each cause that occurred in the United States in 1998. Fetal deaths are excluded. Individual cause-of-death category numbers are those coded according to the 9th Revision of the International Classification of Diseases (ICD-9).
2. American Association of Poison Control Centers (AAPCC), http://www.aapcc.org, 1999. AAPCC is a nationwide organization of poison centers (70 center members) that collects and analyzes national poisoning data to report in an annual survey known as the Toxic Exposure Surveillance System (TESS). Deaths may have been attributed to a single agent or multiple agents. These data do not reflect deaths in which the manner of death was ruled as "Other/Unknown." These data exclude homicides.
3. Substance Abuse and Mental Health Services Administration: Drug Abuse Warning Network (DAWN) Annual Medical Examiner Data, www.samsha.gov, 1999. These data were collected from 139 DAWN-participant medical examiner's offices, located in 40 metropolitan areas throughout the United States. Deaths may have been attributed to a single agent or multiple agents. These data do not reflect deaths in which the manner of death was ruled as "Other/Unknown." These data exclude homicides and deaths in which AIDS was reported.

of the possible diagnoses that must be considered by the physician. For the most efficient treatment of the patient, it is important for the physician to try to determine the nature or identity of the drug or drugs used. A history obtained from an alert patient can be helpful, though in general, the patient history is not reliable at least 50% of the time.[64] This means that observing the patient's symptoms becomes key in eliminating or including various toxins. Toxic agents can produce a myriad of symptoms, such as respiratory depression, shock, seizures, arrhythmias, hyperthermia, or hypothermia. The size of pupils, the respiration rate and heart rate, electrocardiogram, and the condition of organ systems are all important signs that can provide information about the nature of the toxic substance. For this reason, medical toxicologists often group drugs and toxins according to similarities in clinical presentation. These groupings, collectively known as *toxidromes*, are listed in Table 51-9.[65] As seen, many of the drugs found in each category differ from others within the group by structure or use. Symptoms can be subtle or mixed. (Remember that most poisonings involve more than one agent.)

If the physician suspects the presence of one or more drugs, laboratory tests may be ordered to confirm the presence of the drug or drugs and, when appropriate, to determine the amount present. These data can establish the therapy to be used. Numerous immunoassay methodologies provide rapid testing for a selected number of therapeutic and illicit drugs. While there are limitations to these methods, for many cases these rapid-screening tests enhance patient management. Additional clinical laboratory tests, such as electrolytes, bilirubin, creatinine, and glucose, may be ordered to rule out disease states that can also cause alterations in mental status and to assess organ function if a toxin is present.

Rehabilitation and Monitoring

According to the National Household Survey on Drug Abuse (NHSDA), approximately 2.7 million individuals sought treatment for drugs or alcohol abuse in 1998.[66] Urine **drug screens** are often performed during the initial evaluation of patients seeking substance abuse treatment. It is important to recognize that many of these patients also self-medicate with drugs other than the one for which they are seeking rehabilitation. Once treatment has commenced, drug screens may continue in order to appraise the patient's compliance with the program. For example, in rehabilitation monitoring of opiate abusers, a negative opiate screen is a prerequisite

TABLE 51-9   THE MOST COMMON TOXIC SYNDROMES

Anticholinergic Syndromes

Common signs	Delirium with mumbling speech; tachycardia; dry, flushed skin; dilated pupils; myoclonus; slightly elevated temperature; urinary retention; and decreased bowel sounds. Seizures and dysrhythmias may occur in severe cases
Common causes	Antihistamines, antiparkinsonian medications, atropine, scopolamine, amantadine, antipsychotic agents, antidepressant agents, antispasmodic agents, mydriatic agents, skeletal-muscle relaxants, and many plants (notably Jimson weed and Amanita muscaria)

Sympathomimetic Syndromes

Common signs	Delusions, paranoia, tachycardia (or bradycardia if the drug is a pure alpha-adrenergic agonist), hypertension, hyperpyrexia, diaphoresis, piloerection, mydriasis, and hyperreflexia. Seizures, hypotension, and dysrhythmias may occur in severe cases
Common causes	Cocaine, amphetamine, methamphetamine (and its derivatives 3,4-methylenedioxyamphetamine, 3,4-methylenedioxymethamphetamine, 3,4-methylenedioxyethamphetamine, and 2,5-dimethoxy-4-bromoamphetamine), and over-the-counter decongestants (phenylpropanolamine, ephedrine, and pseudoephedrine). In caffeine and theophylline overdoses, similar findings are observed, except for the organic psychiatric signs, resulting from catecholamine release

Opiate, Sedative, or Ethanol Intoxication

Common signs	Coma, respiratory depression, miosis, hypotension, bradycardia, hypothermia, pulmonary edema, decreased bowel sounds, hyporeflexia, and needle marks. Seizures may occur after overdoses of some narcotics, notably propoxyphene
Common causes	Narcotics, barbiturates, benzodiazepines, ethchlorvynol, glutethimide, methyprylon, methaqualone, meprobamate, ethanol, clonidine, gamma-hydroxybutyrate (GHB)

Cholinergic Syndromes

Common signs	Confusion, CNS depression, weakness, salivation, lacrimation, urinary and fecal incontinence, gastrointestinal cramping, emesis, diaphoresis, muscle fasciculations, pulmonary edema, miosis, bradycardia or tachycardia, and seizures
Common causes	Organophosphate and carbamate insecticides, physostigmine, edrophonium, and some mushrooms

for continued participation in methadone maintenance programs.[67] In addition to voluntary drug treatment admissions, certain populations may also be screened for drug use in order to assess the need for drug rehabilitation. These populations include pregnant women and recently incarcerated persons.

Drug usage surveys such as the NHSDA indicate that the heaviest use occurs in persons between 18 and 30 years of age; for females, these are the peak childbearing years.[66] It is therefore important to identify and treat pregnant drug abusers to minimize potential drug-induced complications to the mother and fetus. In many facilities this process of identification involves urine drug screening, especially if the woman has not received prenatal care.[68, 69] Several studies have demonstrated that self-reporting leads to underestimating the true exposure rate. In studies evaluating cocaine use by pregnant women, there were more than twice as many positive urine results for the cocaine metabolite than there were those who admitted to using cocaine.[70]

Immunochemical screening methods for detection of drug use during and after pregnancy are usually performed on urine obtained from either the mother or infant. While maternal urine may be the most convenient specimen for the detection of drugs, false negative test results are a significant problem since elimination is variable and in most cases only

reflects recent drug use. Neonate urine has been shown to reflect less recent drug use as long as cutoffs are lowered to increase sensitivity. However, urine can be difficult to reliably collect in a neonate as it involves the use of special collection bags that may gap, leak, and irritate the infant's skin.[71] Therefore, improvements in the detection and treatment of maternal drug abuse became the goal of many researchers involved in perinatal care. Toward that end, the use of meconium, the neonate's first bowel movement, was introduced in the late 1980s as an alternative specimen to maternal or neonatal urine for the detection of gestational drug abuse.[61]

MEDICOLEGAL CHALLENGES

Technologists in the clinical toxicology laboratory may become involved in the medicolegal system because results may be subpoenaed for legal proceedings. In these circumstances the technologist may be required to testify under oath regarding the validity of analytical results. Such testimony usually involves a detailed discussion of the analytical procedures used to conduct the test in question, as well as all other laboratory procedures and policies that might be involved.

Laboratories performing drug testing for purposes of investigating death, crime, impaired driving, drugs in the workplace, and athletic performance must perform these tests not only according to good laboratory standards of accuracy and precision but also with impartiality. The methods used by such laboratories, as well as the resulting data, must be legally admissible and defensible. To make sure this occurs, several governmental and professional agencies administer and enforce the policies, procedures, and proficiency testing to be used by forensic laboratories. These agencies include the Substance Abuse and Mental Health Services Administration (SAMHSA), College of American Pathologists (CAP), and the Drug Enforcement Agency (DEA). For some settings, the methodology to be used for all testing is defined by these regulatory agencies. Additionally, these agencies establish the concentrations used to establish a positive result, that is, the cutoff concentration. If the concentration of the analyte is equal to or greater than this administratively established concentration, the result is considered positive. Current protocols for medicolegal testing require both screening and confirmation testing. First, specimens are introduced to a rapid, less specific screening procedure such as immunoassay, colorimetry, or gas chromatography to obtain qualitative results. It is expected that the use of these less specific methods will be more cost-effective since most samples are expected to be negative. All presumptive positive specimens are then confirmed and quantified, using a more sensitive and specific methodology such as gas chromatography-mass spectrometry or high-performance liquid chromatography. For workplace and performance testing, additional procedures are followed before the result is finally validated as positive. These procedures include the evaluation and interpretation of the data by a qualified medical review officer (MRO). It is common to require forensic laboratories to present documents including standard operating procedures, instrument maintenance logs, and the specimen's chain-of-custody during legal testimony (see Chapter 3).

BIOLOGICAL AND CHEMICAL AGENTS OF MASS DESTRUCTION

The use of biological and chemical agents in warfare is not a modern invention. The first documented use of a chemical agent occurred during the Athenian and Spartan Wars (431 BC) when sulfur was burned beneath the city walls of Plataea and Belium. One of the earliest historical uses of biological warfare dates to 1348 AD when Tartar warriors catapulted plague-infected corpses over the city walls of Kaffa in the Crimea.[72, 73] Since these times, man has continued to employ poisons and pathogens in domestic and international acts of warfare and terrorism.

Increasingly, hospitals are being requested to develop and implement strategies for emergency response to victims of biological and chemical mass destruction. Planning tactics include laboratory implementation of diagnostic testing for specific agents, rapid-response victim management and treatment, education and increased awareness of personnel, and organized exercises in emergency preparedness involving hospitals, military, and governmental agencies (e.g., Centers for Disease Control and Prevention, Federal Emergency Management Agency, National Disaster Medical System, Federal Bureau of Investigation, local law enforcement). Furthermore, laboratories must establish protocols for specific specimen handling, biosafety requirements, awareness of reference laboratories with higher-level capabilities, protection for healthcare personnel, and pathways of communication to local and federal authorities and the public.

Fig. 51-5 lists many successful or potential biological and chemical agents of mass destruction. These agents are disseminated by water, air, soil, or vector transmission and may result in injury, illness, disease, and death. The effects can be acute or long-term, and recovery depends on the agent, exposure dose, and treatment. Biological agents are especially threatening because of their:

1. Low cost
2. High rates of morbidity and mortality
3. Pathogenicity to humans, animals, and plants
4. Potential for gene manipulation
5. Ease of preparation and dispersal

The NATO Handbook on Biological Terrorism prioritizes 31 biological agents based on these five attributes. For example, anthrax is designated as "high priority" based on the World Health Organization (WHO) estimate that the release of 50 kg of anthrax spores 2 km upwind of a city populated with 500,000 people would result in 125,000 infections (25%) and 95,000 deaths (19%).[73] In addition, many of these agents are used in combination by terrorists, thereby increasing the effectiveness of the attack by complicating the diagnosis and treatment.[74-76]

HERBALS

As the use of alternative medicines rise in this country, reports of adverse and toxic reactions are increasing as well. A misconception exists among many individuals that "natural" products are safe, or at least less toxic, when in fact some of our most potent toxins are "natural." For this reason, plus the fact that many physicians do not endorse the use of alternative medicines, patients tend to underreport the use of such compounds.[77] These products range from dried materials used to brew teas for consumption, to tinctures, to capsules. Recommendations regarding dosage, preparation, and usage vary considerably and depend on the training of the herbalist. Many herbal preparations are sold over-the-counter or bought overseas. As with conventional medications, patients may not understand the proper use of a product and may, for example, ingest a material that was intended to be applied as a salve.[78] Most are not pure products, but rather mixtures of several products. For most, little research has been done to determine the active compounds or the mechanism of action.[79]

Many natural products are toxic independently (Table 51-10), whereas others are contaminated with toxic materials. Herbals, like other drugs and toxins, act at multiple sites to produce a myriad of effects. Patients using comfrey (*Symphytum spp.*), coltsfoot, chaparral (*Larrea tridemata*), mistletoe, and germander have experienced liver dysfunction

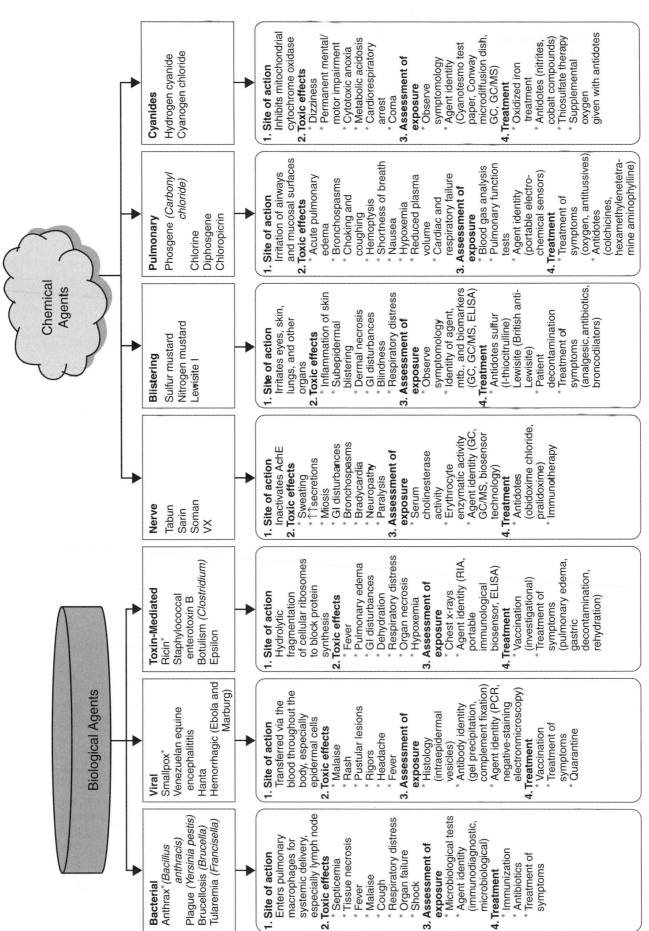

Fig. 51-5 Biological and chemical warfare. Abbreviations: Acetylcholinesterase (AchE); especially (esp.); gastrointestinal (GI); increased (↑); gas chromatography-mass spectrometry (GC/MS); enzyme-linked immunosorbent assay (ELISA); radioimmunoassay (RIA); respiratory (resp.); function (fxn.); treatment (tx). *For biological agents, the site of action, toxic effects, assessment of exposure, and treatment are discussed for the designated agent (*). *(From Jortani SA, Snyder JW, Valdes RV, Jr: The role of the clinical laboratory in managing chemical or biological terrorism, Clin Chem 46:1883, 2000; Budavari S et al, editors: The Merck Index: an encyclopedia of chemicals, drugs, and biologicals, ed 12, Whitehouse Station, NJ, 1996, Merck Research Laboratories; O'Brien T et al: The development of immunoassays to four biological threat agents in a bidiffractive grating biosensor, Biosensors and Bioelectronics 14:815, 2000.)*

TABLE 51-10 HERBALS OF TOXICOLOGICAL IMPORTANCE

Site of Toxicity	Herbal Preparation
Gastrointestinal tract and liver	Kava kava, chaparral, coltsfoot, germander, Chinese teas, mistletoe, comfrey, Jin bu huang
Heart	Ginseng, ephedra, astragalus, salvia, licorice, plantain, oleander, bitterroot
Kidney	Licorice, dandelion, *Aristolochia fangchi*, *Acorus calamus*
Hematopoiesis	Red clover, tang-kuel, yarrow, salvia, pau d'arco, feverfew, ginger, gingko
CNS	Ephedra, tang-keui, yohimbe, valerian, nutmeg, Jimson weed, mandrake, khat, kava kava, ginseng

Herbal Preparation	Reported Drug Interactions
St. John's wort	Cyclosporine, tacrolimus, protease inhibitors, digoxin, theophylline, warfarin, oral contraceptives
Ginseng	Warfarin, heparin, aspirin, nonsteroidal antiinflammatory drugs, corticosteroids
Valerian	Thiopental, pentobarbital, ethanol
Alfalfa	Warfarin
Aloe	Digoxin, diuretics
Feverfew	Aspirin, warfarin
Ma huang	Beta-blockers, caffeine, theophylline, decongestants, methyldopa
Kava kava	Alcohol, sedatives

as a result of alkaloids present in these materials.[80] After using these compounds, patients have experienced effects from mild alterations in liver function tests to more serious conditions, including veno-occlusive disease (Budd-Chiari syndrome), hepatitis, and death. Caffeine, kola, and ephedra are commonly found in products purported to promote weight loss or to increase energy, such as ma huang and guarana. Excessive use of these materials can cause any of the symptoms associated with the sympathomimetic toxidrome, including hypertension and cardiac arrhythmias. Because of its aldosterone-like activity, licorice (*Glycyrrhiza glabra*) can cause hypertension and hypokalemia. As you can see from Table 51-10, the list of potentially toxic herbals is extensive. Some of the plants are cultured commercially; however, the practice of harvesting plants in the wild has led to cases of toxicity when another plant has been misidentified as the intended herb.[81-83]

In other cases, toxicity results from unexpected contaminants such as lead, arsenic, cadmium, ethanol, and mercury. One surprising cause of mercury toxicity was found when women in US states bordering Mexico began to demonstrate neurological symptoms. Eventually, heavy metal screening revealed excessive levels of mercury as the toxin. The source was determined to be an herbal beauty cream originating in Mexico.[84-87]

Both the TDM and toxicology laboratory should be aware of serious drug–herbal-supplement interactions (see Table 51-10). When used with warfarin, products containing feverfew, garlic, gingko, ginger, and ginseng have caused prolonged bleeding times. The interaction of St. John's wort with immunosuppressive drugs and protease inhibitors lead the FDA to issue an advisory cautioning against the use of this alternative medicine with prescription drugs. Licorice, ginseng, plantain, and hawthorn may interfere with digoxin pharmacodynamically or with drug monitoring.[88] Another complication of herbal toxicity is the lack of laboratories that can successfully identify these toxins. Most herbals are not detected by routine clinical testing, although methods for the analysis of some of the more toxic metabolite or components are beginning to appear in the literature. Despite these problems, it must be remembered that some of our conventional drugs (e.g., aspirin, taxol, quinine, digoxin) originated from herbal practices. These products have benefited society tremendously. By conducting rigorous clinical studies, the safety and effectiveness of other herbals and supplements will be identified.[89] The take-home lesson for the toxicologist with respect to alternative medicine is to expect the unexpected and to stay informed.[90]

TREATMENT AND ANTIDOTES

Treatment of the poisoned patient begins by stabilizing the patient's ABCs—airway, breathing, circulation—and includes assisted ventilation, supplemental oxygen, intravenous access, and maintenance of blood pressure.[91-93] Supportive therapy is continued until the body is cleared of the drug. Once stabilized, the patient must be decontaminated of any remaining or unabsorbed toxin.

Here it becomes useful to know the route of entry of the toxin. Skin decontamination may involve washing with soap and water or using vitamin E–laced oils for some pesticides. Treatment options for gastrointestinal decontamination of ingested agents include inducement of emesis (vomiting) with syrup of ipecac, gastric lavage with large bore oral or nasal tubes, administration of activated charcoal, or whole-bowel irrigation. Other toxins are eliminated more rapidly if urine flow is increased (forced diuresis). This is often accomplished by the intravenous administration of a diuretic such as mannitol. In addition, because of a lower concentration in the kidney under diuretic conditions, the potential for nephrotoxicity of some agents (such as cisplatin) is diminished.

Although it is theoretically possible to trap ionized toxins in the urine by altering the urinary pH, the risks associated with this outweigh the benefits in many cases; therefore, use of this decontamination process tends to be restricted to cases involving barbiturates or salicylates. Hemodialysis or hemoperfusion may be also effective. Hemodialysis is useful in removing water-soluble toxins that have a low molecular weight, low volume of distribution, and low protein binding. Chelating agents such as ethylenediaminetetraacetate (EDTA), deferoxamine (DFO), and British antiLewisite (BAL) are used to bind and remove metals. The history of poisons is intertwined with that of antidotes. Unfortunately, compared with the number of toxins encountered, there are relatively few antidotes available. Some of the more commonly encountered antidotes are presented in Table 51-7. The use of these antidotes, as with the previously discussed treatments, must be considered carefully because many have their own set of risks, precautions, and contraindications.[93]

ANALYTES
Analgesics

Acetaminophen is used therapeutically for its antipyretic and analgesic activity, but it has very little anti-inflammatory activity. For most individuals, this drug is a safe alternative to aspirin. Acetaminophen-containing products became very popular following the recognition of a relationship between the occurrence of Reye's syndrome in children and the use of aspirin.

When taken in therapeutic doses, most of the acetaminophen dose is metabolized to nontoxic glucuronide and sulfate metabolites. A small amount is metabolized by several CYP450 isoenzymes (CYP450 3A4, 1A2, 2E1, 2A6, 2D6). Unfortunately, some of these P450s produce a toxic metabolite, *N*-acetyl-*p*-benzoquinone imine (NAPQI).[94] Some NAPQI is produced under therapeutic conditions but is rapidly removed by glutathione before significant damage can be done. In an overdose, excess NAPQI is produced because there is not *enough* glutathione to remove the metabolite.

The hepatotoxic effects of acetaminophen overdose have received much attention, but other organ systems may be affected, including the kidney and central nervous system.[95] In fact some patients have had acetaminophen-related renal failure without hepatoxicity.[96]

Symptoms of toxicity are often delayed and may initially be mistaken for influenza, so poisoning may not be suspected. Left untreated, toxicity progresses by day 3 or 4 to more serious events, including jaundice, bleeding, neurological changes, hepatic necrosis, and death. The risk for hepatotoxicity increases with the use of any drug that induces the CYP 2E1 isoenzyme (e.g., co-ingestion of ethanol). If overdose is determined within 24 hours, an antidote, *n*-acetylcysteine (Mucomyst) is given.[97]

The toxicokinetic picture can be complicated. First, acetaminophen is often combined with other toxic drugs such as codeine or caffeine. The drug is also available in time-released or long-acting formulas. Interpretation of serum levels is more difficult when these formulas have been used.

The preferred specimen for analysis is serum with levels quantified using either immunoassay or HPLC. The therapeutic range is 10 to 20 µg/mL; toxicity is likely when levels are greater than 150 µg/mL at 4 hours or more after ingestion. If the time of ingestion is known to be greater than 4 hours and the ingestion is acute, a single quantitative determination may be adequate. This result is evaluated using the Rumack-Matthew nomogram or another similar to that seen in Fig. 51-6. If the time of ingestion is unknown, serial measurements are recommended, initially and approximately 2 to 3 hours after decontamination. If the patient is

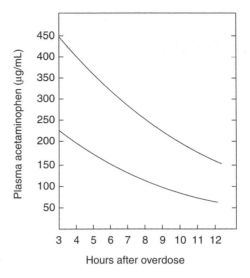

Fig. 51-6 Plasma acetaminophen concentration in relation to time after an acute overdose. Liver damage is likely to be severe above upper line, severe to mild between lines, and clinically insignificant under lower line. *(From Prescott LF et al: Cysteamine, methionine, and penicillamine in the treatment of paracetamol poisoning, Lancet 2(7977):109, 1976.)*

thought to have taken acetaminophen chronically and toxicity is suspected, levels should be determined in two samples collected 3 to 4 hours apart, and the $t_{1/2}$ should be calculated. The patient's renal and liver function should also be monitored.

Salicylates are most commonly ingested as aspirin (acetylsalicylic acid). This compound is rapidly metabolized to the active drug, salicylic acid. The incidence of pediatric poisonings involving salicylates decreased following the recognition of a relationship to Reye's syndrome. At that time, medical personnel and parents were discouraged from using the drug to treat children who had fevers. Today, the number of aspirin-related poisoning episodes is about one-third the number of poisonings with acetaminophen. For children salicylate poisonings are usually acute and involve an overdose, whereas for adults, chronic toxicity may be more common and can go unrecognized for some time. Even at therapeutic doses, salicylates cause direct uncoupling of oxidative phosphorylation and direct stimulation of the CNS, resulting in hyperventilation and respiratory alkalosis. Also, because they disrupt the Kreb's cycle, these drugs cause metabolic acidosis. It is not uncommon to find patients with symptoms of chronic intoxication (ringing in the ears, nausea, unsteady gait). In overdose, gastric emptying slows, so half-life increases by about tenfold. The drug has a low volume of distribution (VD), so decontamination using charcoal or dialysis is effective. As with acetaminophen, salicylate is often found in combination with other drugs (diphenhydramine (Benadryl®), caffeine) and often formulated as a time-released preparation.

Serum is the preferred sample, although the compound can be detected in urine. The therapeutic range depends on use: 20 to 100 µg/ml for analgesia and 100-µg/mL for antiinflammatory activity. The reported toxic range is >300 μg/mL. Levels should be measured initially or after decontamination and approximately 3 hours later to ensure successful decontamination. Methods include colorimetric (Trinder reagent), enzymatic, GC, or HLPC. Patients should also be monitored by blood-gases, pH, electrolytes, and liver function tests.

DRUGS OF ABUSE

The analytes measured within this group (Table 51-11) include families of drugs such as the benzodiazepines and opiates, as well as specific drugs such as lysergic acid diethylamide (LSD) and phencyclidine (PCP). Typically, testing is requested to assist in determining whether the patient's symptoms are caused by one of these drugs (as opposed to trauma or disease) or if substance abuse is expected. Because most **abused drugs** are illegal or are used illegally, drugs of abuse testing serves as a good example in which clinical toxicology testing may transition to the forensic arena. Serum is not used; instead, urine is the sample of choice (hence the term *drugs of abuse in urine* [*DAU*]). When interpreting the results from these tests (Table 51-11), the clinician must remember that most drugs appear in urine as a combination of parent drug and metabolites. Some drugs/metabolites are detectable in the urine for a few hours (LSD), whereas others are excreted for days to weeks (cannabinoids). Since most methods are designed to measure specific metabolites, nothing can be concluded about the active drug in the body (if any remains). This sometimes causes confusion when clinicians obtain a report that a drug is present in the urine, but the patient does not show clinical symptoms of intoxication.

Most clinical laboratories use immunoassay-based methods for DAU testing to provide rapid turnaround times demanded by emergency departments. These assays may cross-react with other metabolites or even with other drugs. Further testing to confirm the presence of the drug should be available either in-house or through a reference lab.

Amphetamines. Amphetamine, methamphetamine, and their derivatives (methylenedioxyamphetamine, methylene-dioxymethamphetamine [see Club Drugs, below]) are sympathomimetic amines that stimulate the CNS, producing excitement, alertness, euphoria, loss of appetite, and reduced sense of fatigue. Both psychological and physiological addiction can occur with amphetamine use. Amphetamines have been used therapeutically to treat narcolepsy, obesity, and attention deficit/hyperactivity disorders. Because of the high potential for abuse, the Code of Federal Regulations Controlled Substance Act categorizes most amphetamines as Schedule II substances. Routes of amphetamine administration include oral ingestion, injection, inhalation, and insufflation. Side effects at low doses include irritability, anxiety, insomnia, blurred vision, hypertension, and cardiac palpitation. Acute toxicity results in agitation, hyperthermia, convulsions, coma, and respiratory and cardiac failure. Amphetamines are rapidly absorbed from the gastrointestinal tract and widely distributed throughout the body. In the liver, amphetamines are metabolized to more polar forms to be

TABLE 51-11   DRUGS OF ABUSE (DAU)

Drug Group	Drugs in Group	Window of Detection	Metabolite Used in Assay	CUT-OFF (ng/mL)	
				Screen	GC/MS
Cannabinoids (THC)		1-30 days	THC-acid	50	15
Cocaine		<72 hours	Benzoylecgonine	300	150
Phencyclidine		<3 days	PCP	25	25
Amphetamines/ methamphetamines	D-amphetamine, D-methamphetamine, ephedrine, pseudoephedrine, phenylpropanolamine, MDA, MDMA, MDEA, PMA	2-4 days (dose/form dependent)	D-amphetamine D-methamphetamine	1000	500
Opiates	Heroin, codeine, morphine, synthetic opioids (methadone, propoxyphene, fentanyl, hydrocodone, etc.)	2-5 days	Morphine sulfate	2000	2000*
Barbiturates	Butabarbital, talbutal, phenobarbital, pentobarbital, secobarbital, amobarbital	1-21 days (dose/form dependent)	Secobarbital	200	
Benzodiazepines	Oxazepam, nordiazepam, diazepam, flurazepam, etc.**	~72 hours	Nordiazepam	100	
LSD		<12-24 hours	LSD	0.5	

*Codeine and morphine only; must assay for 6-acetylmorphine also (heroin metabolite).
**Detected benzodiazepines will vary.
The drugs in the shaded box above are known as the NIDA 5. The methods of detection and of quantifying the cutoffs are dictated by a committee of the National Institutes of Drug Abuse that oversees testing in the workplace.

excreted. Depending on urinary pH, amphetamines are mostly eliminated from the body within 48 hours. These drugs are detected using various methods, including immunoassays and gas chromatography (see Method of Analysis section on the CD-ROM). Methods are available to distinguish among the racemic forms.

Barbiturates. Barbiturates are CNS depressants used medicinally as anxiolytic, anticonvulsant, anesthetic, and muscle-relaxant agents. Barbiturates are controlled as Schedule II, III, and IV drugs. These drugs bind to the chloride channel molecule of the GABA receptor, inducing sedation, euphoria, and mood alterations. Oral and parenteral administrations are the most common ways to take barbiturates. Depending on their duration of action, barbiturates are categorized as ultrashort-, short-, intermediate-, or long-acting drugs. Once absorbed, the major pathways of hepatic biotransformation include oxidation and glucuronide conjugation. Undesirable effects include drowsiness, mental impairment, dysarthria, and ataxia. At elevated levels, barbiturates can cause coma and cardiovascular and respiratory depression. Immunoassays are used to screen for drugs found in the barbiturate class. Chromatographic methods, including GC, GC/MS and HPLC, are used to identify and quantify specific barbiturates.

Benzodiazepines. Benzodiazepines have a pharmacological response similar to barbiturates and are used for the same applications. Most benzodiazepines are classified as Schedule IV drugs; flunitrazepam, however, is categorized as a Schedule I drug. Benzodiazepines are commonly given orally or parenterally. The side effects of these drugs are similar to, but milder than, those of barbiturates. Physical dependence and withdrawal symptoms (including insomnia, agitation, irritability, muscle tension, psychosis, and seizure) may occur with long-term use. Hepatic metabolism reduces benzodiazepines to active and inactive compounds with a half-life equal to or longer than that of the parent drug. The antibodies used in the immunoassays designed to screen for drugs found in the benzodiazepine class are often targeted to nordiazepin. For other benzodiazepines, the degree of cross-reactivity varies considerably. For example, some immunoassays do not detect the presence of flunitrazepam, whereas others may do so if the concentration is sufficient. Chromatographic methods, including GC, GC/MS and HPLC, are used to identify and quantify specific benzodiazepines.

Cannabinoids. Δ^9 tetrahydrocannabinol (THC) is one of at least 61 cannabinoids found in the hemp plant, from which marijuana originates. Binding to the CB1 receptor, THC is the primary psychoactive compound of marijuana that produces the euphoric and relaxant effects for which it is abused.[98] Principal routes of administration are inhalation and ingestion. THC is classified as a Schedule I drug since it has no acceptable medicinal use and a high abuse potential. Generally, THC is believed to be nonlethal when used alone, although some patients exhibit adverse effects such as tachycardia, respiratory anomalies, and behavioral and mental impairment. Tolerance and mild withdrawal symptoms may be experienced following prolonged use. THC is highly lipophilic, rapidly metabolized to more than 20 metabolites. The primary urinary metabolite, 11-nor-Δ^9-tetrahyrdocannabinol-9-carboxylic acid (THC-COOH), is used to identify THC use. Approximately 70% of a THC dose is excreted in feces and urine within 72 hours; however, in frequent users, half-lives greater than 10 days may occur. THC and its metabolites are detected using immunoassay and chromatographic techniques.

Cocaine. Cocaine is a potent CNS stimulant used as a local anesthetic in surgical procedures of the eyes, nose, and throat. Cocaine binds to the dopamine reuptake transporter of the CNS. Because of its high risk for psychological and physical addiction, cocaine is classified as a Schedule II drug. It is available as a hydrochloride salt, which is usually snorted or injected, or as a base that is smoked. The vasoconstrictive action of cocaine can result in myocardial infarcts, subdural hemorrhages, cardiac dysrhythmias, and stroke. Other signs of acute toxicity include intense paranoia, bizarre and violent behavior, hyperthermia, pulmonary dysfunction, and sudden collapse. Cocaine is rapidly metabolized by enzymatic and nonenzymatic processes to its major metabolites, ecgonine methyl ester (EME) and benzoylecgonine (BE), respectively. When ingested with ethanol, the unique cocaine metabolite cocaethylene is formed. Most of a cocaine dose is excreted in the urine within 24 hours as unchanged parent (1% to 9%), EME (32% to 49%), and BE (35% to 54%).[99] Cocaine and its metabolites are detected using immunoassay and chromatographic techniques.

Opioids. Opioids consist of naturally occurring alkaloids of opium (morphine, codeine), synthetic derivatives of opiates (heroin), and other synthetic compounds with actions and analgesic potency similar to that of morphine (methadone, propoxyphene, oxycodone, meperidine, fentanyl). Several types of opioid receptors (mu, μ; kappa, κ; delta, δ, sigma, σ) are located throughout the central nervous system and various tissues. Opioids are prescribed as analgesic, antitussives, and antidiarrheal agents; for relief of acute pulmonary edema; and as suppressants to prevent relapse in heroin addicts (narcotic antagonists such as naltrexone, nalorphine). Opioids are mostly classified as Schedule I (heroin) or Schedule II (morphine, codeine, methadone) drugs. Opioids are abused for their CNS effects, including euphoria, sedation, and relaxation. Routes of administration include intravenous, intranasal, oral, and parenteral. Tolerance, physical dependence, and withdrawal syndromes are closely associated with opioids. Adverse effects include hypotension, pulmonary edema, respiratory depression, coma, and death. Hepatic enzymes rapidly metabolize opioids to more readily excretable forms. Immunoassays are used to screen for drugs found in the opiate class. Chromatographic methods, including GC, GC/MS and HPLC, are used to identify and quantify specific opiates and metabolites.

Phencyclidine. Phencyclidine (PCP, *l*-phenylcyclohexylpiperidine) is a potent hallucinogenic agent and dissociative anesthetic that is classified as a Schedule I substance that has no medical applications. Identified receptors for PCP in the brain either closely resemble or are identical to opioid sigma receptors. PCP antagonizes the glutamate receptors and may block dopamine uptake as well. PCP and its analogs—cyclohexamine (PCE), phenylcyclohexylpyrrolidine (PHP), and thienylcyclohexylpiperidine (TCP)—are snorted, taken orally or intravenously, or smoked in combination with marijuana or tobacco. Tachycardia, psychosis, paranoia, combativeness, mydriasis, and respiratory depression are all documented undesirable effects of PCP. Because of its high lipophilicity, PCP can be stored in the brain and adipose tissue for extended periods. Metabolism occurs principally in the liver through oxidative hydroxylation and conjugation followed by renal clearance. Methods of analysis include immunoassay and gas chromatographic techniques.[99]

Club Drugs

This loose category of drugs (listed in Table 51-12), originally named because of its presence and popularity within the dance club scene, includes 3,4-methylenedioxymethamphetamine (MDMA), gamma hydroxybutyrate (GHB), ketamine, and flunitrazepam.[100] With the exception of ketamine, these club drugs are listed as Schedule I and thus defined as "drugs of abuse with no medical utility." Diphenhydramine and dextromethorphan, two over-the-counter medications, are sometimes included in this group. When taken in high doses, these drugs can cause hallucinations.

3,4-methylenedioxymethamphetamine (MDMA, Ecstasy) is a distant cousin of methamphetamine but does not cause the same physiological and psychotropic effects. Usually taken orally as a tablet or capsule, the drug causes a euphoric sensation about 20 to 40 minutes after ingestion. Most users report no loss of control but find their memory and mental skills decreased when challenged. Side effects include hyperthermia, nausea, tooth grinding, and jaw clenching. Users frequently suck on a pacifier or lollipop to lessen the sore jaw. Dehydration and heatstroke are common side effects of this drug that result in admission to emergency departments. These conditions are further exacerbated by a combination of increased activity without rest and high room temperature in the typical nightclub environment. Several case reports indicate that the hyperthermia and high levels of physical activity have lead to a syndrome of cardiac arrhythmia, rhabdomyolysis, acute renal failure, and disseminated intravascular coagulation similar to that seen with severe heatstroke. To prevent dehydration, Ecstasy lore dictates drinking large quantities of water while under the influence; this in turn has lead to severe water intoxication and hyponatremia.[3,4]

Another consequence of MDMA use is the sudden onset of fulminant liver failure in some users. Although there is evidence of neurotoxicity when animal models are given doses equivalent to that used by humans, evidence of neurotoxicity in humans has not been easily obtained. Evidence suggests that neurotoxicity may become more evident after long-term use.[101] Gas chromatography with mass spectrometry is used to identify the presence of MDMA.

Gamma hydroxybutyrate (GHB), an endogenous chemical, is similar to the neurotransmitter GABA. GHB is a powerful

TABLE 51-12 PHARMACOLOGICAL AND TESTING ASPECTS OF CLUB DRUGS

Drug	Street Names	Metabolites	Sample	Methods of Detection	Window of Detection	Miscellaneous
Methylene dioxy-methamphetamine (MDMA)	Ecstasy, Adam, X, XTC	3,4-methylenedioxy amphetamine (MDA), 4-hydroxy-3-methoxy methamphetamine (HMMA), 4-hydroxy-3-methoxy amphetamine (HMA)	Urine, plasma	Some cross-reactivity of MDA metabolite with amphetamine immunoassays GC; GC-MS	urine ~24 hours plasma ~5 to 6 hours	Metabolized by CYP2B6 and CYP2D6; other similar drugs include MDEA, PMA.
Gamma-hydroxy-butyrate (GHB)	Georgia Home Boy, Gamma-OH, Grievous Bodily Harm		Urine, serum	GC-FID; GC-MS	urine: <12 to 24 hours serum: $t_{1/2}$ <1 hour	Detected levels of GHB will increase in citrate buffered blood.
Flunitrazepam (Rohypnol)	Roofie, Roche, La Roche, Rope	7-Aminoflunitrazepam, N-Desmethy-flunitrazepam, 7-acetamido-flunitrazepam, Norflunitrazepam	Urine, plasma	Some cross-reactivity with benzodiazepine immunoassays; GC-MS	Peaks in urine <6 hours Urinary metabolites detectable up to 28 days	
Ketamine (2-[2-chlorophenyl]-2-methylamino-cyclohexanone)	Special K, Cat Valiums, Vitamin K, KitKat	Norketamine, Dehydronorketamine	Urine, plasma	GC-MS		

Adapted from Gulledge C, Phillips J, Hammett-Stabler C: New kids on the block: an update on selected "club drugs," Therapeutic Drug Monitoring and Clinical Toxicology Division newsletter, 15(4):1, 2000.

sedative/**hypnotic** that causes euphoria and loss of inhibitions, similar to the effects of alcohol. Larger doses cause muscle relaxation and hallucinations.[102] Side effects are related to depression of the central nervous system and may include drowsiness, dizziness, nausea, vomiting, loss of muscle control, amnesia, and unconsciousness. The more serious toxic effects found with higher doses include seizures, bradycardia, and respiratory depression. Chromatographic methods are used to detect the presence of GHB.

Ketamine is used in anesthesia induction before surgery and in veterinary medicine. It is structurally similar to phencyclidine and produces a similar pharmacological effect of dissociation. At higher doses the drug produces a hallucinogenic state, which users equate to a near-death experience. The use of this drug is associated with hallucinations, nystagmus, lethargy, tachycardia, and hypertension. It is most dangerous when combined with ethanol, benzodiazepines, or GHB. Ketamine can be detected using chromatographic methods.

GASES

Carbon monoxide (CO) is one of the leading causes of death in this country (Table 51-8), either through accidental exposure or suicide. CO is a tasteless, odorless gas produced when combustion is incomplete. Carbon monoxide binds tightly to iron in hemoglobin and, in doing so, increases the affinity of the hemoglobin for oxygen. As a result, oxygen is not made available to the tissues of the body. Depending on the dose and duration of exposure, symptoms of CO poisoning range from mild headache to seizures and death. The antidote is oxygen. When available, optimal treatment is achieved using hyperbaric oxygen therapy, in which 100% oxygen can be administered under 2 to 3 atmospheres.[103] The level of CO is determined in whole blood using spectrophotometry (co-oximetry) or GC.

METALS

In many cases, poisoning by heavy metals, including aluminum, arsenic, cadmium, copper, iron, lead, and mercury (Table 51-13), is difficult to diagnose unless a clear history of acute exposure is available. Patients are often exposed to these metals at work or in the home, where the exposure may not be realized for some time. Inhalation of metallic fumes or dusts is the most significant route of occupational exposure. As mentioned earlier, iron from prenatal vitamins remains a common poisoning risk to young children. With heavy metal poisoning, it is important to identify the source of exposure to prevent reexposure or exposure of other individuals. Possible sources include well water, seafood, pressure-treated lumber, paint, and alternative medicines.

In many cases, metals exert toxicity by binding to sulfhydryl groups found in various enzymes and proteins. This action renders the protein inactive. An important feature to remember is that many enzymes and proteins will be affected but some are much more likely to be involved at low doses. For example, cadmium is considered to be extremely nephrotoxic. Very low doses initiate morphological changes in the proximal tubules of experimental animals.[104] But cadmium also causes adverse pulmonary, cardiovascular, and reproductive symptoms. Exposure to most metals produces similar symptoms, with neurological changes (memory loss, mood changes, loss of coordination) and abdominal pain occurring frequently. The optimal specimen type (blood or urine) depends on the metal and whether exposure is thought to be recent, chronic, or acute. The use of metal-free containers is important regardless of the specimen type. Methods used to test for heavy metals include atomic absorption, inductively coupled plasma emission spectroscopy, and mass spectrometry.

Treatment of the patient includes the use of chemicals that bind directly with the metal ions to form stable complexes,

TABLE 51-13   TOXICITY OF HEAVY METALS

Metal	Mechanism	Symptoms	Sample
Arsenic	Binds sulfhydryl groups of enzymes and proteins, uncouples oxidative phosphorylation	Acute: garlic odor, gastrointestinal distress, cardiac arrhythmias, uremia Chronic: weakness, malaise, weight loss, hyperpigmentation, Mee's lines, neuropathy, loss of memory	Urine, hair, nails, blood (if exposure within 4 hours)
Cadmium	Binds sulfhydryl groups; binds carboxyl, cysteinyl, histidyl, hydroxyl, and phosphatyl groups	Gastrointestinal distress, irritability, proteinuria, glycosuria, aminoaciduria, muscle cramps, pulmonary edema, hypertension, loss of memory	Urine, hair
Iron	Corrosive, free radical formation, lipid peroxidation	Bleeding, irritability, tachycardia, metabolic acidosis, fever, hepatic necrosis	Serum
Lead	Binds to sulfhydryl groups	Acute: salivation, vomiting Chronic: hematological (basophillic stippling, hypochromic normocytic anemia), ataxia, nausea, constipation, irritability, convulsions, neuropathies, coma, loss of memory	Whole blood, urine (also erythrocyte protoporphyrin)
Mercury	Corrosive; binds to sulfhydryl, carboxyl, amide, and amine functional groups	Chronic: fine muscle tremors, anorexia, weight loss, fatigue, emotional changes, irritability, loss of memory	Urine

and includes such chelators as ethylenediaminetetraacetic acid (EDTA), British Anti-Lewisite (dimercaprol), or deferoxamine. These complexes are water-soluble and readily excreted by the kidney.

PESTICIDES

Over 1500 active pesticide ingredients are registered with the US Environmental Protection Agency (EPA).[105] Most studies assessing the toxicity of pesticides involve single chemicals. In practice, however, several pesticides are often mixed by the manufacturer or the consumer; in other cases, pesticides may be used sequentially. These practices, as well as exposure to any additives or contaminants, contribute to the difficulty in evaluating toxicity in patients exposed to pesticides. Regional poison control centers and county extension agents are often useful resources for information regarding pesticide products. Additional resources are found via the Internet.[106-109]

Insecticides represent the largest category of toxins found in the home. The three major groups of insecticides, in order of highest to lowest toxicity, are the organophosphates, carbamates, and pyrethroids. Most insecticides found in the home contain pyrethrins and growth regulators rather than organophosphates and carbamates. Insecticides of the organophosphate and carbamate categories are neurotoxins that act by phosphorylating pseudocholinesterase (SchE) and acetylcholinesterase (AchE). When this happens, enzymatic activity is inhibited and the cholinergic neurotransmitter, acetylcholine, cannot be hydrolyzed on its release from the nerve ending. The accumulating acetylcholine continues to stimulate muscarinic and nicotinic receptors throughout the central and peripheral nervous system. Most organophosphates are designed so that the inhibition of the cholinesterases is irreversible. In contrast, the neurotoxic actions resulting from carbamate exposure reverse with time. The clinical signs and symptoms of acute organophosphate poisoning are directly related to the degree of cholinesterase inhibition. Pseudocholinesterase activity decreases more rapidly than that of acetylcholinesterase.[110, 111] Clinical symptoms of acute poisoning are experienced when about 40% of the cholinesterase is inhibited; these symptoms include wheezing and increased bronchial secretions. With moderate to larger exposures, muscle weakness, paralysis, tachycardia, headache, ataxia, and confusion occur. In cases of massive exposure, death occurs when respiration is blocked by a combination of bronchoconstriction, increased bronchial secretion, diaphragmatic contractions, and inhibition of the respiratory centers in the brainstem.

Organophosphate exposure is associated with an additional neurotoxic syndrome known as *organophosphate-induced delayed neuropathy (OPIDN)*. This syndrome is not related to cholinesterase inhibition but to inhibition of neurotoxic esterase (NTE).[112, 113] The clinical presentation of OPIDN occurs several days to weeks after exposure, when the cholinergic symptoms have resolved. Symptoms include mild sensory disturbances, ataxia, weakness, fatigue, reduced tendon reflexes, and muscle twitching and tenderness. In severe cases, it may progress to flaccid lower limb paralysis. Frequently, memory and cognitive abilities are impaired. Histological findings include degeneration of long and large-diameter axons in peripheral nerves and spinal cord. No specific therapy is available; resolution of the symptoms may take months or years, or symptoms may persist permanently. Chronic exposure to some organophosphates can cause long-lasting neurological defects involving vision, memory, and learning. These changes have been observed in humans and in other mammals.

For acute exposure, laboratory testing includes monitoring of blood-gases and acid-base status, renal and liver function, coagulation studies, and measurement of pseudocholinesterase (serum) activity. Pseudocholinesterase activity has the greatest clinical utility if pre-exposure testing has been done as part of occupational monitoring. When baseline studies are not available, assessing the degree of inhibition is difficult, because activity is related to liver function. Additionally, it should be noted that there are other chemicals and drugs known to inhibit cholinesterase.

Rodenticides such as strychnine, arsenic, warfarin, and phosphorus are all toxic not only to the targeted pest but also to nonrodents, including humans. Since these products are usually placed in areas accessible to both the targeted pest and to livestock, pets, and children, these latter groups are most likely to be involved in cases of accidental poisonings. Intentional poisonings of unsuspecting individuals with rodenticides are rare, although there have been reports of the anticoagulant-based rodenticides being used to simulate bleeding disorders.

Superwarfarins have been developed to combat the growing resistance of rats and mice to older rodenticides. These agents include brodifacoum, bromadiolone, chlorophacinone, and difenacoum. The superwarfarins act by inhibiting the synthesis of coagulation factors II, VII, IX, and X. Symptoms of acute ingestion are consistent with those of other coagulopathies and include transient abdominal pain, vomiting, bruising, hematuria, or heme-positive stools. While these patients must be watched closely for bleeding, hospitalization may not be necessary. In cases of intentional chronic ingestion, the patient may present with the complaints of easy bruising and fatigue and may be found to have heme-positive stools or hematuria.[114-116]

Few data are available regarding the pharmacokinetic parameters of these agents in humans. Brodifacoum, chlorophacinone, and difenacoum are 100 times more active than regular warfarin. Half-lives are variable but typically extend up to 120 days. The chemicals are metabolized in the liver via the cytochrome P450 system. Laboratory studies may show a prolonged prothrombin time. The superwarfarins can be measured in serum or plasma, using high-pressure liquid chromatography.[117]

VOLATILES

Ethanol is the most common drug encountered (for a detailed discussion, see Chapter 34). Ethanol follows saturation kinetics, so metabolism changes when the concentration exceeds what the available alcohol dehydrogenase (ADH) can handle. Other enzymes become involved in ethanol metabolism, depending on the concentration and whether exposure is chronic, as with an alcoholic. The acetaldehyde (metabolite) formed is toxic to most tissues. Preferred sample for clinical toxicology is serum or whole blood, but urine, breath, or saliva are also used. Detection is by enzymatic methods or GC. Lethal blood concentration is 350 to 500 mg/dL.

Methanol, isopropyl, and ethylene glycol are also metabolized by ADH to form toxic metabolites. As a result, prevention of toxicity is dependent on early identification and treatment with ethanol or an ADH inhibitor. Increases in anion gap and/or osmol gap that are not explainable by other toxins or pathological processes (e.g., diabetic ketoacidosis, renal failure) may help in recognizing ingestion. With ethylene glycol, calcium oxalate crystals, particularly the mono-hydrate form, are often present and suggestive of poisoning. Serum levels are quantified using gas chromatography. Patients should also be monitored by blood-gases and renal and liver function tests.

References

1. Sidell F: Chemical agent terrorism, www.nbc-med.org, 1996.
2. Garigan TP, Ristedt DE: Death from hyponatremia as a result of acute water intoxication in an Army basic trainee, *Mil Med* 164:234, 1999.
3. Holmes SB, Banerjee AK, Alexander WD: Hyponatraemia and seizures after ecstasy use, *Postgrad Med J* 75:32, 1999.
4. O'Conner A et al: Death from hyponatraemia-induced cerebral oedema associated with MDMA (Ecstasy) use, *New Zeal Med J* 112:255, 1999.
5. Preventing iron poisoning in children, http://vm.cfsan.fda.gov/~dms/bgiron.html, 1997.
6. Opresko DM et al: Chemical warfare agents: estimating oral reference doses, *Rev Environ Contam Toxicol* 156:1, 1998.
7. Aarons L, Graham G: Methodological approaches to the population analysis of toxicity data, *Toxicol Lett* 12:405, 2001.
8. Kroes R et al: Threshold of toxicological concern for chemical substances present in the diet: a practical tool for assessing the need for toxicity testing, *Food Chem Toxicol* 38:255, 2000.
9. Boyes WK et al: EPA's neurotoxicity risk assessment guidelines, *Fundam Appl Toxicol* 40:175, 1997.
10. Wainer IW: Toxicology through a looking glass: stereochemical questions and some answers. In Wong SHY, Sunshine I, editors: *Handbook of analytical therapeutic drug monitoring and toxicology*, Boca Raton, FL, 1996, CRC Press.
11. Hu H: Exposure to metals, *Prim Care* 27:983, 2000.
12. Brown RM: Pharmacology of cocaine abuse. In Redda KK, Walker CA, Barnett G: *Cocaine, marijuana, designer drugs: chemistry, pharmacology, and behavior*, Boca Raton, FL, 1990, CRC Press.
13. Berlin CM, Jr: Advances in pediatric pharmacology and toxicology, *Adv Pediatr* 44:545, 1997.
14. Blaho K, Winbery S, Merigian K: Pharmacological considerations for the pediatric patient, *Optom Clin* 5:61, 1996.
15. Schmucker DL: Aging and the liver: an update, *J Gerontol A Biol Sci Med Sci* 53:B315, 1998.
16. Mulder WJ, Hillen HF: Renal function and renal disease in the elderly: part I, *Eur J Intern Med* 12:86, 2001.
17. Sunaga K, Toshiaki S, Fujimura A: Lack of diurnal variation in glomerular filtration rates in the elderly, *J Clin Pharmacol* 36:203, 1996.
18. Pennie WD et al: The principles and practice of toxigenomics: applications and opportunities, *Toxicol Sci* 54:277, 2000.
19. Park BK, Pirmohamed M: Toxicogenetics in drug development, *Toxicol Lett* 120:281, 2001.
20. Festing MF: Experimental approaches to the determination of genetic variability, *Toxicol Lett* 120:293, 2001.
21. Miller MS et al: Drug metabolic enzymes in developmental toxicology, *Fundam Appl Toxicol* 34:165, 1996.
22. Kreth K et al: Identification of the human cytochromes p450 involved in the oxidative metabolism of "Ecstasy"-related designer drugs, *Biochem Pharmacol* 59:1563, 2000.
23. Ladona MG et al: Cocaine metabolism in human fetal and adult liver microsomes is related to cytochrome P450 3A expression, *Life Sci* 68:431, 2000.
24. Eap CB et al: Cytochrome P450 2D6 genotype and methadone steady-state concentrations, *J Clin Psychopharmacol* 21:229, 2001.
25. Spivack SD et al: Cyp1b1 expression in human lung, *Drug Metab Dispos* 29:916, 2001.
26. Oscarson M: Genetic polymorphisms in the cytochrome P450 2A6 (CYP2A6) gene: implications for interindividual differences in nicotine metabolism, *Drug Metab Dispos* 29:91, 2001.
27. Novak RF, Woodcroft KJ: The alcohol-inducible form of cytochrome P450 (CYP 2E1): role in toxicology and regulation of expression, *Arch Pharm Res* 23:267, 2000.
28. Laurenzana EM, Owens SM: Metabolism of phencyclidine by human liver microsomes, *Drug Metab Dispos* 25:557, 1997.
29. Flockhart DA: Cytochrome P450 drug interactions table, http://medicine.iupui.edu/flockhart, 2002.
30. Tanaka E: Update: genetic polymorphism of drug metabolizing enzymes in humans, *J Clin Pharm Ther* 24:323, 1999.
31. Meyer UA: Pharmacogenetics and adverse drug reactions, *Lancet* 356:1667, 2000.
32. Burchell B et al: Drug-mediated toxicity caused by genetic deficiency of UDP-glucuronosyltransferases, *Toxicol Letters* 112:333, 2000.
33. Ahuja S: *Impurities in pharmaceutical preparations*, New York, 1998, Marcel Dekker, Inc.
34. Stockley I: *Drug interactions: a source book of adverse interactions, their clinical importance, mechanisms and management*, ed 2, Oxford, UK, 1991, Blackwell Scientific Publications.
35. White JR, Campbell RK: Dangerous and common drug interactions in patients with diabetes mellitus, *Endocrinol Metab Clin North Am* 29:789, 2000.
36. Constant J: Pearls and pitfalls in the use and abuse of diuretics for chronic congestive heart failure, *Cardiology* 92:156, 1999.
37. Hylek EM: Oral anticoagulants: pharmacologic issues for use in the elderly, *Clin Geriatr Med* 17:1, 2001.
38. Haji SA, Movahed A: Update on digoxin therapy in congestive heart failure, *Am Fam Physician* 62:409, 2000.
39. Sellers EM, Holloway MR: Drug kinetics and alcohol ingestion, *Clin Pharmacokinet* 3:440, 1978.
40. Schaaf GJ et al: Characterization of biotransformation enzyme activities in primary rat proximal tubular cells, *Chem Biol Interact* 134:167, 2001.
41. Blanchard KT, Clay RJ, Morris JB: Pulmonary activation and toxicity of cyclopentadienyl manganese tricarbonyl, *Toxicol Appl Pharmacol* 136:280, 1996.
42. Costa LG et al: Intracellular signal transduction pathways as targets for neurotoxicants, *Toxicology* 160:19, 2001.
43. Morgan MJ: Ecstasy (MDMA): a review of its possible persistent psychological effects, *Psychopharmacology (Berl)* 152:230, 2000.
44. Goetz CG, Meisel E: Biological neurotoxins, *Neurol Clin* 18:719, 2000.
45. Bromberg MB: Peripheral neurotoxic disorders, *Neurol Clin* 18:681, 2000.
46. Trimble MR, Krishnamoorthy ES: The role of toxins in disorders of mood and affect, *Neurol Clin* 18:649, 2000.
47. Daston GP: Recent advances in reproductive and developmental toxicology, *Inhal Toxicol* 11:535, 1999.
48. Schuppe HC et al: Xenobiotic metabolism, genetic polymorphisms and male infertility, *Andrologia* 32:255, 2000.
49. Ahmed SA: The immune system as a potential target for environmental estrogens (endocrine disrupters): a new emerging field, *Toxicology* 150:191, 2000.
50. Potashnik G et al: Effect of dibromochloropropane on human testicular function, *Isr J Med Sci* 15:438, 1979.

51. Zenzes MT: Smoking and reproduction: gene damage to human gametes and embryos, *Hum Reprod Update* 6:122, 2000.

52. Juberg DR: An evaluation of endocrine modulators: implications for human health, *Ecotoxicol Environ Saf* 45:93, 2000.

53. Geyer SJ: Portrait in history: Percivall Pott, *Arch Pathol Lab Med* 123:661, 1999.

54. Bessems JG, Vermeulen NP: Paracetamol (acetaminophen)-induced toxicity: molecular and biochemical mechanisms, analogues and protective approaches, *Crit Rev Toxicol* 31:55, 2001.

55. Fenton J: *The laboratory and the poisoned patient*, Washington, DC, 1998, AACC Press.

56. Warner A: Cost effective toxicology testing, *Ther Drug Monit Toxicol* 17:35, 1996.

57. Hammett-Stabler CA, Pesce AJ, Cannon D: Urine drug screening in the medical setting, *Clin Chim Acta* 315:125, 2001.

58. Cone EJ, Jenkins AJ: Saliva drug analysis. In Sunshine I, Wong S, editors: *Handbook of analytical therapeutic drug monitoring and toxicology*, Boca Raton, FL, 1996, CRC Press.

59. Woods JR, Glantz JC: Significance of amniotic fluid meconium. In Creasy RK, Resnik R, editors: *Maternal-fetal medicine: principles and practice*, ed 3, Philadelphia, 1994, Saunders.

60. Moore C, Negrusz A: Drugs of abuse in meconium, *Forensic Sci Rev* 7:104, 1995.

61. Ostrea EM et al: Drug screening of meconium in infants of drug-dependent mothers: an alternative to urine testing, *J Pediatr* 115:474, 1989.

62. www.aapcc.org—American Association of Poison Control Centers, May 2001.

63. National Center for Health Statistics; Data Warehouse, http://www.cdc.gov/nchs/datawh/statab/unpubd/mortabs/gmwki.htm, May 2001.

64. Pohjola-Sintonen S et al: Identification of drugs ingested in acute poisoning: correlation of patient history with drug analyses, *Ther Drug Monit* 22:749, 2000.

65. Kulig K: Initial management of ingestions of toxic substances, *N Engl J Med* 326:1677, 1992.

66. Drug abuse statistics, www.drugabusestatistics.samhsa.gov, May 2001.

67. Wolff, K: Addiction medicine. In Karch SB, editor: *Drug abuse handbook*, Bacon Raton, FL, 1998, CRC Press.

68. Lues-Lues RJG: Maternal and fetal considerations of syphilis, *Obstet Gynecol Surv* 50:845, 1995.

69. Dusick AM et al: Risk of intracranial hemorrhage and other adverse outcomes after cocaine exposure in a cohort of 323 very low birth weight infants, *J Pediatr* 122:438, 1993.

70. Das G: Cocaine abuse in North America: a milestone in history, *J Clin Pharm* 33:296, 1993.

71. Casanova OQ et al: Detection of cocaine exposure in the neonate, *Arch Path Lab Med* 118:988, 1994.

72. Cieslak TJ et al: Immunization against potential biological warfare agents, *Clin Infect Dis* 30:843, 2000.

73. Jortani SA, Snyder JW, Valdes RV, Jr: The role of the clinical laboratory in managing chemical or biological terrorism, *Clin Chem* 46:1883, 2000.

74. Simon JD: Nuclear, biological, and chemical terrorism: understanding the threat and designing responses, *Int J Emerg Ment Health* 1:81, 1999.

75. Bradley RN: Health care facility preparation for weapons of mass destruction, *Prehosp Emerg Care* 4:261, 2000.

76. Reutter S: Hazards of chemical weapons release during war: new perspectives, *Environ Health Perspect* 107:985, 1999.

77. Borins M: The dangers of using herbs. What your patients need to know, *Postgrad Med* 104:91, 1998.

78. Brubacher JR et al: Efficacy of digoxin specific Fab fragments (Digibind) in the treatment of toad venom poisoning, *Toxicon* 37:931, 1999.

79. Ko RJ: Causes, epidemiology, and clinical evaluation of suspected herbal poisoning, *Clin Toxicol* 37:697, 1999.

80. Brent J: Three new herbal hepatotoxic syndromes, *Clin Toxicol* 37:715, 1999.

81. Frasca T, Brett AS, Yoo SD: Mandrake toxicity: a case of mistaken identity, *Arch Intern Med* 157:2007, 1997.

82. Anderson IB et al: Pennyroyal toxicity: measurement of toxic metabolite levels in two cases and review of the literature, *Ann Intern Med* 124:726, 1996.

83. Food and Drug Administration: *FDA warns consumers against dietary supplement products that may contain digitalis mislabeled as plantain*, June 12, 1997.

84. Moore C, Adler R: Herbal vitamins: lead toxicity and developmental delay, *Pediatrics* 106:600, 2000.

85. Cadmium and lead exposure associated with pharmaceuticals imported from Asia-Texas, *MMWR* 38:612, 1989.

86. Ernst E: Adverse effects of herbal drugs in dermatology, *Br J Dermatol* 143:923, 2000.

87. Weldon MM et al: Mercury poisoning associated with a Mexican beauty cream, *West J Med* 173:15, 2000.

88. Drug interactions with St. John's wort, *Med Lett Drugs Ther* 42:56, 2000.

89. Goepel M et al: Saw palmetto extracts potently and noncompetitively inhibit human alpha1-adrenoreceptors in vitro, *Prostate* 38:208, 1999.

90. Deng JF et al: The difficulty in handling poisonings associated with Chinese traditional medicine: a poison control center experience for 1991-1993, *Vet Hum Toxicol* 39:106, 1997.

91. Powers KS: Diagnosis and management of common toxic ingestions and inhalations, *Pediatr Ann* 29:330, 2000.

92. Vernon DD, Gleich MC: Poisoning and drug overdose, *Crit Care Clin* 13:647, 1997.

93. Howland MA: Risks of parenteral deferoxamine for acute iron poisoning, *J Toxicol Clin Toxicol* 34:491, 1996.

94. Bessems JG, Vermeulen NP: Paracetamol (acetaminophen)-induced toxicity: molecular and biochemical mechanisms, analogues, and protective approaches, *Crit Rev Toxicol* 31:55, 2001.

95. Collins SP, Gesell LB, Zemlan FP: Neurotoxicity in acetaminophen overdose, *Acad Emerg Med* 8:495, 2001.

96. Eguia L, Materson BJ: Acetaminophen-related acute renal failure without fulminant liver failure, *Pharmacotherapy* 17:363, 1997.

97. Farrell SE: Toxicity, acetaminophen, eMedicine Journal 2: http://www.emedicine.com/EMERG/topic819.htm, 2001.

98. Hillard CI: Biochemistry and pharmacology of the endocannabinoids arachidonylethanolamide and 2-arachidonylglycerolo, *Prostaglandins and Other Lipid Mediators* 61:3, 2000.

99. Baselt RC: *Disposition of toxic drugs and chemicals in man*, ed 5, Foster City, CA, 2000, Chemical Toxicology Institute.

100. Graeme KA: New drugs of abuse, *Emerg Med Clin North Am* 18:625, 2000.

101. Burgess C, O'Donohoe A, Gill M: Agony and ecstasy: a review of MDMA effects and toxicity, *Eur Psychiatry* 15:287, 2000.

102. Kohrs FP, Porter WH: gamma-Hydroxybutyrate intoxication and overdose, *Ann Emerg Med* 33:475, 1999.

103. Tomaszewski CA, Thom SR: Use of hyperbaric oxygen in toxicology, *Emerg Med Clin North Am* 12:437, 1994.

104. Matsuura K et al: Morphological effects of cadmium on proximal tubular cells in rats, *Bio Trace Element Res* 31:171, 1991.

105. *Pesticides industry sales and usage*, US Environmental Protection Agency, publication no. 733-R-99-001, Nov 1999.

106. US Environmental Protection Agency, http://www.epa.gov/.

107. The Ohio State University Pesticide Education Program, http://www.ag.ohio-state.edu/.

108. National Pesticide Telecommunications Network, http://ace.orst.edu/info/nptn/.

109. Health and Safety Information System, http://hsis.fedworld.gov/.

110. Lotti M: The pathogenesis of organophosphate neuropathy, *Crit Rev Toxicol* 21:465, 1992.

111. Lifshitz M, Shahak E, Sofer S: Carbamate and organophosphate poisoning in young children, *Pediatr Emerg Care* 15:102, 1999.

112. Weiner ML, Jortner BS: Organophosphate-induced delayed neurotoxicity of triarylphosphates, *Neurotoxicol* 20:653, 1999.

113. Ray DE: Chronic effects of low level exposure to anticholinesterases—a mechanistic review, *Toxicol Lett* 102-103:527, 1998.

114. Bruno GR et al: Long-acting anticoagulant overdose: brodifacoum kinetics and optimal vitamin K dosing, *Ann Emerg Med* 36:262, 2000.

115. Corke PJ: Superwarfarin (brodifacoum) poisoning, *Anaesth Intensive Care* 25:707, 1997.

116. Tecimer C, Yam LT: Surreptitious superwarfarin poisoning with brodifacoum, *South Med J* 90:1053, 1997.

117. Fauconnet V, Pouliquen H, Pinault L: Reversed-phase HPLC determination of eight anticoagulant rodenticides in animal liver, *J Anal Toxicol* 21:548, 1997.

Internet Sites

http://www.bertholf.net/rlb/Lectures/index.htm—Click on "Clinical and Forensic Toxicology"

http://medicine.iupui.edu/flockhart—Indiana University's Cytochrome P450 Drug Interaction Table

http://www.aapcc.org—American Association of Poison Control Centers

http://www.cdc.gov/nchs/datawh/statab/unpubd/mortabs/gmwki.htm—National Center for Health Statistics

http://www.atsdr.cdc.gov/atsdrhome.html

www.drugabusestatistic.samhsa.gov—Substance Abuse and Mental Health Services Administration (SAMHSA), Office of Applied Studies

http://www.epa.gov/—US Environmental Protection Agency

http://www.ag.ohio-state.edu/—The Ohio University Pesticide Education Program

http://npic.orst.edu/—National Pesticide Information Center

http://ntp-server.niehs.nih.gov/—National Institute of Environmental Health Sciences

http://toxnet.nlm.nih.gov/—TOXNET, US National Library of Medicine

http://www.usdoj.gov/dea/concern/concern.htm—US Drug Enforcement Agency

http://www.bioterrorism.slu.edu/—Center for the Study of Bioterrorism and Emerging Infections at Saint Louis University

http://www.toxicology-info.com/

http://physchem.ox.ac.uk/MSDS/—The Physical and Theoretical Chemistry Laboratory, Oxford University, Chemical and Other Safety Information

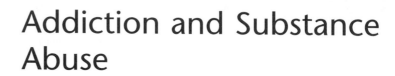

CHAPTER 52

Addiction and Substance Abuse

- *R. Jeffrey Goldsmith*
- *Cheryl Lesar*

Chapter Outline

The addiction process
Theories to explain addiction
Prevalence of addiction among various groups
Pathophysiology of chronic substance abuse
Diagnosis of addiction and substance abuse

Recovery and the treatment process
The preemployment or random drug screen
Why individuals fail drug screens
Change of analyte in disease

Objectives

- Describe the series of steps resulting in addictions.
- Differentiate the causes and factors that result in addiction in young people.

- Describe the method of diagnosis of addiction.
- Describe how drug screens are used to detect drug abuse and monitor rehabilitation.

Key Terms

addiction   The compulsive use of a psychoactive chemical, causing problems in the user's life on a physical, psychological, or sociocultural level. Unconscious psychological defenses like denial are a common feature, distorting the addict's self-awareness and confusing the people around him or her. Addiction is a chronic deteriorating process that leads to death or institutionalization if unchecked. Abstinence allows the mind and body to recover sufficiently to work on the social deficits and deteriorated relationships.

contingency contracts   Behavioral plans that engage the addict in a carefully delineated treatment program. The consequences of failure to follow through are clearly spelled out in the hope that this will encourage the addict to remain in treatment.

craving   An intense urge to use a drug; it may be short lived or tormentingly chronic. Some addicts have environmental triggers of this craving; others have psychological states that evoke the urge, but many don't have craving at all.

drug screens   Qualitative analyses of a body fluid (urine, blood, saliva, and so forth) of a patient in a search for the possible presence of addictive substances. There is usually a brief list of five to ten drugs for which a sample is screened; however, more comprehensive lists are sometimes requested.

recovery   The process of growth and development that occurs after sustained abstinence. Spirituality is an important element in recovery because of the need to transcend the intense self-focus or experience of victimization that many addicts exhibit.

rehabilitation   A comprehensive, multicomponent treatment for alcoholics and addicts who are abstinent and not in withdrawal. It addresses the consequences of alcohol or drug use, the personal problems that are not directly related to the chemical use, and the necessary skills for ongoing abstinence and recovery.

substance abuse   A generic term that covers the pathological use of psychoactive substances. It is not a specific diagnosis and includes both psychological dependence and physiological dependence. For some, this term includes alcohol and drug misuse that would not be covered in DSM-IV and therefore would not be a psychiatric diagnosis.

tolerance   The behavioral and neurochemical adaptation to the drug effects of a psychoactive substance. It allows the person to experience less toxicity from the substance. Everyone can exhibit some tolerance; however, most addicts exhibit a great deal of tolerance.

withdrawal   The central nervous system adjustment to the relatively sudden cessation of a psychoactive substance. There are physical, psychological, and behavioral changes that occur in these states. The symptoms of withdrawal are frequently opposite the acute effects of the substance.

Methods on CD-ROM

Alcohol

Drug screen

Addiction and abuse of alcohol and other drugs affect a significant portion of the population of many countries. Alcohol is the most commonly abused substance in Western civilization, and the patterns of behavior with alcohol are common to other drugs such as marijuana (marihuana), cocaine, opiates, benzodiazepines, and agents, such as glue and petrol (gasoline), that are sniffed. The term *addiction* is defined as the compulsive use of a psychoactive chemical, causing problems in the user's life on a physical, psychological, or sociocultural level. Unconscious psychological defenses against the consequences of addiction, like denial, are common features that distort addicts' self-awareness and confuse the people around them. Addiction is a chronic deteriorating process that leads to death or institutionalization if unchecked. Abstinence from the addictive agent allows the mind and body to recover sufficiently to work on the social deficits and deteriorated relationships that may have predated or resulted from the addiction.

THE ADDICTION PROCESS

It is important to understand that alcohol or other drug use by itself is not addiction. For example, among a national survey of students in ninth to twelfth grades, 79.1% had tried alcohol, 47.1% marijuana, and less than 9% cocaine.[1] If recent drug use by the same group is examined, percentages decrease considerably; only 50.8% had used alcohol, 26.2% marijuana, and 3.3% cocaine in the previous month. Because addiction implies the need to use the drugs frequently, it is clear that not all those who have used the drugs are addicted to them.

For some people, initial occasional consumption of alcohol and/or tobacco leads to the development of the clinical syndromes of alcohol and/or tobacco dependence.[2] Addiction begins when individuals experience desirable effects in a relationship with an object of addiction. This is often

described as *positive reinforcement*. The desirable effects of drugs are probably related to physiological stimulation of brain receptors. For example, the euphoriant and stimulant effects of cocaine are likely caused by stimulation of specific areas of the brain, areas also affected by opiates. This early stage often occurs during a phase of experimentation and risk taking in a young person's life in which many new experiences are tried. This is followed by a middle stage in which **tolerance** is manifested. The term *tolerance* is used to describe the requirement for increased amounts of drug to achieve the desired psychological and physiological states. Tolerance implies using a lot of the drug without toxic effects. In this middle stage some negative consequences of drug abuse occur with psychological pain as a secondary phenomenon. Agitation, nervousness, and worry begin as a result of increased usage, intensifying the pain. The late stage of drug addiction begins when the individual uses drugs to feel normal. This occurs because there is tolerance to the positive reinforcement of the drug and increasing negative reinforcement.

Negative reinforcement, which may include ill health, loss of jobs and friends, as well as the pain and discomfort of the drug withdrawal, encourages the addict to continue abusing the drug. Discontinuance leads to a heightened experience of the pain, and the addict returns to use of the drug to feel better. This is the epitome of the addictive cycle. In the last two phases, the addict loses the ability to regulate the amount of drug consumed once the consumption has begun. This is termed *loss of control*. Not only does the drug use get out of control, but the family functioning and the addict's behavior do too.

Denial develops as a defense mechanism, splitting the positive and negative aspects of an addictive behavior pattern.[3] Everyone intends to behave in a particular way, and there are a variety of culturally determined intentions that make up behavior. The chemicals taken by individuals alter their behavior in such a way that some people behave differently from the way they intend to and from what is culturally determined as appropriate. The discrepancy between the intended behavior and what actually occurs may be explained by excuses and alibis. Explaining away these behavioral discrepancies is termed *denial*. The affected individual wants to believe the denial to avoid the pain of acknowledging the unintended behavior. The person becomes progressively more invested in the denial as a way of understanding his or her world. In other words, because the rest of the world is reacting unfavorably to his or her behavior, the denial becomes a method of rationalizing the behavior. Many modes of treatment involve disrupting the denial so that the person can see his or her actual behavior. This approach leads to a heightened consciousness of pain and a motivation to stop using the agents. It is suggested that it is the pain that is the motivation to stop using a drug. Because the negative consequences of drug abuse appear after a long delay, the individual abusing a drug may already be addicted before these consequences can have an inhibitory effect. Part of the late stage of addiction is the **withdrawal** syndrome, which reinforces **substance abuse**. A partial listing of withdrawal symptoms observed with some of the addicting substances is presented in Box 52-1.

Another aspect of addiction is **craving**. Craving is an intense desire to use a drug. This can occur when the individual is placed in situations that remind him or her of previous drug use or when a particular mood triggers the urge to get high. Some people do not have craving.

THEORIES TO EXPLAIN ADDICTION

A variety of proposed models have been used to explain the addiction process. All the models use the observation of the addict's high affinity for alcohol and drug use and the large quantities consumed. The models differ in how they explain the individual's progress down the path to addiction and the addicted state once it has been achieved. Because the theories suggest different cause-and-effect relationships, each theory in turn dictates different types of treatment interventions. The disease concept is a proposition that addictions are rooted in a biological vulnerability that predisposes the individual to tolerance and loss of control.[4] This hypothesis suggests that abstinence is the only solution, and treatment is directed toward realization of this loss of control. The cognitive/behavioral model of addiction suggests that addicts have different expectancies about their use of alcohol and drugs and get locked into a pattern of use by positive reinforcement (euphoria, being cool socially, feeling less tense), and other negative reinforcements (withdrawal symptoms upon cessation).[4] Treatment is aimed at providing alternative problem-solving skills and coping devices that lead to a sense of self-efficacy. Attachment theory, self-psychology, and affect regulation theory characterize addiction as an attachment disorder induced by a person's misguided attempt to self-repair because of deficits in psychic structure. Vulnerability of the self is the consequence of developmental failures and early environmental deprivation leading to ineffective attachment styles.[5] Treatment is focused on making the usual sense of self less painful and thereby rendering the individual less motivated to use alcohol and drugs as a coping mechanism.

PREVALENCE OF ADDICTION AMONG VARIOUS GROUPS

Evidence from several different national data collection efforts points to a sharp increase of adolescent drug use in the early 1990s after a decade of steady decline. Data from the National Household Survey of Drug Abuse (NHSDA, www.samhsa.gov/oas/nhsda.htm) and the National Parents' Resource Institute for Drug Education (PRIDE, http://www.prideusa.org/), two national surveys that obtain estimates of adolescent substance use, estimate that in 1995 monthly use of marijuana among youth was 8.2%, more than double the 1992 level. Using the PRIDE data, monthly use of any illicit drug by sixth to twelfth graders in 1995 to 1996 was estimated to be 18.3%, up from 10.6% in 1987 to 1988, the first year of the PRIDE survey.[4]

The prevalence of drug use can be categorized on the basis of age and sex. The onset of use of drugs usually occurs in eighth grade. Between the tenth and twelfth grades, large increases in propensity to engage in substance use or abuse occur. There is a strong correlation between use of a substance in tenth grade and future use of the same substance.

BOX 52-1

WITHDRAWAL SYMPTOMS

Alcohol and Sedatives
Tremor
Nausea
Vomiting
Tachycardia
Sweating
High blood pressure
Anxiety
Irritability or depressed mood
Orthostatic hypotension

Tobacco
Craving
Irritability
Anxiety
Difficulty in concentrating
Restlessness
Headache
Drowsiness
Gastrointestinal disturbances

Stimulants and Cocaine
Sleepiness (hypersomnia)
Hyperphagia (abnormally
   increased appetite)
Depressed mood (± suicidal)

Opiates
Lacrimation (tear production)
Rhinorrhea ("runny nose")
Dilated pupils
Piloerection (involuntary
   erection of body hair)
Sweating
Diarrhea
Yawning
Mild hypertension
Tachycardia
Fever
Insomnia
Flulike syndrome with
   myalgia

Caffeine
Craving
Headache
Sleepiness
Irritability

Marijuana
Irritability
Loss of appetite
Insomnia

Although this does not establish addiction, it is consistent with the theory that early use leads to continued heavy use of substances.[4]

After 25 years of age people begin to decrease their drinking and illegal drug use. Heavy drinking and drug use beyond 25 years of age should be taken as potential indicators of addiction. There needs to be careful scrutiny of the behavior and other indications of addiction of individuals in the 18- to 25-year-old group to differentiate the potential drug abuser or addict from the other population.

Table 52-1 describes the various types of alcohol and drug abuse among populations. It can be seen that the heaviest alcohol use occurs in the 18- to 25-year-old age group and decreases in the 26- to 34-year-old group. It is also important to note that males are five times more likely than females to be heavy drinkers. There are also social and cultural differences. This is most striking in the substantial use of tobacco among whites, who are more likely to have smoked than African American and Hispanic populations. Although cocaine use in the United States has received a lot of media attention, actual use of cocaine occurs in less than 3% of the population. Cocaine use historically has been associated with an older population (25 to 40 years of age) although there is currently a shift toward the younger age groups who are more likely to experiment with drugs. Epidemiological studies provide important evidence of a developmental pattern of drug use.[1] Usually a teenager uses alcohol and tobacco before using marijuana. This is especially true for boys, whereas girls sometimes will use one or the other before trying marijuana. Marijuana use often precedes the use of other illegal drugs. Thus highly addictive and illegal drugs are preceded by less addictive and legal substances. The use of legal drugs is a necessary beginning in the addictive process that has something to do with the person's willingness or commitment to use alcohol or drugs. It is possible that these "gateway drugs" sensitize certain parts of the brain. Another hypothesis is that the legal drugs start the individual on the psychological pathway to denial, and this accommodates other drug use.

Misuse of medications is a major cause of morbidity and mortality (see p. 991, Chapter 51).[6] Prescription drug abuse (PDA) covers drugs diverted for addiction purposes (both sale and consumption) by the physician or by the patient, patients inadvertently addicted while taking the medication as prescribed, patients taking medication obtained on the street or from family, and overdoses. Alcoholics and the elderly are prone to PDA when suffering from pain, insomnia, anxiety, or depression.

The addict or drug abuser may use more than one drug.[7] About half of alcoholics are also dependent on other illegal drugs. Eighty percent to ninety-five percent of alcoholics are regular cigarette smokers, which is about triple the national average. In methadone-maintenance patients, at least 50% are also alcohol dependent. In individuals dependent on alcohol or cocaine, very often other drugs will be found; thus the person who is positive for an illegal substance such as cocaine is likely to be positive for alcohol and marijuana.

PATHOPHYSIOLOGY OF CHRONIC SUBSTANCE ABUSE

There are long-term health consequences from smoking, drinking, and substance abuse, such as addiction, cancer, liver cirrhosis, and loss of memory function.[6] Table 52-2 lists some medical problems associated with chronic abuse.[7-9] In addition, direct damage to the central nervous system is often observed in individuals who sniff petrol (gasoline) or glue. The negative effects of female recreational drug and alcohol abuse during pregnancy are well documented.[10] Infants

TABLE 52-2 EXAMPLES OF MEDICAL PATHOPHYSIOLOGY ASSOCIATED WITH CHRONIC ABUSE*

Substance	Disease
Alcohol	Liver cirrhosis
	Cardiomyopathy
	Fetal alcohol syndrome
	Trauma of all types
	Gastrointestinal cancer
	Strokes
	Depression
Cocaine	Nasal septum perforation
	Cardiac arrest
	Seizures
	Panic attacks
	Paranoia
	Premature births
	Neonatal withdrawal
Opiates	Infections, AIDS
	Hepatitis
	Self-poisoning
	Neonatal withdrawal
Tobacco	Emphysema
	Cancer of various types
	Heart attack
	Osteoporosis
	Low birth weight

*These are in addition to withdrawal symptoms.

TABLE 52-1 PREVALENCE OF DRUG USE (PERCENTAGE OF POPULATION)

Males (Age)	Alcohol*	Tobacco	Marijuana	Cocaine
12 to 17	2% to 3%	12%	?	1%
18 to 25	11%	30%	13%	2%
26 to 34	7%	30%	8.6%	1.7%
>34	2% to 3%	24%	2%	0.2%

*Heavy drinkers use five or more drinks per occasion on five or more days in the previous 30 days.

exposed to cocaine are more often premature and can be fussy, difficult-to-manage babies at first. In utero damage has been reported if the vascular effects of cocaine cause a local loss of blood flow to the placenta. This can cause a stroke or organ damage to a fetus. The long-term effects of in utero exposure to cocaine are not known at this time. The fetal alcohol syndrome is characterized by mental retardation, growth retardation, and a variety of craniofacial anomalies.[11] Such babies also exhibit social skill deficits and attentional problems when they are older and perform poorly in school without special attention. It is believed that there is a less severe syndrome, called *fetal alcohol effect*, that affects many more children. Because of the subtlety of this neurological deterioration, it is difficult to say how many individuals are affected.

DIAGNOSIS OF ADDICTION AND SUBSTANCE ABUSE

It can be difficult to diagnose addiction because the chronic use of alcohol or drugs often mimics other psychiatric syndromes. A history of alcohol abuse is an important diagnostic finding. However, the presence of denial is common and often thwarts the clinician, and if the history of alcohol or drug use is not elicited, an erroneous diagnosis is frequently made.

Many people with substance use disorders are vulnerable to other psychiatric disorders and come to addiction treatment services with comorbid psychiatric symptoms.[12] In turn, such psychiatric problems as depression and mania need to be differentiated from medical conditions that may mimic these disorders, such as thyroid disease, Wilson's disease, and others.

A history of alcoholism in a patient's family may place the person in a high-risk group for alcohol or drug dependence.[13] There are multiple components to this vulnerability, which include genetic, physiological, psychological, social, and environmental influences. Alcoholism is believed to be inherited. Studies of the neurobiology of addiction have identified neural pathways in which genetic variation at candidate genes could influence vulnerability.[14]

The presence of withdrawal symptoms is important and, when present, is diagnostic. On the other hand, many people are dependent on alcohol and drugs without obvious withdrawal symptoms, being psychologically dependent. Blackouts and denial are two other phenomena that are important to understand, but they are not considered diagnostic evidence of addiction. Blackouts are true amnestic episodes that are commonly associated with alcoholism and sedative or hypnotic dependence. Although they are not currently diagnostic criteria, they are highly suggestive of dependence. Denial is a common psychological defense and is used by the alcoholic or addict to prevent awareness of the addiction, which deflects the fear of losing control. Denial can be recognized only as such after the addiction is identified; therefore it is not a diagnostic criterion.

Diagnosis and treatment of prescription-drug abuse hinge on the recognition of what is happening. Demanding prescriptions or running out of pills before the proper date may be signs of addiction or selling pills on the street. Chronic daily use of a medication that is habituating, predominantly sedatives and narcotics, is a setup for physical dependence and withdrawal symptoms upon sudden discontinuation. Visits to several doctors on a regular basis can be a sign of drug-seeking behavior or an opportunity for inadvertent overmedication. Each one of these situations is handled differently depending on the patient and the physicians involved. **Drug screens** can be crucial in the confirmation that a patient is using a drug not prescribed by the physician or is using it beyond the prescribed cutoff date. A quantitative analysis may be useful when the patient is suspected of escalating the dose on his own, or getting prescriptions from other doctors surreptitiously when the drug is known to be present but the amount is in question. In part, this unreliable history occurs because alcoholics and addicts are highly stigmatized; people with these disorders are accustomed to considerable negative feedback and disguise their disability until they feel safe acknowledging it. The criteria listed in Box 52-2 for the diagnosis of substance abuse are primarily subjective ones and therefore more difficult to apply.

Attempts to employ quantitative laboratory data often meet with mixed success (see Chapter 34). Combination of tests that include γ-glutamyltransferase, mean corpuscular volume, and aspartate aminotransferase can have a diagnostic sensitivity and specificity for alcoholism in the 70% to 95% range. Carbohydrate-deficient transferrin (CDT) has recently emerged as a new biochemical marker to measure excessive alcohol consumption. Transferrin is a glycoprotein involved in transporting iron to body tissues.[15] The carbohydrate content of transferrin is usually lower in individuals who are actively drinking alcohol, therefore the term *carbohydrate-deficient transferrin* was coined. Alcohol consumption of four to seven drinks per day for at least 1 week can significantly elevate CDT levels in alcohol-dependent individuals.

The positive drug screen is not diagnostic for addiction. The use of alcohol and drugs is a very common phenomenon in the United States in the early twenty-first century. The positive drug screen indicates only that these substances were used within a certain time of the collection of body fluids. A positive drug screen is an important finding. Final diagnosis must be made on clinical grounds by a clinician and physician taking a history and observing the signs and

---

BOX 52-2

DIAGNOSTIC CRITERIA OF ADDICTION

Tolerance
Loss of control
Narrowing of lifestyle
Use despite reasons not to use
Withdrawal symptoms

symptoms of addiction. This clinical observation is especially important when serious legal consequences are possible.

RECOVERY AND THE TREATMENT PROCESS

Denial develops as a defense mechanism when positive drug effects, often experienced early in addiction, are challenged by the negative consequences of addictive behavior. Even court-enforced monitoring may not remove the denial, and the treatment intervention may fail. The influence of ambivalence is important for people considering whether to enter or continue in substance abuse treatment. People use denial as a defense against their ambivalence. Resistance is at the core of what makes it difficult for people to achieve consistently "good" mental health.[3] Therapists using resistance reduction strategies ask clients about their perceived benefits of drug use rather than focusing exclusively on the cost of their behavior. Interviewing in this way provides clients the opportunity to conduct therapeutic work in the safe surrounds of a known behavior and a nonjudgmental environment. Because a resistance reduction strategy does not ask the client to give up anything, they also have less need to resist therapeutic interventions.[3] Families can help increase awareness, and external coercion by courts and other agencies can help improve retention of the patient in treatment. When the addict appreciates that the alcohol or drug use is out of control and that it makes life unmanageable, the addict is more likely to commit to a program of abstinence. With the commitment to abstinence comes a greater cooperation from the patient to reverse the problems of addiction; this is the essence of **recovery**. **Rehabilitation** programs attempt to rebuild the sectors in the addict's life that have been underdeveloped or undermined by the addiction. Spiritual help must be rallied and efforts made to prevent relapse by exploring the triggers to relapse and avoiding situations that could precipitate the relapse. Relapse prevention depends on the discovery of alternative, nondrug coping mechanisms for life's problems.

Both inpatient and outpatient programs to stop the addiction cycle have considerable success. Although many return to use of drugs or alcohol, more than half of the patients completing treatment (50% to 80%) remain abstinent for at least a year.

Strategies of rehabilitation involve the use of contracts and drug screens to work with ambivalent motivations. In this particular circumstance the addict agrees, or contracts, to fulfill a series of rehabilitation steps that may include attending meetings of groups such as Alcoholics Anonymous. In general, the contract specifies that if the person prematurely leaves treatment or is found to be using drugs by history or by screening, he or she will have some consequences, such as violation of probation, the loss of his or her job, or termination from treatment.

Drug screening is a common component of rehabilitation in general, and contracts in particular. Screens are frequently ordered on a weekly basis, but may be used more often. Outpatient treatment may require drug screens on an as-needed basis. The screens usually test for a group of the most commonly abused drugs, but less common drugs are added by name if there is specific concern. Detoxification medication frequently causes a positive screen, as do narcotic analgesics, certain antiseizure medications, and hypnotic drugs used for insomnia. Because addicts often use somatic complaints to obtain these medications from physicians unnecessarily, it is wise to have a physician experienced with the addictions assess positive drug screens and the medication that addicts claim to need. The information is used to confront the addict if surreptitious drug use is suspected. By doing so, the addict has a chance to stop a relapse early, before serious damage occurs.

THE PREEMPLOYMENT OR RANDOM DRUG SCREEN

Many employers use the preemployment drug screen to weed out those potential workers whom they believe will be a risk to their company. The literature has reported costly side effects of employee drug abuse such as decreased productivity and increased use of health benefits.[15] Various substances are measured in preemployment screens, depending on the situation. Urinary alcohol is commonly measured in many programs. By law, those individuals employed by the federal government or who are under the aegis of the Department of Transportation will be screened for those drugs specified by the Substance Abuse Mental Health Service Administration, formerly National Institute of Drug Abuse, including opiates, cocaine, barbiturates, marijuana, and phencyclidine. Increasingly, many employers also screen for illegal substances in individuals already employed. These screens are performed "for cause," that is, because of actions that raise the suspicion of drug abuse, randomly, or at prescheduled times.

The purposes of intraemployment drug screens are similar to the preemployment screens. Random drug screens are used to increase the likelihood of detecting individuals who are using illegal drugs. In the case of transportation workers, the time and place of the drug screen is usually specified. For other groups such as the military, the screening is often on a random basis.

WHY INDIVIDUALS FAIL DRUG SCREENS

Even individuals who know in advance that they will be tested for drugs of abuse still fail drug screens. There are several explanations. The first is that the person did not understand the physiological aspects of drug testing. Many people are not familiar with the drug half-lives and do not appreciate how long drugs remain detectable in the blood and urine after the time of last use. Secondly, an individual who is tested may be in denial about his own addiction and not comprehend that the drug testing is in place to pick up drugs in his body, only those in someone else's body. The rationale is that drug testing is to catch an addict: because I am not an addict, it is not going to catch me. Lastly, the addicted individual may have no intention to use drugs around the time of the announced drug screen; however, loss of control may cause him or her to use drugs at the inopportune moment.

Loss of control may come about in several different ways, one of which is that drug use may be a mechanism of coping with psychological distress. As the drug screen itself becomes a psychological stressor, a drug is used in an attempt to deal with the added tension of the situation. Drug use may occur impulsively when there is a craving, as at a party just preceding the drug screen.

Individuals may not intend to use the drug but do so because of their inability to refuse the drug when offered in a particular setting. The loss of control also occurs with the experience of withdrawal symptoms. Such an individual will feel compelled to use the drug to reduce those symptoms. Possible psychological reasons why an individual may fail a drug test deal with guilt and the working of the unconscious in certain neurotic individuals.

When individuals test positive on a drug screen, someone must be responsible for determining whether the positive result is for a properly prescribed medicine. Therefore, drug screens should be reviewed by a medical review officer (or knowledgeable physician) who can interpret the drug screen in light of the person's drug and medical history.[16] This is particularly important when dealing with positive results in a setting where disciplinary action may take place. The medical review officer can establish if the positive test was the result of prescription drugs, agents such as poppy seeds, or indeed truly illegal drug use.

CHANGE OF ANALYTE IN DISEASE

A drug screen is often used as part of the diagnostic and treatment process. What is meant by a drug screen is referred to in Chapter 51. In general, drug screens use untimed urine specimens obtained from the patient at random intervals, when certain changes in behavior occur, or at specified intervals. There are many different uses for drug screening in drug addiction treatment programs. The identification of

drug use is an important function of drug screening given the unreliability of the alcohol or drug history given by patients.

The use of drug screens can also be critical in the confrontation of active denial in these patients. Although the purpose is to identify alcohol or drug abuse, the data are also used to confront the person's denial. The drugs that are screened for, based on the earlier discussion, include alcohol, marijuana, cocaine, opiates, and so forth. It must be kept in mind that some agents such as LSD cannot be screened using current technology.

Drug screening is a very powerful tool to enforce rehabilitation **contingency contracts** that explicitly require abstinence from certain drugs. Without drug screening the contracts are often unenforceable. Relapse prevention programs use drug screening to monitor ongoing abstinence. The patient in the relapse prevention program has made a commitment to abstinence; however, with certain drugs like nicotine and cocaine, this commitment can be shaken by the experience of craving. Finally, drug screening is a legal requirement of the treatment in methadone maintenance clinics. Patients receiving methadone are required by law to get drug screening, and the results are frequently used to determine the future doses of methadone. If the methadone patient is still using opiates in addition to the prescribed methadone, programs often change the methadone dose to see if that induces the illegal opiates to be discontinued. The drugs to be screened may be only one, such as alcohol, or several depending on the program. It must be realized that many addicts are multidrug users and this information is important in the use and interpretation of drug screens.

An important component of drug screens may be the need for confirmation of a positive result (see p. 1004, Chapter 51). Certainly positive results from employment drug screens must be confirmed, because livelihoods are at stake, and results from certified laboratories require confirmation.

References

1. Kann L et al: Youth risk behavior surveillance—United States, 1997, *MMWR* 47:1, 1998.
2. Anthony JC, Echaegaray-Wagner F: Epidemiologic analysis of alcohol and tobacco use, *Alcohol Res Health* 24: 201, 2000.
3. Shaffer HJ, Simoneau G: Reducing resistance and denial by exercising ambivalence during the treatment of addiction, *J Subst Abuse Treat* 20:99, 2001.
4. Kenkel D, Mathios AD, Pacula RL: Economics of youth drug use, addiction and gateway effects, *Addiction* 96:151, 2001.
5. Flores PJ: Addiction as an attachment disorder: implications for group therapy, *Int J Group Psychother* 51:63, 2001.
6. Bedell SE et al: Discrepancies in the use of medications: their extent and predictors in an outpatient practice, *Arch Intern Med* 160:22129, 2000.
7. Benzer DC: Medical consequences of alcohol addiction. In Miller NS, editor: *Comprehensive handbook of drug and alcohol addiction*, pp 551-571, New York, 1991, Marcel Dekker.
8. Engel C, Benzer DG: Medical complications of drug addiction. In Miller NS, editor: *Comprehensive handbook of drug and alcohol addiction*, pp 573-598, New York, 1991, Marcel Dekker.
9. Geller A: Neurological effects of drug and alcohol addiction. In Miller NS, editor: *Comprehensive handbook of drug and alcohol addiction*, pp 599-621, New York, 1991, Marcel Dekker.
10. Pollard I: Substance abuse and parenthood: biological mechanisms—bioethical challenges, *Women Health* 30:1, 2000.
11. Sokol RJ, Clarren SK: Guidelines for use of terminology describing the impact of prenatal alcohol on the offspring, *Alcohol Clin Exp Res* 13:597, 1989.
12. Marsden J et al: Psychiatric symptoms among clients seeking treatment for drug dependence. Intake data from the National Treatment Outcome Research Study, *Br J Psychiatry* 176:285, 2000.
13. Leshner AI: The disease of addiction, *Lippincott's Prim Care Pract* 4:249, 2000.
14. Enoch MA, Goldman D: The genetics of alcoholism and alcohol abuse, *Curr Psychiatry Rep* 3:144, 2001.
15. Montoya ID, Carlson JW, Richard AJ: An analysis of drug abuse policies in teaching hospitals, *J Behav Health Serv Res* 26:28, 1999.
16. Swotinsky RB, editor: *The medical review officer's guide to drug testing*, New York, 1992, Van Nostrand Reihnhold.

Internet Sites

http://www.usdoj.gov/dea/—US Drug Enforcement Administrations (DEA)

http://www.edc.org/hec/—Higher Education Center for Alcohol and Drug Prevention, a program from the US Department of Education

http://www.health.org/ and http://www.samhsa.gov/—Substance abuse and Mental Health Services Administration (SAMHSA), National Clearinghouse for Alcohol and Drug Information

http://www.samhsa.gov/oas/nhsda.htm—SAMHSA National Household Survey on Drug Abuse Data

http://www.prideusa.org/—National Parents' Resource Institute for Drug Education (PRIDE)

http://www.niaaa.nih.gov/—National Institute on Alcohol Abuse and Alcoholism (NIAAA)

http://www.nida.nih.gov/—National Institute on Drug abuse (NIDA)

http://www.whitehousedrugpolicy.gov/—Office of National Drug Control Policy (ONDCP)

http://www.asam.org/Frames.htm—American Society of Addiction Medicine

http://www.aaap.org/—American Society of Addiction Psychiatry

http://www.casacolumbia.org/newsletter1458/newsletter.htm—National Center on Addiction and Substance Abuse at Columbia University

CHAPTER 53

Classifications and Descriptions of Proteins, Lipids, and Carbohydrates

- *Lawrence A. Kaplan*
- *Herbert K. Naito*
- *Amadeo J. Pesce*

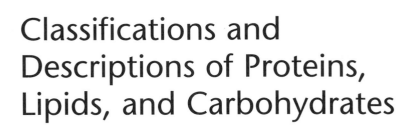

Chapter Outline

Part 1: Proteins
Definition and classification
Chemical properties
Physical properties
Biological properties

Part 2: Lipids
Definition and classification
  Simple lipids
  Conjugated lipids
  Derived lipids
Chemical and physical properties
  Melting point
  Solubility
  Specific gravity
  Alcohol groups of steroids
  Triglyceride composition

Biological properties

Part 3: Carbohydrates
Definition and classification
  Simple monomeric carbohydrates (saccharides)
  Derived monosaccharides
  Complex carbohydrates
Chemical properties
Physical properties
Biological properties

Part 4: Nucleic Acids
Definition and classification
  Purine and pyrimidine bases
DNA and RNA
  DNA and RNA binding affinity

Objectives

- Describe how proteins are classified.
- List the unique chemical properties of proteins.
- Outline some of the biological properties of proteins.
- Describe how lipids are classified.
- Outline some of the biological properties of lipids and their location in specific tissues.
- Describe how carbohydrates are classified.

- Understand how the chemical and physical properties of carbohydrates are related to their biological properties.
- Understand the basic structure of the predominant purine and pyrimidine bases.
- Describe how nucleosides and nucleotides are defined.
- Outline the polymeric structure of DNA and RNA.

Key Terms

aldose   The chemical form of monosaccharides in which the carbonyl group is an aldehyde.

apoprotein   Polypeptide chain not yet complexed to its specific prosthetic group.

carbohydrates   Chemicals with the general formula of hydrated carbon, $(CH_2O)_n$, that are aldehyde or ketone derivatives of polyhydric alcohols. Commonly called *sugars*.

compound (conjugated) proteins   Polypeptide chain complexed with other chemical classes such as lipids (lipoproteins), carbohydrates (glycoproteins), or nucleic acids (nucleoproteins).

conjugated lipids   Esters of fatty acids and alcohols containing additional chemical moieties. Group includes phospholipids, sphingolipids, sterols, bile acids.

denaturation   Unfolding the tertiary structure of a protein that often renders it insoluble, causing it to precipitate out of solution.

derived lipids   Lipids derived from the hydrolysis of simple and conjugated fats; these include the fatty acids.

furanose   Five-membered rings of monosaccharides formed by intramolecular reaction between the carbonyl group and a hydroxyl group; present in alpha or beta stereoisomeric forms.

ketose   The chemical form of a monosaccharide in which the carbonyl group is a ketone.

nucleosides   Purine or pyrimidine bases linked to the 5-carbon sugar molecules ribose or deoxyribose through a β-*N*-glycosidic bond to the 1 position of the pyrimidine ring or the 9 position of the purine ring.

nucleotides   Nucleosides with phosphate groups attached at the 3' and/or 5' positions of the sugar molecule.

peptide bond   The covalent amide bond between a primary amino group of one amino acid and the carboxylic acid group of a second amino acid.

primary structure   The linear sequence of amino acids in a protein, defined by the genetic code resident in DNA.

prosthetic group   A nonprotein chemical group that is bound to a protein and is responsible for the biological activity of the protein. The functional complex between protein and a prosthetic group is called a *holoprotein*, and the protein without the prosthetic group is called an *apoprotein*.

pyranose   Six-membered rings of monosaccharides formed by intramolecular reaction between a carbonyl group and a hydroxy group, present in an alpha or beta stereoisomeric form.

quaternary structure   The three-dimensional spatial arrangement of polypeptide chains, resulting from the combining of more than one polypeptide chain into a larger, stable complex.

Schiff's base   Covalent complex between a primary amine and carbonyl function of an aldose.

secondary structure   The spatial arrangement of a linear chain of amino acids in a polypeptide; common structures include the beta-plated sheet, alpha-helix, and random coil.

sialic acids   *N*-acetyl derivatives of neuraminic acid that are covalently linked to many proteins.

simple lipids   Esters of fatty acids with various alcohols, including the triglycerides and some steroids.

simple proteins   Polypeptide chain consisting only of amino acid groups.

tertiary structure   The intramolecular folding of a polypeptide chain onto itself, resulting from interactions between side-chain groups of individual amino acids.

zwitterion   Molecule containing two ionized groups of opposite charge. (Pronounced tsvit'-er-í-on.)

This chapter is not intended to provide a complete biochemical review of the analytes measured in the chemistry laboratory. (For this, refer to the excellent biochemistry texts listed in the bibliography.) Instead, this chapter focuses on those properties of proteins, lipids, carbohydrates, and nucleic acids that affect how the analytes may be measured.

Part 1: Proteins

LAWRENCE A. KAPLAN

DEFINITION AND CLASSIFICATION

Proteins are linear polymers of alpha-amino acids. There are 20 natural amino acids with the general structure shown in Fig. 53-1. These exist as the L-stereoisomeric form with the amino group placed on the alpha-carbon atom next to the carboxylic acid group. The pK_a of the carboxylic acid group is approximately 1.8 to 2.4, whereas the pK_a of the alpha-

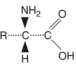

Fig. 53-1   General structure of amino acid of *l*-stereoisomeric form. *Heavy lines*, bonds coming out of plane of page; *dotted lines*, bonds extending behind plane of paper.

amino group is approximately 8.53 to 10.53. This means that at pH less than 2.53, the carboxylic acid will be in the nonionized form (COOH), whereas the alpha-amino group will remain ionized at pH values less than 9.53 (Fig. 53-2). At physiological pH (approximately 7.4), both groups are ionized. A compound (such as an amino acid) with two opposite charges is called a **zwitterion** ("hybrid ion" or "hermaphrodite ion").

The side chain groups of the 20 amino acids are listed in Table 53-1, along with the pK_a values of all ionizable groups.

TABLE 53-1   CLASSIFICATION AND PROPERTIES OF SIDE CHAIN (R GROUPS) FOR NATURALLY OCCURRING AMINO ACIDS

NH_2 | R group (R—CHCOOH)	L-Amino Acid (Symbol)	Amino Acid Molecular Weight	PK$_A$* (25°C)		Secondary Groups
			Primary —COOH	Primary —NH$_2$	
Nonpolar (Hydrophobic)					
H—	Glycine (gly), G	75.07	2.34	9.60	—
CH_3—	Alanine (ala), A	89.09	2.34	9.69	—
CH_3 CH— CH_3	Valine (val), V	117.15	2.32	9.62	—
H_3C CH—CH_2— H_3C	Leucine (leu), L	131.18	2.36	9.60	—
CH_3CH_2—CH— CH_3	Isoleucine (ile), I	131.18	2.36	9.68	—
—CH_2—	Phenylalanine (phe), F	165.19	1.83	9.13	—

H_2C—CH_2
H_2C CH_2
    N
    H
	Proline (pro), P	115.13	1.99	10.60	—

CH_3—S—CH_2CH_2	Methionine (met), M	149.21	2.28	9.21	—
Neutral Polar (Hydrophilic)					
$OHCH_2$—	Serine (ser), S	105.09	2.21	9.15	—
CH_3CH— | OH	Threonine (thr), T	119.12	—	—	—
O ‖ NH_2—CCH_2—	Asparagine (asp), N	132.12	2.02	8.80	—
O ‖ NH_2—CCH_2CH_2—	Glutamine (gln), Q	146.15	2.17	9.13	—
$HSCH_2$—	Cysteine (cys), C	121.16	1.96 (30°)	10.28	8.18 (SH)
HO—⟨ ⟩—CH_2—	Tyrosine (tyr), Y	181.19	2.20	9.11	10.07 (OH)
C—CH_2— ‖ CH N H	Tryptophan (trp), W	204.23	2.38	9.39	—
Acidic Polar (Hydrophilic)					
$HOOCCH_2$—	Aspartic acid (asp), D	133.10	1.88	9.60	3.65 (COOH)
$HOOCCH_2CH_2$—	Glutamic acid (glu), E	147.13	2.19	9.67	4.25 (COOH)
Basic Polar (Hydrophilic)					
$H_2NCH_2CH_2CH_2CH_2$—	Lysine (lys), K	146.19	2.18	8.95	(10.53) (E—NH_3)

H_2N—C—N—$CH_2CH_2CH_2$—
        NH
        ‖
        H
	Arginine (arg), R	174.20	2.17	9.04	12.48 (guanidinium)

HC═—CH_2—
N   NH
    C
    H
	Histidine (his), H	155.16	1.82	9.17	6.00 (imidazolium)

From Cohn EJ, Edsall JT: Proteins, amino acids and peptides, New York, 1943, Reinhold Co.
The pK$_a$ values will be slightly different in a protein molecule.

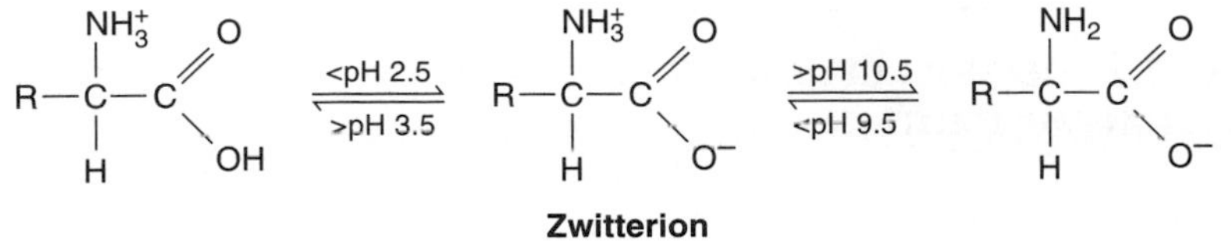

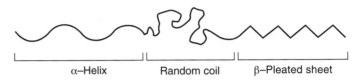

Fig. 53-2   Various ionized and nonionized forms of amino acids present at various pH levels. When two opposite charges are present on same molecule, molecule is called a *zwitterion.*

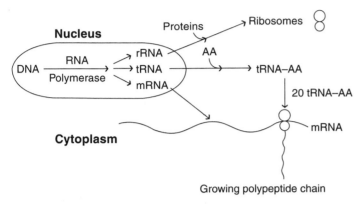

Fig. 53-3   Scheme of synthesis of proteins. *AA,* amino acid; *DNA,* deoxyribonucleic acid; *tRNA,* transfer ribonucleic acid; *mRNA,* messenger ribonucleic acid; *rRNA,* ribosomal ribonucleic acid (18S and 28S forms); *tRNA-AA,* activated amino acid covalently bound to amino acid-specific tRNA.

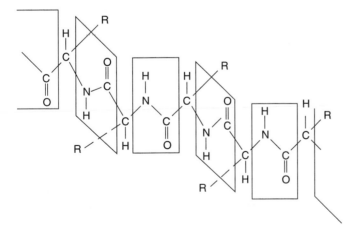

Fig. 53-4   Spatial relationships of a polypeptide bond. *C,* carbon atom; *N,* nitrogen atom; *H,* hydrogen atom; *O,* oxygen atom. *(From Orten JM, Neuhaus OW:* Human biochemistry, *ed 10, St Louis, 1982, Mosby.)*

These side-chain groups can interact with one another to determine the overall chemical, physical, and biological properties of the polypeptide chain.

The amino acids are covalently linked together by the protein-synthesizing machinery of cells. The actual order or sequence of amino acids in a protein chain is predetermined by the genetic code within the cell. The sequence of genetic

Fig. 53-5   Scheme of three possible polypeptide chain conformations defining secondary structure of proteins.

information in DNA is transcribed into messenger RNA, which is translated in the cytoplasm into protein (Fig. 53-3). The specific sequence of amino acids for protein is called its **primary structure**.

The amino acids are linked together by the **peptide bond**. As shown in Fig. 53-4, this bond has a specific arrangement in three-dimensional space. The linear polypeptide chain can exist in three possible conformations, alpha-helix, beta-pleated sheet, and random coil (Fig. 53-5). These conformations are called the **secondary structure** of the protein.

When a polypeptide chain is in solution, it is flexible enough for the molecule to bend, allowing the side chain groups to interact with one another. The types of interactions are listed in Table 53-2. Although the interaction energy of each side group is small, the net energy of all these interactions is great enough to stabilize proteins in a folded, convoluted, three-dimensional spatial arrangement called the **tertiary structure** (Fig. 53-6). Each protein's unique tertiary structure confers on it specific biological properties.

The folded polypeptide chains are often organized as aggregates with identical or different polypeptides. The specific number and type of these polypeptide chains determines the specific properties of the entire complex. The spatial arrangement of these multichain proteins is called the **quaternary structure** of the protein. Usually the biological properties of such quaternary proteins consisting of subunit chains is the sum of each individual chain.

Proteins are generally classified into two major groups, **simple proteins** and **compound (conjugated) proteins**, with several subdivisions within each group. This classification scheme is based on the physical properties and chemical composition of the protein.

I. *Simple proteins*—Generally not associated with other major chemical classes
   A. Globular proteins—Relatively symmetric water-soluble or saline-soluble proteins
      1. Albumin—Major serum protein

TABLE 53-2   TYPES OF INTRAMOLECULAR SIDE-CHAIN INTERACTIONS OF PROTEIN R-GROUPS

Type of Bone	Schematic*
Covalent	
Disulfide (cystine)	$-S-S-$
Lysinonorleucine (in collagen)	$-(CH_2)_3-CH_2-\overset{H}{N}-(CH_2)_4-$
Noncovalent	
Electrostatic	
Hydrogen	
Hydrophobic	
Van der Waals	

*Wavy line, *Polypeptide chain.*

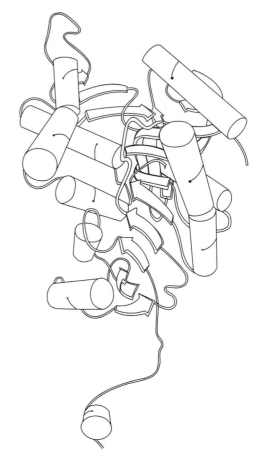

Fig. 53-6 Scheme of tertiary structure of a protein. *Cylinders,* α-helix; *flat arrows,* β-pleated sheet; *lines,* random coil secondary structure of lactate dehydrogenase. *(From Orten JM, Neuhaus OW:* Human biochemistry, *ed 10, St Louis, 1982, Mosby.)*

2. Globulins—Most other serum proteins
3. Histones—Basic proteins found associated with nucleic acids
4. Protamines—Strongly basic proteins found associated with nucleic acids
B. Fibrous proteins—Asymmetric proteins that are insoluble in water or dilute salts; highly resistant to most proteolytic enzymes
   1. Collagens—Major proteins of connective tissue; high in hydroxyproline content
      2. Elastins—Found in elastic tissue such as tendon and arteries
      3. Keratins—Major proteins in animal hair, nails, hooves, and elsewhere
II. *Compound (conjugated) proteins*—Combined with other non–amino acid biochemicals; considered to consist of two components: the protein, called the *apoprotein*, and the nonprotein prosthetic group, the ability of the **prosthetic group** and apoprotein to dissociate varying from group to group
   A. Nucleoproteins—The prosthetic groups are the nucleic acids (DNA or RNA)
   B. Mucoproteins—In which large amounts (more than 4% by weight) of complex carbohydrates are covalently linked to the protein
   C. Glycoproteins—Also contain covalently linked carbohydrate residues but usually less than 4% by weight
   D. Lipoproteins—Contain cholesterol, triglycerides, and phospholipids associated with highly water-insoluble proteins
   E. Metalloproteins—Include proteins that contain metals strongly bound to the protein, either as the ion

or as complex metals, such as the flavoproteins and hemoproteins

F. Phosphoproteins—Contain high concentrations of phosphate groups covalently linked to protein

The biological functions of the proteins are extraordinarily varied, but many functions (see later discussion) are specific for only one or two of these classes of proteins.

CHEMICAL PROPERTIES

The chemical properties of proteins are based on the sum of their parts, that is, the constituent amino acids and prosthetic groups. The peptide bond is chemically reactive and is the basis of the most popular, specific method for quantifying total protein in serum. This is the biuret reaction. The amino acid side-chain groups are also chemically reactive, though only a few of these reactions are used in the chemistry laboratory. The amino groups at the *N*-terminus of the polypeptide chain and those of lysine and the guanidino groups of arginine can react with several compounds to produce an intense fluorescence. These same groups can react with Ninhydrin to give a blue color. Both of these reactions have been used to quantify total protein.

The phenolic group of tyrosine and the indole group of tryptophan react with the oxidizing reagent of the Folin-Wu or Lowry reactions to form a blue color. This method is employed with dilute solutions or microanalysis.

PHYSICAL PROPERTIES

The aromatic amino acids (tryptophan, phenylalanine, and tyrosine) give most proteins an absorption spectrum with the unique absorption maximum at 278 to 280 nm. The absorption at 280 nm is used to estimate the concentration of proteins in solution. In addition, complex proteins, such as hemoglobin, which have prosthetic groups with unique absorption properties, can be individually quantitated without extensive purification on the basis of their specific absorption spectra. The Soret absorption band of hemoglobin at 415 nm is used extensively to quantitate the concentration of hemoglobins.

Polypeptide chains vary widely in molecular size. The smallest polypeptides, such as the endorphins or the hypothalamic hormones, contain 5 to 25 amino acids, whereas the largest proteins, containing several subunits, can have molecular weights in the millions of daltons. Although separation of protein on the basis of different molecular weights can be done, it is a method rarely used in the chemistry laboratory.

The density of most proteins falls within a fairly narrow range, averaging about 1.33 g/mL. Lipoproteins represent an important exception because the lipid content of these proteins gives them an unusually low density, allowing the various classes of lipoproteins to be separated from each other and from other proteins on the basis of their density. This technique is used mainly in specialized laboratories.

An important physical property of proteins is the net charge on the protein molecule. The net charge on a protein is the sum of all ionic charges of the amino acids and the carbohydrate and the prosthetic groups of the protein. Since the various chemical groups are ionized at different pH levels, the net charge of a protein varies with pH. The pH at which a protein carries no net charge is called the *isoelectric point* (*pI*); the isoelectric point of a protein is the point at which the number of positively charged groups equals the number of negatively charged groups. At a pH greater than the pI, the protein will be negatively charged, whereas at a pH less than the pI, it will be more positively charged. At physiological pH most serum proteins are negatively charged.

Since proteins differ in the number and type of constituent amino acids, they also differ in their pIs. Therefore, at different pH levels, proteins will carry different net charges. This difference in net charge is the basis of many procedures for separating and quantifying classes of proteins or individual proteins. The most common procedures are electrophoresis, ion-exchange chromatography, and isoelectric focusing. After separation, individual proteins are detected spectrophotometrically or by use of specific stains.

Proteins found in body fluids are readily water-soluble but can become insoluble in the presence of a wide range of denaturing or precipitating agents. These include organic solvents (such as acetone and acetonitrile), heavy metals (such as tungstic acid), certain salts (such as zinc hydroxide and ammonium sulfate), and strong acids (such as sulfosalicylic acid, trichloroacetic acid, and mineral acids). The **denaturation** of proteins from solution by the use of one or more of these chemicals is the basis for a few routine clinical analyses. Cerebrospinal fluid and urine protein measurements are commonly performed by turbidimetric analysis. In addition, protein precipitation steps are often included as part of purification schemes for analytes before analysis.

BIOLOGICAL PROPERTIES

All proteins fulfill some physiological or biological function. The known functions of proteins cover a wide range of activities and are listed in Table 53-3. Often the known biological property of a protein is the basis of a method for its detection and quantification.

Of the important physiological functions of proteins, the most important to the clinical chemistry laboratory are the transport, receptor, and catalytic functions. Many serum proteins function as specific transporters of small molecules. Most transport proteins are globular proteins. Examples are thyroid-binding globulin (TBG), which binds thyroxine; transcortin, which binds cortisol; and albumin, which transports free fatty acids, unconjugated bilirubin, calcium, and many other endogenous and exogenous compounds. The specific binding properties of these transport proteins have been used as the basis for procedures to measure the serum concentrations of cortisol, TBG saturation, and other analytes. The lipoproteins function as transporters of lipids in serum (see Chapter 33).

Many cellular proteins act as intermediary information processors for hormone molecules. Each protein, called a

TABLE 53-3   BIOLOGICAL FUNCTIONS OF PROTEINS

Function	Example
Transport of small molecules	Transcortin (cortisol), thyroxine (TBG)
Receptors	Estriol receptors (cytoplasmic), insulin receptors (surface)
Catalytic	All enzymes
Structural	Collagen
Nutritional (source of calories and amino acids)	Albumin
Oncotic pressure	Albumin
Host defense versus foreign antigens	Antibodies (all classes)
Hormonal	Thyroid-stimulating hormone (TSH)
Coagulation	Fibrinogen

receptor, binds a specific hormone and then acts to transmit the hormonal message to the cell. Receptor proteins are usually glycoproteins. Assays for specific receptors, such as estrogen and progesterone receptors, are valuable for the management of certain types of cancers.

An important property of some proteins is their ability to catalyze biochemical reactions. The serum concentrations of these proteins, called enzymes, are important in determining the nature of a disease process. Most proteins exhibiting catalytic properties are globular or metalloproteins. An enzyme is most often measured by monitoring the biochemical reaction it catalyzes. The conditions of the enzyme assay are defined so as to give maximum enzymatic activity and sensitivity of analysis (see Chapter 54).

One of the most important biological properties of proteins is their ability to act as antigens (see Chapter 11). An antigen inserted into an immunologically competent host will stimulate the synthesis of antibodies. Antibodies are also globular proteins. An antibody raised against a specific antigen will be able to bind specifically to that antigen. This antibody-antigen interaction is the basis of many assays for the sensitive and specific measurement of proteins and other molecules that cannot be detected by other means.

Proteins play a major role both intracellularly and in tissues. For example, connective tissue is composed primarily of collagen and mucoproteins. The proteins forming the cytoplasmic endoskeleton also fall into this group.

Part 2: Lipids

HERBERT K. NAITO

DEFINITION AND CLASSIFICATION

Lipids (fats) constitute a wide range of organic compounds that differ greatly in their chemical and physical properties and in their physiological roles. They include a variety of substances, such as fatty acids, sterols, triacylglycerides (more commonly called *triglycerides*), phosphorus-containing compounds (phospholipids), fat-soluble vitamins, bile acids, waxes, and other complex fats. As a consequence, it is difficult to provide a uniform and clear-cut definition of lipids that is broad enough to encompass all these diverse compounds. In general, however, one can say that lipids are substances that are insoluble in water but soluble in organic solvents such as alcohol, chloroform, ether, acetone, hexane, and benzene. Even with this general definition, there are some exceptions, such as phospholipids, which are somewhat insoluble in acetone. In addition, some phospholipids, such as phosphatidyl serine, phosphatidyl inositol, and phosphatidyl ethanolamine, have a limited but significant ability to dissolve in water.

There is no generally agreed-on system for the classification of lipids, but for simplicity, the following commonly used classification of lipids may be used.

Simple Lipids

Simple lipids are esters of fatty acids with various alcohols.

Neutral fats. Neutral fats are esters of fatty acids and glycerol (triglycerides). Because they are uncharged, cholesterol and cholesterol esters are also called *neutral lipids*. However, they are structurally steroids and not neutral fats.

The neutral fats contain mixtures of triglycerides, which are esters of glycerol and fatty acids (such as stearic, palmitic, or oleic acid). The general formula for such a fat is:

$$
\begin{array}{c}
H_2C-O-\overset{\displaystyle O}{\underset{\|}{C}}-R_1 \\[6pt]
HC-O-\overset{\displaystyle O}{\underset{\|}{C}}-R_2 \\[6pt]
H_2C-O-\overset{\displaystyle O}{\underset{\|}{C}}-R_3
\end{array}
$$

If $R_1 = R_2 = R_3$ (where R = fatty acid), then the fat is a simple triglyceride. If the Rs are not equivalent, the fat is a mixed triglyceride. Naturally occurring fats usually exist as mixtures of mixed triglycerides.

The fats then are triesters of the trihydric alcohol (glycerol) and of certain but not all organic acids. Since all three glycerol alcohol radicals are esterified, they are termed *triacylglycerides*, or more commonly called *triglycerides*. A simple ester would be formed by the combination of an acid and an alcohol:

$$CH_3COOH + C_2H_5OH \rightarrow CH_3COOC_2H_5 + H_2O$$

A fat is formed by the combination of a fatty acid (usually of relatively high molecular weight) with the alcohol glycerol.

Being esters, the fats are readily hydrolyzed:

$$H_2C-O-C-C_{15}H_{31}$$
$$\underset{O}{\|}$$

$$HC-O-C-C_{15}H_{31} + 3H_2O \rightarrow 3C_{15}H_{31}COOH + \begin{matrix} CH_2OH \\ CHOH \\ CH_2OH \end{matrix}$$
$$\underset{O}{\|}$$

$$H_2C-O-C-C_{15}H_{31}$$
$$\underset{O}{\|}$$

| **Tripalmitin** | **Palmitic acid** | **Glycerol** |

This hydrolysis is accomplished by use of acid, alkali, superheated steam, or an appropriate enzyme (such as pancreatic lipase). In acid hydrolysis, the free fatty acid is liberated. When alkali is used, a soap is formed, and the process is called *saponification*:

$$C_3H_5(O-CO-C_{17}H_{35})_3 + 3NaOH \rightarrow$$
Stearin

$$3C_{17}H_{35}COONa + C_3H_5(OH)_3$$
Sodium stearate   Gylcerol
(a soap)

The fats we eat are mostly triglycerides that contain even-numbered fatty acids because of their mode of biosynthesis. These range from butyric (C_4) to lignoceric (C_{24}) and probably higher fatty acids (see Table 53-5). Odd-numbered fatty acids do occur naturally.

Waxes. Waxes are esters of fatty acids with higher molecular-weight-alcohols than glycerol. Examples are carnauba wax, wool wax, beeswax, and sperm oil. Industrially, they are used in the manufacture of lubricants (sperm oil), polishes (carnauba wax), ointments (lanolin, which contains wool wax), candles (spermaceti), and so on.

Aside from cholesterol, the common alcohols found in waxes are cetyl alcohol ($C_{16}H_{33}OH$), ceryl alcohol ($C_{26}H_{53}OH$), and myricyl alcohol ($C_{30}H_{61}OH$).

Conjugated Lipids

Conjugated lipids are esters of fatty acids and an alcohol, plus additional chemical groups such as alcohols, phosphate, and sugars (Table 53-4).

Phospholipids. Phospholipids are lipids having, in addition to fatty acids and glycerol, a phosphoric acid residue, nitrogen-containing bases, and other constituents. These lipids include phosphatidyl choline (lecithin), phosphatidyl ethanolamine, phosphatidyl inositol, phosphatidyl serine, sphingomyelins, and plasmalogens. Phosphatidyl ethanolamine, phosphatidyl serine, and phosphatidyl inositol (lipositol) are also known as *cephalins*.

This class of complex lipids is also called *glycerophosphatides*, *phosphoglycerides*, *glycerol phosphatides*, or more commonly *phospholipids*. Keep in mind that not all phosphorus-containing lipids are phosphoglycerides; that is, sphingomyelin is a phospholipid because it contains phosphorus, but it is better classified as a sphingolipid because of the nature of the backbone structure to which the fatty acid is attached. In phospholipids, one of the primary OH groups of glycerol is esterified to phosphoric acid; the other OH groups are esterified to fatty acids. The parent compound of the phospholipids is phosphatidic acid, which contains no polar alcohol head group. The phospholipids are constituents of all animal and vegetable cells. They are present in abundance in brain, heart, kidney, eggs, soybeans, and so on. In addition to carbon, hydrogen, and oxygen, the compounds contain the elements nitrogen and phosphorus. In lecithin and cephalin, the nitrogen-phosphorus ratio is 1:1; in sphingomyelin it is 2:1.

$$H_2-C-O-C-R_1$$
$$\underset{O}{\|}$$

$$H-C-O-C-R_2$$
$$\underset{O}{\|}$$

$$H_2-C-O-P-OH$$
$$\underset{OH}{|}$$

Phosphatidic acid

Phosphatidic acid. Phosphatidic acid is important as an intermediate in the synthesis of triglycerides and phospholipids, but it is not found in any quantity in tissues. Phosphatidic acid is the simplest type of phospholipid. Phosphatidic acid is derived from glycerophosphoric acid by esterification of the two remaining OH groups with fatty acids.

Lecithins. On hydrolysis, a typical lecithin forms glycerol, 2 mol of fatty acids, phosphoric acid, and the nitrogenous base, choline. Most lecithins have a saturated fatty acid in the C-1 position and an unsaturated fatty acid in the C-2 position. The structural formula may be written as follows:

$$H_2-C-O-C-R_1$$
$$\underset{O}{\|}$$

$$H-C-O-C-R_2$$
$$\underset{O}{\|}$$

$$H_2-C-O-P-O^-$$
$$\underset{O-CH_2-CH_2-\overset{+}{N}(CH_3)_3}{|}$$

Lecithin
(phosphatidyl choline)

The lecithins, like cholesterol, are common cell constituents that occur principally in animal tissue, having both structural (as part of cell membranes) and metabolic

TABLE 53-4   CLASSIFICATION OF PHOSPHATIDES AND GLYCOLIPIDS

Name	Main Alcohol Component	Other Alcohol Components
Glycerophosphatides		
Phosphatidic acid	Diglyceride (= glycerol diester)	
Lecithin	Diglyceride (= glycerol diester)	Choline
Cephalin	Diglyceride (= glycerol diester)	Ethanolamine, serine
Inositide	Diglyceride (= glycerol diester)	Inositol
Plasmalogens (acetyl phosphatides)	Glycerol diester and enol ether	Ethanolamine, choline
Sphingolipids		
Sphingomyelins	*N*-Acylsphingosine	Choline
Cerebrosides	*N*-Acylsphingosine	Galactose,* glucose*
Sulfatides	*N*-Acylsphingosine	Galactose*
Gangliosides	*N*-Acylsphingosine	Hexoses,* hexosamine,* neuraminic acid*

These components are not present as phosphoric esters but rather in glycosidic linkage; for this reason, cerebrosides, sulfatides, and gangliosides are called gly-colipids.

functions. Although not found in depot fat, they make up a considerable proportion of the liver and brain lipids. They also occur in the plasma as part of the lipid-protein complexes called *lipoproteins*; thus they are important for the formation of these macromolecules, which play an important role in fat transport. Lecithins play an important role in the esterification of free cholesterol to form ester cholesterol. Lecithins are an important constituent of functional lung surfactant.

Cephalins. The cephalins resemble the lecithins in structure except for the component corresponding to choline. There are three main fractions: the ethanolamine cephalins, serine cephalins, and inositol cephalins. The cephalins differ from lecithins in their insolubility in ethanol or methanol.

Phosphatidyl ethanolamine. Phosphatidyl ethanolamine differs from lecithins in that ethanolamine replaces choline. Both alpha and beta cephalins are known. This is one of the more abundant cephalins found in higher plants and animals.

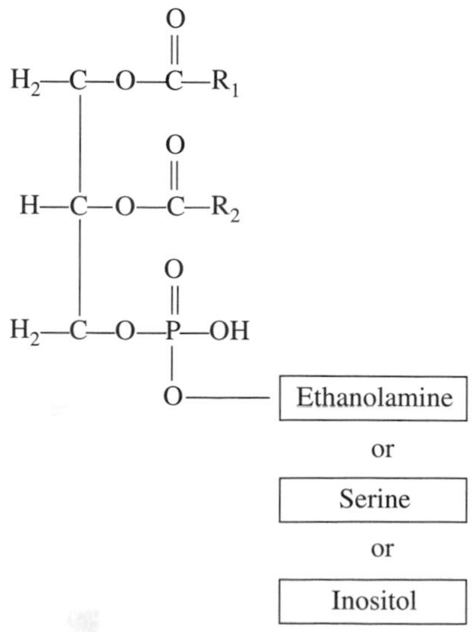

$$
\begin{array}{c}
\quad\quad\quad O \\
\quad\quad\quad \| \\
H_2{-}C{-}O{-}C{-}R_1 \\
\quad| \\
\quad\quad\quad O \\
\quad\quad\quad \| \\
H{-}C{-}O{-}C{-}R_2 \\
\quad| \\
\quad\quad\quad O \\
\quad\quad\quad \| \\
H_2{-}C{-}O{-}P{-}OH \\
\quad\quad\quad\quad | \\
\quad\quad\quad\quad O
\end{array}
$$

Ethanolamine

or

Serine

or

Inositol

Phosphatidyl serine. Phosphatidyl serine, which contains the amino acid serine rather than ethanolamine, has been found in tissues such as the brain.

Phosphatidyl inositol. Phosphatidyl inositol is found in phospholipids of brain tissue and of soybeans and in other plant phospholipids as well. The inositol is present as the stereoisomer myoinositol.

Plasmalogens. Plasmalogens constitute as much as 10% of the phospholipids of the membranes of nerves and muscles. They are also found in the liver and other organs. Structurally, the plasmalogens resemble lecithins and cephalins but give a positive reaction when tested for aldehydes with Schiff's reagent (fuchsin-sulfurous acid) after pretreatment of the phospholipid with mercuric chloride. These phospholipids contain long-chain fatty aldehydes in place of fatty acids. Thus the basic units of this class of compounds include glycerol, phosphorus, fatty aldehyde, and ethanolamine.

Sphingolipids. The amino dialcohol group sphingosine characterizes all sphingolipids. It serves as a structural unit for substitution, just as the trihydroxyalcohol glycerol does in glycerides. Sphingosine is a long-chain C_{18} compound that contains a *trans*-double bond, an NH_2 group on C-2, and two OH groups (on C-1 and C-3). Sphingolipids are especially abundant in the brain. Some storage diseases are characterized biochemically by the accumulation of certain sphingolipids. There are four major categories (see Table 53-2): sphingomyelins, cerebrosides, sulfatides, and gangliosides.

Sphingomyelins. Sphingomyelins are found in the brain and other organs. Stearic, lignoceric, and nervonic acids are the sole fatty acids present in brain sphingomyelins, whereas palmitic and lignoceric acids are the fatty acids in lung and spleen sphingomyelins. A typical formula is shown at the top of p. 1033.

Sphingomyelin

$$CH_3—(CH_2)_{12}—CH=CH—\underset{\underset{H}{|}}{\overset{\overset{HO}{|}}{C}}—\underset{\underset{NH}{|}}{\overset{\overset{H}{|}}{C}}—CH_2—O—\underset{\underset{O^-}{|}}{\overset{\overset{O}{\|}}{P}}—O—CH_2—CH_2—N^+(CH_3)_3$$

Sphingosine

$$\begin{array}{c} | \\ C=O \\ | \\ (CH)_{22} \\ | \\ CH_3 \end{array}$$

Phosphoryl choline

Fatty acid

and its two important constituents are:

$$CH_3—(CH_2)_{12}—CH=CH—\underset{\underset{H}{|}}{\overset{\overset{HO}{|}}{C}}—\underset{\underset{NH_2}{|}}{\overset{\overset{H}{|}}{C}}—CH_2OH \qquad CH_3(CH_2)_{22}—COOH$$

Sphingosine   **Lignoceric acid**

Cerebrosides. Cerebrosides contain galactose or glucose, a high-molecular-weight fatty acid, and sphingosine. Thus cerebrosides have the following basic structure:

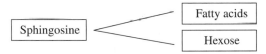

Cerebrosides are structurally similar to sphingomyelins. They may also be classified with the sphingomyelins as sphingolipids. Individual cerebrosides are differentiated by the type of fatty acid in the molecule: *kerasins* contain lignoceric acid; *cerebrons* contain a hydroxylignoceric acid (cerebronic acid); *nervons* contain an unsaturated homologue of lignoceric acid called *nervonic acid*; and *oxynervons* apparently contain the hydroxyl derivative of nervonic acid as a constituent fatty acid.

$$CH_3—(CH_2)_{22}—COOH$$
Lignoceric acid

$$CH_3—(CH_2)_{21}—CH(OH)—COOH$$
Cerebronic acid

$$CH_3—(CH_2)_7—CH=CH—(CH_2)_{13}—COOH$$
Nervonic acid

$$CH_3—(CH_2)_7—CH=CH—(CH_2)_{12}—CO(OH)—COOH$$
Oxynervonic acid

Cerebrosides are found in many tissues other than the brain. In Gaucher's disease, the cerebroside content of the reticuloendothelial cells (as in the spleen) is very high. The cerebrosides are in much higher concentration in myelinated than in nonmyelinated nerve fibers.

Sulfatides. Sulfatides are sulfate derivatives of the galactosyl residue in cerebrosides.

Gangliosides. Gangliosides are glycolipids occurring in the brain (in ganglionic cells). The main components are sphingosine, fatty acids, and branched-chain carbohydrates with as many as seven sugar residues. The construction of

gangliosides is similar to that of cerebrosides, but the carbohydrate moiety is far more complex. The various gangliosides are different primarily in the number of sugar residues.

Derived Lipids

Derived lipids are compounds derived from the hydrolysis of simple and conjugated fats. These include the compounds described below.

Fatty acids. Fatty acids are straight-chain carboxylic acids (both saturated, containing no double bonds, and unsaturated, containing one or more double bonds). More than 100 different kinds of fatty acids have been isolated from various lipids of animals, plants, and microorganisms. All possess a long hydrocarbon chain and a terminal carboxyl group. Fatty acids are obtained from the hydrolysis of fats or can be synthesized from two carbon units (acetyl radicals). Fatty acids that occur in naturally occurring fats usually contain an even number of carbon atoms (because they are synthesized from two carbon units) and are straight-chain derivatives.

Some generalizations may be made about the fatty acids present in lipids of higher plants and animals. Nearly all have an even number of carbon atoms and have chains that are between 14 and 22 carbon atoms long; those having 16 or 18 carbons are by far the most abundant. In general, unsaturated fatty acids predominate over the saturated type, particularly in the neutral fats and in cells of poikilothermic (cold-blooded) organisms living at lower temperatures. Unsaturated fatty acids have lower melting points than saturated fatty acids. Most neutral fats rich in unsaturated fatty acids are liquid down to 5° C or lower. In most unsaturated fatty acids in higher organisms, there is a double bond between carbon atoms 9 and 10; additional double bonds usually occur between C-10 and the methyl end of the chain. In fatty acids containing two or more double bonds, the double bonds are never found in conjugation but are separated by one methylene group. The double bonds of nearly all the

TABLE 53-5 COMMON UNSATURATED FATTY ACIDS, NUMBER OF DOUBLE BONDS, AND LENGTH OF CARBON CHAIN

Fatty Acid	Number of Double Bonds	Number of Carbons
Palmitoleic	1	16
Oleic	1	18
Linoleic	2	18
Linolenic	3	18
Arachidonic	4	20

naturally occurring unsaturated fatty acids are in the *cis* configuration. The most abundant unsaturated fatty acids in higher organisms are oleic, linoleic, linolenic, and arachidonic acids (Table 53-5).

Alcohols. Straight-chain alcohols and cyclic alcohols (such as the sterols) are a subclass of derived lipids.

These compounds are widely distributed in plant and animal tissues, either in the free state or in the form of esters (in combination with higher fatty acids). Chemically, they are known as *phenanthrene derivatives*, or more correctly *cyclopentanoperhydrophenanthrene derivatives*.

Steroids. The best known steroid is cholesterol. It is present in all animal cells and is particularly abundant in nervous tissue and liver. Varying quantities of this steroid are found admixed in animal fats but not in vegetable fats. The structure of a cholesterol molecule is illustrated in Fig. 53-7.

The steroids may be classified into the following groups:

Sterols
    Bile acids
    Substances obtained from cardiac glycosides
    Substances obtained from saponins
    Sex hormones
    Adrenocorticosteroids
    Vitamin D

Cholesterol is the precursor of many other steroids in animal tissues, including the bile acids, detergent-like

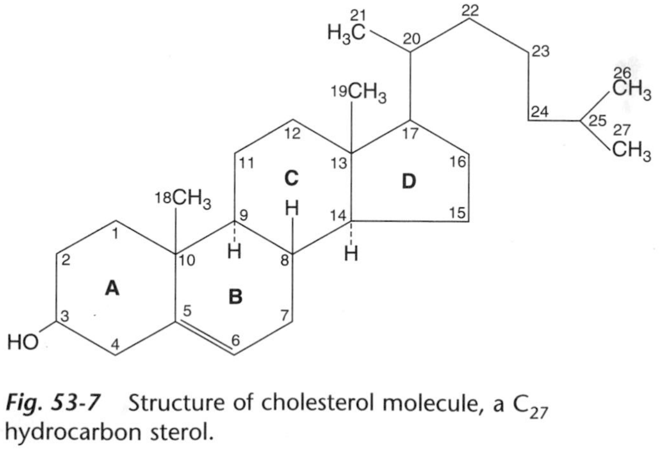

compounds that aid in emulsification and absorption of lipids in the intestine; the androgens, or male sex hormones; the estrogens, or female sex hormones; the progestational hormones; and the adrenocortical hormones.

Cholesterol, a member of a large subgroup of steroids called the *sterols*, is a steroid alcohol containing a hydroxyl group at carbon 3 of ring A and a branched aliphatic chain of eight or more carbon atoms at carbon 17. Sterols occur either as free alcohols or as long-chain fatty acid esters of the hydroxyl group at carbon 3; all are solids at room temperature. Cholesterol melts at 150° C and is insoluble in water but readily extracted from tissues with chloroform, ether, or hot alcohol. Cholesterol occurs in the plasma membranes of animal cells and in the lipoproteins of blood. Cholesterol is found only in animal tissues and fluids, never in plants.

Other similar steroids are phytosterols, which are steroids derived from plants. Among these are stigmasterol, campesterol, and sitosterol.

Fungi and yeasts contain still other types of sterols, the mycosterols. Among these is ergosterol, which is converted to vitamin D.

Bile acids. Bile acids (a C_{24} steroid) are digestion-promoting constituents of bile. They are surface-active agents, which means that they lower surface tension and thus can emulsify fats, an important step in the formation of micelles. Bile acids also activate gastrointestinal lipases. For these reasons, bile acids play an important physiological role in the digestion and absorption of fats.

The major primary bile acids are cholic acid and chenodeoxycholic acid, which are made in the liver by the enzymatic cleavage of the terminal three carbons on the cholesterol molecule (a C_{27} hydrocarbon). Thus the bile acids are one of the end products of the metabolism of cholesterol; however, it should be noted that bile acid constitutes the acidic sterol fraction of the bile, which is about 50% to 60% of the total steroid excreted. The remainder of the steroid output in the bile is in the form of neutral steroids, such as cholesterol.

Hydrocarbons. The hydrocarbons are both aliphatic and cyclic compounds.

Vitamins. Vitamins and their structures are presented in Chapter 39.

Other compound lipids. Sulfolipids, aminolipids, and lipoproteins may also be placed in this category.

CHEMICAL AND PHYSICAL PROPERTIES
Melting Point

The melting point of fatty acids is influenced by the chain length and degree of chain unsaturation. Increasing the chain length and decreasing the number of unsaturated double bonds will increase the melting point of fatty acids. The melting points of fatty acids and other lipids can be used to identify the compound, but this property is not routinely used in analysis.

Solubility

The relative insolubility of lipids in aqueous solutions is an important property of lipids. The major consequence of this insolubility is that analyses of lipids often require a prior

Fig. 53-7 Structure of cholesterol molecule, a C_{27} hydrocarbon sterol.

treatment of the sample to extract the lipid into a more lipid-soluble medium, such as methanol, chloroform, or ether.

Specific Gravity

The specific gravity of all fat is less than 1 g/mL. Consequently, all fats float in water and refrigerated serum samples containing increased amounts of lipid-containing lipoproteins will often have a distinct fat layer floating on top of the aqueous serum. This characteristic has made it possible for lipoproteins to be selectively separated from more dense proteins and for individual lipoproteins to be separated from one another on the basis of varying proportions of lipid content.

Alcohol Groups of Steroids

The chemically reactive alcohol group of steroids is the basis of many assays for quantitating cholesterol. The hydroxyl group can be specifically oxidized by the enzyme cholesterol oxidase. Monitoring of this reaction is the basis for enzyme assays for cholesterol.

Triglyceride Composition

The chemical composition of triglycerides (i.e., glycerol esterified by three fatty acids) is the basis of all methods of quantitating triglycerides. These techniques are based on the quantitation of glycerol released from triglycerides after chemical or enzymatic hydrolysis of the fatty acid esters. The glycerol can be chemically or enzymatically oxidized to form measurable chromogens.

BIOLOGICAL PROPERTIES

The most important biological properties of lipids are structural, nutritional, and hormonal (see Chapter 43). Almost all classes of lipids are used as structural components of membranes. The triglycerides are essential components in the formation of the bimolecular protein-lipid–lipid-protein membranes. Cell membranes also contain varying amounts of steroids, phospholipids, and other complex lipids.

Triglycerides also function as an important source of calories and as a source of carbon atoms for the synthesis of other macromolecules.

Part 3: Carbohydrates

LAWRENCE A. KAPLAN

DEFINITION AND CLASSIFICATION

The earliest carbohydrates were found to have the empirical formula of $(CH_2O)_n$. Thus these chemicals were simply defined as compounds consisting of hydrated (H_2O) carbon, hence the name *carbohydrate*. Subsequently the existence of complex carbohydrates containing other chemical moieties was noted. Thus carbohydrates can be covalently linked to proteins, lipids, and nucleic acids. The various classes of carbohydrates are discussed later.

Simple Monomeric Carbohydrates (Saccharides)

Saccharides are also known as *sugars*, and their common names all end with the suffix *-ose*, meaning "sugar." The

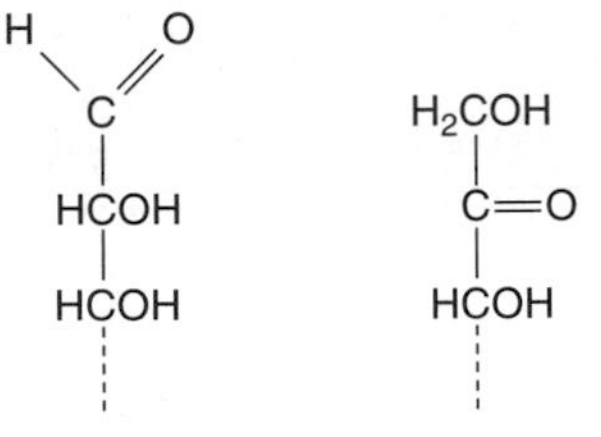

Fig. 53-8 Structural differences between aldoses and ketoses, which are aldehydes and ketones, respectively.

smallest sugar units are *monosaccharides*, in which n in the formula $(CH_2O)_n$ is from 3 to 8. If $n = 3$, the sugar is a triose; if $n = 4$, a tetrose; and so on. The monosaccharides are straight carbon chains in which each carbon atom except one carries a hydroxyl group (—OH); the one remaining carbon atom has a carbonyl group. If the carbonyl group is on the first or last carbon atom, the carbonyl group is an aldehyde and the monosaccharide is called an **aldose**. If the carbonyl group is on an internal carbon atom, it is a ketone, and the monosaccharide is called a **ketose** (Fig. 53-8). Thus a 4-carbon aldose is an *aldotetrose*, a 6-carbon ketose is a *ketohexose*, and so on.

The monosaccharides found in nature are all stereoisomers. Stereoisomerism is physically defined by the ability of a molecule to rotate the plane of incident polarized light. The physical and chemical properties of, for example, all the eight aldohexoses (6-carbon chain) are exactly the same except for their different actions on polarized light. All the monosaccharides in human biochemistry are of the dextroisomeric (D) form. Examples of some monosaccharides are given in Fig. 53-9.

The pentose and hexose monosaccharides also have the ability to form ring structures by intramolecular reaction of the terminal hydroxyl group with the carbonyl function. The six-membered ring forms of the sugars are called **pyranoses**, whereas the five-membered rings are called **furanoses**. The aldohexoses, such as D-glucose, form six-membered rings, whereas an aldoketose, such as D-fructose, forms a five-membered ring (see Fig. 53-9).

Glucose can form two types of six-membered rings. The rings differ in how the hydroxyl group at the number 1 carbon atom is positioned with respect to the plane of the ring. If the hydroxyl group is on the same side of the molecule as the ring oxygen (Fig. 53-9), the isomer is known as the α-D-glucose isomer, whereas if the hydroxyl group is on the opposite side of the ring oxygen, then this isomer is known as the β-D-glucose. Enzymes acting on carbohydrates usually have a specificity directed toward one of the isomers, usually the most common one found, such as β-D-fructose.

Derived Monosaccharides

Derived monosaccharides are formed by reduction or oxidation of the carbonyl groups. The products of reductive reactions are polyols (polyalcohols), such as D-sorbitol or D-mannitol, whereas the products of oxidation are acids, such

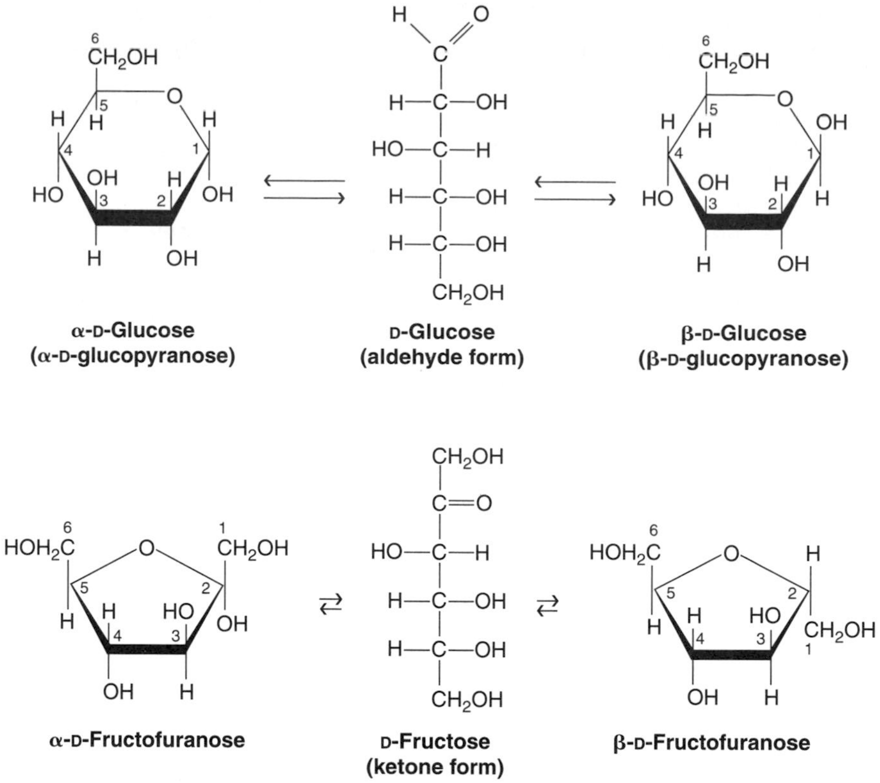

Fig. 53-9 Interrelationships between straight-chain and ring forms of D-glucose and D-fructose, which form pyranose and furanose rings. *(From Orten JM, Neuhaus OW:* Human biochemistry, *ed 10, St Louis, 1982, Mosby.)*

N-Acetylneuraminic acid

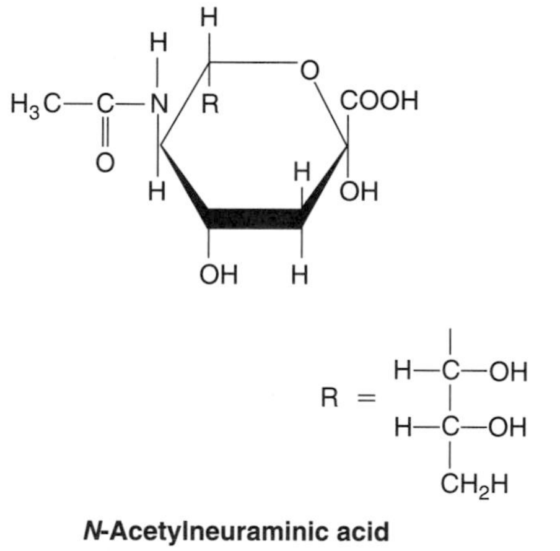

Fig. 53-10 Structure of *N*-acetylneuraminic acid ("sialic acid"). *(From Orten JM, Neuhaus OW:* Human biochemistry, *ed 10, St Louis, 1982, Mosby.)*

as D-glucuronic acid (from D-glucose). Many acid forms of monosaccharides are important constituents of more complex carbohydrates, such as mucopolysaccharides.

An important group of derived monosaccharides is the result of the replacement of a hydroxyl group by an amino group. The term **sialic acid** is used to describe the important *N*-acetyl derivatives of neuraminic acid, which are often found covalently linked to proteins (Fig. 53-10).

Complex Carbohydrates

These molecules are formed by linking two or more monosaccharides by a glycosidic linkage (Fig. 53-11). The simplest disaccharides, important nutritionally, are maltose (two glucose), lactose (milk sugar, one galactose and one glucose), and sucrose (one fructose and one glucose). Oligosaccharides are often defined as carbohydrates containing two to 10 monosaccharide subunits. Polysaccharides are larger polymers of up to 100 million daltons. All three of the most important polysaccharides contain glucose as the monomeric subunit. Cellulose, a structural component of plant walls, consists of glucose units linked by a β-(1→4) glycosidic bond to form long, unbranched chains. Starch, a storage form of glucose in plants, consists of glucose residues connected by α-(1→4) glycosidic linkages, which, unlike the β-(1→4) linkages of cellulose, are amenable to degradation by human hydrolytic enzymes (such as amylase). Starch also differs from cellulose in that it is a branched molecule. Branching points are scattered throughout the molecule formed by α-(1→6) bonds. The two forms of starch are therefore called *amylose* (the straight-chain fraction) and *amylopectin* (the highly branched fraction). Glycogen is the glucose-storage molecule found in animal cells. Glycogen more closely resembles amylopectin than amylose because of its highly branched nature (see Fig. 32-4).

Complex polysaccharides containing hyaluronic acid, chondroitin-4-sulfate, and keratin sulfates as the repeating

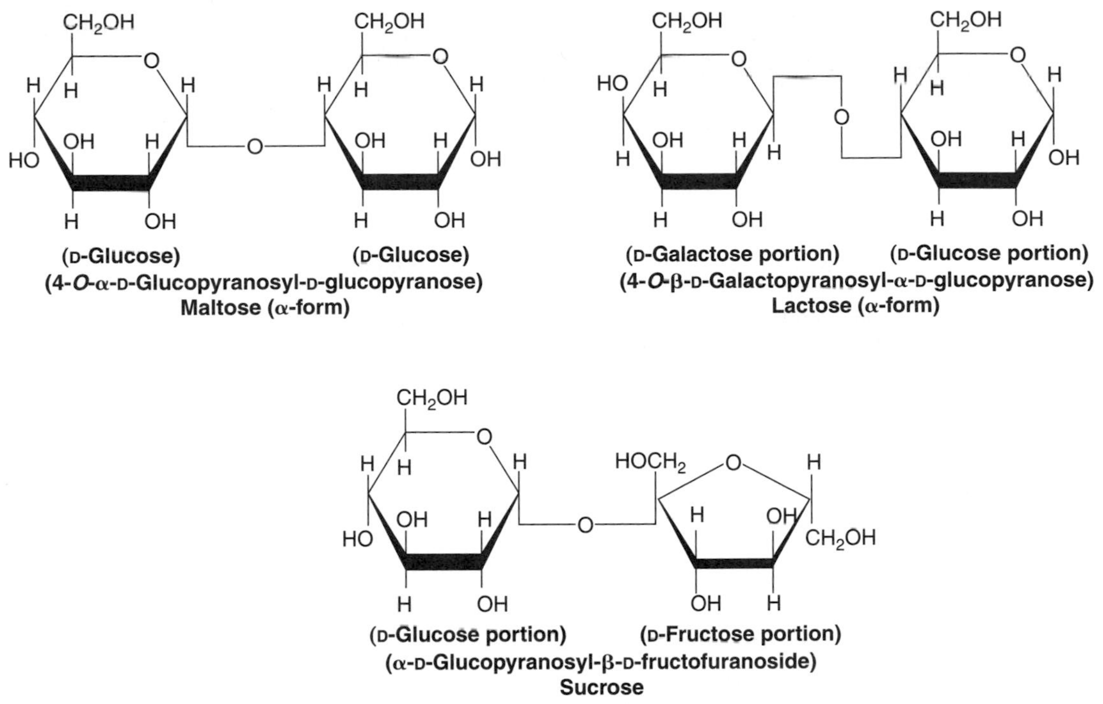

(D-Glucose)   **(D-Glucose)**
(4-*O*-α-D-Glucopyranosyl-D-glucopyranose)
Maltose (α-form)

(D-Galactose portion)   **(D-Glucose portion)**
(4-*O*-β-D-Galactopyranosyl-α-D-glucopyranose)
Lactose (α-form)

(D-Glucose portion)   **(D-Fructose portion)**
(α-D-Glucopyranosyl-β-D-fructofuranoside)
Sucrose

Fig. 53-11   Common disaccharides linked by ?-glycosidic bonds. *(From Orten JM, Neuhaus OW:* Human biochemistry, *ed 10, St Louis, 1982, Mosby.)*

subunits are important constituents of synovial fluid and connective tissue. Heparin is a complex polysaccharide containing D-glucuronic acid-2-sulfate-N-acetyl-D-glucosamine-6-sulfate as the repeating subunit.

CHEMICAL PROPERTIES

The monosaccharides (pentoses and larger) can undergo dehydration in the presence of hot mineral acids to form the cyclic furfural derivatives. Glucose can be dehydrated in this manner to form 3-hydroxymethylfurfural, a reaction that is the basis for a colorimetric assay for glycosylated proteins.

An important chemical property of the monosaccharides is the ability of these compounds to be oxidized or reduced and in turn to reduce or oxidize some other compounds. The ability of reducing aldoses, such as glucose, to be oxidized to the acid form has been the historical basis for chemical assays for glucose. The glucose in turn reduced such compounds as Cu^{++} or $Fe(CN_6)^-$ with the formation of colored complexes of the reduced forms of these compounds (such as Cu^+ and Cu_2O), which is the basis for a confirmation test for the presence of urine glucose.

The enzymatic oxidation of glucose by glucose oxidase is the basis of many of the current glucose assay procedures, whereas the oxidation of glucose-6-phosphate is the basis of the hexokinase assay for glucose.

Aldoses, such as glucose, can react with primary amines to form a **Schiff's base**. This nonenzymatic condensation is the mechanism for the formation of glycoproteins, such as glycosylated hemoglobin, in blood.

PHYSICAL PROPERTIES

The commonly measured monosaccharides and disaccharides are highly water-soluble compounds. Assays for these analytes thus do not require prior extraction or purification. Separation of the monosaccharides by adsorption chromatography is possible, though this is usually performed by specialized metabolic laboratories. The simple monosaccharides, disaccharides, or polysaccharides are not readily distinguished by their spectral or electrophoretic properties.

BIOLOGICAL PROPERTIES

The monosaccharides and disaccharides are the major source of calories for the human body and as such serve as a primary form of nutrition. Polymeric forms of glucose, such as glycogen, serve as a storage for glucose in liver and muscle cells. Complex polysaccharides are found in body fluids and connective tissue.

Part 4: Nucleic Acids
AMADEO J. PESCE

DEFINITION AND CLASSIFICATION
Purine and Pyrimidine Bases

The building blocks of the nucleic acids are the purine and pyrimidine bases. They are part of the structure of ATP and GTP, which function as immediate sources of energy, coenzymes (such as NAD), intracellular messenger molecules, and core components of DNA and RNA. The general structures of purines and pyrimidines are shown in Fig. 53-12.

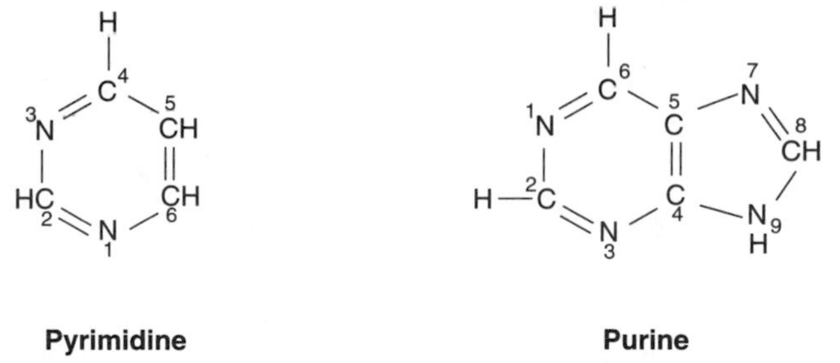

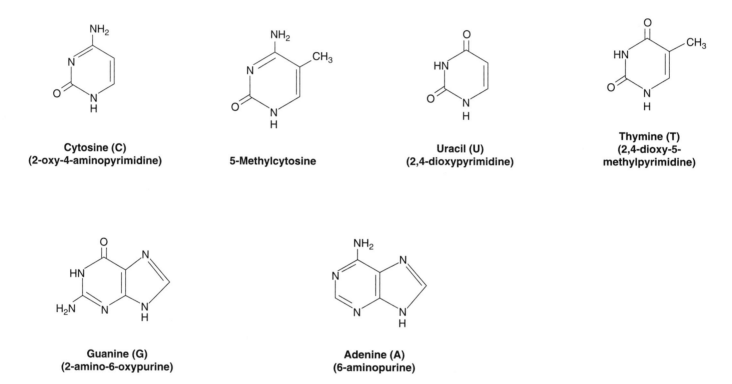

Fig. 53-12 General structures of pyrimidine and purine bases and the IUPAC numbering of the ring positions.

Fig. 53-13 Structures of the most common pyrimidine and purine bases.

The structures of the most commonly observed bases are found in Fig. 53-13. The structure of 5-methylcytosine formed by methylation of cytosine is also presented in Fig. 53-13. These molecules are usually found linked to the 5-carbon sugar molecules ribose or deoxyribose through a β-N-glycosidic bond to the 1 position of the pyrimidine ring or the 9 position of the purine ring (see Fig. 53-14); as such, they are termed **nucleosides**. When the sugar molecules can have phosphate groups attached at the 3' and/or 5' positions (Fig. 53-15), these structures are termed **nucleotides**. The nucleotides can exist as the mono-, di-, and triphosphate forms (Fig. 53-16). The triphosphate forms have regulatory properties and serve as the chemical energy reservoir of the cell. The adenosine and guanosine monophosphate nucleotides can exist in cyclic forms, in which the phosphate is linked to both the 3' and 5' positions (Fig. 53-17).

DNA AND RNA

DNA and RNA are linear polymers of nucleotide bases. There are four natural nucleotides that constitute DNA and four nucleotides that constitute RNA. These nucleotides are linked through phosphate glycoside bonds at the 3' and 5' positions of the 5 carbon ribose or deoxyribose when these molecules are polymerized (Fig. 53-18). The order or sequence of the nucleotides in the DNA chain is the genetic code present within the cell. The sequence of information in the DNA is transcribed into messenger RNA, which is then translated into protein.

The DNA polymer chain has a specific arrangement in three-dimensional spaces. Each chain of the DNA polymer has an opposite or complementary chain. These chains are noncovalently bound to each other through hydrogen bonds, forming a double helix. The bonding is specifically paired,

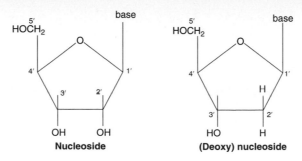

Fig. 53-14 General structures of the ribonucleosides and deoxyribonucleosides and the IUPAC numbering of the sugar positions.

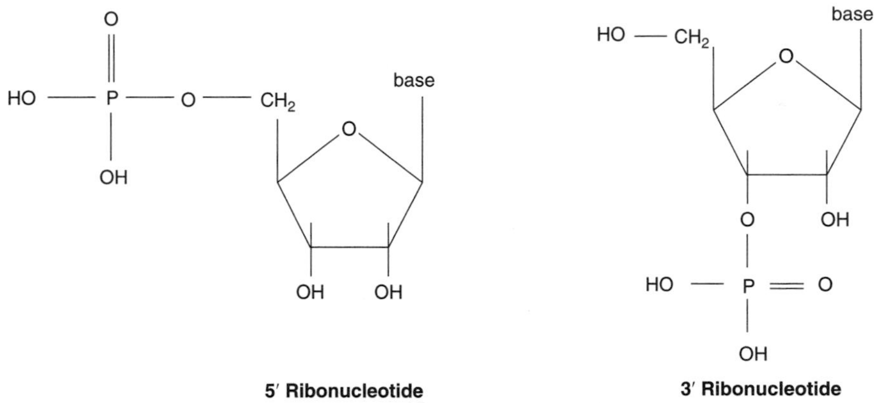

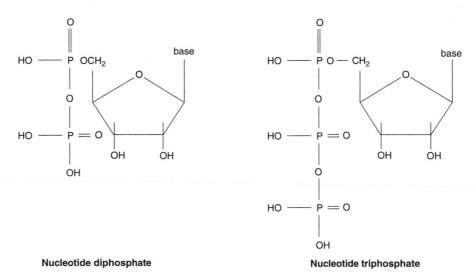

5' Ribonucleotide

3' Ribonucleotide

Fig. 53-15 General structures of the 3' and 5' nucleotides.

Nucleotide diphosphate

Nucleotide triphosphate

Fig. 53-16 5' Nucleotide diphosphate and triphosphate structures.

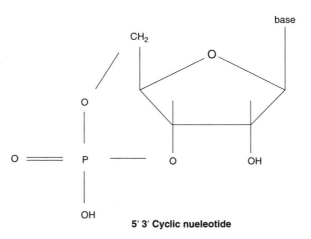

5' 3' Cyclic nueleotide

Fig. 53-17 3',5' cyclic nucleotide structure.

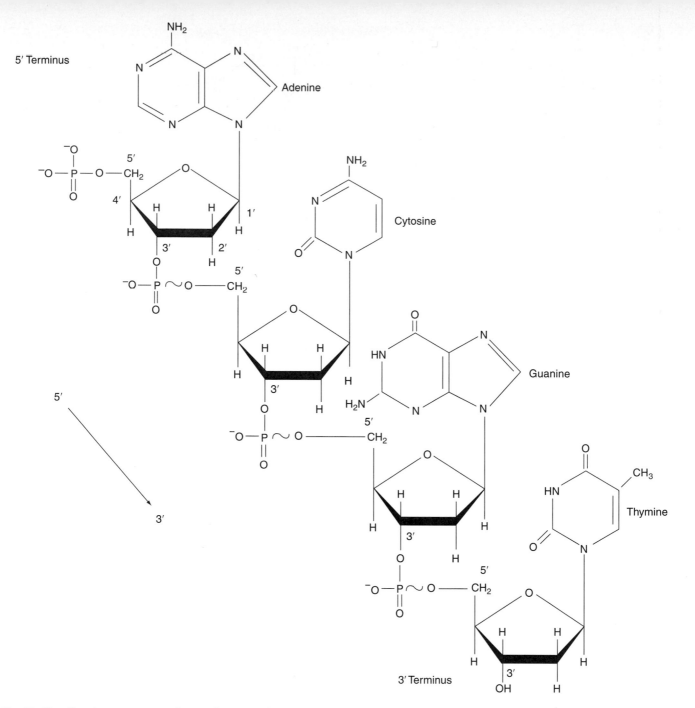

Fig. 53-18 Covalent structure of a single DNA (deoxyribonucleic acid) strand. The polarity of the molecule is shown in the 5′ to 3′ direction by the arrow. *(Reproduced with permission from Roskoski R, Jr: Biochemistry, Philadelphia, 1996, Saunders.)*

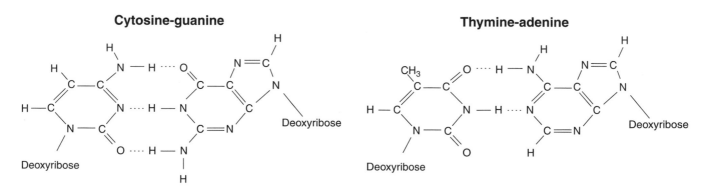

Fig. 53-19 Illustration of complementary base pairing. *(Reproduced with permission from Roskoski R, Jr: Biochemistry, Philadelphia, 1996, Saunders.)*

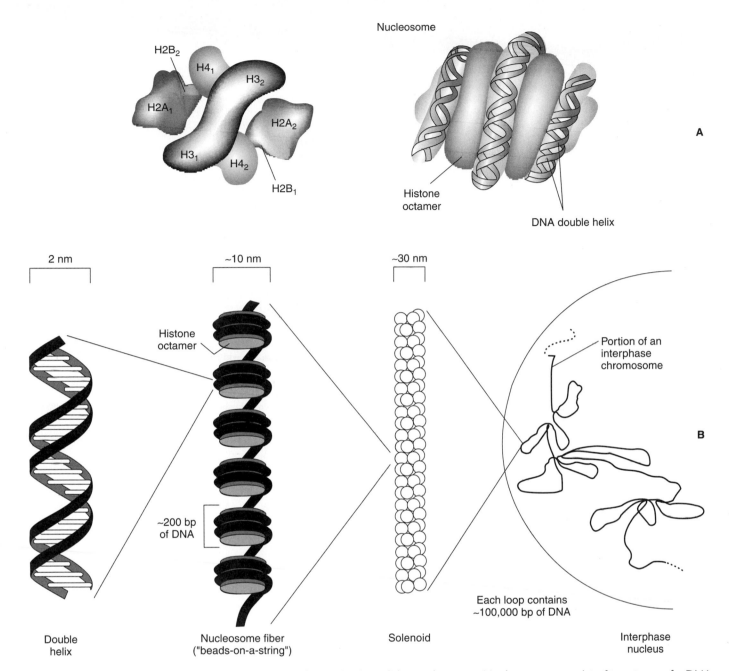

Fig. 53-20   Packaging of human DNA. **A**, Structural organization of the nucleosome. Nucleosomes consist of two turns of a DNA duplex coiled around a histone octamer. The histone octamer of the nucleosome consists of two molecules of each histone H_2A, H_2B, H_3, and H_4. *(Reproduced with permission from Garrett RH, Grisham CM: Biochemistry, Fort Worth, 1995, Saunders College Publishing. Reprinted with permission of Brooks/Cole, an imprint of the Wadsworth Group, a division of Thompson Learning [Fax 800-730-2215].)* **B**, Progressive levels of DNA condensation. *(Reproduced with permission from Thompson MW, McInnes RR, Willard HF: Thompson and Thompson genetics in medicine, ed 5, Philadelphia, 1991, Saunders.)*

with the adenosine hydrogen-bonded to the thymidine molecule and the cytosine molecule hydrogen-bonded to the guanosine molecule (Fig. 53-19). The DNA polymers combine with groups of polycationic proteins termed *histones*, which contain high concentrations of lysine and arginine amino acids. The resulting nucleosome fibers (Fig. 53-20) form very compact structures called *chromosomes*.

DNA and RNA Binding Affinity

The binding affinity of one DNA strand for another is very high, and the laboratory conditions can be modified such that the complementary sequences must be exact for the binding of one DNA molecule to its complementary molecule. This is termed *very stringent binding*. Similarly, the binding between the DNA and its RNA replicate can also be very stringent. These properties are used for a number of nucleic acid assays, as described in Chapters 47 and 48.

Bibliography

General

Devlin TM: *Textbook of biochemistry with clinical correlations*, ed 5, New York, 2002, John Wiley & Sons.

Nelson DL, Cox CT: *Lehninger's principles of biochemistry*, ed 3, New York, 2000, Worth Publishing.

Stryer L, Tymoczko JL: *Biochemistry*, ed 5, New York, 2002, WH Freeman Company.

Voet D, Voet JG, Pratt CW: *Fundamentals of biochemistry, upgrade edition*, New York, 2002, John Wiley & Sons.

Proteins and Amino Acids

Branden C, Tooze J: *Introduction to protein structure*, ed 2, New York, 1998, Garland Press.

Creighton TE: *Proteins: structure*, New York, 1995, WH Freeman.

Kyle J: *Structure in protein chemistry*, New York, 1995, Garland Press.

Lipids

Sebedio JL, Perkins EG, editors: *New trends in lipid and lipoprotein analysis*, Champaign, IL, 1995, AOCS Press.

Cave G, Paltauf F, editors: *Phospholipids: characterization, metabolism, and novel biological applications*, Champaign, IL, 1995, AOCS Press.

Carbohydrates

Brinkley RW: *Modern carbohydrates chemistry*, New York, 1988, Marcel Dekker.

Chaplin MF, Kennedy JF, editors: *Carbohydrate analysis*, ed 2, New York, 1994, Oxford University Press.

Nucleic Acids

Murray RK et al: *Harper's biochemistry*, ed 25, Norwalk, CT, 1999, Appleton & Lange.

Roskoski R, Jr: *Biochemistry*, Philadelphia, 1996, Saunders.

Internet Sites

Proteins

www.friedli.com/herbs/phytochem/proteins.html

http://info.bio.cmu.edu/Courses/BiochemMols/ProtG/ProtGMain.htm

http://www.kumc.edu/research/medicine/biochemistry/bioc800/start.html

http://chemistry.gsu.edu/glactone/PDB/Proteins/Classic/classic.html

www.schoolscience.co.uk/content/5/chemistry/proteins/index.html

Lipids

www.cyberlipid.org/cyberlip/desc0004.htm

Carbohydrates

http://www.chem.qmw.ac.uk/iupac/2carb/

http://ull.chemistry.uakron.edu/genobc/Chapter_17/

Nucleotides

http://www.genome.gov/glossary.cfm?key=nucleotide

http://www.genome.gov/glossary.cfm?key=deoxyribonucleic%20acid%20 (DNA)

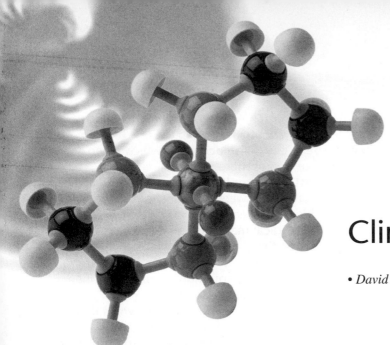

CHAPTER 54

Clinical Enzymology

• *David C. Hohnadel*

Objectives

• Understand the IUB classification of enzymes and why other names are used.
• Describe the differences between apoenzymes, cofactors, and holoenzymes.
• List the major kinetic parameters used to describe enzyme activity.

• Be able to derive the Michaelis-Menten equation.
• Understand how pH, buffers, cofactors, and temperature affect assay kinetics.
• List how reference intervals are influenced by preanalytical variables.

Key Terms

activation energy   The energy required in a chemical reaction to convert reactants to activated or transition-state species that will spontaneously proceed to products.

activators   Inorganic ions that are required cofactors for an enzyme reaction.

active sites   The specific areas on an enzyme where a substrate binds and catalysis takes place.

activity   The amount of substrate for a particular enzymatic reaction that is converted to product per unit time under defined conditions.

allosteric sites, or **regulatory sites**   The sites, other than the active site or sites, of an enzyme that bind regulatory molecules and affect the activity of the enzyme.

apoenzyme   An enzyme without any associated cofactors or with less than the entire amount of cofactors or prosthetic groups.

auxiliary enzyme   In a coupled assay system, an enzyme that links the enzyme being measured with an indicator enzyme.

binding sites   The sites on the surface of the enzyme that serve to bind the substrate or product of the reaction.

bond specificity   The nature of enzyme action that causes the disruption of only certain bonds between atoms.

catalyst   A substance that increases the rate of a reaction without being changed by the reaction.

catalytic site   Another name for active site.

coenzymes   Organic cofactor compounds, such as thiamine pyrophosphate and pyridoxyl-5-phosphate.

cofactors   Nonprotein substances associated with an enzyme that are needed for catalytic activity.

competitive inhibitor   An inhibitor of an enzyme reaction that competes with the substrate by binding at the active site.

constitutive enzymes   Enzymes that are always present during the life of a cell.

coupled assays   Assays with several enzyme reactions leading to an indicator reaction that has an easily measured substance.

denaturation   The loss of the biological properties of a protein, usually as a result of changes in tertiary or quaternary structure.

EC code   The four-number Enzyme Commission code for the systematic classification of enzyme reactions.

ELISA   Enzyme-linked immunosorbent assay.

EMIT   Enzyme-multiplied immunoassay technique.

endopeptidases   Protein-hydrolyzing enzymes that break bonds in the interior of a protein substrate.

end-point assays   Assays in which a single measurement is made at a fixed time.

enzyme kinetics   The study of enzyme reaction rates and the factors that affect them.

enzyme specificity   The degree to which an enzyme will catalyze one or more reactions.

enzyme-substrate complex   An intermediate active complex formed between the substrate and the enzyme during the reaction.

enzymes   Biological materials (proteins) with catalytic properties.

equilibrium constant   The ratio of the concentration of product to the concentration of substrate when the reaction is at equilibrium.

exopeptidases   Protein-hydrolyzing enzymes that break bonds proceeding from one end of the protein substrate toward the center of the substrate.

first-order kinetics   State occurring when the rate of an enzyme reaction is proportional to the concentration of the substrate.

holoenzymes   The complete enzyme-cofactor complex that gives full catalytic activity.

hydrophilic amino acids   Polar, water-loving amino acids.

hydrophobic amino acids   Nonpolar, water-hating amino acids.

inactivation   A reversible denaturation of a protein.

indicator enzymes   Enzymes that produce (or consume) an easily measured substance.

inducible enzymes   Enzymes whose cellular concentrations increase when presented with the appropriate stimulus.

inhibitors   Materials that reduce the catalytic activity of an enzyme.

initial rates   Enzyme measurements made at the start of a reaction just after the lag phase.

international unit of enzyme activity   The amount of enzyme that catalyzes the conversion of one micromole of substrate per minute under defined conditions, $1 \text{ U} = 1.67 \times 10^{-8}$ katal.

in vitro systems   Those systems outside of a living organism, that is, in a test tube.

isoenzymes   Different forms of an enzyme that catalyze the same reaction.

K_m   The symbol for the Michaelis-Menten constant.

katal (kat, K)   An enzyme unit in moles per second defined by the SI system: $1 \text{ K} = 6.0 \times 10^7 \text{ U}$.

kinetic assays   Assays that form increasing amounts of product with time, usually monitored by multiple data points.

labile enzymes   Unstable or easily denatured proteins.

lag phase   The early time in an assay when mixing occurs and temperature and kinetic equilibria are becoming established.

linear phase   Time when an assay is following zero-order kinetics producing a constant amount of product per unit of time.

metalloenzymes   Enzymes that contain very tightly bound metal ions.

Michaelis-Menten constant   A constant related to the rate constants of an enzyme reaction and equal to the concentration of substrate that gives one half the maximal catalytic velocity.

noncompetitive inhibitor   An inhibitor that binds to an allosteric site of an enzyme and does not compete with the substrate by binding at the active site.

optimal assay conditions   Conditions for reaction concentrations of substrates, cofactors, activators, and buffer that produce the maximum rate of enzyme catalysis.

primary structure   The sequence of amino acids of a protein.

prosthetic groups   Cofactors that are so tightly bound that they are considered to be part of the enzyme structure.

quaternary structure   The structural relationship of various enzyme subunits to one another.

reactivation   The restoration of biological properties of a protein after a temporary loss.

regulatory sites   See allosteric sites.

secondary structure   The twisting of amino acids into a semifixed steric relationship in two dimensions.

specific activity   The enzyme activity expressed as units per milligram of protein.

stereoisomeric specificity   The specificity of an enzyme for one form of a D-,L- pair of compounds with an asymmetrical carbon atom.

substrate-depletion phase   The time late in an enzyme assay when the substrate concentration is falling and the assay is not following zero-order kinetics.

substrates   The materials enzymes act upon.

subunits   Single protein chains from enzymes composed of two or more peptide chains in an active form.

Système International d'Unités   An international system of rational and internally consistent units for all types of scientific quantities; SI units.

tertiary structure   The folding of amino acid chains into a three-dimensional structure.

uncompetitive inhibitor   An inhibitor that appears to bind only to the enzyme-substrate complex and not to the free enzyme.

V_{max} The maximum rate of catalysis obtained from variation of substrate.

zero-order kinetics   State occurring when the rate of an enzyme reaction is independent of the concentration of the substrate.

Methods on CD-ROM

Alanine aminotransferase (ALT)
Aldolase
Alkaline phosphatase (ALP)
Amylase
Aspartate aminotransferase (AST)
Cholinesterase
Creatine kinase (CK)

Gamma-glutamyl transferase (GGT)
Lactate dehydrogenase (LD) and lactate dehydrogenase isoenzymes
Lipase
Lysozyme
Prostatic acid phosphatase and prostate-specific antigen

THE NATURE OF ENZYMES

Enzymes are biological materials with catalytic properties; that is, they increase the rate of chemical reactions in cells and in **in vitro systems** that otherwise proceed very slowly. They are large, naturally occurring proteins with molecular weights usually between 13,000 and 500,000 D. Most of the enzymes in cells are **constitutive enzymes**, that is, they are always present, performing some metabolic function. Some tissues, notably the liver, also have enzymes that are not always present but are produced in response to a stimulus. These are **inducible enzymes**. The ingestion of certain drugs causes the liver to produce enzymes capable of metabolizing the drugs to a form that is more easily excreted than the parent compound. The study of these enzymes and the changes in enzyme **activity** that occur in body fluids over time has become a valuable diagnostic tool for the elucidation of various disease states and for testing organ function.

Different tissues or cellular materials contain different amounts or types of enzymes. The hundreds of different enzymes in each cell are attached to the cell walls and membranes and are dissolved in the cytoplasm, or sequestered in the nucleus and other specialized subcellular organelles including microsomes, mitochondria, and lysosomes. Often the determination of one or several enzymes in plasma gives a pattern of activities that is indicative of the tissue or cell type from which the enzymes have been derived. Different cells or compartments within a single cell can even contain different forms of an enzyme that catalyses the same chemical reaction. Assays for these different forms can sometimes be performed to determine the tissue or compartment from which an enzyme has come. A few enzymes are found in plasma or other extracellular fluids where they seem to perform a physiological function, but most enzymes catalyze reactions inside cells or in the lumen of various organs.

Composition and Structure

All enzymes are proteins; that is, they are complex compounds of high molecular weight; they contain amounts of carbon, hydrogen, oxygen, nitrogen, and sulfur that are similar to amounts found in other protein materials; and hydrolysis with strong acid yields a mixture of amino acids and small peptides. Enzymes are distinguished from other proteins that are not enzymes by their catalytic action.

The catalytic behavior of an enzyme is dependent on the **primary**, **secondary**, **tertiary**, and **quaternary structures** of the protein molecule, which are discussed on p. 1027. Changes to the primary amino acid sequence usually result in differences in the three-dimensional structure because the secondary and tertiary folding are different. However, changes to any one of these structures can affect the enzymatic activity of the protein, usually reducing or abolishing it.

Apoenzymes and Cofactors

An enzyme may have nonprotein substances associated with it that are needed for maximal activity. These other materials, called **cofactors**, may be either loosely or tightly bound to the protein portion of the enzyme. Those that are loosely bound can often be removed by dialysis. These materials may be organic compounds such as the oxidized form of nicotinamide adenine dinucleotide phosphate ($NADP^+$) and pyridoxyl-5-phosphate, which are called **coenzymes**, or inorganic ions like chloride (Cl^-) and magnesium (Mg^{2+}), which are called **activators**. Cofactors like the heme portion of peroxidase that are so tightly bound that they are considered to be part of the enzyme structure are termed **prosthetic groups**. Enzymes that have metal ions bound very tightly are called **metalloenzymes**. Two examples of metalloenzymes are ferroxidase, also called *ceruloplasmin*, an enzyme containing a relatively large amount of tightly bound copper, and carbonate dehydratase, also called *carbonic anhydrase*, an enzyme with a large amount of zinc.

The term *coenzyme* is often loosely used when referring to the compound NADH (or NADPH) in a reaction like the lactate dehydrogenase reaction.

$$\text{Pyruvate} + \text{NADH} + \text{H}^+ \overset{\text{LD}}{\rightleftharpoons} \text{L-Lactate} + \text{NAD}^+ \qquad \textit{Eq. 54-1}$$

In a formal kinetic sense, both pyruvate and NADH are substrates for the enzyme reaction, and lactate and NAD^+ are the products. In this case, pyruvate and NADH react with one another on a molar basis. The NADH that reacts is still called a coenzyme, that is, a nonprotein organic material needed for maximal activity, perhaps for historic reasons, although it should be more correctly called a *second substrate*, or *cosubstrate*.

Because it is possible to dialyze away loosely held cofactors from some enzymes and still retain some activity, an enzyme without the associated cofactors is referred to as an **apoenzyme**, and the complete enzyme-cofactor complex is termed a **holoenzyme**. In the clinical use of enzyme assays, the enzyme assay mixture must contain an excess of all the activators and cofactors to ensure that the holoenzyme is the enzyme form being measured, rather than a mixture of apoenzyme and holoenzyme forms.

Catalysts

Enzymes function as biological **catalysts**. They are proteins that have the property of accelerating specific chemical reactions toward equilibrium without being consumed in the process. The material the enzyme reacts with is termed the **substrate**, and a simple enzymatic reaction for one substrate and one product is listed below:

$$\text{E} + \text{S} \underset{k_{-1}}{\overset{k_{+1}}{\rightleftharpoons}} \{\text{ES}\} \underset{k_{-2}}{\overset{k_{+2}}{\rightleftharpoons}} \text{P} + \text{E} \qquad \textit{Eq. 54-2}$$

In this case the enzyme is represented by E, the substrate on which the enzyme acts by S, a postulated enzyme-substrate intermediate complex by $\{ES\}$, and the product of the reaction by P. The forward reaction rate constants are represented by k_{+1} and k_{+2}, whereas the reverse reaction rate constants are represented by k_{-1} and k_{-2}. An example of a single substrate enzyme reaction is the action of the enzyme urease on the substrate urea, although in this case two products are produced:

$$\underset{\textbf{Urea}}{\overset{\overset{\displaystyle O}{\overset{\displaystyle \|}{}}}{\text{H}_2\text{N—C—NH}_2}} + \text{E} \underset{k_{-1}}{\overset{k_{+1}}{\rightleftharpoons}} \{\text{Urea} - \text{E}\} \underset{k_{-2}}{\overset{k_{+2}}{\rightleftharpoons}} \underset{\textbf{Ammonia}}{2\text{NH}_3} + \underset{\substack{\textbf{Carbon} \\ \textbf{dioxide}}}{\text{CO}_2} + \text{E}$$

Water also participates in the reaction but has not been included for clarity. These biological catalysts are like other chemical catalysts in many respects, except that they function in biological systems. Enzyme catalysts, though they are unstable and easily destroyed, have catalytic properties similar to those of other chemical catalysts. These include the following: they are effective in small concentrations; they are unchanged by the reaction; they affect the speed of attaining equilibrium but do not change the final concentrations of the substrates and products of the *equilibrium* state; and they demonstrate a much greater degree of specificity than the usual chemical catalysts for the reactions they accelerate.

It is the first property that makes enzymes such a valuable diagnostic tool. Because they are effective in such small amounts, measurement of changes in enzyme concentrations is a very sensitive way to follow changes that have occurred in various types of tissues.

The amount of enzyme involved in an enzyme assay is very much smaller than the amount of glucose present in an assay for glucose. A conventional chemical assay for enzyme material would be very difficult to produce and require large amounts of sample. Of the several thousand enzymes in plasma, the measurement of the concentration of a single enzyme, even if it is present at a very elevated value, is below the limit of detection for most chemical protein assays. What is easier to measure and is biologically related to many clinical conditions is the amount of catalytic activity of the enzyme and how it changes with time.

The *activity* of an enzyme is the amount of substrate for a particular enzyme reaction that is converted to product per unit time under defined conditions (see p. 1055). The assumption that is made for the use of activity as a concentration is that a given weight of enzyme has a fixed number of units of activity. That is, the specific enzyme activity, in units per milligram of protein, remains constant even when the increase in enzyme activity observed during a particular disorder may come from a different tissue. The increased enzyme activity is assumed to occur because of the presence of more enzyme with the same **specific activity** rather than the presence of another form of the enzyme with a different and perhaps higher specific activity. In practice, activity measurements of enzymes are used as if they were enzyme concentrations.

If the enzyme were acting as a catalyst, it would be unchanged by the reaction, but because of the unstable nature of most enzymes, this property is difficult to demonstrate. It is possible with many current assays to use very short analysis times with sufficient precision to calculate enzyme activity early in an assay period and again after 10 to 15 minutes without showing a decrease in enzyme activity. The amount of substrate converted to product during this time might be 5% to 10% of the initial amount present. Because the enzyme activity determined at both times is unchanged, it is concluded that the enzyme does not participate in the reaction on a molar basis with the substrate and is acting as a catalyst.

Another property of biological catalysts is that they accelerate the attainment of equilibrium but do not shift the final proportions of *S* and *P* in the equilibrium state. One way of considering this process is to examine the effect of lactate dehydrogenase on the conversion of pyruvate to lactate. In the presence of the enzyme LD and the coenzyme NADH, the conversion of pyruvate to lactate occurs rapidly, but without the enzyme the process is so slow that it can hardly be demonstrated.

$$\text{Pyruvate} + \text{NADH} + \text{H}^+ \overset{\text{LD}}{\rightleftharpoons} \text{L-Lactate} + \text{NAD}^+$$

$$\text{Pyruvate} + \text{NADH} + \text{H}^+ \xrightarrow{\text{No enzyme}} \text{No detectable reaction}$$

This is not a one-way process but an approach to the equilibrium concentrations of pyruvate and lactate, because the same enzyme converts lactate to pyruvate with the coenzyme NAD⁺. The speed of the reaction and the conditions employed are not the same in both directions, because they are related to the **equilibrium constant**. It is possible to measure the conversion from either direction, and both methods are widely used to determine LD activity in the clinical laboratory.

Reactive Sites

The Gibbs free-energy change (-ΔG) is the measure of the amount of work a chemical reaction can produce. All reactions that proceed from reactants to products have a net negative free energy (-ΔG). However, the reactants do not become products directly but must absorb enough energy to pass through an activated, or transition, state.

Enzymes lower the energy required for activation to the transition state. Without the enzyme present, even with a favorable negative free energy, that is, with products having a -ΔG lower than that of substrates, the reaction may not proceed to any appreciable extent (Fig. 54-1). The reactants must gain the energy to overcome this **activation energy** barrier to enter the transition state (activated state) and then pass on to products. Without a catalyst present, the reaction will occur only if enough heat or energy can be added to the reaction system. With an enzyme catalyst, the reaction may easily proceed at normal physiological temperatures. Rewriting Eq. 54-2 to account for this transition state in an enzyme-catalyzed reaction, we find that:

$$\text{E} + \text{S} \underset{k_{-1}}{\overset{k_{+1}}{\rightleftharpoons}} \{\text{ES} \rightarrow \text{ES}^* \rightarrow \text{EP}\} \underset{k_{-2}}{\overset{k_{+2}}{\rightleftharpoons}} \text{P} + \text{E} \qquad \textit{Eq. 54-3}$$

in which *ES** is the transition state form of the substrate and *ES* and *EP* are enzyme-substrate and enzyme-product forms with materials bound but not activated. Substantial reductions in the activation energy requirements are often found when enzymes are used as catalysts for the process. For example, the activation energy necessary for the decomposition of hydrogen peroxide is 18,000 cal/mol, but in the presence of the enzyme catalase the activation energy is less than 2000 cal/mol.

One of the most difficult problems enzyme chemists had faced was to explain how an enzyme can reduce the activation energy and at the same time remain unchanged by the reaction. Equation 54-3 schematically shows one general possibility. To better understand the mechanisms of enzyme catalysis, an examination of the details of enzyme structure is necessary.

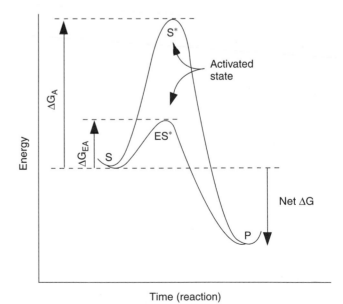

Fig. 54-1 Energy diagram showing reduction in activation energy Δ G$_{EA}$ << Δ G$_A$ that occurs for same reaction with and without enzyme catalyst. *A*, Activated state (also *); *EA*, enzyme activation; *ES*, enzyme substrate; *G*, energy; *P*, product; *S*, substrate.

A wide variety of nonpolar **hydrophobic** and polar **hydrophilic amino acids** are present in enzyme proteins. The external surface of the enzyme for reasons of solubility is believed to be composed of mostly polar but generally unreactive side chains of amino acids. The unreactive amino acid side chains may contain structures like the methyl and isopropyl groups found in alanine and leucine:

$$R—CH_3 \text{ and } R—CH—CH_3$$
$$| $$
$$CH_3$$

Some areas of the enzyme surface contain amino acids with reactive side chains as a part of their structure. The reactive amino acid side chains may contain charged groups like carboxyl and amino groups (i.e., $R—COO^-$ and $R—NH_3^+$) found in aspartic and glutamic acids or lysine and arginine. Noncharged moieties like the hydroxyl and sulfhydryl groups (i.e., $R—OH$ and $R—SH$) found in serine, tyrosine, and cysteine are also reactive. There are other types of reactive groups that are present in amino acids, such as histidine, which has an active nitrogen in a ring structure. The reactive amino acids within an active **catalytic site** bind portions of the substrates, products, activators, and **inhibitors** through ionic and hydrogen bonds. These reactive areas of the enzyme may be on the surface or can exist in more hidden clefts or folds in the enzyme surface and can be involved in the catalytic process itself.

There are only a limited number of places on the enzyme where catalysis can take place. These specific areas are called **active sites**, or *active centers*, and may involve only 5 to 10 amino acids out of a total of 200 to 300 in the entire enzyme. The active site, which has catalytic properties, serves to bind the substrate in a specific way so as to facilitate the breaking and forming of new bonds. The substrate is positioned so that other reactive amino acids at the active site cause this conversion from substrate to product.

The sites on the surface of the enzyme that bind the substrate or product of the reaction are termed **binding sites**. Enzymes, particularly those of a complex structure composed of several **subunits**, often have sites that are far removed from the primary amino acid sequence at the active site but that affect enzyme activity. These sites are called **allosteric sites**, or **regulatory sites**. Although great diversity would be expected among the types of catalytic sites for the many kinds of reactions that enzymes catalyze, some common features have been observed.

The substrate of the reaction binds to the active site and is oriented so that a particular bond is subject to attack (Fig. 54-2). The reactive side-chain moieties of the enzyme interact with the group on the substrate so that the covalent bond to be altered becomes weakened. This bond weakening decreases the activation energy needed for chemical reaction. The weakened bond now undergoes a chemical reaction that breaks the covalent bond and allows new ones to form. The product no longer has the same affinity for the active site as the original substrate and is released from the enzyme.

Changes in the amino acid sequence of a protein could produce different enzymes presumably with different active

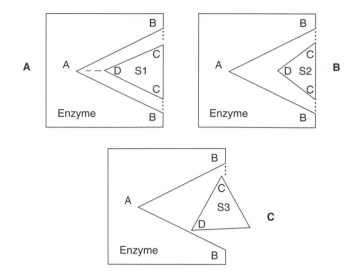

Fig. 54-2 Active site on enzyme is at point *A*, and binding sites are at points *B*. **A**, Correct substrate, *S1*, has complementary binding sites at *C*, and active site can react at point *D* on substrate. **B**, Substrate *S2* has complementary binding sites, but point *D* is too far away for catalysis to take place. If *S2* were present with *S1*, it could act as an inhibitor depending on relative binding constants by preventing *S1* from binding. **C**, Substrate *S3* has only one complementary binding site, *C*, and point *D* is not aligned correctly for catalysis.

and binding sites, or even similar proteins without catalytic activity. Such changes, caused by genetic mutations, are often the cause of inborn errors of metabolism and other diseases of genetic origin (see Chapter 47).

The chemical reactions in which these reactive amino acids take part not only define the enzyme's specific catalytic activity but also determine the sensitivity of the enzyme to losses of activity by such factors as heavy metals, detergents, or even other reactive parts of the same protein molecule. Metals or detergents may bind to active groups and inactivate them. Changes in surface tension, that is, vigorous shaking, may cause unfolding of the protein or **denaturation**. As a result, the spatial relationships of these reactive amino acids with each other are disrupted, preventing the usual reaction from taking place.

Specificity of Reaction

Differences in **enzyme specificity** are believed to be related to physical differences at the active site. Some enzymes react with many related compounds and are said to have a broad specificity. Acid phosphatase is one of the enzymes that exhibits a broad **bond specificity** by hydrolyzing several types of organic phosphate esters, such as β-glycerol phosphate, thymolphthalein phosphate, *para*-nitrophenyl phosphate, and α-naphthyl phosphate. At an acid pH, the enzyme-catalyzed reaction

$$R—O—P + H_2O \xrightarrow{\text{Acid phosphate}} R—O—H + P_i$$

produces an organic alcohol and an inorganic phosphate.

Many enzymes that hydrolyze proteins also exhibit a broad bond specificity, hydrolyzing a large number and variety of peptide bonds within a protein substrate. If the peptide bonds of the substrate that are hydrolyzed are located on the inside of the protein, the enzyme is called an **endopeptidase**, such as pepsin A. Alternatively, carboxypeptidases are enzymes that act on protein substrates cleaving peptide bonds starting from the outside carboxyl end of the substrate and moving toward the middle of the protein. These enzymes are termed **exopeptidases**, and they also demonstrate a broad substrate specificity.

In contrast to the broad specificity of many peptidases, other enzymes are more specific in their action; they will catalyze only a definite reaction with a few substrates. In extreme cases, an almost absolute specificity is demonstrated in which only a single compound will serve as a substrate, such as phosphoenolpyruvate for the pyruvate kinase reaction:

$$
\begin{array}{ccc}
\text{Phosphoenolpyruvate} & & \text{Pyruvate} \\
\text{(PEP)} & & \text{(PYR)} \\
+ & \underset{\rightleftharpoons}{\text{PK}} & + \\
\text{Adenosine diphosphate} & & \text{Adenosine triphosphate} \\
\text{(ADP)} & & \text{(ATP)}
\end{array}
$$

Enzyme specificity should be described for each substrate involved in a reaction. In contrast to the absolute specificity shown for phosphoenolpyruvate in the pyruvate kinase reaction, several natural and synthetic nucleoside diphosphates, such as UDP, IDP, GDP, and CDP will also serve as phosphate acceptors in the reaction in place of ADP. Thus although an absolute specificity is shown for one substrate (PEP), an intermediate degree of specificity is shown for the other substrate (ADP).

An intermediate degree of specificity for each substrate is shown by the hexokinase reaction, in which D-glucose and several other sugars may be phosphorylated, that is, D-mannose, 2-deoxy-D-glucose, and D-glucosamine. However, D-galactose and five-carbon sugars like D-xylose are not substrates. The enzyme can also use a variety of nucleoside triphosphates as phosphate donors, such as ITP and GTP, as well as ATP.

$$
\left.\begin{array}{c}
\text{D-Glucose} \\
+ \\
\text{Adenosine triphosphate} \\
\text{(ATP)}
\end{array}\right\} \xrightarrow{\text{HK}} \left\{\begin{array}{c}
\text{Glucose-6-phosphate} \\
+ \\
\text{Adenosine diphosphate} \\
\text{(ADP)}
\end{array}\right.
$$

Many enzymes demonstrate a **stereoisomeric specificity** for either the L-form or the D-form of a pair of compounds. Hexokinase is absolutely specific for the D-form of glucose; the L-form is not a substrate. Malate dehydrogenase acts only on the L-form of malate, not the D-form. Lactate dehydrogenase acts only on L-lactate, not on D-lactate. However, stereoisomeric specificity does not necessarily mean that the enzyme is absolutely specific, because some forms of lactate dehydrogenase act on hydroxybutyrate as well as lactate, and as mentioned above, hexokinase functions with several D-form substrates.

Subunit Structure

Some enzymes occur in nature in several forms. That is, there may be several types of enzyme that catalyze the same reaction. These are known as **isoenzymes**, or *isozymes*. In a few well-studied enzymes, it has been found that the different forms of isoenzymes occur because the enzymes are composed of two or more different polypeptide chains or subunits bound into an active form. The subunits alone do not have the catalytic properties of the whole enzyme. The isoenzymes may have different kinetic or other physical properties that allow the different forms to be separated or measured. Many of these features have been used to differentiate and characterize the various enzyme forms and to assay for their presence in a sample. Other types or classes of isoenzymes can occur and are considered in the section on isoenzymes (p. 1062), but clinically the most widely used forms are the subunit type of isoenzymes. See Chapter 55 for a discussion of isoenzymes.

Anabolism and Catabolism

The synthesis of all enzymes is assumed to occur by intracellular protein synthetic pathways within the tissues that contain the enzymes. Extracellular enzymes like those involved in the coagulation process are synthesized in the liver and discharged into the plasma. In some cases other organs, that is, the kidney, lung, and pancreas, also contribute to the extracellular enzyme pool. See further discussion on intracellular/extracellular changes in Chapter 55. The large size and complexity of structure of enzymes results in molecular forms that are somewhat unstable and are therefore said to be **labile enzymes**. Many enzymes in vitro lose their catalytic activity with relatively slight changes in pH, temperature, or even salt concentration of the surrounding medium. It is presumed that similar processes occur intracellularly and that constant, though slight, synthesis of enzymes occurs in a steady-state fashion to maintain the required amounts of intracellular enzymes needed for intermediary metabolism.

A loss of enzyme activity can be either reversible and temporary or irreversible and permanent. *Denaturation* is a process whereby biological properties are lost by a protein; that is, enzyme activity is lost. It has been suggested that the denaturation process is an unfolding or "melting" of tightly coiled peptide chains leading to a more disorganized structure.

There is much experimental support for this idea, including increased reactivity of side chains, changes in viscosity, and changes in the sedimentation behavior of the "melted" protein solutions. *Irreversible denaturation* can occur when the enzyme protein chains unfold and are unable to refold to their biologically active form, or when a heavy metal ion (such as mercury or lead) or other material binds tightly at or near the active site. Many other factors and events can lead to denaturation and loss of activity including changes in temperature, the addition of strong acids or bases, exposure to high pressure, treatment with ultraviolet rays, repeated freezing, and the addition of detergents or organic solvents, or the presence of high concentrations of urea or guanidine.

A *reversible denaturation*, or loss of enzyme activity, is called **inactivation**. For example, inactivation can occur if an enzyme solution is allowed to remain for an extended time at room temperature and the enzyme partially loses activity. This temporary activity loss can have several causes including heat instability with the breaking of hydrogen bonds or oxidation of sulfhydryl groups. In both of these cases, there is some loss of the natural structural form. With some enzymes, reducing the temperature of the solution or the addition of a sulfhydryl reducing agent like dithiothreitol may allow the enzyme to refold to the original active form, with reformation of hydrogen bonds or reduction of oxidized sulfhydryl groups, thus producing a **reactivation** of the enzyme and a restoration of lost activity.

Little is known about the mechanism of removal of enzyme proteins from the extracellular fluid compartment. Certainly extracellular proteases hydrolyze the protein material, thus inactivating enzymes that are lost from cells. The degraded inactive proteins are then removed by one of several excretory routes, that is, excretion in bile, the intestine, liver, kidney, or the reticuloendothelial system. In addition, it is known that various enzymes have different half-lives, an indication that several mechanisms of removal may be present.

ENZYME CLASSIFICATION

Many enzymes were first named for their function (such as lactate dehydrogenase), but some have also been named for the type of substrate on which they act: urease hydrolyzes urea, lipase hydrolyzes lipids, and phosphatases act on organic phosphates. Many of the clinically important enzymes are still known by these trivial names that arose from historic circumstances and will continue to pervade the literature because of their simplicity. A systematic convention for the naming of enzymes was developed by the Enzyme Commission (EC) of the International Union of Biochemistry (IUB) and is widely used.

International Union of Biochemistry (IUB) Names and Codes

The IUB systematic name describes the reaction catalyzed. The IUB also recognized that trivial names were important and assigned practical names to many enzymes but no abbreviations. For each individual enzyme the system provides a numeric **EC code** designation consisting of four numbers separated by periods. The first number assigns the enzyme to one of six categories of reaction. The second number denotes the subclass, which is often based on the type of group, such as amino group or hydroxyl group, that takes part in the reaction. The third number indicates the different subsubclass of reaction, often the acceptor group, and the last number is merely the serial number of the particular enzyme in this subsubgroup. For the enzyme lactate dehydrogenase (EC 1.1.1.27), the first number, *1*, indicates that the enzyme is an oxidoreductase; the second number, *1*, indicates that the enzyme acts on the —CH group of donors; the third number, *1*, indicates that the acceptor is NAD^+ or $NADP^+$; and the fourth number, *27*, is merely the serial number of the enzyme in the EC 1.1.1.*x* group (Table 54-1).

Enzyme Commission (EC) Classification

All enzymes are divided into one of six general classes depending on the type of reaction they catalyze. A few clinically important enzymes are listed in Table 54-1 along with the EC code and systematic names.

The first class includes the *oxidoreductases*, those enzymes that catalyze electron transfer or oxidation-reduction reactions, which can be illustrated schematically as follows:

$$A_{red} + B_{ox} \rightleftharpoons A_{ox} + B_{red}$$

An example of an enzyme in this category is lactate dehydrogenase (EC 1.1.1.27). Some common names of enzymes in this category include dehydrogenases, reductases, oxidases, and peroxidases.

The second group of enzymes contains the *transferases*, those enzymes that catalyze the transfer of a group, such as an amino, carboxyl, glucosyl, methyl, or phosphoryl group, from one molecule to another. These reactions can be listed schematically as:

$$A{-}X + B \rightleftharpoons A + B{-}X$$

Alanine aminotransferase (EC 2.6.1.2) is an example of this group. Other common enzymes in this category include kinases and transcarboxylases.

A third group includes the *hydrolases*, which catalyze the cleavage of C—O, C—N, C—C, and some other bonds with the addition of water. These hydrolysis reactions can be illustrated as follows:

$$A{-}B + H_2O \rightleftharpoons A{-}OH + B{-}H$$

An example of this group is acid phosphatase (EC 3.1.3.2). Other common enzymes in this category are amylase, urease, pepsin, trypsin, chymotrypsin, and various peptidases and esterases.

A fourth group contains the *lyases*, which hydrolyze C—C, C—O, and C—N bonds by elimination, with the formation of a double bond or catalyze the reverse reaction, the addition of a group to a double bond. In cases in which the reverse reaction is important the term *synthase* is used in the name.

This type of reaction is illustrated as follows:

$$\begin{array}{ccc} & \overset{\displaystyle O}{\overset{\displaystyle \|}{}}\overset{\displaystyle O}{\overset{\displaystyle \|}{}} & \overset{\displaystyle O}{\overset{\displaystyle \|}{}} \\ R{-}C{-}C{-}OH + H^+ & \rightarrow & R{-}C{-}H + CO_2 \end{array}$$

An examination of the EC listing shows that this and the subsequent groups contain relatively few enzymes that are used in clinical diagnosis.

The fifth group includes the *isomerases*, which catalyze structural or geometrical changes in a molecule. They are also called *epimerases* and *mutases* depending on the type of isomerism involved. This reaction can be illustrated as follows:

$$ABC \rightleftharpoons CAB$$

An example of this group is the enzyme glucose phosphate isomerase (EC 5.3.1.9). It is not commonly used diagnostically.

A sixth and last group consists of the *ligases*, or *synthetases*. In this reaction two molecules are joined, coupled with the hydrolysis of the pyrophosphate in ATP. Many

TABLE 54-1 EXAMPLES OF ENZYME NOMENCLATURE

EC Code	Recommended Name (Trivial)	Abbreviation*	Systematic Name	Other Name or Abbreviation
Oxidoreductases				
1.1.1.27	Lactate dehydrogenase	LD	1-Lactate:NAD⁺ oxidoreductase	LDH
Transferases				
2.3.2.2	γ-Glutamyltransferase	GGT	(5-Glutamyl)-peptide:amino acid 5-glutamyl transferase	—
2.6.1.1	Asparate aminotransferase	AST	1-Aspartate:2-oxoglutarate aminotransferase	Serum glutamic oxaloacetic transaminase, SGOT
2.6.1.2	Alanine aminotransferase	ALT	1-Alanine:2-oxoglutarate aminotransferase	Serum glutamic pyruvic transaminase, SGPT
2.7.3.2	Creatine kinase	CK	ATP:creatine *N*-phosphotransferase	CPK
Hydrolases				
3.1.1.3	Triacylglycerol lipase	LPS	Triacylglycerol acyl hydrolase	Lipase
3.1.3.1	Alkaline phosphatase	ALP	Orthophosphoric-monoester phosphohydrolase (alkaline optimum)	—
3.1.3.2	Acid phosphatase	ACP	Orthophosphoric-monoester phosphohydrolase (acid optimum)	—
3.1.3.5	5'-Nucleotidase	NT	5'-Ribonucleotide phosphohydrolase	—
3.2.1.1	α-Amylase	AMS	1,4,α,-D-Glucan glucanohydrolase	Diastase
3.4.11.1	Aminopeptidase (cytosol)	LAS†	α-Aminoacyl-peptide hydrolase (cytosol)	Arylaminadase, LAP, leucine aminopeptidase
Lyase				
4.1.2.13	Fructose-bisphosphate aldolase	ALS	D-Fructose-1,6,bisphosphate: D-glyceraldehyde-3-phosphate-lyase	Aldolase
Isomerases				
5.3.1.9	Glucose phosphate isomerase	GPI	D-Glucose-6-phosphate: ketol-isomerase	Phosphohexose isomerase
Ligases				
6.3.1.2	Glutamine synthetase	—	L-Glutamate:ammonia ligase (ADP-forming)	—

*Baron DN et al: J Clin Pathol 24:656, 1971 and Baron DN et al: J Clin Pathol 28:592, 1975 are not recommended by the International Union of Biochemistry but are in common use.
†Baron DN et al: J Clin Pathol 28:592, 1975 incorrectly lists (EC 3.4.11.2) the microsomal form of this enzyme as "leucine aminopeptidase."

of these enzymes are involved in DNA, RNA, and protein synthesis; none are currently used in clinical diagnosis. The synthetic reaction type is illustrated as follows:

$$A + B + ATP \rightleftharpoons AB + ADP + P_i$$

An example of this group is the enzyme glutamine synthetase (EC 6.3.1.2), which is rarely used clinically.

Nonstandard Abbreviations

A variety of simple abbreviations containing four or fewer capital letters are also used to represent the enzymes that are routinely measured. These abbreviations are widely used in practice but are *not* part of the IUB system. They are so popular and have become so commonly used that it would be difficult to discard them, and they are listed in Table 54-1.

MEASUREMENT OF ENZYMES

In most enzymatic procedures, the reaction rates are found not to be constant with time. By observing the rate of change of absorbance for a substrate or product at a specific wavelength, the reaction can be followed. Initially, there is a **lag phase** with little change of absorbance per unit time when the reactants are mixed and reach thermal and kinetic equilibrium, then a **linear phase** of constant absorbance change per unit time, and finally a **substrate-depletion phase** with little change of absorbance per unit time (Fig. 54-3).

Enzyme assays must be performed during the linear phase of absorbance change at which a constant amount of activity can be determined for a period of time (Fig. 54-3, *A*). Thus, measurements do not start at zero time but begin after the lag phase has occurred. Measurements can be made at any time

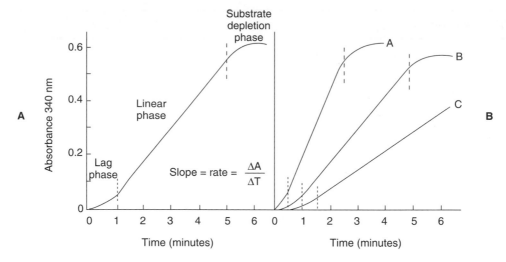

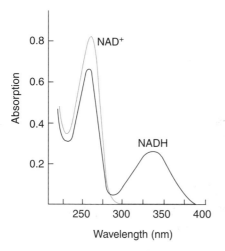

Fig. 54-3 **A**, Typical enzyme reaction with initial lag phase, linear change of absorbance, and final phase of substrate depletion. Enzyme activity is slope of linear phase. **B**, Time course of an enzyme reaction with three different amounts of enzyme present. Curve *A* has a high activity, *B* has a medium activity, and *C* has a low activity. As enzyme activity is increased in an assay system, lag phase decreases, linear phase decreases, and substrate depletion occurs sooner. Δ*A*, Change of absorbance; Δ*T*, change of time.

Fig. 54-4 Absorption spectrum, of 5×10^{-5} M NAD$^+$ in 0.1 M Tris buffer, pH 7.5 (*dotted line*), and absorption spectrum of 4×10^{-5} M NADH in 0.1 M Tris buffer, pH 9.5 (*solid line*).

during the linear phase and can continue up to the substrate-depletion phase.

If the enzyme activity is too great, substrate depletion may occur before the measurements have been completed. Rather than changing the assay time, the most common way to handle samples with high activity is to dilute them twofold or threefold with saline solution or water (Fig. 54-3, *B*). However, not all enzymes demonstrate linearity on dilution, particularly if the enzymes are active at a lipid-water interface, such as lipase (EC 3.1.1.3), or if there are inhibitors present in the sample, such as LD (EC 1.1.1.27) when measured in urine.

One of the more convenient methods of assaying enzyme activity is based on measurement of the absorbance of either the substrates or the products. There are some enzyme systems that involve the conversion of NAD$^+$ to its reduced form NADH, or vice versa. The reduced form, NADH, has a much greater absorption at 340 nm than the oxidized form does, and consequently, reactions that convert one form to the other may be conveniently followed by measurement of the change in absorption at this wavelength. The difference in the absorption spectrum of the reduced and oxidized compounds is shown in Fig. 54-4.

Enzyme Assays

Enzymes currently are measured by either their immunochemical or catalytic properties. The two most commonly employed methods that measure their catalytic properties are the one-point method at a fixed time, sometimes called an *end-point method*, and the multipoint fixed time assay, called the *kinetic method*.

End-point assays are still used in some cases, but in general shorter periods are employed. In these assays a reaction is started and allowed to incubate at a constant temperature for a fixed period, such as 30 minutes. The reaction is then stopped, perhaps by the addition of another reagent, and the amount of product is measured. The assumption in this type of assay is that a constant amount of product is produced throughout the entire assay period.

If the rate of reaction is followed continuously or with many points as a function of time, the assay is termed a **kinetic assay**. Usually the reaction time is short, that is, a few seconds to a few minutes, and there is little danger of enzyme degradation. The term *kinetic assay* is also used to describe enzyme reactions that form increasing amounts

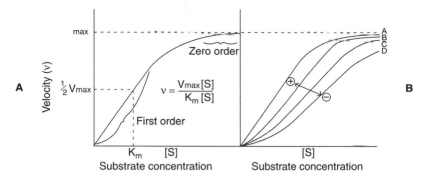

Fig. 54-5 **A,** Relationship of substrate, *S,* to velocity of reaction. At low substrate concentrations, the rate is first order (linearly dependent) with respect to substrate concentration. At high substrate concentrations the rate becomes zero order (independent) with respect to substrate concentration. K_m, Michaelis-Menten constant; V_{max}, maximal rate of reaction. **B,** Relationship between velocity and substrate concentration for an allosteric enzyme. Presence of positive or negative effectors shifts curve toward the + or − side, respectively.

of product with time; the reactions may be monitored as one-point *end-point assays* or *multiple-point* (continuous-monitoring) *assays.* Although this kinetic method terminology is not strictly correct, the continuous or multiple-point assays are superior to the single-point, fixed time assays, because it is easier to demonstrate approximate linearity of the reaction over the entire measurement period.

Principles of Kinetic Analysis

Enzyme kinetics is the study of enzyme reaction rates and the factors that affect them. Initially, many experiments are performed to examine the effects of different assay conditions on measurements of enzyme activity. Eventually, a series of specific conditions are established that give rise to the maximum rate of enzyme activity.

The general enzyme reaction given previously for a *single substrate reaction* may be rewritten slightly for **initial rates**, as in equation 54-4. In this case, the amount of product is very small and the reverse reaction of *P* combining with *E* and forming {*ES*} is ignored, because initial rate measurements are to be made. The initial rate is the rate at the start of the reaction, after the lag phase and during the linear phase in Fig. 54-5*A*, but before substantial product formation.

$$E + S \underset{k_{-1}}{\overset{k_{+1}}{\rightleftharpoons}} \{ES\} \overset{k_{+2}}{\rightleftharpoons} P + E \qquad \textit{Eq. 54-4}$$

For a given quantity of enzyme, the rate of activity that is observed increases with increasing amounts of substrate, as is shown in Fig. 54-5. At low substrate concentrations the rate is linearly dependent on the amount of substrate, that is, *first order*, but at high substrate concentrations the rate is essentially independent of substrate concentration, that is, *zero order*. A mathematical description of the reaction must explain how the reaction can be first order at low substrate concentrations and zero order at high substrate concentrations.

If the enzyme has a limited number of active sites, at a low substrate concentration the rate will be dependent on the amount of substrate present, because there will be a large

effective concentration of unfilled active sites. However, because the total number of sites on the enzyme is limited and the amount of enzyme is constant, then, as the amount of substrate is increased, the sites will become increasingly saturated with substrate until the reaction will appear to be independent of the substrate concentration. At these high substrate concentrations all the enzyme active sites are filled and the reaction proceeds at maximal velocity. Small changes in the substrate concentration after saturation will not affect the reaction rate.

The second step, product formation, is assumed to be the rate-limiting step or the one that determines the overall activity. The equilibrium for the formation of ES complex can be written as follows with the molar concentrations of all the reacting species expressed in brackets:

$$K_{eq} = \frac{k_{+1}}{k_{-1}} = \frac{[ES]}{[E][S]}$$

The equilibrium constant, K_{eq}, is equal to the ratio of the forward over the reverse rate constants. From equation 54-3, the rate of formation of the product *P* is the amount of *[ES]* times the rate k_{+2} at which the enzyme complex is converted to *E* + *P*. Thus the rate of formation of product is:

$$\text{Velocity, or Rate} = [ES] \times k_{+2}$$

Because the rate is the amount of product formed for some period of time:

$$\text{Rate} = \frac{\Delta P}{\Delta T} = [ES] \times k_{+2}$$

and substituting $K_{eq}[E][S]$ for [ES] and rearranging gives:

$$\Delta P = K_{eq} \times [S] \times [E] \times k_{+2} \times \Delta T$$

The amount of product formed is proportional to the amount of enzyme present, the time of the assay, and the amount of substrate present. When a proportionality constant is substituted for the rate constants, the equation becomes:

$$\Delta P = K_1 \times [S] \times [E] \times \Delta T$$

in which ΔP is the amount of product formed during the assay time, [*E*] is the amount of enzyme, [*S*] is the amount of substrate, ΔT is the assay time, and K_1 is a proportionality constant. The enzyme activity, or rate of product formation over time, is then given by:

$$\text{Rate} = \frac{\Delta P}{\Delta T} = K_1 \times [S] \times [E]$$

Usually enzyme assays are performed at a high substrate concentration for a short enough period so that the substrate concentration can be assumed to be constant. The value of this constant substrate concentration can be combined with K_1 to produce a second proportionality constant, K_2, which is the product of K_1 times the substrate concentration. The rate can then be expressed so that it is dependent only on the amount of enzyme present, that is, a zero-order reaction, independent of substrate concentration.

$$\text{Rate} = \frac{\Delta P}{\Delta T} = K_2 \times [E]$$

This rate of reaction, or velocity, is often listed as v, or V_i, or V_o, in the enzyme kinetic literature.

K_m and V_{max}

The enzyme activity, that is, rate, or velocity, is dependent on the substrate concentration when the amount of substrate is low relative to the amount of enzyme present in an assay. This relationship for a single substrate reaction is shown graphically in Fig. 54-5, with the same enzyme concentration assayed at many different substrate concentrations.

At steady state, before much product is present, the rate of formation of the [ES] complex will equal the rate of breakdown. This can be described using the following rate equation:

Formation		Breakdown
$k_{+1}[E][S]$	$=$	$k_{-1}[ES] + k_{+2}[ES]$

By collecting terms and rearranging, the rate constants can be removed and a constant, K_m, is defined.

$$\frac{[E][S]}{[ES]} = \frac{k_{-1} + k_{+2}}{k_{+1}} = K_m \qquad \textit{Eq. 54-5}$$

The rate or velocity of product formation, v, at any time and the free enzyme concentration, $[E]$, are described by:

$$v = k_{+2}[ES] \quad \text{and} \quad [E] = [Et] - [ES]$$

in which $[Et]$ is the total amount of enzyme and $[ES]$ is the amount complexed with substrate. When all the enzyme is present in the form of [ES] (i.e., at very high [S] in a zero-order reaction), the maximum rate, V_{max}, is as follows:

$$v_{max} = k_{+2}[Et]$$

Combining the above three equations gives:

$$[E] = \frac{V_{max}}{k_{+2}} - \frac{v}{k_{+2}} = \frac{V_{max} - v}{k_{+2}}$$

Because from Eq. 54-5:

$$[E] = \frac{K_m[ES]}{[S]} \quad \text{and} \quad [ES] = \frac{v}{k_{+2}}$$

then:

$$\frac{K_m[ES]}{[S]} = \frac{V_{max} - v}{k_{+2}} \quad \text{or} \quad \frac{K_m \times v}{[S] \times k_{+2}} = \frac{V_{max} - v}{k_{+2}}$$

Rearranging gives:

$$K_m \times v = (V_{max} - v)[S] \quad \text{or} \quad v(K_m + [S]) = V_{max}[S]$$

When this equation is solved for v, it gives the *Michaelis-Menten equation*, which is the equation for the rectangular hyperbola shown in Fig. 54-5, *A*.

$$v = \frac{V_{max}[S]}{K_m + [S]} \qquad \textit{Eq. 54-6}$$

[S] is the concentration of substrate, v is the velocity, V_{max} is the maximal rate of reaction when the enzyme is saturated with substrate, and K_m, the **Michaelis-Menten constant**, is that substrate concentration that produces one half the maximal velocity.

At the fixed high substrate concentration found in the usual clinical laboratory assays, the velocity, v, approaches V_{max} and is proportional to the amount of enzyme present, because all other factors are constant. The reaction is said to be zero order with respect to substrate, that is, independent of the concentration of substrate. The common condition used for assaying enzyme activity is a high substrate concentration in which $[S] \cong 10 \times K_m$ or higher. The rate at a substrate concentration of $10 \times K_m$ is given by the following equation:

$$v = \frac{V_{max}(10 \times K_m)}{K_m + (10 \times K_m)} = V_{max}\frac{10 \times K_m}{11 \times K_m} = 0.91\, V_{max}$$

Thus at $[S] = 10 \times K_m$ the rate produced is greater than 90% of V_{max}.

Another way to examine the Michaelis-Menten equation is to see if it is consistent with **first-order kinetics** at low substrate concentrations and **zero-order kinetics** at high substrate concentrations.

At low substrate concentrations in which $[S] \ll K_m$:

$$v = \frac{V_{max}[S]}{K_m + [S]} \cong \frac{V_{max}[S]}{K_m}$$

and because K_m and V_{max} are constants:

$$v = K_1[S]$$

it shows that the rate is dependent only on the first power of the substrate concentration.

At high substrate concentrations in which $[S] \gg K_m$,

$$v = \frac{V_{max}[S]}{K_m + [S]} \cong \frac{V_{max}[s]}{[s]} = V_{max}$$

showing that the rate (v) does not depend on substrate concentration.

As shown in Fig. 54-5, *A*, the relationship of substrate concentration to enzyme activity is a curve that is often similar to a rectangular hyperbola. For multisubstrate enzyme reactions the kinetics are more complex. The presence of activators and inhibitors acting at allosteric or regulatory sites tends to make the curves less linear because of the complex kinetics.

The accurate determination of K_m and V_{max} for each substrate or activator from Michaelis-Menten curves such as those shown in Fig. 54-5, *A*, is very difficult, even if the curves are fairly linear. However, it is necessary to determine these constants so that assays may be established using optimal conditions to correctly measure enzyme activity. If the curve is transformed into a straight line, the K_m and V_{max} can be determined with greater accuracy. The Michaelis-Menten equation may be transformed mathematically and the equation of a straight line obtained in several ways. The K_m and V_{max} can then be graphically determined from the line slopes and intercepts using these transformed equations. Common graphical presentations are shown in Fig. 54-6.

Determination of Enzyme Activity

Units of activity. The results of an enzyme determination are expressed as an *activity* unit in terms of the amount of product formed per unit of time under specified conditions for a given volume of sample, which is often serum. Thus one unit of enzyme activity might be the amount of enzyme that would, under certain specified conditions, cause the formation of 1 mg of the product, P, per minute when 1 mL of the sample was used. In older procedures arbitrary units like these were often employed.

In 1961 the Enzyme Commission recommended the adoption of an **international unit (IU) of enzyme activity**. The IU was defined as the amount of enzyme that would convert 1 micromole of substrate per minute under standard conditions.

$$1 \text{ IU} = \text{micromole/minute}$$

In those instances in which one molecule of substrate is transformed into two or more molecules of a product, the definition is per micromole of product formed.

This unit has been widely adopted, and in some respects it has standardized assay units. It has not reduced the number of reference intervals because if the standard conditions change the apparent enzyme activity changes. For example, if a new buffer is used in the assay, it may affect the enzyme rate and produce a different reference interval.

The **Système International d'Unités** (SI), as originally adopted by the World Health Organization, established the unit of enzyme activity as the **katal (K)**. This is defined as 1 mol/sec of substrate changed. This unit is too large to be useful clinically, and so it has met with little acceptance in the United States although it was recommended by the EC in 1972.

To convert international units to katals:

$$1 \text{ IU} = \frac{\text{Micromole}}{\text{Minute}} \times \frac{10^{-6} \text{ mole}}{\text{Micromole}} \times \frac{1 \text{ min}}{60 \text{ sec}} = 1.67 \times 10^{-8} \text{ K}$$

Thus, 1.0 IU = 16.7 nK (nanokatals). Only the IU have been widely adopted by workers in the field of clinical enzymology. The katal has not gained widespread acceptance.

Standardization by extinction coefficient. Pure human enzyme materials are not readily available, and so enzyme assays cannot be standardized in each laboratory by calibration with pure materials. One standardization method that was used depended on having an accurately calibrated spectrophotometer. Many enzyme assays are followed by spectrophotometric measurements being made at a specific wavelength. With the spectrophotometric method it is usually assumed that at 340 nm, NADH has a molar absorption coefficient, ε, of

$$A/(l \times c) = 6.22 \times 10^3 \text{ L} \cdot \text{mol}^{-1} \cdot \text{cm}^{-1}$$

in which A is the actual absorbance of a solution, l is the light path in centimeters through the solution, and c is the concentration in moles per liter of the absorbing substance. For a 1 cm light path, rearranging for c:

$$c = A \times 10^{-3}/6.22 \text{ mol/L}$$

When the concentration is expressed in micromoles per liter instead of moles per liter, the expression is:

$$c = A \times 10^3/6.22 \text{ }\mu\text{mol/L}$$

From the absorbance change that was measured and the volume of solution used, the number of micromoles of NADH formed or used up during the enzyme-measurement period can be readily calculated.

$$c = \Delta A \times 10^3/6.22 \text{ }\mu\text{mol/L}$$

For example, in the lactate dehydrogenase reaction discussed earlier, if a change in absorbance of 0.06 per minute was observed at 340 nm in a 1 cm curette and a 0.1 mL sample was used with a total assay volume of 3.0 mL, the calculation of activity would be as follows:

$$\text{International units/L} = \frac{0.06 \times 1000 \text{ }\mu\text{mol/mmol} \times 3.0 \text{ mL}}{6.22 \text{ mmol/L} \times 0.1 \text{ mL}}$$

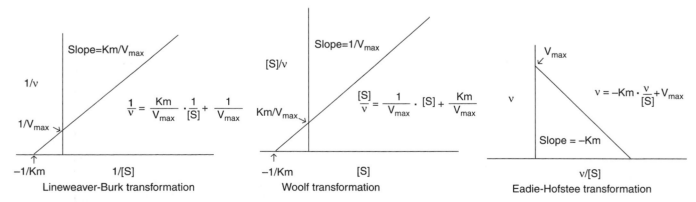

Fig. 54-6   Graphic representation of linear forms of Michaelis-Menten equation.

Standardization by a standard factor. Most current analytical instruments used in the clinical laboratory are highly automated. In some cases they may have spectrophotometric cells with path lengths differing from 1 cm or they may be designed in such a way that the manual standardization method, with an extinction coefficient, cannot be easily used. These automated instruments employ a *K factor* to standardize the calculation of enzyme activity; the K factor for a rate reaction is determined at the time of installation of the automated instrument and whenever the optics of the analyzer have been significantly changed. Several samples of known enzyme activity are used to determine a K factor. K is defined for kinetic rate reactions for a fixed period as:

$$K = (C_u - C_b)/(\Delta A_u - \Delta A_b)$$

in which

C_u is the apparent enzyme activity of the unknown sample
C_b is the apparent enzyme activity of the reagent blank
ΔA_u is the change in absorbance of the unknown sample
ΔA_b is the change in absorbance of the reagent blank

The K is determined and entered into the calibration portion of the software of the automated instrument and used like any other factor for the determination of enzyme activity. This is similar to the assignment of standard values for any other analyte and may be done using a single point or several points to establish a standard curve of enzyme activity.

The enzyme units that have been described express the activity in terms of units per volume of sample. This is a particularly convenient unit of measure in the clinical laboratory to assay enzymes in biological fluids like serum and plasma. To measure an enzyme found in erythrocytes (RBC) or in white blood cells (WBC), another unit of measure is needed. In the case of RBC and WBC enzymes, the enzyme activity can be expressed as units per 10^{10} cells.

In biochemistry laboratories where enzyme purification is important, the activity might be expressed as milligrams of protein or as dry weight of cells or as micrograms of DNA, but these are not convenient units for the clinical laboratory.

Analytical Factors Affecting Enzyme Measurement

The rate of reactions involving enzymes is greatly influenced by temperature, pH, concentration of substrate, and several other factors. Accordingly, all the details of a given procedure must be followed exactly to produce precise and accurate results.

Assays of enzyme activity should be performed under optimal conditions of zero-order kinetics, and so the measured rate is dependent only on the amount of enzyme present. To optimize an assay, such as the lactate dehydrogenase reaction given earlier, a series of reaction assays are set up with increasing concentrations of lactate but with a high fixed NAD^+ concentration and a fixed amount of enzyme. The enzyme rates are then measured, and a graph similar to that in Fig. 54-6 is constructed. A second series of assays is then performed with increasing concentrations of NAD^+ but at the fixed high concentration of lactate determined from the first

experiment, that is, $[S] \cong 10\,K_m$ for lactate, and the same amount of enzyme present. The enzyme rates are again determined and another graph is created to determine the K_m for NAD^+. This same type of experiment is performed for each item of the assay mixture (such as metal ions, pH, buffer) until all the variables have been evaluated for the production of maximal enzyme activity. The final conditions determined from this set of experiments are the **optimal assay conditions**. Experiments to determine optimal assay conditions have been performed for the current clinically important enzymes, and diagnostic kits are commercially available with all the materials at usually optimal concentrations.

pH

Changes in pH considerably affect the enzyme reaction rate. For most enzymes there is a definite pH range at which the enzyme is most active. A pH near the center of this range is usually specified for the measurement of that particular enzyme. The optimal pH is different for different enzymes. Reduced activity is observed at pH values greater or less than the optimal.

A typical pH curve of enzyme activity is given in Fig. 54-7. This is a bell-shaped curve showing changes in enzyme activity versus pH.

At pH values other than the optimal pH, the enzyme activity may be affected because of changes in the structure of the enzyme. These changes may occur at the active site, or may result from conformational changes affecting the three-dimensional structure.

Because the active site of an enzyme often contains ionizable side chains of amino acids, such as $RCOO^-$ or RNH_3^+, a significant change in the pH can lead to the gain or loss of a proton. The result is a substantial change in surface charge at the active site. The active site might, therefore, lose its ability to attract a substrate with an opposing charge. A similar loss of activity occurs if the change in charge is on the substrate molecule rather than on the enzyme. A change of pH might bring about an unfolding of the enzyme and loss of activity if the effect of pH change is to disrupt hydrogen

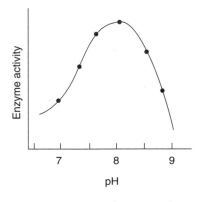

Fig. 54-7 Enzyme activity as a function of pH. Optimal pH range is 7.8 to 8.2; lower activities are observed at pH < 7.8 and pH > 8.2.

bonds and other intramolecular forces holding the enzyme in an active conformation.

Buffer

In many cases, as the enzyme reaction proceeds, products that tend to alter the pH are produced. Most assays include a buffer to maintain the assay pH within the optimal pH range. The buffer chosen should have a pK_a within 1 pH unit of the optimal pH of the enzyme to exert effective pH control.

Buffers not only serve to regulate the pH of an assay, but may also take part in the reaction. Alkaline phosphatase (ALP, EC 3.1.3.1) assays with *p*-nitrophenyl phosphate as a substrate use the buffer 2-amino-2-methyl-1-propanol (AMP) to maintain the pH at 10.2. The enzyme hydrolyzes the substrate into *p*-nitrophenol and inorganic phosphate in a multistep process, part of which involves a temporary phosphorylation of the enzyme. The final and rate-limiting step includes hydrolysis of the enzyme-phosphate bond to regenerate free enzyme. At similar pH values, buffers that are phosphate acceptors in a transphosphorylation process with the enzyme produce rates of alkaline phosphatase activity higher than those of buffers that do not act as phosphate acceptors. Thus AMP buffer produces rates of alkaline phosphatase activity at pH 10.2 higher than those of glycylglycine buffer at pH 10.2 because AMP is a phosphate acceptor. In the case of buffers that do not participate in the reaction, the concentration of buffer that gives maximal enzyme activity at the optimal pH must also be experimentally determined.

It has been found that the buffer and certain salts may have an unusual effect on the K_m. When the buffer-to-substrate ratio is very large, the buffer may compete with the substrate for the enzyme and make the enzyme activity appear to be related to substrate concentration in a nonlinear way. This has been observed with NADH in the LD reaction. Here the buffer-to-substrate molar ratio is 10^4:1 and the rate of reaction is affected by Tris, phosphate, and NH_4HCO_3 buffers and certain salts, such as NaCl and $(NH_4)_2SO_4$, which are often found in the coupling or **auxiliary enzymes** used to prepare assays. There seems to be no effect at buffer concentrations below 0.05 mol/L, which is consistent with several recommendations for optimal LD assay conditions. It would seem prudent to maintain as low a concentration of buffer as possible without compromising pH stability or enzyme rate.

Cofactors

Many enzymes require a nonprotein, often dialyzable, material for maximal activity. Some of these materials are related to vitamin structures. For example, thiamine or vitamin B_1 can be converted to thiamine pyrophosphate, a cofactor in many decarboxylation reactions. Niacin can be converted to nicotinamide adenine dinucleotide, and vitamin B_2, riboflavin, can be converted to flavin adenine dinucleotide. Both of these compounds are involved in many dehydrogenation reactions. Pyridoxine, vitamin B_6, is modified to pyridoxal phosphate, which is used in many transamination reactions.

In analytical assays of transaminase activity, pyridoxyl-5-phosphate is an example of a tightly bound cofactor that is not a substrate. The optimal concentration of a cofactor is determined in the same way as a substrate so that assay conditions can be established with a cofactor concentration of approximately 10 K_m or higher.

Activators and Inhibitors

Many enzymes require specific ions for maximal activity. All phosphate-transferring enzymes, such as hexokinase, require magnesium ions (Mg^{2+}). Other common metal ion activators are manganese (Mn^{2+}), calcium (Ca^{2+}), zinc (Zn^{2+}), iron (Fe^{2+}), and potassium (K^+). Amylase requires chloride (Cl^-) for maximal activity, and there are enzymes that require several ions for maximal activity; for example, pyruvate kinase requires magnesium (Mg^{2+}) and potassium (K^+). In each case, the optimal concentration of the activator must be determined just as the optimal concentration of substrate is determined.

Inhibitors are materials that reduce the catalytic activity of an enzyme. There are many types of inhibitors and several classes of inhibition. Inhibitors may act by removing an activator by chelation; for example, Ca^{2+} and Mg^{2+} are removed by EDTA or oxalate to cause the inhibition of hexokinase. They may also act by binding to the active site to compete with the substrate or by forming a complex at a different site, that is, an allosteric site, which may affect the enzyme activity.

Inhibitors are classed into three main groups. **Competitive inhibitors** bind at the active site and compete with the substrate for binding sites. These materials demonstrate a reversible inhibition that can often be reduced by using a higher substrate concentration.

$$
\begin{array}{ccccc}
E & + S & \rightleftharpoons & \{ES\} & \rightarrow P + E \\
+ & & & + & \\
I & & & I & \\
\Updownarrow & & & \Updownarrow & \\
\{EI\} & + S & \rightleftharpoons & \{ESI\} &
\end{array}
$$

The maximum rate of reaction is not affected if enough substrate is present because of the reversibility of the reactions. The binding of the substrate is affected, and thus the apparent K_m will be higher while the V_{max} remains the same.

Noncompetitive inhibitors bind at an allosteric or regulatory site, which may be at or far removed from the active site. These inhibitors cannot be reversed by the addition of more substrate because they bind at a different location on the enzyme surface.

$$
\begin{array}{ccc}
S & \rightleftharpoons \{ES\} & \rightarrow P + E \\
+ & & \\
E & & \\
+ & & \\
I & \rightleftharpoons \{EI\} &
\end{array}
$$

Because the inhibitor does not compete with the substrate, the K_m will be unaffected, but the amount of E or ES that converts substrate to product will be reduced and the V_{max} will be lessened.

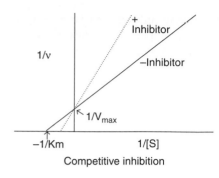

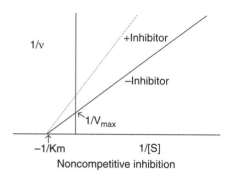

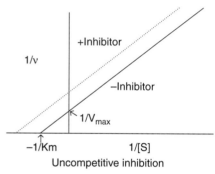

Fig. 54-8 The three types of inhibition are shown by use of Lineweaver-Burk graphic method to demonstrate effect of type of inhibition of K_m and V_{max}.

Uncompetitive inhibitors, a third group of inhibitors, are believed to bind to the enzyme-substrate complex and not to the free enzyme. In this case, at low substrate concentrations, the addition of more substrate increases the inhibition, because it produces more **enzyme-substrate complex** to react with the inhibitor. The result of this type of inhibition is that the V_{max} is reduced and the K_m is increased.

$$
\begin{array}{c}
E + S \;\rightleftharpoons\; \{ES\} \;\rightarrow\; P + E \\
+ \\
I \\
\updownarrow \\
\{ESI\}
\end{array}
$$

The type of inhibition a substance exerts can be determined by examining the results of kinetic studies, with and without inhibitors, using a linear graph of enzyme activity, as is shown in Fig. 54-8. A brief summary of the effects of the types of inhibition is given in Table 54-2. The simple types of inhibition may be classified by examination of the kinetic effect on the K_m and V_{max}.

TABLE 54-2   KINETIC EFFECTS OF INHIBITION

Type of Inhibition	Change in K_m	Change in V_{max}
Competitive	Increased	No change
Noncompetitive	No change	Decreased
Uncompetitive	Increased	Decreased

Coupling Enzymes

Some enzyme reactions of interest, such as alanine aminotransferase (ALT) and aspartate aminotransferase (AST), do not have substrates or form products that can be monitored directly. The initial enzyme reaction may be coupled to a second *indicating enzyme* reaction that, for example, does contain the $NAD^+/NADH$ conversion to make a convenient assay. The AST enzyme reaction can be coupled to the malate dehydrogenase reaction (MD, EC 1.1.1.37):

$$
\text{L-Aspartate} + \alpha\text{-Ketoglutarate} \xrightleftharpoons{AST} \text{L-Glutamate} + \text{Oxaloacetate}
$$

$$
\text{Oxaloacetate} + NADH + H^+ \xrightleftharpoons{MD} \text{L-Malate} + NAD^+
$$

This gives the following net reaction:

$$
\text{L-Aspartate} + \alpha\text{-Ketoglutarate} + NADH + H^+ \rightleftharpoons
$$
$$
\text{L-Glutamate} + \text{L-Malate} + NAD^+
$$

In this case, the substrate for the second reaction, oxaloacetate, is supplied as the product of the first reaction. Oxaloacetate from the AST reaction and the cofactor NADH serve as the substrates for the malate dehydrogenase reaction. This assay would have L-aspartate, α-ketoglutarate, NADH, and the enzyme malate dehydrogenase (MD) present at large excesses so that the rate-limiting item in the assay would be the amount of AST in the sample.

For other enzymes, such as creatine kinase (CK, EC 2.7.3.2), the measurement of the first enzyme requires an intermediate *auxiliary enzyme reaction* and then an **indicator enzyme**. In the measurement of CK, hexokinase (EC 2.7.1.1) is used as an *auxiliary enzyme* and glucose-6-phosphate dehydrogenase (EC 1.1.1.49) is used as an *indicating enzyme*. Both of these additional enzymes have to be present in large excesses to correctly measure CK. It is difficult to establish optimum assays that have more than two coupled reactions because of the large number of components in the assay system and the problems with maximizing all the components without causing inhibition of the limiting reaction.

Temperature

There is no optimal temperature for enzyme assays. Most enzymes show increasing activity as the temperature is raised over a limited temperature range, such as 10° to 40° C; an example is shown in Fig. 54-9.

To minimize any losses of activity if the enzyme cannot be assayed immediately after collection, samples should be stored at refrigerator temperatures, 2° to 6° C, or frozen

TABLE 54-3 ENZYME STABILITY UNDER VARIOUS STORAGE CONDITIONS (LESS THAN 10% CHANGE IN ACTIVITY)

Enzyme	Room Temperature (about 25° C)	Refrigeration (0° to about 4° C)	Frozen (–25° C)
Aldolase (ALS)	2 days	2 days	Unstable*
Alanine aminotransferase (ALT, GPT)	2 days	5 days	Unstable*
α-Amylase (AMS)	1 month	7 months	2 months
Aspartate aminotransferase (AST, GOT)	3 days	1 week	1 month
Ferroxidase I (ceruloplasmin)	1 day	2 weeks	2 weeks
Cholinesterase (CHS)	1 week	1 week	1 week
Creatine kinase (CK)	1 week	1 week	1 month
γ-Glutamyltransferase (GGT)	2 days	1 week	1 month
Isocitrate dehydrogenase (ICD)	1 day	2 days	1 day
Lactate dehydrogenase (LD)	1 week	1 to 3 days[†]	1 to 3 days[†]
Leucine aminopeptidase (LAP)	1 week	1 week	1 week
Lipase (LPS)	1 week	3 weeks	3 weeks
Phosphatase, acid (ACP)	4 hours[‡]	3 days[§]	3 days[§]
Phosphatase, alkaline (ALP)	2 to 3 days[‖]	2 to 3 days	1 month

*Enzyme does not tolerate thawing well.
[†]Depending on isoenzyme pattern in the serum.
[‡]Unacidified.
[§]With added citrate or acetate to pH ~5.
[‖]Activity may increase.

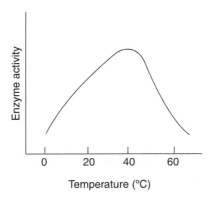

Fig. 54-9 Enzyme activity as a function of temperature of assay. Activity decreases at low temperatures. As temperature is raised, activity increases until rate of denaturation is greater than increase in activity.

(Table 54-3). In a few cases, some forms of enzymes, such as LD_4 and LD_5, have been found to be more stable at room temperature than at refrigerator temperatures. The repeated freezing and thawing of a specimen will often cause denaturation and loss of activity. Above 40° C most enzymes are rapidly denatured and lose almost all activity after a short time. An exception to this general rule is amylase, which seems to be stable up to about 60° C before significant losses of activity occur.

For many enzymes a 1 Celsius degree change in temperature produces about a 10% change in activity. A tolerance of ±0.1 Celsius degree for temperature control of an enzyme analyzer is recommended, because this produces approximately a ±1% change in the activity measured. This amount of variation is small enough to be ignored as an insignificant source of error for most clinical work. A recommendation of ±0.05 Celsius degree for temperature control, which reduces the change in activity to ±0.5%, has also been suggested.

The apparent increase in activity with increasing temperature means that assays that are performed at higher temperatures, such as 37° C, will be more sensitive to slight changes in the amount of enzyme in a sample. The common enzymes employed for clinical diagnosis are less stable at this temperature than at 25° to 30° C, and therefore assays carried out at 37° C must be performed with relatively short assay times, so that enzyme denaturation is minimized.

Arguments for the use of both higher temperatures, that is, 37° C, and lower temperatures, that is, 25° C, have been presented based primarily on scientific and technical reasoning. A reasonable compromise seems to be measurement at 30° C, which is the recommendation of the International Federation of Clinical Chemistry (IFCC). A very accurate gallium standard melting point cell is now available to all laboratories from the National Institute of Standards and Technology. This material has a melting temperature plateau of 29.772° C and can be used to calibrate or check the assay temperature of a wide variety of instruments.

Defining Assay Conditions

Although an optimal set of conditions for the assay of an enzyme can be established, it is clear that not all assays are being performed optimally. At times, the differences between assays may not appear to be significant, and yet the results obtained will be substantially divergent. The effect of various components of an assay upon one another, and thus the result, is even more significant in a **coupled assay**. These assays not only have the concentrations of substrates and activators of the primary reaction to consider, but also must have excesses of the auxiliary and indicating enzymes and their associated activators.

Alanine aminotransferase (ALT) is often measured in an assay that contains an excess of lactate dehydrogenase and NADH, plus L-alanine and α-ketoglutarate and buffer. The usual commercially available kits often specify that about 500 U/L of LD are present as an indicating enzyme and perhaps the animal source of this enzyme. This is not sufficient to define the assay completely, because the K_m of pyruvate varies with the LD isoenzyme type. About four times as many units of LD_1-LD_1 would be required than if LD_5 were used to achieve an equivalent reaction rate. A crude mixture of isoenzymes would be somewhere in between these extremes. Even if the units of LD added to different commercial assays were the same, the measured enzyme rates might vary with each lot of a kit if the indicating enzyme were added without regard to the isoenzyme content. This same kind of variability would occur between manufacturers' kits that contained the same concentrations of substrates, activators, and units of LD if a different source, such as bacterial, of the indicating enzyme were used. It is for this reason that each laboratory must check the reference interval for each enzyme assay, particularly when changing reagent manufacturers.

Enzymes as Reagents

It is possible to measure the serum levels of the substrate of many enzyme reactions by using many of the principles of enzyme kinetics applied in a slightly different way. The enzyme activity at low substrate concentrations is first order, that is, linear with respect to substrate concentration. To measure the concentration of pyruvate in a sample, for example, a special assay mixture is prepared, with only a small amount of the sample added so that the amount of unknown pyruvate in the assay is low, that is, less than the K_m. An assay mixture is used that contains an excess of LD, an excess of the coenzyme NADH, the amount of pyruvate present, and a buffer. The reduction in the amount of NADH in this assay is related to the amount of pyruvate present and the millimolar absorption coefficient of NADH at 340 nm. Alternatively a series of pyruvate standards could be used to calibrate the assay. Other similar enzymatic assays that are commonly used in the clinical laboratory include the determination of glucose, urea, ethanol, cholesterol, triglycerides, and uric acid. Enzymes are sometimes used as components of other assays or assay systems, most commonly in immunometric assays of various designs, and are called **ELISA** or **EMIT** assays (see Chapters 12 and 13). In most cases, the enzymes are used as indicators that a reaction has taken place, by the production of a colored product.

Storage of Enzymes

Most of the enzymes that are used clinically are stable at refrigerator temperatures for 2 to 3 days to about a week and at room temperature for a shorter time. Table 53-3 summarizes data for three temperatures.

Several enzymes deserve particular comment. Acid phosphatase is unstable at all temperatures unless the pH of the serum is reduced to about 5 to 6 with citrate or acetate. Alkaline phosphatase in human serum demonstrates a linear increase in activity dependent on temperature and time. At 96 hours (4 days) there is a 6% increase at room temperature, a 4% increase at refrigerator temperature, and a 1% increase at -20° C. Enzymes in control materials are usually of non-human origin and are much more varied, with some more stable and some less stable than human serum.

The observed biological half-lives of several human enzymes in plasma are given in Table 54-4.

CLINICAL ENZYME MEASUREMENTS

A few enzymes have been used since the turn of the last century to evaluate chronic diseases, but it wasn't until 1954 that LaDue, Wróblewski, and Karmen found a temporary increase in serum aspartate aminotransferase (EC 2.6.1.1) activity after an acute myocardial infarction. After this time, the measurement of changes in plasma enzyme activity gained importance as a means of following the course of a disease or to improve clinical diagnosis. Many investigators began to look for changes in enzyme activity that were specific for a disease state or reflected damage to a particular tissue.

Changes in enzyme activity in the plasma or serum are followed, because it is known that enzymes are primarily intracellular constituents that are released after cell damage or cell death has taken place in a specific organ or tissue. The changes that occur with many diseases or in a particular organ can often be understood by examination of the pattern of several enzyme or isoenzyme changes over a period of hours or days.

Extracellular versus Cellular Enzymes

The enzymes that are found in plasma can be categorized into two major groups. These major subdivisions are the plasma-specific enzymes and the non–plasma specific enzymes.

The plasma-specific enzymes are those enzymes that have a definite and specific function in plasma. Plasma is their

---

TABLE 54-4   PLASMA HALF-LIVES FOR CLINICALLY IMPORTANT ENZYMES

Enzymes	Half-Life (Hours) (Mean ± 2 SD)
LD_1	53 to 173
LD_5	8 to 12
CK	15
AST (GOT)	12 to 22
ALT (GPT)	37 to 57
AMS	3 to 6
LPS	3 to 6
ALP	3 to 7 days
GGT	3 to 7 days

normal site of action, and they are present in plasma at higher concentrations than in most tissues. Among these are the enzymes involved in blood coagulation, as well as ferroxidase, pseudocholinesterase, and lipoprotein lipase. These enzymes are synthesized in the liver and are constantly liberated into the plasma to maintain a steady-state concentration. These enzymes are clinically of interest when their concentration decreases in plasma and some have historically been used as estimates of liver function.

The non–plasma specific enzymes are those enzymes with no known function in plasma. Their concentrations in plasma are usually found to be lower than that in most tissues, and there may be a deficiency in plasma of the activators or cofactors that are necessary for maximum enzyme activity. These enzymes can be further divided into the enzymes of secretion and the enzymes of intermediary metabolism.

The enzymes of secretion are those enzymes secreted from exocrine glands, that is, the pancreas and prostate, and some enzymes from the gastric mucosa and the bones. Enzymes in this group are clinically important when their concentrations are either higher or lower than the reference interval. Elevated values are found when the usual mode of excretion is blocked or when the amount of enzyme produced is increased. Decreases in the amount of enzyme are found when the tissue that ordinarily produces the enzyme is damaged or necrotic. Common examples of this group are amylase, lipase, and acid and alkaline phosphatases.

The other major group of non–plasma specific enzymes are the enzymes of metabolism. The concentrations of these enzymes in tissues are very high, sometimes thousands of times higher than in the plasma. Cellular damage resulting in leakage or necrosis allows a fraction of these proteins to escape into the plasma and causes a sharp rise in the concentration usually observed. Some common examples are creatine kinase (CK), lactate dehydrogenase (LD), alanine aminotransferase (ALT), and aspartate aminotransferase (AST).

Enzymes as Tumor Markers

Excesses of specific proteins are often elaborated into plasma during tumor cell growth. In some cases, these specific proteins are enzymes, such as prostatic acid phosphatase (PAP), or creatine kinase (CK), and have been measured to monitor response to therapy and estimate tumor mass. More specific tumor markers (see Chapter 49) have now replaced these enzymes.

FACTORS AFFECTING REFERENCE VALUES

Several important factors affect the reference intervals for enzyme determinations. If these factors are not accounted for in the interpretation of the results, a misdiagnosis is possible. In the following items a brief comment on the problem and an example are given.

Sampling Time

Because enzymes do not undergo any significant circadian rhythm, sampling time with respect to time of day is un-

important for the determination of enzyme normal or reference intervals. On the other hand, the sampling time with respect to the onset of a clinical condition may be important for detection of a variety of acute and chronic conditions if the changes observed are sufficiently rapid. The classic average time for maximum elevation for a series of enzymes in patients with a myocardial infarction was reported to be as follows: CK-MB, 6 hours; CK, 18 hours; AST, 24 hours; and LD, 48 hours. Not all patients follow this classical pattern, and a spread of several hours is seen for the rapidly changing analytes and several days for the slower changing analytes if a variety of patients are tested.

Age

There are variations in the amounts of enzymes usually present in serum that are the result of differences in age between various subgroups in the population. There are three principal ages to consider as a factor for determining a reference interval for an enzyme assay. These are during the first year of life as various organs, such as liver, are becoming functional, during puberty, and in late middle age when hormonal changes occur.

Perhaps some of the most dramatic changes are seen with the enzyme alkaline phosphatase. Using an alkaline phosphatase method with AMP buffer and *p*-nitrophenyl phosphate substrate at 30° C, the following values can be found: 135 to 270 U/L for children 6 months to 10 years of age, 90 to 320 U/L for children 10 to 18 years of age, and 40 to 100 U/L for adults.

Sex

Differences between the enzyme reference intervals for male and female populations are seen with some enzymes. These differences are most probably related to muscle mass, exercise, or hormone concentration.

An example of these effects is seen with the enzyme creatine kinase; males are reported to have higher reference intervals than females, which is most likely attributable to increased muscle mass. Alcohol dehydrogenase level in gastric mucosa is also reported to be higher in males than in females, allowing males to metabolize ethanol more rapidly. An alcohol load therefore does not adversely affect males as much as females.

Race

Race may also be a factor in a limited number of assays, but data are sparse. Black populations are reported to have higher reference intervals than comparable white populations for creatine kinase, but the effect may be an indirect result of several factors other than race in the two populations.

Exercise

Exercise and movement are important variables in the consideration of reference intervals for several enzymes. Patients who have been at complete bed rest for several days are found to have 20% to 30% lower values for creatine kinase than ambulatory patients. Normal amounts of exercise also elevate creatine kinase. The additional creatine kinase caused by normal exercise is of the MM type, CK_3. Thus the distinction between these elevations and those that are caused by an acute myocardial infarction, which is the MB type, CK_2, is easily accomplished by determination of the isoenzyme pattern, or direct measurement of CK_2. The increases seen after exercise usually disappear after 12 to 24 hours, unless the exercise is extremely strenuous. In ultralong-distance runners, those that run races longer than 26 miles, the CK_2 can be up to threefold higher than the reference interval and the total CK can be up to fortyfold higher than usual. Even when CK isoenzymes are determined, it may be difficult to distinguish a runner with chest pain from a runner with chest pain and a myocardial infarct.

ISOENZYMES
Nomenclature

The multiple natural forms of an enzyme catalyzing the same reaction in a single species are known as *isoenzymes*, or *isozymes*. The EC of the IUB has designated that this term is to apply only to those forms of enzymes arising from genetically determined differences in the amino acid structure, although there is not complete agreement on this designation. Isoenzymes are to be distinguished on the basis of electrophoretic mobility and subscripted with the first form having the mobility closest to the anode (+). For example, CK-BB is subscripted as CK_1, CK-MB as CK_2, and CK-MM as CK_3. Although there exist many reports to the contrary in the literature, isoenzymes should not be labeled on the basis of tissue distribution (i.e., heart type, brain type), because some confusion may arise as a result of differences in the predominant form found in various species. Three groups of multiple enzyme forms have been defined as isoenzymes by the IUB. These are grouped as follows: genetically independent proteins, such as mitochondrial and cytosol forms of CK and malate dehydrogenase; heteropolymers of two or more different subunits, such as CK and LD; and genetic variants in protein structure, such as glucose-6-phosphate dehydrogenases, with more than 50 varieties known in humans.

In a few unusual cases, an enzyme subunit, such as glutamate dehydrogenase, may have catalytic activity by itself. In these cases, the natural enzyme form is made up of several subunits and has a greater activity than the sum of the activities of the separate subunits. In addition, the multiple subunit form of the enzyme often has activators and inhibitors that may more closely control the enzyme activity. A more complex biological structure exists in this case, one whose enzyme activity can be more finely regulated.

The polymeric forms of glutamate dehydrogenase and phosphorylase are not isoenzymes by the IUB definition, because they are polymers of a single subunit and do not differ in amino acid composition. Some additional forms of enzymes that do not fit the strict definition of isoenzymes are those with variations in molecular weight (or length). These forms may occur with the cleavage of different terminal segments of a protein that does not affect the enzyme activity, thus producing various isoenzymes. Hexokinase and carbonate dehydratase are examples of this type of isoenzyme.

Isoforms

An isoenzyme that is released from tissue (e.g., CK-MB) is a single unmodified isoenzyme form. As a part of the normal clearance process of the body, carboxypeptidases in serum cleave the terminal lysine from the CK-M subunit and produce other isoforms of the isoenzyme with slightly different charges. High-resolution electrophoresis or isoelectric focusing can be used to demonstrate the presence of three CK-MM isoforms and two CK-MB isoforms, forming and disappearing with time. The CK-MM isoforms differ only in whether none, one, or two lysines have been removed from the CK-M subunits. The two CK-MB isoforms are the intact CK-MB and the CK-MB in which the M subunit has had a lysine removed. These are of interest as possible early diagnostic markers of acute myocardial infarction (Table 54-5). A more complete description of isoenzymes is given in Chapter 55.

Clinical Significance

Creatine kinase. See Chapters 31 and 55 for a review of the clinical significance of the isoenzymes and isoforms of creatine kinase. For many years, serial measurements of CK, CK-MB, and LD isoenzymes have been used to determine whether a patient has had a myocardial infarction. Measurements of cardiac troponin-I or cardiac troponin-T are replacing these types of enzyme measurements as a more specific and definitive diagnostic assay.

Lactate dehydrogenase. Lactate dehydrogenase (LD) is widely distributed in many tissues. The heart, however, contains an unusual distribution of LD isoenzymes, with an LD_1 concentration greater than LD_2. This LD result is similar to the finding of an unusual distribution of CK isoenzymes, in this tissue. The combination of both CK and LD isoenzyme analyses was considered a powerful method of detecting myocardial infarction, but measurement of LD isoenzymes is rarely performed and both tests are being replaced by measurements of cardiac troponin-I or cardiac troponin-T.

Methods of Analysis

Many older methods of analysis took advantage of slight differences in physical properties or of substrate specificity

---

TABLE 54-5   CK ISOFORMS

Isoform	Subunit	Comment
MM_3	CK-MM	Unchanged isoenzyme
MM_2	CK-MM$_{-L}$	End lysine removed from one M subunit
MM_1	CK-M$_{-L}$ M$_{-L}$	End lysine removed from both subunits
MB_2	CK-MB	Unchanged isoenzyme
MB_1	CK-M$_{-L}$ B	End lysine removed from M subunit

or inhibition patterns of some of the isoenzymes. These methods are rarely used today. The common methods of analysis either take advantage of differences in migration in electric fields or are based on immunological differences in the isoenzyme subunits. These methods are reviewed in more detail in Chapter 55.

The reference method for both CK and LD isoenzyme analysis is electrophoresis. This method is somewhat technique dependent but generally is easy to use and is relatively inexpensive. A large variety of different immunological methods are also available. Because of the ease of use and sensitivity, these methods have generally replaced electrophoresis.

Bibliography

Apple FS: Biochemical markers of thrombolytic success. IFCC Committee on Standardization of Markers of Cardiac Damage, *Scand J Clin Invest Suppl* 230:60, 1999.

Bakerman P, Strausbauch P: *Bakerman's ABC's of interpretative laboratory data*, ed 3, Myrtle Beach, SC, 1994, Interpretative Laboratory Data.

Baron DN et al: Revised list of abbreviations for names of enzymes of diagnostic importance, *J Clin Pathol* 28:592, 1975.

Bowers GN, Jr, Inman SR: The gallium melting-point standard: its evaluation for temperature measurements in the clinical laboratory, *Clin Chem* 23:733, 1977.

Colowick and Kaplan's methods in enzymology series, Philadelphia, Harcourt.

Committee on Standards, Expert Panel on Enzymes: Provisional recommendation (1974) of IFCC methods for the measurement of catalytic concentrations of enzymes, *Clin Chem* 22:384, 1976.

Dufour DR et al: Diagnosis and monitoring of hepatic injury. II. Recommendations for use of laboratory tests in screening, diagnosis, and monitoring, *Clin Chem* 46:2050, 2000.

Enzyme nomenclature: recommendations on enzyme nomenclature of the Commission on Nomenclature and Classification of the Enzymes of the International Union of Biochemistry, New York, 1979, Academic Press.

Enzyme nomenclature, 1992, San Diego, CA, Academic Press. Supplement 1 (1993), supplement 2 (1994), supplement 3 (1995), supplement 4 (1997), supplement 5, *Eur J Biochem* 223:1, 1994; *Eur J Biochem* 232:1, 1995; *Eur J Biochem* 237:1, 1996; *Eur J Biochem* 250:1, 1997; *Eur J Biochem* 264:610, 1999.

Fischbach FT: *A manual of laboratory & diagnostic tests*, ed 6, Philadelphia, 1999, Lippincott, Williams & Wilkins.

Hohnadel DC: Clinical enzymology. In Tilton RC et al: *Clinical laboratory medicine*, St Louis, 1992, Mosby.

Kaplan LA et al, editors: *Clinical chemistry: theory, analysis, and correlation*, ed 3, St Louis, 1996, Mosby.

Mayne PD: *Clinical chemistry in diagnosis and treatment*, ed 6, London, 1994, Edward Arnold.

Pappas NJ, Jr, editor: Theoretical aspects of enzymes in diagnosis. Why do serum enzymes change in hepatic, myocardial, and other diseases? *Clin Lab Med* 9:595, 1989.

Swaroop A: CK isoenzyme variants in electrophoresis, *Lab Med* pp 305-310, May 1989.

Wallach JB: *Interpretation of diagnostic tests*, ed 7, Philadelphia, 2000, Lippincott, Williams & Wilkins.

Wu AHB: Creatine kinase isoforms in ischemic heart-disease, *Clin Chem* 35:7, 1989.

Internet Sites

www.bmb.leeds.ac.uk—Major metabolic pathways in mammalian liver

http://inn.weizmann.ac.il/look_2000/prot.html—Enzyme, metabolic and signaling pathways databases

www.chem.qmul.ac.uk—Nomenclature Committee of International Union of Biochemistry and Molecular Biology

www.genome.ad.jp—KEGG metabolic pathways

http://www.biochem.ucl.ac.uk/bsm/enzymes/index.html—Enzyme Structure Database (deposited in the Brookhaven Protein Data Bank—6562 entries)

http://www.expasy.ch/enzyme—ENZYME Enzyme nomenclature database (ExPASy site, January 27, 2001—3721 entries)

http://biochem.boehringer-mannheim.com/techserv/metmap.htm—Boehringer-Mannheim Biochemical Pathways Chart (updated April 27, 2000)

http://www.enzim.hu/—Institute of Enzymology

CHAPTER 55

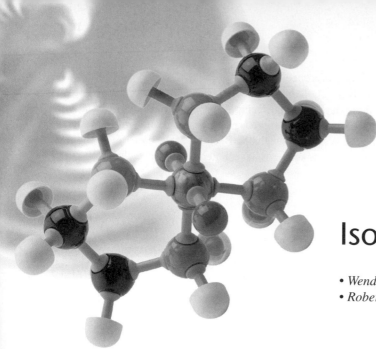

Isoenzymes and Isoforms

- *Wendy R. Sanhai*
- *Robert H. Christenson*

Chapter Outline

Function and characteristics
  Properties of isoenzymes and isoforms
  Structural basis
  Genetic basis
  Posttranslational modifications
  Microenvironmental distribution
  Macroenvironmental distribution
  Lactate dehydrogenase
  Creatine kinase
  Alkaline phosphatase

  Developmental distribution
Change in isoenzyme pattern due to pathological
  processes
Clinical significance of specific isoenzymes
  Creatine kinase (CK)
  Alkaline phosphatase (ALP)
  Lactate dehydrogenase (LD)
  Other isoenzymes
  Fluids other than serum
Modes of isoenzyme analysis

Objectives

- Distinguish between isoenzymes and isoforms
- Define the structural differences of isoenzymes.
- Describe the genetic basis of isoenzymes.
- List the types of modifications that result in isoforms.
- Describe the differences between macro- and microenvironmental distributions of isoenzymes and isoforms.

- Describe the changes in developmental distribution of isoenzymes and isoforms.
- Describe the clinical significance of creatine kinase.
- Identify the methods by which isoenzymes are measured.

Key Terms

dimer   A protein composed of two monomers.
heterodimer   A dimer composed of two different monomers.
heteropolymer   A polymer composed of two or more types of monomers.
homodimer   A dimer composed of two identical monomers.
homologous   Similar in structure, origin, or purpose. Pertaining to different proteins or nucleic acids, either between or within species, that have similar

or identical function. Homologous features are conserved genetically through evolution and result in similar or identical amino or nucleic acid sequences.
homopolymer   A polymer composed of only one type of monomer.
immunoinhibition   Inhibition of enzyme activity by reaction with an antibody.
isoelectric point (pI)   The pH at which the molecule has an overall net charge of zero.

isoenzymes   Multiple forms of an enzyme that catalyze the same biochemical reaction; different isoenzymes may exist within or between species, within an organism, or within a cell. Various isoenzymes may differ chemically, physically, or immunologically.

isoforms   Multiple forms of serum protein that result from posttranslational modifications of the gene product. They are functionally related and may differ only slightly in structure.

macroenvironment   The organ or tissue level; a specific environment that is associated with a specific physiological function.

microenvironment   The cellular level; a specific environment or location that is associated with a specific physiological function.

peptidase   An enzyme that catalyzes the hydrolysis of peptide bond; also called *protease*.

posttranslational modification   A series of in vivo chemical reactions whereby a newly synthesized polypeptide is converted to a functional protein. The changes occur after the protein emerges from the ribosome.

Regan isoenzyme   A specific alkaline phosphatase isoenzyme associated with some cancers.

subunit   The smallest unit of a protein; it may consist of one or more covalently linked polypeptide chains with a distinct secondary (20) structure. Subunits associate in a geometrically specific manner to give rise to a protein's quaternary (40) structure.

tetramer   A protein composed of four monomers.

Methods on CD-ROM

Creatine kinase isoenzymes

Lactate dehydrogenase and lactate dehydrogenase isoenzymes

FUNCTION AND CHARACTERISTICS
Properties of Isoenzymes and Isoforms

Enzymes are proteins that catalyze biochemical reactions (see Chapter 54). **Isoenzymes**, also termed *isozymes*, are genetic variations, arising from multiple gene loci or from allelic genes at a particular locus, that give rise to one or more multiple forms of an enzyme. All isoenzymes possess the ability to catalyze the enzyme's characteristic reaction, and share the same Enzyme Commission (EC) number (see p. 1050). Although isoenzymes of a particular enzyme usually do not differ substantially in molecular size, each isoenzyme has a distinct structure and may have a different affinity for substrates and cofactors. Various isoenzymes of an enzyme can differ in three major ways. They may differ in their enzymatic properties, specifically by their ability to be inhibited by specific agents, in their Michaelis-Menten constants (K_m), and their reactivity with different substrates. Second, they may differ in their physical properties, such as heat stability or **isoelectric point (pI)**. Last, they may differ in their biochemical properties, such as amino acid composition and immunological reactivities.[1] The above differences have been used for measurement of specific isoenzymes.

   Isoforms, in contrast, result from **posttranslational modification(s)** of a parent protein structure. Isoforms may also differ in structure and biochemical properties.

Structural Basis

Improved techniques for analyzing mixtures of proteins show that a particular type of catalytic activity, and hence active site structure within a single species, is frequently due to the existence of several distinct structural forms of isoenzymes.

These different isoenzymes can be distinguished on the basis of differences in physical and chemical properties and 3-dimensional (3D) structure. Although isoenzymes may have quantitative differences in their catalytic properties, they all retain the ability to catalyze a characteristic reaction. Yet, their existence, as multiple forms of enzymes in human tissue, has important implications in the study of human disease and in the understanding of organ-specific patterns of metabolism. For example, variations in enzyme structure may account for differences in sensitivity to drugs and differences in metabolism that manifest themselves as hereditary metabolic diseases.

   The amino acid sequences of isozymes are usually **homologous**, that is, much of the amino acid sequence is similar. Dissimilarities in the amino acid sequences of isoenzymes and the resulting differences in protein structure give rise to differences in catalytic properties, active site structures, pI, charge distribution, hydrophobicity patterns, K_m, pH optima, and therefore, differences in the response of isoenzymes to inhibitors. Such differences can be the basis of identification and measurement of particular isoenzymes.

   The biochemical properties of an isoenzyme are dependent on the number and type of constituent **subunits**. If all subunits are identical in primary, secondary, and tertiary structure, as in AA, BB, AAA, or BBB, the isoenzyme is termed a **homopolymer**. If different subunits are present, as in AB, AAB, or ABBB, the isoenzyme is termed a **heteropolymer**. An example of a heteropolymer is the **dimeric** isoenzymes of cytosolic creatine kinase (CK), which are formed by different paired combinations of two types of subunits, termed *M* (muscle) and *B* (brain), that differ from each other in primary, secondary, and tertiary structure.

Both the CK-MM and CK-BB are homopolymers (**homodimers**); the hybrid CK-MB isoenzyme is a heteropolymer (**heterodimer**).

Genetic Basis

The existence of multiple gene loci and the isozymes derived from them has presumably conferred an evolutionary advantage on the species and has become part of its normal biological pattern. Some of these adaptations are related to the differences in function between and within different types of specialized cells and tissues. Thus the distribution of isozymes is not uniform throughout the body, and wide variations in the activity of different isoenzymes occur between organs, between the cells that comprise a particular organ, and even between the structures that constitute a single cell. The tissue-specific distribution of isoenzymes, and other multiple forms of enzymes, provides the basis for origin-specific diagnosis through isoenzyme measurement.

The presence of different but highly homologous amino acid sequences suggests that some isoenzymes may have arisen through gene duplication, followed by independent mutations of the two genes, resulting in different but homologous primary sequences. In fact, a substantial portion of human enzymes is determined by more than one structural gene locus. The genes that determine a particular group of isoenzymes are not necessarily closely linked on one chromosome, and are sometimes located on different chromosomes. For example, the genes that code for the human salivary and pancreatic amylases both are located on chromosome 1, whereas the genes that code for mitochondrial and cytoplasmic malate dehydrogenase (MD) are carried on chromosomes 7 and 2, respectively. LD, CK, and some forms of alkaline phosphatase (ALP) are among enzymes of clinical importance that have isoenzymes attributable to multiple gene loci.

Certain gene loci may be expressed almost exclusively in a single tissue, some at a particular stage in development. For example, in addition to the two-gene loci that determine the two most common subunits (H and M) of LD, a third LD locus is active only in mature testes. There are four known distinct structural genes that encode for multiple forms of ALP. The isoenzyme of ALP that is normally detectable only in the human placenta is the product of a single structural gene locus, distinct from loci that specify the structures of the other forms of ALP.

A particularly striking example of the localized expression of multiple gene loci is provided by isoenzymes that occur exclusively in specific subcellular organs. Human mitochondria have isoenzymes (having separate gene loci, they are true isoenzymes) for aspartate aminotransferase (AST) and MD that are distinctly different from their functional counterparts in the cytoplasm. The variants are inherited in a Mendelian manner, without corresponding changes in the isoenzymes located elsewhere in the cell.

Posttranslational Modifications

Posttranslational modifications of proteins can give rise to isoforms of an enzyme. These reactions include proteolytic cleavage, protein degradation, and covalent modification of amino acids and can occur intracellularly or after the proteins are released from cells into plasma.

Proteolytic cleavage, a type of protein degradation, is the most common type of posttranslational modification. The reaction is catalyzed by **peptidases**, and involves cleaving peptide chains either from end termini by the action of exopeptidases, or internally by endopeptidases (see p. 1049, Chapter 54). Probably all mature proteins have been modified in this way, since the endoproteolytic removal of their leading amino acid residue occurs shortly after assembly by the ribosome.

The function of protein degradation is threefold: (1) to eliminate abnormal proteins whose accumulation could be harmful to the organism or cell, (2) to permit the regulation of cellular metabolism by eliminating superfluous isoenzymes, and (3) to conserve amino acids within unneeded proteins for synthesis of other proteins. A clinically useful example of the degradation process is seen with the dimeric homopolymer CK-MM.[2,3] After release of intracellular CK-MM into plasma, the *N*-terminal lysine residue of each M subunit can be successively cleaved by an irreversible enzyme reaction catalyzed by a plasma carboxypeptidase.[4] Because lysine residues impart a positive charge to the protein, the three CK-MM isoforms can be separated by serum electrophoresis; the three isoforms are named according to their electrophoretic mobility. $CK-MM_3$ migrates closest to the cathode and is the "tissue" isoform that predominates (>95%) within the intracellular compartment; $CK-MM_2$ shows intermediate migration and is formed after $CK-MM_3$ is released from the cell by cleavage of the terminal lysine from one of the $CK-MM_3$'s two M subunits; $CK-MM_1$ migrates closest to the anode and results from cleavage of the remaining intact terminal lysine from the $CK-MM_2$'s unmodified M subunit.[2,3] A similar enzymatic processing of the M-subunit of CK-MB occurs to allow the formation of $CK-MB_1$ from the tissue isoform $CK-MB_2$.[4] Although unimportant clinically, the B-subunit of CK-MB undergoes terminal lysine cleavage also, giving rise to four CK-MB isoforms.

Covalent modification involves chemical derivatization at the protein's functional groups of side chains and/or at their end terminals. There are more than 150 amino acid side-chain modifications possible; including oxidations/reductions, acetylations, glycosylations, methylations, and phosphorylations/dephosphorylations; that can alter the structural properties of isoenzymes, their catalytic properties and specificities. The result can be a large number of isoforms with different net charges and physical properties, thus allowing separation and identification of the isoform activities.[5] For example, a comparison of heat stability and catalytic properties of ALP from bone, liver, and kidney indicates that these isoforms result from different posttranslational modifications of a single gene product common to them all, termed tissue *non-specific ALP* (*TNALP*).[6] Evidence from selective modifications of enzymes by glycosidases indicates that the differences in the ALP isoforms may be the result of variations in carbohydrate side chains that are enzymatically added to the gene product.[7] The ALP isoforms are difficult to separate by electrophoretic methods because the carbohydrate side chains do not substantially alter the overall charge of the enzyme.

Microenvironmental Distribution

The functional significance of isoenzymes and their differential expression in specific subcellular organelles have lead to intriguing biological questions. The fact that different isoenzymes and isoforms are compartmentalized within the organelles of cells has given rise to theories of specific metabolic processes that presumably conferred an evolutionary advantage for the species. The different structures and net charges of the isoenzymes may influence their interactions with other charged molecules within the cell. For example, the mitochondrial isoenzyme of AST accounts for about 60% of this activity in the parenchymal cells of the liver and cardiac myocytes.

Microenvironmental factors are also important for ALP. All ALP isoenzymes and isoforms are attached to the membranes of cells by a COOH-terminal glycanphosphatidylinositol "anchor."[8] Although the exact function of ALP is unknown, based on the enzyme's location it is hypothesized that ALP may play a relatively nonspecific role in several transport processes by dephosphorylating metabolites, thereby facilitating their passage through the selectively permeable cell membrane.[9] In addition, because the bone ALP isoforms on the cell membrane of osteoblasts are not specific for only one tissue, and because of the association of this ALP with bone mineralization, it has been suggested that ALP functions to promote mineralization by removing inhibitors of crystallization such as inorganic phosphate.[10] Evidence in support of this theory has mainly come from hypophosphatasia, which is characterized by the deficiency of both the enzyme and bone mineralization.[10]

Macroenvironmental Distribution

Tissue-specific differences are found in the distribution of isoenzymes and isoforms (Table 55-1). Although the exact reasons for differential distribution of various isoenzymes and isoforms are not known, it has been proposed that they exist to satisfy particular needs and metabolic demands that have evolved for various tissues. The isoenzymes of LD, CK, ALP, and ACP are included here because they are of major clinical interest.

Lactate Dehydrogenase

Five LD isoenzymes (LD_1 to LD_5) are found in different tissues and although they all catalyze the reversible oxidation/reduction of lactate to pyruvate, they do so with different rates. The enzymes have a molecular weight of 134 kDa and are composed of four polypeptide chains of two types: M or H, each under separate genetic control. The subunit composition of the five isoenzymes, in order of decreasing anodal mobility on electrophoresis in an alkaline medium are LD_1 (HHHH; H_4); LD_2 (HHHM; H_3M); LD_3 (HHMM; H_2M_2);

TABLE 55-1 CREATINE KINASE ACTIVITY IN VARIOUS HUMAN TISSUES

Tissue	ISOENZYME DISTRIBUTION IN U/g OF WET TISSUE (% OF TOTAL ACTIVITY)		
	MM	**MB**	**BB**
Skeletal muscle	3281 (100)	0 to 623 (0 to 19)	0
Heart	313 (78)	56 to 169 (14 to 42)	0
Brain	0	0	157 (100)
Colon	4 (3)	1 (1)	143 (96)
Stomach	4 (3)	2 (2)	114 (95)
Uterus	1 (2)	1 (3)	45 (95)
Thyroid	7 (26)	0.3 (1)	21 (73)
Kidney	2 (8)	0	19 (92)
Lung	5 (35)	0.1 (1)	9 (64)
Prostate	0.3 (3)	0.4 (4)	9.3 (93)
Spleen	5 (74)	0	2 (26)
Liver	3.6 (90)	0.2 (6)	0.2 (4)
Pancreas	0.4 (14)	0 (1)	2.6 (85)
Placenta	1.4 (48)	0.2 (6)	1.4 (46)

From Chapman J, Silverman L: Bull Lab Med 60:1, 1982, National Committee for Mental Health.

LD_4 (HMMM; HM_3); and LD_5 (MMMM; M_4). A different isoenzyme, LD-X or LD-C, having four subunits of X or C is present in postpubertal human testis.

The pH optimum for the lactate-to-pyruvate (L→P) reaction is 8.8–9.8, and the assay is optimized for the LD_1 at 37° C. The reverse (P→L) reaction at 37° C requires a pH optimum of 7.4–7.8. The pH optima for these reactions vary with the source of enzyme (i.e., with the predominant isoenzyme in the sample) and depend on the temperature (temperatures up to $\cong 40°$ C increase the rates of reaction), the substrate, and the buffer concentrations.

Cardiac muscle, kidneys, and erythrocytes show a predominance of the LD_1 and LD_2 isoenzymes, whereas skeletal muscle and liver have a high content of LD_4 and LD_5. The **tetramer** of H chains composing LD_1 has an affinity for pyruvate that is 10-fold less than the affinity of LD_5, a tetramer of M chains. Thus LD_1 preferentially catalyzes the conversion of lactate to pyruvate. It has been suggested that because of its kinetic properties, the LD_1 isoenzyme predominates in tissues that receive a rich oxygen supply, since these tissues undergo oxidative metabolism and ordinarily do not accumulate lactate (or pyruvate) because they can use lactate as a fuel.[11] On the other hand, the LD_5 isoenzyme is the major form in skeletal muscle, which is more dependent on anaerobic glycolysis and accumulates pyruvate under anaerobic conditions. By having the LD_5 isoenzyme, muscle cells are better able to convert P→L and regenerate NAD^+, permitting the energy-producing reactions of the Embden-Meyerhof pathway.

Creatine Kinase (see Chapter 31 for additional details)

CK-MM (CK-3) is the predominant CK isoenzyme in adult skeletal muscle and cardiac tissue. CK-MB (CK-2) is mainly present in cardiac muscle (14%-42% of CK activity), with only a small concentration (up to 3% of the total CK activity) in skeletal muscle. However, CK-MB is not specific for myocardium and proportions of this isoenzyme can reach as high as 10% in some types of noncardiac muscle. The tissue-distribution of CK isoenzymes is listed in Table 55-1. In brain tissue, CK is primarily expressed as the CK-BB (CK-1) isoenzyme. There exists a fourth form that differs from the others both immunologically and by electrophoretic mobility. This isoenzyme, CK-Mt, is located between the inner and outer membranes of mitochondria, and it constitutes (in the heart, for example) up to 15% of the total CK activity. Its structure is determined by a locus on chromosome 15.

Alkaline Phosphatase

The tissue-nonspecific TNALP form of alkaline phosphatase is expressed in virtually all tissues. High activity is particularly noted in mineralizing bone, where ALP is located in the plasma membrane of osteoblastic cells. Intestinal ALP is expressed in the intestinal mucosa and is abundant in the brush borders of epithelial cells. Expression of this enzyme has also been documented in kidney, where it is mainly localized in the distal (S_3) segment of the proximal tubule.[12] Placental ALP is detectable in the serum of pregnant women between 16 and 20 weeks of gestation and becomes undetectable within 3 to 6 days after delivery. It is also present in relatively small amounts in lung and cervix. Placenta-like germ cell ALP has been found in very small amounts, in the testis and thymus of healthy individuals. At birth, ALP in the serum appears to come almost entirely from bone, differing from the pattern observed in the fetus, whose serum contains both bone and fetal intestinal forms. Serum from adults contains many ALP isoenzymes and isoforms, though the major forms released into serum are bone, liver, kidney, and intestinal.[13]

Developmental Distribution

Multiple gene loci and their independent isoenzyme products provide means for the adaptation of metabolic patterns to changing needs of different organs and tissues in the course of development. In addition, differential expression of isoenzymes over time occurs in response to environmental changes and pathological conditions. Gene activation and suppression of the different loci effect such changes. This process is very similar to the shift from the fetal form of hemoglobin to the adult form (see p. 679, Chapter 36). Other alterations in the balance of isoenzymes within the whole organism may derive from changes in the number or activity of cells that contain large amounts of an isoenzyme.

An example of differential expression of isoenzymes over time is seen in the increased number and activity of the osteoblasts responsible for bone mineralization between the early postnatal period and the beginning of the third decade of life. ALP from the active osteoblasts enters the circulation, where elevated levels can be detected in younger people compared with mature adults. An ALP isoenzyme from the

liver also contributes to the total activity of this enzyme in normal plasma, and the total activity of this enzyme increases with age. The reason for latter age-dependent change is unknown.

Changes in the relative proportions of several isoenzymes are noted during the embryonic development of skeletal muscle. The proportions of the electrophoretically more cathodic isoenzymes of LD (LD-5) and CK (CK-MM) increase in this tissue, so the qualitative patterns associated with the differentiated muscle are present by about the sixth month of intrauterine life. Smaller changes in isoenzyme distribution can continue to birth and into early postnatal life. These patterns appear to coincide with energy production demands of fetal tissues.

CHANGE IN ISOENZYME PATTERN DUE TO PATHOLOGICAL PROCESSES

Certain diseases, such as progressive muscular dystrophies, appear to involve a failure of the affected tissue to mature normally or to maintain a normal state. Cancer cells show a progressive loss of the structure and metabolism of the healthy cells from which they arise. Therefore, the isoenzyme pattern of mature, differentiated tissue may be lost or modified if normal differentiation is arrested or reversed, and many examples of isoenzyme changes accompanying such processes have been reported. The isoenzymes and isoforms associated with tumors are often referred to as *oncofetal tumor markers* because their expression is similar to that observed during early embryological development. Interpretation of isoenzyme and isoform patterns of distribution must be performed with caution because the fetal isoenzyme from one tissue may represent the adult isoenzyme form from another tissue.

Examples of changes in isoenzyme distribution can be seen with aldolase, LD, and CK in muscles of patients with progressive muscular dystrophy, which appear to be similar to distributions in embryological development of fetal muscle. The isoenzyme abnormalities in dystrophic muscle have been interpreted as a failure to achieve or maintain a normal degree of differentiation. Isoenzyme patterns in regenerating tissues may also show some tendency to approach fetal distributions. This tendency may result from relaxation or modification of control systems in rapidly dividing cells and may account for some of the isoenzyme changes noted, for example, in muscle in acute polymyositis.

LD activity, in normal adult aortic tissue, involves primarily the LD_3 fraction.[14] However, in atherosclerotic aortic tissue, maximal LD activity is present as the LD_5 fraction. Likewise, myocardial LD activity shifts from predominantly LD_1 to LD_3 during the progression of ischemic heart disease.[14] The LD isoenzymes in serum from patients with lymphoid malignancies are predominantly LD_2, LD_3, and LD_4.[15] A shift to this pattern in serum may indicate the presence of increased numbers of lymphoid cells resulting from malignant proliferation. A shift toward LD_5 expression is observed in many solid tumors, especially in carcinomas of the genitalia or the digestive tract, whereas in some tumors, such as those of germ cell origin, there is a shift toward LD_1 expression.

CK-MB represents a significant proportion of the CK activity in both fetal and adult myocardium, whereas in the fetus, CK-MB is also present as a high proportion of CK activity in skeletal muscle. Thus, while increased amounts of the CK-MB isoenzyme in the sera of normal adults probably represents damage to the heart, in children CK-MB increases may be from either heart or skeletal muscle.

Although CK-BB is the predominant isoenzyme in all early embryonic tissue, expression of this isoenzyme in most adult tissues is associated primarily with the brain and some tissues found in the gut (see Table 55-1). In patients without malignancy, detection of CK-BB in the serum is often associated with a pathological condition affecting the nervous, pulmonary, or gastrointestinal systems.[16] However, the lack of cell differentiation may cause some cells to express significant amounts of CK-BB, which may be detected in the serum.[16]

Human tumors are found to produce increased concentrations of the placental (PL-ALP), intestinal (I-ALP), and germ cell (GC-ALP) isoenzymes and isoforms of ALP. It appears that malignant processes either activate or amplify the expression of an ALP gene that is normally either repressed or expressed at a very low level.

In disorders of bone, increased enzyme production results in elevated levels of bone ALP because of increased osteoblastic activity. Increased serum levels of liver ALP in liver disease, particularly hepatobiliary obstruction, result from increased synthesis and release by hepatocytes, as well as from the release caused by accumulation of bile acids as a result of cholestasis.

CLINICAL SIGNIFICANCE OF SPECIFIC ISOENZYMES

For an enzyme to be clinically useful as a marker of disease, it must have a substantial tissue-to-plasma concentration ratio and a relatively long lifetime in blood. In addition, the release kinetics should accurately reflect the stage of disease and it must be tissue-specific. For all practical purposes, serum and plasma have been the only clinical specimens examined for isoenzyme and isoform markers of specific tissue abnormalities. The most important factors that affect enzyme activities in serum or plasma are those that influence the rate at which enzymes enter the circulation from the cells. These factors can be divided into two main categories: (1) those that affect the rates at which enzymes are released from cells, and (2) those that reflect altered rates of enzyme production, due either to increased synthesis of a particular enzyme by individual cell types or to proliferation of a particular type of enzyme-producing cell.

Normal cell turnover (apoptosis) and characteristic release from living cells is responsible for the "normal" or baseline concentrations in serum that define laboratory reference intervals. Levels beyond the minimum and/or maximum reference values are associated with a variety of pathological abnormalities and form the basis for clinical utility of enzyme determinations. The purpose of the next section is to discuss the major disease states associated with increased levels of isoenzymes and isoforms and to provide a basis for interpretation of abnormal values.

Creatine Kinase

Although the CK-MM, CK-MB, and CK-BB isoenzymes are cytoplasmic, there is creatine kinase (CK) activity in other subcellular locations, particularly in mitochondria. The 85,000-dalton molecular weight of CK precludes its passage across the blood-brain barrier except in cases of severe trauma, and significant increases in serum CK levels usually reflect either skeletal or cardiac muscle release. Measuring the CK isoenzymes can discriminate between skeletal muscle release and cardiac tissue release in most cases. As with most laboratory studies, the complexities of enzyme release and the various clearance mechanisms require that the interpretation of serum enzyme or isoenzyme concentrations be made in the context of the clinical situation. Often, combining multiple serum markers improves the ability to interpret enzyme concentrations and disease diagnosis.

In the past, the combined use of the LD and CK isoenzymes was necessary to yield the necessary information for evaluating patients admitted for the diagnosis of myocardial infarction (MI). A common interpretative problem is encountered when skeletal muscle injury results in significant elevation of CK activity in serum. Because skeletal muscle contains CK concentrations that are eightfold higher per gram of wet tissue than those in cardiac tissue, small areas of skeletal muscle injury or disease can result in serum CK-MB concentrations consistent with substantial damage to the heart. In uncomplicated cases, the use of isoenzyme fractionation can usually differentiate the source of the elevated CK serum activity because skeletal muscle usually consists of greater than 97% CK-MM isoenzyme. Calculation of a relative index, in which CK-MB concentration is the numerator and total CK is the denominator, can help elucidate the source of CK-MB. For cases in which both cardiac and muscle damage is suspected, as in cases of trauma or surgery, interpretation of CK-MB levels is more difficult and troponin measurements are more useful.

It is important to note that an increased proportion of CK-MB content is frequently associated with muscle fiber regeneration. For this reason, certain diseases of skeletal muscle, such as Duchenne muscular dystrophy or polymyositis, often result in serum elevations of total CK and an abnormal increase in serum CK-MB concentrations often to 5% to 15% of the total CK activity. Because the majority of patients with these muscle diseases are not being evaluated for MI, misinterpretation of these CK-MB elevations is infrequent.

Further difficulty in CK isoenzyme and isoform interpretation may be encountered during evaluation of patients undergoing thoracic and other surgery, particularly coronary artery bypass graft surgery. Surgical procedures involving the heart can be expected to cause the release of myocardial enzymes and isoenzymes at concentrations consistent with MI. In such patients the clinician is frequently concerned about perioperative MI either during surgery or during recovery. More specific markers of myocardial injury, such as troponin-I or troponin-T, show greater promise for improving the ability to diagnose perioperative MI.[17,18] Additional information on this subject is found in Chapter 31.

With high-voltage electrophoresis, the CK-MM and CK-MB isoenzymes can each be fractionated into subtypes (isoforms), which differ in their isoelectric points. Isoform formation appears to play a role in normal clearance of the CK-MM and CK-MB isoenzymes from plasma. Of the collective CK-MM and CK-MB isoforms, only MM_3 and MB_2 are found within tissue; upon release into circulation, they are irreversibly converted to their isoforms. The MB_2:MB_1 ratio reflects recent myocardial release and is a sensitive and early marker of MI (see Chapter 31).

CK activity in serum is proportional to muscle mass, and therefore serum CK activity characteristically decreases as a patient's age and muscle mass diminish. Physical activity influences serum CK activity. For example, about 50% to 80% of the asymptomatic female carriers of Duchenne dystrophy show three- to sixfold elevations of CK activity, but values may be normal if specimens are obtained after patients have experienced a period of physical inactivity. Quite high values of CK are noted in viral myositis, polymyositis, and similar muscle disease. However, in neurogenic muscle disorders, such as myasthenia gravis, multiple sclerosis, poliomyelitis and Parkinson's disease, serum enzyme activity is normal. Very high CK activity is also observed in malignant hyperthermia, a familial disease characterized by high fever and brought on by administration of inhalation anesthesia (usually halothane).

Because the liver contains negligible concentrations of CK, patients with primary liver disease (such as Reye's syndrome) and cirrhosis have normal CK activity in their sera. For the same reason, hepatic congestion and hypoxia, which may be accompanied by cardiac disease (discussed in Chapter 31), are not normally characterized by elevations in serum CK values, although they often contribute to the elevations in serum ALT and LD activity.

Serum CK activity demonstrates an inverse relationship with thyroid activity. About 60% of hypothyroid subjects show an average elevation of CK activity that is fivefold above the upper limit of the reference interval; elevations as high as 50-fold may be found. The major isoenzyme present is CK-MM and the presence of CK-MB suggests possible myocardial involvement; hypothyroidism predisposes patients to ischemic heart disease. Troponin measurement in these patients is useful for evaluating myocardial disease.

Alkaline Phosphatase

The value of characterizing ALP isoenzymes and isoforms in serum as a diagnostic aid is becoming more established as improved methods to better differentiate the various ALP forms become available. Most often ALP fractionation is requested to determine whether bone or liver is the source of an elevated level of total serum ALP activity. Specific ALP isoenzyme and isoform measurements, as compared with total ALP measurements, are at least twofold more sensitive for assessment of both bone and liver diseases.

The measurement of bone and liver isoforms so far has proved clinically useful for diagnosing and monitoring diseases such as Paget's disease and hepatobiliary disease. High levels of the bone ALP isoform are seen in several bone disorders including Paget's disease, osteosarcoma; hyperthyroidism; and sometimes osteoporosis. Also, there is an increased production of liver ALP in hepatobiliary diseases. Quantitative measurements of the bone ALP fraction is most important for monitoring patients with bone diseases to evaluate compliance and the response to therapy.

The increased expression of certain ALP genes, mainly variants of placental ALP, as well as the "**Regan**" and "Nagao" **isoenzymes**, is associated with germ cell tumors. These ALP isoenzymes are expressed predominantly in hepatocellular carcinomas or when liver is the site of a metastatic tumor. A significant amount of ALP is expressed in some but not all malignancies, and the explanation of why only some tumors express significant amounts of ALP is unknown.

In the past, the practical implications of ALP isoenzyme and isoform analysis precluded their measurement in many cases. However, the use of improved methods for measuring bone ALP for the monitoring of Paget's disease, osteoporosis, and bone cancer may increase the future use of ALP fractionation.[19,20]

Lactate Dehydrogenase

Although lactate dehydrogenase (LD) isoenzymes have been widely investigated, their clinical usefulness is limited because LD is found in virtually every tissue. Although there is some tissue-specificity for the various isoenzymes, there is considerable overlap in the tissue-specificity of the five isoenzyme forms commonly found in serum. For example, although the LD_5 isoenzyme is frequently used to ascertain damage to skeletal muscle, LD_5 is also the predominant isoenzyme in liver. A similar situation exists for each of the other four isoenzymes, which leads most clinicians to depend on other more specific tests for primary liver, muscle, or cardiac assessment. For several decades an increase in the LD_5 isoenzyme has been observed in the sera of patients with various types of cancer; however, the association of LD isoenzymes with tumors is a nonspecific finding.

Other Isoenzymes

Isoenzymes and isoforms of amylase, AST, and aldolase have been investigated, but only a few laboratories perform fractionation of these isoenzymes and isoforms because their clinical usefulness is not well established.

Fluids Other Than Serum

Some reports indicate that isoenzyme fractionation of several enzymes has significance in cerebrospinal fluid, pleural effusions, urine, and other fluids. For effusions, the main purpose of isoenzyme and isoform studies is to determine the source of the fluid. These fluids are rarely examined for quantitative isoenzyme concentration, and the methods for fractionation

TABLE 55-2   MODES OF ISOENZYME (ISOFORM) ANALYSIS

Technique	Principles of Analysis	Isoenzyme, Isoform
Electrophoresis	Subunits have different charges; isoenzymes are separated in an electrical field.	All
Ion-exchange chromatography	Subunits have different charges; isoenzymes are separated by differential affinity for ion-exchange resin.	CK, LD
Immunoinhibition	Antibody reacts specifically with one subunit type; this property can be used to render an isoenzyme or isoenzymes catalytically inactive or to physically remove an isoenzyme or isoenzymes from solution.	CK, LD, acid phosphatase
Immunoassay	Antibody reacts specifically with one subunit type; extent of reaction is monitored by use of radioisotope, enzyme, or fluorescent tag.	CK, LD, acid phosphatase, alkaline phosphatase, amylase
Heat stability	Individual isoenzyme subunits are rendered catalytically inactive at different temperatures.	Alkaline phosphatase
Catalytic inhibition	Individual isoenzyme subunits bind low–molecular-weight inhibitors with different affinities; such binding results in different inhibition of each isoenzyme.	Acid phosphate (L-tartrate), alkaline phosphatase (urea and L-phenylalanine), cholinesterase (dibucaine)
Substrate specificity	Each isoenzyme subunit binds a substrate with different affinities (K_m), giving each isoenzyme various rates of activity. Also each isoenzyme subunit may bind various substrates with different affinities; different isoenzymes have increased catalytic rates with certain substrates, whereas others have very low activities.	CK, acid phosphatase (α-naphthyl phosphate) LD_1

CK, Creatine kinase; LD, lactate dehydrogenase.

of fluid isoenzymes are occasionally very different from those used for serum. Because available data are so limited, laboratories involved in analyzing these fluids generally determine their own guidelines for clinical consultation and interpretation. Comparison of results with the reference intervals in serum should be discouraged.

MODES OF ISOENZYME ANALYSIS (Table 55-2)

Most of the physical and catalytic differences among individual isoenzymes and isoforms have been used to determine the isoenzyme concentrations in serum. All these methods depend on differences in 3D structure and posttranslational modifications that impart detectable variations to the molecule of interest. More sophisticated methods using specific immunoassays can differentiate between the isoenzymes and isoforms based on the immunological differences of the subunit chains.

ACKNOWLEDGMENTS

The authors are grateful for past contributions by Dr. Kalpana Panigrahi, Dr. John F. Chapman, and Dr. Lawrence M. Silverman.

References

1. Foreback CC, Chu JW: Creatine kinase isoenzymes: electrophoretic and quantitative measurements, *CRC Crit Rev Clin Lab Sci* 15:187, 1981.
2. Panteghini M: Serum isoforms of creatine kinase isoenzymes, *Clin Biochem* 21:211, 1988.
3. Wu ABW: Creatine kinase isoforms in ischemic heart disease, *Clin Chem* 35:7, 1989.
4. Perryman MB, Knell JD, Roberts R: Carboxypeptidase-catalyzed hydrolysis of C-terminal lysine: mechanism for in vivo production of multiple forms of creatine kinase in plasma, *Clin Chem* 30:662, 1984.
5. Rothe GM: A survey of the formation and localization of secondary isoenzymes in mammalia, *Hum Genet* 56:129, 1980.
6. Moss DW: Alkaline phosphatase isoenzymes, *Clin Chem* 28:2007, 1982.
7. Moss DW, Whitaker KB: Modification of alkaline phosphatases by treatment with glycosidase, *Enzyme* 34:212, 1985.
8. Fishman WH: Alkaline phosphatase isoenzymes: recent progress, *Clin Biochem* 23:99, 1990.
9. Harris H: The human alkaline phosphatases: what we know and what we don't know, *Clin Chem Acta* 186:133, 1989.
10. Russell RGG: Excretion of inorganic pyrophosphate in hypophosphatasia, *Lancet* 2:461, 1965.
11. Cahn RD et al: Nature and development of lactic dehydrogenases, *Science* 136:962, 1962.
12. Verpooten GF et al: Segment specific localization of intestinal-type alkaline phosphatase in human kidney, *Kidney Int* 36:617, 1989.
13. Bowers GN et al: Measurement of total alkaline phosphatase activity in human serum (selected method), *Clin Chem* 21:1988, 1975.
14. Wilhelm A: Topochemical variation of LDH and CK isoenzyme patterns in aorta, *Artery* 8:362, 1980.
15. Schapira F: Isoenzymes and cancer, *Adv Cancer Res* 18:77, 1973.
16. Lang H, Wurzburg U: Creatine kinase, an enzyme of many forms, *Clin Chem* 28:1439, 1982.
17. Adams JE et al: diagnosis of perioperative myocardial infarction with measurement of cardiac troponin, *N Engl J Med* 330:670, 1994.

18. Mair J, Dienstl F, Puschendorf B: Cardiac troponin T in the diagnosis of myocardial injury. *Crit Rev Clin Sci* 29:31, 1992.

19. Kaddam IM et al: Comparison of serum osteocalcin with total and bone specific alkaline phosphatase and urinary hydroxyproline:creatine ratio in patients with Paget's disease of bone, *Ann Clin Biochem* 31:327, 1994.

20. Garnero P, Delmas PD: Assessment of serum levels of bone alkaline phosphatase with a new immunoradiometric assay in patients with metabolic bone disease, *J Clin Endocrinol Metab* 77:1046, 1993.

Internet Sites

http://www.chem.qmw.ac.uk/iubmb/misc/isoen.html—IUPAC-IUB Commission on Biochemical Nomenclature (CBN)

http://www.biologie.uni-hamburg.de/b-online/e17/17g.htm—Botany online

http://www.mln.nih.gov/medlineplus/ency/article/003504.htm—Medline Plus: This is for CK isoenzymes, but one can search for other isoenzymes described in this chapter.

http://health.discovery.com/diseasesandcond/encyclopedia/1155.html—Health Discovery Encyclopedia: This is for CK isoenzymes, but one can search for the other isoenzymes described in this chapter.

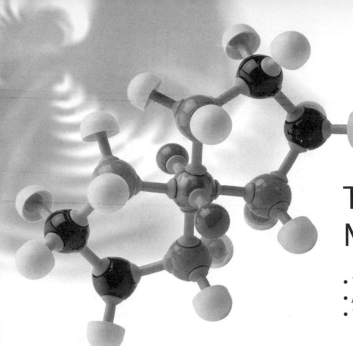

CHAPTER 56

Therapeutic Drug Monitoring (TDM)

- *Wolfgang A. Ritschel*
- *Michael Oellerich*
- *Victor W. Armstrong*

Chapter Outline

Objectives

- Describe the steps involved in the physiological processing of a drug given to a patient.
- Define therapeutic index and therapeutic range.
- Describe the rationale for therapeutic drug monitoring (TDM).

- Describe various dosing regimens and the influence these have on laboratory TDM programs.
- List the factors that may have an influence on the need to perform a TDM analysis stat.

Key Terms

absorption   Uptake of unchanged drug into circulation.

absorption rate constant   Value describing how much drug is absorbed per unit of time.

active transport   Movement of drug across a membrane by binding to a carrier molecule and delivery to the opposite side with expenditure of energy.

bioavailability   The amount of drug in the formulation that the system of the patient can absorb.

biophase   The site of interaction between the drug molecule and its receptor.

bound drug   A pharmacological agent that exists in blood complexed with another molecule (usually protein or lipid).

C_{max} Maximum plasma level of drug.

C_{av}^{ss} Average steady-state concentration.

C_{max}^{ss} Maximum steady-state concentration (peak concentration).

C_{min}^{ss} Minimum steady-state concentration (trough concentration).

compartment   A pharmacokinetic term for the drug concentration, C, and the volume of distribution of that drug.

distribution   Proportional division of drug into different compartments of the body, such as blood and extracellular fluid.

elimination   Final excretion of an agent.

first-order kinetics   The rate of change of plasma drug concentration that is dependent on the concentration itself; that is, a constant proportion of drug is removed with time, or $dC/dt = -k \times C$.

free drug   Pharmacological agent that exists in biological fluids unbound by other molecules.

half-life ($t_{1/2}$)   The amount of time required to reduce a drug level to one half its initial value. Usually it refers to the time necessary to reduce the plasma value to one half of its initial value. The term is also applied to the disappearance of the total amount of drug from the body.

LADME   An acronym for the time course of drug distribution: *l*iberation, *a*bsorption, *d*istribution, *m*etabolism, and *e*limination.

liberation   The process of drug release from the dosage form.

limited fluctuation method of dosing   A method of dosing in which the drug given is not to exceed or to go below specified limits.

maintenance dose   The amount of drug required to keep a desired mean steady-state concentration.

MEC, MIC   The minimum effective concentration, or the minimum inhibitory concentration, for a drug to be active. A drug is effective at any level above this value.

metabolism   The biotransformation of the parent drug into metabolites.

Michaelis-Menten kinetics   A method of transforming drug plasma levels into a linear relationship using the parameters of drug concentration and a constant, K_m.

passive diffusion   The transport of drug by a concentration gradient across the membrane.

peak concentration   The highest concentration reached after a dosage (usually soon after the dose is given).

peak method of dosing   A method whereby the drug must reach a specified maximum level to be effective.

pharmacogenetics   The science concerned with identification and characterization of polymorphic genes encoding, drug metabolizing enzymes, transporters, receptors, and other drug targets.

pharmacokinetics   The quantitative study of drug disposition in the body.

pharmacological effect   The influence of a drug on a patient's biochemical or physiological state (such as lowering of blood pressure and bacteriostasis).

prodrug   A parent compound that is usually not active and must be metabolized to the active form.

receptor   The structure in the body with which the drug interacts, yielding its pharmacological effect. Most often it is located on a cell membrane or other cellular component.

slow release   A dosage form of drug that allows the drug to be slowly placed into solution.

steady state   A condition in which drug input and drug output are equal. This is obtained when, after multiple dosing, the peak concentration and the trough concentration after each dose oscillate within a certain range.

subtherapeutic   A level of drug less than that necessary to have the desired clinical effect.

t   Dosing interval.

t_{max} The time of maximum drug concentration.

terminal disposition rate constant   The overall elimination of drug from the body per unit time.

therapeutic index   The ratio between the plasma concentrations yielding the desired and undesired effects of a drug.

therapeutic range   The relationship between the desired clinical effect of a drug and the concentration of the drug in the plasma.

therapeutic window   A term describing a bell-shaped response curve of drug level versus pharmacological response.

total clearance (Cl_{tot})   A term that describes how much of the volume of distribution of a drug is cleared per unit of time.

toxic   Implies poisonous or deleterious, sometimes fatal, side effects from a therapeutic agent that is present at a level that is too high.

trough concentration   The lowest drug concentration reached, usually before the next dose is given.

zero-order kinetics   The rate of change of plasma concentration, independent of the plasma concentration. A constant amount is eliminated per unit of time, or $dC/dt = -k_0$.

zero-time blood level   A hypothetical blood concentration obtained by extrapolation back to the initial, or zero, time of administration. Usually this yields a maximal value.

Methods on CD-ROM

Anticonvulsant drugs
Carbamazepine
Cyclosporine A
Digoxin
Gentamicin and other aminoglycosides

Lithium
Methotrexate
Procainamide
Theophylline and caffeine

Part 1: Basic Overview of Principles
WOLFGANG A. RITSCHEL

FATE OF DRUG AND NEED FOR THERAPEUTIC DRUG MONITORING
Concept of Therapeutic Range

For many drugs a relationship has been established between the clinical effects and the drug concentration in plasma. In general, to achieve the desired **pharmacological effect** (such as lowering of blood pressure, pain relief, or bacteriostasis) a certain concentration must be reached at the site of interaction between the drug molecule and the **receptor** (cell membrane, cell component) to elicit the clinical effect.

Currently the only qualitative measurements available to assess the drug interactions at the cellular level are measurements of serum drug levels. If the degree of clinical response to a drug is plotted against the logarithm of dose or blood concentration of that drug, a linear curve is obtained. The same semilogarithmic curve is obtained if the drug dose or blood concentration is plotted against the percentage of a given population that has a specific clinical response to the drug. Any dose or concentration that does not result in any measurable or quantifiable effect is **subtherapeutic**. Any dose or concentration larger than the minimum dose or concentration that gives 100% effectiveness is unwarranted and may be **toxic**. (Consider the box at right.)

Similar to the log dose-response curve, there usually is a log dose-toxicity curve (see Chapter 51). Often an overlap is found between the upper portion of the log dose-response curve and the lower portion of the log dose-toxicity curve. For most drugs the **therapeutic range** is a concentration range somewhere in the lower third to middle portion of the log concentration-response curve. The steepness of the log concentration-response curve indicates the magnitude of the therapeutic range. Absolute toxicity is less important than the ratio between the average toxic dose and the average therapeutic dose or concentration (see additional discussion

---

MAJOR CAUSES OF UNEXPECTED SERUM DRUG CONCENTRATIONS OUTSIDE OF THE THERAPEUTIC RANGE

Noncompliance of patient
Inappropriate dosage
Malabsorption
Poor bioavailability of the administered preparation
Drug interactions
Kidney and liver disease
Altered protein binding
Fever
Genetically determined fast or slow metabolism

---

on p. 1085). This ratio, called the **therapeutic index**, is narrow for some drugs (digoxin, lithium compounds) and wide for others. Hence the therapeutic range may also be narrow or wide. It is particularly desirable to monitor drug concentrations for drugs that have a narrow therapeutic range and low therapeutic index (digoxin, lithium, gentamicin), have dose-dependent **elimination** kinetics (phenytoin), or show great individual variability in **metabolism** (tricyclic antidepressants). Thus it is important for the physician to know whether the drug is present in a concentration within the therapeutic range.

The purpose of this chapter is to describe the fate of drugs once administered, to provide some insight into the type of dose regimen used to achieve the therapeutic range, and to describe some basic principles of **pharmacokinetics**.

LADME System to Describe Drug Disposition

It is generally accepted that changes in drug concentrations in the body that occur with time are related to the course of the pharmacological effects. The change of drug concentration with time is described by the **LADME** system, in which the *l*iberation, *a*bsorption, *d*istribution, *m*etabolism, and *e*limination of a drug are considered in sequence.

Liberation, or drug release, from a dosage form.
To be absorbed, a drug must be present in the form of a true solution at the site of absorption. Hence the active ingredient of any dosage form except those that are already true solutions (such as intravenous injection, peroral elixir, peroral syrup, rectal enema, eye drops, and nose drops) has to be released from the dosage form before the drug can be absorbed. The release or liberation is the process of the drug passing into solution. When given orally by tablets, capsules, or suspensions, the drug dissolves in gastric fluid. After intramuscular or subcutaneous injection of suspensions, the drug dissolves in tissue fluid. After rectal administration, suppositories melt in the rectum, and the drug dissolves in rectal fluid. After application of ointments, the drug dissolves in the water of perspiration at the interface between the skin and the ointment. These are a few cases in which liberation is necessary for the drug to be absorbed.

Sustained or controlled-release dosage forms are preparations with **slow release** rates. These are designed for those drugs that do not remain in the body for a long time. Because the drug cannot be absorbed faster than it is released, the apparent absorption rate becomes a function of the release rate and the entire absorption process takes longer, resulting in a prolonged duration of clinical effect.

Absorption. Absorption is the process by which the drug molecule is taken up into systemic circulation. Systemic circulation is usually defined as the bloodstream. The process of absorption must occur whenever a drug is administered *extravascularly*, that is, perorally, orally, intramuscularly, subcutaneously, rectally, topically, and so on. Whenever a drug is given *intravascularly* (intravenously, intraarterially, intracardiacly), no absorption takes place because the drug is directly introduced into the bloodstream.

There are various mechanisms of absorption, including **passive diffusion**, **active transport**, facilitated transport, convective transport, and pinocytosis. Passive diffusion, applicable for about 95% of all drugs, depends on the concentration of nonionized drug being higher on one side of the membrane than on the other. As long as there is a concentration gradient across the membrane, the drug will be absorbed into the region of lower concentration. For weak electrolytes, the drug's pK_a and the pH at the absorption site (such as stomach pH 1.5 to 3, intestines pH 5 to 7, rectum pH 7.8, or skin pH 5) influence the degree of ionization. The pH of blood is 7.4 and rather constant. As a general rule, ionized drug species are passively absorbed much *less* readily than nonionized species. At two pH units below an acid drug's pK_a and two pH units above a basic drug's pK_a, the drugs will be 99% nonionized and have maximal rates of absorption.

The next important absorption mechanism is **active transport**, which requires binding of the drug molecule to a carrier (protein) in the membrane. The carrier delivers the drug to the opposite side of the membrane by an expenditure of energy. The process moves the drug (such as cardiac glycosides, hexoses, monosaccharides, amino acids, riboflavin)

against a concentration gradient. *Facilitated transport* is a similar mechanism, but facilitated transport of a substance (such as vitamin B_{12}) follows the concentration gradient. *Convective transport* is the mechanism of absorption by which small molecules (such as urea) enter systemic circulation through water-filled pores in the membrane. For all these mechanisms the drug must be in true aqueous solution at the absorption site.

A unique absorption mechanism is that of *pinocytosis* of fats and solid particles. Engulfing vesicles form in the cellular membrane and open at the intracellular side, releasing the fat droplets or particles (such as vitamins A, K, D, and E; parasite eggs; fats; and starch).

Distribution. Once drug molecules are absorbed, they distribute within the bloodstream and can (1) be confined to the blood space, (2) leave the bloodstream and enter other extravascular fluids (such as interstitial fluid), or (3) migrate into various tissues and organs. The entire process of transfer of drug from the bloodstream to other compartments is called *distribution*. This process usually takes between 30 minutes and 2 hours but may be completed within a few minutes or may take much longer than 2 hours (distribution time for methotrexate is 15 hours).

Metabolism. Metabolism is the process of biotransformation of the parent drug molecule to one or more metabolites. The metabolites are usually more polar, that is, more water soluble, and can thus be more easily excreted by the kidney. Metabolism occurs primarily in the liver and the kidney but also takes place in plasma and muscle tissue. Usually, but not always, metabolites are less active and less toxic than their parent compounds. However, at this point a group of drugs, known as **prodrugs**, should be mentioned. The prodrug as parent compound is usually not active and must be metabolized to the active form (e.g., the inactive cancer drug cyclophosphamide is biotransformed to the active compound 4-hydroxycyclophosphamide). The active form of prodrugs is either unstable, not readily soluble, or poorly absorbed.

Some drugs form metabolites that are also active. For example, the active drug procainamide is biotransformed to the equipotent metabolite acetylprocainamide. The knowledge of active metabolites is particularly important for TDM to correlate the total concentration of all active forms with pharmacological effects.

Elimination. The final excretion of the drug from the body either as unchanged parent compound or in the form of metabolites is called *elimination*. The major routes of excretion are through the kidney into urine and through the liver into bile and consequently into feces. Other pathways of elimination are through skin (sweat), lungs (expired air), mammary glands (milk), and salivary glands (saliva).

The elimination **half-life** is the time required to reduce the blood level concentration to one half after equilibrium is obtained. After the drug is absorbed and distributed, it takes one half-life to eliminate 50% of the drug, seven half-lives to eliminate 99% of the drug, and 10 half-lives to eliminate 99.9% of the drug.

Effects of biological variation on LADME. If a drug is given in identical amounts by the same route of administration at the same time of day to identical twins, the pharmacokinetic parameters will differ only very slightly. In fraternal twins there will be larger differences. Greater differences will occur within a population group, even if this group is homogeneous with regard to sex, age, body weight, and health. These differences are genetically based variations in drug handling, which may influence absorption, distribution, metabolism, elimination, and drug-receptor interactions. Hence pharmacokinetic parameters for healthy subjects reported in the literature are means with ranges. They are actually valid only for the group studied.

Physiological and pathological factors influencing drug disposition. Apart from biological variations caused by genetic differences, many physiological and pathological factors may alter considerably a drug's disposition.[1]

The most prominent physiological factors are body weight and composition, age, temperature (hyperthermia and hypothermia), gastric emptying time and gastrointestinal motility, blood flow rates (during rest and exercise), environment (high altitude, mountain sickness), nutrition, pregnancy, and circadian rhythm.

Among the most important pathological factors are renal impairment, liver impairment, acute congestive heart failure, burns, shock, trauma, and gastrointestinal diseases.

Blood Levels as Indicators of Clinical Response

The rationale for the use of blood levels as indicators of clinical response is based on the concept that, for those drugs that interact at a receptor site without being changed, the drug concentration at the site of action determines the intensity and duration of the pharmacological effect. Because it is usually not possible to sample at the site of action or **biophase** (such as the cell membrane), the next alternative is to sample whole blood, plasma, or serum, which is the biological fluid in closest equilibrium with the receptor site that can be easily sampled. After the distribution phase is complete, the drug concentration in the central and peripheral **compartments** (i.e., blood) will decline in parallel. At this point a pseudoequilibrium of distribution is obtained regardless of whether the site of action is in the central compartment or in any peripheral compartment. Although the total drug concentration may differ considerably between central and peripheral compartments, the concentration of **free** (unbound) **drug** will be the same. Hence, once the pseudoequilibrium of distribution is reached, a correlation should exist between pharmacological effect and drug concentration in blood. Usually only the total drug concentration is measured, that is, both the free and **bound drug**, in plasma. This is quite acceptable under normal conditions because individual differences in plasma-protein binding seem to be small[2]; in some cases, however, this is not true.[3,4]

Blood Levels after Single Dose of Drug

Most graphical descriptions of a pharmacokinetic response are given as a plot of blood concentration versus time

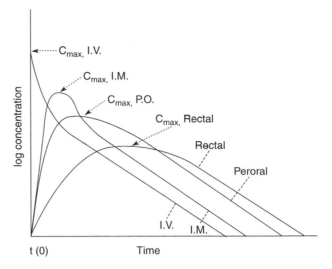

Fig. 56-1   Blood level–time curves of a hypothetical drug upon different routes of administration.

(Fig. 56-1). The shape and course of a blood level–time curve depend on the route of administration and the LADME system.

With rapid intravenous administration, each facet of the drug is instantly in the systemic circulation. If the drug is given by extravascular administration, none will be in systemic circulation at the moment of administration, that is, at time zero. After the drug is released from the dosage form, the blood level–time curve rises with continuous absorption. Once absorbed, a molecule is exposed to distribution, metabolism, and elimination. Because initially a greater proportion is absorbed than is distributed, metabolized, and eliminated, the blood level–time curve rises until input and output are equal. At this time (t_{max}) the **peak concentration** (C_{max}) is reached and the blood level–time curve declines as elimination exceeds absorption (see Fig. 56-1).

Two liberation factors may change the shape of the curve: the rate and the extent of liberation. Drug products from different manufacturers may release the drug at various rates. A slow release may also be intentional, as in the case of slow-release (sustained-release) dosage forms. However, if all the drug is released, the areas under the blood level–time curves of different formulations will be the same. If the drug is not fully released, a so-called **bioavailability** problem might be present and the area under the curve will be reduced (Fig. 56-2). *Bioavailability* refers to the amount of drug systemically absorbed.

The absorption process can be influenced by many factors. Food (when the drug is given orally before, during, or after meals) may have no effect on the absorption, may accelerate or prolong the absorption, or may influence the extent of absorption. For example, the blood level of griseofulvin is greatly enhanced when the drug is given with fat, whereas a tetracycline blood level decreases when the drug is ingested with milk.

The volume of distribution may change in various pathological conditions. If the volume of distribution increases, the blood level decreases and vice versa. In congestive heart

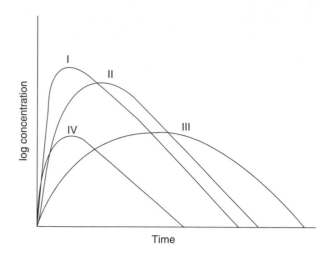

Fig. 56-2 Influence of liberation process on course of blood level–time curves. *I*, Fast-dissolving tablet; *II*, tablet with slower dissolution rate; *III*, sustained-release tablet; *IV*, tablet with poor bioavailability.

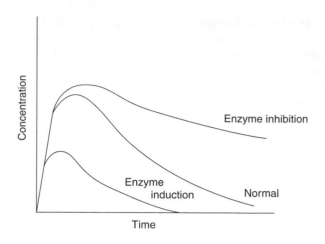

Fig. 56-4 Influence of metabolism processes on course of blood level–time curves. Enzyme inhibition and liver damage may greatly increase blood level, whereas enzyme induction may decrease it.

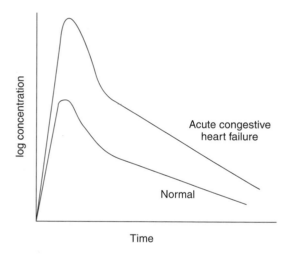

Fig. 56-3 Influence of distribution process on course of blood level–time curves of digoxin. In acute congestive heart failure a higher blood level is observed because of decreased volume of distribution.

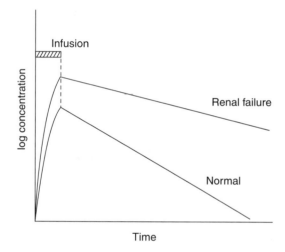

Fig. 56-5 Influence of elimination processes on course of blood level–time curve of gentamicin. In presence of renal failure, peak concentration after short-term infusion is higher and blood level remains elevated with a longer elimination half-life.

failure the volume of distribution for certain drugs is reduced (digoxin, quinidine). The same dose will therefore result in a higher concentration (Fig. 56-3).

For drugs that are extensively metabolized, changes in the course of blood levels may result from impaired metabolism (liver damage) or other drugs given concomitantly that either compete for metabolic pathways (enzyme inhibition) or accelerate metabolism (enzyme induction) (Fig. 56-4).

Elimination of drugs, particularly of those predominantly eliminated through the kidney, may be tremendously prolonged in cases of renal failure and in aged persons. The reduced elimination can result in a manyfold prolonged elimination half-life. Classic examples are the aminoglycosides. Gentamicin's normal half-life of 2 hours may easily be prolonged to 20 hours or more (Fig. 56-5).

Effects of High Levels of Drugs

As stated earlier, for most drugs there is a relationship between drug concentration in the blood and the pharmacological and toxic response. Hence an increase in the blood level is usually associated with an increase in intensity not only of clinical effectiveness but also of toxicity. For most drugs it is desirable either to reach a therapeutic range with the peak concentration or to maintain the blood level throughout the dosage interval within the therapeutic range. A concentration below the therapeutic range is subtherapeutic or ineffective, and a concentration above the therapeutic range is likely to be toxic and cause side effects. However, the therapeutic and subtherapeutic range and the therapeutic and toxic range often overlap (Fig. 56-6). Additionally, an established therapeutic range may be applicable for the

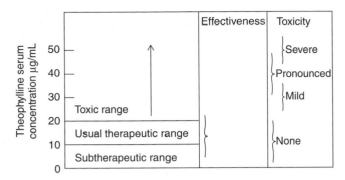

Fig. 56-6 Relationship between serum theophylline concentration and effectiveness and toxicity.

majority of patients but may be too low or too high for an individual patient. One such example is theophylline, for which the usual therapeutic range is between 10 and 20 µg/mL. However, some patients are perfectly controlled with levels as low as 5 µg/mL. On the other hand, whereas most patients do not experience theophylline side effects with levels of 23 µg/mL, some already show toxic signs at this level.

Need for Monitoring of Drug Therapy

Many patients, regardless of whether they are hospitalized or ambulatory, receive more than one drug during any given day,[5] which increases the probability of drug-induced diseases, drug interactions, and side effects. One of the most widely used drugs, cimetidine, has been reported to interact with 21 different drugs.[6] A definite need for drug monitoring is also indicated by the finding that 30% to 50% of dosage administrations in hospitals and nursing homes were in error.[7]

Another reason for drug monitoring is noncompliance with a prescribed dosage regimen. One report states that the percentage of patients failing to take their medication as directed ranges between 20% and 82%.[8]

Drug monitoring for all drugs and all patients is neither possible nor feasible. Furthermore, total drug monitoring is, at least at present, not relevant for all drugs. For other drugs, for which a pharmacological response is easily, quickly, and accurately measured, it is clinically more relevant to monitor directly the clinical response (such as blood pressure, blood glucose, electrolyte excretion) instead of the blood level.

If a patient is responding well to the drug therapy without any signs of toxicity, this dosage regimen should be maintained even though the blood level might be outside the usual therapeutic range. The question, "For which drugs is therapeutic drug monitoring indicated?" can be answered as follows. Monitoring is indicated for many drug groups such as antiepileptic drugs, antiarrhythmic agents, peroral anticoagulants, theophylline, tricyclic antidepressants, lithium carbonate, and aminoglycosides that either show large individual variation or are toxic above the therapeutic range. A flow chart showing the factors underlying the need for monitoring is given in Fig. 56-7.[9]

DOSAGE REGIMENS USED IN ACHIEVING THERAPEUTIC TARGET CONCENTRATION
Prediction of Dosage for Steady-State Therapeutic Levels

Most drugs are not administered as a single dose. Instead most drugs are administered in a series of doses given at specified intervals throughout the entire course of drug therapy. If the drug is administered repeatedly using dosing intervals shorter than the time required to eliminate the drug remaining in the body from the preceding dose, the drug will *accumulate* until a **steady state** is achieved, that is, one in which drug input and output are equal. Steady state is obtained when, with a specific regimen of dosage, the peak concentration (C_{max}^{ss}, or maximum steady-state concentration) and trough concentration (C_{min}^{ss}, or minimum steady-state concentration) after each dose oscillate within a certain range; the goal is to achieve the therapeutic range. By obtaining a blood level–time curve after a single dose, the necessary parameters can be derived to predict the steady state and in turn the dose required to achieve a desired steady state.

The **maintenance dose** required to maintain a desired mean steady-state concentration, C_{av}^{ss}, at a given dosage interval, **t**, depends on the magnitude of C_{av}^{ss} (the required drug concentration in blood to elicit the pharmacological response), the pharmacokinetic parameters of drug disposition, and the patient's body weight. The generalized equation for determining the correct maintenance dose is given in the box on p. 1080.[10]

The dosing interval, *t*, is freely chosen within a wide range, most often at times less than $t_{1/2}$ (half-life). It may have to be increased in renal or hepatic diseases because $t_{1/2}$ is often greatly extended in these cases. In general, at the end of four half-lives (if a dosing interval less than the half-life is chosen) a steady-state level is reached with multiple dosing (Fig. 56-8).

Dosing Regimens

The dosage regimen for multiple dosing maintenance therapy can be designed according to five different methods, depending on the desired target concentration to be achieved or maintained throughout each dosing interval. For monitoring purposes it is necessary to know which method will be used because the optimum blood sampling protocol for laboratory analysis depends on the method in question. Five methods for dosage regimen design follow:

> Minimum effective concentration (**MEC**) or minimum inhibitory concentration (**MIC**) method
> C_{max}^{ss}, or peak, method
> C_{max}^{ss}-C_{min}^{ss}, or limited fluctuation, method
> C_{av}^{ss}, or log dose-response, method
> TW, or **therapeutic window**, method

All methods refer to steady-state concentrations.

MEC or MIC method. For some drugs to be effective it is necessary to reach and maintain a minimum inhibitory concentration (MIC), or a minimum effective concentration

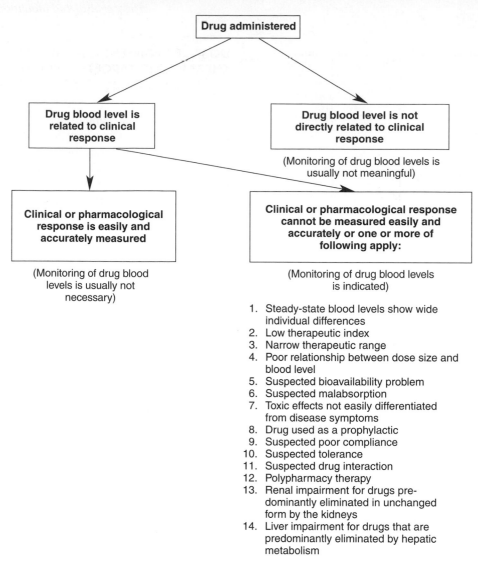

Fig. 56-7 Scheme to identify cases and situations when drug monitoring is indicated. *(Modified from Pippenger CE: Ther Drug Monit 1:3, 1979.)*

The figure contains the following flowchart text:

Drug administered

Drug blood level is related to clinical response

Drug blood level is not directly related to clinical response

(Monitoring of drug blood levels is usually not meaningful)

Clinical or pharmacological response is easily and accurately measured

(Monitoring of drug blood levels is usually not necessary)

Clinical or pharmacological response cannot be measured easily and accurately or one or more of following apply:

(Monitoring of drug blood levels is indicated)

1. Steady-state blood levels show wide individual differences
2. Low therapeutic index
3. Narrow therapeutic range
4. Poor relationship between dose size and blood level
5. Suspected bioavailability problem
6. Suspected malabsorption
7. Toxic effects not easily differentiated from disease symptoms
8. Drug used as a prophylactic
9. Suspected poor compliance
10. Suspected tolerance
11. Suspected drug interaction
12. Polypharmacy therapy
13. Renal impairment for drugs predominantly eliminated in unchanged form by the kidneys
14. Liver impairment for drugs that are predominantly eliminated by hepatic metabolism

---

FACTORS DETERMINING AN INDIVIDUALIZED DOSE SIZE*

Maintenance dose (μg) DM ↓ V_d		Total body clearance† (mL/hr/kg) Cl_{tot} ↓ k_e or β	Desired mean steady-state concentration (μg/mL) C_{av}^{ss} ↓ Therapeutic range		Dosing interval (hr) τ ↓ Interval		Body weight (kg) BW ↓ Body composition
Apparent lipid/water partition coefficient	=	Metabolism:	Receptor sensitivity	×	Increase or no	×	Fat/lean mass
pK_a		Liver blood flow rate	Number of receptors		change with		Lean body weight
Total body fluid		Enzyme activity	Neurotransmittance		reduced dose		Total body weight
Total body fat		Subcellular changes	Homeostasis				
Extent of protein binding		Extrahepatic factors					
Tissue blood flow rate		Excretion:					
		Effective renal blood flow rate					
		Glomerular filtration rate					
		Active tubular transport					
		Morphological changes					

*For further information see Ritschel WA: Contemp Pharmacy Pract 5:209, Washington, DC, 1982, American Pharmaceutical Association.
†V_d, Apparent volume of distribution (mL/kg); k_e or β, overall terminal disposition rate constant (hr^{-1}); $Cl_{tot} = V_d \cdot \beta$.

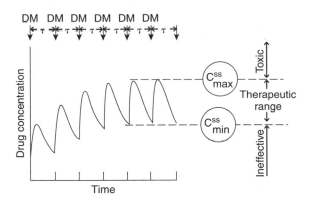

Fig. 56-8 Graph of blood-drug concentrations as function of dose and time. *DM*, Dose; τ, interval between doses; C_{max}^{ss}, concentration maximum at steady state; C_{min}^{ss}, concentration minimum at steady state. In this sample τ is chosen to be equivalent to the half-life of elimination.

(MEC), at steady state. Above the MIC or MEC the drug will be effective regardless of how high a peak level is reached as long as the entire steady-state blood level–time curve is above the required MIC or MEC. If the blood level–time curve falls below the MIC or MEC level, the drug will be ineffective as long as the concentration stays below this level. Drugs such as bacteriostatic antibiotics and other antimicrobial agents (sulfonamides) that have a relatively large therapeutic index are often prescribed at dosages calculated by this method.

C_{max}^{ss}, **or peak, method.** For some drugs it is desirable to reach a certain steady-state peak concentration during each dosing interval. However, for the remainder of the dosing interval it is not required that the drug concentration remain above a minimum level. This is particularly the case with bactericidal drugs, which act only on the proliferating micro-organisms. In these cases it is not desirable to inhibit growth of those microorganisms that have not been killed by the previous dose. Drugs that are often given in dosage regimens based on the C_{max}^{ss}, or **peak method of dosing** include penicillins, cephalosporins, gentamicin, and kanamycin.

C_{max}^{ss}-C_{min}^{ss}, **or limited fluctuation, method.** For some drugs it might be desirable to maintain at steady state an MIC or MEC throughout the dosing interval but never exceed a certain peak value. This is particularly the case if the drug has a narrow therapeutic range. Drugs that might be administered using this **limited fluctuation method of dosing** to compute dosage include gentamicin, kanamycin, streptomycin, isoniazid, and theophylline.

C_{av}^{ss}, **or log dose-response, method.** For drugs whose clinical effect follows a log dose-response curve, drug doses are selected to be in the lower portion of the log dose-response curve. The desired steady-state concentration is then usually in the lower third of the log dose-response curve. For drugs following a log dose response, the intensity of effect (and of toxicity) increases with increasing peak size. Drugs whose dosages are often based on this pattern are digoxin, lidocaine, procainamide, theophylline, quinidine,

bactericidal antibiotics, analgesics, antipyretics, and hypo-glycemic agents.

TW, or therapeutic window, method. With some drugs, such as antidepressants and antipsychotics, the clinical effect increases with dose size only up to a certain point and then actually diminishes as the dose size is further increased. Instead of a therapeutic range there exists a therapeutic window, showing a more or less bell-shaped log dose-response curve.

PHARMACOKINETICS

Pharmacokinetics is the quantitative study of drug disposition in the body. Pharmacokinetics permits (1) describing mathematically the fate of a drug after administration in a given dosage form by a given route of administration, (2) comparing one drug with others or one dosage form with other dosage forms, and (3) predicting blood levels of a drug with different dosage regimens or disease states.

Basically, in pharmacokinetics three types of kinetic processes are used to characterize the fate of drugs in the body: first-order, or linear, kinetics; zero-order, or nonlinear, kinetics; and Michaelis-Menten, or saturation, kinetics.

First-Order Kinetics

Most processes of drug uptake (absorption), diffusion and permeation in the body (distribution), and excretion (urinary elimination) can be described by first-order, or linear, kinetics. This means that the rate of change of concentration of drug is dependent on the drug concentration. When the concentration versus time data are plotted on numeric, or cartesian, graph paper, a concave curve is obtained; when plotted on semilog paper, a straight line is obtained. The relationship is expressed by Eq. 56-1:

$$dC/dt = -k \times C \qquad \textit{Eq. 56-1}$$

in which C is the concentration of the drug, k is the first-order rate constant, and t is time. The minus sign indicates that the drug concentration decreases with time. Drugs are eliminated in a manner that can be described by **first-order kinetics** when a *constant percentage* of drug is eliminated per unit of time. Drugs exhibiting first-order elimination kinetics are antibiotics and sulfonamides, digoxin, lidocaine, procaina-mide, and theophylline. First-order kinetics describes the elimination of most drugs.

Zero-Order Kinetics

If the rate of elimination of a compound from the body is not proportional to the concentration of the drug taken, the elimination usually follows zero-order, or nonlinear, kinetics. This means that the rate of change of concentration is independent of the concentration of the particular drug. In other words, a *constant amount* of drug, rather than a constant proportion, is eliminated per unit of time (elimination depends on the amount per unit of time). When the concentration versus time data are plotted on numeric, or cartesian, graph paper, a straight line is obtained, whereas on semilog paper a convex curve is obtained. The classic example for **zero-order kinetics** is the disposition of alcohol (ethanol).

The relationship can be expressed by Eq. 56-2:

$$dC/dt = -k_0 \qquad \textit{Eq. 56-2}$$

in which the rate of change of concentration, dC/dt, is equal to the zero-order rate constant, k_0, which has the units of amount per unit of time.

Michaelis-Menten Kinetics. In metabolism nearly all biotransformation processes are catalyzed by specific enzyme systems with a limited capacity for the drug. Also in active transport of drugs across membranes the carriers have a limited capacity. Whenever the drug concentration present in a given system exceeds the capacity of the system, the rate of change of concentration is most precisely described by the Michaelis-Menten equation:

$$dC/dt = -(V_{max} \times C)/(K_m + C) \qquad \textit{Eq. 56-3}$$

in which C is the drug concentration, t is the time, V_{max} is a constant representing the maximum rate of the process, and K_m is the Michaelis-Menten constant, the drug concentration at which the process proceeds at exactly one half its maximal rate. Examples of drugs that show saturation-elimination or **Michaelis-Menten kinetics** are phenytoin, high doses of barbiturates, and glutethimide.

Compartment Models

To describe the quantitative processes of a drug in the organism, pharmacokinetics uses the concept of compartments. A compartment is a unit characterized by two parameters: the drug concentration, C, and the volume, V_d. By multiplying the drug concentration by the apparent volume of distribution, the amount, A, of the drug in that compartment is obtained:

$$C \times V_d = A \qquad \textit{Eq. 56-4}$$

A given compartment model is not necessarily specific for a given drug. For example, a drug given intravenously is often described by a two-compartment open model, whereas the same drug given orally or by any other extravascular route may be described by a one-compartment open model. *Open* means that there is input to and output from the compartment.

In reality the human body is a multimillion-compartment system. However, usually there exists in the intact organism easy access to only two kinds of biological fluids, blood (serum, plasma), and urine. Being restricted to blood or urine specimens, the drug has a fate in the body usually described by either a one-compartment or a two-compartment open model. Clinically speaking, the concept of the one-compartment and two-compartment models is usually satisfactory for therapeutic use. The difference between a one-compartment and a two-compartment model is that in the former the distribution occurs instantly whereas in the latter the distribution process needs a measurable time before pseudoequilibrium is obtained.

Terminal Disposition Rate Constant

In the one-compartment open model, the last or terminal portion of the straight (monoexponential) slope of a semilog

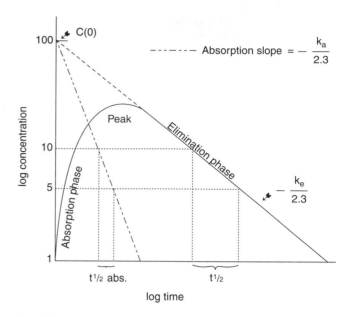

Fig. 56-9 One-compartment model blood level–time curve after extravascular administration, with monoexponential slopes for elimination, k_e, and absorption, k_a. *(From Ritschel WA: Graphic approach to clinical pharmacokinetics, Barcelona, 1983, Prous Science.)*

blood level–time curve gives the overall elimination rate constant, k_e (metabolism, renal excretion, and other pathways of elimination). In the two-compartment model it gives β, the slow-disposition rate constant (Figs. 56-9 and 56-10).

Zero-Time Blood Level

Back extrapolation of the blood level–time curve after intravenous administration results in the **zero-time blood level** C_0. After extravascular administration, the "fictitious" zero-time blood level, C_0, is the intercept of the k_e slope with the ordinate on a semilog plot in the one-compartment model, and the sum of the intercepts A + B of the α and β slopes in the two-compartment model (Figs. 56-9 and 56-10).

Absorption Rate Constant

The k_e slope is extrapolated back to time zero. This yields C_0, a theoretical concentration roughly equivalent to that obtained from an intravenous injection of the same amount of drug. By subtraction of the observed drug concentration during the absorption phase from the concentrations read from the back-extrapolated k_e slope, *residual* points are obtained. When plotted on semilog paper, they are described by a straight line, the slope of which is the **absorption rate constant** k_a (Fig. 56-9) in the one-compartment model.

Elimination Half-Life

Whenever a monoexponential straight line is obtained, a drug's half-life can be calculated. Notice the line describing the terms k_e and β in Figs. 56-9 and 56-10. Other half-lives frequently used are the absorption half-life ($t_{1/2}$abs) and distribution half-life ($t_{1/2}$).

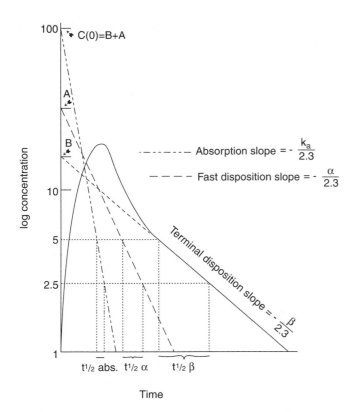

Fig. 56-10 Two-compartment model blood level–time curve after extravascular administration, with monoexponential slopes for slow disposition, β; fast disposition, α; and absorption, k_a. *(From Ritschel WA: Graphic approach to clinical pharmacokinetics, Barcelona, 1983, Prous Science.)*

The terms *half-time*, *half-life*, *plasma half-life*, *elimination half-life*, and *biological half-life* are often used interchangeably. Half-life is equal to the time required for elimination of one half the total dose of drug from the body. The elimination half-life, or plasma half-life, is the time required for the elimination of one half the amount of drug that is in the blood (plasma or serum). In those instances in which the decline of drug concentrations in all tissues does not parallel the decline of drug concentration in plasma, blood, or serum, the half-life and the elimination half-life will be different. Most statements on drug disposition refer to the elimination half-life. In Fig. 56-10 the elimination half-life ($t_{1/2}β$) is depicted graphically.

Volume of Distribution

The volume of distribution is not a real volume and usually has no relationship to any physiological space or body fluid volume. It is simply a term to make the mass-balance equation valid. On intravenous administration the amount of drug in the body is known; however, only the blood can be sampled. Because an amount of drug, *A*, equals the product of concentration and volume (µg/mL × mL), the volume of distribution is the hypothetical volume that would be required to dissolve the total amount of drug to achieve the same concentration as that found in blood.

The volume of distribution is expressed in milliliters. If

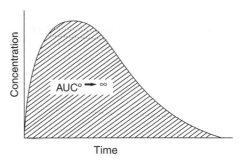

Fig. 56-11 Scheme of total area under the blood level–time curve. $AUC^{0→∞}$, Area under curve from time = 0 to time = ∞. *(From Ritschel WA: Graphic approach to clinical pharmacokinetics, Barcelona, 1983, Prous Science.)*

this value is divided by the patient's body weight, the distribution coefficient, $Δ'$ is obtained in mL/g (or L/kg).

Area Under Blood Level–Time Curve

The integral under a blood level–time curve is a measure of the total amount of drug in the body. The area under the blood level–time curve can be calculated from time zero to infinity, AUC, or may be approximated by plotting the curve on graph paper and cutting out the area and weighing it. The AUC is shown in Fig. 56-11.

Total Clearance

The **total clearance** in pharmacokinetics describes how much of the volume of distribution is cleared of the drug per unit of time, regardless of the pathway for the loss of drug from the body. In effect it is the sum of all clearances by different pathways. The total clearance is the product of the apparent volume of distribution and the **terminal disposition rate constant**.

Steady State

Steady state refers to the accumulation of drug in the body in multiple dosing when input and output are equal within a dosing interval. The magnitude of accumulation depends on the drug's elimination half-life and the dosing interval. The smaller the dosing interval for a given dosage, the greater the accumulation and the smaller the fluctuation around the mean serum value. At steady state the drug concentration oscillates around a mean steady-state concentration, C_{av}^{ss}, with a definite maximum steady-state concentration, C_{max}^{ss}, and a minimum steady-state concentration, C_{min}^{ss}. Only in the case of an intravenous constant rate infusion are C_{max}^{ss}, C_{min}^{ss}, and C_{av}^{ss} identical.

APPLICATION OF PHARMACOKINETICS TO TDM
Clinical Assessment

Clinical (physician) estimation of patient response is the first and most important task in therapeutic monitoring. It must be remembered that therapy requires an approach that considers all aspects of a patient's condition, including the disease symptoms; the disease itself; other diseases present; and the patient's physical condition, age, nutritional status, and psychological aspects. Furthermore, it must be remembered that clinical pharmacokinetics is only a tool that can assist with but never substitute for clinical evaluation.

Application. The clinical evaluation of patient response is composed of the evaluation of vital signs and change of symptoms in response to the drug therapy, such as blood pressure, pulse rate, electrocardiogram, measurement of edema, and urinary output. Furthermore, supportive laboratory analyses may be required, such as serum glucose and electrolyte levels. In all these cases the pharmacological response is evaluated *clinically*, either as direct measurement of pharmacological effect or as a measurement of body constituents, but *not* by the measurement of drug concentration in biological fluid.

Limitations. Sometimes the clinical evaluation might be difficult because of the presence of two or more disease states with similar or overlapping symptoms, polypharmacy (many drugs given simultaneously), or unexpected results. Unexpected results that might occur are that (1) the patient is not responding as expected, showing either no effectiveness or limited effectiveness of therapy, or (2) the patient may exhibit unexpected toxicity or side effects.

A drug may be less effective than expected because (1) the drug has a low bioavailability, (2) the patient is not complying with the prescribed drug regimen, (3) a malabsorption syndrome exists and less of the drug than expected is being absorbed. A patient may exhibit unexpected toxicity or side effects because of drug interactions, enzyme induction, enzyme inhibition, renal or hepatic impairment, edema, dehydration, and so on. In these cases it is advisable, when possible, to request drug monitoring in biological samples (see Fig. 56-7 and the box on p. 1075).

Assessment by Drug Analysis

When the therapeutic target concentration, therapeutic range, or toxic concentration is known, therapeutic drug monitoring can be used to support the clinical evaluation. When a patient is treated with drugs of low therapeutic index, such as aminoglycosides, digoxin, and a lithium compound, or when unexpected side effects or toxicity are occurring (Fig. 56-7), therapeutic drug monitoring should be used.

Basis for monitoring. For monitoring, it is essential to fulfill certain requirements. Otherwise, any evaluation will be in error[11]:

1. The dose size, dosage form, and route of administration must be known.
2. The dosage regimen must be followed.
3. The time between the administration of the last dose and the drawing of the blood sample must be known.
4. The blood sampling time or times must be recorded exactly.
5. The sampling times must be appropriate.

Most of the requirements listed above are self-explanatory. To understand item 5, remember that any samples taken during the absorption or distribution phase are useless for monitoring. Samples taken at peak time allow only an approximation of pharmacokinetic data. Samples taken at peak time and during the terminal elimination phase will result in an overestimation of the elimination rate constant and an underestimation of the elimination half-life.

The optimal sampling times for the various dosage regimen methods are shown in Fig. 56-12. Sampling times of commonly monitored drugs are listed in Table 56-1.[12] A review of the elimination half-lives and the therapeutic ranges of 19 commonly monitored drugs also is given in Table 56-1.[13]

Limitations. The ability to monitor a specific drug in a blood sample can sometimes be limited because (1) accurate information about the times of drug administration and blood drawing is not available, (2) a reliable assay method is not available, and (3) laboratory analysis time is not reasonable. Most difficulties experienced in monitoring are caused by limited or inaccurate information. Precision of the assay must also be considered. The coefficient of variation of an assay can be important when the drug concentration is found to be either at the lower or the upper end of the therapeutic range. The therapeutic ranges reported in Table 56-1 are mean values applicable to the majority of patients; the therapeutic or toxic concentration may be different for a particular patient (Fig. 56-6).

Assessment by Pharmacokinetic Calculations

To evaluate blood samples pharmacokinetically, whether the drug concentration is at steady state must be known. To decide if a steady state has been achieved, the dosage regimen (dose size and dosing interval) and how long this dosage regimen has been in effect must be known. Usually it

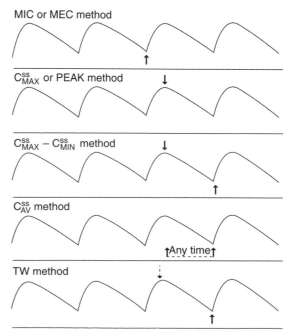

Fig. 56-12 Scheme showing optimal sampling times for monitoring for different methods used for dosage regimens.

is assumed that a steady state is reached when the dosage regimen has been implemented for a time greater than four times the drug's elimination half-life. If the regimen has been in effect for less than $4t_{1/2}$, the number of doses given before the sample was obtained should be known. Using classic pharmacokinetic equations, what the drug concentration should be can be calculated, based on mean pharmacokinetic parameters from the literature and patient information (age, body weight, sex, height, renal status, and so on). The purpose of drug monitoring is to compare the observed drug concentration to the expected or desired one. The observed concentration may be equal to, smaller than, or greater than the desired one. In the latter two cases an adjustment of the dosage regimen may be indicated and recommended.[14]

If C_x (the measured drug concentration) differs from the desired concentration (such as $C_{av\ des}^{ss}$ or $C_{max\ des}^{ss}$), a reason for the deviation should be sought. Some general and probable causes are presented here.

A concentration higher than the expected one could be associated with an increased bioavailability of a drug of generally low bioavailability (e.g., cimetidine increases bioavailability of propranolol), patient noncompliance (i.e., use of more drug or shorter dosage intervals than prescribed), or decreased total clearance (as occurs with renal or liver failure and acute congestive heart failure), or increased protein binding. A concentration lower than expected could result from decreased bioavailability (possibly drug interaction), insufficient drug dosing (longer dosing intervals, missed doses, or noncompliance), increase in the total clearance (drug interaction or enzyme induction), or decreased protein binding.

More Complex Pharmacokinetic Analyses

The preceding equations presented are basic ones. Space and background information do not permit more detail. The purpose of this chapter is to present a general review and to transmit a general understanding of the pharmacokinetic principles involved, including dosage regimens.

TABLE 56-1 COMMONLY MONITORED DRUGS, RECOMMENDED SAMPLING TIMES, HALF-LIVES, THERAPEUTIC RANGES, AND CRITICAL VALUES

Drug	Recommended Sampling Time	Healthy $t_{1/2}$ (Hours)	Therapeutic Range (µg/mL)	Critical Range (µg/mL)
Amikacin	0.5 to 1 hour after dose (trough) and end of dosing interval peak	0.5 to 3.0	Max 20 to 30, Min <5	Max >35, Min >10
Amitryptiline	End of dosing interval	17 to 40	0.120 to 0.250	>0.500
Carbamazepine	End of dosing interval	10 to 60	4 to 11	>15
Cyclosporine	End of dosing interval‡	4.7 to 12.7	0.1 to 0.3	>0.4
Digitoxin	8 to 24 hours after dose	72 to 384	0.01 to 0.025	>0.035
Digoxin	8 to 24 hours after dose	20 to 50	0.0008 to 0.002	>0.0024
Ethosuximide	End of dosing interval		40 to 100	>150
Gentamicin	0.5 to 1 hour after dose and end of dosing interval	0.5 to 3.0	Max 5 to 10 Min <2	Max >12 Min >2
Lidocaine	During infusion	1.2 to 2.3	1.5 to 5.0	>7
Lithium	End of dosing interval	14 to 33	0.3 to 1.3 (mmol/L)	>1.5 (mmol/L)
Phenobarbital	End of dosing interval	50 to 150	10 to 40	>50
Phenytoin	End of dosing interval	20 to 100	10 to 20	>20
Primidone	End of dosing interval	4 to 22	5 to 12	>15
Procainamide	End of dosing interval	3 to 5	4 to 10	>16*
Salicylate	1 to 3 hours after dose	3 to 20	150 to 300†	>400
Tacrolimus	End of dosing interval	5.5 to 16	0.0005 to 0.015	>0.02
Theophylline	Intravenous infusion: 4 to 8, 12 to 24 hours, and 24-hour intervals after start of infusion	3 to 12, nonsmokers	8 to 20	>20
	Oral or intravenous injection; 2 hours after dose			
	Oral sustained release; 4 to 6 hours after dose	2 to 6, smokers		
Tobramycin	0.5 to 1 hour after dose and end of dosing interval	0.5 to 3.0	Max 5 to 10 Min <2	Max >12 Min >2
Vancomycin	1 hour after dose and end of dosing interval	4 to 10	Max 20 to 40 Min 5 to 10	Max >80 Min >20

*Measure both parent and metabolite therapeutic range of combined; critical range >35 for both.
†Anti-inflammatory.
‡For absorption profiling, a 2-hour sampling time with respective therapeutic ranges has been proposed.[18]

Part 2: Practical Aspects of TDM

MICHAEL OELLERICH
VICTOR W. ARMSTRONG

THERAPEUTIC RANGE

Although therapeutic ranges have been empirically established in numerous clinical studies to assist in interpreting drug measurements, drug concentrations must always be interpreted in the context of all clinical data. In contrast to the concept of reference intervals in clinical chemistry, there is no generally accepted concept or protocol on how to establish the therapeutic range of a drug. These therapeutic ranges, therefore, vary somewhat throughout the literature and should be used only as a general guide. They represent the range of drug concentrations within which the probability of the desired clinical response is relatively high and the probability of unacceptable toxicity is relatively low. Clinicians should never assume, however, that a serum concentration within the therapeutic range is safe and effective for every patient. Recommended therapeutic ranges for some commonly monitored drugs are presented in Table 56-1. For most of the drugs listed in this table concentrations are determined in serum or plasma. The exceptions are cyclosporine and tacrolimus, for which whole blood measurements are recommended. Concentrations within the therapeutic range of a drug will produce a pharmacological response in the majority of patients. At concentrations above the upper limit of the therapeutic range an increased incidence of toxic side effects can be expected without as a rule any substantial improvement in the therapeutic effect. The range between the concentration of drug required to produce the therapeutic response and that which produces a toxic effect determines how carefully the dosage of the drug must be monitored. The ratio of these concentrations is called the *therapeutic index* and is expressed as the minimum concentration (or dose) that produces toxicity divided by the minimum concentration (or dose) that gives the therapeutic response in a patient population. When this ratio is 2.0 or less, the compound can be difficult to use in patients without significant toxicity being encountered. Toxic drug concentration values above which there is an enhanced or high probability of adverse effects are listed in Table 56-1.

Therapeutic ranges may require adjustment if other drugs with either synergistic or antagonistic actions are also administered to the patient. A serum concentration of phenytoin considered within the therapeutic range may produce toxic symptoms when other central nervous depressants are present. The existence of pharmacologically active metabolites and alterations in protein binding must also be taken into consideration when interpreting serum concentrations. When certain drugs, such as phenobarbital, are administered over a long period, patients may develop a tolerance to the drug, and the upper limit of the therapeutic range may then be raised.

Target concentrations for cyclosporine or tacrolimus depend on the indication for treatment, time after initiation of therapy, and concurrent immunosuppressive therapy.[15,16] Thus the therapeutic range for cyclosporine and tacrolimus can be taken only as a general guide. Most transplant centers[15,16] recommend higher target concentrations during the early postoperative period and then tapering of cyclosporine and tacrolimus doses to achieve a lower maintenance concentration range usually 3 to 6 months after transplantation (see also p. 984 and Cyclosporin on CD-ROM). Typically, trough concentrations of drug, measured at the end of a dosing interval, are used for immunosuppressive drug monitoring. Alternatively, abbreviated area under the concentration time curve (AUC) strategies have been proposed to better assess drug exposure.[17, 18] A disadvantage of these approaches in clinical practice is the necessity of exact timing of multiple blood samples. In the case of cyclosporine the use of a single sampling point 2 hours postdose has been suggested as a surrogate for the abbreviated AUC.[18]

For a correct interpretation of drug levels, knowledge of the time interval between the administration of the last dose and blood sampling is imperative. With long-term therapy the blood samples should be taken in the steady state. In practice samples are usually taken after four to five half-lives have elapsed when over 90% of the steady-state concentration has normally been reached (Fig. 56-8). Depending on the clinical question either the peak concentration or the trough concentration taken directly before administration of the next dose is measured. When a drug is given by intravenous infusion, blood samples should be taken after the initial distribution phase is completed, usually around 1 to 2 hours. However, for digoxin and digitoxin the time to equilibrium after oral or intravenous administration is usually 8 to 12 hours. For serum concentrations to best reflect the effect on cardiac activity, samples should be taken when drug equilibrium has been achieved between serum and tissue.[19]

In the case of some drugs such as phenytoin or phenobarbital, the timing of the blood sampling is not important, because the fluctuations between the peak and trough concentrations in the steady state are relatively small. With other drugs such as theophylline, which have a narrow therapeutic range and a short half-life, it may be necessary to obtain blood samples at both the peak and trough levels to determine whether the correct dosage has been used. In the case of multiple daily dosing of the aminoglycosides, both peak and trough values should be monitored to prevent the administration of inappropriately high doses, which might predispose the patient to nephrotoxicity and ototoxicity.[20] Instead of multiple- dose regimens, once-daily dosing of aminoglycosides has been advocated to provide better antibacterial efficacy and less nephrotoxicity than conventional multiple-dose strategies with the same *total* daily dose[21]. There is now debate on the type of TDM during once-daily therapy. Some investigators suggest that only measurement of the trough concentration is required and that the dose should be reduced if the concentration is above 1 to 2 mg/L. Others have recommended that dosage be guided by measurement of one or two aminoglycoside concentrations at fixed time points after the infusion. Dosage is then adjusted according to a nomogram,[21,22] by computer-assisted calculation of the daily AUC,[21] or with the aid of a dose prediction software program.[22,23]

Some of the commoner causes of unexpected serum drug concentrations observed in patients are listed in the box on p. 1075. If these factors cannot be eliminated and if an adequate compliance of the patient can be ascertained, it will be necessary to adjust the dosage of the drug.

TDM in pediatric patients is of particular importance because drug metabolism changes with age[24,25] and many factors listed in the box (p. 1075) can have a disproportionate effect on newborns.[26] In the first 6 months of life hepatic and renal function is immature and a much smaller dose per kg must be given to attain the same therapeutic concentration of a drug. As an example, the half-life of theophylline in the premature newborn is about 30 hours, decreasing in children to 2 to 6 hours before increasing again during puberty to values of 6 to 13 hours in nonsmoking adults. Children going through puberty and receiving drug therapy need to be monitored closely because the activity of the enzyme system is changing a great deal over this period.

DOSE-PREDICTION METHODS

Estimates of the dose required to achieve a drug concentration in the therapeutic range have been tabulated based on the levels found in test populations. The use of this information is termed *population-based pharmacokinetic dosing*. These estimates are in the form of tables or nomograms and allow the clinician to choose a dose based on certain features of the patient (such as age, diseases, smoking habits). Although these procedures are inexpensive, they often have a large prediction error. Therefore, prediction methods that allow estimation of drug clearance from a few drug concentration measurements on an individual have been developed to facilitate individual dosage adaptation.

Adjustment of Dosage at Steady State

Clearance is the most important parameter to be considered in designing a rational dosage regimen. At steady state, clearance can easily be estimated by dividing dosing rate by the average steady-state serum drug concentration. For those drugs having a clearance linearly proportional to dosage, a new dose (DN) to achieve the desired concentration can then be calculated from the actual dosage (DA), the actual steady-state serum drug concentration (CA), and the desired serum drug concentration (CN) according to the following equation:

$$DN = \frac{DA}{CA} \times CN \qquad \textit{Eq. 56-5}$$

For practical purposes, the trough concentrations rather than the average steady-state concentrations are generally employed. The use of equation 56-5 is limited in patients whose LADME parameters are at the extremes of the usual patient range. In those cases, peak and trough levels may not change in a linear manner after a dosage adjustment and more sophisticated methods using a small number of serum concentration measurements are used to estimate the individual pharmacokinetic parameters. These estimates are used to predict the optimal dosing scheme when measurements are made under non–steady state conditions or for those drugs whose elimination cannot be described by first-order kinetics.

Three-Point Method of Sawchuk

The dosage prediction method of Sawchuk requires determination of (1) a predose level, (2) a drug concentration obtained 30 minutes after the end of a constant-rate IV infusion, and (3) an additional concentration measured 1 hour before the next dose.[27] If a one-compartment model is assumed, the elimination-rate constant can be estimated from the slope of the concentration-time curve (Fig. 56-9). The distribution volume, V_d, can then be calculated from the dosage, D; the duration of constant-rate infusion, t; the elimination-rate constant, k; the predose level, C_0; and the theoretical initial concentration, C, according to the equation:

$$V_d = \frac{D}{t \cdot k} \times \frac{(1 - e^{-kt})}{(C \cdot e^{-kt} - C_0 \cdot e^{-kt})} \qquad \textit{Eq.56-6}$$

The clearance, CL, is then the product of the elimination-rate constant, k, and the distribution volume, V_d.

Bayesian Forecasting

The clearance and distribution volume of an individual patient can be derived through application of the Bayes formula to pharmacokinetic parameter estimation.[28] This approach uses previously obtained information on the distribution range of pharmacokinetic parameters within the population combined with data on one or more serum drug concentrations observed on the test individual.

The estimates of the pharmacokinetic parameters in the individual patient are obtained from the Bayes formula. These estimates can be improved by taking into account patient-specific data (such as age, sex, disease, medications). Given a patient data set, a best fit is obtained for possible clearance and distribution volume values. Bayesian drug-dosing programs are now commercially available and have been applied to various drugs.[23,29,30] The prospective value of this Bayesian prediction model has been demonstrated[23] on patients receiving aminoglycosides. Use of the clinical pharmacokinetic service recommendations led to lower direct costs of hospitalization, including reduction of hospital stay, illustrating the cost-savings effect made through rational use of TDM predictive models.[23]

CLINICAL INDICATIONS FOR TDM

For those drugs for which there is knowledge of dose response and toxicity the need for monitoring is dependent on patient clinical status. A set of guidelines for TDM services has been proposed.[31]

Clinical indications for the need to have information on drug concentrations are presented in the box on p. 1088. In the prophylactic application of drugs, for example, it is essential to know if the drug concentration is in the desired therapeutic range to prevent the disease symptoms. One example is determination of theophylline levels to ascertain if they are in the range that prevents asthmatic attacks. A further example is the optimization of immunosuppressive regimens where prophylaxis of acute rejection is required.

Knowledge of drug concentrations is critical for patient management when symptoms resulting from drug toxicity and the underlying disease are similar. Premature ventricular contractions, for example, can indicate either digitalis toxicity or intrinsic heart disease. High levels of either quinidine or procainamide can induce ventricular arrhythmias similar to the ones controlled by these drugs. Tachycardia cannot be used in the diagnosis of a theophylline overdose, because tachycardia is present in patients with severe respiratory obstruction. Toxic doses of phenytoin can cause seizures that are symptomatic of the underlying epilepsy.

Measurement of serum drug levels is required to optimize drug dosage in cases in which drug interactions are suspected, or for those drugs that have a considerable intraindividual and interindividual pharmacokinetic variability. It must be stressed that in many severely ill patients, drug absorption, protein binding, and drug elimination can change effective drug concentration or allow potentially active metabolites to accumulate. Determination of drug concentrations is necessary when a change in bioavailability is suspected or when persistent adverse effects occur. Monitoring is also necessary to avoid toxicity such as that seen in patients undergoing high-dose methotrexate therapy, where severe adverse reactions are usually avoidable if the dosage of the antidote, leucovorin, is adjusted according to methotrexate serum concentrations.

SAMPLING AND FREQUENCY OF DRUG MONITORING
Sampling

For most drugs, either plasma or serum samples are used to determine circulating levels of the drug. However, in the case of cyclosporine and tacrolimus[15,16] whole blood is the preferred matrix. Accurate and precise timing, both in administration of the drug and in obtainment of each blood sample, are of paramount importance in therapeutic drug monitoring. This one variable, time, is often the most difficult to obtain. Quality assurance should be directed to ensuring that this information is obtained. The recommended sampling times of commonly monitored drugs are presented in Table 56-1. The specimen has to be accompanied by a request form providing demographic data on the patient and the collection date and time. Data on dose amount, dose interval, time of last dose, route of administration, and other medication should also be included.

Frequency of Drug Monitoring

In addition to the acute care cases described earlier, the frequency of monitoring will depend on the clinical situation of the patient, the experience of the physician, whether serum concentrations have reached steady state, and the half-life of the drug.

In the case of critically ill patients being treated with drugs, such as the aminoglycosides, that have rapid clearance changes, a daily modification of drug dosage may be necessary. For other drugs such as cyclosporine, the variability in response and thus in dosage requirement means that blood level monitoring of this drug should start immediately after the initiation of therapy. Remember that in these cases failure to achieve adequate blood concentrations can be fatal whereas overdosage can result in severe toxic effects. However, because of cost and convenience factors, monitoring can be relaxed with time. Monitoring of cyclosporine A in the early posttransplantation hospitalization period of liver, heart, and kidney transplants is done four to seven times per week. After the intensive early monitoring, the measurement of cyclosporine blood levels can be gradually reduced; for example, in renal transplant recipients with an uncomplicated course, cyclosporine concentrations should be monitored once a month during the first year and at 1-month to 3-month intervals thereafter.[15] However, there are no hard and fast rules, and measurements should be performed if the clinical signs or symptoms indicate that dosage adjustment might be necessary.

Frequent monitoring is often required when optimizing drug dosage or initiating drug therapy. For example, frequent serum digoxin measurement (daily) early in the course of therapy is desirable in patients with moderate to severe renal failure because of variability in both volume of distribution and elimination associated with diminished renal function. Knowledge of drug concentrations is particularly important when a loading dose is administered. Frequent measurements may be necessary to monitor the appropriateness of a modified dosage regimen or to follow the course of drug interaction–induced changes in serum digoxin concentration.

The frequency of monitoring is usually decreased for outpatients following a course of long-term drug therapy. Frequency is in part dependent on the drug. For theophylline, the narrow therapeutic index and the relationship of serum concentration to both efficacy and toxicity make measurement of serum concentrations an essential part of patient management. Serum concentrations of theophylline should be monitored during the initial phase until the steady state has been reached and then at regular intervals (such as 6 to 12 months) thereafter. Serum concentrations of phenytoin should be measured after initiation of therapy to determine if a therapeutic serum concentration has been achieved.

Measurements can be made 2 weeks to 1 month after initiation of therapy because a steady state is generally reached in this time. In case of dosage changes a subsequent control of the drug concentration should be made after an additional four to five half-lives have elapsed.

The measured concentration should be used with relevant clinical information to decide whether an adjustment in the daily dose is required. In patients with therapeutic failure, signs of drug overdose, or suspected noncompliance, an immediate response to obtain an appropriate measurement of serum drug concentration is indicated.

High-dose methotrexate therapy requires serial monitoring of serum concentrations during the leucovorin rescue phase, because the dose of leucovorin needed depends on the serum methotrexate level. In patients with normal renal function it is usually sufficient to measure serum methotrexate levels at 24, 48, and 72 hours.

Turnaround Times

For many of the drugs listed in Table 56-1 a same-day analytical service is feasible. When dosage adjustment is necessary, the results of serum drug concentration measurements will be required before administration of the next dose. When aminoglycoside levels are ordered as peaks and troughs, it is more accurate and efficient to obtain both specimens during the same dosing interval. The laboratory can then measure both peak and trough levels in the analytical batch to minimize variance. This immediate response often allows the laboratory to give results to the physician on the same day, thus allowing sufficient time to establish a new regimen.

Stat. Analyses

In certain clinical situations a prompt determination of serum drug levels may be necessary. Some of the most important indications for the rapid measurement of serum drug concentrations are indicated in the box on p. 1088, and the drugs most likely to require monitoring in the stat. laboratory are listed in the box below. The drugs requiring analysis in the stat. laboratory can be divided into two categories depending on the urgency of the analysis. In the case of a suspected drug overdose, that is, a potentially life-threatening situation, an immediate analysis should be carried out. One example is measurement of the tricyclic antidepressants that occur in suicide attempts. Drug levels that include parent and metabolite are useful for clarification of intoxication with these drugs.

There are occasions for which analyses outside of the usual routine laboratory working hours are necessary. Examples include treatment with aminoglycosides, where urgent determination of serum drug levels in critically ill patients for whom an individual dosage adjustment is necessary; specific treatment protocols for high-dose methotrexate with leucovorin rescue, which may require the off-hour determination of serum methotrexate concentrations; and cyclosporine and tacrolimus levels, which may be required 6 to 7 days a week, particularly in patients after liver transplantation.

QUALITY ASSURANCE
Quality Control

Quality control programs use commercially available quality control materials and proficiency testing programs for TDM. TDM differs from other clinical chemistry testing in that the level of analyte is achieved by changing the dose. Performance standards based on pharmacokinetic theory and consensus strategy have been proposed.[32] More recently statistical principles for analytical goal setting have been applied to the determination of theophylline concentration in serum.[33]

Critical Value Callback

It is sometimes necessary to communicate urgently a critical drug concentration to the clinician or healthcare provider. Critical values include high concentrations associated with enhanced risk of toxicity for that particular drug (Table 56-1), or low concentrations that are inadequate to achieve the desired therapeutic effect. The usual practice is to exclude analytical error by checking the internal quality control used in the analytical run for the assayed specimen and to exclude possible preanalytical error (such as inverted peak and trough values as the result of sample switching, inappropriate time of sampling, specimen taken from same infusion line used to administer the drug) as possible causes of unexpected serum drug concentrations.

DRUGS TO PREDICT ORGAN FUNCTION

Because drugs are not passive passengers, their metabolism has been used to measure organ function, with the argument being that the inability to metabolize is indicative of organ dysfunction. Drug metabolism has been used to determine liver function under the assumption that the quantitative measurement of capacity of the liver to metabolize certain drugs may serve as an estimate of hepatic function. One liver function test uses the metabolism of the drug lidocaine, which is converted by the hepatic cytochrome P-450 system to the metabolite monoethylglycinexylidide (MEGX). A dynamic liver-function test has been devised[34] based on the measurement of MEGX found in serum before and 15 or 30 minutes after a standardized bolus of lidocaine is given

---

DRUGS FOR WHICH ANALYSES SHOULD BE AVAILABLE IN THE STAT LABORATORY

Stat. Analyses in Suspected Drug Overdose
Theophylline
Digoxin
Phenytoin, phenobarbital, carbamazepine
Salicylic acid, acetaminophen
Lithium, tricyclic antidepressants, barbiturates, benzodiazepines

Other Analyses
Tobramycin, amikacin, gentamicin, netlimicin
Cyclosporin, tacrolimus (FK506)
Methotrexate

(1 mg/kg of body weight injected over 2 minutes). Loss of the ability to metabolize the drug and a decrease in hepatic functional blood flow lead to diminished production of MEGX. The MEGX test is of particular value in the field of liver transplantation[34-38] (see also p. 980) and in assessing hepatic function in critically ill patients at risk of developing multiple organ dysfunction syndrome.[38]

FUTURE PROSPECTS

The number of drugs that must be monitored to optimize therapy continues to grow as new agents are approved for human use. Monitoring is essential for medications with narrow therapeutic indices.[39,40] Additional resources will be needed to monitor those drugs and clinical situations in which the measurement of "free" rather than total drug levels in serum will provide greater therapeutic benefit.[41-43] Finally, individualization of therapy based on understanding the patients' **pharmacogenetics** will play a more important role in drug monitoring. This has been illustrated for the polymorphism of thiopurine methyltransferase where phenotyping/genotyping is used to prevent intolerance to 6-mercaptopurine and azathioprine.[44]

References

1. Ritschel WA: *Handbook of basic pharmacokinetics including clinical applications*, Hamilton, IL, 1986, Drug Intelligence Publications.
2. Borga O et al: Plasma protein binding of tricyclic antidepressants in man, *Biochem Pharmacol* 18:2135, 1969.
3. Reidenberg MM et al: Protein binding from diphenylhydantoin and desmethylimipramine in plasma from patients with poor renal function, *N Engl J Med* 285:264, 1971.
4. Levy G: Relationship between pharmacological effects and plasma or tissue concentrations of drugs in man. In Davies DS, Pritchard DNC, editors: *Biological effects of drugs in relation to their plasma concentrations*, Baltimore, 1973, University Park Press.
5. Stewart RB, Forgnone M, Cluff LE: Drug utilization and reported adverse drug reactions in outpatients, *Drugs Health Care* 2:231, 1975.
6. Ritschel WA: Pharmacokinetics of H₂-receptor antagonists, *Sci Pharm* 50:250, 1982.
7. Barker KN, McConnell WE: How to detect medication errors, *Mod Hosp* 99:95, 1962.
8. Stewart RB, Cluff LE: A review of medication errors and compliance in ambulant patients, *Clin Pharmacol Ther* 13:463, 1971.
9. Bochner F et al: *Handbook of clinical pharmacology*, Boston, 1978, Little, Brown.
10. Ritschel WA: The effect of aging on pharmacokinetics: a scientists' view of the future, *Contemp Pharmacy Pract* 5:209, 1982.
11. Hassan FM, Pesce AJ, Ritschel WA: Pitfalls and errors in drug monitoring: analytical aspects, *Methods Find Exp Clin Pharmacol* 5:567, 1983.
12. Slaughter RL, Koup JR: Clinical pharmacokinetic service. In McLeod DD, Miller WA, editors: *The practice of pharmacy*, Cincinnati, 1981, Harvey Whitney Books.
13. Ritschel WA: *Handbook of basic pharmacokinetics*, ed 2, Hamilton, IL, 1980, Drug Intelligence Publications.
14. Evans WW, Schentag JJ, Jusko WJ: *Applied pharmacokinetics: principles of therapeutic drug monitoring*, Vancouver, WA, 1994, Applied Therapeutics.
15. Oellerich M et al: Lake Louise Consensus Conference on cyclosporin monitoring in organ transplantation: report of the consensus panel, *Ther Drug Monit* 17:642, 1995.
16. Oellerich M et al: Therapeutic drug monitoring of cyclosporine and tacrolimus. Update on Lake Louise Consensus Conference on cyclosporin and tacrolimus, Clin Biochem 31:309, 1998.
17. Mahalati K et al: Neoral monitoring by simplified sparse sampling area under the concentration–time curve: its relationship to acute rejection and cyclosporine nephrotoxicity early after kidney transplantation, *Transplantation* 68:55, 1999.
18. Belitsky P et al: Impact of absorption profiling on efficacy and safety of cyclosporin therapy in transplant recipients, *Clin Pharmacokinet* 39:117, 2000.
19. Matzuk MM, Shlomchik M, Shaw LM: Making digoxin therapeutic drug monitoring more effective, *Ther Drug Monit* 13:215, 1991.
20. Edson RS, Terrell CL: The aminoglycosides, *Mayo Clin Proc* 74:519, 1999.
21. Barclay ML, Kirkpatrick CM, Begg EJ: Once daily aminoglycoside therapy. Is it less toxic than multiple daily doses and how should it be monitored? *Clin Pharmacokinet* 36:89, 1999.
22. Morris RG et al: Some international approaches to aminoglycoside monitoring in the extended dosing interval era, *Ther Drug Monit* 21:379, 1999.
23. van Lent-Evers NA et al: Impact of goal-oriented and model-based clinical pharmacokinetic dosing of aminoglycosides on clinical outcome: a cost-effectiveness analysis, *Ther Drug Monit* 21:63, 1999.
24. Loebstein R, Koren G: Clinical pharmacology and therapeutic drug monitoring in neonates and children, *Pediatr Rev* 19:423, 1998.
25. Soldin SJ, Steele BW: Mini-review: therapeutic drug monitoring in pediatrics, *Clin Biochem* 33:333, 2000.
26. Tenge SM, Soldin S, editors: *Guidelines for the evaluation and management of the newborn infant*, Washington, DC, 1998, NACB.
27. Sawchuk RJ et al: Kinetic model for gentamicin dosing with the use of individual patient parameters, *Clin Pharmacol Ther* 21:362, 1977.
28. Sheiner LB, Rosenberg B, Melmon KL: Modelling of individual pharmacokinetics for computer-aided drug dosage, *Comput Biomed Res* 5:411, 1972.
29. Bottger HC, Oellerich M, Sybrecht GW: Use of aminoglycosides in critically ill patients: individualization of dosage using Bayesian statistics and pharmacokinetic principles, *Ther Drug Monit* 10:280, 1988.
30. Pryka RD et al: Individualizing vancomycin dosage regimens: one-versus two-compartment Bayesian models, *Ther Drug Monit* 11:450, 1989.
31. Warner A, Annesley T, editors: *Guidelines for therapeutic drug monitoring services*, Washington, DC, 1999, NACB.
32. Fraser CG: Desirable standards of performance for therapeutic drug monitoring, *Clin Chem* 33:387, 1987.
33. Jenny RW: Analytical goals for determinations of theophylline concentration in serum, *Clin Chem* 37:154, 1991.
34. Oellerich M et al: Monoethylglycinexylidide formation kinetics: a novel approach to assessment of liver function, *J Clin Chem Clin Biochem* 25:845, 1987.
35. Oellerich M et al: Lignocaine metabolite formation as a measure of pre-transplant liver function, *Lancet* 1:640, 1989.
36. Azoulay D et al: Acute cyclosporine toxicity after liver transplantation is predicted by the lidocaine monoethylglycinexylidide test in the donor, *Liver Transpl Surg* 3:526, 1997.
37. Oellerich M et al: Predictors of one-year pretransplant survival in patients with cirrhosis, *Hepatology* 14:1029, 1991.
38. Oellerich M, Armstrong VW: The MEGX test: a tool for the real-time assessment of hepatic function, *Ther Drug Monit* 23:81, 2001.
39. Oellerich M et al: Pharmacokinetic and metabolic investigations of mycophenolic acid in pediatric patients after renal transplantation: implications for therapeutic drug monitoring. German study group on mycophenolate mofetil therapy in pediatric renal transplant recipients, *Ther Drug Monit* 22:20, 2000.
40. Kahan BD et al: Therapeutic drug monitoring of sirolimus: correlations with efficacy and toxicity, *Clin Transplant* 14:97, 2000.
41. Oellerich M, Muller-Vahl H: The EMIT FreeLevel ultrafiltration technique compared with equilibrium dialysis and ultracentrifugation to determine protein binding of phenytoin, *Clin Pharmacokinet* 9(suppl 1):61, 1984.

42. Zielmann S et al: A rational basis for the measurement of free phenytoin concentration in critically ill trauma patients, *Ther Drug Monit* 16:139, 1994.
43. Soldin SJ: Free drug measurements. When and why? An overview, *Arch Pathol Lab Med* 123:822, 1999.
44. Leipold G et al: Azathioprine-induced severe pancytopenia due to a homozygous two-point mutation of the thiopurine methyltransferase gene in a patient with juvenile HLA-B27-associated spondylarthritis, *Arthritis Rheum* 40:1896, 1997.

Internet Sites

www.iatdmct.org—International Association of Therapeutic Drug Monitoring and Clinical Toxicology

www.sfaf.org—Description of TDM by San Francisco AIDS Foundation

http://www.bertholf.net/rlb/lectures/Lectures/Therapeutic%20Drug%20Monitoring.pps—Microsoft PowerPoint lecture by Dr. Robert L. Bertholf, Associate Professor of Pathology, Chief of Clinical Chemistry and Toxicology

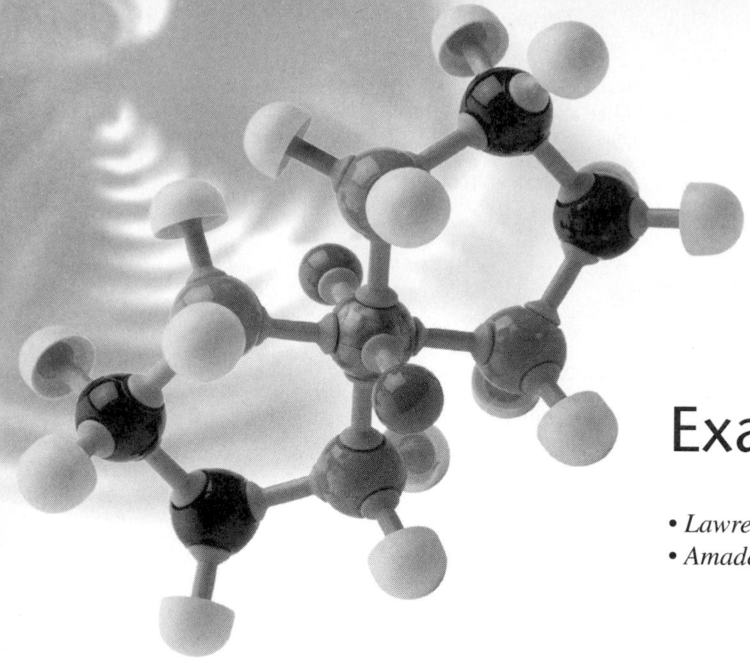

CHAPTER 57

Examination of Urine*

• *Lawrence A. Kaplan*
• *Amadeo J. Pesce*

Chapter Outline

Introduction and clinical utility of urinalysis
Specimen collection
Physical examination of urine
    Volume
    Odor
    Appearance (color and turbidity)
    Specific gravity
    Osmolality
Chemical examination of urine
    Normal constituents
    Reagent-strip testing
    Confirmatory testing
    Urinary pH
    Proteins
    Sugars
    Ketones
    Blood and myoglobin
    Bilirubin
    Urobilinogen

    Nitrites
    Leukocytes
    Porphyrins
    Melanin
Microscopic examination of urine
    Methods
    Standardization
    Crystals
    Organisms
    Cells
    Renal casts
    Fats
Urine cytology
Calculi (lithiasis)
Urine findings in common renal and lower urinary
    tract diseases
Coordinated approach to urinalysis
Quality control

Objectives

• Understand the proper method of collection of
urine specimens for specific testing.
• Discuss the important physical properties of urine
and their relationship to disease.
• Identify the important chemical constituents of
urine, how they are quantified, and how their
presence is confirmed.

• Describe the proper methods of standardization of
urine specimens and common microscopic findings.
• List the urine findings commonly observed in renal
and lower urinary tract diseases.
• Understand quality control procedures for urinalysis.

---

*The authors are grateful for the past contributions of G. Berry
Schumann and Susan C. Schweitzer.

Key Terms

acute tubular necrosis   A disease that involves the destruction of renal tubular epithelial cells and is most commonly associated with reduced blood supply to the renal tubules (ischemia) or toxic exposures.

Addis count   A quantitative urine sediment test in which the number of erythrocytes, leukocytes, and casts are quantified in a timed urine specimen.

aminoaciduria   An excess of one or more amino acids in urine.

amorphous crystals   The granular, noncrystalline precipitate of salts with no pathological importance.

bacteriuria   The presence of bacteria in urine.

bilirubinuria   The presence of bilirubin in urine.

calculus   An abnormal concretion, usually composed of mineral salts, present in the urinary system or other tissues; a renal stone.

catheterization   The passage of a thin, flexible, tubular instrument into the bladder or ureter for the withdrawal of urine.

crystalluria   The presence of crystals in urine.

cylindruria   The presence of casts in urine.

cystitis   Inflammation of the bladder.

cytodiagnostic urinalysis   A specialized urine test combining both physicochemical assessments with a concentrated Papanicolaou-stained urine sediment examination.

dipstick urinalysis   A chemical urine test using test strips for the detection of albumin, glucose, ketone, bilirubin, hemoglobin, bacteria, leukocytes, and other chemical constituents.

dipstick urinalysis testing   The use of a chemical test strip to determine, in a semi-quantitative manner, whether pathological concentrations of various substances are present in the urine.

dysmorphic erythrocyturia   The presence of fragmented erythrocytes in urine sediment indicating renal (glomerular or tubular) hematuria.

erythrocyturia   The presence of erythrocytes in urine.

funguria   The presence of fungus in urine.

glitter cells   Pale-staining, swollen, and degenerated neutrophils found in dilute urine, with cytoplasmic granules that exhibit a characteristic brownian movement.

glomeruli   Coils of blood vessels projecting into the expanded end of the capsule of each of the uriniferous tubules of the kidney.

glycosuria   The presence of glucose in urine.

hemoglobinuria   The presence of free hemoglobin in urine.

hyaline cast   A transparent cast composed of mucoprotein.

hydrometer   An instrument used for determining the specific gravity of a fluid.

ketone   Any compound containing the carbonyl group, —CO—, and having hydrocarbon groups attached to the carbonyl carbon.

melanin   The dark, amorphous pigment of the skin, hair, and various tumors. It is produced by polymerization of oxidation products of tyrosine and dihydroxyphenol compounds and contains carbon, hydrogen, nitrogen, oxygen, and often sulfur.

microscopic urinalysis   A screening urine test requiring a wet unstained urine sediment examination.

myoglobinuria   The presence of myoglobin, an oxygen-binding protein of muscle cells, in urine.

nephritis   Inflammation of the kidney.

nephrosis   A disease of the kidney.

Papanicolaou stain   A differential stain that aids in the identification of nuclear chromatin, cytoplasmic properties (such as keratinization), noncellular entities (such as crystals and casts), and hematopoietic elements.

porphyrins   A group of iron-free or magnesium-free pyrrole derivatives that occur universally in cells. They constitute the basis of the respiratory pigments in animals and plants.

Sternheimer-Malbin stain   A crystal violet and safranin stain used in urinalysis. This stain provides additional contrast for some cells and casts.

urobilinogen   A group of colorless compounds formed from the reduction of conjugated bilirubin by intestinal bacteria; about 1% of the total urobilinogen produced reaches the urine.

yeast   A unicellular nucleated microorganism that reproduces by budding.

INTRODUCTION AND CLINICAL UTILITY OF URINALYSIS

The clinical laboratory examination of urine can provide a wide variety of useful information on an individual's kidneys and the systemic diseases that may affect this excretory organ. Both structural (anatomical) and functional (physiological) disorders of the kidney and lower urinary tract may be elucidated as well as sequential information about the disease, its cause, and prognosis. Careful laboratory examination of urine often narrows the clinical differential diagnosis of numerous urinary system diseases. Usually these laboratory data may be obtained without pain, danger, and distress to the patient. Therefore, properly performed and interpreted laboratory urine tests will always remain an essential part of clinical medicine.

Currently, three types of urinalysis are performed: **dipstick urinalysis** for hospitals, physician offices, and patient home testing; a screening, **microscopic urinalysis**, commonly referred to as a "routine" or "basic" urinalysis; and **cytodiagnostic urinalysis**, a specialized, cytological approach to the urine sediment and correlative **dipstick urinalysis**. The dipstick urinalysis is a front-line test for the detection and monitoring of patients for chemical abnormalities.[1,2] Patients with diabetes often monitor their own condition for signs of glucosuria, proteinuria, and urinary tract infections by home testing of urine.[3]

Microscopic urinalysis provides a cost-effective screening test for the detection of both chemical and morphological abnormalities present in urine. Routine urinalysis procedures depend on two major components: (1) macroscopic, dipstick urinalysis plus, or physicochemical determinations (appearance, specific gravity, and multiparameter reagent-strip measurements of several chemical constituents), and (2) bright-field or phase-contrast microscopic examination of urinary sediment for evidence of hematuria, pyuria, **cylindruria** (casts), **crystalluria**, and so forth. With experience, a urinoscopist may detect many conditions affecting the kidneys and lower urinary tract; many conditions can also be monitored with this easily performed urine test.[4,5]

Cytodiagnostic urinalysis is a more sensitive pathologic test used to examine urine sediment in renal and lower urinary tract disorders.[6-8] However, this procedure is usually reserved for symptomatic patients who are being investigated for possible renal disease and lower urinary tract neoplastic conditions. Cytodiagnostic urinalysis has replaced the quantitative **Addis counts** and provides sequential information regarding the progression or regression of many renal or lower urinary tract disorders.[8]

The purpose of this chapter for medical or clinical chemistry laboratories is to describe briefly the common methodologies employed by most wet, or routine, urinalysis laboratories. Emphasis is placed on the responsibilities of the urinalysis laboratory in the following areas: (1) common procedures and equipment; (2) quality reagents; (3) sensitivity, specificity, and limitations of each procedure; (4) confirmatory tests; (5) accurate identification of urine sediment entities primarily using bright-field microscopy; and (6)

quality control. Also discussed are the technical and diagnostic significance of urinalysis results and the mechanism of diseases that produces urinalysis abnormalities. Remember that all the photoimages referred to in this chapter, including the photomicrographs of urine sediment, are available in color on the accompanying CD-ROM. The CD-ROM also has additional information on many of the subjects covered in this chapter. You are also encouraged to follow the literature for advances in urine laboratory testing and to supplement your knowledge by using the reference list provided at the end of the chapter.

SPECIMEN COLLECTION

Careful attention to collection of the urine specimen and its prompt delivery to the laboratory are crucial for optimum information to be derived from urinalysis.[9,10] Urine should be collected in a clean, sterile container that has a tightly fitting lid to prevent spillage, evaporation, and contamination. Specimen containers should be marked with the patient's name, date, and time of collection.

The first voiding in the morning is usually the most desirable for urinalysis testing, since it provides the most concentrated urine. A clean-catch, midstream collection avoids contamination from the distal area of the urethra. The sample must be free of vaginal secretions and other extraneous debris. Kunin[11] thoroughly describes a variety of collection techniques for urinary tract diseases.

If data from the urinalysis are to be accurate, it is essential that urine be either examined within 2 hours of collection or preserved in some manner, usually by refrigeration ($2°$ to $8°$ C). Appropriate fixatives or preservatives may also be used as long as their effects on the urine and its testing are well understood. If urine is allowed to sit unpreserved at room temperature, it will begin to decompose. Preservatives work by modifying urine so that chemical changes associated with decomposition do not occur and by preventing growth and metabolism of microorganisms. Toluene, phenol, thymol, and acid or basic preservatives are commonly used for urine chemistry determinations, as is excluding light (bilirubin). Ethanol (95%) or commercially available fixatives, such as Mucolexx and Saccomanno, may be used to preserve cell structure. Laboratories should be responsible for ensuring that the correct type and amount of urine preservatives are used for cellular preservation.

Timed urine specimens are frequently used to quantitate various aspects of renal function. The urine collected must reflect excretion over a precisely measured duration of time; specimens must not include urine that is present in the bladder before the timed test begins. The patient should be instructed to obtain a 24-hour urine specimen by discarding the first-voided morning urine on the first day and collecting all subsequent urine up to and including the first-voided morning urine on the second day. Recommended types of specimens for various urine tests are listed in Table 57-1; a more detailed description is provided on the CD-ROM.

When a specimen is received for urine testing, the laboratory workers performing that test must make a decision

TABLE 57-1	PRESERVATION OF URINE FOR COMMONLY MEASURED URINE ANALYTES		
Analyte	**Material To Be Added***	**Sample To Be Used**	**Comments**
Uric acid	10 mL of sodium hydroxide 500 g/L (12.5 M) or 5 g sodium carbonate	Add before 24-hour collection	If unpreserved urine is received, add 0.1 mL of 12.5 M NaOH to 10 mL of well-mixed urine; mix well. May need to warm at 60° C to dissolve precipitate.
Calcium	25 mL of 6 M HCl	Add before 24-hour collection	If unpreserved urine is received, add 0.1 mL of 6 M HCl to 10 mL of well-mixed urine; mix well. May need to warm at 60° C to dissolve precipitate.
Magnesium	25 mL of 6 M HCl	Add before 24-hour collection	If unpreserved urine is received, add 0.1 mL of 6 M HCl to 10 mL of well-mixed urine; mix well. May need to warm at 60° C to dissolve precipitate.
Phosphorus	25 mL of 6 M HCl	Add before 24-hour collection	If unpreserved urine is received, add 0.1 mL of 6 M HCl to 10 mL of well-mixed urine; mix well. May need to warm at 60° C to dissolve precipitate.
Creatinine	None		
Na, K, Cl	None		
BUN	None		
Protein, albumin	None, but keep refrigerated		
Glucose	None, but keep refrigerated		
Amylase	None, but keep refrigerated		

*If more than one preservative (acid, base, or refrigeration) is needed, add none, but keep sample container refrigerated during collection period. In laboratory, split sample for each type of preservative.

as to its acceptability. Specific criteria should be established in the form of written guidelines for the rejection of urine specimens and should include criteria such as visible signs of contamination, incorrect or incomplete labeling, inappropriate type of specimen or preservatives, and time lapse since collection.

PHYSICAL EXAMINATION OF URINE

The physical examination of urine is the initial part of a routine urinalysis. This examination includes assessment of volume, odor, appearance (color and turbidity), and specific gravity or osmolality.

Volume

Urinary volume is influenced by the fluid intake; solutes to be excreted, primarily sodium and urea; loss of fluid by perspiration and respiration; and cardiovascular and renal status. Normally adults excrete 750 to 2000 mL every 24 hours. Conditions that produce an increased or decreased amount of urine are discussed in Chapter 26. Although the volume of a random specimen is clinically insignificant, the volume of specimen received should be recorded for purposes of documentation and standardization.

Odor

Normal fresh urine has an inoffensive odor. An offensive odor can indicate that a specimen is too old for accurate analysis. A foul odor in a specimen that was collected (and not preserved or refrigerated) more than 2 hours earlier indicates an unacceptable specimen. Odor can also provide clues to certain urine abnormalities. An ammonia-like odor is suggestive of urea-splitting bacteria; fruity odors indicate the presence of acetone (**ketone**); a sweet odor is suggestive of the presence of glucose or another sugar; and a foul odor is suggestive of inflammation or the presence of pus. Odor is important in the clinical detection of maple-syrup urine disease (a congenital metabolic defect).

Appearance (Color and Turbidity)

The color of urine is determined to a large degree by its degree of concentration. Normal urine varies widely from colorless to deep yellow. Interpretation of color is subjective and varies with each laboratory examiner. It may be helpful to the technologist to use standardized colored objects in the laboratory as reference points and to use defined colors to describe the urine, avoiding ambiguous terms such as *straw* or *bloody*. Common terms for colors of urine are listed in Table 57-2, and the CD-ROM lists causes of abnormal urine colors.

Red urine is perhaps the most clinically important discoloration; it may be a result of urinary hemoglobin or myoglobin. Intact erythrocytes, hemolyzed erythrocytes, or free hemoglobin (hemolysis) can be responsible for the red color. Hemolysis may occur intravascularly or after the urine has been formed. **Myoglobinuria** is rare and results from crushing damage to muscle. Urinary hemoglobin and myoglobin may not be differentiated by gross inspection or simple tests. Ingestion of beets or certain drugs may redden the urine, and thus such chromogens must be excluded as a source of urine coloration.

Urine characteristic of acute glomerulonephritis is brownish red. It is acidic and contains blood, a combination

TABLE 57-2   COMMON COLORS OF URINE

| Colors | POTENTIAL CAUSES | | | | Clinical Conditions | Commonly Associated Diseases |
	Foodstuffs	Metabolites	Drugs	Organisms		
Yellow to colorless					Polyuria	Diabetes insipidus Diabetes mellitus Chronic renal failure
Yellow	Food color	Urochrome	Quinacrine (Atabrine) Sulfasalazine (Azulfidine) Phenacetin Nitrofurantoin Riboflavin		Healthy	
Yellow-orange	Food color Carotene Rhubarb	Urobilin	Sulfisoxazole and phenozopyridine (Azo Gantrisin) Riboflavin Furazolidone (Furoxone)		Dehydration Jaundice	Liver disease
Yellow-green		Bilirubin-biliverdin	Methylene blue Indican Amitriptyline (Elavil)		Jaundice	Liver disease Biliary obstruction
Yellow-red-brown	Beets Food color Rhubarb	Hemoglobin Myoglobin Porphyrin	Sulfisoxazole and phenazopyridine (Azo Gantrisin) Phenytoin (Dilantin) Pyrvinium pamoate (Povan) Phenazopyridine (Pyridium) Phenolsulfonphthalein Phenindione Amidopyrine	*Serratia marcescens*	Hematuria Hemoglobinuria Myoglobinuria Porphyrinuria Menstrual contamination	Hemolysis Transfusion Burns Renal disease Urological disease
Brown-black		Porphyrin Melanin Methemoglobin Homogentisic acid	Chloroquine (Aralen) Levodopa		Alkaptonuria	Melanoma Ochronosis Phenol poisoning
Blue-green		Indican	Methylene blue	*Pseudomonas* species	Dysuria	Urinary tract infection

producing brownish-colored, acidic hematin. Blood in the urine also may assume a smoky appearance. This can be observed only by shaking the urine while holding it up to a source of light. The "smoke," or turbidity, is actually caused by the presence of erythrocytes suspended in solution. Centrifugation will yield clear urine with a red plug at the bottom of the tube. The smoky appearance of erythrocytes should not be confused with the faint turbidity of other suspensions (such as crystals and cells).

Normally, freshly voided urine is clear. When urine is allowed to stand, **amorphous crystals**, usually urates, may precipitate and cause urine to be cloudy. The turbidity of urine should always be recorded and microscopically explained. Table 57-3 lists common causes of cloudy urine.

Specific Gravity

Urinary specific gravity measurement serves as a partial assessment of the ability of the kidneys to concentrate urine. The normal range is 1.003 to 1.035 g/mL. A value of 1.020 or greater indicates good renal function and increased amounts of dissolved solutes excreted by the kidneys. A specific gravity greater than 1.035 represents the presence of extraneous solutes and should be investigated. Increased specific gravity greater than 1.030 is found in dehydration, diabetes mellitus, congestive heart failure, proteinuria, and adrenal insufficiency. Decreased specific gravity is found in patients with hypothermia and those using diuretics. In a patient with severe kidney disease, urine is produced with a fixed specific gravity that is identical to that of the glomerular filtrate, approximately 1.010. Sediment constituents are often poorly preserved in dilute urine. Therefore a low specific gravity indicates that microscopic examinations of urine may not yield optimally accurate results.

High–molecular-weight substances will affect specific gravity to a greater extent than simple crystalloids will. This becomes significant when urine contains abnormal amounts of larger molecules such as glucose, protein, or x-ray contrast mediums. In cases of pronounced glucosuria or proteinuria,

TABLE 57-3 COMMON CAUSES OF CLOUDY OR TURBID URINE		
Causes	*Methods of Clearing*	*Comments*
Chemical		
Urates	Soluble at 60° C or alkali	Pink sediment
Phosphates and carbonates	Soluble in dilute acid	
Crystals	See specific solubility characteristics	
Mucus	—	Sticky
X-ray contrast media	Soluble in 10% sodium hydroxide	
Lipids	Soluble in ether	Opalescent
Chyle	Soluble in ether	Milky
Cells		
Bacteria	Centrifugation	Foul odor
Fungi	Centrifugation	Sweet odor
Erythrocyte	Centrifugation	Red, smoky
Leukocyte	Centrifugation	
Epithelium	Centrifugation	
Spermatozoa	Centrifugation	

correction factors can be used to adjust the specific gravity to a more representative value; 0.004 is subtracted for every 10 g/L glucose and 0.003 for every 10 g/L protein. The presence of x-ray contrast mediums or preservation is often associated with values of 1.040 or greater.

In previous years a **hydrometer** (urinometer) and a suitable container were used to determine specific gravity. However, hydrometer use is hampered by significant limitations: (1) measurement by hydrometer requires a large volume of urine (10 to 15 mL); (2) hydrometers are calibrated to be used at 20° C; and (3) they cannot be recalibrated. For these reasons, few laboratories employ hydrometers to measure specific gravity.

Most laboratories are now equipped with refractometers that can relate density of a solution to specific gravity (see Chapter 4). There are several advantages to the use of refractometers: (1) they require only a drop or two of urine, (2) they are temperature-compensated, (3) readings are less affected by density than readings by urinometers are, and (4) refractometers have a zero set screw for calibrating the instrument.

In specific gravity methodology, calibration is essential. Instruments should be checked with distilled water on a regular basis. Standardized salt and sucrose solutions can be used for calibration and quality control (see the CD-ROM for a detailed description). The refractometer method is described on the accompanying CD-ROM.

Reagent-strip method. An indirect colorimetric method for estimating specific gravity is available on reagent strips. This method uses a strip that contains a pretreated electrolyte-dye mixture that elicits a pH change based on the ionic concentration of the urine. This test for specific gravity is fast and simple and requires no additional equipment. The manufacturer states that there is no interference with glucose, protein, or radiographic dye. However, sensitivity is poorer than that of the refractometer method (units of 0.005), and urines with a pH of 6.5 or greater require a correction factor with the reagent-strip method.

Falling-drop method. Of historical interest, the falling-drop method is a direct method of measuring specific gravity using a silicone oil in a specially designed column. Specific gravity is related to the time it takes for a drop of urine to fall a distance defined by two optical gates.[9]

Osmolality

The normal kidney is capable of producing urine with a range of 50 to 1200 mOsm/kg (see Chapter 26). Urine ranges from one-sixth to four times the osmolality of normal serum (280 to 290 mOsm/kg). Osmolality is measured by an osmometer (see Chapter 14).

Osmolality is determined by the number of particles per unit mass, whereas the specific gravity is a reflection of the density (size or weight) of the suspended particles. Generally, specific gravity and osmolality are directly related in a linear fashion, although there are important exceptions. For example, if iodinated dyes are administered to a patient for intravenous pyelography, the specific gravity may reach as high as 1.070 or 1.080, though the osmolality will remain within normal limits. The dye particles have a mass that is large enough to raise the specific gravity, but too few molecules are present to notably increase the osmolality.

CHEMICAL EXAMINATION OF URINE

Several chemical constituents are routinely analyzed by urinalysis. Semi-quantitative and qualitative reagent strips and tablet tests are used, as well as quantitative methods for protein, electrolytes, and **porphyrins**.

Normal Constituents

Urine is composed of numerous chemical substances. Table 57-4 lists common chemical constituents measured by urinalysis laboratories.

Reagent-Strip Testing

Reagent-strip tests have enabled urinalysis laboratories to generate valuable semiquantitative chemical results in a rapid, accurate, and efficient manner. In general, properly performed urine test strips are sensitive, specific, and cost-effective.

The urinalysis laboratory is responsible for selecting the most suitable type of reagent strip for its hospital or clinical setting. The following guidelines will ensure the best results:

- Test urine promptly; use properly timed test readings only.
- Beware of interfering substances.
- Understand the advantages and limitations of the test.
- Employ controls.

TABLE 57-4 COMPOSITION OF URINE FROM HEALTHY SUBJECTS

Constituent	Value
Albumin	<15 to 30 mg/L
Calcium	100 to 24 mg/24 hr
Creatinine	1.2 to 1.8 g/24 hr
Glucose	<300 mg/L
Ketones	<50 mg/L
Osmolality	>600 mOsm/L
Phosphorus	0.9 to 1.3 g/24 hr
Potassium	30 to 100 mmol/24 hr
pH	4.7 to 7.8
Sodium	85 to 250 mmol/24 hr
Specific gravity	1.005 to 1.030
Total bilirubin	Not detected
Total protein	<150 mg/24 hr
Urea nitrogen	7 to 16 g/24 hr
Uric acid	300 to 800 mg/24 hr
Urobilinogen	<1 mg/L

TABLE 57-5 PRACTICAL SENSITIVITIES OF COMMERCIAL REAGENT STRIPS

Urine Parameters	Chemstrip*	N-Multistix†
pH	±1 pH unit	±1pH unit
Protein	60 mg/L	50 to 200 mg/L
Glucose	400 mg/L	750 mg/L
Ketones	50 mg/L acetoacetic acid	90 mg/L acetoacetic acid
	400 to 700 mg/L acetone	800 to 1400 mg/L acetone
Bilirubin	5 mg/L	4 to 8 mg/L
Blood	5 intact erythrocytes/μL or hemoglobin from 10 erythrocytes/μL	5 to 20 intact erythrocytes/μL or hemoglobin from 5 erythrocytes/μL
Urobilinogen	4 mg/L	2 mg/L
Nitrite	0.3 mg/L	0.6 to 1 mg/L
Esterase (neutrophils)	6 to 10 leukocytes/hpf	5 to 15 leukocytes/hpf

*Roche Diagnostics, Indianapolis, Indiana.
†Bayer Corporation, Elkhart, Indiana.

Strip tests should be performed on well-mixed urine equilibrated to room temperature. Each chemical parameter must be evaluated within a specific time interval, as suggested by the manufacturer's instructions. The correct number of strips needed for immediate analysis should be removed from the container and the lid tightly replaced. Reagent strips should be stored in a cool (not refrigerated), moisture-free environment. Outdated and air-exposed urine dipsticks must never be used.[12]

TABLE 57-6 USEFUL CONFIRMATORY TESTS

Test	Confirmatory Test	Reason
Protein	Sulfosalicylic acid (SSA) method	Increased specificity and sensitivity
	Protein electrophoresis	Increased specificity
Ketones	Acetest	Increased sensitivity, specificity, and color stability
Bilirubin	Ictotest	Increased sensitivity
Bacteriuria	Culture	Identification and quantification
Abnormal cells, casts	Cytological examination	Increased visualization, quantitation

After dipping the reagent strip into the urine, remove excess urine by gently tapping the strip on the edge of the specimen container. Compare individual reagent-pad reactions with the correct color chart in a properly lighted area. Automated reagent-strip readers (reflectance photometers) are widely available. Table 57-5 lists the sensitivities of two commercially available multiple test strips. Reagent-strip results that are positive may require confirmation with chemical and microscopic methods. Manufacturers' inserts should be reviewed to identify sources of inhibitors and false-positive and false-negative results. Ascorbic acid in urine can interfere with reagent-strip reactions for glucose, hemoglobin, bilirubin, and nitrite. Manufacturers have been encouraged to minimize or eliminate this interference when possible because ingestion of vitamin C supplements is so common.[13] Quality control samples are essential to verify reagent-strip results. Additional information on the chemical basis for reagent-strip testing and interferences are found on the CD-ROM.

Confirmatory Testing

Many laboratory workers equate a confirmatory test with retesting for a given parameter. This confirms nothing; it establishes only the precision for that testing procedure.[9,14] A confirmatory test is one that will establish the accuracy or correctness of the results of another procedure. Examples of confirmatory tests used in urinalysis are quantitative protein analysis, protein electrophoresis, bacterial cultures, and cytological appearance (Table 57-6). A confirmatory test should have either the same or better specificity, be based on a different principle, or have a sensitivity equal to or better than that of the original test.

Urinary pH

Although the standard method for pH measurements uses glass electrodes, urinary pH is usually measured with indicator paper, since small changes in pH are of little clinical significance. Most urinalysis laboratories use multitest reagent strips with two indicators-methyl red and bromthymol blue. These provide a pH range from 5.0 to 9.0 that

TABLE 57-7 COMMON CLINICAL CONDITIONS CAUSING ACIDIC AND ALKALINE URINE

Acidic Urine	Alkaline Urine
Protein diet	Vegetable diet
Starvation	Vomiting
Dehydration	Renal tubular acidosis
Diarrhea	Respiratory and metabolic alkalosis
Diabetic acidosis	Ammonia-producing, urea-splitting
Metabolic and respiratory	bacteria
acidosis	Acetazolamide therapy
Metabolism of fats	Low-carbohydrate diets
Sleep	Chronic renal failure
Acid-producing bacteria	

is demonstrated by a color change from orange (acid) to green to blue (alkaline). The urinary pH range is 4.7 to 7.8. Extremely acidic or alkaline urine usually indicates a poorly collected specimen.

Table 57-7 lists common clinical causes of acidic and alkaline urine. The average American ingests an acid-residue diet high in protein that results in acidic urine (5.0 to 6.5). With alkaline urine (8.0 to 8.5) the clinician should always suspect an unpreserved or old specimen with the presence of urease-producing ammonia bacteria, such as a *Proteus* species. Patients with renal tubular acidosis, a clinical syndrome characterized by an inability to excrete acidic urine, may produce urine with a much higher pH than would be expected on the basis of the acidosis.

The urinary pH is important in the management of renal stones or crystals. Uric acid stones precipitate in acidic urine and are more soluble in basic urines. Alkaline urine will precipitate calcium or calcium phosphate stones, whereas acidic urine will tend to dissolve them. Alkaline urine is desirable during sulfonamide and streptomycin therapy to prevent precipitation of the drugs in the kidneys and the formation of uric acid, cystine, and oxalate stones. The alkaline pH is also maintained during treatment of transfusion reactions and salicylate intoxication. In **cystitis**, the pH is kept acidic to combat **bacteriuria** and to prevent formation of alkaline stones. Technologists should be aware that alkaline urine interferes with the determination of proteins and may alter the urine sediment examination.

Proteins

A healthy person will have a daily protein excretion of about 100 mg/day, a very small fraction of the plasma protein content. The majority of the urine protein is albumin that has crossed the glomerular membrane, but smaller–molecular-weight proteins such as globulins may also be present. Once filtered, proteins are almost completely reabsorbed in the proximal tubule. Proteinuria, therefore, can be the result of either increased filtration or decreased reabsorption (tubular function).

Reagent-strip tests represent a screening procedure for proteinuria. Since the specificity of strip tests is weighted to the detection of albumin, it is highly recommended that the laboratory simultaneously perform a reagent-strip test and an acid precipitation test for the detection of all types of protein. Reagent strips are pH-sensitive and depend on the presence of protein for color generation (Sørensen's protein error). The presence of protein on the strip changes the pH environment of the dye embedded in the pad, resulting in a change in color. Highly buffered, alkaline urine can result in a false-positive test:

$$\text{Tetrabromphenol blue} \xrightarrow[\text{Protein}]{\text{pH 3}} \text{Positive results (green-blue)}$$

$$\text{Tetrabromphenol blue} \xrightarrow[\text{No protein}]{\text{pH 3}} \text{Negative results (yellow)}$$

A positive or faintly positive result should be confirmed with a more specific test such as the trichloroacetic acid or the sulfosalicylic acid tests. A mildly positive test-strip result and a grossly positive turbidity test result may indicate the presence of drugs or Bence Jones proteins.

The sulfosalicylic acid test and semiquantitative turbidity methods are described on the CD-ROM. It lists the sensitivities, types of proteins detected, and sources of false-negative and false-positive results for both the reagent-strip and the sulfosalicylic acid tests. Commercial SSA standards are available.

Sugars

Enzymatic tests. The reagent-strip test is an excellent test that is specific for glucose. It detects the oxidation of glucose to gluconic acid:

$$\text{Glucose} + \text{Oxygen in room air} \xrightarrow{\text{Glucose oxidase}} \text{Gluconic acid} + \text{Hydrogen peroxide}$$

$$\text{Hydrogen peroxide} + \text{Chromogen} \xrightarrow{\text{Peroxidase}} \text{Oxidized chromogen (blue)} + \text{H}_2\text{O}$$

One reagent-strip product uses *o*-toludine as the chromogen for the indicator reaction.

Copper reduction (Clinitest, Benedict's test)

$$\text{Cupric ions} + \begin{array}{c}\text{Glucose}\\ \text{(or reducing}\\ \text{substances)}\end{array} \xrightarrow[\text{Alkali}]{\text{Heat}} \begin{array}{c}\text{Cuprous} + \text{Cuprous}\\ \text{oxide (red)} \quad \text{hydroxide (yellow)}\end{array}$$

The Clinitest tablet (Bayer Diagnostics, Elkhart, Indiana) provides another test for sugar. It is a copper reduction test that measures total reducing substances. In addition to glucose, Clinitest will detect sugars such as galactose, lactose, and pentoses. It also detects ascorbic acid and certain drugs, such as nalidixic acid (NegGram), used to treat urinary tract infections; probenecid, used to treat gout; and cephalosporin, an antibiotic.

Clinitest is an important test in pediatric screening. A negative test-strip result (specific for glucose) but a positive Clinitest result (sensitive for any reducing sugar) may indicate the presence of an inherited metabolic disorder in the newborn.

Clinitest will detect reducing substances at a concentration of 2000 mg/L (200 mg/dL) or greater. Reagent strips will detect glucose at a concentration of 400 to 750 mg/L. Because Clinitest is both less specific and less sensitive than the reagent strip, it cannot be used as a confirmatory test for a positive reagent-strip glucose test. Clinitest should be reserved for patient populations in whom non–glucose-reducing substances need to be detected.

Sugar will appear in the urine because of an increased filtered load, as in diabetes mellitus, or because of decreased tubular reabsorption, as in renal glucosuria. The presence of ascorbic acid may lead to erroneous low results.

Ketones

The term *ketone bodies* includes three discrete but related chemicals: acetoacetic acid, β-hydroxybutyric acid, and acetone (see Chapter 32). Reagent-strip testing for ketones uses a sodium nitroprusside reaction that detects acetone and acetoacetic acid but not β-hydroxybutyric acid, the primary ketone body. It is important to realize that the sodium nitroprusside reagent reacts primarily with acetoacetic acid; acetone has only a 20% reactivity compared with acetoacetate:

$$\text{Acetoacetic acid} + \text{Sodium nitroprusside} + \text{Glycine} \xrightarrow{\text{Alkaline pH}} purple\ color$$

Ketone determinations are important in the monitoring of diabetes and ketoacidosis and should be performed whenever sugar determinations are made.

Blood and Myoglobin

As previously discussed, red urine usually indicates the presence of erythrocytes, hemoglobin, or myoglobin in the urine. Hematuria most often represents a combination of intact erythrocytes (greater than 5 per high-power field), degenerated erythrocytes, and free hemoglobin. Gross hematuria implies hemorrhage or fresh bleeding and in acidic urine results in a red to brown, turbid or smoky appearance. The reagent-strip method for hemoglobin and myoglobin uses the peroxidase-like activity of these proteins:

$$\text{Hydrogen peroxide (H}_2\text{O}_2\text{)} + \text{Chromogen} \xrightarrow{\text{Myoglobin or hemoglobin}} \text{Oxidized chromogen (}blue\text{)} + \text{H}_2\text{O}$$

A positive test indicates the presence of hematuria, **hemoglobinuria**, or myoglobinuria, and a microscopic urinalysis is needed to confirm the presence of erythrocytes. Oxidizing agents such as iodides and bromides in the urine may cause false-positive results; large quantities of ascorbic acid (used in some antibiotics) in the urine may produce false-negative results with some reagent strips.

Myoglobin is a ferrous porphyrin similar to hemoglobin that is commonly seen in urine after crush injuries and muscle trauma. When myoglobin is released in the circulatory system, it is rapidly excreted by the kidney. Like hemoglobin, its presence will produce pink to red urine. Myoglobin-

uria should always be confirmed with rapid immunoassay procedures.

Bilirubin

Dark, yellow to brown, foamy urine is suggestive of the presence of conjugated bilirubin. Normal urine does not contain bilirubin. Jaundiced patients with hepatocellular disease, such as hepatitis, or obstructive disease, such as biliary cirrhosis, may have conjugated bilirubin in the urine. The reagent-strip method for determining bilirubin involves a diazotization reaction:

$$\text{Bilirubin glucuronide} + \text{Diazonium salt} \xrightarrow{\text{Acid}} \text{Azobilirubin (}brown\text{)}$$

Negative results from suspicious urines and questionably positive results, as from highly colored urines, should be confirmed by use of Ictotest tablets (Bayer Corporation, Elkhart, Indiana). The Ictotest employs the same diazotization reaction as the reagent strip. False-negative results may occur if the urine is not fresh, because urinary bilirubin may become hydrolyzed or oxidized when exposed to light.

Urobilinogen

Urobilinogen, a colorless compound, is formed in the intestine by the bacterial reduction of bilirubin (see Chapter 27). Normal urine contains small amounts of urobilinogen. Decreased urobilinogen is found in infants, who lack reducing intestinal bacteria; in patients after administration of antibiotics that suppress intestinal flora; and in patients with obstructive liver disease. Increased urobilinogen is present in hemolytic anemia (increased bilirubin formation) and liver dysfunction.

The reagent-strip tests for urobilirubin differ with the manufacturer. Bayer products use the Ehrlich reaction employing *p*-dimethylaminobenzaldehyde in a simple color reaction with porphobilinogen. The reaction is not specific for urobilinogen, and false-positive findings may result from other Ehrlich reagent-positive compounds (porphobilinogen, PAS). Roche Diagnostics products employ a reaction that is specific for urobilinogen; urobilinogen reacts with a diazonium compound to form a red color. It should be noted that reagent strips will not detect the absence of urinary urobilinogen.

A fresh specimen is essential for the detection of urobilinogen because it is a light-sensitive compound. The preferred specimen for detecting or quantitating urinary urobilinogen is a 2-hour early afternoon specimen. This collection takes into account the diurnal excretion pattern of urobilinogen.

Nitrites

The nitrite test is used in urinalysis laboratories to detect bacteriuria. The reagent-strip nitrite test depends on the reduction of nitrate to nitrite by the enzymatic action of certain bacteria in the urine. Under conditions of acid pH, nitrite reacts with *p*-arsanilic acid to form a diazonium compound, which in turn couples with *N*-(1-naphthyl)ethylenediamine to produce a pink color.[11] The nitrite test should be performed on the first morning specimen or on a urine sample that has been collected at least 4 hours or more after the last voiding to allow the organisms in the bladder time to metabolize the nitrate. Stale urine may have a positive nitrite test result because of bacterial contamination after voiding. The nitrite test is specific for gram-negative organisms; however, some false-negative results will occur in the presence of organisms such as enterococci, streptococci, or staphylococci, which do not form nitrite. The sensitivity of the nitrite test is about 60% when compared with microbiological procedures.[15] Very few cases of false-positive nitrite results occur.

Nitrite testing is of dubious value in hospital clinical urinalysis because there is limited effective control over how and when the urine sample is collected. The nitrite test may have use in a clinic or physician's office because proper control over sampling can be better achieved.

Leukocytes

The presence of leukocytes (pyuria) is a clinically important indicator of inflammation. Reagent-strip tests for pyuria will detect both lysed and intact leukocytes and are based on the presence of intracellular esterases. These enzymes will catalyze the hydrolysis of esters, releasing components that are then used in a color reaction. The intensity of the color reaction is proportional to the number of leukocytes in the specimen. Sensitivities for the two reagent-strip manufacturers are listed in Table 57-5. False-positive results are seen with trichomonads and oxidizing agents. It has not yet been well established whether eosinophils and histiocytes will also give a positive reaction. False-negative values may be seen with high levels of protein and ascorbic acid. Several studies have documented the clinical utility of the leukocyte test as a screening test for pyuria, and many laboratory workers believe a microscopic examination for leukocytes is necessary only on urine specimens that are positive for esterase when tested with reagent strips.[16-19]

Porphyrins

Porphyrins are groups of intermediary products in the biosynthesis of heme and cytochromes, which are produced in the liver and bone marrow (see Chapter 27). Identification of various porphyrins and porphyrin precursors (especially porphobilinogen) is important in the clinical diagnosis of porphyrias, a group of genetic or metabolic disorders. Normal urinary excretion of porphyrins is approximately 2 mg/day. Increased quantities of excreted porphyrins (porphyrinuria) give urine a red or wine color. A screening urinalysis test for porphobilinogen is based on the Watson-Schwartz test (see Methods on CD-ROM).[20] Confirmatory and quantitative tests are available.[9]

Melanin

Normal urine does not contain **melanin**. Melanin is found in the urine of patients with malignant melanoma. Patients with this malignancy will excrete a colorless precursor of melanin (melanogen) that, when exposed to air, will polymerize to form the dark pigment melanin. Screening tests using ferric chloride oxidize melanogen to melanin, which turns urine brown-black.

MICROSCOPIC EXAMINATION OF URINE
Methods

Accurate microscopic identification of urine sediment is important in the early recognition of infectious, inflammatory, and neoplastic conditions affecting the urinary system.[4] It is debatable whether all routine urine specimens require the more time-consuming microscopic analysis. Instead, most laboratory workers agree that a microscopic examination should be performed when the patient is symptomatic, when the physician specifically requests this examination, and when the macroscopic urinalysis is abnormal, in the case of hematuria, proteinuria, or a positive result for pyuria (positive nitrate or esterase result).[11,21]

Several microscopic procedures are available for the sediment examination. Standardized bright-field microscopy is still the most common technique employed.[22] Supravital staining can be combined with bright-field microscopy to enhance cellular detail. Phase-contrast microscopy is probably the best method for rapid urine sediment evaluations without the use of stains. Commercially available standardized slide methods are far superior to conventional glass slide and coverslip methods and serve as a practical alternative to hemocytometer chamber counts.[23]

Currently, automation of urine microscopy has not been widely accepted because of the need to identify and classify numerous urine sediment entities. Systems to partially automate the microscopic urinalysis, using flow cytometry or a flow cell mounted on a microscope stage, are being developed.

Standardization

Standardization of the microscopic urinalysis is essential to reduce ambiguity and minimize subjectivity.[24] Aspects of the microscopic examination that should be standardized are:

1. Volume of urine analyzed
2. Length and force of centrifugation
3. Resuspending volume and concentration of sediment
4. Volume and amount of sediment examined
5. Terminology and reporting format

Bright-field microscopy of unstained urine. Unstained bright-field microscopy uses reduced light to delineate the more translucent formed elements of the urine, such as **hyaline casts**, crystals, and mucus threads.

Accurate identification of leukocytes, macrophages, renal tubular epithelial cells, and viral inclusion-bearing cells may be very difficult in unstained preparations. Cytological techniques, stained preparations, or both should be used to confirm results.[8,25]

Procedure. The urine specimen must be examined while fresh, since cells and casts begin to disintegrate within 1 to 3 hours. Refrigeration (2° to 8° C) for up to 48 hours usually prevents the disintegration of cells and pathological entities. Each specimen is concentrated 10-fold or 20-fold for the purpose of standardization. The examination proceeds as follows:

1. Mix the specimen well.
2. Pour a fixed volume (10, 12, 15 mL) of urine into a graduated centrifuge tube.
3. Centrifuge at 1500 rpm or approximately 80 G for 5 minutes.
4. Remove the supernatant fluid by careful decantation or aspiration to a fixed volume; 1 mL and 0.4 mL are the most common. Resuspend the sediment by gently tapping the bottom of the tube.
5. Place a drop of resuspended sediment on one area of a standardized slide.
6. Examine with low power (100×) and subdued light. Vary the fine focus continuously while randomly scanning the area under the coverslip. During the scan, evaluate the specimen for the presence of squamous and transitional epithelial cells, crystals, mucus, bacteria, **yeast**, and artifacts. Report according to laboratory protocol. Further identification of casts, renal epithelial cells, erythrocytes, and leukocytes can be accomplished using high power.
7. Examine at least 10 low-power fields using subdued light. Count and report the number of casts per low-power field. Be sure to examine the edges because casts are often found along the edge of a coverslip. Abnormal crystals, when present, should also be counted on low power. Bacteriuria, visible at low power, should be reported as at least 2+.
8. Examine at least 10 high-power (440×) fields and report numerical values for erythrocytes, leukocytes, and renal tubular epithelial cells per high-power field.
9. Report all counts (average of 10 fields) and qualitative assessments according to standardized terminology.

Bright-field microscopy with supravital staining. Cellular detail is enhanced with stained sediments.[26] A crystal violet–safranin O stain is often used in the rapid assessment of certain cellular elements.[27] See the CD-ROM for specific details.

Phase and interference microscopy. Many urinalysis laboratories recommend phase microscopy for the detection of more translucent formed elements of the urinary sediment. Sediment, notably hyaline casts, mucus, and bacteria, may escape detection using conventional, unstained, bright-field microscopy. Phase microscopy has the advantage of hardening the outlines of even the most ephemeral formed elements, making detection simple.[24] Even greater morphological detail of formed elements (notably casts and cells) is afforded by interference contrast microscopy.[28-30]

Standardized slide methods. The KOVA system (Hycor Biomedical, Inc. Garden Grove, California), Count-10 and Count-6 (V-Tech, Pomona, California), and the UriSystem (Fisher Scientific, Houston) offer complete standardized procedures that are technically more precise, reproducible, and reliable than conventional bright-field

microscopy.[23] In some laboratories, the hemocytometer continues to be used for quantifying urine sediment entities. Kesson et al[31] provide evidence that chamber counts are more reliable in detecting sediment abnormalities than conventional methods of counting cells under high-power fields.

Semiautomated urinalysis work station. An automated urinalysis instrument called the Yellow IRIS (International Remote Imaging Systems, Chatsworth, California) combines automated microscopy with a dipstick reader and specific-gravity module. This technology may provide more accurate results over standardized manual systems when there are high volumes of test samples and very low concentrations of sediment elements.[32] Manual methods appear to be more sensitive in detecting casts.[33]

Combined cytocentrifugation and Papanicolaou stain. A technique that combines cytocentrifugation and **Papanicolaou staining** has been recommended for more accurate assessment of urine sediment. This more specialized method provides a simple, reproducible, and semiquantitative method for identifying urine sediment entities. Cellular casts, mononuclear cells, tissue fragments, and neoplastic cells may be clearly identified with this method. Although not used in routine laboratories, this technique is growing in acceptance.[6-8]

Crystals (See CD-ROM)

Urinary crystals are commonly seen. Usually crystals are not present when urine is freshly voided, and in general the formation of crystals should be regarded as an artifact of the system of collection. Crystal formation occurs when various chemical constituents become saturated or undergo altered solubilities when urine is stored at cooler temperatures. Certain chemical substances such as albumin prevent crystallization. When heated to 37° C, most crystals disappear. Those still present might have some diagnostic significance when correlated with clinical symptoms.[9]

The types of urinary crystals formed depend on the pH of freshly voided urine. The accompanying CD-ROM lists the common types, properties, and clinical significance of various urinary crystals. Cystine, uric acid, leucine, and tyrosine crystals are the most diagnostically important crystals to recognize. Because of the limited clinical significance of the urinary crystals, most laboratory workers agree that time should not be wasted on their specific identification. Many crystals are induced by various medications, although their clinical significance remains unclear.

Organisms

In a properly collected and processed urine specimen, the presence of organisms is clinically significant. Bacteria, fungi, parasites, and virally infected cells are frequently reported. Organisms seen in urine sediment are microscopically recognized as extracellular or intracellular structures.[25] Bright-field microscopy readily detects extracellular bacteria, fungi, and parasites. Detection of intracellular phagocytized bacteria and fungi, *Toxoplasma* organisms, and viral inclusion bodies usually requires cytological procedures.

Accurate identification of organisms aids in the clinical differential diagnosis of urinary system infections. Stained preparations are important in the evaluation of organisms, identification of associated inflammatory cells, and assessment of epithelial exfoliation and renal cast formation for purposes of localization.[4] Microbiological techniques should be used to confirm and fully classify various urinary organisms.

Bacteria. Urine from healthy individuals is sterile and does not contain bacteria. Some bacteria may be present because of contamination during collection or prolonged storage. If bacteria are seen in centrifuged specimens but not in unspun urine specimens, less than 10^5 bacteria/mL are present. Bacteria in an unspun specimen indicate that greater than 10^5 bacteria/mL are present. The presence of 10^5 bacteria/mL or greater is suggestive of a urinary tract infection. This number corresponds to 10 or more bacteria per high-power field. Identification of bacteria, cocci, or rods can readily be accomplished by bright-field or phase-contrast microscopy. Occasionally, there is difficulty in distinguishing bacteria from amorphous crystals.

Fungi. Fungal urinary tract infections (UTIs) are common in patients with diabetes, those taking birth control pills, or those undergoing intensive antibiotic or immunosuppressive therapy. An associated inflammatory pattern is seen in most UTIs in nonimmunocompromised patients.

Candida albicans is the most common fungus and is identified as budding yeast or mycelia. In general the budding yeast appearance indicates that the fungi are coexisting with the host, whereas the mycelial forms appear during tissue invasion. Yeasts of *Candida albicans* are oval and highly refractile and measure 3 to 5 μm. Often they can be misinterpreted as erythrocytes (7 μm). Unlike erythrocytes, yeasts are not lysed by acids.

Parasites. The presence of parasites in urine usually indicates vaginal or fecal contamination. *Trichomonas vaginalis*, a flagellate, is the most common parasite seen in urine. The incidence of this type of parasitism is very high in women and may be the cause of intense vaginitis. In men the parasite causes an asymptomatic urethritis. Because of the motility of this oval organism, bright-field microscopy is used for simple and rapid identification. Nonmotile trichomonads can easily be mistaken for leukocytes or epithelial cells.

Pinworm ova (*Enterobius vermicularis*) have been found in urine in children because of fecal contamination. Morphologically a pinworm ovum is surrounded by a thick two-layered transparent capsule, and a coiled embryo may be visible inside. Trematode ova of *Schistosoma haematobium* (found in North Africa) and *Schistosoma mansoni* (found in Central America) may also be found in urine.

Virally infected cells. Virus-induced cellular changes have been recognized with increased frequency in urine sediment, especially in immunosuppressed patients. Cytological techniques should be used for the accurate identification of cytomegalovirus, herpes simplex, and *Polyomavirus*, which produce diagnostic intranuclear inclusion cells and are the most common types of urinary system viral infections. Viral inclusion cells must be distinguished from nonviral sources of inclusion cells such as heavy metal exposure (lead and cadmium) and nonspecific degenerative cellular changes. A detailed description of viral inclusion cells can be found in standard textbooks on urine cytology.

Cells

Microscopic identification and evaluation of cells is an important part of urinalysis. Common types of cells normally found in urine include a few erythrocytes, leukocytes, and epithelial cells of renal or lower urinary tract origin. All cells of pathological significance are usually quantified by high-power field examination.

Erythrocytes. Normal urine should never contain more than a few erythrocytes per high-power field.[34] They appear in the urine stream after vascular injury or disorders in the kidney or lower urinary tract. The presence of erythrocytes accompanied by blood casts or dysmorphic erythrocytes is suggestive of renal parenchymal or glomerular bleeding.[35] The detection of urinary dysmorphic erythrocytes, especially acanthocytes, is an important morphologic marker of glomerular or tubular bleeding.[36-38] Quantification aids in diagnosis and patient management. When a urine specimen needs to be obtained from a female patient, it is important that contamination from menstrual flow be avoided.

Erythrocytes measure approximately 7 μm in diameter, have a biconcave disk shape, and often appear pale yellow when bright-field microscopy is used. In hypertonic urine they are smaller and crenated, whereas in hypotonic urine they are larger and swollen. When erythrocytes have been in urine for a considerable time, the hemoglobin may have leaked out of the cells.

On occasion hemoglobin is detected by reagent strip testing in urine in the absence of microscopic erythrocytes in the sediment. Possible explanations for this discrepancy include hypotonic urine or an alkaline urine, both of which can cause erythrocyte lysis. The absence of these conditions is strongly suggestive that the pigment which appears in the urine (hemoglobin or myoglobin) originates from filtration of these substances from the blood.

Leukocytes. The normal excretion rate for leukocytes in the urine is up to 1 leukocyte per 3 high-power fields, 3000 cells/mL, or up to about 200,000 cells/hour. Elevated numbers of leukocytes (pyuria) are associated with numerous urinary tract inflammatory and infectious conditions. Most leukocytes recognized by bright-field microscopy are segmented neutrophils. The identification of lymphocytes, plasma cells, and eosinophils requires special stains.

Little[39] has shown that leukocyte excretion rates in excess of 400,000 cells/hour virtually always indicate urinary tract infection. This rate corresponds to more than 10 neutrophils per high-power field. Patients with active upper urinary tract infections frequently have more than 50 neutrophils per high-power field or have a leukocyte excretion rate in excess of 2 or even 3 million/hour.

Renal tubular epithelial cells (see CD-ROM). Various types of renal tubular epithelial cells line the nephron, and

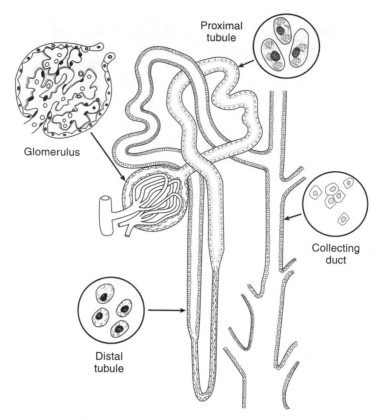

Fig. 57-1 Location of renal tubular epithelial cells.

senescent or diseased cells are constantly being shed into the urine (Fig. 57-1). Since they represent actual renal exfoliation, the presence of more than two renal tubular epithelial cells per high-power field indicates active renal tubular damage or injury.

Considerable difficulty exists in the accurate identification of renal tubular cells, particularly in distinguishing them from other mononuclear cells commonly found in urine. By bright-field microscopy they are polygonal and slightly larger than leukocytes. For accurate identification of various types of renal tubular cells (convoluted versus collecting duct) and sheets or fragments, cytological techniques are required.[8,25]

Oval fat bodies. Oval fat bodies are renal tubular epithelial cells that are filled with absorbed lipids or that have undergone degenerative cellular changes. Oval fat bodies are often associated with proteinuria and lipiduria and are characteristically seen in patients with nephrotic syndrome or diabetes mellitus.

Transitional epithelial cells. A few transitional (urothelial) cells can be found in normal urine. Large numbers of transitional cells, however, may be present with inflammatory conditions in the bladder, **catheterization**, or pathological processes such as malignancy.

By bright-field microscopy, transitional cells appear round to oval, measure 40 to 60 μm, and have a centrally located nucleus. The cytoplasm borders of these cells appear thickened and crisp. When the nuclei of transitional cells

become enlarged or irregular, cytological techniques should be suggested for the purpose of detecting a urinary system malignancy.

Squamous epithelial cells. Squamous epithelial cells line the distal portion of the lower urinary tract and the female genital tract. Squamous cells are the largest of the epithelial cells found in urine. They have abundant flat cytoplasm with small nuclei. Frequently one or more corners of these cells may be folded. Squamous cells in urine usually indicate contamination (vaginal in women, urethral in uncircumcised men) or squamous metaplasia of the bladder and represent the least significant type of epithelial cell found in urine.

Tissue fragments in urine. Any clumps or chunks of solid-appearing material in urine specimens should be noted. This material is identified during the initial inspection of the specimen because of its large size. It is often white or tan. Precise identification of such material is important for an accurate diagnosis. This involves transfer of the observed material to an appropriate fixative to preserve it for a cytological or histological evaluation. Renal papillary necrosis and bladder tumors are most frequently responsible for shedding large tissue fragments into the urine.

Spermatozoa. Spermatozoa may be easily recognized in the urine of a man after ejaculation or in the urine of a woman as a vaginal contaminant after coitus. Identification of spermatozoa is of limited clinical significance, and their presence is usually not reported.

Renal Casts

Renal (urinary) casts are formed cylindrical structures that are organized in the nephron. Casts are significant because of their localizing value. Casts are composed of uromucoid (Tamm-Horsfall mucoprotein), which is always present in urine, usually in solution. Uromucoid is produced by the renal tubular epithelial cells of the ascending limb of the loop of Henle. Casts are formed as a result of urine stasis allowing uromucoid to precipitate. Other factors contributing to cast formation include an increased concentration of protein, salts, and a low urine pH. Since the precipitation of this protein depends on the concentration and composition of urine, casts are more likely to be formed at the distal portion of the nephron and in the collecting ducts of the kidney where the urine is more concentrated. Casts may form in the proximal convoluted tubules in patients with Bence Jones proteins (multiple myeloma).

The appearance of these cylindrical formed elements in urine reflects the shapes (long versus short, straight versus convoluted) and diameter (thin versus broad) of the renal tubular lumens in which they originally were formed. Their number and measurable properties of size, form, and compositions are valuable clues to intrinsic renal parenchymal disease.

Microscopically, casts are characterized by the appearance of the matrix (hyaline, granular, or waxy), the cellular constituents (erythrocytes, leukocytes, or renal tubular epithelial cells), or particulate matter embedded in the matrix (fine or coarse granules or fibrin).

Accurate identification of casts, especially the cellular types, is often difficult when unstained bright-field microscopy (wet preparation) is used. A skilled microscopist is essential to avoid misinterpretations. Phase-contrast and interference-contrast microscopy, as well as special stains, can be used to improve visualization. The cytocentrifugation-Papanicolaou technique is a superior method for the accurate identification of casts in urine specimens of patients with renal disease.

For diagnostic purposes, renal casts are classified as physiological or pathological. Table 57-8 lists the common types, properties, and clinical significance of casts.

Fats

Fats are found in the urine of patients who have fat emboli after bone-crushing injuries, fatty degeneration of the kidney, or nephrotic syndrome. Fat will appear on top of urine and is the last part of voided urine. Vacuolated epithelial cells may be found in the urinary sediment. Oil Red O or Sudan III fat stains should be used for accurate identification of fat droplets in urine.

URINE CYTOLOGY

Urinalysis laboratory workers should be able to recognize abnormal mononuclear cells suggestive of malignancy. These should be referred for urine cytology. Holmquist[26] has advocated the use of supravital stains for malignant cell detection and suggests a role for the urinalysis laboratory in cancer screening.

CALCULI (LITHIASIS)

Urinary calculi are precipitates, concretions, or crystalloids embedded in a binding substance of mucus and protein. Bacteria and epithelial cells also may be included in the calculi.[40] Although the cause of calculus formation remains controversial, the detection and identification of calculi are important for diagnosis of urinary system conditions. Calculi formation in the kidney or lower urinary tract can be the source of gross hematuria and can cause serious anatomical damage and excruciating pain for the patient. Knowledge of the specific composition of a passed or surgically removed calculus may aid the physician in effectively treating lithiasis and preventing future stone formation.

Calculus (stone) analysis for chemical constituents is a complex laboratory procedure. Urinary system calculi are usually composed of calcium oxalate, calcium oxalate mixed with calcium phosphate, ammonium magnesium phosphate, uric acid, or cystine. Most laboratories refer specimens for calculi analysis to more specialized laboratories.

URINE FINDINGS IN COMMON RENAL AND LOWER URINARY TRACT DISEASES

Numerous primary and secondary conditions and diseases occur in the kidney and lower urinary tract. An accurate diagnosis of urinary system disease requires correlation of abnormal urine findings with the patient history, physical examination, symptoms, signs, renal function tests, and other laboratory data. To be classified as abnormal, urine sediment must meet at least one of the following criteria:

1. More than five erythrocytes or leukocytes per high-power field (400×)
2. More than two renal tubular cells per high-power field (400×)
3. More than three hyaline casts, more than one granular cast, or the presence of any pathological cast per low-power field (100×)
4. More than 10 bacteria per high-power field (400×)
5. Presence of fungus, parasites, or viral inclusion cells
6. Presence of pathological crystals (such as cystine) or a large number of nonpathological crystals (such as uric acid)

A summary of urinalysis abnormalities found in common renal and lower urinary tract disease is shown in Table 57-9. Diagnostic findings of both the macroscopic and microscopic examination are also listed for quick review.

COORDINATED APPROACH TO URINALYSIS

Urinalysis continues to be one of the most commonly requested and demanding clinical laboratory procedures.[14] Laboratories involved in the examination of urine must define new responsibilities for both the rapid, routine assessment of urine and the more time-consuming, specialized interpretive tests.[41]

Current, rapid dipstick technology and standardization of bright-field microscopy provide a quality program for the analysis of urine specimens from asymptomatic individuals.

TABLE 57-8 COMMON RENAL (URINARY) CASTS

Types	Characteristic Morphological Appearance	Significance	Associated Diseases
Physiological			
Hyaline	Transparent cylinder	Exercise, dehydration, and fevers	Nonspecific
Granular (fine)	Semitransparent cylinder containing fine refractile granules	Exercise, dehydration, and fever; accumulation of plasma proteins	Nonspecific
Pathological			
Cellular			
Erythrocytic	Semitransparent or granular cylinder containing distinct erythrocyte stroma	Renal parenchymal bleeding, glomerular leakage	Glomerular disease, interstitial hemorrhage (infarction)
Blood	Red-brown granular cylinder, but intact erythrocyte stroma not seen	Same as above	Same as above
Leukocytic	Transparent granular or waxy cylinder containing segmented neutrophils	Renal inflammation	Tubulointerstitial inflammation (pyelonephritis), glomerular disease
Renal tubular epithelial	Semitransparent granular or waxy cylinder containing intact or necrotic renal tubular epithelial cells	Renal tubular damage	Renal tubular injury, acute tubular necrosis, acute allograft rejections, tubulointerstitial disease
Bacterial	Semitransparent or granular cylinder containing bacteria	Renal infection	Acute pyelonephritis
Fungal	Semitransparent or granular cylinder containing fungi	Renal infection, probably sepsis	Acute pyelonephritis, papillary necrosis
Noncellular			
Granular (coarse)	Semitransparent cylinder containing coarse refractile granules	Cellular degeneration, accumulation of plasma proteins	Nonspecific
Waxy	Sharply defined, highly refractile, homogenous cylinder with broken-off borders and indentations	Cellular degeneration	Nonspecific
Fibrin	Transparent or granular cylinder containing thin long fibrils	Leakage of coagulation products	Glomerular disease, thrombosis
Fatty	Semitransparent or granular cylinder containing large highly refractile vacuoles or droplets	Lipiduria	Nephrotic syndrome
Bile	Deep yellow, transparent, granular waxy cylinder	Leakage of bile salts	Liver dysfunction, tubulointerstitial disease
Crystal	Crystalline inclusion in a semitransparent or granular cylinder	Cellular degeneration and malabsorption or excretion	Nonspecific
Other			
Broad	Width of cylinder two to six times that of other casts; waxy and granular most common types	Tubular dilatation and stasis	Advanced renal disease

However, if symptomatic patients are to receive a more comprehensive urine examination, more definitive evaluation and confirmation procedures are required.

A coordinated approach to the urinalysis is depicted on the CD-ROM. Proper use of this approach requires that the clinician and urine technologist understand the roles of the routine laboratory, which offers urinalysis, and the specialized laboratory, which offers a comprehensive sediment examination. After the collection of urine and macroscopic analysis, the physician or laboratory must differentiate between results from symptomatic and asymptomatic patients. Emphasis must be placed on the urinalysis technologist's ability to recognize the results that require additional follow-up testing. This coordinated approach represents a flexible system in which technical responsibilities can be shared and additional laboratory confirmation procedures can be integrated into the system (see the CD-ROM). Communication among physicians, the laboratory technologist, and the medical director is essential to resolve inconclusive results and reestablish credibility of the urine examination.

TABLE 57-9   URINALYSIS ABNORMALITIES FOUND IN COMMON URINARY SYSTEM DISEASES

Conditions	Diagnostic Physicochemical Findings (Macroscopic Urinalysis)	Diagnostic Urine Sediment Findings (Microscopic Urinalysis)
Renal		
Acute glomerulonephritis	Decreased urine volume, increased turbidity (smoky), proteinuria (<2 g/24 hr), hematuria (often gross)	Erythrocytic and blood casts, erythrocytes (often dysmorphic), neutrophils, mixed cellular casts, renal epithelial cells, occasional leukocytic or renal tubuloepithelial casts
Nephrotic syndrome	Lipiduria, significant proteinuria (>4.5 g/24 hr)	Fatty and waxy casts, doubly refractile oval fat bodies (Maltese cross with polarized light), lipid-laden renal tubuloepithelial cells
Chronic glomerulonephritis	Occasional lipiduria, decreased and fixed specific gravity, proteinuria (>2 g/24 hr), hematuria	Pathological casts, especially broad types
Acute tubular necrosis	Decreased urine volume, decreased specific gravity, minimum proteinuria, hematuria	Intact and necrotic renal epithelial cells, renal epithelial fragments, pathological casts
Acute pyelonephritis (tubulointerstitial inflammation)	Occasional odor, increased turbidity, minimum proteinuria, positive nitrite reaction	Leukocyte casts, neutrophils, especially in clumps; bacterial, granular, and waxy casts; renal tubuloepithelial cells
Diabetes mellitus	Proteinuria, glycosuria, ketonuria	Fatty and waxy casts, oval fat bodies, renal epithelial cells, leukocytes
Systemic lupus erythematosus	Proteinuria	Pathological casts, renal epithelial cells, neutrophils, erythrocytes
Cystinosis	Minimum proteinuria or hematuria	Cystine crystals
Acute allograft rejection	Decreased urine volume, minimum proteinuria, hematuria	Renal epithelial cells, renal epithelial casts, lymphocytes, pathological casts, especially renal epithelial casts
Viral nephropathy (cytomegalic inclusion disease)	Minimum proteinuria, hematuria	Mononuclear cells (occasional giant cell forms) with prominent intranuclear or cytoplasmic inclusions
Lower Urinary Tract		
Bacterial urinary tract infection	Occasional odor, increased turbidity, positive nitrite reaction, occasional hematuria	Bacteria, neutrophils, reactive transitional epithelial cells, absence of cast formation
Fungal urinary tract infection	Increased turbidity, occasional hematuria	Fungi, neutrophils and lymphocytes, reactive transitional epithelial cells
Viral urinary tract infection	Occasional hematuria	Viral inclusion bodies, neutrophils, transitional cells
Eosinophilic cystitis	Hematuria	Eosinophils (numerous), reactive transitional epithelial cells, absence of cast formation
Transitional cell carcinoma	Hematuria	Increased numbers of malignant transitional epithelial cells with high nuclear-to-cytoplasmic ratio, hyperchromasia, and chromatin clumping; cells occur singly and as tissue fragments

Modified from Schumann GB: Urine sediment examination, *Baltimore, 1980, Williams & Wilkins.*

QUALITY CONTROL

An effective quality control program is essential to ensure accuracy in urinalysis. A program of quality assurance that covers all aspects of urinalysis and is similar to that used in other areas of the clinical laboratory must be implemented to achieve more reliable urinalysis results.[14]

Commercial quality control preparations are available for the assessment of specific gravity and reagent-strip testing. These preparations may be in tablet, strip, liquid, or lyophilized form. Hoeltge and Ersts[31] describe a 3-year experience using a synthetic-urine control prepared in their laboratory. Currently there is no ideal commercial preparation for urine sediment elements. Quality control of sediment evaluation should focus on standardized techniques and policies.

A suggested urinalysis quality control schedule is found on the CD-ROM. It is important that reagents are dated when they are received by the laboratory and used before expiration. Urine control solutions should retain their utility if they are stored in tightly lidded containers, refrigerated, and protected from light.[11] New lot numbers should always be recorded and validated. A laboratory manual containing operating instructions and documentation of equipment maintenance should be maintained and reviewed yearly. Finally, the importance of technologists pursuing continuing education and maintaining familiarity with references cannot be overemphasized.[42]

References

1. Bonnardeau A, Sommerville P, Kaye M: A study on the reliability of dipstick urinalysis, *Clin Nephrol* 41:167, 1994.
2. Kennedy TJ, McConnell JD, Thall ER: Urine dipstick vs. microscopic urinalysis in the evaluation of abdominal trauma, *J Trauma* 28:615, 1988.
3. Free AH, Free MA: Rapid convenience urine tests: their use and misuse, *Lab Med* 9:9, 1978.
4. Schumann GB: *Urine sediment examination*, Baltimore, 1980, Williams & Wilkins.
5. Fairley KF, Birch DF: Microscopic urinalysis in glomerulonephritis, *Kidney Int* 44:9, 1993.
6. Eggensberger DL et al: Cytodiagnostic urinalysis: three-year experience with a new laboratory test, *Am J Clin Pathol* 91:202, 1989.
7. Marcussen N et al: Analysis of cytodiagnostic urinalysis findings in 77 patients with concurrent renal biopsies, *Am J Kidney Dis* 20:618, 1992.
8. Schumann GB, Schumann JL, Marcussen N: *Cytodiagnostic urinalysis of renal and lower urinary tract disorders*, New York, 1995, Igaku-Shoin.
9. Bradley M, Schumann GB, Ward PCJ: Examination of urine. In Henry JB, editor: *Todd-Sanford clinical diagnosis by laboratory methods*, ed 16, Philadelphia, 1979, Saunders.
10. *Urinalysis and collection, transportation, and preservation of urine specimens: approved guideline*, ed 2, GP16-A2, Villanova, PA, 2001, NCCLS.
11. Kunin CM: *Detection, prevention and management of urinary tract infections*, ed 2, Philadelphia, 1974, Lea & Febiger.
12. Cohen HT, Spiegel DM: Air-exposed urine dipsticks give false-positive results for glucose and false-negative results for blood, *Am J Clin Pathol* 96:398, 1991.
13. Zweiss MH, Jackson A: Ascorbic acid interference in reagent-strip reactions for assay of urinary glucose and hemoglobin, *Clin Chem* 32:674, 1986.
14. Schweitzer SC, Schumann JL, Schumann GB: Quality assurance guidelines for the urinalysis laboratory, *J Med Technol* 2:567, 1986.
15. Monte-Verde D, Nosanchuk JS: The sensitivity and specificity of nitrite testing for bacteriuria, *Lab Med* 12:755, 1981.
16. Shenoy UA: Current assessment of microhematuria and leukocyturia, *Clin Lab Med* 5:317, 1985.
17. Kusumi RK, Grover PJ, Kunin CM: Rapid detection of pyuria by leukocyte esterase activity, *JAMA* 245:1653, 1981.
18. Gillenwater NY: Detection of urinary leukocytes by Chemstrip-L, *J Urol* 125:383, 1981.
19. Avent J, Schumann GB, Vars L: Comparison of the Chemstrip leukocyte test with a standardized Papanicolaou-stained urine sediment evaluation, *Lab Med* 14:163, 1983.
20. Race GJ, White MG: *Basic urinalysis*, Hagerstown, MD, 1979, Harper & Row.
21. Schumann GB, Greenberg NF: Usefulness of microscopic urinalysis as a screening procedure: a preliminary report, *Am J Clin Pathol* 71:452, 1979.
22. Ferris JA: Comparison and standardization of the urine microscopic examination, *Lab Med* 14:659, 1983.
23. Schumann GB, Tebbs RD: Comparison of slides used for standardized routine microscopic urinalysis, *J Med Technol* 3:54, 1986.
24. Winkel P, Statland BE, Jörgenson K: Urine microscopy: an ill-defined method examined by a multifactorial technique, *Clin Chem* 20:436, 1974.
25. Schumann GB, Weiss MA: *Atlas of renal and urinary tract cytology and its histopathologic bases*, Philadelphia, 1981, Lippincott.
26. Holmquist N: Detection of cancer with urinary sediment, *J Urol* 123:188, 1980.
27. Sternheimer R: A supravital cytodiagnostic stain for urinary sediment, *JAMA* 231:826, 1975.
28. Brody LH, Webster MC, Kark RM: Identification of elements of urinary sediment with phase contrast, *JAMA* 206:1777, 1969.
29. Haber MH: Interference contrast microscopy for identification of urinary sediment, *Am J Clin Pathol* 57:316, 1972.
30. Haber MH: *Urinary sediment: a textbook atlas*, Chicago, 1981, American Society of Clinical Pathologists.
31. Kesson AM, Talbott JM, Gyory AZ: Microscopic examination of urine, *Lancet* 2:809, 1978.
32. Roe CE et al: Evaluation of the Yellow IRIS™: an automated method for urinalysis, *Am J Clin Pathol* 86:661, 1986.
33. Elin RJ et al: Comparison of automated and manual methods for urinalysis, *Am J Clin Pathol* 86:731, 1986.
34. Bard RH: The significance of asymptomatic microhematuria in women and its economic implications: a ten-year study, *Arch Intern Med* 148:2629, 1988.
35. Thal SM et al: Comparison of dysmorphic erythrocytes with other urinary sediment parameters of renal bleeding, *Am J Clin Pathol* 86:784, 1986.
36. Kuster S, Ritz E: Fragmentocytes in the diagnosis of renal hematuria-observations in the 19th century, *Nephrol Dial Transplant* 9:569, 1994.
37. Stapleton FB: Morphology of urinary red blood cells: a simple guide in localizing the site of hematuria, *Pediatr Clin North Am* 34:561, 1987.
38. Kohler H, Wandel E, Brunck B: Acanthocyturia-a characteristic marker for glomerular bleeding, *Kidney Int* 40:115, 1991.
39. Little PJ: A comparison of the urinary white cell concentration with the white cell excretion rate, *Br J Urol* 36:360, 1964.
40. Mandel N: Urinary tract calculi, *Lab Med* 17:449, 1986.
41. Schumann GB, Schumann JL, Schweitzer S: Coordinated approach to the urine sediment examination, *Lab Management* 1:45, 1983.
42. Schweitzer SC, Schumann JL, Schumann GB: A model for educating future urine technologists, *J Med Technol* 2:251, 1986.

Bibliography

Brunzel NA: *Fundamentals of urine and body fluid analysis*, Philadelphia, 1994, Saunders.
McBride LJ: *Textbook of urinalysis and body fluids: a clinical approach*, Philadelphia, 1998, Lippincott Williams & Wilkins.

Ringsrud KM, Linné JJ: *Urinalysis and body fluids: a colortext and atlas*, St Louis, 1995, Mosby.
Strasinger SK, Di Lorenzo MS: *Urinalysis and body fluids*, ed 4, Philadelphia, 2001, FA Davis.

Internet Sites

http://www.ec.upstate.edu/path/Urinalysis/frame.htm—Microscopic Evaluation of Urine Sediment, part of a Pathology course offered by the Department of Pathology to second year medical students. Created and maintained by Jannie Woo, PhD, wooj@upstate.edu, Department of Pathology, Copyright 2000, SUNY Upstate Medical University.
http://www-medlib.med.utah.edu/WebPath/TUTORIAL/TUTORIAL.html —Tutorial from Web Path, the Internet Pathology Laboratory

http://www-medlib.med.utah.edu/WebPath/TUTORIAL/URINE/URINE.html —Urinalysis—Helps students learn the basics of urinalysis
http://www.vh.org/Providers/CME/CLIA/UrineAnalysis/UrineAnalysis.html—Urinalysis tutorial from the virtual hospital—Ruthanna Hyduke, MA, Department of Pathology, University of Iowa Hospitals and Clinics
www3.sympatico.ca/dionrich/Homeng.htm—The Microscopic Examination of Urine—by Michael Dion of Rosemont College in Montreal, Canada

www.lhsc.on.ca/lab/renal/—Pfizer's urinalysis in perspective, link to microphotographs of urinary casts

www.cpmc.columbia.edu/whichis/private/aim/31HEMAT.html—Chapter 31 Microhematuria—Lecture by Dr. Tatyana Z. Morton, MD, Presbyterian Health Care, Columbia University

www.kidney.org/—Kidney Foundation

www.kidney.org/affiliates/ajkd_execsum.pdf—Kidney Foundation—Clinical practice guidelines

www.kidney.org/general/aboutdisease/brochures.cfm—Kidney Foundation disease brochures

www.bayerdiag.com/indcx_flash.phtml—Bayer Diagnostics

www.bayerdiag.com/news/breaking_02.html—Bayer Diagnostics—new dipsticks

Appendixes

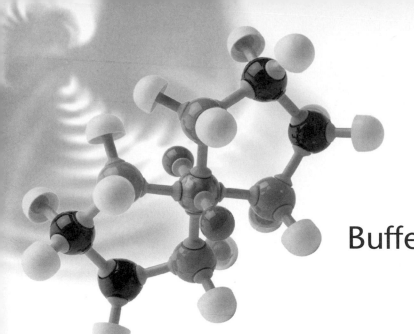

APPENDIX A

Buffer Solutions*

Buffer solutions (or buffers) are solutions whose pH value is to a large degree insensitive to the addition of other substances. It is important to realize, however, that the pH value of a buffer solution does not change only when acids or bases are added or on dilution but also when the temperature changes or when neutral salts are added. In accurate work, therefore, it is important to check the pH value electrometrically after all the ingredients have been added. The extent to which the pH values of buffer solutions vary when acids or bases are added or the temperature changes is shown in the table that follows. In general, dilution to half the concentration changes the pH value by only some hundredths of a unit (buffer No. 1 in the table opposite is an exception in that the change amounts to approximately pH 0.15); addition of 0.1-molar neutral salt solution may change the pH value of approximately 0.1.

---

*This appendix has been compiled by F. Kohler, Department of Physical Chemistry, University of Vienna, and taken from CIBA-Geigy AG, Basel, Switzerland.

In the table the solutions are classified into general buffers (mostly in use for the last 50 years), universal buffers with a low buffering capacity but a wide pH range, and buffers for biological media with a moderate pH range but containing stable ingredients (phosphate and borate, for example, often undergo side reactions with biological media). An important property is often the transparency to ultraviolet light. Occasionally it is desirable to have a volatile buffer, which can be readily removed[1] (examples are buffers Nos. 20 and 21), but the use of very volatile systems makes close control of the pH essential. Most of the pH data found in the literature relate to the Sørensen scale, and it should be noted that the values given in the table opposite are on the conventional pH scale.

Both stock and buffer solutions should be prepared distilled water free of CO_2. Only standard reagents should be used. If there is any doubt as to the purity or water content of solutions, their molarity must be checked by titration. The amounts x of stock solutions required to make up a buffer solution of the desired pH value are given in the second table in Appendix B, p. 1116.

References

1. For a list of volatile buffers see Michl H: In Heftmann E, editor: *Chromatography*, part 1, New York, 1961, Reinhold, p 250.

No.	Name	pH Range	Temperature	pH Change Per °C
General Buffers				
1	KCl/HCl (Clark and Lubs)[1]	1.0 to 2.2	Room	0
2	Glycine/HCl (Sørensen)[2]	1.2 to 3.4	Room	0
3	Na citrate/HCl (Sørensen)[2]	1.2 to 5.0	Room	0
4	K biphthalate/HCl (Clark and Lubs)[1]	2.4 to 4.0	20° C	+0.001
5	K biphthalate/NaOH (Clark and Lubs)[1]	4.2 to 6.2	20° C	
6	Na citrate/NaOH (Sørensen)[2]	5.2 to 6.6	20° C	+0.004
7	Phosphate (Sørensen)[2]	5.0 to 8.0	20° C	−0.003
8	Barbital-Na/HCl (Michaelis)[3]	7.0 to 9.0	18° C	
9	Na borate/HCl (Sørensen)[2]	7.8 to 9.2	20° C	−0.005
10	Glycine/NaOH (Sørensen)[2]	8.6 to 12.8	20° C	−0.025
11	Na borate/NaOH (Sørensen)[2]	9.4 to 10.6	20° C	−0.01
Universal Buffers				
12	Citric acid/phosphate (McIlvaine)[4]	2.2 to 7.8	21° C	
13	Citrate-phosphate-borate/HCl (Teorell and Stenhagen)[5]	2.0 to 12.0	20° C	
14	Britton-Robinson[6]	2.6 to 11.8	25° C	at low pH 0 at high pH −0.02
Buffers for Biological Media				
15	Acetate (Walpole)[7-9]	3.8 to 5.6	25° C	
16	Dimethylglutaric acid/NaOH[10]	3.2 to 7.6	21° C	
17	Piperazine/HCl[11,12]	4.6 to 6.4 8.8 to 10.6	20° C	
18	Tetraethylethylenediamine*[12]	5.0 to 6.8 8.2 to 10.0	20° C	
19	Trismale[7,13]	5.2 to 8.6	23° C	
20	Dimethylaminoethylamine*[12]	5.6 to 7.4 8.6 to 10.4	20° C	
21	Imidazole/HCl[14]	6.2 to 7.8	25° C	
22	Triethanolamine/HCl[15]	7.0 to 8.8	25° C	
23	*N*-Dimethylaminoleucylglycine/NaOH[16]	7.0 to 8.8	23° C	−0.015
24	Tris/HCl[7]	7.2 to 9.0	23° C	−0.02
25	2-Amino-2-methylpropane-1,3-diol/HCl[7,13]	7.8 to 10.0	23° C	
26	Carbonate (Delory and King)[7,17]	9.2 to 10.8	20° C	

From Geigy scientific tables, ed 8, Basel, Switzerland, 1981, CIBA-Geigy AG.
*Can be combined with tris buffer to give a cationic universal buffer (see reference 12).

Table References

1. Clark and Lubs: *J Bact* 2:1, 1917.
2. Sørensen SPL: *Biochem Z* 21:131, 1909, 22:352, 1909; *Ergebn Physiol* 12:393, 1912; and Walbum LE: *Biochem Z* 107:219, 1920.
3. Michaelis L: *J Biol Chem* 87:33, 1930.
4. McIlvaine TC: *J Biol Chem* 49:183, 1921.
5. Teorell and Stenhagen: *Biochem Z* 299:416, 1938.
6. Britton and Welford: *J Chem Soc*, 1937, 1848.
7. Gomori G: In Colowick and Kaplan, editors: *Methods in enzymology*, vol 1, New York, 1955, Academic Press, p 138.
8. Walpole GS: *J Chem Soc* 105: 2501, 1914.
9. Green AA: *J Am Chem Soc* 55:2331, 1933.
10. Stafford et al: *Biochim Biophys Acta* 18:319, 1955; Krebs, HA, unpublished, 1957.
11. Smith and Smith: *Biol Bull* 96:233, 1949.
12. Semenza et al: *Helv Chim Acta* 45:2306, 1962.
13. Gomori G: *Proc Soc Exp Biol* (NY) 68:354, 1948.
14. Mertz and Owen: *Proc Soc Exp Biol* (NY) 43:204, 1940, quoted by Rauen HM, editor: *Biochemisches Taschenbuch*, ed 2, part 2, Berlin, 1964, Springer, p 90.
15. Beisenherz et al: *Z Naturforsch* 8b:555, 1953.
16. Leonis J: *CR Lab Carlsberg*, Sér Chim 26:357, 1948.
17. Delory and King: *Biochem J* 39:245, 1945.

APPENDIX B

Preparation of Buffer Solutions

When not otherwise specified, both stock and buffer solutions should be prepared with water free of CO_2. Only standard reagents should be used. If there is any doubt as to the purity or water content of solutions, their molarity must be checked by titration. The amounts x of stock solutions required to make up a buffer solution of the desired pH value are given in the table on p. 1116.

	STOCK SOLUTIONS		
Buffer No.	A	B	Composition of the Buffer
1	KCl 0.2-N (14.91 g/L)	HCl 0.2-N	25 mL A + x mL B made up to 100 mL
2	Glycine 0.1-molar in NaCl 0.1-N (7.507 g glycine + 5.844 g NaCl/L)	HCl 0.1-N	x mL A + (100 − x) mL B
3	Disodium citrate 0.1-molar (21.01 g $C_6H_8O_7 \cdot 1H_2O$ + 200 mL NaOH 1-N per liter)	HCl 0.1-N	x mL A + (100 − x) mL B
4	Potassium biphthalate 0.1-molar (20.42 g $KHC_8H_4O_4$/L)	HCl 0.1-N	50 mL A + x mL B made up to 100 mL
5	Same as No. 4	NaOH 0.1-N	50 mL A + x mL B made up to 100 mL
6	Same as No. 3	NaOH 0.1-N	x mL A + (100 − x) mL B
7	Monopotassium phosphate $^1/_{15}$-molar (9.073 g KH_2PO_4/L)	Disodium phosphate $^1/_{15}$-molar (11.87 g $Na_2HPO_4 \cdot 2H_2O$/L)	x mL A + (100 − x) mL B
8	Barbital sodium 0.1-molar (20.62 g/L)	HCl 0.1-N	x mL A + (100 − x) mL B
9	Boric acid, half-neutralized, 0.2-molar (corr. to 0.05-molar borax: 12.37 g boric acid + 100 mL NaOH 1-N per liter)	HCl 0.1-N	x mL A + (100 − x) mL B
10	Same as No. 2	NaOH 0.1-N	x mL A + (100 − x) mL B
11	Same as No. 9	NaOH 0.1-N	x mL A + (100 − x) mL B
12	Citric acid 0.1-molar (21.01 g $C_6H_8O_7 \cdot 1H_2O$/L)	Disodium phosphate 0.2-molar (35.60 g $Na_2HPO_4 \cdot 2H_2O$/L)	x mL A + (100 − x) mL B
13	To citric acid and phosphoric acid solutions (ca. 100 mL), each equivalent to 100 mL NaOH 1-N, add 3.54 cryst. orthoboric acid and 343 mL NaOH 1-N, and make up the mixture to 1 liter	HCl 0.1-N	20 mL A + x mL B made up to 100 mL
14	Citric acid, monopotassium phosphate, barbital, boric acid, all 0.02857-molar (6.004 g $C_6H_8O_7 \cdot 1H_2O$, 3.888 g KH_2PO_4, 5.263 g barbital, 1.767 g H_3BO_3/L)	NaOH 0.2-N	100 mL A + x mL B
15	Sodium acetate 0.1-N (8.204 g $C_2H_3O_2Na$ or 13.61 g $C_2H_3O_2Na \cdot 3H_2O$/L)	Acetic acid 0.1-N (6.005 g/L)	x mL A + (100 − x) mL B

From Geigy scientific tables, *ed 8, Basel, Switzerland, 1981, CIBA-Geigy AG.*

	STOCK SOLUTIONS		
Buffer No.	**A**	**B**	**Composition of the Buffer**
16	ββ-Dimethylglutaric acid 0.1-molar (16.02 g/L)	NaOH 0.2-N	(a) 100 mL A + x mL B made up to 1000 mL (b) 100 mL A + x mL B + 5.844 g NaCl made up to 1000 mL (NaCl $\triangleq$ 0.1-molar)
17	Piperazine 1-molar (86.14 g/L)	HCl 0.1-N	5 mL A + x mL B made up to 100 mL
18	Tetraethylethylenediamine 1-molar (172.32 g/L)	HCl 0.1-N	5 mL A + x mL B made up to 100 mL
19	Tris acid maleate 0.2-molar (24.23 g tris[hydroxymethyll]aminomethane + 23.21 g maleic acid or 19.61 g maleic anhydride/L)	NaOH 0.2-N	25 mL A + x mL B made up to 100 mL
20	Dimethylaminoethylamine 1-molar (88 g/L)	HCl 0.1-N	5 mL A + x mL B made up to 100 mL
21	Imidazole 0.2-molar (13.62 g/L)	HCl 0.1-N	25 mL A + x mL B made up to 100 mL
22	Triethanolamine 0.5-molar (76.11 g/L) containing 20 g/L ethylenediaminetetraacetic acid disodium salt ($C_{10}H_{14}O_8N_2Na_2\cdot2H_2O$)	HCl 0.05-N	10 mL A + x mL B made up to 100 mL
23	N-Dimethylaminoleucylglycine 0.1-molar (24.33 g $C_{10}H_{20}O_3N_2\cdot{}^3/_2H_2O$/L) containing NaCl 0.2-N (11.69 g/L)	NaOH 1-N 100 mL made up to 1 liter with A	x mL A + $(100-x)$ mL B
24	Tris 0.2-molar (24.23 g tris[hydroxymethyl]aminomethane/L)	HCl 0.1-N	25 mL A + x mL B made up to 100 mL
25	2-Amino-2-methylpropane-1,3-diol 0.1-molar (10.51 g/L)	HCl 0.1-N	50 mL A + x mL B made up to 100 mL
26	Sodium carbonate anhydrous 0.1-molar (10.60 g/L)	Sodium bicarbonate 0.1-molar (8.401 g/L)	x mL A + $(100-x)$ mL B

The table gives the amounts (x mL) of the stock solutions listed in the first part of Appendix B required to make up a buffer solution of the desired pH value.

pH	1	2	3	4	5	6	7	8	9	10	11	12	13	14	15	16a	16b	17	18	19	20	21	22	23	24	25	26	pH
1.0	54.2																											1.0
1.2	36.0	11.1	9.0																									1.2
1.4	23.2	26.4	17.9																									1.4
1.6	14.7	36.2	23.6																									1.6
1.8	9.3	43.9	27.6										74.4															1.8
2.0	5.9	50.7	30.2										68.8															2.0
2.2	3.8	56.5	32.2									98.8	64.6															2.2
2.4		62.3	34.1	41.0								94.5	61.3	1.6														2.4
2.6		68.4	36.0	34.1								90.0	58.9	3.6														2.6
2.8		74.7	37.9	27.8								85.1	56.9	5.7		7.0												2.8
3.0		81.0	39.9	21.6								80.3	55.2	7.8		13.3												3.0
3.2		86.2	42.1	15.9								76.0	53.9	9.9		20.7	14.4											3.2
3.4		90.3	44.8	10.9								72.0	51.8	11.7		26.3	20.9											3.4
3.6			47.8	6.7								68.4	50.7	13.5	10.9	32.4	26.8											3.6
3.8			51.2	3.3								65.1	49.7	15.3	16.6	36.2	32.4											3.8
4.0			55.1	0.0								62.0	48.6	17.5	23.9	39.3	36.6											4.0
4.2			60.0		3.0							59.1	47.5	19.7	33.5	41.3	40.3											4.2
4.4			66.4		6.7							56.4	45.4	21.9	44.9	43.5	43.1											4.4
4.6			74.9		11.1							53.7	44.3	24.1	56.6	45.7	45.7	94.3										4.6
4.8			85.6		16.5							51.2	43.2	26.3	67.8	48.4	48.3	91.5	94.3									4.8
5.0			100.0		22.6							49.0	42.0	28.6	76.8	51.3	51.5	87.8	91.5									5.0
5.2					28.8	87.1	99.2					46.9	40.8	31.0	84.0	55.0	53.6	83.6	87.8	3.2								5.2
5.4					34.4	78.0	98.4					44.7	39.7	33.4	89.3	58.8	63.6	77.6	83.1	5.0								5.4
5.6					39.1	70.3	97.3					42.4	38.4	35.8		63.9	68.7	71.8	77.6	7.3	94.3							5.6
5.8					42.4	64.5	95.5					40.0	37.0	38.3		69.5	73.6	66.5	71.7	9.7	91.7							5.8
6.0					45.0	60.3	92.8					37.4	35.6	40.8		74.1	78.5	61.8	66.4	12.4	88.0							6.0
6.2					46.7	57.2	88.9					34.5	34.2	43.3		83.5	83.3	58.2	61.7	15.2	83.3	43.4						6.2
6.4						54.8	83.0					31.4	32.9	45.8		87.4	87.4	55.5	58.0	17.9	77.9	40.4						6.4
6.6						53.2	75.4					27.9	31.7	48.3		90.0	91.0		55.3	20.8	72.0	36.5						6.6
6.8							65.3					23.5	30.6	50.9		91.8	93.2			22.2	66.6	31.4		86.4				6.8
7.0							53.4	53.3				19.0	29.6	53.4		93.0	94.9			23.7	61.9	25.4	86.2	80.6				7.0
7.2							41.3	55.0				13.8	28.8	55.8		93.8	95.8			25.2	58.1	19.6	79.6	72.8				7.2
7.4							29.6	57.6				9.8	28.1	58.2			96.8			26.7	55.3	14.6	71.3	63.2	44.7			7.4
7.6							19.7	60.8				6.8	27.6	60.5						28.6		10.2	62.0	52.1	42.0			7.6
7.8							12.8	65.2	53.0			4.6	27.0	62.8						31.2		6.6	52.0	41.1	39.3			7.8
8.0							7.4	70.6	55.4				26.3	65.0						33.9			42.0	31.4	33.7	43.9		8.0
8.2							3.7	75.9	58.0				25.2	67.2					46.4	36.9			31.9	22.9	27.9	41.6		8.2
8.4								81.2	62.1				24.0	69.3				45.5	43.9	39.9			22.5	15.9	22.9	38.4		8.4
8.6								86.2	66.9	94.7			22.6	71.3				43.2	40.9	42.7	45.4		16.0	10.3	17.3	34.8		8.6
8.8								90.1	73.6	92.0			21.4	73.2				40.0	36.8		42.8		11.7		13.0	30.7		8.8
9.0								93.2	83.5	88.4			20.2	75.1				35.8	31.8		39.2				8.8	23.3		9.0
9.2									95.6	84.0			19.0	77.0				30.8	26.2		34.7				5.3	17.7	10.0	9.2
9.4										78.9	87.0		18.1	78.8				25.0	20.4		29.3					13.3	18.4	9.4
9.6										73.2	75.5		17.1	80.4				19.4	15.2		23.6					9.2	29.3	9.6
9.8										67.2	65.1		16.5	81.8				14.3	10.8		19.0					5.2	42.0	9.8
10.0										62.5	59.6		16.0	83.1				10.0	7.4		13.1					4.1	53.4	10.0
10.2										58.8	56.4		15.5	84.3				6.9			9.2					2.3	63.7	10.2
10.4										55.7	54.1		14.7	85.4							6.2						73.1	10.4
10.6										53.6	52.3		13.5	86.5													81.2	10.6
10.8										52.2			11.7	87.8													87.9	10.8
11.0										51.2			9.1	89.3														11.0
11.2										50.4			5.5	91.3														11.2
11.4										49.5			1.3	94.5														11.4
11.6										48.7				99.0														11.6
11.8										47.6																		11.8
12.0										46.0																		12.0
12.2										43.2																		12.2
12.4										39.1																		12.4
12.6										31.8																		12.6
12.8										21.4																		12.8

From Geigy scientific tables, ed 8, Basel, Switzerland, 1981, CIBA-Geigy AG.

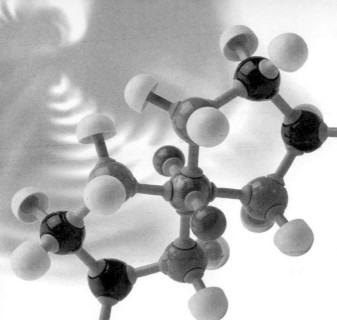

Concentrations of Common Acids and Bases

Compound	Molecular Weight	Specific Gravity	Weight %	Normality	mL/Liter for 1N* Solution
HCl	36.46	1.19	36.0	11.7	85.5
HNO_3	63.02	1.42	69.5	15.6	64.0
H_2SO_4	98.08	1.84	96.0	35.9	28.4
CH_3COOH	60.03	1.06	99.5	17.6	56.9
NH_4OH	35.04	0.90	58.6	15.1	66.5
H_3PO_4	98.00	1.69	85.0	44.1	22.7
Thioglycolic acid	92.12	1.26	80.0	10.9	91.3
HCOOH	46.03	1.21	97.0	25.5	39.2
	46.03	1.19	88.0	22.7	44.1
$HClO_4$	100.50	1.67	70.0	11.65	85.7
Pyridine	79.10	0.98	100.0	12.4	80.6
2-Mercaptoethanol	78.13	1.14	100.0	14.6	68.5

From Brewer JM, Pesce AJ, Ashworth H: Experimental techniques in biochemistry, Engelwood Cliffs, NJ, 1974, Prentice-Hall, Inc.
To calculate concentration (c) from the weight percent (w) of a compound, use the formula:

$$\frac{10\ ws}{M} = c$$

M, Molecular weight; s, specific gravity.
*Remember, the normality (N) is not the same as the molarity (M) for sulfuric and phosphoric acid.

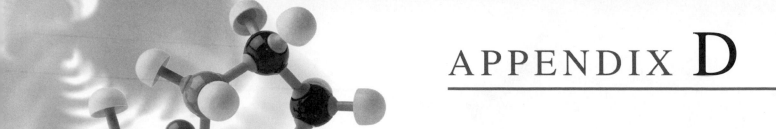

APPENDIX D

Gases in Common Laboratory Use—Technical Information

Product	Formula	State	CYLINDER SPECIFICATIONS				THERMOPHYSICAL PROPERTIES		
			CGA No. Valve Outlet	Highest Purity Grade (%)	Cylinder Size (Cubic Feet)	Approximate Cylinder Pressure (psi)	Molecular Weight	Vapor Pressure at 21.1° C (psig)	Specific Gravity at 21.1° C (1 atm)
Acetylene	C_2H_2	Dissolved gas (in acetone)	510/300	99.6	3 to 5	250	26.04	635	0.095
Air		Compressed gas	346/677	Mixture	200 to 500	2200 to 6000	28.96		1
Carbon dioxide	CO_2	Liquefied gas	320	99.999	2 to 6	274 to 838	44.01	839	1.53
Carbon monoxide	CO	Compressed gas	350	99.99	2 to 6	315 to 1602	28.01	*	0.97
Helium	He	Compressed gas	580/677	99.9999	200 to 300	2200 to 2640	4.003	*	0.138
Hydrogen	H_2	Compressed gas	350	99.9995	2 to 200	323 to 2200	2.02	*	0.0695
Methane	CH_4	Compressed gas	350	99.992	12	780 to 2000	16.04	*	0.555
Nitrogen	N_2	Compressed gas	580/677	99.999	30 to 200	2200 to 2640	28.01	*	0.967
Oxygen	O_2	Compressed gas	540	99.995	30 to 200	2200 to 2640	32.0	*	1.105
Propane	C_3H_8	Liquefied gas	510	99.98	12	109	44.1	109	1.55

Data derived from the Airco Industrial Cases catalogue, Murray Hill, NJ, 1977.
SA, Simple asphyxiant.
*Above critical temperature at 21.1° C.

THERMOPHYSICAL PROPERTIES			HAZARDOUS PROPERTIES			
			FLAMMABILITY			
Critical Temperature (°C)	*Critical Pressure (psia)*	*Specific Volume (cf/lb)*	*Flammable Limits in Air (vol %)*	*Ignition Temperature (°C)*	*Physiological Properties*	*Threshold Limit Value (ppm)*
35.1	890	14.7	2.3 to 100	305		SA
		13.3			Oxidant	
31.0	1071	8.74			Inert	5000
−140.0	507.4	13.8	12.5 to 74	651.1	Toxic	50
−267.8	33.2	96.7				SA
−239.98	190.8	192	4 to 75	585		SA
−82.1	673	23.7	5 to 15	538		SA
−146.9	492.9	13.8			Inert	SA
−118.4	736.9	12.1			Oxidant	
96.8	617.4	8.5	2.1 to 9.5	468		SA

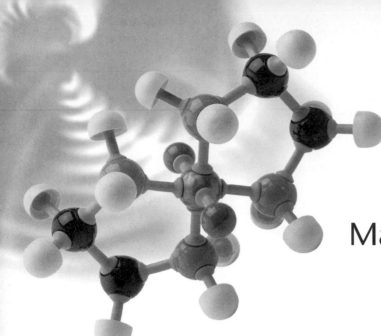

Major Plasma Proteins*

Protein	Molecular Weight	Concentration, mg/100mL	Electrophoretic† Mobility	Biological Function
Prealbumins				
Thyroxine-binding (TBPA)	55,000	10 to 40	7.6	Thyroxine transport
Retinol-binding (RBP)	21,000	3 to 6		Vitamin A transport
Albumin	66,300	3500 to 5500	5.92	Maintain osmotic pressure, transport of bilirubin, free fatty acids, anions, and cations, cell nutrition
α_1 Globulins				
α_1 Acid glycoprotein (α_1 S)	40,000	55 to 140	5.7	Unknown, inactivates progesterone
α_1 Antitrypsin (α_1 AT)	54,000	200 to 400	5.42	Antiserine type of protease
α_1 Glycoprotein (9.55, α_1M)	308,000	3 to 8	α_1	Unknown
α_1 Glycoprotein B (α_1B)	50,000	15 to 30	α_1	Unknown
α_1 Glycoprotein T (α_1T)	60,000	5 to 12	α_1	Unknown, tryptophan-poor
α_1 Antichymotrypsin (α_1X)	68,000	30 to 60	α_1	Chymotrypsin inhibitor
α_1 Lipoproteins, high density (HDL)	28,000	254 to 387	α_1	Lipid transport
α_2 Globulin				
G_0 Globulin (Gc)	51,000	40 to 70	α_2	Vitamin D transport
Ceruloplasmin (Cp)	134,000	15 to 60	4.6	Copper transport, peroxidase activity
α_2 Glycoprotein, histidine rich (HRG)	58,000	5 to 15	α_2	Unknown
Zn-α_2-glycoprotein (Znα_2)	41,000	2 to 15	4.2	Unknown, binds Zn^{2+}
α_2 HS-glycoprotein (α_2HS)	49,000	40 to 85	4.2	Unknown, binds Ba^{2+}
α_2 Macroglobulin (α_2M)	725,000	150 to 420	4.2	Inhibitor of thrombin, trypsin, and pepsin
Transcortin (TC)	49,500	<7	α_2	Cortisol transport
Haptoglobins (Hp)				
Type 1-1	100,000	100 to 200	4.1	Binds hemoglobin, prevents loss of iron
Type 2-1	200,000	160 to 300	α_2	
Type 2-2	400,000	120 to 260	α_2	
α_2 Lipoproteins (VLDL)	250,000	150 to 230	Pre-β	Lipid transport
Thyroxine-binding protein (TBG)	58,000	1 to 2	α_2	Thyroxine transport
β Globulins				
Hemopexin (Hpx)	57,000	50 to 100	3.1	Binds heme
Transferrin (Tf)	76,500	200 to 320	3.1	Iron transport
β Lipoproteins (LDL)	250,000	280 to 440	3.1	Lipid transport
C4 Complement component (C4)	206,000	40 to 80	β_1	Complement system
β_2 Microglobulin ($\beta_2\mu$)	11,818	Trace	β_2	Common portion of the HLA transplantation antigen
β_2 Glycoprotein I (β_2 I)	40,000	15 to 30	1.6	Unknown

Protein	Molecular Weight	Concentration, mg/100mL	Electrophoretic[†] Mobility	Biological Function
β_2 Glycoprotein II (GGG)	63,000	12 to 30	β_2	C3 activator (activates properidin)
β_2 Glycoprotein III (β_2III)	35,000	5 to 15	β_2	Unknown
C-Reactive protein (CRP)	118,000	1	β_2	Opsonin, motivates phagocytosis in inflammatory disease
C3 Complement component (C3)	180,000	55 to 180	β_2	Complement system
Fibrinogen (ϕ, Fib.)	341,000	200 to 600	2.1	Blood clotting
γ Globulins				
Immunoglobulin M (IgM)	950,000	60 to 250	2.1	Antibodies, early response
Immunoglobulin E (IgE)	190,000	0.06	2.1	Reagin of the allergy system
Immunoglobulin A (IgA)	160,000	90 to 450	2.1	Tissue antibodies
Immunoglobulin D (IgD)	160,000	15	1.9	Cell surface and plasma antibodies
Immunoglobulin G (IgG)	160,000	800 to 1800	1.2	Antibodies, long range

From Natelson S, Natelson EA: Principles of applied chemistry, *vol 3, New York, 1980, Plenum Publishing Corp.*
*Does not include clotting factors, complement factors, or enzymes except fibrinogen, C3, and C4 of complement, which occur in substantial concentrations.
[†]Tiselius moving boundary electrophoresis in Tiselius units (cm^2 V^{-1} sec^{-1} $\times$ 10^5, at 0° C, ph 8.6, and ionic strength 0.15).

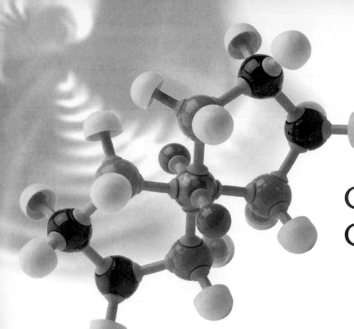

Conversions Between Conventional and SI Units

Conventional Units		× Factor	= SI Units	Conventional Units		× Factor	= SI Units
Gram	g/mL	$\dfrac{10^{15}}{mw}$	pmol/L	Milligram	mg/100 mL	10^{-2}	g/L
	g/100 mL	10	g/L		mg/100 mL	$\dfrac{10^{-2}}{mw}$	mol/L
	g/100 mL	$\dfrac{10}{mw}$	mol/L		mg/100 mL	$\dfrac{10}{mw}$	mmol/L
	g/100 mL	$\dfrac{10^4}{mw}$	mmol/L		mg/100 mL	$\dfrac{10^4}{mw}$	μmol/L
	g/d	$\dfrac{1}{mw}$	mol/d		mg/100 g	10	mg/kg
	g/d	$\dfrac{10^3}{mw}$	mmol/d		mg/100 g	$\dfrac{10}{mw}$	mmol/kg
	g/d	$\dfrac{10^9}{mw}$	nmol/d		mg/d	$\dfrac{1}{mw}$	mmol/d
					mg/d	$\dfrac{10^3}{mw}$	μmol/d
Microgram	μg/100 mL	$\dfrac{10}{mw}$	μmol/L	Milliliter	mL/100 g	10	mL/kg
	μg/d	$\dfrac{1}{mw}$	μmol/d		mL/min	1.667×10^{-2}	mL/s
	μg/d	$\dfrac{10^3}{mw}$	nmol/d	Millimeters of mercury	mm Hg	1.333	mbar
Picogram	pg	$\dfrac{10^3}{mw}$	fmol		mm Hg	0.133	kPa
	pg/mL	$\dfrac{10^3}{mw}$	pmol/L	Minute	min	60	s
					min	0.06	ks
Milliequivalent	mEq/L	$\dfrac{1}{valence}$	mmol/L	Percent	%	10^{-2}	1(unit)
	mEq/kg	$\dfrac{1}{valence}$	mmol/kg		% (g/100 g)	10	g/kg
	mEq/d	$\dfrac{1}{valence}$	mmol/d		% (g/100 g)	10^{-2}	kg/kg
					% (g/100 mL)	10	g/L
					% (g/100 mL)	$\dfrac{10}{mw}$	mol/L
					% (g/100 mL)	$\dfrac{10^4}{mw}$	mmol/L
					% (mL/100 mL)	10^{-2}	L/L

Modified from Campbell JM, Campbell JB: Laboratory mathematics, ed 3, St Louis, 1983, Mosby.
d, Day; Eq, equivalent; g, gram; L, liter; min, minute; mw, molecular weight; Pa, pascal; s, second. f, Femto (10^{-15}); p, pico (10^{-12}); n, nano (10^{-9}); μ, micro (10^{-6}); m, milli (10^{-3}); k, kilo (10^3).

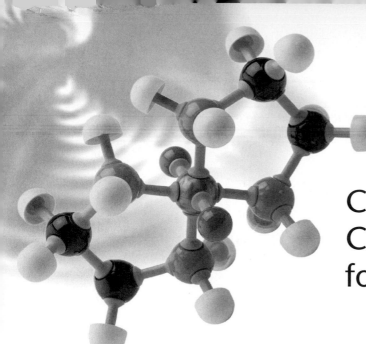

Conversions Between Conventional and SI Units for Specific Analytes

Analyte	Conventional Units	MULTIPLY BY		SI Unit
		Conventional to SI	*SI to Conventional*	
Acetominophen	μg/mL	6.61	0.151	μmol/L
Albumin	g/100 mL	144.9	0.0069	μmol/L
Ammonia	μg/100 mL	0.59	1.7	μmol/L
Anticonvulsant drugs				
Carbamazepine	μg/mL	4.32	0.23	μmol/L
Ethosuximide	μg/mL	7.08	0.14	μmol/L
Phenobarbital	μg/mL	4.31	0.23	μmol/L
Phenytoin	μg/mL	3.96	0.25	μmol/L
Primidone	μg/mL	4.58	0.22	μmol/L
Valproic acid	μg/mL	6.93	0.14	μmol/L
Bilirubin	mg/100 mL	17.1	0.059	μmol/L
Bromide	μg/mL	0.0125	80	mmol/L
Calcium	mg/100 mL	0.25	4	mmol/L
Chloride	mEq/L	1	1	mmol/L
Cholesterol	mg/100 mL	0.026	38.7	mmol/L
Cortisol	μg/100 mL	0.0276	36.2	μmol/L
Creatinine	mg/100 mL	88.4	0.0113	μmol/L
Digoxin	ng/mL	1.28	0.781	nmol/L
Estriol	μg/L	3.47	0.288	nmol/L
Ferritin	μg/L	2.2	0.445	pmol/L
Folic acid	μg/100 mL	22.7	0.044	nmol/L
Gentamicin	μg/mL	2.22	0.45	μmol/L
Glucose	mg/100 mL	0.055	18	mmol/L
Haptoglobin	mg/100 mL	0.118	8.47	μmol/L
HDL cholesterol	mg/100 mL	0.026	38.7	mmol/L
hCG	U/L	—	—	—
5-HIAA	mg	5.23	0.19	μmol/L
Ig A	mg/100 mL	0.0625	16	μmol/L
D	mg/100 mL	0.054	18.5	μmol/L
E	ng/mL	0.005	200	nmol/L
G	mg/100 mL	0.067	15	μmol/L
M	mg/100 mL	0.011	91	μmol/L
Insulin	pg/mL	0.174	5.74	nmol/L
	μU/mL	7.25	0.138	nmol/L
Iron	μg/100 mL	0.179	5.58	μmol/L
Ketones (acetoacetate)	mg/L	0.111	9.01	mmol/L

| Analyte | Conventional Units | MULTIPLY BY | | SI Unit |
		Conventional to SI	SI to Conventional	
Lead	μg/L	4.83	0.207	nmol/L
Lithium	mEq/L	1	1	mmol/L
LDL cholesterol	mg/100 mL	0.026	38.7	mmol/L
Magnesium	mg/100 mL	0.41	2.43	mmol/L
Phosphorus	mg/100 mL	0.323	3.1	mmol/L
Phenylalanine	mg/L	6.05	0.165	μmol/L
Potassium	mEq/L	1	1	mmol/L
Quinidine	μg/mL	3.09	0.324	μmol/L
Salicylate	mg/100 mL	0.0724	13.8	mmol/L
Sodium	mEq/L	1	1	mmol/L
TIBC	μg/100 mL	0.179	5.58	μmol/L
Theophylline	μg/mL	5.55	0.180	μmol/L
Thyroid-stimulating hormone	mU/L	—	—	—
Thyroxine	μg/100 mL	12.9	0.078	nmol/L
Transferrin	mg/100 mL	0.11	9.09	μmol/L
Triglycerides	mg/100 mL	0.0114	87.5	mmol/L
Urea	mg/100 mL	0.166	6.01	mmol/L
Urea N	mg/100 mL	0.356	2.81	mmol/L
Uric acid	mg/100 mL	59.5	0.0168	μmol/L
Vanillylmandelic acid	mg	5.03	0.20	μmol
VLDL cholesterol	mg/100 mL	0.026	38.7	mmol/L
Vitamin B_{12}	pg/mL	0.738	1.36	pmol/L
Gases	mm Hg	0.133	7.51	kPa
Enzymes	U/L	1.67×10^{-8}	0.6×10^{8}	katal/L

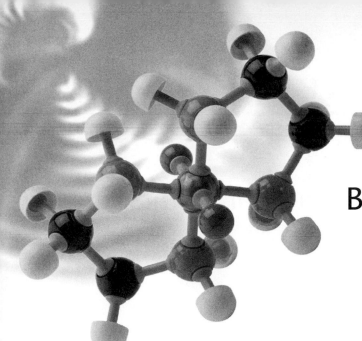

Body Surface of Children

NOMOGRAM FOR DETERMINATION OF BODY SURFACE FROM HEIGHT AND MASS*

Height	Body Surface	Mass

Height	Body Surface	Mass
cm 120 — 47 in	1.10 m²	kg 40.0 — 90 lb
46	1.05	85
115 — 45	1.00	35.0 — 80
44	0.95	75
110 — 43	0.90	70
42	0.85	30.0 — 65
105 — 41	0.80	60
40		25.0 — 55
100 — 39	0.75	
38	0.70	50
95 — 37		20.0 — 45
36	0.65	40
90 — 35		
34	0.60	35
85 — 33		
32	0.55	15.0 — 30
80 — 31	0.50	
30		
75 — 29	0.45	25
28		
70 — 27	0.40	10.0 — 20
26		9.0
65 — 25	0.35	8.0
24		7.0 — 15
60 — 23		6.0
22	0.30	
55 — 21		5.0
20	0.25	4.5 — 10
50 — 19		4.0 — 9
18		3.5 — 8
45 — 17	0.20	
16	0.19	3.0 — 7
0.18		
40 — 16	0.17	6
15	0.16	
0.15	2.5	
14	0.14	5
35 —	0.13	
13	0.12	2.0 — 4
12	0.11	
30 —	0.10	1.5 — 3
11	0.09	
0.08		
cm 25 — 10 in	0.074 m²	kg 1.0 — 2.2 lb

From Geigy scientific tables, ed 8, Basel, Switzerland, 1981, CIBA-Geigy AG.
*From the formula of Du Bois and Du Bois: Arch Intern Med 17:863, 1916: $S = M^{0.725} \times H^{0.725} \times 71.84$, or $\log S = \log M \times 0.425 + \log H \times 0.725 + 1.8564$ (S, body surface in cm²; M, mass in kg; H, height in cm).

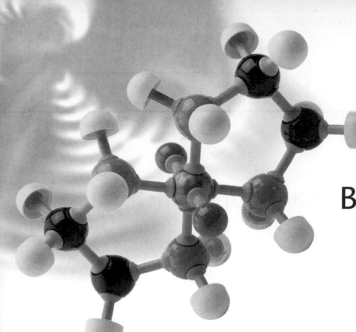

APPENDIX I

Body Surface of Adults

NOMOGRAM FOR DETERMINATION OF BODY SURFACE FROM HEIGHT AND MASS*

Height	Body Surface	Mass

Height:
cm 200 — 79 in
78
195 — 77
76
190 — 75
74
185 — 73
72
180 — 71
70
175 — 69
68
170 — 67
66
165 — 65
64
160 — 63
62
155 — 61
60
150 — 59
58
145 — 57
56
140 — 55
54
135 — 53
52
130 — 51
50
125 — 49
48
120 — 47
46
115 — 45
44
110 — 43
42
105 — 41
40
cm100 — 39 in

Body Surface:
2.80 m²
2.70
2.60
2.50
2.40
2.30
2.20
2.10
2.00
1.95
1.90
1.85
1.80
1.75
1.70
1.65
1.60
1.55
1.50
1.45
1.40
1.35
1.30
1.25
1.20
1.15
1.10
1.05
1.00
0.95
0.90
0.86 m²

Mass:
kg 150 — 330 lb
145 — 320
140 — 310
135 — 300
130 — 290
125 — 280
120 — 270
115 — 260
110 — 250
105 — 240
100 — 230
95 — 220
90 — 210
85 — 200
80 — 190
75 — 180
70 — 170
65 — 160
60 — 150
55 — 140
50 — 130
45 — 120
40 — 110
35 — 100
kg 30 — 66 lb

From Geigy scientific tables, ed 8, Basel, Switzerland, 1981, CIBA-Geigy AG.
*From the formula of Du Bois and Du Bois: Arch Intern Med 17:863, 1916: $S = M^{0.725} \times H^{0.725} \times 71.84$, or $\log S = \log M \times 0.425 + \log H \times 0.725 + 1.8564$ (S, body surface in cm²; M, mass in kg; H, height in cm).

Index

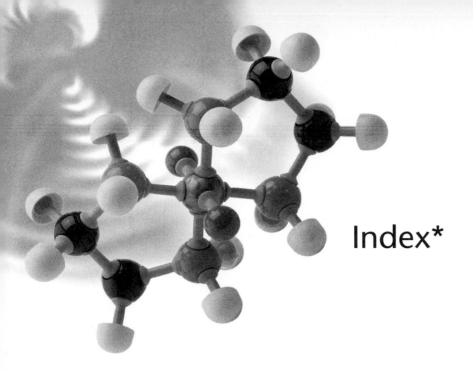

Index*

A

A bands, 568
A. *See* Alanine
Abdominal paracentesis fluid, 780
Abeta-lipoproteinemia, 626
Abnormal chromosomes
 pathological disorders associated with, 915
Abnormalities, 362, 364, 387
 examples of identified genetic, 996*t*
Absorbance, 37, 84, 85, 430
 blank, *432*
 delta, 432
 percentage of transmittance and, *428*
 relationship between transmittance and, 87-88, *88*
 true, 87
Absorbance detection, 148-149
Absorbance error, 429*t*
 absorbance v., *429*
Absorbance variance, 428
Absorption, 553, 1074
 calcium, 554
 carbohydrate, 554
 fat, 554
 iron, 554
 protein, 554
 sodium, 554
 vitamin D, E, A, and K, 554
Absorption process, 86-87
Absorption rate constant, 1074, 1082
Absorption spectrophotometer, 428
Absorption spectroscopy, 87-94, *88*

Absorption spectrum, 84, 86, *1052*
 of oxyhemoglobin, *87*
Absorptive phase, 605
absorptivity, 84
 molar, 85, 88
Abused drugs, 989
Acamprosate, 654
Accelerating voltage, 171
Acceptance regions for rank sum T, 355, 355*t*
Accession number, 324
Accuracy, 340, 348, 402
 control required by CLIA'88, 397-398
Acetaldehyde-modified hemoglobin, 653
Acetaminophen, 1007
Acetone bodies, 265
Acetylcholine, 792
Achlorhydria, 550
Acid-base balance, 466-467, 483
Acid-base control, 463
Acid-base disorders, 469-474
 classes of disorders, 473*t*
 definitions, 469
Acidemia, 462, 470
Acidosis, 441, 457, 462, 470, 471-473
Acinar, 535
 causes of acinar cell loss, *545*
 diagram of, *537*
Acromegaly, 581, 590, 809, 821
ACTH, 825, 877, 892-893
 stimulation tests, 897
ACTH excess, 824
Actin, 566, 569

---

*NOTE: Page numbers in *italics* indicate figures; *t*, tables.

Summation circuit, 188, 196
Support, 130
Surfactant, 463, 466, 762, *763*
 composition of, *762*
Sustrate-depletion phase, 1045
Synapse, 788, 793
Syncytium, 567
Syndrome of inappropriate antidiuretic hormone
 secretion (SIADH), 443, 453
Synergistic effects, 990, 997
Synovial fluid, 780, 784
 normal, 784
 pathological classification of, 785*t*
 physical and chemical characteristics of, 784*t*
Synthase, 1050
Synthesis, 608, *608*
Synthetic pathway, 664
Syringe, 4, 13-14
System maintenance, 334
Systematic analytical error, 404
Systematic error, 341, 403
 estimation of, from comparison-of-methods study,
 416
Système International d'Unités (SI), 4, 1045, 1055
Systemic bias, 381
Systemic involvement, 648
 cancer, 648
 central and peripheral nervous system, 648
 endocrine effects, 649
 heart, 648
 hematopoietic effects, 649
 immune effects, 649
Systemic lupus erythematosus, 780, 785

T

t, 1074
T$_3$, 828, 843
 or cytomel suppression test, 843
T$_4$, 828, 843
Table maintenance, 323
Tachycardia, 574, 658, 666
Tacrolimus (FK506), 973, 976, 984-985
Tandem mass spectrometry, 172, *184*, 184-185
Tapes, 332
Target value, 381
Tay-Sachs disease, 909, 921, *921*
TBEP (tris[2-butoxyethyl] phosphate), 65, *65*, 69
TBG. *See* Thyroxine-binding globulin (TBG)
T-cells, 973
TDM. *See* Therapeutic drug monitoring (TDM)
Technetium 99m, 567
Technical supervisor, 50

Teflon, 10
Teflon tubing, 10
Temperature, 1058
Terminal disposition rate, 1074, 1082
Tertiary structure, 1025, 1045, 1046
Test menu, 288
Test method, 404, 405
Test repertoire, 288, 295
Test results comparison of, 62-63
Test utilization, 60
Testes, *865*
 disorders of the, 867
 early development, 864
 mature, 865
 structural organization, 865
 normal, 864
Testicular feminization syndrome, 850, 870
Testicular hyperfunction, 870
Testing system, 381
Testis determining factor, 911
Testosterone, *820*, 850
 synthesis and secretion of, 866
 transport of, 866
Tests
 performed average cost per, 60
Tetramer, 1065
Thalassemia, 658, 662, 676
 classification of, 688
 definition of, 688
α-Thalassemia, 676, 688, 689
 laboratory findings in, 688*t*
β-Thalassemia, 676, 689
Thallium 201, 567
Theophylline
 Calibration curve for, using internal standard
 technique, *135*
 method selection and, 410*t*
 recommended values for, 1100
 specimen, 1111
 therapeutic ranges, 1111
Theoretical plate number, 108, 114-115
Therapeutic dose, 990, 997
Therapeutic drug monitoring (TDM), 1073-1091
 basic overview of principles, 1075-1079
 clinical indications for, 1087
 clinical settings requiring, 1088
 concept of therapeutic range, 1075-1076
 fate of drug and need for, 1075-1079
 sampling and frequency of drug monitoring,
 1088
Therapeutic lifestyle change, 620
Therapeutic range, 1074, 1086

Analyte	EXPECTED ADULT REFERENCE OR THERAPEUTIC RANGE		Clinical Correlation Range (Page)
	Conventional Units	SI Units	
Fat absorption	<5% of ingested fat is excreted	—	535, 549
Folic acid (S)	1.9-14 ng/mL	4.3-31.7 nmol/L	722
Follicle-stimulating hormone (FSH)	Women		492
	Follicular 2-11 mIU/mL		
	Ovulation 7-25 mIU/mL		
	Luteal phase 2-10 mIU/mL		
	Postmenopausal 20-120 mIU/L		
	Men 2-10 mIU/mL		492
Gamma-glutamyl transferase (S)	Age and gender related; see CD-ROM		492
Gastric fluid analysis	Basal and maximum acid output; see Table, p. 557		535, 549
Glucose (S)	700-1050 mg/L	3.9-5.8 mmol/L	580
Glycosylated hemoglobin (A_{1c}) (B)	4% to 6%		580
Haptoglobin (S)	600-2000 mg/L	7.0-31.8 μmol/L	675
Hemoglobin F (B)	0.6-1.0% of total hemoglobin		675
Hemoglobin separation and quantitation (B)	(see p. 692)		675
High density lipoprotein cholesterol (S); see Cholesterol			
Homocysteine (S)	95th percentile	13-18 μmol/L	603, 722
(P)	(upper limit)	10-15 μmol/L	
Immunoelectrophoresis; see interpretation, Chapter 12			960
Immunoglobulin quantitation (S); age dependent, see CD-ROM			960
	Adult levels:		
IgA	1.4-3.5 mg/mL	8.7-21.9 μmol/L	
IgD	0-0.14 mg/mL	<0.76 μmol/L	
IgE	<300 ng/mL	<1.5 nmol/L	
IgG	8.0-16 mg/mL	53-106 μmol/L	
IgM	0.5-2.0 mg/mL	0.56-2.2 μmol/L	
Insulin (S)	<25 μU/mL (1042 pg/mL)	0.17 pmol/mL	580
Iron (S)	400-1600 μg/L	7.16-28.6 μmol/L	657
Lactate dehydrogenase (S)	90-320 P→L U/L (method dependent)	$1.5\text{-}3.3 \times 10^{-6}$ katal/L	566
Lactate dehydrogenase isoenzymes (S)	LD, 17%-31%; LD_2, 35%-48%; LD_3, 15%-29%, LD_4, 4%-9%; LD_5, 3%-10%		566, 1064
Lactic acid (S)	<250 mg/L	<2.8 mmol/L	462
Lead (B)	<600 μg/L adult	2.9 μmol/L	708, 989
	<100 μg/L child	<0.48 μmol/L	
Lecithin/sphingomyelin ration (A)	>2.0 indicates fetal lung maturity		753
	>55 mg/g albumin indicates fetal lung maturity		
Lipase (S)	<200 U/L turbidimetric	$<3.3 \times 10^{-6}$ katal/L	535
	<60 U/L colorimetric	$<1.0 \times 10^{-6}$ katal/L	
Lipoprotein electrophoresis (P)	Children MF 55% ± 5% β 12% ± 3% pre-β 33% ± 3% α		603
	Adults (18-65) M 65% ± 8% β 12% ± 4% pre-β 23% ± 4% α		
	Adults (18-65) F 60% ± 6% β 8% ± 4 % pre-β 32% ± 5% α		
Lithium (S)	0.4-1.5 mmol/L	0.4-1.5 mmol/L	787, 1073
Luteinizing hormone (LH)	Women		753, 849
	Follicular 1-20 mIU/mL		
	Ovulatory peak 26-75 mIU/mL		
	Luteal phase 1-21 mIU/mL		
	Postmenopausal 26-95 mIU/mL		
	Men 1.4-11 mIU/mL		
Magnesium (S)	18-29 mg/L	0.75-1.21 mmol/L	507

A, Amniotic fluid; B, whole blood; P, plasma; S, serum; U, urine.
*A more complete list and description of methods of analysis can be found in
Clinical chemistry: a managerial and scientific infobase, Cincinnati, 2003, Pesce-Kaplan Publishers, v 5.0.

Continued on next page.

| Analyte | EXPECTED ADULT REFERENCE OR THERAPEUTIC RANGE | | Clinical Correlation Range (Page) |
	Conventional Units	SI Units	
Methotrexate			
24 hours post dose		>10 µmol/L	1073
48 hours post dose		>1 µmol/L	
72 hours post dose		>0.1 µmol/L	
Myoglobin (range of upper limits, 97.5th percentile value, manufacturer dependent)	M 67-86 µg/L F 50-63 µg/L		566
Osmolality (S)	282-300 mOsm/kg serum	—	441
(U)	50-1200 mOsm/kg urine	—	
Oxygen saturation (B)	95%-100% arterial	60%-85% venous	462
Phosphatidylglycerol (A)	Positive result indicates fetal lung maturity		753
Phosphorus (S)	25-48 mg/L	0.81-1.55 mmol/L	507
Porphobilinogen (U)	<4 mg/day excreted in urine	<18 µmol/day	657
Potassium (S)	3.6-5.0 mEq/L	3.6-5.0 mmol/L	441
Procainamide (S)	4-10 µg/mL	17-42 µmol/L	566
	20-30 mg/mL both procainamide + metabolite N-acetylprocainamide	82-126 µmol/L	
Prostate specific antigen (S)	<4.0 µg/L	0.125 nmol/L	960
Pyruvic acid (S, P)	<8.8 mg/L	<0.10 mmol/L	462
Salicylates (S)	<100 µg/mL as anticonvulsant	<0.72 mmol/L	989
	150-300 µg/mL as anti-inflammatory	1.09-2.17 mmol/L	
Schilling test	Excretion >8% to 15% for stage 1 and 2 tests		549
Serum protein electrophoresis	See CD-ROM		960
Sodium (S)	135-145 mEq/L	135-145 mmol/L	441
(U)	40-220 mEq/24 hrs	40-220 mmol/24 hr	
Theophylline (S)	10-20 µg/mL	55-111 µmol/L	1073
Thyroid-stimulating hormone (TSH)	0.4-4.5 mU/L (method dependent)		827
Thyroxine (total)	40-120 µg/L	51-154 nmol/L	827
Total ketones (S)	5-40 µg/L		580
Triglycerides (P)	See Table 33-3, p. 620		603
Troponin I	<0.1 ng/mL (upper limit)	<4.1 pmol/L (upper limit)	566
Urea (S)	50-170 BUN mg/L (method dependent)	1.8-6.1 mmol/L	477
	60-200 BUN µg/L (conductivity)	2.2-7.2 mmol/L	
	80-260 BUN µg/L diacetyl monoxime	2.9-9.4 mmol/L	
Uric acid (S)	36-77 mg/L males	214-458 µmol/L males	477
	25-68 mg/L females	149-405 µmol/L females	
(U)	250-750 mg/24 hrs for average diet	1.49-4.46 mmol/24 hrs	
	<450 mg/24 hrs for low purine diet	<2.68 mmol/24 hrs	
	<1g/24 hrs for high purine diet	<5.95 mmol/24 hrs	477
Urine protein (U)	<150 mg/day	—	
	<100 mg/g creatinine	—	
Vitamin B$_{12}$ (S)	160-950 pg/mL (microbiologic)	118-700 pmol/L	722
	199-732 pg/mL (competitive binding)	147-542 pmol/L	
Vitamin C	See Ascorbic acid		

A, Amniotic fluid; B, whole blood; BUN, blood urea nitrogen; P, plasma; S, serum; U, urine.
*A more complete list and description of methods of analysis can be found in
Clinical chemistry: a managerial and scientific infobase, Cincinnati, 2003, Pesce-Kaplan Publishers, v 5.0.